Neurology
A Queen Square Textbook

Neurology
A Queen Square Textbook
Second Edition

Edited by

Charles Clarke
Robin Howard
National Hospital for Neurology & Neurosurgery
University College London Hospitals NHS Foundation Trust
Queen Square, London WC1

UCL HOSPITALS

Martin Rossor
Simon Shorvon
University College London Institute of Neurology
Queen Square, London WC1

UCL

WILEY Blackwell

This edition first published 2016 © 2016 by John Wiley & Sons, Ltd
First Edition © 2009 by Blackwell Publishing Ltd

Artwork for some figures in chapters 2 and 13 © 2016 by Elsevier. Please refer to individual captions.

Registered Office
John Wiley & Sons, Ltd, The Atrium, Southern Gate, Chichester, West Sussex, PO19 8SQ, UK

Editorial Offices
9600 Garsington Road, Oxford, OX4 2DQ, UK
The Atrium, Southern Gate, Chichester, West Sussex, PO19 8SQ, UK
111 River Street, Hoboken, NJ 07030-5774, USA

For details of our global editorial offices, for customer services and for information about how to apply for permission to reuse the copyright material in this book please see our website at www.wiley.com/wiley-blackwell.

Editors' note
This book is designed as a general guide to clinical diagnosis and treatment and does not include all information necessary for every clinical situation. Prescribing information should be interpreted in the light of professional knowledge, checked and supplemented as necessary by specialised publications and by reference to prescribing product literature, and information services such as the British National Formulary (www.bnf.org).

Publisher's note
Every effort has been made to contact relevant copyright holders but if any have been overlooked, the publisher will be pleased to make the necessary arrangements at the earliest opportunity.

Library of Congress Cataloging-in-Publication Data

Names: Clarke, Charles (Charles R. A.), editor. | Howard, Robin (Neurologist), editor. | Rossor, M. (Martin), editor. | Shorvon, S. D. (Simon D.), editor. | Institute of Neurology, Queen Square. | National Hospital for Neurology and Neurosurgery (London, England)
Title: Neurology : a Queen Square textbook / edited by Charles Clarke, Robin Howard, Martin Rossor, Simon Shorvon.
Other titles: Neurology (Clarke)
Description: Second edition. | Oxford, UK ; Hoboken, NJ : John Wiley & Sons, Inc., 2016. | Includes bibliographical references and index.
Identifiers: LCCN 2016023787 (print) | LCCN 2016024981 (ebook) | ISBN 9781118486177 (cloth) | ISBN 9781118486153 (pdf) | ISBN 9781118486139 (epub)
Subjects: | MESH: Nervous System Diseases
Classification: LCC RC346 (print) | LCC RC346 (ebook) | NLM WL 140 | DDC 616.8–dc23
LC record available at https://lccn.loc.gov/2016023787

A catalogue record for this book is available from the British Library.

Wiley also publishes its books in a variety of electronic formats. Some content that appears in print may not be available in electronic books.

Cover images: front cover - © iStockphoto / back cover - courtesy of Charles Clarke
Cover design by Meaden Creative

Set in 9/11pt Minion by SPi Global, Pondicherry, India
Printed and bound in Singapore by Markono Print Media Pte Ltd

1 2016

Contents

Editorial Team

Principal Editors

Dr Charles Clarke FRCP
Honorary Consultant Neurologist
National Hospital for Neurology & Neurosurgery

Dr Robin Howard PhD FRCP
Consultant Neurologist
National Hospital for Neurology & Neurosurgery

Professor Martin Rossor MD FRCP FMedSci
Professor of Clinical Neurology
UCL Institute of Neurology

Professor Simon Shorvon MD FRCP
Professor of Clinical Neurology
UCL Institute of Neurology

International Editors (First Edition)

Professor Frederick Andermann OC MD FRCP(C)
Professor of Neurology & Paediatrics
McGill University
Montreal, Canada

Dr Nadir Bharucha MD FRCP FRCP(C)
Professor of Neurology
Bombay Hospital Institute of Medical Sciences
Bombay Hospital, India

Professor Raymond Cheung MD PhD FRCP FAAN
Professor of Neuroscience & Neurology
Director, Acute Stroke Services
Department of Medicine
University of Hong Kong, China

Professor Peter Kaplan FRCP
Professor of Neurology
Johns Hopkins University School of Medicine
Baltimore, USA

Professor Jürg Kesselring MD
Head, Department of Neurology & Neuro-Rehabilitation
The Rehabilitation Centre
Valens, Switzerland

Professor Philip Thompson PhD FRACP
Professor of Neurology
University Department of Medicine
University of Adelaide &
Department of Neurology
Royal Adelaide Hospital, Australia

Specialist Advisory Editors

Dr Matthew Adams FRCR
Consultant Neuroradiologist
National Hospital for Neurology & Neurosurgery

Professor Sebastian Brandner MD FRCPath
Professor of Neuropathology
UCL Institute of Neurology

Mr Neil Kitchen MD FRCS (SN)
Consultant Neurosurgeon
National Hospital for Neurology & Neurosurgery

Professor Martin Koltzenburg PhD MD
Professor of Neurophysiology
UCL Institute of Neurology

Professor Tarek Yousry Dr. med. Habil FRCR
Professor of Neuroradiology
UCL Institute of Neurology

Authors

Mr James Acheson MRCP(UK) FRCS FRCOphth
Consultant Neuro-Ophthalmologist
National Hospital for Neurology & Neurosurgery

Dr Matthew Adams FRCR
Consultant Neuroradiologist
National Hospital for Neurology & Neurosurgery

Dr Doris-Eva Bamiou MD PhD FRCP
Consultant Physician in Neuro-Otology
National Hospital for Neurology & Neurosurgery

Professor Kailash Bhatia MD DM FRCP
Professor of Clinical Neurology
UCL Institute of Neurology

Mr Robert Bradford MD FRCS
Consultant Neurosurgeon
National Hospital for Neurology & Neurosurgery

Professor Sebastian Brandner MD FRCPath
Professor of Neuropathology
UCL Institute of Neurology

Mr Fion Bremner PhD FRCOphth
Consultant Neuro-Ophthalmologist
National Hospital for Neurology & Neurosurgery

Professor Adolfo Bronstein MD PhD FRCP
Consultant Physician in Neuro-Otology
National Hospital for Neurology & Neurosurgery

Professor Martin M. Brown MD FRCP
Professor of Stroke Medicine
UCL Institute of Neurology

Dr Diana Caine PhD
Clinical Neuropsychologist
National Hospital for Neurology & Neurosurgery

Dr Jeremy Chataway PhD FRCP
Consultant Neurologist
National Hospital for Neurology & Neurosurgery

Mr David Choi PhD FRCS (SN)
Consultant Neurosurgeon
National Hospital for Neurology & Neurosurgery

Dr Charles Clarke FRCP
Honorary Consultant Neurologist
National Hospital for Neurology & Neurosurgery

Professor John Collinge CBE MD FRCP FRS
Professor of Clinical Neurology
UCL Institute of Neurology

Dr Carla Cordivari MD FRCP
Consultant in Clinical Neurophysiology
National Hospital for Neurology & Neurosurgery

Dr Carmel Curtis PhD MRCP(UK) FRCPath
Consultant Microbiologist
National Hospital for Neurology & Neurosurgery

Dr Rosalyn Davies PhD FRCP
Consultant Physician in Neuro-Otology
National Hospital for Neurology & Neurosurgery

Dr Beate Diehl MD PhD FRCP
Senior Lecturer in Clinical Neurophysiology
UCL Institute of Neurology

Professor John Duncan DM FRCP FMedSci
Professor of Clinical Neurology
UCL Institute of Neurology

Dr Mark Edwards PhD FRCP
Senior Lecturer in Neurology
UCL Institute of Neurology

Dr Sofia Eriksson MD PhD
Consultant Neurologist
National Hospital for Neurology & Neurosurgery

Dr Simon Farmer PhD FRCP
Consultant Neurologist
National Hospital for Neurology & Neurosurgery

Dr Naomi Fersht PhD MRCP(UK) FRCR
Consultant Clinical Oncologist
National Hospital for Neurology & Neurosurgery

Dr Thomas Foltynie PhD MRCP(UK)
Senior Lecturer in Clinical Neurology
UCL Institute of Neurology

Professor Nick Fox MD FRCP FMedSci
Professor of Neurology
UCL Institute of Neurology

Professor Gavin Giovannoni PhD FRCP FRCPath
Honorary Reader in Clinical Neuroimmunology
UCL Institute of Neurology

Dr Elizabeth Graham FRCOphth FRCP DO
Consultant Medical Ophthalmologist
National Hospital for Neurology & Neurosurgery

Dr Richard Greenwood MD FRCP
Consultant Neurologist
National Hospital for Neurology & Neurosurgery

Miss Joan Grieve MD FRCS (SN)
Consultant Neurosurgeon
National Hospital for Neurology & Neurosurgery

Miss Ulrike Hammerbeck MCSP
Clinician Scientist
UCL Institute of Neurology

Professor Michael Hanna MD FRCP
Professor of Clinical Neurology
UCL Institute of Neurology

Professor Marwan Hariz MD PhD
Professor of Functional Neurosurgery
UCL Institute of Neurology

Professor Simon Heales PhD FRCPath
Professor of Clinical Chemistry
National Hospital for Neurology & Neurosurgery

Dr Nicholas Hirsch FRCP FRCA FFICM
Consultant Neuroanaesthetist
National Hospital for Neurology & Neurosurgery

Professor Henry Houlden PhD MRCP(UK)
Professor of Neurology & Neurogenetics
UCL Institute of Neurology

Dr Robin Howard PhD FRCP
Consultant Neurologist
National Hospital for Neurology & Neurosurgery

Dr Gordon Ingle MD FRCP
Consultant Neurologist
National Hospital for Neurology & Neurosurgery

Dr Valeria Iodice MD PhD
Consultant Neurologist
National Hospital for Neurology & Neurosurgery

Professor Rolf Jäger MD FRCR
Professor of Neuroradiology
UCL Institute of Neurology

Dr Paul Jarman PhD FRCP
Consultant Neurologist
National Hospital for Neurology & Neurosurgery

Professor Eileen Joyce PhD MRCP(UK) FRCPsych
Professor of Neuropsychiatry
UCL Institute of Neurology

Mr Neil Kitchen MD FRCS (SN)
Consultant Neurosurgeon
National Hospital for Neurology & Neurosurgery

Professor Matthias Koepp MD PhD
Professor of Clinical Neurology
UCL Institute of Neurology

Dr Prasad Korlipara PhD FRCP
Consultant Neurologist
National Hospital for Neurology & Neurosurgery

Professor Dimitri Kullmann DPhil FRCP FMedSci
Professor of Clinical Neurology
UCL Institute of Neurology

Dr Robin Lachmann PhD FRCP
Consultant in Metabolic Medicine
National Hospital for Neurology & Neurosurgery

Dr Siobhan Leary MD FRCP
Consultant Neurologist
National Hospital for Neurology & Neurosurgery

Dr Alexander Leff PhD FRCP
Reader in Cognitive Neurology
UCL Institute of Neurology

Professor Roger Lemon PhD FMedSci
Sobell Chair of Neurophysiology
UCL Institute of Neurology

Professor Patricia Limousin MD PhD
Professor of Clinical Neurology
UCL Institute of Neurology

Dr Nicholas Losseff MD FRCP
Consultant Neurologist
National Hospital for Neurology & Neurosurgery

Dr Michael Lunn PhD FRCP
Consultant Neurologist
National Hospital for Neurology & Neurosurgery

Professor Linda M. Luxon CBE FRCP
Consultant Physician in Neuro-Otology
National Hospital for Neurology & Neurosurgery

Dr Hadi Manji MD FRCP
Consultant Neurologist
National Hospital for Neurology & Neurosurgery

Dr Manjit Matharu PhD FRCP
Senior Lecturer in Neurology
UCL Institute of Neurology

Professor Christopher Mathias DPhil DSc FRCP FMedSci
Professor of Neurovascular Medicine
UCL Institute of Neurology

Professor Simon Mead PhD FRCP
Professor of Neurology
UCL Institute of Neurology

Professor David Miller MD FRCP FRACP FMedSci
Emeritus Professor of Clinical Neurology
UCL Institute of Neurology

Dr Catherine Mummery PhD FRCP
Consultant Neurologist
National Hospital for Neurology & Neurosurgery

Dr Elaine Murphy MRCP(I) FRCPath
Consultant in Inherited Metabolic Disease
National Hospital for Neurology & Neurosurgery

Dr Paul Nandi FRCP FRCA FFPMRCA
Consultant in Pain Medicine & Neuroanaesthesia
National Hospital for Neurology & Neurosurgery

Dr Jalesh Panicker MD DM FRCP
Consultant Neurologist in Uroneurology
National Hospital for Neurology & Neurosurgery

Dr Matthew Parton PhD FRCP
Consultant Neurologist
National Hospital for Neurology & Neurosurgery

Dr Gordon Plant MD FRCP FRCOphth
Consultant Neurologist
National Hospital for Neurology & Neurosurgery

Dr Diane Playford MD FRCP
Reader in Neurological Rehabilitation
UCL Institute of Neurology

Professor Niall Quinn MD FRCP
Emeritus Professor of Clinical Neurology
UCL Institute of Neurology

Professor Shamima Rahman PhD FRCP
Consultant in Mitochondrial Medicine
National Hospital for Neurology & Neurosurgery

Dr Jeremy Rees PhD FRCP
Consultant Neurologist
National Hospital for Neurology & Neurosurgery

Professor Mary Reilly MD FRCP FRCP(I)
Professor of Clinical Neurology
UCL Institute of Neurology

Dr Jonathan Rohrer PhD MRCP(UK)
MRC Clinical Scientist
UCL Institute of Neurology

Professor Martin Rossor MD FRCP FMedSci
Professor of Clinical Neurology
UCL Institute of Neurology

Dr Fergus Rugg-Gunn PhD MRCP(UK)
Consultant Neurologist
National Hospital for Neurology & Neurosurgery

Professor Josemir Sander MD PhD FRCP
Professor of Neurology & Clinical Epilepsy
UCL Institute of Neurology

Dr Jonathan Schott MD FRCP
Reader in Clinical Neurology
UCL Institute of Neurology

Dr Paul Shanahan MRCP(I)
Consultant Neurologist
National Hospital for Neurology & Neurosurgery

Professor Simon Shorvon MD FRCP
Professor of Clinical Neurology
UCL Institute of Neurology

Dr Katie Sidle PhD FRCP
Consultant Neurologist
National Hospital for Neurology & Neurosurgery

Dr Robert Simister PhD MRCP(UK)
Consultant in Neurology and Stroke Medicine
National Hospital for Neurology & Neurosurgery

Dr Valerie Stevenson MD MRCP(UK)
Consultant Neurologist
National Hospital for Neurology & Neurosurgery

Professor Sarah Tabrizi PhD FRCP FMedSci
Professor of Clinical Neurology
UCL Institute of Neurology

Dr Christopher Taylor MRCP(UK) FRCA FFICM
Consultant Neuroanaesthetist
National Hospital for Neurology & Neurosurgery

Professor Alan Thompson MD FRCPI FRCP FMedSci
Professor of Clinical Neurology and Neurorehabilitation
National Hospital for Neurology & Neurosurgery
UCL Institute of Neurology

Dr Ahmed Toosy PhD MRCP(UK)
Clinical Senior Lecturer in Neurology
UCL Institute of Neurology

Dr Christopher Turner PhD FRCP
Consultant Neurologist
National Hospital for Neurology & Neurosurgery

Professor Matthew Walker PhD FRCP
Professor of Clinical Neurology
UCL Institute of Neurology

Dr Nick Ward MD FRCP
Reader in Clinical Neurology
UCL Institute of Neurology

Professor Thomas Warner PhD FRCP
Professor of Clinical Neurology
UCL Institute of Neurology

Professor Jason Warren PhD FRACP
Professor of Neurology
UCL Institute of Neurology

Dr Tim Wehner MD
Consultant Clinical Neurophysiologist
National Hospital for Neurology & Neurosurgery

Professor David Werring PhD FRCP
Professor of Clinical Neurology
UCL Institute of Neurology

Dr Elena Wilson MD FRCP FRCR
Consultant Clinical Oncologist
National Hospital for Neurology & Neurosurgery

Professor Nicholas W. Wood PhD FRCP FMedSci
Galton Chair of Genetics
UCL Institute of Neurology

Dr Tim Young PhD MRCP(UK)
Consultant Neurologist
National Hospital for Neurology & Neurosurgery

Beginnings

A conversation with Professor Ian McDonald

Ian McDonald[1] kindly agreed to write the foreword for the first edition of this book. Sadly, he died shortly before it was completed. We met one sunny morning in 2004 and talked, sitting together on a bench in Queen Square.

I explained what I had in mind: an integrated, practical textbook from the National Hospital and the Institute of Neurology. 'That is quite splendid', Ian responded, in his inimitable way. 'Of course', he continued: 'a book like this has never been produced and I think no one has been able to draw together the different personalities here – and that will not be at all easy …'. Ian went on: 'Charlie Symonds[2] once told me that he had suggested a similar project to the National Hospital Medical Committee in the 1930s'. Dr Charles Symonds, who had been recently appointed to the staff had received an immediate veto from his senior colleague Dr Samuel Kinnier Wilson.[3] 'Symonds, there is no place for *that*. I have already written the definitive book, and there is no need for another,' Kinnier Wilson is said to have responded, acidly.

During the last five decades, neurology has progressed immeasurably. Queen Square has become a truly international centre. The editors integrated this international dimension, drawing on clinical experience and perspectives for the first edition from Australia, Canada, China, Europe, India and the United States. We thank our international editors for their comments and guidance.

This book came to fruition slowly and was quite a challenge. The authors are busy, distinguished in specialist fields, but they came together to produce the first edition, and now the second. The editors are most grateful to them all.

We hope *Neurology: A Queen Square Textbook* in this second edition continues to achieve its object – to reflect the clinical practice of neurology as we know it and to illustrate the approach we teach and follow at the National Hospital for Neurology & Neurosurgery and the Institute of Neurology, Queen Square.

We all valued Ian McDonald's encouragement and hope that if he were still with us, he would feel the finished product was worthy of the institutions and teachers that have guided our thoughts and practice over the years.

Charles Clarke
Queen Square
London WC1

1. Ian McDonald (1933–2006) was Professor of Neurology at Queen Square from 1978 to 1998, and was well known for his work on multiple sclerosis.
2. Sir Charles Symonds, KBE, CB (1890–1978) was appointed physician to The National in 1926. A selection of his many papers entitled *Studies in Neurology* was published in 1970.
3. Dr Samuel Kinnier Wilson (1878–1937) was appointed physician to The National in 1912. He had written the seminal paper on progressive hepatolenticular degeneration shortly before this. *Neurology*, his well-known textbook, was published posthumously in 1940.

Foreword to the First Edition

Queen Square in Bloomsbury, London, is known the world over as a centre for neurology and clinical neuroscience. Like many institutions, The National, initially The National Hospital for the Relief and Cure of the Paralysed and Epileptic, was founded through the hard work and generosity of people with a broad sense of charitable intent, especially the Chandler family – Johanna Chandler, her sister Louisa and their brother Edward. The doors of the original building opened in Queen Square in 1860. Dr Jabez Spence Ramskill was the first physician appointed, followed shortly by Dr Charles Brown-Séquard. Since 1860 there has been an unbroken record of progress across the clinical neurosciences. The names of all those who contributed in those early years are too numerous to mention, but amongst those who stand out today in an historical perspective are Dr Charles Brown-Séquard, Dr John Hughlings Jackson, Sir William Gowers, Sir David Ferrier, Sir Victor Horsley, Sir Gordon Holmes, Dr Samuel Kinnier Wilson, Sir Francis Walshe, Sir Charles Symonds and Dr Macdonald Critchley.

The National Hospital has undergone many changes and revolutionised its approach, for example towards neurological rehabilitation and brain injury, and has developed close and inseparable links with the UCL Institute of Neurology, which has helped to promote research at Queen Square in both basic and clinical sciences. Both Hospital and Institute are now involved in advancing an extensive range of developments in translational medicine that are transforming the treatment of neurological diseases. These developments are reflected in this book.

The UCL Institute of Neurology

The UCL Institute of Neurology was established in 1950 and has been part of University College London since 1997. The Institute provides research and teaching of the highest quality in neurosciences, and professional training for clinical careers in neurology, neurosurgery, neuropsychiatry, neuroradiology, neuropathology and clinical neurophysiology. With its concentration of clinical and applied scientific activity, the Institute provides a unique national resource for both postgraduate training and research in the basic neurosciences and its associated clinical disciplines. The Institute currently holds active grants for research into the causes and treatment of a wide range of neurological diseases, including movement disorders, multiple sclerosis, epilepsy, brain cancer, stroke and brain injury, muscle and nerve disorders, cognitive dysfunction and dementia; the work of the Institute's clinical academic staff remains closely integrated with The National Hospital.

The National Hospital for Neurology & Neurosurgery today

The National, now part of University College London Hospitals NHS Foundation Trust, is a thriving hospital, largely refurbished behind the 1890 façade. The hospital receives over 1000 new outpatient referrals each month and has over 200 beds, a dedicated ITU, extensive rehabilitation services and all ancillary departments in the most substantial specialist neurological hospital within the UK. The hospital provides the surrounding district general hospitals with specialist services. Many of the consultant staff continue to hold appointments that are linked to both general hospitals, the UCL Institute of Neurology and The National itself. This maintains unique contact between the disciplines of research and clinical practice.

Neurology: A Queen Square Textbook

This book, the first of its kind to come from these two institutions, has a distinctly clinical flavour. It has been written very largely by clinicians, each in the forefront of their field, and focuses on the practical aspects of diagnosis, treatment and patient care. The book also provides an introduction to the basic sciences of neurology, of increasing importance in medical practice. It has been a pleasure to be one of the contributing authors.

Professor Roger Lemon PhD FMedSci
Sobell Chair of Neurophysiology & Director, UCL Institute of Neurology (2002–2008)

Foreword to the Second Edition

I am delighted to be asked to celebrate the publication of this second edition of *Neurology: A Queen Square Textbook*. When I first learnt about this project some 10 years ago I had some misgivings – it seemed to me that neurology had become so specialised that it would be difficult to assemble a coherent book that spanned the whole of the field. I am glad to have been proved wrong, for this work really does encompass the scope of neurology in the twenty-first century.

In the past, neurologists by and large dealt with *all* neurological conditions; today specialisation has taken over and to be a neurologist without a special interest is a rarity. It is thus fitting that the four editors combine vast and broad clinical experience with specialist academic expertise. From the National Hospital for Neurology & Neurosurgery, Charles Clarke, who was the driving force behind the initiation of the project over 10 years ago, is a general neurologist, much of whose work has been in UK district general hospitals. He prides himself on being a 'general practitioner of practical neurology'. His colleague Robin Howard, who works jointly at St Thomas' Hospital in London and the National, is also a highly experienced general neurologist; his specialist interests are intensive care neurology and neuromuscular disease.

From the UCL Institute of Neurology, Martin Rossor has developed his interests in cognitive impairment to establish a unit in Queen Square specialising in dementia, a subject of major importance, long neglected. Simon Shorvon has been consultant neurologist at the hospital since 1983; his specialist expertise is in epilepsy, a field in which he has an international reputation.

This book epitomises this combination of practical experience and academic specialisation, and collaboration between institute and hospital, where as part of our daily workload we continue the tradition of teaching, both as a national centre and internationally to Queen Square postgraduate students from all over the world.

The editors and the authors are experienced and distinguished writers who have devoted time to draw together their practical experience. Each chapter has been carefully edited, so essential for a good finished product. I know that this book has been produced within an atmosphere of cordiality and friendship. The text reflects this.

Here, even at a glance, the reader can understand how large a subject neurology has become and how scientific advances, many pioneered within the UCL Institute of Neurology, have become translated into clinical practice. One can find here well-illustrated neuroanatomy, detailed assessments of common conditions such as stroke and dementia, up-to-date aspects of neurogenetics and ion channels, the philosophy and practicalities of rehabilitation, and rarities such as metabolic disorders of copper, unusual muscle diseases or little-known varieties of headache.

As a measure of its authority, *Neurology: A Queen Square Textbook* has become a standard text for the UK neurologists-in-training exit examination. It is already over 5 years since the first edition was published and while neurology and neuroscience continue to advance, I fully endorse the move to complete this new edition without delay.

> A man would do nothing if he waited until he could do it so well that no one could find fault in what he had done.[1]

This book to my mind really does achieve its purpose and, like my predecessor Roger Lemon, I am delighted to be a contributing author.

Professor Michael Hanna MD FRCP
Professor of Clinical Neurology
Director, UCL Institute of Neurology

1. John Henry Newman, a nineteenth-century English clergyman.

Preface

All Editors, Authors and Specialist Advisory Editors of *Neurology: A Queen Square Textbook* hold or recently held consultant or equivalent posts at the National Hospital for Neurology & Neurosurgery and/or the UCL Institute of Neurology, Queen Square.

The National Hospital is part of University College London Hospitals NHS Foundation Trust, and the Institute of Neurology part of University College London.

Twenty-three Co-ordinating Authors organised individual chapters, encouraged and liaised with over 70 contributors and with them wrote this book.

The Specialist Advisory Editors gave invaluable advice and guidance in their respective fields. To ensure a worldwide perspective, for the first edition our International Regional Editors, all of whom had close connections with Queen Square, provided guidance and comment.

This book is an attempt to provide a fresh and up-to-date approach to the fascinating subject of neurology. We encouraged each author to relate their own clinical experience but, in order to achieve a degree of consistency, we took a robust overview of the important specialities within neurology and their relevance. Each chapter has been coordinated by an expert in the field, to give the reader an overall grasp of each major subject, indicating where developments within neurosciences fit into a broader picture.

On spelling and use of the English language, whilst appreciating that as a living, multicultural tongue there are wide varieties, we have opted for British English – the sort of way we write our letters, and continue to spell 'neurone' with its terminal -e. On medical conditions named after famous figures, we appreciate that many publishers no longer use the apostrophe to describe the disease named after Alzheimer, Wilson, Parkinson and so on. Our authors by and large did not follow this; thus we have left matters much as they signed off their chapters.

The limited size of this book means that it has not been possible to provide references for all material. With the growth of information technology, a wealth of detailed sources is readily available.

We are most grateful to all those who have helped in this joint venture.

Charles Clarke
Robin Howard
Martin Rossor
Simon Shorvon
Queen Square
London WC1

Acknowledgements

We know that the skills of clinical practice are handed down, both by teachers and role models. The editors wish to thank all those who have taught, advised and inspired them in many aspects of neurology and its related disciplines, in neuroscience and in research. When we came to list these many individuals, we soon realised we would be unable to mention each by name. Instead, we trust that all who read this book will understand how much the editors and authors owe to others. We hope we can pass on that knowledge and experience.

We thank those who contributed to the first edition and have moved on, reflecting for most retirement, promotion or in the case of Philip Lee, his death at an early age. Those contributing to the first edition were Peter Brown, Adrian Casey, Sohier Elneil, Clare Fowler, Richard Frackowiak, Peter Goadsby, Andrew Lees, Giovanna Mallucci, Jon Marsden, Geoffrey Raisman, Mary Robertson, Geoffrey Schott, Anette Schrag, Susan Short, Shelagh Smith, David Thomas, Emma Townsley, Michael Trimble and Gelareh Zadeh. Each made a valued contribution.

We thank our publishers, Wiley Blackwell, and especially Rob Blundell, Claire Bonnett and Nick Morgan, as well as Kathy Syplywczak and Jan East for their unstinting patience.

The authors have worked hard and provided the substance of the book, for no personal reward and, despite numerous requests for text, diagrams and amendments, have remained firmly behind this project. We are most grateful to all who have contributed.

Secretarial help has been invaluable, and amongst those who have contributed over and above their normal duties, we thank especially Claire Bloomfield and Wyn Jagger.

The Rockefeller Library provided its valuable resources, both historical and current. The Audio Visual Services Unit was most helpful with the sourcing of some figures and photographs.

Royalties from *Neurology: A Queen Square Textbook* pass directly to The National Brain Appeal (National Hospital Development Foundation), the registered UK charity (No. 290173) that supports projects at Queen Square.

Charles Clarke
Robin Howard
Martin Rossor
Simon Shorvon
Queen Square
London WC1
June 2016

CHAPTER 1

Neurology Worldwide: The Epidemiology and Burden of Neurological Disease

Simon Shorvon
UCL Institute of Neurology

Neurological disease casts a heavy shadow over the lives of the patient, their family and friends and over society. In a recent survey, in Europe about one-third of all burden of disease was caused by brain disease – 23% of the years of healthy life is lost (YLL), 50% of years lived with disability (YLD) and 35% of disability-adjusted life years (DALYs). The aim of all neurological services must be to alleviate the suffering associated with the disease, and to realise this aim the rational planning of such health services requires epidemiological knowledge in five broad areas:

1 Epidemiology of the condition – its frequency and distribution within a population, its causation, mortality and co-morbidity.
2 Broad impact of the disease (the 'burden of illness') on individuals, families, health services and societies and also its financial cost.
3 Effectiveness and cost-effectiveness of diagnosis, investigation and treatment.
4 Existing health care resources – their distribution and priorities, and the potential for prevention.
5 Prognosis and outcome, via cohort studies and case–control studies.

The last three areas are outside the scope of this chapter; here an overview of selected issues related to the epidemiology and burden of neurological illness is given and, as this book is based on practice at Queen Square, here too I emphasise studies from the National Hospital for Neurology and Neurosurgery and the UCL Institute of Neurology. These set the scene for the more detailed consideration of neurological disease contained in the rest of the volume.

Epidemiology of neurological disease

It is self-evident that knowledge of epidemiology is important to underpin any decision about the provision of health care resources. It is also clear that epidemiological data (on frequency, distribution, mortality, etc.) are of little practical value unless related to an intervention or therapeutic advance. Sadly, however, in practice, even where reliable data exist, these are used only inconsistently in planning health care. Neurological disease is one example of this depressing fact, for the amount of education and expenditure is far below its estimated impact. In many, indeed perhaps most, health care settings, the provision of facilities for neurological care is often surprisingly fragmented and inappropriately targeted, even where, as in the United Kingdom, there is a nationwide health service.

Frequency and distribution of neurological disease

Incidence and prevalence rates are the most common measures of frequency used in medicine.

Incidence is a measure of the rate at which new cases occur in a specified population during a specified period. The incidence rate is usually calculated as the number of new cases occurring per 100 000 of the general population per year.

Prevalence is defined as proportion of a population that are cases at a point in time. The prevalence rate is usually calculated as the number of existing cases per 1000 of the general population. Point prevalence is calculated as the number on a particular day (prevalence day) and period prevalence is calculated as the number in a population over a specified period of time. Lifetime prevalence is defined as the risk of acquiring the condition at any time during life and is another important figure.

For many neurological diseases, information on even these basic measures is incomplete. Furthermore, the frequency of many neurological disorders varies markedly in different geographical regions, differs in urban when compared with rural settings, may differ with ethnicity, and is often linked to lifestyle and socio-economic factors.

In most neurological illnesses there are also striking differences in frequency at different ages, and so the age distribution of the population will affect the frequency, and some diseases have marked gender differences. For these reasons, age-specific or sex-specific rates, or frequency estimates in restricted age ranges, are generally more informative than crude rates. For instance, the annual incidence of stroke in a general population is about 190/100 000/year, but in the population over 65 years the rate is 1100/100 000/year. Similarly, the incidence and prevalence of Parkinson's disease in the general population are 20/100 000/year and 2/1000, and in those over 65 years are 160/100 000/year and 10/1000.

Changes in age structure in populations will impact on the number of patients with neurological diseases that have age-specificity. In most developing countries, the population has a far greater proportion of children and young adults than in developed countries. Figure 1.1 shows age structures in a typical developed (Sweden) and

Neurology: A Queen Square Textbook, Second Edition. Edited by Charles Clarke, Robin Howard, Martin Rossor and Simon Shorvon.

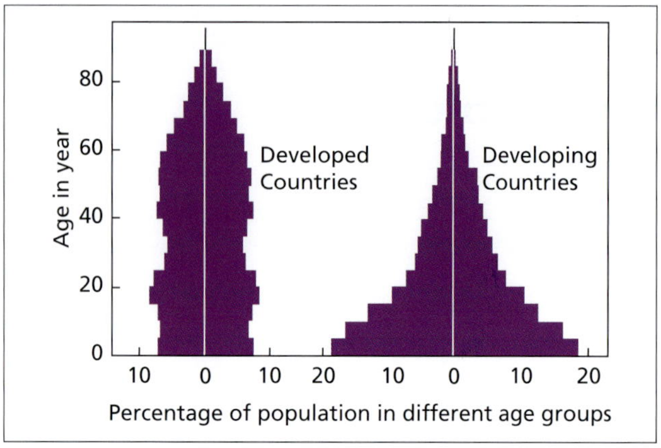

Figure 1.1 Age structure in developed and developing countries.

developing country (Costa Rica). However, globally, the number of people over the age of 65 years is estimated to double by 2030 and so the number of people with degenerative neurological disease is rapidly increasing. It is also important to recognise that although worldwide human populations are growing in an exponential fashion, growth rates vary widely among different countries and regions and the concept of 'doubling time' is a useful way of quantifying this. Doubling time – the time it is predicted to take for a population to double in size – depends not only on population size and mortality rates, but also on the number of children per woman (Table 1.1) and other social and health care parameters.

The approximate non-standardised figures for the prevalence and incidence of neurological disorders in a developed country are shown in Table 1.2. This table illustrates another important point – that for chronic diseases, as are many neurological diseases, the incidence rates may be low but the prevalence rates are high. This is important for health service planning, as the facilities required for incident cases are very different from prevalent cases. The former require provision for investigation and acute therapy and the latter largely for follow-up, social care, long-term therapy and rehabilitation.

The results of age-adjusted incidence and prevalence figures in a population of 100 230 persons in a selection of general practices served by the National Hospital for Neurology and Neurosurgery, London, from a research project published by the author in 2000 are shown in Tables 1.3 and 1.4. The incidence rates of 625 neurological disorders during a single year of observation were reported. Six per cent of the population in whom lifetime prevalence was surveyed had had a neurological disorder. In the United Kingdom, diseases of the nervous system accounted for 7.6% of all GP consultations between 1981 and 1982. The frequency of disability in private households amongst those over 16 years of age in the United Kingdom in 1971 was comprehensively delineated in the Harris Report in 1971. Disabilities relevant to neurology – CNS disorders, muscular dystrophies, congenital malformations of the spine and hydrocephalus, cerebral birth injury, senility as a cause of cognitive disability – occurred with a prevalence of 78/1000. The UK Office for Population Censuses and Surveys (OPCS) survey of disability 16 years later graded disability according to severity as well as overall frequency. The prevalence of complaints relevant to neurology was 13% for 'CNS disorders', 2% each for dementia and mental retardation, and 6% for back complaints. In a later study, 'CNS complaints' accounted for 7% of disability overall but for 16% of conditions with

Table 1.1 Population size in selected developing and developed countries – doubling time.

Country	Approximate population size (millions)	Fertility (mean number of children per woman)	Doubling time* (years)
Yemen	15	7.2	20
Nigeria	107	6.2	23
Pakistan	138	5.6	25
Iran	68	4.7	26
Philippines	73	4.1	30
Mexico	95	3.1	32
Bangladesh	122	3.6	35
India	970	3.5	36
Brazil	160	2.5	48
China	1236	1.8	67
USA	268	2.0	116
France	59	1.7	204
Japan	126	1.5	289
UK	60	1.7	433
Italy	57	1.2	NPG
Germany	82	1.3	NPG
Russia	147	1.3	NPG

NPG, no population growth.
*Doubling time is the predicted time it will take for the population to double in size. The doubling time depends on population size, age structure, number of children per women and mortality rates. These figures were taken from the Population Reference Bureau, and predate improvements in child health, reductions in mortality rates amongst children and young adults and the HIV epidemic.

a high severity score. Roughly similar figures are found elsewhere. Population-based estimates from the United States, for instance, report point prevalence rates of neurological conditions (excluding headache, back pain and discs, mental retardation, psychosis, non-neurological visual and hearing loss and nervous system trauma) of 36/1000.

Ethnic differences in disease were shown by Stewart *et al.* in 1999 who studied stroke in a multi-ethnic region of London. A stroke register was used with 12 sources of case ascertainment. The population size was 234 533 with 72% Caucasian, 21% black (11% Afro-Caribbean, 7.5% West African and 2.5% mixed) and 3% South Asian. Incidence rates were standardised for age and sex. The crude annual

Table 1.2 Annual incidence and point prevalence figures of common neurological disorders. The table includes only those conditions with an incidence above 1/100 000/year; whole populations considered, without age standardisation, and excludes shingles.

Disorder	Incidence (per 100 000 persons/year)	Point prevalence (per 100 000 persons)
Migraine	370	12 100
Acute stroke	190	900
Epilepsy	50	710
Febrile convulsions	50	
Dementia	50	250
Chronic polyneuropathy (all types)	40	24
Transient ischaemic attacks	30	
Bell's palsy	25	
Parkinson's disease	20	200
Meningitis	15	
Subarachnoid haemorrhage	15	
Metastatic brain tumour	15	
Primary brain tumour	5	6
Trigeminal neuralgia	4	1
Multiple sclerosis	4	90
Motor neurone disease	2	4
Acute post-infectious polyneuropathy	2	1
All muscular dystrophies	1	6

Source: data derived from Kurtzke 1982; Hopkins 1993; Zakrzewska and Hamlyn 1999; Hughes 2002; Hirtz *et al.* 2007.

incidence rate of stroke was 130 (120–141)/100 000/year and the age-adjusted rate (to a standard European population) was 125 (115–135)/100 000/year. The rate in the black population was significantly higher with an incidence rate of 221 (177–276)/100 000/year. The rate, not surprisingly, increased with age. The study also looked at social class and found higher rates in those less than 64 years in lower social classes. This sort of study generates hypotheses about causation (as yet not explained) and provides data for rational health care planning (partially implemented).

Table 1.3 The National Hospital for Neurology and Neurosurgery (NHNN) record linkage study: age- and sex-adjusted incidence rates for neurological conditions (MacDonald et al. 2000) compared with previously reported rates.

Conditions	NHNN linkage study: age- and sex-adjusted rate (95% CI)/100 000/year	Previously reported incidence rates/100 000/year
Stroke		
First cerebrovascular episode	205 (183–230)	200
Second cerebrovascular episode	42 (33–55)	28–35
Intracranial haemorrhage	10 (5–17)	5% of stroke, i.e. 10
Seizure disorders		
Epilepsy	46 (36–60)	24–53
Single seizures	11 (7–18)	20
Tumours		
Primary CNS tumours (benign and malignant)	10 (5–18)	7; 15
Parkinson's disease	19 (12–27)	12–20
Compressive mononeuropathies – all except carpal tunnel syndrome (CTS)	49 (39–61)	40
Arm – all excluding CTS	24 (17–33)	
Leg – all	20 (14–29)	
Polyneuropathies		
Diabetic polyneuropathy	54 (33–83)	40
All excluding diabetic and alcoholic	15 (9–23)	11
Shingles	140 (104–184)	71; 131; 400; 480
Other conditions		
Post-herpetic neuralgia	11 (6, 17)	13; 34; 9% of shingles
Bacterial CNS infection (overall)	7 (4–13)	10; 11
Essential tremor	8 (4–14)	24
Trigeminal neuralgia	8 (4–13)	2; 4

(continued)

Table 1.3 (continued)

Conditions	NHNN linkage study: age- and sex-adjusted rate (95% CI)/100 000/ year	Previously reported incidence rates/100 000/ year
Benign CNS tumour	7 (3–13)	10
Multiple sclerosis	7 (4–11)	2–8
Traumatic brain injury	7 (3–12)	4–6
Subarachnoid haemorrhage	7 (3–12)	10–15
Subdural haematoma	6 (3–12)	
Cluster headache	6 (3–10)	6–14
Cranial nerve disorder (excluding II, III, IV, VI, Bell's palsy or trigeminal neuralgia)	6 (2–10)	

Note: Other conditions that were encountered in the study, but which occurred with an incidence of 1–5/100 000: aseptic meningitis, metastatic CNS tumour, presenile dementia, neonatal encephalopathy, other congenital CNS abnormalities, brachial neuritis, Guillain–Barré syndrome, myasthenia gravis, primary malignant CNS tumour, transient global amnesia, spinal cord injury, acute cervical myelopathy, cranial nerve injury, demyelinating conditions (excluding MS), HIV encephalopathy, idiopathic myelopathy, motor neurone disease, spondylitic myelopathy, truncal mononeuropathy, diabetic amyotrophy, focal dystonia, non-cervical disc or cada equina damage, optic neuritis, spinal malformation.

In addition, a small number of cases of the following diseases were also found in this study: cerebellar degeneration, dementia of uncertain cause, frontal dementia with anterior horn cell disease, neurosarcoid with cord involvement, neurofibromatosis, tuberous sclerosis, communicating hydrocephalus, aqueduct stenosis, cerebral cyst, tonsillar herniation with Chiari malformation, syringomyelia, myotonic dystrophy, myositis, idiopathic neurogenic bladder, tubercular meningitis, meningococcal meningitis, syphilis, streptococcal meningitis, *Streptococcus pneumoniae* brain abscess, *Listeria* meningitis, cryptococcal meningitis, and an unidentified ventriculitis.

The collection of epidemiological statistics relating to neurological disorders is difficult; existing figures are probably underestimates and most biases lead to under-ascertainment. Such issues apply to epidemiological studies in all areas, but in addition to the varied general issues there is a particular problem for neurology that requires mention. This is the difficulty of 'case definition' (and thus case ascertainment). Many neurological disorders are defined on clinical criteria, with the inevitable subjectivity this entails. Thus, boundaries exist in which symptoms are occurring without formal diagnosis – for instance, the boundaries between ageing and Alzheimer's disease and between chronic headache and migraine. Similarly, in epilepsy, the inclusion of febrile seizures, single seizures and acute symptomatic seizures within a definition of epilepsy will more than double the apparent incidence rates. In neurological disorders that are only mildly symptomatic in their early stages, such as migraine, some neuropathies, some dementing illnesses and Parkinson's disease, only 'the tip of the iceberg' cases are known to health care professionals. Severity also varies markedly in many neurological conditions, and the inclusion of mild cases will lead to high prevalence rates with relative little impact on burden of illness. Studies of epilepsy from the National Hospital provide examples of this – with over 60% of patients with epilepsy entering long-term remission and thus having only a minor impact on health services. However, any method using hospital statistics will greatly underestimate the true number of cases as many minor or static neurological conditions are cared for outside the hospital setting. Case finding methods also need to be tailored to the disease's spectrum of severity and frequency.

Similar considerations apply when considering rarer conditions, especially those requiring complex medical care where a sound estimate of frequency is important. A study of the prevalence and causation of dementia in those under 65 years, carried out by Harvey *et al.* in 2003 in West London, is one example. In this population of 567 500 people, the prevalence of dementia in those aged 30–64 years was 0.54/1000 (0.45–0.64). For those aged 45–64 years, the prevalence was 0.98/1000 (0.81–1.18). From the age of 35 onwards, the prevalence of dementia was found to approximately double with each 5-year increase in age. On the basis of these figures, it was estimated that in 2003, there were 18 319 (15 296–21 758) people with dementia under the age of 65 in the United Kingdom. Using diagnostic algorithms, 34% had Alzheimer's disease, 18% vascular dementia, 12% frontotemporal dementia, 7% dementia with Lewy bodies and 19% had other causes which included Huntington's disease, multiple sclerosis, corticobasal dementia, prion disease, Down's syndrome (probably underestimated), Parkinson's disease and others.

Neurology is also distinguished from other areas of medicine by the large number of uncommon conditions within its purview (neurology has the highest number of conditions listed in the International Classification of Diseases), and therefore large populations must be studied to obtain accurate population-based data with appropriate statistical reliability. Sampling error increases with rarer events and for many of the uncommon neurological diseases there are few reliable data.

From the perspective of health services, figures of prevalence and incidence of the cases receiving treatment are important, as it is these cases that consume resources, not untreated (usually mild) or cases before diagnosis. In 1998, a large study of epilepsy was published by Wallace *et al.* amongst a population of 2 052 922 persons in England and Wales of the numbers with epilepsy receiving antiepileptic drugs. This provided accurate age-specific rates shown in Figure 1.2.

Causation

Epidemiological studies are also vital for studying the causes of disease. The attribution of causation to neurological disease is rarely a simple matter. Most neurological diseases are multifactorial in nature, being the result of complex interactions between genetic and environmental influences. The balance between the two varies. The genetic influences can be very strong – for instance, in single gene disorders with high penetrance (e.g. Huntington's disease). In others the genetic influence is the result of more complex epigenetic and epistatic interactions (e.g. epilepsy), and in other diseases identifiable Mendelian genetic influences do exist but are seen in some families cases only (Alzheimer's disease for instance is familial in about 10% of cases). The environmental influences are predominant in many diseases, for instance head injury or cerebrovascular disease. An interaction between genetic and environmental factors occurs in other diseases, for instance

Table 1.4 The National Hospital for Neurology and Neurosurgery record linkage study: 'lifetime prevalence' of neurological conditions (MacDonald et al. 2000) compared with previously reported rates.

Conditions	'Lifetime prevalence'/1000 population (95% CI)	Previously reported point prevalence (PP) rates/1000
Stroke	9 (8–11)	5
Transient ischaemia	5 (4–6)	2; 6
Epilepsy	4 (4–5)	5
Congenital neurological deficit	3 (3–4)	3, 2/1000 between 7 and 10 years; CNS malformation 0.7, Down's syndrome 0.5
Parkinson's disease	2 (1–3)	1; 2 (1); 2
Multiple sclerosis	2 (2–3)	1; 2
Diabetic polyneuropathy	2 (1–3)	3
Compressive mononeuropathies (except CTS)	2 (2–3)	0.4
Subarachnoid haemorrhage	1 (0.8–2)	0.5
Polyneuropathy (excluding diabetic and alcoholic)	1 (0.8–2)	0.4
Single seizures	1 (0.9–2)	
Bacterial meningitis	1 (0.8–2)	Abscess 0.02, meningitis 0.05
Other meningitis or encephalitis	1 (1–1)	
Aseptic meningitis	0.9 (0.6–1)	
Essential tremor	0.8 (0.5–1)	3 (1)
Polio	0.7 (0.4–1)	
Severe head injury	0.6 (0.4–1)	1
Optic neuritis	0.6 (0.3–1)	0.1
Benign CNS tumours	0.5 (0.3–1)	0.6 in brain, 0.1 in cord
Intracranial haemorrhage	0.5 (0.2–0.8)	

CTS, carpal tunnel syndrome; HTLV 1, human T-lymphotrophic virus type 1; MS, multiple sclerosis; PN, peripheral nerve.
'Lifetime prevalence' was here defined as a history of the condition at any point up until the survey in this population.
Note: Other prevalent conditions encountered in the study, which occurred with a prevalence of less than 0.5/1000 were: other movement disorders, viral encephalitis, spondylitic and compressive myelopathy, cluster headache, subdural haemorrhage, malignant CNS tumours, peripheral nerve or plexus injury, demyelinating condtions other than MS, cauda equaina lesions, dystonia, benign intracranial hypertension, myelopathy, spinal cord injury, narcolepsy, motor neurone disease, aqueduct stenosis and hydrocephalus in adults, HTLV myelopathy , transient global amnesia, mononeuropathy (excluding carpal tunnel syndrome), trigeminal neuralgia, post-herpetic neuralgia, muscular dystrophies, myasthenia gravis, eye-movement disorders, brachial neuritis, Guillain–Barré syndrome, Horner's syndrome, pupillary abnormalities, sacral plexitis/plexopathy.

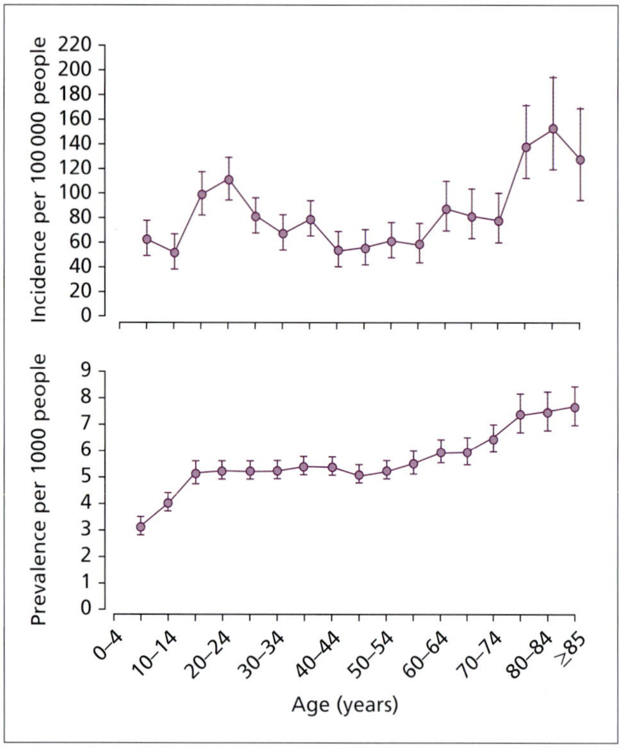

Figure 1.2 Standardised prevalence and incidence rates of treated epilepsy in a population of 2 052 922 persons in England and Wales in 1995. (Bars indicate 95% CI.) Prevalence of treated epilepsy: overall 5.15/1000 people (95% confidence interval [CI] 5.05–5.25) Source: Wallace *et al.* 1998. Reproduced with permission of Elsevier.

the interaction of smoking and genetic susceptibility in Parkinson's disease, or geographic location and genetic susceptibility in multiple sclerosis. The latter is an interesting example as there are often unexplained geographical variations which may reflect either environmental or genetic influences or both. In most neurological diseases, even the common diseases, the primary causes are not clearly understood. Factors which play a part in causation can be divided into the following:

- Predisposing factors (e.g. age, sex, genetic susceptibility);
- Enabling factors (e.g. poor nutrition, housing, inadequate medical care);
- Precipitating factors (e.g. exposure to infectious or noxious agent);
- Reinforcing factors (e.g. repeated or prolonged exposure).

It should be noted that the epidemiological approach to causation is very different from the laboratory approach which studies mechanisms. Cause and mechanism of disease are not necessarily the same (this was a distinction which Hughlings Jackson recognised in relation to epilepsy).

Most neurological diseases are the result of multifactorial causal influences, each of which on their own would not result in the disease, but together have resulted in the disease. In such multifactorial disease, it is often helpful to define 'risk factors' which can be defined as factors that are positively associated with the development of a disease but which on their own are not sufficient to cause the disease. Risk factor studies rely in particular on case–control methodologies, and these can give important clues as to relative importance of different risk factors. The use of hazard ratio (HR) and odds ratio (OR) calculations allow meaningful comparative statistics to be drawn up.

The value of risk factor analysis can be demonstrated by the example of epilepsy resulting from cerebrovascular disease. In one study, a history of stroke has been found to be associated with an increased lifetime occurrence of epilepsy (OR 3.3; 95% confidence interval (CI) 1.3–8.5). Among the other vascular determinants, only a history of hypertension was associated with the occurrence of unprovoked seizures (OR 1.6; 95% CI 1.0–2.4). The risk of unprovoked seizures rises to 4.1 (95% CI 1.5–11.0) in subjects having a history of both stroke and hypertension. Haemorrhagic stroke (subarachnoid haemorrhage and, to a lesser extent, primary intracerebral haemorrhage) are followed by a higher risk of seizures. The cumulative probability of developing seizures after a first stroke is about 6% after 1 year and rises to 11% at 5 years, with significant differences across stroke subtypes. A study by Cleary *et al.* in 2004 compared the frequency of stroke after the development of late-onset seizures, and found late-onset seizures to be a risk factor for stroke as important as high cholesterol or blood pressure. A total of 4709 individuals who had seizures beginning at or after the age of 60 years were compared with 4709 randomly selected matched controls with no history of seizures. Log-rank testing, adjusted for matching, showed a highly significant difference in stroke-free survival between the two groups ($P < 0.0001$) and the relative hazard of stroke at any point for people with seizures compared with the control group was 2.89 (95% CI 2.45–3.41).

The Human Genome project also has added a new dimension to the study of causation of neurological illness, and will in the future also influence studies of the burden of disease. Over 200 Mendelian neurological conditions have been identified and here genomics has had a major impact in understanding the epidemiology and causal mechanisms of disease. Most such diseases are rare and it is clear that the genetic influence on the common neurological diseases is complex and may vary from population to population. To date, around 100 genome-wide association studies of common neurological diseases have been initiated. Eventually, it is to be hoped that such studies will provides estimates of disease heritability, provide unbiased populations for conventional disease-burden studies, and help define the clinical and therapeutic relevance of genetic variants.

The co-morbidities of neurological disease are another area in which risk factor analysis is revealing, but the nature of the association can be complex and not necessarily causal. Some of the causal influences on a disease may also be causal influences on co-morbidity – for instance, smoking resulting in vascular disease causing stroke also increases the risk of renal disease, and thus results in a non-causal association between renal disease and stroke. The treatments of some diseases also result in co-morbidities (e.g. behavioural effects caused by antiepileptic drugs) as does the social handicap of some neurological disorders. The psychiatric co-morbidity of cerebral neurological disorders is particularly complex with genetic, environmental, shared underlying causes and also treatment and direct cerebral damage all potentially contributing. Psychosis, depression and anxiety for instance occur much more frequently in patients with epilepsy than in matched non-epileptic persons, and the relationship of psychiatric disease and epilepsy has been shown to be 'bidirectional'. One explanation of such a bidirectional relationship is that both conditions share risk factors, and particularly genetic risk factors, and several recent studies have found the same copy number variations (CNVs) in epilepsy, autism, schizophrenia, mental retardation and attention deficit hyperactivity disorder.

Mortality

The mortality rate of any condition is defined as the number of persons with that condition dying during a specified period divided by the number of persons in the same population. This information is of limited value, particularly in chronic neurological disease, without a knowledge of the underlying rate of death in patients without the condition or of age distribution. Therefore, mortality is often expressed as the ratio between the observed and expected numbers of death – this measure is known as the standardised mortality ratio (SMR). Expected deaths are calculated by measuring the death rates of a reference population with an age distribution that is similar to the study population. When there is no difference in mortality between the study and reference population the SMR is 1. The 95% CI provides an estimate of the significance of the calculated SMR. Another useful measure is the proportional mortality ratio, which is the percentage of deaths that are due to any one cause. Life expectancy, defined as the median survival, is linked to age and is often lowered in neurological disease when compared with a healthy population, but statistics are complex to derive and there are few studies of this in neurological disease.

Taking epilepsy as an example, in a UK cohort study, reported by Gaitatzis *et al.* in 2006, we followed a cohort of 564 newly diagnosed cases of epilepsy for 11–14 years and found an overall SMR of 2.1 (95% CI 1.8–2.4). The study also calculated the hazard ratio (HR), or risk of mortality in a particular group with a particular risk factor compared with another group without that particular risk factor. For epilepsy overall, it was 6.2 (95% CI 1.4–27.7; $P = 0.049$). Rates varied with the cause of epilepsy: cerebrovascular disease (HR 2.4; 95% CI 1.7–3.4; $P < 0.0001$), CNS tumour (HR 12.0; 95% CI 7.9–18.2; $P < 0.0001$), alcohol (HR 2.9; 95% CI 1.5–5.7; $P = 0.004$) and congenital neurological deficits (HR 10.9; 95% CI 3.2–36.1; $P = 0.003$). An older age at the time of diagnosis was also associated with significantly increased mortality rates (HR 1.9; 95% CI 1.7–2.0; $P < 0.0001$). Life expectancy has also been calculated in the same population based on the Weibull distribution. This depends on age at time of diagnosis and aetiological group, and of course reductions in life expectancy diminish over time. In our study of epilepsy, overall reduction in life expectancy, at the time of diagnosis, was found to be up to 2 years for people with a diagnosis of idiopathic or cryptogenic epilepsy, and up to 10 years in people with symptomatic epilepsy.

Mortality rates can be a useful way of quantifying treatment, but it is equally important in some neurological conditions to consider quality of life. This was well shown in a study of survival after radiotherapy in patients with glioma by Davies *et al.* in 1996. Radiotherapy is known to prolong life if only to a modest extent (in one trial to 38 weeks with radiotherapy compared to 14 weeks with steroids alone). However, the side effects of radiotherapy can be severe, and the trade off between survival and quality of life is important to consider. It was found that the clinical status before radiotherapy was a good indicator of the duration of disability-free life after radiotherapy. The authors showed clearly that for those already disabled by the tumour, radiotherapy offered little physical gain and even if not severely disabled the treatment could cause severe adverse effects.

Other measures and rates

Other epidemiological measures and rates can be derived, for instance related to childbirth or co-morbidity, and are of importance in certain health care areas:

- *Birth rate* is usually defined as the number of live births per mid-year population;
- *Fertility rate* is usually defined as the number of live births per number of women aged 15–44 years;
- *Infant mortality rate* is defined as the number of infant (<1 year) deaths per number of live births;
- *Stillbirth rate* is defined as the number of intrauterine deaths after 28 weeks per total births;
- *Perinatal mortality rate* is the number of stillbirths + deaths in first week of life per total number of births.

Such epidemiological data can be used to investigate causation and assist prevention, but the issues are often complex.

This is well illustrated in a study of fertility in epilepsy amongst a general population of 2 052 922 persons in England and Wales, carried out from Queen Square and reported by Wallace *et al.* in 1998. Age-specific fertility rates were defined as the number of live births per 1000 women-years at risk, in each age category. Fertility was about 30% lower among women with treated epilepsy, with an overall rate of 47.1 live births per 1000 women aged 15–44 per year (42.3–52.2), compared with a national rate of 62.6 in the same age group. The standardised fertility ratios were significantly lower between the ages of 25 and 39 years in women with epilepsy ($P < 0.001$; Figure 1.3). The reasons for these lower rates are complicated. There are undoubtedly social effects: women with epilepsy have low rates of marriage, marry later, experience social isolation and stigmatisation. Some avoid having children because of the risk of epilepsy in the offspring, and some because of the teratogenic potential of antiepileptic drugs. Other patients have impaired personality or cognitive development. However, there are other biological factors that could lead to reduced fecundity. These include genetic factors and adverse antiepileptic drug effects. The lowering of fertility is a worrying finding which is another and important source of disadvantage for women with epilepsy. If there are potentially preventable causes, these should be sought.

Many neurological conditions take a chronic course, so long-term follow-up is important to our understanding of their prognosis and resource implications. Epidemiologically based prospective cohort studies are the optimal method of study to assess the full impact of the disease.

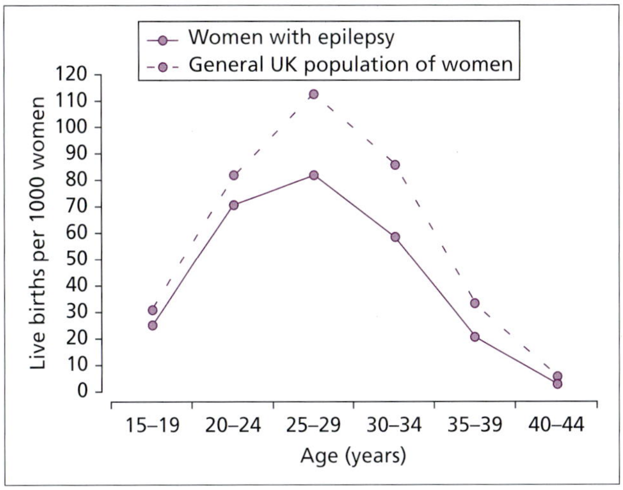

Figure 1.3 Comparison of age-specific fertility rates in women with treated epilepsy and general UK population of women in 1993 (study of a population of 2 052 922 persons). Source: Wallace *et al.* 1998. Reproduced with permission of Elsevier.

Burden of illness

Although the study of the epidemiology of disease provides figures on incidence, prevalence, risk factors and distribution within a population, such information is of limited practical value in terms of population health unless linked to a treatment (or prevention) programme and resource utilisation. A problem that lies at the heart of care provision is the need to focus interventions where needed.

Definitions

The words 'burden of illness' in their widest sense incorporate all negative impacts of illness, although they are often used to denote only the financial costs of illness where costs are understood to encompass the full social costs, both subjective hard to quantify elements as well as objective more easy to quantify measures. These cost of illness studies have the advantage of attempting to quantify a range of negative effects in monetary terms and thus allow comparisons to be drawn. Their disadvantages are obvious – notably the inherent inaccuracies and absurdities of trying to define quality of life issues in terms of monetary loss. Utility measures (e.g. quality-adjusted life years, QALYs, and disability-adjusted life years, DALYs) have also been derived to try to quantify burden more widely, and a particularly important project has been the Global Burden of Disease project sponsored by the World Health Organization (WHO) and World Bank. The burden of illness on individuals and on carers are not comprehensively accounted for in such studies which focus on broad categories biased towards societal and economic considerations.

Cost of illness studies

The principal concern of physicians is to provide individual care, but as health care costs are rising so fast, and even the richest economies are seeking to limit expenditure, clinicians are necessarily now involved in factoring in economic considerations when making therapeutic decisions. This has led to cost of illness studies, which although important are bedevilled with methodological problems that limit their usefulness and validity.

The perspective taken in the analysis is of primary importance in any study of cost of illness. The cost (and burden) for individuals has quite different parameters to the burden for families, for health services or for society in general. Most cost of illness studies are carried out from the point of view of society, with social costs estimated in terms of lost employment, lost productivity and premature death.

Costs are usually divided into two types: direct and indirect. In outline, the direct costs are defined as any resource utilisation required in the care of the illness. These include medical costs such as primary care, hospital outpatient, hospital inpatient, investigation, drugs and non-medical costs such as residential care, community care, training and rehabilitation. Indirect costs are defined as the costs resulting from lost economic production and include premature mortality, dependency, unemployment and underemployment. There are various categories of cost, and any comprehensive analysis should include opportunity costs and transfer payments. Estimation of indirect costs may use the 'human capital' approach which ascribes a monetary value to a person in terms of their potential productivity. In health economic analysis the willingness to pay approach has become popular, which defines costs in terms of how much a person would be willing to spend. This has the advantage of accounting for intangible as well as tangible effects. Both methods are difficult to carry out and both are open to a wide variety of biases and criticisms. With all neurological disorders, the indirect costs are greatly in excess of the direct costs. In one study of epilepsy in 1994, for instance, direct costs accounted for only 13% of all costs in spite of relatively narrow definition of cost.

There are four common methodologies for carrying out economic appraisal:

1. Cost minimisation analysis, which compares interventions where the outcomes are the same;
2. Cost-effectiveness analysis, where outcomes are compared using a single natural measure (e.g. in epilepsy, cost per 50% reduction in seizure frequency);
3. Cost–utility analysis, which is particularly useful for comparing costs between diseases, in which different outcomes can be accounted for and costs are compared in terms of their effects on a utility measure (e.g. the effect on QALYs);
4. Cost–benefit analysis, which measures outcome in terms of economic benefit – accounting for both direct and indirect costs. The latter analysis is the most comprehensive, but in neurology there have been few examples of robust cost–benefit studies. With the increasing availability of expensive therapies and investigations, however, there is a pressing need for good economic appraisal.

Ethical issues relate also to cost-effectiveness. The primary responsibility of a doctor is to the individual patient and not to society. Therapies which are not 'cost-effective' from the epidemiological or societal point of view, may be nevertheless beneficial in an individual – and here the societal and clinical perspectives may clash (indeed, many cultures that purport to put society before the individual usually apply hypocritically different standards to the rulers and the ruled). The impact of social policy, for instance in relation to financial benefits and social support, on the burden of illness is another area that can greatly influence the individual burden.

WHO burden of illness studies

In recent years, the WHO and World Bank have evolved a more comprehensive series of measures of the impact of disease. The best known are the QALY and DALY. The DALY uses a methodology that focuses on disability whereas the QALY focuses on quality of life. These were formidable efforts, involving the WHO in 40 person-years of effort and the collection of data on 483 separate sequelae in 107 diseases and 14 million death certificates. It has to be said, as will be quite obvious to all, that reducing the impact of illness into a one-dimensional measure presents as many methodological difficulties as do studies quantifying illness in monetary terms. The Global Burden of Disease study provides comparative statistics on the impact of disease from 107 countries. To what extent this effort is worthwhile, finally, in helping set priorities has been seriously questioned.

The DALY is an indicator that is most useful in making comparisons between diseases and between regions, and in Table 1.5 some comparative figures are shown for neurological and psychiatric disease. On the basis of this analysis, neuropsychiatric disease accounted for about 15% of the global burden of disease (and 34% of the global burden of disability). For instance, cerebrovascular disease accounts for about 10% of the global burden of neuropsychiatric disease, dementia 2% and epilepsy 1%.

A recent study of disease burden focusing on Europe showed that three of the five highest DALY scoring medical conditions were psychiatric or neurological (stroke, unipolar depression and dementias) and, furthermore, the greatest proportion of DALYs caused by neuropsychiatric diseases were in the highest income group of European countries.

Table 1.5 Disability-adjusted life year (DALY; in thousands) calculations for year 2000 for neurological and psychiatric conditions. Disability-adjusted life year is an indicator of the time lived with a disability and the time lost due to premature mortality. The figures for Europe were separately calculated (Olesen and Leonardi 2003).

	DALYs				
Condition	Europe	Developed countries*	India	Sub-Saharan Africa	World
Neurological and psychiatric conditions (all)†	53 009	24 682	23 949	15 788	165 082
Cerebrovascular disease	10 316	5166	5223	5487	45 770
Unipolar depression	4091	6721	10 064	6193	60 166
Bipolar disease	1541	1673	2867	1785	16 722
Schizophrenia	1609	2151	2041	611	14 614
Epilepsy	633	427	848	526	4712
Alcoholism	4435	4611	1113	2387	18 973
Dementia	4531	3286	1192	453	10 135
Parkinson's disease	428	523	167	63	1278
Multiple sclerosis	303	222	253	140	1569

*Defined as 'established market economies'.
†This category excludes cerebrovascular disease.
Source: World Health Organization (1996).

The personal burden of neurological disease – stigma

The burden of illness of any neurological disease includes aspects that are less directly related to economic factors. Psychological, social, educational, employment and legislative aspects can have a major impact. Some of these are proportionate and rational (e.g. driving restrictions in epilepsy or stroke) but others are not, and a particular issue for patients with neurological disease is the stigma attached to the disease.

Stigma deserves special mention, for it is important in many neurological disorders and yet its consequences are overlooked in burden of illness studies. It is often divided into three categories: enacted (actual experience of discrimination), felt (the fear of discrimination) and self (for instance, devaluation or shame or withdrawal as a personal response to perceived discrimination). There are complex interactions and society will often construct a 'stigma theory' about a disease – to explain the dangers the person represents and which imputes a wide range of imperfections on the basis of the disease. The impact of stigma in neurological disease and epilepsy provides an example. The fact of 'being epileptic' is often more devastating than the simple occurrence of occasional epileptic seizures. In 1989, in Britain, the felt stigma of epilepsy was found to be nine times less common than enacted stigma. The stigma is reflected in the belief that sufferers are retarded, weak, slow, antisocial, physically unattractive or aggressive. Such beliefs are most prevalent in developing societies, and in the United States, for instance, in a number of states, up until 1956, people with epilepsy were prohibited from marrying and could be sterilised, and until the 1970s were excluded from restaurants and theatres. In a large study published in 1999 and 2000, amongst more than 5000 persons with epilepsy in Europe, 51% reported feeling stigmatised and 18% highly stigmatised.

The impact of even non-serious illness can be significant. A study from Dunedin, New Zealand, of tension headache and migraine showed significantly poorer social, mental, physical and emotional functioning than matched non-headache controls. Although equal numbers of those with and without migraine were in employment, 80% of women with migraine were earning £30 000 or less compared with 67% of controls. Nearly half of those with migraine reported that their headaches impaired their social activities. The burden of disease resulting from migraine was considered equal to that of asthma.

Relative costs – developing countries

Ill health has an economic burden that can impose high and regressive cost burdens on the patient and family in all countries. However, in poorer countries the proportion of family income spent on health may be particularly high, not least as ill health results also in unemployment and underemployment. In Sri Lanka, for instance, where health services are free at the point of delivery, it has nevertheless been estimated that the total cost of all illness amounts to 10% of household incomes, and it is likely that neurological illnesses, because of their generally chronic and disabling nature, are particularly onerous. Tuberculosis (TB) is a serious chronic illness which has been well studied from the health economic point of view. In Thailand, it has been reported that TB results in 15% of poor households having to sell material property and 10% taking out loans. In India, amongst patients with TB, 67% of rural patients and 75% of urban patients incurred TB-related debts. Eleven per cent of school children with parents with TB had to discontinue their studies and another 8% had to take up employment. What applies to TB will no doubt also apply to chronic neurological diseases. The impact of diseases depends primarily on the economic position of the family (the lower the economic status, the greater the impact) and the social or family networks and community support available.

Treatment gap

It is also largely economic factors that lie at the heart of failure of treatment. Taking the example of epilepsy again, the concept of the 'epilepsy treatment gap' was devised to provide a numerical measure of the extent of failure of therapy by Farmer and Shorvon in 1989. The treatment gap was defined as the percentage of patients with active epilepsy in a population who do not receive antiepileptic drugs and was an estimate based on prevalence and drug supply figures for that country. Surprising and disturbing results were obtained – in Pakistan, the Philippines and Ecuador treatment gaps of 94%, 94% and 80%, respectively, were ascertained in this study (and considered to be underestimates if anything, resulting from low estimates of prevalence and assumptions of low drug dosages). Since then, prospective population-based studies have largely confirmed similar large treatment gaps in epilepsy in different countries, for instance 62% in China and 73–78% in India. Another study has shown that 41% of people with epilepsy in China have never received antiepileptic drugs. A similar methodology has been widely applied to other countries, for instance recent studies from Georgia and Brazil found about two-thirds of people with active epilepsy had not received appropriate antiepileptic treatment in the month prior to the survey. There are various reasons for these deficiencies of treatment including cost, availability (not least the availability of drugs in pharmacies), cultural factors, lack of medical facilities, and lack of understanding of the potential and role of therapy. Closing the 'treatment gap' has become a priority for health services in many countries, and these findings were a primary stimulus for the highly successful joint WHO and the International League Against Epilepsy (ILAE) campaign to improve epilepsy care – the Global Campaign Against Epilepsy. One intervention study carried out in China 6 months after a Global Campaign survey and found that treatment gap could be reduced by about 20% with relatively simple measures. The campaign is an example of how epidemiological data can be translated into societal action.

References

Cleary P, Shorvon S, Tallis R. Late-onset seizures as a predictor of subsequent stroke. *Lancet* 2004; **363**: 1184–1186.

Harris AI. *Handicapped and Impaired in Great Britain*. London: HMSO, 1971.

Harvey RJ, Skelton-Robinson M, Rossor MN. The prevalence and causes of dementia in people under the age of 65 years. *J Neurol Neurosurg Psychiatry* 2003; **74**: 1206–1209.

Hirtz D, Thurman DJ, Gwinn-Hardy K, Mohamed M, Chaudhuri AR, Zalutsky R. How common are the 'common' neurologic diseases? *Neurology* 2007; **68**: 326–337.

Hopkins A. *Clinical Neurology – A Modern Approach*. Oxford: Oxford University Press, 1993.

Hughes RAC. Peripheral neuropathy: regular review. *BMJ* 2002; **324**: 466–469.

Kurtzke JF. The current neurologic burden of illness and injury in the United States. *Neurology* 1982; **32**: 1207–1214.

MacDonald BK, Sander JWAS, Shorvon SD. The incidence and lifetime prevalence of neurological disorders in a prospective community based study in the United Kingdom. *Brain* 2000; **123**: 665–676.

Olesen J, Leonardi M. The burden of brain disease in Europe. *Eur J Neurol* 2003; **10**: 471–477.

Shorvon SD, Farmer PJ. Epilepsy in developing countries: a review of the epidemiological, socio-cultural and treatment aspects. In: *Chronic Epilepsy: Its Prognosis and Management*. Trimble MT, Reynolds EH, eds. Chichester: John Wiley, 1989: 10–16.

Stewart JA, Dundee R, Howard RS, Rudd AG, Wolfe CDA. Ethnic differences in incidence of stroke: prospective study with stroke register. *BMJ* 1999; **318**: 967–971.

Wallace H, Shorvon SD, Tallis R. Age-specific incidence and prevalence rates of treated epilepsy in an unselected population of 2,052,922 and age-specific fertility rates of women with epilepsy. *Lancet* 1998; **26**: 1970–1973.

World Health Organization. *The Global Burden of Disease*. Geneva: WHO, 1996.

Zakrzewska JM, Hamlyn PJ. Facial pain. In: *Epidemiology of Pain*. Crombie IKCPR, Linton SJ, LeResche L, *et al.* eds. Seattle: IASP, 1999: 171–202.

Further reading

Baker GA, Brooks J, Buck D, Jacoby A. The stigma of epilepsy: a European perspective. *Epilepsia* 2000; **41**: 98–104.

Cockerell OC, Hart YM, Sander JW, Shorvon SD. The cost of epilepsy in the United Kingdom: an estimation based on the results of two population-based studies. *Epilepsy Res* 1994; **8**: 249–260.

Cockerell OC, Shorvon SD. The economic cost of epilepsy. In: Shorvon SD, *et al.* (eds) *The Treatment of Epilepsy*. Oxford: Blackwell Science, 1996: 114–119.

Davies E, Clarke C, Hopkins A. Malignant cerebral glioma. I: Survival, disability and morbidity after radiotherapy. *BMJ* 1996; **313**: 1507–1512.

Davies E, Clarke C, Hopkins A. Malignant cerebral glioma. II: Perspectives of patients and relatives on the value of radiotherapy. *BMJ* 1996; **313**: 1512–1516.

Gaitatzis A, Johnson AL, Chadwick DW, Shorvon SD, Sander JW. Life expectancy in people with newly diagnosed epilepsy. *Brain* 2004; **127**: 2427–2432.

Jacoby A, Snape D, Baker GA. Epilepsy and social identity: the stigma of a chronic neurological disorder. *Lancet Neurol* 2005; **4**: 171–178.

Lhatoo SD, Johnson AL, Goodridge DM, MacDonald BK, Sander JW, Shorvon SD. Mortality in epilepsy in the first 11 to 14 years after diagnosis: multivariate analysis of a long-term, prospective, population-based cohort. *Ann Neurol* 2001; **49**: 336–344.

Li X, Breteler MB, de Bruyne MC, Meinardi H, Hauser WA, Hofman A. Vascular determinants of epilepsy: the Rotterdam study. *Epilepsia* 1997; **38**: 1216–1220.

Lomidze G, Kasradze S, Kvernadze D, Okujava N, Toidze O, de Boer HM, *et al.* The prevalence and treatment gap of epilepsy in Tbilisi, Georgia. *Epilepsy Res* 2012; **98**: 123–129.

Luce BR, Elixhauser A. *Standards for the Socio-Economic Evaluation of Health Care Services*. London: Springer-Verlag, 1990.

Martin J, Meltzer H, Elliot D. *The Prevalence of Disability Among Adults*. London: HMSO, 1988.

Mathers CD, Vos T, Lopez A, Ezzatti M. *National Burden of Disease Studies: A Practical Guide*. Geneva: World Health Organization (Global Program on Evidence for Health Policy), 2001.

Murray CJL, Lopez AD. Global mortality, disability, and the contribution of risk factors: Global Burden of Disease Study. *Lancet* 1997a; **349**: 1436–1442.

Murray CJL, Lopez AD. Alternative projections of mortality and disability by cause 1990–2020: Global Burden of Disease Study. *Lancet* 1997d; **349**: 1498–1504.

Murray CJL, Salomon JA, Mathers CD, Lopez AD. *Summary Measures of Population Health: Concepts, Ethics, Measurement and Application*. Geneva: World Health Organization, 2002.

McCormick A, Rosenbaum M. *Morbidity Statistics from General Practice 1981–82*. London: HMSO, 1990.

Noronha AL, Borges MA, Marques LH, Zanetta DM, Fernandes PT, de Boer H, *et al.* Prevalence and pattern of epilepsy treatment in different socioeconomic classes in Brazil. *Epilepsia* 2007; **48**: 880–885.

Russell S. The economic burden of illness for households in developing countries: a review of studies focusing on malaria, tuberculosis and human immunodeficiency virus/acquired immunodeficiency syndrome. *Am J Trop Med Hyg* 2004; **71** (Suppl 2): 147–155.

Waldie KE, Poulton R. The burden of illness associated with headache disorders among young adults in a representative cohort study. *Headache* 2002; **42**: 612–619.

Wang WZ, Wu JZ, Wang DS, Dai XY, Yang B, Wang TP, *et al.* The prevalence and treatment gap in epilepsy in China: an ILAE/IBE/WHO study. *Neurology* 2003; **60**: 1544–1545.

Wang W, Wu J, Dai X, Ma G, Yang B, Wang T, *et al.* Global campaign against epilepsy: assessment of a demonstration project in rural China. *Bull World Health Organ* 2008; **86**: 964–969.

Wiseman V, Mooney G. Burden of illness estimates for priority setting: a debate revisited. *Health Policy* 1998; **43**: 243–251.

Worldwatch Database. Worldwatch Institute. www.worldwatch.org

World Health Organization. *Investing in Health Research and Development. Report of the Ad Hoc Committee on Health Relating to Fugure Intervention Options*. Geneva: WHO, 1996.

CHAPTER 2

Nervous System Structure and Function

Charles Clarke[1] and Roger Lemon[2]

[1]National Hospital for Neurology & Neurosurgery

[2]UCL Institute of Neurology

BASIC NEUROSCIENCE

Introduction

The complexity of the nervous system must have posed daunting challenges for clinical neurology as our discipline began to develop in the late nineteenth century. However, despite the truly remarkable descriptions of the intricacies of axonal and dendritic networks by Santiago Ramón y Cajal in Spain in the 1890s, using light microscopes (Figures 2.1 and 2.2), the cortical mapping by Korbinian Brodmann in Berlin in the early twentieth century and later the fine detail of neuro-anatomical pathways by Alf Brodal in Oslo and many others in the 1940s, it remained evident that a rudimentary knowledge of neuro-anatomy, and little of neuroscience could provide a robust basis for most day-to-day neurological practice. Many neurologists in the past have had a sketchy knowledge of pathways and disease mechanisms, an indication of the reliability of simple observation of symptoms and signs. It is something of an enigma that trainees in the twenty-first century, alongside the explosion in scientific knowledge still need to know how to use the basic clinical tools developed over 100 years ago – but they can no longer practice neurology with these alone.

Knowledge is increasing rapidly: advances in imaging, neurogenetics, neurochemistry, neurotransmitter technology, immunology and molecular biology have added new dimensions to clinical practice, to the relevance of neuronal and glial ultrastructure and function and complexities of neuro-anatomy. By looking at ultrastructure, imaging, genetics, chemistry and neuronal activity we begin to understand conditions as diverse as Alzheimer's disease, Parkinson's disease, myasthenia gravis, polyneuropathies and headache – itself the most common neurological complaint the world over. This chapter provides a brief overview of how the nervous system is organised and, where appropriate, how abnormalities found on examination are explained.

The functional unit: the neurone

The neurone (>100 billion within the human brain) is the functional unit of the nervous system. Neuronal specificity, size and cell type vary greatly. One α-motor neurone of the lower thoracic cord has an axon over 1 m in length and innervates between several hundred and 2000 muscle fibres, to form a motor unit. By comparison, some spinal or intracerebral interneurones have axons under 100 μm long which terminate on a single neuronal cell body. A summary of neuronal ultrastructure follows.

The neurone is constituted by its nucleus, cytoplasm, neuronal membrane and cytoskeleton (Figure 2.3). Neurotransmission and intrinsic modification of the neurone itself are its functions, to facilitate transfer of information, and to adapt to and record change. The combination of axonal electrical activity and synaptic neurotransmitter release provides the basis for most interneuronal transmission; the release of neuromodulators is also an important role. The integrity of intraneuronal and glial structure and function is also essential; glia play a part in synaptic transmission, re-uptake of neurotransmitters and the general control of the extracellular environment in which the neurones are located. Neuronal plasticity means the ability of neurones to adapt, to change, singly, in sequence and/or in groups and is a particularly well-developed aspect of the mammalian nervous system. Plasticity has a pivotal role in both learning and recovery from injury.

From the neurone cell body (soma, perikaryon) extend neurites (i.e. axons, up to 1 m long), and dendrites that are rarely longer than a few millimetres. Most axons branch repeatedly to establish synaptic connections with other neuronal cell bodies. In this way one neurone is able to make divergent connections with many other neurones within the central nervous system (CNS).

The dendritic and soma membrane represents the main region through which the neurone receives its synaptic input. Some neurones receive many thousands or even hundreds of thousands of such inputs. The neuronal membrane is the 5-nm thick barrier enclosing cytoplasm, excluding substances bathing the neurone. This membrane, a bi-layer of phospholipid has typically a polar hydrophilic head and an insoluble non-polar hydrophobic tail. Neuronal membrane proteins are responsible for the interaction between the neurone and its environment. These proteins are:

- Ion channels, usually either ligand-gated or transmitter-gated
- Receptors, and
- Cell adhesion molecules.

The cytoskeleton consists of microtubules, neurofilaments and microfilaments. Microtubules are some 20 nm diameter, hollow-walled strands of α and β tubulin – polymers of globular microtubule associated proteins (MAPs). For example, tau is an axonal MAP; dynein and kinesin are motor proteins (also known as

Neurology: A Queen Square Textbook, Second Edition. Edited by Charles Clarke, Robin Howard, Martin Rossor and Simon Shorvon.

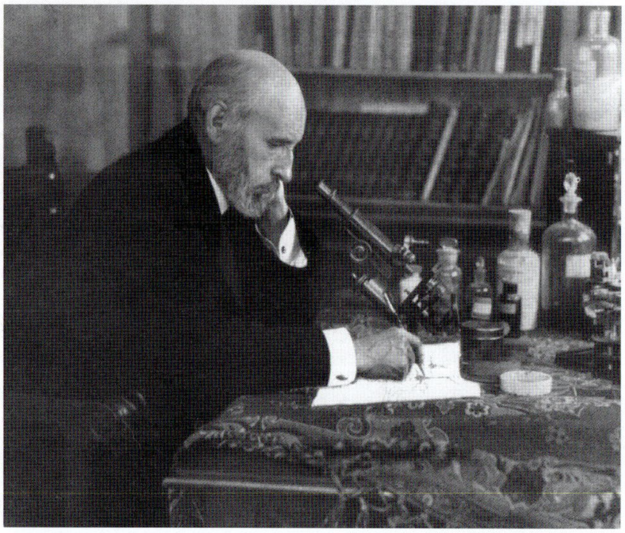

Figure 2.1 Professor Santiago Ramón y Cajal (1852–1934) working at his light microscope in 1915. (With kind permission of the Instituto Cajal, Madrid.)

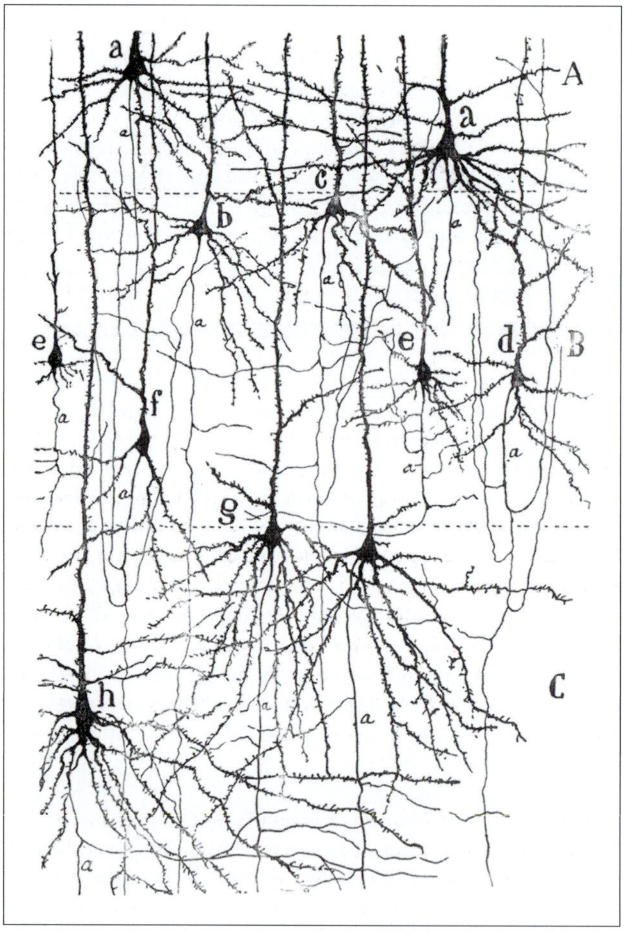

Figure 2.2 Fine detail of neo-cortical pyramidal neurones (Cajal). (a,b,c) Small pyramids; (d,e) medium neurones; (f), bitufted neurones; (g,h) large neurones. (With kind permission of the Instituto Cajal, Madrid.)

molecular motor or motor molecules) that convert chemical energy in adenosine triphosphate (ATP) into mechanical energy (movement).

Neurofilaments are 10 nm thick (intermediate filaments of all other cells), braided, tight, physically strong protein strands. They form a peri-nuclear network and provide structural integrity. Microfilaments are 5 nm thick, braided duplexes of actin (42–44 kDa). They are critically involved in neurone shape.

Neuronal replication is the exception, although neurogenesis has been clearly shown to take place in the olfactory neuro-epithelium, hippocampus and hypothalamus. However, studies of neuronal dynamics show that in all neurones the intraneuronal contents are continually being reformed and degraded. For example, the cofactor ubiquitin molecule interacts with degraded proteins via hydrophobic residues – complexes of more than five ubiquitin molecules are broken down by an ATP-dependent multi-enzyme system, the 26S proteasome. Failure to remove degraded proteins is of signal importance in many neurodegenerative diseases (e.g. Alzheimer's disease; Chapter 8), and myopathies such as inclusion body myopathy (see Inclusion body myopathy, Chapter 10).

Amyloid and tau in Alzheimer's disease

As an example of a disease mechanism, still to be fully unravelled, in Alzheimer's neurofibrillary tangles develop; these are filamentous inclusions within the soma and dendrites adjacent to it. Paired helical and 15-nm straight insoluble protein filaments become visible. These are isoforms of tau, the microtubule binding protein that in health is soluble. This structural change in the cytoskeleton is likely to impair axonal transport, neurotransmission and eventually viability of the neurone.

In the second pathological hallmark of Alzheimer's, the extracellular senile plaque, deposits of amyloid are surrounded by dystrophic neuronal elements. Amyloid is the name given to pathological β-pleated sheets of aggregates of fibrillar peptides that stain with Congo red and are doubly refractive in polarised light. Aβ amyloid, a 4-kDa peptide cleaved from amyloid precursor protein (APP) is the main constituent of histological amyloid.

APP is one member of a larger family of amyloid precursor-like proteins, APLP1 and APLP2. APP is encoded by a gene in the long arm of chromosome 21; it exists in three main isoforms of 695–770 aminoacids. Neuronal APP is the source of most extracellular Aβ amyloid in Alzheimer's disease. APP synthesis takes place in the rough endoplasmic reticulum. It is glycosylated in the Golgi apparatus and offered to the internal surface of the neurone as an integrated membrane protein. A fraction of APP within the plasmalemma remains within the neurone from which are generated various forms of Aβ ($A\beta_{1-40}$, $A\beta_{1-42}$, truncated $A\beta_{17-40}$ peptides). Putative mechanisms of neurotoxicity of Aβ fragments and the genetics of Alzheimer–APP gene mutations (chromosome 21), presenilin 1 and 2 (chromosomes 14 and 1), and allelic forms of ApoE (chromosome 19) are discussed in Chapter 8 (see Alzheimer's disease).

Neurotransmission

Electrical synapses

Between mammalian neurones, the electrical synapses, found, for example, in the giant squid, have largely been replaced by chemical transmission systems. Electrical synapses do, however, persist in the human CNS and are found at gap junctions, where the synaptic cleft is some 3 nm wide. Connexin protein complexes (see Myelin) span these narrow gaps, coupling adjacent cells electrotonically with pores

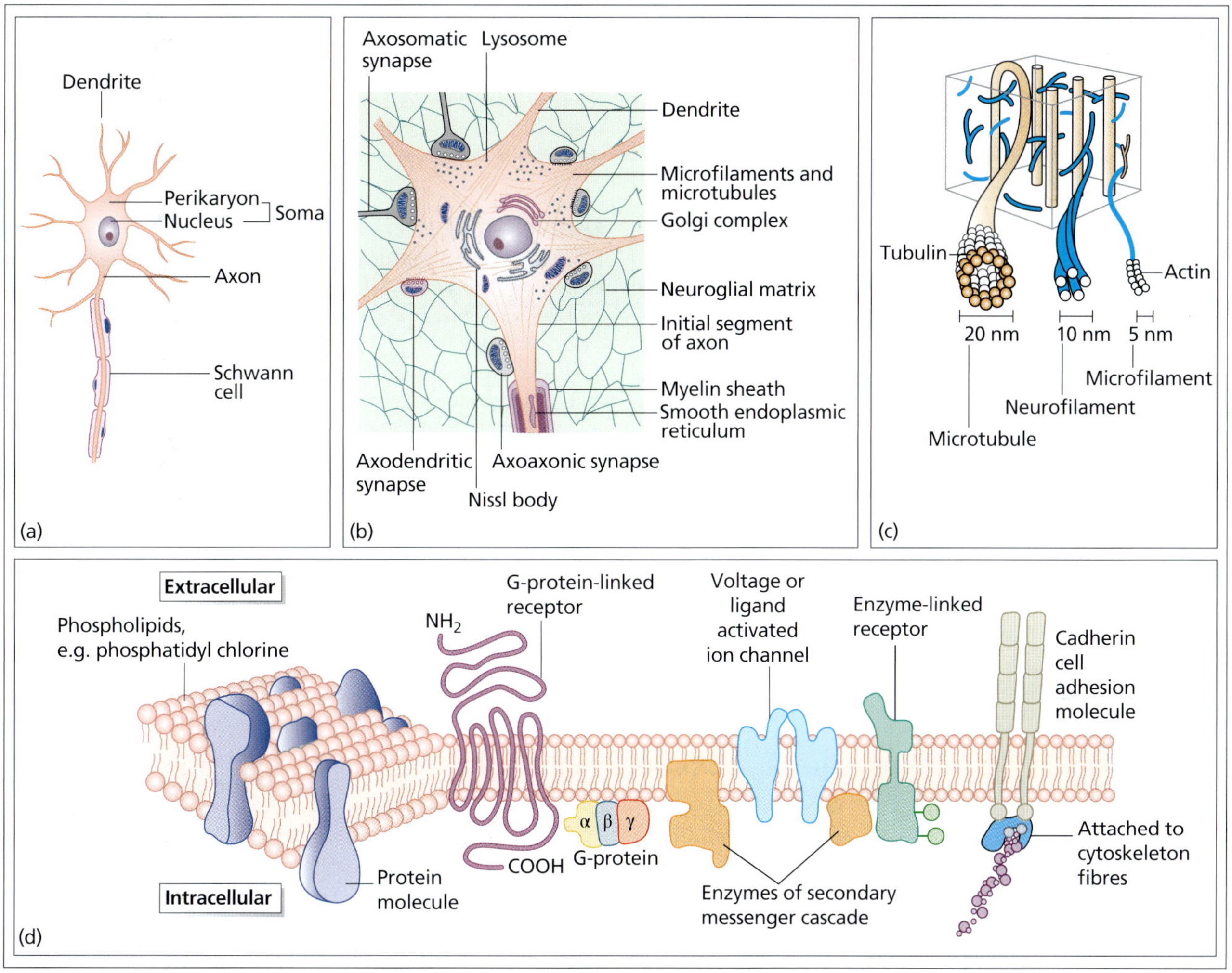

Figure 2.3 Motor neurone. (a) Soma, axon and Schwann cell; (b) ultrastructure; (c) cytoskeleton; (d) neuronal membrane.

some 2 nm in diameter. These pores are large enough for the passage of all major cellular ions and many organic molecules. Electrical transmission is bi-directional, and slow. Gap junctions occur between glial cells, epithelial cells, smooth and cardiac muscle cells, and in some nuclei in the brain (e.g. the inferior olivary nucleus). During brain development, transmission via gap junctions between neighbouring neurones coordinates growth and maturation.

Chemical synapses

In a chemical synapse, the synaptic cleft is some 20–50 nm wide and filled with an adherent matrix, ensuring its stability. The presynaptic element, usually an axon terminal, houses mitochondria, synaptic vesicles and larger secretory granules – the dense-core vesicles seen on electron microscopy. Either side of the synaptic cleft specialised areas of accumulated protein comprise membrane differentiations, with an active zone on the presynaptic side opposite the post-synaptic density. The postsynaptic density houses receptors. Receptors make possible intracellular events, changes in membrane potential or secondary chemical events and are sensitive to interactions with neurotransmitters and neuromodulatory agents released by the presynaptic neurone.

Types of CNS synapse

CNS synapses are classified as axodendritic (axon → dendrite), axosomatic (axon → cell body), axo-axonic and dendro-dendritic (Figure 2.3). Gray's type I and II synapses are terms also used (Figure 2.4):

- *Gray's type I* usually excitatory. Asymmetrical membrane differentiation, with postsynaptic membrane thicker and more complex than presynaptic.
- *Gray's type II* usually inhibitory. Symmetrical membrane differentiation.

Peripheral nervous system synapses

Synaptic transmission is also involved throughout the peripheral nervous system, from autonomic nerve fibres to smooth and cardiac muscle and transmission from motor nerves to striated skeletal muscle fibres via neuromuscular junctions, the specialised cholinergic synapses facilitating fast reliable neuromuscular transmission. Their peripheral site and accessible micro-anatomy have made possible the detailed study of neuromuscular transmission.

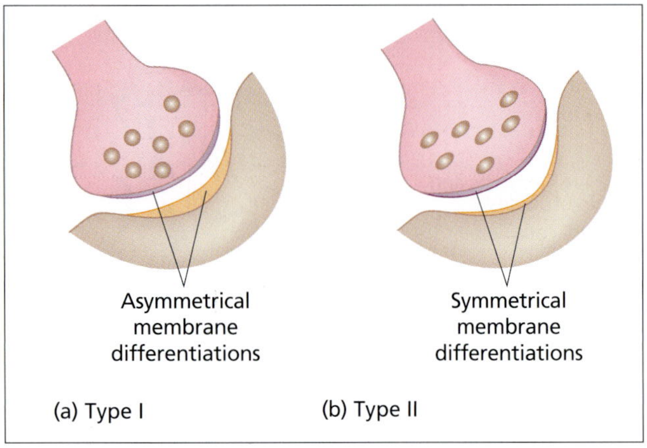

Figure 2.4 Gray's type I and II synapses.

Neuromuscular junction

At the motor end-plate presynaptic active zones are closely aligned to the postsynaptic membrane densely packed with acetylcholine receptor sites (Figure 2.5). Acetylcholine, liberated by an action potential leads to acetylcholine release from synaptic vesicles into the synaptic cleft. Depolarisation of the motor end-plate follows.

Neurotransmitters

Effective chemically mediated synaptic transmission requires transmitters to be synthesised, transported, liberated appropriately, metabolised and/or recycled. Neurotransmitters fall into one of four categories (Table 2.1).

Neurotransmitters are synthesised in several ways. Glutamate and glycine are ubiquitous amino acids, abundant in all cells including neurones. Gamma-aminobutyric acid (GABA) and amine neurotransmitters are made only by neurones that release them, via

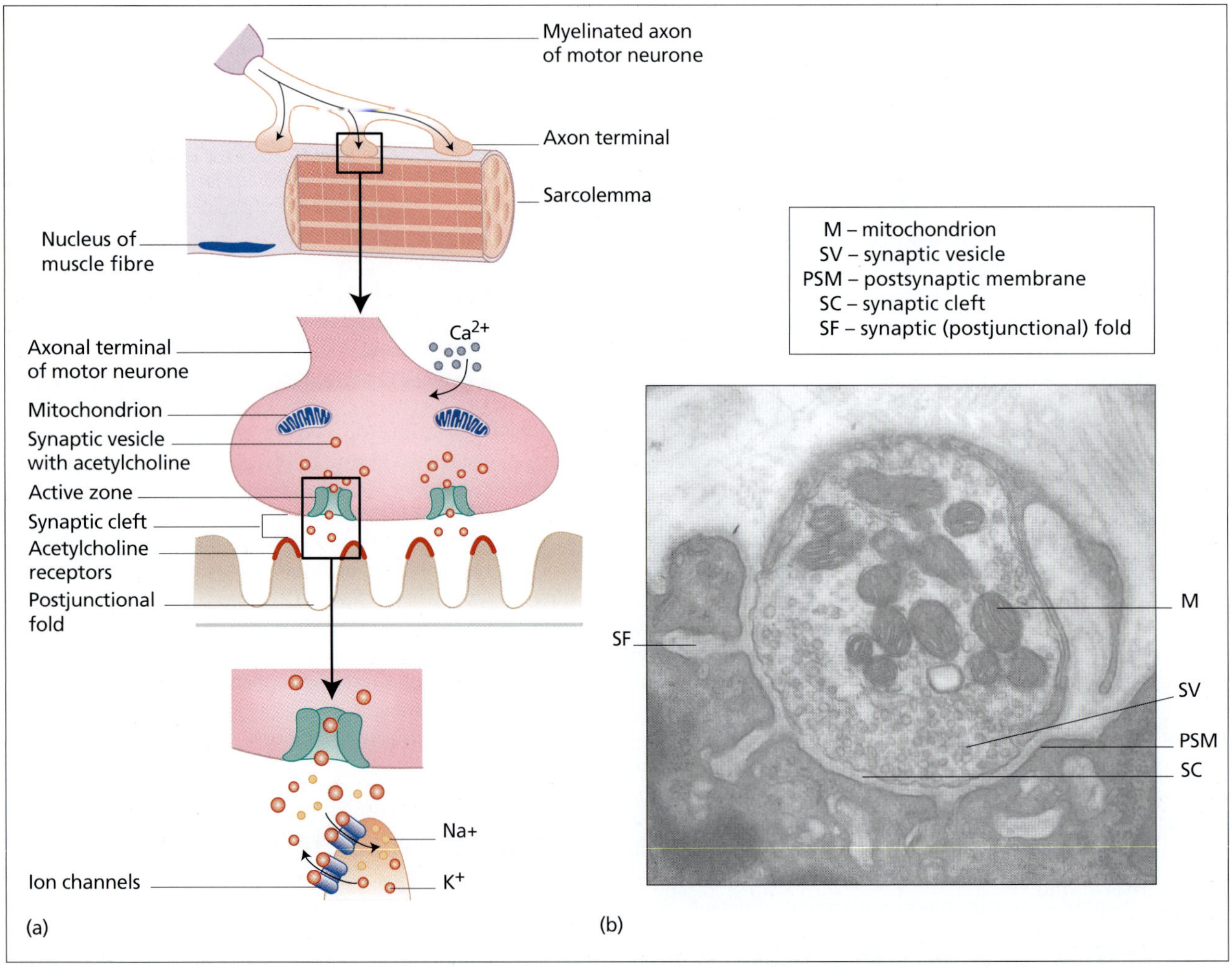

Figure 2.5 Neuromuscular junction. (a) General arrangement and detail. (b) Electron micrograph of neuromuscular junction from mouse flexor digitorum brevis. Courtesy of Professor Tom Gillingwater, Centre for Integrative Physiology, University of Edinburgh. Source: Gillingwater and Ribchester (2001). Reproduced with permission of John Wiley & Sons.

Table 2.1 Principal neurotransmitters.

Amino acids	Amines	Peptides (many others)	Gases
γ-Amino-butyric acid (GABA)	Acetylcholine (ACh)	Cholecystikinin (CCK)	Nitric oxide (NO)
Glutamate (Glu)	Dopamine (DA)	Dynorphin	Carbon monoxide (CO)
Glycine (Gly)	Adrenaline (epinephrine)	Enkephalins (Enk)	
	Noradrenaline (norepinephrine)	*N*-acetyl-aspartyl-glutamate (NAAG)	
	Histamine	Neuropeptide Y	
	Serotonin (5-HT)	Somatostatin	
		Substance P	
		Thyrotropin-releasing hormone (TRH)	
		Vasoactive intestinal peptide (VIP) and vascular endothelial growth factor (VEGF)	

Purines, ATP and adenosine are also neurotransmitters.

specific enzymes and precursors. Synthesising enzymes for both amino acid and amine neurotransmitters are transported to the axon terminal where they direct transmitter synthesis, locally and promptly. Once synthesised, transporter proteins concentrate amino acid and amine transmitters within synaptic vesicles.

Peptide neurotransmitters are strung together by ribosomes within the rough endoplasmic reticulum (ER) and cleaved to form active molecules in the Golgi apparatus (GA). Secretory granules bud off the GA and are carried to the axon terminal by axoplasmic transport.

Amine and amino acid transmitters are stored in and released from synaptic vesicles. Peptide neurotransmitters are stored in and released from secretory granules. These may coexist in the same neurone, to be released under different conditions.

Transmitter release

Neurotransmitter release into the synaptic cleft is triggered by the arrival of an action potential at the axon terminal, where depolarisation of the terminal membrane causes voltage-gated calcium channels to open. Vesicles release transmitters by exocytosis at an active zone into the synaptic cleft; the vesicle membrane is recovered by endocytosis.

Secretory granules (dense core vesicles) also release neurotransmitters by exocytosis, but typically not at active zones. Peptide neurotransmitters are not released by every action potential, but typically by high frequency trains of action potentials. Peptide release is typically slow (50 ms), while amino acid and amine release is rapid.

Transmitter-gated ion channels and G-protein-coupled receptors

Neurotransmitter–receptor binding – the key–lock analogy is simple but valuable – alters the shapes of receptor proteins and hence their function. There are two types of receptor. Transmitter-gated ion channels consist of protein subunits that open an ion pore, and change shape in response to neurotransmitter. For example, the ACh-gated ion channel at the neuromuscular junction, permeable to both Na^+ and K^+, is triggered to produce an excitatory post-synaptic potential (EPSP) in response to ACh. Both ACh and glutamate-gated channels trigger EPSPs when activated (i.e. they are excitatory). Glycine-gated and GABA-gated channels, permeable to Cl^- ions and tending to hyperpolarise the resting membrane potential, are inhibitory, triggering inhibitory post-synaptic potentials (IPSPs). Amino acid and amine neurotransmitters deliver fast synaptic transmission via transmitter-gated ion channels.

G-protein-coupled receptors are involved in a more diverse, slower and longer lasting mechanism of chemical synaptic transmission in response to amino acid, amine and peptide neurotransmitters. Receptor proteins activate G-proteins that travel along the intracellular face of the post-synaptic membrane. These in turn activate effector proteins – membrane-located G-protein-gated ion channels or enzymes that synthesise second messengers. Binding of odorants to receptors within the olfactory system is an example G-protein-gated transmission.

Glia

Within the CNS, four types of glial cells support neuronal activity: astrocytes, oligodendrocytes, microglia and ependymal cells. Schwann cells are the neuroglia of the peripheral nervous system, investing some peripheral axons with myelin. Neurones and glia are biologically interdependent.

Astrocytes

These are microscopically star-shaped shaggy cells from which protrude several dozen, fine astroglial processes that make intimate contact with neurones (Figure 2.6). Intermediate filaments within astrocyte cytoplasm lend tensile strength to the brain and cord. Glycogen granules within astrocyte cytoplasm provide intermediate energy (glucose) to surrounding neurones. Astrocytes are engaged in recycling glutamate and GABA and scavenging potassium ions following neurotransmission; they have an essential role in controlling the composition of the extracellular fluid. Glial limiting membranes – from astrocytic processes – cover the pial surface of the brain and with ependyma line the ventricles. Vascular processes of astrocytes are in intimate contact with CNS capillaries. Astrocytes retain the capacity to multiply, and do so following neuronal injury to form glial scars (gliosis). Neoplastic proliferation leads to astrocytomas (see Astrocytomas, Chapter 21).

Oligodendrocytes (oligodendroglia)

One oligodendrocyte lays the myelin sheaths of 30–40 CNS axons, the inner and outer surfaces forming the spiral sheaths seen as minor and major dense lines on extracellular matrix. The axon is exposed between oligodendroglial segments at each node of Ranvier. Paranodal pockets – collections of cytoplasm – are visible at each end of each myelin lamination (see Schwann cells).

CNS myelination commences *in utero* and continues for some 20 years in humans. The effect of the ensheathing myelin lamellar spiral is to facilitate both saltatory conduction and axonal integrity.

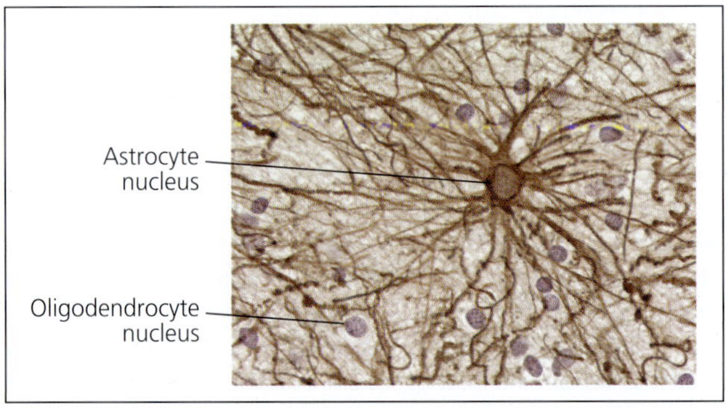

Figure 2.6 Astrocytes. Source: FitzGerald 2010. © 2016 Elsevier. Reproduced with permission of Elsevier.

The nature of CNS demyelination (i.e. the breakdown of normal rapid axonal saltatory conduction), seen typically in multiple sclerosis, is discussed in Chapter 11 (see Mechanisms). Neoplastic proliferation leads to oligodendrogliomas (see Oligodendrogliomas, Chapter 21). Within grey matter, modified oligodendroglia are seen as satellite cells – involved in interneuronal ion transfer. Many CNS axons remain unmyelinated – typically small <0.2-μm diameter fibres.

Microglia

Some cells of neuro-epithelial lineage develop into phagocytes, known as microglia. When stimulated by neuronal injury, demyelination or vascular CNS damage, these motile scavengers increase in size and number.

Ependyma

Ependyma are ciliated cells that line the cerebral ventricles and central cavity of the cord, together with astrocytic glial limiting membrane. Their function is to define the integrity of the parenchyma–CSF interface. Ependymal cilia are involved in CSF propulsion. Neoplastic proliferation produces ependymomas (Chapter 21).

Schwann cells

A sequence of Schwann cells ensheaths each myelinated axon of a peripheral neurone. Like CNS oligodendroglial sheaths, ultrastructural major and minor dense lines are seen, and paranodal sockets of cytoplasm at the end of each Schwann cell, recognised by Ranvier in the 1880s. The mesaxon is the mesenteric membrane, displaced centrifugally as the spiral layering of the Schwann cell develops (Figure 2.7). One main function of the Schwann cell is to make possible saltatory conduction. Modified Schwann cells, known as satellite cells, are found within posterior root ganglia and others known as teloglia at enclosed peripheral sensory nerve endings.

Myelination is an active lifelong process. Remyelination is the response to peripheral nerve injury. The effects and mechanisms of peripheral nerve demyelination are discussed further in Chapter 10.

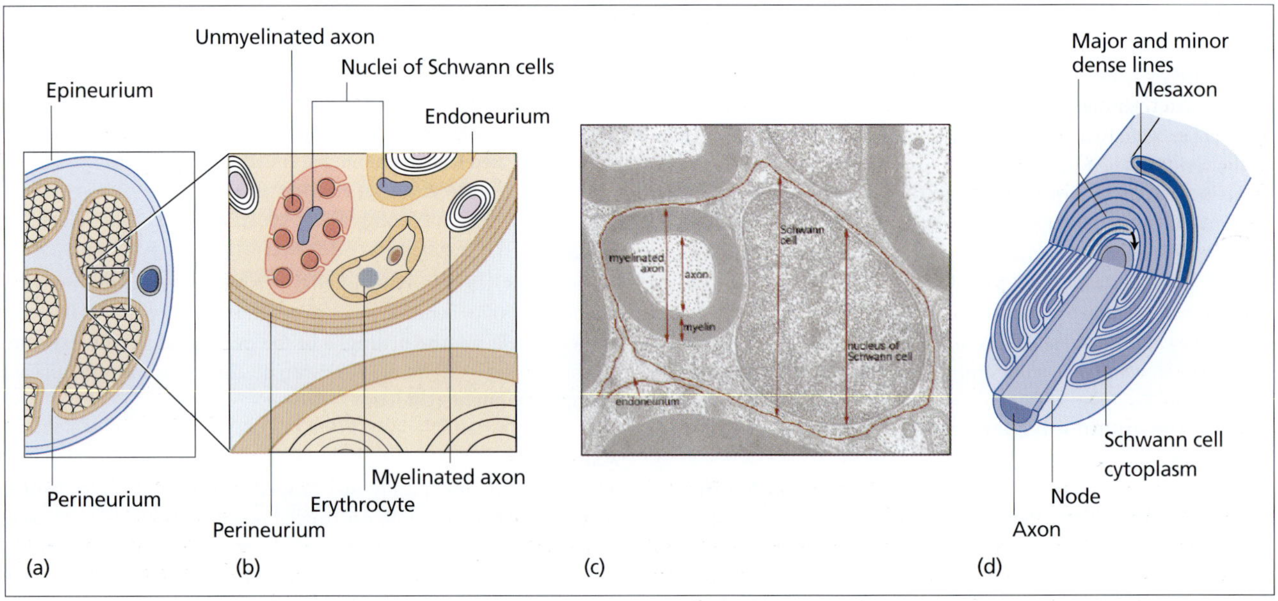

Figure 2.7 Peripheral nerve and Schwann cells. (a) Nerve trunk (transverse section). (b) Detail of (a). (c) Electron micrograph of Schwann cells and axons. Courtesy of Professor Sebastian Brandner, Institute of Neurology. (d) Spiral myelin sheath of Schwann cell.

Table 2.2 Fibre types within peripheral nerves from various mammalian data.

Fibre type	Diameter (mm)	Conduction velocity (m/s)	Function
Aα (mixed)	13–22	17–120	α-motor neurones, muscle spindle primary endings, Golgi tendon organs, touch
Aβ (mixed)	8–13	40–70	Touch, muscle spindle secondary endings, joint position
Aγ (mixed)	4–8	15–40	Touch, pressure, γ-motor neurones
Aδ (mixed)	1–4	5–15	Pain, crude touch, pressure, temperature
B (mixed)	1–3	3–14	Preganglionic autonomic
C (mixed)	0.1–1	0.2–3	Pain, touch, pressure, temperature, post-ganglionic autonomic
Ia (afferent)	12–20	70–120	Muscle spindle primary endings
Ib (afferent)	11–19	66–120	Golgi tendon organs
II (afferent)	5–12	2–50	Touch, muscle spindle secondary endings
III (afferent)	1–5	4–20	Pain, pressure, temperature, crude touch
IV (afferent)	0.1–2	0.2–3	Pain, touch, pressure, temperature

Peripheral nerve fibre types

The complex classification (Table 2.2) of fibre types, assembled largely from mammalian data, is seldom used in clinical practice, but it is of value when a particular fibre type is studied. In the cat, conduction velocity up to 15 m/s is achieved in unmyelinated fibres and up to about 120 m/s in myelinated fibres; there is much variation between species. Afferent fibres are classified on a numerical system I–IV, while the A–C classification includes mixed nerves. Peripheral nerve ultrastructure is outlined in Figure 2.7; pathological features are discussed in Chapter 10.

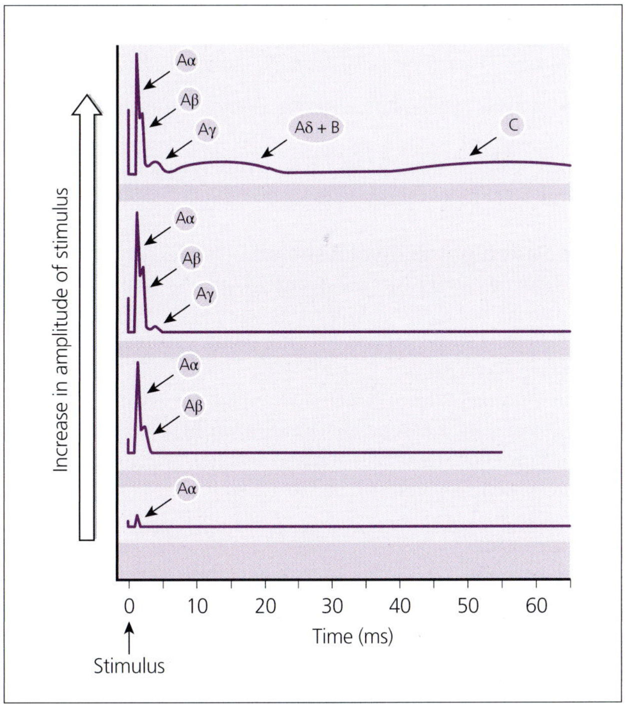

Figure 2.8 Recruitment of nerve fibre types with increasing stimuli. Responses from a typical mixed (motor and sensory) nerve (e.g. sciatic).

Myelin and saltatory conduction

The degree of myelination and fibre diameter are the principal factors determining conduction velocity. The contribution of each nerve fibre type to a compound action potential has been outlined earlier (Figure 2.8). In disease, mechanisms that alter nerve function are divided broadly into axonal (i.e. those that affect the axon itself), and demyelinating, where the intregrity of myelin is compromised.

Myelin was a word coined by Virchow, simply for a fatty substance obtained from various tissues; it was adopted by Schwann to describe the 'white substance' of peripheral nerves. CNS myelin provides similar conduction properties, but there are specific neurochemical characteristics that differentiate it from peripheral nerve myelin. Some functional features of peripheral nerve myelin are outlined here:

- Rapid conduction along both peripheral nerves and within the CNS is achieved by saltatory conduction.
- In the myelinated nerve fibre the axonal membrane is adapted at regular sites. Of note, at each node of Ranvier voltage-gated sodium channels are concentrated; these are involved in action potential propagation. Fast and slow potassium channels are involved in membrane repolarisation.
- Depolarization of the axonal membrane at each node of Ranvier is induced by an initial influx of sodium ions, leading to a voltage-dependent massive influx of more sodium ions, and a new wave of depolarisation to be propagated in saltatory fashion (i.e. jumping) to the next node of Ranvier.
- Depolarisation is also achieved in unmyelinated fibres, but by sodium channels distributed along the whole length of the axon.

Table 2.3 Myelin protein characteristics.

	Approximate percentage*	Mass (kDa)	Chromosome†
Glycoproteins			
P0	65	28	1
PMP22	4	22	17
MAG	1	100	19
Periaxin	5	170	7 (mouse)
E-cadherin	<0.5	130	16
Basic proteins			
MBP	10	14–21.5	18
P2	5	14.8	8
Other proteins			
CNP	<0.5	46/48	17
PLP/DM20	<0.5	30/25	X
Cx32	<0.5	32	X

* Of myelin proteins.
† In humans.

Myelin saves space and conserves energy – to achieve a given mean conduction velocity an unmyelinated axon would require a diameter some 40 times greater than a myelinated one and would consume 5000 times more energy.

Composition of the myelin sheath

Peripheral myelin is the differentiated plasma membrane of a Schwann cell. It is a lipid-rich, tightly packed spiral surrounding the axon (Figure 2.7) penetrated by cytoplasmic channels (Schmidt–Lanterman incisures).

Gene cloning of the principal myelin proteins and their association with specific neuropathies has thrown light on their role in myelin formation, their function and maintenance. Some features of these proteins are outlined in Table 2.3.

Glycoproteins

Protein zero (P0) P0, a major protein of peripheral nervous system myelin is expressed in all myelinating Schwann cells. The role of the P0 molecule is cell adhesion, promoting and maintaining tight compaction of myelin. One of its domains contributes to the intraperiod line.

Peripheral myelin protein 22 (PMP22) This is also concerned with adhesion between lipid and protein molecules. PMP22 is also found widely outside the peripheral nervous system.

Myelin associated glycoprotein (MAG) MAG is believed to participate in signal transduction during glial differentiation, axonal recognition, adhesion and neurite outgrowth. MAG is located in the Schmidt–Lanterman incisures, paranodal loops at nodes of Ranvier, in external and internal mesaxons and the peri-axonal Schwann cell membrane itself.

Periaxin The primary localisation of this peripheral nervous system-specific myelin protein is close to the peri-axonal membrane (rather than an integral membrane protein; cf. P0, MAG and PMP22).

Epithelial cadherin (E-cadherin) Cadherins are calcium-dependent adhesion proteins. In Schwann cells, E-cadherin is the major adhesive glycoprotein in non-compacted regions of the myelin sheath.

Basic proteins

Myelin basic proteins Both central and peripheral nervous systems contain peripheral membrane polypeptides known as myelin basic proteins (MBPs). MBPs are believed to participate with P0 in the major dense line and compaction.

Protein P2 P2 is a fatty acid-binding protein, with postulated roles in the assembly, maintenance and remodelling of myelin.

Other proteins

Cyclic nucleotide phosphodiesterases (CNPs) are concentrated in the outer perimeter of the myelin sheath, the outer mesaxon, Schwann cell surface membrane and peri-axonal region. Proteolipid proteins (PLPs) are localised in compact myelin and thought to have a structural role in the intraperiod line. Connexin 32 (Cx32) is a component of gap junction channels. It is found at paranodal regions and at Schmidt–Lanterman incisures.

Myelination and axon–Schwann cell interactions

In a developing nerve, a bundle of naked axons is surrounded by a single Schwann cell layer. Schwann cell–axon contact triggers Schwann cell proliferation. The axons become segregated and as maturation continues a one-to-one relationship develops – each Schwann cell investing a single axonal segment. The Schwann cell elongates and rotates as myelin develops about the axis of the axon, to form the nodal spiral structure seen on microscopy.

The precise nature of the axonal signal for myelination remains obscure. However, when Schwann cells receive the signal to myelinate, various transcription factors (Oct-6, Krox-20, Sox-10) participate in gene expression to ensure the particular myelinating phenotype of the individual Schwann cell.

Sensory nerve endings

A single nerve fibre has the same type of endings on each of its terminals, comprising a physiological sensory unit that receives information from a receptive field. In the skin, each receptive field covers some 5 mm^2 on a finger tip and 2 cm^2 on the upper arm. Sensory units of different modalities frequently supply the same patch of skin (Figures 2.9 and 2.10).

Nerve endings are:

- Free
- Follicular
- Encapsulated, or
- Merkel–neurite complexes
- Muscle spindle flower spray and annulospiral endings.

Free nerve endings (naked axons) that have lost both perineural and myelin sheaths form a dermal and subepidermal network and innervate joints, ligaments and capsules. Some are thermoreceptors, others nociceptors. Some nociceptors (from finely myelinated Aδ fibres) respond fast to severely painful stimuli (e.g. pinching). Others, from slowly conducting C fibres, are

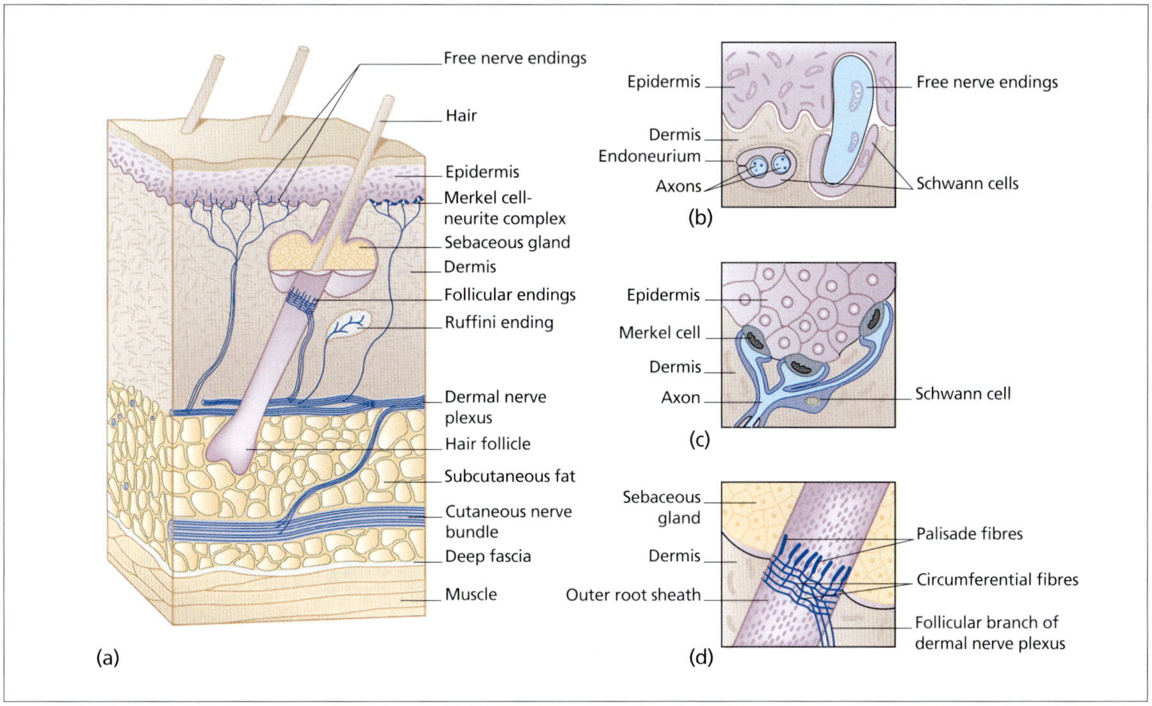

Figure 2.9 Examples of nerve endings in hairy skin. (a) General arrangement. (b) Free nerve endings. (c) Merkel cell–neurite complex. (d) Palisade and circumferential nerve endings. Source: FitzGerald 2010. © 2016 Elsevier. Reproduced with permission of Elsevier.

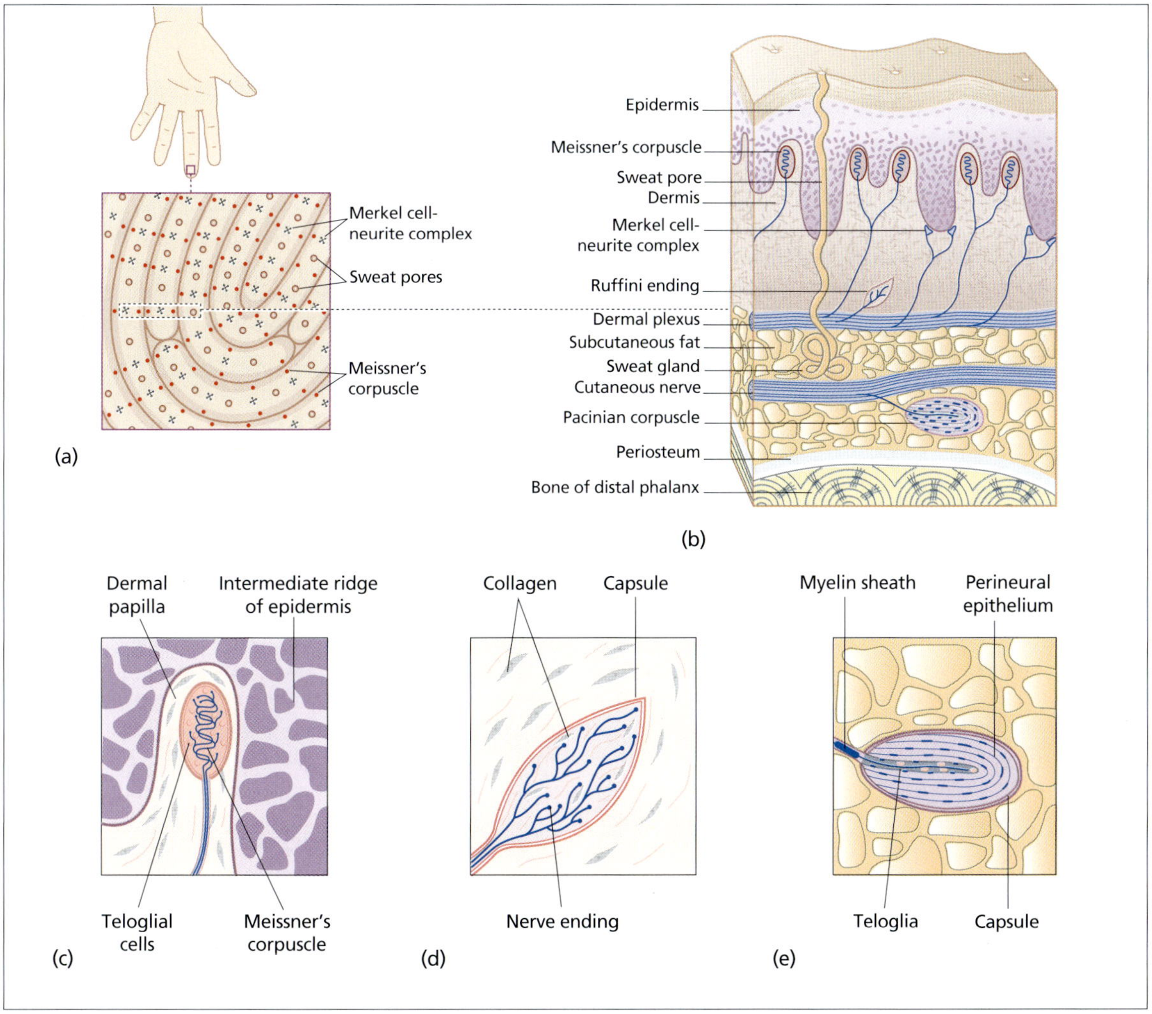

Figure 2.10 Example of nerve endings in non-hairy skin. (a) Finger tip: Meissner's corpuscles and Merkel cell–neurite complexes. (b) Section through skin of finger tip. (c) Meissner's corpuscle. (d) Ruffini ending. (e) Pacinian corpuscle. Source: FitzGerald 2010. © 2016 Elsevier. Reproduced with permission of Elsevier.

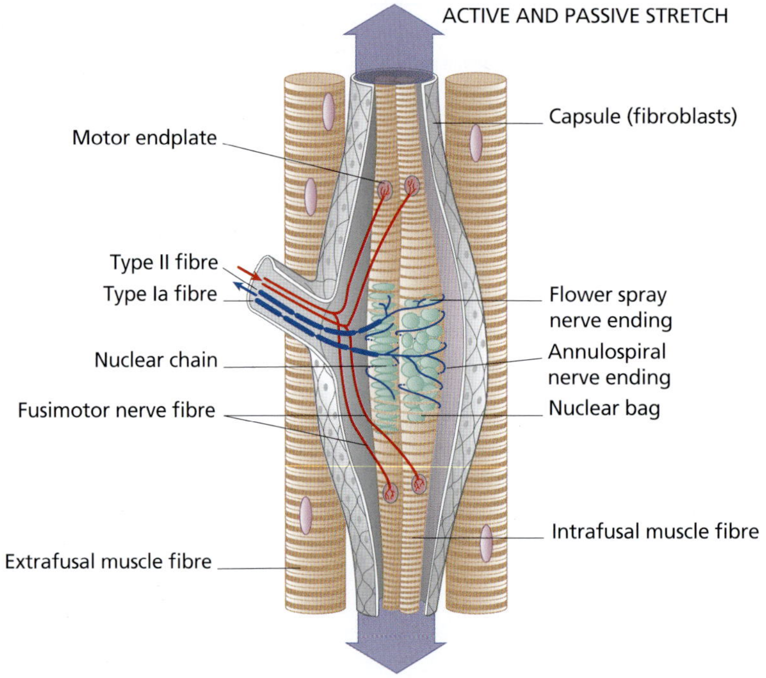

Figure 2.11 The muscle spindle. Source: FitzGerald 2010. © 2016 Elsevier. Reproduced with permission of Elsevier.

polymodal nociceptors, capable of sensing mechanical stimuli, heat, cold and chemical irritants. The axon reflex is mediated by C fibres.

Follicular nerve endings fire when a hair is being bent. A circumferential rim of nerve terminals surround an inner palisade, adjacent to each follicle.

Meissner's and Pacinian corpuscles and Ruffini endings are encapsulated by an inner membrane of modified Schwann cells (teloglia), a middle perineural layer and an outer coat of connective tissue. These mechanoreceptors are separated into four subtypes (Johansson-Vallbo classification):

- Meissner's corpuscles, most numerous on finger pads, detect delicate changes in texture (to 20 μm in elevation) and are rapidly adapting.
- Pacinian corpuscles are subcutaneous, 2–3 mm in diameter and are plentiful (approximately 300) in each hand and foot and also embedded in the periosteum in the limbs. They are exquisitely sensitive to vibration, object detection and release.
- Ruffini endings in the skin respond to shearing stress (skin movement).
- Merkel–neurite complexes are expanded nerve terminals applied to Merkel cells (tactile menisci) within skin basal epithelium that respond to sustained pressure.

The pathophysiology of individual types of sensory nerve terminal is in its infancy, but presumably changes within these sensitive structures cause sensory symptoms that will in due course be recognised clinically.

Muscle spindle motor supply, annulospiral and flower spray endings

Primary type Ia sensory fibres with annulospiral endings surround each intrafusal muscle fibre. Secondary type II fibres (flower spray endings) lie beside each annulospiral ending. Fusimotor fibres are Aγ calibre and innervate contractile intrafusal fibres of the muscle spindle, whereas Aα extrafusal fibres innervate skeletal muscle (Figure 2.11).

Golgi tendon organs

Type Ib afferents form an entwining network around tendons. Golgi tendon organs signal force of contraction and effect negative feedback on agonist–antagonist muscle groups. An important function is to restrict joint oscillation.

THE WORKING BRAIN

Introduction

Neurones and glia are the structural and functional units of all parts of the nervous system. The remainder of this chapter outlines the structure of different regions of the brain and cord, the connections between them and how these operate. Some understanding of neuro-anatomy is assumed, and is readily available from reference texts.

The approach here is to take a typical activity, to trace its origins, describe its features and outline neuro-anatomical pathways and control systems. Movement is discussed first, because it has a pivotal role in clinical assessment.

Mechanisms of movement

Skilled, coordinated, fast and appropriate movement is highly developed in humans. Almost all parts of the nervous system become involved – alertness, cognition, volition, mood, all special senses, sensory stimuli, the motor cortex and associated cortical motor and sensory areas, the spinal reflex arc, cerebellum, basal ganglia, motor nerves, neuromuscular junction and, obviously, muscles themselves.

The essential objects of movement are feeding, survival and reproduction. In humans, movement assumed signal further importance with the development and progressive use of tools to an extent that far exceeds the capacity of any other species.

Three central systems of motor control

All movement is the product of activity within a highly interconnected network. Each final motor pathway that generates eye, head, body and limb movement is under the control of three major interrelated systems within the brain:

- Cortical
- Striatal (basal ganglia), and
- Cerebellar.

The major output from these systems is the corticospinal tract. This pathway originates from motor, somatosensory and limbic areas of the cortex; because all its fibres pass through the pyramids in the medulla, it is often referred to as the pyramidal tract. The tract is particularly well-developed in humans. Clinically, interruption of these fibres is recognised by abnormal physical signs – weakness and loss of skilled movement, and abnormal reflex activity, as seen in hemiplegia. The clinical signs associated with malfunction of the basal ganglia and cerebellum are fundamentally different.

These systems can also be thought of as comprising two motor loops: the cortex–basal ganglia–cortex and the cortex–cerebellum–cortex loops, with the corticospinal outflow providing the major conduit for activity that leads to limb movements generated within these two motor loops.

The corticospinal (pyramidal) system originates in the cortex and delivers information to cranial nerve nuclei and all levels of the spinal cord, including anterior horn cells (spinal motor neurones). Defective function is recognised by abnormalities in the patterns of skilled movement and weakness, and by the appearance of spasticity and reflex change.

The striatal (extrapyramidal) system facilitates fast fluid movement via servo loops between cortex and basal ganglia. To the clinician, slowness (bradykinesia), stiffness (rigidity, rather than spasticity), rest tremor and various disorders of movement (dyskinesias) are the hallmarks of dysfunction in this system.

The cerebellum and its connections have a role in the coordination of smooth, programmed movement and balance. Ataxia (limb and/or truncal) and action tremor are the cardinal features.

It is reasonable and useful clinically to describe signs and syndromes as 'extrapyramidal', meaning slow and parkinsonian, but be wary of the term 'extrapyramidal pathway'. This is because areas such as the basal ganglia that are involved movement disorders are also closely connected to other motor systems. For example, the main basal ganglia output pathway influencing movement is first via its return projections from thalamus to cortex, but thence through the corticospinal 'pyramidal' tract.

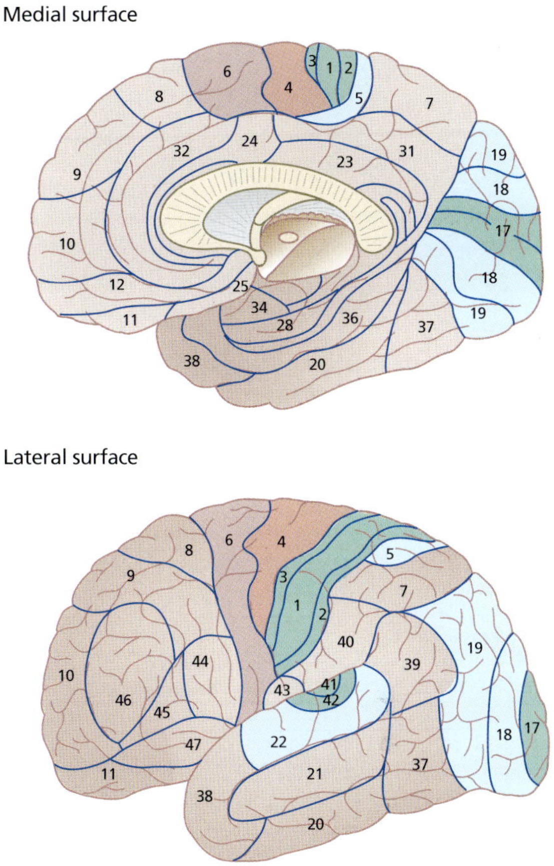

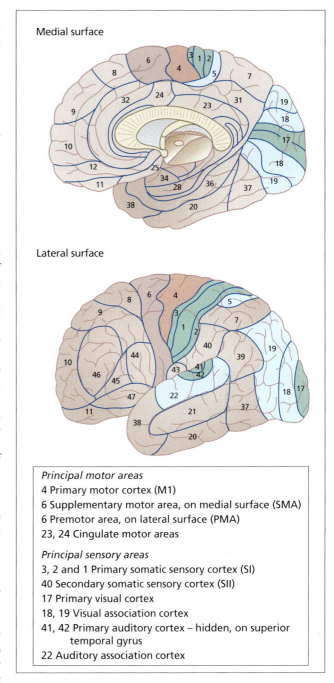

Principal motor areas
4 Primary motor cortex (M1)
6 Supplementary motor area, on medial surface (SMA)
6 Premotor area, on lateral surface (PMA)
23, 24 Cingulate motor areas

Principal sensory areas
3, 2 and 1 Primary somatic sensory cortex (SI)
40 Secondary somatic sensory cortex (SII)
17 Primary visual cortex
18, 19 Visual association cortex
41, 42 Primary auditory cortex – hidden, on superior temporal gyrus
22 Auditory association cortex

Figure 2.12 Cortical areas (after Brodmann 1906). Source: FitzGerald 2010. © 2016 Elsevier. Reproduced with permission of Elsevier.

Corticospinal (pyramidal) system

Penfield's human cortical electrical stimulation experiments in the 1930s explored and mapped areas 4 (primary motor cortex, M1) and 6 (premotor area + supplementary motor area; PMA + SMA), developing the earlier work of Fritsch and Hitzig in the 1870s and individual observations by Ferrier, Sherrington, Campbell and others in the late nineteenth and early twentieth centuries. Brodmann's cortical areas are shown in Figure 2.12 and the cortical contribution to the corticospinal pathway in Figure 2.13, noting the contributions from primary somatosensory cortical areas 1, 2 and 3 – and all cortical sensory areas concerned with movement towards or away from an object. A significant cortico-spinal projection also arises from the cingulate gyrus (areas 23 and 24).

Each corticospinal tract is made up of around 1.1×10^6 fibres and is one of the longer and most compact fibre systems in the human CNS. Some two-thirds of these axons originate from cortical areas 4 and 6, where the cell bodies are located in lamina V of the cortex. Most of the remainder derive from parietal areas, including the somatosensory cortex, posterior parietal cortex and area SII. The course of the fibres through the internal capsule, cerebral peduncle, pons and medulla is shown in Figure 2.14.

The term corona radiata describes the radially arranged fan-like sheet of nerve fibres that continues caudally as the internal capsule.

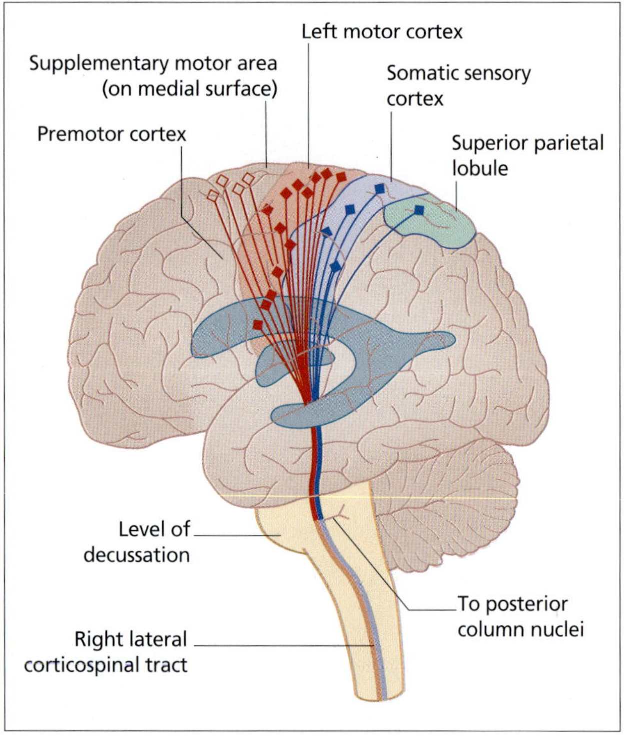

Figure 2.13 Left hemisphere: cortical contributions to pyramidal tract. Source: FitzGerald 2010. © 2016 Elsevier. Reproduced with permission of Elsevier.

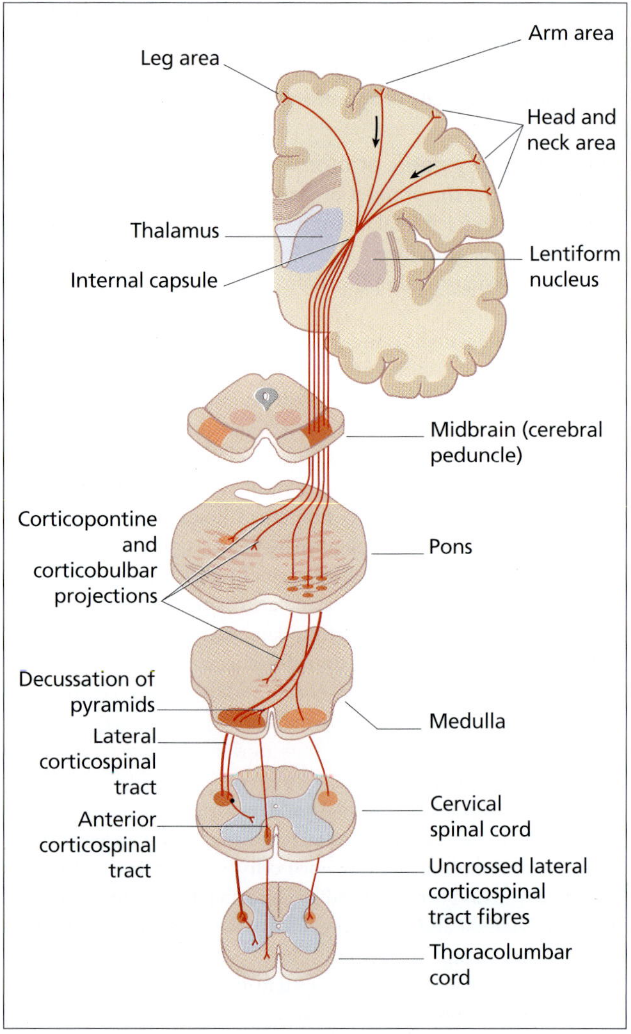

Figure 2.14 Motor cortex and corticospinal (pyramidal) pathways. Source: FitzGerald 2010. © 2016 Elsevier. Reproduced with permission of Elsevier.

The area dorsal to the corona radiata, deep to the cortical mantle is known as the centrum semiovale. Pyramidal describes the roughly triangular cross-section of this tract in the medulla but, as discussed earlier, has come to be used functionally (and interchangeably) with corticospinal to describe the pattern of physical signs with disease of this pathway. The majority but not all (around 75%) pyramid fibres continue into the spinal cord. After decussation, fibres congregate within the cord in the lateral corticospinal tract and terminate along the whole length of the cord, and in all layers of the spinal grey matter, including synapses on motor neurones in the anterior horn. Of corticospinal fibres, 10% remain uncrossed, their neurones of origin outlining an ipsilateral somatotopic map, but of little apparent clinical significance.

The comparative anatomy of the motor pathways indicates that in humans the corticospinal system, as the major descending pathway, has to some extent replaced other descending systems. For example, the rubrospinal tract, which arises from the magnocellular divisions of the red nucleus, is vestigial in humans.

Movement direction and movement synergy Neurones in area 4 are known to show patterns of activity that implicate them in the control of key parameters of movement, such as force, direction and timing of movements. The motor areas probably function to activate particular synergies of muscular action to bring about highly specific movements such as particular types of grasp. These synergies depend in part on the pattern of innervation by the direct cortico-motoneuronal projections from primary motor cortex to specific groups of motor nuclei at spinal level.

Plasticity In all primates, small cortical lesions cause initial paralysis, slowing, or clumsiness depending on lesion size, of a limb, or part of a limb, followed by recovery within hours or days. This recovery is explained by changes in neighbouring cortical cell columns (i.e. plasticity). In the cord, local interneuronal mechanisms underpin movement synergies that function to provide individual skilled movements under the influence of different cortical signals. At a clinical level, following a hemiparesis, the early return of some fine finger or toe movement is a pointer to good recovery of function – a signal that a plastic process of compensation for the damage is under way.

Afferents to the primary motor cortex

The primary motor cortex does not act in isolation as the generator of fast skilled movement. Substantial afferent connections arrive from:

1 The opposite cortex via the corpus callosum. Most prominent are the dense links between cell columns controlling axial muscles, while the least dense are between distal parts of the opposite limbs. This might be expected – head and trunk posture cannot be under unilateral control, whereas the opposite is the case for fine hand movement.

2 Somatosensory cortex. Cutaneous cell columns (areas 1, 2 and 3b) pass forward via short association fibres deep to the central sulcus. Typically, the more complex the subserved movement function (e.g. hand movements), the denser the connections. Proprioceptive cell columns in area 3a receive afferents from muscle spindles and synapse via short association fibres with area 4.
3 Cerebellum, via contralateral dentate nucleus and motor areas of the thalamus. Cerebellar impulses determine synergy and timing of cortical neuronal discharges. The cerebellum receives a dense multimodal input of all sensory modalities, including vision.
4 Supplementary motor area (area 6) on medial surface of hemisphere. This part of area 6 is especially involved in motor planning, motor memory, intention and responds to internal cues. For example, the supplementary motor area is activated via the frontal lobe when a movement is intended. A major function of the supplementary motor area is programming motor sequences already within motor memory via a loop through the basal ganglia and projecting to area 4. Unilateral damage to the supplementary motor area causes contralateral akinesia.
5 Premotor cortex (PMC, area 6 on lateral aspect of hemisphere). The PMC, some six times the size of area 4, is in general responsive to external cues, and seen to be active on functional magnetic resonance imaging (fMRI) when motor sequences follow visual or sensory cues (e.g. reaching for an object in view or feeling the tactile shape of an object). The lateral PMC represents one of the major pathways through which vision is able to control fine movements.

Basal ganglia and 'extrapyramidal' movement disorders

The term basal ganglia describes neighbouring areas within the deep forebrain and midbrain involved in the control of movement. In practical terms this includes:

- The striatum (caudate nucleus, putamen of lentiform nucleus, nucleus accumbens).
- The globus pallidus – lateral and medial parts, divided by the medial medullary lamina. These parts of the globus pallidus are often known as internal (GPi) and external (GPe). The GPi has as an anatomical extension, the pars reticularis of the substantia nigra.
- The subthalamic nucleus.
- The pars compacta of the substantia nigra.

The pathways between these structures are outlined here. The subject is made difficult by many factors: the sheer complexity of the circuitary, difficulty distinguishing differences in ultrastructure between different parts of the basal ganglia and difficulty recognising somatotopic differentiation in these structures, although such organisation exists. It is also frequently impossible to attribute a specific symptom or physical sign to a single structure. In other words (cf. the cerebral cortex), individual diseases do not appear to affect one discrete area, and thus localisation of one function to a particular zone is often not possible.

There was a relative paucity of interest in disorders of movement until the second half of the twentieth century. Advances in knowledge of the functions of neurotransmitters, levodopa therapy, stereotactic surgery, deep brain stimulation and fMRI and have brought a different focus to this field, which continues to expand rapidly.

Extrapyramidal, the term coined by Kinnier Wilson in the 1920s, is a loose but valuable term for the clinical features of these disorders, but it is in theory no more than a clinical pointer towards a motor disorder distinct from one with hallmarks of corticospinal (pyramidal) or cerebellar disease. The words 'extrapyramidal syndrome' are usually used to describe a condition with slowing, stiffness and/or tremor seen in idiopathic Parkinson's disease and in other akinetic-rigid syndromes. However, extrapyramidal is also used, although less frequently, to include other disorders of movement, such as chorea, hemiballismus or dystonia. As previously noted, 'extrapyramidal syndrome' should not extend to 'extrapyramidal pathway'.

Basic circuits within the basal ganglia

The clinical focus is upon the complex motor loops, with dysfunction typified by Parkinson's disease.

Motor loops Several neuronal servo-loops commence and end in the motor and frontal areas of the cerebral cortex. They all involve cortical projections to the striatum (putamen + caudate nucleus) and return projections to the cortex via the thalamus. Within each loop there exist two interrelated motor pathways: direct and indirect pathways. Transmission through the loops is controlled by activity in the nigrostriatal pathway, from the pars compacta of the substantia nigra to the lateral globus pallidus, where axons make two principal types of synapse, on excitatory D_1 (dopaminergic, direct pathway) and inhibitory D_2 (indirect pathway) receptors. Matters have become more complex with the discovery of several more dopaminergic receptor D subtypes.

In normal subjects, the nigrostriatal tract is tonically active, selecting preferentially the excitatory, direct pathway and leading, via the loop back to the cortex, to activation of the supplementary motor area before a movement. This early activation of the cortex is thought to underlie the electrical readiness potential (*Bereitschaftspotential*). Other projections to the motor cortex interact with those from the cerebellum to modulate motor cortex output to the spinal cord.

Activation of the cortex (i.e. the intention to move):

- Stimulates (glutaminergic) putamen neurones (tonically facilitated by nigrostriatal D_1 input), which
- Inhibit (GABAergic) medial globus pallidus neurones, which
- Release (disinhibit) ventral lateral nucleus (VL) thalamic neurones, which
- Activate the supplementary motor area.

The sequences can be seen in Figure 2.15.

The indirect pathway engages the subthalamic nucleus via:

- Striatonigral that inhibit putamen neurones, which
- Inhibit the lateral globus pallidus (GPL), and
- Act on the subthalamic nucleus (STN).

The STN acts on the medial pallidum (somatotopically) to suppress unwanted movement. Destruction of the STN results in uncontrollable movements (see Hemiballismus, Chapter 6). However, high frequency stimulation of the STN relieves tremor and rigidity in Parkinson's disease.

Normal functions of the motor loop The basal ganglia do not initiate movement but they are active when action is generated by specific cell assemblies in the motor cortex:

- Scaling strength of muscle contraction and in collaboration with the supplementary motor area
- Programming appropriate movement sequences and suppressing others, and
- Controlling speed of movement.

The putamen is believed to act as a store of memorised, acquired motor programmes, with an ability to sequence appropriately movements intended and pass information to the supplementary motor area.

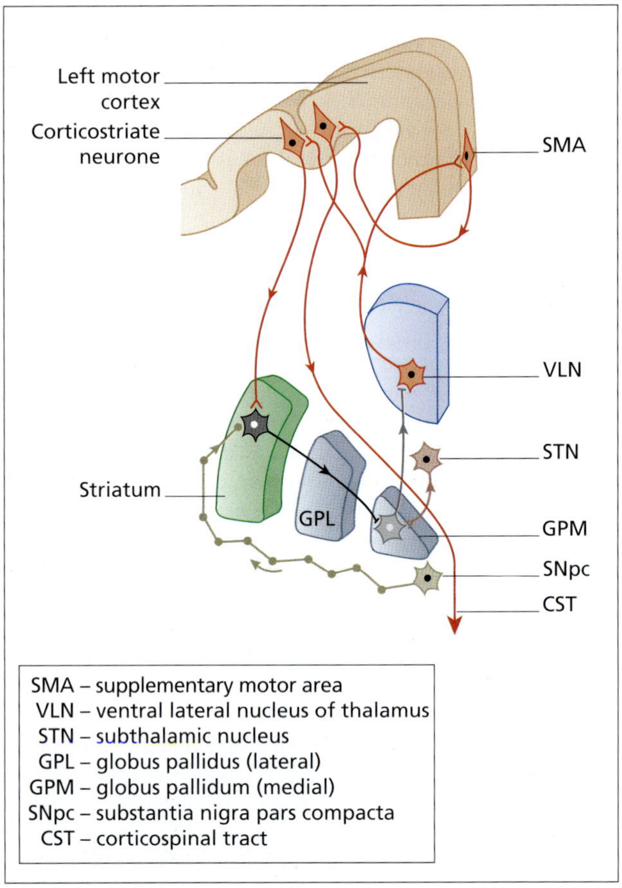

Figure 2.15 Striatal motor loops. Source: FitzGerald 2010. © 2016 Elsevier. Reproduced with permission of Elsevier.

Other basal ganglia circuits

- *Cognitive loop:* motor (volitional) intention
- *Limbic loop:* emotional correlates of movement, and
- *Oculomotor loop:* voluntary saccadic movements.

Cognitive loop A large projection of fibres from the prefrontal cortex reaches the head of the caudate nucleus. Increased activity in the head of the caudate, and anterior putamen, globus pallidus and ventral anterior (VA) thalamic nucleus, occurs when new movements are performed by the opposite hand, suggesting a role in motor learning. The VA nucleus projects to:

- The premotor cortex in an 'open cognitive loop'
- The prefrontal cortex in a 'closed cognitive loop'.

These connexions with the caudate point to the role of the cortex in forward planning of motor intentions. As a corollary, when a motor task has become automatic (i.e. entirely learnt), the motor loop of the basal ganglia appears to take over.

Parkinson's patients have particular problems with new fiddly movements; they are unable to sequence and initiate them. Exceptional activity in this cognitive loop perhaps explains rare temporary release phenomena: immobile patients with severe Parkinson's respond dramatically to great emotional stimulation – 'they can run down the fire escape'. These 'paradoxical' movements may involve cerebellar circuitry.

Limbic loop This describes a loop from:

- Inferior prefrontal cortex, via
- Nucleus accumbens
- Ventral pallidum
- Medio-dorsal nucleus of thalamus, to
- Inferior frontal cortex.

This pathway is concerned with the visible expression of emotion – portrayed in facial expression or in more general postures with emotional content such as submission, dominance or aggression.

The stooped (simian) posture and facial masking of Parkinson's disease can be explained by diminution of activity in this richly dopaminergic pathway – features reversed, at least in part, by levodopa.

Oculomotor loop This loop runs from:

- Frontal eye field and posterior parietal cortex (area 7), to
- Caudate nucleus, to
- Pars reticularis of substantia nigra (SNpr), to
- VA nucleus of thalamus, to
- Frontal eye field and prefrontal cortex.

An inhibitory GABAergic projection reaches the superior colliculus from SNpr. These inhibitory synapses are on neurones controlling saccades. Ocular fixation is accompanied by repetitive impulses (tonic activity) in SNpr. In other words, the eyes are held in one position of fixation by this tonic activity.

When a deliberate saccade takes place ('I want to look right'), the superior colliculus is disinhibited by the activated oculomotor loop. The superior colliculus neurones discharge, reinforcing the direct motor loop and facilitating rapid (almost instantaneous, 70–100 km/hour) conjugate eye movement. Put another way, the sequence is:

- Release of superior colliculus neurones
- Gaze flicks to new target
- SNpr resumes tonic activity
- Gaze vigilance returns.

Slow eye movement (oculomotor hypokinesia) is evident in Parkinson's disease, although it is a minor clinical issue because axial movement (e.g. head turning) is slow. Ocular hypokinesia is explained by loss of dopamine in SNpr, and faulty disinhibition of superior colliculus neurones.

Cerebellum

Cerebellar disease is recognised by physical signs of action tremor, nystagmus, truncal and/or gait ataxia and scanning speech (see Physical signs, Chapter 17).

Phylogenetically, functions of the cerebellum in fish were closely allied to the lateral line organs that comprise the fish vestibular system – controlling the fish's horizontal and vertical posture in water. In quadrupeds, connections with the spinal cord became prominent, facilitating improvement in agility of gait, running and turning. In bipeds, with emerging lateralised skills rich linkages developed between cerebellar lobes and cerebral cortex. These newer cerebellar pathways became intimately concerned with coordination of ipsilateral limbs in addition to the earlier vestibular and spinal connexions.

There are three main zones of the cerebellum (Figure 2.16). Each sends its main output to a distinct nucleus or nuclei:

1. Vestibulocerebellum is the central strip (vermis + fastigial nucleus), with primarily sensory afferents from the vestibular system. Output: fastigial nucleus and brainstem vestibular nuclei.
2. Spinocerebellum describes regions adjacent to the vermis, with major sensory input from the spinal cord. Output: nucleus interpositus.
3. Pontocerebellum (neocerebellum – lateral lobes) receives a massive neuronal input from the contralateral pontine nuclei, the main input of which comes from the cerebral cortex. Output: dentate nucleus. The neocerebellum is most developed and largest in humans.

Cellular anatomy The cerebellar cortex has an outer molecular layer, an inner granular layer, with the piriform layer between the two (Figure 2.17). The granular layer consists of billions of small 6–8 μm diameter neurones (granule cells) with short dendrites. These dendrites receive excitatory synapses from mossy fibres that run to the cerebellar cortex, giving off collateral branches to the deep cerebellar nuclei. Granule cell axons pass to the outer molecular layer, dividing to form parallel fibres, running parallel to the cerebellar folia, to make excitatory synaptic contacts with dendrites of Purkinje cells whose cell bodies lie in the piriform layer.

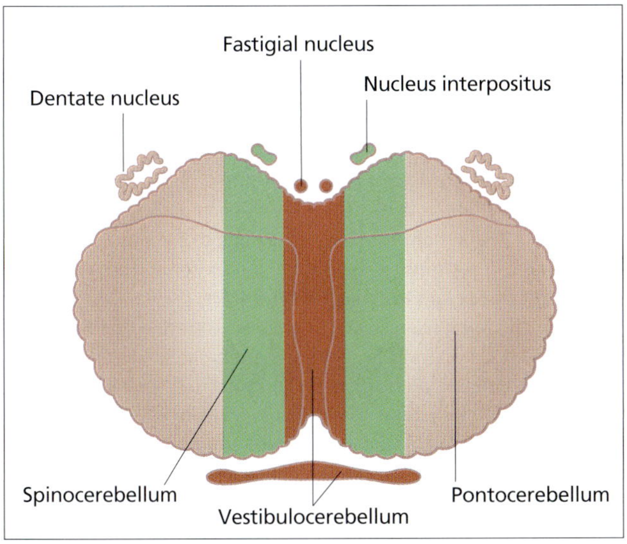

Figure 2.16 Zones of the cerebellum. Source: FitzGerald 2010. © 2016 Elsevier. Reproduced with permission of Elsevier.

Purkinje cells, large neurones with extensive dendritic trees, are interwoven by numerous parallel fibres. Each parallel fibre makes successive single (one-per-cell) synapses with 300–500 individual Purkinje cells. The action of each parallel fibre is excitatory – although many thousand parallel fibres need to act simultaneously to depolarise a single Purkinje cell.

From the contralateral inferior olivary nucleus, each Purkinje cell dendritic tree receives a single climbing fibre. This fibre makes synaptic contact with thousands of dendritic spines of a single Purkinje cell. A single action potential in a climbing fibre triggers a short burst of action potentials from each Purkinje cell, which then becomes temporarily unresponsive to the effects of parallel fibre inputs. Purkinje cell axons leave the cerebellar cortex, the only efferent axons to do so, to reach the deep cerebellar nuclei (dentate, inferior olivary, interpositus), upon which they exert a uniformly inhibitory action.

The molecular layer contains three further, largely inhibitory cell types: basket cells, stellate cells and Golgi cells.

Somatotopic representation in the cerebellum Positron emission tomography (PET) and fMRI have confirmed the somatotopic representation deduced from animal studies (Figure 2.18). Corresponding fMRI activity for hand movement in humans is shown in Figure 2.19.

Afferent cerebellar pathways The scope and complexity of these pathways is summarised here:

- From muscles and skin (trunk and limbs), information from the posterior spinocerebellar and cuneocerebellar (cuneiform nucleus) tracts enter via each ipsilateral inferior cerebellar peduncle. The massive similar trigeminal input (from the head) enters via all three peduncles.
- Afferents monitoring activity in spinal reflex circuits, in the anterior spinocerebellar tracts loop into each superior peduncle via the pons.

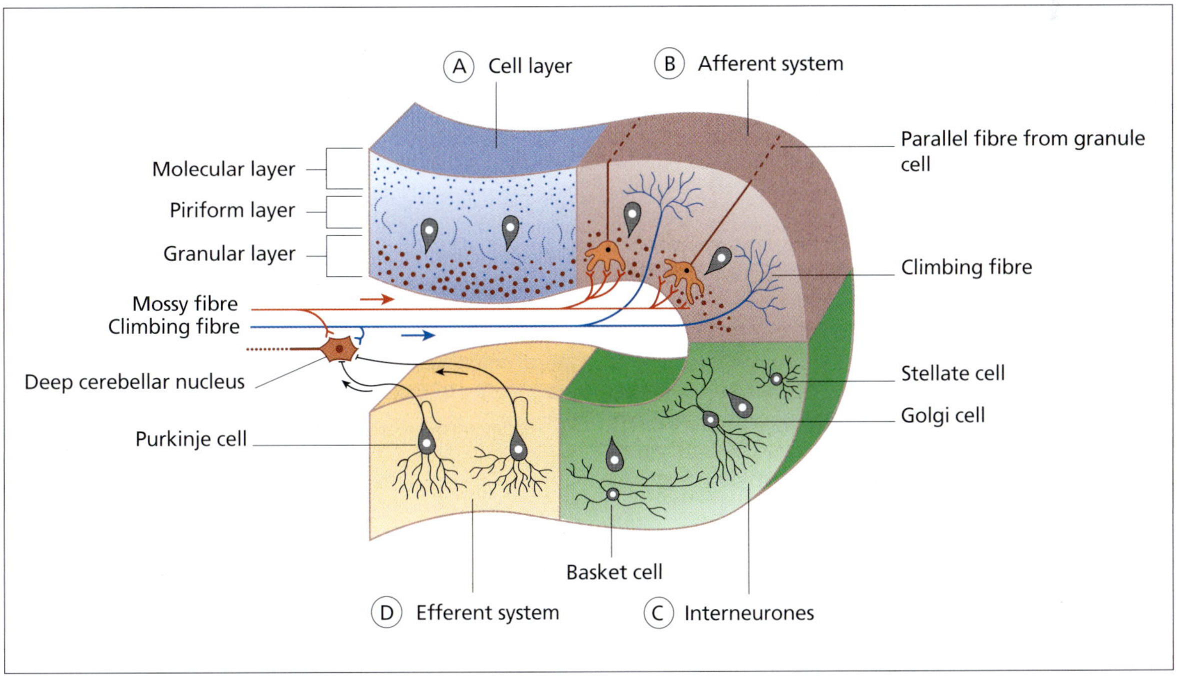

Figure 2.17 Cerebellar cortex cell systems. Source: FitzGerald 2010. © 2016 Elsevier. Reproduced with permission of Elsevier.

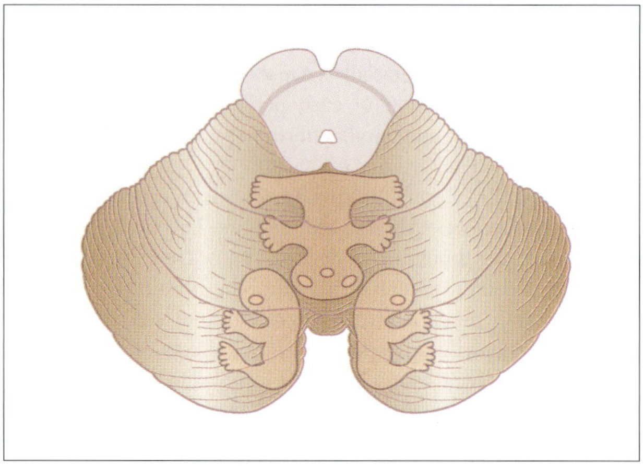

Figure 2.18 Cerebellum: somatotopic maps. Source: FitzGerald 2010. © 2016 Elsevier. Reproduced with permission of Elsevier.

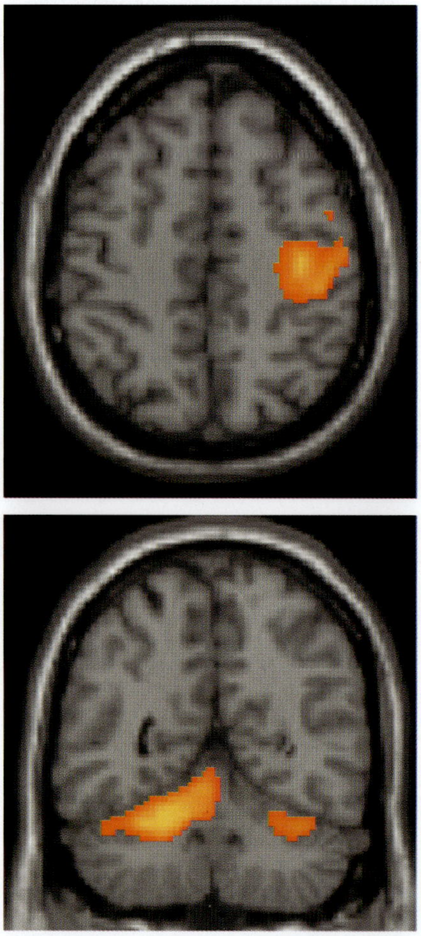

Figure 2.19 Cortical and cerebellar fMRI: voluntary activity of left hand. Courtesy of Dr Alex Leff, UCL Institute of Neurology.

- Vestibular, auditory and visual pathways make up the tecto-cerebellar tracts to enter the ipsilateral superior peduncle.
- The pontocerebellar tract, bringing massive mossy fibre input from the cerebral cortex, enters the contralateral middle cerebellar peduncle.
- The olivocerebellar tract enters the contralateral inferior peduncle (climbing fibre input).
- Reticulocerebellar tracts enter via the inferior peduncles.
- Aminergic fibres (serotonin and noradrenaline) enter all three cerebellar peduncles from the brainstem – excitatory transmission in mossy fibres and climbing fibre terminals.

Olivocerebellar tract, learning, the red nucleus and novelty detection

The inferior and accessory olivary nuclei receive fibres from the ipsilateral sensorimotor (cerebral) cortex. These project as climbing fibres to each contralateral cerebellar cortex in a somatotopic order (accessory nuclei to an anterior cerebellar map, principal nuclei to posterior). When primates are trained to carry out a repetitive motor activity, Purkinje cells show increased simple spike activity – an indication of increased mossy fibre and parallel fibre input. If the task is interrupted (e.g. if activity is physically obstructed), bursts of Purkinje cell complex spikes appear, caused by climbing fibre input. At least, they do so initially. If the obstruction is sustained, these complex spike bursts diminish and eventually disappear. This is one example of the role of the cerebellum in learned movement, for which there is much evidence both in animals and in humans. The system acquires, or adapts to new motor activity. Additional connections to the olivary nuclei come from the visual association cortex and the spino-olivary tract.

Finally, the red nucleus receives collaterals from (cerebral) cortical fibres descending to the olive, and from cerebellar efferents en route to the thalamus. The principal output from the red nucleus is inhibitory to the ipsilateral olive. There is evidence to suggest that if an imbalance occurs between movement intended (cerebral cortex) and movement learned or organised (cerebellum), the red nucleus modulates cell groups within the olive to achieve harmony, and it detects novelty in an organised action. The coarse tremor seen in lesions of the red nucleus can be thought of as a breakdown of this harmonic, over-correcting each part of a movement, and failing to learn to control it.

Efferent pathways The vestibulocerebellum projects to the vestibular system, the spinocerebellum to the cord and the neocerebellum to the red nucleus, thalamus and motor cortex.

From each fastigial nucleus in the vestibulocerebellum, via the inferior peduncles, axons reach both (right and left) vestibular nuclei (Figure 2.20). Output from the medial and superior vestibular nuclei passes to the medial longitudinal fasciculus, and thus control conjugate lateral gaze. From lateral vestibular nuclei (of Dieter), efferent fibres pass to the vestibulospinal tracts; these help control balance and axial stability. Some fastigial outputs pass directly to the spinal cord, for control of head and neck movements.

From each nucleus interpositus (spinocerebellum) axons travel in the superior peduncle, ending largely in the contralateral reticular formation (posture, gait) and red nucleus (motor learning).

In the neo-cerebellum, outflow from the dentate nucleus makes up the majority of the superior peduncle (dentatorubrothalamic tract), and crosses in the brainstem before reaching both red nucleus and motor thalamus. The latter sends onward projections to the cortex.

Clinical correlates In contrast to the complexity of cerebellar micro-anatomy, physical signs of cerebellar disease are distinct, relatively straightforward to recognise but often hard to attribute to individual pathways (Chapters 6 and 17). A lesion of one lateral lobe (e.g. tumour or infarction), causes rebound and past pointing

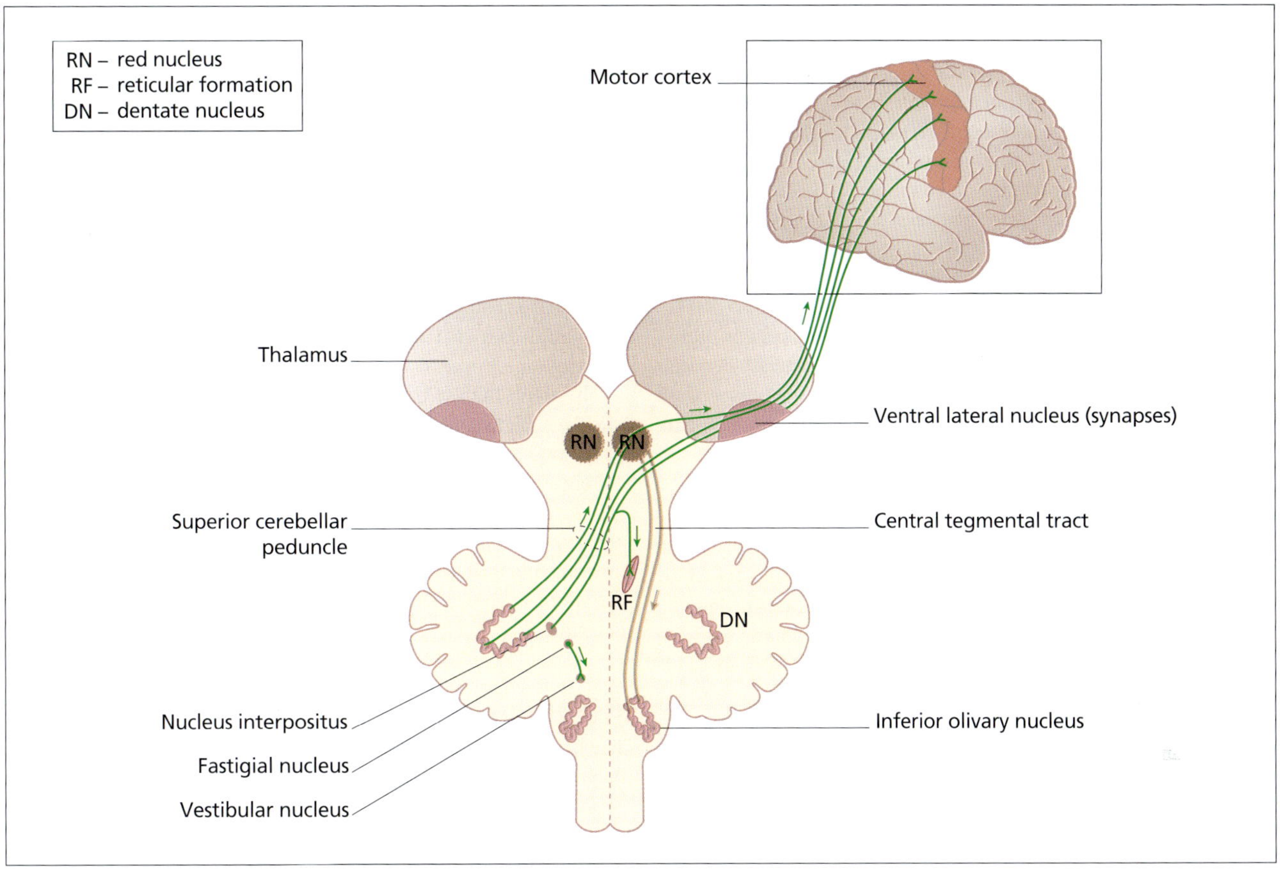

Figure 2.20 Cerebellar efferents. Source: FitzGerald 2010. © 2016 Elsevier. Reproduced with permission of Elsevier.

of the outstretched upper limb – a clinical correlate of the effect of obstruction to a programmed activity described above. Vermis lesions (see Medulloblastoma, Chapter 21) affect primarily vestibular connexions. Truncal ataxia is often an early sign.

Anterior cerebellar lobe lesions (often bilateral, and typically caused by alcohol) cause gait ataxia, often with pronounced head tremor (titubation). In chronic alcohol damage, substantial loss of all major neurone types develops (granular, Purkinje and molecular layer cells). Depression of tendon reflexes – an unusual cerebellar sign, and of little usual clinical value – is explained by loss of tonic stimulation of fusimotor neurones connected via pontine reticulospinal fibres. Nystagmus (coarse, fast phase towards the side of the lesion, and dramatic when it occurs) is an inconstant feature of cerebellar lesions.

Finally, the cognitive affective cerebellar syndrome is of interest, if rarely diagnosed. This syndrome comprises diminished reasoning, inattention, poor memory and flattening of affect, sometimes seen transiently after major cerebellar lesions (e.g. following surgery or massive cerebellar infarction). One explanation, is temporary reduction in blood flow to cerebral cortical association areas, possibly because of diminution of expected impulses of cerebellar origin to the thalamus, and thence to prefrontal cortical areas.

Sensation and sensory pathways

The neurologist usually deals with sensation in its five clinical modalities: touch, nociception, temperature, joint position and vibration sense. The neuroscientist has a wider perspective, looking at sensation first as conscious or non-conscious. Conscious sensation is perceived largely at cortical level. Non-conscious sensation is processed within the cortex too, but also within the cerebellum, via the vestibular system, in the reticular formation and widely within the CNS. It is sometimes hard to say precisely whether a sensation is conscious or non-conscious. For example, vertigo, the illusion of movement, is clearly conscious. However, the precise posture of the head in relation to the trunk is usually non-conscious, whereas the position of limb in relation to an object is usually conscious. Partly because of this problem, and in part because of the complexity of the nervous system, it is often hard to say where a particular sensory modality is localised or how it is perceived. Some of the essentials of the sensory pathways are summarised here. Circuitary within the spinal cord is dealt with in more detail in Chapter 16 (see Anatomy and physiology of spinal maldevelopment).

Conscious and non-conscious sensation

Conscious sensations are exteroceptive and proprioceptive. Exteroceptive sensations stimulate surface somatic receptors (e.g. touch, nociception, temperature) or telereceptors (vision, hearing, olfaction). Proprioceptive (conscious) sensations arise from joints, muscles, bones and the labyrinth (vestibular system). For example, vestibular pathways to the cortex enable us to perceive whether we are stationary or moving, and to discriminate between constant movement, deceleration and acceleration.

Non-conscious sensations are of two kinds:

- Afferent proprioceptive information (e.g. from muscles, joints, tendons, labyrinth) reaching the cerebellum, cortex, reticular formation and elsewhere, and
- Enteroception (e.g. afferents from the gut, heart or blood vessels).

Somatic sensory pathways in the cord and brain

Two major pathways deliver sensory information to the thalamus and thence to the cortex:

- Spinothalamic pathways (nociceptive);
- Posterior columns → medial lemnisci (touch, position, movement).

Each system consists of first, second and third order neurones. They have the following features in common:

- The cell bodies of first order neurones are in the posterior root (dorsal root) ganglia
- Second order neurones decussate before reaching the thalamus
- Third order neurones project from thalamus to cortex
- There is somatotopic organisation throughout the system, and
- Transmission can be controlled (inhibited/enhanced) between first to second, and second to third order neurones (see Gate control in this chapter, and Neurostimulation procedures: gate theory, Chapter 23).

Dorsal root ganglia – first order neurones

The arrangement of spinal nerves, dorsal and ventral roots, laminae of the posterior horn and named cell groups are illustrated in Figure 2.21. The complexity of information outlined in the figure is exemplified by the fact that a single nerve root ganglion serving a limb contains around 100 000 neurones, each enshrouded by satellite cells (modified Schwann cells).

Termination of dorsal root afferents

In the dorsal root entry zone, afferent fibres separate into medial and lateral streams. The lateral stream (Aδ and C fibres) divides into short ascending and descending branches within the posterolateral tract of Lissauer. They then synapse in lamina I (marginal zone), lamina II (substantia gelatinosa) and in III–V.

The medial stream (type I and II mechanoreceptors) divides into ascending and descending branches in the posterior columns. The shorter branches synapse in laminae II, III, IV, V and VI. The longer branches run throughout the posterior columns of the cord to the gracile and cuneate nuclei in the medulla.

Posterior column → medial lemniscus pathway

The fascicles of the posterior columns of the cord are formed partly by axons of dorsal root ganglia (first order neurones) and partly by axons of second order neurones in the dorsal horn of the spinal grey matter. These axons all project to the gracile and cuneate nuclei in the brainstem, whose axons then decussate in the medulla to form each medial lemniscus (ribbon) that terminates in the lateral part of the ventral posterior nucleus of the thalamus. Thalamo-cortical neurones (third and fourth order) then project to the somatic sensory cortex.

Spinothalamic pathway

The anterior and lateral spinothalamic tracts consist of second order neurones passing from laminae I, II, III, IV and V of the posterior grey horn to the opposite thalamus. The two tracts merge in the brainstem to form the spinal lemniscus and then enter the ventral posterior nucleus of the thalamus. Third order thalamic neurones project to the somatic sensory cortex (Figure 2.22).

Other ascending sensory pathways

The two sensory pathways described above dominate the clinical neurology of sensation. Other sensory pathways dealing more with non-conscious sensation are mentioned briefly here.

Spinocerebellar pathways (four on each side) are concerned with non-conscious proprioception and interactions between spinal motor neurones and interneurones (i.e. the excitability of reflex arcs), and movements involving balanced activation of agonist and antagonist muscles:

- Posterior spinocerebellar tract
- Cuneocerebellar tract
- Anterior spinocerebellar tract
- Rostral spinocerebellar tract.

The spinotectal tract passes information from the spinal cord to the superior colliculus, thus relating orientation of the trunk and head towards a visual stimulus. This information is important in orientation reflexes to visual stimuli.

The spino-olivary tract sends tactile information to the inferior olivary nucleus and thence to the opposite cerebellar cortex. This pathway is believed to have a role in motor learning.

Spinoreticular fibres originating in dorsal roots accompany the spinothalamic pathway in the cord. Their functions are arousal and reporting on the content of a stimulus, for example whether it is noxious (pin-prick) or pleasurable (stroking). This is in contrast to the more analytical nature of the spinothalamic pathway which determines the precise nature, intensity and location of a stimulus.

The brainstem

The brainstem's complexity can be understood by considering first its principal fibre systems, its cell columns (nuclei) and traversing connections:

- Principal efferent (motor) pathways
- Principal afferent (sensory) pathways
- Cranial nerve nuclei
- Reticular formation
- Autonomic, basal ganglia, cerebellar and vestibular traversing connections.

As landmarks, five guidelines are helpful:

1. Motor pathways lie in general ventrally.
2. Sensory pathways lie dorsally.
3. Cranial nerve nuclei (two longitudinal columns) denote different levels in the superior–inferior (rostral–caudal) plane.
4. Reticular formation (RF) nuclei tend to lie laterally; some (magnus raphe, median raphe) are midline.
5. Traversing connections are found in all layers of the brainstem.

See also Chapter 4 (see Figure 4.19).

Brainstem functions

Another approach to the intricacy of the region is to consider that phylogenetically the brainstem was almost the entire brain of distant invertebrate ancestors. For example, the RF connected olfaction to reflex movements associated with alertness, respiration, autonomic function and feeding, and hence survival. As more advanced creatures evolved, cranial nerve nuclei, cortical regions and the cerebellum developed, each to serve specialised functions, such as vision and hearing. The brainstem, in addition to any earlier role became by default the conduit for many pathways to and from those destinations, adding to its complexity.

The reticular formation, a major part of the brainstem, has no single overriding function, in the sense that there is no clinical condition recognisable when it is damaged. However, changes within the RF have prominent effects, principally on respiratory control, sleep and wakefulness, cardiovascular control, patterns of primitive movement, sphincters and mood.

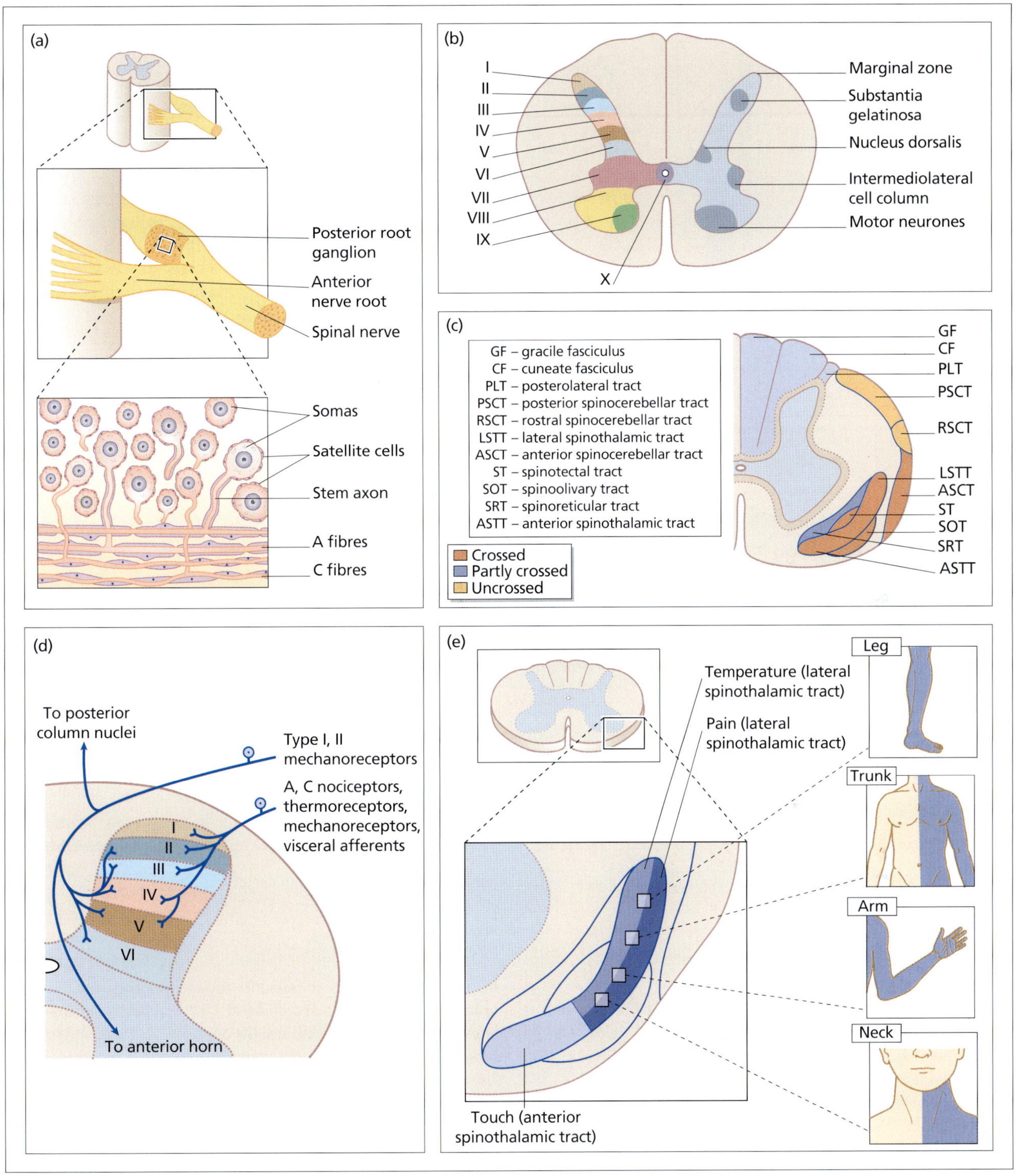

Figure 2.21 Sensatory pathways: spinal cord. (a) Posterior root ganglion. Note T-shaped bifurcation of stem fibres of ganglion cells. (b) Laminae (I–X) and named cell groups at mid thoracic level. (c) Ascending pathways at upper cervical level. (d) Targets of primary afferent neurones in the posterior grey horn. (e) Sensory modalities in spinothalamic pathway at upper cervical level. ASCT, anterior spinocerebellar tract; ASTT, anterior spinothalamic tract; CF, cuneate fasciculus; GF, gracile fasciculus; LSTT, lateral spinothalamic tract; PLT, posterolateral tract; PSCT, posterior spinocerebellar tract; RSCT, rostral spinocerebellar tract; SOT, spino-olivary; SRT, spinoreticular tract; ST, spinotectal tract. Source: FitzGerald 2010. © 2016 Elsevier. Reproduced with permission of Elsevier.

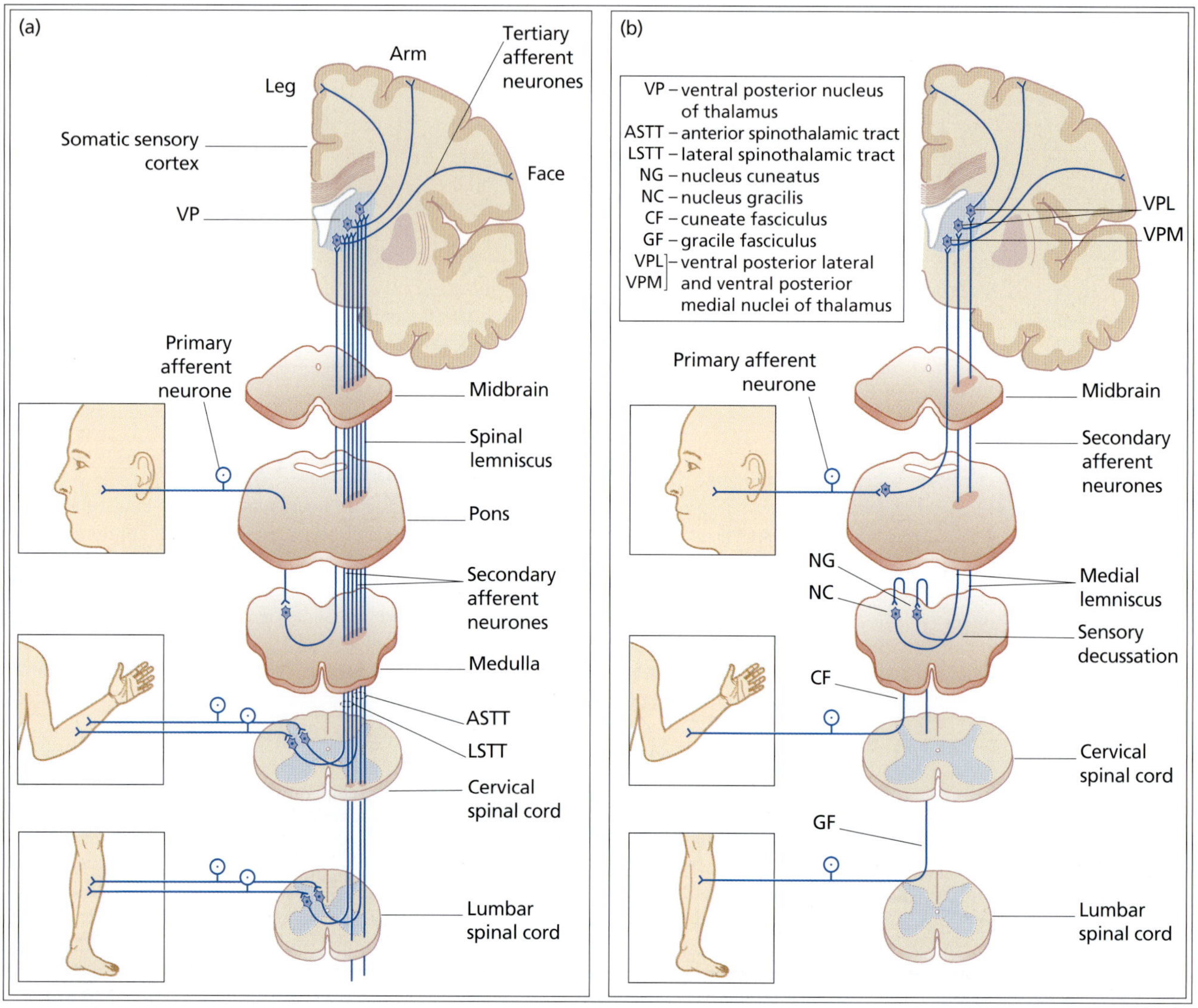

Figure 2.22 (a) Spinothalamic pathway. (b) Posterior column → medial lemniscal pathway. ASTT, anterior spinothalamic tract; CF, cuneate fasciculus; GF, gracile fasciculus; LSTT, lateral spinothalamic tract; NC, nucleus cuneatus; NG, nucleus gracilis; VP, ventral posterior nuclei of thalamus. Source: FitzGerald 2010. © 2016 Elsevier. Reproduced with permission of Elsevier.

Motor fibres

The cerebral peduncle carries all cortical efferent fibres to and/or through the brainstem (corticofugal fibres). These tightly packed motor fibres supply, medially to laterally (Figure 2.23a):

- Eye movements
- Face
- Upper limbs
- Trunk, and
- Lower limbs.

Within the ventral pons motor fibres come to lie in separate bundles. Those for eye movements and face leave to reach their nuclei. The remaining bundles then recongregate in the upper medulla as the pyramidal tract (medullary pyramids). Upper limb (UL) fibres remain medial; lower limb (LL) fibres lateral. A high proportion of these cortico-fugal fibres project to the ipsilateral pontine nuclei; this is the pathway mediating the output of the cerebellar–cortical loop.

Crossing of motor fibres (pyramidal decussation) takes place below the medullary pyramids, so named because of the triangular cross-section of each. Topographical order is maintained: UL medial and LL lateral. UL fibres cross higher in the medulla than LL fibres. This makes it possible, though seldom seen, for tiny brainstem lesions to cause bilateral UL weakness (sparing LLs), or even weakness of one UL and the opposite LL. However, paraparesis or tetraparesis is a more common result of a pyramidal tract lesion.

Motor fibres to cranial nerve nuclei

These corticobulbar motor fibres pass caudally in the genu (knee) of the internal capsule. Depending on the cranial nerve nucleus for which they are destined, a proportion of fibres cross the midline. These proportions vary: some cross completely, some not at all and others in a ratio of about 50 : 50. Understanding these innervation arrangements explains common clinical phenomena.

- Motor nuclei V (mastication muscles) receive 50% of fibres from each cerebral hemisphere. Thus, an internal capsule stroke usually causes no perceptible jaw deviation.
- Nuclei VII are supplied differentially (i.e. upper facial nuclear neurones are supplied 50 : 50 from each hemisphere and lower facial neurones are innervated by crossing fibres). Thus, lesions of the UMN facial motor pathway spare the upper face (i.e. the

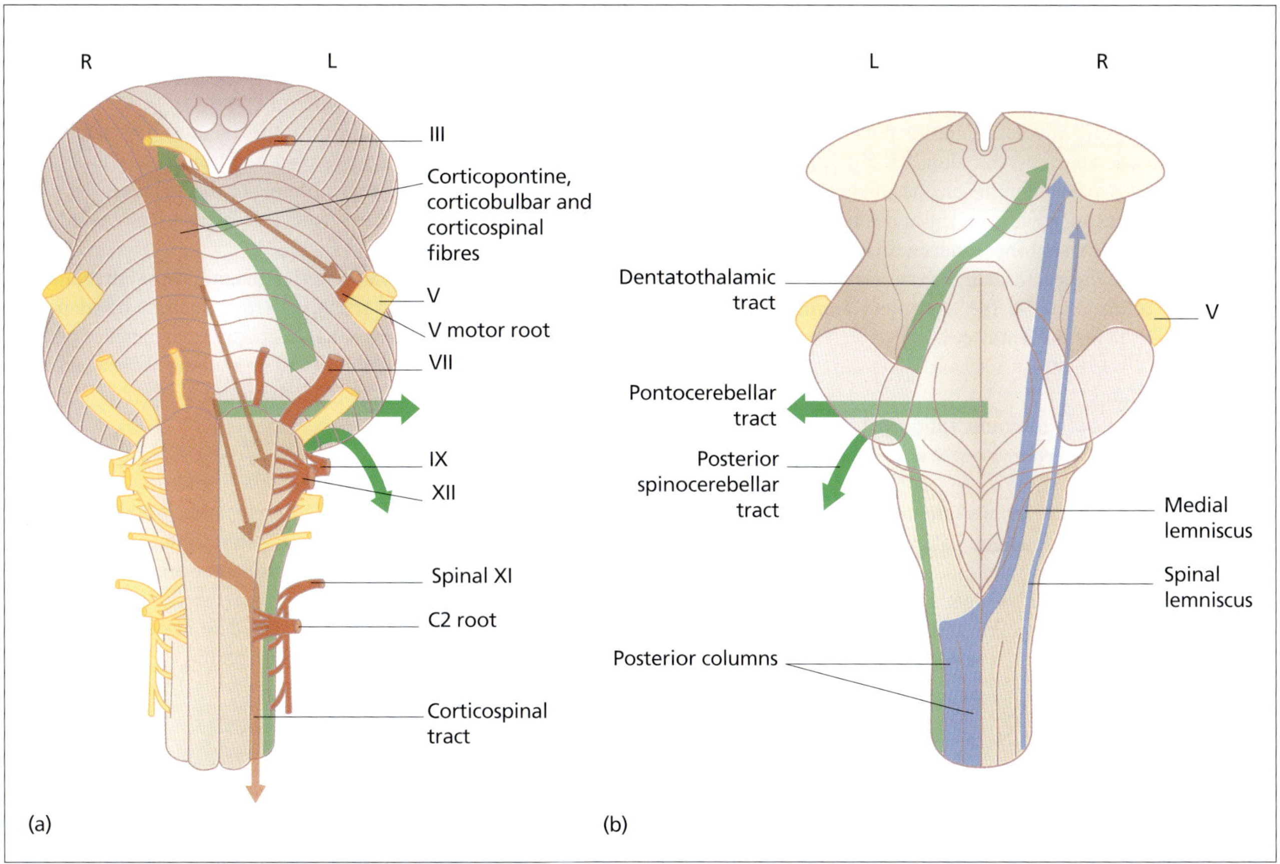

Figure 2.23 Brainstem main efferent (a) and afferent (b) pathways. Source: FitzGerald 2010. © 2016 Elsevier. Reproduced with permission of Elsevier.

familiar fact that a unilateral stroke causes lower but not upper facial weakness).

- IX, X, XI, XII motor nuclear neurones (in nucleus ambiguus and hypoglossal nucleus) are supplied variably by corticobulbar fibres in different individuals (i.e. sometimes 50 : 50, but sometimes less symmetrically). Thus, following an internal capsule stroke, usually there is usually no unilateral palate, tongue or vocal cord weakness (i.e. innervation is 50 : 50 from each side). However, on occasions when unilateral deviation of the tongue is seen in a hemiparesis, it is because the supranuclear innervation of the XIIth nucleus is largely contralateral – there is no need to consider an additional lower motor neurone (nuclear) brainstem lesion (see Pseudobulbar palsy, Chapter 13). The hypoglossal nuclei also receive projections from the RF (see Motor nuclei of V and supratrigeminal nuclei), cortical speech areas and cerebellum.
- For the XIth motor nucleus, uncrossed supranuclear fibres innervate the XIth nuclear neurones for sternomastoid of the same side. Crossed fibres innervate the XIth nuclear neurones for trapezius on the opposite side. In the normal situation as the left hand reaches out to the left (right motor cortex, left anterior horn cells), the head follows, turned to the left, by the right sternomastoid, with left scapula supported and controlled by the left trapezius. With a left hemiparesis the right sternomastoid and the left trapezius become weak.

Sensory pathways within the brainstem

The two sensory systems traverse the brainstem, to merge just before entering the thalamus (Figure 2.23b):

- *Spinothalamic tracts:* pain and temperature sensation (spinal lemniscus)
- *Posterior (dorsal) columns:* light touch, two-point discrimination, light touch, kinesthesia (medial lemniscus).

Matters are complicated by the massive Vth nuclei and their connections.

Spinothalamic tracts

The cell bodies giving rise to the spinothalamic tract are in the dorsal horn and receive ipsilateral primary afferents. The axons of these spinothalamic tract cells cross the midline in the cord (within one to three segments of their point of entry) to form each spinothalamic tract. This ascends from the cord and comes to lie laterally in the medulla (with LL fibres lateral to UL fibres) until it merges with the medial lemniscus in the upper midbrain.

The descending sympathetic pathways lie close to the spinothalamic tracts in the brainstem.

Clinical correlate When a spinothalamic lesion in the brainstem causes loss of pain and temperature in the opposite limbs, an ipsilateral Horner's syndrome is also frequently present.

Posterior column → medial lemniscus

Cell bodies lie in the cuneate (UL) and gracile (LL) nuclei in the medulla. Axons decussate there and form the medial lemniscus. This ribbon-like structure ascends and rotates in the brainstem, maintaining LL fibres laterally and UL fibres medially, to coalesce with the spinothalamic tract .

Vth nerve central pathways

The massive Vth nerve input enters the brainstem in the mid pons. Touch sensation and the corneal reflex afferents pass to the pontine Vth nucleus, and decussate to the opposite Vth pontine nucleus. Pain and temperature afferents enter the pons, but not the pontine Vth nucleus itself. They descend alongside the spinal Vth nucleus, enter the nucleus when they reach the medulla and upper cord and then decussate, to synapse on the opposite Vth spinal nucleus. The quintothalamic tract (or secondary, ascending tract of the Vth nerve) completes the route to the thalamus for nociceptive and temperature information as the trigeminal lemniscus, the tract lying lateral to the medial lemniscus.

Clinical correlates

- The corneal reflex is the most subtle sign of an emerging Vth nerve lesion (see Trigeminal nerve sensory and motor examination, Chapter 4).
- Peripheral Vth nerve lesions are usually recognisable from sensory loss, numbness and/or pain within the cutaneous distribution of V_1, V_2 and V_3.
- Central lesions affecting the spinal nucleus of V produce circumoral sensory loss (onion skin distribution, see Figure 2.54, and Trigeminal nerve lesions, Chapter 13).
- Facial numbness on one side with spinothalamic sensory loss in the contralateral limbs is diagnostic of a dorsolateral brainstem lesion. This crossed sensory loss can occur with a lesion anywhere between upper cervical cord and mid pons.
- When a cavity develops within the medulla (syringobulbia), bizarre patterns of facial and upper cervical sensory loss can be seen when the crossing central fibres of the spinal nucleus of V and quintothalamic tract are damaged. These are often dismissed initially as non-organic.

At a more general level, with such a magnitude of afferent information, the face is highly sensitive. Trigeminal-mediated pain is exquisitely painful, such as toothache and trigeminal neuralgia. The importance of the trigeminovascular system in headaches is considered in Chapter 12 (see Anatomy and physiology of headache).

Cranial nerve nuclear columns

A summary of the embryological development begins to explain the layout (Figure 2.24). Seven nuclear columns (four afferent, three efferent) contribute to the nuclear masses of the brainstem and cord. Motor cranial nerve nuclei are derived from two of these columns:

- III, IV, VI and XII arise from a paramedian nuclear mass known as the general somatic efferent (GSE) column.

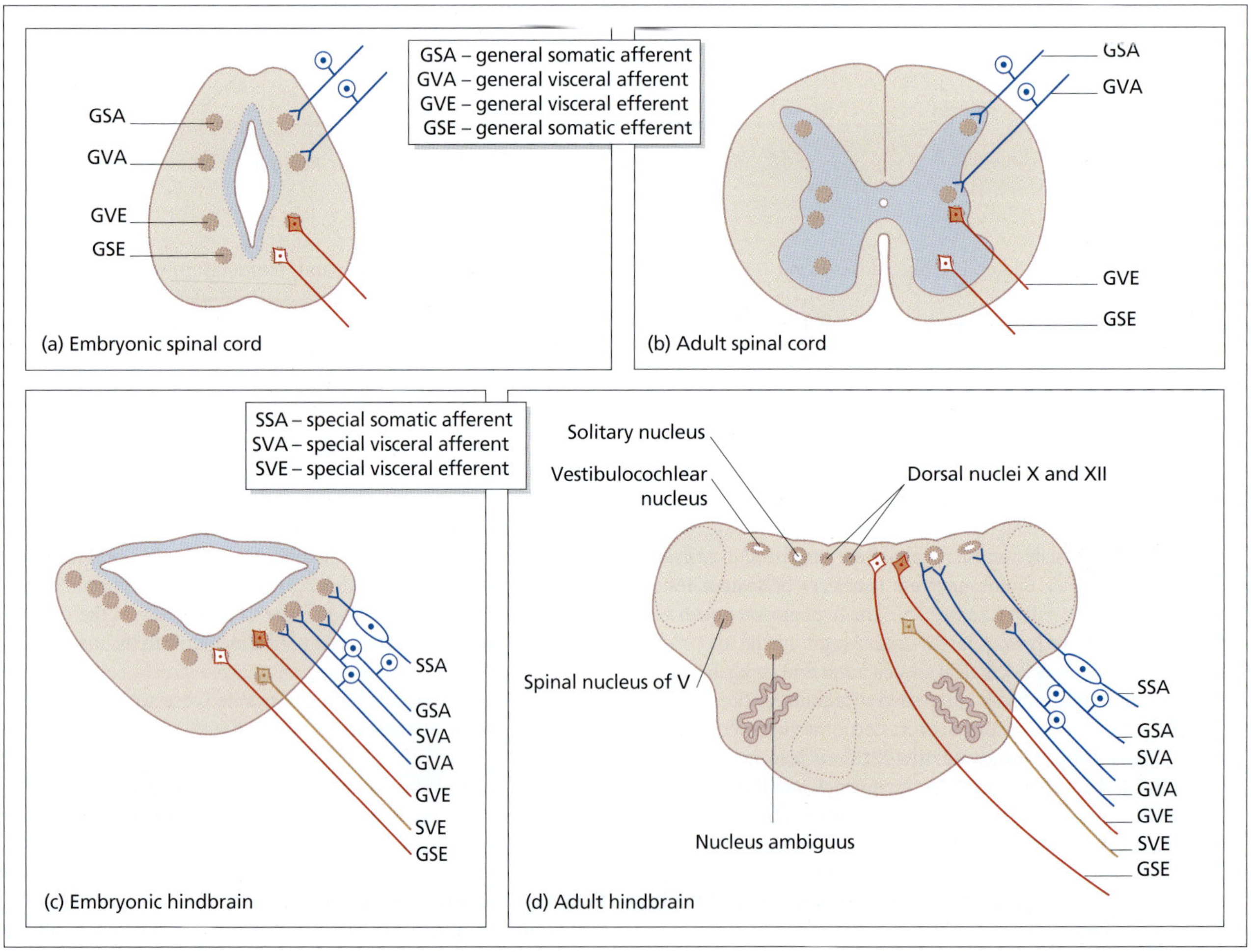

Figure 2.24 Seven nuclear columns: embryonic and adult cord and hindbrain. Source: FitzGerald 2010. © 2016 Elsevier. Reproduced with permission of Elsevier.

- V (motor), VII, IX and X (nucleus ambiguus) and XI (spinal accessory nucleus) arise from ventrolateral cells known as the special visceral efferent (SVE) column.

As the fetus develops, GSE column nuclei III, IV, VI and XII remain close to the midline. The SVE nuclei move laterally along the lateral margin of the fourth ventricle.

Of the main afferent nuclei:

- The Vth nerve nuclei are described later (see Cranial nerves and VIII: vestibulocochlear nerve).
- The vestibular nuclei (SSA) occupy a wide area in the pons, extending through the medulla to upper cervical cord (see Cranial nerves and V: trigeminal nerve).
- The nucleus of the tractus solitarius (SVA) receives taste fibres and relays gustatory reflexes.

Reticular formation

The biological role of the RF can be understood from its origins as a polysynaptic, slow conducting, central pathway that:

- Linked olfactory and limbic systems, and
- Coordinated autonomic and reflex activity.

Phylogenetically, as vision and hearing assumed important roles together with olfaction, direct lateralised pathways of these special senses bypassed the RF. In mammals, the older pathways were superseded by fast direct linkages between cortex and sensorimotor systems. In humans, the RF means the polysynaptic, modulating, neuronal network within the brainstem, although the system extends further – caudally into the cord and rostrally to thalamus and hypothalamus. It is of importance in:

- Respiratory control
- Sleep, wakefulness, arousal and mood
- Cardiovascular control
- Pattern generation of some reflex motor activities (e.g. chewing, swallowing, conjugate gaze)
- Micturition, bowel and sexual function
- Sensory modulation (see Neuro-stimulation procedures: gate theory, Chapter 23), and
- Autonomic and reflex activity generally.

Aminergic neurones are prominent in the RF:

- Serotoninergic RF neurones form a ubiquitous network throughout the raphe nuclei
- Dopaminergic neurones occupy substantia nigra and ventral tegmental nuclei
- Noradrenergic neurones are congregated in the locus coeruleus (floor of 4th ventricle) and through the pons, medulla and midbrain
- Adrenergic neurones occupy principally the medulla, and
- Enkephalins are also involved (peri-aqueductal grey matter).

Essential anatomy

This is outlined in Figure 2.25. The raphe nuclei (raphe, pronounced 'raffay'; Greek: a seam) are the major source of serotoninergic neurones in the neuraxis.

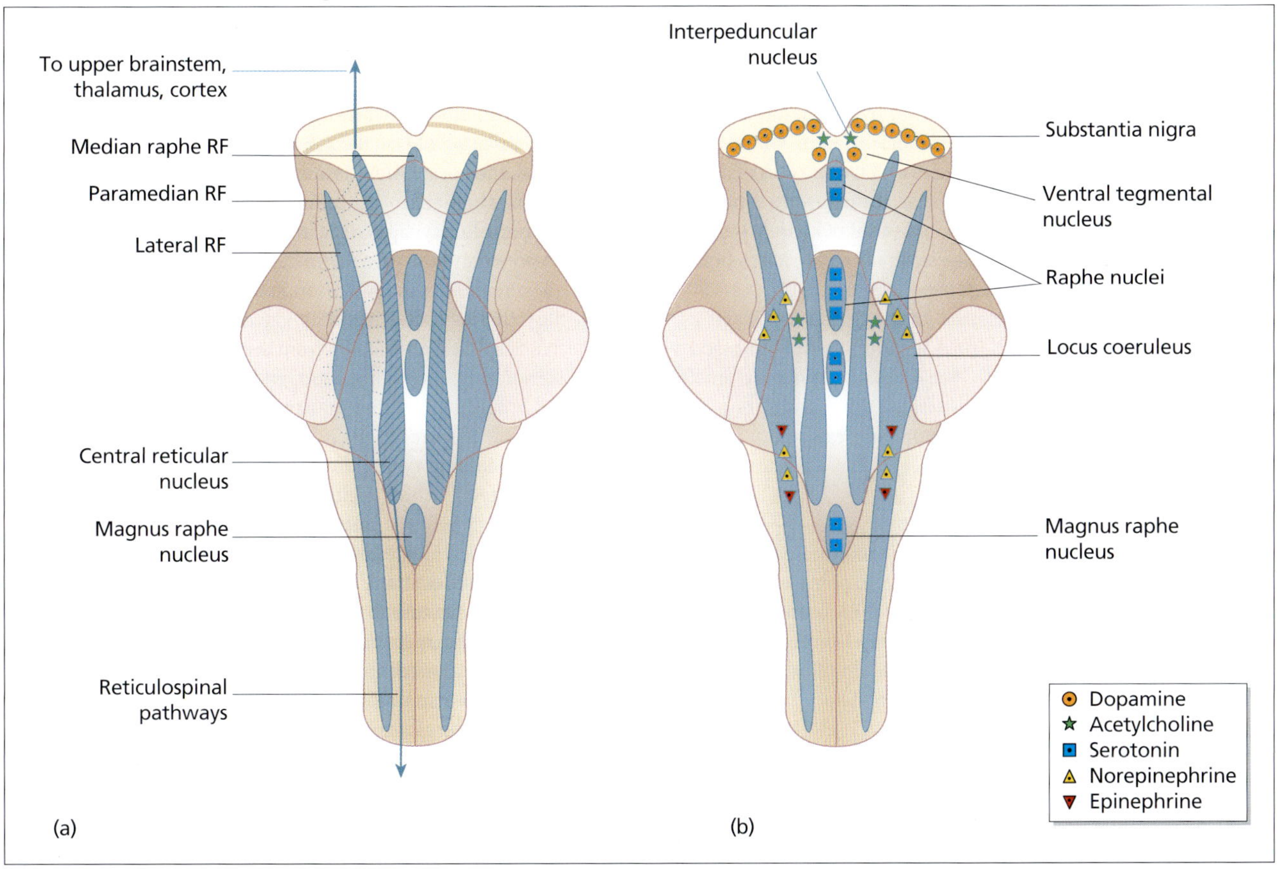

Figure 2.25 Reticular formation: (a) subdivisions (nuclei); (b) principal neurotransmitter cell groups. Source: FitzGerald 2010. © 2016 Elsevier. Reproduced with permission of Elsevier.

Alongside the median raphe nuclei lie the paramedian RF (magnocellular and gigantocellular neurones) on each side. Each paramedian network blends into the lateral RF (parvocellular neurones).

The lateral RF is largely afferent, receiving input from all sensory pathways, especially:

- Olfactory system (via median forebrain bundle, next to the hypothalamus)
- Visual pathways (via superior colliculus)
- Auditory pathways (via superior olivary nucleus)
- Vestibular pathways (via medial vestibular nucleus), and
- Somatic sensory and trigeminal system (spinoreticular tracts, pontine Vth nuclei).

The paramedian RF is a smaller efferent polysynaptic distributive pathway to:

- Thalamus
- Spinal cord (via pontine and medullary reticulospinal tracts), and
- Cardiovascular and respiratory regulators.

Respiratory control

This is achieved via:

- Dorsal and ventral respiratory nuclei
- Medullary chemosensitive area, and
- Carotid chemoreceptors.

Cyclical respiration is modulated by the dorsal and ventral respiratory nuclei in the medulla. The dorsal nucleus is mainly inspiratory (efferent connections to respiratory muscles) and the ventral, expiratory. A third medial paracentral nucleus adjacent to the locus coeruleus is involved in initiating and driving respiratory rhythms. The dorsal respiratory nucleus receives excitatory impulses from the medullary chemosensitive area. These cells in the lateral RF at the level of the IXth nerve nucleus and 4th ventricle choroid plexus are exquisitely sensitive to hydrogen ion concentration: any increase in hydrogen ion concentration stimulates the dorsal respiratory nucleus. Sampling of pCO_2 also takes place here.

Carotid chemoreceptors (glomus cells at the carotid bifurcation) are exquisitely sensitive to changes in arterial pO_2, and/or a rise in arterial pCO_2. Impulses pass via the sinus nerve (a branch of IX) to stimulate the dorsal respiratory centre.

The ventral respiratory nucleus is largely expiratory. It acts as an inhibitory oscillator during normal breathing and is engaged via GABAergic internuncials with the dorsal respiratory nucleus. During increased ventilation (e.g. exercise) the ventral respiratory nuclei activate anterior horn cells supplying expiratory accessory and abdominal muscles.

Sleep, wakefulness and mood

In animal models, destruction of raphe midbrain neurones or depletion of serotonin results in prolonged insomnia. The ascending reticular activating system is a term that harnesses this concept of cortical activation. Activation is seen on electroencephalogram (EEG) during waking from sleep – high amplitude slow (delta) waves are replaced by fast (alpha) waves. The principal cellular candidates for this role are:

- Cholinergic neurones near the coerulean nuclei, or
- Histaminergic neurones in the tuberomamillary nuclei.

Following arousal the alert state is sustained by continuing activation by these neurones and by activation of the basal nucleus of Meynert in the basal forebrain. Inactivity within the ascending reticular activating system is inherent in the mechanisms of coma.

The limbic system and RF are mentioned in Chapter 22 (see Neuropsychiatic aspects of movement disorders) in the relation to mood and the orexin–hypocretin system in Chapter 20 (see Hypersomnias of central origin).

Cardiovascular control

The solitary nuclei in the medulla receive afferents from baroreceptors in the carotid sinus and aortic arch. The barovagal and barosympathetic reflexes modulate blood pressure and cardiac output (see Cardiovascular system; Orthostatic hypotension, Chapter 24).

Patterns of primitive movements

These movements are primitive only in phylogenetic terms:

- Conjugate gaze – pontine centres for lateral and vertical gaze
- Chewing – supratrigeminal premotor pontine nucleus
- Respiration – medullary respiratory nuclei
- Swallowing, coughing, sneezing, vomiting, crying, salivation, and
- Locomotor pattern generators.

Micturition control

A micturition control centre (MCC or M centre) lies in each paramedian pontine reticular formation (PPRF). Axons from magnocellular neurones pass directly to parasympathetic (motor) neurones at S2–4 in the cord.

The essential anatomy of cortical and subcortical influences on micturition are included here (Figure 2.26). Neurones in lateral peri-aqueductal grey matter (LPAG) receive fibres from the sacral posterior grey horn and project excitatory fibres to the M centre. The ventral posterior nucleus of the thalamus also receives sacral fibres. The LPAG also receives excitatory fibres from the pre-optic nucleus (PON).

Gate control: Sensory modulation

The anatomy and role of the RF in pain control, also known as supraspinal antinociception, is summarised in Figure 2.27. Gating (see Neuro-stimulation procedures: gate theory, Chapter 23) involves control of synaptic transmission between one neurone or set of neurones and the next. While the gate theory of pain is sometimes questioned, it remains a useful model.

Tactile sensory transmission is gated at the posterior column nuclei. Nociceptive transmission from the trunk and limbs is gated in the posterior grey horn of the cord, and from the head and neck in the spinal V nucleus. One crucial structure in the cord is the substantia gelatinosa (Figure 2.21b), rich in excitatory glutaminergic neurones and inhibitory GABAergic and enkephalinergic neurones.

Unmyelinated C fibres mediate dull, intense, prolonged, poorly localised pain, largely via excitatory substantia gelatinosa interneurones and thence via lateral spinothalamic tracts to the thalamus. Short, sharp, well-localised pain is mediated by finely myelinated Aδ fibres. These synapse directly on dendrites of relay neurones of the lateral spinothalamic tract.

Large A (mechanoreceptor) afferents from hair follicles and skin synapse on anterior spinothalamic relay cells and send collaterals to inhibitory (GABAergic) gelatinosa cells. These then synapse on lateral spinothalamic tract relay cells.

Gating of C fibre activity can be enhanced by stimulating A fibre afferents or enhancing RF inhibition from the magnus raphe nucleus (MRN), for example by rubbing, transcutaneous electrical nerve stimulation (TENS), implanted stimulators, inducing sleep and some pain-modulating drugs such as gabapentin. All are believed to increase central gating of pain.

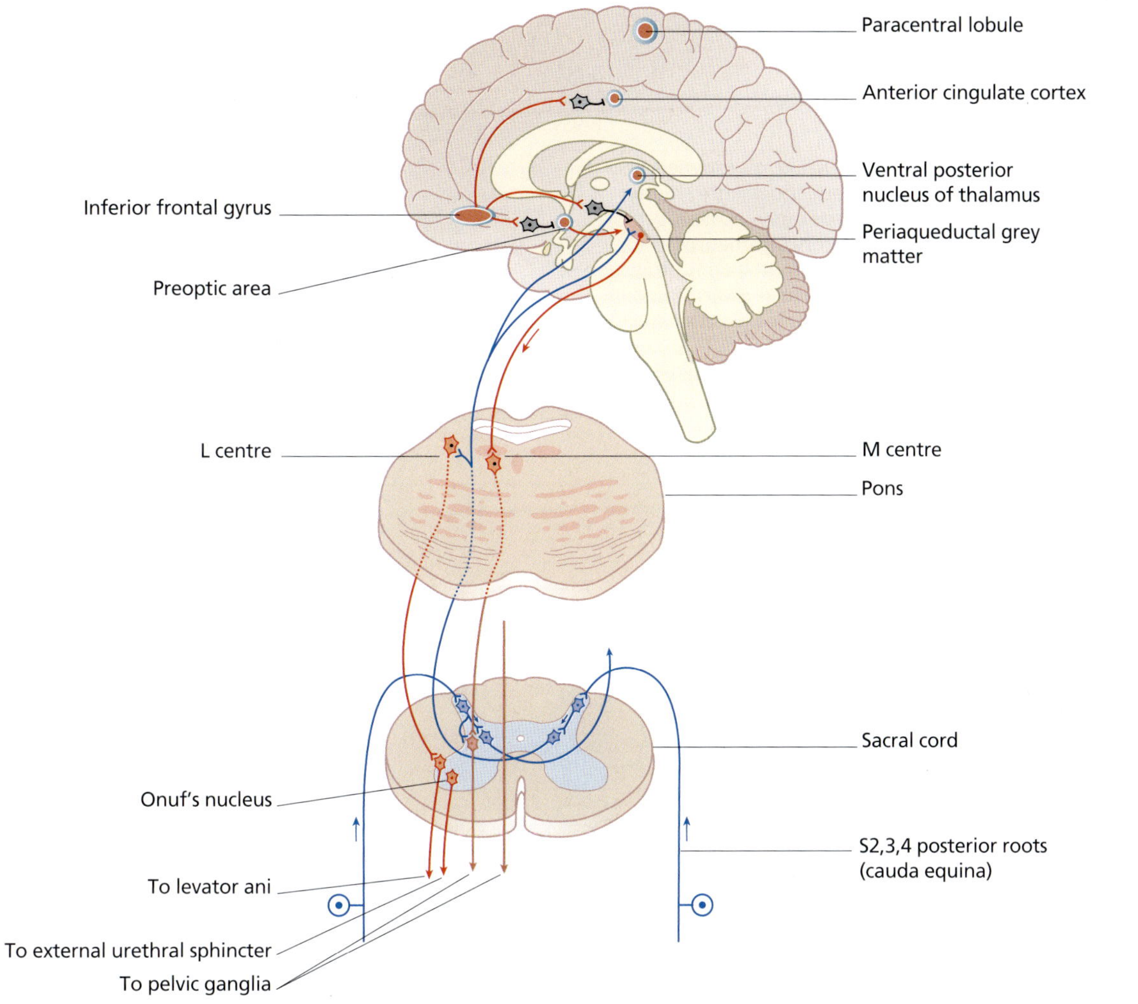

1 As intravesical pressure increases, bladder detrusor and trigone stretch receptors are activated (S2, 3 and 4).
2 Spinoreticular fibres relay impulses to thalamus, midbrain and pons. Right PPRF L centre, LPAG, and RACC are activated.
3 Sympathetic activity increases + parasympathetic activity inhibited. Bladder compliance increases. Bladder continues to fill.
4 Spinoreticular fibres via PPRF L centre activate Onuf's nucleus (sacral cord). External sphincter tone increases: micturition is prevented.
5 Urgency is perceived when bladder becomes full. If time and/or place are unsuitable, the inferior frontal gyrus becomes activated, RACC is suppressed. M centre, LPAG and PON are suppressed.
6 Voluntary micturition is accomplished, when appropriate, by M centre activation and relaxation of the external sphincter accompanied by increase in intravesical pressure/active (voluntary) contraction of abdominal muscles.

Figure 2.26 Neuroanatomy of micturition control and passing urine. Source: FitzGerald 2010. © 2016 Elsevier. Reproduced with permission of Elsevier.

Limbic system, hippocampus and related structures

The limbus (Latin: a rim) was coined by Broca in the late nineteeth century to describe cortex bounded by the corpus callosum. The hippocampus takes its name from Greek, originally for a horse + monster (ιπποϛ + καμποϛ) and later the seahorse, which the hippocampus resembles in coronal cross-section.

The limbic system includes:

- Hippocampi, mamillary bodies and septal area
- Insulae, cingulate and parahippocampal gyri, and
- Amygdala – subcortical nuclear masses adjacent to each temporal pole.

Other subcortical regions nearby are the nucleus accumbens, medial dorsal nucleus of the thalamus, hypothalamus and part of the reticular formation. The orbital cortex (frontal cortex above the orbit), the temporal pole, the corpus callosum, choroid plexus and lateral ventricle are also nearby (Figure 2.28).

The parahippocampal gyri are the main interfaces between hippocampi (known as allocortex) and the cerebral neocortex. The entorhinal cortex is the anterior section – area 28. This is

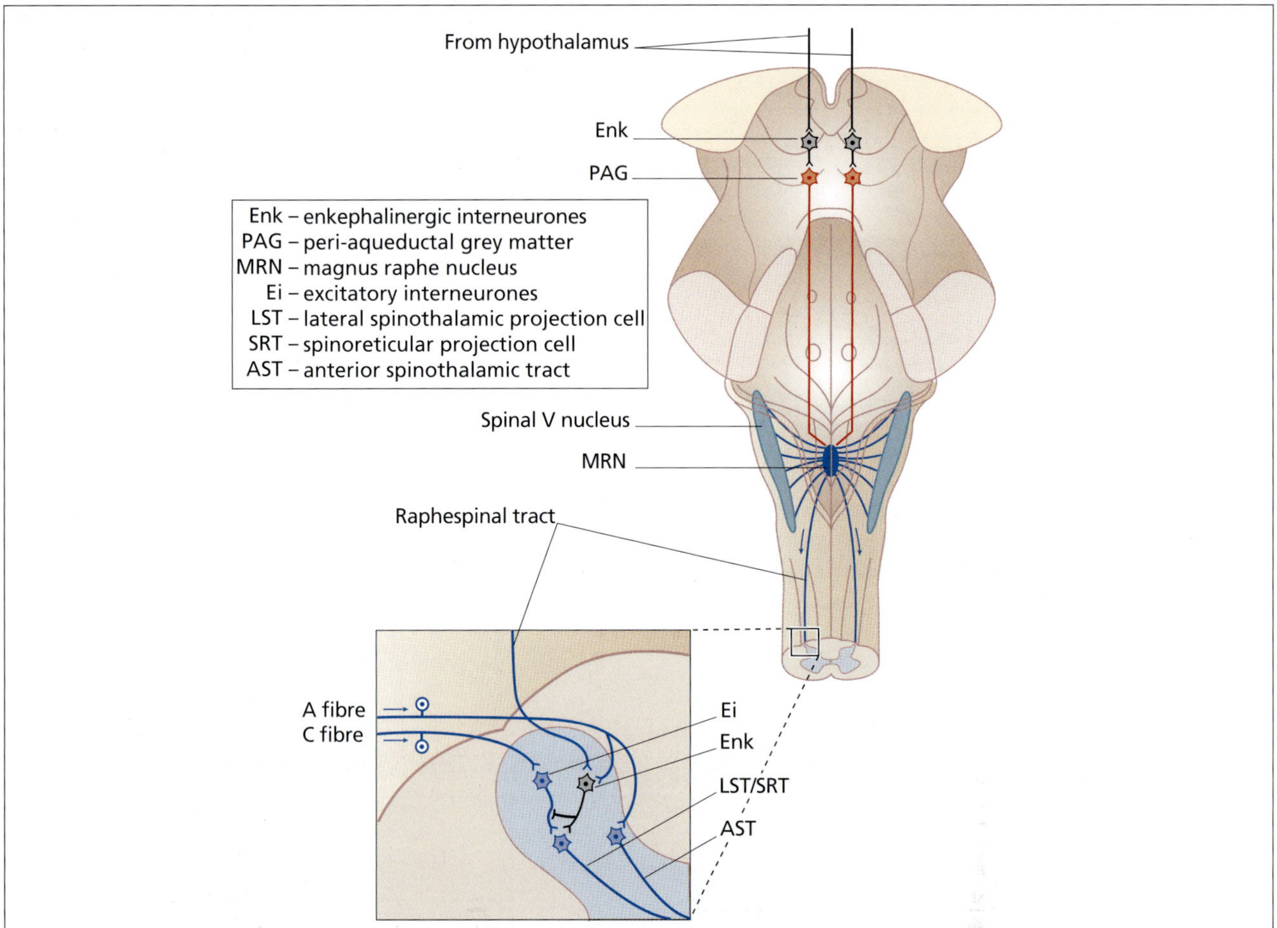

1. The magnus raphe nucleus (MRN) in the medulla is the origin of raphe–spinal fibres in the tract of Lissauer that synapse in the substantia gelatinosa of the cord at all levels.
2. Many RF raphe–spinal fibres are serotonergic. They excite inhibitory interneurones in the posterior grey horn of the cord.
3. Peri-aqueductal grey matter (PAG) projects to the MRN.
4. Hypothalamic and enkephalinergic interneurones exert tonic inhibition on PAG neurones. Inhibitory impulses from the hypothalamus disinhibit (release) PAG excitatory neurones.
5. Passage of purely tactile information – into AST – is not impeded.
6. The cortico-spinal tracts also terminate widely in the dorsal horns, including the substantia gelatinosa; one important function is supraspinal control of sensory input.

Figure 2.27 Anatomy of sensory modulation.

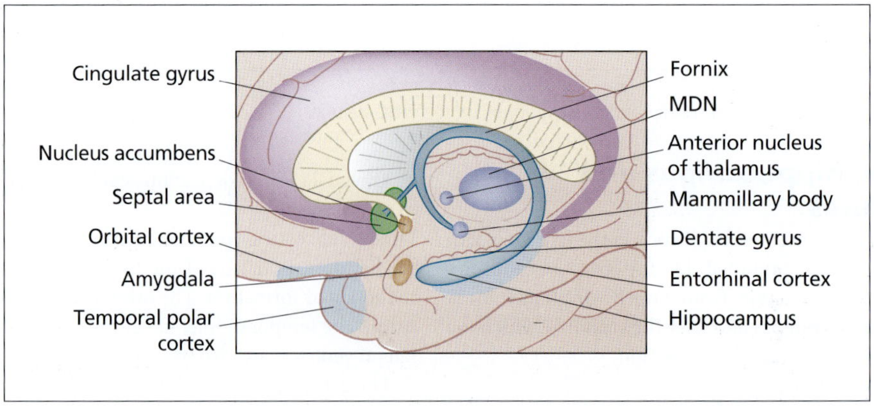

Figure 2.28 Limbic and subcortical areas: medial view. Source: FitzGerald 2010. © 2016 Elsevier. Reproduced with permission of Elsevier.

six-layered cortex, exchanging fibres between the four neocortical association areas and the hippocampus. Each fornix, looping over the medial dorsal thalamic nucleus into the mamillary body, provides a second route between neocortex and hippocampus.

The planes, contours and nomenclature of the hippocampal formation (subiculum, dentate gyrus, hippocampus) are complex. Looking from above, picture a horseshoe lying tilted in the floor of the lateral ventricle. One (lateral) arm is the hippocampus. The other arm twists into the loop of the fornix to follow the contour of the thalamus (Figure 2.29).

The coronal cross-section of the hippocampus – the seahorse-like outline – has its head in the lateral ventricle and a tail leading to the entorhinal cortex. The dentate gyrus is surrounded by the seahorse's head.

Additional terminology comes from the ancient descriptive name for the hippocampus, Ammon's horn (Ammon was the Egyptian ram deity; *cornu* means horn), hence cornu ammonis (CA) zones which divide the hippocampus into four (Figure 2.29d). Pyramidal cells are the main cell types seen in the subiculum and hippocampus and granule cells in the dentate nucleus. Inhibitory GABAergic interneurones are present throughout the area.

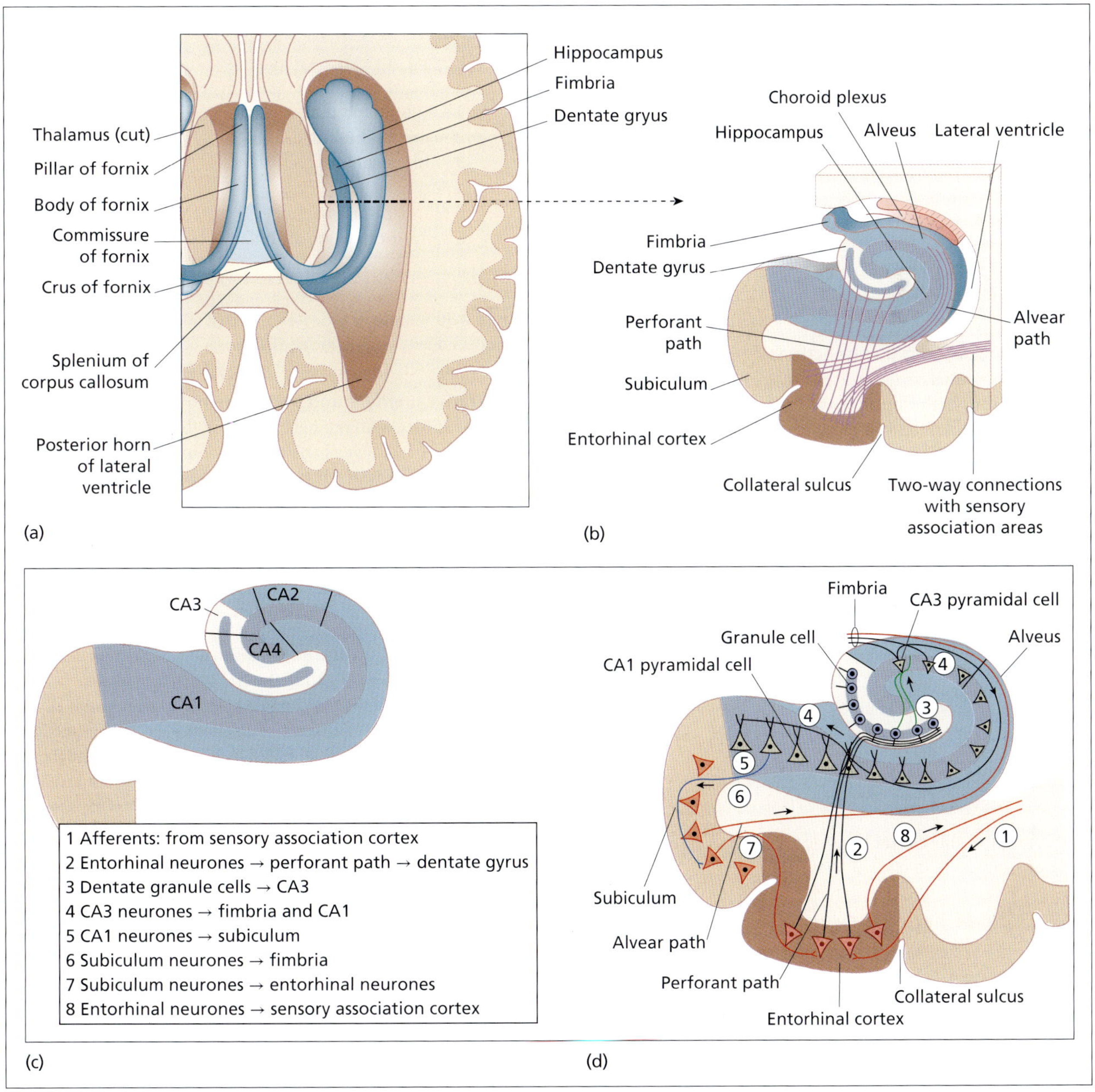

Figure 2.29 (a) Hippocampus and surrounding structures (from above). (b) Coronal section from subiculum to lateral ventricle. (c) Ammon's horn: CA1, CA2, CA3, CA4. (d). Basic hippocampal wiring (1–8). Source: FitzGerald 2010. © 2016 Elsevier. Reproduced with permission of Elsevier.

This region is intimately involved in memory, arousal and mood – and in epilepsy (see Hippocampal sclerosis, Chapter 7). This summary outlines majority views in a complex field. Much original work was derived from clinical observation in humans. Extrapolation from primate studies, and more recently fMRI, have added insights into these areas. Their relevance in epilepsy, memory and mood – and in dementia – is dealt with in Chapters 7 (see Hippocampal sclerosis) and 8 (see Memory).

Afferent hippocampal connections

The perforant path passes from the entorhinal cortex to dendrites of dentate nucleus granule cells. The alvear path passes from the subiculum to the alveus, the ventricular face of the hippocampus. Mossy fibres, the axons of granule cells synapse in CA3 pyramidal cells. CA3 pyramidal cell axons pass into the fimbria, giving rise to Schaffer collaterals between CA3 and CA1. CA1 projects to the entorhinal cortex. Visual, visuo-spatial and auditory afferents also reach the region:

- Auditory fibres from the superior and middle temporal gyri to hippocampus
- Visuospatial data from area 40 (supramarginal gyrus), and
- Visual association data (object shape and colour/facial recognition) from the occipito-temporal region to the perirhinal cortex (adjacent to the entorhinal) and thence to the hippocampus.

Diffuse afferent connections also reach the hippocampus (Table 2.4) largely via the fornix.

Efferent hippocampal connections

First, the entorhinal cortex projects to neocortical association areas. Secondly, axons in the fornix (Latin: vault or arch) project forwards from the subiculum and hippocampus itself. Components of the fornix are:

- Fimbriae (Latin: thin projections, forming a fringe).
- The crus (cross) arches up below corpus callosum, joins opposite the fornix to form the trunk and hippocampal commissure.
- The trunk divides into the two pillars of the fornix.
  Each pillar divides around the anterior commissure:
- Precommissural fibres pass to the septal area
- Postcommissural fibres pass to the anterior hypothalamus, mamillary body and medial forebrain bundle.

Each mamillary body (Latin: mamilla = nipple) projects to the anterior nucleus of the thalamus, thence to the cingulate cortex.

Papez's circuit (1937; Figure 2.30) is the loop:

$$\text{Hippocampus} \rightarrow \text{fornix} \rightarrow \text{cingulate cortex}$$
$$\rightarrow \text{entorhinal cortex} \rightarrow \text{hippocampus.}$$

The concept of this circuit has stood the test of time, though with more anatomical than clinical relevance.

Table 2.4 Diffuse afferents to the hippocampus.

Neurotransmitter	Source	Clinical association
Cholinergic	Septal nuclei	Memory
Noradrenergic	Coerulean nuclei	Arousal
Dopaminergic	Ventral tegmentum	Movement/thought disorder
Serotinergic	Raphe nuclei	Mood

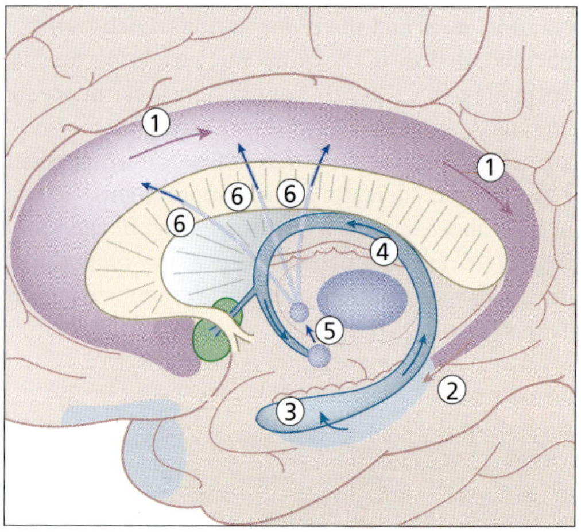

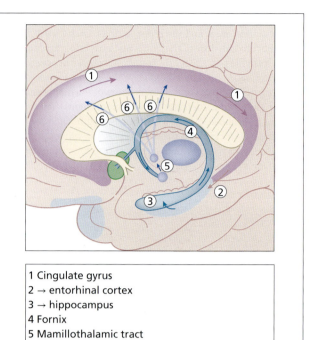

1 Cingulate gyrus
2 → entorhinal cortex
3 → hippocampus
4 Fornix
5 Mamillothalamic tract
6 Anterior nucleus of thalamus → cingulate cortex

Figure 2.30 Papez's circuit. Source: FitzGerald 2010. © 2016 Elsevier. Reproduced with permission of Elsevier.

Declarative memory and long-term potentiation

Data-based (declarative) memory, the ability to retain and retrieve new facts, is lost when the anterior hippocampus is damaged. Procedural memory is preserved (e.g. thread a needle, assemble a jigsaw, ride a bicycle). The hippocampus is not involved in procedural memory – there is growing evidence that the cerebellum is a principal structure involved in these procedural or motor memories.

Long-term potentiation (LTP) is a phenomenon seen widely within the nervous system but especially within the dentate gyrus and hippocampus. As its name implies, target cells remain sensitive to a fresh stimulus a long time (hours) after stimulation.

LTP can be demonstrated in animals both in perforant path → dentate granule cells and Schaffer collateral → CA1 connections. A brief, several millisecond stimulus to either Schaffer collaterals or perforant path induces this long-lasting sensitivity in target neurones following GABA receptor activation. New synapses appear within minutes, while existing synapses expand. It is believed that LTP is of fundamental importance in learning. LTP is enhanced by opioid peptides, norepinephrine and dopamine released within the perforant path.

ACh muscarinic activity within the hippocampus is also significant in learning. Hyoscine in small doses blocks memory for lists and numbers. Hyoscine (scopolamine) became known as 'the truth drug' – of 007 James Bond, CIA and KGB repute. Hyoscine frequently distorts recall and has hallucinogenic effects – making it of no value for extracting secrets from detainees. Physostigmine blocks the effect of hyoscine. This was the original basis for development of anticholinergic therapy in Alzheimer's disease.

Insula, cingulate cortex and parahippocampal gyrus

The insula can conveniently be divided into three:

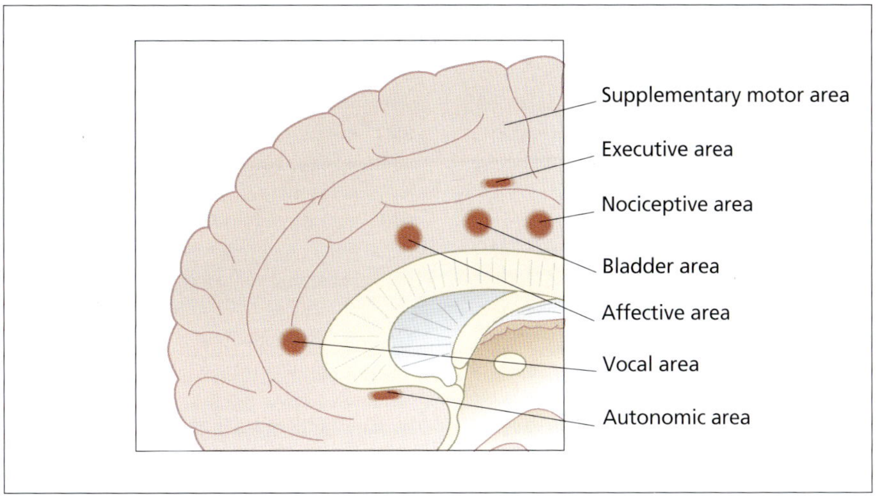

Figure 2.31 Anterior cingulate cortex (medial view): six functional zones. Source: FitzGerald 2010. © 2016 Elsevier. Reproduced with permission of Elsevier.

1 *Anterior:* a cortical centre for pain
2 *Posterior:* connects with the amygdala and entorhinal cortex (emotional responses to and memories of pain), and
3 *Central:* language functions.

The cingulate cortex, part of Papez's circuit merges into the posterior parahippocampal gyrus behind the splenium. The anterior cingulate (part of the rostral limbic system – amygdala, ventral striatum and anterior insula) has six functional zones (Figure 2.31):

1 *Executive:* connected to dorsolateral prefrontal cortex (DLPFC) and supplementary motor area.
2 *Nociceptive:* afferents from thalamus (medial dorsal nucleus).
3 *Affective* (emotional): happy thoughts activate this area on fMRI – and the amygdala switches off. Anterior cingulectomy was once performed for aggressive psychopathic behaviour.
4 *Micturition:* activity seen on bladder filling.
5 *Vocalisation:* active during decisions about syntactic construction. Reduced regional blood flow is seen in some cases of stammering.
6 *Autonomic:* respiratory and cardiac – responses to emotion, sweating and blushing.

Amygdala

Amygdala is Greek for an almond. This is a substantial nuclear group anterior to the caudate nucleus tail. Fear and anxiety are mediated via the amygdala – a glance at afferent and efferent pathways of Tables 2.5 and 2.6 indicates widespread connections and potential pathways for everyday experiences (e.g. feeling unwell, hypotensive and sweaty at the sight of blood).

Kindling is a term used, often conjecturally to describe development of seizure activity in an area of brain contralateral to or distant from an epileptic focus. At a neurophysiological level, it means a group response within neurones that increases following a uniform strength stimulus. This phenomenon is unique and, as far as is known, confined to the amygdala and hippocampus.

Nucleus accumbens

Stimulation of these areas of the ventral striatum (nucleus accumbens, ventral olfactory tubercle, ventral caudate and putamen) leads typically to a sense of well-being akin to a shot of heroin, attributed to excessive dopamine release flooding the prefrontal cortex and nucleus itself. Most stimulant drugs increase dopamine levels in these areas. Ninety-five per cent of nucleus accumbens neurones are spiny GABAergic projection neurones; 5% are cholinergic neurones (non-spiny, also known as aspiny neurones).

Septal region

Afferents to the septal nuclei come from:

- Hippocampus (via fornix)
- Brainstem, via medial forebrain bundle (monoaminergic neurones)
- Amygdala, via the diagonal band of Broca, and
- Olfactory tract, via medial olfactory striae.

Efferents travel in two principal pathways:

1 Striae medullaris → habenula nucleus → habenulo-interpeduncular tract → interpeduncular nucleus, and
2 Septohippocampal tract.

The interpeduncular nucleus participates in sleep–wake cycles (with the locus coeruleus).

The septohippocampal tract is believed to have a role in generating temporal cortex theta EEG activity, by synchronous discharge of hippocampal pyramidal neurones.

Stimulation of the septal region in humans produces pleasurable sexual sensations and/or orgasm. In animals, destructive lesions cause extreme anger – known as septal rage.

Basal forebrain

This region lies between the olfactory tracts and infundibulum (caudally) and the amygdala. The magnocellular basal nucleus of Meynert is the largest single nuclear group here, its cholinergic neurones extending throughout the cortex (Figure 2.32). These magnocellular basal nuclei, septal nuclei and neurones in the diagonal band of Broca are known as basal forebrain nuclei. The floor of the basal forebrain, the anterior perforated substance, is traversed by branches of the anterior cerebral arteries. The basal forebrain nuclei exert tonic cholinergic activity within the cortex, thus maintaining wakefulness, and facilitating perceptive activity. Cholinergic activity is believed to enhance LTP in pyramidal cells of the cortex.

Table 2.5 Amygdala afferents – to the lateral nucleus.

Type	Subcortical origin	Cortical origin
Touch	VP nucleus of thalamus	Parietal cortex
Hearing	MGB	Superior temporal gyrus
Vision	LGB	Occipital cortex
Smell		Piriform lobe
Memory		Hippocampus/ entorhinal cortex
Cardiac	Hypothalamus	
Pain	RF	Insula
Cognitive		Orbital (frontal) cortex
Attention/anxiety	Locus coeruleus	Basal nucleus of Meynert

LGB, lateral geniculate body; MGB, medial geniculate body; RF, reticular formation; VP, ventral posterior (nucleus).

Table 2.6 Amygdala efferents – from the central nucleus.

Pathway/distant target nucleus	Effect
PAG	Pain suppression (antinociception)
PAG	Freezing with fear
Locus coeruleus	Wakefulness/arousal
Medullary norepinephric neurones (to lateral grey horn)	Increase in pulse and blood pressure
Hypothalamus/dorsal nucleus of vagus	Slowing of pulse/syncope
Hypothalamus (corticotrophin RF)	→Cortisol secretion
Parabrachial (thence to respiratory) nuclei	Hyperventilation/apnoea

PAG, peri-aqueductal grey matter; RF, reticular formation.

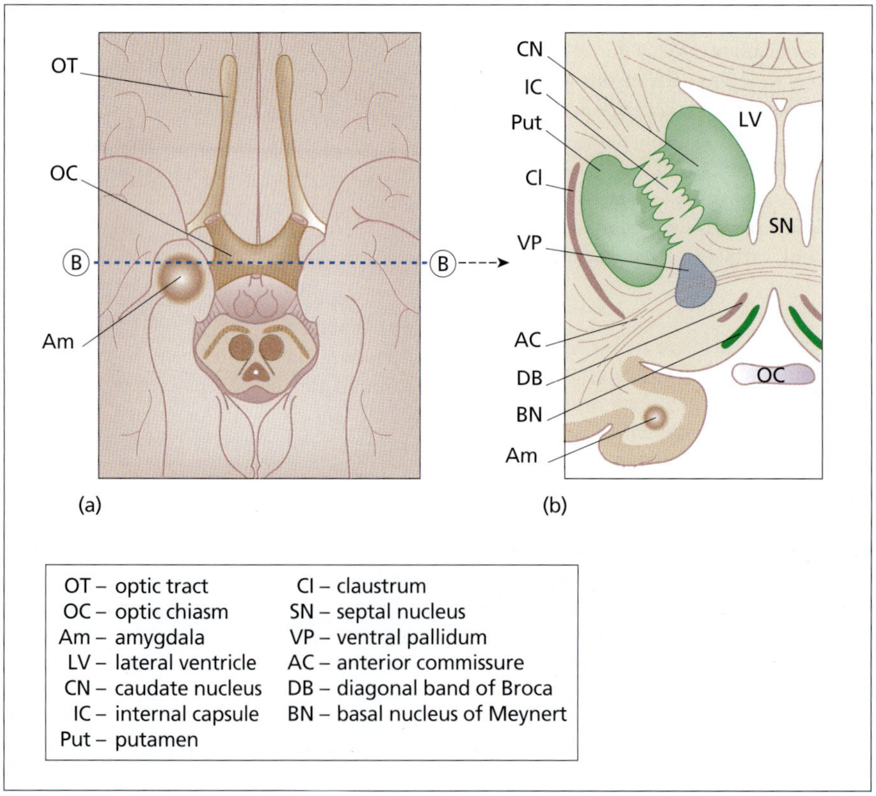

Figure 2.32 (a) Basal forebrain (from below) (b) Basal forebrain nuclei. (Coronal section at BB.) Source: FitzGerald 2010. © 2016 Elsevier. Reproduced with permission of Elsevier.

The thalamus

The paired conjoined thalami are among the larger nuclear masses of the brain. They are complex relay stations. In contrast to this complexity, the clinical neurology is relatively sparse, but of increasing relevance with the development of stereotactic surgery and neurostimulation.

Divisions and connections are shown in Figure 2.33. It can be simplified by noting the large 'Y', of thalamic white matter – the internal medullary lamina – that divides the nuclei into three cell groups:

1 Anterior (within the 'Y')
2 Medial dorsal, and
3 Lateral nuclei.

Lateral nuclei are divided into ventral and dorsal tiers. The medial and lateral geniculate bodies lie posteriorly. The reticular nucleus surrounds each thalamus laterally, separated by an external medullary lamina traversed by thalamocortical fibres. The three groups of thalamic nuclei, somewhat uninformatively named are:

1 Relay (specific) nuclei
2 Association nuclei, and
3 Non-specific nuclei.

Principal connections are shown in Table 2.7.

Cortical connections

Four, largely afferent connections from thalamus to cortex run in the anterior, posterior, inferior and superior thalamic peduncles in a cruciform arrangement:

1 Anterior thalamic peduncle → cingulate gyrus and prefrontal cortex via internal capsule (anterior limb).
2 Superior thalamic peduncle → motor, premotor and sensory cortex via internal capsule (posterior limb).
3 Posterior thalamic peduncle → occipital, posterior parietal and posterior temporal cortex via internal capsule.
4 Inferior thalamic peduncle → anterior temporal and orbital cortex.

Each fan of these sensory fibres forms part of the corona radiata between internal capsule and cortex.

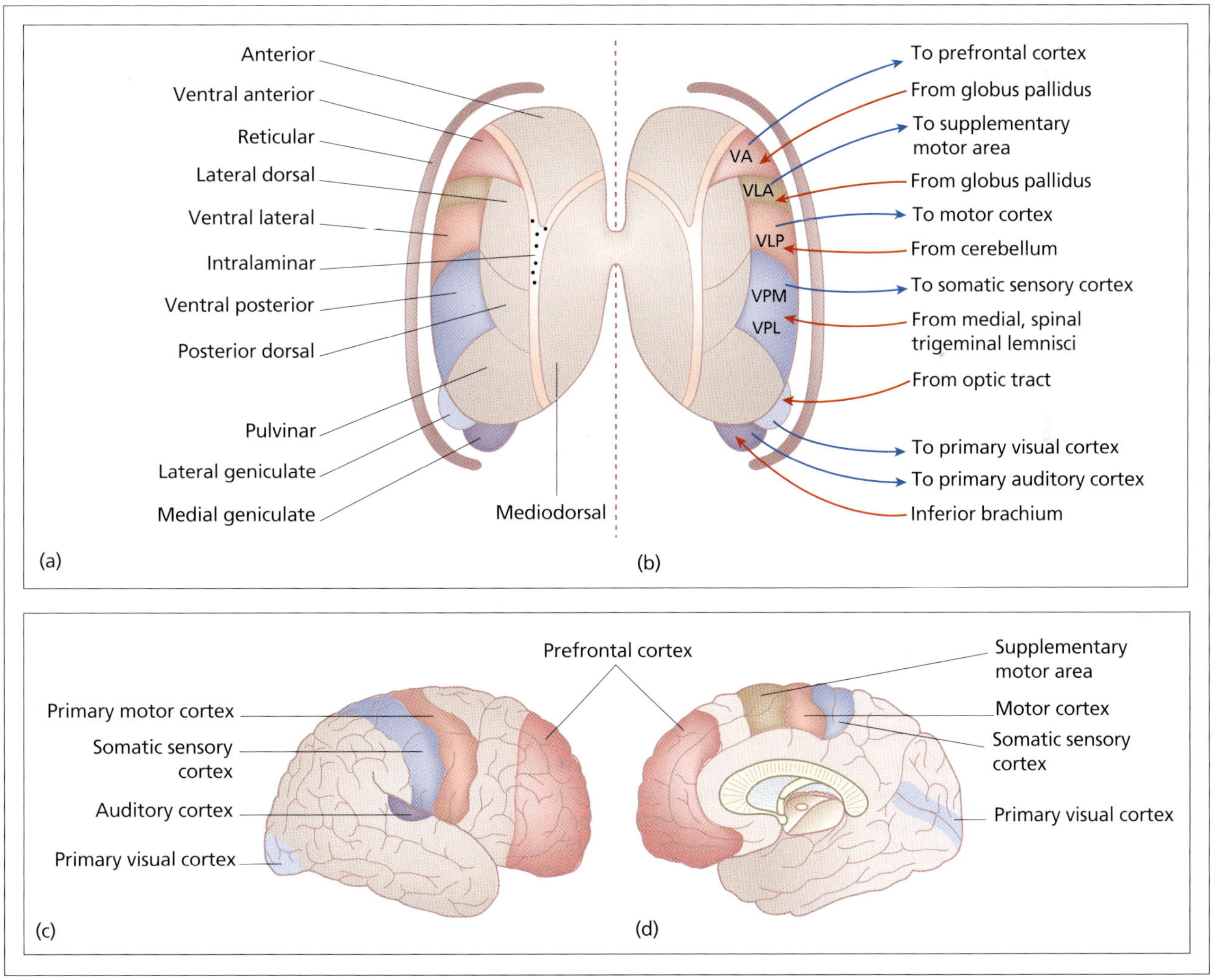

Figure 2.33 Thalamic nuclei and connections (from above). (a) nuclei; (b) connections of relay nuclei; (c) hemisphere – lateral view; (d) hemisphere – medial view. VLA, ventral lateral anterior; VLP, ventral lateral posterior; VPM, ventral posteromedial; VPL, ventral posterolateral. Source: FitzGerald 2010. © 2016 Elsevier. Reproduced with permission of Elsevier.

Table 2.7 Thalamic nuclei: sources and destinations of principal pathways.

Source	Thalamic nucleus	Destination
Mamillary body, hippocampus	Anterior	Cingulate gyrus
Globus pallidus	VA	Prefrontal cortex
Globus pallidus	VLA	Supplementary motor area
Cerebellum (dentate nucleus)	VLP	Motor cortex
Head somatic afferents	VPM	Somatic sensory cortex (S1)
Trunk + limb somatic afferents	VPL	Somatic sensory cortex (S1)
Inferior colliculus (auditory)	Medial geniculate body	Primary auditory cortex
Superior colliculus (vision)	Lateral geniculate body	Primary visual cortex
Parietal lobe	Lateral dorsal	Cingulate cortex
Superior colliculus + parietal lobe	Pulvinar + lateral dorsal	Visual association cortex
Reticular formation, basal ganglia	Intralaminar	Cortex, basal ganglia
Thalamus, cortex	Reticular nucleus	Thalamus

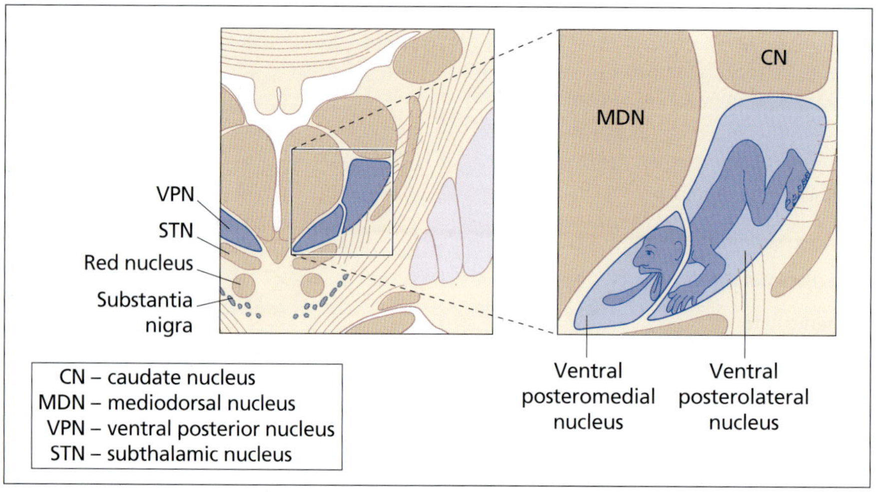

Figure 2.34 Thalamus (coronal section): ventral posteromedial and ventral posterolateral (VPM/VPL) nuclei – somatotopic projection. Source: FitzGerald 2010. © 2016 Elsevier. Reproduced with permission of Elsevier.

Specific (relay) thalamic nuclei

These nuclei of the ventral tier are connected to distinct motor and sensory areas of the cortex:

- Anterior and VA nucleus (Table 2.7).
- The anterior part of the VL receives fibres from the pallidum and relays them to the supplementary motor area.
- The posterior part of VL receives fibres from the opposite superior cerebellar peduncle (from the dentate nucleus) and relays to the motor cortex.
- Ventral posterior nucleus (VP). This receives all axons of the medial, spinal and trigeminal lemnisci and projects to the somatosensory cortex. The somatotopic arrangement is shown in Figure 2.34. The medial part (VPM) deals with the head; the lateral (VPL) with the limbs and trunk. Within each part of the VP there is segregation of sensory modalities – proprioception at the front, nociception at the back, with touch in the middle.
- The ventral intermediate nucleus (VIM), located between VL and VPL provides a direct route for somatosensory input to the motor cortex. VIM is of significant importance in the functional neurosurgical treatment of tremor (see Surgery for Parkinson's disease, Chapter 6).

Within the VP there is no evidence of gating (cf. the substantia gelatinosa) or modulation – the system is either off (no pain) or on (intense pain). This may explain the persistent and untreatable pain of the thalamic syndrome, when a stroke disconnects VP from the sensory cortex (see Central post-stroke pain, Chapter 23).

- The medial geniculate body is an auditory system nucleus.
- The lateral geniculate body is a nucleus of the visual system.

Association thalamic nuclei

These are connected to association areas of the cortex:

- The lateral dorsal nucleus is connected to the cingulate cortex (memory).
- The medial dorsal nucleus is connected to entire prefrontal cortex, olfactory and limbic systems (mood, executive function, cognition, memory, associations of smells).
- The pulvinar and lateral posterior nucleus project to the visual and parietal association cortices, having received fibres from the lateral geniculate. Also, a direct pathway, from optic tract via superior colliculus reaches the visual cortex, without relaying through the lateral geniculate – involved in attention within the visual field, but outside conscious perception.

Non-specific thalamic nuclei

These nuclei are non-specific in the sense that they are not directly involved with individual sensory modalities. The intralaminar nuclei are the rostral termination of the reticular formation. Aminergic afferents reach the region from the midbrain raphe nuclei and the locus coeruleus. Prolongation of such excitatory aminergic activity in thalamocortical fibres is one effect of tricyclic drugs, and a possible mode of their action in chronic pain. There is widespread onward connection from intralaminar nuclei to the cortex.

The shield-shaped reticular nucleus connects to all thalamic nuclei. Each thalamocortical fibre connects to a reticular nucleus neurone via a collateral. Reticular nucleus cells respond by a GABAergic inhibitory response to the corresponding thalamic nucleus – terminating a sensory stimulus (Figure 2.35). During sleep–wake cycles, thalamocortical neurones are constantly inhibited during sleep and constantly active (disinhibited) during wakefulness. This inhibition may explain the effect of sleep and sedation on pain.

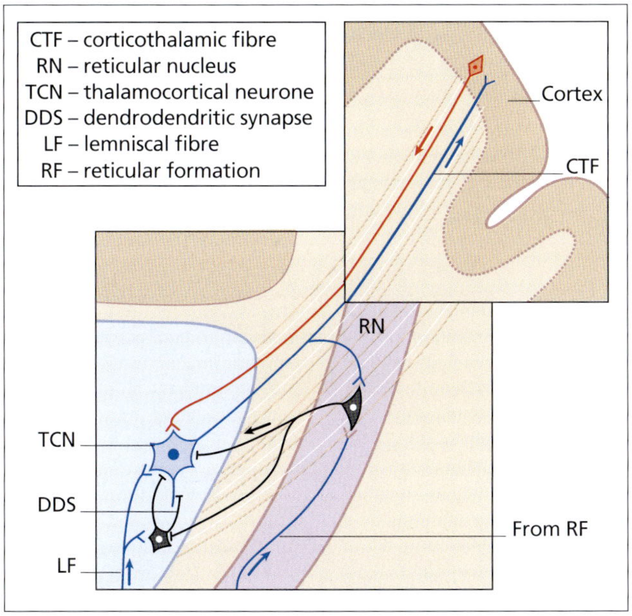

Figure 2.35 Reticular nucleus: connections between cortex and specific thalamic nuclei. Source: FitzGerald 2010. © 2016 Elsevier. Reproduced with permission of Elsevier.

Hypothalamus and pituitary gland

The multiple paired nuclei of each hypothalamus (about 4 g apiece in humans) lie each side of the 3rd ventricle. They are involved in two allied neuro-effector control systems:

1 Autonomic nervous system, and
2 Pituitary axis.

The hypothalamus is a central neural effector of basic survival, with roles in:

- Temperature homeostasis
- Regulation of food and water intake
- Defence, arousal and sleep–wake cycles, and
- Sexual activity.

The hypothalamus mediates control of all endocrine and all autonomic activity.

The essential nuclear anatomy and blood supply are outlined in Figure 2.36 and the three groups of nuclei are listed in Table 2.8. The median forebrain bundle (aminergic fibres) merges with and lies lateral to the lateral nucleus of the hypothalamus on each side.

Arterial and capillary supply

Delicate perforating branches of the anterior communicating artery supply the hypothalamic region. Hypophyseal branches of the internal carotid artery supply the pituitary itself:

- *Superior hypophyseal artery:* anterior pituitary.
- *Inferior hypophyseal artery:* posterior pituitary.

Each hypophyseal arterial system forms a second capillary portal system that surrounds the neuroendocrine cells. Hormones are liberated into venous blood, draining into the cavernous sinus. These fenestrated portal capillaries are outside the blood–brain barrier.

Neuroendocrine cells

These neurones, specific to the region, both conduct action potentials and also liberate into the bloodstream peptide and other hormones, the latter having been synthesised in the endoplasmic reticulum and stored in Golgi complexes. The peptides are attached to long-chain polypeptides – neurophysins. Cell bodies of neuroendocrine cells lie in the region of the pre-optic nuclei and tuber cinereum. The principal nuclei that also contribute to this system are:

- Supra-optic
- Paraventricular
- Ventromedial, and
- Arcuate nuclei.

Small neurone (parvocellular) axons in the tubero-infundibular tract reach the median eminence, where releasing (RH) and inhibiting hormones (IH) are liberated. Large neurone (magnocellular) axons form the hypothalamo-hypophysial tract that passes to the posterior pituitary.

Anterior pituitary axis

The anterior pituitary axis hormones are listed in Table 2.9. All RH/IHs, with the exception of prolactin IH, are peptides. Prolactin IH is dopamine. The complex control systems for these hormones, include:

- Traditional feedback loops
- Depolarisation by action potentials entering from the limbic system and reticular formation (e.g. arousal effects)

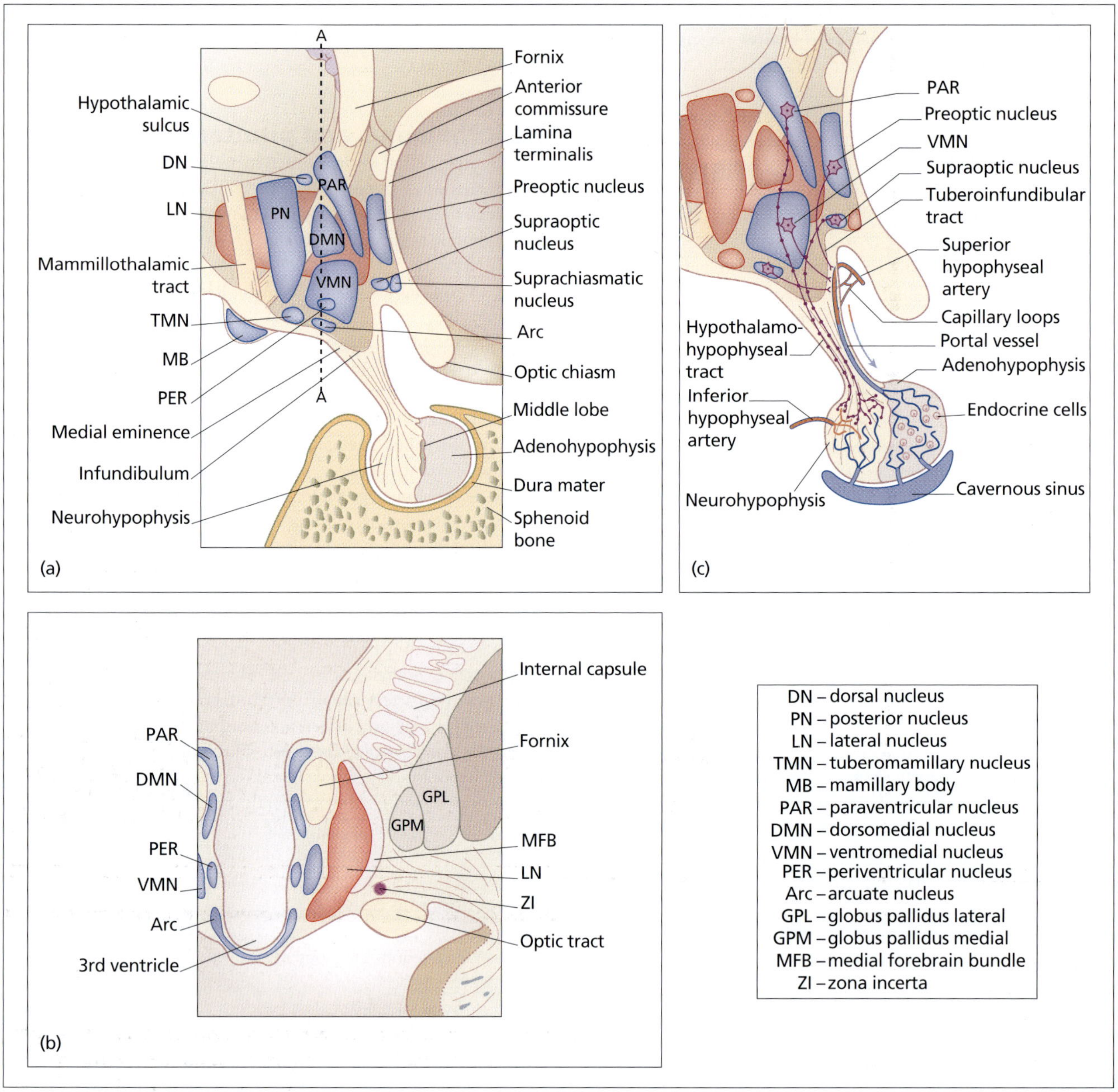

Figure 2.36 (a) Hypothalamic nuclei and pituitary, viewed from right. (b) Coronal section through A–A. (c) Blood supply to pituitary. Source: FitzGerald 2010. © 2016 Elsevier. Reproduced with permission of Elsevier.

Table 2.8 Hypothalamic nuclei.

Anterior	Middle	Posterior
Pre-optic	Paraventricular	Posterior
Supra-optic	Peri-venricular	Mammillary body
Suprachiasmatic	Dorsomedial	Tuberomammillary
	Lateral	Dorsal
	Ventromedial	
	Arcuate	

Table 2.9 Pituitary and hypothalamic releasing/inhibiting hormones (RH/IH).

Anterior lobe hormone	RH/IH
ACTH	Corticotrophin RH
FSH/LH	Gonadotrophic hormone RH
Growth hormone	Growth hormone RH and IH
Prolactin	Prolactin RH and IH
Thyrotropin	Thyrotropin RH

ACTH, adenocorticotrophic hormone; FSH, follicle-stimulating hormone; LH, luteinising hormone.

- Hyperpolarisation by local GABAergic neurones
- Inhibition by opiate-releasing neurones (numerous in the hypothalamus), and
- Activation directly of anterior pituitary endocrine cells by opiates and endorphins.

Posterior pituitary axis

Each hypothalamo-hypophyseal tract passes from large (magnocellular) neurones of the supra-optic nucleus and paraventricular nucleus to the posterior pituitary (neurohypophysis). There are also contributions from periventricular neurones (opiate and peptide neurotransmission) and brainstem (aminergic) neurones.

Vasopressin (antidiuretic hormone) and oxytocin are secreted by specific neurones in both supra-optic and paraventricular nuclei; these hormones are housed in axonal secretory granules (Herring bodies) before being released into the capillary system within the posterior pituitary itself.

Circumventricular organs

This term refers to six groups of specialised neurones and glial cells adjacent to the ventricular system that have an intimate relation to fenestrated capillaries:

1 Neurohypophysis
2 Median eminence
3 Vascular organ of the lamina terminalis (VOLT)
4 Subfornical organ
5 Area postrema
6 Pineal gland.

Functions are outlined in Table 2.10.

Sympathetic and parasympathetic hypothalamic activity

Posterior hypothalamic stimulation produces noradrenergic sympathetic effects:

- Heart rate ↑
- Blood pressure ↑
- Pupil dilatation
- Gut stasis.

Table 2.10 Circumventricular organs.

Organ	Function	Comment
Neurohypophysis	ADH secretion	See text
Median eminence	Anterior pituitary hormone release and inhibition	
VOLT + SFO	Facilitate ADH secretion	Axons to supra-optic and paraventricular nuclei (feedback loop: low blood volume → kidney → renin → angiotensin II → VOLT/SFO → ADH)
Area postrema	Chemoreceptor (emetic) centre	Reflex vomiting (situated at obex of 4th ventricle)
Pineal gland (body)	Melatonin	Sleep–wake cycles

ADH, antidiuretic hormone; SFO, subfornical organ; VOLT, vascular organ of the lamina terminalis.

Anterior hypothalamic stimulation produces muscarinic parasympathetic effects:

- Heart rate ↓
- Blood pressure ↓
- Pupil constriction
- Peristalsis.

The axonal pathway projects from anterior and posterior hypothalamus to autonomic nuclei in the brainstem and cord – via the dorsal longitudinal fasciculus in the midbrain and pons.

Temperature regulation

Thermosensitive neurones in the hypothalamus respond to core temperature changes. Spinoreticular tracts also deliver information to these hypothalamic neurones from skin thermal receptors. The autonomic effector sympathetic system alters skin blood flow and sweating via the posterior nucleus of the hypothalamus – axons pass direct to the lateral horn of the cord. Increase in core temperature is achieved by:

- Skin vasoconstriction
- Abolition of sweating
- Shivering/muscular activity, and
- Behavioural responses (e.g. crouching, huddling, extra clothing).

Hypothalamic temperature-sensitive neurones also respond to exogenous pyrogen, setting the central thermostat to a higher level, and are also involved in the production of central pyrexia (see Initial sssessment and management of coma, Chapter 20).

Water intake and thirst

The zona incerta, a strip of cells beside each lateral nucleus of the hypothalamus, controls thirst. Lesions of this region lead to neglect of drinking, and in animals stimulation leads to thirst and excessive water intake. Many other mechanisms also contribute to osmotic homeostasis (e.g. serum sodium and glucose levels and renal function).

Appetite and satiety

Balance in activity between the lateral and ventromedial hypothalamic nuclei constitutes, in theory at least, a satiety system in humans. In experimental models:

- Lateral hypothalamic (feeding centre) stimulation leads to overeating
- Lateral hypothalamic destruction leads to lack of interest in food
- Ventromedial hypothalamic (satiety centre) stimulation inhibits eating
- Ventromedial hypothalamic destruction (bilateral) leads to gross obesity.

Serotoninergic activity down-regulates the appetite set point, and vice versa, selective serotonin re-uptake inhibitors (SSRIs) and other antidepressants tend to increase appetite.

Mood, sexual arousal, wakefulness and memory

Mood Aggression or docility are features of experimental lateral/ventromedial hypothalamic imbalance. Obese animals with ventromedial lesions become aggressively enraged. Underweight, ventromedially stimulated animals are docile. Hunger stimulates arousal. In human behaviour this may explain why some people become angry when they are not fed at the time they expect to be.

Sexual arousal Specific neurones (INAH3 cells) in each pre-optic nucleus are more numerous in males than in females. This is an area rich in androgen receptors, activated by testosterone and which when experimentally stimulated induces male sexual activity.

In females, neurones rich in oestrogen receptors are found in the ventromedial nucleus: experimental stimulation induces sexual arousal.

Wakefulness The suprachiasmatic nucleus is involved in setting sleep–wake cycles via putative pineal gland connections.

Arousal is mediated via richly histaminergic neurones in the posterior hypothalamus (the tuberomammillary nucleus). These project widely (medial forebrain bundle, cortex, brainstem, cord). Hypersomnolence in humans is seen when the posterior hypothalamus is damaged bilaterally.

Memory The mammillary bodies are stations on Papez's circuit (fornix → mammillary bodies → mammillothalamic tract → anterior nucleus of thalamus). Mammillary body destruction produces a dramatic amnestic syndrome.

Generally, for an area so intimately involved in activities essential for life, lesions of the hypothalamus are surprisingly unusual in practice. The area appears resilient. One reason is simple: bilateral hypothalamic destruction is necessary to produce clinical effects.

Cranial nerves

Olfactory nerve and its cortical connections

This afferent system, far more highly developed in many animals than in humans, comprises:

- Olfactory neuronal epithelium
- Olfactory nerves
- Olfactory bulb and tract, and
- Olfactory cortical areas and connections.

Olfactory epithelium

This epithelial layer covers about one-fifth of the upper nasal cavity. Basal stem cells, unique among neurones in mammals, transform in a regular 4–8 week cycle into fresh highly specialised bipolar neurones. These neurones lie between sustentacular (supporting) cells (Figure 2.37). Their dendrites are ciliated processes containing olfactory receptors that line the receptive area. Afferent axons traverse the cribriform plate, guided by olfactory ensheathing cells, a specialised form of glia.

There are two chemosensory systems within the nasal mucosa, the olfactory system and trigeminal afferents that respond to irritants (e.g. ammonia) and to the sensation of coolness, either to cold itself or to compounds such as menthol. The trigeminal system is not mentioned further here.

Olfactory bulb and tract

Each bulb consists of some 50 000 mitral cells that make synaptic contact with epithelial bipolar neurones in several thousand glomeruli, surrounded by glia. Active glomeruli, stimulated by receptive bipolar cells, inhibit neighbouring glomeruli through a GABAergic pathway via periglomerular cells. Mitral cells are also under the influence of deeper granule cells, with which they make dendrodendritic contact. Stimulated granule cells suppress other mitral cells, selectively, again via GABAergic synapses.

Cortical connections

Each afferent pathway from the nasal cavity remains entirely ipsilateral (Figure 2.38). The olfactory tract divides in the anterior perforated substance into medial and lateral striae. Lateral olfactory stria afferents pass to each piriform lobe of the anterior temporal cortex that includes part of the amygdala, uncus and parahippocampal gyrus, and thence to the posterior orbitofrontal cortex. Each medial olfactory stria contains efferent axons from each anterior olfactory nucleus, bipolar neurones arising within each olfactory tract. Some of these efferent axons travel to the septal area via the diagonal band of Broca. Others cross the midline in the anterior commissure, to stimulate granule cells and thus inhibit mitral cell activity therein – providing a directional cue to the source of olfactory stimulation.

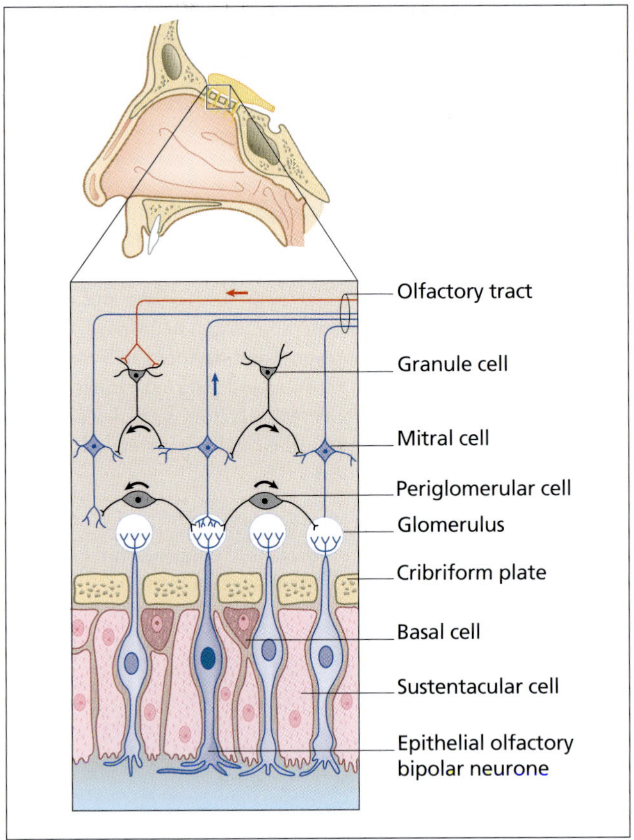

Figure 2.37 Cells of the olfactory system. Source: FitzGerald 2010. © 2016 Elsevier. Reproduced with permission of Elsevier.

The perception and intimate complexity of different aromas is achieved by groups of cortical neurones that respond to particular sequences of action potentials. The widespread central connections of the olfactory cortex make possible association of particular smells with individual memories, both visual and topographical, recent or distant. Anosmia is discussed in Chapter 13 (see Olfactory nerve).

Neurotransmission in the olfactory system

The assessment of anosmia occupies but little space in an outpatient clinic; testing of discrimination of the sense of smell is frequently omitted or simply accepted as normal. However, advances in the neurobiology of olfaction have expanded understanding and have explained how the cortex achieves recognition of such complex afferent data.

The cilia of the bipolar neurones lining the olfactory epithelium lie at the start of a complex sequence:

- Odorant molecules bind to odorant receptor proteins
- G-protein (G_{olf}) stimulation follows
- Cilial adenyl cyclase is activated
- ATP is liberated and cyclic AMP (cAMP) generated
- Cation channels open (Na^+ and Ca^{2+}channels)
- → Opening of Ca^{2+}-activated Cl^- channels, and thus

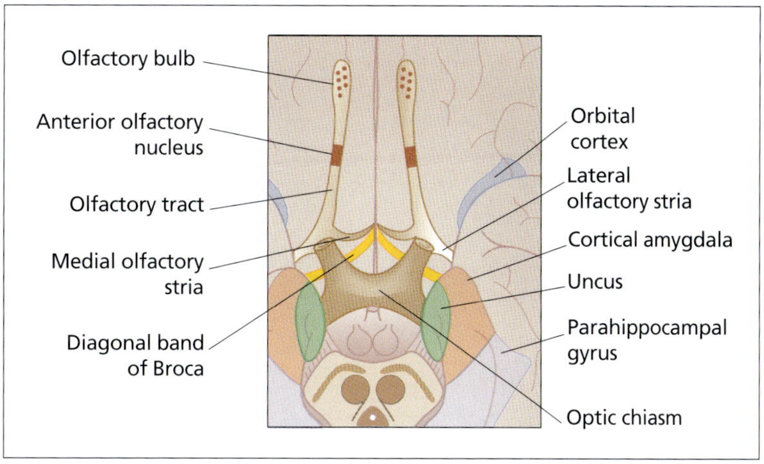

Figure 2.38 Olfactory tract region, from below. Source: FitzGerald 2010. © 2016 Elsevier. Reproduced with permission of Elsevier.

- → Membrane depolarisation and an excitatory action potential and propagation along the axon of a bipolar cell.

There are around 1000 odorant receptor genes. These are expressed on individual bipolar cells (i.e. there are around 1000 receptor cell subtypes, a large number, but vastly insufficient to account for the appreciation, in humans of about 100 000 different smells, and for the exceptional sense of smell in some mammals).

In olfactory neurones, the single second messenger is cAMP (i.e. the channels are cAMP-gated). Each receptor subtype is broadly tuned – each responds to various similar odorants – and, correspondingly, each odorant can stimulate more than one receptor subtype. Thus, each bipolar cell yields potentially ambiguous information. A further selection process takes place at the level of the glomeruli.

Each olfactory bulb contains some 2000 spherical glomeruli 50–200 μm in diameter. The endings of around 25 000 primary olfactory bipolar receptor axons end in the glomeruli, forming synapses with about 100 second order olfactory neurones. The association between individual receptor subtypes and a particular glomerulus is precise. Receptor neurones expressing one gene, although scattered throughout the epithelium, converge on several glomeruli in each olfactory bulb.

Within each glomerulus there is excitation and inhibition (e.g. see Olfactory epithelium) and thence it is the temporal coding of afferent impulses that determines the particular perceived smell by cortical receptive fields. Olfactory cortical neurones recognise a particular 'tune' of impulses as an individual smell.

The projection of each afferent olfactory pathway is direct to phylogenetically ancient regions of the cortex, in contrast to most other sensory tracts that passes first to the thalamus before reaching the cortex. From the olfactory cortex, there are projections to areas throughout the brain.

Finally, not all olfactory perception is at a conscious level. Pheromonal perception in humans undoubtedly exists – probably accounting for part of sexual attraction. For example, pheromones are of critical importance in lepidoptera, enabling attraction to take place over several kilometres in moths between males and females. There is evidence to support the existence of a vomero-nasal receptor organ in humans in the lateral nasal mucosa. Central pathways in humans remain unknown and the neurochemistry of pheromonal activating systems conjectural.

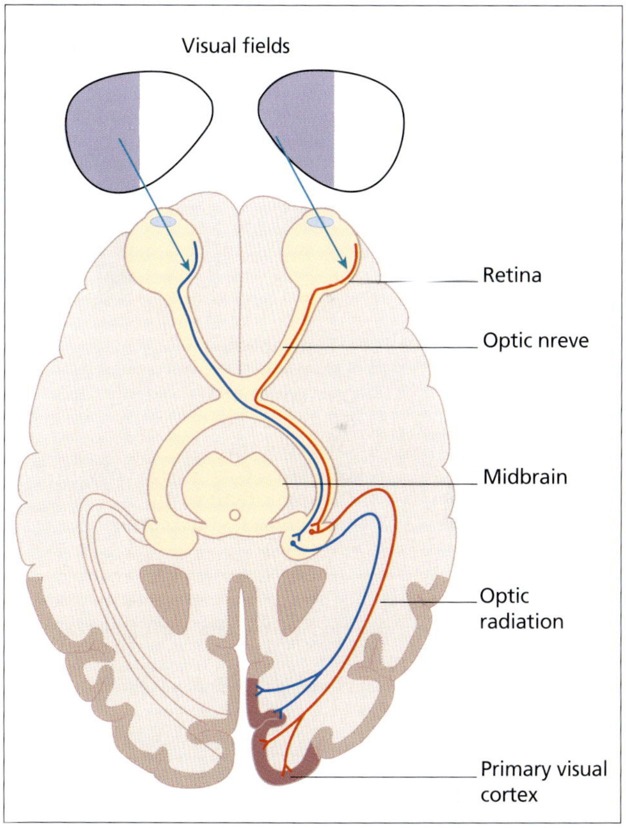

Figure 2.39 Essential anatomy of visual pathway. Source: FitzGerald 2010. © 2016 Elsevier. Reproduced with permission of Elsevier.

Optic nerve and visual system

The visual pathway is summarised in Figures 2.39 and 2.40. Typical field defects are summarised in Figure 2.41 and are discussed further with clinical aspects in Chapter 14 (see Visual field defects).

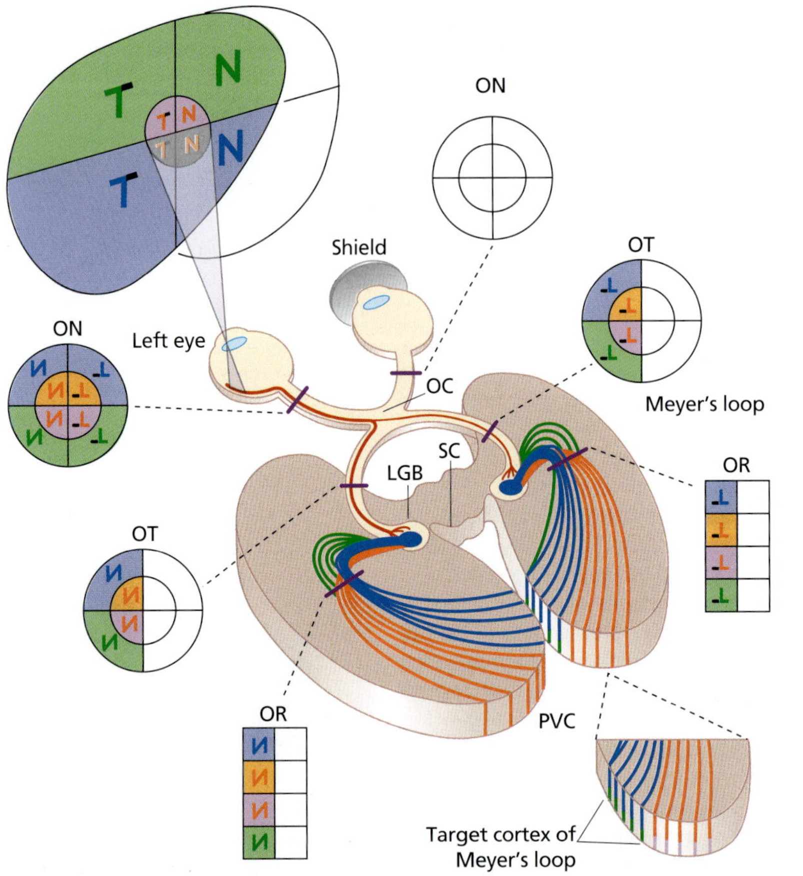

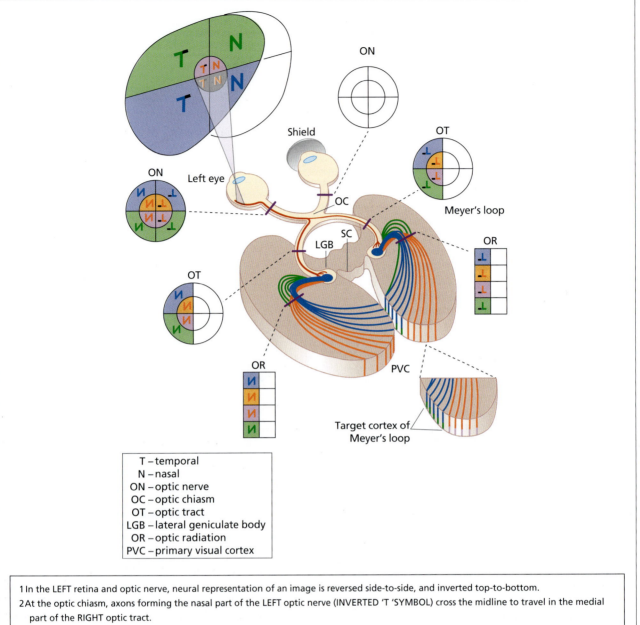

T – temporal
N – nasal
ON – optic nerve
OC – optic chiasm
OT – optic tract
LGB – lateral geniculate body
OR – optic radiation
PVC – primary visual cortex

1 In the LEFT retina and optic nerve, neural representation of an image is reversed side-to-side, and inverted top-to-bottom.
2 At the optic chiasm, axons forming the nasal part of the LEFT optic nerve (INVERTED 'T 'SYMBOL) cross the midline to travel in the medial part of the RIGHT optic tract.
3 At the optic chiasm, axons forming the temporal part of the LEFT optic nerve (INVERTED 'N 'SYMBOL) continue in the lateral part of the LEFT optic tract.
4 Each optic tract synapses in the corresponding lateral geniculate body. (But see also medial and lateral *roots* of the optic tracts, in text.)
5 Each optic radiation is a fan like structure, with foveal (second order) axons passing to the posterior regions of the primary visual cortex.
6 The blank intervals within each optic radiation are filled with second order axons from the shielded RIGHT eye.
7 Meyer's loops, from the upper visual field of EACH eye, run forward to loop into each temporal lobe. These Meyer's loop axons reach their targets in the lower medial part of each primary visual cortex.

Figure 2.40 Detail of visual pathway; RIGHT eye shielded. Source: FitzGerald 2010. © 2016 Elsevier. Reproduced with permission of Elsevier.

The following sections focus on individual regions and functional aspects of this complex and highly developed special sense.

Retinal structure

The eight retinal cell and fibre layers are shown in Figure 2.42:

- Photoreceptors (2) – rods and cones – are applied to the pigment epithelium (1), adjacent to the choroid.
- Ganglion cells (7) are the source of action potentials conducted by axons that form the retinal nerve fibre layer (8) and pass into the optic nerve.
- Two sets of retinal neurones – horizontal cells and amacrine cells – are arranged transversely.

The essential circuitary is shown in Figure 2.43.

Photoreceptors and bipolar cells Cone photoreceptors are sensitive to bright light, colour and shape. They are clustered in and around

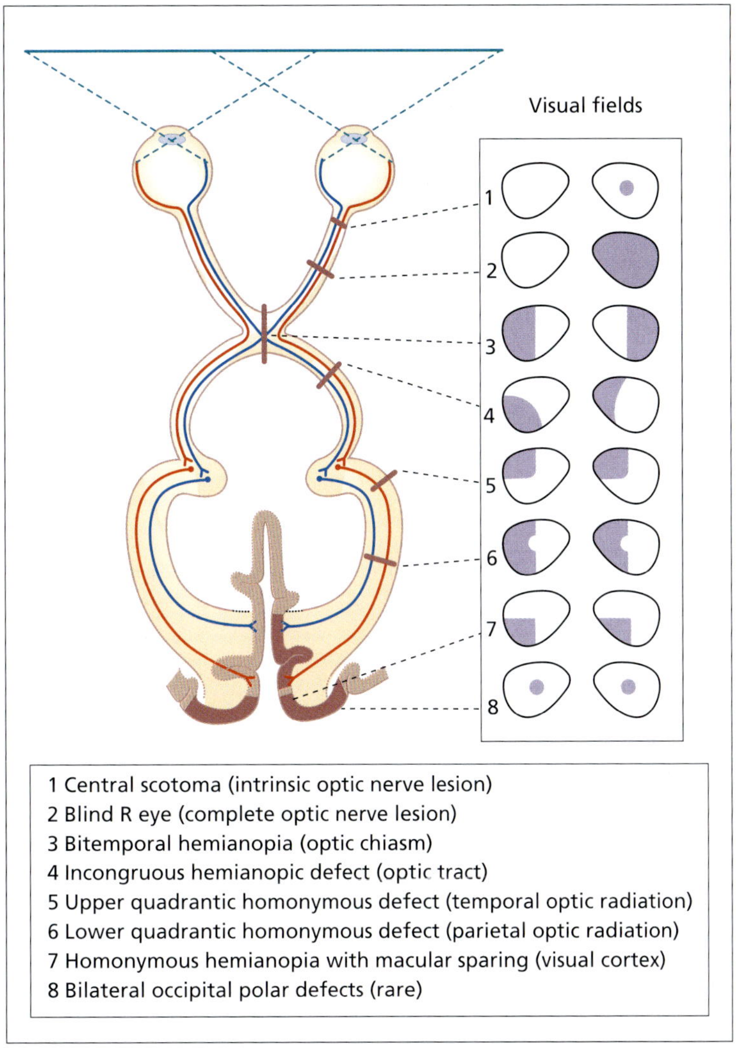

Figure 2.41 Visual field defects: examples of typical lesions.

the fovea. Photoreceptor end-feet synapse with bipolar cells and horizontal cells processes. Cone bipolar cells are either:

- ON bipolars, that is, switched ON (depolarised) by light, or inhibited by neurotransmitters released when light levels fall. They synapse and converge on ON cone ganglion cells.
- OFF bipolars have an opposite response. They synapse and converge on OFF ganglion cells.

Horizontal cells extend dendrites between photoreceptors and bipolar cells with which they make inhibitory contacts. Bipolar cells (and hence retinal ganglion cells) outside the immediate zone of excitation are inhibited. This restricts retinal activity to the area under direct photic stimulation, a feature known as centre–surround antagonism.

Rod photoreceptors are active in conditions of low illumination and are insensitive to colour: dimly lit objects are perceived in shades of grey. Like cones, rods display centre–surround antagonism, between white and black and synapse with ON and OFF bipolar cells.

Rod bipolar cells activate ON and OFF rod ganglion cells via amacrine cells. Amacrine cells have 6–10 dendrites that emerge from one aspect of each cell body. Over one dozen types of amacrine cell are recognised, with different transmitters (e.g. ACh, dopamine, serotonin). Their action is to turn ON or OFF groups of ganglion cells. Functions include enhancement of contrast and detection of subtle movement by retinal rods.

Ganglion cells, of either ON or OFF variety, are activated by bipolar neurones. An ON ganglion cell is activated by a point light source and inhibited via horizontal cells and appropriate bipolars by a surrounding ring of light, known as annular inhibition. An OFF ganglion cell reacts in reverse, being inhibited by a point source and excited by an annulus of light.

Colour recognition within the retina – red, green and blue Colour opponency is the response that characterises specific ganglion cells. Ganglion cells are either:

- ON-line for green + OFF-line for red
- ON-line for red + OFF-line for green
- ON-line for blue + OFF-line for yellow.

Colour recognition is achieved by individual cones sensitive to specific wavelengths of electromagnetic energy.

Heterogeneity of rods, cones and ganglion cells The majority of both rod and cone ganglion cells are parvocellular (small, P cells) – small receptive fields receptive to shape and colour. A minority are magnocellular ganglion cells (large, M cells) – large fields, particularly receptive to moving objects.

The specialised region of cones is the fovea and its central 100 μm, the foveola – the area that has the highest sensitivity for object discrimination and colour appreciation (Figure 2.44). Several anatomical features of the foveola enhance sensivity:

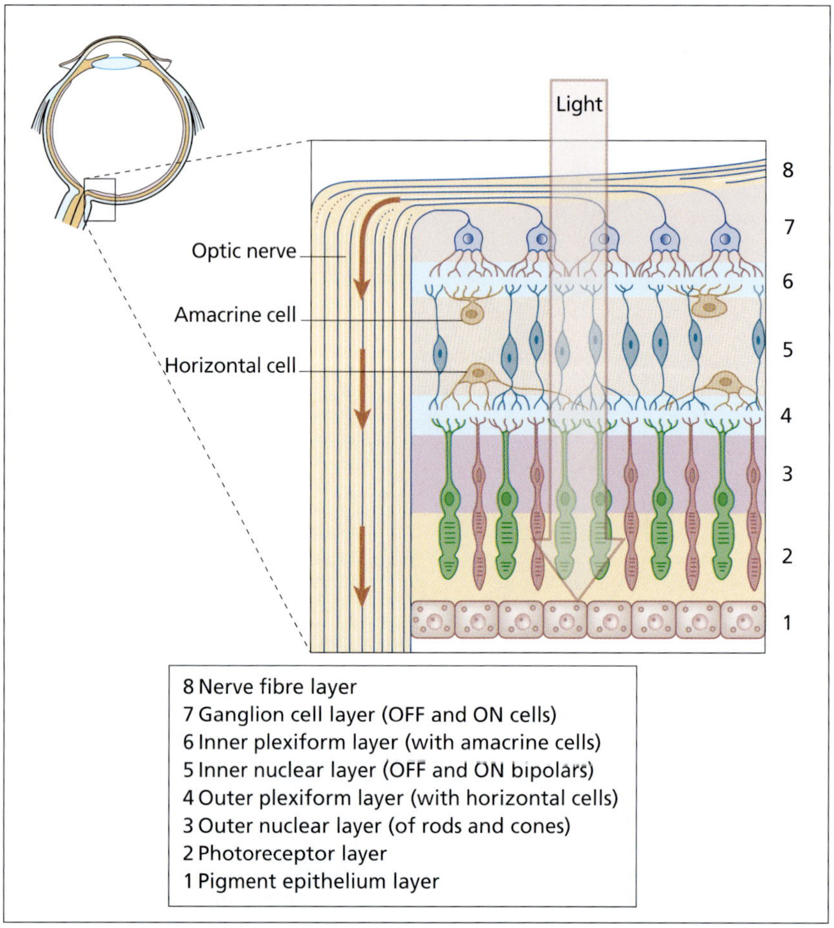

Figure 2.42 The eight retinal layers. Source: FitzGerald 2010. © 2016 Elsevier. Reproduced with permission of Elsevier.

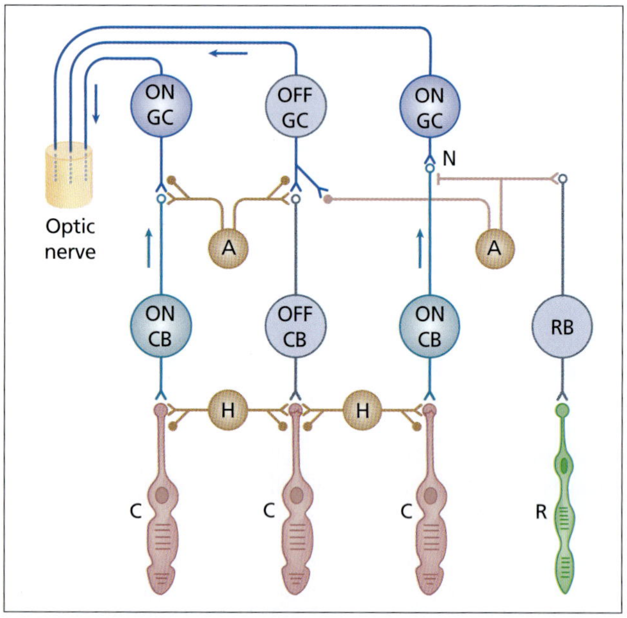

Figure 2.43 Circuit diagram of retina. A, amacrine cell; C, cone; CB, cone bipolar; GC, ganglion cell; H, horizontal cell; N, nexus (gap junction); R, rod; RB, rod bipolar. Source: FitzGerald 2010. © 2016 Elsevier. Reproduced with permission of Elsevier.

- Midget cones in the foveola have one-to-one synaptic contacts with midget bipolar cells and ganglion cells. Outside the foveola sensitivity is less acute.
- Superficial layers of the retina have long neurites; cell bodies surround the fovea rather than covering the cones. This allows light to strike midget cones directly.

Optic nerve, chiasm and optic tract

Each optic nerve (a CNS structure rather than a peripheral nerve) contains between 800 000 and 1.5 million ganglion cell axons, with a supporting infrastructure – astrocytes, oligodendrocytes, blood supply and meningeal sheath. The chiasmal decussation, optic tract and optic radiation are illustrated in Figure 2.40.

Each optic tract (comprised of uncrossed temporal-half and crossed nasal-half retinal axons) divides into a medial and a lateral root. The medial root of each optic tract enters the midbrain. It carries:

- Fibres serving the pupillary light reflex – passing to the pretectal nucleus
- Fibres from retinal M cells – scanning movements – to the superior colliculus
- Fibres to the reticular formation (parvocellular) – arousal function, and
- Fibres relaying from superior colliculus, to pulvinar and visual association cortex – the extrageniculate visual pathway.

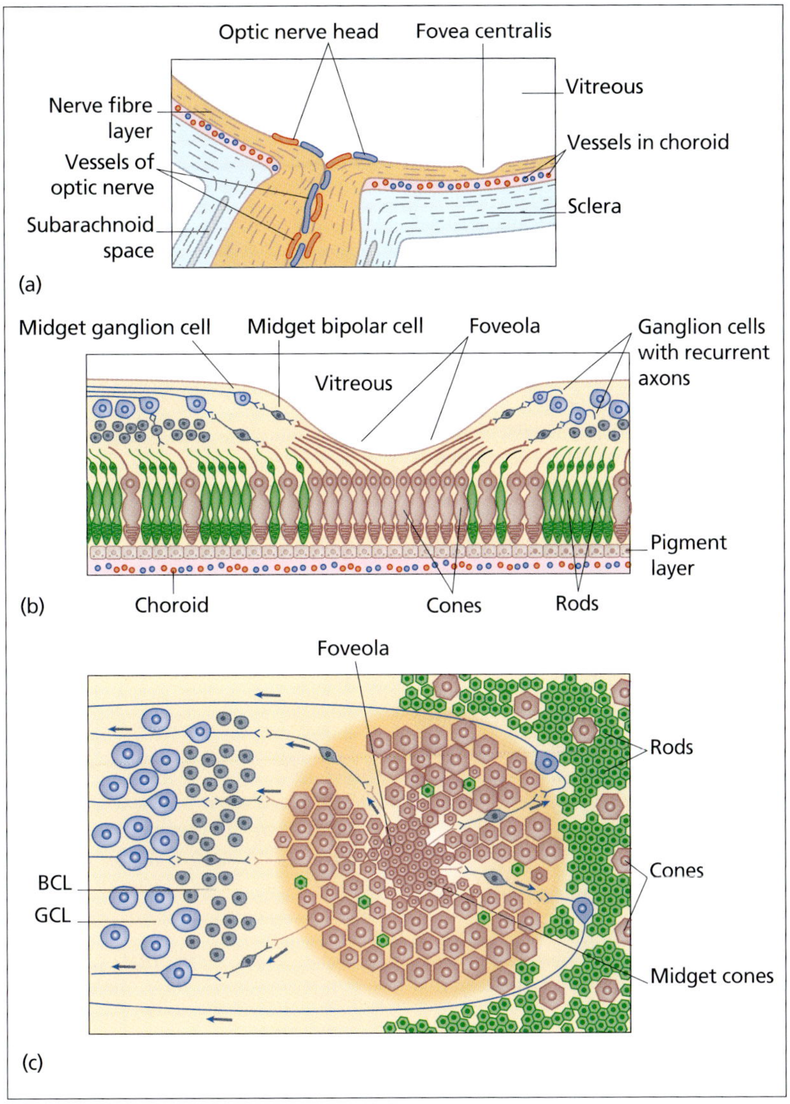

Figure 2.44 (a) Fovea and optic nerve, in section. (b) and (c) Fovea and foveola: section and surface diagram. BCL, bipolar cell layer; GCL, ganglion cell layer. Source: FitzGerald 2010. © 2016 Elsevier. Reproduced with permission of Elsevier.

The axons of lateral root of the optic tract synapse in the lateral geniculate body (LGB) of the thalamus. The LGB is six-layered:

- Three cellular laminae receive crossed fibres and three uncrossed
- The two deepest laminae (magnocellular) receive axons from retinal M ganglion cells (movement detection)
- The four outer laminae are parvocellular, receive axons from P ganglion cells (detail and colour).

Optic radiation

The optic radiation (*syn.* geniculocalcarine tract), its ordered somatotopic arrangements and cortical targets are also shown in Figure 2.40. The radiation is the most prominent white matter bundle in the posterior part of the brain. Important features:

- The radiation enters the posterior (retrolentiform) part of the internal capsule, runs beneath the temporal cortex and alongside the posterior horn of the lateral ventricle.
- Meyer's loop – forward-sweeping fibres in the anterior temporal lobe. These are from the upper part of the visual fields and run to the lower half of the occipital cortex.

Occipital cortex

The optic radiation is seen macroscopically as a pale stripe (stria) of myelinated fibres within the primary visual or striate cortex (Brodmann area 17) before synapsing with spiny stellate cells of cortical layer IV. Francesco Gennari (1752–1797) was a medical student in Padua when he described the occipital striae that bear his name.

The spiny stellate ganglion cells are arranged in alternating ocular dominance columns (alternating inputs between left and right eyes). Thus, impulses from identical points on each retina arrive in the striate cortex in side-by-side columns. Further differentiation is achieved by a hierarchy of cell groups:

- Spiny stellate cells produce simple responses – to fine slits of light in a particular orientation.
- Some pyramidal cells produce complex responses – to broad slits (bars), orientated at a particular angle and either stationary or moving broadside in one direction across the visual field.
- Other pyramidal cells are hypercomplex, responding to L-configurations.

The mechanism of this hierarchy is explained by convergence:

- Several simple cell axons converge on to complex cells, and
- Complex cell axons converge on to hypercomplex cells.

The primary visual cortex can be thought of as a complex pixellated screen, detecting not only position, but shape and movement. Area 17 (V1) does not interpret what we see. For example, area 17 does not itself recognise a face or describe an object. Recognition (i.e. perception) is achieved by connections with the visual association cortex, with the temporal lobes and with memory. The value of vision is also enhanced by eye movement, and by moving the head, limbs and/or trunk in relation to visual stimuli. The cortical eye fields are intimately involved in these processes.

Visual association cortex and V1–V5 terminology

Brodmann areas 18 and 19, also known as peristriate or extrastriate (*syn.* visual association) cortex contain cortical cell columns concerned with feature extraction. This means that certain cell groups respond to geometry (i.e. shape), some to perception of height/depth (stereopsis) and others to colours with ability to differentiate between many hues. The regions contain cell groups that recognise these particular attributes of objects. Afferents arrive primarily from area 17. There are also direct thalamic projections from the pulvinar.

The V1–V5 nomenclature, based more on functional imaging than the descriptive anatomy of the Brodmann system, is now widely used (Table 2.11). The lateral and medial parts of area 19 (V4, V5) contain specialised connections known as 'where' and 'what' visual pathways:

- 'What' is the ventrally placed, medial stream of object recognition (V4)
- 'Where' is the lateral, dorsally situated stream concerned with location (V5), with projections to the posterior parietal lobe.

'What' Three principal types of visual recognition take place in this region (Figure 2.45):

1 Recognition of forms, shapes and categories of objects (generic or canonical identification) takes place in the lateral zone.
2 Human face recognition (generic identification – 'this is a face') takes place in the mid zone.
3 Colour recognition takes place medially.

More sophisticated recognition of individual objects and faces involves area 20 (inferotemporal cortex) and area 38 (temporal pole cortex). Objects and faces that are threatening generate activity via areas 20 and 38 in the amygdala and inferofrontal cortex.

Table 2.11 V1–V5 and Brodmann areas: primary visual and visual association cortex.

V Region	Brodmann area
V1	Brodmann area 17
V2	Brodmann area 18
V3	Brodmann area 19
V4	Identification modules in fusiform gyrus in area 19 (anteromedial)
V5	Movement dedection modules in area 19 (anterolateral)

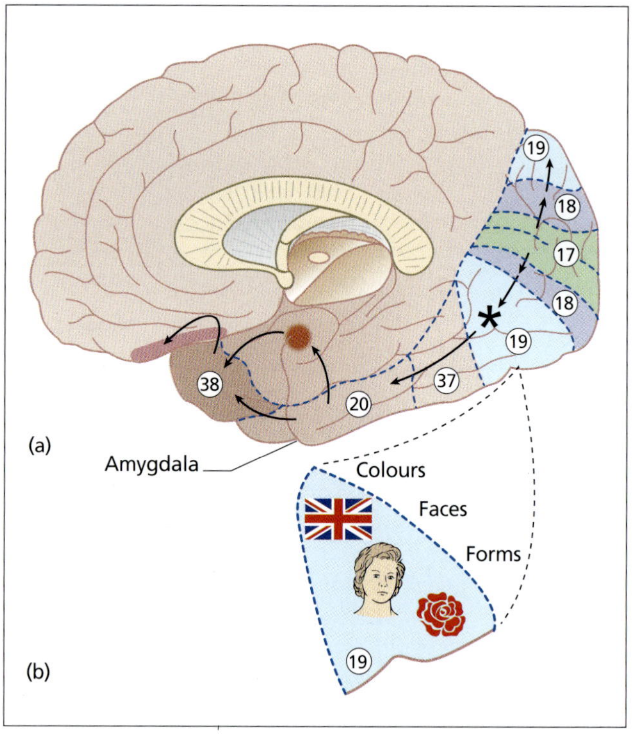

Figure 2.45 'What' visual pathway – right hemisphere, medial surface. (a) Asterisk: visual identification area (fusiform gyrus) in left visual field. (b) Detail of area 19 (ventral portion) – colours, faces and forms. Source: FitzGerald 2010. © 2016 Elsevier. Reproduced with permission of Elsevier.

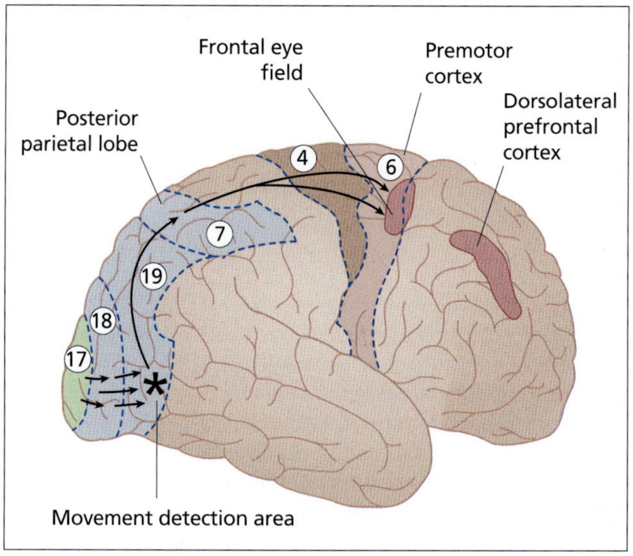

Figure 2.46 'Where' visual pathway – right hemisphere, lateral surface. Asterisk: movement detection area in 19. Right frontal cortical eye field activates conjugate saccades towards left field. Source: FitzGerald 2010. © 2016 Elsevier. Reproduced with permission of Elsevier.

'Where' The lateral part of area 19 is particularly responsive to movement in the contralateral hemifield (Figure 2.46). The main projection is to area 7 (posterior parietal cortex), long known as the area affected in disorders of spatial recognition such as astereognosis (see Sensory abnormalities: patterns at different levels, Chapter 4). Area 7 is involved in:

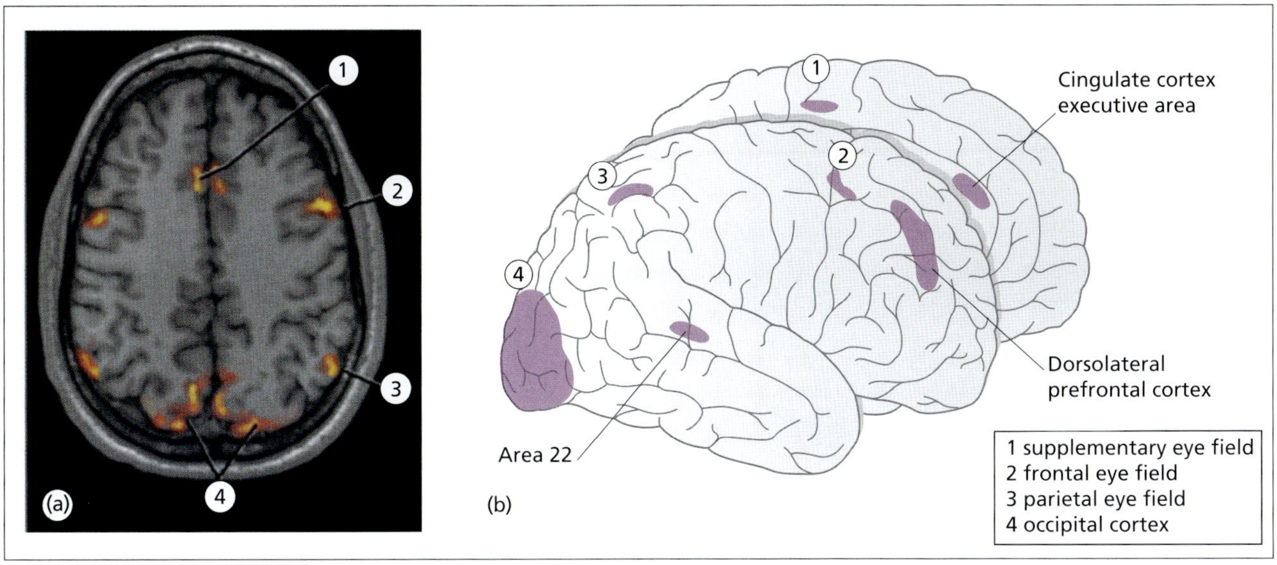

Figure 2.47 Functional MRI (a) and diagram (b) showing cortical eye fields. Source: FitzGerald 2010. © 2016 Elsevier. Reproduced with permission of Elsevier.

Table 2.12 Seven cortical areas involved in saccades: afferents, efferents, functions.

Eye field	Afferents	Efferents	Functions/comments
DLPFC	Visual association cortex	SC, ipsilateral FEF, SEF, CCx	Voluntary saccades, approach and withdraw decisions
CCx	DLPFC, FEF, SEF	SC, ipsilateral FEF	Emotional significance of object; paying attention
SEF	DLPFC, PEF, Area 22	SC, ipsilateral FEF	Motor planning, multiple saccades
FEF	DLPFC, opposite FEF, PEF	SC, opposite PPRF, ipsilateral CCx	Voluntary saccades
Area 22	Auditory association area, PEF	Ipsilateral SC, neck movement	Saccades to sound source
PEF	'Where' pathway, pulvinar, DLPFC	Ipsilateral FEF, SC	Reflex (responsive) saccades
OC	Visual pathway	All cortical eye fields and SC	Interpretion and visual pursuit

CCx, cingulate cortex; DLPFC, dorsolateral prefrontal cortex; FEF, frontal eye field; OC, occipital cortex; PEF, parietal eye field; PPRF, paramedian pontine reticular formation; SC, superior colliculus; SEF, supplementary eye field.

- Movement perception
- Stereopsis (three-dimensional vision)
- Spatial sense (relative position of objects to each other).

Area 7 also receives fibres from the pulvinar known as blindsight fibres. Fibres project to the ipsilateral frontal eye field and premotor cortex. Functional imaging shows increased cortical activity in area 7 in response to a moving object in the contralateral hemifield (covert attention). During saccadic gaze and/or limb movement towards the object, both area 7 and area 5 are activated (overt attention).

Cortical eye fields

Conjugate eye movement is controlled by discrete regions within the grey matter. These are shown in Figure 2.47, Table 2.12. The complexity is evident. fMRI has been of value here, confirming clinical data, and variability between individuals.

Three different mechanisms are involved in driving conjugate (i.e. yoked) gaze (jugum = Latin: the yoke of a pair of oxen):

- *Scanning:* saccades (i.e. rapid movement from one target to another)
- *Tracking:* smooth pursuit of a target across the visual field
- *Compensation:* maintenance of gaze during head movement via vestibulo-ocular fixation reflex.

Voluntary saccades are initiated in the frontal eye fields. Smooth pursuit movements originate in the occipital and parietal cortices (Table 2.12). Velocity detectors in the upper pons receive information via the medial root of the optic tract. Fixation is achieved by visual pursuit modulated by input from the vestibular system (head and neck movement) and smooth ocular movements by the cerebellar flocculus.

Automatic scanning movements are generated by retinal action potentials in the medial portion of the optic tract, via the pulvinar and area 7. These are also influenced by the cerebellar vermis and

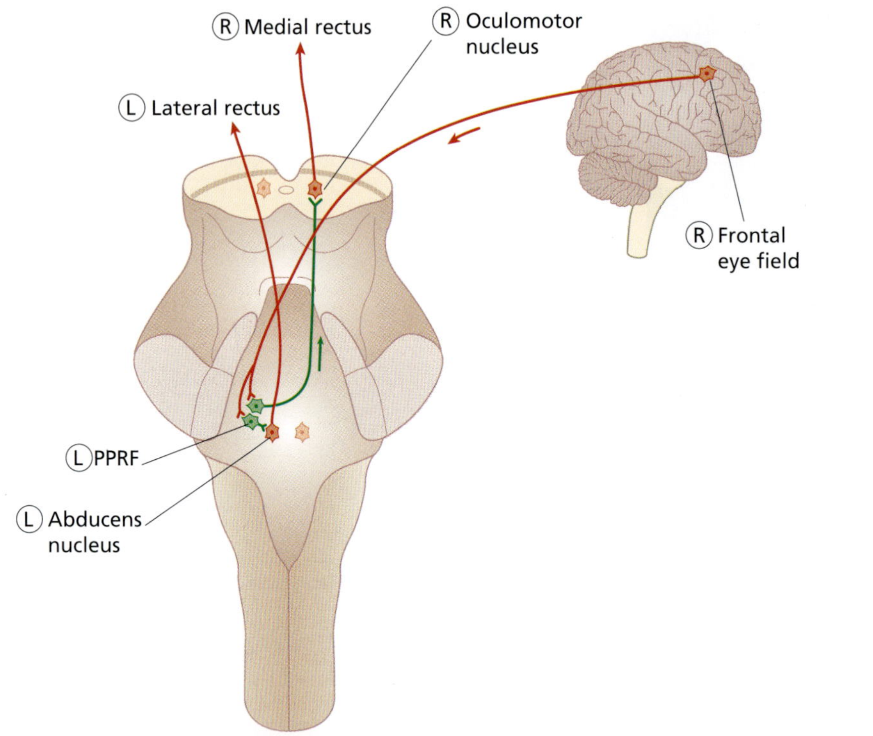

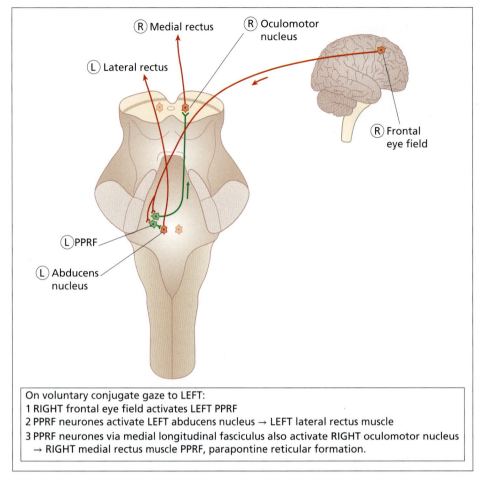

On voluntary conjugate gaze to LEFT:
1 RIGHT frontal eye field activates LEFT PPRF
2 PPRF neurones activate LEFT abducens nucleus → LEFT lateral rectus muscle
3 PPRF neurones via medial longitudinal fasciculus also activate RIGHT oculomotor nucleus → RIGHT medial rectus muscle PPRF, parapontine reticular formation.

Figure 2.48 Voluntary conjugate eye movement (midbrain: posterior view) Source: FitzGerald 2010. © 2016 Elsevier. Reproduced with permission of Elsevier.

vestibular system. This explains some automatic movements (e.g. hands being in position to catch a rapidly moving ball before it becomes visible).

Eye and pupil movement below the level of the cortical eye fields consists of:

- Conjugate gaze mechanisms within the brainstem
- Pupillary light reflexes
- Individual cranial nerves III, IV and VI and the muscles supplied
- Near and far responses.

Gaze centres in the brainstem

Horizontal (lateral) gaze centres lie in the right and left PPRF adjacent to each abducens nucleus (Figure 2.48). Upward gaze is controlled by the rostral interstitial nucleus (RiN) close to the pretectal nucleus (IIIrd nucleus level). This lies at the rostral end of the medial longitudinal fasciculus (MLF). This bundle connects each PPRF and abducens nucleus with the portion of the IIIrd nucleus that supplies the medial rectus – thus yoking together abduction in one eye with adduction in the other. The downward gaze centre is ventral to the RiN at the same level

The light reflex: pupil constriction

The pathway from retinal ganglion cell to post-ganglionic parasympathetic fibres and onwards to the iris (sphincter pupillae) is shown in Figure 2.49. The sympathetic pathway (pupil dilatation) and the near reflex are mentioned in the following section.

III, IV and VI: third, fourth and sixth nerve nuclei and nerves

Essential anatomy is summarised here (Figure 2.50). Lesions of these nerves and nuclei are discussed in Chapters 4, 14, 15 and 20.

Oculomotor nucleus and IIIrd nerve

This compound nucleus, adjacent to the peri-aqueductal grey matter at superior colliculus level consists of neurones that supply:

- Five striated muscles: medial, superior, inferior recti, inferior oblique and levator palpbebrae superioris
- Muscles supplied by the parasympathetic system: ciliaris (ciliary muscle) and sphincter pupillae, via the Edinger–Westphal nucleus.

The oculomotor (III) nerve passes through the midbrain tegmentum, emerges into the interpeduncular fossa, crosses the apex of the petrous temporal bone, enters the cavernous sinus and leaves in two divisions within the superior orbital fissure. Parasympathetic fibres travel in the lower division and leave in the branch to the inferior oblique muscle. They synapse in the ciliary ganglion, pierce the sclera and, via the short ciliary nerves, reach ciliaris and sphincter pupillae.

Trochlear nucleus and IVth nerve

The nucleus is at the level of the inferior colliculus. Each IVth nerve then decussates, emerges from the back of the brainstem, passes around it and enters the cavernous sinus (just below III), entering the orbit through the superior orbital fissure to reach the superior oblique muscle.

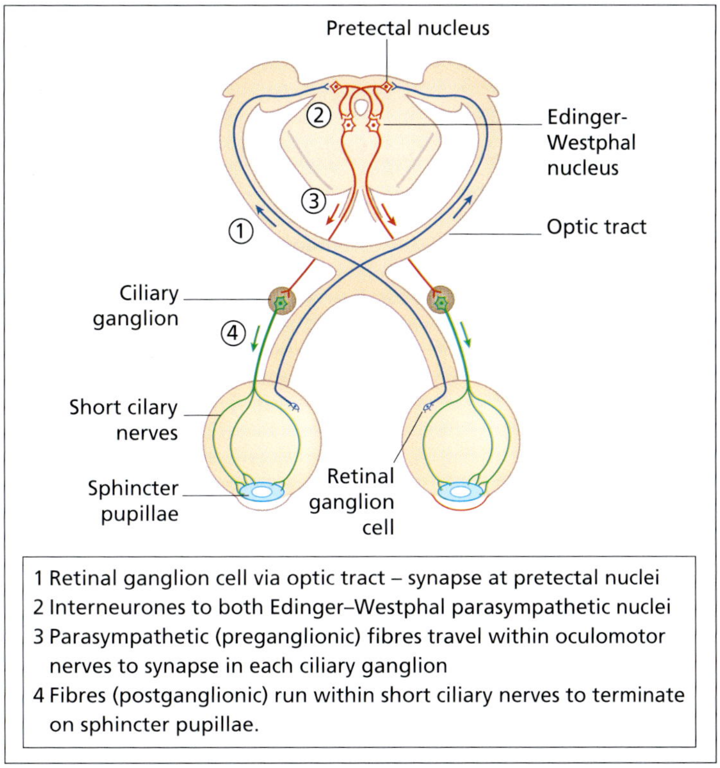

Figure 2.49 Pupillary constriction to light (midbrain at level of superior colliculus). Source: FitzGerald 2010. © 2016 Elsevier. Reproduced with permission of Elsevier.

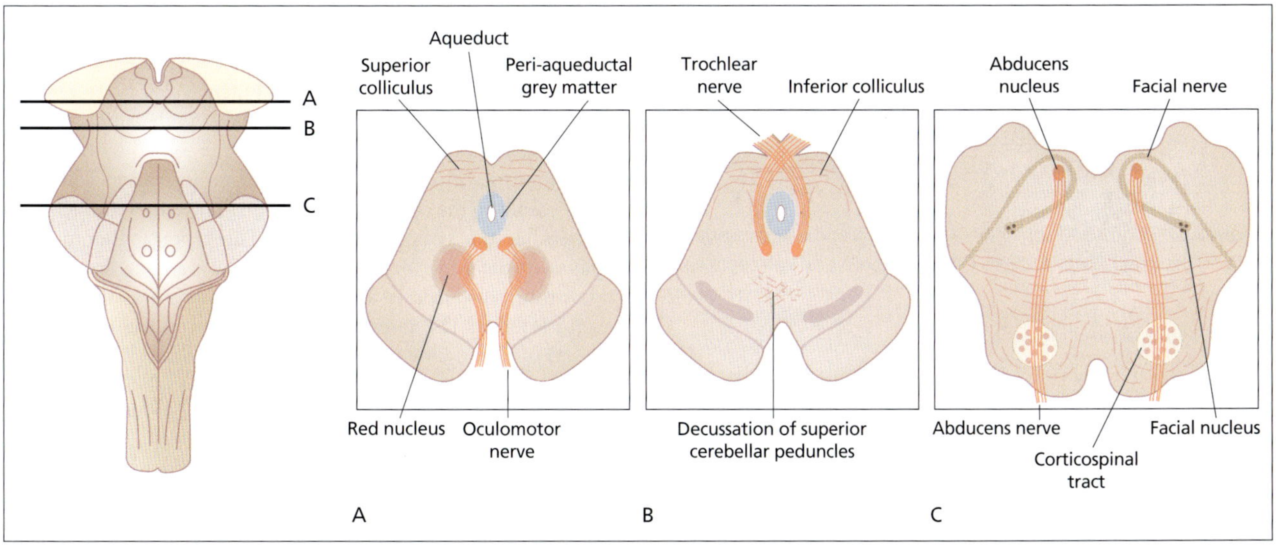

Figure 2.50 Origins of III, IV and VI: transverse sections of brainstem. Source: FitzGerald 2010. © 2016 Elsevier. Reproduced with permission of Elsevier.

Abducens nucleus and VIth nerve

Each VIth nucleus, lower in the brainstem than III and IV, lies in the mid pons at the level of the facial nucleus. The nerve runs a long intracranial course, initially beside the basilar artery, thence over the petrous temporal bone. Within the cavernous sinus it lies beside the internal carotid artery (Figure 2.51). Like III and IV, VI passes through the superior orbital fissure. VI innervates the lateral rectus muscle.

Ocular muscle motor units and sensory connections These motor units contain 5–10 muscle fibres (cf. 500 or more in biceps and large striated limb muscles) and comprise A, B and C muscle fibres:

- A fibres (fast twitch) are involved in saccades
- B fibres (slow twitch) are used in smooth pursuit, and
- C fibres are involved in maintaining the visual axes and are tonically active, when awake.

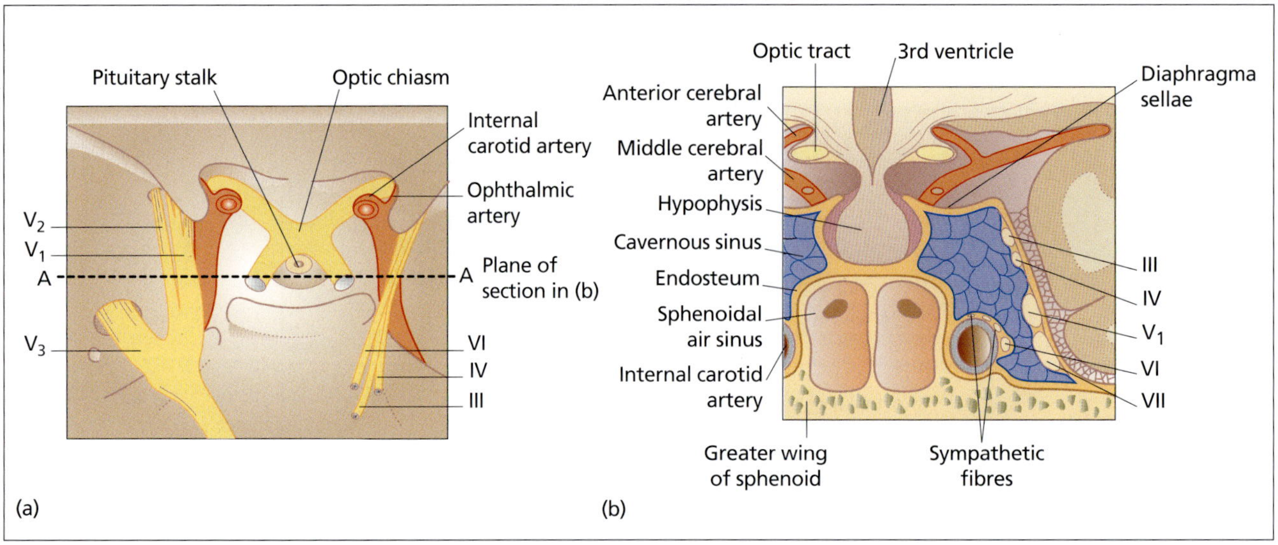

Figure 2.51 III, IV, VI, and V within cavernous sinus. (a) Middle cranial fossa from above (cavernous sinus removed). Right: relations of V. Left: relations of III, IV and VI. (b) Coronal section through pituitary (AA). Source: FitzGerald 2010. © 2016 Elsevier. Reproduced with permission of Elsevier.

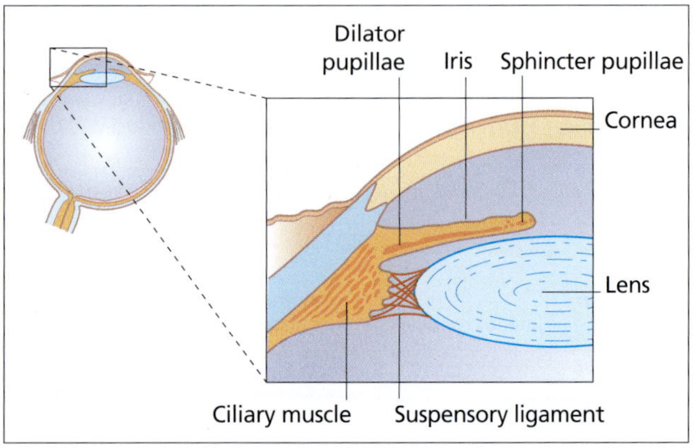

Figure 2.52 Dilator and sphincter pupillae, lens and ciliary muscle. Source: FitzGerald 2010. © 2016 Elsevier. Reproduced with permission of Elsevier.

Proprioceptive pathways from the extraocular muscles extend widely – to the mesencephalic nucleus of V and to the cuneate nucleus in the medulla. Peripheral afferent projections from the neck muscles and output projections from the vestibulocerebellum to these nuclei assist coordinated simultaneous movements of the neck and head in response to changes in gaze.

The near response

Three responses combine to enable gaze to focus on a near object:

1 Covergence of the ocular axes is brought about by contraction of the medial recti
2 The ciliary muscle contracts – the lens bulges passively, the thicker lens shortening its focal length (Figure 2.52), and
3 Sphincter pupillae contract – concentrating light through the central part of the lens.

Retinal impulses pass via the lateral geniculate body to the occipital cortex, thence to the visual association cortex which analyses stereoscopically the object in view. Thence, the efferent pathway reaches the Edinger–Westphal nucleus and vergence cells within the reticular formation.

The far response

To bring a distant object into focus, the ciliary muscle must be inhibited – allowing the suspensory ligament to become tight and flatten the lens. Sympathetic impulses cause this relaxation of the ciliary muscle via β_2 receptors. This dilates the pupil (contraction of dilator pupillae) via α_1 receptors.

Sympathetic pathway to the eye and face

The sympathetic system originates in the hypothalamus. Central efferents decussate in the midbrain and are joined by ipsilateral fibres running within and from the reticular formation. The pathway descends in the cord, emerges in the first ventral thoracic root and reaches the sympathetic chain. These preganglionic fibres synapse in the superior cervical ganglion. Postganglionic fibres run within adventitia of branches of the internal and external carotid arteries. The internal carotid system is accompanied by two sets of fibres. One joins V_1 in the cavernous sinus, but leaves this nerve in the short and long ciliary nerves to the smooth muscles of the eye (dilator pupillae, ciliaris and levator palpebrae superioris). The second forms a plexus around the internal carotid artery. Branches reach the skin of the forehead and scalp. Horner's syndrome is discussed in Chapter 14 (see Horner's syndrome).

External carotid sympathetic fibres are intimately related to all branches of the external carotid artery: superficial and middle temporal, facial, maxillary, middle meningeal, posterior auricular and lingual arteries.

V: trigeminal nerve, sensory and motor nuclei

The trigeminal nerve and its nuclei form a massive sensory input via the ophthalmic (V_1), maxillary (V_2) and mandibular (V_3) divisions. The sensory cutaneous distribution is shown in Figure 2.53.

The Vth nerve also carries sensation from:

- The eyes
- Dura mater of anterior and middle cranial fossae
- Adventitia of cerebral and basilar vessels

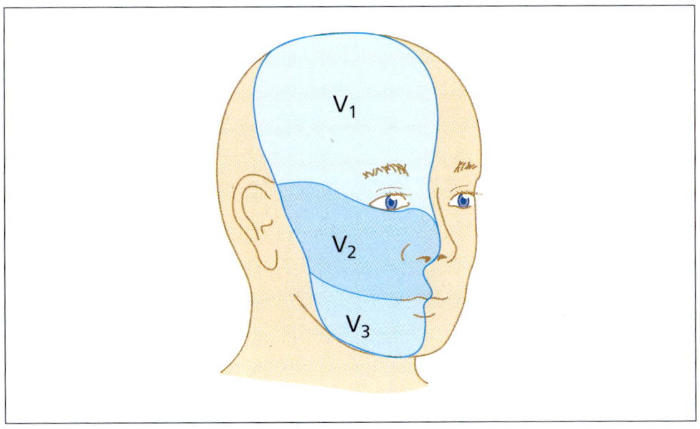

Figure 2.53 Cutaneous distribution of the three divisions of Vth nerve. Source: Patten 1996. Reproduced with permission of Springer Science + Business Media.

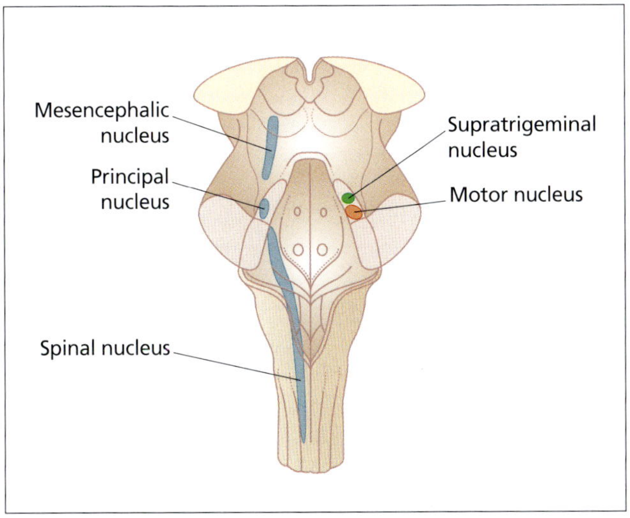

Figure 2.54 Trigeminal nuclei within the brainstem. Source: FitzGerald 2010. © 2016 Elsevier. Reproduced with permission of Elsevier.

- Paranasal sinuses
- Teeth
- Oral and nasal mucous membranes, and
- Facial and masticatory muscles.

Motor nucleus of V and supratrigeminal nuclei

Each Vth motor nucleus in the tegmentum of the pons supplies muscles of mandibular arch origin (Figure 2.54). Supranuclear connections run from each motor cortex to both these V motor nuclei, but largely to the contralateral. Within the reticular formation are the supratrigeminal nuclei, lying at the upper poles of the Vth motor nuclei. These generate masticatory rhythms. Muscles supplied via V_3 are:

- Temporalis
- Masseter
- Pterygoids and digastric
- Infrahyoid muscles, and
- Tensor tympani and tensor palati.

Paralysis of one motor root causes deviation of the opening jaw to that side. The motor root is the efferent arc of the jaw jerk, a monosynaptic reflex.

Sensory Vth nuclei

There are three sensory Vth nerve nuclei (Figure 2.54):

1 Mesencephalic nucleus
2 Principal (pontine), nucleus, and
3 Spinal nucleus.

Mesencephalic Vth nucleus

Peripheral processes enter the sensory root via the trigeminal mesencephalic tract. The mesencephalic nuclear neurones are unique – they are cell bodies of primary sensory neurones (Figure 2.55). Their peripheral origins are the stretch receptors of masticatory muscle spindles (V_3) and stretch receptors of peri-odontal ligaments of the teeth (V_2, V_3) and some fibres from the eye and eye muscles (V_1). Central processes of the mesencephalic afferents descend through the tegmentum of the pons (tract of Probst). Most terminate in the supratrigeminal nucleus; others reach the main part of the motor nucleus, the pontine Vth nucleus and even the dorsal nucleus of the vagus

Principal (pontine) Vth nucleus

These paired nuclei are homologues of the spinal gracile and cuneate nuclei. They process touch discrimination from the mouth, nose and face.

Spinal Vth nucleus

These paired nuclei extend from the pons to spinal level C3. Each main spinal Vth nucleus (pars caudalis) receives pain and temperature afferents from the entire trigeminal area and beyond.

Each nucleus is microscopically a continuation of the outer laminae (I–III) of the posterior horn of the cord. Pain modulation is similar to the situation in the cord – enkephalinergic and GABAergic connections in the substantia gelatinosa and serotoninergic fibres from the reticular formation (magnus raphe nucleus).

Each Vth spinal nucleus receives input from three principal sources:

1 Gasserian ganglion (trigeminal afferents)
2 IX and X, and
3 Three (C2–5) cervical posterior roots (C1 is vestigial or absent).

Trigeminal afferents are the central processes of Gasserian ganglion neurones. Topographical representation within the nucleus is linear (mouth rostral) but layered, like an onion centred on the mouth (Figure 2.56). Peripheral fibres carry pain, temperature and touch centrally (facial skin, teeth, sinuses, cornea, temporo-mandibular joints, dura of anterior and middle fossae). Afferents from IX and X (middle ear, Eustachian tube, pharynx, larynx) also reach the spinal fifth nucleus; their cell bodies are within the inferior sensory ganglia of IX and X. Cervical afferents (dura of posterior fossa and cord, cervical joints) ascend through the hypoglossal canal.

Trigeminovascular system – innervation of cerebral vessels V_1 lies close to the internal carotid artery in the cavernous sinus. Afferent V_1 fibres and autonomic fibres accompany the carotid artery, follow its branches and form a network throughout the intracranial vasculature. The role of this important system in the pathogenesis of headache is discussed in Chapter 12.

Trigeminothalamic tract, lemniscus, cortical projection and reticular formation

The spinal Vth nucleus gives rise to the lower part of the trigeminothalamic. This crosses the midline, ascends in the pons and carries pain, temperature and touch. Within the pons the tract is joined by fibres from the principal (pontine) Vth nucleus to form the trigeminal lemniscus – the ribbon of

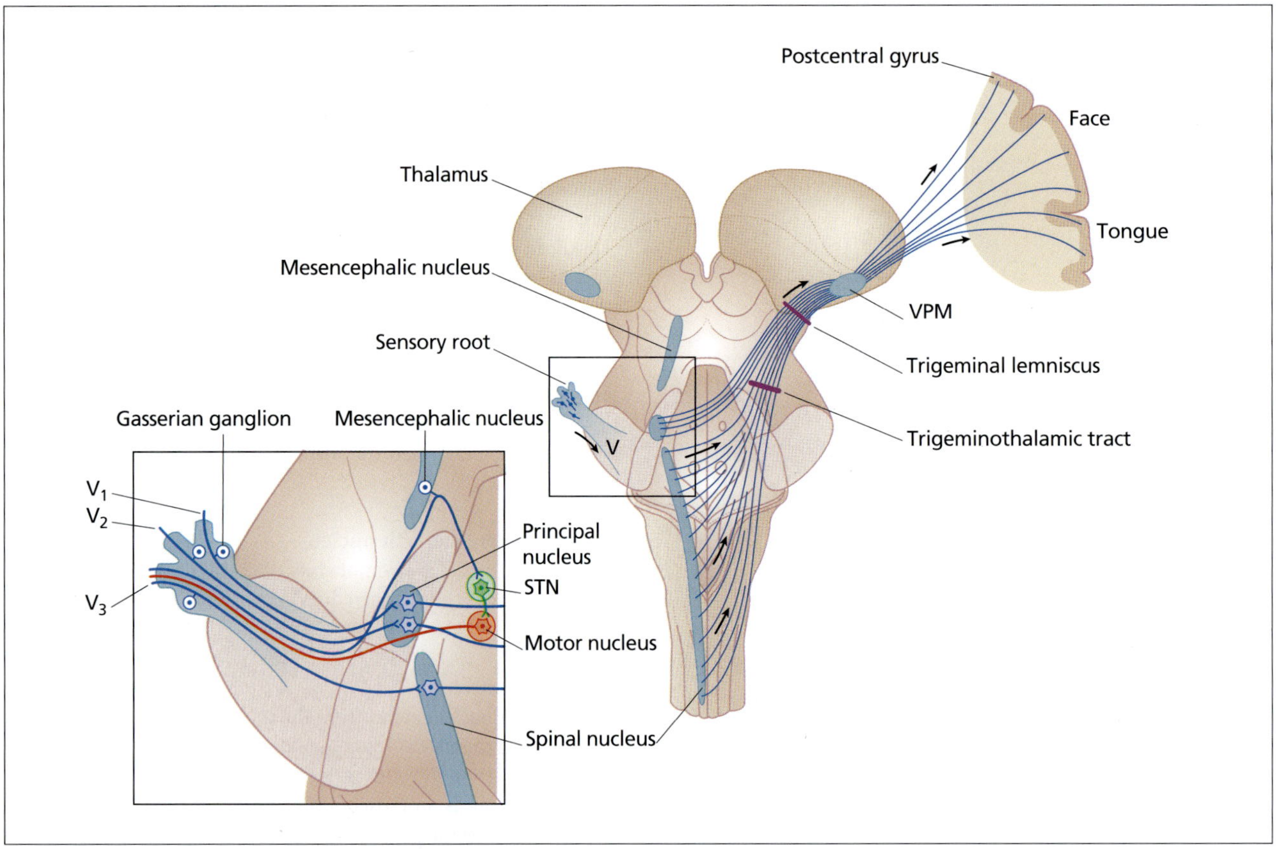

Figure 2.55 Trigeminal pathways within the brainstem. STN, supratrigeminal nucleus; VPM, ventral posteromedial nucleus of thalamus. Source: Patten 1996. Reproduced with permission of Springer Science + Business Media.

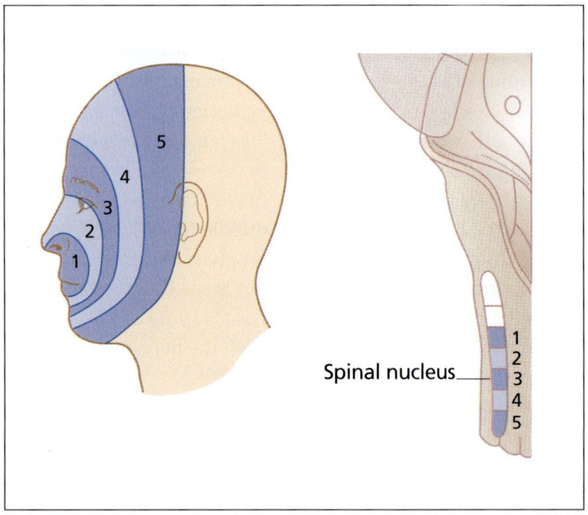

Figure 2.56 Spinal Vth nucleus: distribution. Source: FitzGerald 2010. © 2016 Elsevier. Reproduced with permission of Elsevier.

trigeminal fibres that terminates in the ventral posterior medial nucleus of the thalamus (Figure 2.55). Thence, third order afferents pass from the thalamus to the substantial facial area of the somatic sensory cortex.

Trigeminoreticular fibres synapse in the lateral RF (parvocellular neurones). They are believed to mediate arousal, for example slapping or irritating the face.

The jaw jerk and other masticatory reflexes Spindle afferents from jaw muscles make direct synaptic contact with Vth motor nuclear neurones. Supranuclear lesions of the Vth motor nucleus (see Pseudobulbar palsy, Chapter 13) are accompanied by an exaggerated jaw jerk, a monosynaptic stretch reflex.

Other masticatory muscle reflexes such as jaw closing in response to food in the mouth, jaw opening, chewing, and snapping are mediated via the pattern-generating supratrigeminal motor nuclei. While of no diagnostic significance, they perhaps explain potential hazards of being bitten, by stuporose patients and sleepy animals.

The corneal reflex The afferent pathway is via pain fibres in the nasociliary branch of V_1. The efferent pathway is via VIIth nerve innervated muscles – bilateral blinking (Chapters 4, 13 and 20). The clinical reality is that the patient feels and usually reports the unpleasant stimulus. Visible lacrimation and conjunctival injection follows in a normal eye. All these features diminish when there is a Vth nerve lesion. The upper five-sixths (or so) of the cornea are innervated by the ophthalmic division (V_1), and the lower sixth, from about 5 to 7 o'clock by the maxillary (V_2). Depression of the corneal reflex is an early sign of a Vth nerve lesion – of importance in the diagnosis of cerebello-pontine angle lesions before non-invasive imaging.

VII: facial nerve

The facial nerve arises from the VIIth nucleus in the pons and before leaving the brainstem loops around the abducens (VI) nucleus, known as the internal genu, creating the facial colliculus

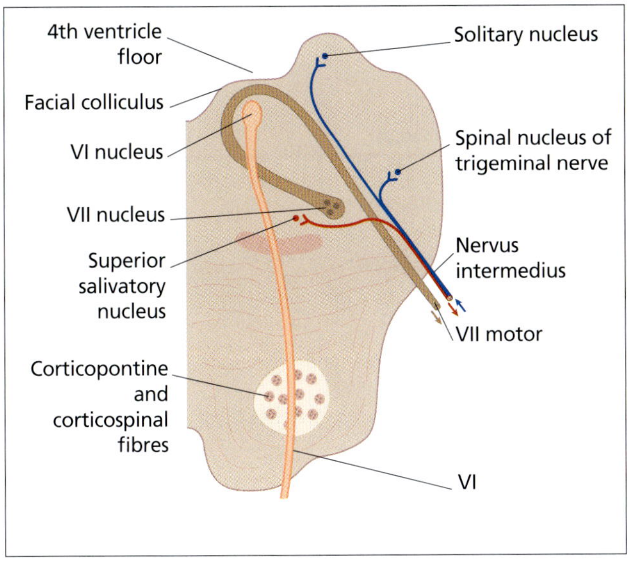

Figure 2.57 Facial nucleus, facial and abducens nerves (pons – cross-section). Source: FitzGerald 2010. © 2016 Elsevier. Reproduced with permission of Elsevier.

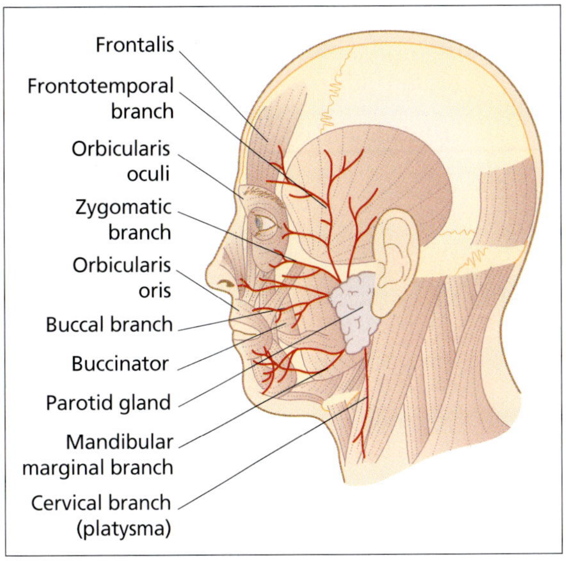

Figure 2.58 Principal facial branches of VIIth nerve. Source: FitzGerald 2010. © 2016 Elsevier. Reproduced with permission of Elsevier.

Table 2.13 Reflexes involving V, VII, VIII and II.

	Corneal reflex	Jaw jerk	Pout reflex	Blink (light)	Blink (noise)	Stapedius
Receptor	Cornea	Masseter (spindles)	Lips	Retina	Cochlea	Cochlea
Afferent	V_1	V_3	V_2, V_3	Optic nerve	Cochlear nucleus	Cochlear nerve
1st synapse	V spinal nucleus	V motor nuclei	V principal nucleus	Superior colliculus	Inferior colliculus	Cochlear nucleus
2nd synapse	VII nucleus (+ pain and lacrimation V)	(Monosynaptic reflex)	VII nucleus	VII nucleus	VII nucleus	VII nucleus
Muscle	Orbicularis oculi	Masseter	Orbicularis oris	Orbicularis oculi	Orbicularis oculi	Stapedius (Chapter 14)

in the 4th ventricle floor (Figures 2.57 and 2.58). The nerve leaves the skull via the stylomastoid foramen – its only constituent. Principal motor branches supply muscles of facial expression. A small motor branch supplies the stapedius. VII also carries sensory taste fibres from the anterior two-thirds of the tongue via the chorda tympani.

Supranuclear connections allow the facial muscles to respond both in volitional and emotional activities, and bilaterally in many common habitual situations – smiling, blinking, frowning – and in several reflex actions (Table 2.13). Part of each VIIth nucleus supplying the upper face, principally frontalis, receives supranuclear fibres from each hemisphere. The face muscles are exquisitely responsive to emotional states, and to all sensory input; the limbic contribution is from the nucleus accumbens in the ventral basal ganglia.

Nervus intermedius, greater petrosal nerve and chorda tympani

Distal to the internal genu, the nervus intermedius (part of VII) acts as one stage of a complex conduit, for efferent parasympathetic and afferent special sensory fibres (Figure 2.59):

- The parasympathetic root arises from the superior salivatory nucleus to form motor components of:
  - the greater petrosal nerve → pterygopalatine ganglion → lacrimal and nasal glands, and
  - the chorda tympani → submandibular ganglion → submandibular and sublingual glands.
- The special sensory root consists of cell bodies that lie in the geniculate ganglion. Afferent fibres from taste buds in the anterior two-thirds of tongue travel in the chorda tympani. Those from taste buds in the hard palate travel in the greater petrosal nerve. Central processes enter the gustatory nucleus, part of the nucleus solitarius that also receives fibres from IX. Thence, second order neurones project via the thalamus, to anterior insular and cingulate cortex.
- Some geniculate ganglion cells also receive sensory impulses from skin around external auditory meatus (see Bell's palsy, Chapter 13).

VIII: vestibulocochlear nerve

The vestibulocochlear nerve contains primarily afferent axons of bipolar neurones whose cell bodies lie within the petrous temporal bone. Peripheral processes of these neurones are in contact with specialised neuro-epithelium of the labyrinth and cochlea.

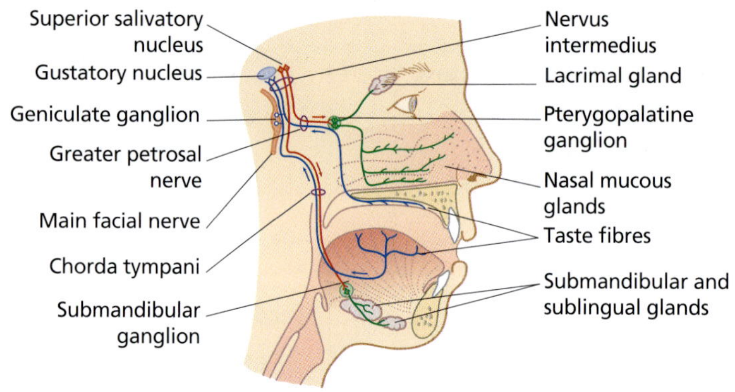

Figure 2.59 Nervus intermedius, greater petrosal nerve and chorda tympani. Source: FitzGerald 2010. © 2016 Elsevier. Reproduced with permission of Elsevier.

The two components of VIII (vestibular and cochlear) enter the junction between pons and medulla at the cerebellopontine angle.

The neuro-otological system is complex – an entire subspecialty is devoted to it (Chapter 15). Vertigo, meaning the illusion of movement, hearing loss and tinnitus are the prominent symptoms. Essential peripheral neuroanatomy and central connections are shown in Figure 2.60.

Vestibular system

The dense petrous temporal bony labyrinth contains perilymph, an extracellular fluid that provides a fluid housing for the membranous labyrinth that encloses the organs of balance. These are washed by endolymph – potassium ion rich, sodium ion poor, similar to intracellular fluid.

Each labyrinth (Figure 2.60a) houses five sensory organs within the utricle, saccule and three semicircular canals. Each utricle and each saccule contains a macula. Each canal contains a crista within an ampulla:

- Maculae (two) are sensory organs of static head position
- Cristae (three) are sensory organs of head movement.

The vestibular ganglion lies in the internal auditory meatus. Peripheral processes are applied to the five sensory organs. Central vestibular nerve axons enter the brainstem to synapse at the lateral, medial, superior and inferior vestibular nuclei (VN). Other connections are shown in Figure 2.60d.

The static labyrinth In the erect posture:

- The utricular macula is essentially horizontal
- The saccular macula is essentially vertical.

Hair cells in these maculae are in contact with vestibular nerve fibres via ribbon synapses (Figure 2.60b). Stereocilia (about 100/cell) and a longer process, a kinocilium (one/cell) projects into otoconia (ear sand), a gelatinous matrix of calcium carbonate crystals. Each macula has a central groove, a striola. Cilia are arranged either side of each striola. Depolarisation takes place whenever kinocilia are parted from stereocilia.

The maculae respond to:

- Linear acceleration (e.g. walking)
- Vertical acceleration (e.g. falling), and
- Tilting.

The roles of the static labyrinth are to indicate head position in relation to the trunk, and to alter centre of gravity of the body to maintain upright or other postures. The system is adapted to work within and to compensate for the Earth's gravitational field; weightlessness causes problems during space travel.

The kinetic labyrinth In the kinetic labyrinth, the ciliated, cellular arrangement of the static labyrinth is replicated in the cristae of the three semicircular canals, their ampullae and each cupula (Figure 2.60c). The cupula is a gelatinous projecting part of each crista within an ampulla – bathed in endolymph. Into each cupula, kinocilia project from hair cells.

The three cupulae are quite exquisitely sensitive to angular acceleration and deceleration. Endolymph remains relatively static. Each crista billows and deflects as this miniature sail-like organ is thrust against endolymph as head velocity changes in a particular plane.

Vestibular nuclei and central connections Central axons of each vestibular nerve synapse at the lateral, medial, superior and inferior VN in the brainstem (Figure 2.60d).

The lateral vestibulospinal tract arises from the lateral VN (nucleus of Dieter). Fibres descend in the anterior funiculus of the cord to synapse with a complex variety of limb, neck and trunk α and γ motor neurones concerned with posture. The flocculonodular lobe of the cerebellum has two-way connections with all vestibular nuclei. There also connections to the vomiting centre in the area postrema in the obex of the 4th ventricle.

The medial vestibulospinal tract arises in the inferior and medial VN, descends in the medial longitudinal fasciculus and ends in the cervical cord. Head and eye-righting reflexes are dealt with by this system; there are connections with the kinetic labyrinth.

Central second order neurones from the VN reach the contralateral VP nucleus of the thalamus. Third order neurones project to the various cortical areas – close to the facial area in the somatosensory cortex, to the insula and temporoparietal cortex.

Vertigo is the illusion of movement characteristic of vestibular pathology. The specific cortical location of this common symptom is unclear. Electrical stimulation of somatosensory cortex sometimes

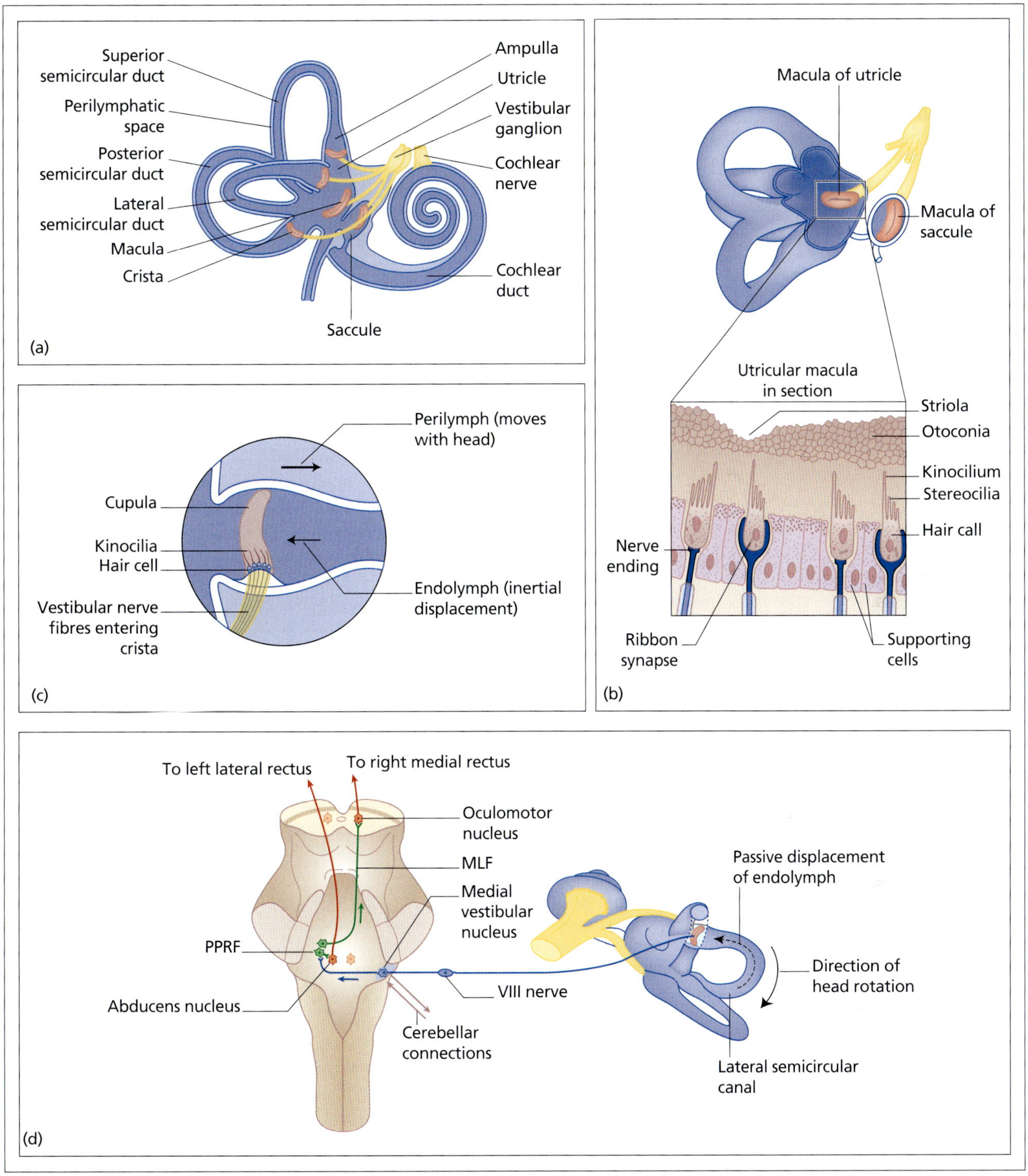

Figure 2.60 Vestibular system. (a) Five vestibular sense organs. (b) Cells of static labyrinth. (c) Kinetic labyrinth: crista in ampulla of semi-circular canal. (d) Head rotation and conjugate lateral gaze. MLF, medial longitudinal fasciculus; PPRF, parapontine reticular formation. Source: FitzGerald 2010. © 2016 Elsevier. Reproduced with permission of Elsevier.

induces it, and vertigo can occur with focal seizure activity in the temporoparietal cortex, though it is uncommon as an epileptic event. It is common knowledge that vertigo is sometimes followed by nausea and vomiting. Any prolonged new vestibular imbalance can be followed by intractable vomiting and profound malaise; this happens for example in seasickness. The neuro-anatomical explanation is vestibular stimulation of the vomiting centre (see Area postrema).

One relevant feature of the vestibular system – and a reason why vertigo, nystagmus and dizziness have relatively poor localising value – is that right–left imbalance in the system, at any level, produces symptoms and/or signs. (Nystagmus is discussed in Chapters 4 and 15.)

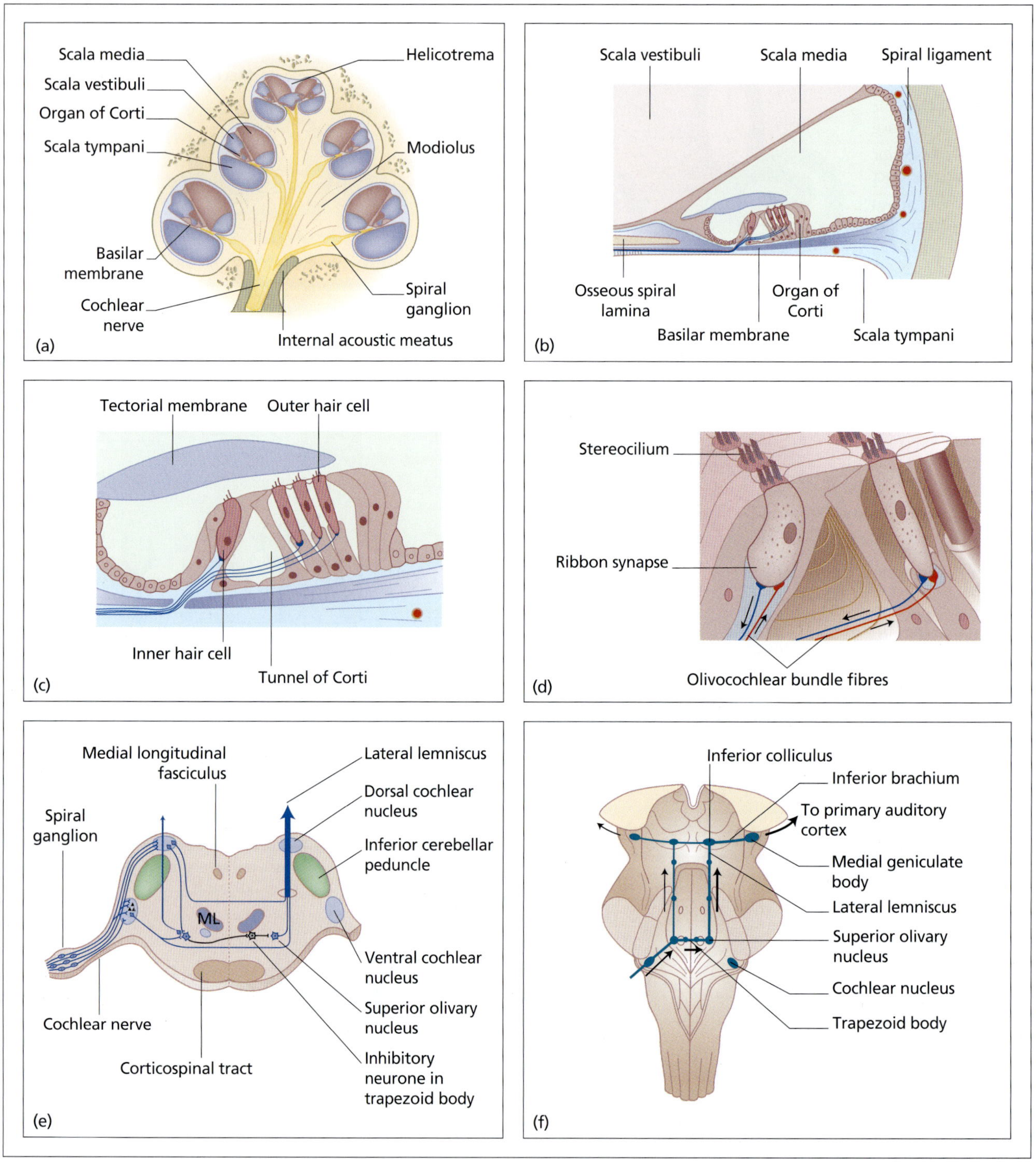

Figure 2.61 Auditory system. (a) Cochlea (in section). (b), (c) and (d): Organ of Corti, hair cells and ribbon synapses. (e) Cochlear nerve, ventral cochlear nucleus (midbrain – cross-section); (f) Central connections to primary auditory cortex (from behind). ML,medial lemniscus. Source: FitzGerald 2010. © 2016 Elsevier. Reproduced with permission of Elsevier.

Auditory system

Sound quantity, quality, position, timing and relevance are detected via:

- Cochlea and cochlear nerve
- Cochlear nuclei and central pathways, and
- Auditory cortex.

Secondary projections interpret the emotional content of sound and music and determine actions in response to sounds.

The afferent system is illustrated in Figure 2.61. Auditory efferents are mentioned in Chapter 15.

Cochlea Hair cells, from which protrude stereocilia, form the principal auditory neuro-epithelium. They lie within the organ of Corti (spiral organ). The complex terminology is summarised as follows:

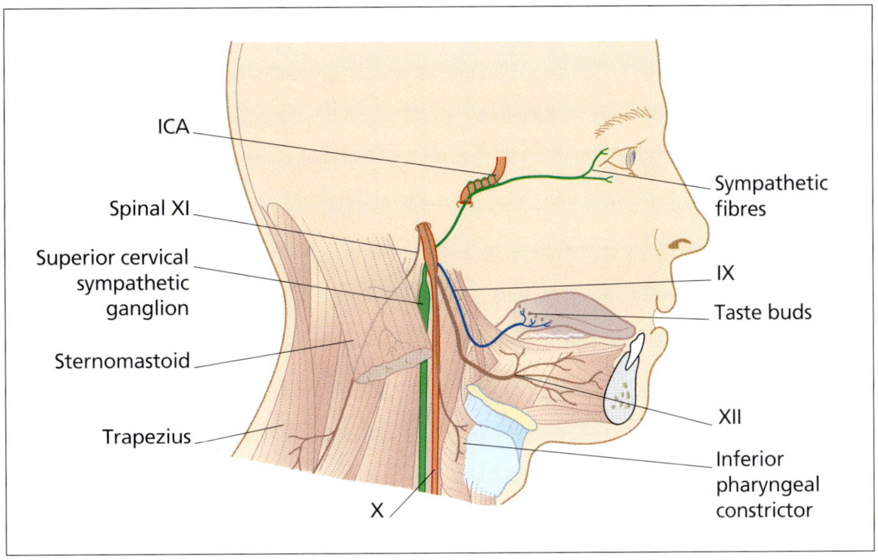

Figure 2.62 Distribution of IX, X, XI, XII and superior cervical ganglion. ICA, internal carotid artery. Source: FitzGerald 2010. © 2016 Elsevier. Reproduced with permission of Elsevier.

- The modiolus is the central bony pillar of the cochlea – it is in the line of the internal auditory meatus.
- The osseous spiral lamina projects from the modiolus. The cochlear spiral has two and half turns and is about 1 cm both in height and diameter.
- The basilar membrane is fixed to the tip of the spiral lamina. It extends across the cavity of the bony cochlea and is attached to the spiral ligament.
- The scala vestibuli and the scala tympani are the upper and lower chambers of the cochlea. They are filled with perilymph. They communicate via the helicotrema.
- The scala media lies above the basilar membrane and is filled with endolymph – and separated from the scala vestibuli by the vestibular membrane.
- The organ of Corti lies on the basilar membrane. The organ contains a central tunnel (tunnel of Corti) containing perilymph diffusing through the basilar membrane.

The arrangement of inner and outer hair cells, tectorial membrane and ribbon synapses is shown in Figure 2.61. Their nerve supply (the cochlear nerve) is via bipolar spiral ganglion cells in the osseous spiral lamina. One inner hair cell has some 20 afferent fibres in contact with it.

Auditory transduction The snug fit and sensitive articulation of the ossicles – 'the footplate of the stapes rests on the oval window' – transmits vibrating pressure waves through the tympanic membrane to the basilar membrane. The basilar membrane is tonotopic:

- Low frequency waves produce resonance where the fibres are longest – at the apical turn of the cochlea
- High frequency waves (high-pitched sounds) cause short fibres in the basal part of the cochlea to resonate.

Cochlear nerve and central connections

Myelinated axons from some 25 000 large bipolar neurones form the cochlear nerve. The pathways are illustrated in Figure 2.61. The sequence is:

- Inferior and superior cochlear nuclei (termination of first order fibres)
- Trapezoid body (second order fibres), superior olivary nucleus to inferior colliculus, and
- Inferior brachium via medial geniculate body to auditory cortex.

The primary auditory cortex is located in Heschl's gyrus on the anterior surface of the temporal lobe. In humans, destruction of this region on one side causes no perceptible deafness but an initial inability to localise sound. Hearing loss is produced rarely by central lesions – potential imbalance is compensated by bilateral representation. The usual focus of clinical neurology is the distinction between conductive and sensorineural deafness (Chapters 4 and 15).

Acoustic reflex pathways Biologically important auditory automatic pathways include:

- Startle and waking responses, via the reticular formation.
- Dampening of sounds (e.g. the sound of one's own voice) via tensor tympani (V) and the stapedius reflex (see Audiological investigation, Chapter 15). The stapedius reflex consists of a contraction of stapedius muscle in response to loud noise. Hyperacusis occurs when the muscle is paralysed (e.g. in Bell's palsy; Chapter 13).
- Head turning and eye turning in response to sounds.
- Pleasurable experience (e.g. of music and rhythm).
- Automatic responses to the call or command of a dominant mate or pack leader.

IX, X, XI and XII: glossopharyngeal, vagus, accessory and hypoglossal nerves

These four cranial nerves are grouped together. These notes indicate their intricacy, multiple nuclei and complex pathways both afferent and efferent. Their distribution is shown in Figure 2.62 and the complex nuclear arrangement in Figures 2.63 and 2.64.

XI: spinal accessory nerve

The spinal accessory (XI) is the motor nerve to extrafusal and intrafusal fibres of trapezius and sternomastoid. The nuclear column (α and γ motor neurones) is in the anterior grey horn (lateral column) of the upper five segments of the cord, from which rootlets emerge (Figure 2.63b). The curious route of this nerve is upwards through the foramen magnum, then back, down and out through

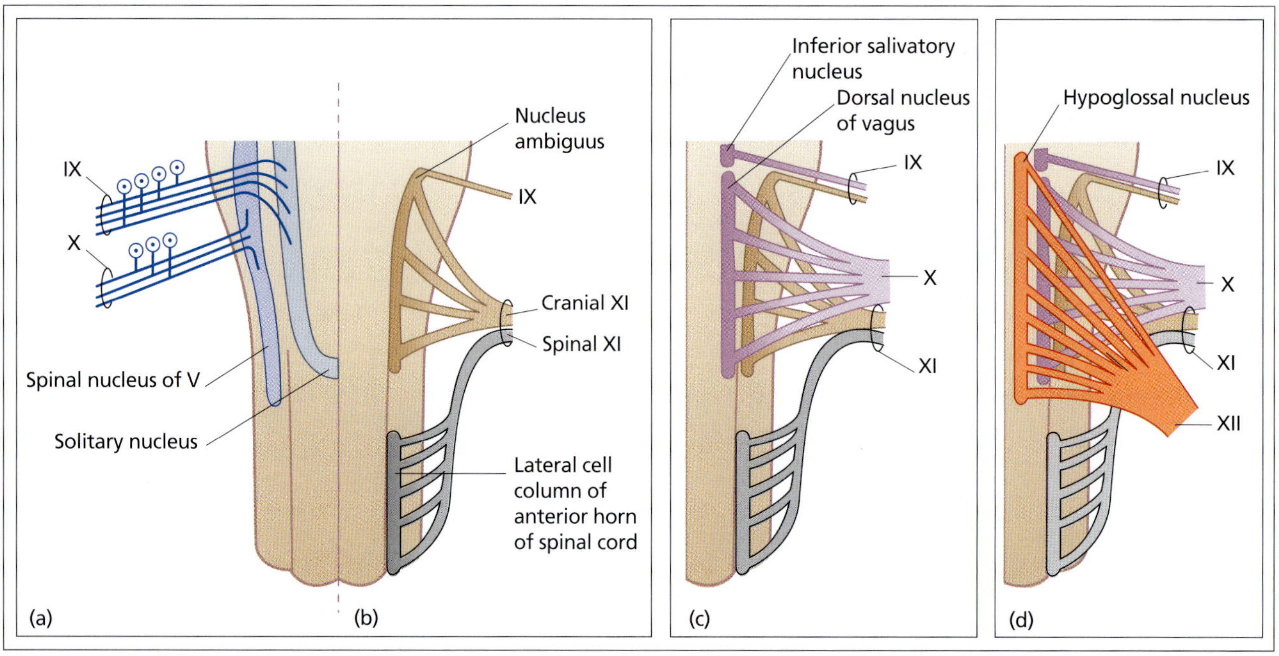

Figure 2.63 Nuclei of IX, X, XI and XII. (a) to (d) Brainstem – anterior views. (a) Sensory nuclei for IX and X. (b) Motor nuclei of IX, cranial XI and spinal XI (special visceral efferent column, contributing to IX and cranial XI). (c) Inferior salivatory nucleus and dorsal nucleus of vagus (general visceral efferent column) contributing to IX and X. (d) Hypoglossal nucleus (somatic efferent column) and XII. Source: FitzGerald 2010. © 2016 Elsevier. Reproduced with permission of Elsevier.

the jugular foramen. Some afferent twigs (cervical and thoracic nerves) combine with spinal XI as it pierces the trapezius, giving rise to a situation believed to be unique for the nerve supply of a muscle: muscle efferents (spinal XI) and muscle afferents (cervical and thoracic twigs) travel by separate pathways.

This anomaly may explain the pain that follows section of motor roots of XI, or spinal XI in the posterior triangle of the neck, where the nerve is superficial and readily damaged during lymph node biopsy (see Accessory nerve, Chapter 13).

Cranial accessory XI, glossopharyngeal IX and vagus X – and their nuclei

Groups of medullary neurones known as the nucleus ambiguus and the solitary nucleus contain some of the cell bodies of nerves IX, X and cranial XI.

The nucleus ambiguus (Figures 2.63 and 2.64) provides special visceral efferent fibres of IX and cranial XI supplying:

- Pharynx (constrictor muscles)
- Stylopharyngeus and levator palati
- Larynx (intrinsic muscles), and
- Oesophagus (striated muscles of the upper third, via the recurrent laryngeal nerve).

The solitary nucleus (Figures 2.63a and 2.64b) merges with its opposite number to form the commissural nucleus. The four functional regions of the solitary nucleus are:

1. Gustatory – afferents from tongue, epiglottis and palate
2. Dorsal respiratory
3. Baroreceptor – afferents from carotid sinus and aortic arch, and
4. Visceral afferent – afferents from gut and respiratory tract.

The cranial (accessory) nerve XI arises from the nucleus ambiguus in the medulla and leaves the skull through the jugular foramen. Cranial XI shares a dural sheath with spinal XI, without exchanging fibres and becomes incorporated into the vagus.

Glossopharyngeal nerve IX

The IXth nerve, almost entirely sensory, leaves the skull via the jugular foramen to reach the mucous membrane of the pharynx and the ear. The tympanic branch of IX that leaves above the jugular foramen, supplies the tympanic membrane. Some central processes synapse with the spinal Vth nucleus. Some of the tympanic branch fibres are parasympathetic – they supply the parotid gland via the lesser petrosal nerve and otic ganglion. The oropharynx and posterior third of the tongue (touch) are supplied by fibres passing to the commissural nucleus. These provide the afferent limb of the gag reflex. Taste fibres (gustatory neurones in the circumvallate papillae of the tongue) terminate centrally in the gustatory nucleus. The carotid branch of IX contains two sets of fibres. One arises in baroreceptor neurones of the carotid sinus and passes to the solitary nucleus. The second arises in glomus cells (chemoreceptors) within the carotid body that terminate centrally in the dorsal respiratory nucleus. Stylopharyngeus muscle is supplied by branchial efferents of IX from the nucleus ambiguus.

Vagus nerve X

The vagus (Latin: wandering) is the largest visceral afferent and a major parasympathetic nerve. Some fibres arise from the dorsal nucleus of the vagus (Figure 2.63c) and others from the nucleus ambiguus. Other cell bodies (for afferent fibres) lie within the solitary nucleus. XII rootlets in the medulla are in series with cranial XI and IX. The nerve emerges from the skull through the jugular foramen with cranial XI and IX. In the jugular foramen are the two small sensory ganglia of the vagus: the jugular and nodose ganglia.

A summary of branches of the vagus follows:

- *Parasympathetic (efferent) neurones* to the heart, lungs and gut originate from the dorsal nucleus of the vagus and nucleus ambiguus.
- *General visceral afferent fibres* from the heart, lungs and gut have cell bodies within the nodose ganglion. Central synapses are in the commissural nucleus. These pathways serve:

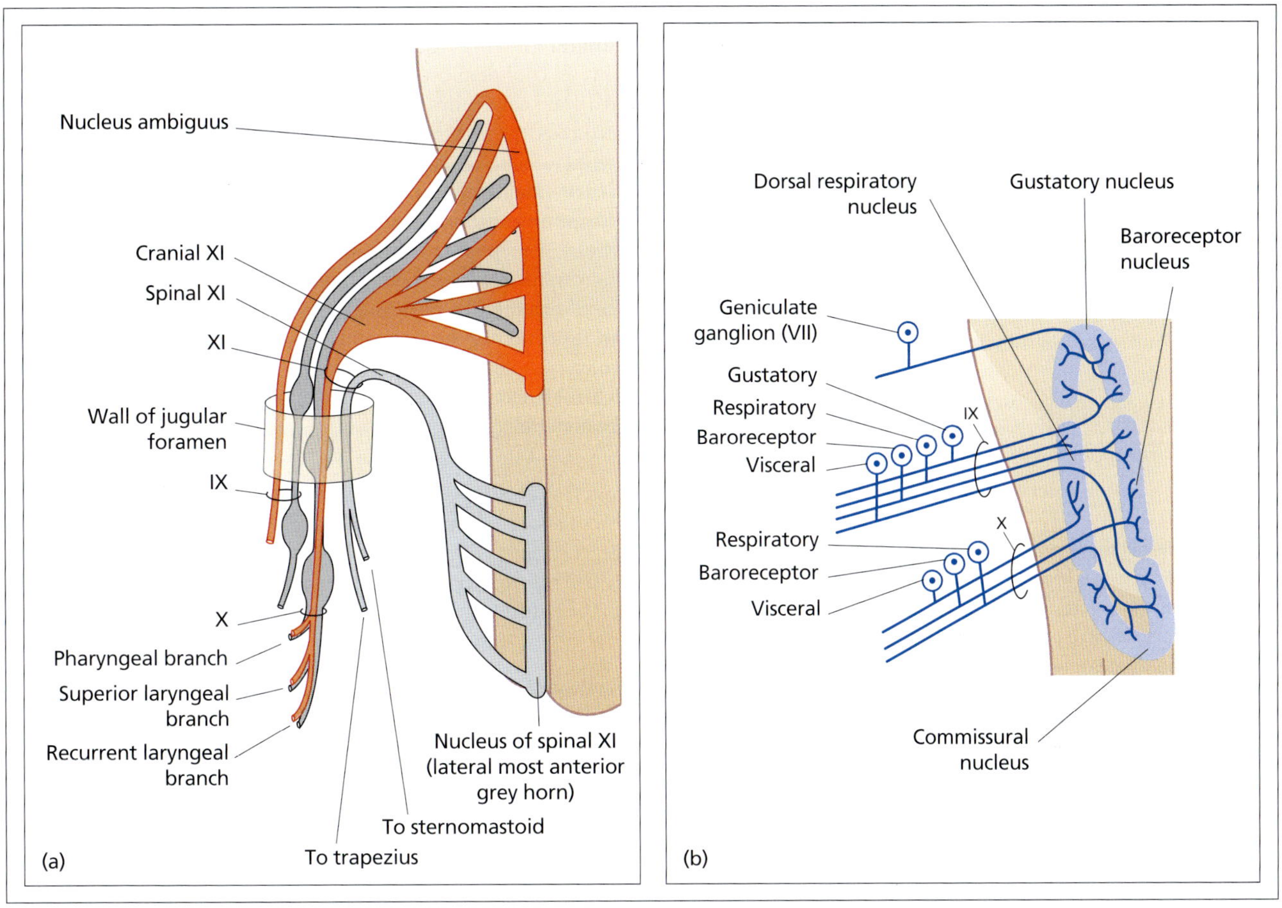

Figure 2.64 (a) Nucleus ambiguus (special visceral afferent column): fibres within IX, X, cranial XI. (b) Solitary nucleus: four functional areas.

 - The cough reflex
 - The Hering–Breuer reflex (inhibition of the dorsal respiratory centre by pulmonary stretch receptors, preventing lung overinflation)
 - The Bainbridge reflex (increase in heart rate following right atrial distension), and
 - Gut afferents signalling satiety (to the hypothalamus).
- *Special viscerent efferent neurones* in the nucleus ambiguus supply pharyngeal and laryngeal muscles, levator palati and muscles (striated) of the upper third of the oesophagus.
- *The auricular branch* supplies skin of the external auditory canal. A meningeal branch supplies meninges of the posterior fossa. Both have cell bodies in the jugular ganglion. Central processes also pass to the spinal nucleus of V (Figure 2.63a).
- *Chemoreceptors* of the aortic bodies, baroreceptors of the aortic arch and taste buds of the epiglottis, are also supplied. The latter synapse in the gustatory nucleus.

XII: hypoglossal nerve

The motor nerve to the tongue originates from the XIIth nucleus, in the same cell column as III, IV and VI, in the 4th ventricular floor (Figure 2.63d). Nerve rootlets leave the medulla between the pyramid and olive, form two fascicles and exit the skull via the anterior condylar foramen (hypoglossal canal), just below the jugular foramen. The nerve passes between the jugular vein and internal carotid artery at the skull base to reach the muscles of the tongue.

The hypoglossal nerve, like its fellow lower cranial nerves, has connections with others. It receives twigs from the vagus, from upper cervical roots, cervical sympathetic (see superior cervical ganglion) and has connections with the lingual nerve, a branch of V_3. Styloglossus, hyoglossus, genioglossus and geniohyoid are the muscles supplied.

A unilateral XIIth nerve lesion is followed by deviation of the tongue to that side and several weeks later by wasting and fasciculation. The surface of the normal tongue when protruded often flickers slightly. Lateral tongue deviation is the obvious physical sign. The larynx is also drawn to the side opposite a hypoglossal palsy on swallowing (Chapters 4 and 13).

Autonomic nervous system

The autonomic, self-regulating sympathetic and parasympathetic system is a diffuse neural network.

- *Controlling centres* (hypothalamus and reticular formation) connect to
- *Preganglionic neurones* (grey matter of brainstem and cord) that project via
- *Preganglionic fibres* that leave the CNS, to synapse at
- *Peripheral autonomic ganglia* (multi-polar neurones), the origins of
- *Post-ganglionic fibres* (unmyelinated) that form terminal networks to reach
- *Target tissues.*

Chapter 24 outlines issues of particular clinical relevance and includes schematic diagrams of the system.

Sympathetic system

The sympathetic outflow is thoracolumbar. Preganglionic neurones are located in the lateral grey horn at lower thoracic, L1, L2 and usually L3 levels. From these spinal neurones, preganglionic fibres leave the cord via corresponding anterior spinal nerve roots to form each paravertebral sympathetic chain.

Thereafter, preganglionic fibres reach sympathetic ganglia by four routes:

1 Some ascend, to synapse in cervical (superior, middle) and stellate ganglia.
2 Others descend to synapse in lumbar and sacral sympathetic ganglia.
3 Some synapse locally at a nearby ganglion. Postganglionic fibres within T1–L2 spinal nerves supply T1–L2 vessels, skin and sweat glands.
4 Some traverse the sympathetic chain, to leave as lumbar/thoracic splanchnic nerves (preganglionic) and reach mesenteric, coeliac, renal and pelvic ganglia.

Sympathetic activity dilates the pupils, increases sweating, increases blood pressure and heart rate, diverts blood from skin and gut to skeletal muscle and closes sphincters.

Parasympathetic system

Parasympathetic preganglionic outflow is cranial and sacral. Fibres emerge via:

- IIIrd, VIIth, IXth and Xth cranial nerves
- Sacral nerve roots.

Cranial parasympathetic III, VII, IX and X fibres and subsequent ganglia

Preganglionic fibres synapse at four cranial ganglia, and mural and intramural ganglia:

- Ciliary ganglion, via III to the pupil (see Near reflex in Optic nerve and visual system)
- Pterygopalatine ganglion, via VII to the lacrimal and nasal glands (secretion)
- Submandibular ganglion, also via VII to submandibular and sublingual glands
- Otic ganglion, via IX to the parotid gland, and
- Mural and intramural ganglia, via X to heart, lungs, oesophagus, pancreas, gallbladder, stomach, bowel.

Sacral parasympathetic fibres and ganglia

From the cord lateral grey matter of S2, S3 and S4 (at L1 vertebral level within the conus), preganglionic fibres lie in the cauda equina within S2–4 ventral nerve roots. They leave the region via sacral vertebral foramina to emerge as pelvic splanchnic nerves. These synapse at:

- Pelvic ganglia (paired) that supply the detrusor muscle and tunica media of the internal pudendal vessels and cavernous tissue of the clitoris/penis, and
- Mural ganglion cells in the distal colon and rectum.

Neurotransmission within the autonomic system

Data about neurotransmitters for one target organ may not hold for another: there is variation at local level.

Neurotransmission at sympathetic and parasympathetic ganglia

This is cholinergic throughout. Preganglionic neurones liberate ACh at axodendritic synapses. Ganglion cell receptors are nicotinic.

Neuro-effector junction transmission at target tissues

Neurotransmitters are secreted along terminal dendrites at target tissues (e.g. pupils, blood vessels, secretory glands). The chief neurotransmitter at sympathetic neuro-effector junctions is noradrenaline (i.e. postganglionic transmission is noradrenergic). An exception is the sympathetic supply to eccrine sweat glands, which is cholinergic. The chief neurotransmitter at parasympathetic neuro-effector junctions is ACh (i.e. postganglionic transmission is cholinergic).

Junctional receptors at target tissues

Two factors influence the effect of physiological stimulation of target organs:

1 The nature of postjunctional receptors, and
2 The nature of prejunctional receptors.

Sympathetic system receptors For noradrenaline, two varieties of α-adrenoceptor and two varieties of β-adrenoceptor are known to exist:

- *Postjunctional α_1-adrenoceptors:* these initiate contraction of dilator pupillae, arteries and arterioles, sphincters and vas deferens.
- *Prejunctional α_2-adrenoceptors:* these inhibit transmitter release at both sympathetic and parasympathetic terminals.
- *Postjunctional β_1-adrenoceptors:* in the heart these increase the force of ventricular contraction. In the kidney they increase renin secretion in response to a fall in blood pressure.
- β_2-Receptors respond to circulating and locally available noradrenaline. Postjunctional β_2-receptors relax smooth muscle, such as in bronchi and the pupil. Prejunctional β_2-receptors on adrenergic terminals promote noradrenaline release.

Parasympathetic junctional receptors These are muscarinic in action. Stimulation:

- Slows the heart rate (vagal tone increases)
- Causes bladder emptying, pupillary accommodation for near vision, intestinal peristalsis, and
- Initiates glandular secretion (e.g. lacrimation).

Other autonomic neurotransmitter systems

The complexity of the autonomic system is compounded by at least three further neurotransmitter lineages, known as non-adrenergic non-cholinergic (NANC) neurones:

- Dopamine is liberated from small interneurones in sympathetic ganglia, exerting a mild inhibitory effect on adrenergic neurones.
- Nitric oxide is important in the parasympathetic system as a powerful arterial dilator.
- Vasoactive intestinal polypeptide (VIP) is known to be active as a neurotransmitter in salivary and sweat glands. VIP acts as a co-transmitter to ACh and is a vasodilator, increasing blood supply to target organs already stimulated by muscarinic parasympathetic activity.

Acknowledgements

The late Professor MJ Turlough FitzGerald, Emeritus Professor, Department of Anatomy, National University of Ireland, Galway, kindly agreed that figures and information from the award-winning textbook *Clinical Neuroanatomy and Related Neuroscience* (FitzGerald MJT, Folan-Curran J, 4th edition, 2002; WB Saunders, Edinburgh) were made available for use in our first edition. This cooperation proved invaluable. Details from figures in the subsequent *Clinical Neuroanatomy and Neuroscience* (FitzGerald MJT, Gruener G, Mtui E, 6th edition, 2012; Elsevier Saunders) have been used here, again with permission of Professor FitzGerald's family. The *Queen Square Textbook* authors and editors are most grateful for this continuing cooperation.

Further reading

Bear MF, Connors BW, Paradiso MA. *Neuroscience: Exploring the Brain.* Baltimore, MD: Lippincott, Williams & Wilkins, 2001.

Brodal A. *Neurological Anatomy in Relation to Clinical Medicine*, 2nd edn. New York/London: Oxford University Press, 1969.

FitzGerald MJT, Gruener G, Mtui E. *Clinical Neuroanatomy and Neuroscience*, 5th edn. Philadelphia, PA: Elsevier Saunders, 2007.

Garbay B, Heape AM, Sargeuil F, Cassagne C. Myelin synthesis in the peripheral nervous system. *Prog Neurobiol* 2000; **61**: 267–304.

Gillingwater TH, Ribchester RR. Compartmental neurodegeneration and synaptic plasticity in the Wlds mutant mouse. *J Physiol* 2001; **534**: 627–639.

Harnsberger HR, Ross J, Macdonald AJ, Osborn AG. *Diagnostic and Surgical Imaging Anatomy: Brain, Head and Neck, Spine*, 2nd edn. Amirsys (Lippincott), 2010.

Iles RK. Cell and molecular biology. In *Clinical Medicine*, 6th edn. Kumar P, Clark M, eds. Edinburgh: Elsevier Health Sciences, 2005.

Lemon RN. Descending pathways in motor control. *Annu Rev Neurosci* 2008; **31**: 195–218.

Nicholls JG, Martin AR, Wallace BG, Fuchs, PA. *From Neuron to Brain*, 4th edn. Sunderland, MA: Sinauer Associates, 2001.

Patten J. *Neurological Differential Diagnosis*, 2nd edn. London/New York: Springer, 1996.

CHAPTER 3

Mechanisms of Neurological Disease: Genetics, Autoimmunity and Ion Channels

Dimitri Kullmann[1], Henry Houlden[1] and Michael Lunn[2]
[1] UCL Institute of Neurology
[2] National Hospital for Neurology & Neurosurgery

Many neurological diseases share pathological processes that require an understanding of genetics or immunity. This chapter considers these from the perspective of the molecular lesion rather than the clinical manifestation. The following sections deal with genetic disorders and neuro-immunology, before examining abnormalities of ion channels, which can be affected by either inherited mutations or autoantibodies.

Genetics

Advances in genetics have had an enormous impact on the field of the inherited neurological disorders, possibly more so than in other areas of medicine. This reflects the wide phenotypic spectrum of neurological conditions and the increasing number of Mendelian genes that have been identified in these disorders. Genetic diseases can be divided into five main categories:

1 Abnormalities in the structure or complement of chromosomes (chromosomal disorders)
2 Mutations or other defects affecting a gene
3 Nucleotide repeat expansions
4 Mendelian disorders that are likely to be caused by digenic or epistatic inheritance, and
5 Conditions in which genetic and environmental factors interact (multifactorial disorders).

Modes of inheritance

Many neurological disorders follow single Mendelian gene inheritance, in both childhood and adult life. It is therefore essential to take a detailed family history and investigate appropriately.

A disease that is determined by a gene on one of the 22 autosomal chromosomes is said to be inherited as an autosomal trait. In the uncomplicated situation such traits affect both males and females alike and, according to the nature of the gene or mutation, may be either dominant or recessive. Similarly, traits determined by genes on one of the sex chromosomes may be either dominant or recessive, but here the effects on individuals of different sexes can vary greatly depending on which sex chromosome carries the gene and whether it acts in a dominant or recessive manner. Such traits are said to be sex-linked or often X-linked, because the vast majority involve genes on the X rather than the Y chromosome. A further form of inheritance is maternal, inherited from the mitochondrial genome; this is transmitted only from the mitochondria and often leads to extreme variability in disease phenotype.

Autosomal dominant inheritance

A dominantly inherited version of a gene, or allele, manifests in the heterozygous state. That is, a person who exhibits the effects of such a gene variant needs to possess it in only a single dose, as one member of the gene pair. When dealing with dominant alleles, an affected individual usually possesses both the mutant gene and its normal counterpart. Occasionally, a person may be found to be homozygous for a dominant allele, but this is extremely rare. An autosomal dominant trait affects both males and females alike and may be transmitted equally by either sex to their offspring of both sexes. When dealing with a condition in which the reproductive capacity is not limited, most affected individuals will have an affected parent, and the trait can often be traced from one generation to another within the family. Similar pedigrees can often be seen in large families with many of the more common autosomal dominant conditions that do not affect reproduction or survival until at least middle age, such as in Huntington's disease and myotonic dystrophy.

A person heterozygous for a dominant gene possesses both a normal and a mutant gene and will therefore produce gametes of two types in equal numbers, which bear one or the other allele. The partner will typically produce gametes only containing the normal allele. On average, half of their children will be affected, although of course with the small size of modern families the true proportion of affected offspring may deviate from this rule.

Autosomal dominant conditions can be very variable in their expression. In other words, the same allele can result in clinical manifestations that exhibit very varied degrees of severity in different individuals. For example, neurofibromatosis type 1 may cause a variety of very severe manifestation such as pseudoarthrosis of the tibia, mental handicap, intracranial tumours, scoliosis or even sarcomatous changes within neurofibromas. Yet, within the same family the gene can also be expressed mildly, resulting in no more than a few café-au-lait spots. When the degree of expression of the gene is very mild then such an individual may pass as normal and remain undetected – the gene is then said to be non-penetrant. It is lack of penetrance of the gene that gives rise on occasions to so-called skipped generations within affected families, when penetrance is defined only in terms of clinical manifestations. However minimal the clinical manifestation,

Neurology: A Queen Square Textbook, Second Edition. Edited by Charles Clarke, Robin Howard, Martin Rossor and Simon Shorvon.

any individual carrying the gene in question has a 50% risk of transmitting the gene to any offspring and there is unfortunately no way of predicting how severely any offspring might be affected.

Another feature of dominant traits, which frequently complicates genetic advice, is the occurrence of new or *de novo* mutations. When dealing with a condition that is typically associated with a significant reduction in fitness, the affected individual is often a sporadic case within the family. Such cases are frequently the result of new mutations, which occurred in either the maternal or paternal gametes, both parents being normal, so that the risk to siblings is very small. An example of such a condition is tuberous sclerosis, a disorder classically associated with a triad of clinical manifestations: mental handicap, epilepsy and adenoma sebaceum. As over 80% of patients exhibit mental handicap, few affected individuals lead normal lives. Emerging evidence suggests that the rate of new dominant mutations correlates with paternal age, and a significant paternal age effect has been demonstrated in a variety of conditions including Apert's syndrome, myositis ossificans and Marfan's syndrome.

Sometimes, an autosomal allele manifests more frequently in one sex than the other, a phenomenon referred to as sex influence. When in the extreme situation only one sex is affected then the phenomenon is known as sex limitation. This effect is probably mediated by hormonal influences. Sex-limited traits are not common, but this mode of inheritance has been suggested for male pattern baldness, thought to be autosomal dominant in males but autosomal recessive (see next section) in females. Females therefore transmit the trait when heterozygous but are bald only when homozygous.

Autosomal recessive inheritance

Disorders inherited in this way affect both sexes equally. Unlike autosomal dominant disorders, however, autosomal recessive conditions manifest only when the responsible gene variant is present in double dose (i.e. in the homozygous state). Thus, affected individuals usually have parents who are both heterozygous for the allele in question, but are clinically unaffected. Similarly, all the offspring of an affected person are usually healthy (although they are all heterozygous), so long as their other parent is not heterozygous for the same gene. As most of the recognised recessive traits are rare, however, this is not very likely in the absence of consanguinity. In the rare event that both parents are homozygous for the same recessive gene, then all of their children would be homozygotes and therefore affected. The pedigree pattern of an autosomal recessive trait is thus quite different from that of a classic autosomal dominant one. Characteristically, the disorder cannot be easily traced from generation to generation within the family; instead, affected individuals are often in the same generation, typically brothers and sisters. If a person is heterozygous for a particular abnormal gene then their gametes will be of two types and will contain either the mutant gene in question or its normal allele. On average therefore, one-quarter of the offspring of two heterozygotes will inherit a double dose of the recessive gene in question and be affected. Half of the offspring will be heterozygotes like the parents, and one-quarter will be normal homozygotes.

The gene variants responsible for most autosomal recessive conditions are rare in the general population. Two people related by blood are naturally more likely to carry a recessive allele in common than two strangers who are unrelated, because the former may have both inherited the allele from some common ancestor. It follows therefore that the two heterozygous parents of a person with an autosomal recessive trait are often found to be blood relatives (consanguineous marriage). The chance that two first cousins will inherit the same gene variant from their common ancestors is 1 in 8. The chance that two unrelated individuals carry the same allele is much smaller, but depends on the frequency of the allele in the population as a whole. Thus, the rarer the allele the more likely it is that the parents of an affected child will be found to be cousins. Sometimes, however, an affected child has inherited two different recessive mutations of the same gene from unrelated parents. This is known as compound heterozygosity.

Often, a condition that appears to be homozygous can in fact result from homozygosity of any one of many different recessive genes. For example, in profound early-onset deafness one of no fewer than 32 different loci may be involved. Thus, two deaf parents who both seem to have an autosomal recessive form of deafness may have children with normal hearing if the parents' problems are caused by involvement of different loci. In some 88% of the marriages of deaf individuals the other partner is also deaf. This is because people with a problem such as deafness are more likely to mix with other individuals having the same handicap, both in institutions catering for their special needs and socially.

Individuals heterozygous for a recessive gene are usually phenotypically normal. However, a situation where heterozygote identification is of value is when a relatively small and well-defined population has a high incidence of a recessive disorder (the gene frequency being high) and hence heterozygote tests will identify high risk marriages and thus enable accurate genetic advice to be given, coupled where possible with effective prenatal diagnosis. The best example of such a situation is Tay–Sachs disease (a severe recessive disorder producing blindness, progressive mental deterioration and death in early childhood) amongst the Ashkenazi Jewish community.

Sex-linked inheritance

Sex-linked inheritance is the mode of inheritance exhibited by genes carried on one or other of the sex chromosomes and can therefore be referred to as X-linkage or Y-linkage. Y-linked inheritance is extremely rare and mainly affects fertility. X-linked recessive traits are those determined by genes on the X chromosome that only manifest in the homozygous or hemizygous state. Females have two X chromosomes and therefore if they bear a mutant recessive defect on one of them it will be counteracted by the normal allele on their other X chromosome. Thus, females manifest such gene variants only in the homozygous state, which is extremely rare. Most females bearing such genes are therefore healthy female carriers of the trait who are themselves unaffected but who are at risk of having affected sons. As males have only one X chromosome they will always manifest an X-linked allele, even if it is recessive, as they have no normal allele to counteract it so all males who inherit such genes are affected. These diseases are transmitted within families either by healthy female carriers, if the disease is serious and leads to early death of affected males (such as Duchenne muscular dystrophy, Lesch–Nyhan syndrome and Lowe's syndrome), or by both female carriers and affected males, if the disease does not appreciably affect fertility and allows survival into the reproductive period (such as Fabry disease and Becker-type muscular dystrophy).

Occasionally, a woman may show manifestations of a disorder known to be an X-linked recessive trait, for example, some known carriers of Duchenne muscular dystrophy show manifestations of the disease, ranging from mild calf pseudohypertrophy to moderately severe proximal muscle weakness. In fact, such manifestations can result in diagnostic confusion and suggest a limb girdle form of muscular dystrophy, in the absence of a family history. The distinction between the two situations has important implications.

An X-linked dominant trait manifests both in the hemizygous male and in the heterozygous female. The mutant gene is transmitted by affected females to half of their daughters and by affected males to all of their daughters. The trait is also transmitted by affected females to half their sons, but all the sons of affected males are normal. There is thus an excess of affected females in such families. Examples of conditions showing this less common mode of inheritance are vitamin D-resistant rickets and the oral-facial-digital syndrome. Some rare X-linked dominant traits, such as incontinentia pigmenti, are believed to be lethal in the hemizygous affected male. In such a situation all affected individuals are female and occur in a direct line of descent. Affected females have a deficiency of live-born sons and an excess of abortions (which may be shown to be male fetuses).

Mitochondrial disorders

This group of conditions is caused by dysfunctional mitochondria. More than 70 different polypeptides interact on the inner mitochondrial membrane to form the mitochondrial respiratory chain. The vast majority of subunits are synthesised within the cytosol from nuclear gene transcripts, but 13 essential subunits are encoded by the 16.5 kilobase (kb) mitochondrial genomic DNA (mtDNA).

Mitochondrial diseases are, in about 15% of cases, caused by mutations in the mtDNA that affects mitochondrial function. Other causes of mitochondrial disease are mutations in nuclear mitochondrial genes, whose gene products are imported into the mitochondria, and a variety of acquired disorders. mtDNA defects are transmitted by maternal inheritance. Deletions generally occur *de novo* and thus cause disease in one family member only, with no significant risk to other family members. mtDNA point mutations and duplications, however, may be transmitted to several individuals down the maternal line. The father of a proband is not at risk of having the disease-causing mtDNA mutation, but the mother usually carries the mitochondrial mutation and may or may not have symptoms. An affected male does not transmit the mtDNA mutation to his offspring.

Included in this group are progressive disorders of childhood and adult life, which may affect the central nervous system (CNS), muscle, or both, as well as other systems. Commoner neurological diseases caused by mitochondrial point mutations include myoclonic epilepsy with ragged red fibres (MERRF), mitochondrial encephalomyopathy, lactic acidosis, and stroke-like episodes (MELAS), and Leber's hereditary optic neuropathy. Chronic progressive external ophthalmoplegia (CPEO) is usually the result of a large deletion. Mitochondrial disorders can present with quite variable features. For instance, the m.3243A>G point mutation may cause MELAS, CPEO, diabetes mellitus or deafness.

An important determinant of disease severity is the variable proportion of mutant mtDNA occurring in cells, known as heteroplasmy. A female harbouring a heteroplasmic mtDNA point mutation may transmit a variable amount of mutant mtDNA to her offspring, resulting in considerable clinical variability among siblings within the same family. mtDNA heteroplasmy complicates prenatal genetic testing and the interpretation of test results for mtDNA disorders. Unfortunately, molecular testing is often unable to predict the severity of the condition, as the degree of heteroplasmy varies from tissue to tissue, and can only be an approximate guide to the likelihood of clinical problems occurring.

Expanded repeat disorders

Repeats of simple nucleotide sequences occur frequently throughout the genome, and the vast majority are not associated with any disease. In 1991, an expansion in a trinucleotide (CAG) repeat in the androgen receptor gene was identified as the cause of Kennedy's disease or spinal and bulbar muscular atrophy 1 (SBMA). The repeat, which normally consists of 13–30 CAGs, lengthens to 40 or more CAGs in patients with this disease. Over the last 25 years, over 20 further disorders have been found to be caused by expanded trinucleotide repeats, including Huntington's disease and a number of spinocerebellar ataxias (Table 3.1). More recently, an expanded hexanucleotide repeat (GGGGCC in the *C9orf72* gene) has been

Table 3.1 Disorders caused by expanded trinucleotide repeats. (a) Polyglutamine disorders caused by a gain-of-function mechanism. The repeat unit is (CAG)n in all these disorders.

Disease	OMIM number	Gene product	Normal repeat length	Expanded repeat length	Main clinical features
HD	143100	Huntingtin	6–34	36–121	Chorea, dystonia, cognitive decline
SCA1	164400	Ataxin1	6–44	39–82	Ataxia, cognitive impairment
SCA2	183090	Ataxin2	15–24	32–200	Ataxia, axonal neuropathy
SCA3	109150	Ataxin3	13–36	61–84	Ataxia, parkinsonism
SCA6	183086	CACNA1A	4–19	20–33	Ataxia
SCA7	164500	Ataxin7	4–35	37–306	Ataxia, maculopathy
SCA17	607136	TBP	25–42	47–63	Ataxia, cognitive decline, chorea
SBMA	313200	Androgen receptor	9–36	38–62	Motor weakness, swallowing, gynaecomastia
DRPLA	125370	Atrophin	7–34	49–88	Ataxia, seizures, dementia

DRPLA, dentatorubral pallidoluysian atrophy; HD, Huntington's disease; SBMA, spinobulbar muscular atrophy; SCA, spinocerebellar atrophy.

Table 3.1 (b) Other unstable repeat disorders.

Disease	OMIM number	Repeat unit	Gene product	Normal repeat length	Expanded repeat length	Main clinical features
Loss-of-function mechanism						
FRAXA	309550	(CGC)n	FMRP	6–60	>200	Mental retardation
FRAXE	309548	(CCG)n	FMR2	4–39	200–900	Mental retardation
FRDA	229300	(GAA)n	Frataxin	6–32	200–1700	Sensory ataxia, cardiomyopathy
RNA mediated toxicity						
DM1	160900	(CTG)n	DMPK	5–37	56–10 000	Myotonia, weakness, cardiac involvement, diabetes, cataracts
DM2	602668	(CCTG)n	ZNF9	10–26	75–11 000	Similar to DM1, more proximal weakness
FXTAS	309550	(CGC)n	FMR1	6–60	60–200	Ataxia, tremor, parkinsonism
C9ORF72	105550	(GGGGCC)n	C9ORF72	1–29	Usually >1000	ALS, FTD can present as CBD
Unknown pathogenic mechanism						
SCA8	608768	(CTG)n	SCA8 RNA	16–34	>74	Ataxia, cognitive decline
SCA10	603516	(ATTCT)n		10–20	500–4500	Ataxia, tremor, dementia
SCA12	604326	(CAG)n	PPP2R2B	7–45	55–78	Ataxia and seizures
HDL2	606438	(CTG)n	Junctophilin	7–28	66–78	Similar to HD
SCA31	117210	(TGGAA)n	BEAN	1	2.5–3.8 kb	Ataxia and neuropathy
SCA36	614153	(GGCCTG)n	NOP56	1	650–2500	Ataxia, tongue fasciculations, deafness

ALS, amyotrophic lateral sclerosis; CBD, corticobasal degeneration; DM1/2, myotonic dystrophy types 1 and 2; DRPLA, dentatorubral pallidoluysian atrophy; FRAXA/E, fragile X mental retardation; FTD, frontotemporal dementia; FXTAS, fragile X tremor/ataxia syndrome; HD, Huntington's disease; SBMA, spinobulbar muscular atrophy; SCA, spinocerebellar atrophy.

shown to be the most common cause of familial amyotrophic lateral sclerosis and frontotemporal dementia in many populations.

The CAG codon is normally translated as a glutamine residue, and abnormal CAG repeats therefore result in expanded polyglutamine tracts in the respective proteins. These disorders often exhibit anticipation, where disease severity worsens in successive generations, and this correlates with an increase in the number of repeats. The expansion is also greater when inherited from the paternal line and interruptions in the expansion can modify the age at onset. Although the expanded polyglutamine tract itself can be toxic, it is in the context of the full-length protein that the distinctive selective neuronal loss occurs. Some nucleotide triplet expansion diseases cause polyalanine tracts. Triplet, penta- and hexanucleotide repeat expansions have also been identified in non-coding regions, typically causing a loss of gene function or toxic effects at the mRNA level.

How heritable are neurological conditions? Lessons from twins

Monozygotic ('identical') twins share the same genetic inheritance but their environments differ increasingly as they age. This unique aspect of twins makes them an excellent model for understanding how heritable a disorder may be and how genes and the environment contribute to certain traits, especially complex behaviours and diseases. Identical or monozygotic twins share nearly 100% of their genes, which means that most differences between twins (such as height, susceptibility to boredom, intelligence, depression, etc.) are brought about by environmental factors. Fraternal or dizygotic twins share only about 50% of their genes and therefore act as a powerful control sample.

To illustrate this, if one of a pair of twins is affected by schizophrenia, the risk to a monozygotic twin is approximately 50%, while that to a dizygotic twin is only about 10–15%. This difference is evidence for a strong genetic component in susceptibility to schizophrenia. However, the fact that the monozygotic twin of an affected individual does not develop the disease 100% of the time indicates that other factors are involved. In migraine with aura the correlation of liability has been estimated at 68% in monozygotic twin pairs, with no significant difference between males and females. Similar twin studies have provided evidence that genetic factors have a role in many other neurological disorders (Table 3.2).

Mutation versus polymorphism

Every individual has over 20 000 genetic variants in the protein-encoding exons and flanking intronic regions. The vast majority of these variants are thought to have no deleterious consequences (benign polymorphisms), but some of these genetic changes can be associated with human disease. Disease-causing genetic mutations are rare and proving the pathogenicity of a genetic variant is often difficult. The criteria to identify a sequence variant as a pathogenic mutation include the following:

- The variant causes a change to the encoded protein, through an amino acid substitution, insertion or deletion, or through a nonsense change (frameshift and premature stop codon).
- The affected amino acid is conserved across species.
- The variant occurs in more than one family and segregates with the disease.
- The genetic variation is absent in normal controls.

Not all of these criteria are always satisfied. Other factors can help clarify the status of candidate variants, such as the putative gene function and pathway being defective in other neurological disorders with similar features, and evidence from gene expression in affected tissues.

Table 3.2 Examples of monozygotic twin concordance rates for different neurological disorders.

Alzheimer dementia	60–80%	Twin studies
Autism	70–90%	Twin studies
Epilepsy	80%	Twin study
Frontotemporal dementia	42%	Family history data
Multiple sclerosis	25–76%	Twin studies
Migraine with aura	68%	Twin study
Restless legs syndrome	40–90%	Twin studies

Ethnic diversity can confound the search for disease-causing mutations, because the frequencies of individual polymorphisms vary across populations, some of which are under-represented in available databases. In addition, truly normal control series are difficult to identify for some age-dependent disorders.

The discovery process

In the early days of gene discovery the disease gene was identified by the nature of the disorder. For example, a known enzyme deficiency was shown to be caused by a genetic defect in the gene coding for that enzyme. Subsequently, many new disease genes were identified from analysis of rare large families, groups of smaller but clinically identical families or sibling pairs, and candidate or genome-wide association studies. Initially, linkage analysis or homozygosity mapping was carried out to identify the genetic region, followed by sequencing of candidate genes within this region using the Sanger method. This approach was, and still is in some areas, very effective, but it is very expensive and time consuming.

Recently, the technical barriers to identifying disease-causing mutations and rare variants have been overcome with next generation sequencing (NGS), where one of the most promising avenues is whole exome sequencing of all protein-encoding regions (exomes) and intron boundaries. Even more complete is whole genome sequencing (introns and exons). Next generation sequencing platforms produced by various companies use different technologies, but in general are high-throughput, producing thousands or millions of sequences at the same time. In finding mutations and risk variants this method offers four critical advantages over the traditional linkage and positional cloning approaches: cost, speed, the use of relatively little DNA and the capacity to use genetically less informative samples. A large number of samples that were previously unsuitable for gene identification can now be used to find novel mutations. Although exome sequencing is a relatively new method, it has already been used to identify mutations that cause Mendelian forms of disease (Figure 3.1). Although this technique generates enormous

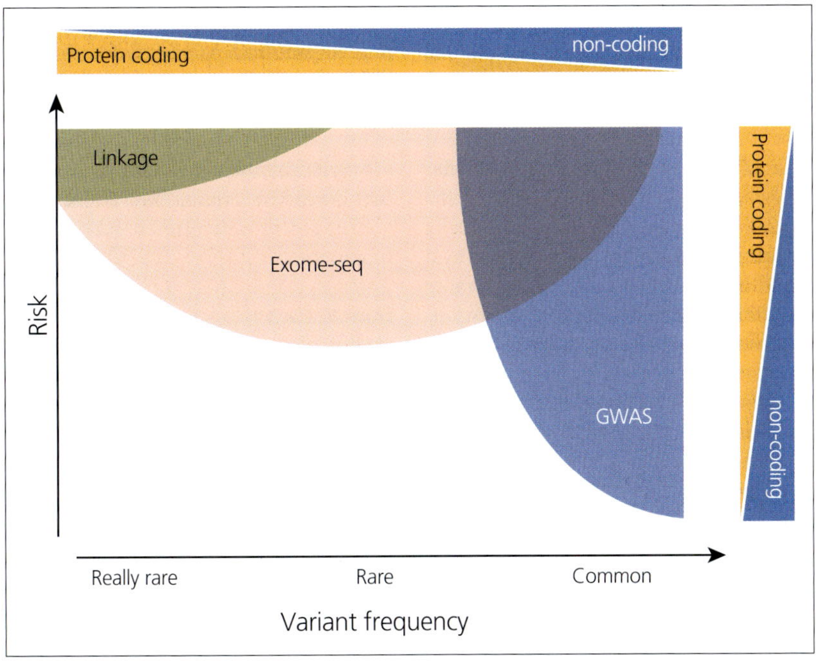

Figure 3.1 Exome sequencing will identify the Mendelian variants previously found using linkage as well as a proportion of variants identified using genome-wide association studies (GWAS).

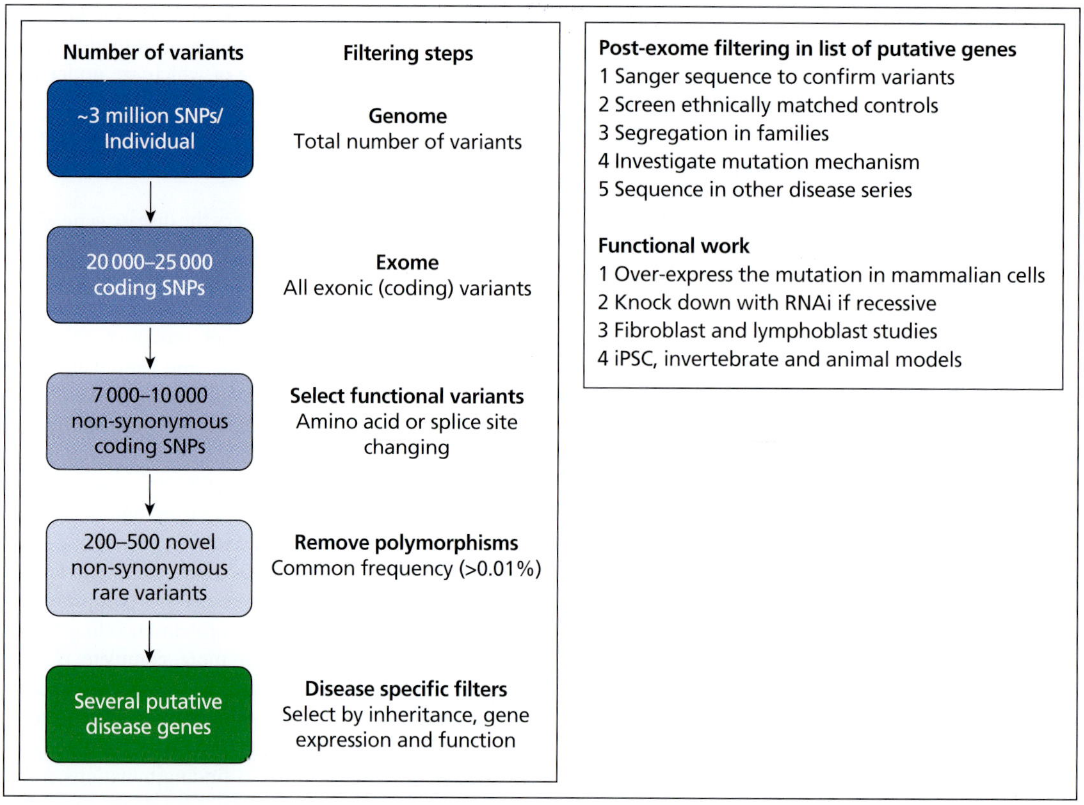

Figure 3.2 Filtering and functional analysis strategy for next generation sequencing data. SNP, single nucleotide polymorphism.

amounts of data, it does not overcome the challenge of differentiating between normal genetic variability and pathogenic mutations, and so it is important to analyse a large number of affected individuals, compare them with unaffected individuals, and interpret the data in the context of gene expression and gene network data (Figure 3.2).

Next generation sequencing typically involves exome sequencing of several affected and unaffected family members, where possible including affected cousins or other distant relatives. In the first instance DNA is extracted and a genome library made from each individual; after this libraries are enriched for exome regions, pooled and sequenced. The most difficult part of NGS is the data analysis which involves the need for a powerful computer cluster to align sequences, remove duplicates and annotate the data sequence and variants. When investigating disease-causing mutations, common polymorphisms and non-coding amino acid changes are then removed to leave a list of unique or very rare (<0.01% of the population) variants that are either heterozygous or homozygous. Another important issue is the degree of exome coverage, because sequencing has an inherent error rate. A high quality exome sequencing data set can achieve average exome-wide coverage of 30-fold, meaning that a typical sequence will have been read 30 times. Difficult regions to sequence are the GC rich exon 1 and repeat-rich regions.

Practical considerations

When considering genetic testing of an individual it is important to understand the practical and financial considerations. Moreover, although genetic factors have a role in an increasing number of diseases, the yield and implications are very different in, say, Parkinson's disease, than in classically inherited disorders such as Charcot–Marie Tooth (CMT) disease. In the Neurogenetics Laboratory at The National Hospital for Neurology and Neurosurgery we have a three-tier approach to genetic screening (Figure 3.3):

1 Initial screening of the common genetic defects or disease genes, which can often also be screened at low cost (Figure 3.4)
2 Secondary screening of the rarer disease-associated genes using a gene panel approach, and
3 Diagnostic exome sequencing (Figure 3.5).

As a way to increase the chance of obtaining a genetic cause, many patients and families are enrolled in research programmes to sequence multiple individuals in the family. This can increase the diagnostic yield, but all research results must be first confirmed in a diagnostic laboratory before they are released to patients.

Ethical considerations: predictive versus diagnostic

Predictive (presymptomatic) genetic testing is often offered to individuals at risk, typically in the late-onset autosomal dominant inherited conditions. Our experience of predictive testing mainly comes from Huntington's disease and other life-limiting conditions. More recently, patients with other conditions such as CMT or DYT1 dystonia are increasingly being referred for testing. The genetic counselling required for predictive testing is considerably different from that required for diagnostic testing, and requires a specialist team consisting of a neurogeneticist (or neurologist and clinical geneticist), clinical nurse specialist, local and actively involved diagnostic laboratory, and access to other specialists in fields such as psychiatry. For some conditions, at least two outpatient visits are required before a result is given on the third clinic

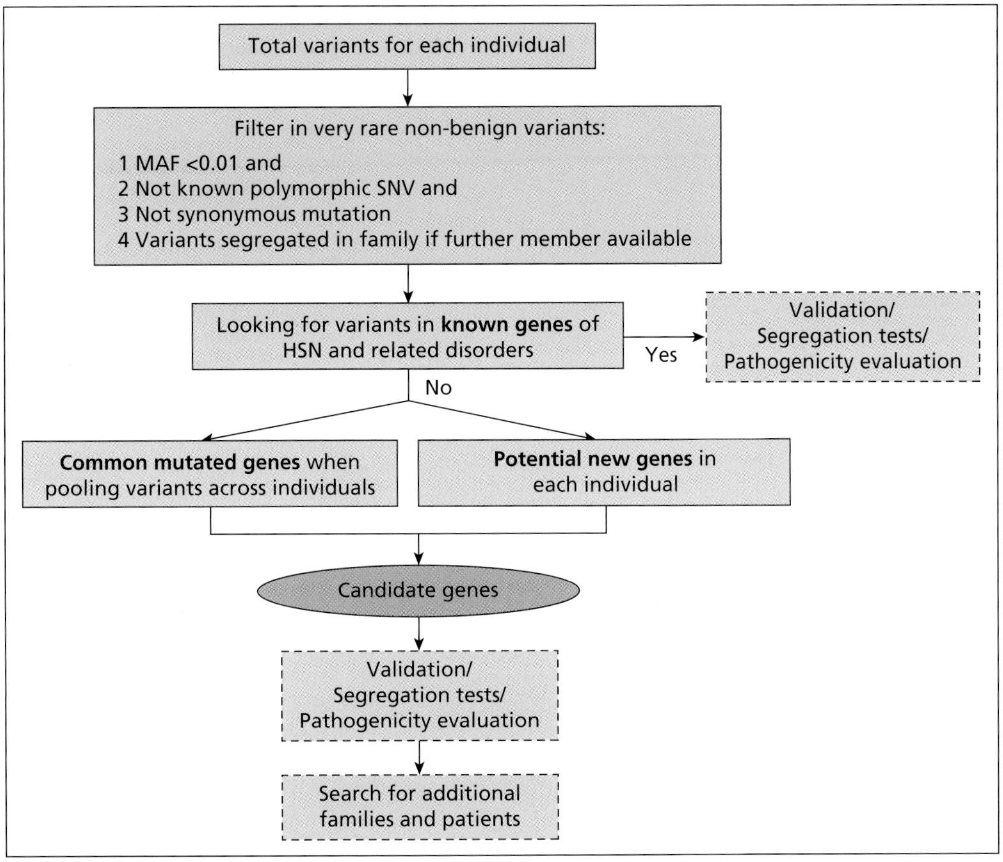

Figure 3.3 Analysis strategy as applied to diseases such as hereditary sensory neuropathy (HSN). MAF, minor allele frequency; SNV, single nucleotide variant.

visit to ensure that the individual fully understands the serious implications of having a positive test result. Important considerations before a result is given are as follow:

1 Does the individual really wish for testing and can the person give full consent?
2 Do the individual and family understand all the implications (and limitations)?
3 Issues involving family, work, insurance, wider life, and
4 Disclosure and confidentiality issues.

Prenatal diagnosis is often undertaken in patients who have had a positive predictive test result or are in the early stages of the disease. In the past, prenatal testing was usually undertaken in recessive childhood-onset disorders, but prenatal testing is now frequently carried out in adult-onset dominantly inherited disorders. Testing is usually carried out at 10 weeks' gestation with chorionic villus sampling. More recently, pre-implantation diagnostic testing has become more readily available. This relies on *in vitro* fertilisation and selective implantation of mutation-negative embryos into the uterus. At present, various logistical and cost limitations mean that only about 20% of procedures result in a pregnancy going to term.

Incidental findings in diagnostic exome and genome sequencing

Exome and genome sequencing reveal information on virtually every gene in the human genome, delivering disease predisposing variants on putatively every allele. Therefore, even if no primary genetic result is obtained and the familial neurological disease gene is not identified, there are multiple and potentially hundreds of incidental results that can be offered to individuals and families. Whether all or some of these incidental results should be returned leads to complicated ethical and practical issues. Which incidental results should be returned? How can they best be used to improve health?

The lack of clear guidance for returning incidental results from exome and genome sequencing is compounded by challenges to how to communicate genetic results clearly. Recently, the American College of Medical Genetics and Genomics (ACMG) and the European Society of Human Genetics (ESHG) have issued recommendations on the return of incidental results from exome and genome sequencing. The ACMG recommended that from exome and genome sequencing, mutations in a list of 57 known disease-associated genes should be reported as the minimum. The ESHG made the subtly different recommendation that the results from only specific genes or sets of genes should be returned to patients, and genetic variants with limited or no clinical utility should be filtered out (if possible neither analysed nor reported). These recommendations have proven to be controversial and there are still divergent views on whether and, if so, what incidental results should be offered for return, issues of informed consent, and providing results for adult-onset conditions to the parents of children who undergo exome and genome sequencing.

The majority of individuals who have undergone exome or genome sequencing so far are of Northern European descent and

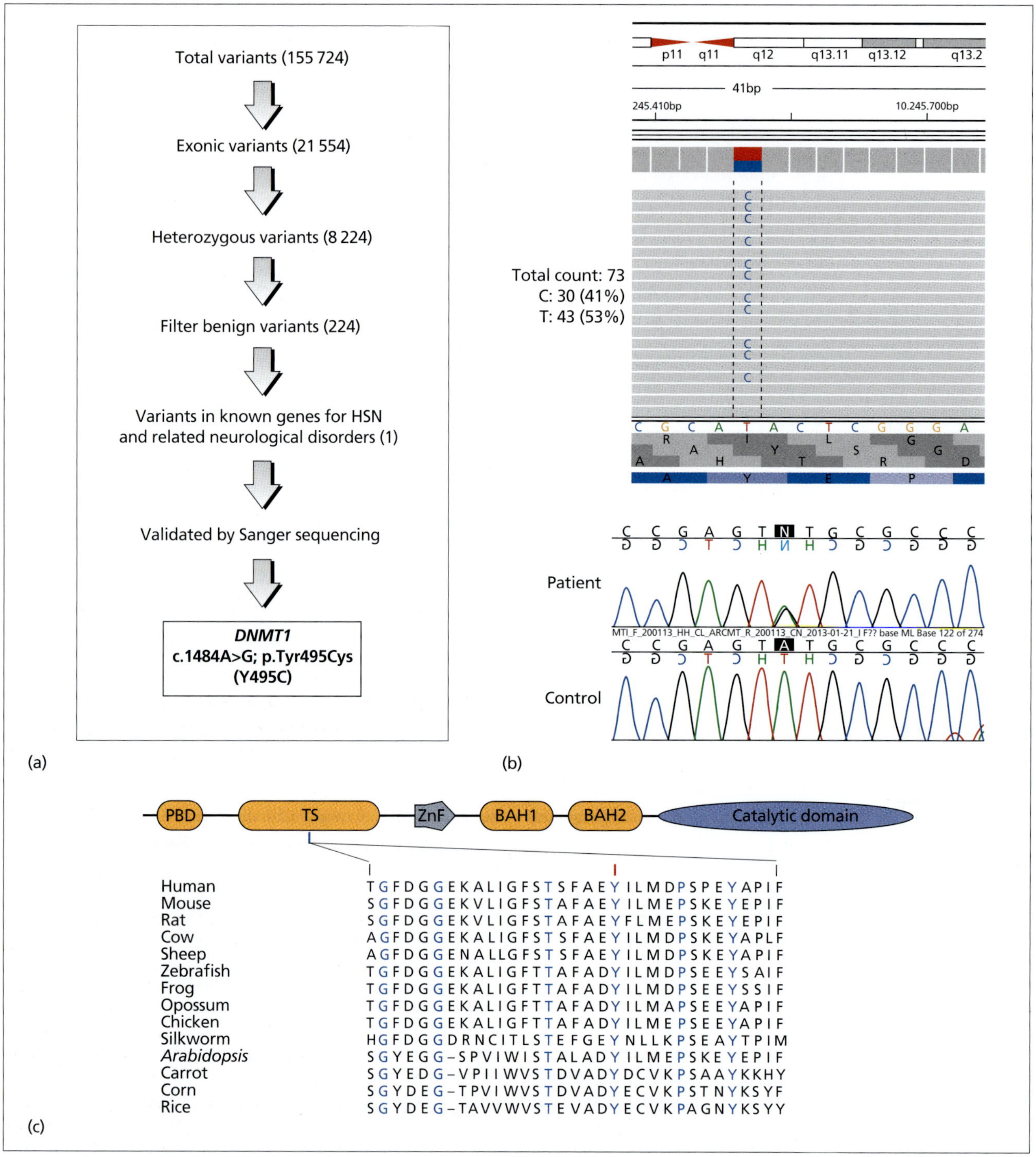

Figure 3.4 Analysis strategy as applied to an autosomal dominant disease such as hereditary sensory neuropathy (HSN) identifying the *DNMT1* gene. (a) Filtering of exome data, total variants refers to exon and flaking intronic changes. (b) Exome viewer shows the proportion of A to G as in a dominant mutation. (c) Sanger sequencing to confirm the variant. (d) Species conservation of this mutation.

we therefore still have a great deal to understand about other population genetic variants and incidental findings. In large-scale exome sequencing in 500 European and 500 African descent adult participants, the number of incidental findings were lower than expected: 3.4% for European descent and 1.2% for African descent of the high-penetrance actionable pathogenic or likely pathogenic variants. Although these data suggest there will be fewer significant variants to discuss and address with patients, the exome or genome will still contain variants of different risk potency for human disease, and other factors such as response to drug treatments.

The diagnostic efficiency of exome and genome sequencing far outweighs the drawbacks of using this technology. Careful

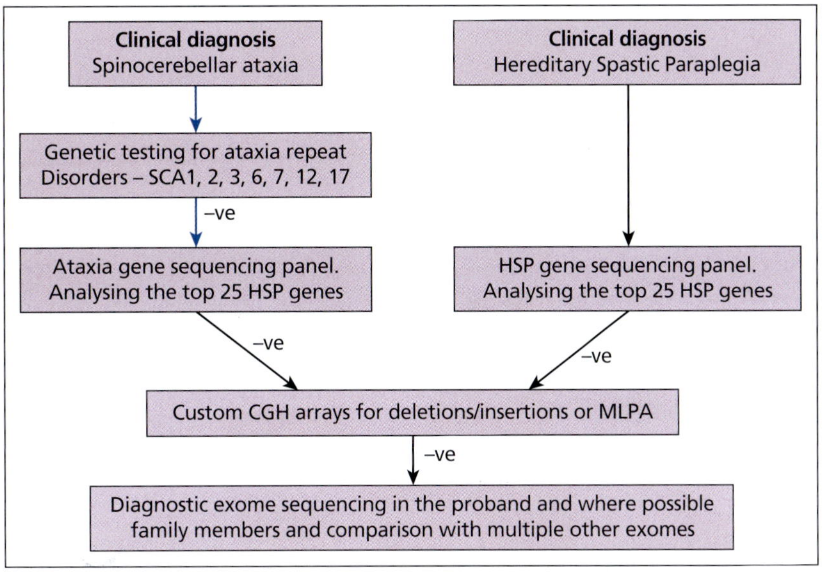

Figure 3.5 The approach to diagnostic testing in disorders such as ataxia where the initial genetic analysis can identify around half of the cases and the extremely heterogeneous, hereditary spastic paraplegia (HSP) where a gene panel and exome approach are initially required. CGH, comparative genomic hybridisation; MLPA, multiplex ligation-dependent amplification.

consideration needs to be given when returning results to patients and families where the main focus must be on identifying the cause of their neurological disease as opposed to delivering uninterpretable incidental findings.

Autoimmunity

Fundamentals

The immune system is a dynamic tissue with a series of elements that perform a specific set of actions to maintain homeostasis of an organism. At its most fundamental, the immune system distinguishes the self from non-self organisms and acts to delete, disable or inactivate foreign invaders. In more complex functionality it also distinguishes damaged, irreparable or altered self from normal tissue to maintain a healthy homeostatic state, interacting closely with physiological and biochemical processes. Where surveillance or activity fail, infection or neoplasia can thrive; where active components become misdirected autoimmune disease (the horror autotoxicus of Ehrlich) may be the result.

The immune system has a number of tools at its disposal, varying in complexity, specificity and phylogenetic developmental diversity, which act in conjunction with one another in a complex interdependent immunological 'soup'. Interference in one aspect of the immune system inevitably causes imbalance in other aspects, although elements of redundancy and shared functionality provide a safety backup system. Therapeutic interventions can have unintended effects because of interference with a balanced system (sometimes already disturbed by disease processes), and these may be severe or life threatening. As therapeutics become increasingly potent and specific so we will see more specific 'lesional' pathologies as fallout from immunotherapeutics. When and if these events occur (not always predictably) they will inevitably teach us about how the immune system works, unfortunately at the expense of those exposed to them.

The CNS and peripheral nervous system (PNS) are afforded some special protection by and from the immune system resulting in a number of diseases caused by invading pathogens (e.g. meningitis), unsuppressed opportunists (toxoplasmosis or progressive multifocal leukoencephalopathy, PML) or autoimmune diseases (multiple sclerosis and Guillain–Barré syndrome). Each of these diseases are discussed in the relevant chapters but the purpose of this chapter is to introduce some broad concepts of disease to assist in understanding at a more general level. Readers who wish to study the specifics of immunology and its relation to disease are referred to excellent up-to-date textbooks of immunology and autoimmune disease.

Components of the immune system

The immune system is a highly developed and as yet imperfectly understood homeostasis mechanism protecting us from pathogens, inflammation and tumours. A detailed description of all its elements is beyond the scope of this chapter. A basic understanding of the components of the immune system, how they interact and how they are modified to regulate immunity in the CNS and PNS is crucial to the understanding of immune diseases. Failure of one or more components or failure of the regulation of normal homeostasis results in disease through pathogen invasion, inflammation or autoimmunity. Modulation of components of the immune system is the basis of immunotherapeutics, a rapidly developing field. Some therapeutics are relatively non-discriminatory (e.g. steroids and cyclophosphamide), whereas newer biologic agents are highly specific and exceedingly potent (e.g. rituximab and alemtuzumab). The ability to lesion the immune system so specifically increases our understanding of individual component functions, but can result in unintended opportunist infection (e.g. PML) or other autoimmune dysregulation (e.g. glomerulonephritis following alemtuzumab use).

Innate immune system

The innate immune system (IIS) refers to the germ line complex of recognition molecules and receptors, effector molecules and cells that provide the immediate recognition and response to invasion and which perform a crucial role in immunohomeostasis

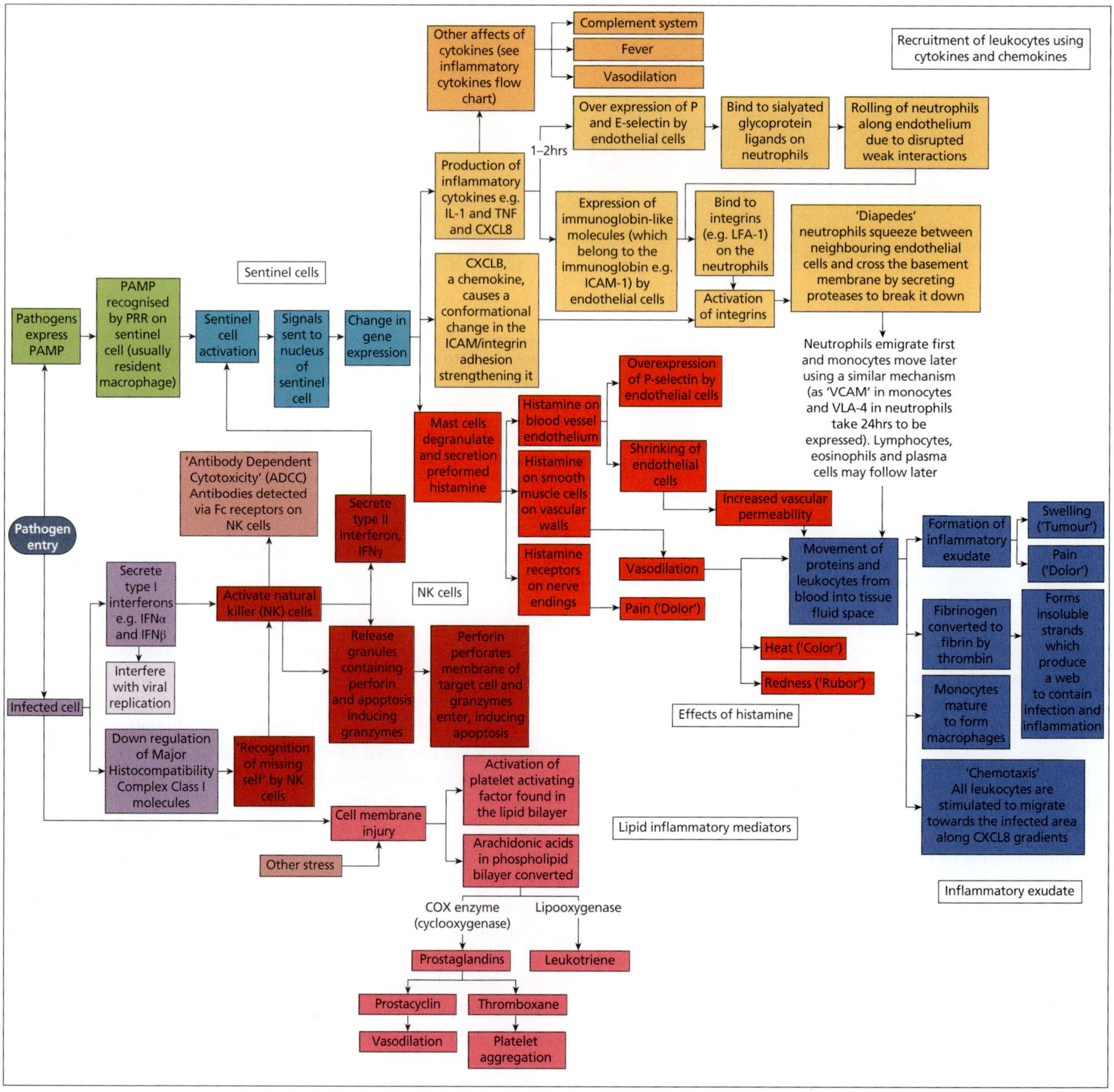

Figure 3.6 Innate immune system. Source: Architha Srinivasan (own work) used under the terms of the Creative Commons Licence CC-BY-SA-3.

(Figure 3.6). The IIS was considered to predate phylogenetically the acquired and adaptive immune system, but adaptive cell components utilise elements of the IIS, and each system interacts with the other such that they must have developed, for a large part, in parallel. The IIS, being the first line of defence, has elements that are concentrated at epithelial surfaces. The CNS and the PNS are sites of relative immune privilege and as such are relatively protected from invasion but also maintained in a state of immune hyporesponsiveness where innate reactions are not so florid. Nevertheless, the IIS has a crucial role in defence against neurological diseases. More importantly, its activity, inactivity or maldirection has important roles in the genesis of some diseases. Modification of the the IIS can be important in the control and treatment of neurological disease.

The IIS is crucial in the early response to invasion by pathogens. When one considers the doubling time of most bacterial pathogens is 20–30 minutes and an adaptive immune response requires days to develop, control and restriction of invasion at an early stage is critical to survival of the organism. The IIS generates the cardinal features of inflammation (rubor, calor, dolor and tumour, or redness, heat, pain and swelling), which engage all the elements of the immune system in containment and control. It is also important in the later stages of disease where the clearance of non-specific debris from cell death an inflammation result in suppression and cessation of inflammation.

The components of the IIS include the following:

1 Physical barriers with tight junctions in epithelial and endothelial surfaces, for example the blood–brain and blood–nerve barriers.

2 Pathogen recognition molecules that are secreted, on the cell surface or cytosolic. These are non-adaptive peptides that recognise components of invading pathogens. They include Toll-like receptors, lectins (e.g. mannose binding proteins), defensins, cathelcidins, collectins and others. The diversity of these recognition molecules restricts the ability of pathogens to adapt and evade them. Furthermore, the pathogen-associated molecular patterns that pathogen recognition molecules target are usually so crucial to pathogen survival that mutation results in death of the pathogen.
3 Enzymes released extracellularly, or more usually into lysosomes, which result in death of endocytosed or nearby organisms (e.g. proteases, lysozyme and NADPH oxidase).
4 Signalling molecules such as cytokines, which attract cells of the innate and adaptive immune system to sites of inflammation or attack (e.g. interleukins 1 and 8, IL-1 and IL-8) as well as cytokines that turn down the response and turn off the response (IL-10).
5 The complement cascade, crucial to the opsonisation of pathogens and chemo-attraction. A further discussion of complement is beyond the scope of this chapter but its importance in disease is critical both in the immediate innate response to pathogen invasion and also through tissue damage caused in disease. The complement cascade is the focus of significant therapeutic interest as inhibition of the cascade almost entirely abrogates paroxysmal nocturnal haemoglobinuria and may also be effective in Guillain–Barré syndrome. A major consequence of inhibition of the system is the potential for severe and life-threatening infection with infectious organisms such as meningococci.
6 Cells recognising and presenting antigens to the adaptive immune system, such as macrophages, dendritic cells and epithelial cells.
7 Cells releasing killing substances (mast cells, neutrophils, natural killer cells).
8 Phagocytic cells (macrophages and monocytes) which endocytose pathogens and opsonised materials. These also phagocytose apoptotic effector cells, a process called efferocytosis, before they are able to spill their remaining toxic contents. This functions to turn off responses and maintain immunological homeostasis.

Adaptive immune system

The adaptive or acquired immune system refers to cells of the lymphoid lineage and the genetically modifiable displayed and secreted molecules from those cells. The cellular components are B cells, which display and secrete immunoglobulin, and T cells, which display T-cell receptors and associated complexes. T cells include both effector cells, providing cell-mediated cytotoxic responses as well as antibody-dependent cellular cytotoxicity, and helper cells interacting with B cells and cells of the innate immune system. The secretion of affinity-matured antigen-specific immunoglobulins by B cells is their primary function and these mark out pathogens and debris for clearance. The adaptive immune system would function poorly without the innate immune system, and likewise the innate immune system requires the backup of the adaptive system to complete the clearance of suppressed foreign material.

Lymphoid cells are generated in the primary lymphoid tissues of the thymus gland (T cells) and the bone marrow (B cells). Lymphoid cells originate from the haematopoietic stem cells by a process of asymmetric division. During very early development the daughter cells migrate to the liver but during late embryonic and postnatal development further differentiation, selection, deletion and anergy takes place in the thymus and bone marrow. The secondary lymphoid tissues (lymph nodes and spleen) are the sites of antigen presentation to the lymphoid cells and B- and T-cell interaction resulting in activation, antigen affinity processing and expansion, following which escape to the peripheries releases cells to sites of activity.

T cells T cells orchestrate many of the functions of the adaptive immune response. T cells mediate their own activity, provide help to B cells and participate in cell-mediated immunity, destroying invading pathogens and neoplastic or potentially neoplastic cells. T cells derive their specificity from a cell-specific, genetically encoded, surface-bound, multi-subunit T-cell receptor (TCR) which recognises peptides presented in the context of major histocompatibility complex (MHC) class 1 or 2 on the surface of antigen presenting cells (APCs) following intracellular processing. About 95% of TCRs are of the α/β lineage and the remainder are γ/δ T cells. γ/δ T cells are not well understood and may be more involved in processing non-peptide-like antigen, possibly encountered on epithelial surfaces. They develop and mature through slightly different processes to the α/β, driving some autonomous development through various checkpoints in the thymus. They expand very little in lymphoid tissue but may undergo considerable expansion in the periphery (Figure 3.7). It is thought that γ/δ T cells are more involved than α/β T cells in the pathogenesis of inflammatory neuropathies such as chronic inflammatory demyelinating polyradiculoneuropathy (CIDP) where the driving stimulus may be carbohydrate-rich invading pathogens.

During development, mononuclear cells of the lymphocyte lineage first become committed to being T cells and they then begin the process of TCR gene rearrangement. They are presented with antigen in the thymus as they transit through interactions in the thymic cortex and then medulla. T cells that have no recognition of self MHC are deleted (positive selection). Following commitment from double positive ($CD4^+/CD8^+$) to single positive ($CD4^+$ or $CD8^+$) cells, they are presented with antigen. Those with strong affinity for self antigens are deleted, which protects against autoimmunity (negative selection). Those with rather weaker interactions may become anergic. Those that do not have a recognition event are rescued from pre-programmed apoptosis, matured and moved to the secondary tissues.

The TCRs on all T cells are non-covalently linked to the CD3 molecular complex. The five subunits of the CD3 complex transduce activating signals through the T-cell membrane following interaction with the peptide–MHC complex on APCs. Both CD4 and CD8 are associated with the intracellular src-family tyrosine kinase Lck, which is responsible for T-cell activation. CD4 and CD8 are also non-covalently associated with accessory molecules, which serve to determine the specific actions of the T cell as a helper or cytotoxic T cell. There are about 15 of these present on the surface of T cells which also serve as co-receptors and factors in T-cell adhesion and activation, such as CD2, CD27, CD28, CD134, and CD137.

Once matured, T cells are released to patrol the peripheries, and mostly are found in secondary lymphoid tissues. The classic mature T cells are either cytotoxic or modulatory/regulatory. Cytotoxic T cells are CD8-positive and see antigen presented in the context of MHC 1. Conversely, CD4 cells recognise antigen presented in the context of MHC II and are conventionally referred to as T-helper cells. However, CD4 cells can be also cytotoxic in graft rejection. Further blurring the distinction into cytotoxic and modulatory cells, CD8 cells can participate in normal physiological

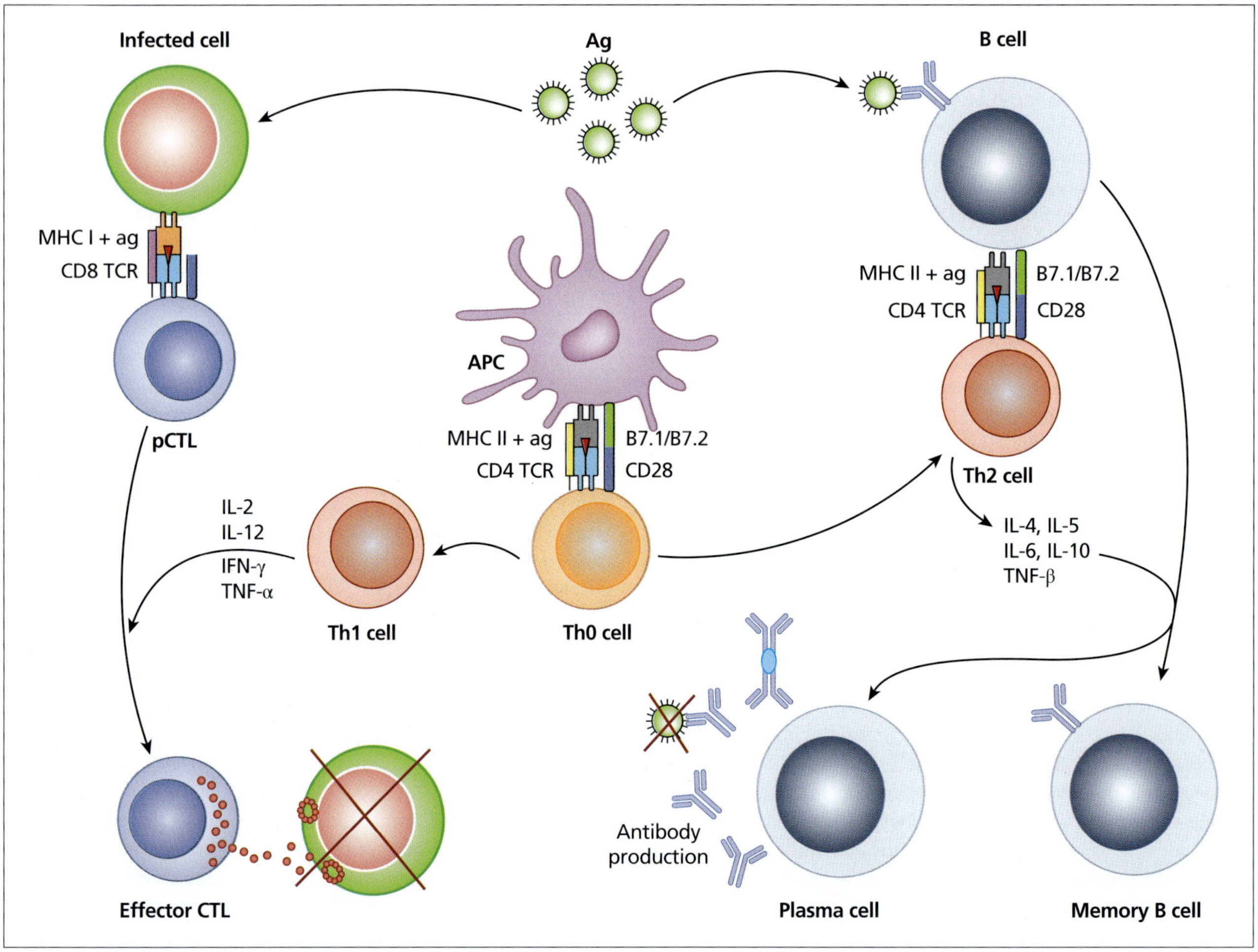

Figure 3.7 Basic stimulation and maturation initiation of B and T cells. Antigen is displayed on the surface of antigen presenting cells (APC) and in the presence of co-stimulatory signals matures T_h cells which in turn assist in B-cell activation and T-cytotoxic responses. Maturation of both T-cell receptors and B-cell surface antibody through gene rearrangement matures specificity of responses. Immune responses are effected directly through B and T-cell mechanisms or the chemotactic recruitment of other cells and cytokines deliver appropriate immune responses. APC, antigen-presenting cell; IFN, interferon; IL, interleukin; MHC, major histocompatibility class; Th, T-helper; TNF, tumour necrosis factor. Source: De Haes 2012. Used under the Creative Commons licence CC-BY-3.

inflammation and have some helper roles. In addition, CD4 cells not only provide 'help' to modulate B-cell responses, but also act as regulatory T cells (T_{reg}) and T-suppressor (T_{sup}) cells. Th1, Th2, Th9 and Th17 responses are determined by different states of differentiation of CD4 cells from a Th0 state by the cytokine milieu. Th1 cells are traditionally 'inflammatory' driving T-help for delayed hypersensitivity reactions and some B-cell help. Th2 responses are more humorally directed, especially stimulating IgE and eosinophils. Th9 responses (driven by IL9) are thought to be tumour directed, but their actions and development remain under investigation. Th17 responses are thought to be those involved in many autoimmune diseases and previously classed as Th1. They are generated by IL-1β and IL-23 or IL-6 and express IL-17, IL-22, IL-26 and γ-interferon.

Memory T cells can be generated expressing CD27 and these may have extremely long survival.

B cells B cells are generated throughout postpartum life from haematopoetic stem cells (HSCs) in the bone marrow. HSCs are forced into B-cell commitment by the suppression of Notch signalling. What induces this signal to force B-cell development is not known. Once a lymphocyte is committed to B-cell lineage it is moved to secondary lymphoid tissues where antigen exposure leads to the antigen-dependent development stage.

A number of stages of development are recognised, defined by the B-cell immunoglobulin gene rearrangements and the displayed cell surface markers. (Figure 3.8). These cell surface markers can be utilised as cell-specific biologic therapeutic targets, most notably CD20, which is displayed on the B-cell lineage from pre-B cells to mature B cells and is the target of rituximab. Plasma cells are CD20-negative hence the resistance of some humoral disease to rituximab treatment. Pro-B cells are also CD20-negative, hence the ability of the B-cell lineage to repopulate after rituximab treatment. CD19 is present on developing B cells from the pro-B cell stage. It is part of a multimolecular cell surface complex involved in the signalling of T-cell help during B-cell maturation. It is also a useful surrogate cell marker to assess the CD20 population (which appears at the following pre-B cell stage) after depletion of this population with anti-CD20 antibodies.

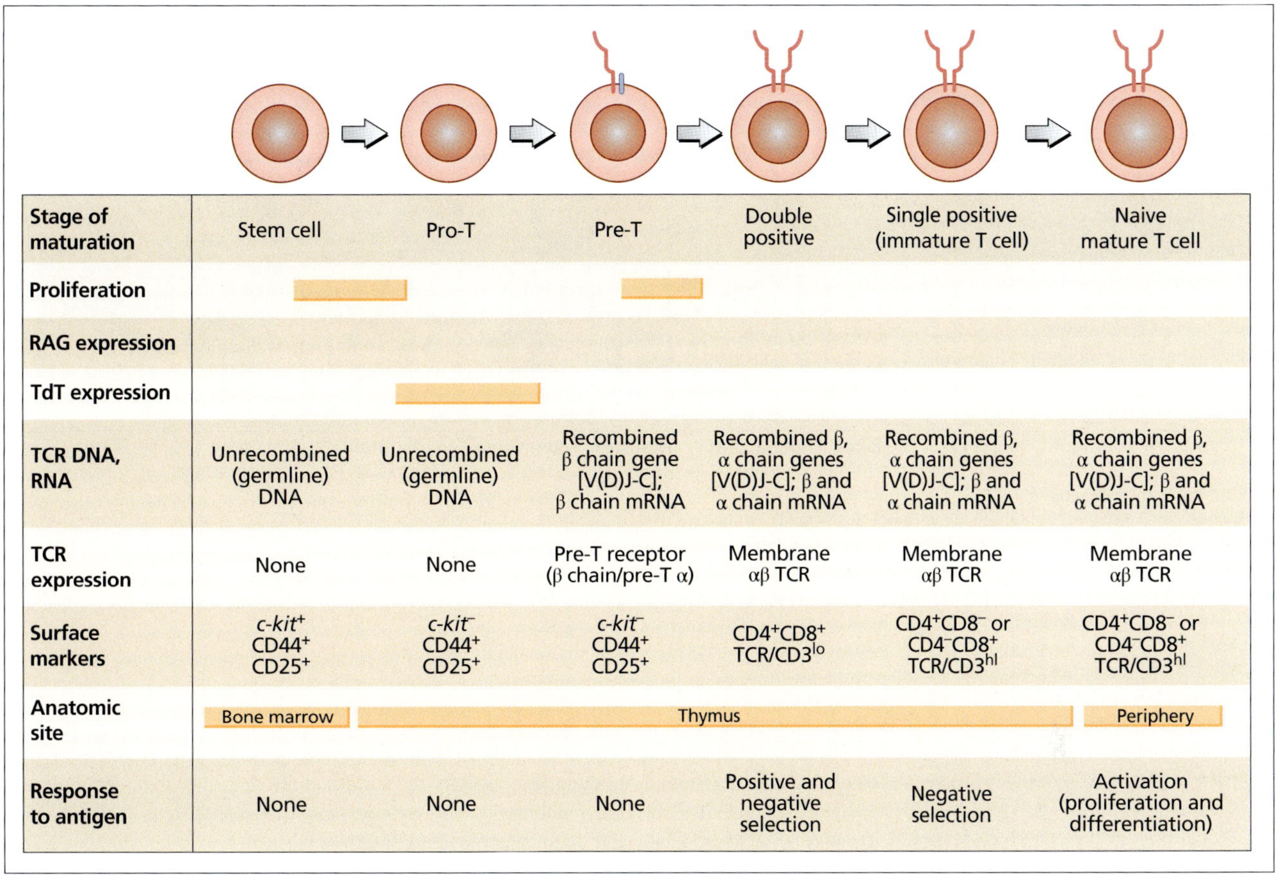
Stage of maturation
Stem cell
Pro-T
Pre-T
Double positive
Single positive (immature T cell)
Naive mature T cell
Proliferation
RAG expression
TdT expression
TCR DNA, RNA
Unrecombined (germline) DNA
Unrecombined (germline) DNA
Recombined β chain gene [V(D)J-C]; β chain mRNA
Recombined β, α chain genes [V(D)J-C]; β and α chain mRNA
Recombined β, α chain genes [V(D)J-C]; β and α chain mRNA
Recombined β, α chain genes [V(D)J-C]; β and α chain mRNA
TCR expression
None
None
Pre-T receptor (β chain/pre-T α)
Membrane αβ TCR
Membrane αβ TCR
Membrane αβ TCR
Surface markers
c-kit+ CD44+ CD25+
c-kit− CD44+ CD25+
c-kit− CD44+ CD25+
CD4+CD8+ TCR/CD3lo
CD4+CD8− or CD4−CD8+ TCR/CD3hi
CD4+CD8− or CD4−CD8+ TCR/CD3hi
Anatomic site
Bone marrow
Thymus
Periphery
Response to antigen
None
None
None
Positive and negative selection
Negative selection
Activation (proliferation and differentiation)

Figure 3.8 Information about the human immune syatem and its inner working. Source: http://immunologynow.com/post/67762750179/t-cell-maturation.

The germ line rearrangements that determine immunoglobulin class and antigen specificity, as well as the cell surface display of the cell defining immunoglobulin, occur throughout B-cell development. Immunoglobulins are made up from the rearrangement of genes coding for a pair of heavy chains and a pair of light chains, which assemble to make a complete immunoglobulin molecule. Heavy chains (IgH) are made from a constant region (μ, γ, α, ε or δ) joined to one of a large number of variable (V-), fewer diverse (D-) or a few joining (J-) segments. Light chains are either κ or λ and have V- and J- but no D- segments. The heavy chains reorganise and assemble before the light chains, with kappa light chains the default position and lambda light chains used where kappa light chain rearrangement fails. When the complete immunoglobulin molecule is assembled it is displayed on the cell surface, which signals the final maturation stages of mature B cells.

All mature B cells display CD19 and CD20 surface markers, but other markers differentiate specific functions. Most B cells are conventional CD5 (B2) cells. B cells displaying CD5 ($CD5^+$ – B1a and B1b cells) probably originate earlier in B-cell ontogeny and are not as tightly regulated as conventional $CD5^-$ B cells. $CD5^+$ B cells release low affinity IgM 'natural' antibody to a number of self antigens and these probably function in an immunoregulatory capacity, their IgG binding (rheumatoid factor) activity being an example. Common antigens recognised by $CD5^+$ elaborated IgM antibodies include insulin, single-stranded DNA, thyroglobulin and possibly myelin-associated glycoprotein. $CD5^+$ B cells probably react more quickly than conventional B cells, facilitating a quick but low affinity humoral response. However, it is unclear whether the IgM elaborated can become pathogenic through affinity maturation as might be postulated in the IgM-associated anti-myelin associated glycoprotein (anti-MAG) paraproteinaemic demyelinating neuropathies.

Mature B cells migrate to secondary lymphoid tissues, with transmural migration through the high endothelial venules facilitated by CD44 and CD62-L (L-selectin). Once in secondary lymphoid tissues IgM and IgD are displayed on the B-cell surface marking these as mature naïve B cells.

Mature B cells can be activated by a number of cytokines and cellular signals: CD25 (IL2R), present on other activated B cells, T cells and monocytes, CD23, a low affinity IgE receptor, and CD80 and CD86 which are the receptors for the TCR associated molecule CD28, which augments the B to T cell synaptic help interaction. Also involved in maturation are CD19, CD20 and CD21 helping to transmit extracellular to intracellular signals. CD40, the cognate partner for CD154 (CD40-L), which is displayed in T cells, is arguably one of the most important signals in B cell antigen-dependent development. The surface immunoglobulin displayed on each B cell provides the antigen specificity and links to intracellular signalling proteins in complex with CD79a and CD79b heterodimers.

Activated B cells move to the mantle zone of germinal centres and under the influence of cytokines undergo class switching to the appropriate Ig class. Many of the follicular B cells undergo apoptosis and it is only the ones with strong affinities that survive this process

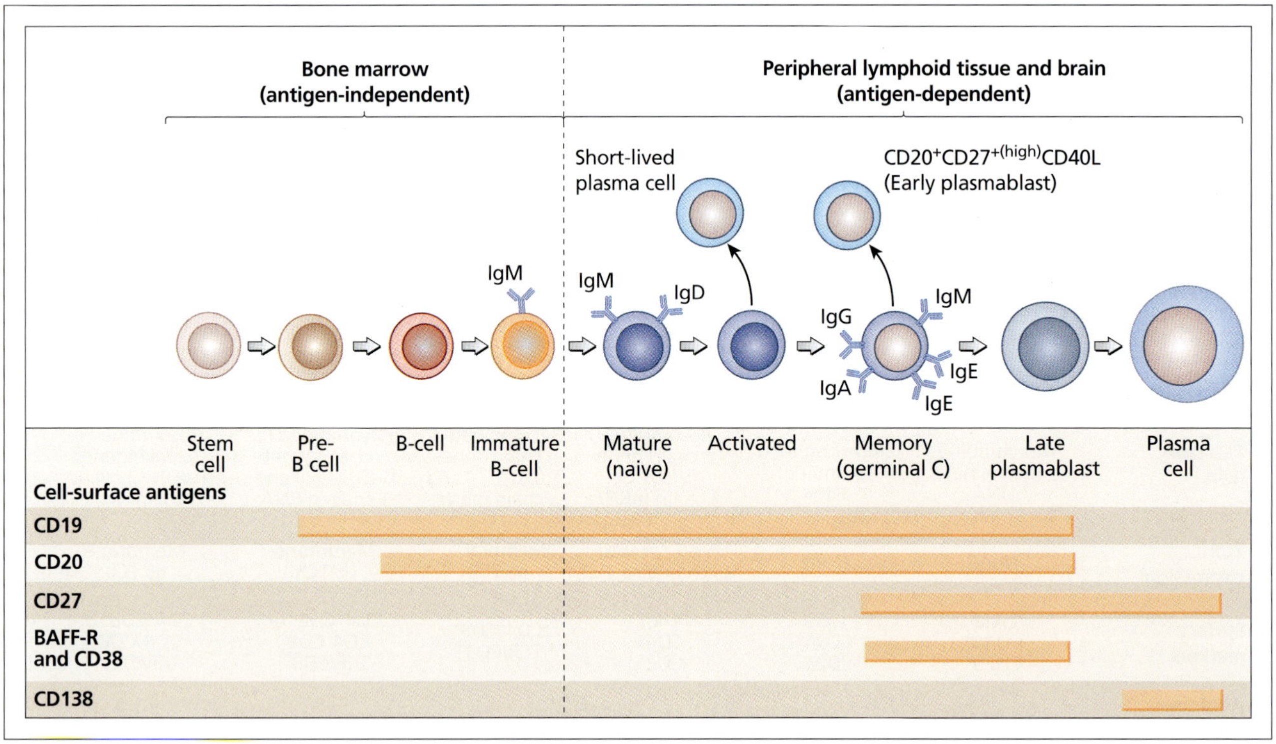

Figure 3.9 B-cell maturation from stem cells to plasma cells is accompanied by surface markers and surface antibody display that identifies the lineage maturity of the cells. These markers may be exploited in diagnosis of lymphomas as well as targeted by therapies such as rituximab, directed at the CD20 surface marker. Source: Dalakas 2008. Reproduced with permission of Nature Macmillan.

before leaving the germinal centre. The final pathway for differentiation is to plasma cells (Figure 3.9). Without T-cell help B cells become short-lived plasma cells secreting low-affinity antibodies. With T-cell help mature activated B cells are driven to memory B cells with a half-life of many years, or $CD138^+$ plasma cells, which secrete antibody in excess but have a shorter half-life of months. Both these cell types are $CD20^-$ and hence a humoral response once set and matured may persist even after rituximab is used therapeutically.

Interactions of B and T cells Within the adaptive immune system the interactions of B and T lymphocytes and APCs through immunological synapses are critical not only to maturation and activation, but also regulation and suppression. Failure of any of these processes can result in immunodeficiencies (e.g. systemic enterovirus infection, PML), autoimmunity through impaired tolerance (Guillain–Barré syndrome) or damage through overactivation of responses (pneumococcal meningitis). The critical co-dependency of the B–T cell interaction can be exploited in many autoimmune diseases, where reduction of one arm of the immune system often affects the other.

APCs set up the activation of the adaptive immune response with APCs presenting antigen to naïve T cells, which when activated provide T-cell help to B2 cells. Once activated, however, a number of processes central to turning off the T-cell response are put in motion. CD28 is down-regulated and CTLA4 expressed; CTLA-4 has a higher affinity for CD80 and CD86 than CD28 and reduces CD28 stimulation. In parallel PD-1 (programmed cell death 1) is expressed, which is the negative signalling homologue of CD28. Programmed cell death pathways are set in motion as soon as T cells become activated and later expression of Fas and the tumour necrosis factor (TNF) receptor 2 result in apoptosis through suicide or homicide. The failure of cell death pathways (especially the Fas pathway) has been implicated in the maintenance of chronic relapsing autoimmune conditions such as CIDP.

Cytokine network Cytokines are hormone-like molecules elaborated by the cellular components of the immune system to coordinate cellular networks and direct cell types in activity and anatomical location. They function as pro-inflammatory up-regulators of the immune system (most cytokines), chemoattractants (chemokines) and negative regulators of the immune response (some cytokines and prostaglandins). They are important also as they can be targets for therapeutic intervention; a number of biological agents exist to interfere with cytokines (e.g. TNF inhibitors and anti-IL-6 agents).

The interleukin designation of many of the known cytokines has simplified the classification; however, some cytokines retain their descriptive terminology such as TNF or the interferons.

In T-cell maturation and response, cytokines are elaborated on the basis of the antigen–APC–T-cell interaction, the local cytokine mileu and the T cells that are anatomically localised to act. Cytokines are crucial in the initial antigen presentation event, and the subsequent inflammatory events that ensue rely on the elaborated cytokines. For example, Th1 cells produce interferons, TNF and IL-2 but not IL-4, and drive delayed type hypersensitivity responses. They are involved in localised inflammatory processes such as rheumatoid arthritis and granuloma formation. Th2 cells produce IL-4 and IL-10 and are responsible for more humoral-based processes with more widespread activity. Asthma and host defence against attack are mediated by Th2. Pro-inflammatory attack and some host defence mechanisms may be mediated by Th17 responses. These are more recently described and previously thought to have been part of the Th1 response. They remain poorly understood. Th17 responses are driven by IL-21, IL-6, IL-1β and possibly IL-23. Th17 inhibition is the focus of active and ongoing research.

A 40-strong family of small protein cytokines known as chemokines are responsible for cellular adhesion and migration of cells to areas of immune need and are referred to as CXC chemokines, identified by a specific protein motif. IL-8 and the peptide C5a might also be considered in this group.

Negative regulation of the immune system is also promoted by cytokines. Transforming growth factor β (TGF-β), prostaglandins, IL-10 and IL-35 all down-regulate components of the immune system.

Protection of neural tissues – the blood–brain and blood–nerve barriers

Intrathecal antibody synthesis and the blood–brain barrier

The blood–brain barrier (BBB) describes the complex concept of a physically impermeable structure that divides the systemic body compartment from that of the CNS across which fluids, solutes and cells can selectively pass resulting in a unique CNS milieu (Figure 3.10). There is a misconception that this provides immunological privilege to the CNS; in fact it enables a more controlled environment to exist within the environment of the body as a whole in which an additional degree of immunological control can be exerted. This results in the relative resistance of complex CNS machinery to immune attack but also generates the environment in which a unique set of autoimmune diseases can occur and unique immune responses result in both damage and damage limitation.

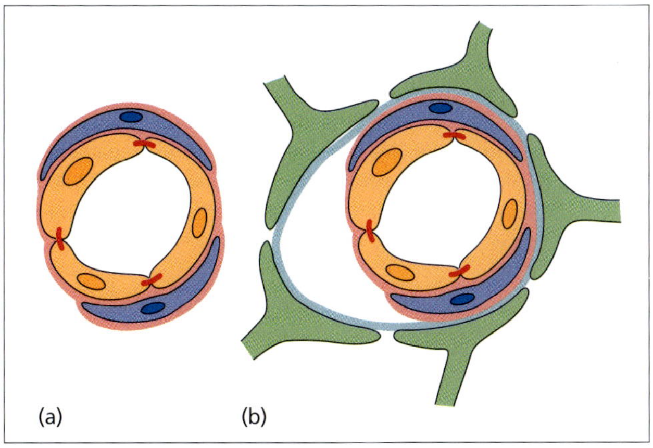

Figure 3.10 The blood–nerve barrier (BNB) (a) and the blood–brain barrier (BBB) (b) have similar structures and function very similarly. Capillary endothelial cells (orange) are joined by tight junctions (red) and with pericytes (blue) and basement membrane form a passively impermeable barrier to the passage of cells and molecules. In the brain, beyond the pericapillary space is the glia limitans (light green) supported by astrocyte foot processes (dark green) which form a second layer of physical barrier. Permitted solutes and molecules cross the barriers by active receptor bound or vesicular transport. The function of the BBB and BNB is very similar in terms of molecular exclusion and transport permission. Source: Adapted from Kanda 2013 with permission of BMJ.

The blood–nerve barrier (BNB) is less well described and understood, as the endoneurial space of the peripheral nerve is less amenable to study, especially in terms of its fluid and solute constituents. It is accepted that the BNB is more 'leaky' that the BBB, and that it undoubtedly modifies any immune responses that would be prone to occur if nerves were not 'hidden' behind it. However, it will not be discussed further here. Further descriptions are to be found in Chapter 10.

In clinical neurology the invasiveness of a cerebrospinal fluid (CSF) examination and the appearance of the CSF as an entirely colourless, translucent ('gin clear') fluid have often consigned it to the position of a 'less useful' body fluid in the diagnosis of disease. This was perhaps true when analytical techniques were only able to identify basic cell types and molecules in relatively large concentrations ('CSF total protein'). Advances in qualitative and quantitative techniques of CSF analysis are beginning to reveal the CSF as an increasingly useful fluid from which to identify biomarkers with relevance to diagnosis, prognosis and response to treatment but discussion of most of this emerging field is beyond the remit of this chapter. However, there is a very solid basis for the use of the CSF as a biomarker in many diseases of the CNS and PNS that are discussed here.

Analysis of CSF solutes

In health, the CSF is maintained as a protein-poor solvent in which are dissolved proteins derived mainly from brain tissue. These are produced in the most part from physiological and pathophysiological processes of release and cellular decay and recycling. Perhaps of most interest in the clinical investigation of the CSF are normal levels of CSF antibodies, amyloid beta, tau and phosphotau proteins (as a baseline from which change indicates disease), and asialotransferrin (as an easy analyte as a marker of CSF as a fluid). Many other proteins contribute to 'total' CSF protein (e.g. transthyretin) but have less use, at present, in the assessment of health or disease.

In the most basic of clinical CSF analysis, CSF total protein is measured by one of a large number of methods. However, 'CSF protein' contains contributions from CNS and systemic compartments (if there is a dysfunctional BBB) and is a very non-specific measure. The measurement of specific protein is much more useful. No albumin is produced in the CNS and so any albumin detected in the CSF is there as the result of direct BBB transport and control or as a result of 'leakage' through a dysfunctional barrier. CSF albumin is easily measured and its ratio to the serum albumin is constant in health. This ratio (CSF_{alb} : $serum_{alb}$) is known as the albumin quotient (Q_{alb}) and is a method-independent measure of BBB permeability. In health, all the IgG in the CSF is actively transported across the BBB (as are other immunoglobluins). A raised CSF IgG in comparison to the serum (raised CSF_{IgG} : $serum_{IgG}$) or the IgG quotient (Q_{IgG}) can be used similarly. The IgG index (Q_{IgG} : Q_{alb}), which is the ratio of these ratios, can define the permeability characteristics of the BBB, helping to define the pathogenesis of processes occurring inside or outside the CSF space with, or without, humoral drive.

Other CSF solutes can also be measured. Most are present in very small quantities and the current dynamic range of most assays as well as inter-individual differences in response is unable to distinguish solute profiles on an individual patient basis. However, some solutes released in large quantities (e.g. a-beta amyloid proteins, *tau*, neurofilament proteins, S-100β and 14-3-3 protein) are easily measured. The profiles of these solutes, assayed in the correct clinical context, can provide biomarker support for the diagnosis of Alzheimer's disease versus frontotemporal lobar dementias and degenerative brain diseases versus 'worried well' (Chapter 8). The collection of CSF samples and their immediate handling are crucial to these assays as considerable pre-process changes can occur as a result of interaction with plastic ware and at room temperature. Furthermore, assays should be carried out in recognised quality controlled laboratories where variances in assays are minimised.

Platforms for assays of low concentration solutes continue to develop. ELISA can be both sensitive and specific. However, multiplex assay systems with enhanced development techniques, mass spectrometry and 'single molecule detection' techniques will advance the field rapidly in the near future.

CSF cells The CSF is essentially an acellular fluid. The CNS is patrolled by a tightly regulated system of microglia generally maintained in a state of active patrol but hyporesponsiveness. Very few cells are found circulating in normal CSF. Most laboratories will quote <5 white cells per cubic millimetre as a normal range, but any cells in the CSF should provoke suspicion of an ongoing process, even if very non-specific. Cells are nearly always lymphocytes, and the identification of macrophages or neutrophils is almost certainly disease related and useful in diagnosis.

Cell counts are not reliable for the identification of other cell types and formal cytology or flow cytometry studies are necessary to provide positive identification. In malignant meningitis, cell type can both make the diagnosis and prompt a search for the primary process or other disseminated disease. In haematological malignancies, where the cell type may be lymphocytic, and where accurate diagnosis depends upon the lymphocytic type, clonal molecular flow cytometry can provide an accurate diagnosis as long as sufficient CSF is provided containing sufficient cells.

Red cells in the CSF are always abnormal, although the most common cause for these is a traumatic lumbar CSF tap.

Other CSF constituents Pathogens can be isolated from the CSF by a variety of methods. Direct visualisation of bacteria or fungi can be immediately useful. Polymerase chain reactions (PCR) for viruses are highly specific and variably sensitive. It must be remembered that PCR depends upon the primers chosen, the strain of the virus and the copy number within the fluid. A negative result should not always be taken as negative and alternative or repeated tests might be useful. Culture studies can grow both bacteria (especially TB) and fungi at a later date and the possibility of such pathogens should be considered at the time of sampling; the request for special cultures will be required as well as adequate volumes of fluid.

The use of immunoglobulin in the CSF covers total IgG, the comparison of serum and CSF oligoclonal banding patterns and specific immunoglobulins in disease. The total IgG level was discussed earlier and is quickly measured. The oligoclonal banding pattern of the CSF in relation to the serum is a more lengthy process but can identify the relative production of monoclonal or oligoclonal humoral responses from within the CSF. This is useful in diagnosis of inflammatory CNS diseases. However, it remains a mystery as to the antigenic targets of oligoclonal bands in any disease and particularly in multiple sclerosis; the identification of a target antigen in this and other diseases would be a huge contribution towards explaining pathogenesis. Attempts have been made to identify virus-specific oligoclonal bands in the CSF with limited success. These techniques have been superseded by PCR and whole genome, next generation sequencing techniques with greater and highly specific coverage for expected or unexpected pathogens.

Immune diseases of the nervous system

The immune system probably has roles in the causation, pathogenesis, resistance to and recovery from a vast number of diseases in the nervous system. Furthermore, clinical diagnosis is greatly assisted by the analysis of 'immune' biomarkers (antibodies, cells, cell-related factors and aberrantly released molecules), which are measured in immunology laboratories. The immune system is critically involved in the resolution (and occasionally the worsening) of infectious diseases but this is not described further here.

Immunology is a part of every chapter of this textbook and diseases may be described as B- or T-cell mediated, complement-dependent or cytokine-driven. It is not possible to make clean divisions of diseases in relation to their involvement of the immune system as each involves the interaction of many players in the 'immunological soup'. As duplication and redundancy of function both exist, the analysis of a single component of the immune system is unlikely to provide the explanation for any one disease. In treatment options, the balance of immune components in disease can be likened to the interaction of strings in a child's cat's cradle; removing any one significant string often leads to the collapse of the structure although sometimes, under particular tension, the disturbance of the wrong string may lead to exacerbation of the immune response in the opposite arm (e.g. the provocation or worsening of demyelinating diseases with inhibitors of TNF-α).

There follows some brief examples of diseases that are discussed later in the book where the immune pathogenesis is felt to be polarised in one direction or another.

Antibody-mediated neurological diseases

Antibody-mediated neurological diseases can be divided into those where the antibody defines the disease and probably is primarily responsible for the pathogenesis of that condition, and diseases where antibodies are markers for the disease without necessarily being causative. There are a number of diseases where there is good theoretical argument for the antibody identified to be pathological (e.g. in the stiff person syndrome associated with anti-GAD antibodies) but where good evidence supporting the theoretical mechanism does not yet – and may not – exist.

Neurological disease with pathogenic autoantibodies Diseases of the PNS and CNS exist with good evidence for predominant antibody-mediated pathogenesis. The fulfilment of the Witebsky postulates is only partial in most of these diseases, largely because the generation of antibodies in animal models in response to immunisation is limited because of self-tolerance. However, myasthenia gravis, Guillain–Barré syndrome, Lambert–Eaton myasthenic syndrome, the surface receptor based autoimmune encephalitides and perhaps stiff person syndromes are examples of a B-cell mediated disease with more or less evidence for a predominant humoral pathogenesis.

The neurological disease with the best evidence for an antibody pathogenesis is autoimmune myasthenia gravis. Antibodies to the post-synaptic acetylcholine receptor result in a complement-dependent disruption of the post-synaptic neuromuscular junction complex which results in fatigable weakness. However, the initiation of the humoral autoimmune antiacetylcholine receptor antibody response remains obscure.

In the acute motor axonal form (AMAN variant) of the Guillain–Barré syndrome the initiation of the antibody response resulting in the disease is understood. Some strains of *Campylobacter jejuni* elaborate human ganglioside-like epitopes on their lipooligosaccharide coat. Infection in individuals who probably both have impaired self tolerance mechanisms and in whom sufficient adjuvant stimulation exists are able to make antibodies to their peripheral nerve gangliosides. Subsequently, these antibodies have both complement dependent and independent effects to alter electrophysiological membrane characteristics at the node of Ranvier and neuromuscular junction, to damage cell structure of axons and myelin and to impair the normal repair mechanisms that result in recovery. Similar mechanisms may exist in the more common demyelinating Guillain–Barré syndrome, acute inflammatory demyelinating polyradiculoneuropathy.

Increasing evidence is emerging that some CNS diseases are directly antibody mediated. Antibodies to neuronal cell surface receptors have recently been described and their number is increasing. Antibodies to the voltage-gated potassium channel complex are mostly explained by antibodies to two of the complex components: LGI1 and Caspr2. Antibodies to LGI1 are responsible for the syndrome of limbic encephalitis with facio-brachial seizures, and those to Caspr2 with Morvan's syndrome (peripheral nerve hyperexcitability with psychiatric and sleep disturbance). Both of these conditions usually respond to broad-spectrum humoral immunosuppression. Antibodies to *N*-methyl-D-aspartate (NMDA) receptors, and more recently AMPA and GABA receptors, have increasingly well-defined phenotypes along with good theoretical, *in vitro* and *ex vivo* models of disease.

Antibodies to the water channel protein, aquaporin-4, and possibly to myelin oligodendrocyte glycoprotein (MOG), are associated with Devic's disease (neuromyelitis optica). The support for an antibody pathogenesis for these diseases largely rests upon there being a putative antigen at a feasible site, antibody binding experiments and response to immunotherapy.

Neurological disease associated with systemic disorders and systemic autoantibodies Several diseases are associated with antibodies that may have systemic effects, including effects on the nervous system, or have antibodies that are central to the diagnosis but which have questionable relevance in the pathogenesis.

The connective tissue diseases have a number of neurological manifestations which may or may not be related to the presence of the antibodies described as a part of the syndromes and sometimes more or less essential in the diagnostic criteria. The anti-neutrophil cytoplasmic antibodies (ANCA) are associated with some vasculitides. Although they may activate neutrophils and are necessary for the diagnosis in some diseases, for example in Wegener's granulomatosis (granulomatosis with polyangiitis), they are not essential to the pathogenesis or the pathology. Antibodies to the extractable nuclear antigens (ENA) are associated with a number of other connective tissue diseases such as primary and secondary Sjögren's syndrome which have associations with some neurological syndromes (e.g. sensory neuronopathy).

Antibodies to phospholipid and cardiolipin are associated with the antiphospholipid syndrome which may cause a catastrophic disorder of coagulation that may involve the CNS. In some cases this resembles multiple sclerosis and making the distinction between causation and association may be very difficult and lead to inappropriate therapies.

Paraneoplastic diseases overlap between humoral and T-cell mediated disease with the presence of antibodies defining the syndromes, and suggesting associated tumour types, but frequently T cells mediating irreversible damage to neural structures. These are discussed further here.

A paraneoplastic syndrome is a disease or symptom that is the consequence of the presence of cancer in the body, but not directly caused by the presence of cancer cells. The diseases are caused by immune factors presumably released by, or in response to, a tumour that cause damage to the end tissue and subsequently result in the phenotypic symptoms and signs. The agents causing the damage are presumed to be antibodies, T cells or other soluble molecules but these are often difficult to demonstrate. A number of well-known paraneoplastic antibodies are described (e.g. anti-Hu, anti-Yo and anti-Ri) which are associated with a group of phenotypically recognisable disorders such as sensory ganglionopathies, limbic encephalitis and the opsoclonus myoclonus syndrome. They are also associated with a number of underlying tumour types such as small cell cancers, breast and ovarian tumours but neither the antibody nor the tumour types co-segregate with one another (Table 3.3).

Many of the antibodies first described are to intracellular antigens and mechanisms of pathogenesis remain unexplained; in these the antibody may be an epiphenomenon and the disease mechanism T-cell mediated. These syndromes tend to be difficult to treat, and although identification and successful resection of the tumour may result in limitation of further progression, reversal or recovery is seldom seen. Increasing numbers of paraneoplastic syndromes are now being described where antibodies to surface antigens and receptors are present and where the antibody appears to have a direct effect. The first of these syndromes was the Lambert–Eaton myasthenic syndrome where voltage-gated calcium channel antibodies are almost certainly pathogenic. More recently, antibodies to surface channels in the encephalitides associated with antibodies to voltage-gated potassium channels, NMDA receptors and glycine receptors have been identified with a number of distinct phenotypical diseases associated with them.

T-cell mediated neurological disease

T-cell mediated neurological disease is more difficult to define as the specific targets of T-cell receptors are more difficult to isolate. In clinical practice, T-cell mediated diseases are generally less reversible than B-cell mediated disease and perhaps because of this less responsive to current immunotherapy. However, increasing numbers of therapies are emerging that target key components of the T-cell immune response, especially cytokines.

Paraneoplastic diseases are described above and a number of these have T-cytotoxic mechanisms of cell injury (e.g. the anti-Hu, -Yo and -Ri associated syndromes).

The final common path to tissue damage in cerebral and peripheral nerve vasculitis involves T-cell infiltration of tissue and destruction of tissues associated with the T-cell infiltrate and the inflammatory milieu elaborated by those cells. The targeting of particular blood vessels has yet to be explained.

Multiple sclerosis is probably the most common and best described of the CNS neurological disorders, once again with perivascular T-cell infiltrates and myelin and subsequently axonal destruction in plaques of inflammation. Whether this process or a neurodegenerative underlying process is the primary mechanism of disease and whether underlying viral pathogens drive the initiation of inflammatory responses remains an ongoing debate.

Table 3.3 Antibody-related paraneoplastic syndrome.

Name	Antigenic target	Function	Syndrome	Associated neoplastic tissues	Associated with tumour (%)
Intracellular paraneoplastic antigens					
Hu (ANNA1)	RNA-binding proteins	Neuronal development	Encephalomyelitis, LE, BE, PCD, sensory neuronopathy, gastrointestinal pseudo-obstruction	SCLC	98
Yo (PCA1)	Purkinje cell cytoplasmic target	Unknown	PCD, rare peripheral neuropathy	Ovary, breast	99
Ri (ANNA2)	Intracellular target unknown	Unknown	BE, opsoclonus myoclonus	Breast	96
CV2 (CRMP5)	Collapsin response mediator protein 5	Neuronal development and cellular plasticity in Purkinje cells	Hu-like. Also chorea, optic atrophy, myelopathy, neuropathies (various)	SCLC, thymoma	95
Ma2	40 kDa protein	Regulation of apoptosis	LE, BE	Testicular	96
Amphiphysin	Amphiphysin	Synaptic function	SPS, PERM, sensory neuronopathy	Breast, SCLC	95
Sox-1	Sry-related HMG box 1	Y-chromosome related DNA binding protein – neuronal differentiation	LEMS	SCLC	Unclear (no higher in paraneoplastic disease than tumour alone)
Recoverin	Retinal recoverin	Retinal calcium binding protein	Autoimmune retinopathy	SCLC, cervix, Müllerian tumour, endometrium, uterine	Uncommon – unclear percentage
GAD	Glutamic acid decarboxylase	Conversion of Glutamate to GABA	SPS	Infrequent or chance. Associated with type 1 diabetes	N/A
Zic4	Zinc finger binding protein 4	Neuronal development	PCD – often coexist with Hu	SCLC, gynaecological cancers	Unclear (no higher in paraneoplastic disease than tumour alone)

Cell surface paraneoplastic antigens

Tr (DNER)	Delta notch-like epidermal growth factor-related receptor		PCD	Hodgkin's lymphoma		
VGKCh (LGI1)	Leucine rich, Glioma inactivated-1	Implicated in glioma metastasis. Transmembrane protein with unclear function	LE with faciobrachial seizures and serum hyponatraemia	Various tumours described – links not strong		<10
VGKCh (Caspr2)	Contactin associated protein-2	Paranodal structure	Morvan's syndrome and neuromyotonia	Thymoma		30–40
VGKCh (LGI1-Caspr-2 negative)	Unknown	Unknown	Epilepsies – phenotype and relevance unclear	Unknown		
VGCaCh	Voltage-gated calcium channel	Presynaptic transmitter release	Lambert–Eaton myasthenic syndrome	Small cell lung		>95
NMDAR	*N*-methyl-D-aspartate receptor	Glutamate receptor involved in plasticity responsible for learning and memory	Encephalitis with psychiatric features, dystonic movement disorder, stupor, dysautonomia and cognitive impairment	Ovarian teratoma Sometimes post inflammation/ infection		~30–60
AMPAR	α-Amino-3-hydroxy-5-methyl-4-isoxazolepropionic acid receptor	Non-NMDA glutamate receptor involved in CNS plasticity, learning and memory	LE	Thymoma, lung, breast		50
GlyR	Glycine receptor	Inhibitory transmission in the spinal cord and brainstem linked to Cl^- conductance	Atypical SPS and PERM	Thymoma, breast, lymphoma		10
$GABA_B$	Gamma aminobutyric acid receptor	Inhibitory receptor linked to K^+ conductance	LE and seizures	Lung		~50–70
AQP4	Aquaporin-4	Water channel	Neuromyelitis optica	None	Rare	
MOG	Myelin oligodendrocyte protein	CNS adhesion molecule responsible for myelin sheath completion and maintenance	NMO spectrum disorders	Unknown	Very rare	

ANNA, antineuronal nuclear antibody; BE, brainstem encephalitis; LE, limbic encephalitis; NMDA, *N*-methyl-D-aspartate; PCD, paraneoplastic cerebellar degeneration; PERM, progressive encephalitis with rigidity and myoclonus; SCLC, small cell lung carcinoma; SPS, stiff person syndromes.

In the PNS there is evidence that CIDP is a T-cell mediated disease with evidence for deficiencies in the autoimmune regulator protein AIRE, reduced T-regulatory mechanisms, failure of Fas-Fas ligand lymphocyte down-regulation and mixed Th1 and Th2 cytokine profile up-regulation in the serum and the endoneurium. There is also evidence for B-cell mediated pathways.

Cytokine-driven processes

Primary cytokine processes are less well described. A clear example of cytokine dysregulation occurs in the POEMS syndrome (polyneuropathy, organomegaly, endocrinopathy, M-protein and skin changes). Although there is a paraprotein in this disorder, it does not appear to play an obvious part in the pathogenesis. In addition, although plasma cells are frequently expanded, it appears that the central processes driving the disease are unregulated vascular endothelial growth factor (VEGF) and IL-6 production, possibly exacerbated by hypoxia-induced factor 1α (HIF-1α). This unregulated cytokine drive results in proliferation, migration and maturation or B cells and increasing amounts of cytokine production resulting in multisystem symptomatology. Once again, interference with these processes within the pathway can result in stabilisation of the disease as long as there is not an essential requirement for the ablated aspect of the pathway (e.g. VEGF).

Interfering with the immune system as a treatment for disease

The immune-mediated neurological diseases present opportunities for effective therapy. Immunotherapies work by a number of different mechanisms and sometimes more than one is required to effect a response. Sometimes, immunosuppression may be required in infection to modulate an overactive and damaging immune response. For example, in the treatment of HIV, TB meningitis or cysticercosis, antimicrobial treatment can result in a devastating immune response resulting in more damage than the primary infection.

Broadly, the mechanisms of action of drugs that modulate the immune system can be classified as follows:

- *Immunomodulatory*: intravenous immunoglobulin (IVIg) acts as an immunomodulatory agent by multiple mechanisms, plasma exchange by non-specific removal of soluble immune factors, and interferons by supplementation and modulation of the cytokine network. The mechanisms of IVIg action are poorly understood. Mechanisms interfering with B- and T-cell interactions, macrophage activity and complement are highly important but anti-idiotype activity is unlikely to be a major mechanism. Plasma exchange non-specifically removes low molecular weight solutes including cytokines and antibodies (especially IgG) and can be quick and effective in its action in appropriate diseases (e.g. Guillain–Barré syndrome, systemic vasculitides and the antibody-mediated autoimmune encephalitides). Interferons modulate the immune response by unknown mechanisms.
- *Immunosuppressive:* steroids, oral immunosuppressants (azathioprine, methotrexate, mycophenolate, ciclosporin) or intravenous agents such as cyclophosphamide, depress immune responses more or less non-selectively. These agents are the backbone of the current immunotherapeutic pharmacopoeia. Steroids work quickly and effectively to suppress B- and T-cell mediated responses and sensitise cells to the effects of other immunosuppressants, particularly cyclophosphamide. However, their medium and long-term adverse event profiles limit their long-term use and in most circumstances the clinician is looking to stop or substitute these agents as quickly as possible. Azathioprine, methotrexate and mycophenolate are easy to use with appropriate regular blood monitoring for adverse effects but they are rather slow to work. Cyclophosphamide is an excellent immunosuppressant and with cautious dose restriction, pulsed therapy and metabolite protection of the bladder epithelium by mesna toxicities are much less than with oral medication.
- *Replacement:* for example, IVIg in hypogammaglobulinaemic disorders. RNA enteroviruses are lytic and immunity relies on humoral rather than cytotoxic clearance. Patients with hypo- or agammaglobulinaemic disorders are susceptible to systemic RNA virus infection that may result in meningoencephalitis. Stabilisation relies upon supplementation of polyvalent immunoglobulins from donors with the normal commensal exposure to common viruses to maintain clearance.
- *Specifically targeted ablative therapies* (e.g. anti-CD20 and anti-CD52 monoclonal antibodies): these therapies are increasingly important in the treatment of immune-mediated disease, sometimes in combination with other immunosuppressants (e.g. rituximab and methotrexate in rheumatoid arthritis). The ability to directly interfere with, ablate or block a specific molecule in the immune system as a very powerful tool. Idiosyncratic and predictable but rare complications are the limiting factor in both the risks of initiating therapy and in long-term use. For example, PML is a known, usually fatal, complication of rituximab, natalizumab and others. Appropriate predictive testing and limitation of the length of exposure reduce the risks. However, for some diseases where death or severe disability is not an outcome then the use of these medications is probably not ethical, but in diseases with potentially worse prognosis they can be very powerful.
- *Specifically targeted molecules interfering with cytokine and chemokine networks* (e.g. anti-TNF, anti-VEGF and anti-IL-6 therapies): some of these therapies are targeted toxins (e.g. the '-cept' drugs, such as etanercept). Others are antibodies with anticytokine therapeutic activity such as bevacizumab which acts as an anti-VEGF agent, or tocilizumab which is anti-IL-6.[1]

Inherited mutations of ion channels

Although rare, monogenic neurological channelopathies provide unparallelled insights into the mechanisms of neurological diseases. The clinical manifestations of some channelopathies are indistinguishable from common disorders whose aetiology is unknown, in particular primary generalised epilepsies and migraine. Thus, neurological channelopathies potentially identify signalling pathways and circuits involved in diseases that account for a large fraction of neurological practice. More broadly, they open a window onto the fundamental workings of the human brain, spinal cord, nerve and muscle.

A common feature of many channelopathies is that they cause discrete paroxysms, while the development of the nervous system is generally unperturbed, and affected individuals function normally

[1] The naming of the biological agents follows an organised schema. The last consonant describes the activity of the agent; for example, 'mab' is a monoclonal antibody and 'cept' a conjugated toxin. The penultimate syllable describes the structure and origin, such that 'xi' is a chimeric and 'zu' a humanised monoclonal. The second syllable describes the target activity, thus 'tu' is a tumour, li(m) the immune and 'ci' the circulatory system. Lastly, the first syllable is any euphonious collection of letters to make the drug name recognisable.

between attacks. In common with many other genetic diseases, ion channel mutations tend to present early in life. Some channelopathies are self-limiting, for instance causing neonatal seizures that remit spontaneously. Other disorders may not resolve and some present as attacks that give way to a fixed or progressive impairment, as seen in some muscle or cerebellar channelopathies. Among possible explanations for the developmental evolution of symptoms are changes in the expression of individual channels, maturation and compensatory alterations in CNS circuits, and excitotoxic damage to affected neurones and muscle cells.

Although most currently known channelopathies are dominantly inherited this pattern may, to some extent, reflect the difficulty of identifying families with recessive disorders, especially where penetrance is incomplete. Furthermore, some symptoms of channelopathies, such as migraine or seizures, are common and occur far more frequently as idiopathic disorders without clear Mendelian inheritance, so it is difficult to justify extensive sequencing of candidate genes in a patient without affected first degree relatives. A further difficulty is that some ion channel mutations have variable manifestations, even when the same mutation is inherited by different members of an affected family, consistent with an interaction with modifying genes or environmental factors.

Channelopathies

Channelopathies can present in any area of clinical neurology (Figure 3.11).

Migraine

Two out of the three genes identified in dominant familial hemiplegic migraine (FHM) encode ion channels.

Epilepsy

Ion channel mutations can cause both focal and generalised seizure disorders, which range in severity from benign neonatal convulsions to early-onset epileptic encephalopathies. An important breakthrough was the realisation that an autosomal dominant pattern of inheritance occurs in some families where several individuals have febrile and other types of seizures. Febrile seizures are generally considered a benign and common self-limiting condition. In families with generalised epilepsy with febrile seizures plus (GEFS+), such seizures may persist beyond early childhood, or may be accompanied by non-febrile seizures. Mutations of at least four ion channel genes cause GEFS+ (Figure 3.12). Other epilepsy syndromes caused by ion channel mutations include malignant migrating partial seizures of infancy, Ohtahara syndrome, autosomal dominant nocturnal frontal epilepsy, rolandic epilepsy

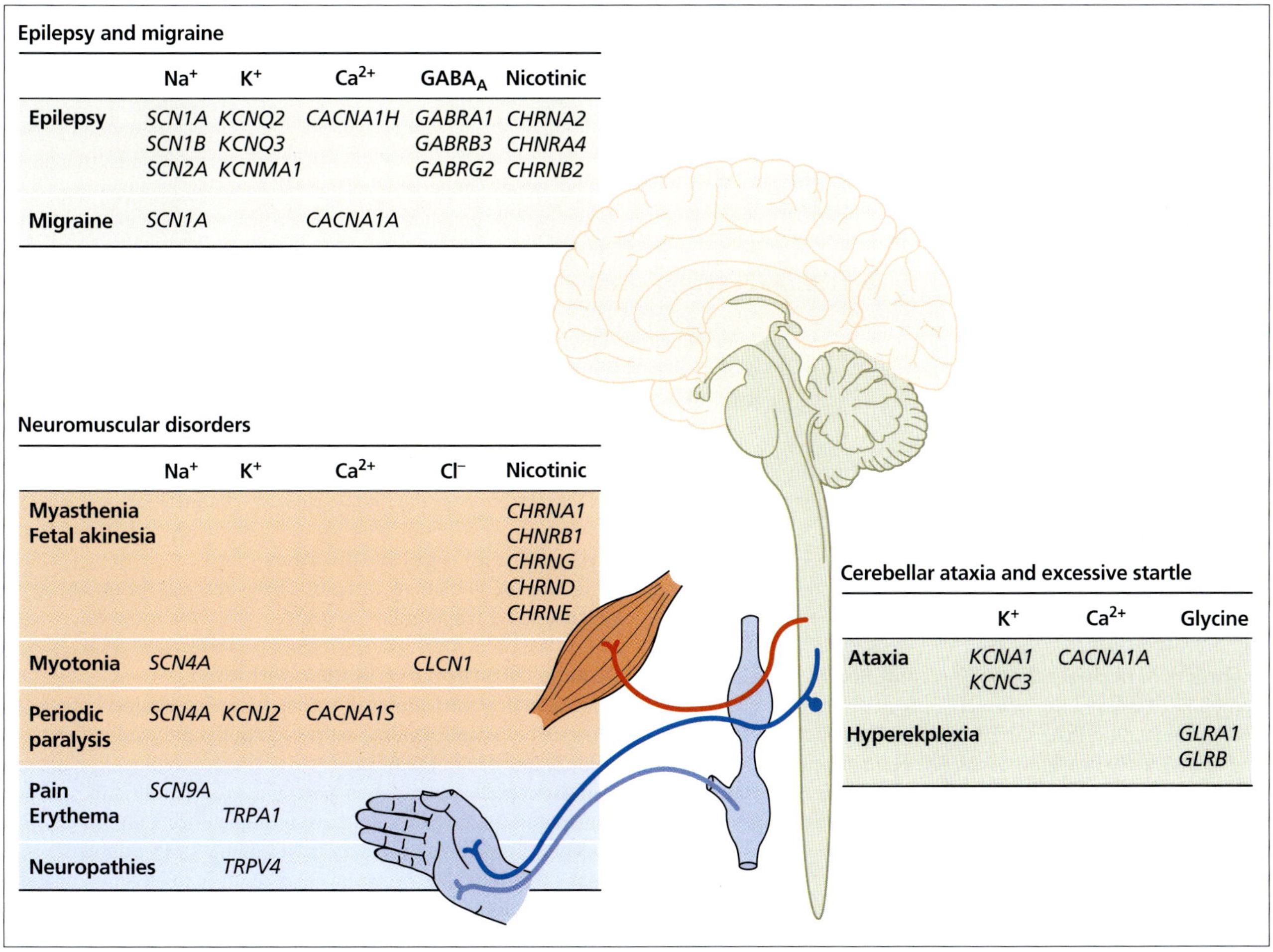

Figure 3.11 Summary of the main ion channel classes, genes, and manifestations. Source: Adapted from Kullmann 2010, with permission of Annual Reviews.

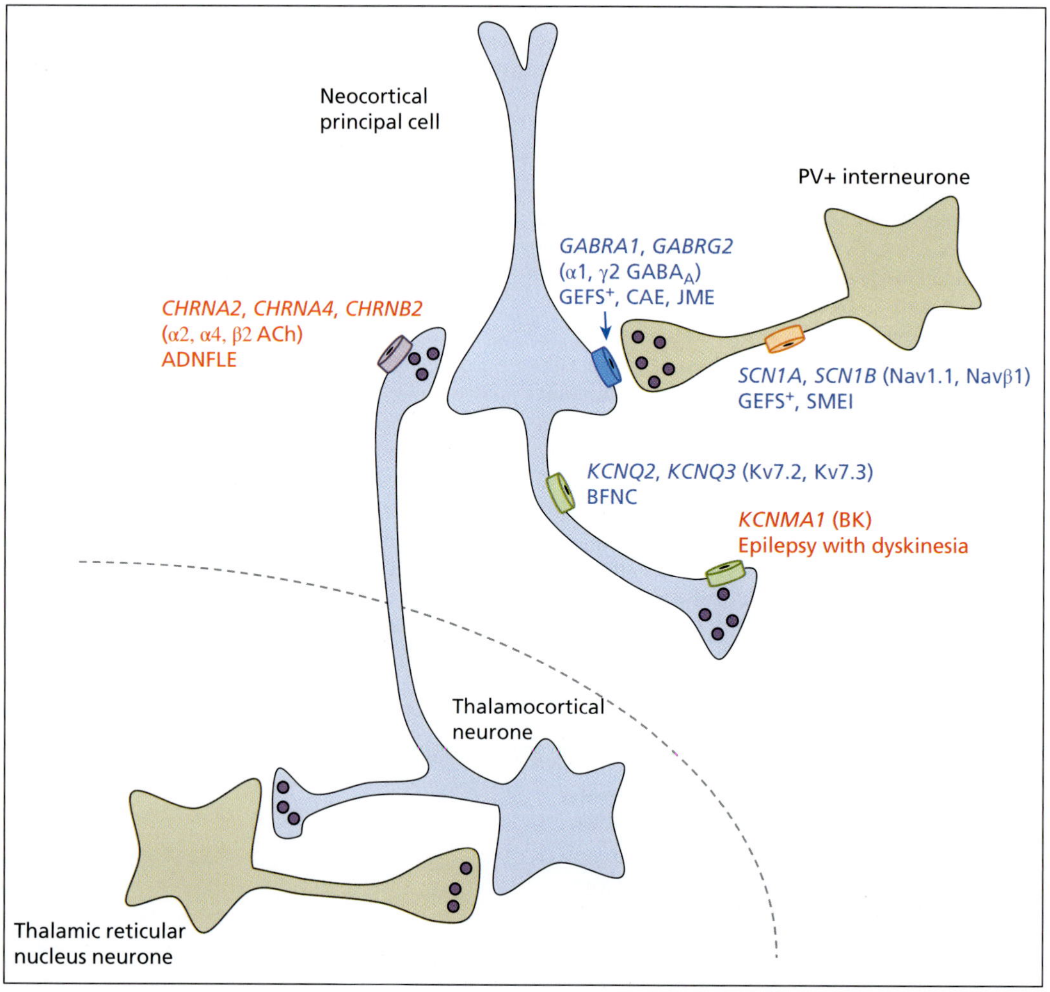

Figure 3.12 Epileptic channelopathies. The tentative roles of different ion channels implicated in epilepsy are indicated schematically, with gain and loss of function in red and blue, respectively. The locations of several channels are inferred mainly from rodent studies. Gene names are indicated in italics. ADNFLE, autosomal dominant nocturnal frontal lobe epilepsy; BFNC, benign familial neonatal convulsions; CAE, childhood absence epilepsy; GEFS+, generalised epilepsy with febrile seizures plus; JME, juvenile myoclonic epilepsy; PV, parvalbumin; SMEI, severe myoclonic epilepsy of infancy. Source: Adapted from Kullmann 2010, with permission of Annual Reviews.

(epilepsy with centrotemporal spikes), and Landau–Kleffner syndrome (a childhood epilepsy syndrome with language regression).

Movement disorders and ataxia

Channelopathies can cause paroxysmal dyskinesia, ataxia and hyperekplexia (exaggerated startle reaction).

Disorders of peripheral nerve and autonomic function

Mutations of one sodium channel gene can cause either paroxysmal pain or congenital insensitivity to pain. Some potassium channel mutations lead to neuromyotonia. Although not considered further in this review, CMTX (an X-linked hereditary neuropathy) is caused by mutations of connexin32. Connexins make up gap junction proteins, a type of intercellular channel.

Muscle disease

Channelopathies can result in congenital myasthenic syndromes, periodic paralysis or myotonia (Figure 3.13). Although myotonic dystrophy, the most common myotonic disorder, is not usually considered a channelopathy, it may have similar mechanisms because mutations of the *DMPK* gene in this disorder alter the processing of mRNA that encodes the muscle chloride channel.

Psychiatric and cognitive disorders

Mutations of glutamate receptors have recently been linked to autism and schizophrenia.

Disease causation in channelopathies

Understanding the features of a channelopathy requires knowledge of the cell type and regional expression of the mutated ion channel subunit, but also of the normal role of the ion channel in neuronal or muscle excitability, action potential propagation and synaptic transmission. Mutations can have multiple effects on ion channel biogenesis, trafficking and operation (Figure 3.14). Premature stop codons and splice site mutations may result in mRNA degradation, while other mutations can give rise to non-functional subunits that fail to assemble normally. Other, typically missense, mutations alter trafficking and voltage- or ligand-dependent gating. Larger scale deletions and duplications of entire exons or genes have recently been reported.

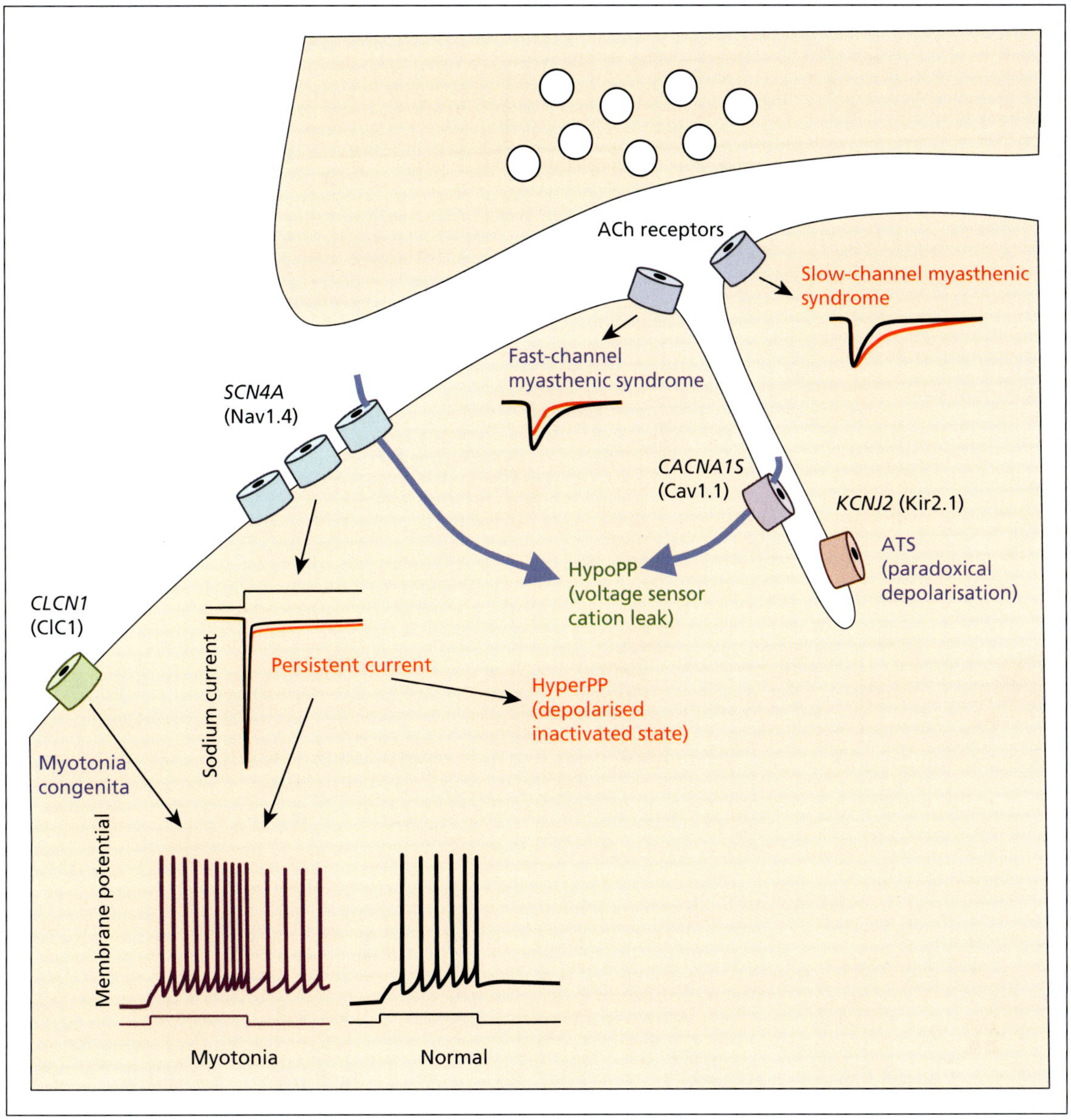

Figure 3.13 Muscle channelopathies. Gain- and loss-of-function mechanisms that underlie muscle channelopathies are indicated in red and blue, respectively. The slowed end-plate current and persistent sodium current that occur in slow-channel myasthenic syndrome and hyperkaelemic periodic paralysis (HyperPP), respectively, can lead to a vacuolar myopathy. The abnormal cation leak via the voltage-sensing pore of Cav1.1 or Nav1.4 that occurs in hypokalaemic periodic paralysis (HypoPP) represents a gain of abnormal function (green). ATS, Andersen–Tawil syndrome. Source: Adapted from Kullmann 2010, with permission of Annual Reviews.

Rather than listing all the known channelopathies we here group them according to the type of channel involved, and attempt to classify them as gain- or loss-of function.

Potassium channels

Voltage-gated potassium channels Voltage-gated potassium channels are the largest family of ion channels. They are composed of four homologous pore-forming subunits, as well as four intracellular beta subunits and normally contribute to regulating excitability or terminating action potentials. Each subunit of a voltage-gated potassium channel typically contains six trans-membrane α-helices, of which the S4 segment acts as a voltage sensor (Figure 3.15). Such channels open upon membrane potential depolarisation. Their activation kinetics vary extensively, and some are also modulated by intracellular messengers such as calcium or sodium.

The pore-forming subunits of inward-rectifying potassium channels, in contrast, lack the voltage-sensing module, and such channels conduct potassium ions preferentially at negative potentials. Thus, they have an important role in stabilising membrane potentials at rest, and only a minor role in repolarising action potentials.

To date, human mutations have been identified in only a few of the genes encoding potassium channels. Dominantly inherited loss-of-function mutations of *KCNA1*, which encodes the Kv1.1 potassium channel, cause episodic ataxia type 1, characterised by paroxysms of dyskinesia but also neuromyotonia. Other potassium channel mutations result in either progressive ataxia or paroxysmal

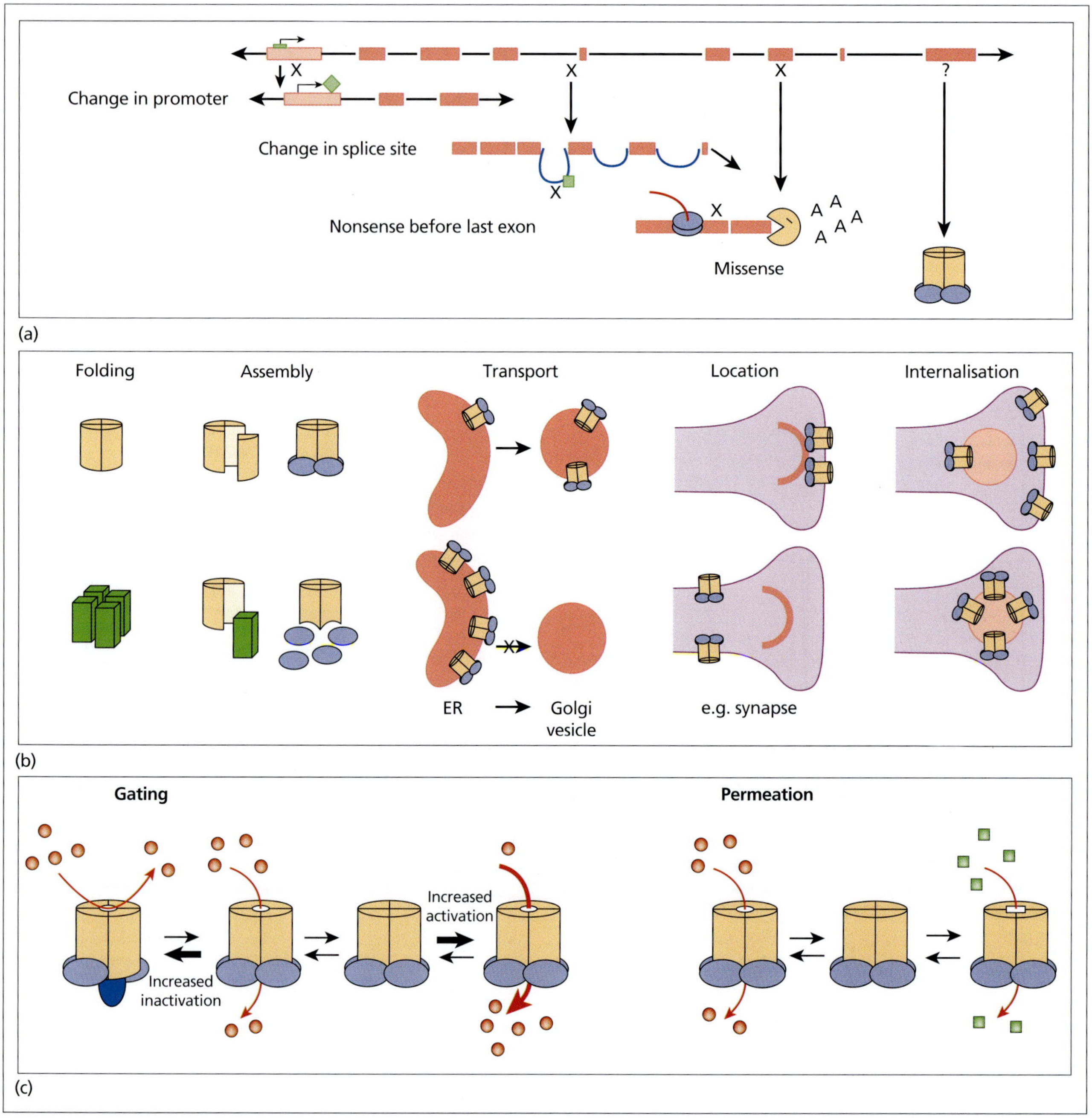

Figure 3.14 Mutations can disrupt ion channel function through many different mechanisms: (a) alterations in transcription; (b) alterations in biogenesis; (c) alterations in function. Source: Kullmann and Schorge 2008. Reproduced with permission of Lippincott Williams & Wilkins.

dyskinesia and epilepsy. The finding that some gain-of-function mutations of a calcium gated potassium channel (*KCNMA1*) or a sodium-gated potassium channel (*KCNT1*) cause epilepsy is at first sight unexpected. A possible explanation is that enhanced repolarisation of the membrane potential reduces inactivation of sodium channels.

Transient receptor potential channels

Transient receptor potential (TRP) channels are closely related to voltage-gated potassium channels. They tend to be less selective for potassium ions (also allowing sodium and, in some cases, calcium ions to flow), and several members are sensitive to temperature and various endogenous and exogenous chemical ligands. Several members of this group of channels have a major role in sensory transduction. Mutations of *TRPV4* can cause a broad range of abnormalities of peripheral nerve development and function, and mutations of *TRPA1* can manifest as a paroxysmal pain disorder.

Sodium channels

Sodium channels open rapidly in response to depolarisation and influx of sodium underlies the upstroke of the action potential. They are structurally homologous to voltage-gated potassium channels, although a single protein with four repeated domains plays the part of the four separate pore-lining proteins of potassium

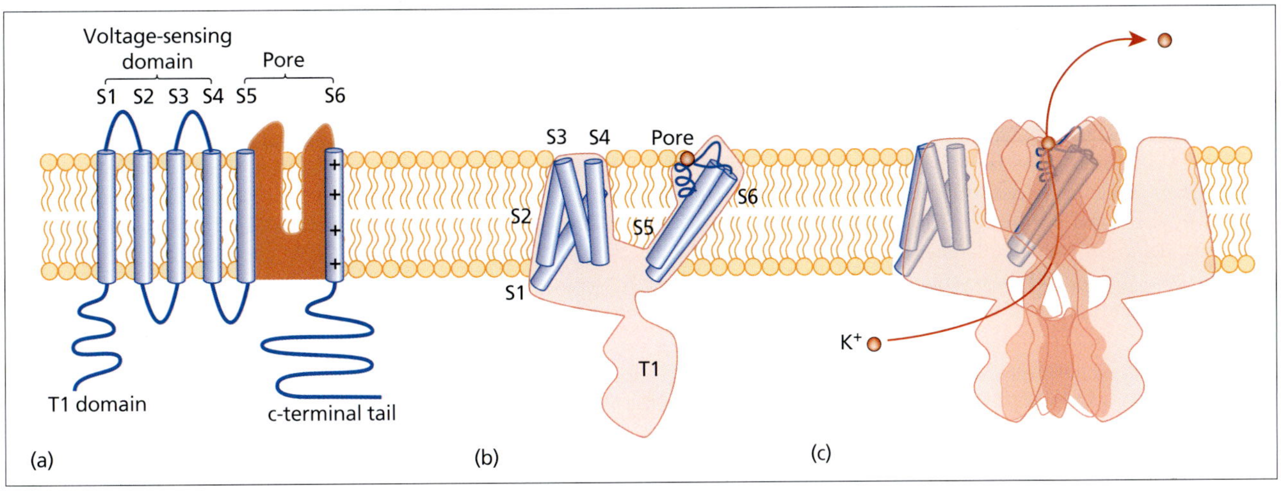

Figure 3.15 Structure of voltage-gated K⁺ channels. (a) Peptide chain showing the six transmembrane segments (S1–6) in the membrane, with the S4 voltage sensor indicated (+). The loop between S5 and S6 forms the pore and selectivity filter. The T1 domain and C-terminal are intracellular. (b) Conformation of a single subunit showing the approximate positions of S1–6 and the selectivity filter (Pore). The T1 domain is important for subunit assembly. (c) Four subunits assemble to make a channel in the membrane. The helices are only shown for one subunit for clarity. The path of a permeating K⁺ ion is indicated. Source: Kullmann and Schorge 2008. Reproduced with permission of Lippincott Williams & Wilkins.

channels. They have one or two associated β subunits with a single trans-membrane segment. An important feature of most sodium channels is that they close rapidly upon sustained depolarisation. Impairment of such fast inactivation occurs in gain-of-function mutations that affect the muscle sodium channel NaV1.4 (encoded by *SCN4A*). Depending on the severity of the impairment in inactivation, muscle fibres are either prone to repetitive firing (myotonia) or can enter a persistent depolarised state, often accompanied by hyperkalaemia (hyperkalaemic periodic paralysis). Paradoxically, loss-of-function mutations of the *SCN1A* gene are an important cause of monogenic epilepsy. A likely explanation is that the encoded α subunit of Nav1.1 is preferentially expressed in cortical interneurones. Impaired excitability of these interneurones predisposes to seizures. A further unexplained finding is that other mutations of *SCN1A* are associated with FHM.

SCN9A, SCN10A and *SCN11A* encode different sodium channels expressed in peripheral nerve. Mutations that impair inactivation cause paroxysmal pain disorders, while recessive loss-of-function mutations manifest as congenital insensitivity to pain.

Calcium channels

Calcium channels have a similar structure as sodium channels although their kinetics are generally much slower. They are divided into three groups according to their kinetics. One of the L-type channels, CaV1.1, has a central role in excitation–contraction coupling in skeletal muscle. P/Q type channels contribute to triggering neurotransmitter release at presynaptic terminals, but are also expressed abundantly in the cerebellar cortex. Low threshold, transiently activating T-type channels have an important role in burst-firing of thalamic neurones. The disease mechanisms of calcium channelopathies are incompletely understood. Hypokalaemic periodic paralysis is caused by mutations of *CACNA1S*, which encodes the muscle calcium channel. However, mutations of the sodium channel gene *SCN4A* can give the same phenotype. Remarkably, almost all mutations of either channel causing hypokalaemic periodic paralysis affect arginine resides in the S4 voltage sensor. These residues are positively charged and sense the trans-membrane potential gradient. Although loss of an arginine residue might be expected to alter voltage activation, hypokalaemic periodic paralysis is actually thought to result from an abnormal cation pathway through a cavity lining the S4 segment, arising from substitution of an arginine residue by a smaller amino acid side-chain. The association of paralysis with hypokalaemia may reflect failure of inward-rectifying potassium channels to stabilise the membrane potential, because these channels fail to conduct when the extracellular potassium concentration is low.

Loss-of-function mutations of *CACNA1A*, which encodes the pore-forming subunit of the CNS calcium channel CaV2.1, cause episodic ataxia type 2, while gain-of-function mutations cause FHM. This channel contributes to triggering neurotransmitter release at synapses throughout the nervous system, and is also abundant in cerebellar Purkinje and granule cells.

Chloride channels

These are unrelated to the voltage-gated channel super-family and are more closely related to some trans-membrane transporters. In skeletal muscle, dimeric ClC-2 channels have a moderate open probability at rest, and have an important role in setting the resting membrane potential. They activate further upon depolarisation. Loss-of-function mutations destabilise the membrane potential and predispose to repetitive discharges. Both dominantly inherited and recessive mutations occur, described as Thomsen and Becker myotonia, respectively. Some cases are compound heterozygotes, where two different recessive mutations occur in an individual, making the task of genetic counselling more difficult.

Ligand-gated ion channels

Fast neurotransmission is mediated by ionotropic receptors, or ligand-gated ion channels. Mutations have been identified in all the main groups.

Acetylcholine receptors Nicotinic receptors (so called because they are activated by nicotine) are either homopentameric or heteropentameric. At the neuromuscular junction ACh opens receptors made up of α1, β1, δ and ε subunits, encoded by *CHRNA1, CHRNB1, CHRND* and *CHRNE*. Mutations of any of these subunits can cause a congenital myasthenic syndrome. These are caused by trafficking or assembly defects, or by a change in receptor kinetics (fast or slow channel syndrome), with different implications for drug treatment. Early in development a γ subunit, encoded by *CHRNG*, takes the place of the δ subunit. *CHRNG* mutations cause multiple pterygium (Escobar's syndrome), thought to be mediated at least in part by impaired fetal motility.

Of the receptor subunits expressed in the CNS, mutations have been identified in *CHRNA4, CHRNA2* and *CHRNB2* (encoding the α4, α2 and β2 subunits, respectively) in autosomal dominant nocturnal frontal lobe epilepsy (ADNFLE). CNS nicotinic receptors mediate fast excitatory transmission to a subset of cortical interneurones, and indirectly modulate excitation of principal cells. Other presynaptic modulatory effects of ACh have also been reported. How the mutations give rise to epilepsy is incompletely understood.

$GABA_A$ receptors These receptors are structurally homologous to nicotinic receptors but are permeable to chloride ions instead of sodium and potassium. They mediate fast inhibitory transmission and are the sites of action of benzodiazepines and several other anticonvulsant, anaesthetic, hypnotic and anxiolytic drugs. Loss-of-function mutations in several subunits have been reported in epilepsy, including *GABRA1, GBRB3* and *GABRG2*, encoding the α1, β3 and γ2 subunits, respectively.

Glycine receptors These are also structurally homologous to $GABA_A$ receptors, and mediate fast inhibition in the spinal cord and brainstem. Dominant or recessive loss-of-function mutations of *GLRA1* and *GLRB* cause familial hyperekplexia.

Glutamate receptors Glutamate receptor mutations were only recently reported. This was a puzzle because these receptors underlie the overwhelming majority of fast excitatory synaptic signals in the brain and spinal cord. They are heterotetrameric receptors, subdivided into three main classes. AMPA (α-amino-3-hydroxy-5-methyl-4-isoxazolepropionic acid) receptors, which open and desensitise very rapidly; kainate receptors, with somewhat slower kinetics; and NMDA receptors. NMDA receptors are permeable to calcium but require not only glutamate but also another ligand (glycine or the D-isomer of serine), as well as membrane depolarisation, to open. This combination of properties explains their role as detectors of the coincidence of presynaptic and post-synaptic activity, which triggers calcium influx leading to synaptic plasticity.

The role of glutamate receptors in synaptic plasticity goes some way to explain why rare mutations of NMDA receptors occur in schizophrenia. One subtype, *GRIN2A* (encoding the NMDA receptor subunit GluN2A), is also associated with rolandic epilepsy and Landau–Kleffner syndrome (paediatric epilepsy with loss of language skills).

Acquired versus inherited channelopathies

Several of the autoimmune disorders associated with (or caused by) antibodies recognising extracellular epitopes affect ion channels: AChRs, P/Q-type Ca^{2+} channels, and glycine and NMDA receptors. Aquaporin 4 is also a transmembrane protein that permits the flow of water between glial cells. As for Caspr2 and LGI-1, these interact with voltage-gated K^+ channels of the Kv1 family, although LGI-1 has also been implicated in modulation of AMPA receptor targeting and function. mGluR1 is a G-protein coupled receptor that is coupled to a cascade that leads to the opening of transient receptor potential channels. Intriguingly, several channels targeted directly or indirectly by autoantibodies are also implicated in inherited diseases. The hereditary channelopathies include mutations of AChRs, P/Q-type Ca^{2+} channels, Kv1.1, and GlyR1 glycine receptors.

In some cases, the phenotype of the hereditary channelopathy overlaps extensively with the acquired autoimmune syndrome affecting the same channel. Thus, several congenital myasthenic syndromes caused by mutations of AChRs are characterised by muscle weakness and fatigability. However, cholinesterase inhibitors, which are effective in myasthenia gravis, are not always effective in the hereditary forms. This can be explained at a molecular level by taking into account the fact that some missense mutations lead to a prolongation of the opening duration of the receptor. For P/Q-type Ca^{2+} channel mutations, in contrast, the hereditary channelopathies are dominated by symptoms attributable to neocortical or cerebellar circuits (hemiplegic migraine, episodic or progressive cerebellar ataxia). The channel is abundant both in the periphery and in the CNS, and a possible explanation for the neuromuscular presentation of Lambert–Eaton myasthenic syndrome is that the channels at the neuromuscular junction are more accessible to circulating antibodies. However, why do missense or truncating mutations of the *CACNA1A* gene that encodes the main pore-forming subunit of P/Q-type channels not detectably affect ACh release at the neuromuscular junction? A possible explanation is that the safety factor for transmission is sufficient to mask subtle derangements that are sufficient to unbalance signalling at probabilistic synapses in the CNS.

The phenotype of hereditary hyperekplexia affecting the GlyR1 subunit is very similar to acquired hyperekplexia. Acquired neuromyotonia caused by anti-Caspr2 antibodies overlaps with the phenotype associated with missense or truncating mutations of the gene encoding Kv1.1. However, these mutations are also associated with disturbed cerebellar coordination, hence the term episodic ataxia type 1, used to describe this channelopathy. Mutations in the *LGI-1* gene, interestingly, lead to a form of non-lesional temporal lobe epilepsy, although the seizures in this condition frequently have auditory features (accompanied by auditory hallucinations or triggered by sounds), and therefore differ from the faciobrachial dystonic seizures associated with autoantibodies against the same protein.

References

Dalakas MC. B cells as therapeutic targets in autoimmune neurological disorders. *Nat Clin Pract Neurol* 2008; **4:** 557–567.

Kanda T. Biology of the blood–nerve barrier and its alteration in immune mediated neuropathies. *J Neurol Neurosurg Psychiatry* 2013; **84:** 208–212.

Kullmann DM. Neurological channelopathies. *Annu Rev Neurosci* 2010; **33:** 151–172.

Kullmann DM, Schorge S. In: *Epilepsy: A Comprehensive Textbook*, vol. **3**, Engel J, Pedley TA, Aicardi J, eds. Lippincott Williams & Wilkins, 2008: 253–266.

Further reading

Genetics

Abrahams BS, Geschwind DH. Advances in autism genetics: on the threshold of a new neurobiology. *Nat Rev Genet* 2008; **9:** 341–355.

Bergoffen J, Scherer SS, Wang S, Scott MO, Bone LJ, Paul DL, *et al.* Connexin mutations in X-linked Charcot–Marie Tooth disease. *Science* 1993; **262:** 2039–2042.

Biesecker LG. Exome sequencing makes medical genomics a reality. *Nat Genet* 2010; **42:** 13–14.

Bundey S, Evans K. Tuberous sclerosis: a genetic study. *J Neurol Neurosurg Psychiatry* 1969; **32:** 591–603.

Caylak E. The genetics of sleep disorders in humans: narcolepsy, restless legs syndrome, and obstructive sleep apnea syndrome. *Am J Med Genet A* 2009; **149A:** 2612–2626.

Choi M, Scholl UI, Ji W, Liu T, Tikhonova IR, Zumbo P, *et al.* Genetic diagnosis by whole exome capture and massively parallel DNA sequencing. *Proc Natl Acad Sci U S A* 2009; **106:** 19096–19101.

Dorschner MO, Amendola LM, Turner EH, Robertson PD, Shirts BH, Gallego CJ, *et al.* Actionable, pathogenic incidental findings in 1,000 participants' exomes. *Am J Hum Genet* 2013; **93:** 631–640.

Gatchel JR, Zoghbi HY. Diseases of unstable repeat expansion: mechanisms and common principles. *Nat Rev Genet* 2005; **6:** 743–755.

Gatz M, Mortimer JA, Fratiglioni L, Johansson B, Berg S, Reynolds CA, *et al.* Potentially modifiable risk factors for dementia in identical twins. *Alzheimers Dement J Alzheimers Assoc* 2006; **2:** 110–117.

Green RC, Lupski JR, Biesecker LG. Reporting genomic sequencing results to ordering clinicians: incidental, but not exceptional. *JAMA* 2013; **310:** 365–366.

Hawkes CH, Macgregor AJ. Twin studies and the heritability of MS: a conclusion. *Mult Scler* 2009; **15:** 661–667.

Helbig I, Scheffer IE, Mulley JC, Berkovic SF. Navigating the channels and beyond: unravelling the genetics of the epilepsies. *Lancet Neurol* 2008; **7:** 231–245.

Ishikawa K, Dürr A, Klopstock T, Müller S, De Toffol B, Vidailhet M, *et al.* Pentanucleotide repeats at the spinocerebellar ataxia type 31 (SCA31) locus in Caucasians. *Neurology* 2011; **77:** 1853–1855.

Kjeldsen MJ, Corey LA, Christensen K, Friis ML. Epileptic seizures and syndromes in twins: the importance of genetic factors. *Epilepsy Res* 2003; **55:** 137–146.

Kobayashi H, Abe K, Matsuura T, Ikeda Y, Hitomi T, Akechi Y, *et al.* Expansion of intronic GGCCTG hexanucleotide repeat in NOP56 causes SCA36, a type of spinocerebellar ataxia accompanied by motor neuron involvement. *Am J Hum Genet* 2011; **89:** 121–130.

La Spada AR, Wilson EM, Lubahn DB, Harding AE, Fischbeck KH. Androgen receptor gene mutations in X-linked spinal and bulbar muscular atrophy. *Nature* 1991; **352:** 77–79.

Majounie E, Renton AE, Mok K, Dopper EGP, Waite A, Rollinson S, *et al.* Frequency of the C9orf72 hexanucleotide repeat expansion in patients with amyotrophic lateral sclerosis and frontotemporal dementia: a cross-sectional study. *Lancet Neurol* 2012; **11:** 323–330.

Mankodi A, Takahashi MP, Jiang H, Beck CL, Bowers WJ, Moxley RT, *et al.* Expanded CUG repeats trigger aberrant splicing of ClC-1 chloride channel pre-mRNA and hyperexcitability of skeletal muscle in myotonic dystrophy. *Mol Cell* 2002; **10;** 35–44.

Mok KY, Koutsis G, Schottlaender LV, Polke J, Panas M, Houlden H. High frequency of the expanded C9ORF72 hexanucleotide repeat in familial and sporadic Greek ALS patients. *Neurobiol Aging* 2012; **33:** 1851.e1–e5.

Ng SB, Buckingham KJ, Lee C, Bigham AW, Tabor HK, Dent KM, *et al.* Exome sequencing identifies the cause of a mendelian disorder. *Nat Genet* 2010; **42:** 30–35.

Ogiwara I, Miyamoto H, Morita N, Atapour N, Mazaki E, Inoue I, *et al.* Nav1.1 localizes to axons of parvalbumin-positive inhibitory interneurons: a circuit basis for epileptic seizures in mice carrying an Scn1a gene mutation. *J Neurosci* 2007; **27:** 5903–5914.

Orr HT, Zoghbi HY. Trinucleotide repeat disorders. *Annu Rev Neurosci* 2007; **30:** 575–621.

Ptácek LJ, George AL, Griggs RC, Tawil R, Kallen RG, Barchi RL, *et al.* Identification of a mutation in the gene causing hyperkalemic periodic paralysis. *Cell* 1991; **67:** 1021–1027.

Rohrer JD, Guerreiro R, Vandrovcova J, Uphill J, Reiman D, Beck J, *et al.* The heritability and genetics of frontotemporal lobar degeneration. *Neurology* 2009; **73:** 1451–1456.

Schäffer AA. Digenic inheritance in medical genetics. *J Med Genet* 2013; **50:** 641–652.

Scheffer IE, Berkovic SF. Generalized epilepsy with febrile seizures plus: a genetic disorder with heterogeneous clinical phenotypes. *Brain J Neurol* 1997; **120:** 479–490.

Singleton AB, Hardy J, Traynor BJ, Houlden H. Towards a complete resolution of the genetic architecture of disease. *Trends Genet* 2010; **26:** 438–442.

Ulrich V, Gervil M, Kyvik KO, Olesen J, Russell MB. Evidence of a genetic factor in migraine with aura: a population-based Danish twin study. *Ann Neurol* 1999; **45:** 242–246.

Van El CG, Cornel MC, Borry P, Hastings RJ, Fellmann F, Hodgson SV, *et al.* Whole-genome sequencing in health care: recommendations of the European Society of Human Genetics. *Eur J Hum Genet* 2013; **21:** 580–584.

Wessman M, Terwindt GM, Kaunisto MA, Palotie A, Ophoff RA. Migraine: a complex genetic disorder. *Lancet Neurol* 2007; **6:** 521–532.

Immunology

Crisp SJ, Kullmann DM, Vincent A. Autoimmune synaptopathies. *Nature Rev Neurosci* 2006; **17:** 103–117.

Mackay I, Rose NR. *The Autoimmune Diseases*, 5th edn. Academic Press, 2014.

Male D, Brostoff J, Roth D, Roitt I. *Immunology*, 8th edn. Elsevier, 2012.

Ransohoff RM, Engelhardt B. The anatomical and cellular basis of immune surveillance in the central nervous system. *Nat Rev Immunol* 2012; **12:** 623–635.

Rimoin DL, Connor JM, Peyritz RE, Korf BR. *Emery and Rimoin's Principles and Practice of Medical Genetics*, 4th edn. Edinburgh: Churchill-Livingstone, 2002.

Witebsky E, Rose NR, Terplan K, Paine JR, Egan RW. Chronic thyroiditis and autoimmunization. *JAMA* 1957; **164:** 1439–1447.

Channelopathies

Browne DL, Gancher ST, Nutt JG, Brunt ER, Smith EA, Kramer P, *et al.* Episodic ataxia/myokymia syndrome is associated with point mutations in the human potassium channel gene, KCNA1. *Nat Genet* 1994; **8:** 136–140.

Cannon SC, Brown RH, Corey DP. A sodium channel defect in hyperkalemic periodic paralysis: potassium-induced failure of inactivation. *Neuron* 1991; **6:** 619–626.

Charlet BN, Savkur RS, Singh G, Philips AV, Grice EA, Cooper TA. Loss of the muscle-specific chloride channel in type 1 myotonic dystrophy due to misregulated alternative splicing. *Mol Cell* 2002; **10:** 45–53.

Claes L, Del-Favero J, Ceulemans B, Lagae L, Van Broeckhoven C, De Jonghe P. De novo mutations in the sodium-channel gene SCN1A cause severe myoclonic epilepsy of infancy. *Am J Hum Genet* 2001; **68:** 1327–1332.

Dichgans M, Freilinger T, Eckstein G, Babini E, Lorenz-Depiereux B, Biskup S, *et al.* Mutation in the neuronal voltage-gated sodium channel SCN1A in familial hemiplegic migraine. *Lancet* 2005; **366:** 371–377.

Du W, Bautista JF, Yang H, Diez-Sampedro A, You SA, Wang L, *et al.* Calcium-sensitive potassium channelopathy in human epilepsy and paroxysmal movement disorder. *Nat Genet* 2005; **37:** 733–738.

Ebers GC, George AL, Barchi RL, Ting-Passador SS, Kallen RG, Lathrop GM, *et al.* Paramyotonia congenita and hyperkalemic periodic paralysis are linked to the adult muscle sodium channel gene. *Ann Neurol* 1991; **30:** 810–816.

Kobayashi H, Abe K, Matsuura T, Ikeda Y, Hitomi T, Akechi Y, *et al.* Expansion of intronic GGCCTG hexanucleotide repeat in NOP56 causes SCA36, a type of spinocerebellar ataxia accompanied by motor neuron involvement. *Am J Hum Genet* 2011; **89:** 121–130.

Kremeyer B, Lopera F, Cox JJ, Momin A, Rugiero F, Marsh S, *et al.* A gain-of-function mutation in TRPA1 causes familial episodic pain syndrome. *Neuron* 2010; **66:** 671–680.

Labrum RW, Rajakulendran S, Graves TD, Eunson LH, Bevan R, Sweeney MG, *et al.* Large-scale calcium channel gene rearrangements in episodic ataxia and hemiplegic migraine: implications for diagnostic testing. *J Med Genet* 2009; **46:** 786–791.

Ogiwara I, Miyamoto H, Morita N, Atapour N, Mazaki E, Inoue I, *et al.* A Met-to-Val mutation in the skeletal muscle Na+ channel alpha-subunit in hyperkalaemic periodic paralysis. *Nature* 1991; **354:** 387–389.

Spillane J, Beeson DJ, Kullmann DM.Myasthenia and related disorders of the neuromuscular junction. *J Neurol Neurosurg Psychiatry* 2010; **81:** 850–857.

Suls A, Claeys KG, Goossens D, Harding B, Van Luijk R, Scheers S, *et al.* Microdeletions involving the SCN1A gene may be common in SCN1A-mutation-negative SMEI patients. *Hum Mutat* 2006; **27:** 914–920.

Yu FH, Mantegazza M, Westenbroek RE, Robbins CA, Kalume F, Burton KA, *et al.* Reduced sodium current in GABAergic interneurons in a mouse model of severe myoclonic epilepsy in infancy. *Nat Neurosci* 2006; **9:** 1142–1149.

CHAPTER 4

The Language of Neurology: Symptoms, Signs and Basic Investigations

Charles Clarke[1], Matthew Adams[1], Robin Howard[1], Martin Rossor[2], Simon Shorvon[2] and Jason Warren[2]

[1] National Hospital for Neurology & Neurosurgery

[2] UCL Institute of Neurology

Knowledge of neuroanatomy and basic neuroscience equips a clinician with the background essential for clinical work. However, there remains a gulf between these scientific aspects of neurology and its language, meaning the words we use to interpret and communicate clinical features in health and disease. The purpose of this chapter is to try to fill that gap and outline the practice of day-to-day neurology:

- To provide a framework for examination, clinical diagnosis and investigation
- To introduce terminology used to capture concepts and patterns – the vocabulary of neurology, and
- To discuss some illustrative patterns essential to recognise.

Facets of the history of neurology and some subtleties of clinical practice are mentioned to provide a brief working overview.

Practical neurology is sometimes straightforward but remarkably difficult at others. Our purpose as diagnosticians is to answer one question: whether or not there is a recognisable disease. In no other branch of medicine is recognition of clinical patterns more important, nor are they more reliable. Despite major advances in imaging, neurogenetics and neuropathology, clinical practice continues to follow a traditional systematic approach:

- Assemble the elements of clinical observation in a structured fashion commencing with the history and symptoms, physical signs found on examination and followed by results of appropriate investigations.
- Recognise by assessing and sifting the layers of information, the site of a lesion, its nature and/or the system affected.

Failure to follow this approach can lead to errors and especially misjudging the seriousness of a problem, either overestimating symptoms – thus leading to alarm and expense or, vice versa, missing a serious disease. Symptoms that do not relate to any serious structural disease are common in practice. These are discussed further in Chapter 22 (see Non-organic disorders in neurology).

Elements of diagnosis

The components of clinical diagnosis in neurology – its essence and singularity – are the clinical history and examination and the interplay between the two. Many people find neurology hard, both because of this interplay and also because of its breadth: few specialties deal with such a wide range of conditions.

In some conditions, such as migraine or epilepsy, we rely on the descriptions of symptoms, that is a narrative from the patient or an eyewitness. There are no physical signs. In other situations, examination has a pivotal role, for example the signs indicating emergence of a spastic paraparesis or a neuromuscular disorder. When one pattern of symptoms might be explained by pathology in different parts of the nervous system or by different mechanisms, interpretation of physical signs is of particular importance. However, despite its sophistication the nervous system has a relatively limited repertoire of symptom complexes. For example, the pain of a headache is often much the same whether the problem is benign or sinister.

Diagnosis is a two-stage process:

1. Do the history and physical signs point to the site of the lesion, or lesions or to a system?
2. Do the time course and character of the findings point to a recognisable disease?

It is the recognition of these patterns that enables reliable diagnosis.

History

The narrative, from the patient, relatives or other witnesses provides primary data. This is vital information. Details of symptoms or events at the onset of a condition are helpful as a first step towards a diagnosis. How to take a present, past and family history is assumed here but there are three areas where difficulties and pitfalls commonly occur.

First, vividness can only be provided by an account taken verbatim, of events. With electronic records and abbreviation overtaking written notes, simple narrative and a clear record of what happened remain important. For example, 'Fitted in bus on way to A&E – bitten tongue' is familiar medical shorthand seen in emergency notes. The inference is that a generalised tonic–clonic seizure took place. The phrase does not indicate what the patient actually said:

> I was standing on the Number 73 bus near King's Cross first thing in the morning taking my mum to the hospital at University College. I felt all dizzy and sick, my eyes went all funny, then my legs went weak and out I went. I came to on the floor, between the seats, in a pool of blood. My mother says I fainted. But then the ambulance came and they said I was shaking. I had bitten my lip quite badly. I was right as rain within one minute but the lady in the ambulance said she thought I had had a fit.

Neurology: A Queen Square Textbook, Second Edition. Edited by Charles Clarke, Robin Howard, Martin Rossor and Simon Shorvon.

From this description – the brief duration of loss of consciousness and transient shaking – syncope seems an obvious answer, and not the generalised tonic–clonic seizure implied by the original medical note. Shorthand and jargon leading to misdiagnosis can have far-reaching consequences.

Secondly, it is important to identify the temporal pattern of symptoms.

- Intermittent events or attacks with full recovery: common causes are epilepsy, migraine, syncope, transient ischaemic attacks. There are other much rarer causes such as paroxysmal dyskinesia.
- Intermittent, with relapses and remissions: multiple sclerosis (MS) is the typical example, but it should not be forgotten that many conditions fluctuate as a result of the patient's affective state and environmental factors.
- Progressive, chronic. Neurodegenerative and neoplastic disorders tend to follow this pattern.
- Acute or subacute and progressive. These are usually infective or inflammatory disorders.
- Acute onset, single insult, with some recovery. Stroke is the prime example. Guillain–Barré syndrome is another.

The long time scale of some neurological conditions can be important – a history of prolonged febrile convulsions in infancy or a head injury long forgotten may be of relevance to episodes of loss of consciousness in adult life.

Other aspects of the history can point to a diagnosis, such as the family history, the latter frequently overlooked.

Thirdly, there is the matter of a physician's attitude, that balance between critical appraisal and sympathy – and a reminder that our principal purpose is to help. Judgmental attitudes not only interfere with diagnosis; they are frequent causes of complaints and the need for second opinions.

Many patients find it difficult to answer unexpected or unfamiliar questions quickly and clearly. There is no such thing as a 'hopeless historian' and if a history is incomplete, it is often as much the fault of the interrogating physician as of the patient. Patients today are also better and more accurately informed than in the past. However, the unsympathetic neurologist is still described too frequently and vividly to be discounted. Whether or not symptoms reflect serious disease, patients do actually suffer from their complaints. That first visit frequently carries a burden – a serious diagnosis is often in mind. Patients and their relatives hang hopes and fears upon single words, phrases and comments made by medical or nursing staff. Furthermore, depression, and psychiatric co-morbidity are features of many neurological conditions and anxiety is common in any clinical situation, serious or apparently trivial.

Nature of symptoms

Textbooks that provided the foundations of clinical practice emphasised the distinction between primary and secondary symptoms, and positive and negative phenomena. This approach needs to be understood, although the classification is not rigid. Most anatomical brain, cord, root and nerve lesions are destructive. They cause negative phenomena such as such as paralysis. Destructive lesions may also cause positive secondary phenomena, typically when neuronal inhibition is released (e.g. exaggerated tendon reflexes, clonus). Positive is also used to describe irritative phenomena, usually electrical such as seizures or myoclonus.

Abnormalities of function can thus be regarded in two ways:

1. Primary (direct) abnormalities, often negative: one part fails to work. Primary abnormalities can also be positive (irritative), for example focal seizures resulting from a cortical glioma, pain in the distribution of a trapped median nerve or hemifacial spasm.
2. Secondary (indirect) abnormalities, usually positive, often indicate over-activity resulting from release of inhibition (e.g. clonus).

Neurological examination

Preliminary assessment

Many features become apparent during conversation, during the narrative history. The neurologist Gordon Holmes wrote in 1946: 'More can often be learned of a patient's disabilities by observing his ordinary actions, as dressing and undressing, walking when apparently unobserved than by specific tests.' We rely heavily on this apparently casual approach unconsciously on a daily basis. It is the way we form an impression when meeting someone new, and gauge our own friends and colleagues. There is much to be learnt from studying this approach before more formal examination. We all use such skills intuitively but can refine them. The following can be readily assessed prior to more formal examination on a couch:

- Greeting, manner, orientation, attention, mental state, mood, personal hygiene, dress
- Cognitive conversational clues – for example a mildly cognitively impaired patient turning towards a relative to answer a simple question
- Speech, language and facial appearance
- Gait and stance
- Clumsiness, weakness of one side
- Involuntary movements
- Patterns of sensory symptoms
- Risk factors, lifestyle, tobacco, alcohol, drug abuse
- Obsessions, religion, illness beliefs, fears
- Degree of disability, aids – both at home and outside, state benefits
- Aspects of daily living, travel, driving, employment, dangerous sports
- Endocrine or general medical clues, such as appearance suggestive of hypothyroidism or hypopituitarism.
- Relations with general practitioners, hospitals and paramedical staff, nursing staff and specialists
- Expectations and ideas about treatment.

Brief neurological examination

It is assumed that the reader can carry out a general examination and understands the rudiments of neurology. Detailed neurological examination for every case is simply impracticable in busy clinical life. In many settings we need to rely on a robust, safe and practical examination tailored to the individual, and to be guided by the history. A man who faints on a bus does not need two-point discrimination to be assessed. A tendency to dwell on excessive detail of examination seemed to beleaguer generations of neurologists. Table 4.1 illustrates a brief neurological examination, completed easily within 5 minutes and readily adaptable to circumstance.

Detailed neurological examination

More detailed examination is sometimes necessary and a full examination is often essential when evaluating a complex cases. The scheme developed at the National Hospital is widely used and

Table 4.1 Brief 5-part neurological examination.

1 Look at the patient	**4 Lower limbs**
General demeanour	Tone
Speech, language, cognition	Power (hip flexion, ankle dorsiflexion)
Gait, heel–toe, possibly	Coordination
Romberg's test	Reflexes
Arm swinging	Plantar responses
2 Head	**5 Sensation**
Fundi	Simply ask, in most: is it normal?
Acuity (if appropriate)	
Pupils	
Eye movements	With an appropriate general examination, including blood pressure this assessment is highly unlikely to miss serious disease
Facial movements	
Tongue	
3 Upper limbs	
Posture of outstretched arms	
Wasting, fasciculation	
Tone, power	
Coordination	
Reflexes	

adapted into Table 4.2. This helps to avoid omitting important data and records information. The order presented here is the way in which most neurologists work; it is helpful to follow it.

Cognition and mental state

Much will have taken place during the clinical history. A written record of the cognitive assessment is useful to document the situation. Many simple screening tests are used to assess basic data such as orientation, recall, naming and reading ability.

More detailed screening tests are also readily available. The Queen Square Cognitive Screening Tests are used widely; there are many others. These assess:

- Orientation and alertness
- Language
- Literacy
- Praxis
- Memory, and
- Right hemisphere function.

These screening tests provide an accurate assessment in a clinic or at the bedside and can be confirmed and explored by further detailed clinical psychometry (see later and Cognitive functions and their clinical syndromes; Neuropsychometry, Chapter 8).

Episodes of disturbed consciousness are discussed in Chapter 7 (see Differential diagnosis of epilepsy), and coma, stupor and similar states in Chapter 20 (see States of impaired consciousness).

Skull, scalp and spine

Skull and scalp examination is often omitted; abnormalities of contour and circumference, old burr holes or gnarled pulseless scalp vessels and skull bruits may be found. One author uses the following technique for listening for bruits, to abolish extraneous noise from eyelid muscles and respiration:

- Ask the patient to close both eyes, gently
- Rest the bell of an old-fashioned stethoscope over one closed lid
- Ask the patient first to open the other eye, and
- To stop breathing, briefly.

Examine the spine and its contour. Assess for scars, stiffness, deformity, pain, spinal bruits and for tufts of hair, dimples, sinuses or suggestions of congenital abnormalities.

Cranial nerves

I: olfaction

Two test substances from a selection of clove oil, peppermint, mint, eucalyptus oil – or simply soap, coffee or an orange – are adequate to determine whether someone can distinguish between odours. More complex olfactory test kits are becoming more widely used, for example in Parkinson's or Alzheimer's disease (see Olfactory nerve, Chapter 13). Ammonia is sometimes available, supposedly to assess trigeminal afferent responses. Such a highly irritant substance should be avoided.

II: vision, pupils and fundi

Visual acuity: a well-lit 3-metre handheld Snellen chart is usually adequate. Correction with the patient's distance lenses or a pinhole (easily fashioned from paper) may be needed. A record of acuity is one hallmark of a careful examination (see also Chapter 14).

Visual field examination to finger confrontation is highly reliable for picking up hemianopic and visual attention defects. When appropriate, follow this by confrontation testing with a 5-mm white and 5-mm red pinhead, or other target. One technique is to ask the patient to cover their left eye and fix the gaze of their right with your own left eye – pupil to pupil. Remember that the visual field is not planar but part of a sphere: move a target along the circumference of a circle, about 50 cm away from the eye. Commence with the pinhead target behind the ear and thus outside the visual field and move it towards the point of fixation. In the normal person both a red and white pinhead will be perceived at around 90° from the visual axis.

There are various manouevres using white and red-headed pins. One suggestion is to ask for a single word response. With the white pinhead, tell the patient to say: 'NOW', when they see the pinhead. With the red pinhead, tell the patient to say ' RED' when they see it.

Central field defects: use an Amsler grid, or, ask the patient to look at newspaper text and indicate any holes in their vision.

Colour vision is speedily assessed with Ishihara plates (still in use after nearly a century), or with detailed 100 Hue Test cards.

Pupil reactions are seen best in low levels of illumination using a bright light shone through the lens, approaching from the temporal side to avoid producing convergence. Subtle abnormalities of the pupillary response to light (e.g. an early Horner's syndrome) can sometimes be picked up by darkening the room. Cross-illumination – a pen torch at right angles to the visual axis – will help light up an iris of a darker shade. Putting these two together (direct and cross-illumination), many a pupil apparently unreactive in daylight, such as in old age (senile miosis) can be seen to constrict. The swinging light test, especially in dim light, can identify a relative afferent pupillary defect. Other abnormalities of the pupils are discussed in Chapters 14 (see Examination) and 20 (see Pupillary responses).

Fundus examination takes experience to perfect. The crux is to develop a suitable personal technique. Suggestions are:

- Have the patient seated, gazing horizontally – not at the ceiling. Suggest that they gaze at some distant specific object. Mention there is no problem if they blink. These manoeuvres avoid one's own clothing or hair falling into the subject's face,

Table 4.2 Detailed neurological examination.

Historical details

Main complaints
History of present illness
Past illnesses
Review of previous opinions, practice notes, etc.
Family history, with details of size of family
Social, personal, alcohol, drugs, tobacco, etc.
Travel, occupation, etc.
Review of systems:
- cardiovascular
- respiratory
- gastro-intestinal
- genito-urinary
- endocrine
- psychiatric history
- allergies – drug and other

Examination

Physical appearance, initial appraisal
Mental state and cognition
Speech, language functions, evidence of higher function problems
Skull and spine
Gait, stance, balance
Hand preference – writing, etc.

Cranial nerves

I. Olfaction
II. Visual acuity
Visual fields – describe/chart

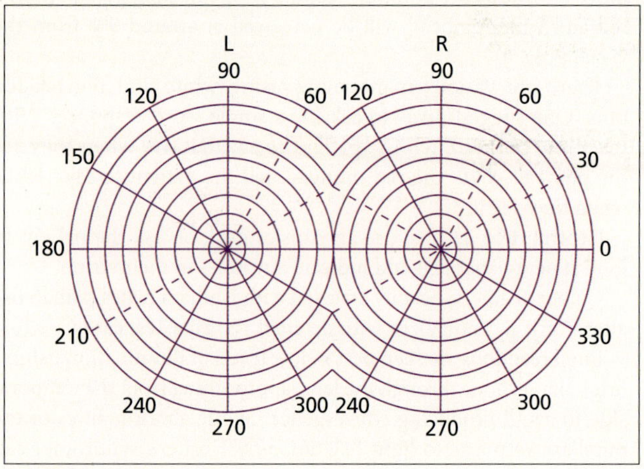

Fundus
Pupils (mm, shape, reactions)
III, IV, VI. Range of ocular movements, nystagmus
Inspection of each eye, proptosis, cornea, primary position of gaze
V. Facial sensation, corneal reflexes. Power: masseter, temporalis. Jaw jerk
VII. Facial symmetry, weakness, abnormal movements, taste
VIII. Hearing, Rinne, Weber, vertigo, nystgamus
IX, X. Swallowing, phonation, gag reflex, pharyngeal sensation
XI. Sternomastoids, trapezii
XII. Tongue appearance, speed, central protrusion, fibrillation

Motor system

Abnormal movements – describe
Posture of upper limbs – describe
Tone
Power
MRC Scale 1/5 and/or describe wasting; fasciculation, muscle consistency
Assess limbs, neck, diaphragm, abdomen
Coordination (finger–nose, heel–shin, alternating movements, foot tapping, etc.)
Reflexes:
- jaw jerk
- biceps jerks
- supinator jerks
- triceps jerks
- finger jerks
- abdominals (upper and lower)
- knee jerks
- ankle jerks
- plantar responses
- other reflexes (state)

Sensation

Assess posterior columns: vibration (128 Hz, VS), joint position (JPS), light touch (LT), 2-point
Assess spinothalamic pathway: pain (PP), hot/cold (TM)
Chart findings: PP, TM, LT, etc.

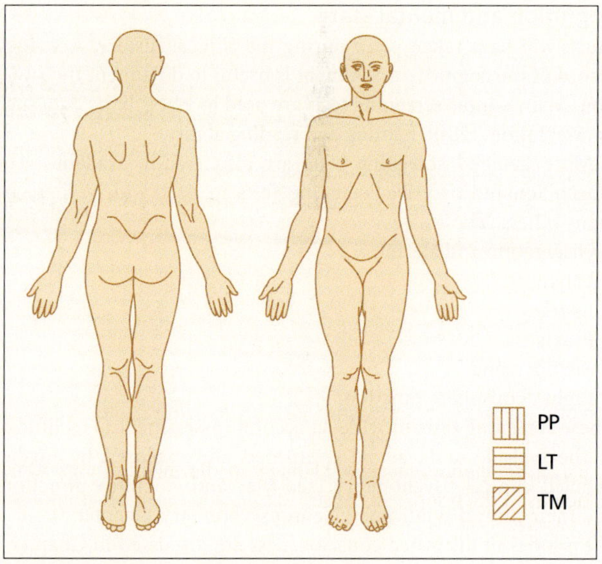

General physical examination

Cardiovascular, BP, respiratory, abdomen, endocrine, skin, nodes, joints

Summary of findings

Formulation

Provisional diagnosis

help fixation and discourage following the ophthalmoscope light source.
- For the left fundus, look through the ophthalmoscope with your own left eye. This encourages the patient to look past your head and to fixate. Do not close your own right eye; if this is hard to achieve, cover it with a free right hand. This helps your viewing left eye to focus on infinity through the ophthalmoscope, and allows your face to relax.

III, IV and VI: eye movements

Recently acquired double vision is a frequent reason for urgent referral and for many doctors a cause of confusion and anxiety. This seems especially so if the 'four formal rules' for diplopia (Table 4.3) are followed rigidly for every case. An alternative, shorthand system relies much on recognition at a glance: every experienced neurologist uses this technique. This simple scheme diagnoses most cases immediately by seeing if the diplopia fits one of four patterns. A tendon hammer shaft is a convenient tool for the patient to follow.

VI: abducens nerve palsy This causes:
- The complaint of double vision with two images side by side (i.e. diplopia with horizontal separation)
- An evident convergent squint
- Double vision that disappears on looking away from the weak lateral rectus muscle and vice versa – worse towards the weak muscle in the obviously squinting eye, and
- No abnormality in reaction to light in the pupil, and no ptosis.

Remember that a lateral rectus palsy can be caused either by a VIth nerve lesion or by disease of the lateral rectus muscle or neuromuscular junction.

III: oculomotor nerve palsy A complete IIIrd nerve palsy causes:
- Ptosis – the upper lid drops, covering the eye completely
- A large pupil unreactive to direct light (the contralateral pupil constricts normally)
- An eye (on lifting the upper lid gently) facing down and out.

Compression of the IIIrd nerve by an enlarging posterior communicating artery aneurysm is a common cause.

The term partial IIIrd nerve palsy usually implies sparing of the pupillary and lid parasympathetic fibres; these lie on the undersurface of the IIIrd nerve and have a separate blood supply. The pupil remains normal. Ptosis is incomplete. The eye faces down and out. A complication of diabetes is a typical cause (see Diabetes mellitus, Chapter 26).

Internuclear ophthalmoplegia Damage to the medial longitudinal fasciculus in the brainstem causes an internuclear ophthalmoplegia (INO):
- Disconjugate horizontal eye movements (i.e. movements not yoked together – the eyes move horizontally at different velocities). One suggestion to help observe disconjugate movement is to look at the centre of the patient's forehead, otherwise there is a tendency for the examiner to fixate on one eye and miss what is happening to movement in the other.
- Incomplete adduction of one eye – and when this is so:
- Coarse jerk nystagmus is seen on lateral gaze in the other eye (i.e. on abduction).

Internuclear ophthalmoplegia is described as left-sided when there is failure of left adduction (i.e. looking to the right). There are various varieties of INO (see Internuclear ophthalmoplegia, Chapter 14).

IV: trochlear nerve palsy A IVth nerve palsy, causes:
- A complaint of double vision on looking down (e.g. descending stairs)
- Twisted images (i.e. one at an angle to the other), known as torsional diplopia
- Head tilt away from side of superior oblique muscle weakness
- No obvious squint.

This is a distinct rarity compared with IIIrd and VIth nerve palsies and INO.

Four rules for diplopia assessment There are numerous other varieties of weakness of the extraocular muscles and the more detailed approach becomes necessary when cases do not fit into the patterns above. The four formal rules established in the early twentieth century are logical and invaluable in such complex cases (Table 4.3). Even using them, some cases of ocular muscle disease (e.g. myasthenia, ocular myopathy) can prove difficult. It is usual to track movements in the shape of an H. Lateral movements are assessed, followed by elevation and depression at about 30° of lateral gaze.

A minor degree of diplopia is an almost normal finding at the extremes of gaze; blurring and false-framing of objects is also easily accomplished, either in error or deliberately, by converging on an object closer than one's natural near point.

Table 4.3 Four rules for recognition of a weak ocular muscle.

1	The false image is usually the less distinct and more peripheral
2	Diplopia occurs in positions that depend upon contraction of a weak muscle
3	The false image is projected in the direction of action of the weak muscle
4	Image separation increases in the direction of action of the weak muscle

V: trigeminal nerve – sensory and motor

Most people with sensory loss in the distribution of one or more trigeminal nerve branches complain of numbness and tingling in a clearly defined zone making detailed assessment of pain, temperature and light touch superfluous (see Figure 4.21 for V distribution). Most people have had temporary partial V_3 sensory loss following a lidocaine injection at the dentist, so this is familiar. Conversely, the loss of corneal sensation found with an early acoustic neuroma, or other lesion at the cerebello-pontine angle (CPA) is usually imperceptible until corneal sensation is actually tested.

Corneal reflex and other aspects of Vth nerve examination Approach the cornea from the lower temporal side to avoid a visual threat, with a pointed wisp of cotton wool. Gently draw down the lower lid. Rest the tip of the cotton wool gently upon the inferolateral cornea – between 6 and 9 o'clock for the right eye. Ask the patient what they feel and observe the surrounding conjunctiva for the normal reddening and tearing. Someone with an early depressed corneal reflex may say 'I can feel you touch me but it isn't painful as on the other side.' When the corneal reflex is depressed, conjunctival reddening and tearing are diminished.

The fine detail of the corneal reflex is that V_2 supplies the lower 60° corneal sector, between about 5 and 7 o'clock; V_1 the supplies the upper 300°. This is occasionally of clinical value.

Neurologists vary in the emphasis they attach to evident blinking which is the VIIth nerve reflex response to corneal nociception during testing the corneal. Many test the corneal reflex to examine the Vth nerve alone. However, the blink (V → VII) response is sometimes valuable in ITU (see Other cranial nerves (blink reflex), Chapter 20).

There are several aspects of Vth nerve examination that relate to the distribution of its three divisions:

- The distribution of V_1 extends to the scalp as far as the vertex via the supra-orbital nerve. Supra-orbital nerve lesions, often traumatic or surgical, can cause persistent headaches and scalp numbness.
- V_3 does not supply the skin of the neck. Patients with non-organic sensory disturbance of the face and neck are sometimes misinterpreted as suffering from a Vth nerve lesion. C2 supplies the posterior scalp, including the area up just in front of the angle of the jaw.
- A slight difference in temperature perception between one side of the face and the other is common. This is rarely of any significance. Brainstem lesions cause onion skin sensory loss (Chapter 2, Figure 2.53 and Chapter 13, Figure 13.2). Complaints of sensory disturbance around the mouth should not be dismissed.

V motor examination Motor lesions of V are unusual, but easy to miss unless jaw deviation to the weaker side on opening the mouth is observed (though a rarely seen sign). Look at the incisor teeth: establish the centre line of the upper and lower incisors and see if the lower incisor centre line remains central or moves laterally as the jaw opens against slight resistance. The jaw jerk should also be assessed.

VII: facial nerve

A complete lower motor neurone (LMN) facial palsy affects all facial muscles on one side, whereas upper motor neurone (UMN) weakness affects lower parts of the face; this spares blinking and wrinkling of the forehead. This difference between UMN and LMN lesions is explained by bilateral innervation of parts of the VIIth nuclei supplying upper facial muscles (see Facial nerve, Chapter 2). There are some subtleties of facial examination. In early UMN facial weakness, all that may be evident is a hint of slowing or delay of a blink, spontaneous grin or grimace. There may be dissociation between voluntary and involuntary movement: formal 'show your teeth' examination can remain normal, while a spontaneous smile is slow on one side.

For LMN examination, divide up the face and suggest definite actions:

- *Frontalis:* 'look upwards' normally produces furrowing of the brow – the response required. A 'wrinkle your forehead' suggestion tends to produce a variable grimace
- *Orbicularis oculi:* try 'screw up your eyes tightly'
- *Alae nasae:* 'wrinkle your nose'
- *Orbicularis oris:* 'now try to whistle gently'
- *Risorius* (and others): 'and now please show me your teeth'
- *Platysma:* men who use a razor find this muscle easy to demonstrate – they tension the skin of the neck. With women, it is said that eversion of the lower lip is the way to demonstrate platysma; another suggestion is to: 'stick out your chin and grunt' – neither seems appropriate. Attempting to copy the examiner usually solves the problem.

Involuntary movement of the face (e.g. myokymia; see later and Other involuntary facial movements (myokymia), Chapter 13), fasciculation and minor degrees of hemifacial spasm can be hard to see. Illuminate the face well, and look closely.

Finally, as a practical point, the gradual emergence of patchy facial weakness is distinctly unusual in Bell's palsy – the most common cause of acute LMN weakness. If LMN facial weakness develops gradually over weeks, suspect a cause other than Bell's. In Bell's (see Bell's palsy, Chapter 13), weakness is usually at its worst within 12 hours; there is frequently pain around the mastoid, hyperacusis and loss of taste.

VIII: auditory nerve

Formal testing is often unnecessary when there is no problem with hearing. If there is a degree of hearing loss, record the distance at which a whisper (or speech) is heard. The Rinne test (Heinrich Rinne, German otologist 1819–1868) is excellent for conductive deafness but of less value for the sensorineural deafness of particular interest to a neurologist.

Here is a simple pragmatic approach to the assessment of hearing:

- Record the distance a whisper is heard from the ear.
- Occlude gently both external auditory meati with the tips of each index finger. Rustle with each middle finger the skin/hair over the mastoid. This provides a rough-and-ready measure of bone conduction. If there is an evident difference between each ear, perceptive (sensorineural) loss is usually present. It is remarkable how accurate this is.

Rinne and Weber tests (Ernst Weber, Leipzig 1795–1878) are discussed in Chapter 15. In practice, suspicion of a cerebellopontine angle lesion (in full, surely?) will be followed by detailed MR imaging and specialised audiometry.

VIII: vestibular nerve

Dizziness, vertigo and nystagmus are dealt with in more detail in Chapter 15 (see Dizziness and vertigo). The basic balance tests are observation of gait and station, and Romberg and Unterberger tests (R+U). Opinions vary about the value of these two named tests. One view is that they are obsolete, pointing out that injuries occur if tests are carried out carelessly. The Romberg test (Moritz Romberg, Berlin 1795–1873) was once used in the diagnosis of tabes dorsalis. In this variety of neurosyphilis, joint position sense became so severely impaired that the patient would lurch wildly on closing the eyes. The Unterberger test ('Stand to attention with arms extended forwards, march on the spot and close the eyes') is a non-specific test developed in 1938 for either vestibular or cerebellar problems. There is turning towards the side of the lesion. One, perhaps cynical, view is that tests show theatrical responses in those with no organic disease – but in these cases particular care must be taken to avoid injury. Most find R+U tests of some value – Romberg's is useful for detection of subtle proprioceptive loss.

With nystagmus a common error is to over-diagnose a few beats of nystagmus at the extremes of lateral gaze. This is normal, not pathological. Nystagmus must usually be sustained, and well within binocular gaze, to be pathological.

IX and X: glossopharyngeal and vagus nerves

Take these nerves together. Observe uvula and fauces with the patient on saying 'Aaah' if there is need to test the gag reflex. Look also for pooling of saliva and residual food remnants. The gag reflex is no longer used alone as a measure of safety for swallowing. Some patients with an intact but hyperactive gag continue to swallow, but do so in a disorganised way and may aspirate; others with a depressed gag are shown on videofluoroscopy to swallow safely without aspirating. If there is a question of bulbar weakness or difficulty swallowing:

- Listen to the voice – this sounds 'wet' in the early stages of bulbar muscle weakness (see Bulbar and pseudobulbar palsy, Chapter 13)
- Ask the patient to cough
- Look for deviation of the palate/uvula (away from the side of the lesion)
- Watch the patient begin to drink a glass of water, if this seems safe and look for spluttering, choking and pooling after a mouthful.

An isolated IXth nerve palsy – a rarity and hard to identify – causes impaired sensation on one side of the pharynx. Tickling the area with a cotton wool bud in the normal person causes discomfort and elicits gagging, via the vagus.

XI: accessory nerve

Examine trapezii and sternomastoids; look for winging of the scapula, weak shoulder shrugging and head turning (see Accessory nerve, Chapter 13).The most common cause of an isolated spinal accessory nerve lesion is attempted biopsy of a node in the posterior triangle of the neck. The nerve is superficial here and easily damaged on its route to trapezius. Muscle weakness is immediate, but weeks or months later, pain around the shoulder and upper scapula may develop, typically intractable and neuralgic in quality.

XII: hypoglossal nerve

Tongue wasting and deviation to the weak side when protruded is the sign of a unilateral XIIth nerve lesion. It is also useful to look at tongue movements. Speed and amplitude of tongue movement are diminished in bilateral pyramidal lesions and commonly early in Parkinson's disease. Tongue fibrillation, seen in motor neurone disease, should be diagnosed only when the tongue rests within the mouth; tongue twitching occurs in normal people when it is protruded.

Gait and disorders of movement

The pattern of walking and abnormal movements will have been noted in the initial appraisal. Reflect on that first impression and analyse it.

Record whether gait is:

- Normal and symmetrical without limp, or abnormal, perhaps in some ill-defined way
- Spastic – narrow-based, stiff, or toe-scuffing
- Hemiparetic
- Extrapyramidal – shuffling, festinant (meaning hurrying), with poor arm swinging, or simply slow
- Apraxic – perhaps with gait ignition failure, or with walking difficulty but with preserved ability to move the legs rapidly while on a bed or seated, with normal imitated bicycling movements
- Ataxic – broad-based, unsteady
- High stepping, foot drop, myopathic, antalgic, neuropathic, or
- Unusual in any other way, for example, affected by dystonia, chorea or myoclonus, or apparently theatrical and non-organic.

It is feasible to categorise most gait problems by observation, but the issue is to avoid missing something subtle yet quite evident. For example, fidgetiness of early chorea can easily pass unnoticed. Early dystonia is easy to miss. Many gait disorders labelled initially as non-organic or even deliberate turn out to be caused by an organic movement disorder. A brief video, now readily available on a mobile phone, can be helpful.

Motor system

Limb function and motor abnormality is a pivotal part of neurological examination. This is an area where eponyms became attached to hard physical signs – Babinski being the lasting example.

Posture of outstretched upper limbs

The posture of the outstretched upper limbs is a useful way to begin. This manoeuvre establishes physical rapport with the patient; examination candidates demonstrate immediately familiarity with neurology. The hands and nails are also readily visible.

Ask the patient to extend the bare arms symmetrically, palms uppermost, and then close the eyes. Upper limb wasting and abnormal movements become evident. Drift with pronation and descent towards the midline is a cardinal sign of an early pyramidal lesion, as valuable diagnostically as an extensor plantar. Postural tremor appears; rest tremor diminishes. Chorea and the asterixis of hepatic disease become apparent. Pseudochorea, the waving movements of denervation (peripheral nerve disease) or parietal lobe disease, may be seen.

Gentle downward pressure at the wrists is then applied, and released. Rebound on one side suggests a cerebellar lesion.

Fatiguability appears as inability to maintain the arm outstretched horizontally, the basis for the arm outstretched duration test in myasthenia.

Non-organic problems are often accompanied by aimless waving around.

Tone

To distinguish between signs of spasticity with pyramidal increase in tone and the stiffness of an akinetic-rigid syndrome requires two distinct examination techniques.

In Parkinson's disease, the extrapyramidal lead pipe rigidity is detectable throughout all passive movements of a joint. Begin with the wrist; take the hand through slow, extension, flexion and rotation movements, so that the wrist joint is moved in all directions. This manoeuvre elicits early signs of stiffness in forearm muscles and cogwheeling. This stiffness becomes more marked when the opposite limb is moved actively (known as synkinesis), a sign that is found in Parkinson but is not specific for the condition. By contrast, in spasticity, the early pronator catch or the beats of emerging ankle clonus will become apparent, but only if sought by brisk rather than slow passive movements – supinating the forearm or dorsiflexing the ankle. Slow passive movements can miss early pyramidal signs because spasticity increases with the rate of passive movement. The catch of increased tone at the ankle becomes apparent before demonstrable sustained clonus is found (i.e. when there are >4 beats of ankle clonus).

Power, muscle bulk and consistency

Various scales have been devised to record weakness, including a 10-point system. The six-point, MRC 0–5 Scale is usually used (Table 4.4) but has two limitations: the inability to record easily slight weakness, and dependence on effort/cooperation. A brief description (e.g. 'I could just overcome hip flexion') deals more effectively with slight weakness than 4^+ and 4^-. 'Give-way' weakness implies poor effort, or can be caused by pain. Skilled hand and foot movement assessment is important: ask the patient to play an imaginary piano and/or touch sequentially with the tip of the thumb the fingertip of the fifth, fourth, ring and index finger, back and forth – and ask them to wriggle the toes. These are good tests of pyramidal function.

Fatiguability should be assessed by repeating a movement if the story suggests this might be present. The slow relaxation of myotonia should also become apparent – provided one remembers to consider it.

Focal or general muscle wasting, fasciculation and muscle consistency should be assessed.

Table 4.4 Six Medical Research Council grades of weakness.

5	Normal power
4	Active movement against gravity and resistance
3	Active movement against gravity
2	Active movement with gravity eliminated
1	Flicker of contraction
0	No visible muscle contraction

Note: these UK Medical Research Council grades (0/5 to 5/5) were designed to record changes in power during poliomyelitis. Although more applicable to lower motor neurone weakness they remain widely used throughout neurology.

Coordination – cerebellar signs

Signs of early cerebellar disease (Chapter 17) may have been noted during initial assessment, such as dysarthria, tremor or an ataxic gait. Rebound on testing upper limb posture is seen. Proceed by looking for dysmetria (past pointing) and action tremor. It is important to appreciate that unsteadiness and shakiness do not equate to cerebellar disease or cerebellar damage – sometimes a pitfall in legal cases following head injury.

Dysmetria: ask the patient to place their forefinger on the point of a tendon hammer shaft, held at the limit of their reach, and then to touch the tip of their nose. For the return cycle, move the tendon hammer to a different position. The finger–nose test is a not a measure of speed, though one still, frequently hears: 'Do this as fast as you can.' Rapid movements can obscure early cerebellar signs.

Follow with other cerebellar test sequences. In early disease, one test will frequently be more abnormal than others. For example:

- Circular polishing of the dorsum of the opposite hand with a single finger.
- Alternating forearm pronation and supination. Demonstrate this test: with forearm vertical, make rotational back-and-forth movements. Next, repeat with the forearm horizontal and palm uppermost. Next, show how pronation–supination is combined with tapping the fingertips of one hand on the dorsum of the other. The clumsy word dysdiadochokinesia is used to describe this abnormality, to distinguish it from dysmetria. Practical tests, such as screwing in a light bulb, are also sometimes helpful.

In the lower limb heel–shin test, ask the patient to:

- Raise one leg, touch the opposite ankle with the heel, and then
- Repeat this circular sequence of movement (i.e. raising the leg again). Simply gliding one heel up and down the opposite shin can miss early ataxia.

Foot tapping against the examiner's palm is another test to elicit lower limb incoordination. In cerebellar disease, tendon reflex abnormalities are rarely of much diagnostic value. Knee jerks with a pendular pattern, meaning slow and swinging when the shins are dangled vertically over the couch, and absent reflexes are seen.

Cerebellar dysarthria is usually evident without resorting to asking for pronunciation of 'West Register Street' – which is in Edinburgh, or 'baby hippopotamus' but these appear to remain entrenched.

The nystagmus of cerebellar disease rarely occurs without other cerebellar features. Finally, remember that midline cerebellar (vermis) lesions may cause gait and trunk ataxia without signs in the limbs.

Table 4.5 Tendon reflexes.

Symbol	Description	Inference
0	Absent with reinforcement	Usually pathological
+/–	Present with reinforcement	Sometimes normal, but may be pathological
+	Present	Normal
+ +	Brisk	Normal
+ + +	Very brisk	Pathological if tone is increased but can be a normal finding
CL	Clonus	>3 beats of ankle clonus = pathological; 2 beats may be normal

Do not miss the slow relaxing reflexes of hypothyroidism.

Table 4.6 Spinal levels of tendon reflexes.

Spinal level	Reflex
C5–6	Supinator
C5–6	Biceps
C7	Triceps
C8	Finger jerks
L(3)–4	Knee
S1	Ankle

Tendon reflexes

Strictly, these are the deep tendon reflexes (DTRs of US texts). The full-size tendon hammer, with a 33 cm (13 in) shaft, is the preferred tool; miniature versions are discouraged. A soft rubber O-ring is preferable to hard one. Make sure the patient is relaxed – with the head and trunk supported comfortably. The 0 to + + + and CL nomenclature is shown in Table 4.5. Minor degrees of reflex asymmetry are common in normal people, as are relatively reduced knee jerks compared with ankle jerks, and sometimes vice versa. Table 4.6 indicates spinal levels of the tendon reflexes. Reinforcement, the method of attempting to elicit tendon reflexes that are at first sight absent, is achieved by several actions. One is to ask the patient to clench their teeth and then relax; another is to clench the hands. The original Jendrassik manoeuvre is to hook the fingers each hand together and pull firmly (Ernö Jendrassik, 1858–1921, Budapest). Areflexia without other physical signs is not in itself an absolute abnormality, but is usually pathological.

Extensor plantar (Babinski) and Hoffmann reflexes Joseph Babinski (1857–1932, Paris) wrote the 26-line description entitled the *phénomène des orteils* (toe phenomenon) in 1896. The extensor plantar response is an indication of an UMN lesion of the brain or spinal cord. Babinski is said to have used a bodkin, a sharp instrument, originally an arrowhead; an orange-stick is now usual. The crux of the matter is that if a reproducible upgoing toe can be produced by any reasonable stroking action on the sole, then this is abnormal. There are over a dozen additional ways to elicit a similar phenomenon, many eponymous, such as Chaddock, Gordon, Oppenheim and Gonda signs; none rivals the original Babinski.

Extensor plantars are exceptional in the normal adult, but are occasionally found. Johann Hoffmann (1857–1919, Heidelberg) described finger reflex hyper-reflexia on flicking the thumb or forefinger. This is little used by most neurologists today; in practice, other UMN signs are usually evident.

Superficial abdominal reflexes Superficial abdominal reflexes are elicited by gentle stroking in each upper and lower quadrant with an orange-stick. This evokes a local subcutaneous muscle twitch in the normal subject. The stimulus should not be sharp. Superficial abdominal reflexes are lost with pyramidal lesions and hard to elicit or absent in the obese, or following abdominal surgical scars. The preservation of upper abdominal reflexes with absent lower abdominal reflexes helps confirm a thoracic level in cord compression; the umbilicus is at T10.

Respiration, diaphragm and abdominal muscles Respiration and the diaphragm can be assessed by observing inspiration and expiration and abdominal muscles. Selective weakness of the diaphragm causes paradoxical upward movement of the umbilicus on inspiration; this is well seen with the patient supine during sniffing. If there is any question of respiratory failure, assess and monitor vital capacity (erect and supine), blood gases and chest X-ray.

Lower and upper motor neurone lesions

Features differentiating LMN and UMN lesions are outlined in Table 4.7. In UMN (pyramidal) lesions, the pattern of weakness is of value diagnostically. In the lower limbs, there is weakness of hip flexors, knee flexors and ankle dorsiflexors compared with their antagonist muscles, while in the upper limbs there is relative weakness of all extensors and of finger abduction. Weakness is usually accompanied by reflex changes but in early UMN lesions, not all features of Table 4.7 need be present. In a very early lesion, loss of finely skilled finger and toe movements, or simply drift of an outstretched arm can be the only sign of abnormality.

Sensory system

Sensory abnormalities are rarely found when the patient is articulate and there are no sensory complaints or other signs.

Focus sensory examination anatomically:

- Assess first the posterior columns, meaning here vibration (VS) and joint position sense (JPS). Then move to the spinothalamic tracts. This is an anatomical approximation, but it is useful.
- Test VS at the ankles using a 128-Hz tuning fork. Familiarise the patient with the test by placing the heel of the vibrating fork on the sternum.
- Test toe and then finger JPS – holding the sides of the digit, take it through the smallest movements.
- Quantification of JPS is achieved by recording responses at the toes, ankles and knees and similarly in the upper limbs. VS can also be recorded similarly, to include its absence at the ankles, knees or even at the xiphisternum or clavicles. If the latter two high levels of apparent sensory loss are recorded, an organic problem is rare.
- Examine spinothalamic sensation first with cold metal and then with a disposable sharp object, not a needle or pin.
- Test light touch with a finger tip or cotton wool. Avoid stroking or tickling; these are spinothalamic modalities. Touch tests with fine hairs of various calibres are obsolete for clinical purposes.
- Chart areas of sensory loss or altered sensation. In loss of sensation move from the anaesthetic area to that of normal sensation. In hypersentivity states move from normal skin towards hypersensitive skin.
- Two-point discrimination (0.5 cm on finger tips, 2 cm on feet) is useful for completeness if circumstances warrant it. A paperclip can be bent to make a two-point tool if discriminator forceps are not available.

Table 4.7 Lower (LMN) and upper motor neurone (UMN) lesions.

Feature	Lower motor neurone	Upper motor neurone
Focal muscle wasting	Visible	Absent
Fasciculation	Visible	Absent
Fibrillation potentials	Recordable on EMG	Absent
Tone	Flaccid/normal	Increased/spastic type
Weakness pattern	Root, nerve or distal	Pyramidal + reduced dexterity
Tendon reflexes	Depressed/usually absent	Exaggerated*
Clonus	Absent	Present
Abdominal reflexes	Present	Absent
Plantar responses	Flexor (normal)	Extensor

* Tendon reflexes can be temporarily depressed or absent following an acute UMN lesion.

Two areas of sensory examination require particular attention:
1 Determination of a thoracic sensory level in a possible compressive cord lesion, and
2 Charting dissociated sensory loss in a possible central cord lesion, such as syringomyelia.

In an early compressive cord lesion, a distal sensory disturbance may not be a complaint. If signs of a mild spastic paraparesis are found during motor and reflex testing, check sensation on the thorax and abdomen with care. Move up from the lower limbs, to the lower abdomen using a cold tuning fork blade. Ask if sensation changes. In the normal person, there is often an apparent slight increase in cold perception as one reaches the groin, again at the lower costal margin and around the clavicle. At other levels, diminished sensation distally may well be pathological. The level of a cord lesion can be determined in this way and tested subsequently with a sharp object and light touch. Be aware that on the thorax, a sensory level on the back is typically higher by a segment or so than on the front of the chest.

In syringomyelia, sensory loss may also pass unrecognised. Painless burns or painless minor injuries should be noted. The areas of dissociated spinothalamic loss on the trunk and upper limbs can be bizarre, conforming to no obvious pattern, because the syrinx involves crossing spinothalamic fibres in the cord central grey matter. Look also for loss of sensation to a sharp object on the posterior scalp (C2).

Generally, when complex sensory loss is found, note the initial findings and return after an interval to re-examine sensation.

Formulation and diagnosis

Drawing together historical data and physical signs is an essential part of assessment but frequently skimped. To conclude that a fall with loss of consciousness and residual weakness is 'collapse ?cause' or 'probably a fit', an evident hemiparesis is 'a CVA' or that a complex headache history is 'migraine' (all common comments in A&E notes) are not formulations any medically qualified person should reach. A structured approach is essential, teasing out features from the history and building on the signs found, to reach either a diagnosis or at least a direction for investigations. Such attention to detail can be hard in an emergency, but it is in acute neurology that many mistakes occur. For example, cases of sudden headache are discounted as benign when the reality is a subarachnoid haemorrhage. A careful history and thoughtful appraisal usually provides the correct answer and safe management. Another common error is the distinction between a seizure and syncope; seizures are overdiagnosed. Mistakes occur if one fails to adopt a structured approach.

As a generalisation, the history often points towards a pathological process, while examination either simply confirms suspicions or suggests anatomical localisation.

Difficulties with the history and examination

When a diagnosis is unclear, try to sort out relevant and entirely secure details within the history and examination. Establish whether or not physical signs are hard (certain). For example, a definite historical fact is a clear witnessed account of a tonic–clonic seizure and unequivocal physical signs are sustained ankle clonus and extensor plantars. Separate these from the less clear such as vague weakness, or dizziness without vertigo. Also, be prepared to recognise, accept and record uncertainty: it may be unclear whether the blackout was a fit or faint. It is obvious that this is advice easier to write than to practice.

While it is sometimes taxing to formulate a possible diagnosis, and one risks making an error, it is essential to try.

Diagnostic tests in clinical neurology

In clinical neurology, and in medicine generally, the substantial majority of investigations do not alter the course of a disease. However, we are surrounded by technology, by defensive practice and the need to provide reassurance that all has been done to exclude sinister conditions. It is essential to be aware of the cost–benefits and to target studies for some real purpose. However, there is often an uncritical approach which results in waste and sometimes confusion. The principal investigations of neurology are outlined here.

Imaging

There has been a revolution in imaging. The first patient was imaged by computerised tomography (CT) in 1971 in London and before the 1980s, CT scanning was sparsely available. At that time, carotid and vertebral angiography, air encephalography and myodil myelography were the standard investigations in specialist units. The human brain was first imaged by magnetic resonance (MR) in Nottingham, UK in 1978. Standard, high resolution MRI is now readily available and even functional MRI (fMRI) is now used in clinical practice. Some basic principles of imaging techniques are mentioned here.

Neuroimaging has a vital role in clinical neurosciences. It offers a range of powerful diagnostic tools, providing *in vivo* information about the structure, function and physiology of the nervous system and the pathologies that afflict it. In addition, there is an ever-expanding range of image-guided therapeutic procedures that enable neuroradiologists to be at the heart of patient treatment, not simply diagnosis. In order for clinicians to utilise radiology departments effectively and efficiently it is essential that they are familiar with the various imaging modalities, their potential risks and benefits and the therapeutic options now available.

Conventional radiography (plain X-rays)

Conventional radiography continues to have a limited role in imaging the skull, spine and skeleton and other radio-opaque structures such as metallic implants and ventricular shunts. However, overlapping structures are superimposed and soft tissue contrast is poor. This presents a problem for imaging the central nervous system (CNS) as it is encased in bones, masking the soft tissues of the brain and spinal cord.

Computerised tomography

Computerised tomography (CT) uses ionising radiation to produce thin tomographic images (slices) that overcome many of the problems inherent in plain X-rays caused by superimposition of tissues. Conventional CT scanners employ a circular assembly consisting of a fan beam of X-rays placed opposite a curvilinear array of detectors. This assembly rotates rapidly around the subject and covers the region of interest either by stepwise acquisition of multiple slices (sequential scanning) or by moving in a continuous spiral (helical scanning). Modern scanners have multiple rows of detectors allowing several slices to be acquired simultaneously, reducing scan times to the order of seconds or minutes.

CT relies on different tissues stopping (attenuating) X-rays to different degrees to provide image contrast. The image is composed of a matrix of volume elements (voxels), akin to pixels in a

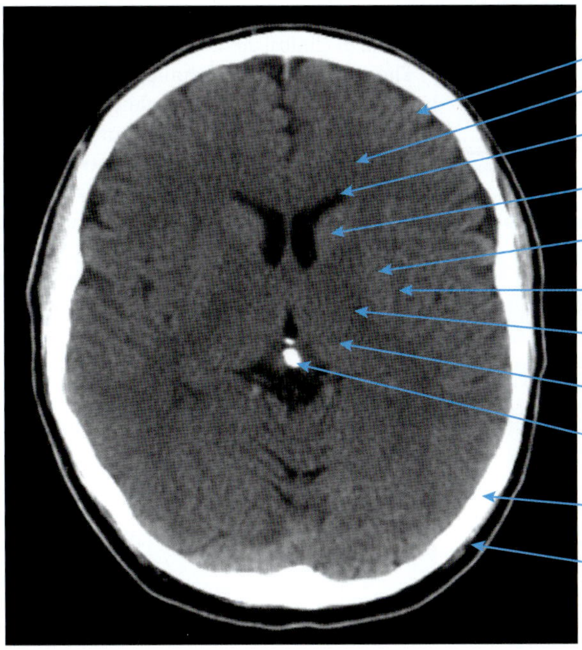

Figure 4.1 Axial computed tomography (CT) image using brain windows. Note that grey matter appears slightly brighter than white matter due to its higher attenuation values. The highly attenuating bone and calcified pineal gland appear white, cerebrospinal fluid (CSF) in the frontal horn appears dark and the poorly attenuating subcutaneous fat and air around the head are black.

two-dimensional digital image, but with an additional depth dimension equal to the slice thickness. Each voxel is assigned a value, in Hounsfield units (HU), reflecting its ability to attenuate the incident X-rays. Grey-scale images are constructed from the voxel matrices, with high attenuation voxels depicted towards the brighter, white end of the spectrum, and low attenuation voxels towards the darker end. These grey-scale images can then be 'windowed' in order to optimise contrast within the tissues of interest (Figures 4.1 and 4.2). The words attenuation and density are often used interchangeably, with high attenuation value voxels described as being hyperdense and low attenuation voxels as hypodense.

Current detector arrays are also able to acquire cube-shaped isotropic voxels that can be manipulated to reconstruct images in any plane (multiplanar reformatting, MPR) and allow 3-D images such as maximum intensity projections (MIPs) and volume renderings (Figure 4.3). Iodine-based contrast media can be used to increase tissue contrast, highlight pathologies such as tumour and infection, obtain relatively selective images of the vessels in CT angiography produce measures of tissue perfusion and, when injected intrathecally, allow detailed depiction of the theca and its contents in CT myelography (Figure 4.4).

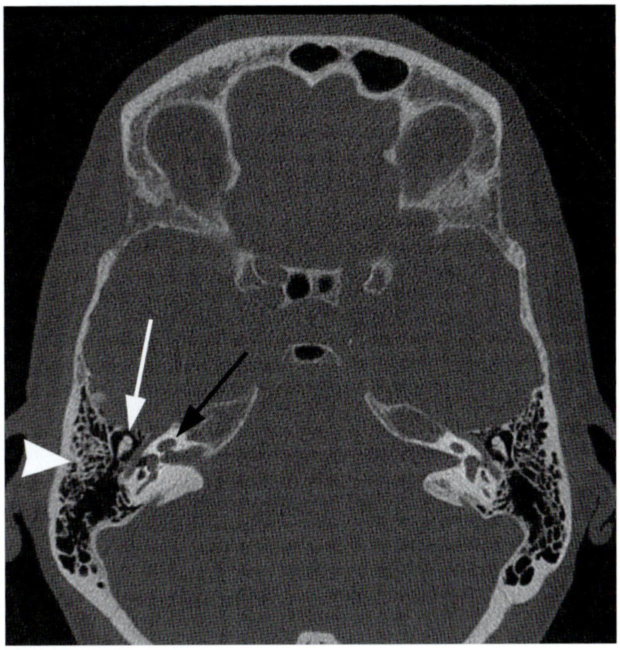

Figure 4.2 Axial CT of the petrous temporal bones using bone windows and processing algorithms to optimise bony detail. Note that the bony architecture of the middle and inner ear, such as the ossicles (white arrow), cochlear (black arrow) and trabeculations of the mastoid (arrowhead) are all well seen but soft tissue contrast is lost and the brain parenchyma appears homogeneously grey.

Magnetic resonance imaging

Clinical MRI utilises strong magnetic fields and radiofrequency pulses to generate a signal from protons in water molecules. By convention, high signal voxels are depicted as bright (often described as hyperintense) and low signal voxels as dark (hypointense). A variety of pulse sequences can be used to interrogate different physical properties of the water protons and image contrast can therefore be generated in multiple ways. The two most commonly used MRI sequences produce images based mainly on the variations in T1 and T2 relaxation times of water protons in different tissues, generating T1-weighted (T1-w) and T2-weighted (T2-w) images, respectively (Figure 4.5a,b). Other commonly used sequences include Fluid Attenuated Inversion Recovery (FLAIR; Figure 4.5c), diffusion-weighted imaging (DWI; Figure 4.6) and sequences that are particularly sensitive for detecting blood degradation products such as T2 gradient-echo (T2*) and susceptibility-weighted imaging (SWI;

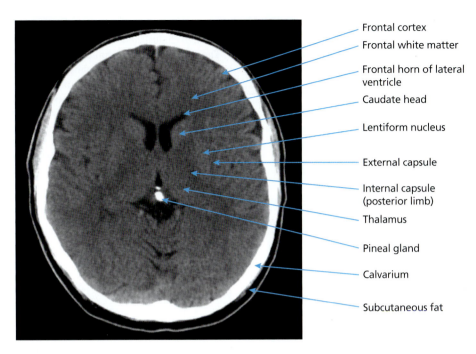

Figure 4.7). Chelates of gadolinium can be used as contrast media with similar roles to those of iodine-based agents used in CT and several types of magnetic resonance angiography (MRA) are available for selective vascular imaging (Figure 4.8).

Advanced MRI

In addition to the routine sequences there are many other sequences grouped under the umbrella term 'advanced MRI' that have been developed to probe tissue structure, function, physiology and biochemistry. The major techniques that have translated from the research to clinical arenas are outlined here.

The advanced MRI technique most used in clinical practice is perfusion MR. Of the many techniques available, dynamic susceptibility contrast (DSC) and dynamic contrast-enhanced (DCE) perfusion have gained the most traction clinically. As their names suggest, both involve the dynamic acquisition of images during injection of a contrast bolus and provide a number of measures of tissue perfusion. Clinically, perfusion MR is mainly used for the assessment of cerebrovascular disease (Figure 4.9), for estimating histological tumour grades (principally gliomas) and differentiating tumour from therapy-induced radionecrosis. A third technique, arterial spin labelling (ASL) magnetically tags water in flowing blood rather than using an injection of potentially harmful contrast and is likely to find increasing clinical application in the future.

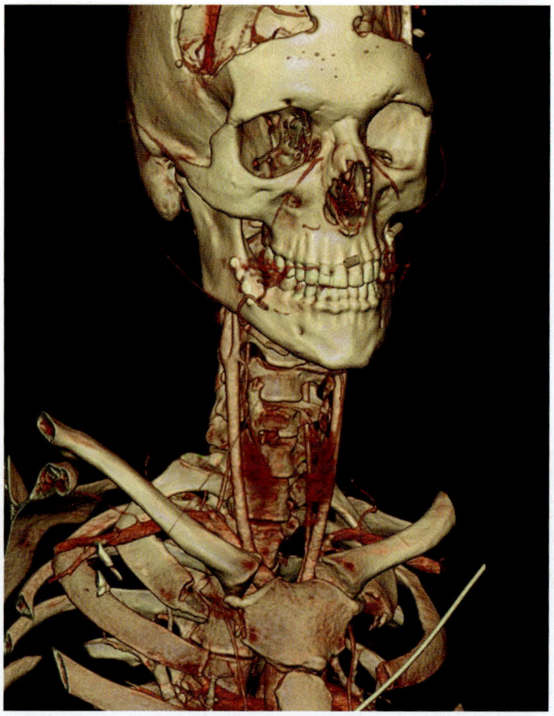

Figure 4.3 Volume rendered image (VRT) produced from a CT angiogram showing the anatomical relationship of the neck vessels and adjacent bones.

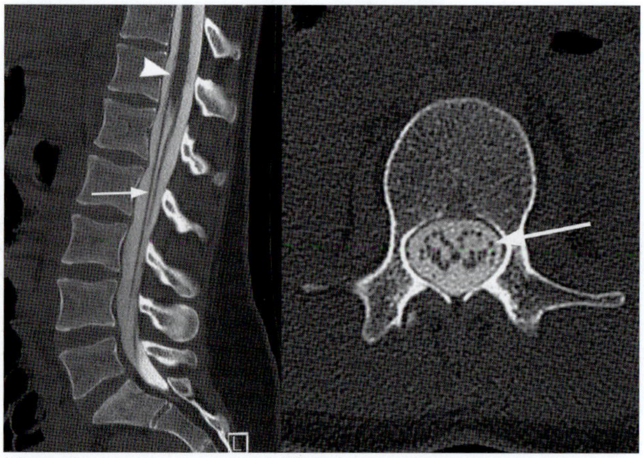

(a) (b)

Figure 4.4 CT myelogram, sagittal (a) and axial (b) images. Intrathecal contrast injection creates high attenuation CSF, outlining contours of the vertebral canal, spinal cord (arrowhead) and nerve roots (arrow).

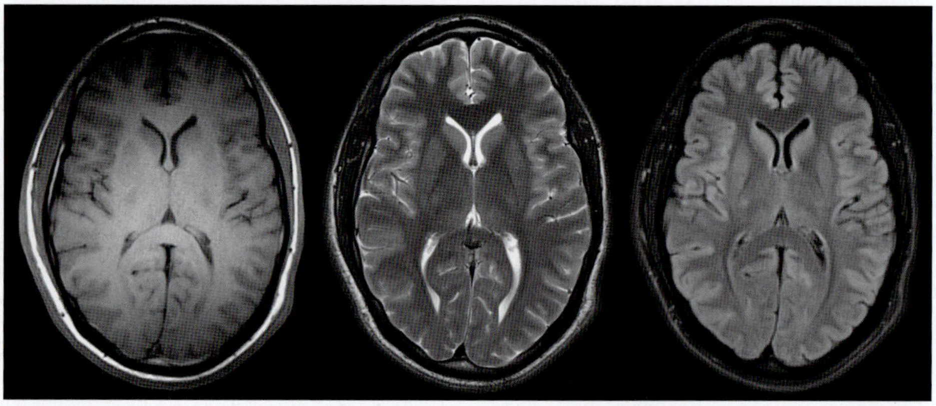

(a) (b) (c)

Figure 4.5 Axial MR (a) T1-weighted (T1-w,), (b) T2-weighted (T2-w,) and (c) Fluid Attenuated Inversion Recovery (FLAIR) images of normal brain at the level of the basal ganglia. On the T1-w image white matter appears hyperintense compared to grey matter and CSF appears very hypointense. This image contrast is reversed on the T2-w image with grey matter appearing hyperintense to white matter and CSF appearing very bright. Note that FLAIR images are essentially T2-w, with grey matter appearing hyperintense to white matter. However, the signal from bulk water is nulled, making CSF appear dark and increasing the conspicuity of T2-hyperintense pathologies, such as multiple sclerosis (MS) plaques, particularly around ventricular margins and other CSF spaces.

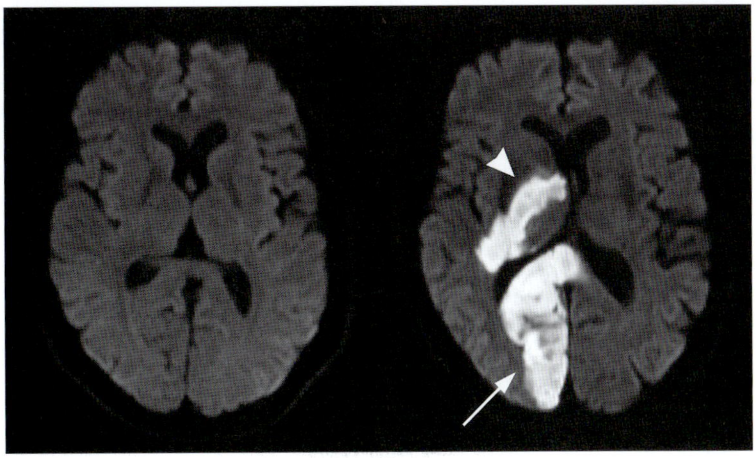

(a) (b)

Figure 4.6 Axial MR diffusion weighted imaging (DWI). (a) Normal brain: the contrast in DWI is partly generated by the diffusivity of water molecules. Voxels in which water is free to diffuse, such as CSF, are depicted as dark and those in which there is restricted diffusion are depicted as bright. Structures such as cell membranes act as natural barriers to diffusion in normal brain parenchyma, which has an intermediate diffusivity and appears mid grey. (b) Acute ischaemic infarction: the archetypal pathology exhibiting restricted diffusion, caused by interstitial pathways for water diffusion being impeded by cell swelling (cytotoxic oedema). In this example, acute infarcts are seen in both posterior cerebral (arrow) and anterior choroidal artery (arrowhead) territories.

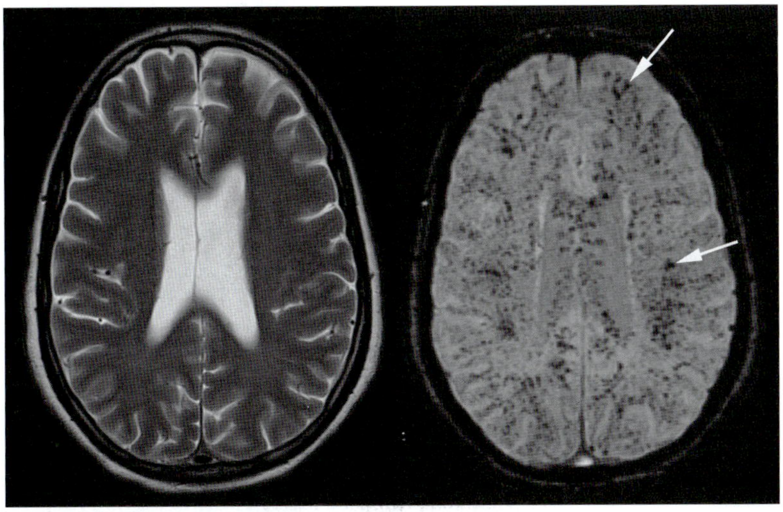

(a) (b)

Figure 4.7 Axial MR susceptibility weighted imaging (SWI): disseminated intravascular coagulation. SWI is particularly sensitive to paramagnetic substances that include many blood breakdown products and other sources of iron. (a) Routine T2-w images. (b) SWI image shows multiple punctate foci of hypointensity (two are arrowed) that are microhaemorrhages not visible on the T2-w image.

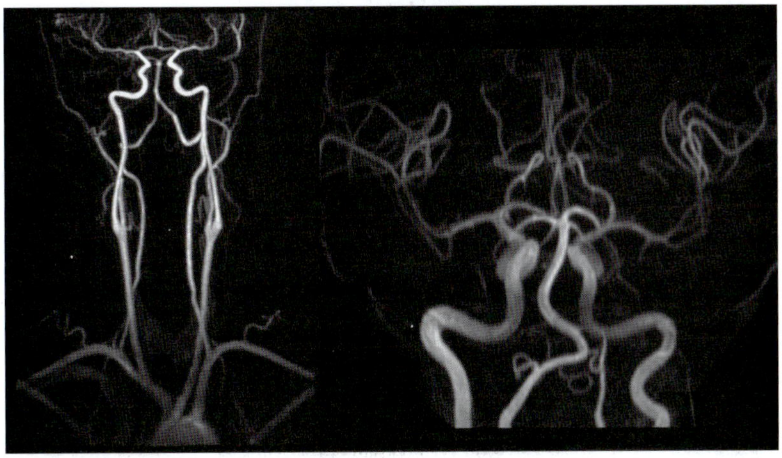

(a) (b)

Figure 4.8 Magnetic resonance angiography (MRA). (a) Contrast-enhanced MRA is the preferred MR method for imaging extracranial neck vessels. (b) Time-of-flight (TOF) is the sequence of choice for imaging intracranial arteries.

Functional MRI and other MR modalities Functional MRI (fMRI) measures changes in blood oxygen levels, known as the BOLD effect, as a surrogate marker of brain activity. A variety of paradigms such as finger tapping and silent word generation tasks can be used to localise eloquent cortex such as the primary motor and language areas (Figure 4.10). The main clinical use of fMRI is for pre-operative planning when functionally important cortex is expected to lie close to the surgical field.

Diffusion tensor imaging (DTI) exploits the anisotropy of *in vivo* diffusion (i.e. the fact that water diffusion has a directional component dependent on the structure and organisation of the tissue it passes through), to provide information about tissue integrity at a cellular and microstructural level and to allow anatomical modelling of highly anisotropic structures such as white matter tracts (Figure 4.11). The images from white matter tractography can be combined with fMRI to produce more complete functional maps, incorporating both eloquent cortex and its associated white matter projections.

Proton MR spectroscopy (MRS) is used to produce a biochemical profile of tissue with the relative proportions of target metabolites such as creatine, *N*-acetyl aspartate, choline, lactate and lipids being used as markers of neuronal viability, membrane turnover and metabolic status. The hope that MRS would allow pathologies to be identified by their specific biochemical profiles has not been realised but it may serve as a useful adjunct in imaging certain diseases such as metabolic disorders and tumours.

Magnetic field strength, advantages and safety issues The majority of current clinical scanners use either 1.5 Tesla (1.5 T) or 3 Tesla (3 T) magnets. Higher field strength 3 T magnets are able to generate better signal-to-noise ratios than their 1.5 T counterparts, which offer several advantages including the potential for higher resolution and/or faster imaging. However, higher field strengths are in general more prone to artefacts and more stringent MR safety rules need to be applied.

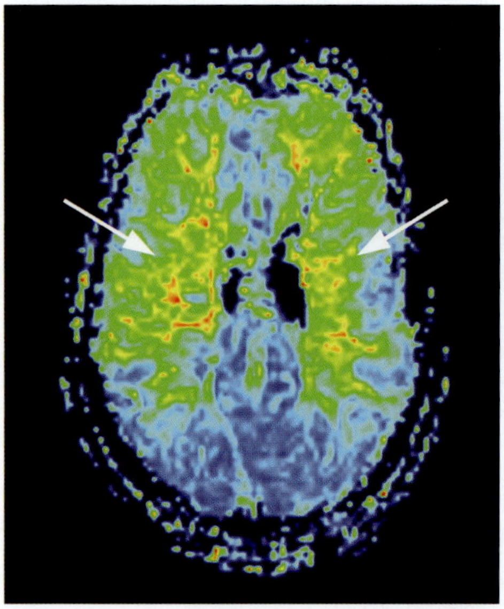

Figure 4.9 Perfusion MR. A dynamic susceptibility (DSC) study of a patient with moyamoya disease showing abnormal perfusion in the middle cerebral artery and deep border-zone territories bilaterally (green and orange voxels highlighted with white arrows).

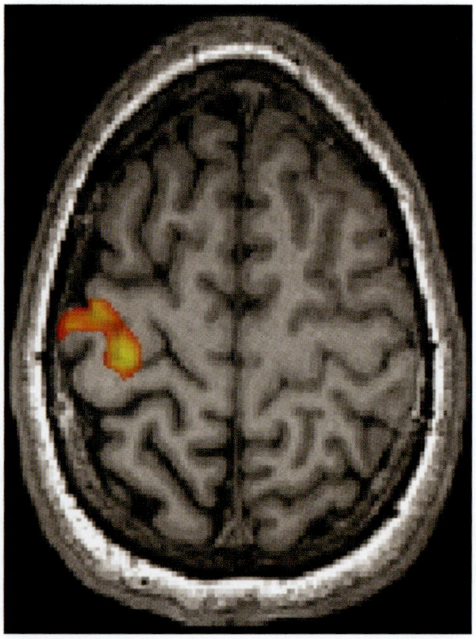

Figure 4.10 Functional MR image: orange and red voxels represent activation of the hand motor area.

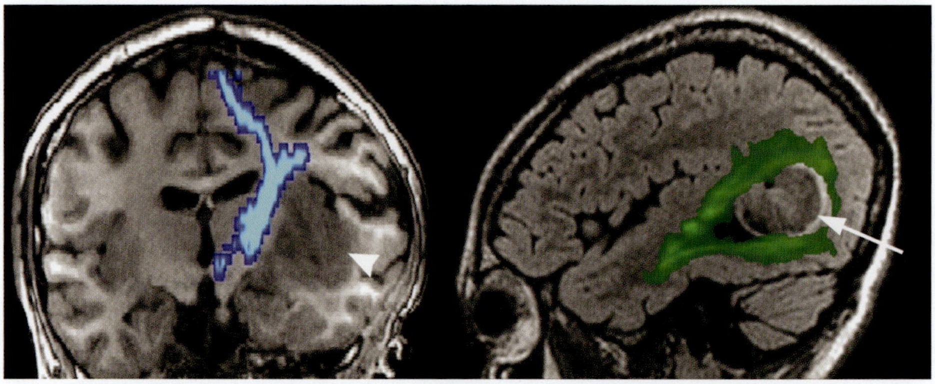

(a) (b)

Figure 4.11 White matter tractography derived from diffusion tensor imaging. (a) Corticospinal tract outlined in blue and deflected medially by an insular tumour mass (arrowhead). (b) Optic radiation (in another patient) outlined in green and splayed around a posterior temporal tumour (arrow).

The advantages of MRI include the fact that it does not use ionising radiation, it is able to generate very good contrast between many tissues and a diverse range of sequences can be employed to provide information not only on structure, but also the chemical composition, physiology and function of tissues. In general, it is unimpeded by the presence of bone and is therefore better suited to imaging the spinal cord and posterior fossa than CT. These benefits are weighed against relatively long scan times, poorer patient tolerance, the requirement for greater specialist physics support to maintain and optimise the scanners and greater overall expense compared with CT. In addition, the movement of ferromagnetic materials within the very strong magnetic fields and heating caused by radiofrequency pulses have safety implications that preclude some patients with metallic implants or foreign bodies from undergoing MRI and require the use of specially designed MR-compatible equipment in and around scanning areas.

Positron emission tomography Positron emission tomography (PET) is a technique that images the spatial and temporal distribution of positron-emitting radioisotopes. Radionuclides such as ^{18}F, ^{11}C and ^{13}N can be tagged to injectable pharmaceutical agents to provide *in vivo* assessment of perfusion, glucose metabolism and DNA synthesis. Combination PET-CT and PET-MR scanners are now available and allow simultaneous acquisition and fusion of structural and functional imaging.

The most commonly used PET tracer is 2[^{18}] fluoro-2-deoxy-D-glucose (FDG) which accumulates in the brain via the same pathway used to take up glucose and can be used as a marker of regional cerebral metabolism. It has a range of potential clinical applications including tumour, dementia, cerebrovascular and epilepsy imaging. In the context of CNS tumours it has been used to discriminate between high and low grade neoplasms, between post-therapy radionecrosis and residual tumour and to localise occult malignancy elsewhere in the body when a paraneoplastic syndrome is suspected. It has been used to identify Alzheimer's very early in the disease course and certain patterns of hypometabolism may help discriminate between different dementia aetiologies. In cases of intractable epilepsy, interictal and ictal PET imaging may be used to localise epileptogenic foci preoperatively where structural MRI has failed.

Single-photon emission computed tomography Single-photon emission computed tomography (SPECT) generates images using gamma-emmitting radioisotopes bound to specific ligands and injected as radiopharmaceuticals. A gamma camera rotating around the patient acquires images from multiple projections, allowing tomographic images to be reconstructed in any plane using similar principles to conventional CT.

The two most common neurological uses of SPECT are perfusion and striatal dopamine transporter imaging. Perfusion SPECT is most commonly performed using ^{99m}technetium (^{99m}Tc) based tracers that pass freely across the blood–brain barrier and are distributed in the brain proportional to blood flow. In pathologies where vascular supply to the brain is compromised this allows regional perfusion to be mapped and, when used in conjunction with a vasodilator challenge using agents such as acetazolamide, may be used to assess cerebrovascular reserve. In the absence of cerebrovascular disease the coupling of blood flow to metabolism and neuronal activity also allows brain function to be studied. Different patterns of regional hypoperfusion have been associated with different dementia types and may have a role in discriminating between them when structural imaging in non-specific. Early post-ictal SPECT has been used to localise epileptogenic foci in a similar way to PET.

Imaging with (^{123}I) ioflupane, tradename DaTSCAN, is another SPECT technique now commonly used in neuroimaging. (^{123}I) ioflupane selectively binds to presynaptic dopamine transport receptors in the striatum and can be used to detect loss of functional dopaminergic neurones (Figure 4.12). Its main licensed role is in distinguishing between essential tremor, in which (^{123}I) ioflupane uptake is preserved, and extrapyramidal syndromes in which tracer uptake is reduced such as idiopathic Parkinson's disease, multiple system atrophy and progressive supranuclear palsy. Its other licensed use is in differentiating Alzheimer's disease from dementia with Lewy bodies, striatal uptake being reduced in the latter. However, DaTSCAN is unable to discriminate between the various pathologies in which striatal dopaminergic neurones are reduced.

Ultrasound Ultrasound is safe, well tolerated by patients and has the additional advantage that most machines are portable, allowing scanning at the bedside where required. In neonates, ultrasound can

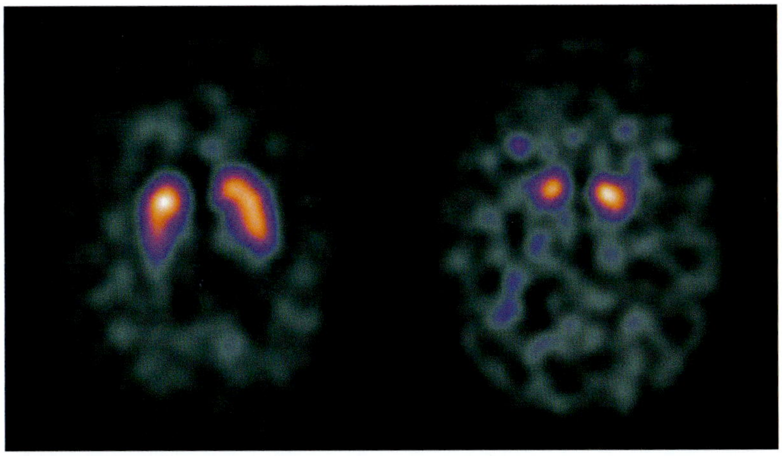

(a) (b)

Figure 4.12 Ioflupane (^{123}I) SPECT scans (DaTSCAN). (a) Normal scan showing symmetrical comma-shaped uptake in the striatum. (b) Parkinson's disease: markedly reduced tracer uptake in the putamina, with preservation of uptake in the more anteriorly positioned caudate heads ('full stops').

be used to image the brain and spine but as bones develop and fontanelles close its role in neuroimaging becomes limited. Duplex ultrasound, known as carotid Doppler, is commonly used to assess the extracranial carotid arteries, principally for detecting atherosclerotic stenoses in patients presenting with transient ischaemic attack (TIA) and ischaemic stroke. Transcranial Doppler (TCD) can be used to obtain velocity and spectral information from intracranial vessels, most commonly via limited acoustic windows in the temporal region. It has a number of applications, the best established being vasospasm monitoring in patients following aneurysmal subarachnoid haemorrhage and assessment of vascular stenoses and occlusions in the context of ischaemic stroke. Elevated middle cerebral or internal carotid artery TCD velocities have also been shown to be an important predictor of stroke in children with sickle cell disease and can be used to guide the use of prophylactic blood transfusions.

Digital subtraction catheter angiography Digital subtraction catheter angiography (DSA) is considered the gold standard for imaging vascular anatomy. It is an invasive procedure in which iodinated contrast is injected directly into the vessels of interest, usually through a catheter introduced via femoral artery puncture. It allows specific vascular territories to be imaged selectively and can separate arterial, capillary and venous phases, yielding information about haemodynamics as well as vascular anatomy and structure (Figure 4.13). The unrivalled spatial and temporal resolution of DSA means it remains the most sensitive investigation for detecting subtle structural vascular abnormalities such as small aneurysms and for demonstrating arteriovenous shunts, particularly those associated with dural arteriovenous (AV) fistulae. However, in addition to the hazards associated with ionising radiation and iodinated contrast media, DSA also carries risks related to peripheral arterial puncture such as pseudoaneurysm formation and retroperitoneal bleeding and the risk of neurological deficit caused by embolus. Complication rates of diagnostic cerebral angiography are low, the risk of permanent neurological deficit is approximately 0.5%. Patients should be selected and consented carefully.

Interventional neuroradiology Interventional neuroradiology encompasses all image-guided therapeutic procedures, but in neuroradiology it commonly refers to endovascular techniques used to treat vascular pathologies. Since the landmark ISAT trial published in 2002, endovascular treatment of aneurysms has become established as a safe and effective alternative to surgical clipping and is now the preferred route of management for the majority of aneurysmal subarachnoid haemorrhage cases. The technique uses platinum coils delivered via intra-arterial catheters to alter flow and promote thrombosis from within the aneurysm, obviating the need for craniotomy. It should be noted that not all aneurysms are suitable for coiling and selection of cases is best carried out by multidisciplinary teams involving both neuroradiologists and neurosurgeons. Many craniospinal AV malformations and dural fistulae are also amenable to endovascular treament and certain tumours such as meningiomas and paragangliomas are sometimes embolised to reduce vascularity pre-operatively.

Spinal procedures constitute another subgroup of interventional neuroradiology, the most common interventions being image-guided injections and vertebroplasty–kyphoplasty. Perineural or peri-articular injections of local anaesthetic and steroid, usually under CT or fluoroscopic guidance, can provide diagnostic information to localise the source of a patient's symptoms and also provide effective relief of pain.

Vertebroplasty and kyphoplasty are designed to treat painful vertebral insufficiency fractures by introducing cement or a balloon respectively into the vertebral body percutaneously.

Clinical neurophysiology

Measurement of central and peripheral electrical function has a useful role: the usual tests are outlined here.

Electroencephalography

Electrical potentials generated by largely synchronous activity of millions of neurones are recorded simultaneously from scalp electrodes in various montages usually via 16 channels. The precise sources of the rhythms first described by Berger in 1929 remain contentious. The main role of electroencephalography (EEG) is in the investigation of epilepsy and diffuse brain diseases, in ITU in states of altered consciousness and in sleep disorders. It has been widely used in other situations, such as in headache, and in cognitive or psychiatric disorders, but it is rarely of particular value.

Videotelemetry, which combines prolonged EEG recording with simultaneous film of the patient, is very helpful in the assessment of attacks of uncertain nature and for localisation of seizures prior to epilepsy surgery (see Neurophysiology for assessing patients for epilepsy surgery, Chapter 7). Sometimes, the video is more useful than the EEG, and where there is diagnostic uncertainty, a home video (often from a mobile phone) of an attack can be extremely useful.

Specially placed EEG electrodes are also sometimes used, such as nasopharyngeal, sphenoidal and intracranial grid and strip

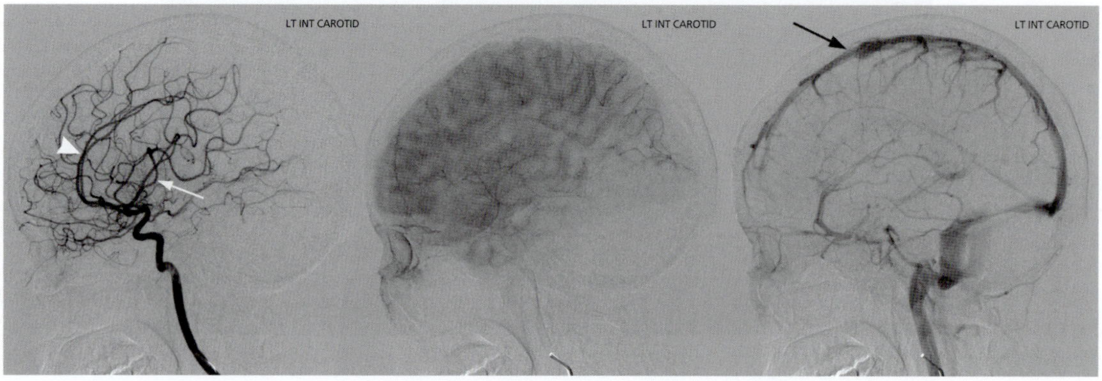

Figure 4.13 Digital subtraction catheter angiogram. From left to right, the three images illustrate arterial, capillary and venous phases of a left internal carotid artery injection, in lateral projection. Note landmarks such as the anterior cerebral artery (arrowhead), branches of the middle cerebral artery (white arrow) and the superior sagittal sinus (black arrow).

electrodes and intracerebral depth electrodes to localise a seizure focus prior to potential surgery. EEG sleep studies and EEG monitoring in coma are discussed in Chapter 20 (see Coma; Sleep and its disorders; Psychogenic unresponsiveness). The principal features of the EEG are summarised here; more detailed discussion of the value of EEG in epilepsy is found in Chapter 7 (see Electroencephalography).

Alpha, theta, delta and beta activity in normal subjects Alpha activity seen prominently in normal subjects over the occipital lobes is an 8–14 Hz (usually 11 Hz) roughly sinusoidal waveform with amplitude some 150 μV. Typically, alpha rhythm attenuates on eye opening. Amplitude of alpha rhythm is usually slightly higher over the non-dominant hemisphere.

Theta activity of 4–7 Hz is also seen, bilaterally and usually symmetrically. In normal subjects theta activity is more prominent below the age of 30 and during drowsiness. In many brain diseases excessive theta activity appears non-specifically.

Delta activity is a slower frequency, less than 4 Hz. Delta activity lower than 1 Hz is recorded from frontal electrodes during the first non-REM sleep period. Historically, the appearance of localised delta activity when awake was used in the diagnosis of hemisphere tumours.

Beta activity describes a rhythm faster than 14 Hz recorded normally from frontal electrodes. Excess beta activity is an effect of drugs such as barbiturates and benzodiazepines.

EEG artefacts Non-pathological waveforms are usually straightforward to recognise. The most common are due to eye opening – high amplitude frontal activity from scalp muscle contraction and eye movement or various sleep phenomenon. These need to be distinguished from frontal intermittent rhythmic delta activity (FIRDA), an EEG abnormality seen in raised intracranial pressure and deep midline lesions.

Epilepsy Spikes, or spike-and-wave abnormalities (Figure 4.14), are hallmarks of epilepsy but it is emphasised that over 50% of patients with epilepsy have a normal EEG between seizures. Epileptic activity is described as generalised when it is bilateral and focal (localised) when recorded over one or several neighbouring electrodes, such as over a temporal lobe. Hyperventilation, photic stimulation and sleep may enhance EEG epileptic activity and are commonly routinely employed.

'Sharp waves' describe waveforms that are not sinusoidal and may occur in patients who have seizures but in whom epileptic spikes are not seen. Sharp waves are sometimes seen in the normal population and are not diagnostic of epilepsy.

The value of EEG in the management of seizures, in the choice of anticonvulsant drugs and in status epilepticus is discussed in Chapters 7 (see Status epilepticus) and 20 (see Status epilepticus, EEG monitoring).

Diffuse and focal brain disorders Recognisable EEG abnormalities appear in several diffuse and focal brain disorders:

- Periodic lateralised epileptic discharges (PLEDS): herpes simplex encephalitis, cerebral abscess, severe anoxic brain damage or occasionally cerebral infarction.
- Repetitive generalised sharp waves at 0.5–1 second intervals: non-specific, but seen in some prion disease cases.
- High voltage stereotyped slow wave complexes, every 3–10 seconds: subacute sclerosing pan-encephalitis (SSPE).
- Triphasic slow wave complexes: metabolic disorders, typically in hepatic coma.

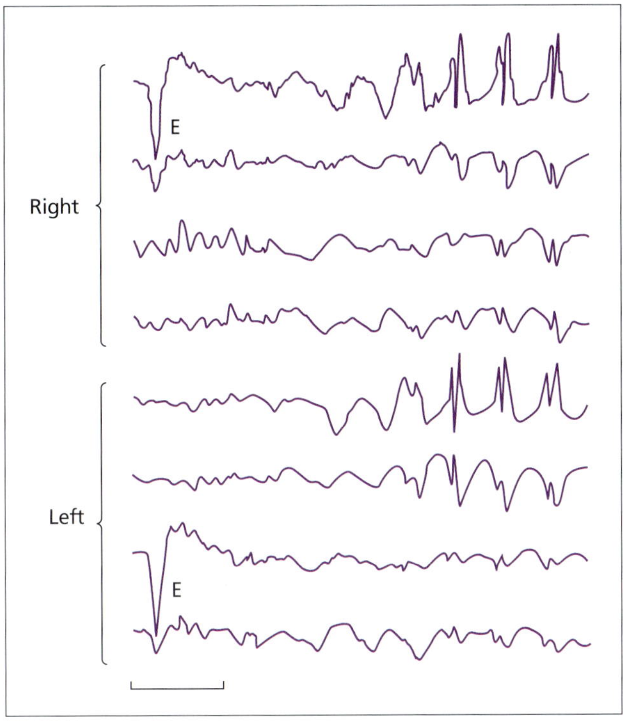

Figure 4.14 Normal electroencephalopgram (EEG) followed by frontal spike and wave activity. E, eye movement artefact.

Brainstem death The EEG is isoelectric (flat) in brainstem death and may also be so in deep coma (e.g. with barbiturates and hypothermia). An isoelectric EEG is not necessary to confirm brain death (see Brainstem death, Chapter 20).

Clinical interpretation of EEG reports Difficulties surround EEG reports. Reporting is not standardised, traces can be hard to interpret and many clinicians will be unfamiliar with how to report an EEG. Conclusions can only be reached within a clinical context. Some useful questions are:

- Is there generalised epileptic activity?
- Is there localised epileptic activity?
- Is there generalised abnormal slow wave activity? If so, how specific is it?
- Is there localised slow wave activity? If so, where is it?
- Could slow wave activity (theta, delta) reported be seen in the normal population?
- Is beta activity reported abnormal?
- Are 'sharp waves' reported truly pathological?
- In coma, is there EEG responsiveness to stimulation?

Responses to these questions, which will sometimes require discussion with a neurophysiologist, help a clinician reach a conclusion in a clinical context. In an effort to standardise EEG reporting, computerised and fractal analysis and pictorial EEG brain mapping have been tried, but none has proved generally useful. EEG records are usually now paperless but written reports by the clinical neurophysiologist and technician remain the usual way results are presented.

Magneto-encephalography and transcranial magnetic brain stimulation

These are largely research tools used in the study of seizures and degenerative brain diseases. Transcranial magnetic brain stimulation is used in central motor conduction velocity measurement.

A copper coil (the magic halo) is placed over the scalp. A current induces a magnetic stimulus sufficient to discharge cortical motor neurones. Muscle contraction is recorded from surface electrodes on an appropriate limb.

Clinical neurophysiological studies of nerve and muscle

Techniques of measurement and data interpretation from studies of peripheral nerves and muscle continue to advance. This is a brief overview of a complex subject.

Electromyography

A concentric needle electrode (CNE) is inserted into voluntary muscle. Amplified recordings from muscle (electromyogram, EMG) are viewed on an oscilloscope and heard through a speaker. Three main features are recorded:

1 Normal motor unit recruitment
2 Denervation and reinnervation changes, and
3 Myopathic, myotonic, myasthenic and changes such as myokymia, cramps, hemifacial spasm, or continuous motor unit activity.

Much depends upon the precise observations of the clinical neurophysiologist. Printouts of EMG traces are somewhat unhelpful compared with practical experience in an EMG laboratory. DVD clips of EMG recordings are useful.

Normal motor unit recruitment Normal muscle at rest is silent electrically although noise from motor end-plates may be heard if the CNE is placed nearby. End-plate noise is a steady 'shhhuush', not unlike noise within a seashell held to the ear. These are high-frequency 10–30 μV brief (<1 ms) potentials. When a single anterior horn neurone fires, all muscle fibres connected to it contract. The contraction of each muscle fibre of the motor unit is not synchronous because of slight differences in conduction along pre-terminal branch axons, giving each motor unit action potential (MUAP or MAP) a compound broad-based waveform lasting up to 12 ms.

The interference pattern is the term used in EMG reports for the appearance and sound during muscular contraction of voluntarily activated individual motor units running together. During a gentle voluntary contraction, a single motor unit can be distinguished both audibly and on the oscilloscope. Initially, this single motor unit fires quite slowly at a rate of approximately 5 impulses per second, but at an increasing rate as voluntary contraction increases. It is then joined by a second motor unit, recognisable by its own waveform, then a third and so on. As voluntary contraction increases, more units are recruited and overlap so that individual units are no longer identifiable. This 'interference' between the units with increasing force of contraction produces the characteristic picture and sound known as a full interference pattern.

Chronic partial denervation If one anterior horn cell (A) fails, for example in motor neurone disease, adjacent anterior horn cells B and C produce sprouting axons that re-innervate muscle fibres originally supplied by A. In chronic partial denervation, the EMG reflects this:

- Decreased number of motor units on voluntary contraction
- Motor units are of larger amplitude than normal
- The mean duration of each muscle action potential increases; new axonal sprouts conduct impulses more slowly than normal
- Motor units may be of abnormal complexity (polyphasic); reversals of polarity are seen.

The EMG hallmarks on an oscilloscope of chronic partial denervation are thus reduced numbers of polyphasic, long duration, high voltage muscle action potentials.

Fibrillation, positive sharp waves, fasciculation and insertion activity When a muscle is denervated, spontaneous contraction of individual fibres begins to occur, typically after some 7–14 days in limb muscles. These contractions produce tiny spontaneous fibrillation potentials of amplitude <10–200 μV (Figure 4.15). These have a triphasic or biphasic waveform with duration <5 ms and an initial positive deflection, displayed by convention in a downgoing direction. These movements of fibrillating subcutaneous fibres in a limb are invisible to the naked eye. However, in the tongue, involuntary movement of denervated fibres (tongue fibrillation) beneath the thin mucosa may be clearly visible. Positive sharp waves are biphasic potentials with a longer duration (<10 ms) than fibrillations and usually with amplitudes of 10–200 μV, though occasionally, when there are also chronic neurogenic changes, up to 2 mV.

Fasciculation describes the visible twitching of a muscle seen in various situations. In normal people, benign fasciculation is common in calf muscles and in other muscles. This is sometimes cause for concern. In denervated muscle, fasciculation potentials with waveforms of dimensions similar to motor unit potentials are produced by spontaneous discharges of motor units. These cause visible twitching (fasciculation), often widespread in motor neurone disease. Typically, this visible involuntary movement flits from place to place, moving on as soon as a twitch catches the examiner's eye.

Insertion activity describes the brief, <2 second volley of muscle activity provoked by the CNE impaling a muscle fibre. This volley becomes prolonged in denervated muscle, which develops exquisite sensitivity to mechanical distortion: showers of fibrillation potentials and positive sharp waves continue for several seconds after CNE insertion. The term 'increased insertion activity' describes these features.

Myopathic EMG changes Myopathic muscle has, on average, fewer than normal fibre numbers in each motor unit. As each motor unit

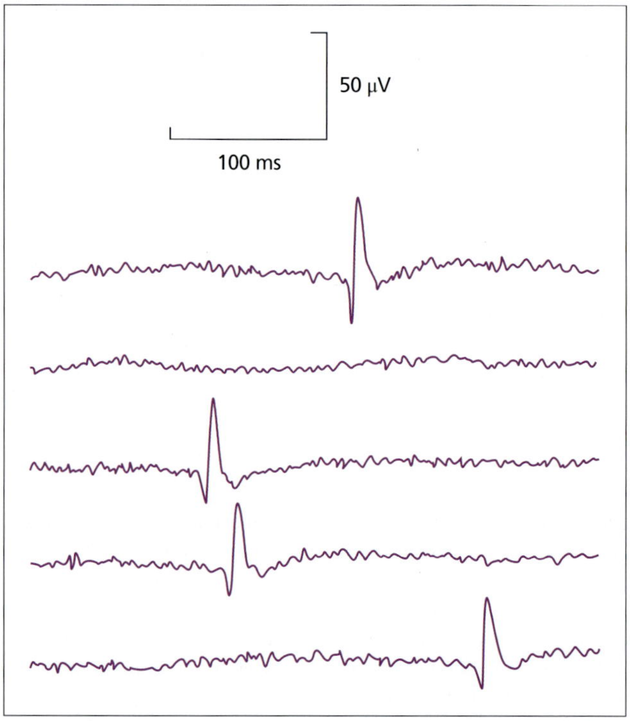

Figure 4.15 Fibrillation potentials from denervated voluntary muscle. Source: Hopkins 1993. Reproduced with permission of Oxford University Press.

shrinks, muscle action potentials become smaller in amplitude and of shorter duration. Surviving fibres may become sufficiently separated so that the spikes they generate do not summate to form the smooth contour of the normal motor unit. Damaged motor units are inefficient, generating less tension than their normal counterparts. Thus, for a given force, additional units must be summoned into activity. The myopathic EMG is characterised by:

- Individual units of low amplitude, of short duration and of polyphasic form
- Rapid motor unit recruitment to a full interference pattern at lower than normal voluntary effort, and
- A recognisable crackly pattern on the loudspeaker.

Myotonic EMG changes Myotonic muscle (see Dystrophia myotonica; Chapter 10) responds to mechanical or electrical stimulation with high frequency action potentials lasting 2–5 seconds. The discharge frequency, initially up to 150 Hz diminishes as the seconds pass producing a whine likened to a dive-bomber of propeller-driven vintage pulling out of its steep descent. Such obvious EMG findings are of less critical diagnostic value than one might expect: myotonia is usually picked up clinically when power is tested, but it can the missed. A softer sound can sometimes be heard through a stethoscope resting over a contracting myotonic muscle.

Complex repetitive discharges (also known as pseudomyotonic discharges) are abnormal discharges that commence and end abruptly. These are the complex polyphasic high frequency waveforms seen in both chronic neuropathic and myopathic disorders.

Hemifacial spasm, cramps, myokymia, neuromyotonic discharges and stiff person syndrome Hemifacial spasm (Chapter 13) is believed to be caused by ephaptic transmission (i.e. transmission between adjacent facial nerve fibres). EMG shows isolated bursts of high frequency motor unit discharges of normal waveform. There is no denervation.

Muscle cramps in normal people are also seen as repetitive high frequency motor unit potential discharges typically at frequencies of 35–70 impulses per second. In myophosphorylase deficiency (see McArdle's disease, Chapter 10), cramps occur but these discharges are not found.

Myokymia (see Other involuntary facial movements (myokymia), Chapter 13) refers to two facial phenomena:

- Quivering facial movements around the eye, common and invariably innocent, often caused by fatigue
- Worm-like wriggling movement, persistent and usually around the chin; this occurs in brainstem gliomas and MS.

Myokymic discharges are rhythmic grouped repetitive discharges of the same motor unit at burst frequencies of 5–60 impulses per second separated by a brief pause.

Neuromyotonic discharges are high frequency >150 impulses per second discharges of a single motor unit, indicating sustained electrical activity.

In stiff person syndrome (see Stiff person syndrome, Chapter 6), continuous normal motor unit activity or low-frequency activity is found simultaneously in opposing muscle groups, as one might expect from the stiffness. The stiffness and pattern of firing is reduced by agents acting either peripherally or centrally (curare, IV diazepam, general anaesthesia).

Peripheral nerve conduction studies

Five electrophysiological measurements are of principal value in the study of neuropathies and peripheral nerve entrapment:

1 Motor conduction velocity (MCV)
2 Sensory conduction velocity
3 Distal motor latency (DML)
4 Sensory (nerve) action potentials (SAPs or SNAPs), and
5 Compound muscle action potentials (MAPs or CMAPs).

Accurate electrode placement and attention to detail is essential. Additional information is gained from repetitive muscle stimulation (e.g. in myasthenia). Central conduction is assessed by recording somatosensory evoked potentials (SEPs) and magnetic stimulation of the motor cortex (MEPs).

Unlike EMG in which the CNE records normal or pathological physiological responses from muscle fibres, peripheral nerve conduction studies (NCS) are carried out using supramaximal electrical stimulation. This measures conduction in the fastest myelinated nerve fibres. While NCS are useful, conduction measurement is a blunt instrument compared with the finesse of EMG methodology and interpretation. Motor conduction measurement is illustrated in Figure 4.16. Tables 4.8 and 4.9 illustrate normal values from nerves commonly tested.

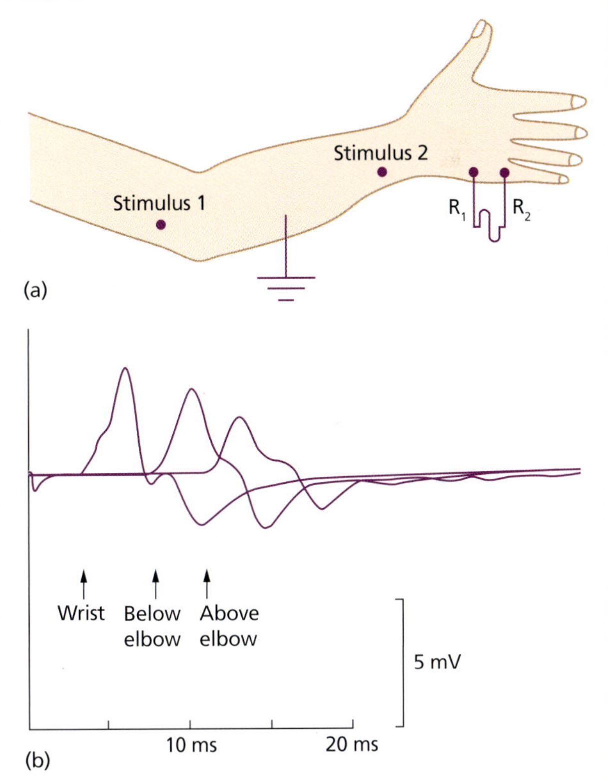

R_1 and R_2: recording electrodes – abductor digiti minimi (ADM).
Stimulus 1 and 2: supramaximal stimuli above elbow and above wrist.
Traces: muscle action potentials (MAPs) from ADM from Stimulus 1, from Stimulus 2, and below elbow (stimulus not shown).
MAP amplitude from stimulation at wrist = 4.0 mV
MAP amplitude from below elbow = 3.0 mV
MAP amplitude from above elbow = 2.1 mV
MCV (calculated: distance/time) from below elbow → wrist = 52 m/s
MCV across elbow segment = 21 m/s
Conclusion: motor conduction block across elbow segment.

Figure 4.16 Ulnar nerve motor conduction studies: compression of nerve at the elbow. Source: Hopkins 1993. Reproduced with permission of Oxford University Press.

Table 4.8 Motor nerve conduction studies: normal values.

Motor nerve	Recording electrode	Amplitude (mV)*	Conduction velocity (m/s)	Distal latency (ms)*
Median	Abductor pollicis brevis	≥4.0	≥49	≤4.4
Ulnar	Abductor digiti minimi	≥6.0	≥49	≤3.3
Radial	Extensor indicis	≥2.0	≥49	≤2.9
Peroneal	Extensor digitorum brevis	≥2.0	≥41	≤6.5
Peroneal	Tibialis anterior	≥5.0	≥44	≤6.7
Tibial	Abductor hallucis brevis	≥4.0	≥41	≤5.8

*Distal latencies depend on distal distances used. Amplitudes are given as baseline to negative peak.

Table 4.9 Sensory and mixed nerve conduction studies: normal values.

Nerve	Electrodes	Amplitude (mV)	Conduction velocity (m/s)
Median*	Digit II → wrist	≥10	≥50
Ulnar*	Digit V → wrist	≥4	≥50
Radial	Snuffbox → wrist	≥15	≥50
Sural	Dorsum → ankle	≥7	≥40
Superficial peroneal	Foot → ankle	≥4	≥40
Medial plantar*	Medial foot → ankle	≥2	≥40

*Orthodromic technique used in United Kingdom. Amplitudes for all sensory or mixed nerve studies given as peak-to-peak values.

Polyneuropathy In axonal neuropathies, MCV is initially well preserved and there is primarily a reduction in CMAP amplitude. SAPs are lower than normal in amplitude. In demyelinating neuropathies, nerve MCV is markedly slowed. Slowing of motor nerve conduction below 38 m/s in the upper limbs and 30 m/s in the lower limbs cannot be explained by axonal dropout of fastest conducting fibres alone and is an unequivocal neurophysiological indicator for demyelination. SAPs are lost or diminished (see Chapter 10).

Entrapment neuropathies Increased distal motor latency in distal neuropathies such as in carpal tunnel syndrome, slowing of nerve conduction across the site of entrapment with diminution of relevant sensory action potential are hallmarks of nerve entrapment. Overall, MCV is preserved. Denervation occurs in affected muscles when entrapment is severe.

F waves These are small-amplitude muscle responses to a peripheral stimulus produced by antidromic discharges of anterior horn cells. Prolonged F wave latency or loss of F waves are seen in root lesions and in acute inflammatory polyneuropathies (Table 4.10).

H reflexes The H reflex, named after Paul Hoffmann (German neurophysiologist, 1884–1962, Freiburg), is generated by electrical stimulation of proprioceptive afferents. Usually the tibial nerve is stimulated at the knee, and muscle contraction of triceps surae (gastrocnemius and soleus) recorded. This is the neurophysiological correlate of a monosynaptic stretch reflex via anterior horn cells. H reflexes are delayed when peripheral conduction is slowed, such as in polyneuropathies or in (when testing the tibial nerve) an S1 root lesion.

Table 4.10 F and H waves: normal average values. Values depend on limb length and age.

Nerve	Minimum latency (ms)
Median	F ≤31
Ulnar	F ≤32
Tibial and peroneal	F ≤56
Tibial	H ≤34

Neuromuscular transmission studies

Repetitive stimulation: myasthenia and myasthenic–myopathic syndromes In myasthenia gravis, a surface electrode, for example on proximal muscles such as trapezius or a facial muscle, is positioned so that supra-maximal stimulation of the accessory or facial nerve evokes the largest demonstrable response. The nerve is then stimulated repetitively at 3 Hz for several seconds. In myasthenia, the responses decrease in amplitude over time (Figure 4.17). If repetitive nerve stimulation does not produce a decrement in a rested muscle, repetition after exercise for 30 or 60 seconds may do so.

In Lambert–Eaton myasthenic syndrome (LEMS), the converse is seen – facilitation (increase) of the motor response with high frequency stimulation as the train of stimulation proceeds. The amplitude of an initial response to low-frequency stimulation is lower than normal. However, repetitive stimulation or brief voluntary contraction for 10 seconds produces an increment in amplitude three to four times that of the initial response.

Jitter phenomenon in myasthenia gravis In myasthenia gravis, the phenomenon known as jitter can be recorded by single fibre studies. The single fibre electrode has a very small pick-up surface. Within a weakly contracting muscle, the voltage of one recorded muscle fibre potential is used to trigger the oscilloscope sweep. Action potentials from another fibre in the same motor unit are recorded but with some delay. In normal muscle, the time difference between discharges from the two fibres remains close to constant and is typically less than 50 μs. In myasthenia, abnormal neuromuscular transmission causes variation in depolarisation time and thus in the inter-discharge interval; the second potential is seen to 'jitter' along the screen (Figure 4.18). Blocking, where one of the pair of muscle fibres intermittently fails to depolarise at all, is an expression of a more severe abnormality of neuromuscular transmission and is the

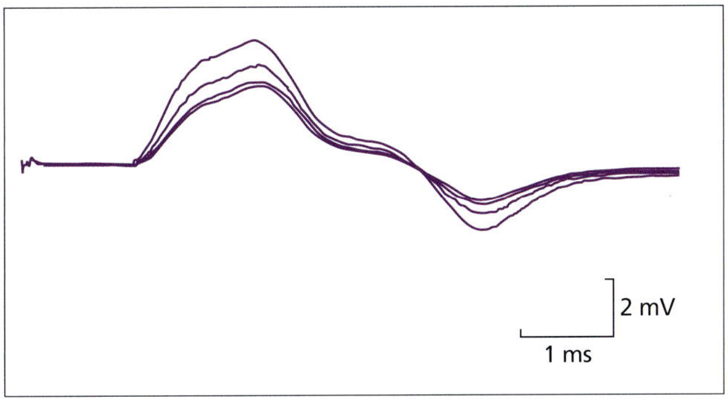

Figure 4.17 Myasthenia gravis. MAP recorded from ADM. 3 Hz stimulation at wrist. First response is 4.1 mV in amplitude. Second response is 3.2 mV. Third and fourth responses (superimposed) are 2.4 mV in amplitude. Decrement = 59% – typical of myasthenia. Source: Hopkins 1993. Reproduced with permission of Oxford University Press.

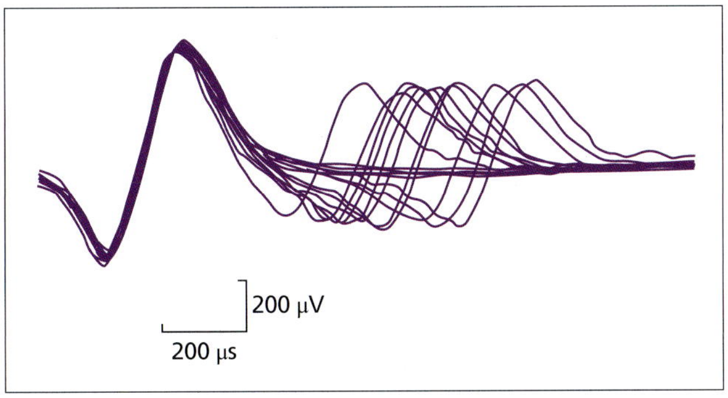

Figure 4.18 Jitter recorded in myasthenia gravis. Source: Hopkins 1993. Reproduced with permission of Oxford University Press.

basis of the myasthenic decrement on repetitive stimulation, and of clinical weakness and fatiguability.

Cerebral-evoked potentials

Evoked potentials record the time for a visual, auditory or other sensory stimulus to reach the cortex. Visual evoked potentials measure amplitude and latency of a repetitive pattern visual stimulus to the cortex. Their value in day-to-day practice is chiefly to confirm previous retrobulbar neuritis, which leaves a permanently prolonged latency despite clinical recovery. Brainstem auditory evoked potentials and somatosensory evoked responses are discussed in Chapters 11 (see Visual evoked responses) and 15 (see Baseline audiometric tests).

Specialised blood and urine tests

Diagnostic data gained from routine blood tests are not dealt with here. Table 4.11 outlines some tests that may be unfamiliar to a newcomer to neurology and provides a reference base. Frequently, it is necessary to consult a clinical pathologist, microbiologist, neurogenetics laboratory or other specialist unit about specialised tests, their yield, relevance and cost (see appropriate chapters).

Cerebrospinal fluid examination

CSF is the clear, colourless, almost acellular fluid around the brain, cord, nerve roots and within the ventricles. Examination provides information about these, the meninges, integrity of the blood–brain barrier and intracranial pressure. Before non-invasive imaging, lumbar puncture (LP) and CSF examination were performed frequently. Eponyms of that era such as the 'paretic Lange' used in the diagnosis of neurosyphilis and the 'colloidal gold reaction' are consigned to history. Today, indications for CSF examination are more specific. However, the reality in observed clinical practice overall is that LP remains overused and its risks underestimated. These notes outline the value, risks and procedure of LP and CSF examination. Cervical puncture is now rarely performed; it is not considered here. Ventricular CSF is sometimes examined in a neurosurgical setting, via a ventricular catheter.

Indications for LP and CSF examination

Principal indications for LP are:

- Diagnosis in an emergency in most cases of suspected meningitis and encephalitis
- Studies of blood products within CSF following suspected subarachnoid haemorrhage (on occasion)
- Measurement of CSF pressure (e.g. idiopathic intracranial hypertension, low pressure headache, CSF leaks)
- Removal of CSF therapeutically (e.g. idiopathic intracranial hypertension, CSF leaks)
- As an aid to diagnosis by assay of CSF constituents in various neurological conditions (e.g. MS, neurosyphilis, sarcoidosis, Behçet's disease, chronic infection, neuro-inflammatory and neuro-immunological disorders, neoplastic meningeal involvement, polyneuropathy and some cases of dementia)
- Intrathecal injection of contrast media and drugs.

In suspected CNS infection, meticulous attention should focus on examination for cells, cell types and microbiological tests. Close liaison between clinician and microbiology laboratory is essential. In addition to cell counts on fresh CSF, bacterial stains (Gram, Ziehl–Neelson), stains for fungi (India ink and others) and specific microbiological techniques (e.g. polymerase chain reactions for bacterial antigens, syphilis serology) are invaluable (Table 4.12).

Table 4.11 Some specialised tests in neurological diseases.

Clinical problem	Laboratory tests	Comments
Wilson's disease and rare cases of cord disease	Serum copper and caeruloplasmin	Extrapyramidal disorders below 40, liver disease; unexplained cord disease with normal B_{12}
Huntington's disease	CAG repeat assay	Chorea and extrapyramidal disease below 40 (see Chapter 6)
Hereditary neuropathies and ataxias	Various genetic tests, depending on features	See Chapters 10 and 17
Acquired neuropathies	Antiganglioside antibodies	See Chapter 10
Paraneoplastic syndromes	Antineuronal antibodies	See Chapters 8, 17, 21
Mitochondrial disease	Muscle biopsy, neurogenetic tests	See Chapter 10
Neurology with coeliac disease	Anti-endomysial and antigliadin antibodies	See Chapter 17
Leukodystrophy	Enzyme studies and genetic tests	See Chapter 19
Aminoacid metabolic disorder (e.g. homocystinaemia)	Urinary and blood amino acids	Homocystinaemia (cystathionine synthase deficiency); see Chapter 19
Adrenoleukodystrophy	Urinary very long chain fatty acids	See Chapter 19
Stiff person syndrome	Anti-GAD antibodies	See Chapter 6
Myasthenic syndromes	Anti-acetylcholine receptor, anti-MuSK antibodies, etc.	See Chapter 10
Myopathies, dystrophies	Creatine kinase, striated muscle antibodies, genetic tests	See Chapter 10
Devic's syndrome	Aquaporin 4 antibodies	See Chapter 11
Porphyrias	Urinary porphyrins	See Chapter 19
Autoimmune limbic encephalitis	Voltage-gated potassium channel antibodies, thyroid microsomal antibodies and other antibodies, depending on clinical context	See Chapter 8

Repeated CSF examination may be necessary in chronic infections such as TB. Paired CSF and blood sugar estimations are valuable in suspected infections.

Clinical and laboratory procedures for CSF spectrophotometry (e.g. rapid transport of specimens) should be clearly established if estimations of CSF methaemoglobin and bilirubin are to be made following suspected subarachnoid haemorrhage. For any specific CSF test, such as oligoclonal band (OCB) and immunoglobulin G (IgG) estimations, requests should be clearly stated with the initial CSF specimens. Parallel blood samples (e.g. sugar, OCB) should be taken when these are appropriate.

Informed consent, risks of LP, CSF removal and intrathecal drugs The LP procedure should be explained to the patient and its potentially painful nature. Written consent should be sought and if possible obtained.

The principal risks of LP relate first to the removal of CSF because this changes the pressure relationships within the system. Coning can occur. CSF often continues to leak into the tissues around the lumbar dura where it was punctured. This leads to low pressure (low volume) headaches (see Low pressure headaches, Chapter 12) and exceptionally to intracranial subdural haematoma.

Secondly, there are local complications at the site of LP:

- Local infection and meningitis
- Trauma – local pain, nerve root damage
- Bleeding
- Spinal epidural haematoma
- Arachnoiditis (see Arachnoiditis, Chapter 16).

Inappropriate intrathecal injection of drugs, such as antibiotics and cytotoxics, can have fatal consequences. Such tragedies are typically due to inexperience. LP should not be performed without clear risk appraisal, especially in the presence of raised intracranial pressure.

Table 4.12 Normal CFS appearance and constituents.

Observation/measurement		Comment
Appearance	Crystal clear, colourless	Crystal (gin) clear when held to light
Pressure	60–150 mm CSF	Patient must be relaxed, recumbent with needle patent for CSF to oscillate in manometer
Cell count	$<5/mm^3$. *No* polys: mononuclears only	One polymorph/mm^3 *just* acceptable
Protein	0.2–0.4 g/L	Slightly raised protein <0.7 g/L rarely pathological
Glucose	$^2/_3$ to $^1/_2$ of blood glucose	CSF glucose $<^1/_2$ blood glucose suspicious
Culture	Sterile	Do not accept contaminants
IgG	<15% of total CSF protein	Usually only on request
Oligoclonal bands	Absent	Parallel blood sample

Contraindications to LP

- Suspicion of a mass lesion within the brain or spinal cord. Caudal herniation of the unci and cerebellar tonsils (coning) may occur if an intracranial mass is present and the pressure below is reduced by removal of CSF. Spinal cord compression may worsen, or even develop, if an unsuspected cord tumour is present. Such complications can develop within minutes of LP. Unconscious patients and those with papilloedema must have CT or brain MRI before LP.
- Any cause of suspected raised intracranial pressure, without careful consideration.
- Local infection near the LP site.
- Congenital abnormalities in the lumbosacral region (e.g. meningo-myelocoele).
- Platelet count below 40×10^9/L and other clotting abnormalities; anticoagulant drugs. Anticoagulation should be reversed before an LP is performed.

These contraindications are relative: there are circumstances when LP is carried out despite them, for example when there is papilloedema and benign intracranial hypertension is suspected. The rare issue of unsuspected and symptomless low cerebellar tonsils, which can descend further through the foramen magnum following lumbar CSF removal, will probably in future dictate that before LP, a brain MRI will be needed except in an emergency.

LP technique

The patient is placed on the edge of a bed or trolley in the left lateral position with knees and chin as close together as possible. The spine should be as horizontal as possible. An experienced assistant is invaluable. Several pillows are useful to help with the patient's alignment and comfort.

The third and fourth lumbar spines are felt and marked. The fourth lumbar spine usually lies on a line joining the iliac crests. Using sterile precautions, 2% lidocaine (lignocaine) is injected into the dermis, raising a bleb in the skin of either third or fourth lumbar interspace. Deeper injection of local anaesthetic should follow. The LP needle (22 gauge atraumatic disposable) is pushed through the skin in the midline. The needle is pressed steadily forwards, slowly and slightly towards the head, the operator feeling with the needle tip for the spinal interspace, pausing and/or re-aiming the needle if local resistance is encountered or substantial pain provoked. In difficult cases, radiological help may be necessary and LP carried out under screening control. When the LP needle tip is felt to penetrate the tense dura mater, the stylet is withdrawn and a few drops of CSF allowed to flow.

The CSF pressure is then measured by connecting a manometer to the shaft of the needle. Normal pressure is 60–150 mm of CSF. The CSF fluid level in the manometer oscillates slowly with respiration and transiently with the pulse and rises briefly on coughing or gentle pressure on the abdomen, assuming the bore of the needle is freely patent. CSF specimens are collected in three sterile containers. An additional fluoride sample for CSF sugar level, with a simultaneous blood sample, should be taken when relevant such as in meningitis. Some 5–15 mL CSF is usually removed for diagnostic tests (Table 4.12).

CSF pressure and naked-eye appearance should be recorded in the notes: clear, cloudy, colourless, yellow (xanthochromic), red – and if red, whether or not the colour begins to clear after the first or subsequent sample. Patients are asked to lie flat for 24 hours after LP to avoid subsequent headaches, and to drink plenty, manoeuvres of uncertain value and based on doubtful evidence. Analgesics may be needed for post-LP headaches and occasionally treatments for prolonged low pressure headaches (e.g. epidural autologous blood patches; see Low pressure headaches, Chapter 12). Post LP headaches often last several days but may continue for weeks or occasionally longer.

Biopsy of brain, nerve and muscle

CNS tissue is less accessible to biopsy than, for example, the liver, lung or intestinal mucosa and all biopsies in neurology require specialised techniques. Careful attention to detail, for collection of specimens, transport and processing is essential. Detailed assessment of biopsies of muscle, nerve, brain and meninges are not considered here, but some general observations may be helpful.

Biopsy of brain or of brain lesions, with or without meningeal biopsy, is carried regularly for diagnosis of brain tumours, for other mass lesions and other specific indications. Stereotactic procedures are employed increasingly (see Surgical management, Chapter 21). If there is any question of an infective process, specimens for microbiological study should be collected in appropriate media with close liaison between operating theatre and laboratory. Brain biopsy is also of some value in diagnosing the causes of dementia and for rarities such as Rasmussen's disease, Whipple disease or vasculitis. Biopsy should where possible be directed at structurally abnormal tissue, seen on imaging. Biopsy of MRI-normal brain has a low diagnostic yield. Blind biopsy of frontal regions is sometimes undertaken, where no imaging abnormalities are seen, but the chance of making a positive diagnosis in this situation is low. Meningeal biopsy is sometimes valuable in the diagnosis of chronic infection or inflammatory diseases, such as sarcoidosis. The principal risks are those of infection, haemorrhage or damage to the surrounding brain. In competent hands, morbidity is below 2%.

Peripheral nerve biopsy (sural or radial) is commonly performed in the diagnosis of chronic neuropathies, and sometimes in vasculitis. The risks are few: infection is rare but painful paraesthesiae sometimes follow in the distribution of the nerve fascicles removed. A numb patch on the lateral aspect of the dorsum of the foot is to be expected following sural nerve biopsy and following radial nerve biopsy at the wrist, a small patch in the snuff box. Detailed microscopical studies are carried out, including electron microscopy. While many nerve biopsies do not alter management, any misgivings are brought roundly into focus by finding unexpected steroid-responsive chronic inflammatory demyelinating polyradiculoneuropathy (see Nerve biopsy; Chronic inflammatory demyelinating polyradiculoneuropathy, Chapter 10) or the occasional diagnosis of leprosy.

Muscle biopsy (deltoid or quadriceps) is a standard procedure for cases of inflammatory muscle disease, dystrophies, mitochondrial disease and metabolic myopathy with appropriate specialised stains and biochemical assays. All muscle biopsies need to be processed by specialised laboratories with ready access to electron microscopy. Open muscle biopsy rather than needle biopsy is now usual in most neurology units.

Neuropsychological testing

The Mini Mental State Examination and Queen Square Cognitive Screening Tests have already been mentioned. More detailed testing of cognition is of value. However, there is variation in reporting, and in the scope of testing. In part, this is because of the disciplines with which neuropsychology has an interface such as neurology and psychiatry and its use in non-medical settings for assessing behaviour. The tests performed are specialised and their precise details outside the knowledge of a general neurologist. Reports tend to vary in emphasis, some dwelling on potential psychiatric diagnoses, others on treatment, while others, more within the ambit of neurology focus upon cognitive function. It is in the latter field that neurologists find most value.

Intellectual function overall

The Wechsler Adult Intelligence Scale Revised (WAIS-R) is divided into subtests (David Wechsler, US psychologist, 1896–1981). The Verbal IQ with the National Adult Reading Test (NART) provides a measure of the premorbid optimal level of function, on the basis that reading vocabulary is relatively resistant to neurodegenerative and other processes that degrade other cognitive functions.

Performance IQ gives a measure of present overall cognitive, especially, non-verbal ability.

Memory Many tests to investigate different aspects of episodic memory are available:

- The Paired Associates Learning Test studies verbal memory and assesses learning of new associations between pairs of items, usually words.
- Story Recall addresses sequencing and importance of items within an incident.
- The Topographical Recognition Memory Test and Rey Figure Tests assess awareness and recall of spatial issues.
- The Recognition Memory Test is available in verbal (words) and visual (faces) versions, assessing identification of previously presented items among novel distractor items, in each domain.

Tests for verbal and non-verbal memory are useful in the localisation of damage to either the dominant or non-dominant temporal lobe, and especially medial temporal lobe structures such as the hippocampus, for instance in the work-up for possible epilepsy surgery.

Language Spontaneous speech is assessed for fluency, articulation, prosody and nominal impairment, content of speech and grammatical correctness.

The Graded-Difficulty Naming Test measures nominal ability (i.e. ability to name pictured items of varying familiarity).

Literacy and calculation Reading, spelling and calculation are assessed, for both speed and efficiency. The Graded-Difficulty Spelling and Graded-Difficulty Calculation Tests record the levels of attainment achieved.

Perceptual function Many tests focusing upon perceptual tasks are available: Silhouettes, Object Decision and Incomplete Letters – which are, for example capitals E, N and K in fragmented form. The Number Location Tests and the Visual Object and Space Perception (VOSP) battery study spatial perception.

Frontal and executive function Although included together, tests of frontal lobe and executive function are not synonymous.

Generally, these address ability to solve problems and test judgement. Unfortunately, many executive function tests are less reliable than one would wish for distinguishing whether or not a problem has an organic substrate. The Wisconsin Card Sorting Test is often used, testing ability to display flexibility and choice in the face of challenges. After seeing a number of stimulus cards, the participant is given additional cards and asked to match each to a stimulus card, and not informed whether one match is correct before progressing to the next.

The Hayling Sentence Completion Test consists of two sets of 15 sentences apiece, each with the last word missing. A sentence is read aloud; the participant has to complete it, using either a typical or a nonsensical concluding word, to provide a measure of response inhibition and lateral thinking

The Behavioural Assessment of Dysexecutive Syndrome (BADS) is a battery of six tests and also questionnaires that require planning, initiation, monitoring and behaviour adjustment to various demands:

1. Rule Shift Cards (testing perseveration)
2. Action Programme (practical problems, e.g. extracting a cork from a narrow tube)
3. Key Search (finding a lost key in a field)
4. Temporal Judgement (judgement/abstract thinking, e.g. a dog's life expectancy)
5. Zoo Map (formulation/implementation of plans), and
6. Modified Six Elements (ability to time-manage).

Attention Various tests of attention are used. Counting the number of letters A in a patchwork of letters is one of the simplest.

Formulation and conclusions

The formulation carried out by the neuropsychologist draws together the results. Problems with concentration and attention must be given appropriate weighting, especially when pain, depression and anxiety are present. The neurologist needs to know whether non-organic factors might have influenced the test results and thus close liaison with the individual psychologist is important. Interpretation of the tests needs to account for the clinical context.

Terminology, or vocabulary of clinical neurology

Names for patterns of symptoms and signs can be called the vocabulary of clinical neurology – terms and phrases used to describe particular conditions. This is an overview of some important patterns seen in clinical practice.

Focal cortical disorders

The cortical mantle is highly developed and differentiated in humans. Dementia (i.e. acquired progressive global cognitive impairment), with its various causes and particular modular features that frequently involve episodic memory and other specific aspects of cognition, is a common cortical problem (see Cognitive functions and their clinical syndromes, Chapter 8). This section outlines features of the principal focal lesions of the frontal, temporal, parietal and occipital cortex.

While cortical localisation by clinical assessment is greatly assisted by brain imaging, a general working knowledge of the cortex is essential. This section summarises some basic aspects within this field, but the reader should be aware of its complexity, the wide variation in approach between the disciplines of neurology, neuropsychiatry and psychology and that there is variation between individual brains. Many cortical functions are not strictly localised or depend upon interactions between the cortex and subcortical structures; beware theories that appear highly specific or didactic. In general, the more complex the behaviour or function, the less localised it is. The concept of a neural network, sometimes widely dispersed, is often a more accurate model.

Language (and speech) disorders

Within a cultural group, language is that combination of sounds or writing with symbolic meaning necessary for interactive communication. A phoneme is the shortest unit of language, corresponding to individual consonant and vowel sounds.

A phoneme may have a different meaning in different languages. The phoneme 'we' the English pronoun sounds like 'oui' (yes) to a person speaking French.

- Dysphasia describes any disorder of language; aphasia is also often used, but see later.
- Dysgraphia describes disorders of written language, generally used to refer to a spelling deficit unless qualified as 'motor dysgraphia'.
- Dyslexia is a disorder of reading ability; in day-to-day parlance, dyslexia is often used to refer to the common developmental problem rather than the less common acquired reading deficit caused by a focal brain lesion.
- Dysarthria is disordered motor production and/or coordination of speech sounds (articulation). Anarthria is complete inability to articulate.
- Dysphonia is a disorder of voice production, that is the speech abnormality caused by passage of expired air over poorly vibrating or paralysed vocal cords. Aphonia is complete inability, or apparent inability to produce sounds.

Aphasia should refer only to complete loss of language function, and dysphasia to some disorder of language function. The prefixes dys- (for disordered) and a- (for no or none), for aphasia/dysphasia and related communication problems are often used interchangeably, if incorrectly, in practice and while there is some dispute about this point, we have adopted common usage – that they mean the same. We have also adopted the same practice for apraxia/dyspraxia, acalculia/dyscalculia and other focal cognitive deficits.

The study of cerebral localisation commenced with recognition in the nineteenth century that the left hemisphere was the seat of language in the majority of people. In 1861, Paul Broca (1824–1880 Paris), described non-fluent (expressive) aphasia in a patient with a tumour in the left third frontal convolution. In 1873, Carl Wernicke (1848–1905, Breslau) described fluent jargon aphasia (speaking unintelligible words) in a patient with a lesion more posteriorly placed, in the angular gyrus. Classic concepts that outlined the system as a whole such as those of Lichtheim (Ludwig Lichtheim, 1845–1928, Breslau) posited cortical modules for conceptual meanings, connected by pathways to a posterior (temporal) centre for processing phonemes, passing information via the arcuate fasciculus to an anterior (frontal) centre for programming and delivering speech output.

Difficulty naming objects – nominal aphasia – became established as a screening test, a common denominator for lesions over a wide area of the posterior frontal, temporal and lower parietal regions of the dominant hemisphere. Word retrieval in nominal aphasia correlates with frequency of a word in everyday life. Thus, slightly unusual objects, for example the winder button (stem button) rather than the wristwatch itself are preferable when asking the question: 'What is this called?'

This section summarises features of four basic varieties of aphasia, derived originally from the concepts of Lichtheim and others. Mixed and incomplete varieties of aphasia are common, and terms such as fluency, while useful descriptively, have limited value for understanding the physiology of these disorders.

Non-fluent aphasia (Broca's aphasia, motor or anterior aphasia) This is the most common variety of aphasia following stroke. The hallmark is the slow, incomplete and laboured production of language, with a major breakdown of grammatical output:

- The patient is fully aware of the problem and often distressed.
- Grammar and syntax are lost. Tenses of verbs are incorrect. Adjectives and conjunctions are lost more than the nouns for common objects.
- Perseveration is common.
- Prosody (normal rhythm) is lost.
- Ability to repeat phrases is lost.
- Comprehension is relatively preserved but complex multiple commands will usually reveal some lack of understanding.

The lesion is around the left, third (inferior) frontal convolution, lower (inferior) motor cortex and nearby temporal insula. The closeness of the motor strip to Broca's area explains why contralateral UMN facial weakness and hemiparesis/hemiplegia are frequently seen. There may also be facial apraxia – dissociation between the idea and production of a non-verbal facial movement such as whistling. Cortical dysarthria, also known as speech apraxia describes the situation when this apraxia extends to speech itself, causing slurring and hesitancy.

Fluent aphasia (posterior, sensory or Wernicke's aphasia) The essence of this variety of aphasia is production of fluent speech that lacks meaning. Patients typically appear to have little insight into an evident problem and are talkative. They look bewildered and tend to be agitated. Phonemic and semantic confusions are common and sometimes prominent. Neologisms (new, meaningless words) are formed with outpourings of meaningless jargon. Prosody tends to remain normal. Ability to repeat phrases is lost; comprehension is lost.

Patients are sometimes mistaken for being psychiatrically ill. This is the aphasia subtype that is most likely to be mistaken for 'confusion' by the casual observer; occurrence of jargon and preserved alertness are clues to the correct diagnosis. If a patient with Wernicke's aphasia recovers, which is unusual, they say they were unaware they had been speaking nonsense. Also, they had been unable to grasp what others had been saying, as if they had been listening to an incomprehensible language.

Conduction aphasia Reduced ability to repeat spoken words or phrases but with reasonable comprehension are features of conduction aphasia, seen with a lesion of the arcuate bundle between posterior and anterior language areas, and posteriorly situated lesions in the cortical language area. The pattern consists of:

- Fluent speech, with nominal dysphasia, semantic confusions with phonemic errors but characteristic attempts at self-correction, often repeated
- Poor repetition - particularly marked for phrases
- Relatively preserved comprehension.

Transcortical aphasias, motor and sensory Preserved ability to repeat spoken words, phrases and sometimes longer passages is the striking feature of transcortical aphasias. The arcuate fasciculus remains intact. Transcortical motor aphasia (TMA) describes a non-fluent aphasia caused typically by a lesion in the left anterior superior frontal region. Patients with TMA have sparse spontaneous speech, with phrases that are short but grammatically correct. These patients have lost the ability to generate new verbal messages: a condition also called dynamic aphasia, because the language disorder is only evident under certain conditions, in particular where novel language output is required. However, they retain the ability to repeat words, phrases or sentences. Repetition is believed to be preserved because the arcuate fasciculus remains intact. Comprehension remains reasonably normal.

Transcortical sensory aphasia (TSA) is caused typically by lesions behind Wernicke's area in the temporal–occipital–parietal region, or more ventrally and anteriorly in the dominant temporal lobe. Patients with TSA have poor comprehension but fluent and reasonably grammatical speech, with preserved repetition. However, they tend to have marked anomia and produce semantic paraphasia (i.e. they do not use words that are correct, but substitute words of similar content, such as pear for apple, pen for writing paper, substituting approximate words or relying on circumlocutions such as 'thingy'). This condition closely resembles the aphasia of semantic dementia, in which a primary breakdown of verbal semantic memory leads to loss of vocabulary and single word comprehension caused by selective degeneration of the anterior temporal lobe.

Mixed transcortical aphasia (MTA) is characterised by both severely reduced language output and by impairment of comprehension, but with preservation of the ability to repeat words and phrases. Patients with this unusual form of transcortical aphasia have a major disability, with difficulty producing propositional language and understanding what is being said to them. However, they can repeat phrases and even complex sentences, and finish a familiar poem or song, once they hear the beginning of the composition. Generally, in MTA, both Broca's and Wernicke's areas and the arcuate fasciculus between them remain intact. The surrounding regions are believed to be damaged, isolating these areas.

Agraphia and acquired alexia Written symbol comprehension depends on the integrity of the dominant angular gyrus. Lesions in this cortical region cause acquired alexia usually with agraphia. Isolated alexia without agraphia is seen with either anterior occipital lobe lesions and/or lesions of the splenium of the corpus callosum.

Temporal lobe lesions

Many small (<2 cm) unilateral temporal lobe lesions are silent in terms of cognitive abnormalities. Epilepsy is common (see Partial seizures, Chapter 7). Upper quantrantic hemianopia is seen when the forward-looping fibres (Meyer's loop; see Optic radiation, Chapter 2) are damaged. A lesion in the more posterior dominant anterior temporal lobe often causes a posterior (Wernicke) aphasia, or less commonly (particularly if bilateral) 'word deafness', that is selective inability to understand spoken (but preserved understanding of written) speech, caused by damage or disconnection of auditory areas in or near Heschl's gyrus.

Non-dominant anterior temporal lobe lesions particularly when they involve more ventral cortex are sometimes associated with inability to recognise faces (prosopagnosia). Unilateral mesial temporal lobe lesions can also produce subtle changes in memory, more marked for verbal material in the dominant and faces and topographical features in the nondominant hemisphere, but often silent clinically until revealed by specific neuropsychological tests.

Bilateral temporal lobe lesions, such as those that follow herpes simplex encephalitis cause profound loss of memory for recent events. Bilateral temporal lobe injury in primates causes hypersexuality, hyperphagia, hyperactivity and aggressive behaviour (Klüver–Bucy syndrome: Heinrich Klüver, US neurologist, 1898–1979; Paul Clancy Bucy, US neuropathologist, 1904–1992). Sometimes, in humans, there are elements of this such as episodic temper dyscontrol but the usual outcome is aimlessness, diminished libido and impaired potency.

Frontal lobe lesions

As in the temporal lobes, many frontal lesions remain silent, though this is likely in part to reflect our limited ability to measure complex behavioural changes reliably. Frontal cortical areas have multiple connections with subcortical structures including the basal ganglia and limbic systems and these distributed networks mediate a range of emotional, social and motivational behaviours. Lesions involving the dorsal frontal convexities are more likely to cause impassivity and apathy (more medial lesions may cause mutism) while lesions of the orbitofrontal cortex are more likely to produce disinhibition; however, anatomical localisation is imprecise.

Lesions involving the dominant inferior frontal gyrus cause anterior (Broca's) aphasia. Substantial damage such as traumatic frontal brain injury, direct or contra-coup) causes a highly disabling lack of social control. Examples of this are:

- Abandonment of the usual social inhibitions – from somewhat inopportune, often rude comments to profound disturbances such as urination, exposure or masturbation in public.
- Inappropriate jollity (*witzelsucht*) – jokes and tales often overlong and unwanted, and/or loss of empathy.

- Apathy (abulia), lack of initiative and poor planning (dysexecutive problems).
- Irritability, anger or the converse, inappropriate placidity in the face of irritation.
- Poor planning, distractability or conversely obsessional behaviour.
- Continuing one action when another is appropriate, known as motor perseveration.
- Utilisation behaviour (environmental dependency). The subject sees a tool, such as a stethoscope during a consultation and begins to use it.

These frontal lobe features may be accompanied by release of primitive behavioural programmes dating from early infant development, such as grasp, rooting or sucking reflexes. Deep bilateral frontal lesions, such as small vessel disease in the elderly, can lead to gait apraxia and failure to initiate walking (gait ignition failure), often with sphincter disturbance.

Alleged brain damage associated with behavioural change has become a common plea in claims following minor head injury, when headaches and moodiness are common The patient and relatives are asked leading questions about features such as impulsivity, temper, socialisation, fiscal ability, multi-tasking, planning, prioritisation, depression and anxiety – all of which are common problems in stressful situations. There is no evidence that these complaints are caused by brain injury following a minor blow to the head, when imaging is normal.

Frontal lobe seizures are described in Chapter 7 (see Frontal lobe epilepsy).

Occipital lobe lesions

Field defects of occipital lobe lesions are mentioned in Chapter 14 (see Visual cortex). Neglect or even denial of virtually complete visual loss (cortical blindness or Anton's syndrome) are sometimes seen following bilateral occipital lobe infarction. An explanation for the phenomenon known as blind sight (perception of objects when the occipital cortex is destroyed) is the preservation of anterior visual pathways via the lateral geniculate bodies that are below the level of awareness. Epilepsy, with episodes of flashing lights or, rarely, more formed features, can occur with occipital lobe lesions.

Parietal lobe lesions

These areas are concerned with the integration into perception of complex visual and somatosensory information, such as awareness of body parts in space and their relation to objects. A complex nomenclature has evolved to describe these perceptual defects. Attempts to associate precise parietal lobe areas to particular functions are bedevilled by variation between individuals, and because the brain is not divided into discrete compartments. The following are seen with lesions of either parietal lobe:

- Attention defects in the contralateral visual field and neglect of the opposite side of the body. Lower quadrantic homonymous field defects occur when the optic radiation is damaged.
- Astereognosis – inability to recognise common objects placed in the palm despite apparently normal peripheral sensation.
- Agraphaesthesia – inability to recognise numbers drawn on the palm with the examiner's finger. However, the range of normal graphaesthesia is so wide that this sign is only useful if there is clear asymmetry between the palms.
- Pseudo-athetosis (waving about) and/or drift of an outstretched contralateral hand.
- Contralateral cortical sensory loss manifesting as impaired two-point discrimination despite intact elementary peripheral sensation.

Sensory epilepsy is sometimes a feature of parietal lobe lesions.

Dominant parietal lesions Inability to execute a skilled movement despite no discernable weakness may be seen – apraxia. For example, the patient may not respond to verbal suggestions such as 'Imitate combing your hair' or 'Pretend to turn a key in a lock': this is 'ideational' apraxia, inability to execute learned motor programmes. Alternatively, the patient may have particular difficulty imitating a meaningless gesture made by the examiner: 'ideomotor' apraxia. Typically, they are bewildered, moving the hand in a non-purposive way or attempting to 'close in' on the examiner's hand.

Lesions of the dominant parietal lobe may produce impairment of literacy skills: alexia (impaired reading), agraphia (impaired writing/spelling) and acalculia (impaired arithmetic). The constellation of these with addition of finger agnosia (inability to name individual fingers) and right–left disorientation is often referred to as Gerstmann's syndrome (Josef Gerstmann, 1887–1969).

Auditory short-term verbal memory is conveniently measured at the bedside as a digit span; normally, a string of 7 (±2) digits can be repeated forwards while a string of 5 (±2) digits can be actively reversed. These measures assess working memory, meaning the short-term memory store used in everyday life when repeating a phone number. Working memory impairment frequently accompanies delirium but, if it occurs in a clear sensorium, has potential localising value as a dominant parietal sign. A discrepancy of >2 digits between forward and reverse digit span is a useful marker of executive dysfunction.

Neglect of contralateral limbs is typically less prominent with dominant than non-dominant parietal lesions.

Non-dominant parietal lesions Patterns include:

- Neglect of the opposite limbs. Neglect can extend to denial that the limbs are the patient's own.
- Inability to construct or draw shapes such as a house or a clock face. The left side of a picture drawn (such as numbers 1–5 on a clock face) tend to be omitted by a right-handed patient with a right parietal lesion. This difficulty with reproducing visual designs is often termed 'constructional apraxia'.
- Visual apperceptive agnosia – inability to perceive objects under degraded viewing conditions or from an unusual angle.

Motor abnormalities: brain and spinal cord

The patterns of abnormality within the motor system are both distinct and recognisable. Features of hemiparesis (and hemiplegia) and paraparesis, cerebellar syndromes and disorders of movement are summarised here.

Hemiparesis

Weakness of the limbs of one side resulting from a pyramidal tract lesion is known as hemiparesis, the term paresis indicating that weakness is not total (cf. hemiplegia, when there is total loss of power following a stroke). The signs of an early hemiparesis, sometimes before weakness becomes evident, are scuffing of the toe of one shoe, drift of one outstretched upper limb on examination or a trace of impaired fine finger and/or toe movement. Thereafter emerge the five principal features of a pyramidal lesion:

1 Increase in tone
2 Weakness in a typical pattern, with upper limb extensors weaker than flexors, and lower limb flexors weaker than extensors
3 Progressive loss of fine movement
4 Unilaterally exaggerated tendon reflexes, and
5 Extensor plantar response (Babinski) and absent abdominal reflexes.

These features gradually develop as a hemiparesis progresses or emerge following the sudden hemiplegia of a stroke. However, in either case, not all these features of a UMN lesion are required to make a firm diagnosis.

As a corollary, to find weakness alone as the sole feature of a hemiparesis is highly unusual and raises the question of whether or not the problem has an organic basis.

Cerebellar syndromes

Features of cerebellar disease are well-defined and straightforward to recognise compared to our knowledge of the complexity of cerebellar function (Table 4.13). Perform examination correctly to elicit early cerebellar signs.

In established cerebellar disease there are several practical points. The first relates to clinical urgency. If an expanding mass lesion of the cerebellum is strongly suspected or found on imaging, there needs to be speedy liaison with a neurosurgeon. While all mass lesions of the brain are potentially serious, many brain tumours above the tentorium can be dealt with in an expectant manner. With cerebellar tumours the rapidity of progression and development of tonsillar herniation over several hours can catch out the unwary.

Secondly, when a severe cerebellar syndrome is part of a multisystem degenerative disease, pyramidal features can be masked. Extensor plantars may be the only pyramidal sign. Finally, ascribing ataxia of stance and gait of midline cerebellar lesions as non-organic has happened all too frequently. The causes of cerebellar syndromes are given in Chapter 17 (see The ataxic disorders).

Disorders of movement

The broad distinction is between akinetic-rigid syndromes and dyskinesias; the principal disorders are listed in Table 4.14. No amount of written description surpasses looking at a disorder of movement, either in the flesh or on video. The types of movement disorders are considered in more detail in Chapter 6 (Movement).

Some presentations cause diagnostic difficulties regularly. First, when an akinetic-rigid condition becomes apparent, early idiopathic Parkinson's disease tends to be over diagnosed. The reality, evident some years later, is that sometimes the cause is a less common akinetic-rigid syndrome. Parkinson's disease is almost always asymmetrical. Parkinson's disease should be diagnosed with caution if rest tremor is not apparent. Progressive supranuclear palsy or multiple systems atrophy tend to be symmetrical from the onset, although the poverty of movement is similar to that seen in Parkinson's disease. Early Wilson's disease should be considered in an akinetic-rigid syndrome beginning below the age of 40.

Benign essential tremor (BET) can cause difficulty. Usually in BET, tremor is seen when the limbs adopt a particular posture. However, there are forms of BET that mimic benign tremulous Parkinson's disease in the early stages. To complicate matters, occasionally action tremor is seen in BET, raising the possibility of cerebellar disease. The passage of time usually sorts out these difficulties.

Early chorea is also easy to miss, being mistaken for restlessness and normal fidgeting. A minor degree of dystonia can also escape recognition. Lower limb myoclonus can look remarkably like the ankle clonus of spasticity.

Finally, the diagnosis of a psychologically determined movement disorder is fraught with difficulty, and frequently wrong when made early. In movement disorder clinics, a substantial proportion of those labelled as functional, somatoform or conversion hysteria, whichever term is chosen, turn out to have organic disease.

Table 4.13 Principal features of cerebellar syndromes.

Lateral cerebellar lobe lesions
Rebound
Action tremor
Past-pointing
Dysdiadochokinesis
Dysarthria
Nystagmus (towards lesion if vestibular connections involved)
Vermis lesions
Ataxia of stance, trunk and gait, sometimes with negative Romberg test (a test primarily of proprioception)

Table 4.14 Principal disorders of movement.

Akinetic-rigid syndromes
Idiopathic Parkinson's disease
Parkinsonism-plus syndromes
Drug-induced parkinsonism (e.g. phenothiazines)
Post-encephalitic parkinsonism
MPTP-induced parkinsonism
Childhood akinetic-rigid syndromes
Dyskinesias
Tremors
Chorea
Hemiballismus
Myoclonus
Tics
Dystonias
Paroxysmal dyskinesias
Drug-induced dyskinesias

MPTP, 1-methyl 4-phenyl 1,2,3,6-tetrahydropyridine.

Paraparesis

Spastic paraparesis, meaning lower limb weakness of cord or, rarely, cortical origin, is one of the pivotal diagnoses of neurology. Prior to the era of MRI, clinical examination had a major role in differentiating between cord compression, a potential neurosurgical emergency, and other causes of paraparesis.

As with a hemiparesis, the clinical picture begins with subtle features:

- Scuffing the toes of shoes, often worse on one side
- Stiffening of gait (spastic gait) with retention of a narrow base

- Noticeable beats of ankle clonus (e.g. on a step or kerbstone)
- Changes in lower limb sensation.

Spinal pain is a common feature of cord compression. For example with a thoracic meningioma, pain at the level of the tumour, develops with an emerging spastic paraparesis and a sensory level, rising from below to the site of compression. The patient complains of numbness or altered sensation commencing in the feet that marches upwards over weeks or months. Brown-Séquard features (pyramidal signs on one side, spinothalamic on the other) may become apparent.

These features apply equally to tetraparesis (*syn.* quadriparesis).

The five principal features of a pyramidal lesion may not all be present. Pain may not be present in cord compression. Marked asymmetry can sometimes cause difficulty. Seek out subtle signs.

Two questions arise when signs of spastic paraparesis are found:

1 Is the paraparesis caused by spinal cord compression?
2 Is the paraparesis the result of a condition in which it is part of the clinical picture?
   - Multiple sclerosis
   - Motor neurone disease
   - Subacute combined degeneration of the cord
   - Syringomyelia
   - Cortical lesions such as a parasagittal meningioma, hydrocephalus and other brain lesions can occasionally present as a paraparesis.

Paraparesis is also caused by many rarities, such as vascular anomalies of the cord, adrenoleukodystrophy and copper deficiency (Chapter 16).

There can be many difficulties with the diagnosis of paraparesis, both in the referral process and within neurology. First, in the community and in primary care, the emergence of difficulty walking is sometimes not taken seriously, and early features of a paraparesis can pass unrecognised unless a neurological examination is carried out. The onset of any gait disturbance demands an explanation. A second issue, within neurology, is misinterpretation of lower limb signs, thinking that they are pyramidal in origin when they are not:

- Parkinson's disease affecting predominantly the lower limbs can be mistaken for spinal cord disease.
- Cortical myoclonus in the lower limbs can be mistaken for pyramidal ankle clonus.
- Stiffness of inflammatory muscle disease, such as polymyositis can be mistaken for spasticity.
- Brisk but normal lower limb reflexes are misinterpreted as pathological, thus prompting investigation for a paraparesis.

Brainstem syndromes

Brainstem anatomy is outlined in Chapter 2 (see The brainstem). Figure 4.19 is a helpful diagram: think of the level within the brainstem and of the dorso-ventral plane. The usual hallmark of a brainstem lesion is the coexistence of features of damage both to motor and/or sensory fibres passing through it and to cranial nerve nuclei. Syndromes involving oculomotor nerves III, IV and VI indicate upper or mid brainstem disease affecting the area dorsally. Mid and lower brainstem disease affects cranial nerve nuclei VII–XII.

Bulbar and pseudobulbar palsy are terms used to describe common lower brainstem syndromes (see Bulbar and pseudobulbar palsy, Chapter 13). Both cause dysarthria, dysphagia, drooling and respiratory problems. Bulbar palsy describes disease of the lower cranial nerves (IX, X, XII), that is the nerves of the medullary bulb,

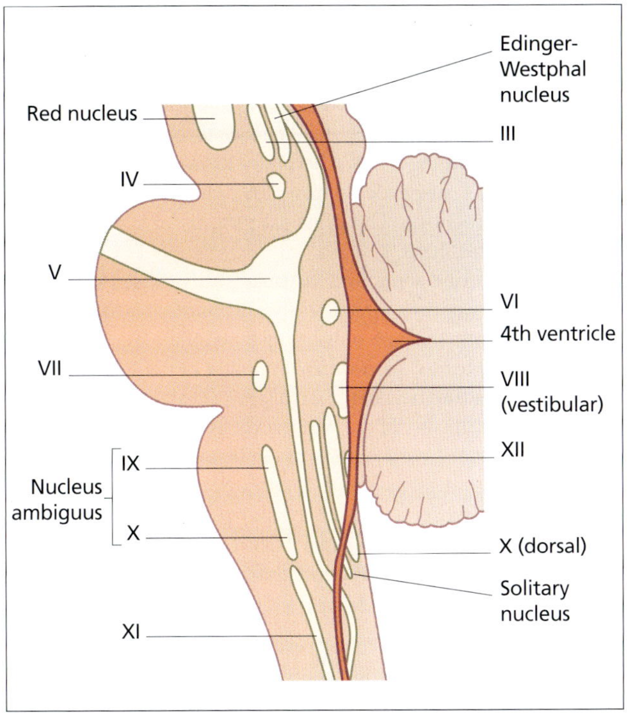

Figure 4.19 Brainstem: lateral schematic view. Source: Hopkins 1993. Reproduced with permission of Oxford University Press.

their nuclei and muscles supplied. Pseudobulbar palsy is shorthand for UMN lesions of lower cranial nerve nuclei. MS, brainstem stroke and motor neurone disease cause pseudobulbar palsy, the latter usually both bulbar and pseudobulbar. Advanced Parkinson's disease and other extrapyramidal syndromes also cause poverty of movement of the bulbar muscles.

Anterior horn cell disease

The anterior horn is the ventral grey matter in the spinal cord. It contains the motor neurones, that are flowing out of the spinal cord, through the spinal roots, to innervate muscles. Anatomically, the neurones are somatotropically organised (medial innervation of proximal muscles and lateral innervation of distal muscles), and the pattern of weakness depends on the level of the spinal root(s) affected. There are relatively few diseases that afflict the anterior horn; are all serious. The most common are: motor neurone disease (MND), the spinal muscular atrophies, Kennedy's disease, poliomyelitis and some viral diseases (notably West Nile virus, see Chapter 9). The conditions produce lower motor neurone signs of wasting and weakness in the affected muscles (see Anterior horn cell diseases, Chapter 10). Motor neurone disease is the most common anterior horn disorder in western neurological practice, often characterised by prominent fasciculation with additional upper motor neurone signs. Typically too in all anterior horn cell diseases, initially at least, the pattern of weakness is highly selective, reflecting the somatotropic and root pattern of innervation. For instance, patients with motor neurone disease can present with weakness of one or two finger flexors only before more widespread changes occur. Neurophysiological tests are characteristic with normal conduction velocities, small amplitude CMAPs, normal sensory conduction, larger than normal motor unit potentials, denervation and reinnervation patterns.

Sensory abnormalities: patterns at different levels

Sensory symptoms and signs are difficult to evaluate. The pattern of symptoms may be unfamiliar, examination time-consuming and its results less certain than reflex and motor abnormalities. Eponyms abound, such as positive Tinel, tic douloureux, causalgia, anaesthesia dolorosa, lightning pains, Lhermitte, Brown-Séquard, dissociated sensory loss, suspended sensory loss, sacral sparing, thalamic pain and astereognosis. The principal patterns of sensory disturbance are outlined here.

An approach that some find valuable is to view sensory symptoms in one of two ways. First, if a sensory symptom is the principal complaint, such as the pain of trigeminal neuralgia (see Trigeminal neuralgia, Chapter 13) or nocturnal tingling of the hands in early median nerve entrapment at the wrist (see Carpal tunnel syndrome, Chapter 10), the quality of the symptom is frequently diagnostic. In other situations, the combination of the history, sensory signs and other neurological signs point to an anatomical diagnosis. An example is the sensory signs that point to the level spinal cord compression when the principal feature is spastic paraparesis. Figure 4.20 summarises various patterns of sensory loss.

Peripheral nerve lesions

A lesion of an individual peripheral nerve produces symptoms and signs within its distribution. Nerve section is followed by complete sensory loss. Demarcation is clear-cut. The areas of sensory loss found in individual nerve lesions are discussed in Focal and compressive neuropathies, Chapter 10. In nerve entrapment or partial damage, the quality of sensory disturbance varies between numbness, tingling and painful pins and needles. Jules Tinel (1879–1952, Le Mans and Paris) wrote about gunshot wound nerve injuries in 1917. He described painful tingling in the distribution of a damaged nerve when it was percussed, now known as a positive Tinel's sign. In some cases of carpal tunnel syndrome when the median nerve at the wrist is tapped lightly at the wrist, there is sharp tingling in the thumb and the three and a half fingers innervated by the median nerve.

Neuralgia (see Neuropathic pain, Chapter 23) describes pain of great severity in the distribution of a nerve or nerve root. In trigeminal neuralgia (*tic douloureux*; see Trigeminal neuralgia, Chapter 13), the paroxysmal nature of the pain, its distribution and electric shock-like quality are diagnostic.

Causalgia (see Complex regional pain syndrome, Chapter 23) describes chronic pain after nerve section or crush injury and is sometimes seen after amputation. Anaesthesia dolorosa is spontaneous pain occurring in an anaesthetic area. It is used to describe discomfort or chronic debilitating pain, developing for example after destructive procedures to the trigeminal nerve.

Sensory root and root entry zone lesions

The distribution of spinal dermatomes is shown in Figure 4.21. Unlike peripheral nerves there is some overlap between adjacent dermatomes making the area of sensory loss following a single nerve root lesion smaller than shown. Root pain is typically perceived both within the dermatome and within the myotome but tends to be less demarcated than pain in a peripheral nerve lesion. For example, with an S1 root lesion resulting from a lumbosacral disc, the sensory disturbance is down the back of the leg, typically without clear dermatome demarcation. Stretching of the nerve root by straight leg raising or increasing local spinal CSF pressure (coughing, straining) typically makes matters worse.

When a root is affected within the cord, such as in tabes dorsalis, sudden, irregular, very intense stabbing pains involve one or more spots, typically on the ankle, calf, thigh or abdomen. These are known as the lightning pains of tabes and are seldom seen today.

Neuralgia in a nerve root distribution can follow shingles (see Post-herpetic neuralgia, Chapter 23). This is a persistent distressing burning pain.

Spinal cord lesions

Posterior columns Symptoms, although they may be worse on one side, are often not clearly demarcated. Patients describe various patterns of symptoms:

- Band-like sensations around trunk or limbs
- Limb clumsiness and deadness
- Numbness and burning
- Electric shock-like sensations.

Joint position sense, vibration, light touch and two-point discrimination become diminished below a cord lesion. Stamping gait and pseudochorea of the outstretched hands are the product of failing position sense.

Lhermitte's sign is a sudden electrical sensation down the back and into the limbs produced by bending the head forward, stretching the cervical cord. Lhermitte's is diagnostic of lesions of the posterior columns or occasionally caudal medulla. It is seen in:

- MS, typically in exacerbations
- Cervical myelopathy
- Radiation myelopathy
- Subacute combined degeneration of the cord, and occasionally in
- Cord compression, Behçet's, Arnold–Chiari syndrome and following trauma.

The phenomenon was probably first described by Pierre Marie and Charles Chatelin (Paris, 1917); Jean Lhermitte re-described it in 1920, writing the seminal article some 4 years later.

Spinothalamic tracts A lesion within the spinothalamic tracts of the cord that blocks conduction produces changes in pain and temperature sensation below its level. With progressive compression from outside the cord, such as by an enlarging thoracic meningioma (extramedullary cord compression), the sensory level will tend to commenced in the feet and rise until the level of the tumour is reached. This is because of the lamination of spinothalamic fibres in the cord. The patient may notice loss of spinothalamic sensation, for example being unable to gauge water temperature with their foot. Extramedullary cord compression tends to affect both principal cord sensory pathways (i.e. both posterior column and spinothalamic).

When a lesion is within the cord (intramedullary) such as a syrinx (a central cavity) sensory loss can initially be confined to the spinothalamic pathways. Spinothalamic sensory loss occurs in isolation: the phrase dissociated sensory loss implies that a syrinx or other central cord lesion is suspected. Suspended sensory loss is a term describing another aspect also seen typically with a syrinx. The patch of dissociated sensory loss does not extend to the lower limbs and is thus hanging, on the thorax or abdomen.

Sacral sparing is another phrase used to capture the phenomenon of preserved sacral and perineal sensation when a central cord lesion expands centrifugally, damaging first centrally placed fibres and reaching last the spinothalamic sacral fibres on the periphery of the cord.

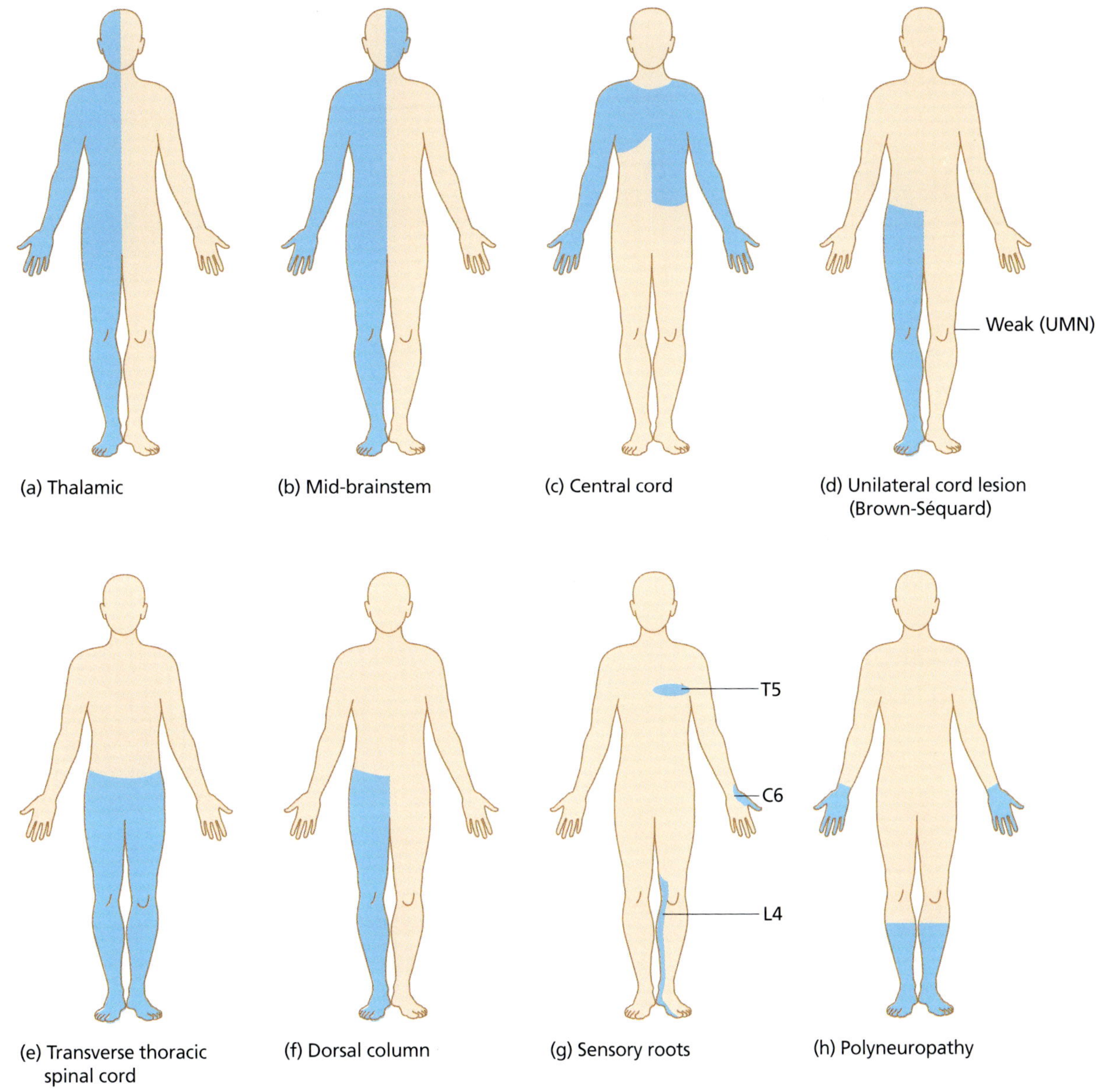

(a) Thalamic lesion: sensory loss throughout opposite side (rare).
(b) Brainstem lesion (rare): contralateral sensory loss below face and ipsilateral loss on face.
(c) Central cord lesion (e.g. syrinx): 'suspended' areas of loss, often asymmetrical and 'dissociated' (i.e. pain and temperature loss but light touch remaining intact).
(d) 'Hemisection' of cord or unilateral cord lesion = Brown-Séquard syndrome: contralateral spinothalamic (pain and temperature) loss with ipsilateral weakness and dorsal column loss below lesion.
(e) Transverse cord lesion: loss of all modalities below lesion.
(f) Isolated dorsal column lesion (e.g. demyelination): loss of proprioception, vibration and light touch.
(g) Individual sensory root lesions (e.g. C6, cervical root compression; T5, shingles; L4, lumbar root compression).
(h) Polyneuropathy: distal sensory loss.

Figure 4.20 Principal patterns of loss of sensation. Source: Clarke 2005. Reproduced with permission of Elsevier.

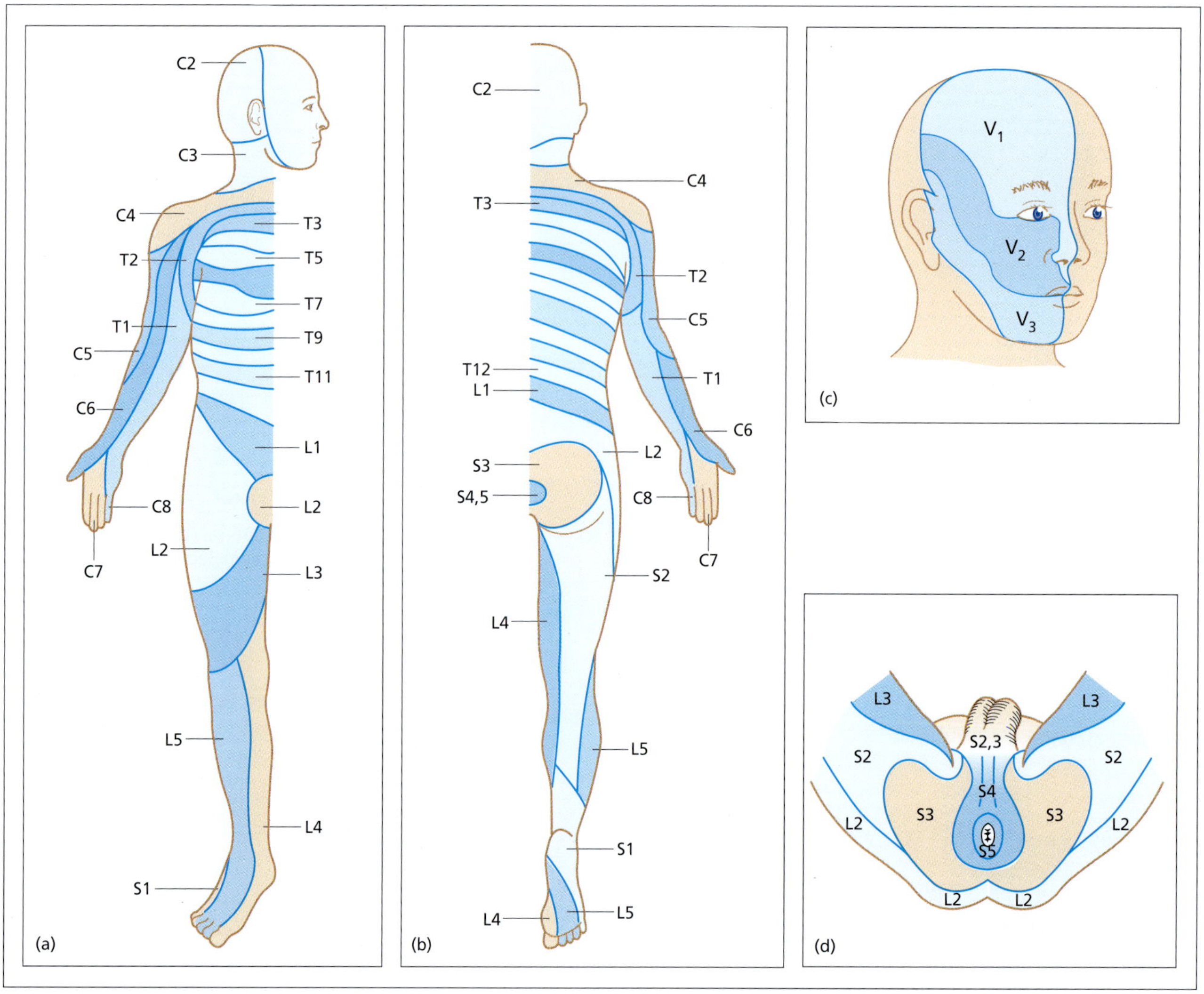

Figure 4.21 (a), (b) and (d) Spinal dermatomes. Source: O'Brien 2000. Reproduced with permission of The Guarantors of Brain. (c) Cutaneous distribution of divisions of Vth nerve. Source: Patten 1996. Reproduced with permission of Springer Science + Business Media. Precise distribution varies amongst published sources, especially for sacral dermatomes, perineum and Vth nerve.

As a cavity develops within one side of the cord, dissociated sensory loss on one side occurs with pyramidal signs such as a spastic lower limb on the other. This carries the eponym Brown-Séquard. Charles-Edouard Brown-Séquard (1817–1894) published a treatise in 1849 on traumatic hemisection of cord. Originally from Mauritius, Brown-Séquard became a physician at the National Hospital. Brown-Séquard findings mean spinothalamic signs on one side with pyramidal and dorsal column signs on the other. They point to a cord lesion, on the same side as the pyramidal and dorsal column loss. The patient may report: 'I cannot feel the bathwater with my left foot, but it's my right that drags.'

Sensory changes in brainstem lesions

Complex patterns of sensory loss occur with lesions in the brainstem, their character depending on the level of the lesion. Trigeminal sensory loss (see V: trigeminal nerve, sensory and motor nuclei, Chapters 2; V. Trigeminal nerve, Chapter 13) and dissociated (spinothalamic) sensory loss in the limbs, are seen, such as in the lateral medullary syndrome (see Vertebral artery, Chapter 5). The site of a brainstem lesion is usually determined more from signs from cranial nerve nuclei and brainstem connections than by the pattern of sensory loss.

Sensory changes following thalamic lesions

Destructive lesions of the complex thalamic nuclei and thalamocortical projections are relatively unusual causes of sensory symptoms. Two principal patterns are found. When the ventral posterior lateral (VPL) and ventral posterior medial (VPM) thalamic nuclei (Chapter 2) are damaged, such as following a thrombo-embolic stroke, contralateral hemi-anaesthesia follows immediately. All sensory modalities are usually affected. Sometimes, however, during the weeks or months following the stroke, highly unpleasant disabling persistent pain (see Thalamic pain, Post-stroke central pain, Chapter 23) develops in the partially anaesthetic limbs. This pain is usually permanent. Spontaneous pain does not develop following cortical lesions, nor following damage within the internal capsule or basal ganglia nuclei outside the thalamus, but does so occasionally when the spinothalamic tract is damaged in the cord or brainstem.

Sensory changes in parietal lobe lesions

Features of parietal lobe lesions such as astereognosis (i.e. the inability to perceive the shape of an object in the hand) are mentioned earlier in this chapter. Attacks of tingling or odd altered sensation caused by sensory epilepsy can occur with parietal tumours. Negative sensory symptoms, meaning complaints of sensory loss, are unusual. It is more typical that a patient says that a hand or limb 'doesn't work properly' or 'doesn't feel quite right'.

Mononeuropathy, polyneuropathy, root lesions

These notes summarise features of peripheral nervous system conditions, dealt with in detail in Chapters 10, 13 and 16.

Mononeuropathy

Common isolated single nerve lesions (mononeuropathies) are distinct and easy to recognise once seen. Ulnar, median, radial, common peroneal (lateral popliteal), lateral cutaneous nerve of the thigh and sural nerve lesions are the most common. Most are caused by entrapment but there are other causes such as nerve tumours and vasculitis. Cranial nerve lesions are discussed in Chapter 13.

Multiple mononeuropathy

This means the occurrence of two or more peripheral nerve lesions. Principal causes worldwide are leprosy, diabetes, hereditary neuropathy with liability to pressure palsies (HNPP), and vasculitis such as polyarteritis.

Polyneuropathy

Polyneuropathy (formerly known as peripheral neuropathy and polyneuritis) describes conditions in which nerves die back, usually symmetrically to cause peripheral sensory loss, muscle weakness and wasting with loss of tendon reflexes. It is sometimes hard to characterise a neuropathy from its phenotype and thus to distinguish between genetic and acquired neuropathies.

Abnormal myelin is more prone to inflammatory change than normal myelin: both genetic and inflammatory neuropathies can coexist.

Neurogenic muscle wasting

The crux of the matter is to distinguish between:

- Generalised muscle thinning, a normal finding in old age, and loss of muscle bulk seen in cachexia
- Widespread wasting seen motor neurone disease, polyneuropathy and some myopathies
- Focal wasting that follows denervation.

Neurological examination seeks out sites of predilection:

- Small hand muscles, supplied by ulnar and/or median nerves (T1)
- Guttering of the forearm flexors
- Wasted anterior tibial compartment – sunken appearance lateral to the leading edge of the tibia
- Wasted extensor digitorum brevis muscles – concave dished appearance of the small oyster-like muscles below each lateral malleolus.

Generalised thinning of muscles with advancing age is common and contributes to a gaunt appearance and spidery hands. However, the muscles are strong on bedside testing. In pathological states, muscles are weak. Muscles that are clinically normal (bulk, consistency and power) are usually electrophysiologically and histologically.

Root lesions

Characteristics of a lesion affecting a nerve root are:

- Radicular pain
- Wasting and weakness of affected muscles
- Sensory loss or referred sensory symptoms, and
- Loss of or depression of one or more deep tendon reflexes.

Two descriptive terms are used. Radiculopathy is often applied to root lesions that are part of an inflammatory, vascular or neoplastic process (i.e. part of a disease), with derivative complex terms such as polyradiculomyelopathy. The phrase 'cervical or lumbar root problem' usually implies a compressive lesion, caused typically by degenerative disc and/or spinal disease. There is no real difference between the two; the shorter English word, root, is preferred to the longer, radiculopathy (from Latin *radix,* a root) but the longer terms remain in widespread use

Root pain or discomfort is caused by distortion or stretching of the meninges surrounding a nerve root and is perceived both in the myotome and the dermatome (Table 4.15). This clinical point is relevant in C7 root compression: pain is felt deep to the scapula (C7 muscles) and the sensory disturbance runs in the C7 dermatome to the middle finger. The triceps jerk is lost. For further discussion see Chapters 10 and 16.

Cauda equina syndrome

The cauda equina (horse's tail) is the leash of roots emanating from the lower end of the cord below vertebral body level L1/L2. Pressure (e.g. central L4/L5 disc) on the cauda equina affects all lumbo-sacral roots streaming caudally. There is loss of bladder and bowel control, numbness of buttocks and thighs with paralysis of ankle dorsiflexion (L4), toes (L4, L5), eversion and plantar flexion (S1). The S1 reflexes are lost (ankle jerks). A cauda equina syndrome from a central disc can progress rapidly over several hours or less, sometimes with little back pain and is a neurosurgical emergency.

Difficulties occur in distinguishing between a cauda equina lesion and a lesion of the conus medullaris, the lowermost part of the cord, such as an MS plaque in the conus. In both, weakness, sensory loss and loss of sphincter control occur. In an acute conus lesion lower limb tendon reflexes can be lost, as in a cauda equina lesion. Extensor plantar responses and patterns of sensory loss typical of a cord lesion, such as a sensory level in the abdomen or Brown-Séquard signs usually enable distinction clinically. Theoretically the two conditions may coexist; urgent MR imaging is likely to settle the matter and indicate any surgical emergency.

Myopathy

Muscle disease tends to produce symmetrical abnormalities. Details and difficulties in the diagnosis of muscle diseases are discussed in Chapter 10 (see Muscle diseases).

Inflammatory muscle disease, such as polymyositis, causes induration, pain and weakness. Dystrophies and most metabolic muscle diseases present typically with weakness alone; pseudohypertrophy (excessively bulky muscles) may be seen. Slow relaxation is a feature of myotonic conditions. Fatiguability is characteristic of myasthenia gravis, and the reverse, an increase in power on exercise is sometimes seen in LEMS.

Table 4.15 Principal limb movements, nerve root values, muscles and peripheral nerves.

Movement	Root	Muscle	Peripheral nerve
Shoulder abduction	C5, (C6)	Deltoid	Axillary
Elbow flexion (supinated)	(C5), C6	Biceps	Musculocutaneous
Elbow flexion (mid-prone)	C5, (C6)	Brachioradialis	Radial
Wrist extension	(C6), C7, (C8)	Triceps	Radial
Tip of thumb flexion (and index finger flexion)	C7, C8	Flexor pollicis and digitorum profundus I, II	Median
Tip of ring and Vth finger flexion	C8	Flexor digitorum profundus IV, V	Ulnar
Thumb abduction	T1	Abductor pollicis brevis	Median
Finger abduction	T1	Dorsal interossei	Ulnar
Finger flexion	(C7), C8, (T1)	Long and short flexors	Median and ulnar
Hip flexion	L1, L2, (L3)	Iliopsoas	Nerve to iliopsoas
Hip adduction	L2, L3, L4	Adductor magnus	Obturator
Knee extension	L3, L4	Quadriceps femoris	Femoral
Ankle dorsiflexion	L4, L5	Tibialis anterior	Deep peroneal
Big toe extension	L5, (S1)	Extensor hallucis longus	Deep peroneal
Ankle eversion	L5, S1	Peroneal muscles	Superficial peroneal
Ankle inversion	L4, L5	Tibialis posterior	Tibial
Ankle plantar flexion	S1, S2	Gastrocnemius, soleus	Posterior tibial
Knee flexion	S1, (S2)	Hamstrings	Sciatic
Hip extension	S1, (S2)	Gluteus maximus	Inferior gluteal

Subacute paralytic conditions

This loose term is used to describe increasing weakness over the course of days, up to an arbitrary period of 3 weeks. Spinal cord compression, poliomyelitis, Guillain–Barré syndrome, vasculitic neuropathies, myasthenia gravis, LEMS, botulism, periodic paralyses and MS are potential causes (Chapters 9, 10 and 11). These cases are often challenging diagnostically.

Respiratory impairment is of critical importance and easy to miss with severe limb weakness. Remarkably, even with widespread knowledge, initial paralytic symptoms are regarded as non-organic in about one-quarter of patients when they first seek help from a doctor.

Unexplained symptoms, abnormal illness behaviour and somatoform disorder

Symptoms that are unexplained or only partially explained by organic disease are features in 20–30% of new cases seen in any general neurology clinic. Many neurologists have been tempted to think that deliberate symptom exaggeration and even fabrication are more frequent than they are believed to be today. The fact is that many patients have real symptoms that are worrying, painful, unpleasant or uncomfortable but which do not reflect any serious underlying disease. For example, unexplained fatigue, give-way weakness or paralysis with non-organic sensory loss are symptoms for which no organic disease is likely to be found. In a more psychiatric context, abnormal illness behaviour is a diagnosis in common use; the phrase suggests that the patient complains about symptoms in a way believed to be disproportionate, but also reflects the attitude and reactions of medical staff, implying unnecessary admissions to hospital, investigations or treatment. For example, about one-third of cases of apparent status epilepticus seen in A&E and some 15% of cases of recurrent seizures referred to epilepsy specialist clinics are believed to be non-organic, but these conditions are treated initially, very largely as if they were seizures, often on the grounds of safety. These matters are discussed in Chapter 22 (see Non-organic disorders in neurology).

One suggestion as an approach to this issue is to accept that the majority of patients do have the symptoms of which they complain. This comment excludes those involved in legal claims, where non-organic features are especially prominent and of more doubtful nature. The second suggestion is to exclude organic disease with all reasonable certainty. Specialised tests may be necessary. The third requirement is to understand the psychiatric diagnoses that might lead to or explain such symptoms. These include:

- Anxiety and depression.
- Somatic symptom disorder, usually implying symptoms in more than one system, often lifelong, such as irritable bowel, chronic fatigue or unexplained pain, with the implication that psychological problems have been somatised.
- Hypochondriasis, meaning a state of fear, distress and anxiety about possible disease.
- Conversion and dissociative disorder: motor or sensory symptoms thought to relate to psychological factors.
- Somatic manifestations of depressive illness or anxiety.

Factitious disorder (symptoms to gain medical attention) and malingering (symptoms for material gain) are also possible, if rare explanations. However, in many cases of apparent illness behaviour, no formal psychiatric diagnosis is apparent.

The approach to anxiety and/or aggressive behaviour needs qualification. Anxiety is ubiquitous; we all experience it. Most symptoms do not reflect serious disease but fear of illness is common. This may all seem obvious, but there remains a tendency to equate anxiety with non-serious problems. The reality is that substantial anxiety occurs as frequently in sinister as in less serious medical conditions. A sympathetic understanding of symptoms of a non-organic nature is essential.

References

Clarke C. Neurological diseases. In *Clinical Medicine*, 6th edition. Kumar PJ, Clark M, eds. Elsevier, 2005.

Hopkins AP. *Clinical Neurology: A Modern Approach*. Oxford Medical Publications, 1993.

O'Brien MD (for the Guarantors of Brain). *Aids to the Examination of the Peripheral Nervous System*, 4th edn. Edinburgh/London: Saunders, 2000.

Patten J. *Neurological Differential Diagnosis*, 2nd edn. London/New York: Springer, 1996.

Further reading

General neurology, examination, classic works

Campbell WW, DeJong RN, Armin F, Haerer AF. *DeJong's The Neurologic Examination: Incorporating the Fundamentals of Neuroanatomy and Neurophysiology*. Philadelphia: Lippincott Williams and Wilkins, 2005.

Holmes G. *Introduction to Clinical Neurology*. Edinburgh: E. & S. Livingstone, 1946.

Nerve conduction and electromyography

Preston DC, Shapiro BE. *Electromyography and Neuromuscular Disorders*, 2nd edn. Philadelphia: Elsevier Butterworth-Heineman, 2005.

Electroencephalography

Goldensohn ES. *EEG Interpretation: Problems of Over-reading and Under-reading*, 2nd edn. Blackwell, 2002.

CSF examination

Royal College of Pathologists of Australia. *CSF Examination Manual* (updated, 2007). www.rcpamanual.edu.au (accessed 7 December 2015).

Neuropsychiatry

Trimble M. *Somatoform Disorders*. Cambridge: Cambridge University Press, 2004.

Neuropsychology screening tests

Warrington EK. *The Queen Square Screening Test for Cognitive Deficits* 2003. (Available from: Students' Office, UCL Institute of Neurology, Queen Square, London WC1N 3BG.)

Imaging

Adams RJ, McKie VC, Hsu, L, et al. Prevention of a first stroke by transfusions in children with sickle cell disease and abnormal results on transcranial Doppler ultrasonagraphy. *New Engl J Med* 1998; **339:** 5–11.

Alexander AL, J Lee, Lazar M, Field AS. Diffusion tensor imaging of the brain. *Neurotherapeutics* 2007; **4:** 316–329.

Bajaj N1, Hauser RA, Grachev ID. Clinical utility of dopamine transporter single photon emission CT (DaT-SPECT) with (^{123}I) ioflupane in diagnosis of parkinsonian syndromes. *J Neurol Neurosurg Psychiatry* 2013; **84:** 1288–1295.

Kaufmann TJ, Huston J, Mandrekar JN, Schleck CD, Thielen KR, Kallmes DF. Complications of diagnostic cerebral angiography: evaluation of 19,826 consecutive patients. *Radiology* 2007; **243:** 812–819.

Molyneux A, Kerr R, Stratton I, Sandercock P, Clarke M, Shrimpton J, *et al.* International Subarachnoid Aneurysm Trial (ISAT) of neurosurgical clipping versus endovascular coiling in 2143 patients with ruptured intracranial aneurysms: a randomised trial. *Lancet* 2002; **360:** 1267–1274.

Willinsky RA, Taylor SM, TerBrugge K, Farb RI, Tomlinson G, Montanera W. Neurologic complications of cerebral angiography: prospective analysis of 2,899 procedures and review of the literature. *Radiology* 2003; **227:** 522–528.

CHAPTER 5

Stroke and Cerebrovascular Diseases

Nicholas Losseff[1], Matthew Adams[1], Martin M. Brown[2], Joan Grieve[1] and Robert Simister[1]

[1] National Hospital for Neurology & Neurosurgery

[2] UCL Institute of Neurology

Epidemiology

Stroke is a major public health problem, being the third most common cause of death after myocardial infarction and cancer, and the leading cause of adult disability. Stroke accounts for 9% of deaths in England and Wales. The incidence of stroke has fallen over the last 10 years and prevalence increased, as a result of more effective primary prevention and treatment. Nevertheless, every year in the United Kingdom about 100 000 people will have their first stroke and about 40 000 patients will have a recurrent stroke. About 12% of patients die within 56 days of their stroke. Stroke is more common than most people realise. Approximately one-quarter of 45-year-old men will have a stroke before they reach the age of 85 (Table 5.1). Stroke is a very labour-intensive and expensive condition to manage, mainly because of the long length of stay in hospital. The mean length of stay in an acute hospital bed after stroke is about 16 days. Around half of all stroke survivors are left dependent on others for everyday activities: if a patient can return home, the burden on carers is significant. It is clear that new models of care are significantly reducing various aspects of this burden as time goes on and more stroke patients are treated expediently in hyperacute and multidisciplinary units.

About 5% of the UK National Health Service budget is spent on looking after stroke patients in England and Wales. The cost of looking after an individual patient with stroke is around £14 000 just for the acute phase. When longer term and informal care costs are included, this increases considerably. Stroke will become increasingly expensive in the future because the prevalence will increase as the population of elderly people in many parts of the world continues to rise.

Stroke is also an important condition in young people and can occur at any age, including *in utero* and in the neonatal period – it is a major cause of cerebral palsy, in childhood and young adult life. One-quarter of all strokes occur in people below the age of 65.

The incidence and types of stroke vary in different racial groups. Asian people appear to have a higher incidence of intracranial atherosclerosis than Caucasians and the incidence rates of first ever stroke are higher in black people of African or Caribbean descent than Caucasian populations living in the same cities. However, whether these differences reflect genetic or social and environmental factors is uncertain.

Clinical approach to stroke

Stroke can be briefly defined as an acute focal neurological deficit resulting from vascular disease. The World Health Organization provides a longer definition: 'rapidly developing clinical signs of focal (or global) disturbance of cerebral function, with symptoms lasting 24 hours or longer, or leading to death, with no apparent cause other than of vascular origin.' This definition has become outmoded as treatment and understanding have evolved. In 2013, the Stroke Council of the American Heart Association/American Stroke Associated recommended an updated definition that would better reflect current practice, and seeks to provide a single terminology for brain, retinal and spinal cord events. This updated definition of stroke includes ischaemic stroke as well as stroke secondary to intracerebral haemorrhage, cerebral venous sinus thrombosis and subarachnoid haemorrhage. The new definitions incorporate clinical and tissue criteria and try to address difficulties with current terminology. The guiding philosophy behind these changes is that the duration of the clinical event should be of secondary importance to the evidence from imaging (or pathology). In the new terminology central nervous system (CNS) infarction is defined as cerebral, spinal cord or retinal focal ischaemic injury. This is based on either pathological, imaging, or other objective evidence of focal ischaemic injury in a defined vascular distribution *or* on clinical evidence of ischaemic injury lasting greater than 24 hours or until death, with other aetiologies excluded. Whereas an ischaemic stroke is to be defined as "an episode of neurological dysfunction caused by focal brain, spinal or retinal infarction" (as above). Silent CNS infarction has imaging or neuropathological evidence of infarction without a history of acute neurological dysfunction attributable to the lesion. The term transient ischaemic attack (TIA) will remain and will apply to clinical events lasting less than 24 hours and without evidence of CNS infarction. Hence, the diagnosis of TIA will depend substantially on the imaging modality used to evaluate the clinical event, as around one-third of clinical TIA's show acute infarction on diffusion weighted imaging (DWI) despite the fact they last less than 1 hour and the proportion increases to over 50% in those whose TIA lasts more than 3 hours. These infarcts are often small and not seen on computed tomography (CT) scan, but are nevertheless associated with an increased risk of subsequent stroke. Thus, MRI with DWI sequences is the

Neurology: A Queen Square Textbook, Second Edition. Edited by Charles Clarke, Robin Howard, Martin Rossor and Simon Shorvon.

Table 5.1 Cumulative probability (%) of a 45-year-old person having a stroke before the age listed in the left-hand column.

Age	Men	Women
65	3	3
75	10	6
85	24	18
90	33	28

imaging of choice for suspected TIA or minor stroke. In keeping with the above, intracerebral haemorrhage is defined as a focal collection of blood within the brain parenchyma or ventricular system that is not caused by trauma, and stroke caused by intracerebral haemorrhage as "rapidly developing clinical signs of neurological dysfunction attributable to a focal collection of blood within the brain parenchyma or ventricular system that is not caused by trauma". Silent intracerebral haemorrhage is defined as "a focal collection of blood products without history of acute neurological dysfunction".

The use of the term "stroke" should be restricted to a description of the clinical event experienced by the patient. Appearances on brain imaging should not be described as showing a stroke – but concordant with the above – the scan may show infarction or haemorrhage, which may either have been responsible for a stroke or may have been asymptomatic. Also, to say someone has had a stroke is not sufficient as a medical diagnosis. Accurate diagnosis requires the cerebral circulatory disturbance to be defined in terms of pathology (ischaemia, infarction or haemorrhage), its anatomical location within the brain (e.g. left middle cerebral artery territory), and the underlying mechanism (e.g. cardio-embolism). One task of the stroke physician is to make an accurate pathophysiological diagnosis in these terms to guide appropriate management. This requires a basic knowledge of the clinical and radiological patterns that different stroke syndromes produce and the underlying pathophysiology of stroke.

Those patients with acute neurological disturbances that may be the result of stroke require immediate assessment in hospital for consideration of reperfusion therapy (e.g. thrombolysis). Equally, patients with a recent history of TIA require urgent investigation and treatment to prevent a recurrence. The fact that a patient with a TIA appears to recover fully gives a false sense of security that there is no urgency for assessment. However, in a UK population-based study in Oxfordshire, the average risks of recurrent stroke at 7 days, 1 month and 3 months after TIA were 8%, 12% and 17%, respectively. In patients with specific risk factors for recurrence, the 7-day risk may be as high as 31%. The need to emphasise these aspects of acute stroke and TIA has led to the use of the term 'brain attack' to emphasise to the public the urgency of the situation. It also has the value of emphasising that acute focal neurological events have a differential diagnosis, in that stroke mimics will need to be distinguishable from stroke and TIA. The older term, cerebrovascular accident (CVA) should be avoided completely. Stroke is not accidental; the term CVA implies a negative approach to the patient and their illness.

The underlying pathology responsible for the persistent symptoms of stroke is either infarction or haemorrhage. Haemorrhage is subdivided according to location into intracerebral haemorrhage

Table 5.2 Underlying pathology of stroke.

Pathology	Anatomical subdivision
Infarction	Small vessel (lacunar) infarction
	Total or partial territorial infarction
	Border-zone infarction
Intracranial haemorrhage	Lobar
	Deep/basal ganglia
	Posterior fossa
Subarachnoid haemorrhage	Aneurysm, AVM
Cerebral venous thrombosis	Vein, venous sinus

AVM, arteriovenous malformation.

and subarachnoid haemorrhage (Table 5.2). In about 85% of cases, stroke is secondary to infarction. When infarction involves only a small volume of the tissue in the subcortical white matter (<1.5 cm in diameter on brain imaging) secondary to occlusion of a penetrating artery, the resulting death of tissue is known as a lacune or a lacunar infarct. The underlying pathology responsible for lacunar infarction is often referred to as small vessel disease. This may also lead to asymptomatic changes on imaging of the deep white matter known as leukoaraiosis, discussed in more detail later. Lacunes are generally found in subcortical white matter or the basal ganglia (Figure 5.1). Larger infarcts usually involve a wedge of both cortical and subcortical white matter and result from occlusion of the trunk or branches of the major cerebral arteries, most commonly the middle cerebral artery (MCA). The size of infarction resulting from arterial occlusion will depend on the adequacy of the collateral supply via the circle of Willis and pial collateral vessels. Infarction may therefore affect all or only part of the territory of the occluded artery. Occasionally, infarction occupies the border-zones between arterial supplies, particularly if the infarction follows an episode of generalised reduction in cerebral blood flow (e.g. after cardiac arrest) or results from occlusion or near-occlusion of the ipsilateral internal carotid artery. It is then known as border-zone or watershed infarction.

About 10% of acute strokes are caused by intracerebral haemorrhage (i.e. within the substance of the brain). When the bleeding occurs from deep penetrating arteries, often secondary to small vessel disease, the centre of the haemorrhage is usually located within the basal ganglia, particularly the lentiform nucleus or the deep white matter tracts. More superficial haemorrhages are known as lobar haemorrhages and are more commonly caused by vascular malformations or cerebral amyloid angiopathy. In about 5% of cases, intracranial bleeding occurs primarily within the subarachnoid space. Subarachnoid haemorrhage is distinctive in that there may be no focal damage to the brain if the patient only has meningeal irritation (e.g. headache and/or neck stiffness). Subarachnoid haemorrhage is therefore not always classified as a form of stroke. However, the arguments are stronger in favour of including subarachnoid haemorrhage within the definition of stroke, because subarachnoid haemorrhage may be accompanied by intracerebral

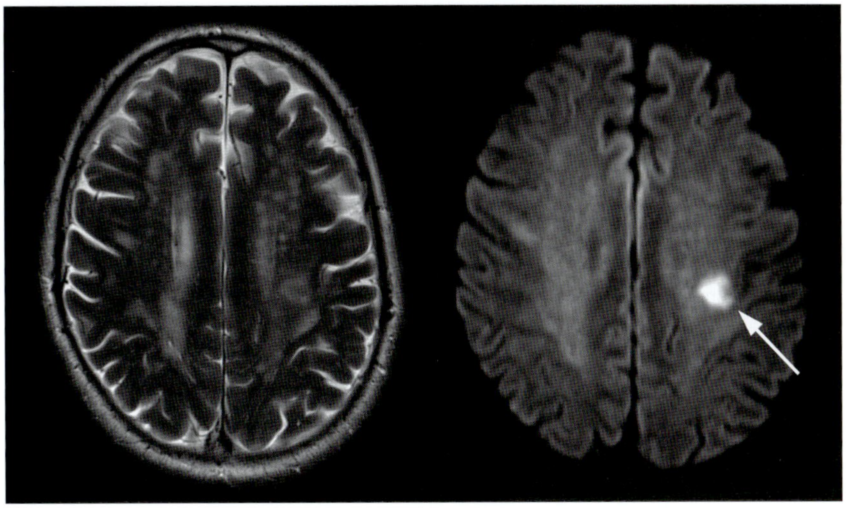

Figure 5.1 Subcortical infarct. Extensive background small vessel disease is seen on T2-weighted imaging (a) but diffusion weighted imaging (DWI) (b) reveals the acute subcortical infarct (arrow).

haemorrhage with focal deficits. Also, subarachnoid bleeding frequently causes constriction of the intracranial arteries, known as vasospasm, which can result in cerebral infarction with focal symptoms identical to those seen in other causes of ischaemic stroke.

The well-known vascular risk factors (e.g. hypertension, diabetes and smoking) are not in themselves causes of stroke, but instead promote the development of the underlying pathological processes (e.g. atherosclerosis) responsible for stroke. Their importance is therefore to provide targets for interventions to prevent stroke, rather than in diagnosis.

The majority of strokes result from arterial pathology but a small proportion, less than 1%, result from cerebral venous thrombosis. Although rare, this is an important cause to recognise because of the need for specific investigations and treatment. Cerebral venous thrombosis may cause isolated cerebral infarction, haemorrhagic infarction, intracerebral haemorrhage or subarachnoid haemorrhage. Patients with venous thrombosis can also present with raised intracranial pressure and epileptic seizures without focal cerebral features.

It is usually impossible to distinguish reliably between infarction and intracranial haemorrhage from the history and examination. Headache can occur in both, although the features of very sudden onset of severe headache and neck stiffness in subarachnoid haemorrhage are usually distinct. Cranial imaging is the only reliable method to distinguish between infarction and haemorrhage. Imaging also plays a major part in confirming the anatomical location of the pathology. The location may also provide clues to likely mechanisms. Other investigations are required to establish the underlying mechanism of the infarction or haemorrhage in order to plan appropriate treatment and prevention.

Medical assessment of the stroke patient on admission should concentrate on establishing the diagnosis in terms of pathology, anatomy and mechanism. It is important that initial assessment and the response to treatment and therapy should include an assessment of the patient's functional abilities, as well as their neurological examination. Validated scoring systems have been developed specifically for use in stroke patients. The most widely used scores for neurological impairment, based on the standardised neurological examination, are the Scandinavian Stroke Scale and the National Institutes of Health Stroke Scale (NIHSS). The most widely used functional outcome scores are the Barthel Index and the Modified Rankin Scale. A number of schemes have also been developed to assist in classifying subtypes of stroke. These include the Oxfordshire Community Stroke Project Classification, which divides stroke on clinical features alone into total anterior cerebral infarction (TACI, usually total MCA territory infarction), partial anterior territory infarcts (PACI), lacunar infarcts (LACI) and posterior cerebral infarction (POCI). However, this classification is not particularly accurate in the first few hours after onset and only predicts the size of infarction on imaging in about three-quarters of patients. A more specific approach, originally developed for use in a clinical trial, is known as the TOAST Classification. This divides ischaemic stroke on the basis of detailed investigations, into athero-thrombotic, cardio-embolic, small vessel occlusion, other determined cause and undetermined cause. Other more detailed classification systems have been proposed, but are not widely used.

Ischaemic stroke

Important vascular anatomy

Heart and great vessels

The left ventricle gives rise to the ascending aorta and then to its arch. Arising from the arch from right to left are the innominate, the left common carotid and the left subclavian arteries. The innominate bifurcates into the right subclavian, which gives off the vertebral and the right common carotid artery. The left subclavian gives rise to the left vertebral (Figure 5.2). Multiple anatomical variations of this common arrangement have been described. The most common anomalies are a common origin of the left common carotid and the brachiocephalic truck or origin of the left common carotid from the left brachiocephalic trunk. Very rare anatomical arrangements can allow the left and right common carotid arteries to arise from a common trunk and this may very occasionally explain an unusual pattern of brain infarction.

It therefore makes sense that embolic material arising from the heart or ascending aorta can enter any vessel or combination of

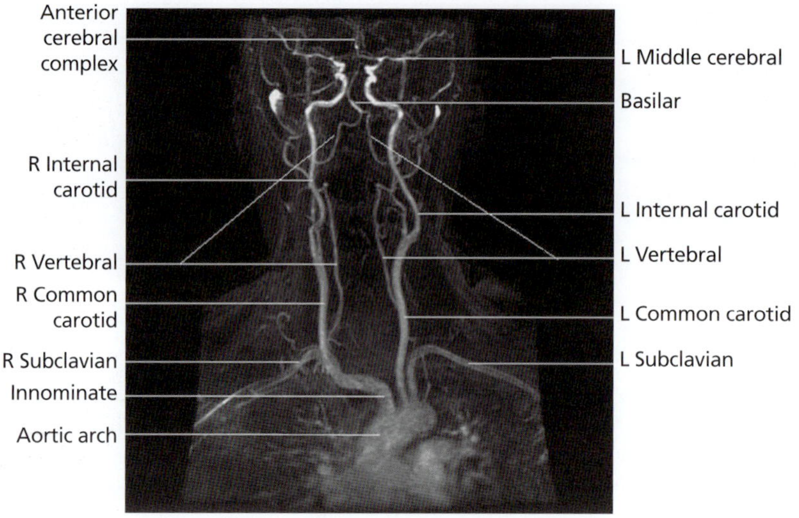

Figure 5.2 Contrast enhanced magnetic resonance angiogram (MRA) of the heart, great vessels, cervical and intracerebral circulation. L, left; R, right.

vessels. An innominate plaque of atherosclerosis may cause embolism within the right carotid and right vertebral territory or even very occasionally within the left carotid territory.

Extracranial and intracranial arteries

The internal carotid arteries (ICAs) begin in the neck at the carotid bifurcation, usually near the angle of the jaw, and ascend cranially. Note that it is the common carotid pulse that is palpated in the neck. The ICAs travel behind the pharynx but give off no branches in the neck. This makes them readily identifiable on angiography and distinct from the external carotid arteries which do branch. The ICAs enter the skull through the carotid canal in the petrous bone and then pass through the cavernous sinus. The cavernous carotid pierces the dura and then gives off the ophthalmic artery. The supraclinoid portion of the carotid gives off the anterior choroidal and posterior communicating artery before bifurcation into anterior and middle cerebral arteries. The external carotids give branches to the neck, face and scalp. Some of these are easily palpated (e.g. the superficial temporal artery). The external carotids can act as a collateral blood supply to the hemisphere via meningeal branches, especially in the event of ICA occlusion. Often, the only clinical symptom of this is a throbbing unilateral temporal headache caused by diversion through superficial channels. Biopsy this at your peril.

The anterior choroidal arteries are small and course posteriorly along the optic tract. They give off branches to a zone between the other internal carotid branches (anterior and middle cerebral artery) and the posterior circulation. They supply perforating branches to the globus pallidus, posterior limb of the internal capsule, temporal lobe, thalamus and lateral geniculate body.

The anterior cerebral arteries (ACAs) course medially then run posterior over the corpus callosum. They supply the anterior and medial portions of the hemispheres, basal frontal lobes and caudate. Within the cortical territory of the ACA is the leg area of the motor homunculus. The two ACAs are usually joined together by an anterior communicating artery (ACOM) and there are various anatomic variations that dictate the pattern of ischaemic damage. In carotid occlusion the ACA territory is often spared because of collateral supply from the ACOM. If there is no ACOM then this mechanisms fails. Sometimes, both anterior cerebral arteries are supplied by a single carotid, so carotid occlusion may infarct both ACA territories or neither.

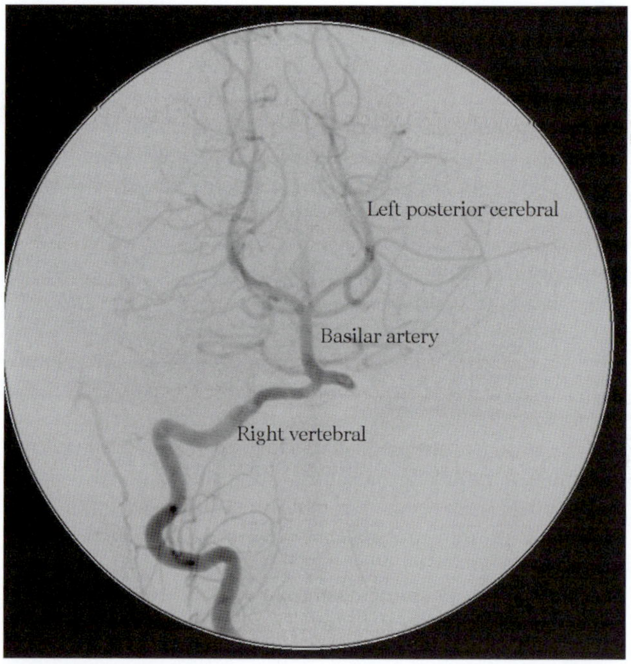

Figure 5.3 Vertebrobasilar circulation (catheter angiogram).

The MCAs course laterally after their origin; the proximal MCA trunk gives off numerous penetrating lenticulo-striate arteries to the basal ganglia and internal capsule. Near the Sylvian fissure the MCA usually trifurcates into small anterior temporal branches and large superior and inferior trunks. The superior trunk supplies the lateral portion of the hemisphere above and the inferior trunk the portion below the Sylvian fissure. Amongst its cortical supply the MCA supplies the arm area of the homunculus.

The vertebral arteries arise from each subclavian and are unusual in that they anastomose to form a larger artery, the basilar artery (Figure 5.3). The vertebral arteries course upwards and backwards entering the transverse foramina at C5 or C6. They run up through the intravertebral foramina exiting to pierce the dura and enter the foramen magnum. Their intracranial portions anastomose at the ponto-medullary junction to form the basilar artery. In the neck the vertebral arteries give off many spinal and muscular branches. The intracranial vertebral gives rise to the posterior and anterior spinal arteries, penetrating branches to the medulla and the posterior inferior cerebellar arteries. The basilar artery then runs up in the midline giving off the bilateral anterior and inferior, superior cerebellar arteries and also penetrating branches to the brainstem. At the ponto-mesencephalic junction the basilar terminates into posterior cerebral arteries (PCAs). The PCAs give off perforating branches to the midbrain and thalamus, course around the cerebral peduncles and then supply occipital and inferior temporal lobes. The anatomy of the vertebral circulation is more varied than that of the carotid. Commonly, one vertebral is hypoplastic or may terminate in the posterior inferior cerebellar artery (PICA).

The ACAs, MCAs and PCAs are connected via communicating vessels and all these vessels together form the circle (or pentangle) of Willis. In most cases, the posterior and anterior communicating vessels on both sides form a complete circle but, in some individuals, the circle is interrupted by absence of one or more of the communicating arteries. The most common abnormality in 5–10% of people is the fetal PCA pattern in which the P1 segment linking the basilar with the PCA is missing on one side. In these cases, the ipsilateral PCA territory is entirely supplied by the internal carotid artery. This fact is important to remember when investigating patients with PCA infarcts.

Venous anatomy

The cerebral veins may be divided into the venous dural sinuses and the superficial and deep venous systems. The dural sinus walls are formed by the layers of the dura itself and are situated at the junction of the falx and tentorium. The intracranial veins drain into the sinuses which then drain into the jugular veins. The ophthalmic and facial veins drain into the cavernous sinuses which lie symmetrically in the parasellar region. The important venous sinuses are the midline sagittal and straight sinus and the transverse sinuses (Figure 5.4).

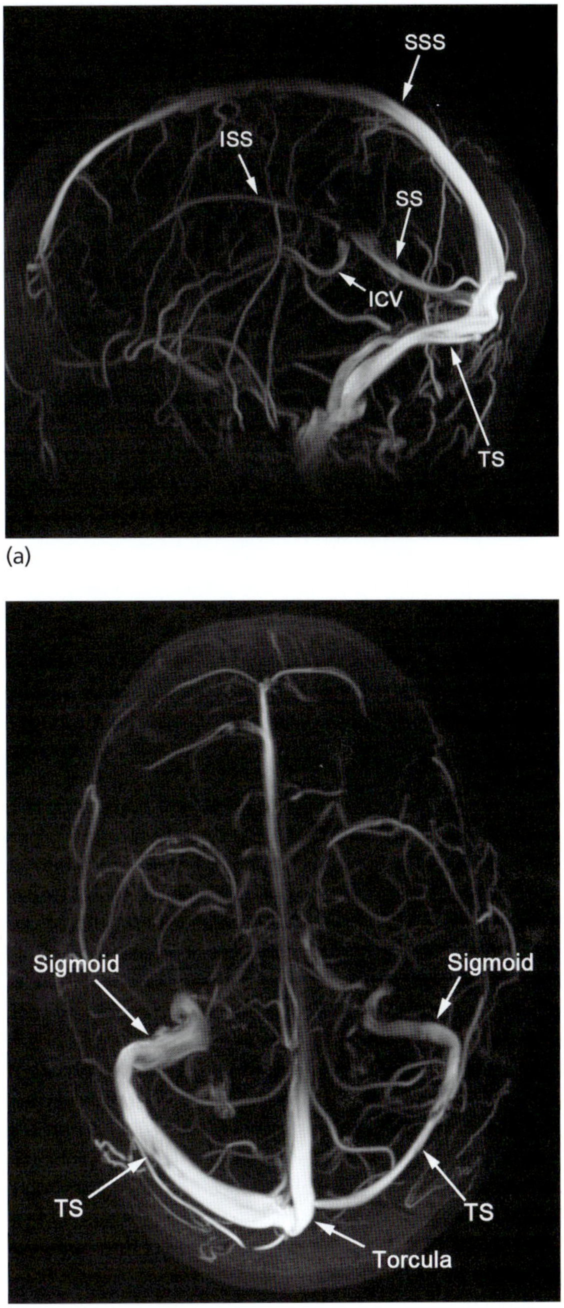

ICV internal cerebral vein
ISS inferior sagittal sinus
Sigmoid sigmoid sinus
SS straight sinus
SSS superior sagittal sinus
Torcula torcula herophili
TS transverse sinus.

Figure 5.4 Sagittal (a) and axial (b) images from a MR venogram illustrating intracranial venous anatomy.

Pathophysiology of ischaemic stroke

Thrombosis, embolism and hypoperfusion

There are three potential mechanisms of ischaemic stroke:

1 Thrombosis
2 Embolism, and
3 Hypoperfusion (haemodynamic failure).

While these are inter-related, each mechanism can produce distinct clinical syndromes. It is important to think about these mechanisms when assessing patients as ultimately this guides treatment.

The effect of a localised blood vessel occlusion on blood flow in the area supplied by the vessel will depend on the following factors: the extent of the occlusion, the time that the occlusion lasts, and the adequacy of collateral circulation. The resulting focal symptoms will depend on the area of the brain in which blood flow is reduced below the level sufficient to impair neuronal activity. Consider how these factors interact: one patient has a 95% internal carotid stenosis on which a thrombus forms and occludes the vessel. There may be no symptoms if this thrombosis remains localised (i.e. does not embolise to the brain) and the collateral circulation to the hemisphere above the occluded carotid is adequate. Conversely, even if the thrombosis remains localised, the absence of an effective collateral circulation may result in infarction of the whole of the carotid territory. If the collateral circulation is poor, then the most vulnerable areas will infarct; these are the areas with the poorest perfusion pressure and furthest away from the occluded artery. An example is shown in Figure 5.5 as a linear areas of infarction in the border-zone between the anterior and middle cerebral artery territory. The occluded carotid artery is very unlikely to recanalise as the obstruction is principally hardened atheroma.

Another scenario is this: on the roughened surface of the 95% stenosis, platelets activate to form a white thrombus which embolises to the brain. The thrombus may lodge in the origin of the anterior cerebral artery and have no effect because the territory has an adequate collateral circulation via the anterior communicator.

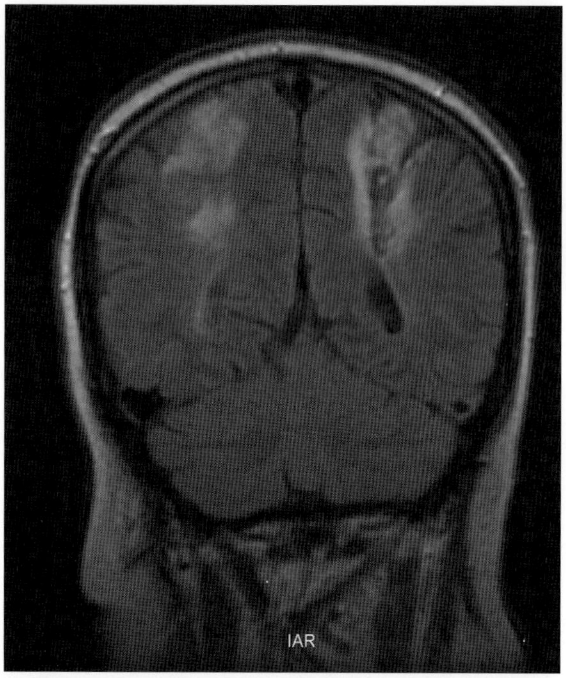

Figure 5.5 Coronal MR FLAIR image of bilateral border-zone infarction following carotid occlusion

Maybe it lodges at the origin of the MCA for an hour before it lyses. The meningeal collaterals over the surface of the hemisphere maintain some cortical areas for the time but the lenticulostriate perforators arising from the MCA origin are all blocked and the deep territory fails rapidly as there is no collateral blood supply. The deep territory has irreversibly infarcted but the superficial collateralised territory is hanging on. Unfortunately, the patient develops a pneumonia and becomes hypotensive: the tenuous collaterals can no longer perfuse the hemisphere. The entire hemisphere infarcts.

Stenosis and occlusion are distinct. Occlusion of a vessel may occur without pre-existent stenosis or other localised disease. This is usually a result of embolism from the heart or a more proximal arterial stenosis. For example, atrial fibrillation and atherosclerotic stenosis of the internal carotid artery are both risk factors for intracranial occlusion upstream (e.g. MCA occlusion).

Thrombosis is difficult distinguish from embolism, but hypoperfusion may be more easily recognisable. However, it is important to think about the macroscopic mechanisms of ischaemia. It is unlikely that an occluded atheromatous carotid will recanalise with thrombolysis, but if the patient has border-zone ischaemia, then keeping up their blood pressure may help. Conversely, thrombolysis of fresh red cardio-embolic thrombus obstructing the proximal MCA is a practical proposition.

Patterns of stroke are discussed in detail later. The adequacy of collateral circulation depends not only on systemic perfusion pressures, but many factors including the anatomy of the circle of Willis and other collateral pathways and the degree of acquired small and large blood vessel disease, particularly the effects of atherosclerosis, diabetes and hypertension.

Microscopic and metabolic changes

The brain is metabolically a highly active organ. Although it accounts for only 2% of body weight, it uses 20% of cardiac output when the body is at rest. Brain energy use is also dependent on the degree of neuronal activation. The brain uses glucose exclusively as a substrate for energy metabolism by oxidising this to carbon dioxide and water. This metabolism allows conversion of adenosine diphosphate to adenosine triphosphate (ATP). A constant supply of ATP is essential for neuronal integrity and this process is much more efficient in the presence of oxygen. Although ATP can be formed by anaerobic glycolysis, the energy yielded by this pathway is small and it also leads to the accumulation of lactic acid. The brain needs and uses approximately 500 mL oxygen and 100 mg glucose each minute, hence the need for a rich supply of oxygenated blood containing glucose. Cerebral blood flow (CBF) is normally approximately 50 mL/minute for each 100 g of brain. By increasing oxygen extraction from the blood adequate compensation can be made even if blood flow is reduced to approximately 20–25 mL per 100 g/minute. Sophisticated systems exist that allow the cerebral circulation to maintain constant levels of CBF in the face of changing systemic blood pressure, usually called autoregulation. In the healthy state, CBF remains relatively constant when mean arterial blood pressure is 50–150 mmHg.

As cerebral blood flow falls, metabolic paralysis ensues and this may be reversible. However, if prolonged, infarction is inevitable. When CBF falls below 20 mL/100 g/minute, oxygen extraction starts to fall and changes may be detected on electroencephalography (EEG). At levels below 10 mL/100 g/minute, cell membrane functions are severely disrupted. Below 5 mL/100 g/minute, cell death is inevitable within a short time.

When neurones become ischaemic, a cascade of biochemical changes potentiate cell death. These pathophysiological changes have been of considerable interest to those developing treatments to lessen the damage caused by ischaemic stroke. In the ischaemic brain, ion channels fail, potassuim ions move out of the cell into the extracellular space and Ca^{2+} moves in, where it further compromises the ability of the cell to maintain ionic homeostasis and leads to mitochondrial failure. Hypoxia leads to the generation of free radicals which peroxidise fatty acids in cell membranes causing further cell dysfunction. Anaerobic glycolysis results in lactic acidosis further impairing cellular metabolic functions. Excitatory neurotransmitter activity (e.g. glutamate) is greatly increased in areas of brain ischaemia because of increased release and failure of uptake mechanisms. These neurotransmitters are themselves toxic at these increased levels by causing further calcium and sodium ions influx into cells through their actions on NMDA receptors. Hence, ischaemia triggers a vicious cascade of events leading to cell electrical failure and then death. At some point the process becomes irreversible even after reperfusion of tissues. Even if the severity of ischaemia is inadequate to cause necrosis, it may trigger apoptosis.

Ischaemic penumbra

The degree of ischaemia caused by blockage of an artery varies, partly depending on collateral supply. At the centre of an infarct the damage is most severe but at the periphery collateral flow may allow continued delivery of blood, although at a lower rate. This zone may become dysfunctional secondary to electrical failure although not dead and is referred to as the ischaemic penumbra. In any solar or lunar eclipse there is an umbra (the dense shadow) and the penumbra surrounding it. It is this outer zone that is further at risk following the onset of stroke. Sophisticated imaging can now define areas of irreversible brain damage and areas in which perfusion is suboptimal but where irreversible infarction has not taken place. The penumbra is the area of brain with the potential to survive. It is entirely likely that high-quality simple supportive management in the acute stage aimed at maintaining normal physiological parameters decreases the degree of this further secondary brain damage.

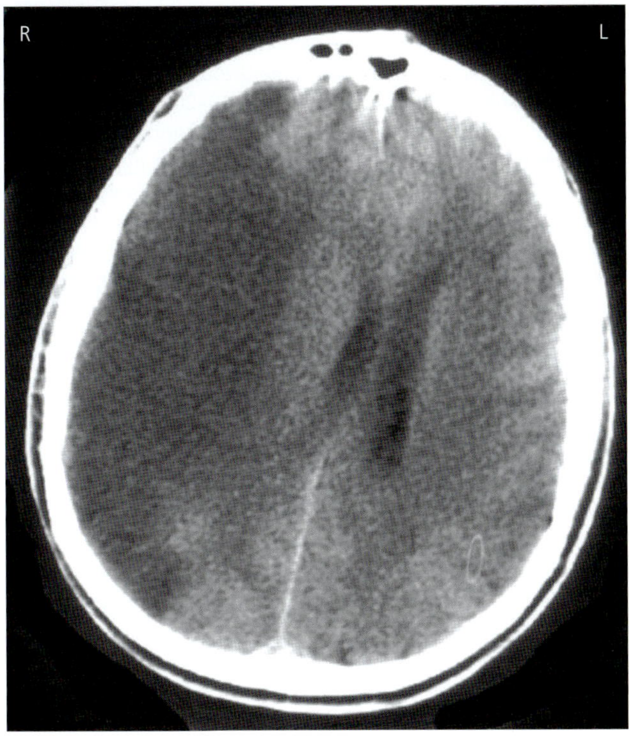

Figure 5.6 Unenhanced computed tomography (CT): Cytotoxic oedema in middle cerebral artery (MCA) distribution leading to brain swelling.

Pressure changes

Energy failure results in cytotoxic oedema where water accumulates inside cells. This is the radiological hallmark of early cerebral infarction and its distribution obeys vascular territories, unlike vasogenic oedema (extracellular accumulation) which spreads along white matter tracts. Significant brain swelling follows cytotoxic oedema increasing intracranial pressure and further decreasing CBF compromising the penumbra and surrounding brain (Figure 5.6). Large MCA infarction associated with significant mass effect is known as malignant MCA infarction because ultimately coning may occur with brainstem compression or there may be important local pressure effects (e.g. posterior cerebral artery occlusion from stretching of the artery across the tentorium). Similarly, oedema of cerebellar infarction may lead to brainstem compression.

Risk factors and causes of ischaemic stroke

Ischaemic stroke is the result of vessel occlusion from *in situ* thrombosis, embolism or haemodynamic failure. Embolism may be from artery to artery (30–40%) or from the heart (30–40%). In 25% of cases, disease of the walls of small penetrating intracranial blood vessels is responsible for lacunar infarction.

It should be recognised that risk factors are not direct causes of stroke, but instead are for the most part demographic factors, pre-existing diseases or lifestyles of individuals that promote diseases of the heart or blood vessels. Hence, the main risk factors for stroke are the risk factors for atherosclerosis and heart disease (Table 5.3). Non-atherosclerotic vasculopathies and primary haematological disease are much less common.

Both the clinical syndromes and risk factors of lacunar stroke and large vessel occlusion overlap. The effect of more than one risk factor on an individual's risk of stroke is multiplicative, not additive. Stroke is therefore often associated with a combination of risk factors coming together rather than a single entity. It should be borne in mind that the presence of a risk factor does not imply causation. For example, stroke can only be attributed to the effects of smoking in about half the smokers with stroke, while a hypertensive patient presenting with symptoms suggestive of stroke may in fact have another neurological condition mimicking stroke.

Table 5.3 Major risk factors for stroke.

Age
Hypertension
Smoking
Diabetes mellitus
Atrial fibrillation
Heart disease
Dyslipidaemia
Alcohol
Obesity
Symptomatic and asymptomatic carotid stenosis
Drug misuse

Age, hypertension, smoking, lipids and drug misuse

The incidence of stroke rises dramatically with age, doubling each decade past 55 years. Half of all stroke occurs in the over-70 age group. At least 25% of the adult population have hypertension >140/90 mmHg. After age, this is the most important and modifiable risk factor. The Framingham data show a linear relationship between risk of stroke and arterial hypertension and this effect is seen across all levels of blood pressure.

Smoking remains a leading preventable cause of death and an independent risk factor for stroke, especially in young adults where smoking increases the risk of stroke by four times the risk in non-smokers. In older patients, it particularly predisposes to carotid stenosis. Diabetes mellitus increases the risk of stroke by about two- to fourfold when compared with those without diabetes. The excess diabetic risk is independent of age and blood pressure status. High total cholesterol and low-density lipoprotein (LDL) correlate with atherosclerosis. Although low levels of high-density lipoprotein (HDL) correlate well with coronary artery disease, the relationship is less clear for cerebrovascular disease where elevated LDL concentrations have been shown to be more strongly linked with disease progression. Alcohol consumption demonstrates a J-shaped relationship; heavy drinking being associated with a higher risk of all stroke, both ischaemic and haemorrhagic. The presence of asymptomatic carotid disease carries a greater cardiovascular than cerebrovascular risk. Asymptomatic stenosis of greater than 75% carries an annual stroke risk of only 2% or less. In contrast, if the stenosis is recently symptomatic, the annual risk increases to 15% and is even higher if the stenosis is greater or the symptoms very recent. This is discussed in greater detail in the section on secondary prevention. Plaque structure rather than the degree of narrowing is important, with ulcerated heterogeneous plaques being more likely to rupture or allow thrombosis on their surface. Drug-related stroke is an increasing problem and may be multi-factorial. The mechanisms of stroke after drug misuse are very broad (Table 5.4).

Table 5.4 Mechanisms of stroke associated with drug misuse.

Complications of parenteral administration (e.g. heroin, cocaine)
Infective or non-bacterial (marantic) endocarditis – infarction or haemorrhage from associated mycotic aneurysm
Direct embolisation of particulate matter – infarction via right to left shunt (e.g. patent foramen ovale or pulmonary shunt) or from direct carotid administration
Acute severe hypertension (TIA, infarction or haemorrhage)
Arterial vasospasm (infarction or TIA), e.g. crack cocaine, cocaine, amphetamine, possibly cannabis
Arterial dissection
Hypersensitivity vasculitis: associated with amphetamine, heroin, cocaine and crack cocaine (headache encephalopathy, stroke-like episodes, seizures) – all rarely proven

TIA, transient ischaemic attack.

Table 5.5 Cardiac causes of stroke.

High risk	Atrial fibrillation (especially combined with other risk factors)
	Valvular heart disease
	Prosthetic heart valves
	Bacterial endocarditis
	Non-infective (marantic) endocarditis (Chapter 21)
	Cardiac surgery
Low risk	Myocardial infarction
	Ventricular/atrial aneurysm
	Cardiomyopathy (e.g. amyloid, alcohol, cocaine)
	Septal abnormalities (e.g. ASD, patent foramen ovale, atrial septal aneurysm)
Rare	Intracardiac lesions (myxoma, fibroelastoma)

ASD, atrial septal defect.

Another effect of drugs of abuse is rupture of a coincidental underlying aneurysm or arteriovenous malformation. This is a common cause of intracranial cerebral haemorrhage (ICH; either subarachnoid or parenchymal) in users of stimulant drugs (e.g. amphetamine, crack and cocaine). All patients with drug-related subarachnoid haemorrhage (SAH) or ICH need careful evaluation to exclude such causes based on the pattern of haemorrhage. In some patients, induction of antiphospholipid antibodies has been associated with cocaine and heroin. Whether they confer a specific risk is not clear and it must be noted that antiphospholipid antibodies are also associated with infection and vasculopathies of many causes.

Cardiac disease

Heart disease may be divided into high or low risk (Table 5.5). Atrial fibrillation remains the most important cause of cardio-embolism. Atrial fibrillation is a common cardiac disorder, with up to 5% of over-60-year-olds affected. Atrial fibrillation is an important risk factor for stroke, with a general risk of about 4% per year in patients who have not had prior embolic symptoms and about 12% per year in patients with prior TIA or stroke. Other coexistent risk factors (e.g. age, hypertension or left ventricular dysfunction) also increase the risk. Sick sinus syndrome through atrial dysfunction may also result in embolism. As many as 10–20% of patients with valvular heart disease have a stroke as the abnormal valve surface promotes thrombosis and embolisation. The most important used to be rheumatic mitral stenosis but this is now overtaken by endocarditis on native or prosthetic valves. The manifestations of endocarditis are protean and include ischaemia, ICH and SAH, encephalopathy and meningitis. Endocarditis is much more common on prosthetic valves and often resistant to treatment. Non-infective endocarditis was first described by Libman and Sacks; the condition spans simple valve thickening to frank vegetations containing platelets and fibrin. Systemic lupus erythematosus (SLE), antiphospholipid syndrome and malignancy are potential causes.

After myocardial infarction (MI), there is a systemic embolism rate of about 3%. Most emboli will affect the brain. Most thrombi arise in the ventricle after anterior MI. Left ventricular thrombi can be detected in approximately 30% of patients after anterior MI. The thrombi develop within 3 days and embolism occurs on average 2 weeks after MI. Stroke is therefore rarely the presenting feature of MI, but this can occur in patients who have had an asymptomatic (silent) MI. The risk of stroke associated with impaired cardiac function and heart failure is substantial.

Paradoxical embolus resulting from venous thrombosis entering the arterial circulation is an increasingly recognised and potentially important cause of stroke. However, in patients with a potential route for paradoxical embolism and stroke (e.g. patent foramen ovale), it is often not clear if emboli have been formed *de novo* in the heart or arose in the venous circulation (e.g. from deep vein thrombosis) to cause paradoxical embolism, whether the stroke is related to arrhythmia, or whether the stroke is unrelated to the cardiac abnormality. However, a classic triad is recognised that suggests true paradoxical embolism:

1. Deep vein thrombosis has been demonstrated prior to the stroke or there is a good reason for a venous thrombus (e.g. thrombophilia)
2. The stroke happens at a time when shunting and paradoxical embolus are possible (e.g. during a Valsalva), and
3. The stroke syndrome is typically cardio-embolic (e.g. posterior cerebral artery occlusion or small cortical infarct).

The most common potential intracardiac shunt is patent foramen ovale (PFO). However, this is present in about 25% of the population, making its presence difficult to put into context. In young apparently idiopathic stroke, the incidence of PFO approaches 50%. Recent studies suggest PFO alone after stroke carries a small 2% risk per year of further stroke. However, this seems to be increased to 15% by the concomitance of an atrial septal aneurysm (ASA), suggesting that this is an important co-factor. Isolated ASA without PFO is a very rare occurrence and hence no reliable prognostic information pertains to this group.

Stroke and the blood

Many haematological conditions can lead to stroke (Table 5.6), especially when other risk factors are present.

Sickle cell disease may produce stroke in childhood by intracranial stenosis and occlusion of the terminal carotid and proximal MCA. A channel of friable collaterals may form at the skull base (secondary Moyamoya syndrome, see later). In adults with sickle cell disease, ischaemic stroke is more frequently caused by small vessel disease or occlusion and often several other risk factors are

Table 5.6 Haematological causes of stroke.

Important	Sickle cell disease
	Polycythaemia of any cause
	Thrombocythaemia
	Antiphospholipid antibody syndrome
Rare	Thrombotic thrombocytopenic purpura
	Paroxysmal nocturnal haemoglobinuria
	Leukaemia and myeloma
Uncertain (except by cerebral venous thrombosis or paradoxical embolus)	Activated protein C resistance ± factor V Leiden mutation
	Protein C
	Protein S
	Antithrombin III deficiencies
	Prothrombin G20210 mutation
	Other thrombophilias
Other causes of hypercoagulability	Malignancy (especially stomach cancer)
	Vasculitis
	Homocystinuria
	Drugs (e.g. contraceptive pill, intravenous immunoglobulin)
	Nephrotic syndrome
	Disseminated intravascular coagulation

present. There are many neurological phenomena associated with sickling and stroke is only one of them. Migrainous symptoms are common in patients with sickle cell disease.

Of the hypercoagulable states, thrombophilia is commonly tested for in younger patients but rarely proven as a cause of arterial stroke. Cerebral venous thrombosis is a far more likely mechanism of stroke associated with thrombophilia, but the latter may be relevant if there has been paradoxical arterial embolism. The most common detectable abnormality in the population is activated protein C (APC) resistance; the others are very rare. Resistance to APC is one of the most commonly identified venous thrombo-embolic risk factors but there is no clear relationship to arterial stroke. APC resistance is inherited in a dominant fashion and in most patients associated with a single point mutation in the factor V gene (factor V Leiden). Patients may be homozygous or heterozygous. It is much more important to request a full blood count looking for polycythaemia and thrombocythaemia than a thrombophilia screen. Beware marginally high RBC and platelet counts which may be easy to dismiss but are common in JAK 2 positive myeloproliferation.

Antiphospholipid antibodies and syndrome

One distinct haematological condition is the antiphospholipid antibody syndrome (APAS) in which arterial stroke is well documented. This is not the same as having antiphospholipid antibodies which may occur in association with other vasculopathies including atherosclerosis. In most cases, the finding of antiphospholipid antibodies in a patient with stroke is unrelated to the stroke, and follow-up studies show antiphospholipid antibodies are not associated with an increased risk of recurrent stroke. However, in a small proportion of patients antiphospholipid antibodies appear to have a pathogenic role in arterial and venous thrombosis. Ischaemic stroke is the most common arterial thrombotic event with APAS. Other neurological manifestations include neuropsychiatric features, movement disorders and migrainous headaches often with aura. There may be recurrent fetal loss and livedo reticularis. Antiphospholipid antibodies may be inferred by the presence of a circulating lupus anticoagulant (a functional test of coagulation) or IgM/IgG cardiolipin or beta 2 glycoprotein 1 antibodies (immunologic assays). These antibodies may be present in patients with systemic lupus erythematosus, chronic infection and neoplasia but a rarer subgroup has primary APAS with no other associated disease. Where relevant all antibody tests and the lupus anticoagulant need to be checked as relevant positivity may occur only in one test. Levels of antibodies can fluctuate considerably and the diagnosis cannot be made unless the antibodies remain present for more than 3 months.

Table 5.7 Non-atherosclerotic vasculopathies which can cause stroke.

Idiopathic/traumatic arterial dissection
Drug misuse
CADASIL
Mitochondrial disease
Arterial dissection secondary to identifiable collagen disease
Fibromuscular dysplasia
Vasculitis
Collagen vascular disease
Sneddon's syndrome
Susac's syndrome
Cervical/cranial irradiation
Moyamoya syndrome
Associated with acute or chronic meningitis and viral infection
Syphilis, malaria
HIV infection

CADASIL, cerebral autosomal dominant arteriopathy with subcortical infarcts and leukoencephalopathy.

Non-atherosclerotic vasculopathies and other rare cases of stroke are discussed elsewhere in this chapter (Table 5.7) and in Chapter 26.

Clinical syndromes of cerebral ischaemia

Transient ischaemic attacks

We have tended to distinguish TIAs from completed stroke on an arbitrary basis but the pathophysiology behind the cause may be identical (e.g. severe carotid stenosis) and both require urgent specialist assessment and investigation. The term brain attack, used by some to describe the acute presentation of TIA and stroke, emphasises urgency. Careful history, examination and sophisticated neuroimaging often reveal that what has been labelled as a TIA is in fact associated with infarction. It is nevertheless useful to distinguish transient as opposed to persistent symptoms and signs, as the differential diagnosis of transient events is different.

The symptoms of transient ischaemia are usually negative, maximal at onset and last typically for a few to 30 minutes. The definition of TIA allows the symptoms to persist for up to 24 hours. We often think of transient ischaemia as indicating atherosclerosis within a specific arterial territory but TIAs may occur in the setting of multiple risk factors without imaging evidence of vasculopathy; or they may occur secondary to a haematological cause (e.g. polycythaemia). High-frequency attacks (several a week) are likely to be brought about by embolism from severe stenosis of a large artery; very high-frequency attacks (several a day) tend to follow from intermittent haemodynamic failure above a critically stenosed artery with poor flow. Such haemodynamic attacks may be distinguished by their diurnal variation (more common in the morning) and at times when blood flow is diverted elsewhere in the body (e.g. after eating or on exercise). Sometimes they present with limb jerking, similar to a focal motor seizure, which may then give way to weakness.

As a general rule, if a patient has more than three TIAs there should be an identifiable reason for them. If there is not a good reason evident after thorough investigation, then the diagnosis should be questioned. Common sites often ignored are found by examining the heart in detail (by trans-oesophageal echocardiography, TOE), the aortic arch (also best seen on TOE), the great vessels, the vertebral arteries and their origins and the intracranial circulation. None of these sites is covered by carotid duplex and adequate investigation requires both echocardiography and CT or MR angiography.

TIAs are associated with a high rate of subsequent stroke: one-third of all untreated patients subsequently have a stroke. The immediate risk is high: 20% of strokes occur within a month and 50% within a year.

Within the carotid circulation (Table 5.8) the retinal circulation may be affected leading to transient monocular blindness (amaurosis fugax). This is usually described as a curtain or shutter coming down over one eye. Blindness usually lasts several minutes only; very occasionally, cholesterol emboli (a Hollenhorst plaque) may be seen after or during an attack. Hemisphere ischaemia is suggested by sudden onset contralateral weakness or dysphasia, when the dominant hemisphere is affected. The symptoms of hemisphere ischaemia usually last up to 20 minutes. Sensory loss in isolation is less common.

Within the vertebrobasilar circulation, attacks may cause diplopia, facial or tongue numbness, dysarthria, vertigo and bilateral visual loss. In some cases it is not possible to decide whether anterior or posterior circulation has been affected: an innominate stenosis with embolism (rare) may produce attacks with mixed features.

It is very unusual for isolated vertigo (Chapter 15) to be caused by vertebrobasilar ischaemia but not impossible – after all, infarction may be asymptomatic. Isolated vertigo is usually the result of an isolated vestibulopathy.

TIAs are usually considered unlikely to be caused by haemorrhage. However, better availability of MRI and blood sensitive acquisition sequences (such as T2* weighted imaging or susceptibility weighted imaging, SWI) reveals that microhaemorrhage or small cortical or sulcal bleeds can be associated with transient neurological symptoms and are often linked with uncontrolled hypertension (Figure 5.7) or cerebral artery amyloidopathy.

Table 5.8 Symptoms of transient ischaemia and other symptoms not of transient ischaemia.

Symptoms of transient ischaemia	
Carotid territory	Monocular visual loss
	Unilateral weakness
	Dysphasia
Vertebrobasilar	Diplopia
	Vertigo/dysequilibrium
	Bilateral visual loss
	Bilateral weakness
Either	Headache
	Dysarthria
	Hemianopia
	Unsteadiness
	Sensory loss
Symptoms not usually suggestive of transient ischaemia	
Syncope	
Isolated amnesia	
Drop attacks	
Generalised weakness	
Confusional states	
Isolated vertigo	

Alternative diagnoses

About one-quarter of people attending specialist cerebrovascular clinics with possible TIAs have alternative diagnoses (Table 5.9). The most common is migraine with focal symptoms. These are either part of an aura preceding headache (not usually confused with TIAs), or without headache (commonly confused) or following a migrainous headache – the extremely rare hemiplegic migraine. Stroke itself and TIAs are not infrequently accompanied by headache. Some serious conditions may cause both migrainous symptoms and infarction (e.g. cervical artery dissection, APS and giant cell arteritis).

The two main pointers toward migraine are positive phenomena and spread. Visual aura may consist of zigzag lines and scintillating scotomas. Sensory aura is tingling rather than numbness and in a mouth–hand distribution. Patients may complain of weakness but this is usually vague. Symptoms evolve slowly – taking several minutes for the visual disturbance to maximise, or for the tingling to spread from the hand to the face (the typical distribution). True hemiplegic migraine (Chapter 12) is a rare familial channelopathy and quite distinct from other forms of migraine.

Other commonly confused conditions are transient global amnesia and epilepsy. Transient global amnesia (TGA) is sometimes precipitated by Valsalva activated straining (e.g. immersion in cold water, travel or emotional stress). Hanging up curtains is a common precursor. Generally, in TGA, acute anterograde amnesia develops and patients usually appear bewildered and ask repetitive questions such as 'Where am I?' and 'What's going on?' There is no loss of personal identity as in a fugue state. The attacks last several hours and after recovery the patient has little recollection of the event.

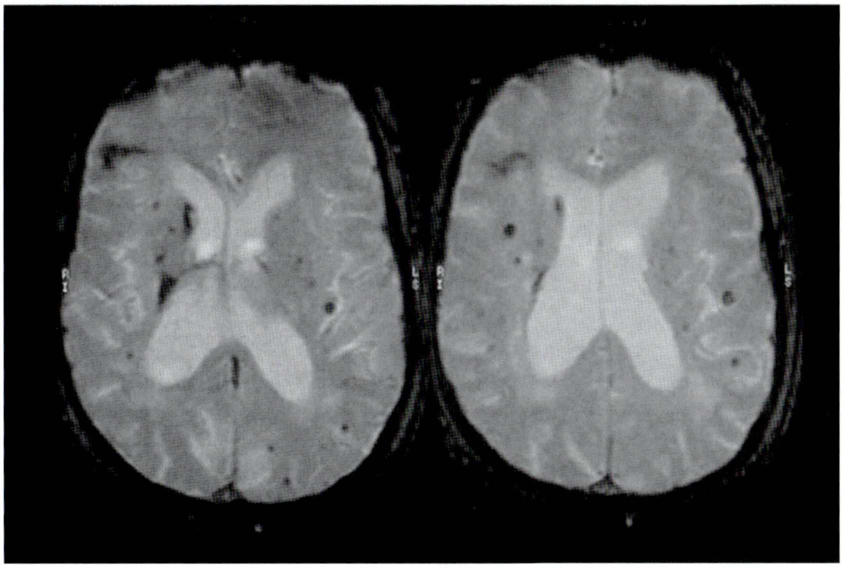

Figure 5.7 Multiple microhaemorrhages on MR T2*.

Table 5.9 Differential diagnosis of transient ischaemia.

Migraine
Transient global amnesia
Epilepsy
Multiple sclerosis
Mass lesions, subdurals
Hypoglycaemia
Syncope

TGA is a heterogeneous disorder but in general is benign and not associated with a subsequent stroke risk. There does seem to be a subgroup of patients who have lost cognitive reserve (e.g. from chronic small vessel disease or otherwise silent Alzheimer pathology) who may present with TGA, and even rarer transient epileptic amnesia. Patients should be investigated with imaging and for vascular risk factors.

In addition, other serious intracranial pathology may cause transient symptoms such as tumours, subdural haematomas and multiple sclerosis. Hypoglycaemia may masquerade as all sorts of transient neurological disturbances, including hemiparesis but this is rare in practice. Syncope can sometimes produce confusing clinical pictures including focal deficits.

Investigation when true transient ischaemia is thought possible is the same as for completed stroke and is discussed later.

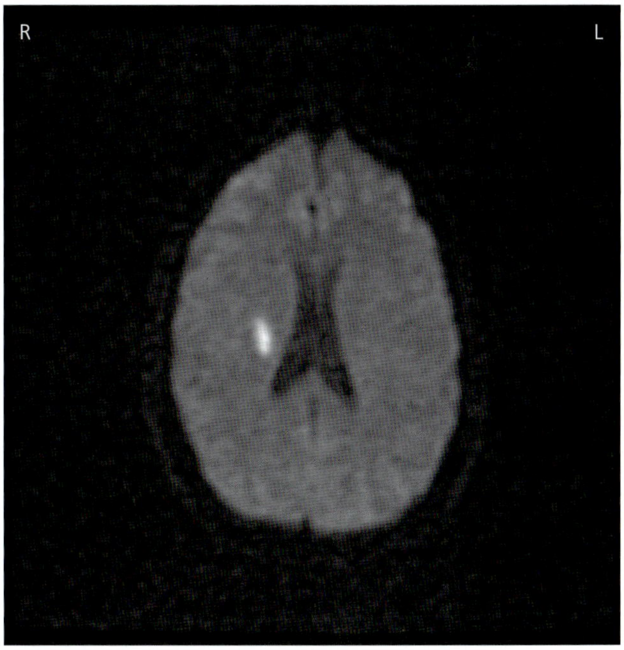

Figure 5.8 Diffusion weighted MRI following lacunar infarction.

Lacunar stroke

Lacunes are small, subcortical or brainstem infarcts ranging from 1 to 15 mm in size. They need to be distinguished from the dilated peri-vascular spaces commonly visible on MRI. This is easy with MR FLAIR imaging: although both may be white on T2, lacunes are cavities and therefore black with a hyperintense rim. Lacunar infarction is caused by occlusion of small penetrating vessels most commonly arising from the MCA and basilar artery (Figure 5.8). Lacunes may be silent. They may be preceded by TIAs in some 20%; sometimes these are high-frequency attacks refractory to all treatments (capsular warning syndrome). Lacunar TIAs tend to be briefer and more stereotyped than large vessel TIAs. The two pathologies underlying vessel occlusion are usually lipohyaline change and/or microatheroma. Although lacunar infarction is also associated with carotid stenosis, it does not commonly happen as an embolic syndrome. The major risk factors for lacunar stroke are hypertension, diabetes and hypercholesterolaemia. Occlusion of small penetrating vessels is commonly asymptomatic but if eloquent structures are involved then the syndromes are fairly stereotypic. The most common sites for lacunar infarction are the putamen, pallidum, pons, thalamus, caudate, internal capsule and corona radiata.

Table 5.10 Common lacunar syndromes.

Pure motor
Sensorimotor
Pure sensory
Ataxic hemiparesis
Dysarthria/clumsy hand

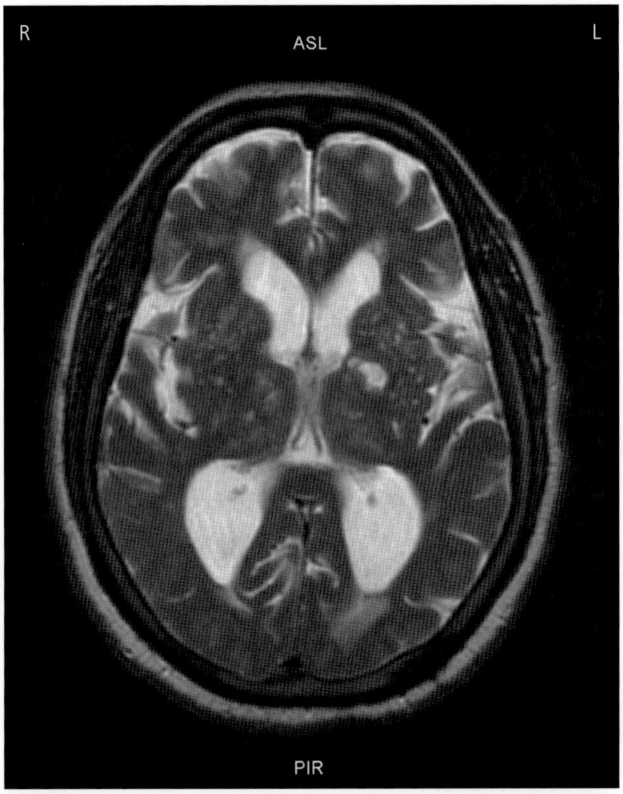

Figure 5.9 Axial T2 MRI showing multiple lacunes in the deep grey and capsular white matter with periventricular abnormal signal reflecting diffuse small vessel disease.

The principal clinical feature of lacunar infarction is that patients lack cortical signs. Cortical signs include dysphasia, neglect syndrome, apraxia, hemianopia and conjugate eye deviation. It is difficult to tell clinically whether infarction has taken place affecting deep hemisphere structures or brainstem structures as the syndromes overlap. One is tempted to think that a profoundly dysarthric patient must have had brainstem infarction but this is unreliable. There are many lacunar syndromes but those commonly seen in practice are pure motor hemiparesis, pure sensory hemiparesis, sensorimotor hemiparesis, ataxic hemiparesis and clumsy hand-dysarthria syndrome (Table 5.10).

CT may not detect some smaller lacunar infarcts especially in the brainstem; MRI is much more sensitive. Often patients with lacunar infarction may have widespread changes (Figure 5.9) and it can be difficult clinically to identify the symptomatic lesion without DWI. Appropriate patients should also have evaluation of the extracranial carotids, looking for significant stenosis. The large carotid endarterectomy trials have shown that carotid stenosis is a risk factor for lacunar stroke. Those with severe carotid stenosis benefit from endarterectomy, in terms of secondary prevention but the mainstay of secondary prevention is control of hypertension, diabetes, antiplatelet agents and statins where appropriate.

If sufficient damage from repeated penetrating vessel occlusion takes place, global problems appear. These patients often have diffuse peri-ventricular change on CT and MR imaging, known as leukoaraiosis and atrophy. They may develop gait apraxia (gait ignition failure, marche à petit pas) and postural instability with a predisposition to falling backwards, and dementia of a subcortical type with prominent lack of initiation and poor attention. Patients with small vessel disease may also be at greater risk of Alzheimer's disease (Chapter 8) and the two often coexist. These syndromes are distinct from multiple cortical stroke. Leukoaraiosis can also be found coincidently without overt symptoms or signs in those over 50 years especially with appropriate risk factors. There is an increased incidence of depression and subclinical cognitive impairment in these patients.

Rarer causes of lacunar syndromes

APAS can present with lacunar infarction; often these patients also have a history of migrainous phenomena and headaches. Anticoagulation is often prescribed although there is not much evidence to support this practice. CADASIL (cerebral autosomal dominant arteriopathy with subcortical infarcts and leukoencephalopathy) presents in a similar fashion (see later, and Chapter 26).

Large vessel occlusion

The pattern of infarction after large vessel occlusion will depend on many factors. The common risk factors listed above are important, but compared to lacunar infarction the emphasis skews towards large vessel stenosis and heart disease as sources of embolism.

The main clinical distinction between large vessel occlusion and lacunar infarction in the carotid circulation is the presence of cortical signs (eye deviation, dysphasia, neglect syndromes, hemianopia). The hemiparesis produced by MCA occlusion affects the arm more than the leg because of cortical involvement (the leg cortex is in anterior cerebral artery territory).

Internal carotid artery disease

The major cause of this is atherosclerosis, with stenosis in the distal common carotid artery extending to the proximal ICA and external carotid artery. Occlusive disease of other arteries commonly accompanies ICA stenosis; coexisting myocardial ischaemia and limb ischaemia are common. Atherosclerosis in the ICA produces its symptoms either by embolism, thrombus formed on ulcerated plaque, haemodynamic failure from severe stenosis (>95%) or carotid artery occlusion.

An important clue to a potential ICA stenosis is transient monocular blindness, amaurosis fugax (the ophthalmic artery is the first branch above the ICA origin). Occasionally, the patient may develop a low flow retinopathy or global ischaemic ocular syndrome from a combination of small vessel and critical ICA stenosis. This may cause haemodynamic retinal symptoms including bleaching out of colours in sunlight and persistent after images from bright lights. Although a bruit may mark the presence of ICA stenosis and is an independent risk factor for stroke, the ICA flow can be so severely diminished that a bruit is absent. Embolism is most likely to produce a partial or complete MCA syndrome and is discussed later. Haemodynamic failure above a critical stenosis can lead to border-zone infarction. Horner's syndrome may be present when the artery is acutely thrombosed. Carotid occlusion occasionally presents with a stuttering deficit, sometimes over many weeks.

Narrowing and thrombotic occlusion of the carotid siphon in the distal ICA is less frequent than at the origin but is usually caused by atherosclerosis. This may be more common in the Asian population. In younger patients, distal stenosis and occlusion may be caused by vasculitis, dissection or Moyamoya disease.

Middle cerebral artery occlusion

Total MCA occlusion The MCA may be affected by embolism or thrombosis *in situ*. Patients with severe intracranial atherosclerosis have a high incidence of stroke because of thrombosis *en plaque*. People of Asian and African descent seem particularly affected by intracranial stenosis. In Caucasians, while MCA occlusion is common, MCA stenosis is rare.

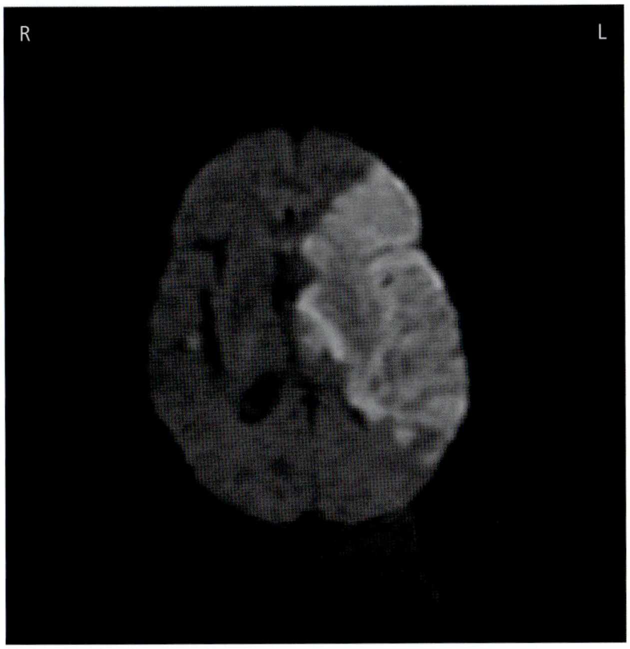

Figure 5.10 Diffusion weighted MRI showing complete MCA territory infarction.

If the main trunk occludes and there are inadequate collaterals then the whole territory infarcts (Figure 5.10). The clinical picture produced is sometimes known as 'front-to-back' infarction with conjugate eye deviation (frontal lobe damage), aphasia (dominant hemisphere), hemiplegia, hemisensory loss and hemianopia (parietal and temporal lobe damage). Neglect syndromes where the patient is unaware of the hemiplegic side occur acutely with both non-dominant and dominant hemisphere damage but generally only persist with non-dominant damage. Patients with complete MCA syndromes can develop fatal brain swelling (malignant MCA oedema) which peaks at 4–5 days and can lead to herniation and coning. In appropriate cases surgical decompression is required (Figure 5.11).

MCA branch occlusions These produce fragments of the syndromes described earlier. Upper branch occlusion affecting frontal structures produces hemiparesis, hemisensory loss, ocular deviation and non-fluent motor dysphasia (expressive) where the patient understands (intact temporal lobe) but cannot produce speech. Lower branch occlusions can affect the temporal lobe resulting in fluent dysphasia (receptive) where production of speech is good but incoherent and the patient does not understand (Chapters 4 and 8).

MCA distal embolism Small cortical branches occluded (e.g. by emboli) may present only with weakness or isolated cortical signs, difficult to distinguish from the effects of a lacunar infarct.

MCA deep infarction (striato-capsular infarction) This tends to occur when collateral circulation protects the cortex but deeper structures (the striatum and capsule) become infarcted (Figure 5.12). This pattern of infarction is also seen with MCA stenosis and when emboli obstruct the lenticulo-striate perforators and then break up. Patients have unilateral motor and sensory loss but also exhibit cortical signs (unlike pure lacunar infarction). These cortical signs resolve more quickly than when the cortex itself is damaged. Striato-capsular infarction should prompt a search for cardiac and ipsilateral carotid sources of embolism.

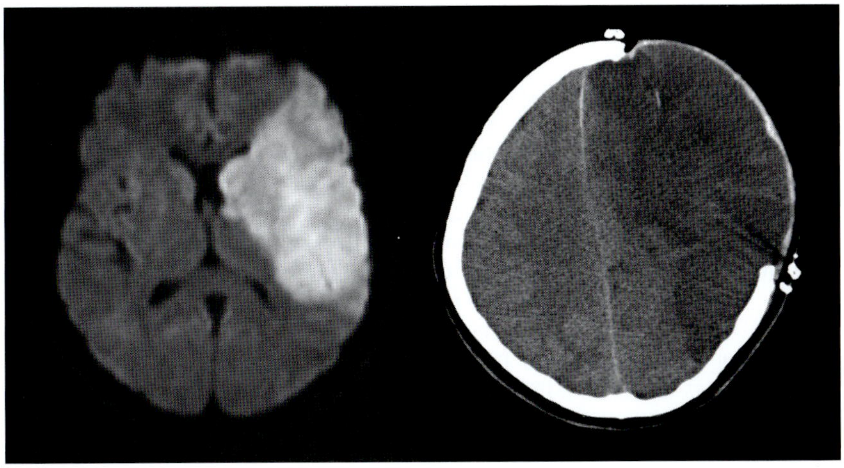

(a) (b)

Figure 5.11 Malignant middle cerebral artery (MCA). (a) A large acute left MCA infarct is seen on DWI. (b) CT at 5 days post infarct shows severe swelling and decompressive craniectomy.

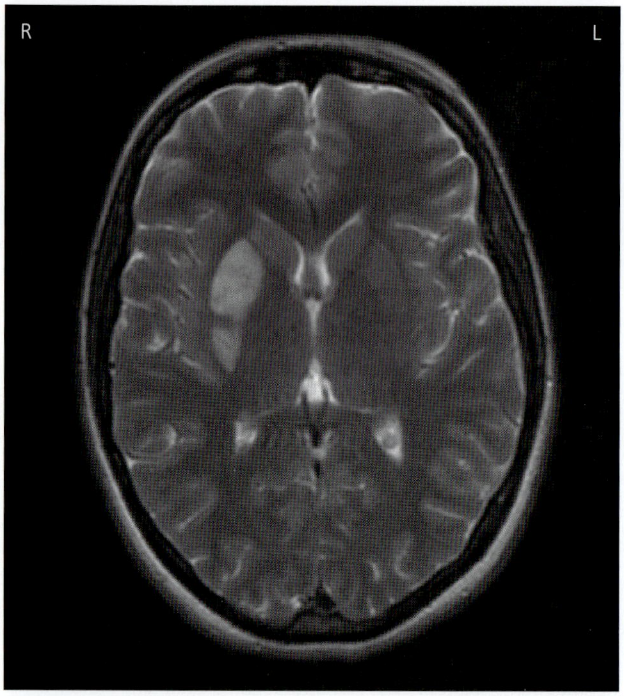

Figure 5.12 Axial T2 MRI of striato-capsular infarction.

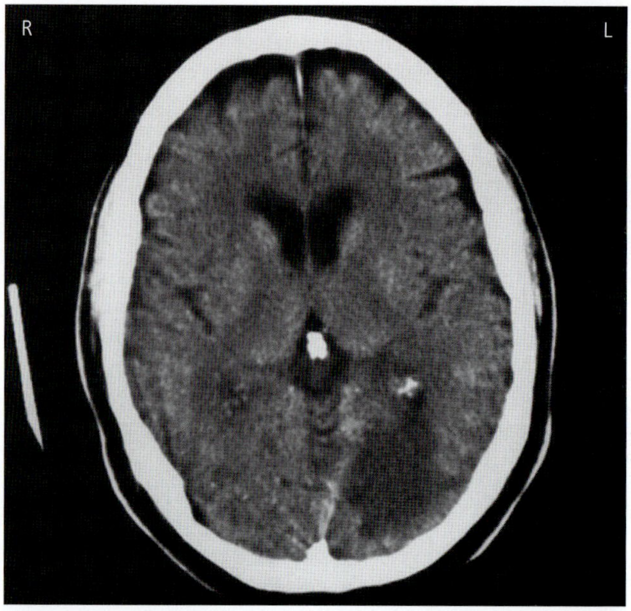

Figure 5.13 Unenhanced CT showing area of infarction following posterior cerebral artery (PCA) occlusion.

Anterior cerebral artery occlusion

This territory is far less often affected than that of the MCA. Although the same risk factors apply, ACA territory infarction should raise the level of awareness for unusual aetiologies at play. This also occurs in the setting of SAH, secondary to vasospasm. The clinical features of ACA occlusion are contralateral hemiplegia. The leg is most affected as the cortical representation of the leg lies within the territory. Some patients may have motor neglect and apraxia.

Anterior choroidal artery occlusion

Syndromes include hemiparesis (face, arm and leg), prominent hemisensory loss and hemianopia, often temporary. However, unlike hemianopia associated with complete MCA infarction, other cortical signs may be subtle and transient.

Posterior cerebral artery

Occlusion of these arteries is commonly embolic. More patients with PCA syndromes are in atrial fibrillation than with other large vessel occlusions (Figure 5.13). The PCA supplies principally the occipital cortex: an isolated hemianopia is common. When infarction is more anterior, affecting parieto-occipital areas, neglect syndromes may accompany the hemianopia. The PCAs also supply the thalami and posterior-medial temporal lobes. If these structures are involved the patient may present with confusion, dysphasia (thalamic) or memory impairment (thalamic or temporal). If both PCA territories are infarcted, as may happen when an embolus lodges at the top of the basilar, cortical blindness and confusion ensues. Sometimes, these patients may be left with tunnel vision and may recognise small but not large objects. Memory impairment, especially for new information, may be severe.

Vertebral artery

The most common pattern produced by occlusion of or embolism from the vertebral arteries is infarction of the dorsolateral medulla within the territory of the posterior inferior cerebellar artery causing a lateral medullary syndrome (Wallenberg's syndrome). This results in a Horner's syndrome, dissociated (temperature and pain) sensory loss on the ipsilateral side of the face and the opposite side of the body, nystagmus, ataxia of the ipsilateral limbs, and ipsilateral palatal and vocal cord paralysis. Vertebral embolism or occlusion may also result in more extensive infarction of the brainstem and cerebellum; these syndromes are discussed next. The most common site for atheroma to affect the vertebral artery is at its origin from the subclavian.

Basilar artery

Whereas the middle and posterior cerebral arteries are more often affected by embolism than *in situ* thrombosis, the opposite is true of the basilar artery. This is because the basilar is wider than its two feeding vertebral arteries and it can be affected by severe atherosclerosis on which *in situ* thrombus can form (Figure 5.14). Basilar thrombosis may also result from propagation of thrombus from one of the vertebral arteries (e.g. after vertebral artery dissection) and can also occur without obvious precipitants, especially in younger adults. The basilar thrombus may obstruct blood flow into perforating vessels supplying the central brainstem structures or the two upper cerebellar arteries. A number of clinical pictures may be encountered. In the medulla, lower cranial nuclei may be affected giving rise to a lower motor neurone type bulbar palsy. Upper motor neurone impairment of the same structure may cause a pseudobulbar palsy, with brisk facial reflexes, brisk jaw jerk and a spastic tongue. This is often accompanied by spontaneous laughter or crying (emotional lability). Above the medulla, pontine infarction can cause a VIth nerve palsy, gaze paresis, internuclear ophthalmoplegia and pinpoint pupils. Emboli may also lodge at the top of the basilar causing midbrain infarction with loss of vertical eye movement, pupillary abnormalities, coma or locked-in syndrome.

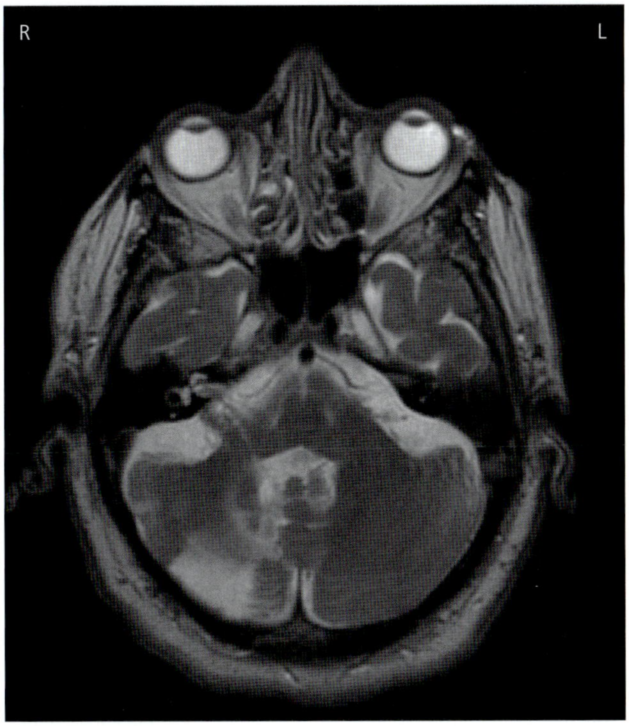

Figure 5.14 Axial T2 MRI: cerebellar infarction following basilar thrombosis (basilar artery: now patent).

Involvement of the origin of one or both of the posterior cerebral arteries may lead to a hemianopia or cortical blindness. All these syndromes will be accompanied by quadriparesis to some degree, which may be very asymmetric.

Border-zone syndromes and ischaemic encephalopathy

The brain is particularly vulnerable to a global decrease in perfusion. Most frequently, this is caused by cardiac disease (arrhythmia or pump failure) and hypoxaemia, although hypovolaemia alone may result in these syndromes. Hypoxia without ischaemia (i.e. without reduction in blood flow) does not lead to cerebral infarction. The usual circumstance in which these patients are encountered is following cardiac arrest, severe blood loss and cardiopulmonary bypass in which embolism may also occur. Acutely in the non-anaesthetised non-comatose patient, global perfusion failure results in non-focal brain dysfunction (confusion, attentional deficits, light-headedness). Following a profound insult a number of watershed syndromes brought about by damage to the border-zone regions are recognised.

The area particularly vulnerable to reduction in perfusion pressure is the parieto-occipital cortex that lies at the superficial border-zone between MCA and PCA territories. This is the area furthest from the heart. Infarction of this region results in abnormalities of behaviour, memory and vision. The visual abnormalities are complex and include inability to see all the objects in a field of vision, incoordination of hand and eye movement such that the patient cannot locate objects in the visual field, and apraxia of gaze in which the patient cannot gaze where desired. Other areas of vulnerability are the deep border-zones within the subcortical white matter of the centrum semi-ovale, and border-zones between the ACA and MCA, and the hippocampi, where infarction may result in a Korsakoff-type syndrome. In severe cases, necrosis can follow within the basal ganglia, cerebellum and brainstem. The term watershed is often used to mean border-zone, though strictly speaking a watershed is a line dividing two drainage basins, which is a poor analogy with perfusion anatomy. Unilateral patchy deep border-zone ischaemia in the centrum semi-ovale is characteristic of ipsilateral internal carotid artery occlusion or severe stenosis and may be seen in patients presenting only with TIA or minor stroke.

Vascular dementia

Dementia (i.e. cognitive deficits in multiple domains) can follow multiple cortical or subcortical lacunar infarcts (multi-infarct dementia). Typically, patients have a stepwise deterioration associated with other features of stroke. In diffuse small vessel disease, the onset may be more subtle with the more gradual onset of cognitive impairment (Chapter 8) often accompanied by gait apraxia where patients exhibit failure to initiate gait, postural instability (often falling over backwards) and a shuffling small-stepped gait. Patients with diffuse small vessel disease may have prominent attentional difficulties in excess of discrete cortical patterns of dysfunction and often present with periods of encephalopathy associated with new infarction. Multiple cortical infarcts, from large vessel occlusions, are much rarer as a cause of dementia. In addition, it is important to note that patients with vascular disease (clinically and radiologically) are at an increased risk of Alzheimer's disease and it is the combination of the two pathologies that causes dementia in many patients with vascular disease (mixed dementia). This can be distinguished to some extent on clinical and neuropsychological ground, but it is often difficult to separate the effects of the two diseases.

Intracranial haemorrhage

Intracranial haemorrhage may be intracerebral, subarachnoid, subdural or extradural. This section deals principally with intracerebral haemorrhage (ICH), both supratentorial and infratentorial haemorrhage.

Approximately 10% of stroke is caused by brain haemorrhage with an annual incidence of 10–15/100 000 population. The incidence increases significantly after the age of 55 years and doubles with each decade to the age of 80. However, there has been a small but progressive decline in the incidence of both stroke and brain haemorrhage in the last three decades, because of an improvement in the management of risk factors and secondary prevention; the control of hypertension in primary care has been of particular importance.

Despite being less common than ischaemic stroke, haemorrhage has a significant impact because the subsequent mortality is so high. In one study of over 1000 stroke cases, 30-day mortality for supratentorial and infratentorial ischaemic stroke was 15% and 18%, respectively. Mortality following supratentorial and infratentorial haemorrhage was 58% and 31%.

Spontaneous ICH results from intracerebral arterial rupture, particularly perforating vessels, or less frequently from the venous system. The haematoma expands following the path of least resistance, usually along white matter tracts, and occasionally into the ventricular system. Neurological deficit results both from direct tissue destruction and indirectly from local compression and mass effect, usually in proportion to both the volume of haematoma and its rate of expansion. Intraparenchymal haemorrhage can occur at any site, although some areas are more susceptible than others. Eighty per cent of such intraparenchymal haemorrhages occur within the cerebral hemispheres and some 20% are infratentorial.

Traditionally, brain haemorrhage has been thought to have a sudden devastating presentation. While it is true that patients who present in coma or who have vomiting, headache and neck stiffness are more likely to have had a haemorrhage than ischaemic event, it is wrong to believe that patients with less severe stroke syndromes can be diagnosed on clinical grounds to have had ischaemic strokes. This is particularly illustrated by the recognition of microhaemorrhage with T2* and SWI imaging which occasionally reveals minute bleeds as the underlying cause of clinical syndromes previously thought to have been caused by ischaemia.

Risk factors

The most important risk factor associated with brain haemorrhage is hypertension, found in 40–60% of patients. Hypertension leads to disease of the small perforating arteries (hypertensive arteriopathy), which is an important cause of leukoaraiosis on imaging as well as promoting rupture of these vessels. Compared with brain haemorrhages from other causes, this type of bleed is more frequently fatal, a reflection of both its high incidence and its tendency to occur in critical locations. Hypertensive bleeds occur in deep white matter (36%), pons (11%) and cerebellum (8%), regions that are supplied by the lenticulo-striate branches of the MCA or the paramedian perforating branches of the basilar artery. The underlying weakness of these vessels is usually caused by hyaline degeneration of arterioles promoted by long-standing hypertension, but can also result from fibrinoid necrosis in patients with malignant hypertension or eclampsia. Identical pathology can be seen in elderly patients without known hypertension.

Other conditions important in the aetiology of brain haemorrhage are aneurysms (20%), vascular malformations (5–7%), coagulopathies (5–7%), tumours (1–11%), sporadic cerebral amyloid angiopathy and secondary haemorrhage into a recent infarct (haemorrhagic infarction) (Table 5.11). It is important to recognise that hypertension is a risk factor for haemorrhage from all these pathologies and thus a history of hypertension is not sufficient to diagnose a hypertensive bleed. Non-medicinal use of cocaine and amphetamines may cause haemorrhage, although there is often an underlying vascular malformation in these cases.

Aneurysms are saccular or fusiform arterial deformities, the result of protrusion of the intima through a structural defect in the arterial muscular layer. Typical circle of Willis aneurysms, also known as berry aneurysms, most commonly cause SAH, although this is associated with intraparenchymal bleeding in 30% of patients. Mycotic aneurysms usually form in smaller cortical arteries when septic emboli lodge in the vessel. This is usually seen in the context of infective endocarditis, where up to 17% of patients develop cerebral emboli. Usually, these mycotic aneurysms thrombose, if the infection is treated adequately, and no further intervention is required. Rarely, the mycotic aneurysm continues to enlarge or ruptures; surgical intervention is necessary to clip and/or resect it. Arterial invasion by tumour or severe atherosclerosis occasionally leads to aneurysm formation, although rupture is rare. Other vascular malformations that cause brain haemorrhage include arteriovenous malformations (AVMs), cavernous malformations and capillary telangiectasia. Developmental purely venous anomalies were also thought to cause haemorrhage: however, the current understanding is that it is the cavernous malformation commonly associated with the venous anomaly that is the source of bleeding.

Table 5.11 Causes of brain haemorrhage.

Hypertension
Anticoagulants
Amyloid angiopathy
Arteriovenous malformations
Aneurysms
Cavernous haemangiomas
Amphetamine/cocaine ingestion
Infective endocarditis
Tumours
Disseminated intravascular coagulation
Venous thrombosis
Cerebral vasculitis, malaria
Malaria

One of the most important and potentially treatable causes is anticoagulation, especially when poorly controlled and combined with other risk factors. Any patients on anticoagulants with new focal neurology must be assumed to have bled until proven otherwise with urgent cranial imaging. In those that have bled, anticoagulation should be immediately reversed. The mechanism by which anticoagulation promotes cerebral haemorrhage is uncertain. It is possible that what would be an asymptomatic microbleed in the non-anticoagulated patient becomes macroscopic and symptomatic in an anticoagulated patient. Certainly, cerebral haematomas associated with anticoagulation are larger and continue to enlarge for longer in patients on anticoagulants. Other causes of coagulopathy, including thrombocytopaenia, leukaemia and liver and renal failure, may also cause similar problems. Patients with coagulopathy are also much more likely to bleed into cerebral infarcts.

An increasingly important and recognised condition causing ICH is sporadic cerebral amyloid angiopathy (CAA). This is a common age-related cerebral small vessel disease, characterised by progressive deposition of amyloid-β in the wall of small cortical and leptomeningeal arteries. Population-based autopsy studies show that the prevalence of CAA is 20–40% in non-demented, and 50–60% in demented elderly population. Deposition of amyloid-β causes injury to the vessel wall, which in moderate to severe disease may rupture, causing cerebral microbleeds, cortical superficial siderosis or larger symptomatic ICH. Although CAA is most often recognised by the occurrence of spontaneous lobar ICH in the elderly, it can also cause transient focal neurological deficits, disturbances of consciousness and progressive cognitive decline.

CAA is also associated with transient focal neurological episodes (sometime called 'amyloid spells'), which can resemble TIAs, migraine auras or focal seizures. Patients often complain of recurrent, brief (minutes), stereotyped attacks of paresthesias or numbness (spreading smoothly over contiguous body parts), visual symptoms (sometimes migraine aura-like), face or limb weakness or dysphasia. Although these symptoms may clinically suggest TIAs, increasing data suggest that 'amyloid spells' in CAA are more often associated with intracranial bleeding.

The radiological demonstration of haemorrhagic manifestations of the disease in the brain (especially using T2*-GRE or SWI MRI) allow the *in vivo* clinical radiological diagnosis of CAA (Figure 5.15). The diagnosis of CAA currently relies on the demonstration of multiple haemorrhagic lesions in strictly lobar brain

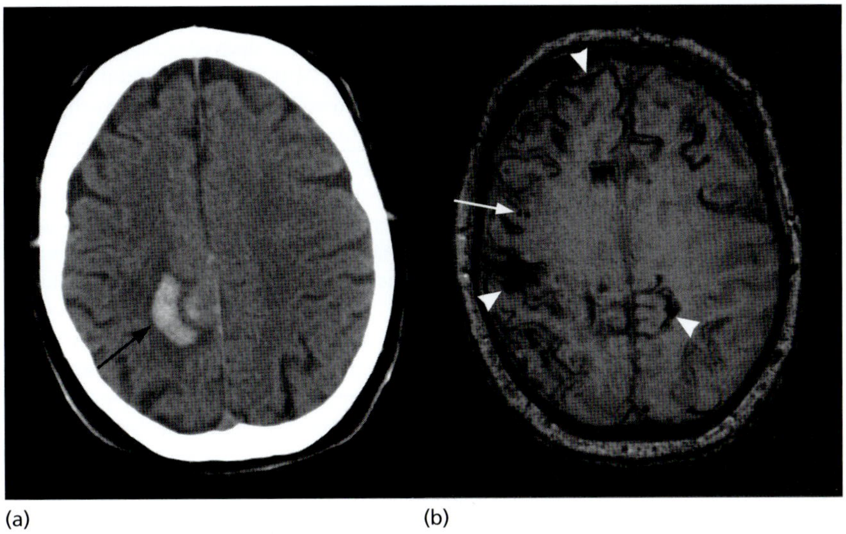

Figure 5.15 Cerebral amyloid angiopathy: a small lobar haemorrhage (black arrow) with adjacent subarachnoid haemorrhage is seen on CT (a) and susceptibility weighted imaging (b) shows multiple areas of superficial haemosiderin deposition (arrowheads) and peripheral microhaemorrhages (white arrow) typical of cerebral amyloid angiopathy.

areas – the Boston criteria, including both cerebral micro-bleeds, as well as ICH, although pathological validation for microbleed-only patients is limited.

Clinical syndromes of intracranial haemorrhage

The rupture of a vessel or microaneurysm results in the sudden development of haematoma, of variable size. These haematomas characteristically then slowly enlarge over the next few hours, and sometimes continue to enlarge over a matter of days especially in patients on anticoagulants, leading to progressive focal neurological deficit and then deterioration of conscious level secondary to mass effect. Haemorrhage may be divided into a number of categories depending on location. These are deep (centered on basal ganglia structures), lobar, pontine and cerebellar. In all sites, hypertension remains the most important risk factor and while amyloid angiopathy classically gives rise to lobar and not deep haemorrhage, hypertension is still the most important risk factor in lobar haemorrhage.

Deep haemorrhage

Haematomas may be centred on the putamen, caudate or thalamus. In putaminal haemorrhage, the picture is of contralateral hemiparesis and conjugate deviation of the eyes towards the side of the haematoma (Figure 5.16). Cortical function may be impaired. If the mass effect becomes critical then signs of herniation ensue. These haematomas may rupture into the ventricles leading to intraventricular haemorrhage. In the case of putaminal haemorrhage the presence of ventricular blood implies a very large haematoma with a poor prognosis. Caudate haemorrhage is much rarer and small haematomas may readily rupture into the ventricles. When the lesion is large the picture is similar to putaminal haemorrhage but if small, haematomas may mimic subarachnoid haemorrhage with acute headache and meningism with little in the way of focal signs. Thalamic haemorrhage predominantly produces sensory change in the contralateral limbs. If local midbrain compression occurs the eyes may be forced into downward gaze with small poorly reactive pupils. Thalamic haemorrhage in the dominant hemisphere may produce dysphasia with notable naming difficulties.

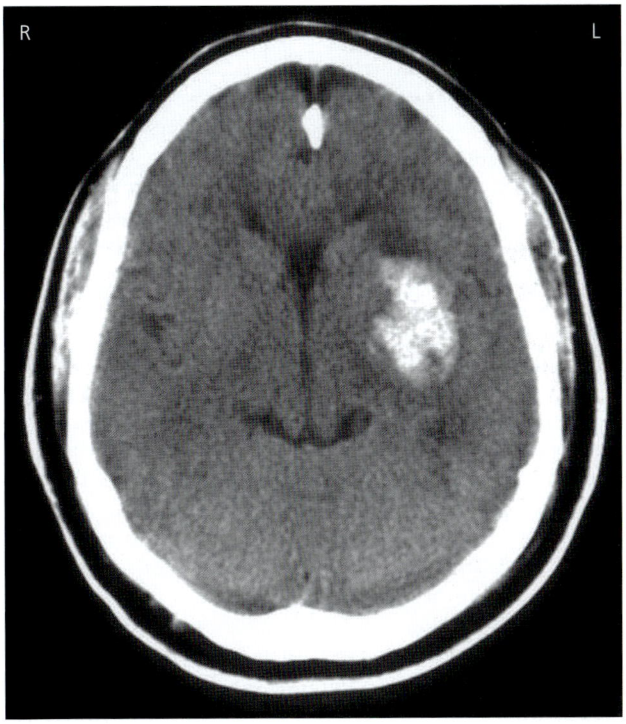

Figure 5.16 Unenhanced CT showing large putaminal haematoma.

Lobar haemorrhage

These cortical lesions produce signs appropriate to their location. In the frontal lobe, ipsilateral eye deviation and contralateral hemiparesis is common. In the posterior frontal and fronto-parietal region, hemisensory loss is found, associated with dysphasia when the lesion is within the dominant hemisphere. Parietal lobe haemorrhage causes hemisensory loss and neglect/inattention syndromes. Bleeding into the dominant temporal lobe results in a fluent dysphasia with poor comprehension secondary to damage to Wernicke's area.

Lobar haemorrhages are more likely to be associated with structural abnormalities (e.g. a vascular malformation) than deep haemorrhages. Alternatively, amyloid, trauma, haemorrhagic transformation of infarction and a haemorrhagic tumour should be considered within the differential diagnosis.

Infratentorial haemorrhage

The classic picture in pontine haemorrhage is coma associated with pinpoint pupils, loss of horizontal eye movements and quadriparesis. Hyperpyrexia and irregular respiratory patterns ensue. Although a large haematoma here is often fatal, the outcome may be surprisingly good in some patients.

Cerebellar haemorrhage accounts for some 10% of all brain haemorrhages. It is important to recognise that cerebellar haematomas may result in secondary fatal brainstem compression and hydrocephalus. Posterior fossa craniectomy to decompress the brainstem can be life-saving and patients may make an excellent functional recovery, even from deep coma. The usual picture is of acute headache and vomiting with unilateral ataxia. Unilateral gaze paresis in association with ataxia or in isolation may occur and also skew deviation. When brainstem compression is present from the onset or develops later, the picture suggests a pontine haemorrhage, with the patient either presenting or deteriorating into coma. Emergency CT scanning is essential.

Intraventricular haemorrhage

This mimics SAH (see later) with headache, vomiting, neck stiffness and depression of consciousness. There may be associated pyramidal signs, particularly if associated with a parenchymal haematoma. This may be caused by extension of blood following deep haemorrhage, aneurysmal rupture or a subependymal angioma. This is particularly the case with caudate haemorrhage as this nucleus lies adjacent to the ventricular margin.

Specific issues in intracerebral haemorrhage

Brain imaging is mandatory, without delay. Although MRI is greatly superior to CT at refining the pathophysiological diagnosis, it is not currently available for most patients in the emergency situation. The appearances of haemorrhage on CT are also easier to interpret than on MRI, especially in non-expert hands and CT is therefore often the preferred imaging technique at presentation. Acutely, a CT is essential to distinguish infarction from haemorrhage or reveal mimics of the stroke syndrome such as tumour or subdural haematoma. Haemorrhages seen on MRI undergo complex changes depending on the image sequence, the proportion of oxyhaemoglobin, deoxyhaemoglobin and methaemoglobin, and its distribution; this may make interpretation difficult. However, signal loss on susceptibility weighted MRI is more specific and sensitive to new and old haemorrhages than the older MRI sequences.

In appropriate patients it is necessary to exclude an aneurysm or underlying vascular malformations with angiography. In some cases, CT or MR angiography might be sufficient, but these may miss small lesions and catheter angiography is still required in a small proportion of cases. The decision to perform catheter-based angiography should be made after discussion with an interventional neuroradiologist and/or vascular neurosurgeon. If performed in the acute situation, consideration should be given to repeating angiography once the mass effect of the haematoma has resolved. In 10% of cases where initial angiography is normal, a small arteriovenous malformation is demonstrated on delayed imaging. This is caused by occlusion of the arteriovenous malformation by the mass effect of the acute haematoma. In this situation either the angiogram should be delayed or repeated following resolution of the haematoma. MRI is often a useful complementary investigation in order to exclude underlying parenchymal lesions. Again this is best performed after some days once there has been resolution of some of the blood products.

Following a brain haemorrhage, the general supportive management issues are just as important as in ischaemic stroke. Medical treatment is aimed at correcting any underlying systemic disorder such as severe hypertension or coagulopathy, as well as preventing or limiting secondary complications such as pulmonary emboli, MI and pneumonia. Aspirin (often taken as an over-the-counter preparation) or any other medication with antiplatelet (clopidogrel, non-steroidal anti-inflammatory agents) or antithrombotic actions (dipyridamole) should be stopped. Early intensive lowering of blood pressure was shown to be safe in the second INTERACT trial, while secondary analyses suggested that this might improve outcome. Until recently, there were no specific haemostatic drugs that had been shown to alter outcome. Initial trials of recombinant activated factor VII showed that this pro-coagulant appeared to reduce haematoma size and improves outcome when given within 4 hours of onset; however, phase IIb/IIIa studies have been negative. Further trials are needed to explore similar products. Frequent neurological assessments, as well as serial CT scans, are necessary particularly early in the clinical course when management can be modified accordingly.

Anticoagulant-related haematomas often present as slowly evolving lesions. It is essential, even if they are small at initial imaging, to reverse warfarin immediately as delay may have devastating consequences. This maxim includes patients with prosthetic valves as the risk–benefit ratio is much in favour of anticoagulation reversal for a period of 2 weeks, after which the rebleeding rate is considerably lower. The rate of systemic embolism from thrombus on the prosthetic valve during this period is small.

Neurosurgical practice in relation to evacuating intracerebral haematomas varies. The middle of the road approach that the authors follow is to evacuate life-threatening cerebellar haematomas large enough to cause brainstem compression and hydrocephalus and superficial lobar haematomas that are causing marked mass effect. Few neurosurgeons will tackle deep-seated basal ganglia haematomas unless under exceptional circumstances, in the main because the associated morbidity is significant. The optimal management of this form of stroke beyond organised care is unclear from the evidence and the results of the two Surgical Trial in Intracerebral Haemorrhage (STICH) trials suggested no significant benefit to surgical evacuation. In these two prospective randomised studies of over 1000 patients, there was no overall benefit from early surgery when compared with initial conservative management.

Prognosis of intracranial haemorrhage

The prognosis of brain haemorrhage depends primarily on the location and size of the haematoma. These factors are closely followed by the patient's age, the cause of the haemorrhage and the development and severity of post-haemorrhagic complications such as cerebral oedema, hydrocephalus and raised intracranial pressure, as well as systemic complications such as pulmonary embolus, MI and pneumonia. In gauging prognosis and discussing possible outcome with a patient or their relatives, it is worth pointing out that improvement following haemorrhage tends to be more delayed than following infarction, and that there are some cases where eventual recovery is good following resolution of the haematoma.

Subarachnoid haemorrhage

The main cause of non-traumatic SAH is rupture of an intracranial aneurysm. This accounts for 85% of cases. SAH is a devastating condition with an overall case fatality of 50% (including pre-hospital deaths), with 30% of survivors being left dependent, with major neurological deficits. In spite of many advances in diagnosis and treatment over the last decades, the case fatality rate has changed little, if at all.

Non-aneurysmal peri-mesencephalic haemorrhage is seen in 10% of cases and carries a good prognosis with less frequent neurological complications. The remaining 5% of cases are caused by rare conditions, including AVMs (including spinal AVMs), cerebral vasculitides, tumours, dural arteriovenous fistulae, dural sinus thrombosis, carotid or vertebral artery dissections, coagulopathy and drugs.

The annual incidence of SAH in the United Kingdom is approximately 10/100 000, increasing consistently with age until the sixth decade, with a peak incidence at 55–60 years. There are marked variations in the incidence of SAH worldwide. The incidence is lowest in the Middle East and highest in Japan, Australia and Scandinavia, especially in Finland where SAH incidence is around three times that of the rest of the world. The age-specific rates for SAH tend to be higher in those of Afro-Caribbean origin than Caucasian. There is female preponderance, with male : female ratio of around 1 : 1.8.

Risk factors

The risk of aneurysmal rupture depends on the size and location of the aneurysm. The International Study of Unruptured Intracranial Aneurysms (ISUIA) documented a 5-year cumulative rupture rate for all aneurysms of the anterior circulation (except posterior communicating [PCOM] artery aneurysms) of 0%, 2.6%, 14.5% and 40% if sized less than 7, 7–12, 13–24 and more than 25 mm, respectively. The same risks for posterior circulation and PCOM artery aneurysms were 2.5%, 14.5%, 18.4% and 50%, respectively.

Most cases of aneurysmal SAH are sporadic; however, there is considerable evidence to support the role of genetic factors in the development of intracranial aneurysms. There is a strong association between intracranial aneurysms and heritable connective tissue diseases, although these form a small proportion of any case load, in the order of 5%. These conditions include autosomal dominant polycystic kidney disease, Marfan's syndrome, pseudoxanthoma elasticum, Ehlers–Danlos syndrome and α_1-antitrypsin deficiency. Familial intracranial aneurysms account for 7–20% of patients with aneurysmal SAH. Approximately one-third of asymptomatic members of affected families will have evidence of intracranial aneurysms on angiography. In a study of 8680 individuals, the prevalence of asymptomatic aneurysms in the subgroups with and without a family history was 10.5% and 6.8%, respectively. The relative risk of siblings of SAH patients having a haemorrhage is six times that of the general population, with a threefold increased risk in parents – an overall fourfold increased risk in first degree relatives. Familial aneurysms tend to rupture at a smaller size than sporadic cases and often display genetic anticipation, with haemorrhages occurring at progressively younger ages in successive generations. The occurrence of aneurysms at identical and/or mirror sites is more frequent in familial cases and appears to be a function of the degree of kinship between affected individuals.

Environmental factors have been extensively studied and cigarette smoking is the only factor consistently identified, raising the risk 3–10 times that of non-smokers. This also appears to be a dose-dependent effect. The SAH risk decreases with the number of years since giving up smoking, with excess risk largely disappearing 2–4 years after cessation of smoking. Hypertension is almost certainly important but to a lesser degree, although there is conflicting evidence over its role as it is a common co-morbid condition. It seems that hypertension and smoking act as synergistic risk factors. The risk of SAH in hypertensive smokers is nearly 15 times that in the non-smoking non-hypertensive population. There is a strong temporal association between snorting cocaine (and other methods of ingestion) and both haemorrhagic and ischaemic cerebrovascular events. The use of sympathomimetic drugs, such as cocaine and methamphetamine, tend to increase the incidence and decrease the age at which aneurysmal rupture occurs; aneurysmal size at rupture also tends to be smaller.

Clinical features

The cardinal clinical feature is the sudden onset of a thunderclap headache. Headache is present in the majority of patients. This is usually of unique severity and sudden onset and is often accompanied by nausea and vomiting (77%). Thunderclap headache, although a cardinal feature, is non-specific and only 1 in 10 of those presenting with a sudden explosive headache will turn out to have had an SAH. There are no highly reliable features from the history that distinguish benign thunderclap headache from SAH. Exceptionally, bacterial meningitis can present with SAH.

Signs of global or focal dysfunction may be found depending on the severity and location of SAH. Consciousness is frequently altered, with confusion and lethargy in 30%, transient loss of consciousness in one-third and coma in 17%. In these patients, a history of headache may be lacking. Signs of meningeal irritation are found in most but not all patients and it is a common error for these either not to be elicited or misinterpreted in patients with acute headache. Neurological abnormalities are seen in 64% of cases with focal signs such as hemiparesis, IIIrd or VIth nerve palsies in 21%. Focal deficits may be caused by intraparenchymal extension of blood or later by vasospasm with resultant ischaemia and infarction.

Symptoms do sometimes help to localise the aneurysm. Anterior communicating artery (ACOM) aneurysms may present with frontal symptoms (bilateral lower-limb weakness, bilateral extensor plantars, incontinence and abulia) and electrolyte disturbance is not uncommon. Both anterior choroidal (although uncommon) and MCA aneurysms may present with hemiparesis, aphasia or visuospatial neglect, while peri-callosal artery and distal ACA aneurysms present with a contralateral lower-limb monoparesis. A IIIrd nerve palsy suggests an aneurysm of the PCOM artery (Figure 5.17), or less commonly of the superior cerebellar artery. A painful pupil-involving IIIrd nerve palsy is usually a warning of potential imminent rupture of a PCOM artery aneurysm and should be investigated without delay.

Retinal and preretinal (subhyaloid) haemorrhages are seen in 25% of SAH patients. There are three types of haemorrhage that can occur alone or in combination with SAH:

1. Retinal haemorrhages may surround the fovea.
2. Subhyaloid preretinal haemorrhages are seen in 11–33% of cases as bright-red blood near the optic disc.
3. Terson's syndrome, consisting of haemorrhage within the vitreous humour, occurs in approximately 4% of SAH cases and usually bilaterally (Figure 5.18).

Subhyaloid and vitreous haemorrhages are associated with a high mortality rate. Patients with Terson's syndrome who survive should

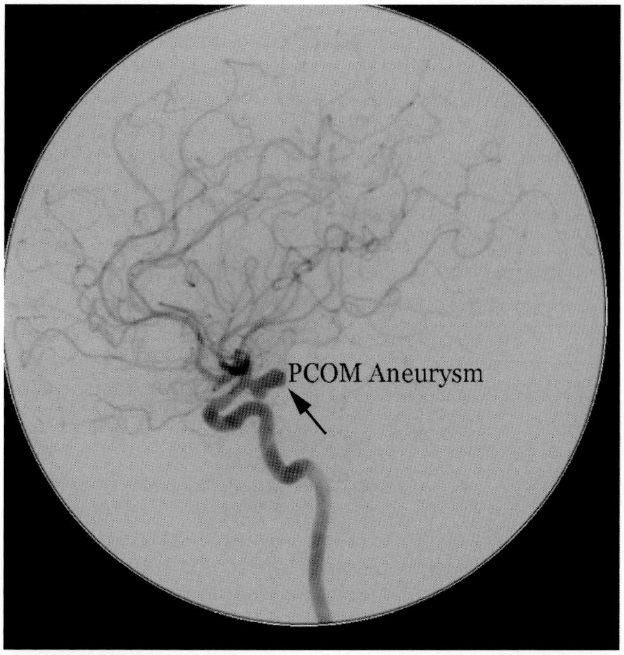

Figure 5.17 Large bi-lobed posterior communicating (PCOM) artery aneurysm (catheter angiogram).

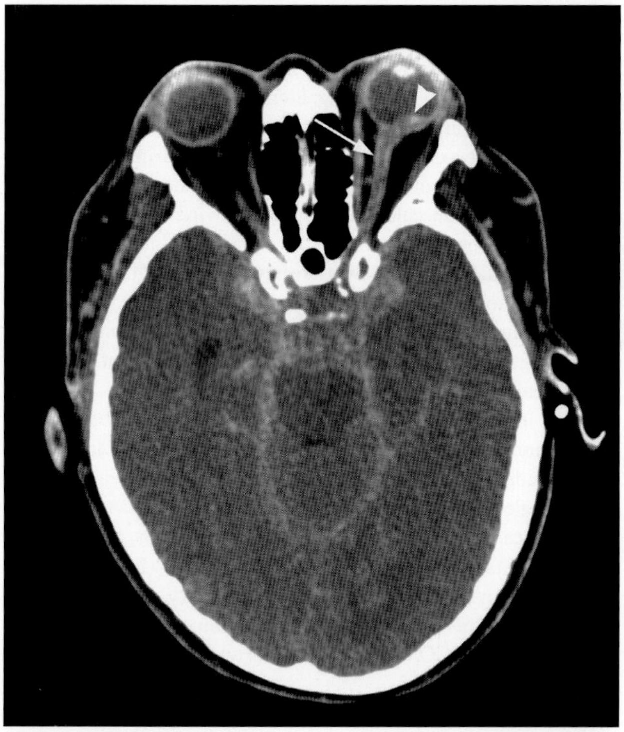

Figure 5.18 Terson's syndrome: CT of a patient with a subhyaloid haematoma (arrowhead) following extensive subarachnoid haemorrhage (Terson's syndrome). Blood is also seen tracking along the optic nerve sheath (white arrow).

be followed for the long-term complications of raised intra-ocular pressure and for retinal detachment.

Many retrospective studies comment on unusual or acute headaches predating the definite SAH by several days to weeks. These headaches have been thought to represent warning leaks, intramural haemorrhage or aneurysmal enlargement and are sometimes called sentinel headaches. This may occasionally be the case. An alternative explanation is recall bias. A prospective study examining 148 patients with sudden onset headaches of thunderclap type showed that only 25% went on to SAH. Of these SAH patients, only two could recall a similar headache previously.

SAH tends to be misdiagnosed – as migraine or benign acute headache syndrome – typically when the headache is not catastrophic in severity, but simply sudden. Some of these SAH cases remain ambulant – and in these low back pain and sciatica resulting from local irritation by blood products can develop within 4–10 days of the haemorrhage. At the other end of the spectrum a small proportion of SAH cases are found dead, or are seen to die rapidly, within minutes or hours from massive haemorrhage.

Investigation

CT is mandatory in those with suspected SAH, generally revealing diffuse blood of a symmetrical distribution around the basal cisterns, Sylvian fissures and cortical sulci (Figure 5.19). Modern generation CT will demonstrate the presence of blood in 95% of patients scanned within 48 hours. However, blood is rapidly cleared from the cerebrospinal fluid (CSF) and the CT pick-up rate gradually decreases to 80% at 3 days, 50% at 1 week and 30% at 2 weeks. When asymmetrical or localised, the distribution of blood may suggest the location of the aneurysm in up to 70%. This is particularly important in the 10–15% of patients who harbour multiple aneurysms, when it may help to guide intervention towards the aneurysm that has bled. Intraventricular haemorrhage is characteristic of ruptured ACOM artery aneurysms; intracerebral haemorrhage is most commonly seen with PCOM artery and MCA aneurysms. Head CT can also demonstrate hydrocephalus, cerebral ischaemia or infarction, midline shift or a rebleed.

If clinical suspicion is strong and the CT is normal, lumbar puncture preferably by an experienced operator should be performed assuming there are no contraindications. If clinically appropriate this should be delayed for 12 hours from the ictus to allow time for xanthochromia (yellow discoloration) to develop. Xanthochromia of the supernatant, which is positive in almost all SAH patients between 12 hours and 2 weeks, is diagnostic. This must be determined by spectrophotometry rather than visual inspection. Negative CSF is very helpful in excluding SAH but bloodstained CSF may result from a traumatic tap. A decrease in the number of red cells from bottles one to three is a very unreliable way of supporting a traumatic tap instead of SAH. It should be remembered that patients may have had both SAH and a traumatic tap.

Conventional MRI is not sensitive to acute haemorrhage as there is too little methaemoglobin for haemorrhage to be easily differentiated from CSF. Visualisation of blood products by MRI improves over 4–7 days following SAH. MRI is therefore excellent for demonstrating subacute and previous SAH, when the diagnostic yield from CT falls.

In patients with either diagnostic CT and/or lumbar puncture, or when results of these tests are equivocal, some form of arterial imaging is necessary to search for a ruptured aneurysm or other lesion. Digital subtraction angiography (DSA) has been the gold standard investigation until recently, but non-invasive alternatives, including CT and MR angiography, are gaining popularity. DSA should demonstrate the aneurysmal site, type, size, orientation,

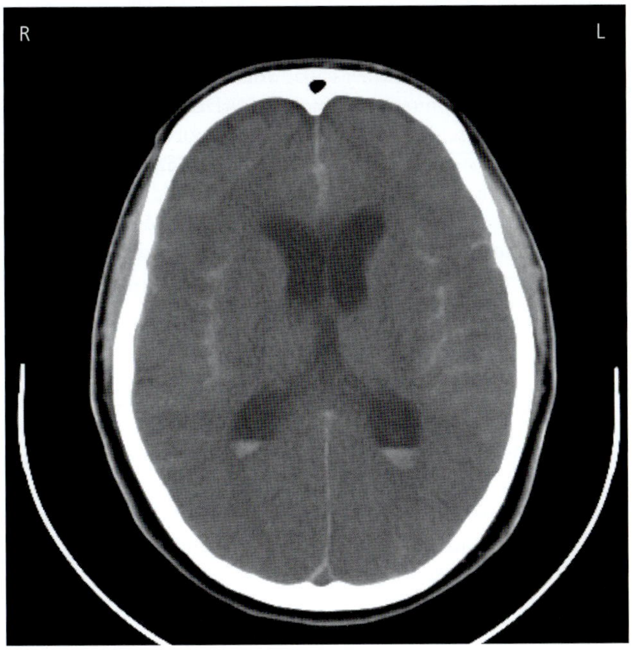

Figure 5.19 Unenhanced CT showing diffuse subarachnoid and intraventricular blood.

neck intraluminal calcification and thrombus, the relationship between aneurysm and parent vessel, collateral flow through the circle of Willis, the presence of adjacent perforators and the state of the cerebral vasculature, including other aneurysms. In the case of multiple aneurysms, identification of the ruptured lesion may be difficult. The distribution of blood and location of any focal intraparenchymal haematoma on CT are more useful for identification. In situations where the CT reveals diffuse blood or the haemorrhage had been diagnosed on lumbar puncture, and multiple aneurysms are found subsequently, the aneurysm most likely to have ruptured is usually the largest, has greater irregularity, mass effect or associated local vasospasm.

Recent advances in three-dimensional CT angiography have meant that it now has a sensitivity and specificity approaching that of percutaneous catheter angiography (sensitivity 77–97% and specificity 87–100%). Imaging time is significantly reduced, allowing acquisition of the entire CT volume in 30–45 seconds during the first arterial pass of an intravenous contrast injection, with minimal patient movement artefact. Its non-invasive nature may obviate the need for cerebral angiography with its inherent risks, at least as a first line investigation. MR angiography also reveals most aneurysms greater than 3 mm in diameter. The sensitivity of MR angiography for identification of aneurysms is 85–90%, with a specificity greater than 90% when compared with DSA as the gold standard, with an excellent intra-observer consistency and good-to-excellent inter-observer reproducibility. However, MRI times are significantly longer than CT. This is particularly relevant in this group of patients who are often in great pain and restless.

Despite thorough investigation, 10–15% of SAH cases have a normal angiogram. Of these, 65% will have a distinctive pattern of subarachnoid blood lying in the prepontine or peri-mesencephalic cisterns. These patients tend to be younger, non-hypertensive, of better clinical grade and more often male than SAH patients with angiograms positive for aneurysms. The aetiology of the SAH in these cases is unclear but the cause may be venous haemorrhage. The overall prognosis tends to be good, partly because rebleeding is rare and few patients develop delayed ischaemic deficit. However, the diagnosis should only be entertained with caution as 10% of vertebrobasilar aneurysms present with a similar distribution of blood. Repeat imaging should be considered carefully because these aneurysms can be obscured by vasospasm, hypoperfusion, poor angiographic technique or thrombosis. Such re-imaging at 2–4 weeks finds previously undetected aneurysms in 2–5% in these cases.

Initial management

General supportive care should be instituted. Stabilisation of the patient, with optimisation for aneurysm treatment, together with prevention of secondary cerebral insults is achieved by ensuring adequate ventilation and oxygenation, normovolaemia and haemodynamic stability and control of intracranial pressure. Frequent neurological examination is required in order to identify any neurological deterioration requiring further investigation or management.

Bed rest is generally recommended until aneurysm treatment is undertaken. Aspirin should be stopped, if it is being taken. Nimodipine, a calcium-channel antagonist, has been shown to reduce the risk of cerebral infarction by 34% and as a result, poor outcome following SAH by 40%. An oral dosage of 60 mg 4-hourly is currently used. With a ruptured aneurysm prior to surgery or coiling, gentle volume expansion with slight haemodilution may help to return the circulating volume to normal and prevent or minimise the effects of vasospasm; however, hypertension should be avoided. Once the aneurysm has been secured, hypertension is allowed (see later), but there is no agreement on the safe range. Hyperglycaemia and hyperthermia are both associated with a poor outcome and should therefore be corrected. These problems are more often seen in poor grade patients, and their effect on outcome may therefore not be independent of presenting clinical condition. Analgesia is often required.

Aneurysm treatment

Currently, the two main treatment options for securing an aneurysm are microvascular neurosurgical clipping and endovascular coiling. Traditionally, craniotomy and clipping has been the method preferred, although the optimum timing of surgery has been debated. The rebleeding rate from aneurysms is particularly high during the first 2 weeks, and then declines. This early high rebleed rate, which may have devastating complications, together with more recent improvements in microsurgical techniques, is the reason why early intervention is generally favoured. Securing the aneurysm will also facilitate the treatment of complications such as cerebral vasospasm. The Guglielmi Detachable Coil (GDC) has been available since 1991 and has been increasingly used in clinical practice. Detachable platinum coils are delivered endovascularly into the aneurysm. Once the correct position within the aneurysm has been achieved, the coil is detached from the wire. Multiple coils of various lengths and thicknesses are often packed into the aneurysm to exclude it from the circulation. The results of the International Subarachnoid Aneurysm Trial (ISAT) showed that patients treated by endovascular means have a 24% better chance of survival, free of disability, at 1 year than those treated surgically. The risk of epilepsy was substantially lower in patients who underwent endovascular coiling, but the risk of rebleeding was slightly higher. Also, in patients who underwent cerebral angiography, the rate of complete occlusion of the aneurysm was greater with surgical clipping. ISAT was a landmark study that validated the technique of endovascular coiling in patients suitable for either treatment method. However, many aneurysms are not equally suitable for either microsurgical clipping or endovascular coiling. In individual cases, several factors – such as patient's age, and overall medical condition and the aneurysm's location, size, morphology and relationship to adjacent vessels – need to be analysed by a multidisciplinary team to decide on the most appropriate treatment.

Management of complications

Neurological complications are common and include symptomatic vasospasm (46%), hydrocephalus (20%) and rebleeding (7%). Untreated, 15–20% of patients will rebleed in the first 2 weeks, carrying with it a significant mortality (50–75%) and risk of permanent neurological disability. There is an initial peak of rebleeding in the first 48 hours of approximately 4%, which rapidly plateaus to 1–2% per day until 40 days post-haemorrhage. After 6 months there is a long-term risk of further haemorrhage of 3% per year in patients whose aneurysm has not been excluded from the circulation. The risk of rebleed is increased with poor clinical grade, posterior circulation lesions, hypertension, elderly patients and abnormal clotting.

Cerebral vasospasm is multi-factorial in origin. The mechanisms include the liberation of spasmogenic metabolites during clot lysis in the basal cisterns and impairment of cerebral vasodilatation related to endothelial dysfunction and structural changes within the arterial wall. Symptomatic vasospasm, often leading to delayed ischaemic deficit, occurs in 20–30% of patients and is at its worst 3–14 days following the haemorrhage. The severity and distribution of vasospasm are related to the amount and site of subarachnoid blood. Basal subarachnoid blood tends to be a more important risk factor for vasospasm than intraventricular blood or diffuse blood over the cortex. Other predisposing factors include increasing age of the patient, high systolic blood pressure, poor clinical grade, decreased conscious level, the presence of a motor deficit or hydrocephalus, while patients with vertebral aneurysms, predominantly intraventricular haemorrhage or a negative CT, have a lower risk of developing symptomatic vasospasm. Diagnosis of vasospasm can be difficult and is often made after exclusion of other causes of neurological deterioration such as hydrocephalus, electrolyte disturbance, seizures or a rebleed. Elevated velocities on transcranial Doppler can be useful in confirming clinical suspicion. Once identified, patients are treated with hypervolaemia and induced hypertension in an attempt to improve cerebral blood flow. In those patients refractory to medical treatment, transluminal balloon angioplasty at the site of the most severe vasospasm, or vasodilator infusion (e.g. papaverine) can be used to improve both angiographic appearances and the patient's clinical condition.

Symptomatic hydrocephalus caused by diminished CSF absorption is seen in 10–35% of patients. Acutely, hydrocephalus is treated by a period of external ventricular drainage but, in the longer term, 10–15% of patients will require a permanent ventriculo-peritoneal shunt.

The highest risk of seizures is within the first 24 hours of initial bleeding, occurring at presentation in 3–18% of individuals. Epilepsy persists in 6–15% of survivors and is associated with intraparenchymal haematoma, vasospasm, MCA aneurysms, poor clinical grade, systemic hypertension, peri-operative complications, rebleed, early seizures, shunt-dependent hydrocephalus, neurological deficit and blood load.

The most common medical complications of SAH include pulmonary oedema in 23% (either cardiogenic or neurogenic), cardiac arrhythmias in 35% and electrolyte disturbances in 28% of patients. Hyponatraemia (Chapters 20 and 26), is caused either by cerebral salt-wasting, with low-intravascular volume, or the syndrome of inappropriate antidiuretic hormone (SIADH), with normal or increased intravascular volume; both, if left untreated, have a high morbidity and mortality. The distinction is important because cerebral salt-wasting is treated by aggressive fluid administration and sodium supplements, while treatment of SIADH involves fluid restriction. Fluid restriction of patients with cerebral salt wasting will worsen their hypovolaemia and will predispose them to vasospasm (Chapter 20).

Outcome

Pre-hospital mortality is 3–26%, with an overall mortality of 45–60% in the first 30 days following SAH. Overall morbidity is some 25–33%, caused in the majority of patients by vasospasm, although initial deficits and intervention also contribute. The major predictive factors for a poor outcome are level of consciousness on admission, age and amount of blood on presenting CT. More than 50% of survivors report problems with memory, mood or neuropsychological function. Despite this, half to two-thirds of patients surviving SAH are able to return to work 1 year after presentation. Prompt physical and neuropsychological assessment for rehabilitation are important. The recent National Confidential Enquiry Audit into the management of patients with SAH, shows significant improvements in care over the last decade but there are still ongoing issues with misdiagnosis of this patient group in primary and secondary care, delay and poor organisation of care transfers, and variability in radiological practice.

Arteriovenous malformations

Arteriovenous malformations (AVMs) form part of the larger group of structural cerebral vascular malformations (CVMs). Also included within this group of developmental vascular anomalies of the CNS are cavernous malformations, developmental venous anomalies and capillary telangiectasia. AVMs are characterised by a complex tangle of abnormal arteries and veins that lack a capillary bed but are linked either by one or more direct fistulas creating an arteriovenous shunt, or through a mass of dysplastic vessels within the nidus. Although considerably less common than intracranial aneurysms, with a prevalence of 0.14–0.5%, AVMs are an important cause of haemorrhage in patients under 40 years old. They are thought to arise from developmental derangements of the cerebral vascular system during the 40–80 mm stage of embryogenesis.

Presentation

Some 65% of individuals with AVMs present with haemorrhage at a peak age of 25–40 years. These figures may under-represent the true incidence of haemorrhage as clinically silent haemorrhage is diagnosed by imaging or at surgery in as many as 10% of patients: haemosiderin staining is seen surrounding the lesion. It has been postulated that episodes of acute headache, seizures or other acute neurological symptoms may also represent episodes of otherwise silent haemorrhages. Risk factors for haemorrhage include increasing age, previous haemorrhage (particularly in the preceding 12 months), deep site (basal ganglia and posterior fossa especially), small size, diffuse nidus, deep venous drainage, a single draining vein and associated aneurysms. Haemorrhage may be intracerebral, subarachnoid or intraventricular. Most supratentorial haemorrhages are lobar in location, but they also occur in the basal ganglia

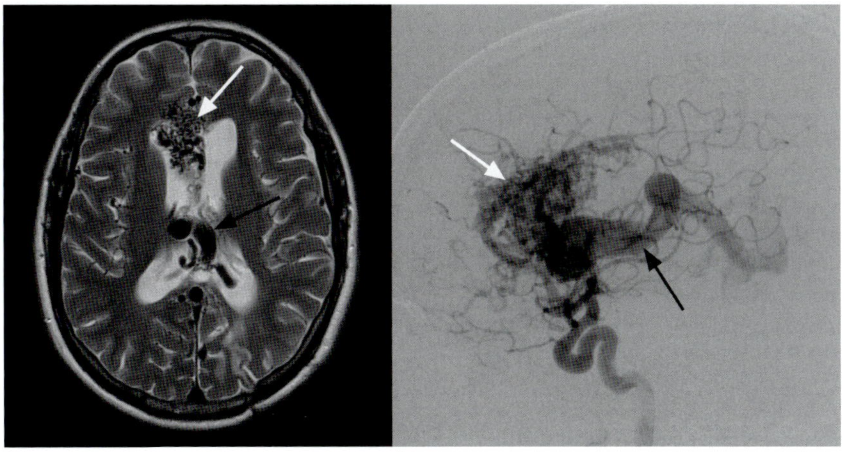

Figure 5.20 Arteriovenous malformation (AVM). (a) T2-w and (b) digital subtraction angiography (DSA) images of an arteriovenous malformation highlighting the nidus (white arrow) and dilated draining vein (black arrow).

or thalamus. In the posterior fossa, AVMs are the cause of most cerebellar haemorrhages in normotensive patients less than 40 years old. Pial-based AVMs may cause direct SAH. In most instances, however, SAH results from the rupture of an intraparenchymal bleed through the pial surface. In contrast to aneurysms, SAH from an AVM is rarely associated with vasospasm and recurrent haemorrhage within the first 2 weeks of AVM rupture occurs in only 1% of patients.

Alternative presenting symptoms in patients with AVMs include seizures in 20–30%, particularly if the lesion is large, involves the cortical surface or temporal lobe or there has been previous haemorrhage or surgery. Frontal lobe AVMs commonly present with generalised seizures, motor strip AVMs can cause Jacksonian seizures and medial temporal lobe AVMs are often associated with complex partial seizures. Patients may also present with non-haemorrhagic focal neurological symptoms. Most commonly seen in lesions within the MCA distribution, the focal symptoms are dependent on the location of the AVM. Large basal ganglia lesions may present with slowly progressive dementia, hemiparesis or visual field defect, while occasionally brainstem AVMs produce motor or sensory deficit with or without cranial nerve involvement, sometimes with patterns resembling multiple sclerosis. The cause of neurological deficit is often uncertain: recurrent haemorrhages, multiple micro-infarcts, decreased perfusion because of arterial stenoses, venous hypertension and steal phenomena have all been noted as mechanisms. Patients with AVMs often complain of headaches although, as a primary presentation, they are unusual (12%). Pain tends to be well localised, unilateral and throbbing and is often difficult to distinguish from other types of vascular headache or migraine. Headaches occur more frequently in AVMs that have a significant dural or pial component and despite treatment of the lesion, they often persist following treatment. Cranial bruits are present in as many as 25% of cases and again are more common with dural AVMs. With widespread MRI, many asymptomatic AVMs are now discovered coincidentally.

Natural history

Knowledge of the natural history of a disease is a prerequisite for evaluating the influence of any treatment on the course of that disease. This is especially true when the risks of therapy may be profound. Advances in treatment for AVMs are developing more rapidly than advances in our knowledge of their natural history. It has become increasingly difficult to identify large groups of untreated patients with AVMs for prospective study because of the availability of so many treatment options. Although it is possible to quote expected mortality and morbidity figures for AVMs on the basis of size, location and angioarchitecture, estimating the risks associated with a specific AVM is much more difficult. It is therefore important that the management of any patient with an AVM should be evaluated and planned carefully by an experienced multidisciplinary team of neurosurgeons, neuroradiologists and neurologists.

The treatment of AVMs is primarily intended to eradicate or lessen the risk of future haemorrhage. Untreated AVMs do have a significant risk of mortality and morbidity, most commonly associated with haemorrhage. In one prospective study, the annual mortality rate was 1% and that of severe morbidity 1.7%, these rates being constant over some 24 years. The long-term risk of AVM rupture for patients with symptomatic AVMs is estimated to be 2–3% per year. The risk appears higher in children and probably in those patients who have had a previous haemorrhage. Factors associated with AVM haemorrhage include small size, deep location, intranidal aneurysms, deep venous drainage and draining vein stenosis. A single haemorrhage is associated with 10–13% mortality and 30% serious morbidity. There is controversy whether or not treatment of high risk components within an incurable AVM (e.g. venous aneurysms) modifies the bleeding risk.

Management

In any patient where treatment is considered, MRI and formal angiography in expert hands is performed to define the angioarchitecture and to give precise anatomical localisation (Figure 5.20). This allows the risks of treatment or conservative management to be defined as accurately as possible. A variety of anatomical and physiological factors such as AVM size and location, number and distribution of arterial feeders, pattern of venous drainage and flow through the AVM nidus influence the technical difficulty and consequent risk of surgical, endovascular or radiosurgical treatment. The Spetzler–Martin AVM grading is commonly used (Table 5.12). This stratifies surgical risk specifically in association to the size,

Table 5.12 Example of surgical risks according to Spetzler–Martin grade.

Grade	No deficit (%)	Minor deficit (%)	Major deficit (%)
I	100	0	0
II	95	5	0
III	84	12	4
IV	73	20	7
V	69	19	12

venous drainage and eloquence of surrounding brain and is frequently used in this decision-making process.

Many factors influence whether or how an AVM should be treated including age and co-morbidity, presentation, AVM location, size, morphology and complexity, expected natural history and treatment risks. Management plans for these lesions should only be made by a multidisciplinary team that can balance risk of treatment against expected natural history. Following rupture of an AVM, the risk of early rebleeding is significantly lower than that observed in aneurysmal rupture. Consequently, AVM treatment should be considered carefully and can often be delayed to allow the patient to recover and undergo treatment under optimal conditions.

Treatment modalities include operative resection, endovascular embolisation and stereotactic radiosurgery, either alone or in combination. Surgical removal of an AVM is the most definitive treatment offering the best chance of lasting cure. Surgery for accessible lesions, particularly if small with single arterial supply and venous drainage, is the treatment of choice. Nevertheless, surgery carries significant mortality and morbidity. Patients should be carefully selected. Complete surgical resection should be confirmed by formal angiography postoperatively.

Endovascular embolisation of AVMs is a rapidly evolving technique. The present agent of choice is *N*-butyl cyano-acrylate (NCBA) which is a medical glue. It is successful in eradicating approximately 20% of lesions. Procedural risk can be high. Between 2% and 17% have major or minor morbidity and mortality is 1–4%. The overall risk of an ischaemic complication per procedure is around 10%. Inadvertent glue deposition in normal cerebral vessels can cause infarction. Catastrophic AVM rupture from glue placement in a draining vein (raising intranidal pressure) is also a significant complication. However, endovascular treatment can be an extremely useful adjunct to surgery and radiosurgery, by reducing blood flow and eliminating surgically inaccessible arterial feeders pre-operatively. Sequential endovascular treatments can incrementally reduce the size of an AVM, making it amenable to definitive surgical or radiosurgical treatment. In some patients, endovascular treatment is useful in palliation, particularly for refractory headaches or progressive neurological deficit. However, recanalisation of previously embolised segments can certainly occur in the long-term.

Stereotactic radiotherapy (Chapter 21), in particular LINAC or gamma knife radiosurgery can be used in selected patients to provide a single high dose of stereotactically localised radiation to the AVM nidus. The usual radiation dose is 20 Gy. This is administered to the margin of the nidus. This radiation causes endothelial damage, smooth muscle cell proliferation, progressive sclerosis and subsequent thrombosis of nidal vessels over time. The success of stereotactic radiosurgery depends on AVM size and radiation dose delivered. Several studies have demonstrated AVM obliteration in 80% with nidal size less than 2–3 cm diameter or 10 mL volume by 2 years. A small percentage will go on to thrombose between 24 and 36 months. The patient remains at risk of haemorrhage during this time. Delayed radiation injury, such as radiation necrosis of cortical tissue or cranial nerve palsy, is related to the radiation dose, volume treated, patient age and AVM flow characteristics. Radiation-induced tumours are very rare and generally occur many years after treatment. Radiation-related complications are correlated with the volume of normal brain tissue that receives greater than 12 Gy.

Conservative management (i.e. no intervention whatever) may be the best option in those patients with a low life-long risk of haemorrhage (e.g. asymptomatic older patients), given that all available treatment modalities have risks and the uncertainty about their benefits. Younger patients with a history of haemorrhage are now almost always offered some form of treatment. AVM cases should probably not take aspirin, nor probably non-steroidal anti-inflammatory drugs unless there is good reason. A recent trial into the benefits of interventional treatment in unruptured AVM's was suspended as a result of excess morbidity in the treatment arm, though this is not surprising given the low but cumulative risk of rupture. Many years follow-up will be needed to see there is a point at which the risk is reversed.

Cavernous malformations

Cavernous malformation (CM), also called cavernous angiomas, cavernomas or cavernous haemangiomas, have a prevalence around 0.5% in the population (Figure 5.21). A retrospective review of MRI scans reported a detection rate of 0.4–0.9%. They are uncommon in children and have a peak incidence in the fourth and fifth decades of life. Overall, they account for 10% of all symptomatic intracranial vascular abnormalities. They can be familial and are often multiple.

Grossly, CMs are well-circumscribed, lobulated, raspberry-like lesions that vary from a few millimetres to several centimetres in diameter. Microscopically, they consist of a tangle of intertwined cluster of sinusoidal vascular channels that have one layer of endothelial lining and a variable layer of fibrous adventitia. Radiological evidence of previous haemorrhage, usually silent, is common, and there is often thrombosis within the dilated venules.

CMs are commonly asymptomatic but they may present with seizures or haemorrhage. Occasionally there is a progressive development of a neurological deficit, most likely to be caused by recurrent small bleeds. The frequency of haemorrhage among those who present either incidentally or with seizures is 0.4–2% per year. Among those presenting with symptomatic haemorrhage, the annual recurrent risk of haemorrhage is higher: 4–5% in the subsequent year. The risk of haemorrhage does appear to be dependent on location; there is a higher risk associated with deep lesions – brainstem, cerebellum, thalamus and basal ganglia. CMs are most readily seen on MRI as a combination of high and low T1 and T2 signal with surrounding haemosiderin (Figure 5.21). They are angiographically occult.

Surgery is usually considered only in patients with multiple haemorrhagic episodes and sometimes in those with poorly controlled seizures. Most surgeons have a high threshold for advising surgery for CMs; but excision, even for those CMs in critical

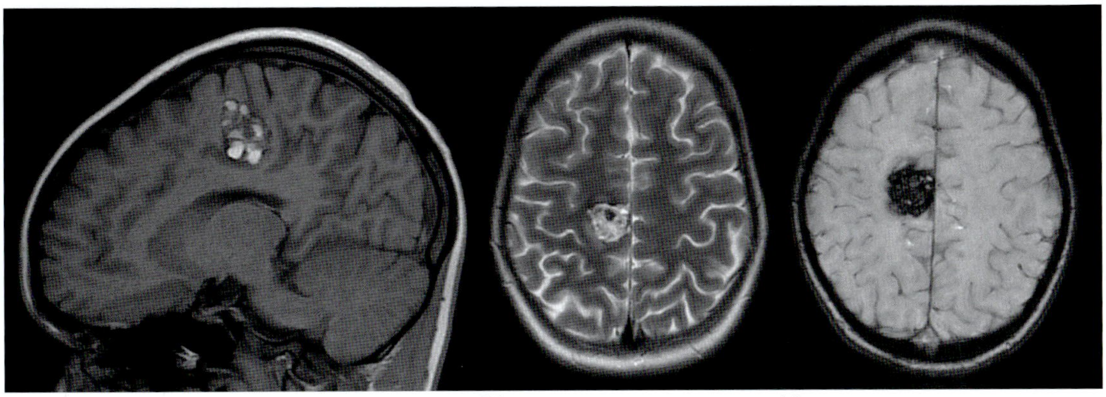

(a) (b) (c)

Figure 5.21 Cavernoma. From right to left: (a) T1 sagittal, (b) T2 axial and (c) susceptibility weighted (SWI) images showing a lobulated lesion in the right frontal lobe typical of a cavernoma. Note the central regions of T1 and T2 hyperintensity, hypointense margins and internal septations and marked hypointensity on SWI.

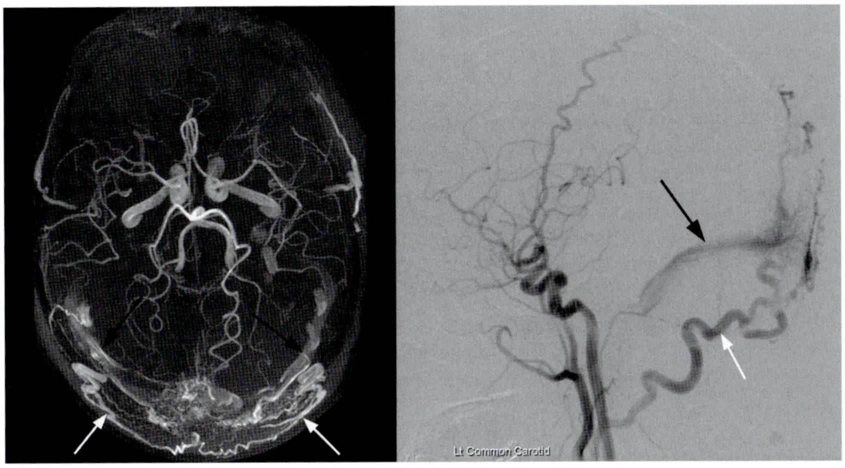

Figure 5.22 Dural fistula. Axial MRA and lateral common carotid digital subtraction angiography (DSA). Enlarged occipital arteries (white arrows) are seen contributing to the occipital arteriovenous fistula with shunting into the transverse sinuses (black arrows).

locations, often has an acceptable morbidity. Radiosurgery has also been carried out but it is unclear whether it alters the natural history. The concept that CMs tend to bleed in clusters supports the decision to treat CMs with stereotactic radiosurgery. Some studies suggest a reduced haemorrhage rate, usually after a 1–3 year latent period.

Dural fistulae

Dural arteriovenous fistulae (DAVF) are rare and can be found from adolescence to old age. They are most common in young adult women. They consist of an arteriovenous fistula with multiple arteries converging on a single venous structure. They are primarily fed by dural arteries but high-flow lesions can recruit pial branches. Different patterns of venous drainage are seen, for example drainage into a sinus with or without flow restriction or drainage into cortical veins either directly or by reflux from a venous sinus.

DAVFs are thought to be acquired lesions probably a result of venous thrombosis, usually silent, with development of collaterals. They may be located anywhere within the intracranial dura, although most are found adjacent to major dural venous sinuses, particularly the transverse sinus. Symptoms and signs differ greatly but are in the main caused by the pattern of venous drainage. Significant symptoms include haemorrhage, neurological deficit and intracranial hypertension. The overall risk of haemorrhage is approximately 2% per year; much depends on site and haemodynamics of the lesion. Rather than bleeding, common features are audible bruits, cranial nerve palsies and ocular signs such as papilloedema.

Head CT rarely detects a DAVF, although dilated veins may suggest its presence. MRI may demonstrate dilated feeding vessels and veins but is neither sensitive nor specific. Six vessel catheter angiography (i.e. including the external carotid arteries) is necessary to detect and delineate a fistula accurately and is the optimal investigation (Figure 5.22).

Treatment of DAVFs has evolved over the last three decades. Cortical venous drainage is a risk factor for haemorrhage. Action is required in these cases. Patients without cortical venous drainage and without threat of visual loss from papilloedema have a benign natural history and may require no therapy. Treatment of these patients is justified only if the risk of complication is low. Sometimes palliation is necessary. The primary treatment has been surgical disconnection of the fistula and resection of the dural segment and venous sinus. Not surprisingly, this carries a high risk of substantial blood loss and morbidity. Recently, there has been less emphasis on resection of the venous sinus. This has proved as effective as sinus resection and the risk of venous infarction is lower. Therapeutic embolisation can be used for either palliation or attempted cure. This can be achieved via transarterial and/and transvenous routes. DAVFs can also be treated with stereotactic radiosurgery with or without endovascular embolisation of accessible feeding vessels. Partial prior endovascular treatment aims to reduce the risk of haemorrhage prior to the later obliteration of the DAVF by stereotactic radiosurgery.

Investigation of stroke and TIAs

Stroke investigation is aimed at identifying risk factors and confirming or refuting the clinical diagnosis. Investigation nearly always improves the clinician's understanding of the pathophysiology of the stroke or transient ischaemic syndrome. This then guides acute treatment and secondary preventative measures. It is facile to separate completed stroke from TIAs when considering appropriate investigation. The aetiologic spectrum is identical, although management may be very different.

Basic investigations for all: simple tests

In all patients, basic blood screening should include full blood count to look for anaemia, polycythaemia, thrombocythaemia and thrombocytopenia. Polycythaemia is an important risk factor for stroke and care should be given to clarify marginal results. Anaemia of chronic disease may be a marker for endocarditis. Exceptionally, haematological malignancies may be complicated by stroke. Basic coagulation analysis should be undertaken in patients with haemorrhage and is especially important in those receiving anticoagulants or any other medication. Urea and electrolytes guide homeostatic management in the acute phase and may also reveal end-organ damage from hypertension. Patients with significant electrolyte disturbance may present with global or focal dysfunction. Plasma glucose is an essential triage test; diabetes is common and hypoglycaemia can cause focal signs. Hyperglycaemia is also associated with severe stroke. Rarely, hyperosmolar non-ketotic diabetic coma presents as a stroke. Basic lipid analysis for cholesterol and fasting triglycerides should be performed in all. Syphilis and HIV serology should be performed if the patient has been at risk at any time. Erythrocyte sedimentation rate (ESR) and C-reactive protein (CRP) are non-specific screening tests for inflammatory arterial disease and endocarditis. Serum proteins and immunoglobulins are necessary to exclude myeloma or other gammopathy. Multiple blood cultures and repeated urine examinations should be carried out if there any question of endocarditis. Thyroid function tests should be performed in all patients especially those with atrial fibrillation. In all patients, chest X-ray and electrocardiography (ECG) should also be carried out. The principal point of chest radiology is to establish the presence of a normal cardiac silhouette and look for consolidation. The ECG changes of note are left ventricular hypertrophy secondary to hypertension, previous or acute coronary syndrome (possible cardiogenic embolus) and, most importantly, atrial fibrillation or other unsuspected dysrhythmia.

Imaging

Neuroimaging is essential. Although MRI is greatly superior to CT, it is not currently widely available as a routine acute investigation. Initial CT is performed to distinguish infarction from haemorrhage or reveal mimics of the stroke syndrome such as tumour or subdural haematoma. In the early stages, depending partly on time interval, the size of infarction and the skill of the radiologist, CT may be negative. Only 50–70% of infarcts are ever visible with CT. It has become generally accepted that CT can diagnose a haemorrhage >0.5 cm accurately (i.e. exclude it) and indeed it is preferable to conventional MRI in the acute phase. However, patients with microhaemorrhage on susceptibility weighted MRI may present with minimal impairments when CT and conventional MRI are normal. The very early CT changes of stroke are subtle, but the ability to read these is crucial in making decisions about the suitability of a patient for thrombolysis. The very early stages of cytotoxic oedema in the MCA territory are indicated by loss of the insular ribbon, and effacement of the sulci with obscuration of the lentiform nucleus, shown in Figure 5.23. The evolution of CT changes following MCA infarction is shown in Figure 5.24.

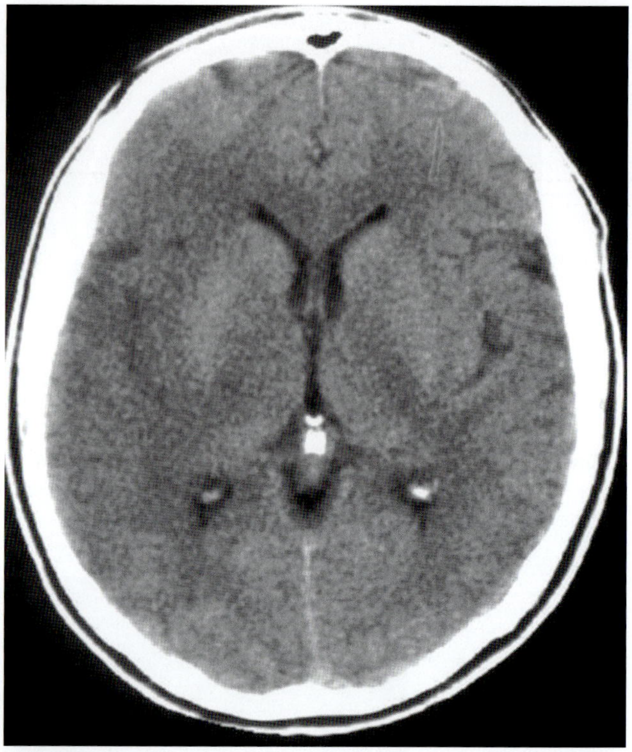

Figure 5.23 Early partial right hemisphere infarction on unenhanced CT following right MCA occlusion. There is effacement of right temporal sulci, obliteration of the Sylvian fissure, with slight hypoattenuation of the cortex, right temporal lobe and of the insula.

CT can indicate clearly large vessel occlusions (e.g. a dense outline of the MCA), pointing to a central cause for embolism, or multiple haematomas suggestive of amyloid angiopathy or vasculitis. The size of the infarct or haemorrhage will provide useful information relating to prognosis and the presence or likelihood of subsequent brain swelling. A small infarct in the territory of a lenticulo-striate penetrating vessel suggests a completed vascular syndrome, but if the anatomy suggested a more proximal MCA source then this would indicate the whole MCA territory is at risk. The role of CT in the diagnosis of SAH is discussed earlier.

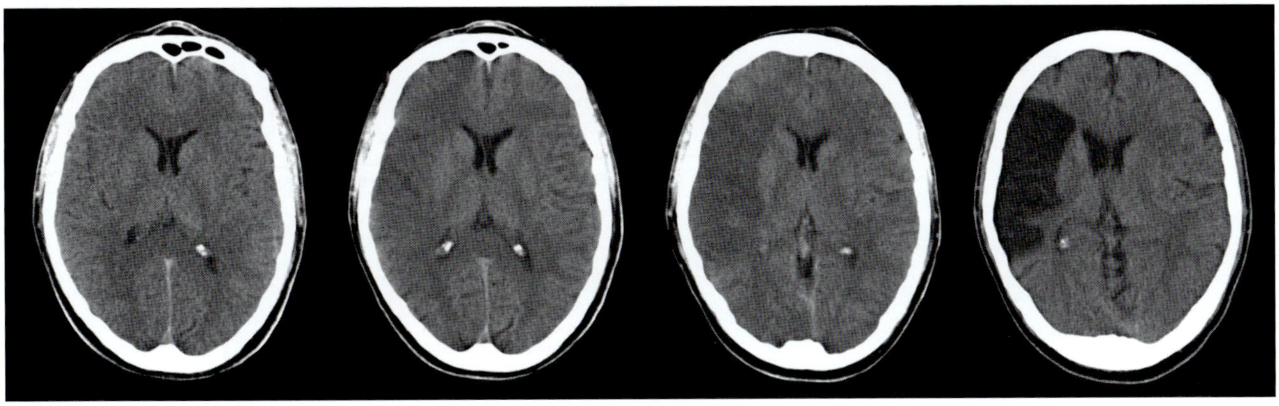

Figure 5.24 Evolving MCA infarct. Serial CT illustrating typical evolution of a right MCA infarct (from right to left: 3 years prior, day 1, day 2 and 3 months after symptom onset). The earliest features are loss of normal grey–white matter differentiation affecting the right insular ribbon and cortices of the adjacent frontal and temporal lobes with local sulcal effacement. On day 2 the infarct has a lower attenuation and is better defined with increased mass effect. After 3 months it has matured to encephalomalacia with associated volume loss and ex vacuo dilatation of the adjacent frontal horn.

MRI is a far more sensitive investigation than CT for both stroke and non-stroke pathology. It is especially superior in the posterior fossa and for revealing small areas of infarction secondary to penetrating vessel occlusion. Sophisticated multimodal imaging can also be used to distinguish acute from chronic infarction and may demonstrate microhaemorrhage. These techniques are likely to become critical to safe delivery of hyperacute treatments such as thrombolysis. MRI has high sensitivity to detect cerebral venous thrombosis and can be used in conjunction with MR angiography to detect dissections of the carotid and vertebral arteries. The two most useful MR sequences are diffusion weighted imaging and blood sensitive sequences such as T2* and susceptibility weighted imaging. Diffusion weighted imaging (DWI) maps the constant diffusion of water. This rapidly becomes abnormal after ischaemia returning a 'light bulb signal' indicative of restricted diffusion resulting from cytotoxic oedema. This usually indicates completed infarction but this is not absolute; some reversible diffusion changes have been demonstrated. Older infarcts may also appear bright on DWI ('T2 shine-through'), but these can be distinguished from acute infarcts by examining the apparent diffusion coefficient (ADC) images that show acute infarcts as dark. DWI can be matched with clinical examination, MR perfusion imaging and MR angiography to ascertain whether there are salvageable areas of brain. In addition, DWI commonly refines the pathophysiological diagnosis of stroke, by separating into time intervals different areas of infarction and demonstrating acute multi-territory changes suggestive of cardiac embolus, not apparent on conventional MRI.

MR susceptibility weighted sequences help demonstrate areas of microhaemorrhage not visible on conventional MR or CT. The distribution of these microhaemorrhages may point to amyloid (superficial location) or severe hypertensive arteriopathy (deep location). Patients with microhaemorrhage are at higher risk of primary intracerebral haemorrhage and have a more severe form of small vessel disease than those without haemorrhage.

In patients with haemorrhage in whom a non-hypertensive aetiology is suspected, it is necessary to exclude an AVM. In some this can be adequately achieved with MRI and/or MR angiography delayed until resolution of the haematoma. However, many such patients will require catheter angiography.

Conventional MR sequences are also useful in the diagnosis of cervical artery dissection (see carotid and vertebral dissection). MRI is sensitive and specific when used to image in cross-section the carotid artery from the bifurcation to the skull base. The vertebral artery is harder to image accurately and false positives are common and secondary to the vertebral venous plexus returning a 'dissection type' signal. Contrast enhanced MR angiography is also helpful here.

Whatever imaging modality is available, information derived should be used to build up the pathophysiological profile and to guide management. Most importantly, the imaging abnormalities must be concordant with the clinical picture. For example, the presence of acute or old infarction in non-symptomatic vascular territories should focus further investigation toward a central embolic source. Also, extensive asymptomatic small vessel disease is a risk factor for cerebral haemorrhage and helps refine a decision away from anticoagulation in a patient in atrial fibrillation.

Imaging also has a critical role in managing patients with stroke who may benefit from neurosurgical intervention. Imaging for stroke should happen at presentation as accurate diagnosis is a key component of a range of interventions that improve outcome. For pragmatic reasons in some services this has been delayed up to 24 hours. In all situations immediate (i.e. at 3 a.m.) imaging is recommended in a number of circumstances (Table 5.13).

Table 5.13 Recommendations for immediate imaging in stroke based on National Institute for Health and Care Excellence (NICE) guidance 2008.

Indications for thrombolysis or early anticoagulation treatment
On anticoagulant treatment
A known bleeding tendency
A depressed level of consciousness (Glasgow Coma Scale below 13)
Unexplained progressive or fluctuating symptoms
Papilloedema, neck stiffness or fever
Severe headache at onset of stroke symptoms

Source: National Institute for Health and Clinical Excellence 2008. Reproduced with permission of NICE.

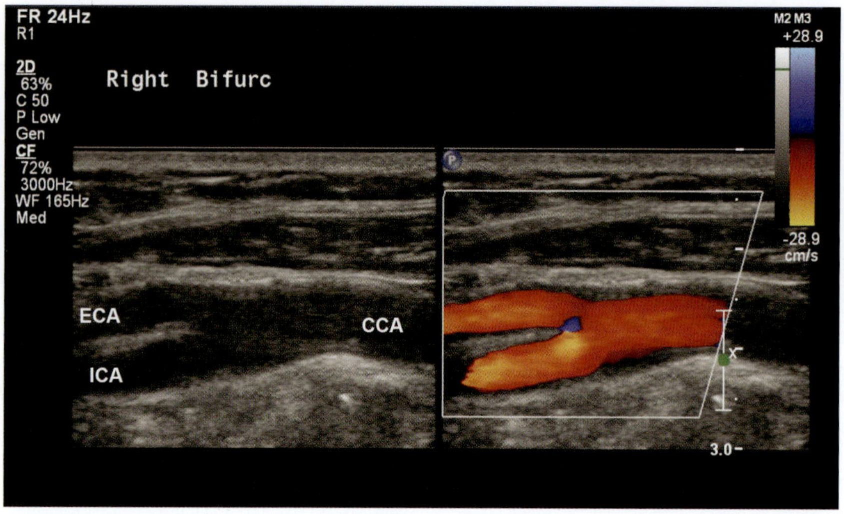

Figure 5.25 Carotid Doppler. Colour Doppler ultrasound image of a normal carotid artery bifurcation. The greyscale image on the left is labelled to show the common carotid (CCA), internal carotid (ICA) and external carotid (ECA) arteries. The colour Doppler image on the right demonstrates flow within the vessel, depicted red.

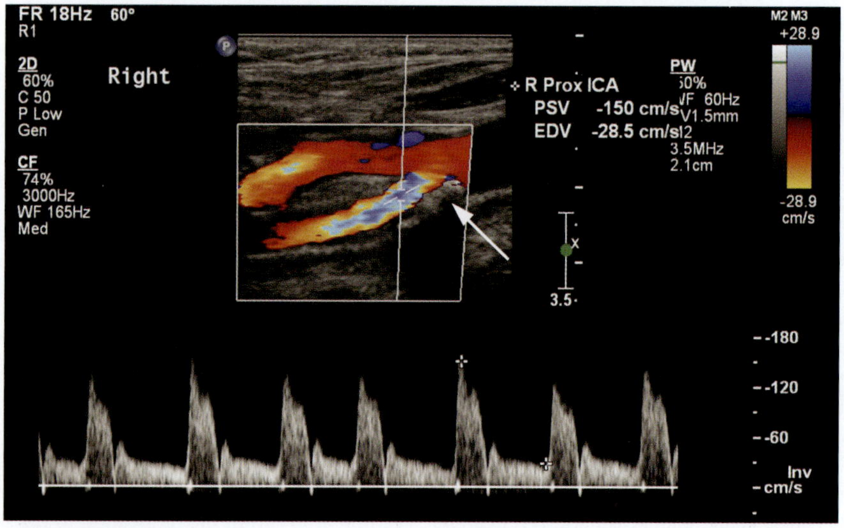

Figure 5.26 Carotid Doppler stenosis. Colour Doppler image showing stenosis of the internal carotid artery due to atheroma (arrow). Elevated peak systolic velocities of 150 cm/s are shown on the spectral trace below the colour image.

Many of these recommendations relate to the simple yet important principle that any patient with a depressed level of consciousness may need urgent neurosurgical intervention. One of the most important recommendations is that patients on anticoagulants should be imaged immediately.

Guided investigations following basic profile

Imaging, simple tests and the clinical profile should build up the pathophysiological diagnosis sufficiently to direct further investigation. Ischaemic stroke within the carotid territory should prompt the search for carotid stenosis. This is obviously essential in those in whom secondary preventative surgery would be considered. The emphasis is on non-invasive imaging, in preference to invasive techniques such as catheter angiography. MR angiography, CT angiography and duplex imaging are all useful. If any of these is completely normal then the screen is adequate with regard to stenosis at the carotid bifurcation. If any suggests carotid stenosis greater than 50% or occlusion then it is very useful to carry out a confirmatory non-invasive test. If they are concordant one can assume that the information is accurate. In patients in whom the information is non-concordant it may be necessary to perform a third non-invasive modality before formal catheter angiography. It should be appreciated that catheter angiography carries the risk of causing stroke, fatal or severely debilitating, especially in those with severe atherosclerosis, and it has other hazards (see later).

Ultrasound of the neck vessels in real time 'B' mode provides images in several arterial planes, as well as allowing measurement of blood flow velocity and wave patterns by utilising the Doppler shift (Figure 5.25 and Figure 5.26). It is accurate in experienced hands, at the carotid bifurcation, the major area of interest in patients with carotid territory stroke or TIA. It has a good sensitivity and specificity for occlusive lesions, but has limitations. It only visualises the mid-cervical portions of the carotid and vertebral arteries. It is not possible to see the distal internal carotid artery, although distal stenosis can be suspected from changes in spectral patterns. Often the vertebral origin is difficult to image and small clots, localised dissection and ulcers are difficult to image at any site. Calcification may obscure the visualisation of a stenosis. Arteries may be misidentified. For example, a carotid occlusion may be reported as trickle flow by mistaking a small branch of the cervical artery for the carotid. The combination is better than either alone. B-mode imaging allows individual arteries to be identified and provides information about the arterial wall (e.g. intimal-media thickness or composition of an area of atherosclerosis). Duplex can highlight areas of stenosis by combining B mode imaging with colour-flow. The severity of the stenosis of an artery above a certain threshold can then be determined from increases peak systolic and diastolic blood flow velocity measured by analysis of the Doppler signal. Duplex is widely available and non-invasive but there are some difficulties. It is operator dependent and requires considerable experience. It is not completely sensitive or specific for high-grade stenosis and does not always correlate with measurements of stenosis made by angiography.

Doppler can also be applied transcranially (TCD) through the temporal 'window' and the foramen magnum and has significantly advanced the study of stroke. TCD can accurately detect atherosclerotic lesions in the intracranial ICA, MCA, intracranial vertebral artery and the mid and proximal basilar artery. TCD may be used to detect emboli, acutely image intracranial vessel thrombosis and in some centres it has been used in combination with thrombolysis as a mechanical aid to clot dissolution. TCD may also be used to detect systemic right to left shunts (e.g. through a PFO). Agitated saline can be injected into a vein and the MCA insonated for arrival of small bubbles with a Valsalva manoeuvre.

Another safe sensitive non-invasive technique is MR angiography (MRA). MRA can accurately visualise the carotid bifurcation but may overestimate the degree of stenosis. MRA of the vertebral origin from the subclavian is subject to artefact in many cases, but the portions of the vertebral artery within the neck and within the intravertebral foramina are well shown. MRA of the intracranial circulation is providing a useful screening tool both for aneurysms and occlusive disease.

CT angiography (CTA) is rapidly taking over as a primary vascular imaging technique at admission of a patient to hospital. It is rapid and can be obtained at the time of emergency initial imaging. This aids immediate decisions with regard to acute treatments and is an accurate technique to detect acute intracranial occlusion by thrombus and is also sensitive to underlying stenosis throughout the cervical and intracranial vessels, including the vertebral artery not well seen on Duplex imaging. CTA has a sensitivity of 92–100% in the diagnosis of intracranial stenosis when compared with catheter angiography, and is a very accurate method for the detection of severe carotid atheroma, dissection and occlusion. CTA requires a significant contrast dose and hence impaired renal function is a relative contraindication.

The advent of MRA, CTA and duplex has led to a steady decrease in the indications for catheter angiography but this technique is still useful in selected circumstances. Intra-arterial angiography carries a small but definite risk of causing a stroke. The commonly quoted figure is 1% but inexperienced operators have a higher risk. The catheter or contrast can dissect the femoral artery and/or cause 'trash foot' as a result of dislodging aortic or arterial atheroma. Contrast medium can occasionally precipitate renal failure

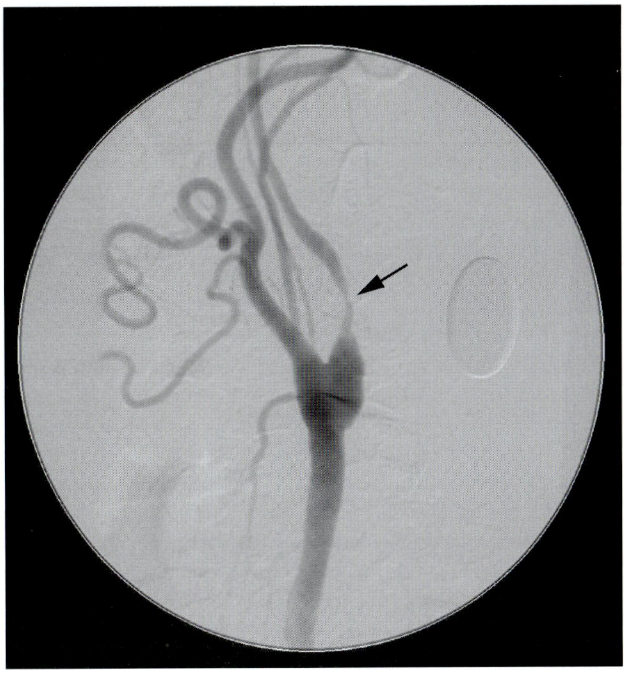

Figure 5.27 Severe left internal carotid artery stenosis (catheter angiogram).

and provoke allergic reactions. Some patients develop alarming but usually temporary blindness after vertebral injections. The decision for angiography should be made carefully in a multidisciplinary setting. The non-invasive tests must have been carried out first and usually a therapeutic decision must follow catheter angiography if this is to be performed. It is necessary to perform angiography in a number of vascular situations. In occlusive carotid disease, angiography may clarify discordant results from non-invasive tests (e.g. MRA suggests a 90% stenosis but duplex 50%). It may clarify sites not visible on non-invasive testing or subject to artefact (Figure 5.27). Catheter angiography is able to detect smaller aneurysms than MRA and is necessary following SAH when MRA is negative. It can be used to screen for underlying vascular malformations when MRI and MRA are normal and is often the only way of detecting dural fistulae. Despite the sophistication of MR venography, the venous phase of a catheter angiogram is superior and can clarify anatomic variants less clearly interpretable on MR. Currently, as CT angiography continues to improve it is taking over from catheter angiography in an increasing number of cases.

The degree of carotid stenosis is defined currently by three different methods and it is important to know which method is being discussed as the values differ; so does the evidence on which intervention is based. All three methods measure the diameter of the stenosis at the site of the maximal narrowing of the artery but the proportional stenosis that they produce is then calculated from different estimates of what the normal artery should have measured at that point, as the denominator. The European Carotid Surgery Trial (ECST) method used an estimate of the normal luminal diameter at the site of stenosis. In the North American Symptomatic Carotid Endarterectomy Trial (NASCET) it is based on comparison with the distal internal carotid artery diameter. In the common carotid method, it is based on the common carotid diameter. These produce different measurements. The NASCET method produces a lower percentage stenosis than the ECST or common carotid methods for the same lesion at the carotid bifurcation.

Both CT and MR can be also be used to measure regional cerebral perfusion after injection of contrast agents, as can PET and SPECT after injection of radioisotopes, while the newer technique of MR arterial spin labelling can be used to measure cerebral blood flow without using injected contrast. However, none of these techniques have entered routine practice except in a small number of enthusiastic units. The use of these techniques in selecting patients for therapy is discussed later.

Cardiac investigations

In patients with suspected cardiogenic embolus, transthoracic echocardiography can define wall motion abnormalities or the presence of atrial or ventricular thrombus. In selected patients with prosthetic valves, suspected aortic root disease and right to left shunts TOE provides better visualisation than the transthoracic mode. If cardiogenic embolus is still strongly suspected despite normal chest X-ray, ECG and echocardiogram, then sometimes Holter monitoring may be useful to reveal paroxysmal atrial fibrillation; monitoring may need to be prolonged and implantable rhythm monitoring devices are increasingly being used to pick up infrequent episodes of paroxysmal atrial fibrillation. Echocardiography has a high yield in patients with known cardiac disease, with systemic embolic phenomena and when the stroke pathophysiology points to cardiac embolism (e.g. PCA occlusion). TOE is undoubtedly superior to transthoracic insonation, particularly as the left atrium is directly anterior to the oesophagus. TOE also visualises the proximal aorta (e.g. for atherosclerosis). If previous blood cultures have been negative, consider repeating them to exclude bacterial endocarditis.

Special investigations

Thrombophilia assessment is rarely useful in arterial stroke with the exception of antiphospholipid antibodies. It should be noted that antiphospholipid antibodies can be associated with many sorts of vasculopathy and they are not uncommonly seen coincidentally in patients with atherosclerosis. Venous thrombophilia may be relevant in the rare circumstance of a positive family history of thrombosis associated with embolic stroke through a PFO. Autoantibodies may mark a systemic vasculitis. In appropriate circumstances, screening for common mitochondrial and NOTCH III (CADASIL) mutations, leukocyte galactosidase A for Fabry's disease, homocysteine, syphilis and HIV serology should be carried out. Very occasionally, if a vasculitic or an infective aetiology is suspected it will be necessary to examine the CSF. Urine toxicology screening should be carried out if drug misuse is suspected.

Management of acute stroke

Over the last two decades, stroke has changed from being seen as untreatable, to a condition where there is now a range of options for acute interventions, shown conclusively to improve outcome. In the first few hours after ischaemic stroke, measures are designed to restore blood flow (reperfusion), preserve the ischaemic penumbra (neuroprotection) and prevent early recurrence (antiplatelet treatment). Admission to a stroke unit and multidisciplinary rehabilitation are vitally important and are complementary to medical treatments. It is now well-recognised that rehabilitation should start as soon as possible after onset of stroke (Chapter 18), aiming to optimise recovery, enhance neural plasticity and facilitate functional adaptation to any residual impairments as far as possible. Active rehabilitation consists of measures designed to facilitate and enhance recovery from impairments, such as task specific training and measures to improve independence (e.g. the provision of walking aids or modified utensils). Key to successful rehabilitation requires the setting of achievable goals as in any learning or relearning exercise. Successful stroke unit care also pays critical attention to the prevention of complications and the prevention of recurrent stroke.

An early accurate diagnosis of the underlying pathological cause and mechanism of stroke should have been made to guide appropriate therapy. At the most basic level it is essential to distinguish between haemorrhage and infarction by brain scanning. Therefore, CT or MRI scan should be performed immediately on admission of the patient to hospital. The more that is understood about the pathophysiology of the stroke at admission, the more the effectiveness of the interventions. Some initial supportive treatment remains generic (e.g. assessment of swallowing and prevention of aspiration). If initial treatments are given without clear knowledge of the underlying pathology, apart from the distinction between haemorrhage and infarction, then it should be borne in mind that interventions such as thrombolysis, designed to lyse a clot, are unlikely to be effective if the cause of ischaemia is arterial occlusion by atheromatous debris or a dissecting haematoma. On the other hand, identification of the mechanism of stroke may lead to specific therapies (e.g. antibiotics for bacterial endocarditis or intra-arterial clot retrieval), in addition to more generic treatments.

Organised care in a stroke unit

One of the most important aspects of stroke treatment is quite simple. It is to treat patients in an organised stroke unit. The trials of stroke unit care show that about 1 in 12 patients are saved from death or being dependent by being cared for on an organised stroke unit rather than in a general medical ward. The same benefits cannot be achieved by providing a mobile stroke team visiting general medical wards in hospital, nor by visiting patients in their own homes. More patients are discharged from stroke units to their own homes without increasing average length of stay. The benefits of stroke unit care appear to apply equally to elderly and young patients, to both genders and irrespective of whether the stroke is mild, moderate or severe. All patients should therefore be admitted to an acute stroke unit as soon as possible after onset, irrespective of age, gender or clinical severity, for multidisciplinary assessment and treatment. It is likely that all patients benefit from the provision of information, the positive attitudes to stroke and the organised provision of care on an organised stroke unit. From a public health perspective, the benefits of stroke unit care arising from the overall prevention of death, reduction in disability and need for institutional care are considerable when compared with individual pharmacological treatments. Also, organised stroke care is unlikely to harm anyone.

The reasons why organised stroke care benefits patients are complex. Factors identified that characterise stroke unit as opposed to general medical ward care (e.g. a discrete geographical area, multidisciplinary team meetings) are to some extent epiphenomena of a more fundamental difference. This simply is having an effective team that has ownership of the patient's problems and a responsibility to address them. The complex problems of patients with stroke go far beyond the strict medical issues and cannot be effectively addressed by a disjointed approach. It is likely that the benefits from organised care result first from better care of the acute patient (e.g. accurate diagnosis, appropriate use of drugs, prevention of swallowing complications/hypoxia/hypovolaemia, appropriate treatment of pyrexia, hyperglycaemia) leading to less secondary brain damage. Secondly, coordinated goal-orientated rehabilitation and discharge planning is a totally different proposition to more fragmented delivery of rehabilitation. Patients with intracerebral haematomas often gain considerably and as much from organised care as patients with ischaemic stroke. In contrast to ischaemic stroke, they take much longer to start to recover and need careful supportive care during this time.

The benefits of stroke unit care in the randomised trials were maximal when patients were admitted within a week of onset. The benefits are likely to be even greater where patients are admitted acutely for monitoring and provision of acute treatment such as thrombolysis. This has been recently evidenced by health reforms in London, UK, where new regional hyperacute stroke units (HASUs) were commissioned in 2010 to provide immediate 'hyperacute' care for the first 1–2 days after stroke. These large units allowed a critical mass of staffing, expertise and infrastructure to be available and responsive 24/7. The units have produced a considerable decrease in mortality following stroke and a considerable increase in the delivery of intravenous thrombolysis. However, the optimal service delivery model depends on many non-clinical factors (e.g. in the mountainous region of Bavaria the use of telemedicine provides population exposure to appropriate expertise). There are several and increasing strong arguments for patients to be admitted to an acute/hyperacute stroke unit directly from the community or from the A&E department. Several models of service delivery of acute stroke care exist, depending on local circumstances. Some acute stroke units keep patients for 2–7 days before discharging those who require further therapy to a rehabilitation stroke unit. Other units combine acute and early rehabilitation care on one ward, keeping patients for up to 6 weeks before discharging them home or to alternative rehabilitation facilities. These facilities include community rehabilitation centres, community stroke teams providing treatment at home, rehabilitation facilities for care of the elderly and specialised neurological rehabilitation units.

Specific treatments for acute ischaemic stroke

Thrombolysis

'Time is brain' and early treatment is the most important factor for successful thrombolysis. To deliver this on a public health basis requires a considerable coordination of care across agencies and public awareness of the need for immediate treatment. It is essential that 'stroke' is recognised as a medical emergency.

Thrombolysis is one of the most exciting, controversial and complex recent developments in stroke medicine. The first thrombolytic agent to be tried in acute ischaemic stroke in the 1980s was streptokinase, but this agent was found to cause an unacceptable incidence of cerebral haemorrhage and was abandoned. Later trials showed that alteplase, a recombinant tissue plasminogen activator, was far safer. The most convincing benefits of intravenous alteplase were shown in the National Institute of Neurological Disease and Stroke (NINDS) study, which randomised patients within 3 hours of onset of ischaemic stroke, half within 90 minutes of onset. The trial required a CT before treatment, and blood pressure was carefully controlled in those with raised readings, using intravenous drugs if necessary. One in eight patients treated benefited in terms of making a full, or nearly full, recovery and the proportion of patients in Part 2 of the study achieving a Rankin grade 0 or 1 score at 3 months follow-up was 39% after alteplase treatment, compared to 26% after placebo. This benefit was accompanied by a significant risk of symptomatic intracranial haemorrhage after alteplase of 6%, compared to less than 1% in the placebo group. However, this did not lead to a significant difference in mortality rates between the two groups. Most benefit from alteplase was demonstrated in the group recruited within 90 minutes from stroke onset and in those with moderately severe stroke.

Subsequent trials of alteplase randomised patients up to 6 hours after onset of ischaemic stroke, but failed to show the striking benefits of the NINDS 3-hour study. Subsequent meta-analysis, combining the results of all previous major trials of intravenous thrombolysis with alteplase, has shown that there is a clear relationship between the time to treatment and the chances of benefit: the earlier patients are treated the better such that the odds ratio (OR) for a good outcome with alteplase at 3 months (mRS 0/1) is 2.55 for treatment started within 90 minutes of onset when compared with an OR of 1.6 for treatment started between 90 and 180 minutes. These results led to alteplase receiving a licence for use in North America, Europe and elsewhere. The European Union licence has strict conditions, initially limiting use to 3 hours from onset of stroke (now extended to 4.5 hours) and insists that only experienced teams with neurological training should administer the drug. Beyond 4.5 hours from onset, the benefit remains uncertain. The IST-3 trial found a non-significant trend favouring alteplase in the group treated between 4.5 and 6 hours and a 2012 updated meta-analysis of randomised controlled trials comparing treatment with alteplase with placebo given within 6 hours of stroke onset reported a significant benefit of alteplase with an OR of 1.29 in this time window. Although the IST-3 trial did not demonstrate significant benefit of alteplase between 0 and 6 hours compared with placebo it did demonstrate that patients over the age of 80 years benefited from thrombolysis when treated within 3 hours and that this treatment was not associated with increased rates of treatment-related haemorrhage in this older population.

Intravenous thrombolysis should only be offered to patients according to established protocols if they satisfy the inclusion criteria (Table 5.14). Patients treated with thrombolysis outside the strict protocol have an unacceptable rate of complications, especially intracranial haemorrhage. Training and experience are required to diagnose stroke, exclude stroke mimics and interpret CT appearances in acute ischaemic stroke. Established infarction shows on the CT as a well-defined area of low attenuation. However, the early changes of infarction are often subtle. In the MCA territory infarction, these include loss of distinction of the lentiform nucleus and insular ribbon cortex, loss of cortical definition between grey and white matter, and effacement of the sulci. Although not part of the NINDS protocol, most experts would exclude patients with early signs of infarction involving a large proportion of the MCA territory, because such signs imply that ischaemia has already progressed to irreversible infarction (Figure 5.11). Patients and relatives need to accept that although thrombolysis provides a chance of some real benefit, there is also a risk of harm from cerebral haemorrhage. Patients should not be denied thrombolysis if consent cannot be obtained (e.g. because of aphasia). It is essential that the timing of symptom onset should be well established, so that patients are only treated within the guidelines, currently within 4.5 hours of onset. For example, patients who wake from sleep with deficit from an ischaemic stroke are not eligible for thrombolysis with alteplase

Table 5.14 Guidelines for intravenous alteplase in acute ischaemic stroke.

Eligibility
Age 18 years or older
Clinical diagnosis of acute ischaemic stroke
Assessed by experienced team
Measurable neurological deficit
Glasgow Coma Score >8
Timing of symptom onset well established
CT or MRI and blood tests results available
CT or MRI consistent with diagnosis
Time since onset <4.5 hours at start of infusion
Exclusion criteria
Symptoms only minor or rapidly improving
Haemorrhage on pre-treatment CT (or MRI)
Suspected subarachnoid haemorrhage
Active bleeding from any site
Recent gastrointestinal or urinary tract haemorrhage within 21 days
Platelet count less than 100 000/mm^3
Recent treatment with heparin and APTT above normal
Recent treatment with warfarin and INR elevated
Recent major surgery or trauma within the previous 14 days
Recent post-myocardial infarction pericarditis
Neurosurgery, serious head trauma or previous stroke within 3 months
History of intracranial haemorrhage (ever)
Known arteriovenous malformation or aneurysm
Recent arterial puncture at non-compressible site
Recent lumbar puncture
Blood pressure consistently above 185/110 mmHg
Abnormal blood glucose (<3 or >20 mmol/L)
Suspected or known pregnancy
Active pancreatitis
Epileptic seizure at stroke onset
Cautions and limitations
Severe neurological deficit (NIHSS >22)
Visible changes on pre-treatment CT of infarction > one-third of MCA territory
Diabetic retinopathy

APTT, activated partial thromboplastin time; CT, computerised tomography; INR, international normalised ratio; MCA, middle cerebral artery; MRI, magnetic resonance imaging; NIHSS, National Institutes of Health Stroke Scale.

unless they are known to have been gone to sleep without symptoms within the 4.5 hour time window.

Only a proportion of patients will be suitable for thrombolysis, especially because many patients will not reach hospital within 4.5 hours of onset. Nevertheless, changes in service delivery are required to institute thrombolysis (e.g. development of acute stroke teams and protocols to ensure that patients are scanned with alacrity). The proportion of patients reaching hospital in a timely fashion can be increased by joint hospital and ambulance service protocols, involving training of ambulance personnel in the recognition of stroke, so that patients with suspected stroke are taken directly to an acute stroke centre. Education of the public to recognise stroke symptoms and to summon emergency ambulance services immediately is also required.

In the future, selection of patients with persisting penumbra may play a part in selecting cases for thrombolysis. For example, a mismatch between a small volume of infarction shown on DWI and a larger volume of impaired cerebral blood flow shown on perfusion MRI may be an indication of salvageable penumbra, and this could allow the extension of the window for thrombolysis beyond 4.5 hours in patients who arrive late and have persistent mismatch. Alternative thrombolytic agents may also allow the time window to be prolonged. For example, desmoteplase shows promise as an intravenous thrombolytic agent when administered within 3–9 hours of ischaemic onset in patients with MRI perfusion–diffusion mismatch, but the agent needs to be tested in larger randomised trials. CT perfusion imaging is an alternative to perfusion MRI, and may become more widely applicable in the future.

Another experimental approach to improving the effectiveness of thrombolysis is to combine intravenous alteplase with therapeutic transcranial ultrasound applied to the skull and focused on the site of arterial occlusion. Experimental studies have shown that ultrasound improves the activity of clot lysis, presumably by facilitating access of the thrombolytic drug to the core of the thrombus. Clinical trials have suggested an improvement in recanalisation rates with continuous transcranial Doppler ultrasound given for a 2-hour period after administration of intravenous alteplase. Again, larger trials are required to demonstrate the benefit of this approach.

The majority of evidence in favour of thrombolysis relates to the intravenous route of administration. This reflects the ease and rapidity with which an intravenous transfusion can be administered. On the other hand, local arterial infusion of thrombolytic agents has the advantage that a preliminary angiogram can be performed to confirm arterial occlusion, and that the agent can be infused exactly where it is needed. Case series and the PROACT II randomised trial suggest that intra-arterial thrombolysis can be highly effective, even up to 6 hours after onset in selected patients. However, intra-arterial thrombolysis requires specialised facilities and experienced neuroradiologists, limiting its widespread applicability. Moreover, the need to establish arterial access increases the delay to treatment compared with the intravenous route. The idea of giving intravenous thrombolysis first followed by intra-arterial thrombolysis ('bridging' therapy) was therefore introduced, but the dose of intra-arterial agent that can then be used is limited by the increased risk of haemorrhage from the thrombolytic agent. In practice, intra-arterial thrombolysis as a catheter-based approach has been largely replaced by mechanical thrombectomy, which appears to be more effective than intra-arterial therapy.

Mechanical recanalisation

For patients presenting with stroke secondary to proximal intracranial artery occlusion it is becoming clear that a good outcome following treatment will depend on whether this vessel is rapidly recanalised. Control data from the PROACT II study identified that only 22% of untreated stroke associated with proximal MCA

(M1 segment) stenosis was associated with a good outcome (mRS 0–2) and from the SENTIS control group that presentation with terminal ICA occlusion is associated with good outcome in only 5% of occasions. Early recanalisation appears to be the key to recovery and meta-analysis of the available data has shown that good recovery may be twice as likely with demonstrated recanalisation compared with persistent occlusion and that mortality reduces from 42% of patients with proximal occlusion to 14%. As a consequence of such data and the demonstration of only modest efficacy of intravenous alteplase in improving outcomes in the presence of proximal MCA occlusion, there has been substantial interest in the potential benefits provided by mechanical clot retrieval procedures that aim to physically remove persisting clot in proximal intracranial vessels.

In 2013, the results from three randomised controlled trials, MR RESCUE, IMS3 and SYNTHESIS EXPANSION, were reported in the same edition of the *New England Journal of Medicine*. All three studies evaluated the efficacy of endovascular treatments when compared with standard intravenous alteplase treatment for hyperacute ischaemic stroke associated with proximal intracranial artery occlusion. Endovascular treatment was not associated with excess treatment-related risk but did not demonstrate benefit compared to standard treatment. Proponents of endovascular treatment have pointed out that these data may be misleading because of poor patient selection, delayed treatment in the endovascular group or the use in the trials of endovascular technology that has already been superseded. In particular, very few patients were treated in these trials with removable stent systems ('stent retrievers'), which appear to be more effective than earlier devices, perhaps because expansion of the stent across the occluded segment of the artery results in more rapid reperfusion even before the clot is pulled out by stent. Subsequent to these trials five new randomised controlled trials (MR CLEAN, ESCAPE, SWIFT PRIME, EXTEND-IA and REVASCAT) have now clearly demonstrated that early intra-arterial treatment with second-generation mechanical thrombectomy is superior to conventional intravenous thrombolysis in large artery occlusion of the proximal anterior circulation. The largest of these trials, MR CLEAN, enrolled 500 adults within 6 hours of acute ischemic stroke onset caused by a proximal anterior circulation large artery occlusion and randomly assigned them to treatment with intra-arterial therapy or to usual care. Intra-arterial therapy involved mechanical thrombectomy with retrievable stents in 82%, and 90% of subjects in both groups received intravenous thrombolysis prior to randomisation. Compared with conventional therapy, the group assigned to intra-arterial treatment had improved outcomes at 3 months, including functional independence. There was no significant difference between the groups in the rates of symptomatic intracranial haemorrhage or death. When these results were announced the remaining trials were stopped early. Undoubtedly, this will now become the standard of care, though the relative numbers of patients suitable are very small. However, advanced logistics and concentration of expertise are required to deliver and replicate these trail benefits in a clinical setting, and certainly in the United Kingdom this will mean further centralisation of specialised services, as attempts by the non-expert will rapidly negate any possible benefit.

Antiplatelet therapy in acute stroke

Two very large randomised trials have shown that aspirin, given within 48 hours of onset, has a small but significant benefit in reducing the rate of recurrent ischaemic stroke. About 1/100 patients treated with aspirin avoid death or disability without a significant increase in the risk of symptomatic cerebral haemorrhage. Although this benefit seems small, it translates into a substantial cost effectiveness, given the commonness of stroke and the low cost of aspirin. For example, in the United Kingdom it is estimated that if everyone with stroke were given aspirin within 48 hours of onset, preferably after a CT scan to exclude cerebral haemorrhage, then more than 1000 patients would be saved from death or disability every year. Aspirin has not been extensively studied in patients with cerebral haemorrhage, but the majority of experts and emergency physicians consider aspirin contraindicated in any cerebral haemorrhage or if there is substantial acute haemorrhagic transformation within an ischaemic stroke.

Evidence is accumulating that the addition of clopidogel to aspirin may be more effective in secondary prevention immediately after minor stroke or TIA than aspirin alone. In 2013, a large trial of 5170 patients recruited within 24 hours of minor stroke or high risk TIA and randomised to clopidogrel plus aspirin or aspirin alone was reported. The dual therapy group experienced 30% fewer ischaemic strokes and demonstrated an absolute risk reduction of 3.5% at 90 days and no excess haemorrhage. These data are consistent with the degree of risk reduction reported in the Canadian-based FASTER trial reported in 2007 and are likely to lead to widespread change in practice for those with minor stroke and TIA in the acute phase. Antiplatelet therapy for longer term prevention is discussed later.

Anticoagulation in thrombo-embolic stroke

A large number of randomised trials have failed to demonstrate any overall benefit of early anticoagulation (i.e. within the first 2 weeks) with standard heparin, or with low molecular weight heparins, either routinely in acute stroke or in patients with progressive stroke or acute cardioembolic stroke associated with atrial fibrillation. The latter is in contrast to the clear benefit of warfarin in the long-term prevention of stroke from atrial fibrillation. In the acute stroke trials, any reduction in the rate of recurrent ischaemic stroke related to anticoagulation was matched by an increased rate of symptomatic intracranial haemorrhage. The evidence shows that there is no place for the routine use of anticoagulation or subcutaneous heparin in acute stroke. Best practice for preventing immobility-induced venous thromboembolism (VTE) has become clearer since the publication of the CLOTS3 (Clots in Legs Or sTockings after Stroke) trial results. This trial followed on from two earlier trials – CLOTS and CLOTS2, which had demonstrated that below knee or above knee stockings fitted soon after acute stroke made no difference to the risk of development of VTE and in some cases created harm by damaging the skin and impairing distal circulation. Prior to the completion of CLOTS3 these findings left stroke clinicians with difficult and often arbitrary decisions to make about when to start VTE prophylaxis in patients who were immobile but had had a recent large territory stroke or haemorrhage. However, CLOT3 has provided a clearer pathway for all stroke inpatients. This study recruited 2876 patients with acute stroke and randomised them to placebo or intermittent pneumatic compression stockings. Follow-up lower limb Doppler ultrasound found proximal deep venous thrombus in 12.1% of the placebo patients and only 8.5% of patients wearing the stockings. Early mobilisation (e.g. sitting the patient up the day after stroke) and active physiotherapy will continue to play an important part in limiting the risk of VTE.

There may also be a role for the use of heparin in selected patients who are thought to be at high risk of early stroke recurrence. We use low molecular weight heparin in patients with demonstrated thrombus in the heart, or in some patients with acute vertebral or carotid artery occlusion, so long as the patient does not have a large infarct (more than one-third of MCA territory by volume). In these latter cases the risk of symptomatic haemorrhagic transformation may be increased. Anticoagulation is sometimes recommended in patients with carotid and vertebral artery dissection (see later), so long as the dissection is limited to the extracranial portions of the artery. However, this treatment has not been shown to be superior to antiplatelet therapy in small randomised trials. In patients in whom there is a good indication for long-term anticoagulation (e.g. atrial fibrillation), we delay anticoagulation for 2 weeks if the infarct is large.

Neuroprotection

Many neuroprotective drugs, designed to block various components of the biochemical cascade leading to cell death after an ischaemic insult, have been shown to reduce the size of infarction in animal models of ischaemic stroke. To date, none of these agents has fulfilled their promise in randomised trials in human stroke. A number of factors may be responsible for this failure to translate animal research to the bedside, including inability in clinical trials to replicate experimental conditions and inclusion of patients too late – up to 24 hours after onset of stroke. In animal studies of neuroprotection, agents are usually only effective if given within an hour or two after induction of ischaemia.

The only licensed drug with an apparent protective benefit is nimodipine, given after recent SAH. In the British Aneurysm Trial, nimodipine reduced the incidence of cerebral infarction and the proportion of patients with a poor outcome by about 10%. Nimodipine has been shown to have no effect, or even to be harmful, in patients with ischaemic stroke and it is therefore possible that the benefits in patients with SAH arose because the patients can be pre-treated before the onset of ischaemia from vasospasm, or because nimodipine reduces severity of vasospasm.

Maintenance of homeostasis

Although drug therapy to protect the brain against the effects of ischaemia may not be beneficial, it is still logical to maintain the brain's physiological and biochemical environment in normal homeostatic balance, to preserve the penumbra and take all steps to prevent secondary deterioration. However, there is no trial evidence that the measures we recommend below to maintain homeostasis improve final outcome. Oxygen saturation should be monitored routinely and hypoxaemia treated appropriately.

Blood sugar levels are elevated in about one-quarter of all stroke admissions and elevated blood glucose on admission is a risk factor for haemorrhagic transformation of the acute infarct. This includes patients with known and undiagnosed diabetes, and patients in whom elevation in blood glucose appears as a stress response. Mortality, poor outcome and infarct size are increased in patients with raised blood glucose, but whether the larger size of infarction contributes to the high blood glucose, or vice versa, is uncertain. Nevertheless, we recommend avoiding administering intravenous glucose in patients with acute stroke, and we institute insulin therapy on a graded scale when the blood glucose is >10 mmol/L, to maintain optimal levels within 6–9 mmol/L. Equally, hypoglycaemia should be avoided.

The majority of patients with acute stroke have raised blood pressure on admission, often because of pre-existing hypertension and an invariable hormonal or autonomic response to the stroke itself. The blood pressure readings usually fall over the course of the first week. It is not clear whether hypertension in the acute stage is harmful (because it might reduce blood flow in already maximally dilated blood vessels) or beneficial (by reducing oedema and the risk of haemorrhagic transformation). However, the recent large INTERACT-2 trial showed that intensive lowering of blood pressure (target systolic level of <140 mmHg) in patients with spontaneous intracerebral haemorrhage was not harmful and might have been beneficial. However, the situation may be different in ischaemic stroke where the adequacy of collateral blood flow is a critical determinant of outcome. Some trials have shown no benefit but treatment was often started late in these studies and one trial suggested harm from blood pressure lowering. Further trials are therefore in progress. Until the results of these trials are available, we recommend continuing any previously prescribed antihypertensive agents, but do not intervene to lower blood pressure unless the patient is a candidate for thrombolysis, has hypertensive encephalopathy, malignant hypertension or the blood pressure readings are persistently above an arbitrary threshold of 200 mmHg systolic pressure or 110 mmHg for diastolic readings. Over-vigorous lowering of blood pressure in acute stroke can certainly lead to extension of the infarct. In most cases, blood pressure should therefore be lowered using oral agents, although in patients in whom thrombolysis is appropriate, intravenous medication with labetalol is used. This should be given at a dose titrated against the blood pressure. The latter should be closely monitored in any patient receiving hypotensive therapy to avoid precipitous falls in blood pressure, aiming for systolic readings of 150–185 mmHg. Intramuscular agents should be avoided because of their unpredictable effect on blood pressure. In other cases, we would recommend that the institution of medication to treat hypertension should be delayed for 48 hours or more after onset.

Spontaneous hypotension after stroke is rare, but may occur if the patient develops cardiac problems or becomes dehydrated. Hypotension should be corrected promptly by raising the foot of the bed, fluid replacement and stopping hypotensive medication. Occasionally, inotropic medication may be required. A very small number of patients, usually with carotid occlusion or a severe intracranial stenosis, can be very sensitive to blood pressure levels to the extent that they may develop a new symptoms or increase in severity of their signs (e.g. worsening hemiparesis) if their blood pressure falls (e.g. when sitting or standing up). Such patients may benefit dramatically from measures to correct hypotension, Similarly, patients with intracranial vasospasm after SAH may develop focal deficits that respond to measures to increase blood pressure.

Pyrexia is associated with poor outcome of stroke, while animal studies show that even a small fall in body temperature is associated with smaller infarct volumes. Hence, we recommend that all patients should have fever treated vigorously (e.g. with paracetamol) and infections should be treated promptly with antibiotics. In clinical practice, therapeutic hypothermia is difficult to achieve, requires intensive care and is associated with significant complications on rewarming, and has therefore not entered routine clinical practice. However, a large European trial of hypothermia has been started which might affect practice in the future.

Treatment of cerebral oedema

Cerebral infarction is associated with failure of membrane pumps and influx of water into the cells. Cytotoxic oedema is therefore an inevitable consequence of cerebral infarction, and it is this feature that allows infarcts to be seen on CT. All infarcts are associated with a degree of swelling of the ischaemic tissue, which is manifest in larger infarcts on imaging by compression of the sulci and ventricles. The swelling of the infarct may last up to 4 weeks before the oedema resolves. In large hemispheric infarcts, this mass effect can cause transtentorial herniation with compression of the brainstem and is the most common cause of death in the first week after cerebral infarction. Typically, in patients with symptomatic cerebral oedema, the patient appears stable after the onset of symptoms for the first 24–48 hours, and then deteriorates on the second or third day, with progressive impairment of consciousness, coma and respiratory failure. This most often occurs in a patient with a large infarct caused by MCA occlusion, which is then sometimes known as malignant MCA infarction because it is an important cause of death from ischaemic stroke. Direct brainstem compression may also occur in patients with large cerebellar infarcts.

Cytotoxic cerebral oedema secondary to infarction tends to be unresponsive to steroids, but mannitol may provide a temporary respite pending surgical treatment. Paralysis and hyperventilation are rarely of benefit. Instead, decompressive neurosurgery with a large craniectomy should be considered.

Consideration for decompressive hemicraniectomy is National Institute for Health and Care Excellence (NICE) guidance for patients with large territory (>50% of total territory) anterior circulation acute infarction with developing 'malignant' mass effect. This treatment has been demonstrated in recent trials to save life (number needed to treat = 4) if treatment is initiated within 48 hours of stroke onset. Current guidance recommends that eligible patients will be aged 60 years or younger, have a National Institute of Health Stroke Scale (NIHSS) score of above 15, and have reduced level of alertness to give a score of 1 or more on item 1a of the NIHSS (Table 5.15). Trial data suggest that infarct volume of more than 145 mL will inevitably lead to the development of the 'malignant' mass effect syndrome in patients aged 60 years or younger and acute stroke with infarct volumes greater than 145 mL should be actively considered for proactive decompression even before malignant swelling starts to develop. Most recently, data presented from the DESTINY 2 trial has suggested that decompressive surgery is also beneficial for patients of good pre-morbid function and aged >60 years. Our practice is to proactively transfer patients at risk of developing significant mass effect secondary to a large volume ischaemic stroke to our high dependency unit and work closely with neurosurgical colleagues to plan the best time for the procedure in appropriate cases. Such patients will require daily interval brain imaging pending a decision regarding surgery and there is no doubt that unnecessary delay in these patients can lead to secondary infarction resulting from direct pressure effects.

Patients with cerebral haemorrhage may also deteriorate because of oedema and transtentorial herniation, or direct brainstem compression. Occasionally, cerebral infarction, usually in the cerebellum, is associated with the development of hydrocephalus from compression of the aqueduct, although this is much more common following intracranial haemorrhage. Hydrocephalus may require shunting, or evacuation of the infarct or haemorrhage (see earlier).

Management of progressive stroke

About one-third of patients with ischaemic stroke progress in the first day after onset. Acute progression is even more common in patients with cerebral haemorrhage because of continued bleeding

Table 5.15 National Institute of Health Stroke Scale (NIHSS).

Scale	Grade	Observations
1a Level of consciousness (LOC)	0	Alert
	1	Not alert, but arousable with minimal stimulation
	2	Not alert, requires repeated stimulation to attend
	3	Coma
1b LOC questions – *Month? Patient's age?*	0	Answers both correctly
	1	Answers one correctly
	2	Both incorrect
1c LOC commands: *Open/close eyes Grip (non-paretic hand)*	0	Obeys both correctly
	1	Obeys one correctly
	2	Both incorrect
2 Best gaze	0	Normal
	1	Partial gaze palsy
	2	Forced gaze palsy
3 Visual field testing	0	No visual field loss
	1	Partial hemianopia
	2	Complete hemianopia
	3	Bilateral hemianopia (blind, including cortical blindness)
4 Facial palsy	0	Normal symmetrical movement
	1	Minor paralysis (effaced nasolabial fold, asymmetry on smiling)
	2	Partial paralysis (total or near total paralysis of lower face)
	3	Complete paralysis of one or both sides (absence of facial movement in the upper and lower face)
5 Motor function arms (R & L)	0	Normal (extends arm 90° or 45° for 10 s without drift)
	1	Drift
	2	Some effort against gravity
	3	No effort against gravity
	4	No movement
	U	Untestable (joint fused or amputated – scores 0)
6 Motor function legs (R & L)	0	Normal (hold leg in 30° position for 5 s without drift)
	1	Drift
	2	Some effort against gravity
	3	No effort against gravity
	4	No movement
	U	Untestable (joint fused or amputated – scores 0)

(continued)

Table 5.15 (continued)

Scale	Grade	Observations
7 Limb ataxia	0	No ataxia
	1	Present in one limb
	2	Present in two limbs
8 Sensory	0	Normal
	1	Mild to moderate decrease in sensation
	2	Severe to total sensory loss
9 Best language	0	No aphasia
	1	Mild to moderate aphasia
	2	Severe aphasia
	3	Mute
10 Dysarthria	0	Normal articulation
	1	Mild to moderate slurring of words
	2	Near unintelligible or unable to speak
	U	Intubated or other physical barrier (scores 0)
11 Extinction and inattention	0	Normal
	1	Inattention or extinction to bilateral simultaneous stimulation in one of the sensory modalities
	2	Severe hemi-inattention or hemi-inattention to more than one modality

Source: adapted from http://www.ninds.nih.gov/doctors/NIH_Stroke_Scale.

and enlargement of the haematoma. In ischaemic stroke, the causes of early progression are often unclear, but may include extension of the area of ischaemia from thrombus propagation, recurrent embolism, failure of initially adequate collaterals or enlargement of the penumbra from release of cytotoxic chemicals and the local effects of cytotoxic oedema. In patients who deteriorate after a period of stability, a number of other causes need to be considered:

- Metabolic disturbances (e.g. low or high blood sugar, or hyponatraemia)
- Hypotension, or severe hypertension
- Cardiac arrhythmias or MI
- Pyrexia and infections
- Dehydration
- Hypoxia (e.g. from aspiration, infection or silent pulmonary embolism)
- Cerebral oedema or hydrocephalus
- Haemorrhagic transformation of infarction
- Vasospasm after subarachnoid haemorrhage,
- New infarction (often from cardiac embolism) or haemorrhage in a new location.

Patients who deteriorate should therefore be investigated for these possibilities by repeat CT or MRI, chest imaging, search for infection and appropriate blood tests. Management will depend on the findings.

Common medical complications of stroke

- Frank dysphagia, or an unsafe swallow with the risk of aspiration, is very common and occurs in about one-third of patients with hemispheric stroke and two-thirds of those with brainstem stroke. This can easily cause aspiration pneumonia, leading to hypoxia and stroke progression. All patients with acute stroke should therefore have their swallowing assessed as soon as possible, using an agreed protocol. They should be kept nil-by-mouth until their swallowing has been assessed as safe. It is very likely that dehydration and starvation are harmful in the acute stages of stroke and fluid replacement should commence as soon as the patient is admitted if swallowing is not safe. It also makes sense to start feeding patients immediately. Even if a patient can swallow safely, the spontaneous intake of food and liquid is often inadequate because of poor appetite, cognitive impairment, neglect or physical difficulties in feeding. Nurses and carers should therefore have adequate time to help a patient to eat and drink sufficiently. When the oral route is not safe or practical, it is essential to establish other routes. In the short term, it is often convenient to replace fluids via an intravenous line, but this has the disadvantage of immobilising the patient. A nasogastric tube is therefore preferred, with the advantage of allowing feeding as well as fluid replacement, with less risk of cardiac overload or line infection. If nasogastric tube feeding is likely to be required for more than 2 weeks, consideration should be given to inserting a percutaneous endoscopic gastrostomy (PEG) tube. This is usually preferred by patients and has the advantage that a large tube can be used. However, there are some risks of tube insertion, including peritonitis. Overall, there is little difference to the outcome after early PEG feeding compared with a nasogastric tube. It should be borne in mind that nasogastric tubes may increase the risk of gastrointestinal haemorrhage.
- Deep vein thrombosis is usually seen in severely hemiparetic limbs and is very common on radiographic studies. Pulmonary embolus is a rare but important cause of death after stroke. The prevention of venous thromboembolism is discussed in the section on anticoagulation.
- Pressure sores should only occur in those patients who have lain at home undiscovered and immobile for some hours before admission to hospital. In all hospital patients sores should be avoided by frequent turning, careful positioning and the use of appropriate bedding (e.g. an air mattress). Early mobilisation and sitting the patient out of bed as soon as possible after onset also play a part in preventing pressure sores and other complications of immobility.
- Shoulder pain is a common complication of stroke, largely preventable by good positioning of the shoulder and early physiotherapy. In particular, a paralysed upper limb should not be allowed to hang unsupported at the side of the patient, because the weight of the limb leads to subluxation of the shoulder joint and subsequently a painful frozen shoulder. The correct position of a patient in a bed or chair, with the weak limb supported at all times by a comfortable pillow or similar support, is essential. Patients who do experience shoulder pain may benefit from standard rheumatological treatments, including local steroid injections. The paralysed upper limb must never be neglected from motor therapy as it will contract and become dysfunctional and painful.
- Limb swelling of the hand or foot of a hemiparetic limb is common and is partly explained by excessive sympathetic activity.

The patient often complains that the limb is cold, because vasodilatation results in heat loss, even though the limb may feel warm to touch. This type of oedema should be distinguished from oedema secondary to a deep venous thrombosis. Elevation of the limb may help. Diuretics are not indicated.

- Spasticity is a common but not universal feature of the upper motor neurone lesion resulting from infarction or haemorrhage. The increase in tone often develops several days or weeks after the onset of stroke. In the upper limb, the pattern of spasticity usually leads to flexion at each joint, and in the lower limb to extension. Early mobilisation and appropriate physiotherapy probably play an important part in limiting the development of severe spasticity, and particularly the development of contractures. Oral drug treatment has a limited role in treating spasticity in stroke. The problem is that drug treatment often results in generalised muscle weakness and function is rarely improved. However, local injections of botulinum toxin into individual muscles may benefit patients in whom spasticity is causing focal problems.
- Depression is very common after stroke and may reflect a direct neurophysiological cause, as well as reaction to the illness and persistent disability. Depression is associated with poor outcomes and should therefore be treated vigorously and expert psychiatric advice sought if necessary.
- Post-stroke pain (Chapter 23) is characteristically associated with infarction in the thalamus and often develops weeks or even months after the onset of stroke. The pain is often described as a deep burning pain throughout one side of the body, which limits the patient's activities and may lead to severe depression. Standard analgesics are often ineffective, but relief may be obtained with tricyclic antidepressants, particularly amitriptyline taken at night, or anticonvulsants (e.g. gabapentin). Occasionally, transcutaneous nerve stimulation is helpful.
- Dystonia is a rare complication of stroke involving the basal ganglia and usually develops some months after the initial event. Chorea is occasionally seen in patients with the Moyamoya syndrome (see Moyamoya angiopathy), and is also a rare acute manifestation of basal ganglia lacunar infarction.

Secondary prevention

Secondary prevention implies specific evidence-based measures that reduce the risk of future stroke following a defined clinical event. In the case of TIA, this implies preventing, to some degree, the risk of subsequent stroke. Following a stroke, secondary prevention means recommending and adopting measures that have been shown to prevent stroke recurrence. Advice that is not based upon evidence, nor widely agreed, is frequently given to patients in these clinical settings. Much of the evidence related to primary prevention, such as the control of hypertension, also applies to secondary prevention.

Secondary prevention after TIA and stroke

Patients who have had a TIA are at high risk of stroke and those who have had a stroke are at high risk of recurrent stroke. Both are at risk of MI. As a general figure, following either of these events, the risks of stroke or a recurrent stroke are about 5% per annum, but can be as high as 30% in patients with severe carotid stenosis. In general, the older the patient, and the more risk factors present, the greater the risk of recurrence. However, with appropriate management, the risks can be reduced substantially. The EXPRESS study performed by the Oxford Group demonstrated an 80% relative risk reduction when patients with TIA were seen within the 24 hours of referral and commenced immediately on secondary prevention treatments. Scoring systems to grade risk with TIA have been developed (most notably the ABCD2 score; Table 5.16) once the diagnosis of TIA has already been made. High risk patients (ABCD2 >3) should be seen within 24 hours of referral while low risk patients (ABCD2 ≤3) might be seen within 5 working days. Many stroke services have been reorganised around this scoring system, which has the vulnerability that the score and hence the risk stratification are only valid *after* an informed evaluation of the patient, which is the first task of the clinician running the TIA service. Studies have shown that the score is often poorly measured when done outside an expert context. The accuracy of the score can be improved in TIA patients if the findings on CTA or MRI are incorporated in the score, because acute infarction on DWI and the finding of arterial occlusion or stenosis on CTA both independently increase the risk of early stroke.

Table 5.16 The ABCD2 score for transient ischaemic attack (TIA). A TIA is judged to be high risk if the ABCD2 score is 4 or more and as low risk if the score is 3 or less. National guidance in the United Kingdom recommends review by a stroke specialist within one working day of all patients with TIA and ABCD2 score greater than 3.

ABCD2 risk factor	Values	Score
Age	>59 years	1
Blood pressure	Systolic blood pressure >140 mmHg or diastolic blood pressure >90 mmHg	1
Clinical symptoms	Unilateral weakness	2
	Isolated speech disturbance	1
	Other	0
Duration of symptoms	>60 minutes	2
	10–59 minutes	1
	less than 10 minutes	0
Diabetes mellitus	Present	1
Maximum score possible		9
High risk score		4 or greater
Low risk score		3 or less

Source: Johnston et al. 2007. Reproduced with permission of Elsevier.

Evidence from EXPRESS and the FASTER trial performed in Paris demonstrates that for patients with TIA or minor stroke there is much to be saved by effective measures to prevent recurrence. Treatment should be based on addressing risk factors and the results of investigations, together with an assessment of the degree of risk and benefits of treatment in individual patients.

Targets for preventive measures include the following:

- Lifestyle risk factors
- Lowering blood pressure
- Lowering cholesterol by statin therapy and diet
- Optimising treatment of other conditions that promote vascular disease (e.g. diabetes)
- Prevention of cardiac embolism (e.g. valve surgery or anticoagulation for atrial fibrillation)

- Targeted treatment for atherosclerotic stenosis by carotid endarterectomy or stenting,
- Inhibition of platelet aggregation with antiplatelet agents.

In patients with a history of cerebral haemorrhage, prevention should be targeted only at the first four issues and, in general, antiplatelet therapy and anticoagulation are contraindicated. Sources of cerebral haemorrhage, particularly aneurysms and AVMs may require specific treatment as previously described.

Following cardiogenic thrombo-embolism, formal anticoagulation treatment to prevent recurrence should start immediately after a TIA or rapid recovery from a minor stroke. In patients with more severe stroke, we start anticoagulation with warfarin at around 2 weeks after onset. Several trials have shown no benefit to anticoagulation within the first 2 weeks after onset, because any reduction in the numbers of recurrent ischaemic stroke is balanced by cerebral haemorrhage secondary to the therapy in the hyperacute setting. In patients who are very disabled, some preventive measures may need to be delayed, for example for stroke secondary to a symptomatic internal carotid artery stenosis the decision on whether to perform a carotid endarterectomy will usually be deferred until the risks of reperfusion injury in the damaged cerebral hemisphere are reduced and the potential benefit of protective surgery for the remaining anterior circulation territories can be evaluated against the primary injury and associated persisting clinical deficit. Anticoagulants and antiplatelet therapy have a rapid effect at reducing risk in appropriate patients and it is also possible that there is a rapid impact of statins in the stabilisation of acute symptomatic atheromatous plaque disease. However, in general, statin therapy and lowering of blood pressure appear to take several months to be effective at reducing risk, and the maximum benefits are not achieved for up to 1–2 years.

There is much to be gained by effective secondary prevention of stroke: the patient who stops smoking will halve their risk of stroke; a patient with atrial fibrillation taking warfarin will reduce their risk of stroke by two-thirds; antihypertensive therapy will reduce the risk by about 40%, and a patient with stroke secondary to arterial disease taking simvastatin 40 mg/day will have their stroke risk reduced by 30%. Carotid endarterectomy in patients with recent symptoms and severe carotid stenosis may reduce the risk of recurrence by as much as 80%. Antiplatelet therapy is the least effective of these measures and only reduces the risk of recurrent stroke by about 15%. Each of these treatment modalities acts independently. Thus, patients with multiple risk factors stand to benefit considerably from multimodal intervention.

Lifestyle modification

Patients with the relevant risk factors should be strongly advised to stop smoking, eat healthily to reach and maintain a normal weight, to take regular exercise and to reduce excessive alcohol consumption.

Lowering blood pressure

Epidemiological studies have established clearly that the lower an individual's blood pressure, the lower the risk of stroke, even within the normal range. In patients with hypertension, it is therefore likely that the lower the blood pressure is reduced with treatment the better, so long as the patient does not develop unwanted effects. Thus, we suggest that if the patient is at any risk of recurrence and can tolerate the medication, the British Hypertension Society (BHS) guidelines (optimum targets: below 140/90 mmHg in general and below 130/80 mmHg for patients with diabetes) should be followed closely (i.e. the blood pressure maintained at levels lower than these). This may require the use of three or four antihypertensive agents. At one time, there was concern that lowering the blood pressure in patients with prior stroke might be harmful, but the PROGRESS trial established that even patients with a relatively normal blood pressure after a stroke (often achieved with prior medication), benefited from further reduction in their blood pressure using a combination of an angiotensin converting enzyme (ACE) inhibitor and a diuretic.

Most experts believe that the benefits of lowering blood pressure in preventing stroke are related to the degree in reduction of blood pressure, not the drug class used to lower it. However, there is some evidence that β-blockers are less effective than other classes of antihypertensive agent.

Diabetes mellitus

Both type 1 and type 2 diabetes are well-recognised risk factors for stroke, probably because of the association of atherosclerosis and hypertension with diabetes. In keeping with this assumption, vigorous control of hypertension has more benefit in reducing the incidence of stroke in patients with diabetes than tight control of blood sugar levels. However, it is important to maintain HbAc1 levels at less than 7%.

Lowering cholesterol

There is now convincing evidence from the Heart Protection Studies and the SPARCL study that lowering cholesterol with a statin after ischaemic stroke dramatically reduces the risk of recurrent stroke and MI. The lower the achieved level of cholesterol the lower the risk, with an approximately 30% reduction in the risk of recurrent ischaemic stroke and MI associated with a reduction in LDL cholesterol of 1.0 mmol/L. The benefits of statin therapy are therefore greater than those of antiplatelet therapy. All patients with stroke and TIA should therefore be considered for statin therapy, unless they have a total cholesterol of <3.5 mmol/L or LDL cholesterol <1.8 mmol/L.

Anticoagulation

Anticoagulation in acute stroke has been discussed earlier. In contrast to the lack of benefit of heparins in acute stroke, there is good evidence that anticoagulation with warfarin prevents recurrent stroke in patients with cardio-embolic sources of thrombus (Table 5.17). The evidence is best for atrial fibrillation, which is associated with a very high rate of recurrent stroke. In the European Atrial Fibrillation Trial, warfarin reduced the rate of recurrent TIA and stroke from 12% per annum down to 4% per annum, a two-thirds reduction in risk. In contrast, aspirin was much less effective, reducing the rate of recurrence by only about one-sixth. It is likely that warfarin works more effectively than aspirin because it affects the formation of thrombin-based clots in the heart, whereas antiplatelet agents are more effective at preventing thrombus starting with platelet aggregation on atheromatous clots. Thus, warfarin is the treatment of choice in patients with atrial fibrillation following stroke or TIA to prevent recurrence. In the elderly, the risks of intracranial haemorrhage (including subdural haematoma), the need for regular monitoring and the issue of compliance, especially if there is cognitive impairment, need to be considered but the benefits of anticoagulation in these patients is usually so substantial that significant problems with the treatment should be identified before anticoagulation is considered to be contraindicated. Occasional falls or one single fall with injury should not be automatic reasons for long-term withdrawal of anticoagulation. Antiplatelet treatments are not as effective as warfarin, even when

Table 5.17 Indications for anticoagulation in secondary stroke prevention.

Established indications

Cardiac embolism

- Atrial fibrillation
- Mechanical valve prosthesis
- Recent myocardial infarction
- Left ventricular aneurysm
- Dilated cardiomyopathy

Cerebral venous and venous sinus thrombosis

Possible indications

Recent major vessel occlusion

- Internal carotid artery occlusion
- Basilar artery occlusion

Recent extracranial cervical arterial dissection

Severe carotid stenosis prior to surgery or stenting

Crescendo TIAs despite antiplatelet therapy

Thrombophilia and prothrombotic states

Paradoxical embolism

Table 5.18 The CHA_2DS_2.VASC scoring system for assessing risk of stroke in the presence of atrial fibrillation. Maximum total score = 9. The presence of congestive heart failure, hypertension, age 65–74 years, diabetes mellitus, stroke/TIA, or female sex score 1 point each while age >74 years and history of previous thromboembolism score 2 points each.

CHA_2DS_2-VASc score	Risk category	Adjusted stroke risk (%/per year)
0	Low	0
1	Intermediate	1.3
2	High	2.2
3	High	3.2
4	High	4.0
5	High	6.7
6	High	9.8
7	High	9.6
8	High	6.7
9	High	15.2

Source: Adapted from Camm 2012. Reproduced with permission of Oxford University Press with additional data from Lip 2010.

used in intensive combinations of aspirin and clopidogrel, and these treatments can be associated with similar levels of non-CNS-related haemorrhage. Fixed or low dose warfarin therapy is not effective in preventing embolism in patients with atrial fibrillation.

Several novel oral anticoagulant treatments have now been licensed in Europe and in the United States. These medications have the benefit of requiring no blood level testing, fixed dosing and reduced risk of over or under-treatment complications. Rivaroxaban and apixaban are inhibitors of factor Xa while dabigatran is a direct thrombin inhibitor. To date, most vascular networks have adopted a position that recommends these medications for patients with atrial fibrillation only after they have failed with a trial of warfarin for some reason (e.g. because of non-compliance or poor management of International Normalised Ratio [INR] levels.) From the trial data, these drugs have similar efficacy and when compared with warfarin are all non-inferior to warfarin with reported reduction in intracranial haemorrhage rates. They have not been tested in patients with metallic valves or with other prothrombotic conditions such as antiphospholipid syndrome and for these patients warfarin will remain the treatment of choice.

Several scoring systems have been developed to assist clinicians in planning anticoagulation treatment. The CHA_2DS_2.VASC scoring system is widely used to assess risk of stroke in the presence of atrial fibrillation while the HAS.BLED tool may be useful in estimating treatment haemorrhage risk in patients prescribed warfarin (Table 5.18 and Table 5.19). A criticism of these scoring systems is that neither requires evaluation of the contemporary brain imaging and it is likely that incorporation of information from MRI (e.g. prior silent cortical infarcts) and sequences sensitive to haemorrhage (e.g. susceptibility weighted imaging) may add value to risk assessment. Standard practice is to offer anticoagulation for all

Table 5.19 Clinical characteristics comprising the HAS.BLED bleeding risk score.

H - Hypertension	Hypertension' is defined as systolic blood pressure >160 mmHg	1
A - Abnormal renal and liver function (1 point each)	Abnormal renal function is defined as serum creatinine ≥200 mmol/L Abnormal liver function is defined as chronic hepatic disease (e.g. cirrhosis) or biochemical evidence of significant hepatic derangement	1 or 2
S - Stroke	Previous stroke	1
B - Bleeding	Bleeding refers to previous bleeding history and/or predisposition to bleeding (e.g. bleeding diathesis or anaemia)	1
L - Labile INR	Labile INRs refers to unstable/high INRs or poor time in therapeutic range (e.g. 60%)	1
E - Elderly	Age >65 years	1
D - Drugs or alcohol (1 point each)	Drugs/alcohol use refers to concomitant use of drugs, such as antiplatelet agents, non-steroidal anti-inflammatory drugs, or alcohol abuse, etc.	1 or 2
	Total (maximum)	9

Source: Camm 2012. Reproduced with permission of Oxford University Press with additional data from Pisters *et al.* 2010.
INR, International Normalised Ratio.

those with CHA_2DS_2.VASC scores >1 and to consider anticoagulation or antiplatelet agents for those with a CHA_2DS_2.VASC score of 1. Consideration of the HAS.BLED score in conjunction with the CHA_2DS_2.VASC score is most useful in patients with high risk of bleeding. In practice, anticoagulation should be introduced with caution in patients with very frequent falls or a HASBLED score of >2 but anxiety about bleeding, particularly in patients who fall frequently, may become less of an issue in the future when the novel oral anticoagulants are more widely used because these new agents appear to guarantee a therapeutic dose without excessive anticoagulation and with reduced risk of intracranial bleeding.

Anticoagulation is indicated as a life-long treatment for patients who have had heart valves replaced with mechanical prostheses. If such patients have a cerebral haemorrhage while on warfarin, the treatment can be stopped relatively safely empirically, but should in most cases be restarted after 7 days. Other cardiac conditions associated with a high likelihood of the development of cardiac embolism listed in Table 5.17 should be considered for anticoagulation.

Possible indications for anticoagulation after stroke are also listed in the Table 5.17. Evidence that anticoagulation is superior to aspirin in all these disorders is lacking. It needs to be borne in mind that there are significant long-term risks of warfarin therapy, including a risk of intracranial haemorrhage of 1–2% per annum. We therefore usually only recommend anticoagulation for short periods in patients with uncertain indications to cover the period of time when their risk of recurrence is highest (e.g. for a maximum of 6 months after an acute ischaemic event).

The usual target INR for the treatment of atrial fibrillation is 2.5 (range 2.0–3.0). For patients with mechanical prosthetic valves, a higher INR target of 3.5 (range 3.0–4.0) is usually chosen. A target INR of 2.5 is appropriate for most other indications. Analysis of the Atrial Fibrillation Trials suggests that an INR of 2.0 or less is insufficient to prevent thrombo-embolism, while the risk of haemorrhage rises substantially with an INR of >4.0. It is important that anticoagulant clinics, and the patients themselves, are aware of these recommended levels.

The management of patients who are found to have a patent foramen ovale (PFO), in association with TIA or stroke, remains controversial. There appears to be an association between PFO and cryptogenic stroke (i.e. those patients in whom no other cause is evident after full investigations). However, whether the mechanism of stroke in these patients is paradoxical embolism from cryptic deep vein thrombosis, embolism of thrombus formed in the PFO itself, or some unrelated mechanism, is not clear. Nevertheless, careful observational studies have suggested that the rate of recurrent stroke in patients with PFO treated with aspirin alone is as low, as the rate in patients with cryptogenic stroke without PFO, except if the PFO is associated with atrial septal aneurysm, when the risk may be increased. There appears to be little consistent relationship between the risk of stroke treated with aspirin and the size of the PFO. In patients where the PFO is thought to be relevant to the mechanism of their stroke, the PFO can be closed using percutaneous techniques and mechanical devices. The risks of this treatment are low, but not zero, and the long-term consequences of having a prosthesis in the heart are uncertain. None of the three randomised trials completed to date has conclusively shown PFO closure to be of benefit on an intention to treat basis, though subgroup analysis has suggested potential benefit in high risk groups, particularly younger patients with a large PFO. We therefore favour medical management with optimised antiplatelet treatment in the majority of cases but value a multidisciplinary approach to the decision-making process to assist in the identification of patients more suitable for PFO closure. The evidence suggests that warfarin is no more effective than aspirin in these patients provided a full thrombophilia screen in negative.

For non-cardioembolic stroke, a number of randomised trials have shown that warfarin is no more effective than aspirin in preventing recurrent stroke in patients who have had TIA or stroke that has not been attributed to atrial fibrillation or a cardiogenic source (i.e. patients with stroke attributable to atherosclerosis, small vessel disease or cryptogenic mechanisms). Antiplatelet therapy is therefore preferred to anticoagulation in patients with this type of stroke, sometimes known as athero-thrombotic stroke. The danger of warfarin therapy in this group of patients was emphasised by the results of the Stroke Prevention in Reversible Ischaemia Trial (SPIRIT), which was stopped prematurely because of an excess of brain haemorrhage in patients who did not have atrial fibrillation or cardiac embolism randomised to warfarin compared with those randomised to aspirin after a recent TIA or stroke . Most of the haemorrhages occurred in patients over the age of 75 and in those who had moderate or severe small vessel disease (leukoaraiosis) on CT. This trial used a high target range for INR of 3.0–4.0, which may have increased the risk of cerebral haemorrhage; nevertheless, extensive leukoaraiosis should be considered a relative contraindication to warfarin therapy.

Warfarin treatment has been recommended in the past as an option in patients with recurrent stroke or TIA symptoms on antiplatelet agents but perhaps more appropriately recurrent events despite apparently optimal treatment should result in detailed re-evaluation for causation. These further investigations should be determined by the pattern of the recurrence, for example TOE, aortic arch imaging and implantable rhythm monitoring investigations are useful in evaluating unexplained recurrent embolic stroke; up-to-date high resolution intracranial arterial imaging is important for recurrent single territory events; and a wider survey of uncommon causes of small vessel arteriopathy (e.g. CADASIL or Fabry's disease) for progressing small vessel disease .

This process of re-evaluation on the mechanism for stroke despite optimised treatment is particularly important for patients who have recurrent symptoms on warfarin with apparently good INR control. The range of options here is wide. It may be that warfarin control is less good than thought and needs to be optimised, perhaps with a higher target INR. Other possibilities might be that the recurrent events relate to a different vascular process (e.g. large artery disease or small vessel arteriopathy) and for these patients intensification of the warfarin treatment is unlikely to be helpful. It is mandatory in these cases to exclude a symptomatic carotid artery event that might be treated with carotid surgery. For patients with new small vessel events blood pressure and cholesterol control should be optimised but there is a theoretical option to add in an antiplatelet treatment (e.g. low dose aspirin 75 mg/day). In general we would avoid this option wherever possible because there is clear evidence of significant increase in haemorrhage risk in patients on this dual agent combination but in exceptional cases where these options are being considered primarily from a stroke prevention position blood sensitive MRI sequences are increasingly helpful in guiding the evaluation of risk–benefit. In some cases, dual therapy (warfarin plus an antiplatelet) or even triple therapy with warfarin plus two antiplatelet agents is necessary to cover recent stroke in the context of cardiogenic thrombo-embolism and acute coronary artery disease requiring coronary artery stenting and dual antiplatelet cover. In these situations there is no one correct treatment strategy and best practice is for stroke and cardiology clinicians to determine the minimum duration of the antiplatelet treatments, the optimal stent device and to ensure that the patient is aware that there will be an unavoidable period of increased risk of haemorrhage.

Antiplatelet therapy

Aspirin has been the mainstay of treatment to prevent recurrent stroke for many years in patients who are not anticoagulated, and has the advantage of being very cheap. However, it should be borne in mind that antiplatelet therapy has less relative benefit in reducing the risk of vascular events than lowering blood pressure or lowering cholesterol. In a meta-analysis looking at the overall benefit of aspirin after stroke or TIA, the overall relative risk reduction in the combined outcome of stroke, MI or vascular death in different trials was only 13%. Aspirin also has the disadvantage of frequent side effects, particularly at high doses, including gastrointestinal haemorrhage and intracranial haemorrhage, which have incidences of approximately 27 and 5 per 1000 patients per year, respectively. The most common side effect is gastrointestinal irritation, and as many as 25% of patients discontinue aspirin treatment within a year or so of starting. Gastrointestinal side effects are less troublesome at lower doses. There is little evidence for a significant difference in effectiveness at any dose above 30 mg/day, and we therefore recommend using the lowest easily available convenient dose, which in the United Kingdom is 75 mg once daily.

There has been considerable interest in developing alternative, more effective antiplatelet agents than aspirin. The first widely used alternative to aspirin was dipyridamole. Initially, there was doubt about the effectiveness of dipyridamole in preventing stroke, but the Second European Stroke Prevention Study (ESPS-2) showed that dipyridamole in a modified released preparation at a dosage of 400 mg/day had a similar effectiveness to aspirin in preventing recurrent stroke in patients with recent stroke or TIA. The combination of low dose aspirin and dipyridamole was significantly superior to aspirin or dipyridamole alone, with a relative reduction in stroke recurrence, compared with placebo, of 37%. These results have recently been confirmed by the ESPRIT trial. Dipyridamole is a very safe antiplatelet agent, and does not appear to significantly increase the risk of bleeding, even when combined with aspirin. However, it is not well tolerated by a significant proportion of patients because of side effects, particularly headache. These side effects may be minimised by starting with a low dose of dipyridamole and increasing the dose gradually, and may work in some patients over a few weeks, if they persist in taking the tablets. In ESCS-2, nearly 30% of patients discontinued combination therapy because of side effects.

NICE in England, in its 2010 appraisal of antiplatelet agents for the prevention of thrombosis in patients with stroke, recommended that all patients with recent stroke and TIA should be started on clopidogrel with the combination of aspirin and dipyridamole being an option. Clopidogrel is an antiplatelet agent that was developed as a replacement for ticlopidine, an older antiplatelet agent that had the disadvantage of a 1% incidence of neutropenia. Clopidogrel 75 mg/day was compared with aspirin in the CAPRIE trial, and was shown to be slightly better than aspirin in the prevention of the combined outcome of all vascular events in patients with recent stroke, MI or peripheral vascular disease. However, the absolute reduction in vascular events attributed to clopidogrel over and above the benefit of aspirin alone was only 0.5% (i.e. the number needed to prevent one additional event was 200 patients over 2 years). Clopidogrel is slightly better tolerated than aspirin in terms of gastrointestinal symptoms, but has a slightly higher rate of rash and diarrhoea as side effects. The rate of haemorrhage associated with clopidogrel is similar to that of aspirin.

The combination of clopidogrel and aspirin may be more effective than either drug alone in preventing recurrent stroke. In the MATCH trial, clopidogrel plus aspirin was compared with clopidogrel alone in patients with recent stroke considered at a high risk of recurrence. In this trial, there was a significant increase in the risk of life-threatening haemorrhage in patients treated with the combination, without any significant reduction in the rate of ischaemic stroke. In contrast, in 2013, the CHANCE study, a randomised double-blind placebo controlled trial comparing clopidogrel plus aspirin with aspirin alone started within 24 hours of minor stroke or TIA in 5000 Chinese patients, reported a relative risk reduction of 43% in stroke occurrence within 90 days for the dual agent combination compared with aspirin alone. The combination treatment was not associated with excess haemorrhage compared with aspirin as monotherapy. Similarly, in the EXPRESS study, patients with TIA judged to be at high risk of recurrence (e.g. early presentation post index TIA) appeared to benefit from combination therapy with aspirin and clopidogrel without excess haemorrhage at 90 days. If these finding are repeated in the planned Platelet-Orientated Inhibition in New TIA and Minor Ischaemic Stroke (POINT) trial, a rationale for short-term dual agent treatment in the immediate period post minor stroke or TIA will be established. Pending further clarification on the safety and efficacy of combination treatment with aspirin and clopidogrel in stroke patients, dual agent treatment is already used in some departments for high risk TIA, patients post coronary or carotid artery stenting, and in high risk patients planned for carotid endarterectomy secondary to symptomatic significant carotid disease.

Management of carotid stenosis

Symptomatic carotid stenosis

The large randomised trials comparing carotid endarterectomy with medical treatment alone completed over 20 years ago demonstrated that selected patients with recent ipsilateral TIA or non-disabling stroke, who are fit for surgery and have significant carotid stenosis, benefit from carotid endarterectomy to remove the stenosis (Table 5.20). The benefit of surgery is strongly related to the severity of the stenosis and the recentness of symptoms. The risk of recurrent stroke in patients with recent TIA who do not have carotid endarterectomy and are treated medically increases substantially

Table 5.20 Indications for carotid surgery.

History of ipsilateral carotid TIA or stroke with reasonable recovery
Severe stenosis (≥70%, NASCET method, excluding near-occlusion) and symptoms within 6 months
Moderate stenosis (50–69%, NASCET method) and symptoms within 2 months and male gender
Patients must be fit for surgery and an experienced, skilled surgical team available

NASCET, North American Symptomatic Carotid Endarterectomy Trial; TIA, transient ischaemic attack.

above 50% stenosis with increasing deciles of stenosis over the next 5 years. Carotid endarterectomy has a risk of causing a stroke or death at the time of the surgery, in good hands, of 4–6% in recently symptomatic patients, but thereafter removing the stenosis surgically almost abolishes the risk of ipsilateral recurrence, with a subsequent annual rate of stroke of only about 1%. The risks of surgery bear little relationship to the severity of internal carotid artery stenosis. Hence, the benefits of surgery increase with increasing degrees of stenosis above 50% or so, in patients with recently symptomatic stenosis. However, patients with very severe stenosis in which the distal internal carotid artery has collapsed (an appearance referred to as pseudo-occlusion or near occlusion on angiography) have a low risk of recurrent stroke and do not benefit from surgery. Patients with complete carotid occlusion were not included in the endarterectomy trials, but previous studies suggested that surgery for carotid occlusion was hazardous.

The benefits of surgery for carotid stenosis decline with time from symptoms to the operation. Patients with moderate degrees of stenosis (50–69%, measured using the NASCET method) benefit from surgery if it is performed within the first few weeks after recent symptoms, especially if they are male, but not if the surgery is delayed beyond a month or two. Patients with more severe stenosis may benefit from surgery performed up to 6 months after symptoms, but any delay in surgery in these patients will mean that some patients will already have had a stroke while awaiting surgery. It is therefore essential that patients should be referred as soon as possible after TIA and stroke for carotid investigations, and operated on as soon as possible if significant stenosis is detected, the patient is neurologically stable and the patient is at high risk of recurrent stroke on medical therapy alone. Very early surgery can be hazardous and the optimum time to operate is between days 2 and 14 after symptoms.

A number of other clinical features apart from stenosis severity and time from symptoms alter the risk of recurrent stroke: the nature of the symptoms, the sex and age of the patient, their vascular risk factors and whether or not the carotid plaque is ulcerated on angiographic imaging. There are tools available that use these features to calculate the risk of recurrent stroke in recently symptomatic patients and these should be used to select patients for surgery. One issue is that medical therapy has improved substantially since the data that are used to calculate the risks and benefits of endarterectomy in symptomatic patients were collected. The current evidence suggests that medical therapy is now so effective that the benefits of removing the narrowing may not justify the risk of surgery in as many as 60% of patients with a lower risk of stroke currently receiving endartarterectomy. The Second European Carotid Surgery Trial (ECST-2) has recently started with the aim of establishing whether these patients should be managed by drug therapy alone or should be referred for surgery. There is also ongoing research examining whether methods of imaging the composition of carotid plaque, including various ultrasound, MRI and PET techniques, are effective at identifying the 'vulnerable' plaque likely to cause future symptoms. It is likely that in the future, one or more of these techniques will prove useful in selecting patients for endarterectomy.

The main hazard of carotid endarterectomy is stroke during the procedure itself. There is also a small incidence of stroke in the first 2 weeks after endarterectomy, probably resulting mostly from a thrombus formed on the endarterectomy site. Surgery also risks MI, pulmonary embolism and the development of a haematoma at the wound site. Up to 10% of patients develop a cranial nerve palsy, usually a unilateral hypoglossal nerve palsy, but these usually recover and only rarely cause disability (Chapter 13). Performing the operation under local anaesthesia has been shown in a randomised clinical trial to be no safer than operating under general anaesthesia. About 1% of patients develop hyperperfusion syndrome, which usually follows endarterectomy (or stenting) for a very tight stenosis, and may be more common in patients who develop postoperative hypertension. Patients with hyperperfusion syndrome complain of headache and may develop seizures and/or cerebral haemorrhage. Treatment of the hyperperfusion syndrome includes the urgent lowering of blood pressure. In patients with large acute infarcts, there may be a risk of causing reperfusion haemorrhage if the artery is operated on immediately, and it may be wise to wait 2 weeks or more before operating on these patients

Asymptomatic carotid stenosis

Patients investigated for TIA, stroke or other vascular conditions may be found to have a stenosis of one or more internal carotid arteries that is asymptomatic. A number of randomised trials have established that patients found to have carotid stenosis who have never had ipsilateral symptoms, or have had symptoms more than 6 months prior to randomisation, have a very low rate of ipsilateral stroke during follow-up of around 2% per annum. Carotid endarterectomy for asymptomatic carotid stenosis is less hazardous than in symptomatic patients, but carried a risk in these trials of around 3% within 30 days of the operation. Surgery then reduces the risk of ipsilateral stroke to about 1% per annum. The 5-year risk of any stroke or surgical death in the Asymptomatic Carotid Surgery Trial (ACST) fell from about 12% in patients in whom surgery was deferred until a more definite indication appeared (e.g. the stenosis became symptomatic), down to 6.4% in patients who had early endarterectomy. Subgroup analysis of ACST showed that patients over the age of 75 did not benefit from surgery, and the benefit in women was doubtful. The low rate of stroke in patients treated medically means that operating on asymptomatic carotid stenosis as a policy would result in a very large number of patients having unnecessary surgery, while some would be harmed from the operation, and only a small proportion (5%) would gain some benefit by avoiding stroke over the next 5 years. The majority of neurologists have concluded that this does not justify a policy of endarterectomy for asymptomatic stenosis, although exceptions may be made for young patients who are particularly anxious. The earlier carotid endarterectomy trials did not incorporate state-of-the-art medical treatment. It is likely that in asymptomatic patients who are treated with high dose statins, have vigorous control of hypertension and stop smoking, the benefits of endarterectomy will be even less than those demonstrated in the trials. The evidence from non-randomised studies suggest that the risk of stroke in asymptomatic patients has fallen in the last few years to around 1% or even lower in those receiving intensive medical therapy and risk factor modification. However, the risks of endarterectomy have also fallen to around 1%. There are therefore arguments supporting the need for new trials studying the effects endarterectomy compared with medical therapy in patients with asymptomatic stenosis. Several have started recently.

There does not appear to be a close relationship between stenosis severity and risk of future stroke in patients with asymptomatic carotid stenosis. There is therefore no benefit to following up asymptomatic stenosis with regular ultrasound examinations.

The benefits of carotid endarterectomy or stenting for patients with asymptomatic carotid stenosis who require major surgery, especially coronary artery bypass grafting (CABG), is uncertain. Severe carotid stenosis increases the risk of stroke during CABG, but the risk is not necessarily reduced by prior carotid endarterectomy or stenting, and the risk of stroke during treatment of the carotid artery is similar to the risk of stroke during CABG. Hence, a routine policy of screening and treatment of carotid stenosis prior to CABG is probably not justified. Patients who are symptomatic from both their carotid and coronary arteries should have the carotid treated prior to treatment of the coronary arteries.

Carotid stenting

Carotid stenting has become an alternative treatment to carotid endarterectomy for symptomatic carotid artery stenosis (Figure 5.28). Carotid stenting has the advantage of avoiding any incision in the neck and is usually performed under local anaesthesia. It appears less invasive and is therefore often preferred by patients to carotid endarterectomy, given the choice. However, carotid endarterectomy remains the treatment of choice for most patients. Randomised trials comparing endarterectomy with stenting for symptomatic carotid stenosis have consistently shown higher rates of procedural stroke in patients treated by stenting compared with endarterectomy. Stenting appears to be particularly hazardous in elderly patients, contrary to what might have been expected. However, subgroup analysis of the trial data has shown that patients younger than 70 years of age have a similar risk of procedural stroke comparing stenting with surgery, as do patients with less than average severity of white matter lesions on brain CT or MRI. Long-term follow-up in the trials have shown that stenting has a similar effectiveness compared with endarterectomy at preventing recurrent ipsilateral stroke after the periprocedural period. On the basis of this evidence carotid endarterectomy should remain the treatment of choice for symptomatic carotid stenosis in patients suitable for surgery except in younger patients and those with little white matter disease in whom stenting can be considered if appropriate carotid stenting expertise is available. Stenting remains an option in specific situations such as cases where surgery is not appropriate or particularly risky (e.g. 'hostile neck' secondary to previous radiotherapy) or in patients with significant cardiac risk. There are currently insufficient data concerning the safety of stenting compared with endarterectomy for asymptomatic carotid stenosis to form firm conclusions, but trials specifically examining this question are in progress.

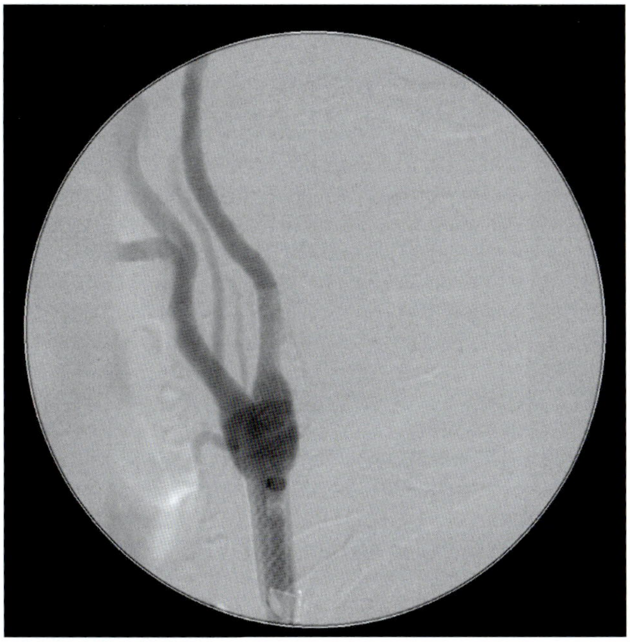

Figure 5.28 Left carotid stenosis; stent passes from CCA into ICA (catheter angiogram).

Vertebral stenosis

Posterior circulation stroke secondary to vertebrobasilar stenosis is not usually treated by surgical methods because of difficulty with access and then stenting is the only available treatment other than medical therapy. In the same way that stroke recurrence in the anterior circulation is highest in the presence of a symptomatic internal carotid artery stenosis so the recurrence rate for posterior circulation events is higher when a vertebrobasilar stenosis is demonstrated. The risk of recurrence is highest with intracranial stenosis and has been shown in one pooled analysis to be 33% at 90 days compared to 16.2% for extracranial vertebral artery stenosis and 7.2% when no stenosis is demonstrable. Current evidence suggests that stenting for proximal vertebral artery stenosis is relatively safe.

Intracranial artery stenosis

Angioplasty and stenting are occasionally used to treat proximal MCA stenoses but treatment at this site has considerable hazards and is usually regarded as a last resort for patients with severe stenosis and recurrent symptoms unresponsive to other treatments. The Stenting versus Agressive Medical Management for Preventing Recurrent Stroke in Intracranial Stenosis (SAMMPRIS) study compared stenting using the Wingspan stent system against intensive medical therapy for recently symptomatic intracranial artery stenosis and was terminated early because of excess stroke and death at 30 days in the stented group (14.7% versus 5.8%). The final results of the trial showed that even with longer follow-up, the patients who were treated with intensive medical therapy alone still had a significantly lower rate of stroke than those allocated stenting. With time, better methods of dilating intracranial stenosis will become available but SAMMPRIS is also notable for the relatively low rate of recurrent stroke in the medically treated group when compared to previous reports of very high recurrence rates in such patients. This low rate of recurrence has been attributed to the intensive blood pressure and cholesterol reduction, short-term dual antiplatelet treatment with aspirin plus clopidogrel and frequent follow-up to encourage compliance with medication and lifestyle measures. The risks for recurrent stroke are highest in the immediate period post stroke or TIA referable to the stenosis, for high grade stenosis and in cases where there is poor collateral supply to the distal territory.

Non-atherosclerotic vascular disease and other rarer causes of stroke

Although the majority of patients with ischaemic arterial stroke and primary intraparenchymal haemorrhage have atherosclerosis, there are several important non-atherosclerotic vasculopathies, including extracranial arterial dissection and conditions associated with vasculitis.

Carotid and vertebral artery dissection

Cervicocephalic dissections of the vertebral or carotid arteries should be especially considered in young patients. Although many disease processes that may be associated with dissection (e.g. Marfan's syndrome, Ehlers–Danlos syndrome and fibromuscular dysplasia), the vast majority occur in apparently normal subjects after trivial neck trauma (e.g. minor whiplash injuries) or apparently spontaneously. The incidence of dissection resulting from major head and neck trauma is surprisingly low at around one case per 10 000 patients with head or neck trauma of sufficient severity to be admitted to hospital. In otherwise spontaneous dissection, hyperextension of the neck during hair washing in the salon or when painting a ceiling, are common preceding events. Whether these apparent precipitants are relevant or not is unclear. In particular, dissection is often attributed to manipulation of the neck, but epidemiological evidence suggests that in many cases it may be neck pain from the dissection that has taken the patient to a chiropractor or other therapists in the first place. New evidence is emerging that many of these patients probably have subtle underlying collagen defects that may make them particularly vulnerable to even normal neck movement. These patients may have fragments of Marfanism. For example, they may be entirely double-jointed, or they may have a relative with Marfan's syndrome.

Fibromuscular dysplasia, a non-atheromatous condition that may involve all three arterial wall layers, can affect many systemic arteries. It is most commonly described in middle-aged women. Bilateral ICA involvement is common, sparing the bifurcation and intracranial carotid artery. In fibromuscular dysplasia, dysplastic fibrous tissue and proliferating smooth muscle cause constricting areas interspersed with areas of dilatation. This is responsible for the characteristic sign on angiography – the 'string of beads' sign. Many of these lesions are benign or present with benign symptoms (e.g. pulsatile tinnitus) but stroke may occur from embolism or occlusion. The recurrence rate of stroke is low. However, patients with fibromuscular dysplasia have a high incidence of intracranial aneurysms and SAH.

Dissection is produced by the subintimal penetration of blood and subsequent extension between the vessel layers resulting in an intramural haematoma, which expands the artery. This may narrow the lumen and lead to occlusion of the vessel but more often the dissection exposes a thrombogenic surface on which intraluminal haematoma develops. This haematoma may then embolise and produce stroke. Occasionally, a free flap of intima may protrude into the lumen of the artery without an evident mural haematoma or there may be only a small tear of the intimal surface leading to thrombosis. The latter mechanism is very difficult to demonstrate in life. The vast majority of cases of dissection affect the extracranial carotid and vertebral arteries and usually start at the level of C1/2, probably because the vertebral and carotid arteries lie close to the transverse process of C1 and are injured during neck rotation. Dissection appears to be less common in older patients, perhaps because atherosclerosis renders the cervical arteries less flexible. Intracranial dissection is much rarer but usually leads to SAH because of the thinness of the muscular wall of the intracranial arteries, which is sometimes catastrophic. Occasionally, intracranial dissection cuts through perforating vessels and present as stroke.

The classic clinical scenario is of the precipitating event to be followed shortly by the development of neck pain and headache. There may be a delay of several days, sometimes weeks before embolisation causes stroke. Patients more often present when stroke has occurred. In some, dissection may never give rise to symptomatic embolisation but in others dissection may be instantly associated with devastating cerebral infarction. Asymptomatic dissection may be recognised by chance during imaging for another indication and is sometimes bilateral in a patient with unilateral symptoms. Although any stroke syndrome may occur as a complication of dissection, the presence of a Horner's syndrome may be particularly alerting. In the carotid circulation, this will be caused by involvement of the ascending sympathetic fibres surrounding the ICA in the neck. In the vertebro-basilar circulation this may result from embolic occlusion of the posterior inferior cerebellar artery with resultant infarction of the dorsolateral medulla where the descending sympathetic tracts lie (lateral medullary syndrome). Some patients present with a painful Horner's syndrome alone brought about by carotid dissection. Occasionally, carotid dissection causes compression of a lower cranial nerve or nerves within the jugular foramen (e.g. a unilateral XIIth nerve lesion causing deviation of the tongue). MRI or CTA provides a sensitive and non-invasive means to confirm dissection. MRI fine-cut axial imaging with sequences that suppress signal from fat through the neck may reveal the characteristic cresentic vessel wall haematoma and flow-related MRI (Figure 5.29). Catheter angiography may show tapering luminal compromise or, rarely, an intimal flap. Carotid imaging is easier to interpret than vertebral imaging; as the vertebral artery is wrapped at some points in a venous plexus this sometimes give the artificial appearance of cresentic haematoma on cross-sectional MRI. The dissection should be followed on MRI and/or CT because about 50% show recanalisation (allowing anticoagulation or antiplatelet therapy to be discontinued) and rarely a false aneurysm develops. These are usually asymptomatic but exceptionally rarely may expand resulting in a retropharyngeal mass effect. Carotid ultrasound may show the characteristic features of a distal stenosis beyond the site of insonation, but is not as sensitive as other techniques. If the artery is completely occluded it may be difficult to confirm a suspicion of

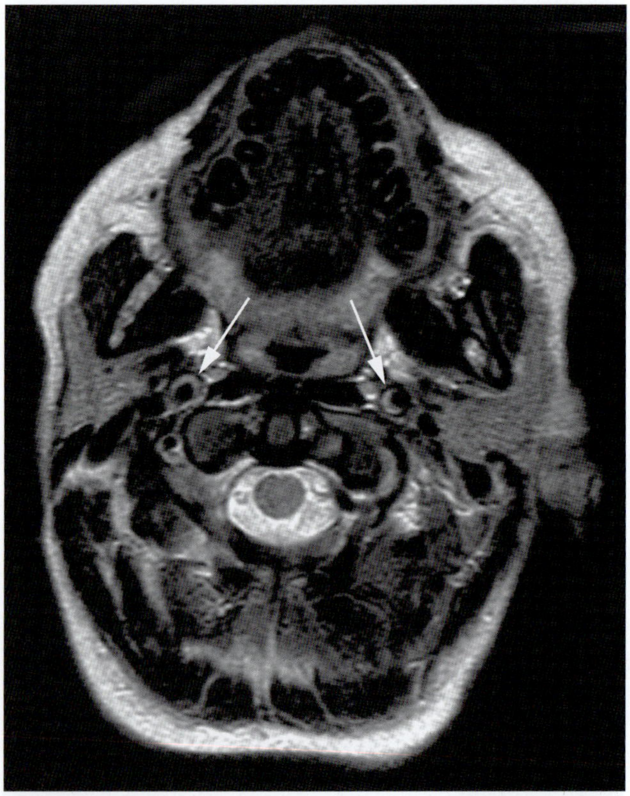

Figure 5.29 Axial T2 MRI through the skull base showing bilateral ICA dissection. Flow voids indicate patency of each arterial lumen; the crescent-shaped hyperintensity is the intramural thrombus on each side (arrows).

dissection – ultrasound does not visualise the site of the mural haematoma, and dissection can only be inferred on MRI if the occluded distal carotid or vertebral artery appears expanded.

There is no agreed protocol for prevention of (further) stroke events associated with a demonstrated acute dissection. Antithrombotic therapy with either anticoagulation or antiplatelet drugs has long been used but the two treatments were only recently compared in the CADISS trial, which enrolled subjects with extracranial carotid or vertebral dissection and randomly assigned them to either antiplatelet or anticoagulant treatment for 3 months. There was no significant difference between the two groups in terms of stroke recurrence, which occurred in 2% of the antiplatelet group and 1% in the anticoagulant group. There were no deaths in either group but one major bleeding occurred in the anticoagulant group.

Because of the very low rate of recurrence, this trial cannot establish which treatment is superior. However, the data are reassuring, and most physicians now use antiplatelets in preference to anticoagulation for secondary and/or primary prevention of stroke following cervical artery dissection, as it is much less complicated to administer and possibly safer. Anticoagulation should definately be avoided in those with a volume of infarction exceeding one third of the MCA territory, large territory cerebellar infarction and in intradural dissection. Stenting in the acute phase is hardly ever necessary but may have a role for recurrent events especially when brought about by haemodynamic and/or perfusion failure. In patients with false aneurysm formation, follow-up to ensure stability with MRI and/or CT angiography or ultrasound is recommended for 2 years. Progressive expansion may need stenting but is rare. The risk of recurrence of symptomatic dissection in the absence of any underlying collagen disorder or obvious precipitant is around 1% per annum.

Vasculitis

Vasculitis is beloved by some in the differential diagnosis of stroke. Although vasculitis may result in stroke (usually from uncontrolled hypertension), it is exceedingly rare for vasculitis to present simply as stroke. Vasculitis may be of infective origin, necrotising, associated with collagen vascular disease, other systemic disease, hypersensitivity, giant cell or miscellaneous. Neurological investigations, other than the occasional cerebral biopsy, are not particularly helpful in the diagnosis of cerebral vasculitis. If MRI is requested with the words: 'Stroke – ? vasculitis', the report is likely to indicate: 'Vasculitis cannot be excluded.' Despite this opinion, contrast enhanced MRI can be helpful in suggesting an inflammatory arteriopathy if there is enhancement of both the meninges and parenchyma and MRI sequences sensitive to blood breakdown products may reveal microhaemorrhagic sequelae of active vessel wall disease. Other clues for a vasculitic process on MRI are that the pattern of acute infarction indicates pathology in vessels of a similar caliber, that there is multi-territory and sequentially appearing signal change, or that there is evidence of both acute ischaemia and parenchymal haemorrhage. In systemic and other vasculitides, the diagnosis is based on the extracranial features and typical serology. It is only when the vasculitis is confined to the nervous system (isolated angiitis) that the diagnosis will require more detailed investigation (see also Chapters 9 and 26).

Infective vasculitis

Infective vasculitis associated with meningitis can occur acutely in the appropriate setting of severe bacterial, fungal, tuberculous or herpes zoster infection. There is nearly always an appropriate proceding history suggestive of a menigo-encephalitis syndrome. After primary syphilis infection, an obliterative endarteritis affecting the small vessels of the brain may occur with a usual latency of 7 years. Headache and encephalopathy predominate in the prodrome before stroke occurs. Evidence of previous infection is easy to screen for in the blood and those with neurological involvement usually have pleocytosis and positive serology in the CSF (Chapter 9). Enhanced MRI may show chronic syphilitic pachymeningitis with thickening of the meninges. Lyme borreliosis can mimic syphilis.

Viral infection may well be responsible for some cases of vasculitis previously considered idiopathic. Hepatitis B and C and herpes zoster are proven examples. Zoster is the most well-described form of viral arteritis to affect the CNS. The classic scenario is of V_1 shingles followed by brain infarction several weeks later. The infarct is usually ipsilateral to the rash and some patients may have encephalitis. The carotid territory is most commonly involved with occlusion at the siphon or MCA. In children, stroke may follow primary zoster infection (chickenpox). Patients with HIV have higher rates of cerebrovascular disease but there are many mechanisms underpinning this, including atherosclerosis secondary to HIV therapy and hypercoagulability.

Parasites may also be associated with endarteritis. Cysticercosis may be complicated by stroke when cysts lodge in the subarachnoid space leading to meningeal inflammation. The major basal arteries may be affected by this process and asymptomatic angiographic stenosis is more common than stroke.

In cerebral malaria caused by *Plasmodium falciparum*, haemorrhagic stroke may accompany the diffuse brain injury, particularly in children.

Systemic vasculitides

Systemic vasculitis has been classified immunopathologically, by the nature of the vessel involved or clinically. Most strokes associated with systemic vasculitis are brought about by uncontrolled hypertension, not cerebral involvement, and patients have usually been unwell for a considerable time. When looking at vasculitis through stroke spectacles, vessel size is a good starting point. Issues relevant to stroke are discussed here.

Large vessel vasculitis These are Takayasu and giant cell arteritis. Both are granulomatous vasculitides. In giant cell arteritis (Chapter 26), the internal elastic lamina of the extracranial medium sized arteries becomes fragmented and invaded by inflammatory cells. It virtually always occurs in those aged over 50 and in 90% is accompanied by an elevated ESR. Patients complain of headache with scalp tenderness associated with malaise, depression, myalgia and sometimes claudication of the jaw muscles while eating. Examination usually reveals thickened tender temporal arteries. Stroke is a very rare complication of the disease but may occur from involvement of the extradural vertebral artery leading to brainstem infarction. A far more common complication without treatment, or at presentation, is anterior ischaemic optic neuropathy (Chapter 14). Diagnosis is established by temporal artery biopsy. Treatment is with high dose prednisolone, and if the diagnosis is correct the response of the systemic symptoms is dramatic and usually occurs within 1 day. Occasionally, the intracranial ICA may be involved.

Takayasu's arteritis was originally described in Japanese girls and women and is often called pulseless disease. There may be a prodromal phase associated with anaemia and raised ESR followed by severe occlusive disease of the aortic arch and its branches, leading to absent neck and limb pulses. Stroke is not a common feature but headache, dizziness and syncope are more frequent. The diagnosis of Takayasu's arteritis may be made by ultrasound showing occluded or stenotic large neck vessels at their origin from the aorta with thickened walls. Characteristic sites of involvement include the proximal common carotid artery, subclavian artery and the innominate artery.

Medium vessel vasculitis Polyarteritis nodosa (PAN) is the principal medium vessel vasculitis. It is important to remember that PAN is usually ANCA negative. PAN affects medium and small arteries. The most common neurological feature is mononeuritis. CNS involvement may occur in 20%, but it is often late in the disease. Presenting features include cerebral infarction, cerebral haemorrhage and SAH.

Small vessel vasculitis Microscopic polyarteritis is usually ANCA positive and affects small vessels, as do Wegener's granulomatosis and Churg–Strauss syndrome. Encephalopathy and peripheral manifestations are common but stroke rare. Exceptional patients have presented with SAH as the first sign of vasculitis.

Collagen vascular disease
Systemic lupus erythematosus (SLE) commonly causes neurological problems. These often have a neuropsychiatric component and are rarely caused by the vasculitis. Encephalopathy, psychosis, seizures, stroke-like focal deficits, myelopathy and neuropathy are all encountered. At pathological examination the histology is often one of non-specific gliosis although thrombosis may be observed especially in those with a lupus anticoagulant and antiphospholipid antibodies. Echocardiography shows a high frequency of valvular disease in SLE, particularly Libman–Sacks endocarditis, which may lead to cerebral embolism. Myocarditis is also a feature of SLE. Response to immunosupression of florid neurological involvement is often poor. Lupus may also cause a terminal carotid occlusive syndrome leading to a Moyamoya angiopathy.

Other vasculitis
Very rarely, true necrotising arteritis can be seen in association with rheumatoid resulting in encephalopathy or small infarcts. Brain infarcts have also been reported in systemic sclerosis along with SAH, but there is a high incidence of hypertension in systemic sclerosis. Sarcoid may occasionally cause a cerebral vasculitis or focal infarction, usually in association with meningeal involvement.

Isolated angiitis of the central nervous system
This rare condition affects small and medium sized intracranial vessels. It may cause a combination of infarcts and haemorrhages. Presentation is usually chronic with prominent headache, leading to encephalopathy and then stroke-like focal dysfunction. Any age may be affected and there is a male predominance. The disorder may be acute over weeks or subacute. Angiography may reveal segmental narrowing of intracranial vessels but this is neither sensitive nor specific. Many patients have normal angiography. The CSF often shows a pleocytosis with oligoclonal immunoglobulin on electrophoresis. Brain imaging may show multiple small vessel infarcts and sometimes haemorrhages, if advanced. Diagnosis is by meningeal and brain biopsy, which typically shows a granulomatous vasculitis. If patients have neither headache nor CSF pleocytosis then biopsy rarely shows vasculitis. Treatment is with steroids and cyclophosphamide.

Thrombotic thrombocytopenic purpura
This is characterised by microangiopathic haemolytic anaemia, thrombocytopenia and systemic microinfarction from platelet-rich thrombi. Renal failure, fever and transient neurological signs, or diffuse encephalopathy, are common. Large vessel infarction and cerebral haemorrhage may also occur. Posterior leukoencephalopathy has been described. The mainstay of treatment is plasma exchange but anticoagulation is sometimes necessary and the decision to do this has to be finely balanced against the risk of haemorrhage.

Behçet's disease
The common neurological manifestations of Behçet's disease are meningitis, encephalitis with multifocal signs, stroke-like events and dural sinus thrombosis. The lesions of Behçet's disease do not conform to arterial territories, suggesting a venous origin, and usually angiography shows no abnormalities. The brainstem is frequently involved.

Susac's syndrome
Susac termed this condition a microangiopathy of the brain and retina. The cochlea is also involved. There is always obliteration of the large retinal arteries causing focal scotomata and stepwise visual loss. Tinnitus and sudden hearing loss are common and the principal neurological features are dementia, pyramidal and cerebellar dysfunction. The disorder usually affects young women.

Sneddon's syndrome
This is characterised by chronic skin lesions, livedo reticularis and stroke. The most important feature is the livedo. Skin biopsy may show distinctive abnormalities in small and medium arteries. Cerebral angiography may show branch intracranial occlusions. Some cases have been attributed to the antiphospholipid antibody syndrome.

Mitochondrial disease
MELAS syndrome (mitochondrial myopathy, encephalopathy, lactic acidosis and stroke-like episodes) is sometimes considered as a differential diagnosis under the young stroke umbrella. Imaging may show multifocal abnormalities most often in the parieto-occipital and temporal lobes. Although the ischaemic lesions affect cortex and underlying white matter, these often cross arterial territories and the arteries supplying these areas are normal on investigation. Other features of a mitochondrial cytopathy are usually present (Chapter 10).

Fabry disease
Fabry disease is an X-linked liposomal disorder in which there is deficiency of α galactosidase A. Typical clinical manifestations include painful neuropathy, stroke and renal failure, but young stroke may be the presenting feature. Angiography shows branch artery occlusion caused by the diffuse arteriopathy associated with sphingolipid accumulation. Imaging usually shows features of small vessel disease with a bias towards infarction in the brainstem and posterior circulation territories.

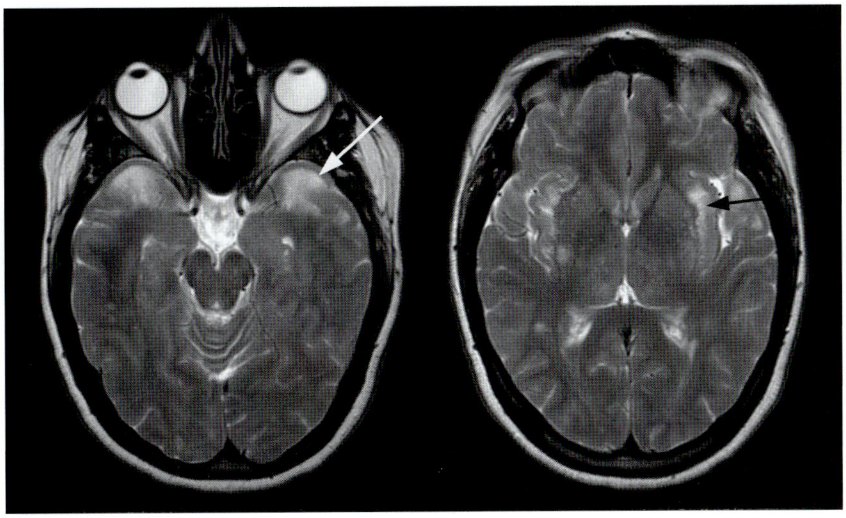

Figure 5.30 CADASIL. T2-weighted images showing multiple small subcortical infarcts in the deep grey nuclei and white matter with confluent high signal in the temporal poles (white arrow) and external capsules (black arrow) typical of CADASIL.

CADASIL and CARASIL

Cerebral autosomal dominant arteriopathy with subcortical infarcts and leukoencephalopathy (CADASIL) is the most common genetic vascular disorder of the brain and, although rare, does crop up from time to time in vascular clinics. The disorder is characterised by migraine headache often with aura and extensive white matter abnormalities and lacunar infarction. Patients may present with depression, migraine, dementia and/or progressive gait difficulty. MRI often shows characteristic involvement of the temporal white matter (Figure 5.30). Although dominantly inherited, many cases appear to present as new mutations. The diagnosis can be obtained through skin biopsy and genetic testing for the underlying mutation of the NOTCH III gene (Chapter 8). CARASIL is the acronym for same descriptor except that for the inheritance being recessive, not dominant. CARASIL is a very rare disorder and has similar neurological symptoms to CADASIL, but is also characterised by premature alopecia and attacks of back pain secondary to vertebral disc degeneration.

Hypertensive encephalopathy

This condition, which is now rare, develops if systemic blood pressure exceeds the upper limit of cerebral autoregulation. Oedema develops in the hyperperfused intracerebral circulation. Patients present with headache, fits, focal TIA-like events, stroke and depressed consciousness. In addition, examination may reveal optic disc swelling and microscopic haematuria characteristic of malignant or accelerated hypertension. The blood pressure is usually very high (e.g. 250/150 mmHg) but may be lower. In these patients the rate of blood pressure elevation has often been rapid and brought about by renal disease. Slower elevation allows autoregulatory mechanisms to compensate to some extent. Brain imaging may show a posterior reversible leukoencephalopathy, as well as focal infarcts or haemorrhage. Eclampsia in pregnancy and the puerperium has similar features.

Migraine and stroke

There is a small but definite increase in stroke incidence in patients with migraine. However, this needs to be interpreted with caution as vascular disease predisposes to migraine headaches and aura. In particular, carotid artery dissection may precipitate a classic migraine attack with visual aura. There are links between antiphospholipid syndrome, sickle cell disease and possibly PFO with migraine, all of which can cause stroke. Other associations include mitochondrial disease and CADASIL. There remain very rare patients who develop infarction at the peak of a typical migraine attack, for which no other reason can be found. The symptoms of these migrainous strokes mimic the features of the patient's aura, and the associated infarction usually involves the occipital cortex. Hemiplegic migraine is a very rare familial channelopathy. Almost all young patients with migraine-like headache who suffer a hemiplegia have had the stroke from a cause unrelated to migraine. Migraine without aura but particularly migraine with aura are independent risk factors for stroke (Chapter 12). This risk appears to be substantially increased in female migraineurs who smoke, are hypertensive and take the oestrogen-containing contraceptive pill.

Moyamoya angiopathy

The term Moyamoya ('puff of smoke') angiopathy refers to an angiographic appearance in which terminal carotid occlusion is associated with the development of a fine and friable network of basal collateral vessels. Moyamoya disease is a distinct condition, prevalent in Japan but also occasionally seen in the West, in which a symmetric progressive and obliterative intracranial arteriopathy develops, causing stenosis and occlusion of the basal vessels, usually the termination of both internal carotid arteries and the M1 segment of the MCA (Figure 5.31). Early or arrested cases may show involvement of only one side, but this can progress to bilateral involvement. The basilar and vertebral arteries are very rarely affected and never in isolation. The term Moyamoya syndrome is used when similar appearances occur in association with identifiable causes such as radiotherapy and sickle cell disease. Moyamoya disease presents most often in children with TIA, ischaemic stroke, chorea, severe migrainelike headaches or seizures. Some patients appear to stabilise clinically in late adolescence, although long-term follow-up studies are lacking. Adults may present with similar symptoms and the likelihood is that the condition starts in childhood and those presenting in adulthood either have a slower rate

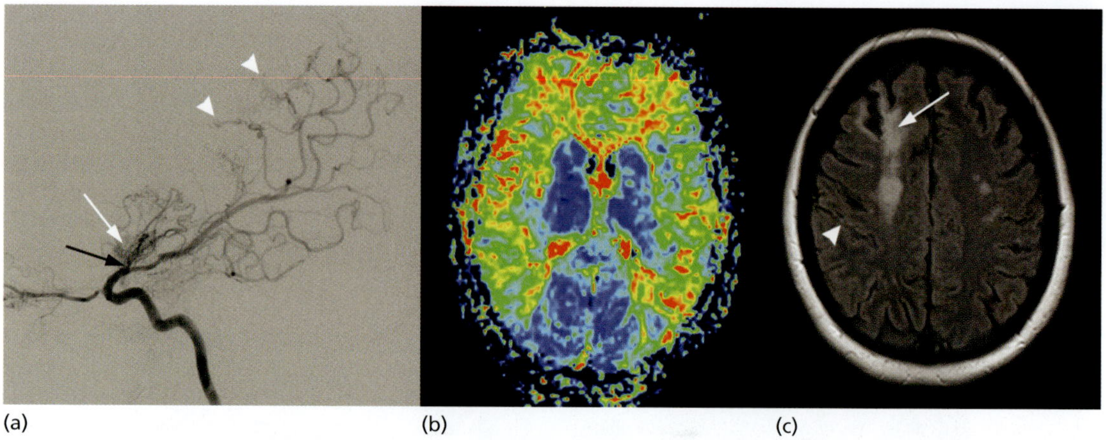

Figure 5.31 Moyamoya. (a) Internal carotid artery digital subtraction angiogram showing occlusion of the vessel just distal to the posterior communicating artery (black arrow) and typical Moyamoya collateral vessels (white arrow). Pial collaterals arise from posterior cerebral artery branches (white arrowheads). (b) Perfusion MRI shows abnormal mean transit time throughout the middle and anterior cerebral artery territories with sparing of the basal ganglia and tissue supplied by the posterior cerebral arteries (blue voxels). (c) Right anterior border-zone infarcts (white arrow) and sulcal hyperintensity ('ivy sign') (arrow head) representing distended pial vessels are seen on FLAIR.

of progression or they develop better collateralisation that only fails when they develop additional vascular disease from smoking, hypertension or atherosclerosis. Adults can also present later in life with ICH from rupture of the friable collaterals. Treatment options include surgical revascularisation, either extracranial–intracranial bypass or synangiosis, a procedure in which vascularised omentum or muscle is juxtaposed to the brain. Children are usually prescribed aspirin, but this should be stopped in adults because of the risk of haemorrhage. Intensive and early control of vascular risk factors, including mild hypertension and elevated cholesterol levels, is key to preventing deterioration in adults.

Cerebral venous thrombosis

Cerebral venous thrombosis is often considered under the umbrella of stroke but is a condition with diverse manifestations that mimic many other neurological disorders. It is increasingly recognised because of enhanced awareness and the use of MRI. Venous thrombosis may be septic or non-septic. Septic causes are increasingly rare but cavernous sinus thrombosis secondary to facial cellulitis and lateral sinus thrombosis secondary to purulent otitis media or mastoiditis are still seen. Septic thrombophlebitis of the cortical veins may also be associated with severe bacterial meningitis.

Aseptic thrombosis can affect the cortical veins, dural sinuses and deep veins. There are numerous potential causes. The most common are raised oestrogen levels in women, associated with pregnancy, the puerperium and the contraceptive pill. There are no reliable estimates of incidence although venous thrombosis may complicate 11/100 000 deliveries. Other factors include dehydration in association with systemic disease, thrombophilia (particularly the factor V Leiden polymorphism), activated protein C resistance and Behçet's syndrome. It has become clear that such external factors pose far more significant risk for recurrent thrombosis than inherited thrombophilias (Table 5.21). In 20% of cases of venous thrombosis no aetiology is uncovered.

The clinical syndrome that results from cerebral venous thrombosis may be acute or subacute. The most frequent manifestations are headaches, seizures, altered consciousness, focal signs and optic disc swelling. Hence, cerebral venous thrombosis should be considered in the differential diagnosis of patients presenting with severe headache, seizure disorders, coma, stroke, acute meningoencephalitis syndromes or isolated intracranial hypertension, mimicking idiopathic intracranial hypertension. Venous sinus thrombosis can cause headache, sometimes thunderclap, as the only feature. Only 50% of patients have papilloedema.

Venous thrombosis results in venous hypertension that leads to raised intracranial pressure. This may give rise to a syndrome of headache with papilloedema and normal CT imaging, initially identical to idiopathic intracranial hypertension. However, as the venous pressure rises, forced local arterial hypertension can lead to cerebral haemorrhage. Alternatively, or in addition, spread of the thrombus to cortical veins results in venous infarction, which is often haemorrhagic and results in focal neurological deficit and depression of consciousness.

Patients with venous sinus thrombosis may be severely ill and such patients often present to neurosurgeons as cases of primary intracerebral haemorrhage in coma. However, the radiological findings are usually distinct from both arterial ischaemic stroke and intracerebral haemorrhage. Venous infarction is characterised on imaging by vasogenic as opposed to cytotoxic oedema. These areas do not confine themselves to vascular territories and are often haemorrhagic. The thrombus in the venous sinuses may be visible on plain MRI although false negatives occur in the hyperacute (first few days) and chronic phases (1–2 months) necessitating flow-related imaging (Figure 5.32). Sometimes, the flow-related imaging can be difficult to interpret, especially whether the transverse sinus on the left is hypoplastic (a common variant) or thrombosed. If sufficient clinical suspicion exists and MR/MRV are negative, we recommend CT angiography or, if necessary, catheter angiography. Depending on local practice, CT angiography may be the investigation of choice. Rarely, venous sinus thrombosis is the result or the cause of dural fistulae and this often needs full intra- and extracranial angiography to diagnose.

The most common sinus involved is the sagittal sinus, followed by the lateral sinuses. Cortical veins may rarely be involved in isolation (Figure 5.33). Imaging proof of isolated cortical venous thrombosis is difficult. Often one has to embark on treatment on the basis

Table 5.21 Causes of cerebral venous thrombosis.

Prothrombotic disorders	Polycythaemia Paroxysmal nocturnal haemoglobinuria Sickle cell Haemolytic anaemia Factor V Leiden Protein C and S deficiency Antothrombin III Prothrombin gene mutation DIC Antiphospholipid syndrome
Malignancy	Visceral carcinoma Carcinoid Lymphoma Myeloproliferative disease
Drugs	Combined contraceptive pill Hormone replacement therapy Heparin-induced thrombocytopenia Ovarian hyperstimulation
Pregnancy and the puerperium	
Systemic inflammatory disease	Behçet's Systemic lupus erythematosus Sarcoidosis Giant cell arteritis Granulomatosis with polyangiitis (Wegener's) Thrombangitis obliterans Inflammatory bowel disease (Crohn's disease and ulcerative colitis}
Severe dehydration	Any cause including exercise
Systemic infection	Septicaemia Endocarditis TB Malaria Aspergillosis
Cardiac	Congenital, CCF
Vascular malformation	Dural AV fistulae
Others	Nephrotic syndrome Head injury Low CSF pressure
Local cranial causes	Extradural infection: facial cellulitis, mastoiditis, sinusitis Intradural: abscess, meningitis Tumour: metastasis, menigioma
Idiopathic	Intravenous cannula

CCF, congestive cardiac failure; CSF, cerebrospinal fluid; DIC, disseminated intravascular coagulation; TB, tuberculosis.

of the clinical presentation and MRI of a presumed venous infarct. Thrombosis of the deep venous system is rare in adults and gives rise to thalamic venous infarction with prolonged coma.

Cavernous sinus thrombosis should be considered a separate entity as it is most commonly caused by local sepsis rather than primary or secondary non-septic hypercoagulable states. It is a serious disease with a high mortality. The veins draining the face are the common portals, hence the view that facial cellulitis is also a very serious condition. The early symptoms are pain, headache, fever, facial oedema then proptosis and ophthalmoplegia (Chapter 14). The principal treatment is antibiotics. Non-septic cavernous sinus thrombosis may follow head injury and thrombosis within dural cavernous arteriovenous fistulae. Cavernous sinus thrombosis rarely presents to stroke neurologists, but is seen more commonly in ophthalmological and emergency medical practice.

The accepted treatment of intracranial venous thrombosis is anticoagulation, whether haemorrhage is present or not. The evidence for this is controversial. Anticoagulants were first given to prevent pulmonary embolism from intracranial thrombosis. Early studies suggested that patients treated with anticoagulants had a 7% mortality compared with 37% if untreated. A small prospective trial and retrospective analysis also suggested a significant survival benefit with anticoagulation and also the safety of heparin in the presence of haemorrhage. Later studies have suggested no advantage to heparin but were weighted toward less sick patients with indolent intracranial hypertension presentations, and better than expected outcomes in the placebo arm. It is the general view from clinical practice that anticoagulation is an essential treatment for these patients. The favoured method is subcutaneous low molecular weight heparin rather than intravenous heparin unless surgery is contemplated. The literature supports the safety of heparin in haemorrhage. In addition to anticoagulation, sepsis must be identified and treated with antibiotics and drainage where appropriate (e.g. mastoiditis). Patients with significant intracranial pressure will need ventilation and occasionally consideration for craniotomy. Our policy following venous thrombosis is to anticoagulate for 6 months, or for longer terms if a persisting reason for hypercoagulability persists. In patients with disc swelling, vision should be monitored using a visual field screen (e.g. Goldmann) at regular intervals. Visual obscuration (Chapter 14) is a sign of incipient optic nerve infarction. Optic nerve fenestration, therapeutic lumbar puncture, lumbo-peritoneal shunting and acetazolamide all have their place in management. Recently, thrombolytic agents delivered by a transvenous endovascular route have been used to treat patients with sinus thrombosis and may be safe with haemorrhage. Early studies show promising results, but our current policy is to reserve this for patients not responding to, or worsening on, heparin.

The outcome of venous thrombosis tends to be polarised. Usually, patients either make a good recovery or die. Good outcome may be seen in up to 85%, death in 12% and the remainder have an intermediate outcome. Mortality is higher with age and in association with infection or cancer. Seizures occurring during the acute phase have a good long-term prognosis with low rate of recurrence. Recurrent thrombosis may be seen in 10–20%, usually in the first year. The necessity for long-term anticoagulation after the first thrombosis is based on identifying ongoing active risk factors and the strategy is identical to that applied to limb venous thrombosis.

Reversible cerebral vasoconstriction syndrome

Reversible cerebral vasoconstriction syndrome (RCVS) is characterised by transient dysregulation of cerebral vascular tone leading to prolonged but reversible constriction of intracranial arteries, with resolution within 3 months. It is an increasingly recognised

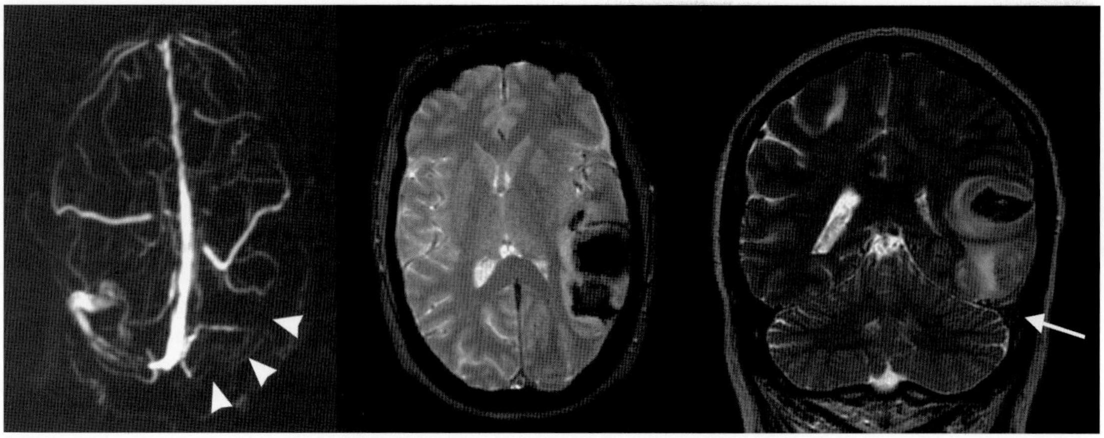

(a) (b) (c)

Figure 5.32 Venous infarct. (a) MR venogram viewed as if looking from above the patient towards the feet. No flow is visible in the occluded left transverse sinus (arrowheads). (b,c) T2*-w axial and T2-w coronal images showing a haemorrhagic venous infarct in the left temporal lobe. Note abnormal signal in the thrombosed left transverse sinus (arrow) immediately below the infarct.

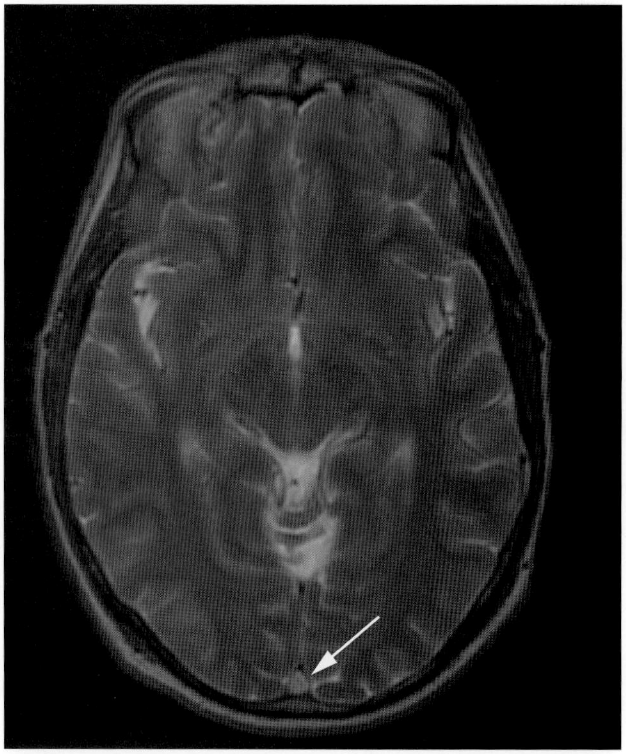

Figure 5.33 Absence of flow in the superior sagittal sinus on T2 MRI due to thrombosis (arrow).

syndrome, and a common medical condition transferred to neurosurgeons.

The most common clinical presentation is with severe acute headache (typically thunderclap), with or without additional neurological symptoms including focal neurology and seizures. Most patients (>90%) will present with recurrent thunderclap headaches. The syndrome may be spontaneous (idiopathic), or may occur secondary to a precipitant (25–60%). Reported precipitants include vasoactive substances, pregnancy or puerperium, catecholamine-secreting tumours, and immunosuppressants or blood products. The most commonly reported precipitants are serotonin selective re-uptake inhibitors, cannabis and cocaine, and over-the-counter nasal decongestants. A trigger immediately prior to the onset of headache is recounted by 80% of patients, including sexual intercourse, straining, physical exertion, urination, high emotional state, showering and head movements.

Complications of RCVS include seizures, SAH and intracerebral haemorrhage during the first 7 days after headache onset when small calibre vessels are affected, followed by ischaemic infarcts during the second week when medium and larger calibre arteries are affected. SAH is of small volume and tends to be localised, overlying the cortical surface.

CT/MR brain imaging at presentation is frequently normal. Angiography shows multifocal segmental narrowing and dilatation, in a 'string of beads' pattern. Serial angiography has found peak involvement of arterial segments 16 days after headache onset, with unsynchronised progression and regression of vasoconstricted arterial segments. Complete reversal of angiographic abnormalities is apparent between 1 and 3 months after presentation. The differential diagnosis for a single thunderclap headache includes primary headache syndromes, aneurysmal SAH, intracranial haemorrhage, cervical or intracranial dissection, hypertensive encephalopathy, post-partum vasculopathy, venous thrombosis, giant cell arteritis and pituitary apoplexy. Recurrent thunderclap headaches are much more likely to be RCVS or primary headache syndromes.

The following diagnostic criteria for RCVS have been proposed:

1 Acute severe headache with or without neurological signs or symptoms
2 Multifocal segmental vasoconstriction of cerebral arteries demonstrated by angiography
3 No evidence for aneurysmal SAH
4 Normal or near-normal CSF analysis (protein <1 g/L, white cells <15 mm^3, glucose normal)
5 Reversibility of angiographic abnormalities within 12 weeks after onset.

Initial management includes cessation of potential precipitants, blood pressure control and medical management of seizures.

There have been no clinical trials evaluating pharmacotherapy in RCVS and open studies have not found any significant clinical benefit with calcium channel blockers or glucocorticoids. Calcium channel blockers (particularly nimodipine) are frequently used as vasodilators, but care must be taken to avoid hypotension and subsequent border-zone infarction in areas perfused by the constricted artery.

The prognosis in RCVS in favourable, with excellent recovery in uncomplicated cases.

Vascular disease of the spinal cord

The spinal cord is most often affected by occlusion of the anterior spinal artery which supplies the anterior two-thirds of the cord. The blood supply is most tenuous in the upper thoracic region of the cord, which is a border-zone region. Although the anterior spinal artery is vulnerable to aortic dissection, most patients with anterior spinal artery occlusion presenting to a neurologist have atherosclerosis secondary to multiple risk factors, especially hypertension and diabetes. The dorsal columns are spared (because of a rich plexal supply) after the anterior spinal artery occludes. The resultant clinical picture is that of acute areflexic paraplegia characterised by dissociated sensory loss, with striking preservation of joint position and vibration sense but marked loss of pinprick and temperature sensation. Paraplegia is also well recognised following aortic surgery. There is a vogue still for anticoagulation of these patients and placement of a lumbar drain but little evidence to support these measure.

The spine can also be affected by AVMs and dural fistulae. Dural fistulae present with symptoms resulting from venous hypertension and cord ischaemia. Bleeding does not occur from spinal dural fistulae, unlike their cranial counterparts. They often present in elderly men with step-wise cauda equina symptoms with prominent exercise exacerbation. MRI virtually always shows dilated draining veins and treatment may be possible with embolisation or surgery. The remainder of spinal AVMs are mostly intramedullary; they present in younger men with cord syndromes, cord or epidural bleeding. Treatment is often difficult, and unsatisfactory. Other features of vascular cord disease are discussed in Chapters 16 and 26.

Stroke: overall conclusions

Stroke is a varied and challenging speciality. There is a diverse age range at presentation and a multitude of systemic issues that need to be dealt with. It is a speciality for those who enjoy multidisciplinary working, both within a medical context and across professions. Stroke is also high risk, patients can become unwell very quickly, and re-admission is common after minor stroke or TIA, because of deterioration and even when all risk factors have been adequately addressed. Well-planned intervention can also go wrong, but the discipline is underpinned by a rich evidence base to guide practice and new trials to answer unknowns are always being constructed.

References

Camm AJ, Lip GY, De Caterina R, Savelieva I, Atar D, Hohnloser SH, *et al.* 2012 focused update of the ESC Guidelines for the management of atrial fibrillation: an update of the 2010 ESC Guidelines for the management of atrial fibrillation. Developed with the special contribution of the European Heart Rhythm Association. *Eur Heart J* 2012; **33**: 2719–2747. DOI: 10.1093/eurheartj/ehs253.

Corrigendum to 'Guidelines: 2012 focused update of the ESC Guidelines for the management of atrial fibrillation: an update. *Eur Heart J* 2013; **34:** 2850–2851; DOI: 10.1093/eurheartj/eht291.

Johnston SC, Rothwell PM, Nguyen-Huynh MN, *et al.* Validation and refinement of scores to predict very early stroke risk after transient ischaemic attack. *Lancet* 2007; **369:** 283–292.

National Institute for Health and Care Excellence (NICE). Clinical Guideline 68. Stroke: Diagnosis and initial management of acute stroke and transient ischaemic attack (TIA). London: National Institute for Health and Clinical Excellence, 2008.

National Institutes of Health. Stroke scale. http://www.ninds.nih.gov/doctors/NIH_Stroke_Scale.pdf (accessed 16 December 2015).

Pisters R, Lane DA, Nieuwlaat R, de Vos CB, Crijns HJ, Lip GY. A novel user-friendly score (HAS-BLED) to assess 1-year risk of major bleeding in patients with atrial fibrillation: the Euro Heart Survey. *Chest* 2010; **138:** 1093–1100.

Further reading

Anticoagulation

Chatterjee S, Sardar P, Biondi-Zoccai G, Kumbhani DJ. New oral anticoagulants and the risk of intracranial hemorrhage: traditional and Bayesian meta-analysis and mixed treatment comparison of randomized trials of new oral anticoagulants in atrial fibrillation. *JAMA Neurology* 2013; **70:** 1486–1490.

Franke CL, de Jonge J, van Swieten JC, *et al.* Intracerebral hematomas during anticoagulant treatment. *Stroke* 1990; **21**: 726–730.

Pereira AC, Brown MM. Aspirin or heparin in acute stroke. *Br Med Bull* 2000; **56:** 413–421.

Arteriovenous malformations

Ruiz-Sandoval JL, Cantu C, Barinagarrementeria F. Intracerebral hemorrhage in young people: analysis of risk factors, location, causes, and prognosis. *Stroke* 1999; **30:** 537–541.

Atrial fibrillation

Lip YH, Frison L, Halperin JL, Lane DA. Identifying patients at high risk for stroke despite anticoagulation. a comparison of contemporary stroke risk stratification schemes in an anticoagulated atrial fibrillation cohort. *Stroke* 2010; **41:** 2731–2738.

Penado S, Cano M, Acha O, Hernández JL, Riancho JA. Atrial fibrillation as a risk factor for stroke recurrence. *Am J Med* 2003; **114**: 206–210.

CADASIL

Desmond DW, Moroney JT, Lynch T, *et al.* The natural history of CADASIL: a pooled analysis of previously published cases. *Stroke* 1999; **30**: 1230–1233.

Carotid stenosis

Rothwell MP, Eliasziw M, Gutnikov SA, *et al.* Analysis of pooled data from the randomised trials of endarterectomy for symptomatic carotid stenosis. *Lancet* 2003; **361**: 107–116.

Causes of stroke

Bamford J, Sandercock P, Dennis M, *et al.* A prospective study of acute cerebrovascular disease in the community: the Oxfordshire Community Stroke Project – 1981–86. 2. Incidence, case fatality rates and overall outcome at one year after cerebral infarction, primary intracerebral and subarachnoid haemorrhage. *J Neurol Neurosurg Psychiatry* 1990; **53**: 16–22.

Cavernous angiomas

Requena I, Arias M, Lopez-Ibor L, *et al.* Cavenomas of the central nervous system: clinical and neuroimaging manifestations in 47 patients. *J Neurol Neurosurg Psychiatry* 1991; **54**: 590–594.

Cerebral amyloid angiopathy

Yamada M. Cerebral amyloid angiopathy: an overview. *Neuropathology* 2000; **20**: 8–22.

Dissection

Brandt T, Hausser I, Orberk E, *et al.* Ultrastructural connective tissue abnormalities in patients with spontaneous cervicocerebral artery dissections. *Ann Neurol* 1998; **44**: 281–285.

Fabry's disease

Brady RO, Schiffmann R. Clinical features of and recent advances in therapy for Fabry disease. *JAMA* 2000; **284**: 2771–2775.

Endovascular treatment of hyperacute stroke

Berkhemer OA, Fransen PS, Beumer D, *et al.* MR CLEAN Investigators. A randomized trial of intraarterial treatment for acute ischemic stroke. *N Engl J Med* 2015; **372:** 11–20.

Broderick JP, Palesch YY, Demchuk AM, *et al.* Interventional Management of Stroke (IMS) III Investigators. Endovascular therapy after intravenous t-PA versus t-PA alone for stroke. *N Engl J Med* 2013; **368:** 893–903.

Ciccone A, Valvassori L, Nichelatti M, *et al.* SYNTHESIS Expansion Investigators. Endovascular treatment for acute ischemic stroke. *N Engl J Med* 2013; **368:** 904–913.

Kidwell CS, Jahan R, Gornbein J, *et al.* MR RESCUE Investigators. A trial of imaging selection and endovascular treatment for ischemic stroke. *N Engl J Med* 2013; **368:** 914–923.

Fibromuscular dysplasia

Ortiz-Fandino J, Terre-Boliart R, Orient-Lopez F, *et al.* Ischemic stroke, secondary to fibromuscular dysplasia: a case report. *Rev Neurol* 2004; **38**: 34–37.

Haematological disorders

Austin S, Cohen H, Losseff N. Haematology and neurology. *J Neurol Neurosurg Psychiatry* 2007; **78**: 334–341.

Hypertension

MacMahon S, Peto R, Cutler J, *et al.* Blood pressure, stroke, and coronary heart disease. 1. Prolonged differences in blood pressure: prospective observational studies corrected for the regression dilution bias. *Lancet* 1990; **335**: 765–774.

Incidence, prevalence and prognosis

Bamford J, Sandercock P, Dennis M, *et al.* A prospective study of acute cerebrovascular disease in the community: the Oxfordshire community stroke project, 1981–1986. 2. Incidence, case fatality rates and overall outcome at one year of cerebral infarction, primary intracerebral and subarachnoid haemorrhage. *J Neurol Neurosurg Psychiatry* 1990; **53**: 16–22.

Inflammatory vascular disorders

Hankey GJ. Isolated angiitis/angiopathy of the central nervous system. *Cerebrovasc Dis* 1991; **1**: 2–15.

Mitochondrial disease and MELAS

Ciafaloni E, Ricci E, Shanske S, *et al.* MELAS: clinical features, biochemistry and molecular genetics. *Ann Neurol* 1992; **31**: 391–398.

Moyamoya syndrome

Chiu D, Shedden P, Bratina P, Grotta JC. Clinical features of moyamoya disease in the United States. *Stroke* 1998; **29**: 1347–1351.

Patent foramen ovale

Mas JL, Arquizan C, Lamy C, *et al.* Recurrent cerebrovascular events associated with patent foramen ovale, atrial septal aneurysm, or both. *N Engl J Med* 2001; **345**: 1740–1746.

Radiology

Jager HR. Diagnosis of stroke with advanced CT and MR imaging. *Br Med Bull* 2000; **56**: 318–333.

Secondary prevention

Antithrombotic Trialists' Collaboration. Collaborative meta-analysis of randomised trials of antiplatelet therapy for prevention of death, myocardial infarction, and stroke in high risk patients. *BMJ* 2002; **324**: 71–86.

Camm AJ, Lip GY, De Caterina R, Savelieva I, Ater D, Hohnloser SH, *et al.* Guidelines: CPG ESCCfP, Document R. 2012 focused update of the ESC Guidelines for the management of atrial fibrillation: an update of the 2010 ESC Guidelines for the management of atrial fibrillation – developed with the special contribution of the European Heart Rhythm Association. *Eur Heart J* 2012; **33:** 2719–2747.

Colhoun HM, Betteridge DJ, Durrington PN, *et al.* Primary prevention of cardiovascular disease with atorvastatin in type 2 diabetes in the Collaborative Atorvastatin Diabetes Study (CARDS): multicentre randomised placebo-controlled trial. *Lancet* 2004; **364**: 685–696.

Dennis M, Sandercock P, Reid J, *et al.* CLOTS (Clots in Legs Or sTockings after Stroke) Trials Collaboration. Effectiveness of intermittent pneumatic compression in reduction of risk of deep vein thrombosis in patients who have had a stroke (CLOTS 3): a multicentre randomised controlled trial. *Lancet* 2013; **382**: 516–524.

Heart Protection Study Collaborative Group. Effects of cholesterol-lowering with simvastatin on stroke and other major vascular events in 20,536 people with cerebrovascular disease or other high-risk conditions. *Lancet* 2004; **363**: 757–766.

Kasner SE. CADISS: a feasibility trial that answered its question. *Lancet Neurol* 2015; **14**: 342.

Lip GY, Nieuwlaat R, Pisters R, Lane DA, Crijns HJ. Refining clinical risk stratification for predicting stroke and thromboembolism in atrial fibrillation using a novel risk factor-based approach: the euro heart survey on atrial fibrillation. *Chest* 2010; **137:** 263–272.

Pisters R, Lane DA, Nieuwlaat R, de Vos CB, Crijns HJ, Lip GY. A novel user-friendly score (HAS-BLED) to assess 1-year risk of major bleeding in patients with atrial fibrillation: the Euro Heart Survey. *Chest* 2010; **138:** 1093–1100.

PROGRESS Collaborative Group. Randomised trial of a perindopril-based blood-pressure-lowering regimen among 6105 individuals with previous stroke or transient ischaemic attack. *Lancet* 2001; **358**: 1033–1041.

Saxena R, Koudstaal PJ. Anticoagulants for preventing stroke in patients with nonrheumatic atrial fibrillation and a history of stroke or transient ischaemic attack. *Cochrane Database Syst Rev* 2004; **2:** CD000185.

Wang Y, Wang Y, Zhao X, *et al.* CHANCE Investigators. Clopidogrel with aspirin in acute minor stroke or transient ischaemic attack. *N Engl J Med* 2013; **369**: 11–19.

Stroke definition

Sacco RL, Kasner SE, Broderick JP, *et al.* An updated definition of stroke for the 21st century: a statement for healthcare professionals from the American Heart Association/American Stroke Association. *Stroke* 2013; **44**: 2064–2089.

Stroke units and organisation

Losseff N, Ames D, Cloud G, Cluckie G, Gompertz P, Grant B, Markus H, Brown MM. Priorities in stroke care: The London stroke strategy. *BMJ* 2009; **338**: b2616.

Stroke Unit Trialists' Collaboration. Collaborative systematic review of the randomised trials of organised inpatient (stroke unit) care after stroke. *BMJ* 1997; **314**: 1151–1159.

Subarachnoid haemorrhage

Broderick JP, Viscoli CM, Brott T, *et al.* Major risk factors for aneurysmal subarachnoid hemorrhage in the young are modifiable. *Stroke* 2003; **34**: 1375–1381.

International Subarachnoid Aneurysm Trial (ISAT) Collaborative Group. International Subarachnoid Aneurysm Trial (ISAT) of neurosurgical clipping versus endovascular coiling in 2143 patients with ruptured intracranial aneurysms: a randomised trial. *Lancet* 2002; **360**: 1267–1274.

Surgical treatment

Mendelow AD, Gregson BA, Fernandes HM, *et al.* Early surgery versus initial conservative treatment in patients with spontaneous supratentorial intracerebral haematomas in the International Surgical Trial in Intracerebral Haemorrhage (STICH): a randomised trial. *Lancet* 2005; **365**: 387–397.

Vahedi K, Hofmeijer J, Juettler E, *et al.* DECIMAL, DESTINY, and HAMLET investigators. Early decompressive surgery in malignant infarction of the middle cerebral artery: a pooled analysis of three randomised controlled trials. *Lancet Neurol* 2007; **6**: 215–222.

Thrombolytic therapy

ATLANTIS, ECASS and NINDS rt-PA Study Group Investigators. Association of outcome with early stroke treatment: pooled analysis of ATLANTIS, ECASS, and NINDS rt-PA stroke trials. *Lancet* 2004; **363**: 768–774.

Berkhemer OA, Fransen PS, Beumer D, *et al.* A randomized trial of intraarterial treatment for acute ischemic stroke. *N Engl J Med* 2015; **372**: 11.

NINDS t-PA Stroke Study Group. Intracerebral hemorrhage after intravenous t-PA therapy for ischemic stroke. *Stroke* 1997; **28**: 2109–2118.

Sandercock P, Wardlaw JM, Lindley RI, *et al.* IST-3 Collaborative Group. The benefits and harms of intravenous thrombolysis with recombinant tissue plasminogen activator within 6 h of acute ischaemic stroke (the third international stroke trial [IST-3]): a randomised controlled trial. *Lancet* 2012; **379**: 2352–2363.

Wardlaw JM, Murray V, Berge E, *et al.* Recombinant tissue plasminogen activator for acute ischaemic stroke: an updated systematic review and meta-analysis. *Lancet* 2012; **379**: 2364–2372.

Transient ischaemic attack

Albers GW, Caplan LR, Easton JD, *et al.* Transient ischemic attack: proposal for a new definition. *New Engl J Med* 2002; **347**: 1713–1716.

Rothwell PM, Giles MF, Chandratheva A, *et al.* Effect of urgent treatment of transient ischaemic attack and minor stroke on early recurrent stroke (EXPRESS study): a prospective population-based sequential comparison. *Lancet* 2007; **370**: 1432–1442.

Venous thrombosis

Bousser MG. Cerebral venous thrombosis: diagnosis and management. *J Neurol* 2000; **247**: 252–258.

CHAPTER 6
Movement Disorders

Kailash Bhatia[1], Carla Cordivari[2], Mark Edwards[1], Thomas Foltynie[1], Marwan Hariz[1], Prasad Korlipara[2], Patricia Limousin[1], Niall Quinn[1], Sarah Tabrizi[1] and Thomas Warner[1]
[1]UCL Institute of Neurology
[2]National Hospital for Neurology & Neurosurgery

Movement disorders are common causes of disability, especially in older people. They either cause poverty of movement or unwanted, involuntary movements. Much early work in the field was pioneered by Kinnier Wilson and Purdon Martin at The National Hospital, and many others elsewhere. David Marsden, in London and Stanley Fahn (the Neurological Institute, New York) founded the Movement Disorder Society and its journal *Movement Disorders*. This chapter provides an overview of the different forms of parkinsonian and dyskinetic disorders.

Parkinsonian (akinetic-rigid) syndromes

Cardinal motor features of parkinsonism

Akinesia is the defining and principal disabling feature of parkinsonism (Table 6.1). It is a symptom complex, comprising slowness of movement (bradykinesia), poverty of movement and small amplitude of movements (hypokinesia), difficulty initiating movement or with simultaneous motor acts and, most specifically, fatiguing and decrementing amplitude of repetitive alternating movements, which distinguish true akinesia from pyramidal or cerebellar slowing. Almost all individuals with parkinsonism also display muscular rigidity to passive movement across a joint. Unlike spasticity, it is fairly equal in flexors and extensors, and may feel like bending a lead pipe; the presence of additional tremor (which may not be visibly evident) can add a ratchety 'cogwheel' feel to the rigidity (tremor alone can cause cogwheeling, but without rigidity).

Tremor is an optional feature of parkinsonism, and indeed of Parkinson's disease (PD) itself. Up to 80% of PD patients will display a tremor at some stage. Classically, this is in the form of a 4–6 Hz rest tremor which, in the hand, is 'pill-rolling' with flexion of the thumb. It typically subsides or lessens with movement, to reappear after an interval when a new static position (e.g. arms outstretched) is achieved ('re-emergent tremor'). A number of patients can additionally, or instead, display a faster postural tremor. A classic rest tremor, particularly if accompanied by a jaw tremor, is a strong pointer to PD or drug-induced parkinsonism, but this combination can also be seen in dystonic tremor. Classic rest tremor is uncommon, and jaw tremor rare, in other degenerative forms of parkinsonism. To the above triad a fourth 'cardinal' motor feature of parkinsonism is sometimes added – postural abnormality. Flexed posture may or may not be evident early in the disease, and postural instability is typically a late feature in PD, so this item is not usually useful for diagnosing PD, although if present early on can point to alternative causes of the syndrome.

Molecular advances have revealed helpful schemata for classifying the principal degenerative parkinsonisms into alpha-synucleinopathies, including PD, dementia with Lewy bodies (DLB) and multiple system atrophy (MSA), and tauopathies, including progressive supranuclear palsy (PSP) and corticobasal degeneration (CBD).

Parkinson's disease

PD has traditionally been, and continues to be, defined as a clinicopathological entity, in which progressive levodopa-responsive parkinsonism, without atypical features (see later), is associated, at postmortem, with neuronal loss and the presence of intracytoplasmic, eosinophilic, alpha synuclein containing inclusions known as Lewy bodies in specific central and autonomic nervous structures. These include particularly the pigmented brainstem monoaminergic nuclei, the substantia nigra (dopaminergic) and locus caeruleus (noradrenergic). However, the pathology is usually much more widespread, also involving serotonergic raphe nuclei, dopaminergic mesolimbic, mesocortical and tubero-infundibular pathways, the cholinergic nucleus basalis of Meynert (NBM), the cerebral cortex, the hypothalamus, the dorsal motor nucleus of vagus, the olfactory tract and sympathetic ganglia. The pathological criteria have been correlated in detail with the classic clinical PD phenotype lending support to the continued use of diagnostic criteria as elaborated in 1988 by the Queen Square Brain Bank (Table 6.1).

The prevalence of PD in most countries is around 180/100 000. Overall, incidence rises steadily with age with an average age at onset of about 60 years, and fewer than 5% of cases starting before age 40. Despite modern treatment, life expectancy is still reduced, with a standardised mortality ratio of about 1.9.

Clinical heterogeneity has long been recognised within 'PD', and the concept of PD as a single entity has been turned upside down with the identification of individuals and familial kindreds carrying any of a variety of genetic mutations now known to be causally related to PD pathogenesis. For example, mutations in two genes (*alpha-synuclein* and *LRKK2*), or duplications or triplications of *alpha-synuclein*, can cause dominantly inherited or sporadic parkinsonism accompanied by Lewy bodies in the brain. On the other hand, mutations of three recessive genes (*parkin, DJ1* and *PINK1*)

Neurology: A Queen Square Textbook, Second Edition. Edited by Charles Clarke, Robin Howard, Martin Rossor and Simon Shorvon.

Table 6.1 UK PDS Brain Bank diagnostic criteria for Parkinson's disease.

STEP 1. Diagnosis of a parkinsonian syndrome
Bradykinesia (slowness of initiation of voluntary movement with progressive reduction in speed and amplitude of repetitive actions) – obligatory
And at least one of the following:
• Muscular rigidity
• 4–6 Hz rest tremor
• Postural instability not caused by primary visual, vestibular, cerebellar or proprioceptive dysfunction
STEP 2. Exclusion criteria for Parkinson's disease
History of repeated strokes with stepwise progression of parkinsonian features
History of repeated head injury
History of definite encephalitis
Oculogyric crises
Neuroleptic treatment at onset of symptoms
More than one affected relative
Sustained remission
Strictly unilateral features after 3 years
Supranuclear gaze palsy
Cerebellar signs
Early severe autonomic involvement
Early severe dementia with disturbances of memory, language and praxis
Babinski sign
Imaging evidence of a cerebral tumour or communicating hydrocephalus
Negative response to large doses of levodopa if malabsorption excluded.
MPTP exposure
STEP 3. Supportive prospective positive criteria for Parkinson's disease
(Three or more required for diagnosis of definite Parkinson's disease)
Unilateral onset
Rest tremor present
Progressive disorder
Persistent asymmetry affecting the side of onset most
Excellent response (70–100%) to levodopa
Severe levodopa-induced chorea
Levodopa response for 5 years or more
Clinical course of 10 years or more

Source: Queen Square Brain Bank.

can present mainly in younger individuals with clinical PD without Lewy bodies. The list of *PARK* genes and loci is increasing exponentially, with more still to be identified. How many of these should still be called PD is a moot point. The phenotypes of these monogeneic 'PDs', especially of *LRKK2* cases, can be indistinguishable from typical sporadic PD. However, patients with *alpha-synuclein* mutations or triplications have somewhat younger onset, shorter survival and a higher incidence of dementia. Although *alpha-synuclein* mutations are rare, excessive levels of otherwise normal *alpha-synuclein*, as a result of gene duplications or triplications, are sufficient to cause dominantly inherited Lewy body parkinsonism. Furthermore, in meta-analyses of thousands of apparently 'sporadic' PD patients, the strongest whole genome association is with common variation in the alpha-synuclein gene. Evidence is emerging that exogenous fibrils of alpha-synuclein can enter neurones (by a form of endocytosis), and promote recruitment of endogenous alpha-synuclein leading to the formation of Lewy bodies. This reinforces the theory that Lewy body pathology is potentially 'transmissible' from one neurone to the next, as has been observed in the clinical trials of fetal cell transplantation for PD. Another rare cause of monogenic autosomal dominant PD are mutations in the *VPS35* gene.

The recessive forms have younger onset, slower disease progression and present with leg tremor more often than sporadic PD. In independent populations mutations in the glucocerebrosidase (*GBA*) gene can cause either familial or seemingly sporadic PD. A mutation in a single copy is associated with an increased risk of PD, and of dementia within PD. Table 6.2 lists the currently identified *PARK* genes and loci. Overall, monogenic PD accounts for about 6–8% of all PD. However, different genetic causes vary in frequency in different populations (e.g. both *GBA* and *LRKK2*-related parkinsonism is particularly common in Ashkenazi Jews and *LRRK2*-related parkinsonsim in North Africans). Overall, incidence rises steadily with age, although recessive forms become less frequent with age.

Molecular advances have introduced alternative schemata for classifying the principal degenerative parkinsonisms into alpha-synucleinopathies (Lewy body diseases and MSA), tauopathies (including PSP and CBD), and others (e.g. cases with parkin mutations). Table 6.3 summarises causes of parkinsonism and other conditions sometimes confused with PD.

PD has been traditionally defined as a motor disorder, but the frequency and importance of premotor and non-motor features is increasingly recognised.

Premotor features of PD

All neuronal systems have built-in reserves which allow a degree of neuronal loss to be tolerated, and which can be compensated for by up-regulation of surviving neuronal function before a threshold is reached at which point symptoms become apparent. Thus, 60–80% of nigrostriatal dopaminergic reserve is lost before the motor features of parkinsonism emerge. Brains with 'subclinical' nigral Lewy bodies have been called 'incidental Lewy body disease'. Sequential fluorodopa positron emission tomography (PET) scans have been used to estimate, by back-extrapolation, the duration of the presymptomatic phase of PD, with estimates varying between 3 and 6 years. However, a number of pathological and clinical observations have questioned this. Thus,, Braak *et al.* (2006), based on examination of Lewy body pathology in a large number of brains of individuals with and without clinical parkinsonism in life, postulated 6 'stages' of PD. In stages 1 and 2, Lewy bodies are restricted to the medulla, pontine tegmentum and anterior olfactory structures, and it is only in stage 3 that the nigrostriatal tract is first involved. Thus, back-extrapolation from fluorodopa PET scans can only, at best, tell us when stage 3 might begin. Clinically, constipation, dysphagia, olfactory impairment, cardiovascular autonomic involvement and REM sleep behaviour disorder (RBD) can

Table 6.2 *PARK* genes and loci.

Park number	Chromosome	Gene	Inheritance pattern	Clinical features	Comments
*PARK1**	4q21	*SNCA*	AD	EOPD	Missense mutations, genomic multiplication
PARK2	6q26.2-q27	*Parkin*	AR	YOPD	
PARK3	2p13	Unknown	AD	Classic PD	Unconfirmed
PARK5	4p13	*UCLH1*	?	Classic PD	Unreplicated mutations in a single sibling pair
PARK6	1p36	*PINK1*	AR	YOPD	
PARK7	1p36	*DJ-1*	AR	YOPD	
PARK8	12q12	*LRRK2*	AD	Classic PD	
PARK9	1p36	*ATP13A2*	AR	Juvenile parkinsonism, pyramidal signs, dementia	
PARK10	1p32	Unknown	Risk factor	Late onset parkinsonism	Unconfirmed
PARK11	2q37	Unknown	Risk factor	Late onset parkinsonism	
PARK12	Xq21-25	Unknown	X-linked	Late onset parkinsonism	Unconfirmed
PARK13	2p12	*HTRA2*	AD or risk factor	Late onset parkinsonism	Unconfirmed
PARK14	22q12-q13	*PLA2G6*	AR	Early onset parkinsonism-dystonia	
PARK15	22q12-q13	*FBXO7*	AR	Juvenile parkinsonism and pyramidal signs	
PARK16	1q32	Unknown	Risk factor	Late onset parkinsonism	Unconfirmed
PARK17	16q11.2	*VPS35*	AD	Classic PD	
PARK18	3q27.1	*EIF4G1*	AD	Classic PD	Unconfirmed
PARK19	1p31.3	DNAJC6	AR	Juvenile onset	
PARK20	21q22.11	SYNJ1	AR	EOPD	
PARK21	3q22.1	DNAJC13	AD	Classic PD	

AD, autosomal dominant; AR, autosomal recessive; EOPD, early onset Parkinson's disease; YOPD, young onset Parkinson's disease (usually before 40 years).
* *PARK4* is an erroneous locus; the family was subsequently proven to have an *SNCA* triplication (i.e. *PARK1*).

precede, by many more years, the appearance of the motor disorder in PD. In RBD there is loss of the usual muscle atonia that accompanies dreaming, such that the individual is able to 'act out' usually frightening dreams, often striking or injuring their bed-partner, and often with vocalisations. In one sleep laboratory study, 38% of 29 men with (at that time idiopathic) RBD went on to be diagnosed with a parkinsonian disorder an average of 3.7 years after the diagnosis and 12.7 years after the onset of their RBD.

The identification of premotor PD features has led to great interest in the detection of cohorts of individuals with premotor features of sufficient sensitivity and specificity for predicting the future development of PD. The main purpose is to enable trials of candidate neuroprotective agents to be applied as early in the disease process as possible, when they may be most likely to modify the neurodegenerative process.

'Typical' motor presentation of PD

Most patients with PD only present to medical attention following the onset of the well-known motor features of the disease. PD is classically an asymmetric disease, remaining so throughout its course. It more commonly starts in the arm, with impaired dexterity on fine tasks, and often with a tremor at rest (e.g. holding a

Table 6.3 Causes of parkinsonism and other conditions sometimes confused with Parkinson's disease.

Idiopathic Parkinson's disease (including DLB)
Genetically determined 'Parkinson's diseases' (see Table 6.2)
Other neurodegenerative diseases
Classically sporadic
• Multiple system atrophy (MSA)
• Progressive supranuclear palsy (PSP)
• Cortico-basal degeneration (CBD)
Genetic
• Dominant
Huntington's disease (HD, Westphal variant)
Spinocerebellar ataxia type 2 (SCA2)
SCA3
Frontotemporal dementia with parkinsonism related to chromosome 17 (FTDP-17)
• Recessive
Wilson's disease (WD)
Neurodegeneration with brain iron accumulation disorders (NBIAs)
• Uncertain
Parkinsonism–dementia–ALS complex of Guam
PSP-like atypical parkinsonism in Guadeloupe
• Other genetic
Dopa-responsive dystonia (DYT5, Segawa disease – older patients) – dominant with incomplete penetrance
Dystonia-parkinsonism in Filipinos (DYT3, XDP,Lubag) – X-linked
Rapid onset dystonia-parkinsonism (DYT12) – dominant
• Reversible drug-induced secondary to dopamine receptor blocking or dopamine depleting drugs
• Toxic, due to MPTP/CO/methanol/manganese
• Post-encephalitic due to encephalitis lethargica/post-strep/ Japanese B encephalitis
• Dementia with Lewy bodies (DLB)
• Vascular parkinsonism/pseudoparkinsonism*
• Post-traumatic due to repeated head trauma ('punch-drunk syndrome') or midbrain compression
• Essential tremor*
• Dystonic tremor*

* Often misdiagnosed as Parkinson's disease even though fatiguing/decrement of repetitive movements not present.

newspaper). Other patients present with a tendency to drag one leg or shuffle. The spouse may have noticed a general slowing down, a change in facial expression or impaired arm swing. Direct questioning may reveal a change in voice or micrographia, but these symptoms as presenting complaints are less common, and raise the possibility of atypical disease. The patient may admit to aching or sometimes pain in the affected limb, and presentation with or development of a frozen shoulder or worsening back discomfort is well recognised.

Examination will reveal akinesia, usually with rigidity and often tremor, which can be difficult to bring out. The patient should be asked to relax their hands in their lap or over the arms of a chair, and deliberately put under stress by being asked to count backwards with the eyes closed, then repeated with the arms outstretched, then with the fingers in front of the nose. Often the earliest tremor to be observed may be an adduction–abduction tremor of the fingers. Sometimes, the only time a rest tremor is observed is on walking, when reduced arm swing, flexed posture (initially of one arm) and gait abnormality can be seen.

Atypical features should also be sought. The 'bedside' examination of eye movements should be normal (except for some limitation of convergence or of up-gaze with normal saccadic velocity), and there should be no evidence of limb or gait ataxia or dysdiadochokinesis, no apraxia and no pyramidal signs. The so-called striatal toe can mimic a Babinski response, but is often present spontaneously or on walking and is not accompanied by other pyramidal features. Sometimes (particularly younger) patients may present with 'dystonic claudication' (exercise-induced leg dystonia) on prolonged walking. Early postural stability or freezing of gait, although sometimes seen in PD, should raise other possibilities. Of note, patients who are unsteady for whatever reason may not swing their arms, and abnormal arm swing is also common in patients with dystonia.

Unilateral PD (stage 1 on the non-linear Hoehn and Yahr scale) progresses, through stage 2 (bilateral), which typically lasts for 5–10 years, until postural instability (stage 3) appears. Over time, fully developed disease (stage 4) develops, and after many years the patient may eventually become chair- or even bed-bound (stage 5). However, this progression is influenced by treatment, so that a patient on chronic levodopa treatment can fluctuate between stage 4 or even 5 when 'off', to stage 2 or 3 when 'on'. Freezing of gait is usually a late feature.

Non-motor features of PD

Beyond the premotor symptoms, a host of other non-motor features occur in, and can be the most disabling features of PD so should be routinely enquired about:

- Sialorrhoea is particularly a problem in later disease; only a few patients can tolerate centrally acting anticholinergics such as scopolamine because of the risk of confusion, but some can be helped by peripherally acting drugs, or botulinum toxin injections. As this is caused by reduced frequency of swallowing rather than excessive saliva production, simple tricks such as chewing gum to promote swallowing can be effective in controlling this problem.
- Drenching sweats usually occur in levodopa-treated patients, often as wearing off or 'off' phenomenon. They are poorly understood and no effective pharmacological treatment exists, other than adequate dopaminergic replacement. Anxiety, and sometimes panic, can also be a major problem, and can occur acutely in the wearing off or off state.
- Urinary urgency and frequency are common, as a result of detrusor hyper-reflexia, and can be helped by a peripherally acting anticholinergic such as trospium.
- Depression, usually minor rather than major, affects about 40% of patients before, at, or after diagnosis. The symptomatology of this minor depression overlaps with abulia, and lack of initiative and drive, which is also common in PD. In numerous studies,

depression has been shown to be the most important factor correlating with impaired quality of life, so it should be actively sought, and treated if found. Clinical depression can be treated with nortriptyline, with an SSRI such as citalopram, or with a serotonergic noradrenergic re-uptake inhibitor (SNRI) such as mirtazapine or venlafaxine.

- Pain is also common in PD. It may be a presenting feature or can arise in established disease, often as a wearing off or off phenomenon, sometimes in conjunction with dystonia. It is usually lateralised to the side more affected by PD.
- Cognitive impairment can occur early in PD but is usually a very mild dysexecutive syndrome which is detectable only when specifically sought using neuropsychological tests. As the disease progresses, other cognitive problems can emerge including more obvious disturbances of memory and attention, and presence of hallucinations and visuospatial deficits. After surviving 20 years of disease, 80% of PD patients will have developed dementia (see Dementia in association with Lewy body pathology).

Many of these non-motor features appear only when the patient's dose of levodopa is wearing off, or in the off state, but can represent the patient's biggest problem. Appropriate management is to take measures to minimise time 'off' (e.g. by appropriate adjustment of dopaminergic medications), rather than necessarily resorting to antidepressants or analgesics. A whole range of neuropsychiatric disturbances resulting from the disease or its treatment can also occur (see later).

Ancillary investigations

Young onset (less than 40 years) patients should always be screened for Wilson's disease with serum copper and caeruloplasmin and slit-lamp examination. Routine magnetic resonance imaging (MRI) of the brain is normal in PD and not necessary in typical cases. A dopamine transporter (DaT) single photon emission computerised tomography (SPECT) scan can sometimes be useful to confirm a nigrostriatal lesion, particularly in those with rest tremor when there is some doubt about the presence of bradykinesia, but in a typical case of PD is unnecessary.

Treatment of PD

No drug has so far been proven to be neuroprotective in PD. When the patient is first diagnosed they may not yet feel in need of symptomatic treatment, and the doctor may not wish to rush into treatment at the first visit. There have been recent suggestions that early initiation of treatment might preserve or restore healthy behaviours such as exercise, and thus have long-term benefit, even without a neuroprotective action, but this is not yet proven. Commonly, PD clinicians still wait until the patient's symptoms are beginning to affect their daily life before starting symptomatic treatment.

Discussion of treatment options has been greatly influenced over the years by what is known about the long-term levodopa syndrome of fluctuations and dyskinesias among patients started on treatment with levodopa as first line, often in high dosages. As a result, many patients and clinicians had developed a form of 'levodopa phobia' which can lead to marked under-treatment. In fact levodopa remains the most effective symptomatic treatment for PD and is therefore discussed first.

Levodopa

Preparations of levodopa combined with the peripheral dopa decarboxylase inhibitors (DDIs) carbidopa or benserazide (co-careldopa, Sinemet; co-beneldopa, Madopar) are still the most potent and effective symptomatic treatment for PD, and remain the 'gold standard'. Levodopa, in competition with other large neutral amino acids, is transferred across the wall of the proximal small bowel, and again across the blood–brain barrier, by an active transport system. Some patients find that protein in meals impairs the effect of a dose of levodopa close to meals, so that timing or size of the dose, or the protein intake, may need adjustment. Once in the brain, no longer protected from the peripheral DDI that cannot follow it, levodopa is metabolised in the surviving presynaptic dopaminergic terminals to dopamine, which is released physiologically (with both tonic and phasic bursts) to stimulate dopamine receptors in striatum.

It is usual to start with half a tablet of 25/100 (DDI/levodopa) strength twice or three times daily for a couple of weeks, then doubling the dose and waiting to judge the effect. If ineffective or insufficiently effective, the dosage can then be increased to 1½ or 2 tablets three times daily, although the ELLDOPA trial showed increasing rates of dyskinesia and wearing off, particularly as the dose increased from levodopa 300 to 600 mg/day. Almost all PD patients will show marked improvement at this dose but, if ineffective, the total daily dosage of levodopa should be further increased to 1–1.5 g/day (if tolerated) before concluding that it has no benefit in a given patient. Lack of response of all of the motor signs to levodopa should prompt the clinician to reconsider the accuracy of the diagnosis.

One should note that there are long duration effects of levodopa, such that a treatment change can take at least 2 weeks for its effect to equilibrate in the brain, and similarly one can see late deterioration up to 2 weeks after discontinuing or reducing the dosage. Initially, benefit is smooth throughout the day, even if a dose is late or missed – the so-called honeymoon period. Over time, however, patients start to notice early morning akinesia, or wearing off of their doses, and around the same time may develop an 'overshoot' from akinesia to dyskinesia when the dose is working. A very rough rule of thumb is that these problems develop in 10% of patients per year of treatment, so that after 5 years about 50% of patients will have them, and after 10 years almost all patients will ultimately experience them, to a greater or lesser degree. In general, younger onset patients develop them earlier and to a more severe degree. Rates reported from clinic-based series are higher than those in community-based studies.

Gradually, a 'threshold' level of dopaminergic transmission in the striatum develops, so that the doses work in an all-or-none fashion, and the patients fluctuate, from on and mobile, to off with recurrence of their parkinsonian features, sometimes over minutes or even seconds. On periods are usually associated with the development of involuntary dyskinetic movements likely as a result of levodopa being taken up by non-dopaminergic neurones and released inappropriately as a false transmitter, and to supersensitivity of postsynaptic dopamine receptors and changes in synaptic plasticity in the striatal output pathways occurring as a result of prolonged non-physiological dopaminergic replacement.

Mobile dyskinesias can be peak dose (occurring mainly at the peak of action of each dose), square wave (occurring throughout the period of benefit) or diphasic (being much more severe at the beginning or at the end of action of a dose of levodopa). Most on period dyskinesias are usually a mixture of chorea and dystonia, but when diphasic (usually in young onset patients) they can be violent and disabling stereotyped or ballistic movements. Some patients develop off period dystonia, which is relatively fixed, usually painful, most commonly affects one leg, and relates to falling, low or intermediate levels of dopaminergic stimulation; paradoxically, this is both caused and relieved by levodopa, disappearing when the patient turns 'on'. Levodopa-induced dyskinesias in PD typically involve limbs more than neck and face, and are more severe on the initially, and more, affected side.

Attempts to treat levodopa-induced dyskinesias by fractionation of doses to give smaller amounts frequently lead to dose failure or unpredictability of effect. Relative to standard preparations, bioavailability of controlled release (CR) levodopa is only 70%; moreover, although providing a longer tail at the end of the dose, CR is absorbed more slowly than standard, leading to delayed 'on' and sometimes only a short on period because the threshold is only briefly exceeded. CR formulations have therefore been disappointing in managing daytime fluctuations, but remain useful at bedtime to improve nights. A (very expensive) levodopa-carbidopa gel (Duodopa) delivered continuously into proximal jejunum via a gastrostomy and jejunal extension tube (PEG-J) can give stable plasma levels and improve fluctuations in patients who are unsuitable for, or unable to tolerate, apomorphine or surgery.

Other side effects of levodopa Levodopa can also cause nausea or vomiting, mainly by stimulating dopamine receptors in the chemoreceptor trigger zone in the area postrema in the floor of the fourth ventricle, functionally outside the blood–brain barrier. It can also cause or aggravate postural hypotension, mainly through a central action. Overall, levodopa is far better tolerated than the alternative symptomatic agents.

Monoamine oxidase B inhibitors

Selegiline and rasagiline are irreversible inhibitors of monoamine oxidase B (MAO-B), the iso-enzyme responsible for catabolising dopamine to homovanillic acid (HVA). Unlike MAO-A inhibitors, they can safely be given together with levodopa. Used alone in early disease, selegiline has been shown, probably through a mild symptomatic effect, to delay the need for levodopa by about 9 months. Symptomatic effects are modest. Oral selegiline is partly metabolised to metamphetamine, so should be given in the morning to avoid insomnia. Zelapar, a buccally absorbed preparation of selegiline, avoids first-pass metabolism and hence this problem. Otherwise, these drugs have very few side effects when given alone, but can potentiate any of the symptomatic side effects of levodopa. Safanamide, a new MAO-B inhibitor (but also dopamine reuptake and glutamate inhibitor), has recently been licensed for use in the United Kingdom and the EU.

Great publicity surrounded the publication of the DATATOP (selegiline) and the TEMPO and ADAGIO trials (rasagiline) which sought to evaluate whether these agents can have neuroprotective properties. The rasagiline trials adopted a delayed start design deliberately to try to disentangle the known symptomatic effects of these drugs (observed in DATATOP) from possible disease-modifying effects. Although small benefits appeared to emerge as a result of earlier introduction of rasagiline at a dose of 1 mg, the data on the 2-mg dose were negative, casting doubt on the overall reliability of the trial findings, and prompting the US Food and Drug Administration (FDA) to conclude that no neuroprotective effects had been demonstrated.

Catechol-*O*-methyl transferase inhibitors

Entacapone (peripheral) and tolcapone (peripheral and central catechol-*O*-methyl transferase [COMT] inhibitor) block the conversion of levodopa to 3-*O*-methyldopa, its principal metabolite. They both extend the elimination half-life of levodopa, and thereby often extend the duration of action of individual doses. They are of no use if given without levodopa, and in the case of entacapone should be given simultaneously with levodopa. Tolcapone is generally the more effective of the two, but is only used as a second line treatment because of a (low) risk of potentially fatal hepatotoxicity, necessitating frequent liver function test monitoring. Both drugs can cause gastrointestinal upset, particularly diarrhoea, and a harmless orange discoloration of the urine. A combined tablet containing levodopa, carbidopa and entacapone (Stalevo) is available.

Dopamine agonists

Dopamine agonists stimulate dopamine receptors directly. Five oral agonists (three ergoline: bromocriptine, pergolide and cabergoline; and two non-ergoline: ropinirole and pramipexole) and one transdermal non-ergoline agonist (rotigotine) have been introduced. Apomorphine is the only dopamine agonist that can be administered subcutaneously and has a rapid time to onset of action. While the oral and transdermal agonists are commonly given before levodopa is introduced, in an attempt to reduce or delay the development of fluctuations and dyskinesias, they undoubtedly have a weaker antiparkinsonian effect. Apomorphine on the other hand is generally reserved for people who have already experienced levodopa-induced complications.

Adverse effects Dopamine agonists stimulate both peripheral and central dopamine receptors.

Peripheral side effects include nausea and, rarely, aggravation of existing cardiac disease or peptic ulceration. The risk of nausea and vomiting (particularly problematic with initiation of apomorphine) can be reduced by the peripherally acting dopamine receptor antagonist domperidone. However, the Medicines and Healthcare products Regulatory Agency (MHRA) has recently determined that because of its potential for causing cardiac problems, not more than 30 mg/day domperidone should be given, for a maximum period of 1 week. Other antiemetics that do not block dopamine receptors are cyclizine, promethazine and ondansetron. Tolerance to nausea usually develops rapidly over 10 days or so, and there is cross-tolerance between levodopa and agonists, and between different agonists. Covering the introduction of an agonist is therefore most important with *de novo* treatment, optional when adding an agonist to levodopa, and unnecessary when switching between agonists (except to switch to apomorphine)

All agonists can cause ankle swelling, sometimes extending to the knees, or higher. In most cases the mechanism is unknown, but evidence of cardiac failure should always be sought. The ergot derivatives, particularly, can cause a tense angry erythematous rash called erythromelalgia. It has long been recognised that ergot agonists can (rarely) cause lung fibrosis, pleuro-pulmonary effusions or (even more rarely) retroperitoneal fibrosis. More recently, they have also been found to cause fibrosis of heart valves (most commonly the tricuspid), analogous to what is seen with carcinoid tumours and fenfluramine treatment. This reaction is thought to be mediated by stimulation of 5HT2B receptors, and to be wholly, or mostly, restricted to ergoline agonists. The vast majority of patients found on echocardiography to be affected are asymptomatic, but because of these problems the ergoline agonists are no longer recommended.

Central side effects include postural hypotension (mainly central), excessive daytime somnolence and a variety of neuropsychiatric manifestations.

While any antiparkinsonian medication can cause neuropsychiatric adverse effects, the oral agonists definitely cause more problems than levodopa. At the milder end of the spectrum, levodopa, agonists and anticholinergics can cause vivid dreams or nightmares, illusions, extracampine hallucinations (delusions of presence) or (typically visual) pseudohallucinations (with retained insight), of animals or people, sometimes Lilliputian, often non-threatening. More problematic are true hallucinations (with loss of insight) and delusions (often paranoid). So-called impulse control disorders (ICDs) are much more common with agonists, and include hypersexuality, pathological and compulsive gambling, shopping or eating. Agonists can also cause morbid jealousy (Othello syndrome). 'Punding' (defined as repeated stereotyped pointless complex behaviours, for instance sorting, or assembling and disassembling items) is more common with patients 'addicted' to excessive doses of levodopa in the 'dopamine dysregulation syndrome'.

All patients considering or taking dopamine agonists must be warned and interrogated about these possible neuropsychiatric effects.

De novo use of dopamine agonists The main advantage of *de novo* agonist monotherapy is that it rarely causes significant motor fluctuations or dyskinesias until, almost inevitably, levodopa is later added. However, over recent years the relative merits of starting treatment with an agonist versus starting with levodopa have gradually altered. Long-term studies have shown that, despite delaying the onset of levodopa-related complications (fluctuations and dyskinesias) by using an agonist first, these problems often start much sooner after levodopa is started, and at the end of 10–15 years there is no difference in outcome irrespective of which treatment was started first. Moreover, if fluctuations and dyskinesias cannot be adequately controlled medically, deep brain stimulation (DBS; see later) can now usually control them very effectively. In addition, the 1 in 8 risk of agonists provoking one or more ICDs has to be factored in. Therefore for many neurologists and patients the pendulum is now swinging back in favour of levodopa.

When first introduced, at low dosage, dopamine agonists can also have a paradoxical effect of worsening parkinsonism by shutting down endogenous dopamine release, before higher dosages that stimulate the postsynaptic D2 receptors are reached. Agonists are often used in suboptimal dosage, commonly because the patient stops increasing the dosage at the end of a 'starter pack', or because of confusion about what is meant by 'minimum effective dose' – this can be construed as the dose that is effective, but is usually the minimum dose that has any useful effect.

If one oral agonist fails to have any useful effect at maximum dosage, there is usually little to be gained by switching to another. If one agonist is poorly tolerated because of somnolence, one may switch to another, although risking the same problem again. If an agonist is poorly tolerated because of hallucinations, delusions or confusion, there is a significant risk of the same with another agonist.

Add-on use of dopamine agonists Dopamine agonists have longer clinical and pharmacological half-lives than levodopa. Hence, when added, they can help to minimise 'troughs' of dopaminergic stimulation and increase on time. Dyskinesias will usually increase, unless the dose of levodopa is reduced to compensate. In general, the less a patient's dopaminergic stimulation is obtained from levodopa and the more from an agonist, the less severe their dyskinesias tend to be.

Apomorphine is the oldest and most effective agonist and has a definite role as 'add-on' therapy to levodopa. It can be given via pen injections to rescue unpredictable off periods, or via continuous infusion to reduce them. The effect of single injections (usually 3–5 mg) is rapid (within 10–15 minutes) and reliable. Infusions (usually 3–6 mg/hour) can be supplemented by on-demand boluses. Apomorphine causes more drowsiness, particularly initially, and less psychiatric morbidity than oral agonists. It can very rarely cause an autoimmune haemolytic anaemia, so periodic haemoglobin, reticulocytes and Coombs testing is mandatory. Patients may also develop tender, inflamed or infected subcutaneous nodules or panniculitis which may cause them to abandon treatment. Infusions are usually given for about 12 hours during the day, but some patients use apomorphine infusions just at night, or 24 hours/day, with a lower rate at night.

Any oral agonists can usually be tailed off and levodopa dosage often reduced, which usually improves dyskinesias.

Anticholinergics

Anticholinergics such as benzhexol were the first drugs used to treat PD. They usually have only a mild symptomatic effect, often restricted to reducing tremor, although when abruptly discontinued patients can dramatically worsen. Because of cortical pathology, and the cholinergic deficit caused by NBM pathology, older PD patients are particularly susceptible to develop hallucinations and organic confusional states when given centrally acting anticholinergics. These agents should be avoided in elderly patients and their use restricted to younger, cognitively intact, usually tremor-dominant patients. Peripheral side effects of anticholinergics are common and predictable; they can cause blurred near vision because of mydriasis (so are contraindicated in narrow angle glaucoma), delayed gastric emptying and constipation. However, they can help sialorrhoea, and also reduce the detrusor hyper-reflexia commonly responsible for frequency and urgency in PD, but can precipitate retention of urine if there is also an element of prostatic obstruction.

Amantadine

This drug was originally used as an anti-influenza medication. Its use in PD was discovered serendipitously. It has several actions: an amphetamine-like effect (releasing presynaptic dopamine stores); a mild anticholinergic effect; a mild dopamine re-uptake inhibition effect; finally, it is also an *N*-methyl-D-asparate (NMDA) glutamate receptor antagonist. Traditionally, amantadine was used as a mild early treatment. Often the effect would wane, at least in part, after 6 weeks or so. The drug commonly causes ankle oedema and livedo reticularis. It can cause hallucinations or confusion, and is excreted by the kidneys, so should be used with caution in renal failure. More usefully, amantadine has also been recognised to have a (sometimes dramatic) antidyskinetic effect in at least some patients on levodopa, without worsening parkinsonism, presumed to be mediated by its NMDA antagonist property. It can also help freezing, even on freezing, in a minority of patients.

Surgery for PD

For some patients with more or less advanced PD, with motor fluctuations, dyskinesias or troublesome tremor, and who are difficult to manage despite the combination of available drugs, functional neurosurgery is an option, and can be most valuable. Lesioning procedures such as thalamotomy and pallidotomy were applied for many years but have been largely replaced in most countries by deep brain stimulation (DBS). DBS uses permanently implanted electrodes in the brain in conjunction with a neuropacemaker implanted in the chest wall that delivers high frequency electrical impulses. The three established brain targets for the treatment of PD with DBS are the ventrolateral thalamus, the internal pallidum (GPi) and the subthalamic nucleus (STN). DBS on each target improves a different range of symptoms.

Thalamic deep brain stimulation Thalamic stimulation was developed in 1987 to treat tremor related to PD or essential tremor, initially contralateral to a previous thalamotomy. In view of the benefits on tremor and the low rate of side effects, bilateral thalamic stimulation was then performed. However, thalamic DBS does not allow reduction in drug dosage. Balance problems and dysarthria are possible side effects, especially after bilateral surgery. Patients are usually asked to stop the stimulation at night to reduce the risk of tolerance and rebound. Benefits on tremor can be maintained for more than 10 years. Nevertheless, some long-term studies have shown that in many patients other symptoms such as gait difficulty, akinesia and dyskinesia progress and are not helped by thalamic DBS. This has led to the search for other brain targets in which DBS can help those symptoms and there has been a decrease in the indications for thalamic DBS. Thalamic DBS still has a place for elderly patients with tremor dominant disease.

Subthalamic nucleus deep brain stimulation Subthalamic nucleus deep brain stimulation (STN DBS) was developed in 1993, following basic research in the MPTP monkey model of PD. Hyperactivity of the STN was identified in their parkinsonian condition and an improvement of symptoms after STN lesions. In patients with PD, STN DBS can improve a large range of off-phase symptoms: limb bradykinesia, rigidity, tremor and gait difficulty including balance and freezing (if they are also dopa-sensitive). Levodopa-induced dyskinesias also improve over time, largely because of drug dosage reduction. 'Off' dystonia improves as well. Dopa-refractory symptoms are not helped and the effect on speech is variable, and it is not unfrequent that speech intelligibility deteriorates over time. Medications are usually reduced after STN DBS. In the early stage, stimulation is increased slowly in parallel with drug reduction to avoid increase of dyskinesias. After 5 years of STN DBS, benefits on appendicular symptoms are maintained; however, the effect on axial features (gait, balance, speech) and the on-phase scores often declines. Side effects are not infrequent: speech problems, possible neuropsychiatric problems (in particular mood changes) and more rarely eyelid opening apraxia and dyskinesias induced by the stimulation.

Internal pallidum deep brain stimulation Internal pallidum (GPi) DBS was developed in parallel with STN DBS but a smaller number of patients have received surgery because most teams opted for STN DBS. The effect on 'off' symptoms is more variable than with STN. The most reliable effect of GPi DBS is on dyskinesia. Nevertheless, although results of a US randomised blinded comparative study have shown only a moderate difference between the results of GPi and STN DBS, another similar Dutch study has shown superiority for STN DBS over GPI DBS. However, GPi DBS seems to be more lenient with the advantage of a lower rate of side effects, and it remains useful particularly for older patients or patients with severe dyskinesias who are at higher risk for adverse effects with STN DBS.

Patient selection for surgery Patient selection aims at identifying those patients likely to benefit from surgery and unlikely to have severe adverse effects. Therefore, it is important to identify the disabling symptoms and assess if they are dopa-sensitive or dopa-induced and how they impact on the patient's daily life. A levodopa challenge is very helpful to assess in detail 'off' symptoms, the response to medications and the severity and type of dyskinesias. Cognitive functions and mood should also be carefully assessed. Brain MRI is carried out to exclude contraindications such as severe atrophy, extensive white matter change and focal lesions. The patient's general condition has to be considered. Patients treated by platelet anti-aggregants or anticoagulants should be able to stop them for 2 weeks before and 2 weeks after surgery. Speech and swallowing have to be considered, because of the risk of deterioration. Patients and their family should be given detailed information about the procedure, its risks and potential benefits, as well as its limitations. Patient and family expectations have to be addressed. The choice of brain target for DBS depends on the profile of symptoms and the risk factors.

Surgery Surgery is performed under stereotactic conditions. The implantation of the electrodes was usually carried out under local anesthesia, but thanks to better imaging modalities it is increasingly carried out in general anaesthesia, especially on brain targets that can be readily visualised pre- and postoperatively, such as the STN and GPi. Brain atlases can provide some guidance, in particular when the target cannot be visualised on MRI, for example the subnuclei of the ventrolateral thalamus (ventral oral posterior [Vop], and ventral intermediate [Vim] nuclei). During awake surgery, different electrophysiological methods can be used, Microelectrode recording techniques are used by many surgeons, although it has been shown that their use can result in higher risk for hemorrhage. In awake patients. intraoperative stimulation allows one to confirm the benefits and to observe side effects. The neuropacemaker and the connectors are always implanted under general anaesthesia. The general risk of surgery includes haemorrhage in 0–4% of patients, according to the technique and the surgeon, and infections of the system occur in about 2–3% of patients.

Stimulator adjustment and long-term management Patients implanted with DBS need life-long follow-up by a specialist team. Stimulation parameters have to be adjusted from time to time, as well as medication. Electrical parameters are similar for all targets: voltage is usually between 2 and 4 V, pulse width usually 60 μs, occasionally 90 μs, but tends to be higher in GPi, and frequency is typically 130 Hz or above. Monopolar stimulation is preferred unless side effects limit the increase in voltage. Adjustment of thalamic DBS is usually straightforward. However, adjustment of STN DBS has to be progressive, in parallel with adjustment of medications. Adjustment of GPi DBS does not have the same immediate effect on the symptoms. The neuropacemaker has to be changed approximately every 3–7 years.

Some side effects, in particular neuropsychiatric problems such as depression, apathy and mania, can occur even a long time after surgery. Infections or skin erosions can also occur late. Some medical equipment, in particular diathermy and monopolar coagulation, should not be used in DBS patients. Brain MRI after implantation can only be performed under restricted conditions of energy delivery and using a receiver–transmitter head coil.

The future Existing DBS procedures, although very helpful, have limitations. They only allow symptomatic improvement, they do not appear to change the progression of the disease and they are ineffective against dopa-refractory symptoms, with the exception of tremor. There is no real alternative at present, although preliminary albeit conflictual reports of DBS in the area of the pedunculo-pontine nucleus have suggested that it might improve gait. There is a renewed interest in stereotactic lesional procedures, and pilot trials are underway using non-surgically invasive techniques such as gamma knife or focused ultrasound to perform thalamotomy or pallidotomy in patients with PD or essential tremor. Dopaminergic cell transplants and intraputaminal delivery of glial derived neurotrophic factor (GDNF) have shown apparent improvement in a minority of patients, and these procedures are under renewed investigation after having been halted previously because of side effects. Further development of potentially disease-modifying and restorative procedures is the challenge for the future.

Dementia in association with Lewy body pathology

It has long been recognised that patients with PD have a higher risk of developing dementia than age-matched controls. Longitudinal studies have found cumulative dementia risks between 42%, and up to 80% with follow-up as long as 20 years. Dementia starting more than 1 year after the onset of parkinsonism is arbitrarily called Parkinson's disease dementia (PD-D).

In contrast, the development of parkinsonism and dementia within 1 year of each other, or a similar type of dementia without spontaneous parkinsonism is termed dementia with Lewy bodies (DLB), and is the most common cause of dementia in the elderly after Alzheimer's disease (AD; see Chapter 8). Mean survival of both DLB and PD-D cases after the development of dementia is only 5 years. Postmortem pathological examination reveals the presence of Lewy body pathology (often accompanied by varying numbers of senile plaques and sometimes of both senile plaques and neurofibrillary tangles) in both cerebral cortex and brainstem. On a pathological basis, it is usually impossible to distinguish patients with a clinical diagnosis of PD-D from patients with a clinical diagnosis of DLB.

Progressive disabling cognitive impairment is a mandatory requirement for the diagnosis of both PD-D and DLB. For probable DLB two, and for possible DLB, one of the following three core features are required:

1 Fluctuating cognition with pronounced variations in attention and alertness
2 Recurrent visual hallucinations, and
3 Spontaneous features of parkinsonism.

Other supportive features of DLB are RBD and, in the absence of spontaneous parkinsonism, severe neuroleptic sensitivity and impaired dopamine transporter uptake in striatum on PET or SPECT scanning.

The management of confusion and hallucinations and of cognitive impairment in PD, PD-D and DLB is challenging. Intercurrent illness should be sought and treated (including infection, constipation, metabolic disturbance or head injury). The number and type of psychoactive (mostly antiparkinsonian) drugs taken should be rationalised, starting with reduction of anticholinergics, then dopamine agonists and amantadine, then MAO-B inhibitors, then COMT inhibitors, leaving the patient on monotherapy with a levodopa preparation in the lowest dose possible. If hallucinations or delusions persist, an antipsychotic drug may be needed. Quetiapine is well tolerated, but not of proven efficacy in this indication. The only drug with class 1 evidence of antipsychotic efficacy, while not worsening underlying parkinsonism, is clozapine. However, because of the risk of bone marrow suppression and the consequent stringent monitoring requirements, it is little used in the United Kingdom in this indication, for which it is considered a second line drug.

The cortical cholinergic deficit in demented, and even in non-demented, PD patients and in DLB, is greater than that in AD. Therefore, the cholinesterase inhibitors are also effective in these indications. Rivastigmine, started at a dose of 1.5 mg twice daily and gradually increased to 6 mg twice daily, or donepezil, started at a dose of 5 mg once a day and increased to 10 mg once a day, can be very helpful in some patients, although responses can be disappointing in others. However, these drugs can worsen any urinary frequency or urgency.

Multiple system atrophy

This sporadically occurring alpha-synucleinopathy was also previously described as Shy–Drager syndrome, striato-nigral degeneration, or (some cases) sporadic olivo-ponto-cerebellar atrophy (sOPCA). It causes varying combinations of parkinsonism (MSA-P, usually poorly responsive to levodopa), cerebellar dysfunction (MSA-C), autonomic failure (orthostatic hypotension, male erectile dysfunction and urinary incontinence or incomplete bladder emptying) and pyramidal signs. Pathology involves varying combinations and locations of neuronal loss and oligodendroglial pathology (ubiquitin and alpha-synuclein positive intracytoplasmic inclusions; GCIs) in striatum (especially posterior putamen), substantia nigra, locus caeruleus, inferior olive, pons and cerebellum, and in the intermediolateral cell columns and Onuf's nucleus of the spinal cord. It is almost invariably sporadic. Prevalence is about 4/100 000, mean age at onset is 57 years (never starting before age 30) and mean survival is about 7 (1–16) years. Often autonomic failure (AF) antedates the other neurology. If isolated AF persists for more than 5 years the term pure autonomic failure is used – such patients usually have Lewy body pathology in autonomic ganglia, and also in substantia nigra, but not enough to cause parkinsonism. Rare cases of MSA or of PD 'convert' from a label of pure autonomic failure after the arbitrary 5-year period.

Other clinical features of MSA include RBD and sleep apnoea (also common, but less so, in PD), increased snoring, nocturnal or daytime stridor, emotional incontinence, myoclonic jerks of the fingers, impaired sweating and heat intolerance, Raynaud's phenomenon, cold dusky hands, disproportionate fixed antecollis, postural instability, dysphagia and a characteristic dysarthria – high-pitched, quivery, strained and hypophonic in MSA-P or slurring cerebellar-type in MSA-C. Frank dementia is rare, and an exclusion criterion for the diagnosis, because patients (usually more elderly) with the combination of dementia, parkinsonism and autonomic failure are much more likely to have Lewy body pathology, and dementia, when it does occur in MSA, is a late feature. Consensus diagnostic criteria for MSA were recently revised. Treatment of MSA is symptomatic. Levodopa can be of minor benefit in the early stages, but can exacerbate postural hypotension and can also cause atypical orofacial dyskinesias. Amantadine is useful in some patients. Symptomatic treatment of the autonomic aspects can be of greater help.

Progressive supranuclear palsy

Progressive supranuclear palsy (PSP) is a tauopathy, usually sporadic, rarely familial. It classically causes axial (hence symmetrical) akinesia and rigidity, early falls (classically backwards without warning), dysarthria (lower pitch, growling, with late groaning), dysphagia, personality change, frontal cognitive deficits and eye features. These include frontalis overactivity, levator inhibition, sometimes blepharospasm, and a characteristic supranuclear gaze palsy (or, more correctly, paresis) which is necessary for the clinical diagnosis and which gives the disease its name. Often the earliest feature is slowing of vertical voluntary saccades, followed by supranuclear limitation of up-gaze (non-specific) or down-gaze (always pathological), followed by similar abnormalities on horizontal saccades. The supranuclear cause of any limitation of voluntary gaze is identified when a complete range of automatic reflex eye movements is demonstrated by the oculocephalic, or doll's head, manoeuvre, such automatic–voluntary dissociation indicating that the oculomotor pathway from the nucleus distally is intact. The latency to initiate saccades is typically normal in PSP, in contrast to CBD (see later).

The pathology of PSP involves neuronal loss and gliosis, with straight neurofibrillary tangles and tufted astrocytes particularly in substantia nigra, dentate nucleus, pallidum, subthalamic nucleus and, to a variable degree, cerebral cortex. An increase in the concentration of the 4 repeat isoform of tau is present.

The prevalence of PSP is about 5/100 000, mean age at onset is 63 years, never starting before 40, and mean survival is 7 years. Although about half of patients with pathologically proven PSP show the classic clinical picture (Richardson's syndrome) with mean survival of 6 years, about one-third have a longer course averaging 9 years (PSP-P) with more PD-like features, including some levodopa response and resting tremor, with falls and gaze palsy developing later on. Other clinical features include emotional incontinence, frontal release signs, a memory retrieval deficit, palilalia and palilogia, other motor perseveration, sitting down 'en bloc' and prominent sialorrhoea. Despite severe postural instability, patients usually fail to widen their base which, combined with 'motor recklessness', causes frequent falls, with injury. Unlike MSA and PD, cardiovascular AF is not a feature of PSP. However, urinary disturbance is common. A small percentage of individuals present with an isolated phenotype of 'pure akinesia and gait freezing', with little other evidence for parkinsonism or gaze palsy, and rarely PSP patients can present with a corticobasal syndrome or withspeech apraxia. Treatment of PSP is symptomatic, and minor benefits can be seen with levodopa and/or amantadine. The mainstay of treatment is supportive and patients should be seen by the multidisciplinary team including dietitians, speech therapists, occupational therapists and physiotherapists.

Corticobasal degeneration

This tauopathy is also largely sporadic, with only very rare familial cases. Nevertheless, it shares with PSP over-representation of the H1/H1 tau haplotype, and consequent excessive concentration of the 4 repeat tau isoform, indicating some shared genetic susceptibility. Many with the disease present to movement disorder specialists with the asymmetric and progressive evolution, usually starting in one arm (but sometimes in a leg), of 'difficulty' using the limb, which progressively becomes useless because of a combination of akinesia, rigidity, fixed dystonia, myoclonus, jerky tremor, cortical sensory loss and, above all, apraxia. Sometimes there is an additional 'alien limb' phenomenon, when the limb wanders off 'with a mind of its own'. Progression is then to the opposite limb or the other limb on the same side, ultimately to all four limbs, and a supranuclear gaze palsy (paresis) gradually develops which classically is the 'mirror-image' of PSP. Thus, there is great difficulty initiating voluntary saccades, with prolonged latency (oculomotor apraxia), but when the eyes finally move they do so with normal velocity. The pathology of CBD includes swollen ('ballooned') cortical neurones predominantly in frontal and parietal areas and neurofibrillary tangles and astrocytic plaques. The prevalence of CBD is unknown, but it is rarer than MSA or PSP. Mean age at onset is 63 years and mean survival is 8 years.

However, the classic clinical picture described can be misleading. Thus, those with CBD can present to dementia specialists with apraxia or a progressive non-fluent aphasia, or disease can present symmetrically, or with falls. Conversely, it may be misdiagnosed in life as PSP. Other diseases can also present with a corticobasal-like syndrome, including vascular lesions, but also prion disease, Alzheimer's disease and disorders with TDP-43 pathology. Some of these are caused by mutations in progranulin, *FUS*, *C9orf72* and other genes. Hence in clinical cases the term corticobasal syndrome is preferred to corticobasal degeneration, as different pathologies can result in same clinical syndrome. New diagnostic criteria have been recently proposed.

Ancillary investigations to distinguish between PD, MSA, PSP and CBD and other conditions

Brain imaging using MRI in MSA patients may reveal, supratentorially, putaminal atrophy, a hyperintense slit-like lateral rim to the putamen, or posterior putaminal hypointensity (Figure 6.1). Infratentorially, pontine atrophy, a 'hot-cross bun' appearance of the pons in cross-section (Figure 6.2), hyperintensity of the middle cerebellar peduncles or cerebellar atrophy may be seen.

In PSP one may see atrophy of the midbrain, as evidenced by the 'hummingbird sign' and an increased pons to midbrain ratio on sagittal cuts (Figure 6.3), and atrophy of the superior cerebellar peduncles on axial cuts (best demonstrated with voxel-based morphometry). In CBD there can be asymmetrical or unilateral frontal and parietal atrophy.

F-dopa PET or dopamine transporter SPECT scans only provide evidence of nigral pathology, so cannot reliably distinguish between these conditions. However, a normal scan can provide useful evidence in favour of psychogenic or drug-induced parkinsonism, or of essential or dystonic tremor, or in distinguishing between dopa-responsive dystonia (normal) and 'juvenile PD' (abnormal). FDG-PET may show a signal void in striatum in MSA (and PSP), and asymmetrical fronto-parietal hypometabolism in CBD. Cardiac ^{123}I meta-iodobenzyl guanidine (MIBG) scanning usually, but not always, reveals evidence of postganglionic cardiac denervation in PD, whereas such scans are usually normal in MSA, PSP and CBD.

Autonomic function tests can reveal evidence of autonomic failure, but not whether it is caused by Lewy body pathology or MSA or be brought about by drug treatment.

Urethral or anal sphincter electromyography (EMG) can show evidence of denervation and reinnervation (increased amplitude, duration and polyphasia) consequent on loss of anterior horn cells in Onuf's nucleus at S2–3. A normal result would argue against MSA, but abnormal results occur also in PD and PSP.

Vascular parkinsonism

Subjects with multiple infarcts or, more commonly, multiple basal ganglia lacunes or deep white matter vascular changes, can present with what is often a poor mimic of PD, or even of true parkinsonism. Typically, spontaneous movements and facial expression are good, posture upright, and while there may be pyramidal slowing of finger movements, there is no classic fatiguing or decrement, and no tremor. The gait can be wide-based or unsteady, and

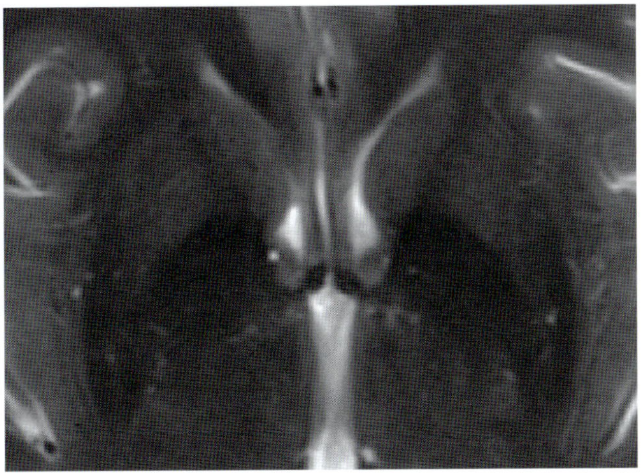

Figure 6.1 Hypointensity in the posterior putamen in multiple system atrophy (MSA) (T2-weighted magnetic resonance imaging; MRI T2W).

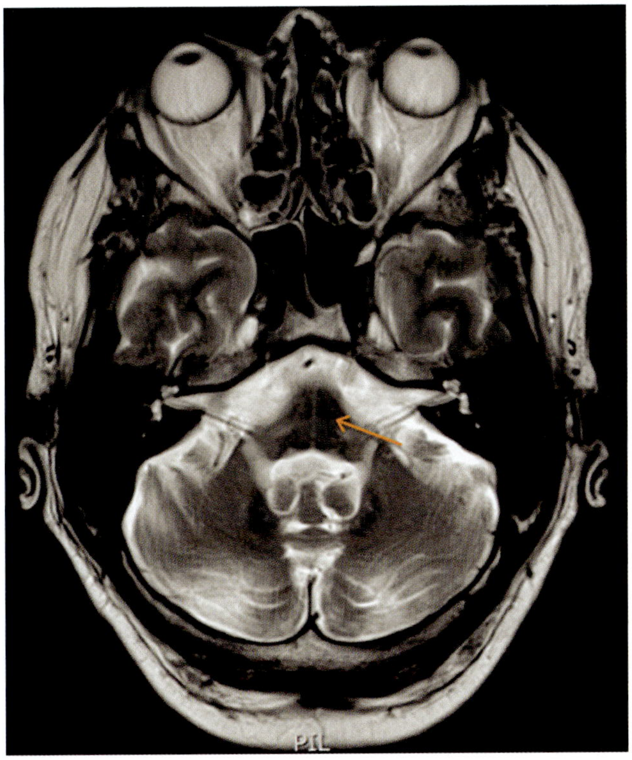

Figure 6.2 'Hot cross bun' appearance (arrow) in the pons in MSA (MRI T2W).

small-stepped (marche à petits pas) rather than shuffling. Start hesitation or gait initiation failure, freezing, and some fatiguing of alternating ankle movements are often present, leading to terms such as lower body parkinsonism or parkinsonian ataxia. True parkinsonism involving upper as well as lower body, in the presence of cerebrovascular disease (CVD) is usually brought about by the co-occurrence of PD – the patient's upper body has levodopa-responsive parkinsonism while their lower half behaves differently, and gait problems and falls often appear or worsen suddenly or

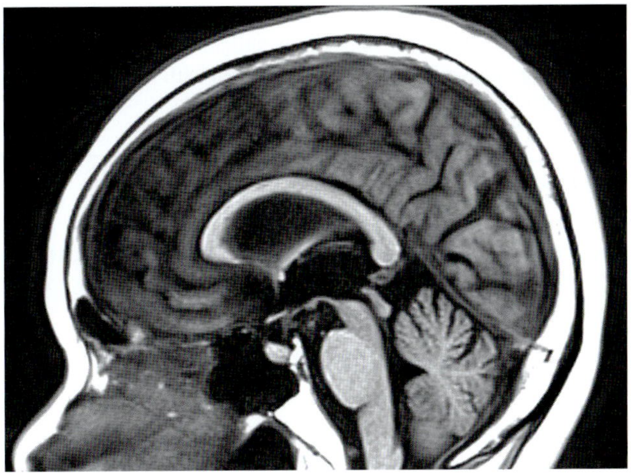

Figure 6.3 Coronal MRI section showing the 'hummingbird' appearance due to midbrain atrophy in progressive supranuclear palsy (PSP) (MRI T2W).

subacutely. However, some cases of apparent true parkinsonism resulting from CVD, with no Lewy body pathology, have been reported, and some of these have responded to levodopa, so that a trial of this drug is probably justified in all cases of CVD with convincing 'parkinsonian' features.

Ethnic or region-specific parkinsonism

X-linked dystonia-parkinsonism ('Lubag') with striatal mosaicism is essentially limited to Filipinos and is caused by a mutation in the *TAF1* gene. Patients may respond to levodopa, and beneficial effects have been seen with DBS. The parkinsonism–dementia–ALS complex in Guam, a disease characterised by tangle pathology rather than Lewy bodies, may be of environmental, rather than genetic, origin, as it is fast disappearing. Atypical parkinsonism on Guadeloupe may be heterogeneous, and at least partly environmentally determined.

Other causes of parkinsonism

Other genetic causes of parkinsonism include the Huntington's disease Westphal phenotype, seen mostly in juvenile onset cases; Wilson's disease; SCAs 1–3, in which tremor and levodopa-responsiveness can be seen; FTDP-17; and other rarer causes (Table 6.2).

Environmental causes include toxins (MPTP, CO, methanol and manganese) and drugs (dopamine receptor blockers, presynaptic dopamine depletors); post-infectious, particularly after Japanese B encephalitis and encephalitis lethargica (which still occurs rarely, with positive antibasal ganglia antibodies); post-traumatic encephalopathy in boxers and other sportspeople; and hydrocephalus and tumour.

The coexistence of parkinsonism and dystonia should prompt imaging looking for the presence of metal deposition in the basal ganglia. A range of conditions can cause neuronal degeneration with brain iron accumulation (NBIA) – listed in Table 6.3 and also discussed in section on dystonia. These can be distinguished using genetic tests. Iron deposition is best revealed during T2* sequence MRI, while CT imaging usefully demonstrates basal ganglia calcification. The presence of abnormal deposition in the absence of evidence to suggest iron, calcium or copper deposition, and especially with the coexistence of cirrhosis, should raise the suspicion of hypermanganesaemia, and can be associated with mutations in the SLC30A10 manganese transporter.

Tremor

Tremor is defined as rhythmic sinusoidal alternating movement. It can be described in several ways (e.g. rest; postural; action or terminal; or intention). Tremor in PD, MSA and PSP has been discussed earlier.

Benign essential tremor

This is commonly inherited as an autosomal dominant trait. Most people with essential tremor (ET) have little or no disability, so never see a neurologist. Published community prevalence figures vary hugely, but an average of studies is 3–400/100 000. Interestingly, despite being very common and inherited with a high penetrance, no gene has been identified to cause the majority of ET. There are a few families linked to some genetic loci and some families carry a genetic disorder restricted to them (e.g. the Lingo gene). Typically, ET involves both arms first, fairly symmetrically, and to a greater degree than any other body parts (neck, legs, voice) which may be subsequently involved. The tremor is usually vertical (flexion–extension) rather than pronation–supination. It often worsens slowly over many years, but even then often does not cause marked functional impairment, although in some cases it does. It often improves after alcohol, and may be helped by β-blockers, primidone, gabapentin and topiramate in some cases. There are a number of other tremor disorders often mistaken as ET: dystonic tremor, enhanced physiological tremor and other conditions that cause postural tremor.

Dystonic tremor

The authors' view of dystonic tremor is that it is poorly defined, under-recognised and often misdiagnosed as ET or as benign tremulous PD. This view is controversial, and not yet generally accepted. The Movement Disorder Society Consensus Statement on Tremor restricts the term dystonic tremor to a tremor in a body part also displaying overt dystonia (e.g. tremulous torticollis). When someone with spasmodic torticollis, for example, also has a tremor of one or both arms, without overt dystonia in those limbs, it is called tremor associated with dystonia. Such an arm tremor usually displays other characteristics: it may be unilateral or asymmetrical, relatively slow, pronation–supination, coming in 'flurries', jerky, position-specific or markedly worsened by certain tasks (e.g. attempting to write), and therefore more commonly disabling than ET; it can be associated with abnormal or reduced arm swing, or a jaw tremor, and about one-third of these patients also display a dominant family history (in taking a family history of tremor it is always useful to ask what shook [e.g. neck] as well as who shook). We would also call this tremor dystonic tremor. Where the patient has tremor with these characteristics, but (as yet) no evident dystonia, we currently label this as atypical tremor, while recognising that many of these subjects may later turn out to have dystonic tremor. Drug treatment is disappointing in older patients, but levodopa and anticholinergics are worth trying in younger subjects.

Both ET and dystonic tremor can be helped by botulinum toxin injections or, in severe cases, thalamic deep DBS or pallidal DBS (if dystonic).

Neuropathic tremor

Some neuropathies, particularly immunoglobulin M dysgammaglobulinaemic neuropathy, can cause a postural (and if severe, even a resting) tremor. The severity of the tremor does not necessarily correlate with the severity of the neuropathy or the degree of deafferentation. In patients with unexplained tremor it is always important to search for any clinical evidence of neuropathy.

Fragile X tremor ataxia syndrome

It has recently been recognised that individuals (usually males) with premutations (55–200 CGG repeats) in the fragile X mental retardation 1 (*FMR1*) gene can, as they get older, present with a relatively slowly (compared with MSA-C) progressive syndrome combining postural or action tremor and ataxia, sometimes with additional parkinsonism, peripheral neuropathy, cognitive impairment and dysautonomia. There can be a family history of, and an increased risk, especially to males, of mental retardation, and premature ovarian failure can occur in females. MRI commonly shows hyperintensity of the middle cerebellar peduncles or of subcortical white matter, and cerebellar atrophy.

Cerebellar (pathway) tremor

Intention tremor

This is caused by brainstem or cerebellar outflow pathway lesions, the most common cause being multiple sclerosis (MS). The tremor is not just action or terminal (features common to many postural tremors), but worsens steadily throughout the whole trajectory of the movement. Symptomatic drug treatment is unhelpful. DBS may transiently help, but its benefits are usually overwhelmed by the progression of MS lesion load.

Holmes tremor

This form of tremor, previously called midbrain tremor or rubral (red nuclear) tremor, is a tripartite tremor incorporating tremor at rest, postural tremor and intention tremor. It is caused by a combination of damage to the cerebello-rubrothalamic and nigro-striatal pathways.

Palatal tremor

This comprises rhythmic (1–2 Hz) contractions of the soft palate, presumably resulting from a dysfunction (essential palatal myoclonus, EPM) or a lesion (symptomatic palatal myoclonus, SPM) involving the connections between dentate nucleus, red nucleus and inferior olivary nuclei (the Guillain–Mollaret triangle). EPM consists of rhythmic contractions of the tensor veli palatini, innervated by the trigeminal nucleus. In SPM, the main muscle involved is the levator palatini, innervated by the facial nucleus and the nucleus ambiguus. EPM is typically associated with clicking, whereas SPM usually persists during sleep and is often associated with hypertrophy of the inferior olive. SPM is often associated with vertical ocular movements (oculopalatal myoclonus) or rhythmic and oscillatory limb movements at a rate of 1–3 Hz. Important causes of SPM include Wilson's disease, stroke and/or tumour and Alexander's disease. A number of EPM cases are of functional (non-organic) origin. Oculomasticatory myorhythmia or oculo-facial-skeletal myorhythmia are believed to be pathognomonic of Whipple's disease. Clonazepam sometimes helps.

Orthostatic tremor

This is a rare condition in which subjects feel unsteady, and often tremulous, while standing still, but not on walking, so that they like to either sit down or to keep moving. It is characterised by 13–16 Hz tremor of the leg muscles, easily recorded on surface EMG which can often be felt or auscultated, but not usually seen. Some cases have additional features of parkinsonism or restless legs. Clonazepam sometimes helps.

Drug and toxin-induced tremor

Tremor can be caused by a number of different drugs or toxins including dopamine-depleting or receptor-blocking drugs, cinnarazine, some calcium-channel blockers, diltiazem (mostly rest tremor), sodium valproate (rest or postural), or beta-agonists, theophylline, caffeine, nicotine, lithium, amiodarone, SSRIs and tricyclic antidepressants, ciclosporin, thyroxine excess, and intoxication with marijuana, cocaine, amphetamines or mercury (postural).

Psychogenic tremor

This is dealt with in Other movement disorders.

Dystonia

Dystonia is a heterogeneous and common movement disorder typically characterised by involuntary muscle spasms leading to abnormal postures of the affected body part. Typically, the spasms in dystonia are mobile and this often leads to a slow writhing of the affected body part as described by the older term 'athetosis'. Co-contraction of agonist and antagonist muscles is the underlying reason for the abnormal posturing in dystonia, and this can be obvious clinically or more easily on simple EMG assessment. Dystonia can be variable in its presentation and in some cases tremor or jerks can be the predominant feature with the abnormal postures being subtle. In fact the recent 2013 consensus statement on classification and definition of dystonia recognises tremor as an integral part of dystonia and includes it within the definition. Dystonia can also often be task, or position-specific (e.g. present only on writing or playing a musical instrument but not with other tasks). Another characteristic feature of dystonia, particularly focal dystonia, is the presence of a sensory trick or *geste antagoniste*, whereby applying a sensory stimulus to a particular area will cause the abnormal posture to resolve. Some non-motor aspects of dystonia have been recognised including abnormalities in specialised sensory function such as spatial and temporal discrimination and psychiatric features such as anxiety and depression.

Epidemiology

There have been few epidemiological studies of dystonia. Most studies have provided estimates based on few cases. A European prevalence study with pooled data from eight countries undertaken to provide more precise rates of dystonia found the crude annual period prevalence rate (1996–1997) for all primary dystonia was 152 per million, with focal dystonia having the highest rate of 117 per million (108–126) of which cervical dystonia was most common (57 per million), followed by blepharospasm (36 per million) and writer's cramp (14 per million). However, the authors pointed out that because of under-ascertainment of cases, these rates were probably an underestimate of the true prevalence of dystonia.

Classifying dystonia

Dystonia can be classified in a number of ways including by age of onset, by distribution and aetiology (Table 6.4). With regard to aetiology there have been major advances in the genetic causes of the dystonias and this list keeps growing. Clinically, however, the most important and useful division is classifying patients broadly into two categories: those with 'primary dystonia'; and those with 'secondary/heredodegenerative' dystonic conditions. Dystonia is the only clinical sign (with the exception of tremor) in primary dystonia, and there is no neurodegeneration. The age of onset (below or above age 28), and distribution (focal, segmental, generalised) can be very useful to decide whether the patient fits into the well-defined phenotypes of primary dystonia (see later), and for picking up patients with unusual phenotypes (e.g. an adult presenting with generalised dystonia, which would be incompatible with typical primary dystonia) and to investigate these patients further to find out the likely secondary/heredodegenerative cause. Clinical features or 'red flags' that should make one consider secondary dystonia rather than primary dystonia are listed in Table 6.5. A new consensus classification has proposed that dystonia be classified by two axes. Axis 1 clinically defines dystonia as either 'isolated' or 'combined' (when associated with other features). Those with combined features may

Table 6.4 Classification of dystonia.

By aetiology	By distribution	By age at onset
Primary (no neurodegeneration; dystonia only ± tremor)	Focal Segmental	Young onset (<28 yrs) Adult onset (>28 yrs)
Dystonia-plus syndromes	Multifocal	
Dopa-responsive dystonia	Hemidystonia	
Myoclonus dystonia		
Secondary		
Symptomatic		
Heredodegenerative		
Paroxysmal		

Table 6.5 Clinical clues in the history and examination suggesting a secondary cause of dystonia.

Abnormal birth/perinatal history
Developmental delay
Continued progression of symptoms
Unusual distribution of dystonia given age of onset (e.g. leg dystonia in an adult, hemidystonia)
Unusual nature of dystonia (e.g. fixed dystonic postures)
Prominent bulbar involvement by dystonia
Additional neurological symptoms (pyramidal signs, cerebellar signs, cognitive decline)
Seizures
Other systems affected (e.g. organomegaly)
Previous exposure to drugs (e.g. dopamine receptor blockers)

further be characterised into a syndrome and particular etiologies are to be considered in Axis II. Psychogenic dystonia is dealt with later in this chapter.

Primary dystonia

In patients with primary dystonia, age at onset appears to be very important in determining the clinical phenotype. Young onset dystonia (before the age of 28 years) most commonly manifests with limb onset dystonia, followed by subsequent generalisation and was referred to in the older literature as dystonia musculorum deformans or Oppenheim's dystonia. It is now known that about 70% of patients presenting in this way will carry a single GAG deletion in the *DYT1* gene on chromosome 9. This condition is more common in Ashkenazi Jews, with a possible founder in Eastern Europe about 3 centuries ago. It has an autosomal dominant inheritance, but a very low phenotypic penetrance such that only 30–40% of gene carriers will ever develop dystonia, and in those who do this will almost always happen before the age of 30 years.

When dystonia appears in adult life, a focal or segmental distribution is commonly seen and the condition does not generalise. These presentations, in order of frequency of occurrence, include cervical dystonia (spasmodic torticollis), cranial dystonia (e.g. blepharospasm, Meige syndrome [blepharospasm and oromandibular dystonia]), writer's cramp, laryngeal dystonia (sometimes called spasmodic or, inappropriately, spastic dysphonia) and other task-specific dystonias. Cranio-cervical dystonia is more common in women than men, with the opposite pattern seen in task-specific writing dystonia. The adult onset focal dystonias are not a forme fruste of the early onset *DYT1* gene-related dystonia, and this gene has been excluded in these disorders,, most of the patients being sporadic. Apart from *DYT1* a number of genes have now been identified causing primary dystonia but also some forms of combined dystonia (where there are other associated features; Table 6.6) and the list is growing. Amongst these is one causing isolated primary cranio-cervical dystonia with onset in the early adulthood is *DYT6*, caused by mutations in the *THAP1* gene. Patients with *THAP1* often have marked laryngeal with cervical or oromandibular dystonia often with spread to the limbs. Other rare causes of cervical/segmental dystonia are due to rare genetic forms due to *CIZ1*, *GNAL* and *ANO3* gene mutations. *DYT7* and *DYT13* have been described in rare families with cranio-cervical segmental dystonia but the genes are yet to be discovered (Table 6.6).

Dystonia-plus syndromes

This category refers to two diseases without evidence of neurodegeneration whose motor manifestations are restricted to dystonia, plus parkinsonism or myoclonus. Some would consider it reasonable to include them with *DYT1* under the heading of primary dystonias.

Dopa-responsive dystonia

Dopa-responsive dystonia (DRD; *DYT5*), previously also called Segawa disease, typically presents in childhood, purely with lower limb dystonia, and parkinsonism may rarely be associated, although the latter can be a presenting feature when onset is at an older age. A diurnal fluctuation in symptom severity with a gradual worsening of symptoms throughout the day was said to be typical of the condition, but is present in only 60% of cases. This condition is inherited in an autosomal dominant manner, with reduced penetrance, and is caused by mutations in the GTP cyclohydrolase 1 gene (*GTPCH1*; *DYT5*), a rate-limiting step in the production of dopamine from tyrosine. Although rare, it is of critical importance to the practising neurologist as it is entirely treatable by small doses of levodopa. This typically leads to complete resolution of symptoms, which is sustained without the development of long-term complications as seen in PD.

It is increasingly recognised that DRD can present with unusual phenotypes such as spastic diplegia, writer's cramp and other focal dystonias including predominant cervical dystonia and even ataxia. In view of this, an adequate trial of levodopa (ideally up to 100–200 mg according to age/weight plus peripheral decarboxylase inhibitor, three times daily), for at least 2 months is strongly recommended in all those with young onset dystonia, especially as genetic diagnosis is time-consuming and not generally available. A phenylalanine loading test and cerebrospinal fluid (CSF) pterin studies can be helpful. It is also important to differentiate patients with DRD from those with young onset Parkinson's disease, who may present with foot dystonia, and in whom the early use of levodopa is not recommended. A DaT SPECT or a fluorodopa PET scan (both normal in DRD) can be useful in this regard. Other inherited defects of the dopamine synthesis pathway (e.g. the recessively inherited tyrosine hydroxylase deficiency) can also cause DRD, but usually as part of a more severe neurological syndrome.

Myoclonus dystonia

Patients with myoclonus-dystonia (*DYT11*), caused by autosomal dominantly inherited mutations in the ε-sarcoglycan gene on chromosome 7q21, present with early onset dystonia in combination with myoclonic 'lightning' jerks. The jerks respond quite dramatically to alcohol. The condition typically starts in childhood, and is mostly inherited through the father because of maternal genomic imprinting. The myoclonus or dystonia mainly affects the head, neck and arms, with the legs usually being spared. The myoclonus worsens during movement (action myoclonus) and is often more prominent than the dystonia. It had been suspected that hereditary essential myoclonus (when myoclonus is prominent) and dominantly inherited myoclonic dystonia, with lightning jerks and dramatic response to alcohol, might often be the same disease, and this has now been confirmed with the discovery of the causative mutations, although other broadly similar cases are mutation-negative. Psychiatric features such as anxiety, depression and obsessive-compulsive disorders are also a feature of the condition in a fair proportion of cases.

Figure 6.4 shows the breakdown of dystonia classification scheme according to clinical presentation and its genetic correlations.

Symptomatic dystonia

Dystonia can be secondary to a number of environmental causes, many of which affect the basal ganglia. Dystonia is commonly seen following brain injury (e.g. perinatally: dystonic/dyskinetic/athetoid cerebral palsy) or following stroke. In such patients a static deficit is commonly seen, although onset can be delayed for months or even years after injury, and progression and late worsening of symptoms is sometimes seen.

Tardive dystonia is dealt with in Other movement disorders.

Heredodegenerative dystonias

Dystonia can be a feature of a wide range of neurodegenerative conditions, which can make selection and prioritisation of the appropriate investigations and reaching the correct diagnosis a difficult task. One aspect of such conditions that can be helpful is that many

Table 6.6 Dystonia genetic conditions.

Gene	Locus	Inheritance	Phenotype	Gene product (gene)
DYT 1	9q32-34	AD	Young onset, generalised	Torsin A (*TOR1A*)
DYT 2	NM	AR	Young onset, generalised	
DYT 3	Xq13.1	XR	Filipino dystonia–parkinsonism	Gene transcription factor (*TAF1*)
DYT 4	NM	AD	Laryngeal ± limb dystonia (1 family)	
DYT 5a *DYT 5b*	14q22.1-2 11p16.5	AD AR	Young onset, dopa-responsive dystonia–parkinsonism	GTP cyclohydrolase 1 (*GTPCH1*) Tyrosine hydroxylase (TH)
DYT 6	8p11.21	AD	Young onset, cranio-cervical or generalised	Thanatos-associated protein 1 (*THAP1*)
DYT 7	18p	AD	Adult onset, focal dystonia (1 family)	Not identified
DYT 8	2q35	AD	*PNKD1*	Myofibrillogenesis regulator 1 (*MR-1*)
DYT 9	1p31	AD	*EID1*/Episodic chorea or ataxia and spasticity	Glucose transporter 1 (*SLC2A1*)
DYT 10	16p11-q12	AD	*PKD1*	*PRRT2*
DYT 11	7q21.3	AD	Myoclonus dystonia	ε-sarcoglycan (SGCE)
DYT 12	19q13.2	AD	Rapid onset dystonia–parkinsonism	Na+/K+ATPase α3 subunit (*ATP1A3*)
DYT 13	1p36	AD	Young onset segmental or generalised dystonia (1 family)	Not identified
DYT 14 = DYT 5a				
DYT 15	18p11	AD	Myoclonus dystonia (1 family)	Not identified
DYT 16	2q31.2	AR	Young onset, generalised dystonia-parkinsonism	Stress-response protein (*PRKRA*)
DYT 17	20p11-q13	AR	Young onset, mixed phenotype (1 family)	Not identified
DYT 18	1p34.2	AD	*EID2*	Glucose transporter 1 (*SLC2A1*)
DYT 19	16q13-22	AD	*PKD2* (1 family)	Not identified
DYT 20	2q31	AD	*PNKD2* (1 family)	Not identified
DYT 21	2q14-q21	AD	Adult onset mixed phenotype (1 family)	Not identified
DYT 22	Reserved			
DYT 23	9q34.3	AD	Myoclonus dystonia	*CACNA1B*
DYT 24	11p14.2	AD	Adult onset cranio-cervical dystonia	Anoctamin 3 (*ANO3*)
DYT 25	18p11	AD	Cranio-cervical dystonia	G protein subunit α_{olf} (*GNAL*)
*CIZ 1**	9q34.11	AD	Adult onset cervical dystonia	Cip-1-interacting zinc protein

AD, autosomal dominant; AR, autosomal recessive; EID, exercise-induced dystonia; NM, not mapped; PKD, paroxysmal kinesigenic dystonia; PNKD, paroxysmal non-kinesigenic dystonia; XR – X-linked recessive.

* Waiting for replication studies and/or not assigned a DYT.

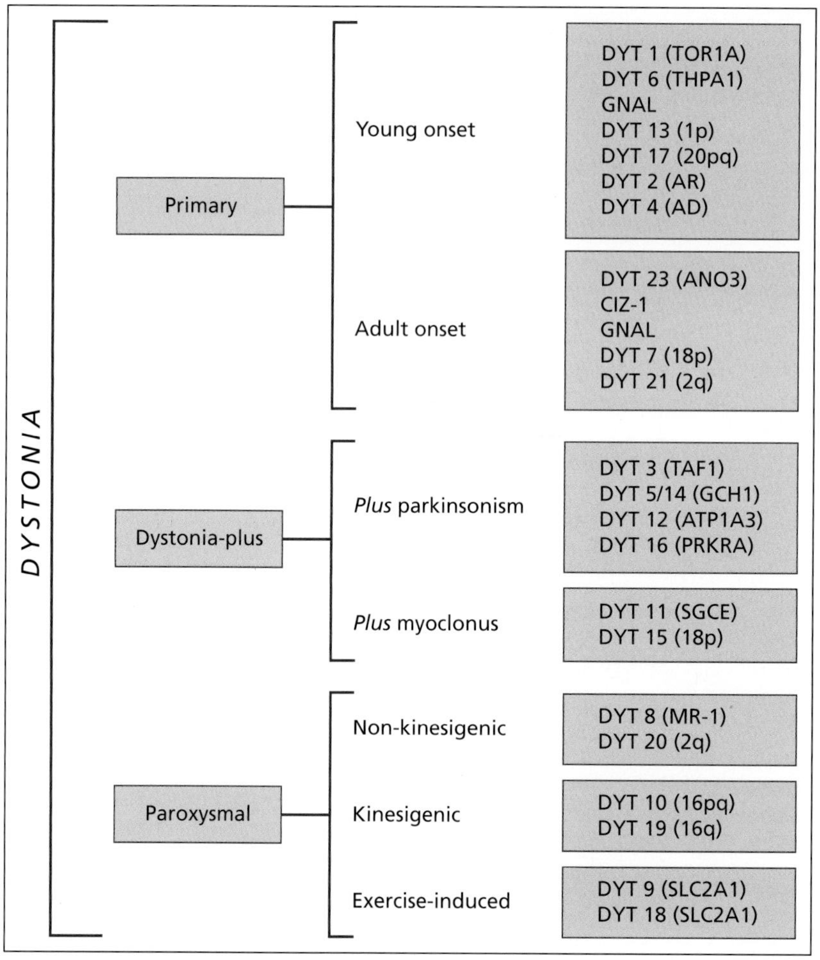

Figure 6.4 Clinico-genetic correlations in dystonia phenotypes.

have syndromic associations which can help guide the investigating clinician. For example, peripheral neuropathy in association with dystonia would make one think of neuro-acanthocytosis or metachromatic leukodystrophy as more likely diagnoses. Prominent facial dystonia or flapping tremor would make one consider Wilson's disease and associated ataxia can point to spino-cerebellar degenerations such as SCA2 or SCA3. Prominent bulbar or severe tongue involvement by dystonia is a strong pointer to secondary dystonia and would favour certain conditions including neurodegeneration with brain iron accumulation (NBIA; formerly known as Hallervorden–Spatz syndrome) and also neuro-acanthocytosis and Lesch–Nyhan syndrome. Appropriate investigation should be carried out. Brain MRI is very important as it may show characteristic changes; for example, the 'eye of the tiger sign' characteristic of NBIA caused by mutations of the pantothenate kinase 2 gene (*PANK2*) (Figure 6.5). A list of some of these conditions, with their associated clinical symptoms, is given in Table 6.7, and the investigations to be carried out as suggested by the syndromic association are given in Table 6.8.

Wilson's disease

Of all the causes of heredodegenerative dystonia, Wilson's disease (WD) is the most important because it is treatable, and fatal if left untreated. It is an autosomal recessive disorder of copper metabolism that most commonly presents in the first two decades of life. It occurs worldwide with prevalence of 1–3/100 000. More than 300 different mutations have been identified distributed across the responsible gene, *ATP7B* on chromosome 13, which encodes a copper-dependent transmembrane protein P type ATPase. The most common in patients of European origin is the H1069Q mutation. The heterozygote carrier rate is 1%.

Clinical presentations

Patients may present with acute liver failure, chronic hepatitis or cirrhosis, most commonly in the first decade of life, and a few present with an acute haemolytic anaemia. Other features include joint and bone abnormalities, azure lunulae of the finger nails, aminoaciduria and cardiomyopathy.

Most cases of neurological WD present with slurred speech and a movement disorder in adolescence, often in association with behavioural disturbances. Approximately half of all cases present with neuropsychiatric symptoms, usually between 14 and 20 years of age.

The 'pseudosclerotic' neurological variant is perhaps the most common, with the onset of a Holmes or wing-beating tremor and some ataxia and dysarthria; in other patients dystonia or an akinetic-rigid syndrome may dominate. Early gait abnormalities are frequent and a mixed movement disorder is common,

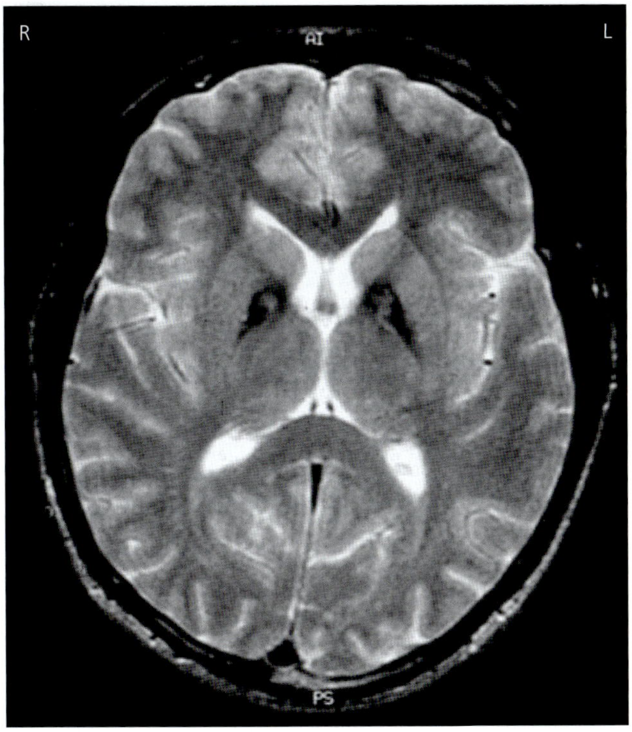

Figure 6.5 Classic 'eye of the tiger sign' (central hyperintensity with surrounding hypointensity in globus pallidus) in a patient with neurodegeneration with brain iron accumulation (NBIA) caused by a *PANK2* mutation (MRI T2W).

Table 6.7 Examples of common hereditary degenerative causes of dystonia and associated syndromic clinical features.

Wilson's disease	Kayser–Fleischer rings, ataxia, cognitive decline
Neurodegeneration with brain iron accumulation (*PANK2*, Hallervorden–Spatz syndrome)	Retinal degeneration, pyramidal signs, oromandibular/bulbar involvement
Neuro-acanthocytosis	Peripheral neuropathy, oromandibular dystonia, epilepsy
Metachromatic leukodystrophy	Peripheral neuropathy, frontal dementia
GM1/GM2 gangliosidosis	Cognitive decline
Glutaric acidaemia	Cognitive decline
Huntington's disease	Cognitive decline, personality change, depression, supranuclear eye movement abnormalities
Ataxia telangiectasia	Supranuclear eye movement abnormalities
Niemann–Pick type C	Vertical gaze palsy, cognitive decline

sometimes with associated risus sardonicus and pseudobulbar palsy. Dysarthria is the most common sign, whereas chorea and athetosis affect only about 10%. If left untreated, fronto-limbic cognitive dysfunction may develop and seizures, myoclonus and

Table 6.8 List of investigations in those suspected of secondary dystonia depending on syndromic associations in Table 6.7.

MRI brain/spine (structural lesions, leukodystrophies, 'eye of tiger' sign in NBIA)
Nerve conduction studies (neuro-acanthocytosis, metachromatic leukodystrophy)
Copper studies, slit-lamp, gene test, ?liver biopsy (Wilson's disease)
White cell enzymes (GM1, GM2, metachromatic leukodystrophy)
Alphafetoprotein, immunoglobulins (ataxia telangiectasia)
Lactate/pyruvate, mitochondrial mutations, muscle biopsy (mitochondrial disease)
Fresh thick blood smear for acanthocytes (neuro-acanthocytosis)
Plasma amino acids, urinary organic acids, aminoacids, oligosaccharides (glutaric academia, GM1, GM2)
Skin biopsy-fibroblast culture, bone marrow biopsy/axillary skin biopsy (Niemann–Pick type C, Kufs)
Phenylalanine loading test/CSF pterin assessments (DRD)
ERG, retinal examination, *PANK2* gene test (positive in some cases of NBIA)

DRD, dopa-responsive dystonia; ERG, electroretinogram; MRI, magnetic resonance imaging; NBIA, neurodegeneration with brain iron accumulation.

pyramidal signs have been reported. Cases presenting later than age 40 are exceptionally rare. Virtually every patient with WD presenting with neurological dysfunction has Kayser–Fleischer (K-F) rings on slit-lamp examination. These are caused by copper deposition on the inner surface of the cornea in Descemet's membrane and have a golden brown or greenish appearance. They can occur in other forms of chronic liver disease but in the context of a neurological presentation in adolescence can be considered pathognomonic for WD.

The histopathological findings in the brain include swollen glia and an increase in astrocytes within the grey matter, often with spongiform change.

Diagnosis

The emergence of parkinsonism, dystonia or a tremor in an adolescent or young adult with slurred speech should always raise the possibility of WD, particularly if there is a family history of hepatic, psychiatric or neurological disorder in childhood. Consanguinity should be enquired about. Suspected cases should be referred to an experienced ophthalmologist for slit-lamp examination.

The combination of a movement disorder with emotionalism, a risus sardonicus and a K-F ring makes the diagnosis highly likely but biochemical confirmation is required. Unfortunately, there is still no one single fail-safe test.

A low serum caeruloplasmin level is consistent with WD and is diagnostic when K-F rings are present. Low levels of caeruloplasmin also occur in hereditary acaeruloplasminaemia and Menkes' disease. Some WD heterozygotes have a reduced caeruloplasmin level, while a few WD patients with decompensated liver disease can have normal levels. In females, the oral contraceptive pill can raise an otherwise low level to within the normal range. In WD, a hepatic copper concentration greater than 250 μg/g dry weight is usual. Serum aminotransferase levels are also usually abnormal. However, a lower hepatic copper value does not absolutely exclude

WD and long-standing cholestasis can also cause high copper levels. The biochemical results therefore need to be taken in the context of the clinical picture and the histological changes. Although genetic testing is not available as a routine service test, in ambiguous cases it can be extremely helpful to at least screen for the more common mutations. Urinary copper, derived from the free non-caeruloplasmin-bound copper circulating in plasma, is elevated in WD. An excretion rate greater than 100 μg/24 hours (0.6 mmol/L in 24 hours) is considered diagnostic but levels above 40 μg/24 hours can be significant in a neurological presentation. Wide-necked bottles with copper-free disposable polyethylene liners are recommended. Urinary copper excretion after penicillamine loading can be a useful ancillary test.

In neurological cases, brain MRI can show high signal abnormalities on T2-weighted images and low intensity lesions on T1 in the putamen, globus pallidus, thalamus, midbrain, pons and cerebellum. White matter abnormalities are also common and cortical atrophic changes also occur. Proton density MRI sequences can be particularly sensitive. Once WD has been diagnosed, screening of all first degree relatives is essential.

Treatment

The first chelation treatment, parenterally administered British anti-Lewisite (BAL), was introduced in 1951. In 1956, John Walshe first reported clinical benefit with penicillamine and half a century of use has confirmed its efficacy in most cases. However, some patients cannot tolerate the drug and about 20% of patients with neurological presentations can deteriorate markedly on its introduction. Regular monitoring with a full blood count and renal function tests is recommended. Adverse events include fever, rash, lymph gland enlargement, neutropenia, thrombocytopenia and proteinuria. Nephrotoxicity, a lupus syndrome, bone marrow suppression, skin changes including elastosis perforans serpiginosa and a myaesthenic syndrome are late complications. Children and pregnant women should be given weekly pyridoxine.

In 1969, Walshe discovered another chelator, trientene, which has proved to be a well-tolerated alternative. It is still generally used as a second line drug, but some now recommend it as the initial treatment of choice in neurological cases, although deterioration can also occur on starting treatment. Pancytopenia has been reported and sideroblastic anaemia may occur if copper deficiency develops.

Oral elemental zinc, which induces intestinal metallothionein which binds copper within the enterocyte, has also been recommended, particularly for asymptomatic and presymptomatic patients and as maintenance therapy after a period of initial chelation.

Tetrathiomolybdate forms a complex with copper and protein and prevents copper absorption when given with food, and has been claimed to be highly effective, but remains investigational. Whichever drug is chosen, regular lifelong monitoring to ensure compliance is essential.

Chocolate, liver, nuts, mushrooms and shellfish contain high levels of copper, so are best avoided. Anticholinergics may modestly help dystonia and some patients with an akinetic-rigid syndrome may have some improvement with levodopa. In patients with hepatic disease who deteriorate despite optimum therapy, liver transplantation, which corrects the underlying pathophysiology, can be life-saving. For refractory or deteriorating neurological disability despite other treatments, a course of intramuscular BAL injections is worth trying. The use of liver transplantation for patients with progressive neurological impairment despite adequate chelation is controversial. Patients with WD surviving into middle age have an elevated risk of hepatic carcinoma.

Paroxysmal dyskinesias

Paroxysmal dyskinesias are defined as intermittent attacks of involuntary movements, usually dystonia, chorea or ballism, with normal neurological examination between attacks. Episodes are induced by trigger factors including sudden movements (paroxysmal kinesigenic dyskinesia; PKD), prolonged exercise (paroxysmal exercise-induced dyskinesia; PED) or alcohol and coffee (paroxysmal non-kinesigenic dyskinesia; PNKD) or sleep (paroxysmal nocturnal dyskinesia; PND). The duration can be seconds to hours. Recently, genetic mutations for all three forms of the primary paroxysmal dyskinesias have been identified. PRRT2 gene mutations underlie the majority of sporadic and familial PKD cases. Mutations of the myofibrillogenesis regulator gene (*MR-1*) on chromosome 2q33-35 have been identified in patients with PNKD. The encoded protein appears to have a role in the detoxification pathway of methylglyoxal, a compound present in coffee and alcoholic beverages, both of which can induce attacks. About 40% of PED cases are caused by mutations of the glucose transporter 1 gene (Glut1). In PND, nicotinic acetylcholine receptor gene mutations occur and this is an example of a ligand-gated channelopathy. For the other forms, various loci have been proposed but genes have not yet been identified. Secondary paroxysmal dyskinesias have also been described and possible causes include demyelination, vasculopathy, infectious disease (HIV, cytomegalovirus), cerebral and peripheral trauma, neurodegenerative disease, hormonal and metabolic dysfunction, neoplasm and cerebral palsy. Anticonvulsants (first choice carbamazepine in PKD), benzodiazepines, barbiturates or acetazolamide can bring relief. PED related to Glut1 gene mutations can benefit by changing to a ketone diet or modified Adkins diet. Triggering factors should be avoided.

Investigation of dystonia

Following a careful history (in particular, drug and family history) and examination, investigation of patients with dystonia should be tailored to the presentation of the patient, and in particular whether the clinical picture suggests primary or secondary dystonia. Common clinical situations are of children or adolescents presenting with a primary focal, segmental or generalised dystonia, or adults presenting with a primary focal or segmental dystonia. For the former category, investigations should include copper studies and slit-lamp to exclude WD, brain imaging (preferably MRI), the *DYT1* or another gene test as appropriate and an adequate trial of levodopa. For adult onset primary dystonia, copper studies and slit-lamp to exclude WD should be performed if presentation is under 50 years of age; brain imaging is not generally required, but if there is fixed or painful cervical dystonia an MRI of the spine should be carried out to exclude structural lesions. More extensive investigations are needed in patients with presumed secondary dystonias (Table 6.5) but this list can be narrowed down by considering pertinent aetiological possibilities according to the presence of associated clinical features as shown in Table 6.7, and an outline of the investigations is given in Table 6.8.

Treatment of dystonia

Drug treatment of dystonia is most appropriate in those with younger onset generalised and/or segmental dystonia for whom botulinum toxin (see later) would be unlikely to control the full extent of the dystonia. First line treatment is with anticholinergics such as trihexyphenidyl. Slow introduction of the drug is very important to avoid side effects, but some, particularly younger, patients can ultimately tolerate very high doses (100 mg/day or more) with good effect. Clonazepam can be useful for the treatment of tremor, jerks and pain associated with dystonia. Other drugs that are sometimes useful include tetrabenazine, baclofen and even dopamine receptor blocking drugs. As mentioned above, all patients with young onset dystonia should receive an adequate trial of levodopa. The treatment of WD has been detailed above.

Botulinum toxin has revolutionised the treatment of patients with focal dystonia. Botulinum toxin cleaves specific proteins involved in vesicular fusion at the presynaptic terminal, thereby blocking the release of acetylcholine, the principal neurotransmitter at the neuromuscular junction. The affected nerve terminals do not degenerate, but the blockage of acetylcholine release is irreversible. Neuromuscular transmitter release recovers by sprouting of new nerve terminals and formation of new synaptic contacts, which takes about 3 months. Transmission is also inhibited at gamma neurones in muscle spindles, which can alter reflex overactivity.

A number of randomised double-blind clinical trials have established the efficacy of botulinum toxin injection treatment for focal dystonia. Treatment is required every 3–4 months, and is expensive, but a 70–80% improvement in symptoms is common in most patients, particularly those with blepharospasm and cervical dystonia. Treatment of those with limb dystonia, in particular writer's cramp, is often more difficult and benefit can be inconsistent. Main side effects of treatment are excessive weakness of the treated muscle or spread of effect to nearby muscles (e.g. paralysis of pharyngeal muscles following sternomastoid injections). Immune-mediated resistance to botulinum toxin is seen in a small proportion of chronically treated patients, particularly those who receive high doses, 'top-up' doses or injections more frequently than every 12 weeks. An alternative toxin, botulinum toxin type B, is available, but antibodies to the commonly used type A toxin can be cross-reactive with type B toxin, and, in addition, a primary immune response to type B toxin can also occur. Botulinum toxin can be helpful for those with generalised dystonia where a particular functional problem can be linked to dystonia in a single or a small group of muscles.

Surgery for dystonia

Although the primary treatment for dystonia is medical, a number of patients, particularly those with generalised dystonia, remain severely disabled and can benefit from surgery. Ventrolateral thalamotomies, and to a lesser degree pallidotomies, were performed from the 1950s for alleviation of dystonia. The results were not consistent and some patients had initial benefit that wore off over time, necessitating several operations. Complications, including dysarthria and dysphagia, were not uncommon, especially in bilaterally operated patients.

Concerns about potential side effects of bilateral lesions, and the beneficial effect of globus pallidus internus (GPi) DBS on dyskinesias in PD patients, led the group of Coubes in France to propose the use of GPi DBS in dystonia. Their early report of successful treatment has been confirmed in larger series of patients and multicentre controlled trials.

Primary generalised dystonia is recognised as being the indication giving the best results and both *DYT1* positive and negative patients can obtain a good effect – up to 70% improvement of the clinical score has been reported. The improvement is gradual and follows a complex time course; the mobile aspects of the dystonia tend to improve more rapidly than the fixed aspects that can take up to 6 months. In consequence it is difficult to adjust stimulation parameters according to acute changes of symptoms. The outcome in those with focal dystonia such as cervical dystonia or writing dystonia is mixed although tremor and jerks associated with cervical dystonia can respond quite well.

Beneficial effect on quality of life has also been reported, while there was little change on cognitive scores and neuropsychiatric measures, in particular on depression. The presence of fixed orthopaedic deformities limits the potential beneficial effect of DBS. Sudden interruption of the stimulation can lead to severe dystonic state in these patients, who may need urgent or prophylactic battery replacement.

Myoclonus dystonia (*DYT11*) can also benefit from GPi DBS. Some forms of secondary dystonia may benefit, but usually not to the same extent as primary dystonia. Neuroleptic-induced tardive dystonia may show major benefit with GPi DBS and some forms of heredodegenerative dystonias such as PANK2-related brain iron accumulation disorders, neuracanthocytosis and others may have some benefit for a limited period of time. In Lubag-related status dystonicus pallidal DBS may be life-saving.

The surgical procedure is similar to that used for PD and is usually carried out in one session under general anaesthesia. Side effects are rare and usually reversible by adjustment of electrical parameters.

Chorea

Chorea is derived from the Greek word *choreia* meaning a dance. Chorea is a state of excessive spontaneous movements, irregularly timed, randomly distributed and abrupt. Severity can range from restlessness with mild intermittent exaggeration of gesture and expression, fidgety movements of the hands or unstable dance-like gait to a continuous flow of disabling and violent movements. Chorea has many causes which can be simply divided into acquired and inherited. This section summarises the assessment and investigation of the choreic patient and focuses on the important causes of chorea seen in clinical neurological practice (Table 6.9).

Assessment of chorea

Assessment of the choreic patient depends on directed history and examination (Figure 6.6; Table 6.10), which will determine the appropriate investigations to consider (Table 6.11). Onset and nature of progression are important features. Abrupt or subacute onset is more suggestive of acquired causes. It is important to take a detailed drug history, to ask about recent throat infections (Sydenham's chorea or PANDAS), pregnancy (chorea gravidarum), rashes or joint aches (systemic lupus erythematosus; SLE), and metabolic history (hyperthyroidism), and to note the symmetry of the chorea, as asymmetric onset suggests a structural or vascular lesion in the contralateral basal ganglia (Figure 6.7). Most inherited causes of chorea have a slow and insidious onset, most commonly noticed by friends or relatives rather than patients themselves. A detailed family history is crucial and particular attention should be paid to a parent who died at a relatively young age.

Huntington's disease

Huntington's disease (HD) is a slowly progressive autosomal dominant neurodegenerative disorder and the most important inherited cause of chorea. Onset is usually in adult life with a mean age of about 40 years, although juvenile and elderly onset are well described.

Table 6.9 Inherited and acquired causes of chorea.

Inherited causes	Acquired causes
Huntington's disease*	Focal striatal pathology:
	Stroke
Neuro-acanthocytosis	Hyperglycaemia
McLeod syndrome	Space-occupying lesions
Dentatorubro-pallidoluysian atrophy	Drug-induced
	Chorea gravidarum
	Thyrotoxicosis
Benign hereditary chorea	Systemic lupus erythematosus/ antiphospholipid syndrome
Spinocerebellar ataxia types 1, 2, 3 and 17	Post-infective:
Mitochondrial disorders	Sydenham's chorea (group A streptococcal infection)
Inherited prion disease	Paediatric autoimmune disorders associated with streptococcal infections (PANDAS)
Huntington's disease-like 2	
Wilson's disease	Herpes simplex encephalitis
Friedreich's ataxia	Polycythaemia rubra vera
	Infective:
Neurodegeneration with brain iron accumulation type 1	AIDS
Ataxia telangiectasia	New variant Creutzfeldt–Jakob disease
Neuroferritinopathy	
Lysosomal storage disorders	
Amino acid disorders	
Tuberous sclerosis	

* The most common cause of inherited chorea – the remainder of these disorders are rare.

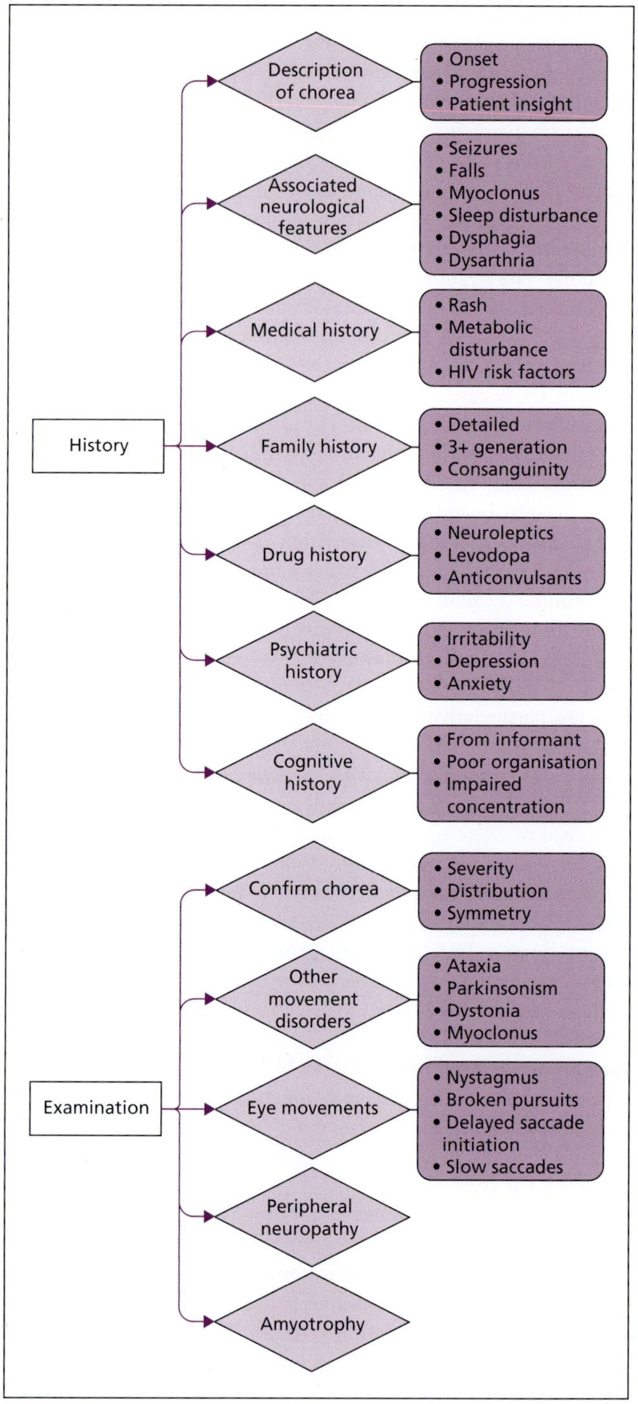

Figure 6.6 Clinical assessment of the choreic patient.

It progresses inexorably, with death occurring 15–20 years from onset. Prevalence is 4–10/100 000 in populations of Western European descent, but HD has been described throughout the world. HD is named after George Huntington who originally described it in 1872. In 1993, the causative gene defect was identified as a CAG repeat expansion, encoding polyglutamine repeats within a novel protein huntingtin. This highly polymorphic CAG repeat is located in exon 1 and ranges between 10 and 28 copies on normal chromosomes, but is expanded to a range of 36–121 on HD chromosomes. Adult onset patients usually have 40–55 repeats, with juvenile onset patients having over 60. CAG repeats above 40 are fully penetrant, although there is a borderline repeat range between 36 and 39 repeats with reduced penetrance.

CAG repeat lengths vary from generation to generation, with both expansion and contraction, but there is a tendency for repeat lengths to increase, particularly when transmitted through the paternal lineage. The instability of the CAG expansion with the tendency to expand during transmission underlies the phenomenon of anticipation. Genetic anticipation describes increasing severity and earlier onset of an inherited disease during intergenerational transmission and is a hallmark of HD and the other trinucleotide repeat disorders. CAG repeat instability during paternal transmission is important in the development of large expansions associated with juvenile HD; approximately 80% of juvenile HD patients inherit the HD gene from their father. There is a correlation between CAG repeat size and age at onset, such that the larger the repeat, the earlier the onset. Most individuals with more than 50 repeats develop the disease before the age of 30 years. CAG repeat number

Table 6.10 Neurological examination findings in the choreic patient.

	Peripheral neuropathy	Cerebellar signs	Amyotrophy	Oculomotor dysfunction	Motor impersis-tence	Tics/ vocal-isations	Parkin-sonism	Dystonia	Myoclonus	Orolingual dystonia	Psychiatric disorders
Huntington's disease				•	•	•	•*	•*	•*		•
Neuro-acanthocytosis	•	•	•			•				•	•
McLeod syndrome	•	•	•			•					•
Friedreich's ataxia	•	•									
Mitochondrial disease	•	•		•				•	•		
Ataxia telangiectasia	•	•		•							
Spinocerebellar ataxias	•†	•		•							•‡
DRPLA		•									
Prion disease		•							•		
Wilson's disease				•		•	•	•			•
NBIA							•	•			
HDL2						•		•	•		•

DRPLA, dentatorubro-pallidoluysian atrophy; NBIA, neurodegeneration with brain iron accumulation.
* Juvenile and Westphal variants of Huntington's disease.
† Typically SCA2.
‡ Typically SCA17.

also appears to govern the development rate of neuropathological changes. However, CAG repeat length does not completely explain variations in age of onset, clinical phenotype or rate of clinical progression, so that other modifying genes obviously have an important role.

Neuropathologically, in the early stages of disease, the brain can look macroscopically normal, but later there is marked cortical atrophy with ventricular dilatation, severe atrophy of the caudate more than the putamen, with atrophy of the internal segment of the globus pallidus and substantia nigra pars reticulata.

Clinical features

HD can produce a varied clinical phenotype. It is important to realise that as the disease progresses, the signs and symptoms change, so disease duration can markedly modify the clinical presentation.

Motor features The onset of HD is often difficult to discern clearly. Many patients report psychiatric problems or mild cognitive symptoms before developing any motor problems. However, the definitive diagnosis of HD is usually made when motor abnormalities are noted on examination. Subtle motor abnormalities seen early in the disease include general restlessness, abnormal eye movements, hyper-reflexia, impaired finger tapping, and fidgety movements of fingers, hands and toes during stress or when walking. Oculomotor abnormalities are a cardinal feature of the disease, and often the earliest motor sign. Saccadic abnormalities are characteristic and include gaze impersistence and distractibility and delayed initiation or slowing of voluntary saccades (vertical worse than horizontal).

As the disease progresses, more obvious extrapyramidal signs develop; chorea is seen in 90% of adult onset patients but can decrease in the late stages, whereas dystonia, rigidity and parkinsonism may dominate the clinical picture in late disease. A key motor abnormality in HD is impaired voluntary motor function with clumsiness, motor impersistence and disturbances in fine motor control and motor speed. Gait disturbance is common, with impaired postural reflexes making patients more prone to falling. Dysarthria and dysphagia are common and should be asked about.

Table 6.11 Investigations to consider in the choreic patient.

Test	Notes
MRI imaging	Stroke or other focal basal ganglia pathology T2* imaging abnormal in iron accumulation disorders T1 basal ganglia hyperintensities in hyperglycaemia FLAIR imaging abnormal in prion disease Deep brain T2 hyperintensities in Wilson's disease
Full blood count	Haematocrit can be elevated in PRV
Red cell mass	Sensitive test required for diagnosis of PRV
Blood film	3 × fresh thick blood films necessary to exclude neuro-acanthocytosis
Erythrocyte membrane chorein levels (western blot)	Neuro-acanthocytosis
Serum caeruloplasmin	Reduced in Wilson's disease
Urinary copper level	Elevated in Wilson's disease
Liver biopsy	Sometimes required to diagnose Wilson's disease
Pregnancy test	Chorea gravidarum in first trimester
HIV test	(Hemi) chorea/ballism can be presenting feature of AIDS
Erythrocyte sedimentation rate and antinuclear antibody	Sensitive tests to reveal SLE
Anti-dsDNA	Relatively specific to SLE
Anticardiolipin and lupus anticoagulant	Antiphospholipid syndrome is risk factor for chorea
Thyroid function tests	Thyrotoxicosis
Antistreptolysin O (ASO) titre	Recent streptococcal infection suggests Sydenham's chorea/PANDAS
Antibasal ganglia antibodies	Associated with post-infective chorea, chorea gravidarum and OCP-induced chorea
Muscle biopsy	Ragged red fibres or respiratory chain abnormalities in mitochondrial disease
Cerebrospinal fluid analysis	Can reveal inflammatory/neoplastic causes

MRI, magnetic resonance imaging; OCP, oral contraceptive pill; PANDAS, paediatric autoimmune disorders associated with streptococcal infection; PRV, polycythaemia rubra vera; SLE, systemic lupus erythematosus.

Cognitive features Cognitive abnormalities are variable but universal in HD. The key cognitive abnormalities seen are impaired executive function with poor planning and judgement, impulsive behaviour, disorganised actions and difficulty coping with multiple tasks. Many patients exhibit psychomotor slowing with apathy, lack of self-care and loss of initiative which can make caring for them difficult. Patients often complain early on of visual and verbal memory problems, in addition to poor concentration and attention.

Psychiatric features The combination of psychiatric and cognitive features causes the greatest disability, functional decline and distress to relatives and HD patients. Psychiatric symptoms are common, particularly depression and anxiety. Irritability is also very common and some patients become aggressive. As the disease progresses, obsessions and compulsions often make life difficult for carers. Psychosis, despite being well-recognised, is relatively rare. The suicide rate in HD is much higher than in the general population. Psychiatric symptoms often cause great

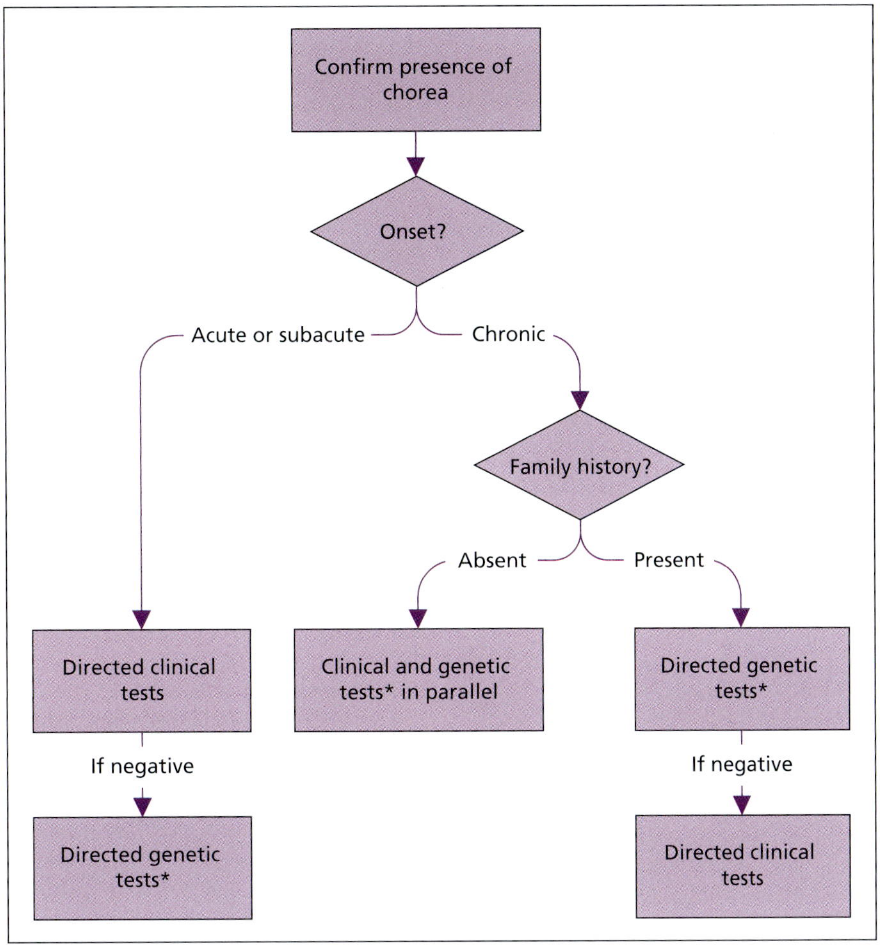

Figure 6.7 Approach to the investigation of the choreic patient. *Genetic testing must always be preceded by detailed expert genetic counselling.

distress to patients and relatives and should be actively managed with the same drugs used in standard psychiatric practice.

Juvenile Huntington's disease

Juvenile HD cases are defined as onset before age 20 years, usually associated with repeat lengths greater than 60. They have more severe disease and shorter life expectancy. The akinetic-rigid form of the disease (Westphal variant) is more common in juvenile HD: patients typically have little chorea and are predominantly rigid and dystonic. Juvenile HD patients also have a higher incidence of seizures and myoclonus than adult onset patients. Younger adult-onset patients with HD (<40 years) can also present with a predominantly parkinsonian phenotype similar to the juvenile HD cases.

Differential diagnosis of Huntington's disease

Huntington's disease phenocopies Before the advent of genetic testing for HD, diagnosis was based on clinical evaluation and neuropathological examination. Now, genetic diagnosis allows definitive confirmation of the disease. Genotype–phenotype studies have increased our understanding of disorders that can present like HD (HD phenocopies) with similar cognitive, psychiatric and motor features, but are HD gene negative (Table 6.12). HD phenocopies occur in approximately 1% of large genetic screens of individuals with clinical signs of HD. An approach to genetic testing of HD phenocopies is suggested in Figure 6.8.

HDL2 (HD-like 2) is caused by a CAG/CTG expansion in the *Junctophilin-3* gene and is very rare, and moreover only reported so far in individuals with African ancestry. In one consanguineous family, a phenocopy syndrome (HDL3) was mapped to 4p16.3, but no causative mutation has been identified. Other dominantly inherited diseases mimicking HD are dentatorubro-pallidoluysian atrophy (DRPLA), another polyglutamine disorder caused by a CAG repeat expansion in the atrophin-1 gene, and spinocerebellar (SCA) 17 – also called HDL4 – caused by a CAG repeat expansion in the TATA-binding gene (*TBP*). SCA1 and SCA3 (Chapter 17) may also mimic HD. Inherited prion disease can cause HD phenocopies: one mutation causes HDL1, an early onset prion disease with prominent psychiatric features. Recently, *C9ORF72* mutation, which is known to cause frontotemporal dementia, was also found to be an important cause of HD phenocopy. Neuroferritinopathy, a very rare, dominantly inherited disorder, caused by mutations in the ferritin light chain, has clinical features overlapping with HD.

Neuro-acanthocytosis

There are several conditions (the neuro-acanthocytoses) in which chorea and other movement disorders are associated with the presence of acanthocytosis of the red blood cells in the peripheral blood.

Table 6.12 Differential diagnosis of Huntington's disease (HD phenocopies).

Condition	Cause
HDL1	Octapeptide repeat insertion in gene encoding prion protein
HDL2	Triplet repeat expansion in gene encoding junctophilin-3
Frontotemporal dementia	Mutations of the C90rf72 gene
SCA17 (HDL4)	Triplet repeat expansion in gene encoding TATA-box binding protein
Inherited prion disease	Mutations in gene encoding prion protein
SCA1	Triplet repeat expansion in gene encoding ataxin-1
SCA3	Triplet repeat expansion in gene encoding ataxin-3
DRPLA	Triplet repeat expansion in gene encoding atrophin-1
Neuro-acanthocytosis	Mutation in gene encoding chorein
Neuroferritinopathy	Mutations in gene encoding ferritin light-chain
NBIA	Mutations in the *PANK2* gene

DRPLA, dentatorubro-pallidoluysian atrophy; NBIA, neurodegeneration with brain iron accumulation.

Autosomal recessive neuro-acanthocytosis is rare, and associated with mutations in the *CHAC* gene leading to production of a truncated protein termed chorein. Onset is typically in the fourth decade with a progressive movement disorder, psychiatric and cognitive changes which mimic HD. The movement disorder comprises chorea, dystonia and tics, with prominent eating dystonia, dystonic tongue protrusion and tongue and lip biting and also sudden head/trunk flexion or extension drops. Psychiatric and cognitive features are similar to HD. Unlike HD, seizures are seen in 50% of patients, and there is commonly a distal amyotrophy or axonal neuropathy with a high creatine kinase. Investigations include analysis of fresh blood films for >3% of acanthocytes. More than one blood film may be necessary to identify these. Genetic testing for mutations in the *CHAC* gene is difficult, so confirmation relies on demonstration of low erythrocyte membrane chorein levels in the blood. McLeod syndrome is a very rare X-linked recessive disorder linked to mutations in the *XK* gene, which encodes the Kell antigen. It usually begins around the age of 45 years and is slowly progressive, with limb chorea and facial tics. Dystonia is less common than in chorea-acanthocytosis and subcortical dementia and psychiatric features tend to occur later in the disease. Axonal neuropathy, cardiomyopathy and haemolytic anaemia can be seen, CPK is often elevated, and acanthocytes are usually found in fresh thick peripheral blood films.

Acanthocytes have also been described in pantothenate kinase-associated neurodegeneration (PKAN, or NBIA type 1) and HDL2 and all these disorders are encompassed under 'core neuro-acanthocytosis syndromes'.

Post-streptococcal autoimmune disorders

Sydenham's chorea and PANDAS (paediatric autoimmune disorders associated with streptococcal infection) can both present with chorea and neuropsychiatric manifestations. Sydenham's chorea is one of the major manifestations of rheumatic fever. It occurs in children, mainly girls, between 5 and 15 years of age and is now rare in the developed world. Widespread chorea, behavioural disturbance and obsessive-compulsive symptoms are common. It is self-limiting and usually resolves within 6 months, with about 20% of cases being

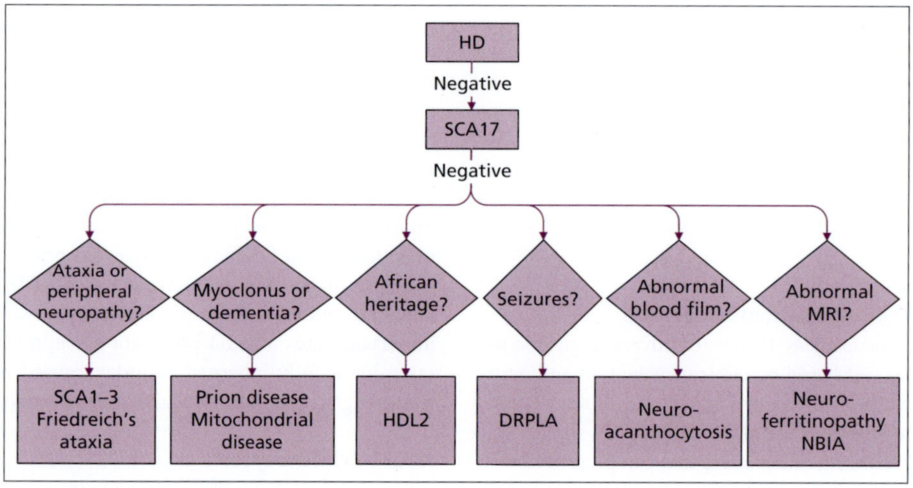

Figure 6.8 Suggested approach to genetic testing in chorea.

recurrent. Antibasal ganglia antibodies can be detected. The mechanism of damage is thought to be molecular mimicry with cross-reaction between anti-streptococcal antibodies and neurones in the basal ganglia. PANDAS is also discussed under tics.

Benign hereditary chorea

Benign hereditary chorea (BHC) is a very rare, dominantly inherited disorder caused by mutations in the gene encoding thyroid transcription factor 1 (*TITF1*). It is usually of early onset and is characterised by very slowly progressive chorea without cognitive decline or other neurological features, but there is clinical heterogeneity within and between families. Some cases of BHC also display dystonia, myoclonic jerks, mild dysarthria, gait disturbances or low–average intelligence, and many cases can also have hypothyroidism or pulmonary abnormalities of varying degrees, leading to the recent application of the term 'brain–thyroid–lung syndrome'. Some cases of BHC are caused by mutations in another gene, *ADCY5,* encoding adenyl cyclase 5.

Drug-induced chorea

Many different medications can cause chorea. The main ones include neuroleptics (tardive dyskinesia), levodopa/dopamine agonists/anticholinergics (most often, but not exclusively, in patients being treated for parkinsonism), anticonvulsants (phenytoin, carbamazepine, valproate, gabapentin), CNS stimulants (amphetamines, methylphenidate, cocaine), benzodiazepines, oestrogens (oral contraceptive pill or, rarely, hormone replacement therapy) and lithium (although this more commonly causes myoclonus or jerky tremor).

Drug management of chorea

Chorea can cause cosmetic embarrassment to some patients but many do not notice the severity of their chorea. Indeed, it is often relatives, rather than patients, who request treatment. Best agreed practice is to use antichoreic medication sparingly as no drug is particularly efficacious, and a balance has to be struck between benefits and side effects. For functionally disabling chorea, drugs such as sulpiride, olanzapine, risperidone and tetrabenazine can be useful by non-specifically damping down movements in general, but they can worsen speech, swallowing and gait and balance, so need careful monitoring.

Tics

Tics are typically relatively brief rapid intermittent stereotyped involuntary movements (motor tics) or sounds (vocalisations). In a sense tics are caricatures of normal movements; the common motor tics being eye blinking, elevation of a shoulder, a facial grimace, and vocal being a sniff or grunt which are all part of our repertoire of normal movements or sounds. Classically, they can be suppressed, at least temporarily, by an effort of will, but at the expense of rising inner tension, often followed by a rebound exacerbation. Most tics are abrupt in onset and duration (clonic tics), but can also be slow and sustained, either dystonic (associated with more sustained muscle contractions) or tonic (if muscle contractions are not associated with any movement, e.g. arm or abdominal tensing).

Gilles de la Tourette syndrome

Gilles de la Tourette syndrome (GTS) is a common and widely recognised variety of tic. The diagnostic criteria for GTS include multiple motor tics and one or more phonic and/or vocal tics, which must last longer than a year. The motor and phonic tics do not necessarily occur together, characteristically wax and wane over time, occur in bouts and are suggestible and suppressible. The maximum age at onset is 18 years. The mean age at onset of motor tics is about 7 years, and vocal tics 11 years, The worst severity is at 10–12 years, and the majority of symptoms disappear in half of the patients by the age of 18 years. Associated behaviours such as obsessive-compulsive behaviour or obsessive–compulsive disorder (OCB/OCD) can be more evident later.

Tics in GTS can be simple (e.g. blinking, eye rolling, head nodding, facial grimacing) or complex (e.g. touching, squatting). Premonitory sensations (also referred to as premonitory urges, mental urges or inner tension) precede both motor and phonic tics in up to 80% of patients; these can be localised (burning feeling in the eye before an eye-blink, or a sensation similar to nasal stuffiness before a sniff – the sensation has been likened to that which occurs before a sneeze). They can be localised (around the area of the tic) or generalised (covering a wide area of the body). New tics appear in response to a new somatosensory sensation, such as a cough (phonic tic) persisting after an upper respiratory tract infection. Tics usually begin in the head and face, and blinking is one of the most common first tics. Simple phonic tics include sniffing, throat clearing, gulping, snorting and coughing. Complex vocal tics include barking, the making of animal noises, inappropriate voice intonations and uttering strings of words. Tics characteristically are suggestible, suppressible, there is rebound after suppression and they have a waxing and waning course. Other important and characteristic features of GTS include echolalia (copying what other people say), echopraxia (copying what other people do) and palilalia (repeating the last word or part of sentence said by the individual). Coprolalia (inappropriate involuntary swearing, often disguised by the patient) is uncommon, occurring in only 10–15%, starting at around 15 years. Many clinicians are under the misapprehension that coprolalia must be present in order to make the diagnosis. Instead of the whole swearword, many individuals say only parts of the word and disguise it (by coughing, saying something, covering their mouths). Copropraxia (e.g. the V sign) also occurs but is rare.

Epidemiology, history and prevalence

GTS has been described worldwide but with apparent different prevalence rates. The male : female ratio is 3 : 1. Clinical characteristics are similar irrespective of the country of origin. In some instances it seems that within families, the affected males have tic symptoms, whereas the females often have OCB. GTS was once considered to be uncommon. However, studies report a prevalence of 0.4–3.8% for youngsters aged 5–18 years, and a figure of 1% worldwide overall prevalence has been calculated. The prevalence of GTS in individuals with learning difficulties or autistic spectrum disorders can be as high as 6–10%. It is important to note that GTS individuals identified in community settings have more behavioural, mental health and educational difficulties than their peers. Many people with GTS never come to medical attention. Among those who do, the correct diagnosis is often missed as many clinicians remain under the misapprehension that coprolalia is necessary for the diagnosis.

Psychopathology and associated co-morbidity

About 90% of GTS individuals have psychiatric co-morbidity. The most common is attention deficit hyperactivity disorder (ADHD), followed by OCB and OCD. Checking rituals, 'evening up', counting rituals and compulsions to touch objects or people may be present, but are not often volunteered and need to be asked about. Anger control problems, sleep difficulties, coprolalia and self-injurious behaviours are more common in those with co-morbidity. Patients with GTS have more depression, anxiety, hostility, obsessional symptomatology and personality disorders than controls.

Assessment

GTS is a clinical diagnosis. Standardised schedules are available to describe the phenomenology, and quantify and qualify associated behaviours and psychopathology, and to monitor response to treatment. Investigations are usually not necessary, but may be helpful in diagnosing alternative causes of tics (see later).

Current aetiological theories

Various causes have been postulated including genetic influences, neuro-immunological reactions to infections, and prenatal and peri-natal difficulties. Complex segregation analysis suggested that GTS was genetic, consistent with a single major gene and autosomal dominant transmission, but with incomplete penetrance. However, much of the genome has been excluded, so the genetics of GTS is much more complicated than previously thought. The term PANDAS (paediatric autoimmune neuropsychiatric disorders associated with streptococcal infections) was coined for children with post-streptococcal OCD and tics. This pathogenic mechanism is somewhat controversial but most centres that have sought them have also found anti-basal ganglia antibodies (ABGAs) in a subgroup of patients with GTS. Streptococcal infection (with group A beta-haemolytic strains) probably does not cause GTS, but individuals can inherit a susceptibility to GTS and to the way they react to some infections.

Multiple phenotypes of GTS

Some clinicians prefer not to make a diagnosis of GTS when the patient presents with only simple motor and phonic tics, when they simply call it a 'tic disorder'. However, several recent studies have demonstrated by hierarchical cluster analysis or principal component factor analysis that there is more than one type of GTS. Moreover one factor (phenotype), replicated by several centres, consists almost solely of simple motor and phonic tics. Other factors include complex tics and associated psychopathologies, as well as aggressivity and self-injurious behaviour. There have been initial suggestions that the varying phenotypes can have different aetiologies.

Other forms of tic disorder

Tic disorders, usually referring to motor tics, are much more common than GTS, although prevalence figures differ, depending on the population studied. They have been reported to occur with a point prevalence of 1–29% of young people. The most common tic disorders can be divided into the following:

1 Transient tic disorder (TTD), in which there are single or multiple motor and vocal tics occurring for at least a month but for no longer than a year
2 Chronic motor or vocal tic disorder (CMTD), in which motor or vocal but not both have been present in excess of a year, or
3 Tic disorder not otherwise specified, such as adult onset tic disorder with an age at onset after 18 years.

Once again, tics are more frequent in those individuals with behavioural difficulties, learning difficulties, and those requiring special education placement or those seen as 'problem children'.

Other diseases that can cause tics

Tics can also be seen in WD, neuro-acanthocytosis, Lesch–Nyhan syndrome, neuroferritinopathy, autism spectrum disorders, and in association with acquired lesions of the caudate nucleus and after chronic neuroleptic drug intake. However, they are usually only a part of the clinical picture, so should not be confused with primary tic disorder. Not all vocalisations are tics – they can be seen in dystonia, HD and tardive dyskinesia, for example.

Investigation of tics

In the typical case (the vast majority) no investigations are necessary. If the presentation is unusual, the following could be helpful: serum copper and coeruloplasmin and slit-lamp examination for WD; ASO titre, throat swab, anti-DNA antibodies and ABGAs for post-streptococcal tics; fresh thick blood films (×3), creatine phosphokinase, nerve conduction studies, MRI, chorein and ChAc gene testing for neuro-acanthocytosis.

Management of GTS and tics

In mild cases, explanation, reassurance and psycho-education may be the only interventions required. When the condition is causing problems, supportive psychotherapy, cognitive–behavioural therapy (CBT) and habit reversal training (HRT) may be useful: HRT specifically targets tics. Ideally, management should be multidisciplinary and treatment should be targeted at symptoms.

In many patients, medication may be required for the treatment of the tics and psychopathologies. The main agents for the tics are the typical and atypical neuroleptics, given in small doses (relative to treating psychosis), for example haloperidol 0.5–3 mg/day or sulpiride 100–400 mg/day. The older 'typical' neuroleptics such as haloperidol, pimozide, sulpiride and tiapride, and the newer 'atypical' neuroleptic such as risperidone have all been shown to be superior to placebo in double-blind trials. Tetrabenazine can also be effective but can often cause depression. Clonidine or guanfacine can help tics, impulse control or ADHD. If these agents are used, baseline ECG is advisable, as is regular monitoring of pulse and blood pressure. Recently, the newer 'atypical' neuroleptics (risperidone, quetiapine, aripiprazole) as well as sulpiride and tiapride have become more popular because of the unacceptable side effects of the older agents. The response to medication in GTS patients is idiosyncratic. Importantly, individuals with this often life-long, generally benign, condition should be warned of the possibility of developing a superimposed tardive movement disorder after chronic treatment with neuroleptic drugs.

Antidepressants, especially SSRIs, are useful for depression (using the standard dose, e.g. 20 mg fluoxetine), whereas the dose for OCB/OCD is higher (e.g. 40–60 mg). Clomipramine (a tricyclic) can be useful in OCB/OCD, but usually has more side effects than the SSRIs and is dangerous in overdose. SSRIs have been reported to cause suicidal ideation and there are now strict guidelines for the use of SSRIs in young people. In some patients, botulinum toxin injections to the affected areas (e.g. vocal cords if loud distressing vocal tics/coprolalia) can improve the tics and the urge to tic. DBS of internal capsule, GPi or thalamus in some carefully selected, severely affected and treatment-resistant patients has apparently helped.

When a patient has GTS + ADHD, one should assess which symptoms are most problematic, and attempt to treat these. Clonidine helps tics, ADHD and sleep. It was once thought that stimulants (e.g. methylphenidate) that improve ADHD increased tics, and were therefore contraindicated, but this is now known not to be the case in most patients. Newer once-daily slow-release preparations can increase compliance. If the ADHD and tics pose equal difficulties, try clonidine; if ADHD is the greatest problem, try stimulants. The next option is to use stimulants with clonidine. Stimulants can also be given with neuroleptics.

Myoclonus

Myoclonus is defined as a sudden brief shock-like involuntary movement caused by muscular contraction or inhibition. Muscle contraction produces positive myoclonus and muscle inhibition causes negative myoclonus or asterixis (e.g. liver flap). Myoclonus can be focal, multifocal, generalised, spontaneous or reflex. It can occur at rest, when maintaining a posture or during action. Myoclonus can be classified as cortical, subcortical, spinal or peripheral, based on the presumed physiological mechanism underlying its generation. Alternatively, based on its aetiology, it can be classified as physiological, essential, epileptic or symptomatic (Table 6.13).

Physiological myoclonus

This includes hypnic jerks (initial phases of sleep), hiccup (physiological myoclonus of diaphragm) and startle response (commonly exacerbated by anxiety).

Essential myoclonus

See Myoclonus dystonia (DYT11).

Epileptic myoclonus

This term is used to denote conditions where myoclonic jerks are part of an epileptic syndrome (see Neurophysiological assessment of movement disorders and Chapter 7). Generalised myoclonus can occur in the syndromes of idiopathic generalised epilepsy or in the secondarily generalised epilepsies which include the progressive myoclonic epilepsies or the static epileptic encephalopathies. Epileptic myoclonus is accompanied by generalised epileptiform discharges, but the myoclonus itself can be focal, segmental or generalised. Focal myoclonus can occur in secondary symptomatic epilepsy as a result of infection, inflammation, vascular disease, trauma or tumours.

Familial cortical tremor (also called benign autosomal dominant familial myoclonic epilepsy)

Clinically, this superficially resembles essential tremor. It is associated with infrequent or rare generalised seizures. It is an autosomal dominant, benign condition characterised by fine shivering-like 'tremor'. It usually presents in the third or fourth decade of life and there is no significant clinical progression. The myoclonus usually responds to valproate, carbamazepine or primidone, and has been mapped in Japanese families to chromosome 8q and in Italians to chromosome 2p.

Epilepsia partialis continua

This is spontaneous, regular or irregular muscle twitching of cortical origin confined to one part of the body and continuing for a period of hours, days or weeks. This condition is further described in Chapter 7.

Secondary myoclonus

This occurs in the context of an underlying neurological or non-neurological disorder brought about by trauma, brain hypoxia or progressive myoclonic encephalopathies. Often there is clinical or pathological evidence of diffuse or focal nervous system involvement.

Non-progressive myoclonic encephalopathies

It is important to recognise metabolic causes (renal or hepatic failure, vitamin E deficiency, increased level of antithyroid autoantibodies), toxic causes (bismuth, methyl-bromide, tethraethyl, chloralose poisoning) or drugs (levodopa, lithium, tricyclic antidepressants, morphine, antibiotics, SSRIs, MAOIs, antipsychotic and anaesthetic agents) that can cause myoclonus. Usually, such myoclonus is multifocal and often stimulus-sensitive, and can include negative myoclonus.

Post-anoxic action myoclonus (Lance–Adams syndrome)

This is a distinct condition secondary to severe cerebral hypoxia (usually after respiratory rather than cardiac arrest) characterised by action myoclonus, usually without other neurological disturbances, after a latent interval of 24–28 hours (Chapter 19). Myoclonus can be positive, triggered by movement, or negative when the limbs are outstretched against gravity. The voice may be fragmented by the myoclonic jerks. It can be multifocal or generalised. It is most commonly cortical reflex myoclonus, but reticular reflex myoclonus and exaggerated startle may also occur. With treatment using clonazepam, sodium valproate or piracetam or levetiracetam, distal myoclonus can be greatly improved, but asterixis in proximal leg muscles ('bouncy legs') may continue to render the patient wheelchair-bound.

Opsoclonus myoclonus

This is a well-delineated syndrome that most often occurs in children with neuroblastoma (a tumour that can remit without treatment) or medulloblastoma, or in adults in association with small cell carcinoma of the lung, breast carcinoma or melanoma. It also can be post-infectious or metabolic (coeliac disease) or drug-related. This syndrome is characterised by rapid involuntary saccadic eye movements (opsoclonus) and sudden involuntary muscle contractions (myoclonus). Ataxia is quite often also present. This syndrome is thought to be mediated by autoantibodies directed against onconeural antigens that are expressed by the tumours and also by neurones. Treatment of the underlying cause often leads to an improvement in the syndrome. In idiopathic cases, steroids and/or immuno-modulatory treatment have been used with some success.

Myoclonus in neurodegenerative disorders

Cortical myoclonus is present in about 15% of patients with DLB or PD-D but is uncommon in PD patients without dementia.

Patients with MSA often display irregular small-amplitude myoclonic movements (mini-polymyoclonus) of the hands and/or fingers on posture (jerky postural tremor) that are stimulus-sensitive, or occur during voluntary movements. A cortical origin can often be demonstrated by back-averaging techniques, and somato-sensory evoked potentials (SSEPs) are sometimes 'giant'.

Myoclonus occurs in most patients with CBD, usually appearing focally in the arm and less commonly in the legs, together with other manifestations such as apraxia, rigidity, dystonia and alien limb phenomenon. It can occur in repetitive rhythmic fashion (jerky tremor) at rest and more commonly when attempting to activate the arm or following somato-sensory stimulation (reflex myoclonus). A cortical origin has been postulated. In contrast to CBD, myoclonus is rare in PSP, another tauopathy.

Table 6.13 Classification of myoclonus.

I. Physiological myoclonus
Sleep jerks (e.g. hypnic jerks)
Hiccough (singultus)

II. Essential myoclonus (± dystonia)
Hereditary (autosomal dominant)
Sporadic

III. Epileptic myoclonus
Progressive myoclonic epilepsy (PME)
Mitochondrial disease
Lafora body disease
GM2 gangliosidosis (Tay–Sachs disease)
Ceroid lipofuscinosis (Batten/Kufs disease)
Sialidosis

Progressive myoclonic ataxia* (PMA)
Mitochondrial disease
Unverricht–Lundborg disease
Spinocerebellar degenerations
Coeliac disease

Other myoclonus epilepsy
First year of life:
  Infantile spasms
2–6 years:
  Lennox–Gastaut syndrome
Older children and adolescents (and adults):
  Photosensitive epileptic myoclonus
  Myoclonus absences
  Juvenile myoclonic epilepsy
Epilepsia partialis continua
Cortical reflex myoclonus

IV. Symptomatic myoclonus
A. Storage diseases
See III (above) PME

B. Spinocerebellar degenerations
Friedreich's ataxia
Ataxia-telangiectasia

C. Other degenerations
Basal ganglia degenerations
Wilson's disease
Dystonia
Hallervorden–Spatz disease
Huntington's disease
Multiple system atrophy
Cortico-basal degeneration
Dentatorubro-pallidoluysian atrophy (DPRLA)

D. Dementias
Creutzfeldt–Jakob disease
Alzheimer's disease
Dementia with Lewy bodies
Parkinson's disease dementia
Frontotemporal dementia

E. Infectious or post-infectious
Subacute sclerosing panencephalitis
HIV
Post-infectious encephalitis

F. Metabolic
Hyperthyroidism
Hepatic failure
Renal failure
Dialysis syndrome
Hyponatraemia
Hypoglycaemia
Non-ketotic hyperglycaemia
Biotin deficiency
Mitochondrial disease

G. Malabsorption
Coeliac disease
Whipple's disease

H. Toxic and drug-induced syndromes

I. Physical encephalopathies
Post-hypoxic action myoclonus (Lance–Adams)
Post-traumatic

J. Paraneoplastic encephalopathies

K. Opsoclonus-myoclonus syndrome
Idiopathic
Paraneoplastic
Infectious

L. Focal nervous system damage
Post-stroke
Post-thalamotomy
Tumour
Trauma
Inflammation

M. Exaggerated startle syndrome
Hereditary/sporadic/secondary

N. Palatal myoclonus (tremor)
Idiopathic/symptomatic

O. Spinal myoclonus
Segmental
Propriospinal

P. Peripheral nervous system
Hemifacial spasm

Q. Psychogenic myoclonus

* Myoclonus and cerebellar features main problem, perhaps with mild mental impairment and epilepsy.
Source: Caviness and Brown 2004. Reproduced with permission of Elsevier.

HD can rarely be associated with myoclonus, usually in individuals with a juvenile onset and longer CAG repeats. Myoclonus is more common in DRPLA, when it is usually associated with epilepsy.

In Alzheimer's disease, myoclonus is usually multifocal but can also be generalised. There can be sporadic large myoclonic jerks or repetitive small ones which may occur at rest, during action or be stimulus-sensitive. Commonly, myoclonus appears in middle and late stages of the disease, affecting about 50% of patients. It may occur at the onset of the disease in patients with earlier age of onset, rapid progression and in familial causes of Alzheimer's disease.

Myoclonus has recently been described in some patients with frontotemporal dementia and parkinsonism linked to chromosome 17 (FTDP-17). Myoclonus is often observed (82–100%) in sporadic, familial and new-variant Creutzfeldt–Jakob disease (CJD) during the course of the disease, in which the jerks are often diffuse, generalised, relatively rhythmic and associated with periodic sharp-wave EEG activity (1–1.5 Hz). They are stimulus-sensitive and can persist during sleep.

Subcortical myoclonus

Rhythmic myoclonus in a brainstem or spinal segmental distribution suggests a focal lesion at or near that segment of the brainstem or spinal cord. Generalised jerks most commonly reflect an origin in the brainstem reticular formation while axial jerks usually suggest a spinal cord lesion.

Startle syndromes

The startle reflex is a bilaterally synchronous shock-like set of movements evoked by sudden stimuli. Its most prominent features are forceful closure of the eyes, raising of flexed arms above the head, and flexion of the neck, trunk, elbows, hips and knees. The auditory startle reflex originates in the caudal brainstem, more specifically in the bulbo-pontine reticular formation. The nucleus reticularis pontis caudalis seems particularly important. Startle syndromes occur in three different groups of disorders with abnormal response to startling events: hyperekplexia, neuropsychiatric startle syndrome and startle-induced epilepsy.

The major form of hyperekplexia is characterised by generalised stiffness noticeable soon after birth, but subsiding during the first years of life, excessive startling to an unexpected stimulus that remains throughout life, and generalised stiffness in response to startle that lasts a few seconds and which commonly produces a fall forwards 'as stiff as a board' while fully conscious. In this form, mutations in the α1 subunit of the glycine receptor gene, *GLRA1*, or related genes have been identified. A minor form of hyperekplexia is characterised by excessive startle only, with latencies of muscle activation longer than in the major form. No definite genetic substrate for this form has been found. Excessive startle also occurs in the context of neuropsychiatric conditions such as anxiety, panic attack, post-traumatic stress disorders or culture-specific disorders such as the jumping Frenchmen of Maine.

Startle epilepsy is an asymmetric tonic epileptic seizure typically induced by a sudden stimulus, mostly observed in young patients with infantile cerebral hemiplegia or those with a structural lesion in the central cortex. Startle is a transient phenomenon in these cases disappearing in adulthood.

Palatal myoclonus

See Palatal tremor.

Spinal myoclonus

Segmental myoclonus involves one or two contiguous spinal segments, whereas in proprio-spinal myoclonus several segments are involved because electrical activity spreads upwards and downwards from a spinal generator via slower proprio-spinal pathways. Spinal myoclonus has been reported in association with spinal cord trauma, vascular disease, disc herniation, drugs and infection. It is usually rhythmic or periodic, involving muscles belonging to one or two spinal segments.

Proprio-spinal myoclonus may also be rhythmic or arrhythmic but is characterised by axial jerks with flexion of the trunk and limbs. It occurs mainly when the patient is relaxed, predominantly when lying on a bed or falling asleep, and may be a cause of insomnia. Jerk duration is usually longer and more variable (50–1000 ms) than in cortical myoclonus. Some reports suggest that a number of those presenting with proprio-spinal myoclonus may have a functional disorder.

Peripheral myoclonus

Peripheral myoclonus is rare and characterised by rhythmic or semi-rhythmic myoclonus secondary to nerve, root or anterior horn cell disease. Hemifacial spasm is the most common example. Peripheral myoclonus can be also multifocal in anterior horn cell disease (as in post-polio syndrome).

Psychogenic myoclonus

Psychogenic myoclonus can occur spontaneously or following an external insult. It may be focal (restricted to a few muscles or limb) or generalised. Jerks usually have an inconsistent character over time, occasionally associated with other unusual neurological symptoms, with sudden onset and offset. There is often underlying psychopathology, the jerks are commonly distractible and can respond to placebo or psychotherapy (see Other movement disorders).

Drug-induced myoclonus

Many different drugs can cause myoclonus. These include antidepressants (especially SSRIs), opiates, antiparkinsonian medications, some antibiotics (especially quinolones), lithium, bismuth, neuroleptics, anaesthetic agents (especially propofol), cholinesterase inhibitors and, perhaps surprisingly, anxiolytics (especially benzodiazepines) and anticonvulsants.

Treatment of myoclonus

The treatment of myoclonus depends upon the underlying disorder. Depending upon its aetiology, myoclonus can be partially or totally reversed, as in drug-induced or metabolic myoclonus, or surgically treatable lesions. Unfortunately, treatment of the underlying disorder is not always feasible.

Most causative conditions are poorly responsive to pharmacological treatment and often require polytherapy but this can cause side effects such as ataxia and drowsiness.

In cortical myoclonus, sodium valproate is particularly effective. This can be combined with piracetam or levetiracetam and both have been shown to be very useful agents. Benzodiazepines and barbiturates are also effective and believed to facilitate GABAergic transmission: clonazepam can be combined with valproate and levetiracetam as polytherapy with these three agents is often successful for cortical myoclonus. Lamotrigine and phenobarbital can also be effective in some cases.

Myoclonus dystonia responds partially to clonazepam, which is also particularly useful in hyperekplexia and in spinal myoclonus. Bilateral pallidal DBS can help severe myoclonus dystonia. Injection of botulinum toxin can help in palatal myoclonus and in hemifacial spasm.

Other movement disorders

Psychogenic (functional) movement disorders

Psychogenic movement disorders (PMD) can take any form although dystonia and tremor are the most common manifestations and psychogenic parkinsonism and chorea are rare. PMD represent 4–25% of all new cases seen in specialist movement disorders clinics.

The diagnosis of a PMD is primarily clinical, although investigations to exclude alternative or additional diagnoses, and specific electrophysiological tests for certain forms of PMD, can have an important role. However, PMD is not simply a diagnosis of exclusion, and positive features suggesting the diagnosis should be sought: marked fluctuations during examination; distractibility; increase with attention or suggestion; incongruence with patterns of recognised movement disorders; the presence of other non-organic signs; discrepancy between objective signs and disability; abrupt onset with rapid progression to maximum severity; inconsistency over time; a history of previous somatisations; and a sustained and substantial response to placebo or psychotherapy. While none of these features is pathognomonic, they allow a classification based on degree of diagnostic certainty (Table 6.14).

Specific PMDs may have additional clinical and investigational features that support the diagnosis. In psychogenic tremor these include co-activation of antagonist muscles; pause in tremor or entrainment of tremor frequency with externally paced tapping movements of the contralateral hand or foot, pause with ballistic movement of the other limband a significant increase of amplitude or change of tremor frequency when the limb is loaded with a weight or the limb is restrained. Subjects may display an excessive attention to self in carrying out simple tasks. In psychogenic myoclonus the presence of a Bereitschaftspotential (premovement potential) preceding myoclonic movements, of prolonged

Table 6.14 Diagnostic criteria for psychogenic dystonia. As only the first two categories provide a clinically useful degree of diagnostic certainty they have been combined to one category of 'Clinically definite'.

Documented
Persistent relief by psychotherapy, suggestion or placebo has been demonstrated, which may be helped by physiotherapy, or the patient was seen without the dystonia when believing him or herself unobserved
Clinically established
The dystonia is incongruent with classic dystonia or there are inconsistencies in the examination, plus at least one of the following three: other psychogenic signs, multiple somatisations or an obvious psychiatric disturbance
Probable
The dystonia is incongruent or inconsistent with typical dystonia, or there are psychogenic signs or multiple somatisations
Possible
Evidence of an emotional disturbance

or variable duration EMG-bursts, and of long latency and variable recruitment in stimulus-sensitive myoclonus all support the diagnosis.

However, in some cases investigations can exclude a psychogenic cause. Thus, in myoclonus, consistent duration of myoclonic bursts less than 70 ms or latency to stimulus-sensitive myoclonus of less than 70 ms or the presence of giant SEPs or cortical correlates of myoclonic jerks on back-averaged EEG exclude a psychogenic aetiology. Similarly, an abnormal DaT SPECT scan excludes a diagnosis of psychogenic parkinsonism. However, the specificity of many tests that are reported to be abnormal in certain movement disorders (e.g. reciprocal inhibition in dystonia) is currently unknown and these tests cannot therefore be relied upon to differentiate them from PMD. In addition, many classic features of movement disorders (e.g. *geste antagoniste* in dystonia or treatment-induced dyskinesias in PD) can be seen in PMD. The perceived difficulty of imitating a movement disorder is not sufficient to exclude this diagnosis, and this is exemplified in rare cases of psychogenic palatal tremor. A diagnosis of PMD should not be made simply because the movement disorder is bizarre. Sometimes it is necessary to observe the patient over time to reach a diagnosis. Clinicians should also be aware of overlay of functional symptoms on a typical organic movement disorder.

The prognosis of long-standing PMD is generally poor, although patients with PMD presenting soon after onset appear to have a better prognosis. Management of PMD should include thorough initial investigations followed by discussion of the diagnosis in a clear but unconfrontational manner emphasising the unconscious origin of PMD. Where appropriate, exploration of psychiatric disorders or psychological factors underlying the disorder, appropriate referral for diagnosis and treatment, initiation of pharmacological and physical therapy, and continued follow-up by a multidisciplinary team (including the neurologist) should be considered. Avoiding both unnecessary drug treatment and perpetuating illness beliefs are clearly important management goals, particularly in complex and long-standing cases.

Movement disorders associated with dopamine receptor blockade or dopamine depletion

Dopamine receptor blocking drugs are commonly used for psychiatric indications (neuroleptics) but also in the treatment of nausea, vomiting, vertigo, unsteadiness and migraine. Dopamine depletors originally included reserpine (for hypertension), but now only tetrabenazine (for hyperkinetic movement disorders) is licensed. All of the following types of movement disorder can be produced by any of these drugs, except that tetrabenazine does not cause tardive movement disorders.

Drug-induced parkinsonism (DIP) occurs frequently. Often mild, it can nevertheless sometimes be severe, and can be asymmetrical. It is reversible, the vast majority of cases remitting within weeks to 3 months, and a dwindling residual between 3 and 12 months of stopping the offending drug. The longer the duration of parkinsonism after withdrawal of the causative drug, the greater the chance that the individual was already in the early stages of PD (or other parkinsonian disorder). Management is to withdraw the causative agent if possible, and if not, to substitute an atypical neuroleptic drug with less anti-D2 dopaminergic effect. Anticholinergics can help. So too can levodopa, but this risks psychiatric relapse, and has limited effectiveness until the causative drug is withdrawn. DaT SPECT scan is normal in pure DIP.

Acute dystonic reactions affect about 2% of individuals exposed to these drugs. They arise within hours of starting the medication and predominantly affect head and neck, with oculogyria and jaw and neck dystonia, sometimes painful. They spontaneously subside over hours, but within seconds to minutes after IV administration of a centrally acting anticholinergic.

Akathisia ('not sitting') can occur early or late in treatment (the latter, tardive akathisia, can persist after drug withdrawal). The patient has an inner compulsion to move, a 'motor restlessness' that causes them to pace up and down or shift from one foot to the other, with rather stereotyped movements. Treatment is unsatisfactory.

Tardive dyskinesia arises after weeks, months or years of treatment, but persists for a variable time period, sometimes permanently. It can begin, or worsen temporarily, after discontinuing the offending drug. Most cases display relatively rapid, predominantly choreiform buccolinguomasticatory movements, with lip-smacking and sometimes tongue protrusion. These are more common with increasing age and female sex.

Tardive dystonia, more common in younger male subjects, phenomenologically resembles idiopathic dystonia, so can take the form of torticollis or axial dystonia for example. However, retrocollis, or opisthotonic trunk movements, are more common than in idiopathic torticollis or axial dystonia, as are 'copulatory' pelvic thrusting movements. Tardive dystonia can often be functionally, as well as socially disabling. The remission rate for this condition is very low – only 14% even 8 years after discontinuation of the offending drug, which nevertheless remains the best prognostic feature.

Although the newer 'atypical' neuroleptic drugs appear to be safer with regard to the provocation of tardive movement disorders than older drugs, there are no entirely safe dopamine receptor blocking drugs and, at least for tardive dystonia, no safe period of use. Unfortunately, centrally acting dopamine receptor blocking drugs continue to be used inappropriately for depression and anxiety and also for gastrointestinal disorders such as nausea or vomiting (e.g. metoclopramide).

Anticholinergics can worsen choreiform tardive dyskinesia, but may improve tardive dystonia. Tetrabenazine can sometimes help both. Paradoxically, just as tardive dyskinesia can present when the offending neuroleptic drug has its dose reduced, or is discontinued, an increase in the dose of the offending drug can improve the movements, but only in the short term, before further aggravating the problem.

Tardive tics, myoclonus and tremor have been described, but are very uncommon.

The neuroleptic malignant syndrome (NMS) is a potentially fatal reaction to the introduction, increase or change of dosage of dopamine receptor blocking drugs (Chapter 19). In its fully developed form it involves the subacute appearance of severe muscle rigidity (sometimes with necrosis and myoglobinuria, leading to renal failure), akinesia, diaphoresis, agitation progressing to stupor and coma, and hyperpyrexia. CPK levels are elevated, often markedly, and a polymorphonuclear leukocytosis is common. Management includes stopping the offending drug, intensive care, cooling, antipyretics, and traditionally the administration of dantrolene and bromocriptine. Mortality in severe cases can still be up to 20%, but is much less in milder cases. The underlying mechanism is thought to be a combination of hypothalamic and striatal dopamine receptor blockade. Rarely an NMS-like syndrome can occur in PD after acute reduction or withdrawal of dopaminergic drugs.

Restless legs syndrome

Restless legs syndrome (RLS) is probably the most common movement disorder, affecting to some degree 3–10% of the population, with most of those needing treatment being over the age of 50 years. It causes unpleasant sensations or an urge to move in the legs (and sometimes other body parts), classically on retiring to bed at night, which is only, and almost instantly, relieved by getting up and walking about. It can also occur when trying to relax when sitting or lying down during the day. Some (younger onset) cases are dominantly inherited. There are associations with iron deficiency, uraemia, pregnancy, peripheral neuropathy and possibly with PD. Serum ferritin is often low (Chapter 19).

Essential criteria for diagnosis are as follows:

1 An urge to move the legs, usually accompanied by uncomfortable or unpleasant sensations in the legs.
2 These symptoms begin or worsen during periods of rest or inactivity such as lying or sitting.
3 Symptoms are partially or totally relieved by movement, at least for as long as the activity continues.
4 Symptoms are worse, or only occur, in the evening or at night.

Supportive criteria are as follow:

1 Positive response to dopaminergic treatment
2 Periodic limb movements during wakefulness or sleep, and
3 Positive family history suggestive of autosomal dominant inheritance.

If drug treatment is needed, dopamine agonists (e.g. pramipexole and ropinirole) are currently favoured over levodopa because chronic levodopa treatment can lead to 'augmentation' – spillover of symptoms to the daytime, an increase in severity of symptoms, and involvement of other body parts. Second line drugs that sometimes help are opiates, gabapentin, carbamazepine and clonazepam. If there is iron deficiency or low ferritin, iron supplementation is indicated.

RLS is commonly associated with periodic leg movements of sleep (PLMS). Several gene associations for RLS (with or without PLMS) and for PLMS (with or without RLS) have recently been discovered.

Painful legs and moving toes

This rare condition (see also Chapter 23) is characterised by slow undulating flexion–extension movements of the toes, accompanied by pain in the legs, usually unilateral. There may be evidence of peripheral nerve or root lesion involving the affected leg. No treatment is effective.

Stiff person syndrome, stiff limb syndrome and encephalomyelitis with rigidity

Stiff person syndrome is characterised by axial rigidity at rest involving mainly trunk (causing hyperlordosis) and sometimes also proximal lower limb muscles. A crucial finding is the presence of continuous motor unit activity in the paraspinal muscles that persists even when trying to relax, so that EMG electrical silence cannot be obtained. The rigidity and continuous motor unit activity lessen, or even disappear, during sleep and after spinal or general anaesthesia, indicating a central source.

Exteroceptive or cutaneo-muscular reflexes are enhanced, habituate poorly and spread as reflex spasms into muscles normally not involved in the reflex. These findings point to enhanced spinal interneurone excitability, caused by defects either within spinal interneuronal networks at a segmental level or their descending control. Polysynaptic reflexes are characteristically exaggerated in both upper and lower limbs as well as the axial (paraspinal) muscles.

Most patients have anti-GAD and/or glycine receptor antibodies in serum and CSF, and some have additional diabetes or other autoimmune disturbances or markers Typically, patients show a useful response to high-dose baclofen and diazepam, and remain ambulant.

The stiff limb syndrome is rarer, and characterised by rigidity, painful spasms and abnormal postures of distal limb/s (more commonly a leg than an arm). Affected patients may show continuous motor unit activity in the affected limb but this may sometime be absent. However, abnormal exteroceptive reflexes can be detected as well as abnormally segmented EMG activity during spasms. Autoimmune markers are infrequent and anti-GAD may be negative but such patients may have antiglycine receptor antibodies. The condition responds poorly to treatment, most patients becoming wheelchair-bound.

A third, even rarer, disorder comprises patients with a rapidly progressive and fatal inflammatory encephalomyelitis with rigidity (PERM), usually with abnormal CSF and additional denervation. Again anti-GAD and glycine receptor antibodies but also amphiphysin and DPPX antibodies should be looked for as well as doing a paraneoplastic screen. There can be an overlap between any of these forms and patients may start with one and change to another form or have combined features.

Neurophysiological assessment of movement disorders

Neurophysiological investigations in movement disorders are objective methods to investigate and support clinical diagnosis of different abnormal movements, and to monitor their severity and the effects of treatment.

Many methods are available, most of them useful for research purposes, but often of limited clinical utility. All electrophysiological tests should be interpreted in conjunction with clinical features but neurophysiology may disclose information that it is not possible to obtain by clinical observation alone.

Neurophysiological assessment of tremor

Tremor is the movement disorder most subjected to neurophysiological study. It can be characterised on the basis of its frequency, pattern of muscle activation, and duration and amplitude of the muscle bursts. Multichannel EMG recording and accelerometer data can be very useful to assess frequency and other characteristics of muscle activation in tremor.

The situation in which tremor occurs (rest, postural, action), and the presence of associated neurological signs, are important to guide the electrophysiological diagnosis of tremor. Tremor frequency can be helpful to some degree. Thus, the upper limit of frequency of physiological or voluntary tremor in healthy subjects is 11 Hz. Tremor above this frequency is always pathological, and most commonly caused by orthostatic tremor with a frequency of 13–18 Hz. Tremor at 5–7 Hz is often seen in patients with PD and essential tremor (ET) and tremor at >9 Hz in patients with enhanced physiological tremor (EPT). Low frequency tremor <4 Hz may be seen in Holmes tremor, dystonic tremor and cerebellar tremor. However, there is considerable overlap in frequency between different tremor disorders. Tremor amplitude is of little value for diagnostic purposes.

Tremor can arise from different sources. External loading (500–1000 g in the hand) typically reduces the tremor frequency in peripheral tremor (physiological tremor, EPT), but not in central tremor (PD, ET).

Cortical tremor (rhythmic cortical myoclonus) can show burst duration as short as 25–50 ms. Otherwise, burst duration is not particularly useful in identifying the anatomical origin of a tremor. Multichannel EMG recording can show a rostro-caudal pyramidal progression of the pattern of muscle recruitment, or rhythmic arrests of muscle tone as in negative cortical myoclonus or asterixis. The pattern of muscle activation between agonist and antagonist muscles (synchronous or alternating) is not very helpful in guiding the diagnosis.

Dystonic tremor is an irregular tremor usually below 7 Hz. It is associated with dystonic postures in the affected extremity or elsewhere, is subject to position- and task-specific worsening, and increases with attempts to move the body part in the opposite direction to the dystonic pattern.

In psychogenic tremor, amplitude often diminishes and frequency can change during distraction (counting, or tapping with the opposite limb). Furthermore, tapping different frequencies with the unaffected hand 'entrains' to the same frequency as that on the tremulous side. Tremor amplitude and frequency usually increase when adding a load to the affected limb.

Neurophysiological assessment of dystonia

Many neurophysiological abnormalities have been found in patients with dystonia, but these are only partially useful for diagnostic purposes in individual patients. Impaired reciprocal inhibition of forearm flexor muscles at intermediate and long latency, reduced cortical silent period duration, and short- and long-interval intracortical inhibition have been seen in different studies in dystonic patients.

More sophisticated analyses of EMG discharges consider EMG–EMG coherence. This may disclose the character of the descending discharges responsible for the abnormal muscle activity in dystonia. An abnormal 4–7 Hz drive is seen in dystonic muscles in patients with the *DYT1* gene mutation, idiopathic torticollis and myoclonus dystonia. In the arms there is evidence of an abnormal cortico-muscular drive in the 15–30 Hz band leading to co-contraction between antagonistic muscles, with the exception of writer's cramp where a discrete peak in EMG–EMG coherence may be seen at 11–12 Hz.

Neurophysiological assessment of myoclonus

Myoclonus is classified according to its physiopathological basis as cortical, reticular or spinal.

Cortical myoclonus

This is usually arrhythmic but can also be rhythmic (cortical tremor). It is characterised by jerks of short duration (typically <50 ms) involving many muscles and usually synchronously in agonists and antagonists. EMG recording from an extremity can demonstrate spread of jerks from the proximal muscle to distal with velocity corresponding to that of alpha motor fibres.

In cortical myoclonus, the EEG often shows multifocal or generalised spike and wave or multiple spike and wave which is usually time-locked to the muscle jerks. However, in some cases the EEG does not show any time-locked abnormality. EEG back-averaging can disclose myoclonus-related EEG activity that cannot be recognised on the conventional polygraph. This technique can determine the precise time interval from the EEG activity to the myoclonus. It also identifies the scalp distribution of the myoclonus-related EEG activity based on simultaneous multi-channel recordings. Back-averaging analysis shows a positive–negative biphasic spike at the central electrode somatotopically representing the muscle from which the myoclonus is recorded. The initial positive precedes the onset of myoclonic EMG discharge in a hand muscle by approximately 20 ms. The more distal the muscle the myoclonus is recorded from, the longer is the EEG–EMG time interval. Myoclonus-related discharge spreads through the motor cortex within one hemisphere, and also transcallosally to the homologous area of the contralateral motor cortex (10–15 ms). Unfortunately, EEG back-averaging analysis is limited by muscle activity in the scalp and also in cases where the jerks are of high frequency, or are infrequent.

In subjects in whom myoclonic EMG bursts are of small amplitude, or repeat rhythmically at high frequency, frequency analysis has advantages over back-averaging. Frequency analysis of EMG–EMG and also EEG–EMG coherence can detect a pathologically exaggerated common drive in distal limb muscles, showing significant coherence in the physiological range (15–60 Hz) but also, in some cases, at much higher frequencies.

Patients with cortical myoclonus may also show giant sensory evoked potentials; the initial components, a post-central negative peak (N20) and a precentral positive peak (P20), are not enhanced; however, the subsequent components (P25, P30, N35) are 3–10 times as large as normal. Long loop reflexes (C-reflexes) obtained by the motor subthreshold stimulation of the median nerve, recording from both thenar muscles, are also enhanced with a latency in the thenar muscle of around 45 ms, and 10–15 ms longer contralaterally because of the transcallosal transit time. Negative myoclonus is produced by a sudden (50–400 ms) interruption of a tonic muscle contraction, associated with an ictal discharge.

In CJD, myoclonus is not stimulus-sensitive and occurs continuously and quasi-periodically in the resting condition every 600–1500 ms. There may be accompanying dystonic posturing. EMG bursts are similar to, or slightly longer than, those of classic cortical myoclonus. Periodic sharp discharges (PSDs) are usually associated with muscle jerks, but can occur independently. EEG spike-wave and EMG activity correlate loosely. On back-averaging, the negative spike-wave is much smaller than the PSD recorded with raw EEG. The time interval between EEG and jerks is 50–85 ms (much longer than required for conduction through the pyramidal tract). Typical cortical reflex myoclonus can be seen in late stages of disease.

In subacute sclerosing panencephalitis (SSPE) sudden movements, followed by a tonic phase ('hung-up jerks'), can be related to periodic high-amplitude EEG discharges occurring every 4–13 s.

Essential myoclonus, myoclonus dystonia (except for SSPE), palatal and oculo-palatal myoclonus are characterised by EMG discharges lasting up to 400 ms. In such cases the EEG does not show any specific correlate to the EMG discharge.

Reticular, or brainstem, myoclonus

This is characterised by generalised jerks with prominent involvement of proximal and flexor muscles. Jerks can be spontaneous or stimulus-induced, particularly with respect to sound.

Jerks originate from the brainstem reticular formation; the first muscle to be activated is trapezius or sternomastoid; subsequently there is spread to the cranial and caudal muscles with different velocities of activation.

Myoclonic jerks can be associated with cortical spikes. However, the lack of correlation between the two suggests that spikes are projected to, but do not originate at the cortex. Evoked potentials are not increased, but there can be an enhanced C-reflex.

The normal human startle response consists of a brief flexion response, most marked in the upper half of the body, elicited by unexpected auditory, and sometimes somaesthetic, visual or vestibular stimuli. Conduction of efferent impulses both upwards and downwards from the generator, possibly in the medial reticular formation, is slow. The shortest latencies are 20–50 ms for the orbicularis oculi muscle. In the quadriceps muscle the latencies of the responses are 100–150 ms.

Electromyographic responses in the intrinsic hand and foot muscles are particularly delayed. However, the auditory startle reflex electromyographic latencies are rather variable. The constant reflex EMG activity in orbicularis oculi is the most important event in the normal auditory startle reflex. If one considers the auditory blink reflex in orbicularis oculi as separate from the startle response, then the earliest muscle recorded is the SCM, with a latency of <100 ms. The activity then spreads up the brainstem from the XIth nerve to the Vth cranial nerve and down the spinal cord (reflex brainstem myoclonus). In physiological startle the stimulus-induced response tends to habituate, and disappears after 4–6 stimuli. Exaggerated startle responses are seen in hyperekplexia, in neuropsychiatric startle syndrome and in stimulus-induced epilepsy and stiff person syndrome.

Spinal myoclonus

Two different patterns of spinal myoclonus are recognised: propriospinal myoclonus and segmental myoclonus. Myoclonus is most often positive, but negative myoclonus also occurs.

Proprio-spinal myoclonus is characterised by arrhythmic sequences or runs of axial jerks producing flexion or extension of the trunk. Bursts of muscle activity vary from 50 ms to 4 s. EMG jerks arise from abdominal or cervical spinal segments and slowly spread rostrally and caudally at <10 m/s. Cranial muscles are not involved, with the exception of the neck. It can be stimulus-sensitive. It is important to keep in mind psychogenic myoclonus and look for premovement potential in these cases.

Segmental myoclonus is described as regular or irregular repetitive jerks, involving a group of muscles innervated by one or two spinal segments.

Further reading

Parkinson's disease and related disorders

Aarsland D, Andersen K, Larsen JP, Lolk A, Nielson H, Kragh-Sorensen P. Risk of dementia in Parkinson's disease: a community-based, prospective study. *Neurology* 2001; **56**: 730–736.

Braak H, Bohl JR, Muller CM, Rub U, de Vos RA, Del Tredici K. Stanley Fahn Lecture 2005: The staging procedure for the inclusion body pathology associated with sporadic Parkinson's disease. *Mov Disord* 2006; **21**: 2042–2051.

Burn DJ, Lees AJ. Progressive supranuclear palsy: where are we now? *Lancet Neurol* 2002; **1**: 359–369.

Chaudhuri KR, Healy DG, Schapira AH. Non-motor symptoms of Parkinson's disease: diagnosis and management. *Lancet Neurol* 2006; **5**: 235–245.

De Lau LML, Breteler MMB. Epidemiology of Parkinson's disease. *Lancet Neurol* 2006; **5**: 525–535.

Deuschl G, Schade-Brittinger C, Krack P, *et al.* A randomized trial of deep-brain stimulation for Parkinson's disease. *New Engl J Med* 2006; **355**: 896–908.

Emre M, Aarsland D, Brown R, *et al.* Clinical diagnostic criteria for dementia associated with Parkinson's disease. *Mov Disord* 2007; **22**: 1689–1707.

Gibb WR, Lees AJ. The relevance of the Lewy body to the pathogenesis of idiopathic Parkinson's disease. *J Neurol Neurosurg Psychiatry* 1988; **51**: 745–752.

Gilman S, Wenning GK, Low PA, *et al.* Second consensus statement on the diagnosis of multiple system atrophy. *Neurology* 2008; **71**: 670–676.

Horstink M, Tolosa E, Bonucelli U, *et al.* Review of the therapeutic management of Parkinson's disease. Report of a joint task force of the European Federation of Neurological Societies (EFNS) and the Movement Disorder Society-European Section (MDS-ES). Part I: early (uncomplicated) and Part II: late (complicated) Parkinson's disease. *Eur J Neurol* 2006; **13**: 1170–1185 and 1186–1202.

Houlden H, Schneider SA, Paudel R, Melchers A, Schwingenschuh P, Edwards M, *et al.* THAP1 mutations (DYT6) are an additional cause of early-onset dystonia. *Neurology* 2010; **74** :846–850.

Kiriakakis V, Bhatia KP, Quinn NP, Marsden CD. The natural history of tardive dystonia: a long-term follow-up study of 107 cases. *Brain* 1998; **121**: 2053–2066.

Li JY, Englund E, Holton JL, *et al.* Lewy bodies in grafted neurons in subjects with Parkinson's disease suggest host to graft disease propagation. *Nat Med* 2008; **14**: 501–503.

Limousin P, Krack P, Pollak P, *et al.* Electrical stimulation of the subthalamic nucleus in advanced Parkinson's disease. *New Engl J Med* 1998; **339**: 1105–1111.

Litvan I, Agid Y, Calne D, *et al.* Clinical research criteria for the diagnosis of progressive supranuclear palsy (Steele-Richardson-Olszewski syndrome): report of the NINDS-SPSP international workshop. *Neurology* 1996; **47**: 1–9.

Mahapatra RK, Edwards MJ, Schott JM, Bhatia KP. Corticobasal degeneration. *Lancet Neurol* 2004; **3**: 736–743.

McKeith IG, Dickson DW, Lowe J, Emre M, O'Brien JT, Feldman H, *et al.* Diagnosis and management of dementia with Lewy bodies. Third report of the DLB consortium. *Neurology* 2005; **65**: 1863–1872.

Nilsson C, Markenroth Bloch K, Brockstedt S, Lätt J, Widner H, Larsson EM. Tracking the neurodegeneration of parkinsonian disorders: a pilot study. *Neuroradiology* 2007; **49**: 111–119.

Paviour DC, Surtees RA, Lees AJ. Diagnostic considerations in juvenile parkinsonism. *Mov Disord* 2004; **19**: 123–135.

Schrag A, Kingsley D, Phatouros C, Mathias CJ, Lees AJ, Daniel SE, *et al.* Clinical usefulness of magnetic resonance imaging in multiple system atrophy. *J Neurol Neurosurg Psychiatry* 1998; **65**: 65–71.

Sheerin UM, Houlden H, Wood NW. Advances in the genetics of Parkinson's disease: a guide for the clinician. *Mov Disord Clin Pract (Hoboken)* 2014; **1**: 3–13.

Vidailhet M, Rivaud S, Gouider-Khouja N, *et al.* Eye movements in parkinsonian syndromes. *Ann Neurol* 1994; **35**: 420–426.

Volpicelli-Daley LA, Luk KC, Patel TP, *et al.* Exogenous alpha synuclein fibrils induce Lewy body pathology leading to synaptic dysfunction and neuron death. *Neuron* 2011; **72**: 57–71.

Wenning GK, Colosimo C, Geser F, Poewe W. Multiple system atrophy. *Lancet Neurol* 2004; **3**: 93–103.

Williams DR, de Silva R, Paviour DC, *et al.* Characteristics of two distinct clinical phenotypes in pathologically proven progressive supranuclear palsy; Richardson's syndrome and PSP-parkinsonism. *Brain* 2005; **128**: 1247–1258.

Zijlmans JC, Daniel, SE, Hughes AJ, Revesz T, Lees AJ. Clinicopathological investigation of vascular parkinsonism, including clinical criteria for diagnosis. *Mov Disord* 2004; **19**: 630–640.

Chorea

Bates G, Harper PS, Jones L, eds. Huntington's Disease, 3rd edn. Oxford: Oxford University Press, 2002.

Cardoso F. Chorea: non-genetic causes. *Curr Opin Neurol* 2004; **17**: 433–436.

Hensman Moss DJ, Poulter M, Beck J, *et al.* C9orf72 expansions are the most common genetic cause of Huntington disease phenocopies. *Neurology* 2014; **82**: 292–299.

Mencacci N, Erro R, Wiethoff S, *et al.* ADCY5 mutations are another cause of benign hereditary chorea. *Neurology* 2015; **85**: 80–88.

Wilson's disease

Ala A, Walker AP, Ashkan K, Dooley JS, Schilsky ML. Wilson's disease. *Lancet* 2007; **369**: 397–408.

Aggarwal A, Bhatt MH. The pragmatic treatment of Wilson's disease. *Mov Disord Clin Pract* 2014; **1**: 14–23.

Kinnier Wilson S. Progressive lenticular degeneration: a familial nervous disease associated with cirrhosis of the liver. *Brain* 1912; **34**: 295–509.

Walshe JM. History of Wilson's disease: 1912 to 2000. *Mov Disord* 2006; **21**: 142–147.

Dystonias

Albanese A, Bhatia K, Bressman SB, *et al.* Phenomenology and classification of dystonia: aconsensus update. *Mov Disord* 2013: **28**: 863–873.

Asmus F, Zimprich A, Tezenas Du Montcel S, *et al.* Myoclonus-dystonia syndrome: epsilon-sarcoglycan mutations and phenotype. *Ann Neurol* 2002; **52**: 489–492.

Charlesworth G, Bhatia KP, Wood NW. The genetics of dystonia: new twists in an old tale. *Brain* 2013; **136**: 2017–2037.

Costa J, Espírito-Santo C, Borges A, *et al.* Botulinum toxin type A therapy for cervical dystonia. *Cochrane Database Syst Rev* 2005; **1**: CD003633.

Coubes P, Roubertie A, Vasyssiere N, Hemm S and Echenne B. Treatment of DYT1-generalised dystonia by stimulation of the internal globus pallidus. *Lancet* 2000; **355**: 2220–2221.

Fahn S, Bressman SB, Marsden CD. Classification of dystonia. *Adv Neurol* 1998; **78**: 1–10.

Fung VSC, Jinnah HA, Bhatia K, Vidailhet M. Assessment of patient with isolated or combined dystonia: an update on dystonia syndromes. *Mov Disord* 2013; **28** :889–898.

Nemeth AH. The genetics of primary dystonias and related disorders. *Brain* 2002; **125**: 695–721.

Nygaard TG, Marsden CD, Fahn S. Dopa-responsive dystonia: long-term treatment response and prognosis. *Neurology* 1991; **41**: 174–181.

Trender-Gerhard I, Sweeney MG, Schwingenschuh P,et al. Autosomal-dominant GTPCH1-deficient DRD: clinical characteristics and long-term outcome of 34 patients. *J Neurol Neurosurg Psychiatry* 2009; **80**: 839–845.

Vidailhet M, Vercueil L, Houeto JL, *et al.* Bilateral, pallidal, deep-brain stimulation in primary generalized dystonia: a prospective 3 year follow-up study. *Lancet Neurol* 2007; **6**: 223–229.

Tics

Robertson MM. Tourette syndrome, associated conditions and the complexities of treatment. *Brain* 2000; **123**: 425–462.

Singer HS. Tourette's syndrome: from biology to behaviour. *Lancet Neurol* 2005; **4**: 149–159.

Tremor

Bain PG, Britton TC, Jenkins IH, Thompson PD, Rothwell JC, Thomas PK, *et al.* Tremor associated with benign IgM paraproteinaemic neuropathy. *Brain* 1996; **11**: 789–799.

Deuschl G. Neurophysiology tests for the assessment of tremor. *Adv Neurol* 1999; **80**: 57–65.

Deuschl G, Bain PG, Brin M. Consensus statement of the Movement Disorder Society on tremor. *Mov Disord* 1998; **13**: 2–23.

Lorenz D, Deuschl G. Update on the pathogenesis and treatment of essential tremor. *Curr Opin Neurol* 2007; **20**: 447–452.

Morgan JC, Sethi KD. Drug-induced tremors. *Lancet Neurol* 2005; **4**: 866–876.

Myoclonus

Caviness JN, Brown P. Myoclonus: current concepts and recent advances. *Lancet Neurol* 2004; **3**: 598–607.

Erro R, Bhatia KP, Edwards MJ, Farmer SF, Cordivari C. Clinical diagnosis of propriospinal myoclonus is unreliable: an electrophysiologic study. *Mov Disord* 2013; **28**: 1868–1873.

Shibasaki H, Hallett M. Electrophysiological study of myoclonus. *Muscle Nerve* 2005; **31**: 157–174.

Psychogenic movement disorders

Edwards, MJ, Bhatia, KP. Functional (psychogenic) movement disorders: merging mind and brain. *Lancet Neurol* 2012; **11**: 250–260.

Hallett M, Fahn S, Jankovic J, Lang AE, Cloninger CR, Yudovsky SC, eds. Psychogenic Movement Disorders. Philadelphia: Lippincott Williams and Wilkins, 2006.

Williams DT, Ford B, Fahn S. Phenomenology and psychopathology related to psychogenic movement disorders. *Adv Neurol* 1995; **65**: 231–257.

Other movement disorders

Bhatia KP. Paroxysmal dyskinesias. *Mov Disord* 2011; **26**: 1157–1165.

Trenkwalder C, Paulus W, Walters AS. The restless legs syndrome. *Lancet Neurol* 2005; **4**: 465–475.

CHAPTER 7

Epilepsy and Related Disorders

Simon Shorvon[1], Beate Diehl[1], John Duncan[1], Matthias Koepp[1], Fergus Rugg-Gunn[2], Josemir Sander[1], Matthew Walker[1] and Tim Wehner[2]

[1] UCL Institute of Neurology

[2] National Hospital for Neurology & Neurosurgery

Definitions

A standard definition of epilepsy is as a disorder of brain characterised by an ongoing liability to recurrent epileptic seizures.

An epileptic seizure is defined as the transient clinical manifestations that result from an episode of epileptic neuronal activity. The epileptic neuronal activity is a specific dysfunction, characterised by abnormal synchronisation, excessive excitation and/or inadequate inhibition, and can affect small or large neuronal populations.

In addition to an ongoing liability to recurrent seizures, epilepsy is also associated with neurobiological, cognitive, psychological and social consequences ('being epileptic'), and with co-morbidities. These aspects can be as significant to an individual as are the epileptic seizures themselves, and can also require management in the clinic setting.

Epidemiology

Epilepsy is a common condition. The incidence of epilepsy is in the region of 80 cases per 100 000 persons per year, with different studies showing rates varying mostly between 50 and 120 per 100 000 per year. Its point prevalence has been found to be 4–10 cases per 1000 persons in most studies, although higher figures are found from settings in resource-poor countries. The frequency of epilepsy is also slightly higher in lower socio-economic classes. The incidence of seizures is age dependent, with the highest rates in the first year of life and a second peak in late life. About 40% of patients develop epilepsy below the age of 16 years of age and about 20% over the age of 65 years. In Western practice, epilepsy accounts for about 20% of all neurological consultations, and in developing countries the proportion is even higher.

An isolated (first and only) seizure occurs in about 20 persons per 100 000 each year. The cumulative incidence of epilepsy – the risk of an individual developing epilepsy in his/her lifetime – is 3–5%. The fact that prevalence is much lower than cumulative incidence demonstrates that in many cases epilepsy remits. In fact, the prognosis is generally good, and within 5 years of the onset of seizures 50–60% of patients will have entered long-term remission. However, in about 20% of cases, epilepsy, once developed, never remits. Fertility rates are reduced by about 30% in women with epilepsy. Standardised mortality rates are also 2–3 times higher in patients with epilepsy than in others in the population. The excess mortality is caused largely by the underlying cause of the epilepsy. Some deaths are directly related to seizures and there are higher rates of accidents, sudden unexpected death and suicides amongst patients with epilepsy when compared with the general population. The rates of death are highest in the first few years after diagnosis – reflecting the underlying cerebral disease (e.g. tumour, stroke). In chronic epilepsy, the excess mortality is partly a result of sudden unexpected death in epilepsy (SUDEP). The rates of SUDEP range from about 1 death per 2500 persons per year in mild epilepsy to 1 death per 100 patients per year amongst those with severe and intractable epilepsy. About 30% of children and 20% of adults with epilepsy have additional learning or neurological disabilities. Epilepsy occurs in about 20% of those with learning disability.

Of adults with newly diagnosed epilepsy, 18% show additional cognitive impairment, 6% motor disabilities (usually hemiplegia due to stroke) and 6% severe psychiatric disorders. About 1 in 15 persons with epilepsy is dependent on others for daily living because of epilepsy and the associated handicaps.

Epilepsy is associated with significant medical, social and secondary handicap. The World Health Organization (WHO) has estimated that epilepsy causes 6.4 million disability-adjusted life years (DALYs) and 1.32 million years of life (YLL) lost worldwide, and amongst neurological diseases is less only than stroke and dementia in its impact.

ILAE classification of seizure type

The International League Against Epilepsy (ILAE) classification of seizure type is the most widely accepted classification scheme for epilepsy. It has undergone a series of revisions since it was first proposed and further revisions are under consideration, and are controversial. Here the well-accepted classification and terminology are used.

The current classification divides seizures into generalised and partial categories (Table 7.1). Generalised seizures are those that arise from large areas of cortex in both hemispheres, in which consciousness is always lost, and are subdivided into seven categories. Partial (or focal) seizures are those that arise in specific often small loci of cortex in one hemisphere. They are divided into simple partial seizures which occur without alteration of consciousness and complex partial seizures in which consciousness is impaired or lost. A secondarily generalised seizure has a partial onset (the aura)

Neurology: A Queen Square Textbook, Second Edition. Edited by Charles Clarke, Robin Howard, Martin Rossor and Simon Shorvon.

Table 7.1 The International League Against Epilepsy (ILAE) classification of seizure type (1981).

I. Partial (focal, local) seizures
A. Simple partial seizures
1. With motor signs
2. With somatosensory or special sensory symptoms
3. With autonomic symptoms or signs
4. With psychic symptoms
B. Complex partial seizures
1. Simple partial onset followed by impairment of consciousness
2. With impairment of consciousness at onset
C. Partial seizures evolving to secondarily generalised seizures (tonic–clonic, tonic, or clonic)
1. Simple partial seizures evolving to generalised seizures
2. Complex partial seizures evolving to generalised seizures
3. Simple partial seizures evolving to complex partial seizures evolving to generalised seizures
II. Generalised seizures (convulsive and non-convulsive)
A. Absence seizures
1. Absence seizures
2. Atypical absence seizures
B. Myoclonic seizures
C. Clonic seizures
D. Tonic seizures
E. Tonic–clonic seizures
F. Atonic seizures
III. Unclassified epileptic seizures

Source: ILAE Commission Report 1989. Reproduced with permission of Wiley.

which spreads to become a generalised attack. Simple partial seizures may spread to become complex partial seizures, and either can spread to become secondarily generalised. The classification is based entirely on clinical and electroencephalography (EEG) phenomenology, but some generalised seizure types occur only in specific types of epilepsy. Partial seizures invariably imply focal brain pathology, although this may not necessarily be demonstrated by conventional clinical investigation. About two-thirds of newly diagnosed epilepsies are partial and/or secondarily generalised.

Partial (focal) seizures

These are defined as partial seizures in which consciousness is not impaired. Complex partial seizures are those in which consciousness is impaired. Both imply focal cerebral disease and seizures can arise from any cortical region, the most common sites being the frontal and temporal lobes.

Simple partial seizures

The symptomatology depends on the anatomical localisation of the seizures. Motor manifestations include jerking, spasm or posturing, speech arrest, dysarthria, choking sensations, version of the head or eyes or, less commonly, rotation of the whole body can occur in epilepsy arising in many cortical areas. Todd's paralysis can occur after a seizure, and is a reliable lateralising sign of epilepsy arising in contralateral motor cortex. Sensory manifestations can take the form of tingling or numbness or pain. Visual phenomena such as flashing lights and colours occur if the calcarine cortex is affected. A rising epigastric sensation is the most common manifestation of a simple partial seizure arising in the mesial temporal lobe. Autonomic symptoms occur such as changes in skin colour, blood pressure, heart rate, pupil size and piloerection.

Complex perceptual or affective 'auras' can take various forms, and are more common in complex partial than in simple partial seizures. They can occur in epilepsy arising from temporal, frontal or parietal foci. There are six principal categories:

- *Dysphasic symptoms* can occur if cortical speech areas (frontal or temporoparietal) are affected and should be distinguished where possible from anarthria (speech arrest) which suggests a frontocentral origin.
- *Dysmnestic symptoms* (disturbance of memory) such as flashbacks, déjà vu, jamais vu, or distortions of memory are most common in mesial temporal lobe seizures although also occur in inferior frontal or lateral temporal lobe seizures.
- *Cognitive symptoms* include dreamy states and sensations of unreality or depersonalisation and occur primarily in temporal lobe seizures.
- *Affective symptoms* include fear (the most common symptom), depression, anger, elation, erotic thoughts, serenity or exhilaration. These are encountered most common in mesial temporal lobe epilepsy (TLE). Laughter (without mirth) is a feature of the automatism of seizures (known as gelastic seizures) which arise in frontal areas, and are a consistent feature of the epilepsy associated with hypothalamic hamartomas.
- *Illusions* of size (macropsia, micropsia), shape, weight, distance or sound are usually features of temporal or parieto-occipital epileptic foci.
- *Structured hallucinations* of visual, auditory, gustatory or olfactory forms, which can be crude or elaborate, are usually caused by epileptic discharges in the temporal or parieto-occipital association areas. Hallucinations of taste, usually an unpleasant taste, are a frequent symptom of TLE. Visual hallucinations can vary greatly in sophistication from simple colours or flashing lights in epilepsy arising in calcarine cortex to complex visual perceptual hallucinations in posterior temporal association areas. Auditory hallucinations and changes in auditory perception also vary in complexity, and most commonly occur in seizures arising in Heschl's gyrus.

Complex partial seizures

These arise from the temporal lobe in about 60% of cases, the frontal lobe in about 30% and from other cortical areas in about 10% of cases. The clinical features reflect the site of onset of the seizures. The complex partial seizure may evolve during its course and in some seizures it is possible to identify three distinct components: the aura, the absence (loss of consciousness) and the automatism. The aura is in effect a simple partial seizure. It is usually short-lived, lasting a few seconds or so, although in rare cases can be prolonged. Many patients experience isolated auras as well as full-blown complex partial seizures. The symptoms in the aura can take any of the forms described above and depend on the anatomical location of the epileptic discharge. Absence is characterised by motor and speech arrest, during which the patient appears vacant (the 'motionless stare').

Automatisms are defined as involuntary motor actions that occur during or in the aftermath of epileptic seizures, in a state of impaired awareness. The patient is usually totally amnesic for the events of the automatism. Sometimes the actions have purposeful elements, are affected by environment and can involve quite complex activity. Automatisms should be distinguished from post-ictal confusion. Automatisms are most common in temporal and frontal lobe seizures. The most common automatisms are as follow:

- *Oro-alimentary automatisms* in which orofacial movements occur such as chewing, lip smacking, swallowing or drooling. These are characteristic of partial seizures of mesial temporal origin.
- *Gestural automatisms* include fiddling movements with the hands, tapping, patting or rubbing, ordering and tidying movements. Complex actions such as undressing are quite common also as are genitally directed actions. These too are most common in mesial TLE.
- *Ambulatory automatisms* involve walking, circling, running and are most common in frontal lobe epilepsy, but do occur in TLE also.
- *Verbal automatisms* include words and sentences, meaningless sounds, humming and whistling. Speech during the seizure suggests that the seizure is arising from the non-dominant hemisphere and dysphasia after the seizure suggests a dominant hemisphere seizure origin. Verbal automatisms can occur in both frontal and temporal seizures.
- *Violent behaviour* can occur in an automatism, it is best considered as a response in an acutely confused person and is especially likely if the patient is restrained. The violent actions of the epileptic automatism are generally never premeditated, never remembered, never highly coordinated or skilful and seldom goal-directed; these are useful diagnostic features in a forensic context.

Partial (focal) epilepsy can also be classified by anatomical location. This is a phenomenological classification, based largely on the clinical and EEG appearances of the seizures, and is obviously important when considering surgical therapy. The most common schemes divide seizures into those arising in frontal, temporal, parietal and occipital lobes and also in the central region (pre- and post-central gyrus) (Table 7.2). Subdivisions are proposed but, because epileptic seizure discharges spread extensively, anatomical classifications are often not as specific as might be hoped. Sixty per cent of partial epilepsies arise in the temporal lobe.

Partial seizures may spread to become generalised. The partial seizure is often experienced as an aura in the seconds before the generalised seizure. The generalised seizure is usually tonic–clonic, tonic or atonic.

The EEG during a complex partial seizure of mesial temporal lobe onset typically shows, at the onset, a rhythmic (5–7 Hz) discharge localised to the anterior mid temporal lobe. In lateral temporal seizures, the ictal onset EEG changes are more likely to have a spiked or high-frequency pattern. Complex partial seizures of frontal lobe epilepsy show ictal EEG onset patterns that are typically generalised or widespread, comprising high-frequency activity or slow rhythms or attenuation. Ictal onset EEG patterns in parietal and occipital seizures vary, in part dependent on pathways of seizure propagation, and there is a higher rate of false localisation and lateralisation.

Generalised seizures

Six forms are defined in the ILAE classification although, in practice, transitional forms or manifestations modified by therapy are common. Consciousness is impaired from the onset of the attack, motor changes are bilateral and more or less symmetric, and the EEG patterns are bilateral and grossly synchronous and symmetrical over both hemispheres.

Typical absence seizure (petit mal seizure)

The seizure takes the form of an abrupt sudden loss of consciousness (the absence) and cessation of all motor activity. Tone is usually preserved, and there is no fall. The patient is not in contact with the environment, is inaccessible and often appears glazed or vacant. The attack ends as abruptly as it started, and previous activity is resumed as if nothing had happened and there is no post-ictal confusion. The patient is often unaware that an attack has occurred. Most absence seizures (>80%) last less than 10 seconds. Blinking, subtle clonic movements, alterations in tone and/or brief automatisms can occur, particularly in longer attacks. The attacks can be repeated, sometimes hundreds of times a day, often cluster and are often worse when the patient is awakening or drifting off to sleep. Absences may be precipitated by fatigue, drowsiness, relaxation, photic stimulation or hyperventilation.

Typical absence seizures develop in childhood or adolescence and are encountered almost exclusively in the syndrome of idiopathic generalised epilepsy. The EEG during a typical absence is diagnostic, showing high voltage, regular, symmetric and synchronous 3 Hz spike-wave paroxysms. The features useful in differentiating a complex partial seizure from a typical absence are shown in Table 7.3.

Atypical absence seizure

This, like a typical absence seizure, takes the form of loss of awareness (absence) and hypomotor behaviour (Table 7.4). However, the duration is longer, loss of awareness is often incomplete and much less marked and associated tone changes are more severe than in a typical absence seizure. The onset and cessation of the attacks are not so abrupt. Amnesia may not be complete and the subject may be partially responsive. The ictal EEG shows usually diffuse but often asymmetric and irregular spike-wave bursts at 2–2.5 Hz, and sometimes fast activity or bursts of spikes and sharp waves. The background interictal EEG is usually abnormal, with continuous slowing, spikes or irregular spike-wave activity, and there is overlap of ictal and interictal EEG features.

Atypical absences occur in the symptomatic epilepsies, and are usually associated with learning disability, other neurologic abnormalities or multiple seizure types. These seizures most commonly form part of the Lennox–Gastaut syndrome and occur at any age.

Myoclonic seizure

This takes the form of a brief contraction of a muscle, muscle group or several muscle groups brought about by a cortical discharge. It can be single or repetitive, varying in severity from an almost imperceptible twitch to a severe jerking, resulting, for instance, in a sudden fall or the propulsion of handheld objects. Recovery is immediate, and the patient often maintains that consciousness was not lost.

Myoclonic seizures occur in idiopathic generalised epilepsy, in the childhood epileptic encephalopathies (e.g. Lennox–Gastaut syndrome) and in epilepsy associated with other forms of learning disability, and in the progressive myoclonic epilepsies. Focal myoclonus can also occur in focal epilepsy of frontal or occipital origin. Epileptic myoclonus needs to be differentiated from non-epileptic myoclonus of spinal and subcortical origin.

Table 7.2 Partial seizures arising in different brain regions.

Brain region of origin	Clinical features
Mesial temporal lobe origin	Tripartite seizure pattern (aura, absence, automatism), although only one feature may be present
	Auras are common and include: visceral, cephalic, gustatory, dysmnestic, affective, perceptual or autonomic auras
	Partial awareness commonly preserved, especially in early stages
	Slow evolution of seizure
	Prominent motor arrest or absence (the 'motionless stare')
	Dystonic posturing of the contralateral upper limb common in the early stages of the seizure
	In seizures arising in the dominant temporal lobe, speech arrest common during the seizures and dysphasia common post-ictally
	Seizures longer than frontal lobe seizures (typically >2 min), with a slower evolution and more gradual onset/offset
	Post-ictal confusion and dysphasia common
	Autonomic changes (e.g. pallor, redness, and tachycardia)
	Automatisms: less violent than in frontal lobe epilepsy, and usually take the form of oro-alimentary (lip smacking, chewing, swallowing), or gestural (e.g. fumbling, fidgeting, repetitive motor actions, undressing, walking, sexually directed actions, walking, running) and sometimes prolonged
	In hippocampal epilepsy, history of febrile seizures, onset in childhood or adolescence, initial early response lost after several years
Lateral temporal lobe onset	Features overlap with mesial temporal lobe onset, with the following differences:
	Motor arrest and absence less prominent
	Aura more likely to take the form of complex perceptual changes, visual and auditory hallucinations
	Tonic posturing more common
	More frequent secondary generalisation
Frontal lobe origin	Frequent attacks with clustering
	Brief stereotyped seizures (<30 s)
	Nocturnal attacks common
	Sudden onset and cessation, with rapid evolution and awareness lost at onset
	Absence of complex aura
	Version of head or eye common
	Prominent ictal posturing and tonic spasms
	Prominent complex bilateral motor automatisms involving lower limbs; often bizarre and misdiagnosed as dissociative seizures
	Absence of post-ictal confusion
	Frequent secondary generalisation
	History of status epilepticus
Parietal and occipital lobe origin	Somatosensory symptoms (e.g. tingling, numbness or more complex sensations – may or may not march)
	Sensation of inability to move
	Sexual sensations
	Illusions of change in body size/shape
	Vertigo
	Gustatory seizures
	Elementary visual hallucinations (e.g. flashes, colours, shapes, patterns)
	Complex visual hallucinations (e.g. objects, scenes, autoscopia, palinopsia, often moving)
	Head turning (usually adversive, with sensation of following or looking at the visual hallucations)
	Visuospatial distortions (e.g. of size [micropsia, macropsia], shape, position)
	Loss or dulling of vision (amaurosis)
	Eyelid fluttering/blinking/nystagmus

Table 7.2 (continued)

Brain region of origin	Clinical features
Central cortical origin	Often no loss of consciousness Contralateral jerking (which may or may not march) Contralateral tonic spasm or dystonia Posturing, which is often bilateral Speech arrest and spasm of bulbar musculature (producing anarthria or a choking, gurgling sound) Contralateral sensory symptoms Short duration and frequently recurring attacks Prolonged seizures with slow progression (and episodes of epilepsia partialis continua) Post-ictal Todd's paresis

Table 7.3 Differentiation between typical absences and complex partial seizures.

	Typical absence	Complex partial seizure
Age of onset	Childhood or early adult	Any age
Aetiology	Idiopathic generalised epilepsy	Any focal pathology or cryptogenic epilepsies
Underlying focal anatomical lesion	None	Limbic structures, neocortex
Duration of attack	Short (usually <30 s)	Longer, usually several minutes
Other clinical features	Slight (tone changes or motor phenomena)	Can be prominent; including aura, automatism
Post-ictal	None	Confusion, headache, emotional disturbance are common
Frequency	May be numerous	Usually less frequent cluster
Ictal and interictal EEG	3 Hz generalised spike-wave	Variable focal disturbance
Photosensitivity	10–30%	None
Effect of hyperventilation	Often marked increase	None, modest increase

Table 7.4 Clinical features differentiating typical and atypical absence seizures.

	Typical absence	Atypical absence
Context	No other neurological signs or symptoms	Usually in context of learning difficulty, and other neurological abnormalities
Consciousnes	Totally lost	Often only partially impaired
Focal signs in seizures	Nil	May be present
Onset/offset of seizures	Abrupt	Often gradual
Coexisting seizure types	Sometimes tonic–clonic and myoclonic	Mixed seizure disorder common, all seizure types

Clonic seizure

Clonic seizures are most frequent in neonates, infants or young children, and are always symptomatic.

Tonic seizure

This takes the form of a tonic muscle contraction with altered consciousness without a clonic phase. Often there is extension of the neck; contraction of the facial muscles, with the eyes opening widely, upturning of the eyeballs, contraction of the muscles of respiration, spasm of the proximal upper limb muscles causing the abduction and elevation of the semi-flexed arms and the shoulders. The ictal EEG may show flattening (desynchronisation), fast activity (15–25 Hz) with increasing amplitude (to about 100 μV) as the attack progresses, or a rhythmic 10 Hz discharge similar to that seen in the tonic phase of the tonic–clonic seizure.

Tonic seizures occur in the setting of diffuse cerebral damage, learning disability, are invariably associated with other seizure types and are the characteristic and defining seizure type in the Lennox–Gastaut syndrome.

Tonic–clonic seizure (grand mal seizure)

This is the 'convulsion' or 'fit'. It is sometimes preceded by a prodromal period during which an attack is anticipated, often by an ill-defined vague feeling or sometimes more specifically, for instance by the occurrence of increasing myoclonic jerking. If an aura then occurs (in fact a simple or complex partial seizure) in the seconds before the full-blown attack, this indicates that the tonic–clonic seizure is secondarily generalised. The seizure takes the form of loss of consciousness, sometimes with the epileptic cry (a loud guttural sound), tonic stiffening (and the patient will fall if standing) initially sometimes in flexion but then in axial extension, with the eyes rolled up, the jaw clamped shut, the limbs stiff, adducted and extended, and the fists clenched. Respiration ceases and cyanosis is common. The eyes remain open and the pupils dilated and unreactive. There are frequently heart rate changes, which are sometimes marked and can take the form of tachycardia or bradycardia and even asystole. This tonic stage lasts on average 10–30 seconds and is followed by the clonic phase, during which convulsive movements, usually of all four limbs, jaw, and facial muscles occur; breathing can be stertorous and arrest of respiration can occur; and saliva (sometimes bloodstained owing to tongue biting) may froth from the mouth. The tongue biting in an epileptic seizure is typically on the lateral aspects of the tongue, and this is said to occur only in an epileptic seizure. The convulsive movements decrease in frequency (eventually to about four clonic jerks per second), and increase in amplitude as the attack progresses. The attack is usually followed by a period of flaccidity of the muscles and consciousness is slowly regained. Confusion is invariable in the post-ictal phase. The patient often has a severe headache, feels dazed and extremely unwell, and often lapses into deep sleep. Petechial haemorrhages around the eyes, lethargy and muscle aching is common. Injuries also occur. Crush fractures of the vertebrae are common. Posterior dislocation of the shoulders is said only to occur in epileptic seizures.

Primary generalised tonic–clonic seizures occur mainly in idiopathic generalised epilepsy. Secondarily generalized tonic–clonic seizures are encountered in many different types of epilepsy including in symptomatic generalised epilepsies, epileptic encephalopathies, various epilepsy syndromes, febrile convulsions and acute symptomatic seizures. They have no pathological or syndromic specificity.

Atonic seizure

The most severe form is the classic drop attack (astatic seizure) in which all postural tone is suddenly lost causing collapse to the ground like a rag doll. The seizures are short and are followed by immediate recovery. Longer (inhibitory) atonic attacks can develop in a stepwise fashion with progressively increasing nodding, sagging or folding.

The seizures are always associated with diffuse cerebral damage, learning disability and are common in severe symptomatic epilepsies (especially in the Lennox–Gastaut sndrome and in myoclonic astatic epilepsy).

ILAE classification of the epilepsies and epilepsy syndromes

An epileptic syndrome is defined as 'an epileptic disorder characterised by a cluster of signs and symptoms customarily occurring together', and the ILAE classification scheme attempts to categorise epilepsy according to syndrome (Table 7.5). This system is under revision, and may change in the future. Some syndromes have single aetiologies and specific features, but others have multiple causes and heterogeneous clinical features. The syndromes are often age specific, and over time in individual patients one epileptic syndrome can evolve into another (e.g. West's syndrome commonly evolves into Lennox–Gastaut syndrome). The same seizure type can occur in very different syndromes (e.g. myoclonic seizures in the benign syndrome of juvenile myoclonic epilepsy and the refractory syndromes of the progressive myoclonic epilepsies).

The classification scheme allows a more comprehensive approach to categorisation than simply classifying by seizure type, but is not widely used in routine clinical practice. The following are the most common syndromes.

Idiopathic generalised epilepsy

This term should be used to denote a common and important category of epilepsy that has a characteristic clinical and electrographic pattern and a presumed genetic basis. Idiopathic generalised epilepsy (IGE) accounts for about 10–20% of all patients with epilepsy. It probably has a strong genetic basis, but no common susceptibility gene has been found, and the occurrence of epilepsy is not simple 'genetic', but also involves epigenetic and epistatic factors, and is also dependent on developmental aspects.

The condition is sometimes subdivided into separate syndromes, although this is contentious and there is a great deal of overlap. The core clinical features are shared to a greater or lesser extent by these syndromes (at least those with onset in later childhood or early adult life). The most important subdivisions are as follow.

Childhood absence epilepsy

This condition, more common in girls, appears in childhood (peak age 6–7 years), and is not associated with learning disability or other neurological problems. It accounts for 1–3% of newly diagnosed epilepsies and up to 10% of childhood epilepsies. The seizures take the form of generalised absence attacks (see earlier). The prognosis is good, and rapid remission on therapy is expected in 80% or more of patients. When followed up after age 18 years, only approximately 20% of previously diagnosed patients are still having seizures.

Juvenile myoclonic epilepsy

This is the most common subtype of IGE, and accounts for up to 10% of all epilepsies. The characteristic seizures are brief myoclonic jerks, occurring in the first hour or so after awakening, and usually in bursts. These are sudden, shock-like jerks, affecting mainly the shoulders and arms, usually but not always symmetrically. It is often

Table 7.5 The International League Against Epilepsy (ILAE) classification of the epilepsies and epilepsy syndromes (1989).

1. Generalised

- Idiopathic generalised epilepsies with age-related onset (in order of age)
  - Benign neonatal familial convulsions
  - Benign neonatal convulsions
  - Benign myoclonic epilepsy in infancy
  - Childhood absence epilepsy
  - Juvenile absence epilepsy
  - Juvenile myoclonic epilepsy
  - Epilepsy with generalised tonic–clonic seizures on awakening
  - Other generalised idiopathic epilepsys not defined above
  - Epilepsies with seizures precipitated by specific modes of activation
- Cryptogenic or symptomatic generalised epilepsies (in order of age)
  - West syndrome
  - Lennox–Gastaut syndrome
  - Epilepsy with myoclonic astatic seizures
  - Epilepsy with myoclonic absences
- Symptomatic generalised epilepsies
  - Non-specific aetiology
    - Early myoclonic encephalopathies
    - Early infantile encephalopathy with burst suppression
    - Other symptomatic epilepsies not defined above
- Specific syndromes
- Epilepsies in other disease states

2. Localisation-related epilepsies

- Idiopathic with age-related onset
  - Benign epilepsy with centrotemporal spikes
  - Childhood epilepsy with occipital paroxysms
  - Primary reading epilepsy
- Symptomatic
  - Epilepsia partialis continua
  - Syndromes characterised by specific modes of precipitation
  - Temporal lobe epilepsies
  - Frontal lobe epilepsies
  - Parietal lobe epilepsies
  - Occipital lobe epilepsies
- Idiopathic

3. Epilepsies and syndromes undetermined as to whether focal or generalised

- With both generalised and focal seizures
  - Neonatal seizures
  - Severe myoclonic epilepsy in infancy
  - Electrical status epilepticus in slow-wave sleep
  - Acquired epileptic aphasia
- Other undetermined epilepsies (not defined above) with unequivocal generalised or focal features

4. Special syndromes

- Febrile convulsions
- Isolated seizures or isolated status epilepticus
- Seizures occurring only when there is an acute metabolic or toxic event due to factors such as alcohol, drugs, eclampsia, non-ketotic hyperglycinaemia

not clear whether consciousness was retained or lost. The myoclonus develops between the ages of 12 and 18 years. In about 80% of cases, generalised tonic–clonic seizures also occur, usually months or years after the onset of myoclonus, and it is these that often trigger the diagnosis. About one-third of patients also develop typical absence seizures, again usually on awakening. About 5% of patients exhibit strong photosensitivity. The myoclonic seizures (and other seizures) can be precipitated by photic stimuli, lack of sleep, alcohol, hypoglycaemia and poor compliance with medication. Complete response to treatment can be expected in 80–90% of cases, but lifelong therapy may be needed.

Epilepsy with grand mal seizures on awakening

This condition overlaps considerably with other generalised epilepsies especially with juvenile myoclonic epilepsy in which most affected people also have generalised tonic–clonic seizures (GTCS) on awakening. The EEG usually has a normal background with bursts of generalised spike-waves or polyspike-waves. Whether this syndrome represents a discrete entity or simply part of the spectrum of other forms of IGE has been the subject of discussion for several decades, without clear resolution.

Benign partial epilepsy syndromes

There are a number of benign partial epilepsy syndromes. As with the IGEs, there is overlap between syndromes and the subdivision is a matter of some contention.

Benign partial epilepsy with centrotemporal spikes

Benign partial epilepsy with centrotemporal spikes (BECTS; *syn*: rolandic epilepsy, benign epilepsy with rolandic spikes) is the most common 'idiopathic' partial epilepsy syndrome, accounting for perhaps 15% of all epilepsies. The peak age of onset is 5–8 years and over 80% of cases have onset at 4–10 years. The condition reflects an age-related genetically determined neuronal hyperexcitability in the rolandic area. The characteristic EEG feature is the high-amplitude rolandic spike, and 10% or more of children with the EEG disturbance do not actually have seizures. The seizures are infrequent, and 50% of children experience a total of less than five attacks in all. Fifty per cent of seizures occur only at night, and the daytime seizures usually occur when the child is tired or bored. The complex partial seizures take a characteristic form, usually beginning with spasm and clonic jerking of one side of the face and throat muscles, then speech arrest and guttural vocalisations. The seizures may evolve to secondarily generalised tonic–clonic attacks. There are no associated neurological disturbances and intellect is normal. The epilepsy ceases in almost all cases, usually by the age of 12 years, without long-term sequalae. There is an excellent response to therapy with carbamazepine or other antiepileptic drugs. The condition is usually quite benign although some children have associated learning difficulties and atypical EEG or clinical features merge into other more severe childhood epileptic syndromes.

Early onset benign occipital epilepsy (*syn*: Panayiotopoulos syndrome)

This syndrome occurs in those aged between 1 and 14 years (mean 4–5 years). The partial seizures take the form of eye deviation, nausea and vomiting, with subsequent evolution into clonic hemiconvulsions. Typically, the seizures are prolonged, often lasting hours, and are infrequent (mean number three). The interictal EEG shows occipital spikes, with a morphology similar to that in BECTS, often continuous and abolished by eye opening (the fixation-off phenomenon). However, it is misleading to consider these as 'occipital lobe' seizures and the spikes may reflect spread. Some seizures consist only of vomiting, of syncopal symptoms or prominent autonomic symptoms. The prognosis is uniformly excellent, and the epilepsy always remits over time without adverse sequelae. This syndrome is often misdiagnosed as migraine.

West syndrome

West syndrome has an incidence of 0.25–0.42/1000 live births. It is defined by the occurrence of infantile spasms and the EEG changes of hypsarrhythmia. The infantile spasms take the form of sudden, generally bilateral and symmetrical contractions of the muscles of the neck, trunk or limbs, tend to cluster and may occur hundreds of times a day. In the most common type, the flexor muscles are predominantly affected, and the attack takes the form of sudden flexion with arms and legs held in adduction (the so-called salaam attacks). The peak age of onset is 4–6 months and 90% develop in the first year of life. Most cases have an underlying cerebral pathology. The most common cause is tuberous sclerosis (7–25% of all cases); neonatal ischaemia and infections (about 15% of all cases); lissencephaly and pachygyria and hemimegalencephaly (about 10% of cases); Down syndrome and acquired brain insults. The prognosis is poor, with most cases developing severe epilepsy, intellectual and psychomotor deterioration. About 5% of children die in the acute phase of spasms. A few patients, especially if treated quickly, recover completely.

Lennox–Gastaut syndrome

This term is used to denote an age-specific epileptic encephalopathy with a characteristic clinical seizure and EEG pattern and learning disability. However, whether it is a specific syndrome or whether the symptoms and EEG changes simply reflect severe childhood epilepsy with learning disability is a source of contention. There are many potential underlying causes and there is no specific histopathological change nor specific treatment. About 1–5% of childhood epilepsies conform to this pattern. The age of onset is between 1 and 7 years and it can develop in patients who earlier had West syndrome, myoclonic astatic epilepsy or neonatal seizures. In one-third of cases no cause is identifiable (cryptogenic Lennox–Gastaut syndrome). About one-third of cases are caused by malformations of brain development. The epilepsy is very severe, with seizures usually occurring many times a day. These take the form of atypical absence, tonic, myoclonic, tonic and tonic–clonic seizures, and later complex partial and other seizure types develop. The most characteristic are tonic attacks, which occur most often in non-REM (but not REM) sleep and in wakefulness. Non-convulsive status (atypical absence status) may last hours or days and be repeated on an almost daily basis.

The EEG shows a characteristic pattern with the presence interictally of long bursts of diffuse slow (1–2.5 Hz) spike-wave activity, widespread in both hemispheres, roughly bilaterally synchronous but often asymmetrical. The background activity is abnormal with an excess of slow activity and diminished arousal or sleep potentials. Learning disability is the other major feature of the condition.

At least 50% of cases have an intelligence quotient (IQ) below 50. The prognosis for control of seizures and for the development of intellectual impairment is poor, and many patients require institutional care in childhood and in adult life, and are dependent for daily activities. Response to treatment is often poor, and the seizure disorder can be exacerbated by over-treatment or therapy with sedating drugs. Carbamazepine and benzodiazepines may exacerbate tonic or atonic seizures.

Febrile seizures

Febrile seizures are seizures that occur in the context of an acute rise in body temperature in children between 3 months and 5 years of age, in whom there is no evidence of intracranial infection or other defined cause. About 3–5% of children will have at least one attack, and 19–41/1000 infants with fever will convulse. The first febrile seizure happens in the second year of life in 50%. In over 85%, the seizures are generalised and are usually brief. The seizure usually occurs early in the febrile illness, and in about one-quarter of cases is the first recognisable sign of the illness.

These essentially benign seizures need to be differentiated from the 5–10% of first seizures with fever in which the seizure is in fact caused by viral or bacterial meningitis, and from other cases where the fever lights up an existing latent predisposition to epilepsy.

About 35% of susceptible children will have a second febrile seizure and 15% three or more. Recurrence is more common if the initial convulsion was at a young age or was prolonged. In about 10–20% of children, subsequent neurodevelopment problems are noted, but these usually reflect pre-existing problems and are not brought about by the convulsions. About 2–10% of children with febrile seizures will later develop epilepsy. The risk is higher in those with pre-existing neurodevelopmental dysfunction. It has been proposed that febrile convulsions sometimes cause hippocampal sclerosis, and by this mechanism subsequent TLE, particularly if the febrile convulsion was prolonged or severe; how frequently this occurs is unknown.

Causes of epilepsy

Epilepsy is a multifactorial condition, and even if there is a predominant cause, genetic and environmental factors often play a part in its development and manifestations. The range of causes differs in different age groups, patient groups and geographical locations. Broadly speaking, genetic, congenital and perinatal conditions are the most common causes of early childhood onset epilepsy, whereas in adult life, epilepsy is more likely to be result from external non-genetic causes, but this distinction is by no means absolute. In late adult life vascular disease is increasingly common. In certain parts of the world, endemic infections such as malaria or cysticercosis are common causes.

A classification of causes is shown in Table 7.6 and the approximate frequencies of different aetiologies in a typical Western population are shown in Table 7.7.

Table 7.6 Aetiological classification of epilepsy.

Main category	Subcategory	Examples of aetiology
Idiopathic epilepsy	Pure epilepsies due to single-gene disorders	Benign familial neonatal convulsions; autosomal dominant nocturnal frontal lobe epilepsy; generalised epilepsy with febrile seizures plus; severe myoclonic epilepsy of childhood; benign adult familial myoclonic epilepsy
	Pure epilepsies with complex inheritance	Idiopathic generalised epilepsy (and its subtypes); benign partial epilepsies of childhood
Symptomatic epilepsy – of predominately genetic or developmental causation	Progressive myoclonic epilepsies	Unverricht–Lundborg disease; dentato-rubro-pallido-luysian atrophy; Lafora body disease; mitochondrial cytopathy; sialidosis; neuronal ceroid lipofuscinosis; myoclonus renal failure syndrome
	Neurocutaneous syndromes	Tuberous sclerosis; neurofibromatosis; Sturge–Weber syndrome
	Other single-gene disorders	Angelman syndrome; lysosomal disorders; neuro-acanthocytosis; organic acidurias and peroxisomal disorders; prophyria; pyridoxine-dependent epilepsy; Rett syndrome; urea cycle disorders; Wilson's disease; disorders of cobalamin and folate metabolism
	Disorders of chromosome structure	Down's syndrome; fragile X syndrome; 4p-syndrome; isodicentric chromosome 15; ring chromosome 20
	Developmental anomalies of cerebral structure	Hemimegalencephaly; focal cortical dysplasia; agyria-pachygyria-band spectrum; agenesis of corpus callosum; polymicrogyria; schizencephaly; periventricular nodular heterotopia; microcephaly; arachnoid cyst
Symptomatic epilepsy – of predominately acquired causation	Hippocampal sclerosis	Hippocampal sclerosis
	Perinatal and infantile causes	Neonatal seizures; post-neonatal seizures; cerebral palsy; vaccination and immunisation
	Cerebral trauma	Open head injury; closed head injury; neurosurgery; epilepsy after epilepsy surgery; non-accidental head injury in infants
	Cerebral tumour	Glioma; ganglioglioma and hamartoma; DNET; hypothalamic hamartoma; meningioma; secondary tumours
	Cerebral infection	Viral meningitis and encephalitis; bacterial meningitis and abscess; malaria; neurocysticercosis, tuberculosis; HIV
	Cerebrovascular disorders	Cerebral haemorrhage; cerebral infarction; degenerative vascular disease; arteriovenous malformation; cavernous haemangioma
	Cerebral immunologic disorders	Rasmussen's encephalitis; SLE and collagen vascular disorders; inflammatory and immunological disorders
	Degenerative and other neurologic conditions	Alzheimer's disease and other dementing disorders; multiple sclerosis and demyelinating disorders; hydrocephalus and porencephaly
Provoked epilepsy	Provoking factors	Fever; menstrual cycle and catamenial epilepsy; sleep–wake cycle; metabolic and endocrine-induced seizures; drug-induced seizures; alcohol and toxin-induced seizures
	Reflex epilepsies	Photosensitive epilepsies; startle-induced epilepsies; reading epilepsy; auditory-induced epilepsy; eating epilepsy; hot-water epilepsy
Cryptogenic epilepsies		

DNET, dysembryoplastic neuroepithelial tumour; SLE, systemic lupus erythematosus.

Table 7.7 Causes of epilepsy and approximate frequency.

Cause	Frequency (%)*
Cryptogenic – unknown presumed symptomatic basis	20–40
Idiopathic – unknown presumed genetic basis	10–20
Provoked – predominate provoking factor	5–20
Symptomatic	
vascular	5–10
perinatal	5–10
neurodegenerative	5–10
hippocampal sclerosis	5–10
neoplasm	5–10
trauma	5–10
infection	1–5
immunological	1–5
developmental anomalies	1–5
neurocutaneous, progressive myoclonic epilepsy, single gene disorders, chromosomal	1–3
Provoked – reflex epilepsy	1–3

* Indicative prevalent frequency in different general clinical settings.

Idiopathic epilepsy

Idiopathic epilepsy is defined as an epilepsy of predominately genetic or presumed genetic origin and in which there is no gross neuroanatomic or neuropathologic abnormalities nor other relevant underlying disease. Although the 'idiopathic' epilepsies are likely to have a strong genetic basis, in most cases epigenetic and epistatic factors, and developmental aspects are probably as important as any individual genetic change in the clinical expression of the condition. Single gene disorders probably underlie only 1–2% of all epilepsies, and usually in these conditions there are additional neurological or systemic features (Table 7.8).

Pure epilepsies resulting from single gene disorder

There is a small number of rare conditions in which epilepsy is the main or only manifestation that is Mendelian in its inheritance pattern. These include the following conditions.

Benign familial neonatal convulsions which start in the first 10 days of life and which usually remit spontaneously, although 10% of patients develop subsequent epilepsy. This is an autosomal dominant condition resulting from mutations of voltage-gated potassium channel genes *KCNQ2* and *KCNQ3*.

Autosomal dominant nocturnal frontal lobe epilepsy (ADNFLE) is caused by mutations in the α_4 and β_2 subunits of the nicotinic acetylcholine receptor. In this condition, frontal lobe complex partial seizures occur exclusively during sleep, sometimes each night and sometimes many times during the night. The seizures are brief, lasting less than 1 minute, and are clustered around the onset and end of sleep. The seizures can be misdiagnosed as parasomnias or even dissociative seizures (in spite of the fact that dissociative seizures never arise from sleep), and are not uncommonly resistant to therapy.

Generalised epilepsy with febrile seizures (GEFS+) is a more heterogeneous form of epilepsy, inherited in an autosomal dominant

Table 7.8 Some single-gene disorders causing epilepsy.

Acute intermittent porphyria
Aminoacidurias (phenylketonuria, maple syrup urine disease, glutaric acidaemia type 1)
Angelman's disease
Arginino-succinicaciduria
Biotinidase deficiency
Carnitine palmitoyltransferase 11 deficiency
Chorea-acanthocytosis (neuro-acanthocytosis)
Cortical dysplasias (e.g. agenesis of the corpus callosum, agyria pachygyria band spectrum, peri-ventricular heterotopia, schizencephaly)
Creatinine synthetase deficiencies
DRPLA
Familial cavernoma
Gangliosidoses (various subtypes) (infantile GM1, GM2)
Glucocerebrosidase deficiency (Gaucher's disease)
GLUT-1 deficiency
Hexosaminindase A deficiency
Huntington's disease
Isovaleric acidaemia
Lafora body disease
Lysosomal storage diseases (e.g. Gaucher's disease, Niemann–Pick disease, sialidoses)
Menkes disease
Mitochondrial diseases (including MERFF, MELAS, Alper's disease, MNGIE)
Mucopolysaccharidoses (various subtypes)
Neuronal ceroid lipofuscinoses (NCL, various subtypes)
Non-ketotic hyperglycinaemia
Organic acidurias (e.g. methylmalonic aciduria, glutaric aciduria, propionic aciduria)
Peroxisomal enzyme deficiencies (various types, e.g. Zellweger syndrome)
Pyridoxamine 5′-phosphate oxidase deficiency
Pyruvate dehydrogenase deficiency
Rett syndrome
Sulfite oxidase deficiency
Neurocutaneous syndromes (e.g. tuberous sclerosis, neurofibromatosis)
Unverricht–Lundborg disease
Urea cycle disorders (e.g. ornithine trans-carbamylase deficiency)
Wolf–Hirschhorn syndrome

List excludes the single gene disorders causing 'pure epilepsy' – see text.
DRPLA, dentato-rubro-pallido-luysian atrophy; MERFF, myoclonic epilepsy with ragged red fibres; MELAS, mitochondrial myopathy, encephalopathy, lactic acidosis and stroke; MNGIE, mitochondrial neurogastrointestinal encephalopathy syndrome; NCL, neuronal ceroid lipofuscinosis.

fashion, with age-specific manifestations and variable penetrance. Febrile seizures are the most constant feature, in which seizures are precipitated by fever and tend to occur throughout childhood, but other afebrile seizures also occur. The phenotype is wide and it is arguable whether this condition deserves to be categorised as a syndrome. Various mutations underlying the epilepsy in these families have been identified in the α or β subunits of the voltage-gated sodium channel genes *SCN1A* and *SCN1B*, and γ_2 subunit of the $GABA_a$ receptor.

Dravet's syndrome (severe myoclonic epilepsy of infancy, SMEI) is a severe epilepsy, developing in early life and with a poor prognosis. Most cases have mutations in the *SCNIA* gene, the same gene that causes the more benign GEFS+, and indeed there are families in which both phenotypes coexist. Seizures occur between the ages of 2 and 9 months, and are often prolonged clonic or tonic–clonic seizures, and are precipitated by fever or even hot baths. Myoclonic seizures develop later and episodes of non-convulsive status epilepticus are common. The prognosis is generally poor with intractable epilepsy, early death, severe retardation or institutionalisation in most patients, but milder cases do occur and sometimes the Dravet mutation is found in patients with less severe epilepsy presenting in adult life.

Pure epilepsies with complex inheritance

These are much more common than the single gene epilepsies. These are divided into idiopathic generalised epilepsies and benign partial epilepsies of childhood, and the more common forms (syndromes) were decribed earlier. Although presumed to have a genetic basis, no common susceptibility genes have yet been identified and almost certainly their clinical forms are dependent on epigenetic and epistatic factors and developmental aspects. To what extent other cryptogenic epilepsies have a genetic basis is less clear (including crypogenic febrile convulsions, cryptogenic West's syndrome, cryptogenic Lennox–Gastaut syndrome). There is often no strong family history in any of these conditions.

Symptomatic epilepsy

Symptomatic epilepsy is defined as an epilepsy predominately caused by a gross neuroanatomical or neuropathological abnormality or a relevant systemic disease, which can be acquired or genetic in origin. Almost any condition affecting the cerebral grey matter can result in epilepsy. The epilepsy usually takes a partial or secondarily generalised form and, in most causative conditions, the epilepsy does not have any particularly distinctive features.

Some symptomatic epilepsies are genetic or congenital in origin, for instance congenital and innate causes of epilepsy which are developmental or genetic (examples include some of the cortical dysplasias, neurocutaneous syndromes, monogenic diseases, chromosomal disorders and progressive myoclonic epilepsies). At least 240 single gene and chromosomal disorders result in neurological disorders in which epilepsy is part of the phenotype. Most are rare or very rare and manifest initially in childhood. Many are inborn errors of metabolism.

After an acute cerebral event, the epilepsy is often divided into 'early' (i.e. seizures occurring within a week of the insult) and 'late' (i.e. epilepsy developing later). There is often a 'silent period' between the injury and the onset of late epilepsy, and the nature of the epileptogenic processes occurring during this period is largely unknown. The occurrence of a silent period raises the possibility that neuroprotective interventions to inhibit these processes could prevent later epilepsy, but to date no effective neuroprotectant agent is available. Antiepileptic drug therapy will prevent early epilepsy but does not reduce the frequency of late seizures. Early seizures are caused by the acute disturbance and have different mechanisms, and are often not followed by late epilepsy – a fact important to emphasise to patients.

Inborn errors of metabolism

Seizures are sometimes the presenting features of inborn errors of metabolism. There are many examples and an increasing number are treatable, especially if detected early.

Epilepsies resulting from inborn errors of metabolism in the neonatal period or early infancy are pyridoxine deficiency, pyridoxamine 5′-phosphate oxidase deficiency, folinic acid-responsive seizures, biotinidase deficiency, GLUT1 deficiency, non-ketotic hyperglycinaemia, series biosynthetase defects, sulfite oxidase deficiencies, Menkes disease, defects of peroxisomal function and beta-oxidation, disorders of glycosylation and infantile neuronal ceroid lipofuscinosis (Chapter 19).

Epilepsies usually presenting in late infancy or early childhood include creatinine synthetase defects, the early causes of progressive myoclonic epilepsy (sialidosis, mitochondrial diseases, neuronal ceroid lipofuscinosis), mitrochondrial disease (especially *POLG1* defects), gangliosidoses, disorders of glycosylation, and peridoxine and pyridoxamine 5′-phosphate oxidase deficiencies.

Epilepsies presenting in adolescence or late childhood include causes of progressive myoclonic epilepsy, Lafora body disease, myoclonic epilepsy with ragged red fibres (MERRF), mitrochondrial disorders, Unverricht–Lundborg disease, late-onset forms of neuronal ceroid lipofuscinoses, late-onset GM1 gangliosidosis (such as Tay–Sachs disease and Gaucher type III), lysosomal storage disease (e.g. Niemann–Pick) and peroxisomal disorders.

Most of these inborn errors of metabolism are single gene disorders, although sometimes a wide variety of mutations in a gene, or even mutations in different genes, can cause a similar phenotype. Most are associated with mental handicap, often severe, and with regression if untreated. Many have associated clinical signs and other congenital anomalies or dysmorphologies, and many are associated with limited lifespan. As genetic understanding advances it is also clear that the phenotype of many conditions is wider than previously realised, and occasional mild cases can present late.

Some of these conditions are treatable, and early detection and therapy in some will prevent regression and deterioration. The treatable causes include pyridoxine deficiency, pyridoxamine 5′-phosphate oxidase deficiency, folinic acid-responsive seizures, biotinidase deficiency, GLUT1 deficiency, non-ketotic hyperglycinaemia, series biosynthetase defects, sulfite oxidase deficiencies, Menkes disease and some aminocidurias.

The investigation of these conditions is discussed in Chapter 19, and also further on in this chapter 'Investigation of epilepsy'.

Progressive myoclonic epilepsy

This form of epilepsy can be caused by various genetically determined neurological disorders (Table 7.9). In most parts of the world, the four most common are mitochondrial diseases, Unverricht–Lundborg disease, dentato-rubro-pallido-luysian atrophy (DRPLA) and Lafora body disease.

Unverricht–Lundborg disease (Baltic myoclonus) is the most benign form. It is an autosomal recessive disorder resulting from dodecamer repeats in the *EPM1* gene coding for the cystatin B protein, a protease inhibitor. The condition is particularly common in

Table 7.9 Causes of progressive myoclonic epilepsy (PME).

Most common causes
Baltic myoclonus (Unverricht–Lundborg disease)
Ceroid lipofuscinoses
DRPLA
Lafora body disease
Mitochondrial disease (MERRF)
Sialidoses
Rarer causes
Alper's disease
Alzheimer's disease
Biotin-responsive progressive myoclonus
Coeliac disease
Gaucher's disease
GM2 gangliosidosis (juvenile type)
Hexosaminidase deficiency
Huntington's disease
Juvenile neuroaxonal dystrophy
Menkes disease
Non-ketotic hyperglycinaemia
Phenylketonuria
Tetrahydrobiopterin deficiencies

In a significant proportion of patients, no cause can be identified.
DRPLA, dentato-rubro-pallido-luysian atrophy; MERFF, myoclonic epilepsy with ragged red fibres.

Finland (where the incidence is in excess of 1/20 000 persons) and other Scandinavian countries as a result of founder effects. Myoclonus develops, usually between the ages of 6 and 15 years, and the condition slowly progresses. Ataxia and tremor later become major clinical features. There is a very slow intellectual decline.

DRPLA is inherited in an autosomal dominant fashion. It is particularly common in Japan (a frequency of 0.2–0.7/100 000 persons) and northern Europe. It is a triplet repeat disorder involving the *DRPLA* gene which is of uncertain function. The condition presents in childhood or adult life and is slowly progressive. Ataxia, choreoathetosis, dementia and behavioural changes, myoclonus and epilepsy occur.

Lafora body disease is an autosomal recessive condition, most common in southern Europe, and characterised by Lafora bodies, periodic acid–Schiff (PAS) positive intracellular polyglucosan inclusions found in neurones, sweat glands and elsewhere. The age of onset is 6–19 years and patients develop progressive myoclonic, tonic–clonic and partial seizures. There is also a progressive and severe dementia, and ataxia and dysarthria also occur. Death occurs within 2–10 years. Up to 80% of patients have a mutation in the *EPM2A* gene, which codes for Laforin, a tyrosine phosphatase protein. A second gene, *EPM2B,* has been identified, which codes for Malin, a ubiquitin ligase protein.

Mitochondrial cytopathy (MERRF) is one of the phenotypes of mitochondrial cytopathy. In 90% of cases, the genetic defect is an A–G transition at nucleotide-8344 in the $tRNA^{lys}$ gene of mtDNA, and some other cases are caused by *T8356C* or *G8363A* mutations. This is a multi-system disorder with a very variable phenotype in which myoclonic seizures are often the first symptom, followed by generalised epilepsy, myopathy, ataxia and dementia. Heteroplasmy is responsible for some of the phenotypic variation.

Epilepsies in neurocutaneous syndromes

The neurocutaneous conditions often result in epilepsy. Tuberous sclerosis complex, Sturge–Weber syndrome and neurofibromatosis (type 1) are the most important. Other rare conditions causing epilepsy include hypomelanosis of Ito, epidermal naevus syndrome (Jadassohn's syndrome), hereditary haemorrhagic telangiectasia, midline linear naevus syndrome, incontinentia pigmenti and Klippel–Trenaunay–Weber syndrome.

Tuberous sclerosis This is a not uncommon condition (1/5800 live births in some studies) and there is a high spontaneous mutation rate (1/25 000). It is inherited in an autosomal dominant fashion. To date, about 300 unique *TSC1* or *TSC2* mutations have been identified. The clinical features of the condition are variable. Epilepsy is the presenting symptom in 80% or more of patients. It can take the form of neonatal seizures, West's syndrome, Lennox–Gastaut syndrome or as adult onset partial or generalised seizures. About two-thirds of patients present before the age of 2 years, with motor seizures, drop attacks or infantile spasms. About 25% of all cases of West's syndrome are caused by tuberous sclerosis. The skin is abnormal in almost all patients, and skin lesions include hypomelanotic macules (87–100% of patients), facial angiofibromas (47–90%), shagreen patches (20–80%), fibrous facial plaques and subungual fibromas (17–87%). CNS tumours are the leading cause of morbidity and mortality. The brain lesions can be distinguished on the basis of magnetic resonance imaging (MRI) studies and comprise: subependymal glial nodules (90% of cases), cortical tubers (70% of cases) and subependymal giant cell astrocytomas (6–14% of cases). Fifty per cent of patients have developmental delay or mental retardation. An estimated 80% of children with tuberous sclerosis have identifiable renal tumours by the age of 10 years. Lesions also appear elsewhere and cardiac and retinal lesions are common.

Sturge–Weber syndrome This is an uncommon sporadic developmental disorder, of uncertain causation. The cardinal features are a unilateral or bilateral port wine naevus, epilepsy, hemiparesis, mental impairment and ocular signs. The port wine naevus is usually but not exclusively in the distribution of the trigeminal nerve. It can cross the midline and spread into the upper cervical dermatomes. In one-third of cases the naevus is bilateral. The epilepsy can be focal or generalised. It is often the earliest symptom, and most patients with Sturge–Weber develop seizures within the first year of life (at least 70%) and almost all have developed epilepsy before the age of 4 years. Adult onset epilepsy can occur occasionally. The early seizures are often triggered by fever. The seizures take the form of partial or multi-focal attacks often with frequent and severe secondary generalisation. Convulsive status occurs in over half of cases. Seizures developing in the neonatal period can be very difficult to control and carry a poor prognosis. The hemiplegia and mental impairment deteriorate in a stepwise fashion following a severe bout of seizures, and this is one of the few situations where clear-cut cerebral damage results directly from epileptic attacks, presumably by ischaemic or excitotoxic mechanisms. Severe learning disability is now less common because of better control of the epilepsy. Status epilepticus particularly often results in a permanent and significant worsening of the neurological deficit. The epilepsy should be aggressively treated to prevent neurological deterioration. Resective surgery (either lesionectomy, hemispherectomy or lobectomy) should be given early consideration.

Cortical dysplasia

Cortical dysplasia (*syn*: cortical dysgenesis, malformations of cortical development) is a term that is applied to developmental disorders of the cortex producing structural cerebral change. In some cases the cause is unknown, but others are caused by identifiable genetic abnormalities and some by environmental influences such as infection, trauma, hypoxia, exposure to drugs or toxins. The clinical features vary, but epilepsy and learning disability are the most common manifestations. Cortical dysplasia is the underlying cause of the epilepsy in up to 30% of children and 10% of adults referred to epilepsy centres with intractable epilepsy. It includes the following conditions.

Hemimegalencephaly In this condition, one cerebral hemisphere is enlarged and is structurally abnormal with thickened cortex, reduced sulcation and poor or absent laminar organisation. Giant neurones are found throughout the brain and in 50% of cases balloon cells too. The condition can occur in isolation, associated with other cortical dysplasias or as part of other syndromes (notably tuberous sclerosis or other rarer neurocutaneous syndromes). Hemimegalencephaly results in severe epilepsy with learning disability, hemiplegia and hemianopia. Surgical therapy (hemispherectomy or hemispherotomy) can cure the epilepsy.

Focal cortical dysplasia There are a variety of subtypes, with different histological appearances influenced by the time of formation at different stages of embryogenesis. In some the cortical lamination is normal, but in others there may be associated widespread macrogyria and polymicrogyria. Epilepsy is the leading symptom, and other clinical features depend on the extent of the lesion and include learning disability and focal deficits.

Schizencephaly This term denotes the presence of clefts in the cortex, stretching from the surface to the ventricle. Schizencephaly can be unilateral or bilateral and is often peri-sylvian in location. The causes are heterogeneous, and include germline mutations of the homeobox gene *EMX2* and environmental insults during development including radiation, infection and ischaemia. Epilepsy is the most common symptom (over 90% of cases), associated usually but by no means always with learning disability or cognitive changes. Focal neurological deficit is common in extensive or bilateral cases.

Agyria pachygyria band spectrum (lissencephaly, pachygyria, agyria and subcortical band heterotopia) These abnormalities of cortical gyration are grouped together as they show an interconnected genetic basis. In all the gyration is simplified and the cortex is thickened. Lissencephaly (literally, smooth brain) is the most severe form, in which gyration is grossly diminished or even absent. Subcortical band heterotopia (*syn*: double cortex syndrome) denotes the presence of a band of grey matter sandwiched by white matter below the cortical grey matter. The band may be thin or thick, and can merge with overlying cortex in which case the cortex takes a macrogryic form. It is caused in about 80% of cases by germline deletions in the DCX (*XLIS*) gene and occurs almost always (but not exclusively) in females. The pachygyria and bands are anteriorly predominant. The genetic anomaly in the other 20% of cases has not been identified.

Macrogyria refers to thickened cortex, and can occur as an isolated phenomenon, is variable in extent and when focal is indistinguishable on clinical or imaging grounds from some forms of focal cortical dysplasia. Isolated lissencephaly is present in 12 per million live births and results in profound retardation, epilepsy and spastic quadrapareisis. In less severe cases, where the lissencephaly is restricted to one region of the brain (albeit usually bilaterally, with an anterior or posterior gradient), the epilepsy and learning disability may be mild. Of cases of isolated lissencephaly, 60–80% are caused by identifiable mutations in the *LIS1* or *XLIS* (also known as the DCX) genes, on 17p13.3 and Xq22.3-q24, respectively, and in 40% the entire gene is deleted. Other forms of lissencephaly have more widespread associations. The best known is the Miller–Dieker syndrome, caused by large deletions of *LIS1* and of several other contiguous genes on 17p13.3, in which the lissencephaly is associated with epilepsy, facial dysmorphism, microcephaly, small mandible, failure to thrive, retarded motor development, dysphagia, decorticate and decerebrate postures. All these conditions usually present in children with epilepsy and learning disability. The clinical severity of the syndrome seems to correlate with the extent of the cerebral anomaly.

Agenesis of the corpus callosum This anomaly occurs in various genetic and congenital disorders. Epilepsy is invariable and is the leading symptom. In Aicardi's syndrome, the corpus callosum agenesis is associated with peri-ventricular heterotopia, thin unlayered cortex and diffuse polymicrogyria.

Polymicrogyria The appearance of small and prominent gyri, separated by shallow sulci, is known as polymicrogyria. It can have a genetic or environmental cause. Epilepsy is the leading clinical feature, associated with learning disability and focal neurological signs and the manifestations vary greatly in severity. Bilateral peri-sylvian polymicrogyria (Kuzniecky syndrome) is a condition in which there is severe upper motor neurone bulbar dysfunction and diplegia as well as severe epilepsy and mental retardation.

Periventricular nodular heterotopia (syn: bilateral peri-ventricular nodular heterotopia, subependymal nodular heterotopia) In this condition, subependymal nodules of grey matter are present, usually bilateral and located along the supralateral walls of the lateral ventricles. It is much more common in females, inherited in an X-linked dominant fashion and many (but not all) of the cases have shown mutations in the *FLN1* (filamin-1) gene. Bilateral peri-ventricular nodular heterotopia usually has a genetic origin, but unilateral cases often do not and are presumably caused by intrauterine vascular or other congenital insults. The clinical presentation can vary from mild epilepsy presenting in older children or young adults to severe infantile or childhood partial epilepsy.

Hippocampal sclerosis

Hippocampal sclerosis is the most common cause of mesial temporal lobe epilepsy which is itself the most common form of partial epilepsy. It is found in over one-third of patients with refractory focal epilepsy attending hospital clinics in whom there is no other structural lesion, but is less frequent in those with mild epilepsy. Hippocampal sclerosis typically is associated with complex partial seizures. There is a clear association with a history of childhood febrile convulsions, and it has been proposed that the febrile convulsions, especially if prolonged or complex, result in hippocampal sclerosis which itself results in subsequent TLE. Serial MRI studies have demonstrated that status epilepticus also can result in hippocampal sclerosis and there is clear evidence from animal experimentation that prolonged partial seizures can cause hippocampal damage and in some cases progression of the hippocampal atrophy and worsening seizures. In other cases, hippocampal sclerosis may be a congenital lesion, and hippocampal sclerosis can also occur after severe brain trauma or vascular damage.

Cerebral palsy, perinatal and prenatal injury

Cerebral palsy is a non-specific term that covers many prenatal and peri-natal pathologies. It is strongly associated with epilepsy. In the US National Collaborative Perinatal Project, a prospective cohort study of infants followed to the age of 7 years, epilepsy was found to occur in 34% of children with cerebral palsy, and cerebral palsy was present in 19% of children developing epilepsy. In the same cohort, the risk of learning disability (associated with cerebral palsy) was 5.5 times higher among children developing epilepsy following a febrile seizure than in children with a febrile seizure alone. Learning disability (IQ <70) is present in 27% of children with epilepsy, and seizures are present in about 50% of children with mental retardation and cerebral palsy. In case-controlled studies, only severe perinatal insults have been found to increase the risk of subsequent epilepsy (examples are perinatal haemorrhage and ischaemic hypoxic encephalopathy). Factors such as pre-eclampsia, eclampsia, forceps delivery, being born with the 'cord round the neck', low birth weight or prematurity have only a very modest association, if any, with the presence of subsequent epilepsy.

Post-vaccination encephalopathy

The role of vaccination (notably pertussis vaccination) in causing a childhood encephalopathy and subsequent epilepsy and learning disability has been the subject of intense study. The UK National Childhood Encephalopathy Study found that children hospitalised with seizures and encephalopathy were more likely to have received DTP (diptheria, tetanus, pertussis) vaccination in the previous 7 days than control children. Although potential methodological biases of this study have been severely criticised, the results from this and other studies have led many authorities to accept that there is a small risk of encephalopathy after pertussis vaccine. Another large study of 368 000 children found no excess risk. Similarly, suggestions that MMR (mumps, measles, rubella) vaccine increases the risks of autism and epilepsy are now thought to be unfounded.

A recent study has shown that many cases of so-called post-vaccination encephalopathy carry the causal mutation of Dravet syndrome (usually an SCN1A mutation) and so the vaccination simply precipitates the encephalopathy which was in all likelihood going to develop anyway.

Thus, conventional medical advice is now that vaccination is safe, and although a small number of children do develop encephalopathic reactions that result in later epilepsy, this number is considerably less than the risk of encephalopathy after the naturally occurring viral illnesses that vaccination prevents. The vaccines that have been thought to be associated with post-vaccination encephalomyelitis are smallpox, measles, DTP, Japanese B encephalitis and rabies.

Cerebral tumour

About 6% of all newly diagnosed cases of epilepsy are caused by cerebral tumours, with the incidence of tumour higher in adults than in children. Seizures occur in about 50% of all brain tumours. Tumours of the frontal and temporal regions are more likely to cause epilepsy than other cortical tumours and epilepsy is rare in subcortical or cerebellar tumours.

Gliomas are most common brain tumour causing epilepsy, and low grade gliomas are more epileptogenic than high grade tumours. Overall, slow-growing or benign tumours account for about 10% of all adult-onset epilepsies. There can be a history of epilepsy for many years. In chronic refractory tumoural epilepsy, oligodendrogliomas account for 10–30%, dysembryoplastic neuroepithelial tumours (DNETs) for 10–30%, astrocytomas for 10–30%, gangliogliomas for about 10–20% and hamartomas for 10–20%. The epilepsy in all, except the DNETs, arises in the surrounding tissue and not the substance of the tumour and this can have implications for surgical therapy. Epileptogenesis can be caused by impaired vascularisation of the surrounding cortex, changes in the excitatory and inhibitory synapisis or other morphological changes.

Ganglioglioma are mixed developmental tumours that are composed of neoplastic glial and neuronal cell types and comprise around 10% of the neoplasms removed at temporal lobectomy. Seizures are the primary presenting symptom in 80–90%. The dysembryoplastic neuroepithelial tumour (DNET or DNT) is a pathological entity only recently differentiated from other forms of 'benign gliomas' and accounts for 10–30% of resected tumours in the temporal lobe. They are benign tumours with only a slight propensity for growth, and epilepsy is usually the only clinical symptom. As these are developmental in origin, they have instrinsic epileptogenesis (in contrast to other cerebral tumours) and are important to identify as partial resection will often control the seizures. Hamartomas are benign tumours which account for 15–20% of tumours removed at temporal lobectomy. These are more common in children.

The hypothalamic hamartoma is usually a benign tumour, confined to the tuber cinereum, which characteristically presents with gelastic seizures, learning disability, behavioural disturbance and later with precocious puberty. The lesions are subtle and can be very easily missed on even high-quality MRI scanning. Gelastic seizures are characteristic of hypothalamic hamartoma but do occur in other midline lesions and also occasionally in TLE. The attacks take the form of sudden laughter associated with other variable motor features (clonic movements, head and eye deviation). The laughter is 'mirthless', in other words not associated with any emotional feelings of joy or happiness, and occurs in situations that do not provoke humour.

Meningiomas are also common causes of adult epilepsy, and epilepsy is the presenting symptom of the tumour in 20–50% of cases. Meningiomas are more likely to cause epilepsy when located over the convexity, parasagittal/falx and sphenoid ridge, or if there is peri-tumoural oedema. There is no relationship between the presence of epilepsy and histological type.

Cerebrovascular disease

Stroke is the most commonly identified cause of epilepsy presenting over the age of 50 years, and occult stroke also explains the occurrence of other cases of apparently cryptogenic late onset epilepsy.

A history of stroke has been found to be associated with an increased lifetime occurrence of epilepsy (OR 3.3; 95% CI 1.3–8.5).

About 5–10% of patients with cerebral haemorrhage develop late epilepsy. The incidence of early epilepsy (seizures in the first week) is higher, up to 30% in some series and about one-third of those with early seizures continue to have a liability to epilepsy. Epilepsy is more common after large haemorrhages and haemorrhages that involve the cerebral cortex and almost always develops within 2 years of the haemorrhage. After cerebral infarction, epilepsy occurs in about 6% of patients within 12 months and 11% within 5 years of the stroke. Epilepsy is more common in cerebral infarcts located in the anterior hemisphere, and involving cortex. Epilepsy can also complicate occult cerebrovascular disease. Late onset epilepsy can be the first manifestation of cerebrovascular disease and, in the absence of other causes, newly developing seizures after the age of 40 years should prompt an urgent screen for vascular risk factors.

Epilepsy develops in 6–15% of survivors of subarachnoid haemorrhage caused by ruptured intracranial aneurysm, with a higher incidence in those with haematoma and cerebral infarction, disability on discharge, and those who have required an external ventricular drain or shunt or surgical treatment.

Arteriovenous malformation

An arteriovenous malformation (AVM) is a congenital malformation comprising a network of arterial and venous channels communicating directly with each other. Between 17% and 36% of supratentorial AVMs present with seizures, with or without associated neurological deficits, and 40–50% with haemorrhage. Smaller AVMs (<3 cm diameter) are more likely to present with haemorrhage than large ones. Conversely, large and/or superficial malformations are more epileptogenic, as are AVMs in the temporal lobe. About 40% of patients with large AVMs have epilepsy, and epilepsy is the presenting symptom in about 20%. The annual risk of bleeding of an AVM is in the region of 2–4% per year, irrespective of whether the malformation presented with haemorrhage, and the average mortality about 1% per year. Venous malformations are congenital anomalies of normal venous drainage and these have a very low risk of haemorrhage or epilepsy.

Cavernous haemangioma (cavernoma)

Cavernous haemangiomas account for 5–13% of vascular malformations of the CNS. At least 15–20% of patients remain symptom-free throughout their lives. Patients present with seizures (40–70%), focal neurological deficits (35–50%), non-specific headaches (10–30%) and cerebral hemorrhage. The seizures are typically partial in nature and often brief, infrequent and minor in form. Family histories can be found in about 10–30% of cavernous haemangiomas, and three different genes (or loci) have been identified. The most common gene with causative mutations is *KRIT1*. This gene contains 16 coding exons and is located on chromosome 7q21.2. Loss of function mutations result in the formation of cavernoma. The other identified genes are *MGC4607* and *PDCD10*, and there are some families without evidence of mutations in any of these three genes and in whom the genetic defect remains obscure.

Other vascular lesions

Cortical venous infarcts are particularly epileptogenic, at least in the acute phase, and may underlie a significant proportion of apparently spontaneous epileptic seizures complicating other medical conditions and pregnancy for instance. Seizures occur in several connective tissue disorders and in patients with cerebral vasculitis. The most commonly encountered is systemic lupus erythematosus. Seizures also occur with cerebrovascular lesions secondary to rheumatic heart disease, endocarditis, mitral valve prolapse, cardiac tumours and cardiac arrhythmia, or after carotid endarcterectomy. Epilepsy is also common in eclampsia, hypertensive encephalopathy and malignant hypertension and in the anoxic encephalopathy that follows cardiac arrest or cardiopulmonary surgery. Unruptured aneurysms can cause epilepsy, especially if large and if embedded in the temporal lobe.

Dementia and degenerative disorders

Epilepsy is a common feature of degenerative neurological disease that involves the grey matter, but is seldom a leading symptom in pure leukodystrophy.

The most common neurodegenerative disorders are the dementias in late life. Six per cent of persons over the age of 65 years have dementia, and the rate increases exponentially as a function of age. Alzheimer's disease is the most common cause of dementia, and patients with Alzheimer's disease are six times more likely to develop epilepsy than age-matched controls. Partial and secondarily generalised seizures occur, and are usually relatively easily treated with conventional antiepileptic therapy. Myoclonus is another common finding in patients with Alzheimer's disease, occurring in about 10% of autopsy-verified cases and is a late manifestation. Five per cent of patients with Huntington's disease have epilepsy, usually in the later stages. Epilepsy is more common in the juvenile type, and occasionally takes the form of a progressive myoclonic epilepsy. Epilepsy, and indeed status epilepticus, can be the presenting feature of Creutzfeldt–Jakob disease (CJD). Generalised tonic–clonic or partial seizures occur in 10% of established cases, and myoclonus in 80%, and can be induced by startle or other stimuli.

Post-traumatic epilepsy

Head trauma is an important cause of epilepsy. It is customary to draw a distinction between open head injury, where the dura is breached, and closed head injury, where there is no dural breach. Post-traumatic seizures are traditionally subdivided into immediate, early and late categories. Immediate seizures are defined as those that occur within the first 24 hours after injury, early seizures are those that occur within the first week and late seizures occur after 1 week.

Closed head injuries are most common in civilian practice, usually from road traffic accidents, falls or recreational injuries, and in different series have accounted for 2–12% of all cases of epilepsy. Traumatic brain injury in the United States has been estimated to have an incidence of 825 cases per 100 000 per year, with about 100–200 per 100 000 per year admitted to hospital. Early seizures after closed head injury occur in about 2–6% of those admitted to hospital, with a higher frequency in children than in adults. Early seizures have not been found generally to be an independent predictive risk factor of late seizures. Of patients requiring hospitalisation for closed head trauma, 2–5% will subsequently develop epilepsy (late post-traumatic seizures). Mild head injury – defined as head injury without skull fracture and with less than 30 minutes of post-traumatic amnesia – is, in most studies, not associated with any markedly increased risk of epilepsy. Moderate head injury – defined as a head injury complicated by skull fracture or post-traumatic amnesia for more than 30 minutes – is followed by epilepsy in about 1–4% of cases. Severe head injury – defined as a head injury with post-traumatic amnesia of more than 24 hours, intracranial haematoma or cerebral contusion – is followed by epilepsy, in most studies, in about 10–15% of patients. The excess risk of epilepsy is highest during the first year, with the time of onset of epilepsy peaking at 4–8 months post-injury, and diminishes during the ensuing years.

Post-traumatic epilepsy is much more frequent after open head injury. This is particularly so in penetrating wartime injuries, with 30–50% of patients developing subsequent epilepsy. Overall, the risk of late epilepsy, if early epilepsy is present, is about 25% compared to 3% in patients who did not have early seizures. The risk of epilepsy after open head injury is greatest if the extent of cerebral damage is large and involves the frontal or temporal regions.

Calculations of the risk of epilepsy in various circumstances following injury have been made. The presence of a dural breach (e.g. with a depressed fracture), an intracranial haematoma and long post-traumatic amnesia (≥24 hours) have been found consistently to increase significantly the risk of subsequent epilepsy. In one series, the risk of seizures by 2 years was 27% in the presence of depressed skull fracture, 24% with subdural haematoma (and 44% if this was severe enough to need surgical evacuation), 23% with intracranial haematoma and 12% with long post-traumatic amnesia.

Antiepileptic drug therapy reduces the risk of early seizures. However, there is no evidence that prophylactic antiepileptic drug treatment after head trauma reduces the long-term risk of epilepsy. It is commomn practice to given antiepileptic drugs for a few weeks after a severe head injury, but then to discontinue the medication if no seizures have occurred.

Epilepsy after neurosurgery

The risk of late postoperative seizures is greater in patients with younger age, early postoperative seizures and severe neurological deficit. The incidence of seizures varies according to the nature of the underlying disease process, its site and extent. A large retrospective study found an overall incidence of 17% for postoperative seizures in 877 consecutive patients undergoing supratentorial neurosurgery for non-traumatic conditions. The patients had no prior history of epilepsy and the minimum follow-up was 5 years. The incidence of seizures ranged from 4% in patients undergoing stereotactic procedures and ventricular drainage to 92% for patients being surgically treated for cerebral abscess. The risk of craniotomy for glioma was 19%, for intracranial haemorrhage 21% and for meningioma removal 22%. All these risks were greatly enhanced if seizures occurred pre-operatively. Among patients developing postoperative seizures, 37% did so within the first postoperative week, 77% within the first year and 92% within the first 2 years. If early seizures occurred (i.e. those occurring in the first week), 41% of patients developed late recurrent seizures.

Studies after unruptured aneurysm show an overall risk of about 14%. The risk of a middle cerebral aneurysm resulting in epilepsy is 19%, and anterior communicating aneurysms and posterior communicating aneurysms carry a risk of about 10%. If the aneurysm has bled, causing an intracranial haematoma, the incidence of epilepsy is higher.

An overall risk of epilepsy following shunt procedures is about 10%, although this depends on the site of the shunt insertion.

It is not clear whether the prophylactic use of anticonvulsants after neurosurgical procedures is worthwhile. Currently, it is usual to prescribe prophylactic anticonvulsant drugs for several months after major supratentorial neurosurgery and then gradually to withdraw the medication unless seizures have occurred.

Bacterial or viral meningitis and encephalitis

CNS infections are a major risk factor for epilepsy. Seizures can be the presenting or the only symptom, or one component of a more diffuse cerebral disorder.

Encephalitis and meningitis result in a sevenfold increase in the rate of chronic epilepsy compared with that in the general population. The increased risk is highest during the first 5 years after infection, but remains elevated for up to 15 years. The risk is much higher after encephalitis (RR 16.2), especially herpes simplex virus 1 (HSV-1) infection, than bacterial meningitis (RR 4.2) or aseptic meningitis (RR 2.3). The incidence of severe HSV-1 encephalitis is about 1 per million persons per year, and seizures are a frequent symptom in the acute phase of severe HSV encephalitis. Most survivors are left with neurological sequelae including severe epilepsy. Epilepsy is also a leading symptom of tuberculoma. In patients presenting simply with epilepsy, it is now usual to treat with antitubercular and antiepileptic drugs (with a short course of adjunctive steroids), and to defer surgery. When medical therapy is initiated without diagnostic confirmation from a biopsy, the patient should be carefully monitored, and if the mass does not decrease in size after 8 weeks of therapy, biopsy should be reconsidered.

Pyogenic brain abscess is an uncommon but serious cause of epilepsy. The estimated annual incidence of brain abscess in the United States is 1/10 000 hospital admissions, and abscess surgery accounts for 0.7% of all neurosurgery operations. Brain abscess can develop in association with a contiguous suppurating process (usually otitis media, sinus disease or mastoiditis, 50%), from haematogenous spread from a distant focus (25%), as a complication of intracranial surgery (15%) and trauma (10%). Commonly isolated organisms are streptococci, including aerobic, anaerobic and microaerophilic types. *Streptococcus pneumoniae* is a rarer cause of brain abscesses, which are often the sequel to occult cerebrospinal fluid (CSF) rhinorrhoea and also to pneumococcal pneumonia in elderly patients. Enteric bacteria and *Bacteroides* are isolated in 20–40% of cases and often in mixed culture. Anaerobic organisms have become increasingly important organisms and in many instances more than a single bacterial species is recovered. Gram-negative bacilli rarely occur alone. Staphylococcal abscesses account for 10–15% of cases and are usually caused by penetrating head injury or bacteraemia secondary to endocarditis. Clostridial infections are most often post-traumatic. Rarely, *Actinomyces* or *Nocardia* are the causative agents in a brain abscess.

Parasitic diseases

Neuro-cysticercosis is the most common parasitic disease of the CNS. Epilepsy is the most common clinical manifestation and usual presenting symptom and neuro-cysticercosis a major cause of epilepsy in endemic areas in parts of Latin America, Asia and West Africa. A solitary cerebral parenchymal lesion is a common form of presentation, but lesions are often multiple. Over time, the cysts shrink progressively and then calcify or disappear completely. Seizures develop when a cyst is degenerating or around a chronic calcified lesion. Where there is a single cyst it is usual to control seizures with antiepileptic drugs and not to use anticysticercal drugs. If anticysticercal drugs are to be used, steroids need to be given in co-medication to prevent sudden rise in intracranial pressure and exacerbation of symptoms.

In endemic regions, a common clinical scenario is the occurrence of a seizure with a single enhancing lesion on CT. The differential diagnosis includes neuro-cysticercosis, tuberculosis, gliomas and other tumours, toxoplasmosis and other infective lesions. Over 90% of the lesions in India are caused by neurocysticercosis, and currently the usual management strategy is to screen the patient for other signs of tuberculosis but if none are present not to give antitubercular therapy. CT is repeated in 12 weeks and if the lesion has not regressed, or has increased, a review of diagnosis including surgical biopsy is the preferred approach. Antiepileptic drugs are given.

Malaria causes a 9–11-fold (95% CI 2–18) increase in the risk of chronic epilepsy – a risk that is at least double the risk of epilepsy after complex febrile seizures.

Inflammatory and immunological disorders

The importance of inflammatory or immunological mechanisms in the precipitation and causation of epilepsy is increasingly being recognised. Inflammatory or immunological reactions can occur in infections or in vascular disease, and also in a range of primarily immunological conditions, in which epilepsy is a prominent feature.

Immune-mediated diseases The most common immunological disease associated with epilepsy is systemic lupus erythematosus (SLE). Seizures are the most frequent neuropsychiatric manifestation, both at disease onset and during the course of the disease, with a frequency ranging from 40% to 85%. In antiphospholipid syndrome, seizures occur in about 9% cases. Seizures also occur less commonly in Kawasaki disease, Henoch–Schönlein purpura, Wegener granulomatosis, in other causes of vasculitis and in scleroderma. Seizures are common in the rare condition of linear scheroderma (Parry–Romberg syndrome). In SLE, the seizures are related to disease activity and can be the only CNS manifestation. Both generalised and focal seizures occur and can be caused either by inflammatory or ischaemic pathologies.

Limbic encephalitis is an increasingly recognised subacute encephalopathic inflammatory disorder of the CNS, sometimes associated with benign or malignant neoplasms, and sometime idiopathic. The first identified condition (in 1960), was Hashimoto encephalitis, but in the last two decades increasing numbers of paraneoplastic and non-paraneoplastic antibodies associated with this condition have been described. Epilepsy occurs in almost all cases of limbic encephalitis regardless of cause. It can vary in form from very slight partial seizures to complex partial seizures or severe generalised seizures. Diagnosis is by MRI, blood and CSF examination and EEG. The range of identifiable antibodies in the serum and CSF includes intracellular antibodies: Hu/ANNA-1, Ma-2, CRMP-5, amphiphysin, glutamic acid decarboxylase (GAD), and extracellular antibodies: voltage gated potassium channel (VGKC) antibodies, *N*-methyl-D-aspartate receptor (NMDAR) antibodies, glycine receptor antibodies, adenylate kinase 5 antibodies, and BR serine/threonine kinase 2 antibodies. Sometimes, epilepsy occurs without encephalopathy associated with VGKC or VGCC, GLu-R3, anti-GAD or anti-GM1 antibodies and in these cases knowing whether the antibodies are pathogenic or not can be difficult.

Hashimoto encephalopathy (now often referred to as STREAT – steroid responsive encephalopathy associated with autoimmune thyroiditis) is one of the most common forms, and is associated with high serum levels of anti-thyroid peroxidase (anti-TPO) antibodies (formerly known as microsomal antibodies). These antibodies are probably not pathogenic but are a marker of some unknown cerebral-binding antibody. As its name suggests, most but not all cases are successfully treated with steroids.

Epilepsy also occurs in inflammatory bowel diseases, including ulcerative colitis, Crohn's disease and Whipple's disease. Ten per cent of people with coeliac disease develop neurological complications including epilepsy, which is often associated with occipital calcification on CT.

Rasmussen encephalitis This is an unusual condition in which chronic inflammation develops slowly and progressively in the cortex of one cerebral hemisphere. It usually begins in childhood although rare adult onset cases are described. The inflammatory process may evolve for up to 10 years or more and the symptoms and signs are usually initially slowly progressive and then eventually stabilise. The cause of the inflammation is quite unclear, but it is presumed to be an autoimmune response, and its remarkable unihemispheric distribution is also completely unexplained. Patients with the condition present with focal and secondarily generalised seizures which can be severe and periods of epilepsia partialis continua (EPC) are common. Associated with the seizures is progressive loss of motor and cognitive skills and speech (if in the dominant hemisphere, sometimes progressing to aphasia). Hemipareisis and hemianopia are common. Diagnosis is suspected on MRI scanning which shows marked unilateral and progressive unihemispheric focal atrophy. Treatment is difficult. Antiepileptic drugs are usually ineffective in controlling seizures. Various attempts to suppress or modulate the immune system, in particular with corticosteroids and/or intravenous immunoglobulin (IVIg) have proved effective in only a minority of cases. Surgery to control seizures can be carried out. Large resections are needed and hemispherectomy and hemispherotomy can be strikingly effective at controlling seizures and improving behaviour and cognition.

Differential diagnosis of epilepsy

Epileptic seizures feature in the differential diagnosis of many transient neurological symptoms. Here, the principal differential diagnoses of the common presentions are described (Table 7.10). There are differences in the common presentations and differential diagnoses in adults, infants and children and we largely confine this description to adult patients.

Table 7.10 The clinical presentations of epilepsy in relation to differential diagnosis.

Loss of awareness
Generalised convulsive movements
Focal convulsive movements
Facial muscle and eye movements
Drop attacks
Transient focal sensory symptoms
Transient visual symptoms
Transient vestibular symptoms
Psychic experiences
Aggressive outbursts
Episodic phenomena in sleep
Prolonged confusional or fugue states

The key to making a correct diagnosis is a detailed history from the individual patient and from a reliable witness who has seen the episodes in question. In individuals attending clinics with 'first seizures', not more than 25% of patients are usually considered to have had an epileptic seizure. The most common diagnostic error is to diagnose a syncopal episode as an epileptic seizure. Undue reliance is often placed on investigations, particularly the EEG and MRI. Inappropriate weight is often given to EEG findings that are 'compatible with epilepsy'.

It is a sound aphorism that the diagnosis of epilepsy is made primarily on the history, and the role of the EEG is to assist in the subsequent classification of the type of epileptic seizures and the epilepsy syndrome. The role of MRI is not to diagnose epilepsy, but to identify any underlying structural cerebral abnormality in those with diagnosed epilepsy.

There is considerable scope for the misdiagnosis or inaccurate diagnosis of epilepsy and epilepsy syndrome, which can have serious consequences. In tertiary referral practice it has been estimated that in about 20% of those with a diagnosis of refractory epilepsy the diagnosis is incorrect.

When taking the history it is a good tactic to first allow the individual and witnesses to give their own freehand account of the points that they consider most important and to then go through the salient points in a systematic manner. It is not uncommon that a dramatic event causes the individual to seek advice and for minor events that may have occurred for some time to have been overlooked. Such minor events may produce important diagnostic clues and so need to be specifically enquired for. For example, episodes of an epigastric rising sensation, déjà vu and premonition suggest temporal lobe focal seizures; brief blank staring spells and flurries of upper limb jerks in the first hour after waking (i.e. myoclonic jerks) suggest a generalised epilepsy. In contrast, a greying of vision or rushing sound in ears suggest syncope.

In those who have had repeated episodes, a video recording of an episode is frequently extremely helpful, conveying more information than can be relayed by even the most careful witness, and has the benefit of being objective. Video recorders, particularly on mobile telephones, have become commonly available. Where diagnosis is uncertain, these video recordings are invaluable.

The clinical examination is usually less rewarding than the history, but is still important. In addition to determining if there are any focal neurological deficits, the individual's mood and mental state need to be assessed. The skin should be examined for evidence of a neurocutaneous syndrome, systemic signs identified and blood pressure checked. If an individual presents with episodes of loss of awareness or falling, a cardiac examination and measurement of lying and standing blood pressure is indicated.

The following clinical presentations can occur.

Loss of awareness and collapse

Whatever the cause, the patient may have amnesia for both the event and its exact circumstances. The main causes are syncope, seizures, psychogenic non-epileptic attacks (dissociative attacks) and cardiac arrhythmias. Transient cerebral ischaemia caused by vascular abnormalities is less common. Microsleeps (very short daytime naps) may occur with any cause of severe sleep deprivation or disruption. Other causes of diagnostic confusion are much less common and include hypoglycaemia or other intermittent metabolic disorders, structural anomalies of the skull base affecting the brainstem, or lesions affecting the circulation of the CSF.

Epilepsy

Several types of epileptic seizure can present with loss of awareness as the only reported feature. These include absences, complex partial, tonic or atonic seizures. Typical absences are sometimes associated with eyelid blinking or twitching, and sometimes small myoclonic facial or limb jerks, or brief facial automatisms such as lip smacking or chewing. Atonic seizures usually give rise to drop attacks but may appear to cause blank spells if the patient is sitting or lying down and so cannot fall. Complex partial seizures may cause loss of awareness with few if any other features. Detailed enquiry must always be made for any associated psychic or motor phenomena that may raise the possibility of a seizure disorder.

Syncope

Syncope is the most common cause of episodes of loss of awareness. A simple faint (*syn:* reflex syncope, vasovagal syncope) usually has identifiable precipitants – for instance from standing for prolonged periods, particularly if associated with peripheral vasodilatation (e.g. hot stuffy weather, crowds, drug or alcohol use), dehydration, frightening, emotional or unpleasant scenes, painful stimuli (blood taking). There is usually a prodromal period which can last seconds or minutes and consist of such symptoms as sweating, feeling of faintness, greying out of vision (due to retinal ischaemia, pathognomonic of syncope) and a rushing sound in the ears. The mechanism of syncope is a sudden fall in blood pressure with rapid resolution (providing an erect posture is not maintained, and there is rapid recovery without confusion.

There are other causes of syncope. Some are caused by valsalva-type restriction of cardiac return (e.g. cough syncope or the syncope from playing wind instruments); impaired baroreceptors resulting from atheroma of the carotid (carotid sinus syncope); postural syncope (e.g. in peripheral neuropathy, suddenly getting up from a decubitus position); autonomic disturbances (e.g. micturition syncope); cardiac syncope (see later). As these are not caused by vasovagal reflex changes, the typical aura of vasovagal syncope may not be present.

Cardiac syncope

Cardiac syncope is caused through cerebral ischaemia because of a sudden reduction of cardiac output. There are sometimes prodromal features similar to simple syncope (due to falling cerebral perfusion). Other prodromal features that should suggest a cardiac cause include a history of palpitations, chest pain or shortness of breath. Attacks resulting from transient complete heart block or asystole are abrupt and short with rapid loss of consciousness. Lack of cardiac output may also be caused by short episodes of ventricular tachycardia or fibrillation. Prolongation of the QT interval may lead to such events and the familial genetic syndromes of prolonged QT interval must not be missed. Patients with mitral valve prolapse and aortic stenosis may present with episodic loss of awareness caused by fluctuating cardiac output or associated arrhythmias. Those with aortic stenosis and hypertrophic cardiomyopathy are especially prone to present with episodes of sudden collapse with loss of awareness during exercise. A cardiological opinion should be sought if there is the possibility of cardiac dysfunction causing episodes of loss of awareness, falls or convulsions (see later). A 12-lead electrocardiogram (ECG) should be carefully inspected, particularly for evidence of prolongation of the QT interval and consideration given to prolonged ECG monitoring with an implanted ECG loop recorder.

Table 7.11 Differentiation of epileptic seizures and dissociative seizures.

	Epileptic seizure	Dissociative seizures
Precipitating cause	Rare	Common, emotional and stress-related
When alone or asleep	Common	May be reported
Onset	Usually short	May be short or over several minutes
Aura	Various, usually stereotyped	Fear, panic, altered mental state
Speech	Cry, grunt at onset; muttering, words in automatisms	Semi-voluntary, often unintelligible
Movement	Atonic, tonic; if clonic, synchronous small amplitude jerks	Asynchronous flailing of limbs; pelvic thrusting; opisthotonos
Injury	Tongue biting, fall; directed violence rare	May bite tongue, cheeks, lip, hands, throw self to ground. Directed violence not uncommon
Consciousness	Complete loss in generalised tonic–clonic; may be incomplete in complex partial	Variable, often inconsistent with seizure type
Response to stimulation	None in generalised tonic–clonic; may respond in complex partial and post-ictally	Often reacts and this may terminate episode
Incontinence	Common	Sometimes
Duration	Few minutes	Few minutes, may be prolonged

Dissociative seizures

Dissociative seizures, sometimes known as non-epileptic attack disorder (NEAD) or pseudoseizures typically gives rise to episodes of two broad types: attacks involving motor phenomena, and attacks of lying motionless with apparent loss of awareness. The duration of the attack is a key diagnostic feature. The motionless attacks are often prolonged, continuing for several minutes or sometimes hours. Such behaviour is very rare indeed in epileptic seizures and there will nearly always be other positive phenomena in epileptic attacks that last for more than a few minutes. In addition, attacks are often precipitated by external events or stress. Patients with dissociative seizures often have a history of abnormal illness behaviour or childhood abuse, or some distinct psychological precipitant. Dissociative seizures are much more common in females than males, and usually commence in adolescence or early adulthood (Table 7.11).

Microsleeps Any cause of sleep deprivation can lead to brief daytime naps, sometimes lasting for only a few seconds. Impaired quality of sleep may also be a factor. The most important is obstructive sleep apnoea, although microsleeps also occur in other sleep disorders. Microsleeps are a common problem when driving, particularly on featureless straight roads and are the cause of many road traffic accidents. There are usually clear warning signs such as the driver feeling a need to close their eyes, yawn, turn the radio volume up or open the windows. These events are of legal significance as a driver who continues to drive despite such warning signs and who causes an accident is likely to be prosecuted for dangerous driving. Narcolepsy can present with short periods of suddenly falling asleep during the day. Systematic enquiry should be made for other symptoms of the narcolepsy cataplexy syndrome, such as loss of body tone precipitated by emotion or laughter, sleep paralysis and hypnogogic hallucinations.

Panic attacks

Panic attacks usually start with feelings of fear and anxiety, associated with autonomic changes and hyperventilation. This leads to dizziness or light-headedness, orofacial and/or peripheral paraesthesia (which may be asymmetric), carpopedal spasm, twitching of the peripheries, blurred vision or nausea. Occasionally, the preludes may be forgotten, and attacks present with loss of awareness. Often, but not always, there is a clear situational precipitant. Panic attacks are almost always longer than seizures. However, none of these features are consistent, and differentiation from epilepsy can be difficult.

Hypoglycaemia

Hypoglycaemic attacks causing loss of consciousness are rare except in patients with diabetes mellitus treated with insulin or less commonly oral hypoglycaemics. Very occasional cases may be seen caused by insulin secreting tumours. There is usually a history of events occurring if meals are delayed or missed and marked prodromal symptoms of anxiety, sweating and unease which improve with taking glucose.

Other neurological disorders

If a head injury causes loss of consciousness, there is amnesia. In accidental head injury, particularly road traffic accidents, it may be difficult to distinguish amnesia caused by the injury from cases in which there was a loss of consciousness that caused the accident. Isolated episodes of loss of awareness may also be caused by abuse of psychotropic drugs or other substances.

Generalised convulsive movements

The differentiation from epilepsy is usually simple, but some conditions with generalised movements mimicking convulsions cause diagnostic confusion.

Epilepsy

A generalised convulsion is generally the most readily diagnosed epileptic seizure (described earlier). The diagnosis is usually clear from the history and a witnessed account. The prodromal symptoms, pattern of convulsions, lateral tongue biting, bloody frothing, apnoea, cyanosis, post-ictal confusion and headache, and injury (for instance, posterior dislocation of the shoulder) are characteristic of tonic–clonic seizures.

Syncope with myoclonic jerking movements

People who faint often have myoclonic twitches of the extremities. This may be associated with limb posturing and stiffening, and is caused by the transient cerebral ischaemia associated with syncope (possibly mediated at subcortical level). With prolonged cerebral hypoperfusion, as can occur if the syncopal person is maintained in an upright posture, the jerking can be severe and occasionally a true convulsion is precipitated (an 'anoxic seizure'). Incontinence of urine may occur, particularly if the bladder is full and tongue biting may occur.

Primary cardiac or respiratory abnormalities presenting with secondary anoxic seizures

Episodes of complete heart block or transient asystole can have syncopal features followed by collapse to the ground and anoxic seizures. More commonly, there is an abrupt collapse with no warning and the person is observed to be pale and witnesses commonly remark that 'they thought the person was dead'. The attacks last for less than 1 minute, but may be followed by a prolonged period of confusion, particularly in elderly patients. There should be a low threshold for obtaining a cardiological opinion in such cases and consideration given to insertion of an implanted ECG loop recorder to identify cardiac arrhythmias.

Involuntary movement disorders and other neurological conditions

The best known is paroxysmal kinesiogenic choreoathetosis. Attacks are usually precipitated by sudden specific movements and last a few seconds to minutes. Paroxysmal dystonia can present with attacks that last for minutes to hours. Patients with involuntary movement disorders such as idiopathic torsion dystonia may show severe acute exacerbations that may mimic convulsive movements. There is no alteration in consciousness in any of these conditions.

Patients with mental retardation often have stereotyped or repetitive movements, which may include head banging or body rocking, and more subtle movements which may be difficult to differentiate from complex partial seizures.

Hyperekplexia

Hyperekplectic attacks are characterised by excessive startle, and the attack can take the form of stiffening and collapse with a sudden jerk of all four limbs. Attacks are provoked by sudden unexpected stimuli, most commonly auditory. Hyperekplexia needs to be distinguished from seizures induced by startle, which commonly arise from the central portions of the frontal lobe. Hyperekplexia usually has a genetic basis and a number of genes have been identified (including *GLRA1, GLRB, SLC6A5, GPHN* and *ARHGEF9*).

Dissociative seizure

Dissociative seizures involving prominent motor phenomena are more common than those with arrest of activity. The movements are varied but often involve semi-purposeful thrashing of all four limbs, waxing and waning over many minutes, showing distractibility or interaction with the environment, and sometimes prominent pelvic movements and back arching. To an experienced eye, the jerking is quite different from the coordinated jerking of tonic–clonic seizures, with its typical evolution and timing, but can be more difficult to differentiate from complex partial seizures of frontal lobe origin, which can take the form of bizarre motor features. The key feature of the latter is that the episodes are usually stereotyped, short, occur during both wake and sleep (dissociative seizures do not occur in sleep) and the associated features and context usually render differential diagnosis easy.

Focal convulsive movements

The differentiation from epilepsy of other conditions in which focal movements occur is more difficult than in those conditions in which generalised movements occur. It can be difficult especially if brief focal attacks occur, but the stereotyped nature of the attack and its context usually assist in differentiating focal epilepsies from the other conditions.

Focal motor seizures

Focal motor seizures involve jerking and posturing of one extremity, which can 'march'. There is often associated paraesthesia. Following the attack, there may be localised transient weakness for seconds or minutes, sometimes longer. Seizures arising in many different brain regions may cause dystonic posturing. The seizures can be very frequent and are stereotyped.

Epilepsia partialis continua is a rare form of epilepsy that often causes diagnostic confusion. In this condition focal motor activity, such as jerking of the hand or part of the face, can persist for hours or days, continue into sleep, sometimes for years. The movements often become slow and pendulous, with some associated dystonic posturing.

Tics

Tics usually present with stereotyped movements in childhood or adolescence, sometimes restricted to one particular action (e.g. eye blinking) but can be multiple in nature. Tics may be confused with myoclonic jerks. However, unlike myoclonic jerks, they can be suppressed voluntarily, although to do so leads to a rise in psychological tension and anxiety which is then relieved by the patient allowing the tics to occur. This is a very useful diagnostic point. Repetitive tics and stereotypies are particularly common in those with intellectual disability.

Transient cerebral ischaemia

Those with transient ischaemic attacks (TIAs) usually present with negative phenomena (i.e. loss of use of a limb, hemiplegia or other deficits), although positive phenomena such as paraesthesiae may occur. TIAs may last for a few minutes, but may persist for up to 24 hours. TIAs are not usually stereotyped or repeated with the frequency of epileptic seizures, and there are usually associated features to suggest vascular disease. There is usually no loss of consciousness.

Tonic spasms of multiple sclerosis

These spasms usually occur in the setting of known multiple sclerosis, but can be the presenting feature, although other evidence of multiple sclerosis will usually be found on examination and investigation. The spasms may last for several seconds and sometimes longer than 1 minute. They can be very difficult to differentiate from focal motor seizures.

Paroxysmal movement disorders

Patients with paroxysmal kinesiogenic choreoathetosis may present with focal motor attacks that are very similar to epileptic seizures, but only occur on the initiation of movement and so usually do not pose diagnostic difficulty. Tremor can occur in a variety of movement disorders and is usually sufficiently persistent and rhythmical to make the non-epileptic nature clear, but may be difficult to distinguish from certain forms of epilepsia partialis continua. Myoclonus of subcortical origin may be suspected from the distribution of involved muscles (e.g. spinal myoclonus may be restricted to specific segments, either unilateral or bilateral). Patients with peripheral nerve entrapment (or other lesions) usually present with weakness but very rarely can present with episodic jerks or twitches.

Transient facial muscle and eye movements

Abnormal facial movements occur in many neurological conditions including partial seizures, tics, dystonias or other paroxysmal movement disorders, drug-induced dyskinesias and hemifacial spasm, and psychological disorders.

Partial seizures

Benign childhood epilepsy with centro-temporal spikes usually presents with seizures in childhood affecting the face, often with unilateral grimacing, hemibody sensory and motor phenomena, or secondarily generalised seizures occurring in sleep. Focal motor seizures may cause twitching of one side of the face which may be restricted to specific areas.

Complex partial seizures can cause automatisms with lip smacking, chewing, swallowing, sniffing or grimacing, with amnesia and impaired awareness. If these features are caused by seizure activity the attacks are usually relatively infrequent. Dystonia or other movement disorder episodes are likely to be more persistent or occur many times per day.

Movement disorders

Hemifacial spasm typically presents in the elderly or middle aged with clusters of attacks of intermittent twitching that initially involve the eye but subsequently can spread to the rest of that side of the face. The twitching of the eyelid can result in forced closure of the eye. Less commonly, the spasms start lower in the face and spread to the eyelid. Facial weakness may develop and continue between attacks.

Bruxism can occur either during the day or in sleep, especially in children with learning disability. Episodes are usually more prolonged than with the automatisms of complex partial seizures, and there are no associated features to suggest an epileptic basis. As with dystonia and other movement disorders affecting the face, there may be evidence of involvement elsewhere, and attacks are usually more frequent than is seen with isolated seizures.

Other neurological disorders

Defects of eye movement control are common in patients with a wide range of neurological disorders. There are usually associated features that indicate a non-epileptic basis. Bizarre eye movements also occur in blindness and may be mistaken for epileptic activity. Careful examination is required to ascertain the precise features of the eye movement disorder, and in particular any precipitating factors or features of cerebellar or brainstem disease.

Drop attacks

Any cause of loss of awareness may proceed to a sudden collapse or drop attack. Epilepsy, syncope and other cardiovascular disorders are common causes of drop attacks.

Epilepsy

Sudden drop attacks are common in patients with learning disability and secondary generalised epilepsies. The falls may be tonic or atonic in nature and frequently cause severe facial injuries if the individual falls forwards. In individuals without learning disability, epileptic drop attacks are rare. However, tonic–clonic seizures that are only partially treated can be modified to take the form of drop attacks.

Cardiovascular causes

If cerebral hypoperfusion is sufficient to cause sudden collapse there is usually loss of awareness (see earlier), but a drop attack may be the dominant presenting symptom. This may occur particularly in posterior circulation hypoperfusion, and other associated symptoms usually make the diagnosis clear.

Movement disorders

Most movement disorders that cause drop attacks have other more prominent features that make the diagnosis clear (e.g. Parkinson's disease). Patients with paroxysmal kinesiogenic choreoathetosis may present with drop attacks if there is lower limb involvement.

Brainstem, spinal or lower limb abnormalities

There are usually fixed neurological signs that give a clue towards the diagnosis. Tumours of the third ventricle, such as colloid cysts, may present with sudden episodes of collapse. Spinal cord vascular abnormalities may present with abrupt episodes of lower limb weakness leading to falls, without impairment of awareness.

Cataplexy

Cataplexy usually occurs in association with narcolepsy, although it may be the presenting clinical feature. There is no loss of consciousness with attacks. Attacks may be precipitated by emotion, especially laughter. Often there is only loss of tone in the neck muscles, with slumping of the head, rather than complete falls.

Metabolic disorders

Periodic paralysis caused by sudden changes in plasma potassium is rare. The condition may be familial or associated with other endocrine disorders or drugs. Usually there is a gradual onset, and the attacks last for hours.

Idiopathic drop attacks

These attacks are most common in middle-aged females. They take the form of a sudden fall without loss of consciousness. Characteristically, the patients remember falling and hitting the ground. Recovery is instantaneous, but injury may occur. The cause is quite unclear, but it may be a spinal reflex.

Vertebrobasilar ischaemia

This condition is over-diagnosed and probably accounts for very few drop attacks. Typically, the attacks occur in the elderly, with evidence of vascular disease and cervical spondylosis. The attacks may be precipitated by head turning or neck extension resulting in distortion of the vertebral arteries and are of sudden onset, with features of brainstem ischaemia such as diplopia, vertigo and bilateral facial and limb sensory and motor deficits.

Transient focal sensory symptoms

Epileptic seizures involving the primary sensory cortex are less common than motor seizures, and the symptoms take the form of spreading paraesthesia. Seizures involving the supplementary sensory areas or medial frontal cortex can cause sensory symptoms. There are usually other epileptic features because of involvement of adjacent or related brain structures. Transient sensory phenomena may also be seen in peripheral nerve compression or other abnormalities of the ascending sensory pathways, hyperventilation or panic attacks and in TIAs.

Lesions of sensory pathways cause persistent symptoms, but diagnostic confusion may arise early on in the natural history, when complaints are intermittent, or if they are posture related. Hyperventilation may be associated with unilateral and localised areas of paraesthesia (e.g. one arm). Intermittent sensory illusions may be experienced in relation to amputated or anaesthetic limbs. Migrainous episodes may also cause localised areas of paraesthesia, but usually have the distinction of a gradual evolution of sensory phenomena, both positive and negative, and associated features of migraine.

Transient vestibular symptoms

Acute attacks of vertigo may occasionally be caused by a seizure in the parietal or temporal lobes. In these cases there are generally associated features that point to cerebral involvement, such as a focal somato-sensory symptoms, déjà vu or disordered perception. The attacks are very short-lived. Peripheral vestibular disease is a much more common cause and gives rise to paroxysmal rotational vertigo, which is longer lasting, and a perception of linear motion and there are often also other symptoms of auditory and vestibular disease such as deafness, tinnitus, pressure in the ear and relation to head position. Migraine also is a cause of transient vestibular symptoms and occasionally resembles epileptic seizures.

Transient visual symptoms

Migraine is a common cause of episodic visual phenomena, and the differentiation from epilepsy can occasionally be difficult. In migraine, the evolution of the visual symptomatology is usually gradual, continuing over several minutes (up to 20 minutes). Fortification spectra are diagnostic of migraine and do not occur in epilepsy. In migraine there may be associated photophobia, nausea and headache but a migrainous visual aura without headache is not uncommon. Epileptic phenomena are usually much shorter, evolving over seconds, and the visual hallucinations are more commonly of coloured blobs rather than jagged lines. In both migraine and epilepsy, the phenomena may move across the visual field, but in epilepsy usually stay unilateral. On occasions, a migraine attack may precipitate an epileptic seizure (this phenomenon is known as migralepsy).

Transient psychic experiences

Intermittent psychic phenomena can on occasions be very difficult to differentiate from epilepsy, especially if short. Again, their context and their stereotyped nature usually allow the diagnosis to be made.

Epilepsy

Partial seizures of temporal lobe origin are commonly associated with fear, déjà vu, memory flashbacks, visual, olfactory or auditory hallucinations. Other features include altered perception of the environment with a distancing from reality or change in size or shape of objects; altered language function; emotions such as sadness, elation and sexual arousal.

Psychic experiences can have some relation to past experiences. They are usually recalled as brief scenes, sometimes in a sequence. They are usually unclear, for example a patient may describe an illusion of someone standing in front of them who they know, but they cannot name or describe them in detail. The déjà vu experiences in an epileptic seizure are very frequently associated with a dreamy sensation and are very intense – and both features help differentiate from non-epileptic déjà vu. A rising epigastric sensation can occur alone or in association with such experiences. Elemental visual phenomena, such as flashing lights or coloured circles, are more often seen in occipital lobe epilepsy.

Migraine

Migrainous psychic phenomena sometimes involve an initial heightening of awareness. The principal features are usually visual illusions which may be elemental or complex. They rarely have the same intense emotional components of temporal lobe illusions or hallucinations. The time course is usually more prolonged than with partial seizures, with an evolution over several minutes and there are associated features of a pounding headache, photophobia and nausea or vomiting. There may be identifiable precipitants, and there is often a relevant family history.

Panic attacks

These are usually associated with feelings of fear and anxiety. Hyperventilation may lead to dizziness and light-headedness. There are often unpleasant abdominal sensations similar to the epigastric aura of partial seizures. In epileptic seizures though the rising sensation extends above the region of the throat and neck – and this is rare in a panic attack, where the sensation is usually confined to the epigastrium and chest. The evolution, associated increases in heart rate and respiration, longer time course and history of precipitating factors usually make the diagnosis clear, but distinction from temporal lobe seizures may be difficult.

Drug-induced flashbacks

These share many of the qualities of psychic temporal lobe seizures. Flashbacks are individualised hallucinations usually related to the circumstances of the drug abuse, often with emotional content of fear or anxiety. A careful history should be taken for substance abuse, especially LSD, psilocybin, peyote and mescaline.

Hallucinations or illusions caused by loss of a primary sense

Hallucinations and illusions of an absent limb are well-recognised in amputees. Similarly, people who lose sight either in the whole or part field may experience visual hallucinations or illusions in the blind field. Such phenomena can be elemental or complex and include evolving scenes. Similar experiences can occur with deafness.

Such experiences resulting from the loss of a primary sense present particular diagnostic difficulty when they occur in the setting of a structural lesion, which could also result in epilepsy. Occipital infarction, for example, can cause visual loss and also gives rise to epileptic seizures. Often the hallucinations caused by sensory loss are usually more prolonged, lasting for minutes or hours, but on occasions can be brief.

Psychotic hallucinations and delusions

Hallucinations and delusions are the hallmark of psychotic illnesses. The following features would suggest a psychiatric rather than epileptic basis: complex nature with an evolving or argued theme, auditory nature involving instructions or third person language, paranoid content or associated thought disorder. Psychotic episodes are usually more long-lasting than isolated epileptic seizures, although intermittent psychosis may be difficult to differentiate. Persistent mood changes may be a helpful guide, but even short temporal lobe seizures can be followed by mood changes lasting for hours or days. Furthermore, flurries of epileptic attacks may themselves cause an organic psychosis lasting for several days. Ruminations and pseudo-hallucinations, in which the patient retains some insight, can occur in affective disorders.

Dissociative seizures

Dissociative seizures can be associated with reports of hallucinations and illusions. Initially, the symptoms may seem plausible, but should be suspected if they are florid and multiple in type (e.g. auditory, olfactory and visual at different times) with evolving stories or patterns of expression and are associated with emotional outburst.

Aggressive outbursts

These are rarely epileptic in nature if they occur in isolation. They are especially common in adults and children with a learning disability. In this setting there is organic brain disease that could lower the overall seizure threshold.

A not infrequent forensic issue is the occurrence of violent, or other, crimes in patients with epilepsy, in which it is a defence claim that the crime was committed in a state of automatism. Certain features are strong evidence against an epileptic basis to the attack:

- Absence of a prior history of epilepsy with automatisms
- Premeditation and evidence of planning or preparation
- Directed violence
- Evidence of complicated and organised activity during the episode
- Recall of events during the episode
- Witness accounts not indicative of a disturbance of consciousness
- Subsequent attempts at escape or concealment of evidence
- Prolonged aggression, and
- Motive.

Other features such as previous offending behaviours or personality disorder are also helpful in differentiating the very rare epileptic violence from the more common criminal behaviour.

Episodic phenomena in sleep

Attacks occurring during sleep present some diagnostic difficulties because they are often poorly witnessed, and the patient has little, if any, recall of the event or the preceding circumstances.

Normal physiological movements

Whole body jerks commonly occur in normal subjects on falling asleep. Fragmentary physiological myoclonus usually involves the peripheries or the face, and occurs during stages 1 and 2 and REM sleep. Periodic movements of sleep may be an age-related phenomenon, being seen in less than 1% of young adults, but occurring with increasing frequency during middle and old age such that they are present in perhaps half of the elderly population. Typically, these movements occur at regular intervals of 10–60 seconds and in clusters over many minutes.

Frontal lobe epilepsy

Frontal lobe seizures can display specific sleep-related characteristics causing diagnostic confusion. Such attacks are often frequent, brief, bizarre and often only occur during sleep. Attacks may include apnoea, dystonic, myoclonic or choreiform movements which can be unilateral or bilateral, and some retention of awareness. The attacks are scattered throughout the night, and usually arise from non-REM sleep. Frequency is highly variable, but some patients have more than 20 attacks in a night. An important clue to the diagnosis is the occurrence of additional secondarily generalised seizures and seizures also occurring in wakefulness. Other features of diagnostic importance are their stereotyped nature, their brief duration, association with spasm or tonic stiffening. The interictal EEG may or may not be abnormal and the MRI can show frontal lesions. The syndrome of ADNFLE is a genetically determined form of frontal lobe epilepsy.

Other epilepsies

Seizures arising in other brain regions can present with nocturnal attacks. The patient may be aroused by an aura, although often this is not recalled when attacks arise from sleep. Complex automatisms, in which the patient gets out of bed and wanders around, can cause confusion with parasomnias. With nocturnal seizures of any type the partner is frequently awoken by particular components, such as vocalisation, but does not witness the onset. Generalised tonic–clonic seizures not uncommonly occur on or shortly after awakening.

Pathological fragmentary myoclonus

Excessive fragmentary myoclonus persisting into sleep stages 3 and 4 may be seen with any cause of disrupted nocturnal sleep.

Restless leg syndrome

The restless leg syndrome (*syn:* Willis–Ekbom disease) is characterised by an urge to move the legs, especially in the evening when lying or sitting. It can be associated with unpleasant paraesthesiae. All patients with restless legs have periodic movements of sleep. These may be severe and can also occur during wakefulness. In addition, there may be a variety of brief daytime dyskinesias.

Non-REM parasomnia

Non-REM parasomnias usually present in childhood or adolescence, and are often familial. The attacks take the form of night terrors or sleep walking. They arise from slow wave sleep, typically at least 30 minutes, but not more than 4 hours, after going to sleep and the timing is often consistent. Attacks can be spaced out by months or years and rarely occur more than once per week, and usually no more than one attack occurs in a single night. They are more likely after stressful events, or when sleeping in a strange bed.

Night terrors involve intense autonomic features (sweating, flushing, palpitations) and a look of fear. Patients may recall a frightening scene or experience, but do not usually recount a vivid dream prior to the attacks. Certainly children do not recall events. They can be difficult to arouse, and confused for several minutes. Vocalisations are common.

Sleep walking may involve getting out of bed and performing complex tasks. Sometimes it is possible to lead the patient back to bed without awakening. They may respond if spoken to, but their speech is usually slow or monosyllabic. Brief abortive episodes are more common, involving sitting up in bed with fidgeting and shuffling (mimicking a complex partial seizure).

Non-REM parasomnias may cause self-injury but rarely directed aggression. They are associated with enuresis.

REM parasomnia

REM parasomnia usually occurs in middle age or the elderly, and shows a marked male predominance. It more often occurs in the later portion of sleep. During REM sleep, patients may have an increase in the frequency or severity of fragmentary myoclonus, thrash about, call out, display directed violence or appear to enact vivid dreams. Attacks may last from seconds to minutes. If awoken, patients can recall part of these dreams. Although REM sleep behaviour disorders can occur in healthy elderly subjects, they are also seen in association with drugs (e.g. tricyclics) or alcohol, or CNS diseases such as multi-system atrophy. REM sleep disorders can be the presenting symptom of these conditions or occur during the course of the CNS disorders.

Sleep apnoea

Patients with sleep apnoea usually present with daytime hypersomnolence. However, the apnoeic episodes can cause episodic grunting, flailing about or other restless activity that can appear to mimic nocturnal epilepsy. Occasionally, the resultant hypoxia precipitates secondary seizures.

Other movements in sleep

Nocturnal body rocking occurs in patients with learning disability, or following head injury. In patients with many different forms of daytime dyskinesias, similar movements may occasionally occur during overnight sleep, usually in the setting of brief arousals.

Prolonged confusional or fugue states

Epileptic seizures usually last for seconds or minutes. After generalised tonic–clonic seizures (or, less often, complex partial seizures) there may be confusion lasting for many minutes, but rarely more than an hour. Such episodes only present diagnostic difficulty if the initial seizure is unwitnessed. Nevertheless, epileptic states can last for longer periods of time, as can other types of cerebral disorder and the differential diagnosis of prolonged epileptic confusional states (non-convulsive status) should include acute encephalopathy, non-convulsive status epilepticus, transient global amnesia, intermittent psychosis and dissociative seizures.

Acute encephalopathy

Virtually any severe metabolic disturbance can cause an acute encephalopathy (e.g. diabetic ketoacidosis; hypoglycaemia; respiratory, renal or hepatic failure; drug ingestion; hyperpyrexia; sepsis). Transient metabolic disturbances are most often seen in treated diabetes mellitus due to insulin-induced hypoglycaemia. Occasionally, metabolic disorders, such as porphyria and urea cycle enzyme defects, present with exacerbations with symptoms lasting for hours or days and give the appearance of an episodic condition. Acute neurological conditions also need to be considered, particularly encephalitis, meningitis, other intracranial infection, head injury, cerebral infarction or haemorrhage. Drug abuse can cause isolated episodes or recurrent bouts, related to intoxications.

Non-convulsive status epilepticus

Patients with complex partial seizures, typical or atypical absences sometimes present with prolonged confusional states caused by complex partial epilepticus or absence status. Such attacks can be the first manifestation of the seizure disorder, or occur in the setting of known epilepsy.

Intermittent psychosis

Although usually more sustained, patients with psychiatric disorders sometimes present with episodes of delusions, hallucinations or apparent confusion, lasting for hours or days.

Transient global amnesia

These episodes typically commence acutely, and last for minutes or hours and involve both retrograde and anterograde amnesia. Patients are able to perform complex activities, but afterwards have no recall of them. There is a lack of other neurological features to the attacks, and consciousness appears to be preserved. During an attack, patients do not appear overtly confused. The attacks involve bilateral medial temporal dysfunction, which in some patients can be on the basis of ischaemia or have an epileptic basis.

Hysterical fugue

A fugue state may arise without an organic physical cause, as a conversion symptom. These episodes may be brief or very prolonged, lasting for days or even weeks. If seen during the episode, inconsistencies are often found on examination of the mental state. There is usually a history of serious psychiatric disturbance or alcohol or drug abuse. In some cases, the question of malingering arises, most commonly in a situation in which the person's state prevents questioning by law officers and when the subject professes no memory of events. The diagnosis is more difficult to identify if the patient is only seen subsequently. The matching of witness accounts and the apparent sequence of events is essential, but it may remain difficult to come to a firm conclusion.

Investigation of epilepsy

The investigation of epilepsy is aimed, broadly speaking, to address two questions: (a) is the diagnosis epilepsy, and if so, what type of epilepsy (seizure type, epilepsy syndrome)?; and (b) what is the cause of epilepsy?

The first question is determined largely by the clinical history (and hence the absolute necessity of a witnessed account and/or a video clip of a seizures). EEG is also a helpful adjunct, although as emphasised later, many patients with epilepsy will have normal findings on routine EEG. ECG and routine blood tests also exclude other conditions which can mimic epilepsy. The second question is addressed most commonly by MRI scanning (and other neuroimaging) and biochemical, haematological and immunological tests. The indications for each test depends on the clinical circumstance.

In addition to these questions, investigation can be directed at finding a surgically treatable epilepsy (see Presurgical assessment). The usefulness of investigations into directing medical therapy is disappointingly limited. It is confined largely to identifying those seizure types and syndromes for which specific therapy is available (a minority of cases). There are no genetic tests currently in clinical practice that can assist in 'personalising' treatment, and claims in this area have often been overstated.

Routine tests to carry out in all cases

On presentation, all cases of epilepsy should have a full blood count, biochemical screening of hepatic and renal function and blood sugar, and screening immunological tests. Other investigations depend on age and context. An ECG and EEG should be carried out in all cases, and MRI in the great majority (see later).

Biochemical, haematological and immunological tests

Other tests depend on the clinical context and Tables 7.12, 7.13, 7.14 and 7.15 list biochemical tests that can be made from serum and/or urine, CSF investigations and serum immunological tests. Some of these are highly specialised and are indicated only in the identification of rare disorders and are not routinely performed. Various haematological conditions include epilepsy amongst the

Table 7.12 Biochemical tests in the investigation of epilepsy (blood and/or urine).

Test	Indication
Acylcarnitines	Fatty acid peroxidation defects, organic acidurias
Amino acids	Glycine, serine, theonine, glutamine, phenylananine, proline, various aminoacidurias
Ammonia	Urea cycle disorders (arginino-succinic acidaemia, carbamoyl phosphate synthetase deficiency, citrullinaemia, ornithine transcarbamylase deficiency), organic acidaemias
Alpha-aminoadipic semialdehyde (α-AASA)	Pyridoxine-dependent seizures (PDE, MoCoF and SUDX deficiencies
Biotinidase activity	Biotinidase deficiency
B12, methymalonic acid and homocysteine	B12 deficiency states, disorders of folate metabolism, and other non-specific clinical settings
Calcium and magnesium	Renal tubular disorders , PDE, neuonatla seizures with hypomagnesaemia or hypocalcaemia, primary disorders of calcium and magnesium balance and endocrine function (e.g. hypoparathyroidism, pseudohypoparathyroidis)
Copper and caeruloplasmin	Menkes syndrome, Wilson's disease
CoQ10	Disorders of CoQ10 biosynthesis, mitochondrial diseases
Creatine and guanidinoacetate	Creatine synthesis disorders (GAMT and AGAT deficiencies)
Creatine kinase	Dystrogycanopathies
Drug/toxic screen (incl. alcohol)	Drug intoxication, poisoning
Electrolytes	Various disorders involving renal function
Folate and RBC folate	Folate deficiency
Glucose	Diabetes, disorders of fat oxidation, glycogen storage disorders, disorders of gluconeogenesis
Glycosaminoglycans	Mucopolysaccharidoses
Homovanillic acid/vanillylmandelic acid ratio	Menkes disease
Lactate	Mitochondrial diseases, PDHc deficiency, biotinidase deficiency, lipoic acid synthetase deficiency, fructose 1,6 diphosphatase deficiency
Liver function tests	Hepatic disorders of various causes, mitorchondrial disorders
Oligosaccharides	Oligosaccharidoses (e.g. sialidosis)
Organic acids	In various organic acidaemias and acidurias such as methylmalonic acidaemia, glutaric acidaemia type 1), Krebs' cycle defects, fatty acid oxidation disorders
Orotic acid, uracil	Some urea cycle defects (e.g. ornithine transcarbamylase deficiency)
Porphyrins	Porphyrias
Pterins	Disorders of biogenic amine metabolism (tetrahydrobiopterin deficiency disorders)
Purine and pyrimidine metabolites	Hypoxanthine, succinyladenosine
Sulfite and sulfocysteine	SUDX deficiency, MoCoF deficiency
Uric acid	Lysch–Nyhan syndrome, MoCoF deficiency
Very long chain fatty acids	Peroxisomal disorders (including Zellweger syndrome)
White cell enzyme activity	Lysosomal storage disease, mucopolysaccharidosis, mucolipidosis, gangliosidosis, leukodystrophies, neuronal ceroid lipofuscinosis, glycoprotein storage disorders

The application of these tests depends on the clinical situation (see text).
Source: adapted from Shorvon 2013. With permission of Oxford University Press.

Table 7.13 Haematological tests in the investigation of epilepsy.

Full blood count and differential	Primary haematological and other conditions
Blood culture	CNS/systemic infection
Blood film	Acanthocytosis Macrocytosis/megaloblastic RBCs – B12 and folate deficiency Sickle cells Blast cells
Vaculoated lymphcytes	Lysosomal storage diorders
Clotting profile	Bleeding tendency

The application of these tests depends on the clinical situation (see text).
Source: adapted from Shorvon 2013. With permission of Oxford University Press.

Table 7.14 CSF examination in the investigation of epilepsy.

General CSF examination (cell count, sugar, protein)	Infection, inflammation
Cytology	Primary or secondary CNS malignancies
Oligoclonal bands (unmatched in serum)	CNS inflammation, autoimmunity, infection, parainfectious process
14-3-3, S-100	Classic Creutzfieldt–Jakob disease
CSF: serum glucose ≤0.5	GLUT1 deficiency
Lactate	Mitochondrial diseases
Serine and glycine	Disorders of serine biosynthesis
Alpha-aminoadipic semialdehyde (α-AASA)	Pyridoxine deficient seizures
5-methyl-tetrahydrofolate (5-MTHF)	Cerebral folate deficiency (idiopathic or secondary) after exclusion of systemic folate deficiency
Pyridoxal 5′-phosphate (PLP)	Pyridox(am)ine phosphate oxidase (PNPO) deficiency

The application of these tests depends on the clinical situation (see text).
Source: adapted from Shorvon 2013. With permission of Oxford University Press.

symptoms but this is seldom the presenting symptom. Specific immunological tests are indicated where limbic encephalitis is suspected or in acute onset of status epilepticus in the absence of any obvious cause. Lumbar puncture is not routinely indicated in patients with epilepsy, and is warranted only when the clinical condition and/or other investigations raise the possibility of an

Table 7.15 Immunological tests in the investigation of epilepsy.

Antibody	Condition
Anti-Hu	Limbic encephalitis associated with SCLC
Anti-Ma2	Limbic encephalitis associated with testicular cancer
Anti-CRMP-5/CV2	Limbic encephalitis associated with SCLC, thymoma
Anti-amphiphysin	Idiopathic or paraneoplastic limbic encephalitis associated with breast cancer and SCLC
Anti-GAD	Limbic encephalitis without neoplasia
Anti-adenylate kinase-5	Limbic encephalitis without neoplasia
Anti-voltage-gated potassium channel (VGKC)	Limbic encephalitis
Anti-NMDA receptor	Paraneoplastic (teratoma) or non-paraneoplastic limbic encephalitis
Anti-AMPA (GluR1/GluR2) receptor	Paraneoplastic limbic encephalitis associated with neoplasia of thymus, breast SCLC
Anti-AMPA (GluR3)	Rasmussen's encephalitis
Anti-$GABA_B$ receptor	Limbic encephalitis, 50% paraneoplastic to SCLC
Antiglycine receptor	Limbic encephalitis
Antigliadin, antireticulin, anti-endomyesial	Coeliac disease
ANA, anti-dsDNA, anti-Sm	Cerebral lupus
Anticardiolipin, lupus anticoagulant	Antiphospholipid syndrome
Antithyroid peroxidase	Hashimoto's encephalopathy (STREAT)
Oligoclonal bands in CSF (unmatched in serum)	Autoimmunity, infection, parainfectious process

The application of these tests depends on the clinical situation (see text).
AMPA, α-amino-3-hydroxy-5-methyl-4-isoxazolepropionic acid; CSF, cerebrospinal fluid; NMDA, *N*-methyl-D-aspartate ; SCLC, small cell lung cancer; STREAT, steroid-responsive encephalopathy with autoimmune thyroiditis; VGKC, voltage gated potassium channel.
Source: adapted from Shorvon 2013. With permission of Oxford University Press.

infectious, inflammatory or autoimmune condition. GLUT-1 deficiency, which is important not to overlook, is also highly suggested by a low CSF glucose in the absence of any other cause.

There are, in addition to these investigations, a variety of histological tests that can be carried out on biopsy material – and these often provide the definitive diagnosis. These include biopsy of liver to detect Wilson's disease, mitochondrial disease and glycogen storage diseases; bone marrow for Niemann–Pick type C; hair for Menkes disease; muscle for mitochondrial disease; skin for Lafora body; neurofibromatosis and other systemic disoders and fibroblast assays for a variety of enzymes. Brain biopsy also can be carried out to diagnose a variety of inflammatory, infectious, structural, metabolic (including mitochondrial) or degenerative disorders.

Electroencephalography

Electroencephalography (EEG) was introduced into clinical practice in the early 1940s, and has since developed into an array of digitally based techniques, integrated with video and other investigative modalities. However, like all investigations, it has limitations which must be recognised, and its applications should be targeted to specific clinical questions. Consideration here will be confined to its applications to epilepsy, and its use in other conditions (e.g. in confusional state, altered state of consciousness, sleep disorders, coma, CJD, subacute sclerosing panencephalitis [SSPE]) is to be found in the relevant sections of this book.

A standard EEG recording takes about 60–90 minutes to complete and about half of this time is necessary to place and remove the recording electrodes. Electrodes are applied using the international 10–20 system. Additional electrodes may be placed depending on the specific question of the study (e.g. anterior temporal and/or superior sphenoidal electrodes to allow better identification or characterisation of epileptiform abnormalities arising from this area, or surface electromyographic (EMG) electrodes to allow correlation of jerks with EEG activity).

The EEG signal is generated by the sum of all inhibitory and excitatory post-synaptic potentials and provides a view of the electrical activity generated in cerebral cortex. It is attenuated, filtered and potentially contaminated by structures between the cortex and the recording electrode: CSF, dura, bone, muscle, blood vessels, and skin. The EEG signal is further influenced by the patient's age, level of consciousness, underlying structural pathology, metabolic alterations and medication effects. It also varies according to brain region. EEG has a high temporal resolution (on the order of milliseconds); however, its spatial resolution is poor. The electric signal of interest needs to be amplified by a factor of 100 000 or more. This leaves the EEG signal vulnerable to both physiological (such as ECG, eye blinks, chewing, tongue movements) and non-physiological (such as electrode artefacts, electrical interference) artefacts. During routine EEG, recording conditions can be optimised and the technical quality of the study can be improved, as the physiologist can identify and eliminate artefacts online. Long-term ambulatory recordings are much more prone to artefacts that cannot be corrected.

Hyperventilation and photic stimulation increase the yield for abnormal EEG findings and should therefore be routinely included in the investigation of patients with suspected seizure or epilepsy, following standardised protocols. Although these procedures are generally safe, certain contraindications (e.g. significant pulmonary and cardiovascular disease, pregnancy) have to be considered. Both hyperventilation and photic stimulation can rarely trigger seizures. For this reason, the patient should provide consent.

Abnormal EEG findings (those that one would not expect in a healthy reference population) can be broadly categorised as non-specific, specific (usually for epilepsy, or rarely for certain neurodegenerative disorders, e.g. CJD or SSPE), or patterns of unclear significance (further discussed later).

EEG in the diagnosis of epilepsy

EEG is the primary investigation in epilepsy. However, it should not be forgotten that the diagnosis of epilepsy is essentially clinical, and EEG has a high false negative rate and a low but important false positive rate. EEGs are liable to misinterpretation when there is insufficient knowledge of the range of normal and non-specific EEG phenomena – this has repeatedly been identified as a common reason for false diagnosis of epilepsy.

The sensitivity of a standard EEG in detecting interictal epileptiform features (discussed later) in patients with epilepsy is of the order of 30–40%. It increases if a substantial amount of sleep is included in the recording. If the initial EEG recording in a patient with a suspected seizure disorder is 'negative' (i.e. does not show any epileptiform discharges), further recordings should aim to record sleep.

The combination of wake and sleep records gives a yield of abnormalities in about 80% in patients with clinically confirmed epilepsy. Sleep EEG can be achieved by recording natural sleep, or by using hypnotics (e.g. chloral hydrate) to induce sleep. Whether sleep deprivation has additional value for induction of epileptiform activity is unclear, but there is some evidence that it specifically activates spikes in IGE. Evaluation of different EEG protocols in young people (<35 years) with possible epilepsy found that sleep-deprived EEG provided significantly better yield than routine EEG or drug-induced sleep EEG, and it may be the most cost-effective protocol for investigation of new onset epilepsy. The incremental yield of subsequent EEGs with sleep reaches a ceiling effect after the third recording, and it is estimated that up to 10% of patients with epilepsy never show epileptiform features on interictal EEG recordings. For these reasons, a 'negative' or normal EEG cannot 'rule out' epilepsy.

The sensitivity of an individual standard EEG is low; its diagnostic value relies on a high specificity. A misinterpreted EEG demonstrating epileptiform discharges where none exist is a common problem. It is potentially damaging with social and employment consequences, impaired quality of life and effects from unnecessary antiepileptic drug exposure. For this reason, most neurophysiologists agree that it is essential to be clear as to whether a particular sharpened waveform represents an epileptiform activity or not. The EEG reader must be thoroughly familiar with all pitfalls of misinterpreting spiky waveforms, which can occur as normal variants or background fluctuations. Sharpened features should only be reported as epileptiform if they are unequivocally so, using clear criteria regarding morphology and topography, and it is imperative that the report clearly communicates the neurophysiologist's assessment.

With conservative interpretation, only a very small percentage of otherwise normal subjects show epileptiform abnormalities in their EEG. The incidence of epileptiform discharges is very low, around 0.5–1% in adults with no known history of epilepsy and about 2–4% in children. In one study incidence was estimated at 4 in 1000 in a population of healthy men, and this includes spikes during photic stimulation only. There is variable follow-up duration reported and one person indeed developed epilepsy during that period. It can be concluded that unequivocal unprovoked interictal epileptiform discharges in adults are highly associated with epilepsy, bearing in mind that epilepsy is a clinical diagnosis. Epileptiform phenomena may also be seen in up to 30% of patients who have neurological disorders or cerebral pathologies (e.g. tumour, head injury, cranial surgery), without a history of witnessed seizures. Thus, an abnormal EEG showing epileptiform activity does not in itself indicate that the subject must have a seizure disorder.

The National Institute for Health and Care Excellence (NICE) guidelines for diagnosis and management of the epilepsies recommend that routine EEG should be performed only if the clinical history of an event suggests that it was an epileptic seizure, and that EEG should not be used if the presentation suggests syncope or non-epileptic attack. In children, EEG is generally recommended after a second seizure, as the diagnostic yield from routine EEG after a single seizure is considered too low to influence management.

Epileptiform phenomena

Transient (isolated) EEG features classified as epileptiform are spikes, sharp waves, and spike or polyspike and wave complexes. They reflect the fundamental electrical abnormality in epilepsy, namely the hyperexcitability of a cortical area. It has been estimated that 6–10 cm^2 of cortex needs to be activated synchronously for an epileptiform discharge to be visible on scalp EEG, and more recent studies found even larger cortical areas of 10–20 cm^2 that have to be activated on intracranial EEG. Although the terms 'spike, sharp wave, and spike wave complex' have been defined by morphology and duration, their distinction has relatively little clinical implications, and neurophysiologists often use them interchangeably. They can all occur as single discharges, or in runs or trains.

Some epileptiform phenomena – 3 per second spike-wave complexes, hypsarrythmia and generalised photoparoxysmal responses – are strongly correlated with clinical epilepsy. Others, such as focal sharp waves in centro-temporal regions, are moderately correlated with clinically evident seizures. The probability therefore that an interictal epileptiform discharge indicates epilepsy relates to the location of the discharge and the age of the person.

The EEG of normal subjects can show a range of spikey, sharpened or rhythmic features that resemble epileptiform activity, particularly in sleep. These 'patterns of unclear significance' include benign epileptiform transients of sleep, wicket spikes, 14 and 6 Hz positive bursts, occipital 6Hz spike and wave bursts, rhythmic mid-temporal theta of drowsiness, midline theta, frontal arousal rhythm and subclinical rhythmic epileptiform discharge in adults (SREDA). These variants mostly have no link with epilepsy, but are a potential source of confusion and EEG misinterpretation.

Location of electrodes and site of epileptic focus, age of patient, the presence of medication, diurnal timing of the EEG and the frequency, severity and type of epilepsy all influence the chance of detecting epileptiform discharges. The timing of EEG in relation to last seizure event may be relevant as one study has found that an interictal EEG within 24 hours of a seizure revealed an abnormality in 51% compared with 34% who had later EEG.

EEG in the classification of epileptic seizures and syndromes

Clinical criteria alone are not necessarily sufficient for characterisation of a seizure or epilepsy type, or infallible. Both epileptiform activity and interictal background cortical rhythms provide information that can complement the history and aid diagnosis. EEG findings contribute to diagnostic refinement at different levels: by establishing whether the seizure disorder is focal or generalised, idiopathic or symptomatic, or part of an epilepsy syndrome. This information can help with prognosis and selection of an anticonvulsant.

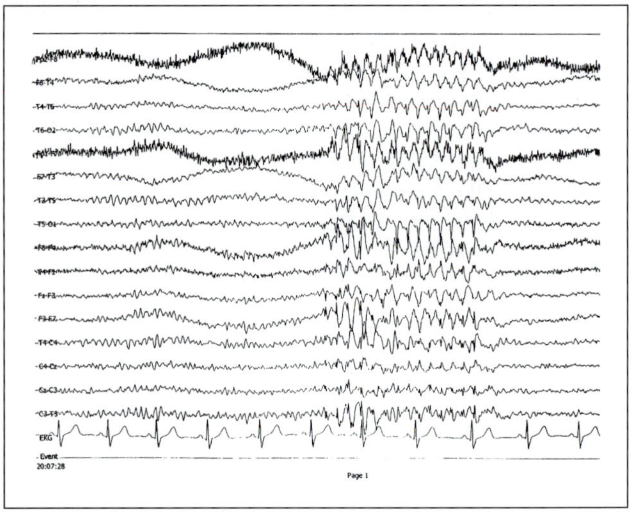

Figure 7.1 Typical spike-wave discharge in a patient with absence epilepsy.

Although division of seizure types into partial (focal) and generalised is a cornerstone of clinical practice, it is important to appreciate there can be EEG (and clinical) overlap between the two. Rapid spread and generalisation of epileptiform activity arising from a frontal lobe focus can mimic idiopathic generalised epilepsy; focal spikes and regional accentuation of generalised spike-wave discharges are well-recognised in IGE syndromes.

Idiopathic generalised epilepsy The typical interictal EEG findings in IGE are generalised spike or polyspike and slow wave complexes (spike-wave complexes) at 3–5 Hz (Figure 7.1), with normal background cortical rhythms. A subset of patients show photosensitivity (defined as a generalised photoparoxysmal response on photic stimulation). In childhood absence epilepsy, there is characteristic bilateral synchronous 3-Hz spike wave, usually lasting 5–10 seconds. Careful analysis of the individual spike wave complexes often reveals that they are slightly faster at the onset of a burst (3.5–4 Hz). During the main portion, they usually slow down to 3–3.5 Hz, and may slow down even further to approximately 2.5 Hz towards the end. Although generally seen in a widespread and symmetric distribution, there may be asynchronies between the two hemispheres of 5–20 ms. In childhood absence epilepsy, runs of 3 Hz spike-wave complexes are often enhanced or provoked by hyperventilation. Background cortical rhythms are normal, but some children show runs of occipital rhythmic delta slowing (up to 40% of cases), which may persist after remission of absences. Photosensitivity is uncommon (less than 10%), and possibly indicative of poorer prognosis. Patients with juvenile absence epilepsy usually show polyspike discharge or spike-wave frequency above 3 Hz. In juvenile myoclonic epilepsy, the interictal EEG characteristics are brief bursts of polyspike (sometimes single spike) and wave discharges up to 6 Hz. Variable asymmetry and slight asynchrony of the discharge is common between the two hemispheres, and interictal focal abnormalities occur in up to 40%. Not all patients with IGE show typical electrographic findings in the first EEG. Childhood or juvenile absence epilepsy is most likely to show diagnostic EEG abnormalities at initial investigation, whereas other syndromes may need serial recordings (including sleep deprivation) to elucidate the diagnosis. This should not delay appropriate treatment.

Ictal EEG patterns in IGE may occur as a prolongation of the interictal epileptiform features (e.g. in typical absence epilepsy). In fact, the longer a run of spike-wave complexes lasts, the more likely it is associated with a transient disturbance in cognition or working memory, and ultimately behavioural arrest. Myoclonic jerks may produce EMG artefacts in the recording, but they can be easier detected if surface EMG electrodes are placed over the extremities. In generalised tonic–clonic seizures, fast rhythmic spikes are commonly seen at the onset, before the ictal EEG becomes obscured by muscle artefacts. In the clonic phase, this activity becomes discontinuous, and is ultimately replaced by rhythmic slow waves with alternating spikes or polyspikes. In the immediate post-ictal phase, the EEG is often diffusely suppressed for several seconds. A period of diffuse irregular slow follows that is gradually replaced by the patient's baseline activity.

In seizures of focal onset, ictal EEG manifestations can be quite variable. In contrast to IGE, the morphology of the ictal pattern is often different from the associated interictal features. A common manifestation is a rhythmic activity that evolves in amplitude, frequency and distribution. This may be preceded by a more widespread or even diffuse attenuation of EEG activity. Diffuse attenuation may be the only ictal EEG manifestation, for example in the epileptic spasms that are characteristic of West syndrome. Repetitive epileptiform discharges can also constitute an ictal pattern, or they may be followed by an evolving rhythmic pattern. Low amplitude circumscribed fast activity is often the earliest ictal manifestation on intracranial EEG, which may be undetectable using scalp recordings. As in generalised tonic–clonic seizures, the ictal scalp EEG may become obscured by EMG and movement artefact (e.g. chewing automatisms). In the post-ictal phase, slowing is commonly seen, often most prominent over the area of seizure origin. Interictal epileptiform abnormalities may become more abundant following a seizure.

Ictal EEG patterns may occur without any behavioral or cognitive alteration (subclinical seizure). Conversely, focal seizures may occur without any detectable scalp EEG change. This is often the case for epileptic auras. However, even more severe focal seizures may occasionally lack a correlate on scalp EEG.

Benign childhood epilepsy syndromes The EEG is the definitive diagnostic test in benign childhood epilepsy with centro-temporal spikes. The defining EEG feature is the occurrence of high-amplitude focal sharp wave discharges in central and temporal regions, either bilateral or unilateral, and potentiated by sleep. A few children show focal discharges in other brain regions or generalised spike-wave activity. Background cerebral rhythms are normal. The EEG is often very abnormal even in the presence of infrequent (or indeed any) seizures. In the occipital variant, named after Panayiotopoulos, the majority of patients show shifting or multifocal spikes or spike and wave complexes with posterior emphasis; however, spikes may be seen over any brain region. The clinician should be alerted to a diagnosis of a benign childhood epilepsy syndrome in a child with infrequent, mostly nocturnal seizures or paroxysmal autonomic symptoms whose routine EEG shows frequent multi-focal discharges.

Lennox–Gastaut syndrome The classic EEG finding in this condition with severe intractable multiple seizure types and learning disability are slow spike-wave complexes that range from 1 to 2.5 Hz. These occur in a generalised or lateralised distribution and become enhanced in non-REM sleep. They may disappear in adolescence and adulthood. Runs of rapid spikes in non-REM sleep are another common finding. The background EEG is often disorganised and excessively slow, reflecting a significant baseline dysfunction of the brain.

Electrical status epilepticus in sleep This rare childhood condition is characterised by the presence of continuous spike and wave discharges in non-REM sleep, combined with rare, if any, EEG abnormalities in the awake state and REM sleep. Most children have seizures, but the hallmark finding is regression of cognition and behaviour. It occurs in a number of childhood epilepsies, including the Landau–Kleffner syndrome of acquired aphasia and epilepsy.

Progressive myoclonic epilepsies These epilepsies show generalised spike and wave discharge, photosensitivity, 'giant' sensory-evoked potentials (SEPs), facilitation of motor-evoked potentials (MEPs) by afferent stimulation and abnormalities of background cerebral activity, typically an excess of slow activity. The background abnormalities are usually progressive, particularly in syndromes with dementia or significant cognitive decline such as Lafora body disease. Some specific features occur in some cases: vertex sharp waves in sialidosis, occipital spikes in Lafora body disease and giant visual-evoked potentials (VEPs) in lipofuscinosis.

Partial epilepsy Broadly speaking, localised EEG changes are more common in TLE than in extratemporal epilepsies (Figure 7.2 and Figure 7.3), and spike, polyspike and/or high-frequency discharges are more likely to occur in foci that are located superficially in neocortex. However, even prolonged interictal EEG can be normal or non-localising in partial epilepsies if the epileptogenic region:

1 Is extensive
2 Is remote from the location of the scalp electrodes (e.g. mesial frontal lobar areas), or
3 Involves too small a neuronal aggregate for synchronised activity to be registered on the scalp.

In partial epilepsies, the most important ictal EEG changes for seizure localisation are those that occur within the first 30 seconds after the seizure onset. Later changes are of limited value for localisation or lateralisation of the epileptogenic region, because the discharge will by then have propagated to other brain areas.

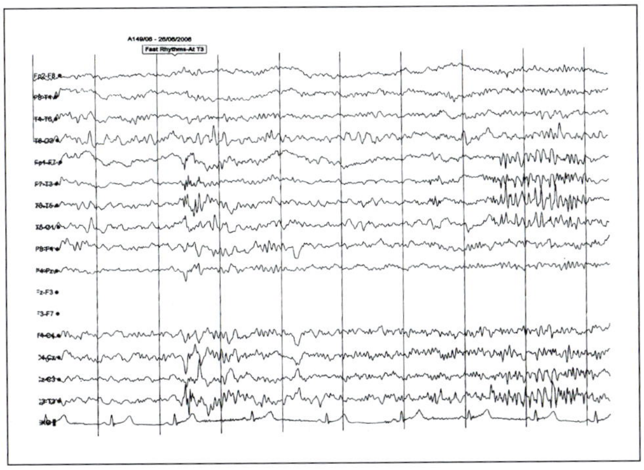

Figure 7.2 High-frequency interictal discharge in a patient with neocortical or lateral temporal lobe epilepsy.

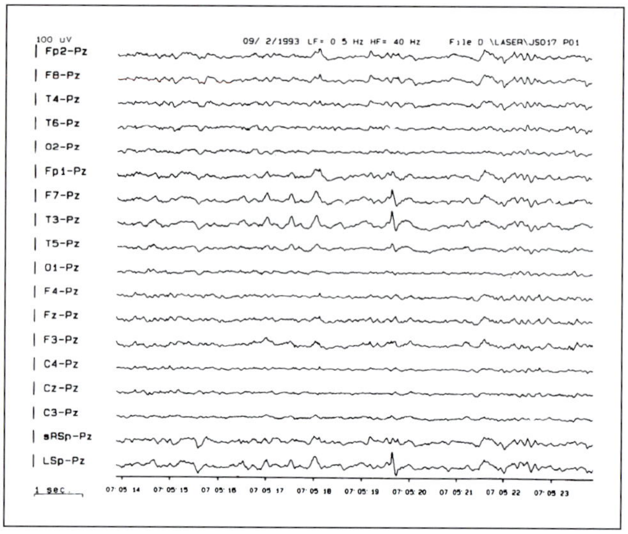

Figure 7.3 Interictal EEG: left mesial temporal lobe epilepsy, referential recording. Focal spikes at electrodes sited near the left anterior temporal lobe (F7 and Sp1) and mid temporal lobe (T3).

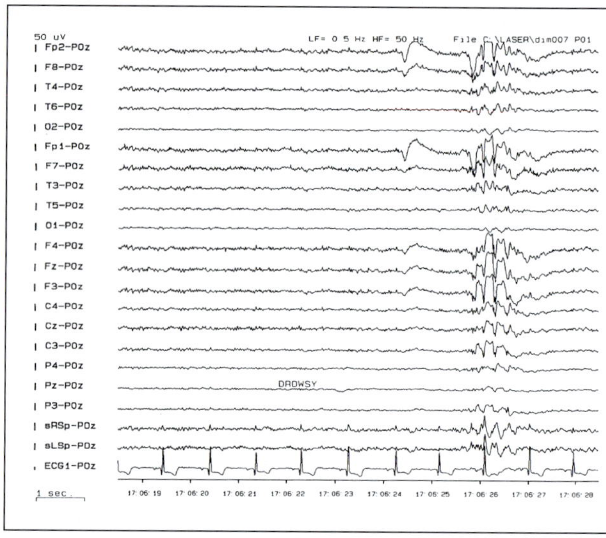

Figure 7.4 Widespread bilateral spike-wave discharge in a man with frontal lobe complex partial seizures (hypermotor semiology).

Temporal lobe epilepsy Mesial TLE associated with unilateral temporal lobe pathology, usually hippocampal sclerosis, shows anterior and mid temporal interictal spikes, and a characteristic rhythmic ictal discharge accompanying seizures in more than 80% of cases. The appearance of a localised scalp EEG pattern may follow the onset of clinical symptoms by 30 s or more. Independent bitemporal interictal spikes are common, but predominate over the pathological temporal lobe in 60% of cases.

In lateral TLEs, interictal spikes tend to be located over the mid and posterior temporal lobar regions; the ictal EEG discharge is typically higher frequency than in mesial TLE, and lateralised in about 50% of cases. In practice, the EEG changes are not specific enough to differentiate lateral and mesial TLE in a reliable fashion and, furthermore, temporal changes can occur in frontal and other extratemporal epilepsies.

Frontal lobe and other extratemporal epilepsies Focal interictal EEG abnormalities are the exception, and there are no specific patterns associated with the subtypes of frontal lobe epilepsy. Many patients show widespread or even generalised abnormalities (Figure 7.4), because of rapid spread to other lobar regions and secondary generalisation. The same is true for ictal changes, the most common pattern in frontal lobe epilepsy being either high amplitude slow or a diffuse fast discharge followed by generalised attenuation and/or bilateral slow activity. In lateral frontal lobe epilepsy, repetive spiking characterises the ictal EEG in about 40% of cases; evolving rhythmic patterns are about as common. The ictal EEG allows localisation or lateralisation in about 70%. In mesial frontal lobe epilepsy, the most common patterns are low amplitude fast activity, and diffuse attenuation of the EEG. In contrast to lateral frontal lobe epilepsy, the localising value is poor, of the order of 25%.

Patients with parietal lobe epilepsy (PLE) tend to have multifocal epileptiform discharges. The most common ictal EEG patterns are paroxysmal fast and repetitive epileptiform activity. As in mesial FLE, the patterns are often nonlocalisable, or may mislocalise. In occipital lobe epilepsy (OLE), rhythmic patterns of variable frequency are seen in about 60%, and paroxysmal fast or repetitive spiking in most other cases. False localisation is relatively common in patients with OLE.

EEG and prediction of seizure recurrence

If the initial EEG shows definite epileptiform discharge, there is a greater risk of seizure recurrence in individuals presenting with the first unprovoked seizure, particularly if idiopathic in type. EEG has distinguished between high and low risk groups in a number of studies: a systematic review showed risk of recurrence at 2 years was 27% if the EEG was normal, but 58% if epileptiform activity was present. Following epilepsy surgery, epileptiform activity on the interictal EEG has been shown to predict seizure recurrence.

EEG and withdrawal of antiepileptic medication

The type of epilepsy syndrome is the most important variable in predicting likelihood of seizure recurrence for patients in remission who are considering withdrawal of medication. EEG can provide supplementary information: presence of spike-wave discharge in patients with IGE and evidence of a generalised photosensitive (photoparoxysmal) response are associated with high risk of recurrence. The prognostic significance of other patterns and abnormalities in other types of epilepsy is less clear.

EEG and antiepileptic drugs

Acute administration of barbiturates and benzodiazepines suppresses interictal discharges, but the effect declines when these drugs are given as chronic therapy. Sodium valproate suppresses generalised spike-wave complexes, and photoparoxysmal responses, and EEG can be used to monitor therapeutic efficacy in patients with childhood absence epilepsy. Lamotrigine may have a similar effect, and ethosuximide also suppresses generalised discharges. Other antiepileptic drugs have variable or inconsistent effects on either focal or generalised epileptiform activity, and EEG is therefore of little or no use in monitoring response to drug treatment. 'Treating the EEG' is generally undesirable.

Antiepileptic drugs can affect background cortical rhythms, but significant slowing does not occur unless there is drug toxicity.

Long-term EEG monitoring

Long-term monitoring (LTM) allows extended EEG recording, which can be undertaken as an ambulatory procedure using a portable recorder, or via hard wired recorders with time-linked video in a hospital setting. Usually, the aim is to document 'attacks' rather than the interictal state. LTM has been shown in several studies to change diagnosis and affect management in >50% of difficult to treat cases. Its principal applications are shown in Table 7.16.

Ambulatory EEG monitoring is most suited to clinical problems that do not require concurrent synchronised video to document clinical features, or for monitoring in a specific environment. It is more susceptible to artefacts than EEG recordings in a laboratory. Ambulatory recording does not have the advantage of inpatient video EEG telemetry units where specialised staff are usually experienced in the identification of subtle clinical events and the diagnostic assessment and care of patients during seizures. Systematic interview and focused examination during and after seizures contributes valuable information about areas of cortex activated during seizures or rendered dysfunctional by the seizure activity. High technical quality of the recording can be easier achieved than with ambulatory EEG, and simultaneous video recordings allow correlation of patient behaviour with EEG phenomena. These units are the safest environment for reduction in medication dose to provoke seizures. Their downside is that they are resource intensive.

Table 7.16 The principal clinical applications of long-term electroencephalogram (EEG) monitoring.

Differential diagnosis of paroxysmal neurological attacks
Distinction between nocturnal epilepsy and parasomnias
Diagnosis of psychogenic non-epileptic seizures
Characterisation of seizure type and the electro-clinical correlates of epileptic seizures
Quantification of epileptiform discharge and seizure frequency
Evaluation in epilepsy surgery candidates
Identification of sleep-related epileptiform discharge/electrical status in children
Electro-clinical characterisation of neonatal seizures
Monitoring of status epilepticus (convulsive, non-convulsive, electrographic)

Source: adapted from Shorvon 2013. With permission of Oxford University Press.

The optimal length of study for LTM depends on the clinical problem, and frequency of attacks; if it is less than once per week in patients who do not take anticonvulsants, LTM is not likely to be beneficial.

Neurophysiology for assessing patients for epilepsy surgery

Interictal and ictal EEG are pivotal investigations in presurgical evaluation, but are generally more important in resective surgical procedures than in functional procedures such as callosotomy and vagal nerve stimulation.

EEG and tonic–clonic status epilepticus

EEG is essential for diagnosis and management of status epilepticus in convulsive (Figure 7.5) and non-convulsive forms. As a minimum standard, EEG should be performed within 12–24 hours for admissions with uncontrolled seizures or confusional states. EEG monitoring should be available during treatment of refractory status. There are generally no specific EEG markers of the different electro-clinical types of status: all show variations of waxing and waning rhythmic patterns, with or without frank epileptiform discharges.

EEG is used in convulsive status epilepticus to:

- Confirm status and exclude pseudostatus
- Differentiate causes of altered mental status – continuing seizures, drug-induced coma or encephalopathy, and
- In the refractory stage to monitor and guide treatment, as clinical manifestations of ongoing seizure activity may then be subtle or absent, even though seizure activity may continue in the brain.

EEG is used as guide to the dosing of anaesthetic treatment in refractory status, with dosing often modulated to obtain burst suppression on the EEG (Figure 7.5), although seizure suppression is deemed sufficient in patients unable to tolerate higher dose

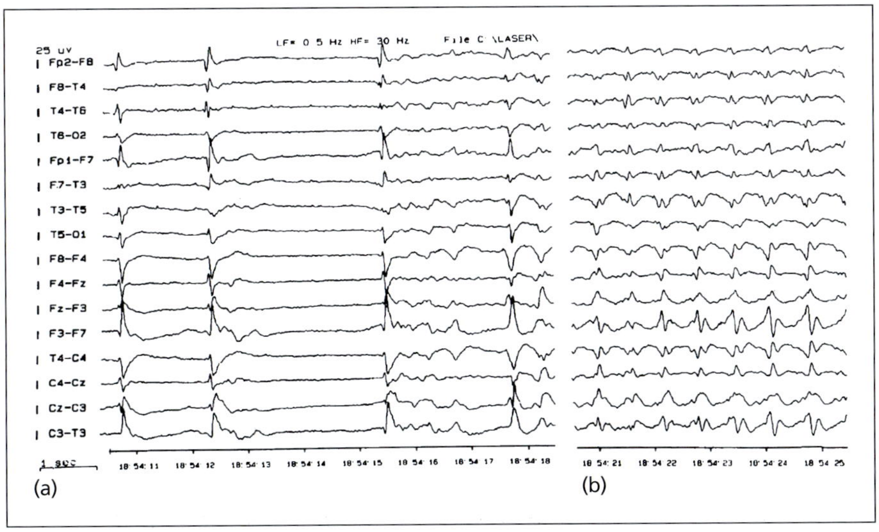

Figure 7.5 Segments from EEG monitoring in convulsive status: (a) burst suppression and some breakthrough discharge; (b) electrographic status.

anaesthesia. EEG may also contribute information of prognostic value, and for instance continuing electrographic status after the convulsive phase is associated with worse outcome in convulsive status epilepticus.

Non-convulsive status epilepticus

This term describes a range of conditions, with variable clinical features and causes. EEG is necessary for diagnosis of non-convulsive status epilepticus (NCSE), especially when the clinical manifestations are subtle. The EEG expression of non-convulsive status depends on cause, and includes any of continuous spike-wave discharge (generalised in absence status epilepticus), discrete localised electrographic seizures, diffuse slow activity with or without spikes, and periodic and/or repetitive epileptiform discharge. Electrographic confirmation of NCSE is often difficult in focal status, as the EEG may, show only subtle changes. In epileptic syndromes, such as Lennox–Gastaut syndrome, when there is overlap of ictal and interictal EEG patterns; and in patients with acute cerebral damage (e.g. caused by infection or trauma), interpretation of EEG is complicated by the fact that the changes of NCSE may be subtle and also because EEG abnormalities can result directly from the primary pathology. EEG can be recorded during acute administration of intravenous benzodiazepine or other antiepileptic therapy, and the rapid resolution of the abnormal EEG patterns, when associated with clinical improvement, can be taken as supportive evidence of a diagnosis of NCSE.

EEG in the intensive care setting

EEG has three main roles in the ICU patient. First, it can be used to distinguish coma from diminished responsiveness resulting from other causes (psychiatric, sedation, neuromuscular, locked-in syndrome); secondly, to detect non-convulsive or clinically subtle seizures (most cases of status in the ICU are non-convulsive or difficult to identify on clinical grounds alone); thirdly, to identify an encephalopathy. EEG is the cornerstone examination for non-convulsive seizures in the critically ill patient in intensive care , but it is difficult to interpret and subject to many errors that can lead to a wrong diagnosis and unnecessary or inadequate treatment. Differentiation between NCSE and a non-specific encephalopathy can be difficult, but the clinical context is critical.

It may be able to add information for the prognostication of patients with severe diffuse brain injury, such as following cardiac arrest. Generalised suppression of the background, absence of EEG reactivity or generalised epileptiform patterns indicate a poorer prognosis. However, there is evidence that a single EEG is not a useful test to predict outcome and has only limited diagnostic accuracy. EEG is also used as an adjunctive test in the determination of electrocerebral inactivity ('brain death').

EEG and cognitive deterioration

Acute confusional states or acute and/or subacute cognitive decline in epilepsy may be caused by frequent subtle or clinically unrecognised seizures; a marked increase in epileptiform discharges; a metabolic or toxic encephalopathy; or non-convulsive status epilepticus. EEG can be very helpful in determining the cause in acute confusional states, but is less likely to be useful in chronic cognitive decline other than to confirm the presence of an organic brain syndrome.

Imaging in epilepsy

X-ray computed tomography

MRI is generally the imaging modality of first choice for epilepsy. However, X-ray computed tomography (CT) is useful in acute situations where MRI is not appropriate and where rapid brain imaging is required. CT is also superior to MRI in the detection of focal cortical calcification and in changes to the skull vault or other bony structures. CT is also helpful when there are contraindications to MRI, such as a cardiac pacemaker or cochlear implants.

CT is not as sensitive or specific as MRI for identifying most of the common epileptogenic abnormalities, such as indolent gliomas, cavernomas, malformations of cortical development (MCD) and lesions in the medial temporal lobe.

Magnetic resonance imaging

Most patients who develop epilepsy or whose chronic epilepsy has not been fully assessed should be investigated with MRI, to detect the underlying cause of the epilepsy (it should be remembered that the role of MRI is not to make a diagnosis of epilepsy per se). The ILAE commission has suggested the following clinical indications for MRI in the investigation of patients with epilepsy, although these will depend on availability and clinical circumstances:

- Focal onset of seizures
- Onset of generalised or unclassified seizures in the first year of life, or in adulthood
- Focal deficit on neurological or neuropsychological examination
- Difficulty in obtaining seizure control with first line antiepileptic drugs, and
- Loss of seizure control or change in the seizure pattern.

In patients with newly diagnosed epilepsy, MRI identifies a causal epileptogenic lesion in 12–14%. In chronic epilepsy, current MRI detects relevant lesions in 50–70%, rising to 75-80% in those with refractory focal epilepsy.

MRI is not required in patients with a definite electroclinical diagnosis of idiopathic generalised epilepsy who go into early remission.

All patients with intractable epilepsy considered for surgery should undergo high resolution structural MRI as the success of surgery is directly related to the ability to pinpoint the site of seizure onset and underlying structural abnormalities. A structural abnormality does not necessarily indicate the site of seizure origin, and clinical EEG and other data need to be correlated with imaging. Postoperative MRI is useful to identify the extent of a cortical resection or the presence of residual pathology, particularly if seizures continue after surgery.

Hippocampal sclerosis The hippocampus is best visualised by acquiring thin slices (1–3 mm) orthogonal to its long axis. The primary MRI features of hippocampal sclerosis are hippocampal atrophy, demonstrated with coronal T1-weighted images, and increased signal intensity within the hippocampus on T2-weighted and FLAIR images (Figure 7.6). Additionally, decreased T1-weighted signal intensity and disruption of the internal structure of the hippocampus may be present. Other MRI abnormalities associated with hippocampal damage include atrophy of temporal lobe white matter and cortex, dilatation of the temporal horn and a blurring of the grey–white border in the temporal neocortex. Atrophy of the amygdala and entorhinal cortex variably accompany hippocampal damage but may also occur in patients with TLE and normal hippocampi. FLAIR images provide an increased contrast between grey and white matter, and facilitate differentiation of the amygdala from the hippocampus.

Visual assessment can reliably detect hippocampal volume asymmetry of more than 20%; however, lesser degrees of asymmetry require quantitative volumetric analysis. The use of contiguous thin slices increases the reliability of measurements and permits localisation of atrophy along the length of the hippocampus. Automated

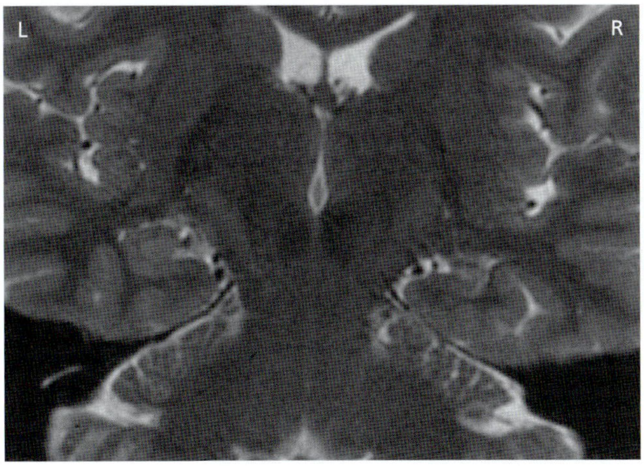

Figure 7.6 Left hippocampal sclerosis. Coronal T2-weighted image showing atrophy and increased T2 signal in the left hippocampus. The right hippocampus is normal.

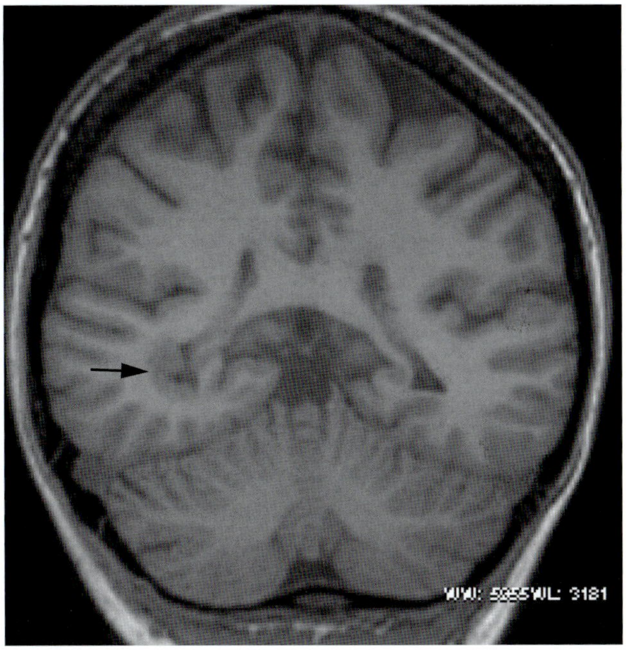

Figure 7.7 Subependymal heterotopia on the right (arrow) in coronal IR_{prep} T1-weighted image. Nodules of grey matter density are shown in the wall of the lateral ventricle.

methods for measuring hippocampal volume are now becoming available, with the advantages of speed and avoidance of human error. However, hippocampal volumes should have a correction applied that takes into account intracranial volume, so that symmetrical bilateral atrophy can be identified. Patients with unilateral hippocampal volume loss, no other imaging abnormality and concordant clinical and EEG data have the optimal outcome after temporal lobe resective surgery. Measurement of T2 relaxation time is another objective way to assess hippocampal damage. The advantage of this technique is that hippocampal T2 (HT2) times are absolute values, which can be compared against control data. Increased HT2 reflects gliosis and neuronal loss. HT2 prolongation also correlates with the hippocampal volume loss. Both volumetry and T2 relaxometry techniques can be used to identify subtle amygdala pathology.

Malformations of cortical development There are many forms of malformations. The MRI features of focal cortical dysplasia are focal cortical thickening, simplified gyration, blurring of the cortical–white matter junction and T2 prolongation in the underlying white matter A thin slice FLAIR acquisition gives the most sensitivity. Type 2B focal cortical dysplasia is the most obvious on MRI, with dysmyelination of white matter extending towards the lateral ventricle. Type 1 and 2A are more subtle and often not evident on MRI. Automated voxel-based iamge analysis can increase the pick-up rate, but with a risk of false positive findings. Complete surgical removal of focal cortical dysplasia is accompanied by a 30–50% remission rate, but the epileptogenic zone may be more extensive than the abnormality visible on MRI. Polymicrogyria with an excessive number of small and prominent convolutions is a frequently identified dysplasia. Several syndromes of region-specific symmetric polymicrogyria have been reported, and some have been linked to specific genetic loci. Schizencephaly is often found in MRI in conjunction with polymicrogyria. Peri-ventricular heterotopia may be unilateral or bilateral and has a characteristic MRI appearance (Figure 7.7).

Primary brain tumour Patients with low-grade primary brain tumours frequently have intractable focal seizures as a presenting symptom. Underlying histopathologies include dysembryoplastic neuro-epithelial tumours (DNT), ganglioglioma, gangliocytoma, and pilocytic and fibrillary astrocytoma. Most lesions have low signal on T1- and high signal on T2-weighted images, and are not usually associated with vasogenic oedema. Complete resection of the neoplasm and overlying cortex results in successful control of seizures in most cases. DNTs are benign developmental tumours with features of a focal circumscribed cortical mass which may indent the overlying skull. Cyst formation and contrast enhancement may occur. Some DNTs calcify and may be more readily demonstrated with X-ray CT. Confident differentiation from low grade astrocytomas and gangliogliomas is not possible by MRI.

Vascular malformation Cavernous haemangiomas (cavernomas) are relatively common lesions which are important to identify as they are often surgically resectable. Most cavernous haemangiomas are not visible on CT but come to light on MRI scanning. The lesions are circumscribed and have the characteristic appearance on MRI (Figure 7.8). The central part contains areas of high signal on T1- and T2-weighted images, reflecting oxidised haemoglobin, with darker areas on T1-weighted images as a result of the presence of deoxyhaemoglobin. The ring of surrounding haemosiderin appears dark on a T2-weighted image. Up to 50% of cavernous malformations are multiple, and can show autosomal dominant inheritance.

AVMs with high blood flow have a different and distinctive appearance with a nidus, feeding arteries and draining veins and the vascular supply can be further characterised by MR angiography or contrast angiography.

Trauma, stroke and infection Focal or diffuse cortical damage can develop as a consequence of trauma, infarction or infection of the CNS. Cerebrovascular disease associated with epilepsy is particularly common in older age groups. Worldwide, neurocysticercosis and tuberculomas are the most common causes of intractable focal epilepsy. These lesions have typical appearances on MRI which evolve with time and which, unless calcified, may resolve.

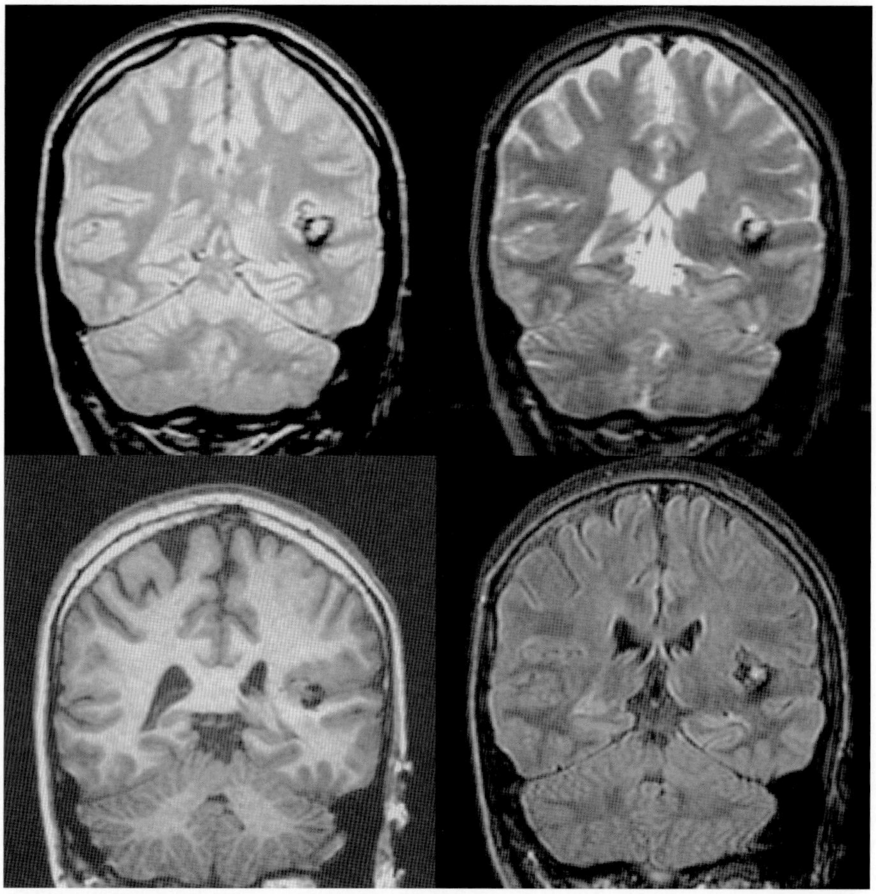

Figure 7.8 Cavernoma on the left (coronal 3.0 T MRI). Proton density (top L), T2-weighted (top R), IR_{prep} T1-weighted (low L), FLAIR (low R). The acquisitions demonstrate heterogeneous hyperintense signal caused by blood products in different stages of evolution, surrounded by a rim of low signal intensity from haemosiderin.

Functional magnetic resonance imaging

Functional MRI (fMRI) can visualise regional brain activity. The areas are detected by measuring changes in blood oxygenation level-dependent (BOLD) contrast that occur during cognitive, sensory and other tasks, and allow the mapping of networks involved in the performance of these tasks. The clinical applications of fMRI are very limited. The most important are in the localisation and lateralisation of cognitive functions of epilepsy patients being evaluated for surgery in order to minimise the risk of causing a fixed deficit. However, the studies require patient cooperation, both in performing tasks and limiting motion, and findings may not be sufficiently sensitive or specific to reliably guide surgical planning, and it is important to choose activation procedures that are appropriate tests of function in the area of brain to be resected and to recognise the limitations. However, localisation of the primary motor and strip, and lateralisation of language are now routinely performed for clinical purposes. Important caveats are that areas that do not activate cannot be assumed to be functionally inert and not all areas that activate are crucial for function.

Tractography

The course of major white matter tracks in the brain can be inferred using tractographic analysis of the directions of diffusion of water in the brain. The principle underpinning this imaging technique is that water preferentially diffuses along axons and myelin sheaths (i.e. is directional not random) and this property allows the orientation of tracts to be visualised. Data are acquired using diffusion imaging and current spatial resolution, within a clinically reasonable imaging time, is approximately $2mm^3$ – many orders of magnitude greater than the size of individual axons. There are a range of software packages for tractography: these can be deterministic and are quick to perform but not so reliable and are prone to error when tracts are curved, or probabilistic, which are more time consuming and computationally intensive.

In clinical epilepsy practice, the main role of tractography is to visualise the optic radiation and corticospinal tracts when planning surgical resection close to these critical structures. This is particularly relevant to anterior temporal lobe resections which are associated with a 5–20% incidence of clinically evident visual field defects which may prevent driving. Demonstration of the optic radiation, which extends anteriorly to a variable extent, allows prediction of the risk and modification of surgical approach to mitigate this (Figure 7.9).

Single-photon emission computed tomography

Single-photon emission computed tomography (SPECT) allows measurements of regional cerebral blood flow changes in the areas affected by epileptic activity. The radioligands currently principally

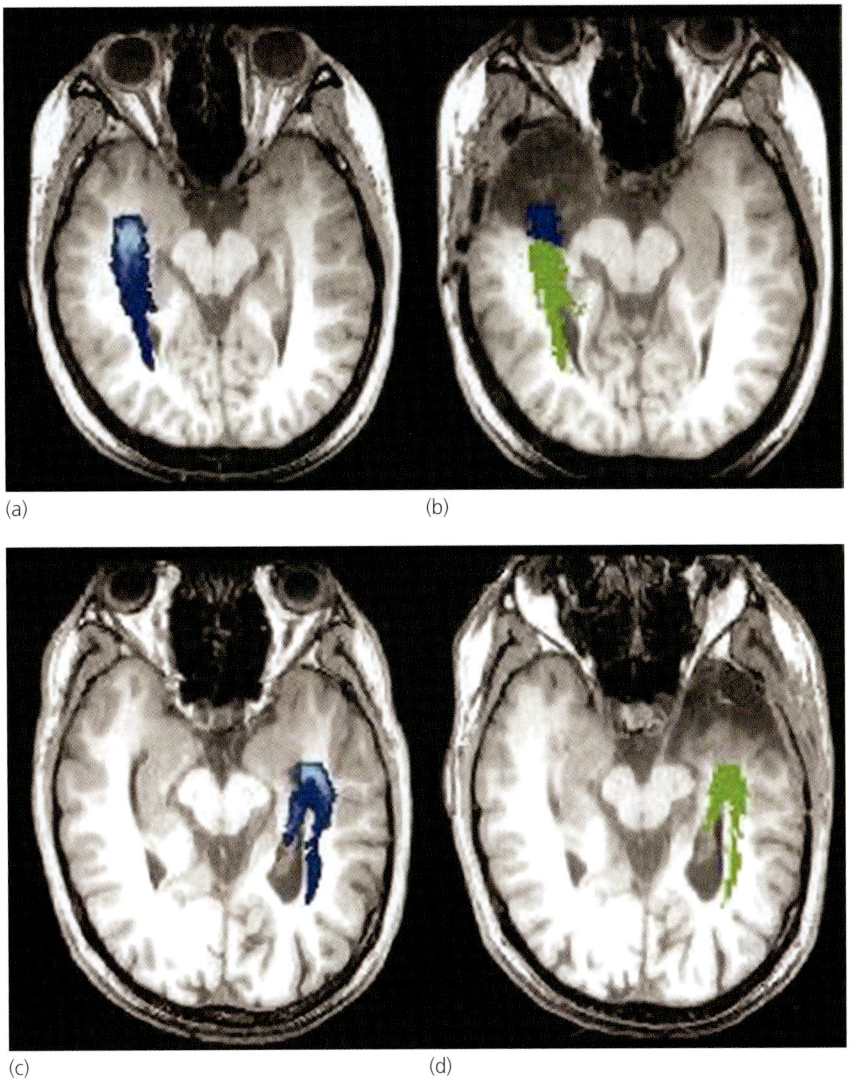

Figure 7.9 Preoperative structural T1-weighted image and optic radiation (a) and postoperative structural T1-weighted image with propagated preoperative tractography (b) show that part of the optic radiation was resected (blue) in patient, who developed a severe visual field deficit (VFD). Corresponding preoperative (c) and postoperative images (d) are shown in a patient who did not develop a VFD. Source: Winston et al. 2012. Reproduced with permission of John Wiley & Sons.

used in SPECT studies are ^{99m}Tc-hexamethyl-propylenamine oxime (^{99m}Tc-HMPAO) and technetium-^{99m}Tc-cysteinate dimer (ECD, bicisate). Currently available stabilised forms of ^{99m}Tc-HMPAO and ECD are stable *in vitro* for several hours, whereas unstabilised ^{99m}Tc-HMPAO needs to be produced immediately before intravenous injection. Seventy-five per cent of ^{99m}Tc-HMPAO is extracted across the blood–brain barrier, reaching peak concentrations within 1 minute after injection. The images can then be acquired up to 6 hours after tracer injection. Both ictal and post-ictal SPECT studies should be performed during simultaneous video-EEG monitoring to determine the relationship between seizure onset and tracer injection. Interictal SPECT images serve as a reference baseline study for the interpretation of ictal images.

Ictal ^{99m}Tc-HMPAO SPECT is highly sensitive and specific in localising seizure onset in intractable TLE. Correct localisation of complex partial seizures may be achieved in over 90% of TLE patients. The use of subtraction ictal SPECT co-registered to MRI (SISCOM) improves the rate of localisation. A characteristic pattern in temporal lobe seizures is an initial hyperperfusion of the temporal lobe, followed by medial temporal hyperperfusion and lateral temporal hypoperfusion. Post-ictal and interictal SPECT injections are easier to perform than ictal injections, but the images are more difficult to interpret and have lower sensitivity and specificity and are not clinically as useful as a stand-alone test.

Extratemporal seizures are often brief and it is therefore difficult to obtain an ictal recording. Accurate localisation of an extratemporal seizure focus may be possible in 90% of the cases using the SISCOM technique. Ictal SPECT demonstrates ipsilateral frontal hyperperfusion in frontal lobe epilepsy. Activations may also be detected in the ipsilateral basal ganglia and contralateral cerebellum. The method provides additional information in patients with unrevealing EEG and MRI results, and can also be used to study the blood flow changes underlying specific clinical features observed in extratemporal seizures. Post-ictal and interictal SPECT is of very limited localising value in extratemporal epilepsy.

Ictal SPECT provides a complementary method for localising seizure foci in patients with intractable focal epilepsy evaluated for surgical treatment. The investigation may be particularly valuable in patients with normal MRI and presumed extratemporal seizures in order to generate a hypothesis that may then be tested with intracranial EEG recordings.

Positron emission tomography

Positron emission tomography (PET) maps cerebral glucose metabolism using ^{18}F-deoxyglucose (^{18}FDG). Interictally, PET shows areas of reduced glucose metabolism that usually include the seizure focus but are more extensive. Regional hypometabolism is best analysed with co-registration of PET scans to MRI. Voxel-based statistical parametric mapping (SPM) and surface reoconstruciton of PET data are useful in clinical evaluation of the data. The spatial resolution of quantitative ^{18}FDG-PET is superior to SPECT. Ictal ^{18}FDG-PET scans are difficult to obtain because cerebral uptake of ^{18}FDG occurs over 40 minutes after injection.

^{18}FDG-PET detects interictal glucose hypometabolism ipsilateral to the seizure focus in 60–90% of patients with TLE. Unilateral, or asymmetric bilateral diffuse regional hypometabolism usually extends medially and laterally in the temporal lobe. ^{18}FDG-PET has some additional sensitivity over optimal volumetric MRI but does not provide clinically useful information if hippocampal atrophy is present. ^{18}FDG-PET is more useful for lateralising than precisely localising the epileptic focus. Unilateral focal temporal hypometabolism in ^{18}FDG-PET predicts a good outcome of surgery for TLE. Absence of unilateral hypometabolism, however, does not preclude a favourable outcome. Symmetric bilateral temporal hypometabolism is associated with higher incidence of postoperative seizures as are areas of severe extratemporal cortical, or thalamic hypometabolism.

^{18}FDG-PET has lower sensitivity for lateralisation of epileptic foci in extratemporal epilepsies than in TLE. The areas of decreased glucose metabolism are also less frequently well-localised. Sixty per cent of the patients with frontal lobe epilepsy show regional hypometabolism in ^{18}FDG-PET, and a relevant underlying structural pathology is found on MRI in 90% of them. The area of hypometabolism may be either diffuse or widespread, or restricted to the co-localising MRI lesion. In a recent Queen Square series, PET scans were normal in 37% patients, showed unifocal hypometabolism in 51% and bilateral hypometabolism in 12%. The TLE group had a higher proportion of abnormal PET scans which were abnormal in 72% with TLE and 52% with frontal lobe epilepsy. PET data gave false lateralisation and/or localisation in 5%. An FDG-PET scan was useful in 53% patients; leading directly to surgery in 6% cases, helping to plan intracranial EEG in 35% and excluding 12% from further evaluation. It was more useful in TLE (66%) than frontal lobe epilepsy (38%). In summary, the place of interictal ^{18}FDG-PET is in determining the lateralisation and approximate localisation of the epileptic focus, especially in the presurgical assessment of patients with normal MRI and when there is not good concordance between MRI, EEG and other data, in order to generate a hypothesis to be tested with intracranial EEG recordings.

Magnetoencephalography Magnetoencephalography (MEG) is a non-invasive neurophysiological technique that measures the magnetic fields generated by neuronal activity. These magnetic fields originate from dipolar intracellular currents associated with dendritic inhibitory and excitatory post-synaptic potentials within sulcal pyramidal neurones orientated tangentially with the cortical surface. MEG is insensitive to radially orientated neurones located on the gyral crown, which comprise approximately one-third of cortical neurones, and which dominate the EEG, and it is because of this that MEG can potentially complement or enhance information provided by EEG. MEG has high temporal resolution, in the milliseconds range, which is comparable to EEG, and favourable to functional MRI which has a temporal resolution of several seconds.

The recorded magnetic field pattern is analysed to determine the localisation of either spontaneous (e.g. epileptic) or evoked (e.g. somatosensory) neuronal activity. The resulting map of magnetic dipoles is typically superimposed on a co-registered MRI scan to facilitate accurate neuro-anatomical localisation.

The utility of MEG has improved recently with the widespread availability of whole head magnetometers comprising up to 275 sensors which produce greater accuracy of dipole localisation and spatiotemporal propagation within an acceptable time period through more extensive spatial coverage.

Although MEG has been used to map somatosensory, motor, auditory and visual specific cortex, the main application of MEG in epilepsy is the characterisation of epileptic foci through the source localisation of interictal epileptiform activity, although, infrequently, ictal abnormalities are recorded by chance. The sensitivity of MEG for the identification of interictal epileptiform discharges, typically spikes, is approximately 50–70%, with 89% localisation accuracy.

MEG is more useful in patients with extratemporal lobe epilepsy because of the improved signal to noise ratio from neocortical generators rather than deep sources. It has been shown that the localisation of interictal MEG dipoles correlate with ictal-onset zones as defined by intracranial EEG and complete resection of these areas predicts good postoperative seizure outcome. At the present time, the information derived from MEG is complementary to data acquired from other investigations including MRI, PET and scalp and invasive EEG recordings but, in future, it is possible that it will be used to guide surgical resection or more commonly, inform placement of intracranial electrodes in patients with complex refractory focal epilepsy.

MEG is also ideally suited non-invasively to explore the occurrence and clinical validity of interictal high frequency oscillations, such as ripples and fast ripples, and this may provide improved localisation accuracy of epileptic foci in a greater proportion of patients, including those without frequent spikes.

Medical treatment

Principles of treatment of newly diagnosed patients

The decision to initiate drug therapy has important implications for a person with newly diagnosed epilepsy. In addition to its biological effects, therapy confers illness status, confirms the state of 'being epileptic', can affect self-esteem, social relationships, education and employment. The decision to treat depends essentially on a balance between the benefits and the drawbacks of therapy, and should be tailored to requirements of the individual patient. The benefits of therapy include the lower risk of recurrence of seizures, and thus of potential injury and even death, and the psychological and social benefits of more security from seizures. The drawbacks of therapy include the potential drug side effects, the psychological and social effects, the cost and inconvenience. Chronic, long-term or subtle side effects are not easily detected, and weigh heavily on the decision to treat. An example is the potential adverse effect on learning in children, and partly because of this pediatricians initiate therapy less early than adult neurologists. The following factors influence the decision.

Diagnosis

It is essential to establish a firm diagnosis of epilepsy before therapy is started. This is not always easy, particularly in the early stages of epilepsy. There is almost no place at all for a 'trial of treatment' to clarify the diagnosis; it seldom does. A good first-hand witnessed account is essential, as diagnostic tests are often non-confirmatory. In practice, the misdiagnosis rate is quite high. For example, about 20% of all patients with apparent epilepsy referred to a tertiary level epilepsy service turn out to have non-epileptic attack disorder.

Risk of recurrence of seizure

The estimation of risk of seizure recurrence is obviously a key factor in deciding whether to initiate therapy. It is now generally accepted that about 50–80% of all patients who have a first unprovoked non-febrile seizure will have further attacks. The risk of recurrence is high initially and then falls over time. In a national UK study, the risk of a recurrence after the first seizure was 44% in the initial 6 months, 32% in the next 6 months and 17% in the second year. It follows therefore that the greater the elapsed time since the first attack, the less likely is subsequent recurrence (Figure 7.10) and in many cases, by the time of presentation, seizures will have already recurred. In a hospital-based study from the United Kingdom, the median number of tonic–clonic seizures occurring before the diagnosis was made was 4 (range 1–36) and the median number of partial seizures was 6 (range 1–180).

If more than one spontaneous seizure has occurred, the risk of further attacks in the future without treatment is, in most clinical circumstances, over 80%, and generally speaking the more seizures that have occurred prior to therapy, the greater the risk of further attacks. The risk of recurrence is influenced by a number of factors:

- *Aetiology* The risk is greater in those with structural cerebral disease, and least in acute symptomatic seizures provoked by metabolic or drug and/or toxin exposure. The risk of recurrence of 'idiopathic' or 'cryptogenic' seizures is approximately 50%. The risk is lowest after acute symptomatic (provoked) seizures providing the provoking factor is removed.

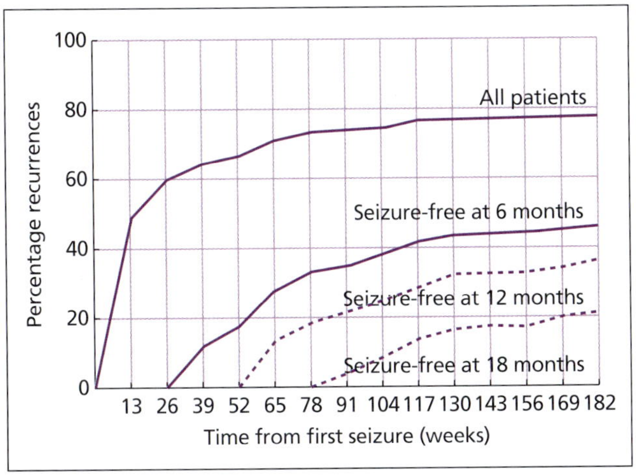

Figure 7.10 Actuarial percentage risk of recurrence after a first seizure (from the National General Practice Study of Epilepsy [NGPSE]). The lines show the risk of recurrence in all patients (n = 564) at the time of the first seizure, and then the subsequent risks for patients still seizure free at 6, 12 and 18 months after the first seizure. Source: Hart et al. 1990. Reproduced with permission of Elsevier.

- *EEG* Evidence in this area is contradictory. While there is consensus that the risk of recurrence is high if the first EEG shows spike and wave discharges, the predictive value of a normal EEG or an EEG with other types of abnormality after a single seizure – and if there is any predictive value – is slight.
- *Age* The risk of recurrence is somewhat greater in those under the age of 16 or over the age of 60 years, probably because of the confounding effect of aetiology.
- *Seizure type and syndrome* Partial seizures are more likely to recur than generalised seizures, again because of the confounding effect of aetiology. Children with most of the benign epilepsy syndromes (e.g. BECTS) have a few seizures only. In the other more severe childhood epilepsy syndromes, recurrent seizures are almost inevitable.

Type, timing and frequency of seizure

Some types of epileptic seizure will have a minimal impact on the quality of life (e.g. simple partial seizures, absence or sleep attacks). The benefits of treating such seizures, even if happening frequently, can be outweighed by the disadvantages. If the baseline seizure frequency is very low, the disadvantages of treatment can be unacceptably high. It would be unusual to treat a person having less than one seizure a year, especially if this was confined to sleep, or a minor or partial seizure.

A protocol for initial treatment

A protocol for the initial treatment in newly diagnosed patients is as follows (the principles are summarised in Table 7.17).

1. Establish diagnosis. There is little place for a 'trial of treatment'. Investigation will usually involve EEG and neuroimaging, and other investigations as necessary. Neuroimaging should be with MRI scanning in all patients with partial-onset epilepsy or epilepsy developing after the age of 15 without good explanation. The MRI must be of high quality, with T1-, T2-weighted and FLAIR sequences. Volumetric scanning is useful as this allows reformatting and quantitation.
2. Identify and counsel about precipitating factors – if these can be avoided, this occasionally obviates the need for drug therapy.
3. Decide upon the need for antiepileptic drug therapy. If therapy is needed, baseline biochemical and haematological parameters should be measured.
4. Advise about the goals, likely outcome, risks and logistics of therapy. Patients should be given clear instructions to seek immediate medical attention if signs of hypersensitivity or idiosyncratic drug reactions develop.
5. Start with monotherapy with the chosen first choice drug, initially at low doses, and titrating up slowly to a low maintenance dose. Emergency drug loading is seldom necessary except where status epilepticus threatens.
6. If seizures continue, titrate the dose upwards to higher maintenance dose levels (guided, where appropriate, by serum level monitoring). In about 60–70% of patients, these simple steps for initial therapy will result in complete seizure control.
7. In remaining patients, alternative monotherapy should be tried with another appropriate first choice antiepileptic drug. The second drug should be introduced incrementally at suitable dose intervals, and titrated to a low maintenance dose, and then the first drug can be withdrawn in slow decremental steps. If seizures continue, the dose of the newly introduced drug should be increased incrementally to maximal doses.

Table 7.17 Principles of antiepileptic drug treatment in patients with newly diagnosed epilepsy.

Aim for complete control without adverse effects
Diagnosis of epileptic seizures should be unequivocal
Seizure type, syndrome and aetiology should be established
Baseline haematological and biochemical investigations should be performed prior to drug initiation
Use one drug at a time (monotherapy), at least initially
Initial titration should be to low maintenance doses
Further upward titration will depend on response and side effects
If first drug fails, alternative monotherapies should be tried
Upward and downward titration should be in slow, stepped doses
Polytherapy should be used only if monotherapy with at least three first choice drugs has failed to control seizures
Patients should be fully counselled about goals, role, risk, outcome and logistics of drug treatment

Source: adapted from Shorvon 2013. With permission of Oxford University Press.

Table 7.18 Assessment and treatment plan in patients with chronic epilepsy.

Assessment
Review diagnosis and aetiology (history, EEG, imaging)
Classify seizures and syndrome
Review adherence to prescription
Review drug history:
Which drugs were useful in the past?
Which drugs were not useful in the past?
Which drugs have not been used in the past?
(also dosage, length of therapy, reasons for discontinuation)
Review precipitants and non-pharmacological factors
Treatment plan
Document proposed sequence of drug 'trials'
Decide what background medication to continue
Decide upon the sequence of drug additions and withdrawals
Decide the duration of drug 'trials'
Decide when to do serum level monitoring
Consider surgical therapy
Consider non-pharmacological measures (e.g. lifestyle, alternative therapy)
Recognise the limitations of therapy
Provide information on above to patients

Source: adapted from Shorvon 2013. With permission of Oxford University Press.

8 If the steps in (7) fail, a third alternative monotherapy should be tried in the same manner. If seizures continue, or recur after initial therapy with 1–3 drugs tried in monotherapy as above.
   - The diagnosis should be reassessed in patients with continuing attacks. It is not uncommon in this situation to find that the attacks do not have an epileptic basis. Investigation should be considered to exclude the possibility of a progressive lesion. The possibility of poor compliance should be explored.
   - Alternative monotherapies or polytherapy should be considered.
   - The patient should be referred for specialist epilepsy advice.

Treatment protocol for patients with chronic epilepsy

When first seeing a patient with chronic uncontrolled epilepsy, a two-stage procedure should be adopted. First, an assessment of diagnosis and previous treatment history should be made. As a second step, a treatment plan should be devised (Table 7.18).

Assessment

The steps in the assessment are summarised in Table 7.18. The review of previous treatment history is an absolutely essential step, often omitted. The response to a drug is generally speaking relatively consistent over time. Find out which drugs have been previously tried, what was the response (effectiveness, side effects), what was the maximum dose and why the drug was withdrawn.

Treatment plan

A treatment plan (schedule) should be formed on the basis of this assessment. The plan should take the form of a stepwise series of treatment trials, each to be tried in turn (if the previous trial fails to meet the targeted level of seizure control). The treatment plan is ideally devised to trial each available antiepileptic in turn, in a reasonable dosage, singly or as two-drug therapy (or, more rarely, three-drug combinations). This will involve deciding which drugs to introduce, which drugs to withdraw and which drugs to retain. Decisions will also be needed about the duration of each treatment trial. There is often nihilistic inertia in much of the treatment of chronic epilepsy which should be resisted, and an active and logical approach to therapy can prove very successful.

Choice of drug to introduce or retain Generally, these should be drugs that are appropriate for the seizure type and that have either not been previously used in optimal doses or that have been used and did prove helpful. Rational choices depend on a well-documented history of previous drug therapy. Other factors are also important – and therapy where possible should be tailored to individual requirements; such factors include co-morbidities, co-medication, obesity, gender, lifestyle, age and presence of renal or hepatic disease.

Choice of drug to withdraw These should be drugs that have been given an adequate trial at optimal doses and that were either ineffective or caused unacceptable side effects. There is obviously little point in continuing a drug that has had little effect, yet it is remarkable how often this is done.

Duration of treatment trial This will depend on the baseline seizure rate. The trial should be long enough to have differentiated the effect of therapy from that of chance fluctuations in seizures.

Trial of therapy It is usual to aim for therapy with either one or two suitable antiepileptic drugs. If drugs are being withdrawn, it is wise to maintain one drug as an 'anchor' to cover the withdrawal period.

Drug withdrawal Drug withdrawal needs care. The withdrawal, or sudden reduction in dose, of antiepileptics can result in a severe worsening of seizures or in status epilepticus – even if the withdrawn drug was apparently not contributing much to seizure control. Only one drug should be withdrawn at a time. If the withdrawal period is likely to be difficult, the dangers can be reduced by covering the withdrawal with a benzodiazepine drug (usually 10 mg/day clobazam), given during the phase of active withdrawal.

Drug addition New drugs added to a regimen should also be introduced slowly, at least in the routine clinical situation. This results in better tolerability, as too fast an introduction of these drugs will almost invariably result in side effects. It is usual to aim initially for a low maintenance dose, but in severe epilepsy higher doses are often required.

Limits of therapy

Drug therapy will fail in about 10–20% of patients developing epilepsy. In this situation, the epilepsy can be categorised as 'intractable' and the goal of therapy changes to defining the best compromise between adequate seizure control and drug-induced side effects. Individual patients will take very different views about where to strike this balance. Intractability is inevitably an arbitrary decision. There are over 10 first line antiepileptic drugs, and far more combinations (with 10 first line antiepileptic drugs there are 45 different two-drug and 36 different three-drug combinations). All combinations cannot therefore be tried.

Choice of drugs and details of antiepileptic drugs

The choice of drugs for use in newly diagnosed and chronic epilepsy is to some extent based on seizure type and syndrome (Tables 7.19 and 7.20). Details of the antiepileptic drugs in current usage are shown in Tables 7.21, 7.22, 7.23, 7.24, 7.25 and 7.26.

Table 7.19 Drug options by seizure type (authors' own practice, modified from NICE).

Seizure type	First line drugs	Second line drugs	Other drugs that may be considered	Drugs to be avoided (may worsen seizures)
Generalised tonic–clonic	Carbamazepine Lamotrigine Levetiracetam Oxcarbazepine Sodium valproate Topiramate	Clobazam Clonazepam Perampanel	Acetazolamide Felbamate Phenobarbital Phenytoin	Tiagabine Vigabatrin
Absence	Ethosuximide Lamotrigine Sodium valproate	Clobazam Clonazepam Topiramate	Phenobarbital	Carbamazepine Gabapentin Oxcarbazepine Pregabalin Tiagabine Vigabatrin
Myoclonic	Levetiracetam Sodium valproate Topiramate	Clobazam Clonazepam Lamotrigine Piracetam Zonisamide		Carbamazepine Gabapentin Oxcarbazepine Pregabalin Tiagabine Vigabatrin
Tonic	Lamotrigine Sodium valproate	Clobazam Clonazepam Levetiracetam Topiramate	Acetazolamide Phenobarbital Phenytoin	Carbamazepine Oxcarbazepine
Atonic	Lamotrigine Sodium valproate	Clobazam Clonazepam Levetiracetam Rufinamide Topiramate	Acetazolamide Phenobarbital	Carbamazepine Oxcarbazepine Phenytoin
Focal with/without secondary generalisation	Carbamazepine Lamotrigine Levetiracetam Oxcarbazepine Sodium valproate Topiramate	Clobazam Gabapentin Perampanel Pregabalin Zonisamide	Acetazolamide Clonazepam Felbamate Phenobarbital Phenytoin Tiagabine	

Antiepileptic drug listed in alphabetical order.
Source: adapted from Shorvon 2013. With permission of Oxford University Press.

Table 7.20 Drug options by epilepsy syndrome seen in adult practice (author's practice).

Epilepsy syndrome	First line drugs	Second line drugs	Other drugs	Drugs to be avoided (may worsen seizures)
Juvenile absence epilepsy	Ethosuximide Lamotrigine Sodium valproate	Topiramate	Clonazepam Clobazam	Carbamazepine Oxcarbazepine Phenytoin Tiagabine Vigabatrin
Juvenile myoclonic epilepsy	Lamotrigine Levetiracetam Sodium valproate Topiramate	Clobazam Clonazepam Piracetam	Acetazolamide	Carbamazepine Gabapentin Oxcarbazepine Phenytoin Pregabalin Tiagabine Vigabatrin
Generalised tonic–clonic seizures only	Carbamazepine Lamorigine Levetiracetam Sodium vaproate Topiramate	Clobazam Clonazepam Oxcarbazepine Perampanel Zonisamide	Acetazolamide Phenobarbital Phenytoin	Tiagabine Vigabatrin
Focal epilepsies: cryptogenic, symptomatic	Carbamazepine Lamotrigine Levetiracetam Oxcarbazepine Sodium valproate Topiramate	Clobazam Clonazepam Gabapentin Perampanel Phenytoin Pregabalin Zonisamide	Acetazolamide Clonazepam Felbamate Gabapentin Phenobarbital Primidone Vlgabatrin	
Benign epilepsy with centrotemporal spikes	Carbamazepine Lamotrigine Oxcarbazepine Sodium valproate	Topiramate Zonisamide		
Benign epilepsy with occipital paroxysms	Carbamazepine Lamotrigine Oxcarbazepine Sodium valproate	Levetiracetam Topiramate		
Lennox–Gastaut syndrome	Carbamazepine Lamotrigine Oxcarbazepine Sodium valproate Topiramate	Clobazam Clonazepam Felbamate Levetiracetam Rufinamide Zonisamide	Phenytoin Phenobarbital Vigabatrin	
West syndrome	ACTH or corticosteroid Vigabatrin	Lamotrigine Sodium valproate Topiramate Zonisamide	Felbamate	

Antiepileptic drug listed in alphabetical order.

Monotherapy versus combination therapy

Single-drug therapy will provide optimal seizure control in about 70% of all patients with epilepsy, and should be chosen whenever possible. The advantages of monotherapy are:

- Better tolerability and fewer side effects
- Simpler and less intrusive regimens
- Better compliance, and
- No potential for pharmacokinetic or pharmacodynamic interactions with other antiepileptic drugs.

Table 7.21 The range of antiepileptic drugs in current use.

Drug	Year of introduction	Main mode(s) of action	Main indication
Acetazolamide	1952	Carbonic anhydrase inhibition	Second line therapy for partial onset and generalised seizures
Carbamazepine	1963	Inhibition of voltage gated sodium channel	First line drug for partial and tonic–clonic seizures
Clobazam	1986	GABA receptor agonist	Second line therapy for partial onset and generalised seizures
Clonazepam	1975	GABA receptor agonist	Second line therapy for partial onset and generalised seizures
Eslicarbazepine acetate	2009	Inhibition of voltage gated sodium channel	Second line therapy for partial onset and generalised seizures
Ethosuximide	1953	Inhibition of T-type calcium channel	Generalised absences only
Felbamate	1993	Inhibition of NMDA glutamate receptor	Second line therapy for partial onet seizures (but because of side effects now rarely used)
Gabapentin	1993	Action on the alpha2-delta subunit of the voltage gated calcium channel	Second line therapy for partial onset seizures
Lacosamide	2008	Inhibition of voltage gated sodium channel (blocks slow inactivation)	Second line therapy for partial onset seizures
Lamotrigine	1991	Inhibition of voltage gated sodium channel	First line drug for partial, absence and tonic–clonic seizures
Levetiracetam	1999	Binding to the synaptic vesicle SV2A protein	First line drug for partial, absence and tonic–clonic seizures
Oxcarbazepine	1990	Inhibition of voltage gated sodium channel	First line drug for partial onset seizures
Perampanel	2012	Selective, non-competitive antagonist of AMPA glutamate receptor on post-synaptic neurones	Second line drug for partial onset seizures
Phenobarbital	1912	GABA receptor agonist	Drug for partial, absence and tonic–clonic seizures, currently used as second line drug
Phenytoin	1938	Inhibition of voltage gated sodium channel	Drug for partial, and tonic–clonic seizures, currently used as second line drug
Piracetam	1967	Binding to the synaptic vesicle SV2A protein	Second line therapy for myoclonic serizures
Pregabalin	2004	Action on the alpha2-delta subunit of the voltage gated calcium channel	Second line therapy for partial onet seizures
Primidone	1952	GABA receptor agonist	As for phenobarbital
Retigabine	2011	Opens neuronal potassium channels KCNQ2 and KCNQ3	Second line therapy for partial onet seizures (but because of side effects now rarely used)
Rufinamide	2007	Inhibition of voltage gated sodium channel	Drop attacks in Lennox–Gastaut syndrome
Stiripentol	2007	GABAergic, enhances action of other drugs possibly via interactions	Second line therapy in SMEI when taken with valproate and clobazam
Tiagabine	1996	Inhibition of post-synaptic GABA reuptake	Second line therapy for partial onet seizures (but because of side effects now rarely used)

(continued)

Table 7.21 (continued)

Drug	Year of introduction	Main mode(s) of action	Main indication
Topiramate	1995	Glutamate reduction; GABAergic; sodium channel modulation; calcium channel modification; carbonic anhydrase inhibitor	First line drug for partial, absence and tonic–clonic seizures
Valproate	1968	Not known	First line therapy for all generalised seizures and also useful in partial onset seizures
Vigabatrin	1989	Inhibition fo GABA transaminase	Second line therapy for partial onset seizures (but because of side effects now rarely used)
Zonisamide	1990	Sodium channel modulation; calcium channel modification; carbonic anhydrase inhibitor; glutamate receptor action; GABAergic	Second line therapy for partial and tonic–clonic seizures

Not considered here are diazepam (introduced in 1965) and lorazepam (introduced in 1975) as these are mainly used in emergency (acute) rather than long-term chronic therapy.
Source: adapted from Shorvon 2013. With permission of Oxford University Press.

Table 7.22 The range of antiepileptic drugs in current use: dosing in adults.

	Initial dose (mg/day)	Drug initiation: usual dose increment (mg/day) stepped up every 2 weeks	Usual daily maintenance dose (mg/day)	Usual maximum dose (mg/day)	Dosing intervals (per day)	Drug reduction: usual dose decrement (mg/day) stepped down every 4 weeks	Maintenance doses can be different when given as co-medication
Acetazolamide	250	250	500–1000	750	1–2	250	No
Carbamazepine*	100	100–200	400–1800	2400	2	200	Yes
Clobazam	10	10	10–30	30	1–2	10	No
Clonazepam	0.25	0.25–0.5	1–4	6	1–2	0.5	No
Eslicarbazepine	400	400	800–1200	1200	1	400	Yes
Ethosuximide	250	250	500–1500	1500	2–3	250	Yes
Felbamate	1200	1200	1200–3600	3600	2–3	600	Yes
Gabapentin	300–400	300–400	1800–3600	3600	2–3	300–400	
Lacosamide	50	50	200–400	600	2	50	Yes
Lamotrigine	12.5–25	25–100	100–400	600	2	100	Yes
Levetiracetam	125–250	250–500	750–4000	4000	2	250–500	No
Oxcarbazepine	300	300	900–2400	3000	2	300	Yes
Perampanel	2	2	8–12		1	2	Yes
Phenobarbital	30	15–30	30–180	180	1	15–30	Yes
Phenytoin	200	25–100	200–400	500	1–2	50	Yes

Table 7.22 (continued)

	Initial dose (mg/day)	Drug initiation: usual dose increment (mg/day) stepped up every 2 weeks	Usual daily maintenance dose (mg/day)	Usual maximum dose (mg/day)	Dosing intervals (per day)	Drug reduction: usual dose decrement (mg/day) stepped down every 4 weeks	Maintenance doses can be different when given as co-medication
Piracetam	4800	2400	12 000–32 000	32 000	2–3	1200–2400	No
Pregabalin	50	50	100–600	600	2	50	No
Primidone	62.5–125	125–250	500–1500	1500	1–2	125–250	Yes
Retigabine	300	300	900–1200	1200	3	300	No
Rufinamide	400	400	2400–3200	32000	2	400	Yes
Stiripentol	50	100	4000		2–3	100	Yes
Tiagabine	4–5	4–15	30–45	50–60	2–3	4–5	Yes
Topiramate	25–50	25–50	75–400	600	2	50	Yes
Valproate	200–500	200–500	400–2000	3000	2–3	200–500	Yes
Vigabatrin	500	500	1000–2000	4000	2	500	No
Zonisamide	50	50	200–600	600	1–2	50	Yes

Values in this table are based on the authors' own practice, and may vary from those published elsewhere.
* Values are for the slow release formulation, which is the formulation of choice, particularly at high doses.
Source: adapted from Shorvon 2013. With permission of Oxford University Press.

Table 7.23 The range of antiepileptic drugs in current use: pharmacokinetic properties.

	Oral bioavailability (%)	Time to peak level (hours)	Half-life† (hours)	Protein binding (%)
Acetazolamide	<90	1–3	10–12	90–95
Carbamazepine	75–85	4–8	5–26[5]	75
Clobazam	90	1–4	10–30 (50[1])	83
Clonazepam	80	1–4	20–55	86
Eslicarbazepine	<100	2–3	13–20	<40
Ethosuximide	<100	<4	30–60[5]	<10
Felbamate	<100	1–4	11–25[5]	20–25
Gabapentin	<65[6]	2–3	5–9	None
Lacosamide	<100	0.5–4	13	15
Lamotrigine	<100	1–3	12–60[5]	55
Levetiracetam	<100	0.5–2	6–8	None
Oxcarbazepine	<100	4–6	8–10[1,5]	38[1]

(continued)

Table 7.23 (continued)

	Oral bioavailability (%)	Time to peak level (hours)	Half-life[†] (hours)	Protein binding (%)
Perampanel	<100	2	105	95
Phenobarbital	80–100	0.5–4	75–120[5]	45–60
Phenytoin	95	4–12	7–42[2,5]	85–95
Piracetam	>90	1	5–6	0
Pregabalin	90	1	5–7	None
Primidone	<100	3	5–18[5] (75–120[1])	25
Retigabine	60	0.5–2	6–10	80
Rufinamide	<85	4–6	8–12	30
Stiripentol	<100	1.5	4–14	99
Tiagabine	<96	1–2[3]	5–9[5]	96
Topiramate	<100	2–4	19–25[5]	13–17
Valproate	<100	0.5–2[4]	12–17[5]	70–95
Vigabatrin	<100	0.5–2	4–7	None
Zonisamide	<100	2–4.5	49–69[5]	40–50

[1] Value for active metabolite.
[2] Phenytoin has non-linear kinetics, and so half-life can increase at higher doses.
[3] Absorption of tiagabine is markedly slowed by food, and it is recommended that the drug is taken at the end of meals.
[4] The time to peak concentration varies according to formulation (0.5–2 hours for normal formulation, 3–8 hours for enteric coated).
[5] Half-life varies with co-medication.
[6] Absorption of gabapentin is by a saturable active transport system, and rate will depend on capacity of the system.
[†] Half-life in healthy adult.
Source: adapted from Shorvon 2013. With permission of Oxford University Press.

Table 7.24 The range of antiepileptic drugs in current use: metabolic properties.

Drug	Major metabolic pathways	Hepatic enzymes	Inhibition or induction of CYP enzymes	Drug interactions	Active metabolite
Acetazolamide	None	No	No	No	No
Carbamazepine	Epoxidation and hydroxylation, and then conjugation	CYP3A4, CYP2C8, CYP1A2 and then UGT (15%)	Induces CYP2B6, CYP2C, CYP3A, CYP1A2	Common	Carbamazepine epoxide
Clobazam	Desmethylation and hydroxylation and then conjugation	Yes	Slight effects only	Minor only	*N*-desmethylclobazam
Clonazepam	Reduction, hydroxylation and acetylation	Yes	Slight effects only	Minor only	No
Eslicarbazepine acetate	Hydrolysis and conjugation	Yes	Inhibits CYP2C9	Common	Eslicarbazepine

Table 7.24 (continued)

Drug	Major metabolic pathways	Hepatic enzymes	Inhibition or induction of CYP enzymes	Drug interactions	Active metabolite
Ethosuximide	Hepatic oxidation then conjugation	CYP3A4, CYP2E1	No	Common	No
Felbamate	hydroxylation and conjunction	CYP3A4 CYP2E1, UGT (10%)	Induces CYP3A4, inhibits CYP2C19	Common	No
Gabapentin	None	No	No	No	No
Lacosamide	*O*-desmethylation	CYP2C19	Inhibits CYP2C19	Some drug interactions	No
Lamotrigine	Only phase 2 glucuronidation	UGT14A (>80%)	No	Common	No
Levetiracetam	Hydrolysis in many body tissues	No	No	Minor only	No
Oxcarbazepine	Reduction to MHD, then conjugation	Aldo-ketoreductase enzymes (not via CYP enzymes), UGT (60%)	Inhibits CYP2C19, induces CYP3A	Some	MHD
Perampanel	Oxidation and glucuronidation	CYP3A	Induces CYP3A	Common	No
Phenobarbital	Oxidation, glucosidation and hydroxylation, then conjugation	CYP2C9, CYP2C19, CYP2E1	induces CYP2B6, CYP2C, CYP3A	Common	No
Phenytoin	Oxidation, hydroxylation, and glucosidation	CYP2C9, CYP2C19, CYP2C18 (possible), UDPGT1A	Induces CYP2B6, CYP2C, CYP3A	Common	No
Piracetam	None	No	No	No	No
Pregabalin	None	No	No	No	No
Primidone	Metabolism to phenobarbital, and then biotransformation as for phenobarbital	CYP2C9, CYP2C19, CYP2E1	Induces CYP2B6, CYP2C, CYP3A (derived phenobarbital)	Common	Phenobarbital
Retigabine	Acetylation and glucuronidation		Nil	No	No
Rufinamide	Hydrolysis	Carboxylesterase enzymes, (not via CYP enzymes)	Induces CYP 3A4	Common	No
Tiagabine	Oxidation then conjugation	CYP3A4	No	Common	No
Topiramate	No* (in polytherapy: hydoxylation or hydrolysis and then conjugation)	CYP enzymes	Inducer of CYP3A4	Some drug interactions	No
Valproate	Oxidation, epoxydation, reduction and then conjunction	CYP2C9, CYP2C19, CYP2B6, UGT (40%)	Inhibits CYP2C9 (and a very weak inhibitor of CYP2C19, CYP3A4)	Common	No
Vigabatrin	None	No	No	No	No
Zonisamide	Reduction, *N*-acetylation and conjunction	CYP3A4	No	Common	No

CYP, cytochrome.
* In monotherapy. In polytherapy, some hepatic metabolism.
Source: adapted from Shorvon 2013. With permission of Oxford University Press.

Table 7.25 The range of antiepileptic drugs in current use: side effects.

Drug	Common side effects	Risk of hypersensitivity
Acetazolamide	Acidosis, drowsiness, anorexia, irritability, nausea and vomiting, loss of appetite, weight loss, enuresis, headache, thirst, dizziness, hyperventilation, flushing, loss of libido, renal stones. Severe hypersensitivity affecting skin and blood	Yes – marked risk
Carbamazepine	Drowsiness, fatigue, dizziness, ataxia, diplopia, blurring of vision, sedation, headache, insomnia, gastrointestinal disturbance, tremor, weight gain, impotence, effects on behaviour and mood, hepatic disturbance, rash and other skin reactions, bone marrow dyscrasia, leukopenia, hyponatraemia, water retention, endocrine effects, effects on cardiac conduction, effects on immunoglobulins	Yes
Clobazam	Drowsiness, sedation, asthenia, ataxia, weakness and hypotonia, diplopia, mood and behavioural change, dependency, withdrawal symptoms	Slight
Clonazepam	Drowsiness, sedation, asthenia, ataxia, weakness and hypotonia, diplopia, mood and behavioural change, drooling and hypersalivation, dependency, withdrawal symptoms	Slight
Eslicarbazepine acetate	Headache, dizziness, somnolence, nausea, diplopia, vomiting, blurred vision, vertigo, fatigue, constipation and diarrhoea	None to date
Ethosuximide	Gastrointestinal symptoms, drowsiness, ataxia, diplopia, headache, dizziness, hiccups, sedation, behavioural disturbances, acute psychotic reactions, extrapyramidal symptoms, blood dyscrasia, rash, lupus-like syndrome, severe hypersensitvity	Yes – marked risk
Felbamate	Severe hepatic disturbance and aplastic anaemia, insomnia, headache, weight loss, gastrointestinal symptoms, vomiting, constipation, rhinitis, urinary tract infection, fatigue, dizziness, lethargy, behavioural change, ataxia, visual disturbance, mood change, psychotic reaction, acne, neurological symptoms	Yes – marked risk
Gabapentin	Drowsiness, dizziness, ataxia, headache, tremor fatigue, weight gain, exacerbation of non-convulsive generalised seizures, pancreatitis, depression, psychosis, headache, myalgia and urinary incontinence; hepatitis, jaundice, movement disorders, thrombocytopenia and acute renal failure	Slight
Lacosamide	Dizziness, headache, nausea, diplopia. Also, depression, confusional state, insomnia, ataxia, memory impairment, irritability, somnolence, tremor, nystagmus, blurred vision, vertigo, tinnitus, vomitinh, constipation, dry mouth, pruritus, asthenia, fatigue	None to date
Lamotrigine	Rash (sometimes severe), blood dyscrasia, headache, ataxia, asthenia, diplopia, nausea, vomiting, dizziness, somnolence, insomnia, depression, psychosis, tremor	Yes – marked risk
Levetiracetam	Somnolence, asthenia, infection, dizziness, headache, irritability, aggression, behavioural and mood changes. The irritability and behavioural change can be severe. Rarer side effects include confusion, psychosis, leukopenia, thrombocytopenia and alopecia	Slight
Oxcarbazepine	Somnolence, headache, dizziness, diplopia, ataxia, confusional state, apathy, agitation, tremor, memory disturbance, rash, hyponatraemia, weight gain, alopecia, nausea, vomiting, gastrointestinal disturbance, hypothyroidism, blurred vision, vertigo, pancreatitis	Yes – but very uncommon
Perampanel	Dizziness, somnolence, ataxia, dysarthria, irritability, aggression, anger, anxiety, confusional state, change in appetite, diplopia, blurred vision, vertigo, nausea, fatigue, weight gain	
Phenobarbital	Sedation, ataxia, dizziness, insomnia, hyperkinesis (children), dysarthria, mood changes (especially depression), behaviour change, aggressiveness, cognitive dysfunction, impotence, reduced libido, folate deficiency and megablastic anaemia, vitamin K and vitamin D deficiency, osteomalacia, Dupuytren's contracture, frozen shoulder, shoulder-hand syndrome, connective tissue abnormalities, rash. Risk of dependency. Potential for abuse	Slight

Table 7.25 (continued)

Drug	Common side effects	Risk of hypersensitivity
Phenytoin	Ataxia, dizziness, lethargy, sedation, headaches, dyskinesia, acute encephalopathy (phenytoin intoxication), hypersensitivity, rash, fever, blood dyscrasia, gingival hyperplasia, folate deficiency, megaloblastic anaemia, vitamin K deficiency, thyroid dysfunction, decreased immunoglobulins, mood changes, depression, coarsened facies, hirsutism, peripheral neuropathy, osteomalacia, hypocalcaemia, hormonal dysfunction, loss of libido, connective tissue alterations, pseudolymphoma, hepatitis, vasculitis, myopathy, coagulation defects, bone marrow hypoplasia	Yes
Piracetam	Dizziness, insomnia, nausea, gastrointestinal discomfort, hyperkinesis, weight gain, tremulousness, agitation, drowsiness, rash	No
Pregabalin	Weight gain, dizziness, drowsiness, irritability, speech disorder, paraesthesia, confusion, fatigue, visual disturbance, increased salivation, taste disturbance, oedema, depression, insomnia, mood swings, asthenia, muscle cramp, rash, pancreatitis, arrhythmia, rhinitis, menstrual disturbances, breast discharge, breast hypertrophy, neutropenia, rhabdomyolysis and renal failure	No
Primidone	As for phenobarbital. Also dizziness and nausea on initiation of therapy	Slight
Retigabine	Dizziness, somnolence, pigmentary changes (blue discoloration) around eyes nails, lips and skin and also in retina, fatigue, asthenia, malaise, oedema, dysuria, urinary hesitation, urinary retention, dry mouth, constipation, memory disturbance, vertigo, paraethesia, tremor, dysarthria, dysphasia, myoclonus, anxiety, psychosis, disorientation, appetite and weight change	
Rufinamide	Headache, dizziness, somnolence, fatigue, nausea, vomiting, diplopia, blurred vision, ataxia, anxiety, insomnia, tremor, oligomenorrhoea, rash, diarrhoea, dyspepsia, conspipation, anorexia, weight loss, rhinitis, ear infection, sinusitis	None to date
Stiripentol	Loss of appetite, weight loss, nausea, vomiting insomnia, drowsiness, ataxia, hypotonia, dystonia, aggressiveness, irritability, agitation, hyperexcitability, hyperkinesis. Side effects are probably mainly due to the increase in plasma concentrations of other anticonvulsants. Nausea and vomiting and weight loss are particularly noted when used in combination with sodium valproate	No
Tiagabine	Dizziness, tiredness, nervousness, tremor, ataxia, concentration difficulties, depressed mood, emotional lability, confusion, hostility, aggression, word-finding difficulties, psychosis, diarrhoea, abdominal pain, nausea, flu-like symptoms, muscular twitching, It also has a strong propensity to induce non-convulsive status epilepticus in patients with generalised epilepsy	No
Topiramate	Parasthesia, somnolence, dizziness, depression, nausea, diarrhoea, fatigue, weight loss, bradyphrenia, insomnia, expressive language disorder, anxiety, confusional state, disorientation, aggression, mood altered, agitation, mood swings, depressed mood, anger, abnormal behaviour, disturbance in attention, memory impairment, amnesia, cognitive disorder, mental impairment, psychomotor impairment, ataxia, tremor, lethargy, hypoaesthesia, dysgeusia, vertigo, tinnitus, gastrointestinal effects, alopecia, pruritus, arthalgia, myalgia, muscle twitching, anhydrosis. Significant rare effects include renal calculi and pancreatitis	No
Valproate	Weight gain, nausea, vomiting, hepatic dysfunction, Tremor, extrapyramidal disorder, somnolence, memory impairment, headache, nystagmus, encephalopathy, lethargy, ataxia, confusional state, agitation, aggression, hyperactivity, hyponatraemia, hyperammonaemia, transient alopecia, curling of hair, angioedema, rash, dysmenorrhoea, polycystic ovaries, haemorrhage, bruising, anaemia, thrombocytopenia, pancytopenia, leukopenia, deafness, oedema, enuresis, reversible Falconi syndrome, osteopenia, osteoporosis, abnormal coagulation, pleural effusion, vasculitis, myelodysplastic syndrome. Hypersensitivity can rarely occur taking the form of toxic epidermal necrolysis, Stevens–Johnson syndrome, erythema multiforme, drug rash with eosinophilia and systemic symptoms (DRESS) syndrome	Yes

(continued)

Table 7.25 (continued)

Drug	Common side effects	Risk of hypersensitivity
Vigabatrin	Irreversible visual field defects, weight gain, somnolence, agitation, aggression, nervousness, depression, paranoid reaction, hypomania, mania, psychotic disorder, irritability, excitation (children), speech disorder, headache, dizziness, paraesthesia, disturbance in attention and memory tremor, dystonia, dyskinesia, hypertonia, blurred vision, nausea, abdominal pain, fatigue, oedema	No
Zonisamide	Weight loss, paraesthesia, renal stones, cholelithiasis, anhidrosis, heat stroke, aggression, suicidal ideation, cholecystitis, renal failure, rhabdomyolysis, myasthenic syndrome, malignant neuroleptic syndrome, metabolic acidosis, renal tubular aciduria, hypokalaemia. Very rarely hypersensitivity reactions which can cause: erythema multiforme, Stevens–Johnson syndrome, toxic epidermal necrolysis, pancreatitis, pneumonitis, agranulocytosis, aplastic anaemia, leukopenia, lymphadenopathy, pancytopenia, thrombocytopenia	Yes

Source: adapted from Shorvon 2013. With permission of Oxford University Press.

Table 7.26 The range of antiepileptic drugs in current use: dosing in children.

Drug	Children – average initial dose	Children – average maintenance dose
Acetazolamide	10 mg/kg/day	250–750 mg/day
Carbamazepine	<1 year, 50 mg/day 1–5 years: 100 mg/day 5–10 years: 200 mg/day 10–15 years: 100 mg/day	<1 year: 100–200 mg/day 1–5 years: 200–400 mg/day 5–10 years: 400–600 mg/day 10–15 years: 600–1000 mg/day
Clobazam	0.25mg/kg/day	0.25–1.5mg/kg/day
Clonazepam	<1 year: 0.25 mg/day 1–5 years: 0.25 mg/day 5–12 years: 0.25 mg/day	<1 year: 1 mg/day 1–5 years: 1–2 mg/day 5–12 years: 1–3 mg/day
Eslicarbazepine acetate	–	–
Ethosuximide	10–15 mg/kg/day	20–40 mg/kg/day
Felbamate	15 mg/kg/day	45–80 mg/kg/day
Gabapentin	10–15 mg/kg/day/kg	3–4 years: 40 mg/kg/day 5–12 years: 25–35 mg/kg/day >12 years: as for adults
Lacosamide	–	–
Lamotrigine	2–12 years: 0.3 mg/kg/day (monotherapy) 0.15 mg/kg/day (with valproate co-medication) 0.6 mg/kg/day (with co-medication with enzyme-inducing drugs)	2–12 years: 1–10 mg/kg/day (monotherapy) 1–5 mg/kg/day (with valproate co-medication) 5–15 mg/kg/day (with co-medication with enzyme-inducing drugs)
Levetiracetam	10–20 mg/kg/day	20–60 mg/kg/day
Oxcarbazepine	4–5 mg/kg/day	20–45 mg/kg/day
Perampanel	–	–
Phenobarbital	Neonates: 1–2 mg/day 1 month–12 years: 1–1.5 mg/kg/day, >12 years: 15 mg/day	Neonates: 3–4 mg/day 1 month–12 years: 3–8 mg/kg/day >12 years: 30–180 mg/day

Table 7.26 (continued)

Drug	Children – average initial dose	Children – average maintenance dose
Phenytoin	1 month–12 years: 1.5–2.5 mg/kg/day >12 years: 50 mg/day	1 month–12 years: 2.5–7.5 mg/kg/day >12 years: 75–150 mg/day
Piracetam	–	–
Pregabalin	–	–
Primidone	1–2 mg/kg/day	10–20 mg/kg/day
Rufinamide	<30 kg: 200 mg	<30 kg not receiving valproate: 1000 mg/day <30 kg receiving valproate medication, 600 mg/day
Stiripentol	50 mg/kg/day	100 mg/kg/day (max 4000 mg)
Tiagabine	– nil –	–
Topiramate	0.5–1 mg/kg/day	5–9 mg/kg/day
Valproate	Neonates: 20 mg/kg 1 month–12 years: 0–15 mg/kg	Neonates: 20 mg/kg 1 month–12 years: 25–30 mg/kg (up to 60 mg/kg in infantile spasms)
Vigabatrin	10–15 kg: 125 mg/day 15–30 kg: 250 mg/day >30 kg: 500 mg/day	10–15 kg: 40 mg/kg/day or 500–1000 mg/day 15–30 kg: 1000–1500 mg/day >30 kg: 1500–3000 mg/day
Zonisamide	2–4 mg/kg/day	4–8 mg/kg/day

–, Not licensed for use in children.
Source: adapted from Shorvon 2013. With permission of Oxford University Press.

Combination therapy is needed in about 20% of all those developing epilepsy, and in a much higher proportion of those with epilepsy that has remained uncontrolled in spite of initial monotherapy (chronic active epilepsy). The prognosis for seizure control in these patients, even on combination therapy, is less good. Nevertheless, skilful combination therapy can make a substantial difference by optimising control of the epilepsy (including situations where it is not possible to obtain full control) and minimising the side effects of treatment. The choice of drugs in combination has not been satisfactorily studied. It has been proposed, but without any substantial supporting evidence, that mixing drugs with differing modes of action has a synergistic effect. Patients need to be advised carefully about the implications of polytherapy in terms of drug interactions, teratogenesis and potential pharmacodynamic effects.

Role of antiepileptic drug level measurements

The measurement of drug levels of some antiepileptic drugs is helpful for a number of reasons. In chronic refractory patients these include assessing optimal doses, assessing toxicity and side effects, assessing interactions with other drugs and compliance. The levels of phenytoin should be regularly measured because of the non-linear kinetics of this drug.

Patient information

All treatment is a balance between benefits (seizure control) and risk (e.g. side effects) and it is important to tell patients of the risks of therapy so that an informed decision can be made. Written information is generally better than simple verbal instruction. Consent to therapy must be informed and patients should be given enough time to discuss and explore the various treatment options.

Treatment of patients with epilepsy in remission

Epilepsy can be said to be in remission when seizures have not occurred over long time periods (conventionally 2 or 5 years). Some 70–80% of patients will be in remission at some point after the initiation of therapy. Many cases of untreated epilepsy also remit and in the long term at least 50% of patients are in remission and off medication.

The clinical management of ongoing therapy in patients in remission is usually straightforward. Drug doses should be minimised, and it is usually possible to avoid major adverse effects. In most cases, little medical input is required with appropriate care provided at primary care level and annual visits to the specialist. The seizure type, epilepsy syndrome, aetiology, investigations and previous treatment should be recorded. Routine haematological or biochemical checks are recommended on an annual basis in an asymptomatic individual. Enquiry should be made of long-term side effects (e.g. bone disease in post-menopausal women) and counselling about issues such as pregnancy made where appropriate. At some point, the calm of this ideal situation is likely to be disturbed by the question of discontinuation of therapy.

Table 7.27 Some factors that increase the risk of seizure recurrence after withdrawal of therapy in patients with epilepsy in remission.

Short duration of seizure freedom prior to drug withdrawal
Age above 16 years
History of myoclonic seizures or secondarily generalised seizures
History of multiple seizure types
Certain epilepsy syndromes (e.g. juvenile myoclonic epilepsy, childhood encephalopathies)
Symptomatic epilepsy
Prolonged period of active epilepsy before achieving seizure control
History of seizures after treatment was initiated
Seizure control requiring multiple drug therapy
EEG showing generalised spike-wave discharges
Presence of learning disability or associated neurological handicaps

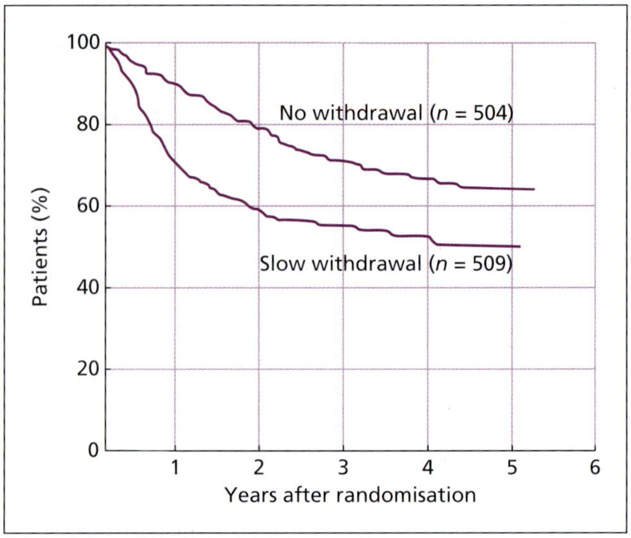

Figure 7.11 Medical Research Council (MRC) drug withdrawal study. Actuarial percentage of patients seizure free amongst those randomised to continuing or to slow withdrawal of antiepileptic drugs. A study of 1013 patients who were seizure free for 2 years or more. Two years after randomisation, 78% of those who continued treatment and 59% of those who withdrew antiepileptic drugs were seizure free. Source: Chadwick et al. 1996. Reproduced with permission of John Wiley & Sons.

Discontinuation of drug therapy

It is often difficult to decide when (if ever) to discontinue drug treatment. The decision should be made by a specialist who is able to provide an estimate of the risk of reactivation of the epilepsy. This risk is influenced by the factors listed in Table 7.27; but it must be stressed that withdrawal is never entirely risk free. The decision whether to withdraw therapy will depend on the level of risk the patient is prepared to accept.

Probability of remaining seizure free after drug withdrawal The best information comes from the Medical Research Council (MRC) antiepileptic drug withdrawal study, which included 1013 patients who had been seizure free for 2 years or more (Figure 7.11). Within 2 years of starting drug withdrawal 59% remained seizure free (compared with 79% of those who opted to stay on therapy). Other studies have had essentially similar findings.

Seizure-free period The longer the patient is seizure free, the less is the chance of relapse. The overall risk of relapse after drug withdrawal, for instance, after a 5-year seizure-free period is under 10%.

Duration of active epilepsy This is probably an under-studied factor. One has a strong impression that the shorter the history of active seizures (i.e. the duration of time from the onset of epilepsy to the onset of remission), the less is the risk of relapse.

Type and severity of epilepsy The type of epilepsy and its aetiology are important influences on prognosis. The presence of symptomatic epilepsy, secondarily generalised or myoclonic seizures, neurological deficit or learning disability greatly lessen the chance of remission, and also increase the chances of recurrence should remission occur. The higher the number of seizures prior to remission, the greater the number of drugs being taken to control the seizures and the presence of two or more seizure types (a surrogate for severity of epilepsy) all increase the risk of relapse.

EEG The persistence of spike-wave complexes in those with IGE is the most useful prognostic EEG feature, indicating a higher chance of relapse. This is especially the case in childhood and juvenile absence epilepsy. Other EEG abnormalities have no great prognostic utility, and the presence of focal spikes or changes to EEG background in adults are of little help in estimating the chances of remission or relapse after drug withdrawal.

Age There is no clear overall relationship between age and the risk of relapse, although there are age-specific syndromes that have specific prognostic patterns. There is a low chance of relapse in the benign epilepsies of childhood or in generalised absence epilepsy. These data simply emphasise the obvious point that the overriding determinant of prognosis is the type and aetiology of epilepsy.

How to withdraw therapy – the importance of slow reduction

When a decision to withdraw therapy is made, the drugs should be discontinued slowly one at a time. Fifty per cent of patients who are going to experience seizure recurrence on withdrawal do so during the reduction phase, and 25% in the first 6 months after withdrawal; this should be explained carefully to the patient. Although not mandated in law, driving restrictions should be recommended during the withdrawal period and the subsequent 6 months.

Recommended rates of withdrawal in routine practice are given in Table 7.22, although in many instances there is no need to proceed so rapidly. In general terms, the slower the withdrawal, the less likely are seizures to recur. If seizures do recur, the drug should be immediately restarted at the dosage that controlled the attacks. About 10% of patients will not regain full remission even if the drug is replaced at the dosage that previously resulted in long remission. Why this should be the case is unclear, but in some patients at least, it seems that recurrence alters subsequent seizure risk.

Management of epilepsy in learning disability

Definition

Learning disability is a descriptive concept, not a disease or illness. Learning disability is defined as a composite of:

- Deficiency in learning with an IQ of less than 70 (i.e. 2 standard deviations below the mean)
- Difficulties with daily living skills, and
- An onset within the developmental period (less than 18 years of age).

It does not infer a particular aetiology. Social functioning is an integral part of the diagnosis. It is different from mental illness; a person with learning disability can also develop mental illness. As a concept, it is also different from learning difficulties, which generally refers to specific learning problems (e.g. dyslexia), rather than a global impairment or intellect and function, although some ambiguity does exist in the use of the terms.

Prevalence of epilepsy in people with learning disability

People with learning disabilities are 30 times more likely to experience seizures than the general population. In most cases, both the cognitive difficulties and the seizures represent overt symptoms of the underlying pathology. The risk of epilepsy increases with more significant intellectual disabilities and additional motor and sensory impairments. Prevalence of epilepsy in people with severe learning disabilities and additional impairments ranges from 50% to 75%. The mortality ratio of people with learning disabilities and epilepsy is also higher than that of people with learning disabilities alone.

Assessment

There are a number of specific issues that complicate the evaluation of epilepsy in people with learning disabilities. Furthermore, assessment is compounded by recollection and communication difficulties, coexistence of mental illness and by related problems that may mimic epileptic seizures.

Communication difficulties – 'management by proxy' People with learning disabilities and epilepsy tend to have consistently poorer adaptive and social skills and more speech difficulties than people with intellectual disabilities alone. In this population, it is common to make a diagnosis and decisions about treatment based on carers' reports: a witness report from a carer or family member is common, a report from the individual is less so. Thus, history and management will commonly progress through another – 'management by proxy'. The degree of this will increase as the individual's communicative skills decrease. This is problematic, as people with learning disability often rely on paid care staff. Even though the content of concerns was found to be similar between families, care staff and clinicians, care staff showed the lowest degree of concern with poorest inter-rater reliability of all three groups, reflecting the level of emotional involvement with the client.

Psychiatric co-morbidity – 'diagnostic overshadowing' People with learning disability and epilepsy are twice as likely to experience mental health problems, particularly affective disorders, than their peers without epilepsy. 'Diagnostic overshadowing' is common with a person's presenting symptoms put down to their learning disability, rather than seeking another, potentially treatable cause. Is the observed strange behaviour caused by epilepsy, mental illness (i.e. depression, psychosis related or unrelated to epilepsy), physical ailment (i.e. pain, deterioration in vision), an attempt at communication, a response to a stressful situation (i.e. change in carers, bereavement) or a side effect of a drug? People with learning disabilities can experience difficulties recognising or communicating their internal experiences and therefore it is particularly important for this group that those around them survey all factors potentially implicated in behavioural change (e.g. antiepileptic drug intoxication).

With an increase in prevalence of nearly all forms of psychiatric disorders, people with learning disability and additional epilepsy are further socially disadvantaged. Other risks include potentially life-threatening accidents and head injuries, which also can result in further brain damage and dependency on others. They often have less effective and cruder coping mechanisms, which can lead to difficulties in the diagnostic and treatment process:

- Non-epileptic attack disorders are more common in people with learning disability who have limited communication skills to express emotional conflicts.
- Self-induced seizures can be stress-avoidance mechanisms with pleasurable auras experienced in photosensitive patients, or providing a sense of control over the unpredictable epilepsies.
- Increased aggression is often reported, when seizures are reduced, either because of complex electrophysiological interactions ('forced normalisation') or less seizure-related sedation and, thus, greater awareness mixed with limited communication skills and ways to express frustration.

Behaviour or seizure? Seizures are paroxysmal episodes of abnormal behaviour. A generalised tonic–clonic convulsion is well defined and does not mimic many other conditions. Other seizure types, however, are less confidently diagnosed and are more dependent on the quality of the verbal description from the individual and witnesses. Patterns of behaviour seen in complex partial seizures, particularly when there are associated ictal or post-ictal automatisms, can be difficult to differentiate from psychiatric disturbances or from non-epileptic attack disorders. Differentiating these in people with learning disability is further complicated by communication issues and the high prevalence of repetitive episodes of manneristic or stereotyped behaviours and motor disorders in this population.

It is not entirely clear how epilepsy is related to challenging behaviour. The results of studies have been at times contradictory, with some finding a relationship and others not. This is perhaps not surprising considering the wide variety of aetiologies and syndromes encompassed under the general umbrella of epilepsy and the fact that it is usually associated with additional impairments. There is a complex relationship between poor impulse control and epilepsy, in particular arising from the frontal lobe in people with learning disability. These people have been found to be more at risk of displaying challenging behaviour or episodic rage and aggression, which appears to be involuntary, can have some features shared with frontal lobe seizures, and most likely is brought about by frontal lobe dysfunction.

Diagnostic difficulties

People with learning disabilities often have difficulties complying with medical procedures. Good planning and communication between the person and staff, carers and/or relatives is important to increase the chance of tolerating an EEG and/or MRI or any other tests. Even though people with learning disability often have diffuse brain abnormalities, and thus are poor candidates for resective curative surgery, both MRI and EEG can provide important diagnostic clarification and prognostic information. People with learning disabilities are often under-investigated and epilepsy often undiagnosed because of therapeutic nihilism by some doctors as well as management-by-proxy disproportionately carried out by carers who are often poorly paid people with little understanding of the complexities of people with learning disabilities or carers from different social backgrounds and little appreciation of health issues.

Treatment

As for all those with epilepsy, antiepileptic medication constitutes the first line of treatment. However, seizures remain poorly controlled in approximately 68% of clients with learning disabilities, despite the fact that around 40% regularly take more than one antiepileptic drug.

There is little evidence-based prescribing in people with learning disability and epilepsy who are usually excluded from most regulatory antiepileptic drug trials. The majority of data come from add-on open non-randomised studies, usually of the novel antiepileptic drugs. Examples are studies using an open non-controlled methodology in populations with learning disability and refractory epilepsy which have shown a 50% reduction in seizures in 33% of patients at 3 months follow-up on vigabatrin, with a reduction in this response by one-third at 5-year follow-up and a 50% improvement in seizure control on lamotrigine in 74% of children, with an associated improvement in quality of life based on subjective clinical judgement. There are a few randomised controlled trials, mainly focusing on the difficult to define epileptic syndrome of Lennox–Gastaut, which is strongly associated with learning disability. Both lamotrigine and topiramate led to significant reduction in atonic (drop) attacks and improvement in global health or reduction in seizure severity as assessed by parents. In West's syndrome, an impressive efficacy for vigabatrin was shown in both open and a limited placebo-controlled trials.

For the majority of people, we therefore apply knowledge on interventions gained in the general population to this special population, but the validity of this approach in this population remains unproven. Seizure reduction, although still the prime aim of epilepsy treatment, should not be the only parameter by which the success of interventions can be assessed. Broader quality of life issues should be considered. This is particularly important in this already disadvantaged group, for whom freedom from seizures can be very elusive. The UK government's 2001 White Paper emphasises the need to involve the person with learning disabilities and to devise individually planned care. It seems vital therefore that we consider the individual's own concerns about their epilepsy if we are to develop more effective, broader treatments enabling people with learning disability and epilepsy, to achieve their aspirations in life unimpeded by their epilepsy.

Management in the elderly

After stroke and dementia, epilepsy is the third most common serious chronic neurological disorder in the elderly with the highest prevalence (1.5%) and incidence (136/100 000). Almost 25% of all new cases of epilepsy occur in those over 65 years of age. These figures are furthermore an underestimate because of the difficulties in the clinical diagnosis of epilepsy in the elderly.

Causes of epilepsy

Stroke is the leading cause of new onset epilepsy after the age of 65 years and accounts for 50–75% of cases where a cause is found. Seizures are more likely to be associated with larger haemorrhagic areas of infarction, with cortical rather than subcortical involvement and to recur if dementia or other neurological disorders are also present. Neurodegenerative disorders, such as Alzheimer's disease, increase the risk of developing epilepsy by tenfold. The third most common cause of seizures in later life are tumours: gliomas, meningiomas, and metastases. Elderly patients do not always show neurological signs, and are less likely than younger patients to present with seizures.

Diagnosis and investigations

NICE has made no specific recommendations for older people. Epilepsy in the elderly, as in other age groups, is a clinical diagnosis and relies upon accurate clinical history and eye witness accounts, which often are not available as many elderly people live alone. The accurate diagnosis is further complicated by co-morbidities and polypharmacy.

The main differential diagnoses of an epileptic seizure at any age are syncope which can be reflex, cardiogenic or orthostatic. A 12-lead ECG is essential in patients presenting with falls or transient loss of consciousness, in order to diagnose, risk stratify and refer urgently those with (often not previously recognised) features of ischaemic heart disease.

Interictal EEG should be interpreted with caution, as it is much less diagnostically helpful in the elderly than in younger people, with up to 40% of elderly people showing non-specific EEG abnormalities, but rarely typical epileptiform activity.

Similarly, non-specific age-related changes on MRI, such as diffuse atrophy and peri-ventricular hyperintensities from hypertension, are common and increase with age.

Medical treatment

There is a very small evidence base concerning the management of newly diagnosed epilepsy in the elderly. The First Seizure Trial Group highlighted old age as a significant predictor of recurrence. Therefore, prescribing an antiepileptic drug to an elderly patient should be considered after one unprovoked seizure, especially if there is a structural lesion on neuroimaging which increases the risk of recurrence, or a high risk of injury from a further seizure.

In general, all commonly used antiepileptic drugs appear similarly effective for seizure control in the elderly, and thus drug choice depends more on tolerability than individual antiepileptic drug efficacy. Antiepileptic drug side effects, such as cognitive disturbance, dizziness and somnolence can contribute to falls and injuries, even if not caused by seizures. Adverse drug events are common in elderly people, particularly sedation from drugs such as barbiturates, phenytoin and topiramate. The co-morbidities of mild cognitive impairment and dementia have implications for carers, especially regarding medication concordance and adherence.

Antiepileptic drugs sometimes also aggravate pre-existing disorders in the elderly, such as dementia, cardiac arrhythmias, polyneuropathy and osteoporosis. Antiepileptic drugs increase already increased risk of fracture in the elderly and in patients taking enzyme-inducing antiepileptic drugs should be prescribed prophylactic vitamin D and calcium.

Pharmacokinetics of antiepileptic drugs differ in old age because of altered volume of distribution, lower protein binding, impaired hepatic metabolism, less enzyme inducibility and slower renal elimination. Drug metabolism depends on the physical status of the patient, co-morbidities and effects of other medications. As renal function declines with age, care is needed when using renally excreted drugs; lower doses should generally be prescribed. Antiepileptic drugs without active metabolites and limited drug interactions are generally preferred.

Certain drugs commonly prescribed to elderly people, such as tramadol, also reduce seizure threshold. Older people seem to be more susceptible to the epileptogenic effects of antipsychotics, antidepressants (particularly tricyclics), antibiotics, theophylline, levodopa, thiazide diuretics and even the herbal remedy, ginkgo biloba, which is the most commonly prescribed herbal remedy in nursing home populations. The vulnerability of elderly patients and the increased likelihood of multiple prescribed medications make them susceptible to drug interactions:

- Potent hepatic enzyme inducers, such as phenobarbital, phenytoin, carbamazepine and primidone, can decrease plasma concentration of warfarin, many psychotropic (amitriptyline, haloperidol, chlorpromazine and clozapine), immunosuppressive, antimicrobial, antineoplastic and cardiovascular/antiarrhythmic drugs (digoxin, β-adrenoreceptor blocking agents, calcium antagonists, verapamil and amiodarone)
- Concomitant prescription of particular drugs (erythromycin, isoniazid, verapamil, diltiazem) inhibit hepatic metabolic pathways and so increase concentrations of antiepileptic drugs.

Elderly patients with medically intractable epilepsy and an underlying structural cerebral lesion should occasionally be considered for surgical treatment. The presurgical work-up is similar to that in younger patients; however, there are limited data on the long-term outcomes of resective epilepsy surgery in elderly patients. The risk of complications is considered higher than with younger patients.

Antiepileptic drug treatment

Currently available antiepileptic drugs are presented in alphabetical order. Data are presented in Tables 7.21, 7.22, 7.23, 7.24, 7.25 and 7.26 which summarise the clinical, pharmacological and pharmacokinetic properties for each drug.

Acetazolamide

Acetazolamide, a carbonic anhydrase inhibitor, which is primarily used in the treatment of glaucoma and for other medical indications, can also be used in epilepsy. It is a broad-spectrum antiepileptic drug but it is used mainly in seizure disorders in the paediatric age group. In the adult population, it can be useful for intermittent use in catamenial epilepsy. One caveat is that many responders develop tolerance to its antiepileptic action if used continuously. Common side effects include paraesthesia of extremities, alterations of taste, nausea and vomiting, diarrhoea, athralgia, loss of appetite, dizziness, fatigue, irritability, thirst and polyuria. Very rarely, rashes including Stevens–Johnson syndrome and toxic epidermal necrolysis may occur. As a carbonic anhydrase inhibitor, acetazolamide is associated with an increased risk of kidney stones. Patients should be advised to increase fluid intake to decrease this risk. Its main clinical relevant interaction is with carbamazepine as acetazolamide may increase its levels.

Benzodiazepines

Benzodiazepines are useful in epilepsy as both a rescue medication for serial seizures or prolonged seizures as well as for long-term treatment. Clobazam, a 1,5 benzodiazepine, can be very useful as an add-on for patients with refractory seizures, either partial or generalised, and may produce long-lasting seizure freedom in up to 30% of patients. Clonazepam can also be used, particularly in myoclonic seizures, but tends to be less well-tolerated. Diazepam, midazolam or lorazepam are not used much nowadays for chronic oral treatment but are useful in the emergency treatment of status epilepticus, serial or prolonged seizures.

The main disadvantages of benzodiazepines are tolerance and related problems of dependency, and a tendency for seizure exacerbation on withdrawal. Common side effects include drowsiness, sedation, ataxia, muscle weakness and hypotonia, mood and behavioural change, and in children drooling and hypersalivation. Hypersensitivity reactions do not usually occur with benzodiazepines. Benzodiazepines are relatively devoid of clinically significant interactions. Clobazam and clonazepam are the best suited for long-term treatment.

Carbamazepine

Carbamazepine, an iminodibenzyl, is a first line drug for initial treatment of partial seizures and tonic–clonic seizures. Carbamazepine is a potent auto-inducer and must be started at a low dose to keep development of transient neurotoxicity at a minimum. The dosage can be increased every 1–2 weeks to a maintenance level that controls the seizures. Even when taking this cautious approach, some people may experience diplopia, nausea, dizziness or headache on initiation of therapy, although these effects are usually transient. Common side effects, apart from these, include drowsiness, ataxia, confusion and agitation (particularly in the elderly), hyponatraemia, neutropenia and idiosyncratic skin rashes. Very rare side effects include hepatitis, Stevens–Johnson syndrome, toxic epidermal necrolysis and cardiac conduction disturbances. Fluid retention may limit the use of carbamazepine in the elderly or those with cardiac failure. In addition, carbamazepine may aggravate bradycardia in patients with heart disease. Hyponatraemia seen with carbamazepine is rarely symptomatic but occasionally leads to confusion, peripheral oedema and an increase in the number of seizures. The associated neutropenia does not usually cause any clinical manifestations.

The use of controlled release preparations are preferable in all situations in routine practice, as they reduce toxicity associated with peak plasma concentrations of the drug.

Carbamazepine, as an enzyme inducer, reduces the levels and effectiveness of several drugs, such as oral contraceptives, steroids, haloperidol, antineoplastic drugs, antihypertensive drugs, tricyclic antidepressants, antipsychotic drugs, theophylline and warfarin. Conversely, other drugs inhibit its metabolism which can result in neurotoxicity: cimetidine, clarithromycin, dextropropoxyphene, diltiazem, erythromycin, imidazole antifungal drugs, isoniazid, tricyclic antidepressants, antipsychotic drugs, verapamil and viloxazine. Interactions of carbamazepine with other antiepileptic drugs are also common. Carbamazepine increases the clearance particularly of ethosuximide, sodium valproate, topiramate and lamotrigine. Inhibition or enzyme induction is seen with phenobarbital, phenytoin or primidone with usually small but unpredictable changes in the plasma concentrations of these drugs.

Eslicarbazepine acetate

Eslicarbazepine acetate is licensed as an add-on medication for focal epilepsy. It is the pro-drug of eslicarbazepine which is the major active metabolite of oxcarbazepine. It therefore has a very similar efficacy and side effect profile to oxcarbazepine, although peak dose effects seen with oxcabazepine are less with eslicarbazepine and so it is claimed to be better tolerated. It inhibits activity of voltage-gated sodium channels and this is likely to be its main mode of action. There are no head-to-head comparisions between this drug and oxcarbazepine or carbamazepine but in a randomised clinical trial response was seen in some people who had not responded to carbamazepine or oxcarbazepine.

Ethosuximide

Ethosuximide, a succinimide, is a first line drug for the treatment of generalised absence seizures in children and young adults. It is not generally effective for other seizures types. The most important side effects are sedation, headaches, malaise, nausea, vomiting, abdominal pain and anorexia. Very rarely, it can cause psychotic episodes with paranoid ideation, aplastic anaemia, systemic lupus erythematosus and Stevens–Johnson syndrome. Ethosuximide-induced headache and abdominal pain can be severe in individual patients. Ethosuximide does not inhibit or induce the metabolism of other drugs but its clearance is reduced by valproate.

Felbamate

Felbamate, a dicarbamate, is an effective drug in partial and in generalised seizures, and has been found to be particularly useful in refractory partial epilepsy. It was also the first antiepileptic drug to have shown efficacy as add-on treatment in refractory Lennox–Gastaut syndrome.

However, its use is currently restricted to very refractory cases only for safety reasons as there is a relatively high rate of hypersensitivity, causing aplastic anaemia or hepatotoxicity. These rare but often fatal reactions affect about 1 in 4000 people exposed. There are other common side effects including insomnia, fatigue, dizziness, lethargy, behavioural change, mood change and psychotic reaction. It interacts with many drugs and dosing is affected by these interactions.

Gabapentin

Gabapentin, an amino acid, is a mild antiepileptic drug occasionally useful as add-on treatment of partial seizures. It is not effective for any other seizure type. Its major indication currently, however, is an analgesic for chronic neuropathic pain. Side effects of gabapentin include nausea, vomiting, peripheral oedema, dizziness, drowsiness, ataxia, tremor, asthenia, emotional lability, weight gain, dysarthria and diplopia. Rare but serious side effects include pancreatitis, depression, psychosis, thrombocytopenia and acute renal failure. Gabapentin can precipitate non-convulsive status epilepticus in some patients with generalised epilepsy. Gabapentin is devoid of drug interactions.

Lacosamide

Lacosamide is licenced as an add-on for focal epilepsy in people over the age of 16 years. It is a sodium channel blocking drug, but it differs from other sodium channel blocking agents in that its effect is mainly on the slow inactivation of the sodium channel.

The most common side effects of lacosamide are dizziness, headaches, nausea and diplopia. It seems better tolerated if no other sodium channel blockers are used concomitantly. No idiosyncratic side effects have yet been associated with this drug. However, it should be used with caution in people with a history of cardiac conduction problems as it is known to increase the PR interval in some people.

No clinically significant drug–drug interactions are known but there are suggestions of pharmacodynamic interaction with traditional sodium channel blockers such as carbamazepine and oxcarbazepine.

Lamotrigine

Lamotrigine, a triazine, is a first line drug for partial and generalised seizures. It is a broad-spectrum drug but may occasionally exacerbate myoclonic seizures particularly as part of Dravet syndrome. The initiation of lamotrigine therapy should be at a very low dosage with a slow upward titration to decrease the risk of the development of skin rash, which is one of the most common and important side effects. The rash may be severe and lead to Stevens–Johnson syndrome in some rare cases, particularly if the medication is not stopped promptly. Other side effects include nausea, fatigue, dizziness, insomnia, tremor, agitation, confusion, hallucinations and blood disorders (including leukopenia, thrombocytopenia and pancytopenia).

Lamotrigine has the potential for various drug interactions. The elimination of lamotrigine is accelerated by enzyme-inducing antiepileptic drugs, such as carbamazepine, phenytoin and phenobarbital, and inhibited by valproate. Therefore, if lamotrigine is used as an add-on then dose and titration schedule needs to be adjusted according to the concomitant medication.

In women, lamotrigine levels may be reduced, occasionally dramatically, with the use of the combined contraceptive pill or during pregnancy and dosage adjustments may be necessary to avoid breakthrough seizures.

Levetiracetam

Levetiracetam, a pyridoline, is a broad-spectrum first line medication for partial and generalised seizures which is well tolerated overall. The most frequent side effects encountered in clinical practice are lethargy, irritability, drowsiness, dizziness, headache, emotional lability, insomnia and anxiety. The irritability and behavioural change can be severe and the drug should be used with caution in patients with pre-existing anxiety.

Levetiracetam should be started at a low dose and titrated upwards every 2 weeks to the initial maintainance dose because of the risk of behavioural change.

No clinically relevant interaction with other drugs has yet been described; however, it is likely that it has pharmacodynamic interactions with other antiepileptic drugs.

Oxcarbazepine

Oxcarbazepine is a structural variant of carbamazepine with a similar efficacy as an add-on drug for refractory partial seizures and as a first line agent in previously untreated patients with tonic–clonic and partial seizures. It also shares many side effects with carbamazepine but overall oxcarbazepine is claimed to be slightly better tolerated. Common side effects include nausea, dizziness, headache, drowsiness, agitation, lethargy, ataxia, impaired concentration, depression, tremor, hyponatraemia, acne, alopecia, skin rash and diplopia. Rare side effects include hepatitis, pancreatitis, arrhythmias, hypersensitivity reactions, thrombocytopenia, systemic lupus erythematosus and Stevens–Johnson syndrome. Hyponatraemia is more marked than with carbamazepine and occasionally leads to confusion and increase of seizures. Cross-sensitivity with carbamazepine in skin rashes is seen about one-third of patients.

Oxcarbazepine has less potential for pharmacokinetic interactions than carbamazepine but nevertheless interactions occur (e.g. with oral contraceptives), and co-medication with oxcarbazepine can significantly lower lamotrigine levels. Oxcarbazepine can lower the levels of ciclosporin.

Perampanel

Perampanel is licensed for the adjunctive treatment of refractory partial epilepsy. It acts by antagonising AMPA receptor function and is the first licensed antiepileptic drug with this mode of action. The most common treatment emerging events so far seen are dizziness, drowsiness, ataxia, lethargy, irritability, weight gain and blurred vision. It has no clinically significant pharmacokinetic effects on other drugs, although its levels can be affected by co-medication with strong inducers of hepatic P450 enzymes, and dose adjustments may be necessary.

Perampanel has an extremely prolonged half-life and can be given in a once a day regimen. It has a marked peak–dose effect (causing dizziness) and so is taken usually just before retiring at night to sleep.

Phenobarbital

Phenobarbital, the oldest barbiturate in the pharmacopoeia, is an effective broad-spectrum antiepileptic against most seizure types, intravenously or with long-term oral use. It is hardly used nowadays in developed countries as a long-term oral drug, although it is still widely used in emergency situations intravenously. In patients controlled at low daily doses, phenobarbital is a cost-effective and well-tolerated medication which is used especially in resource-poor countries. The main disadvantage of phenobarbital is its potential to affect cognition, although at low doses this effect is minimal. Side effects include drowsiness, depression, lethargy, cognitive slowing, Dupuytren's contracture, ataxia and allergic skin reactions. In the elderly, hyperactivity, restlessness and confusion may be seen, while hyperkinesia is a problem in children. Megaloblastic anaemia is a chronic side effect and the use of concomitant folic acid supplementation is recommended.

Phenobarbital interacts with a number of drugs, antiepileptic or otherwise, and this must be taken into account. It has pharmacokinetic interactions with steroids, antibiotics, oral contraceptives, tricyclic antidepressants, antipsychotic drugs, antineoplastic and other drugs. It decreases the levels of carbamazepine, lamotrigine, phenytoin, valproate, zonisamide and ethosuximide.

Phenytoin

Phenytoin, a hydantoin, is an effective oral treatment of partial seizures and tonic–clonic seizures and is also useful intravenously in status epilepticus. However, because of its great potential to cause chronic side effects and pharmacokinetic interactions, it is now not used as first line therapy in many countries. The most common side effects include cosmetic changes as gingival hyperplasia, acne, hirsutism, facial coarsening and neuropsychiatric disturbance, particularly depression, fatigue and cognitive slowing. Other side effects include nausea, tremor, paraesthesias, dizziness, headache, anorexia and skin rash. Rarely, it may cause hepatotoxicity, peripheral neuropathy, Dupuytren's contracture, lymphadenopathy, osteomalacia, megaloblastic anaemia, leukopenia, thrombocytopenia, lupus erythematosus and Stevens–Johnson syndrome. As is the case with phenobarbital, it can cause megaloblastic changes and the use of concomitant folic acid supplementation with phenytoin is recommended in some patients.

It has non-linear pharmacokinetics and this can result in large increases in plasma concentrations even with small dose increments; conversely, levels may fall abruptly even with modest dose reduction. Routine monitoring of plasma levels of phenytoin therefore is recommended (in fact phenytoin is the only antiepileptic drug for which blood level monitoring is essential).

Phenytoin is a potent enzyme inducer, and as such can be expected to lower levels of other drugs such as carbamazepine, phenobarbital, and other antiepileptic drugs, anticoagulants, amiodorone, antihypertensive drugs (including losartan), chloramphenicol, digoxin, statins, steroids, ciclosporin, sulphonamides, imidazole antifungal drugs, tricyclic antidepressants, antipsychotic drugs, antineoplastic drugs and the oral contraceptives. Conversely, the metabolism of phenytoin can be inhibited by enzyme inducers such as allopurinol, chloramphenicol, cimetidine, isoniazid, metronidazol, phenothiazine and sulphonamides.

Piracetam

Piracetam is a -racetam drug, as is levetiracetam, but binds less trongly to the SP1V binding site and has no strong action against partial or tonic–clonic seizures. It was licensed first as a memory enhancer but has been found to have a remarkable effect against myoclonic seizures in some (but not all) patients, and is especially useful in progressive myoclonic epilepsy. It has few side effects and no interactions and is excreted unchanged. It has to be taken in very large doses.

Pregabalin

Pregabalin, a gabapentin analogue, is a second line antiepileptic for partial seizures. It has no indication in any other seizure type. In addition to epilepsy, pregabalin also has use in generalised anxiety disorder and neuropathic pain. Weight gain is a prominent side effect, as are drowsiness and fatique. Like gabapentin, it seems devoid of any clinically significant interactions.

Primidone

Primidone is a barbiturate that is largely metabolised to phenobarbital, and its effects are very similar to those of phenobarbital. It is currently rarely used for the treatment of epilepsy.

Retigabine

Retigabine is licensed as add-on therapy in partial epilepsy. It is the first drug licensed that acts as a modulator of potassium channels. The most common emerging treatment side effects are CNS-related and drowsiness, dizziness, slurred speech, ataxia, tremor and diplopia. It also causes difficulty with micturition in some patients, because of the presence of potassium channels in the bladder wall. An unexpected side effect, noticed soon after licensing, is a blue discoloration of the skin, particularly around the eyes and the nails, and pigmentary changes in the retina. The mechanism of this is unknown but this side effect has severely limited the utility of this drug which is now not widely prescribed.

Rufinamide

Rufinamide is a triazole derivative, unrelated to any other currently used antiepileptic drugs, and it was licensed, under the orphan drug scheme, for adjunctive use in the Lennox–Gastaut spectrum where it has modest effects on drop attacks. It is relatively well tolerated, although has a range of side effects characteristic of sodium channel blocking drugs.

Stiripentol

Stiripentol is licensed, under the orphan drug scheme, for use in Dravet's syndrome in conjunction with sodium valproate and clobazam. It is an aromatic alcohol and is unrelated to any other antiepileptic drug. Its mode of action is unknown and some of its action may well be a result of its potent blocking effects on the metabolism of other antiepileptic drugs. Its positive effects are relatively modest.

Tiagabine

Tiagabine, a GABAergic drug, has a mild to moderate efficacy in the control of partial seizures. It has no indication in other seizure types and indeed is known to exacerbate generalised seizures. The most common adverse events are CNS-related and consist of sedation, tremor, headache, mental slowing, emotional lability, speech impairment, tiredness, depression and dizziness. Rarely, confusion, psychosis and leukopenia may occur. Increases in seizure frequency. Episodes of non-convulsive status also occur, particularly when used in idiopathic generalised epilepsy.

Drugs that induce CYP3A4/5 enzymes can increase the clearance of tiagabine significantly and higher doses are often be required if they are used concomitantly. It needs to be taken three times a day, with meals, because of its short half-life. Because of the side effect profile, and peak dose effects, which especially occur if the drug is taken on an empty stomach, tiagabine is now rarely prescribed.

Topiramate

Topiramate, a sulfamate-substituted monosaccharide, with multiple modes of action, is a antiepileptic drug that is extremely effective against partial and secondarily generalised seizures. However, it has a difficult side effect profile at high doses, with a high incidence of neurological side effects. These can be avoided by using low doses or titrating the dose upwards very slowly. These adverse effects include headache, sedation, impaired memory and concentration, speech disturbance, asthenia, anxiety, depression, sleep disorders, visual disturbances and confusion. Weight loss and paraesthesia are very common. Very rarely, topiramate may cause acute myopia with secondary angle-closure glaucoma. Topiramate is an inhibitor of carbonic anhydrase and as such is associated with an increased risk of renal stones; patients should be advised to increase fluid intake during treatment to decrease this risk.

Enzyme inducers tend to accelerate the clearance of topiramate and higher doses may be required if they are used concomitantly. Topiramate though does not affect the clearance of other antiepileptic drugs to any significant effect.

Valproate

Valproate, a pentanoic acid, is the most effective drug in the treatment of idiopathic generalised epilepsy and is very effective in this syndrome in controlling absences, myoclonus and generalised tonic–clonic seizures. It is also effective against partial seizures. Common side effects include weight gain, tremor, behavioural disturbances, menstrual disturbances, ankle swelling and loss or curling of hair. Cognitive impairment is sometimes seen and encephalopathy has been occasionally reported, possibly because of hyperammonaemia, which is a common result of valproate therapy. Rare cases of hypersensitivity have occurred including cases of fatal hepatotoxicity, especially in infants during polytherapy. Valproate is effective in controlling anxiety and agitation is used in psychiatric practice for this purpose. The use of valproate during pregnancy is associated with an increased risk of teratogenicity and later learning disability even in the absence of malformation, and valproate should therefore be used cautiously if at all in in pregnancy.

Valproate has a complex interaction profile. It mildly inhibits the metabolism of other antiepileptic drugs which is rarely of clinical relevance except when prescribed with lamotrigine, the plasma levels of which are greatly elevated on co-medication with valproate. Interactions with phenytoin and carbamazepine can also be significant. Carbapenem antibiotics cause a profound lowering of valproate levels and this combination should be avoided. Valproate concentrations are also lowered by some antineoplastic drugs. Valproate concentrations can be greatly elevated with co-medication with antidepressant drugs.

Valproate serum level monitoring is not recommended as there is no relationship between clinical effects and the plasma concentration.

Vigabatrin

Vigabatrin, a GABA analogue that binds to and irreversibly inhibits GABA transaminase, the principle metabolising enzyme of GABA, and this results in a marked increase in synaptic GABA. Its use is currently limited by the finding (some 8 years after it was licensed) of irreversible visual field defects in over half of patients on long-term therapy. These are usually asymptomatic in the early stages but can progress and lead to severe visual impairment. It also can cause severe behavioural change and psychiatric disturbance, including agitation and psychosis. Because of these side effects, prescription of the drug is now limited to situations where all other therapy has failed. It also has a niche indication as first line treatment of West syndrome as an alternative to ACTH or steroids.

Zonisamide

Zonisamide is a sulphonamide, which has antiepileptic action against a wide variety of epileptic seizure types including partial seizures and for myoclonic and tonic–clonic seizures. The common side effects of zonisamide include nausea, drowsiness, dizziness, irritability, depression, ataxia, speech disorder, impaired memory and attention, anorexia and weight loss. Less common effects include psychosis and hypokalaemia. There is also a small risk of severe hypersensitivity. Zonisamide is a carbonic anhydrase inhibitor, and is associated with an increased risk of kidney stones; patients should be advised to increase fluid intake during treatment to decrease this risk.

Zonisamide does not cause any significant change in the clearance of other antiepileptic drugs or other drugs such as the oral contraceptive. Drugs which induce CYP3A4, *N*-acetyl-transferases or flucuronidation enzymes may accelerate the clearance of zonisamide and higher doses of zonisamide are sometimes required if used concomitantly with inducing drugs. The drug interactions of zonisamide are complex and the safety of co-medication should be carefully assessed.

Emergency drug treatment

Prolonged convulsions or serial seizures

If a tonic–clonic seizure continues for 5–10 minutes, benzodiazepine therapy, either intravenously (IV), or via the buccal or rectal route, should be given. Undiluted IV diazepam is given at a rate not exceeding 2–5 mg/min, using the Diazemuls© formulation. The adult bolus intravenous or rectal dose is 10–20 mg, and in children the equivalent bolus dose is 0.2–0.3 mg/kg. Intravenous lorazepam is an alternative with some advantages over IV diazepam (longer time of action, less risk of cardiovascular collapse) The dose is 4 mg in adults or 0.1 mg/kg in children.

In out of hospital settings, buccal midazolam 10 mg has become the drug of choice, as an alternative to rectal diazepam and is preferred by patients and carers for ease of use and preservation of dignity.

If clusters of seizures occur, acute therapy after the first seizure can be given to prevent subsequent attacks. Oral clobazam (10–20 mg) is a common choice, and will take effect within 1–2 hours and last for 12–24 hours.

Status epilepticus

Seizures are mostly self-terminating, usually within a couple of minutes; however, on occasions they endure, leading to status epilepticus. Conventionally, status epilepticus is defined as seizure activity that continues for at least 30 minutes, but practically seizures that continues beyond 5 minutes or which repeat without full recovery in between are categorised as a premonitory (pre-status epilepticus) phase, which often progresses to status epilepticus. There have been various estimates of the incidence of status epilepticus, ranging 10–60 per 100 000 person years depending upon the characteristics of the population studied (the incidence is higher in poorer populations).

More than half of the cases of status epilepticus occur in people without a prior history of epilepsy. Usually the cause of the status epilepticus is obvious from the history and imaging. The common causes of *de novo* status epilepticus , in other words in patients without a history of epilepsy, are acute cerebral anoxia (causing myoclonic status epilepticus in coma), alcohol abuse, cerebral tumour, cerebral infection (especially encephalitis), stroke, head injury, fever (febrile status epilepticus in children), drugs or toxins or metabolic disorders. If there is a history of epilepsy, status epilepticus is often caused by reduction or withdrawal of antiepileptic drugs or intercurrent illness. If the cause is not immediately obvious, the status can be a result of uncommon conditions such as mitochondrial disease, inflammatory or immunological disease, unusual infectious causes, drugs or toxins, or genetic disorders. In some cases no cause is found and in many such cases unidentified autoimmune mechanisms are presumed to be present.

About 10–20% of people developing status epilepticus will die in the acute phase, mostly because of the underlying cause. The mortality rate is higher in (20–50%) in those resistant to first line therapy. Neuronal damage, cognitive deficits, focal neurological deficits and epilepsy can also result from convulsive status epilepticus, especially if prolonged and inadequately treated.

Treatment of non-convulsive status epilepticus

In non-convulsive status epilepticus, the approach to treatment depends on the subtype. In typical absence status epilepticus, which responds very well to oral or intravenous benzodiazepines, intensive emergency therapy is rarely needed. The treatment of complex partial status epilepticus is more challenging, and the outcome depends upon aetiology and degree of consciousness. If consciousness is relatively retained, complex partial status has a good prognosis and responds well to oral or intravenous benzodiazepines (in the elderly intravenous valproate or levetiracetam may be better tolerated). In contrast, patients in coma with non-convulsive status epilepticus have a very poor prognosis and aggressive treatment in this group is probably justified, although clinical trials are lacking.

Treatment of convulsive status epilepticus

If tonic–clonic status epilepticus is allowed to persist for more than about 2 hours, there is a substantial risk of seizure-induced cerebral damage. The risk rises the longer the seizures continue. For this reason, the drug treatment of tonic–clonic status epilepticus is best divided into stages:

- Early status epilepsy is defined as the first 30 minutes of seizure activity.
- Established status epilepticus is reached if early stage (benzodiazepine) treatment fails.
- Refractory status epilepticus is reached if seizures continue for more than 1–2 hours after initiating therapy, despite early or established stage therapy.
- Super-refractory status epilepticus is reached when refractory status epilepticus has continued despite 24 hours of anaesthesia.

In addition, the development of status may be preceded by a *premonitory stage* characterised by a crescendo of seizure activity. Treatment with benzodiazepines at this stage is often very effective and can prevent the progression into status epilepticus. The treatment of choice has become buccal midazolam, but benzodiazepines can also be used by other routes, including rectal diazepam and buccal or intramuscular midazolam.

Stage of early status epilepticus

Once status epilepticus has developed, intravenous therapy is required. However, intramuscular midazolam should be considered in situations where intravenous access is delayed or difficult. Intravenous benzodiazepines (preferably lorazepam because of its more favourable pharmacokinetic profile with a longer redistribution half-life) are the initial treatment of choice. Also at this stage, systemic factors need to be considered. Blood should be tested for electrolytes, glucose, full blood count, calcium and magnesium. Intravenous fluids should be administered and glucose and/or thiamine should be given if hypoglycaemia is suspected. Status epilepticus results in respiratory depression and oxygen should be administered.

Stage of established status epilepticus

If intravenous benzodiazepines are not completely effective then loading with another intravenous agent is usually required. Traditionally this has been phenytoin (or fosphenytoin) but valproate or levetiracetam are increasingly being used as alternatives especially as both lack the cardiovascular complications that can accompany a phenytoin infusion.

Stage of refractory status epilepticus

If convulsive status epilepticus continues and has not responded to benzodiazepine and then second-stage therapy, the status epilepticus will be entering a phase of physiological compromise, with the danger of neuronal damage and increasing drug resistance. At this stage the patient should be transferred to an intensive care unit and given an anaesthetic (propofol, thiopentone/pentobarbital or midazolam) to reduce electrographic activity which is the source of cerebral damage. Antiepileptic drug therapy should be continued.

In addition to the treatment of status epilepticus itself, it is also necessary to treat the cause. Refractory status epilepticus has a very different spectrum of causes from drug-responsive status epilepticus; in particular, encephalitis is more frequent and a prior history of epilepsy is less frequent. Antiviral therapies, especially aciclovir, are now well established in the treatment of suspected encephalitis. However, the use of corticosteroids is more controversial. Steroids

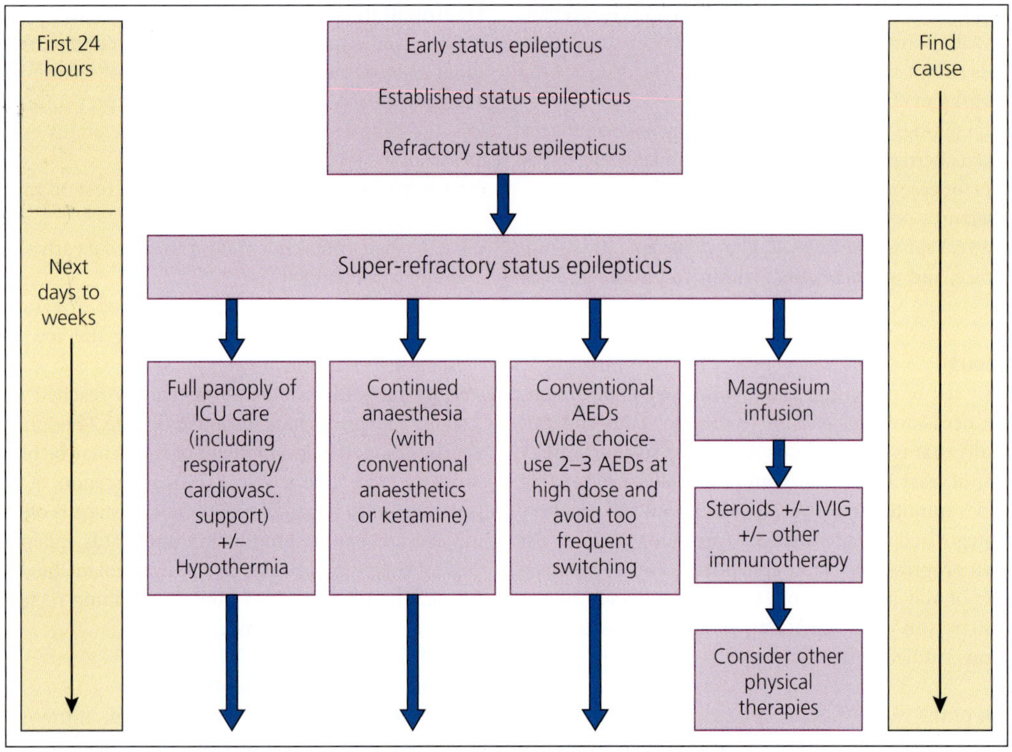

Figure 7.12 The treatment of super-refractory status epilepticus. In parallel to the treatment of seizures outlined, emergency therapy should also be directed where possible at the underlying cause of the status epilepticus. AEDs, antiepileptic drugs; ICU, intensive care unit; IVIG, intravenous immunoglobulin. Data from Shorvon and Ferlisi 2011.

have been recommended in cases of acute viral encephalitis where there is evidence of progressive cerebral oedema. Autoimmune encephalitis (in particular resulting from NMDA receptor antibodies) has increasingly been recognised as a cause of refractory status epilepticus, and may respond to immunosuppressive therapy including high dose methylprednisolone, intravenous immunoglobulin and plasma exchange.

Stage of super-refractory status epilepticus

Super-refractory status epilepticus has been defined as status epilepticus that continues for more than 24 hours after the onset of anaesthetic therapy. General anaesthesia remains the backbone of therapy in refractory super-refractory status epilepticus. The three anaesthetic drugs commonly used are propofol, midazolam and thiopentone. Ketamine is reserved as a second line drug because of the very limited clinical evidence base and the potential neurotoxic effects. It is usual initially to reverse anaesthesia every 24–48 hours initially and if seizures continue then to re-establish it (cycling). Antiepileptic drugs should always be given, so that when the anaesthetic agent is withdrawn there is adequate antiepileptic cover. The choice of drug is rather arbitrary, but one or two drugs in high doses should be given, frequent switches should be avoided, and where possible drugs with low interaction potential and predictable kinetics, low allergenic potential and without renal or hepatic toxicity should be given. Hypothermia, magnesium infusion, pyridoxine infusion (in children), immunological therapy with steroids and or IVIg or plasma exchange should be considered. If the seizures continue, other therapies have been tried including the induction of a ketogenic diet, and the use of electroconvulsive therapy or emergency neurosurgery (Figure 7.12).

A systematic protocol-driven approach is important in this emergency situation. The choice of drug regimen is somewhat arbitrary. A protocol favoured is shown in Table 7.28 and details of the drugs used are given in Tables 7.29 and 7.30.

Epilepsy surgery

Epilepsy surgery is carried out with three objectives: to stop seizures, to ameliorate the seizures or to remove a progressive lesion or one that carries other risks such as haemorrhage. The term applies to an approach to the assessment and the surgery, which differs from surgery carried out for other reasons.

Here we concentrate on the assessment, surgery and outcome of those who have surgery primarily for their epilepsy. These are patients whose epilepsy proves resistant to antiepileptic drugs. Given the conservative estimates that approximately 20% of patients are resistant to treatment with antiepileptic drugs, and 50/100 000 people per year develop epilepsy. Then every year approximately 1/10 000 people develop refractory epilepsy (i.e. 6000 every year in the United Kingdom). In the United Kingdom, approximately 1000 of these patients (3% of the incident cohort) are suitable for presurgical assessment of whom approximately half (500) patients per year are suitable for surgery.

All patients who are being considered for surgery need a detailed presurgical evaluation, this is necessary not only to assess the likelihood of surgical success, but also to establish the suitability

Table 7.28 Protocol for the treatment of status epilepticus in adults.

Stage of early status (0–30 min)

Lorazepam 4 mg IV bolus (can be repeated once)

↓ (if seizures continue after 30 min)

Stage of established status (30–60/90 min)

Phenobarbital IV infusion 10 mg/kg at 100 mg/min

or

Phenytoin IV infusion 15 mg/kg at 50 mg/min

or

Fosphenytoin IV infusion 15 mg PE/kg at 100 mg PE/min

or

Valproate IV infusion 25 mg/kg at 3–6 mg/kg/min

↓ (if seizures continue after 30–90 min)

Stage of refractory status (>60/90 min – general anaesthesia)

Propofol: IV bolus 2 mg/kg, repeated if necessary, and then followed by a continuous infusion of 5–10 mg/kg/hour initially, reducing to a dose sufficient to maintain a burst suppression pattern on the EEG (usually 1–3 mg/kg/hour)

or

Thiopental: IV bolus 100–250 mg given over 20 seconds with further 50 mg boluses every 2–3 min until seizures are controlled, followed by a continuous IV infusion at a dose sufficient to maintain a burst suppression pattern on the EEG (usually 3–5 mg/kg/hour)

or

Midazolam: IV bolus 0.1–0.3 mg/kg at a rate not exceeding 4 mg/min initially, followed by a continuous IV infusion at a dose sufficient to maintain a burst suppression pattern on the EEG (usually 0.05–0.4 mg/kg/hour)

When seizures have been controlled for 12 hours, the drug dosage should be slowly reduced over a further 12 hours. If seizures recur, the general anaesthetic agent should be given again for another 12 hours, and then withdrawal attempted again. This cycle may need to be repeated until seizure control is achieved

Table 7.29 Drugs used in the pre-anaesthetic management of convulsive status epilepticus.

	Route of administration	Adult dose	Paediatric dose
Diazepam	IV bolus (not exceeding 2–5 mg/min) rectal administration	10–20 mg 10–30 mg	0.25–0.5 mg/kg 0.5–0.75 mg/kg*
Midazolam	IM or buccal IV bolus IV infusion	5–10 mg* 0.1–0.3 mg/kg at 4 mg/min* 0.05–0.4 mg/kg/h	0.15–0.3 mg/kg*
Clonazepam	IV bolus (not exceeding 2 mg/min)	1–2 mg at 2 mg/min*	250–500 mg
Fosphenytoin	IV bolus (not exceeding 100 mg PE/min)	15–20 mg PE/kg	
Lorazepam	IV bolus	0.07 mg/kg (usually 4 mg)*	0.1 mg/kg
Phenytoin	IV bolus/infusion (not exceeding 50 mg/min)	15–20 mg/kg	20 mg/kg at 25 mg/min
Phenobarbital	IV bolus (not exceeding 100 mg/min)	10–20 mg/kg	15–20 mg/kg
Valproate	IV bolus	15–30 mg/kg	20–40 mg/kg

* May be repeated.

PE, phenytoin equivalents.

Table 7.30 Anaesthetic drugs used in status epilepticus.

Midazolam	0.1–0.3 mg/kg at 4 mg/min bolus followed by infusion of 0.05–0.4 mg/kg/hour
Thiopentone	100–250 mg bolus over 20 seconds then further 50-mg boluses every 2–3 min until seizures are controlled. Then an infusion of 3–5 mg/kg/hour to maintain burst suppression
Pentobarbital	10–20 mg/kg bolus at 25 mg/min followed by an infusion of 0.5–1 mg/kg/hour increasing to 1–3 mg/kg/hour to maintain burst suppression
Propofol	2 mg/kg bolus followed by an infusion of 5–10 mg/kg/hour to maintain burst suppression

of the patient, to determine the type of operation (including further invasive investigations) and to assess the potential risks.

Who is suitable for presurgical assessment?

The main criterion for selecting patients for presurgical assessment is drug resistance. Thus, there has to have been an adequate trial of medical therapy, but what is adequate? This question has generated a certain amount of debate. Although some studies have suggested that failure to respond (rather than withdrawal because of side effects) to an initial treatment results in an 11% chance of becoming seizure free with subsequent treatments, this is overly pessimistic and long term remission rates on therapy are much greater. Furthermore, patients who are turned down for surgery or refuse surgery have been shown to have a 15–25% chance of becoming seizure free over subsequent years. This is partly because patients seen at time of presurgical assessment are at the nadir of their disease, but also because new antiepileptic drugs have had an impact; adding new antiepileptic drugs in a sequential fashion to the drug regimen of refractory patients can render one-quarter of these patients seizure free.

A generally accepted minimum is that a person should have tried at least 2–3 first line antiepileptic drug treatments at appropriate dosage over a period of 2 years (although some consider this much too soon to contemplate surgical referral). Whether to continue with trials of antiepileptic drugs or to refer directly for surgery depends upon the chance of surgical success and the severity of the epilepsy.

Epilepsy severity is difficult to characterise and to evaluate; it has to be considered on an individual basis and assessed in the light of the likely success and adverse effects of surgery. It is also important to consider the morbidity and mortality attached to even infrequent seizures. SUDEP has a particularly high incidence in patients evaluated for but refused surgery – over 1% per year. Nevertheless, it has to be established that reducing the frequency or stopping the seizures will result in a significant improvement of quality of life. In people with multiple problems (e.g. epilepsy and severe psychiatric disease or severe learning difficulties), the epilepsy may only contribute a small amount to the person's disability. Indeed, during the presurgical period it is paramount to ascertain the expectations that carers, family and the patient have of surgery. Only too often, people feel that epilepsy surgery will resolve all problems, and so are disappointed if seizure freedom has had little impact on their lives. Counselling is therefore necessary so that all involved can have realistic expectations.

Another consideration is the risk of operation. The risks of surgery may be unacceptable, even in cases where the chance of seizure freedom is high. Risks depend not only upon the type of operation (e.g. removal of eloquent cortex or memory problem following dominant temporal lobe resection), but also on the health of the individual (e.g. surgery in patients with other medical conditions). The immediate risks of operation have to be considered in relation to longer term benefits and this is often a difficult equation (e.g. the mortality of the operation may be offset by the reduction in the chance of SUDEP, or the loss of memory following an operation may be offset by the risks to memory of continued seizures).

Presurgical assessment

The goals of the presurgical assessment are to identify the epileptogenic zone (defined as the minimum area of cortex that has to be removed in order to render a patient seizure free), and assessment of the risks associated with its removal. It is a multidisciplinary process, involving the neurologist, neurophysiologist, neuropsychologist, neurosurgeon, psychiatrist and radiologist.

There are two main strategies for the surgical treatment of seizures. The first involves curative resective surgery, in which the aim of the surgery is the removal of the epileptogenic zone. This can be restricted to a focal lesion or may involve lobar or multi-lobar resection (e.g. hemispherectomy). The second approach is palliative, aimed at decreasing the frequency or severity of seizures but not removing the epileptogenic zone.

The assessment of the epileptogenic zone relies upon the convergence of findings from a range of presurgical investigations including clinical history, seizure semiology, scalp EEG, neuroimaging and neuropsychometry. Discordance between these may lead to a lesser chance of surgical success and also points to the need for further investigation such as invasive EEG recordings. The relative weight that is lent to each of these investigations varies depending on the type of operation and the pathogenesis of the epilepsy and in many instances is either controversial or undetermined. Although it is good clinical practice to consider each piece of information independently (i.e. unbiased by results of other investigations), in practice it is not uncommon to reassess a certain finding in the context of all available data.

Clinical history

The clinical history contains a number of details that are critical in preoperative assessment. The age of the patient is relevant as surgery has a greater neuropsychological impact on older patients. Further, there is some evidence to suggest that the longer someone has had mesial TLE, the less chance that there will be of long-term seizure freedom following resection. Handedness gives an indication of hemisphere dominance. Antecedent history is of relevance, for example a history of febrile seizures is a good prognostic factor for surgery in those with hippocampal sclerosis, but a poor prognostic factor in those undergoing frontal lobe resection. The semiology of the seizures is critical (see below). In temporal lobe resections, a history of secondary generalised seizures is predictive of poorer outcome. It is also important to have details of social support and psychiatric concerns.

Psychiatric history

A psychiatric assessment is necessary prior to surgery. First, there are relative contraindications to surgery including active depression or psychosis that will need treating. It is also important to ascertain whether the person is able to give fully informed consent. The additional presence of dissociative seizures is a relative contraindication, as they can often worsen after resective surgery. The risks of post-resective depression and/or psychosis also need to be estimated. Patients may require additional psychiatric support both peri- and postoperatively. About one-quarter of patients have transient mood disturbances in the first year following surgery and approximately 10% may require treatment for depression. A proportion also develop frank psychosis. There are also other personality changes and organic mental disorder which follow resective surgery, particularly on the temporal or frontal cortex.

Neuroimaging

High-quality MRI has become a cornerstone of preoperative assessment. The presence of an identifiable well-defined lesion has a considerable impact on the surgical approach and the prognosis for surgery. If it can be shown that a lesion is the substrate for the epilepsy, then complete resection of that lesion stands a high chance of rendering the patient seizure free, while failure to resect or incomplete resection carry a poorer prognosis. The presence of an identifiable lesion on MRI also increases the chance of surgical success compared to 'MRI-negative' patients. At a minimum, the MRI investigation should involve T2-weighted sequences, proton density sequences, FLAIR sequences and T1-weighted volume acquisition (partition size less than 1.5 mm). Finer cuts and also other sequences may also be helpful, for example gradient echo or susceptibility-weighted imaging to look for blood products in association with cavernomas or arteriovenous malformations.

The role of FDG-PET, other PET ligands and ictal SPECT remains less certain, but they are useful in MRI-negative patients, on occasions when there is discordance between other investigations and in patients in whom there are extensive or multiple pathologies (e.g. tuberous sclerosis).

Ictal SPECT may be helpful when seizure semiology, interictal and ictal EEG and other imaging modalities are uninformative and can add to help guide intracranial evaluation, or confirm the ictal onset zone in patients with discordant imaging and neurophysiology findings (in order to avoid intracranial evaluation), and in patients with extensive or multiple pathologies (e.g. tuberous sclerosis). It is very resource intensive, and thus practical only in patients with a high frequency (daily or near daily) of suitable seizures.

Functional MRI can be used to identify eloquent cortex and to lateralise language. In this latter capacity, it has largely replaced the Wada test. It is likely that as a non-invasive investigation, fMRI will be increasingly used as a method for correlating structure with function such as in the assessment of memory, but currently it is not reliable enough for these purposes.

Electroencephalography and other neurophysiological investigations

The interictal EEG is useful and can be of prognostic relevance (e.g. atypical epileptiform abnormalities in patients with hippocampal sclerosis predicts poorer outcome). Interictal epileptiform abnormalities can usually be localised with higher precision than ictal patterns. Adding selected interspaced electrodes to the standard 10–20 system may improve the localising yield and allow sublobar classification of interictal and ictal EEG changes.

However, ictal video-EEG telemetry to record seizures is the pivotal investigations in presurgical evaluation, although there are occasional cases with clear-cut pathology, typical history and interictal EEG findings in whom recording habitual seizures during video EEG telemetry may not be essential. The hope is that this is concordant with neuroimaging, as discordance reduces the chance of a good outcome and can necessitate invasive EEG recordings.

Drug reduction and other activation procedures such as sleep deprivation are often employed to facilitate the occurrence of seizures in video-telemetry settings. This may be helpful even in some patients with frequent daily seizures (e.g. if habitual seizures have no localising behavioral or EEG features). Drug reduction carries a small risk of secondary generalisation, seizure clusters and status epilepticus, and may therefore be contraindicated in some patients. In any case, patients need to consent, and benzodiazepines have to be available for rapid intravenous or mucosal application to abort seizure clusters or prolonged convulsions. Experienced nursing staff are needed to ensure patient safety during a seizure.

The assessment of the patient in the ictal and post-ictal period can provide valuable localising information about the patient's cognitive state, for example level of awareness, impairment of language function out of proportion to impairment of consciousness (ictal/post-ictal aphasia), visual field deficits, areas of inattention or extinction and subtle post-ictal paresis. Detailed analysis of the behavioural manifestations during an attack may yield further localising or lateralising information.

In addition, some patients may be able to provide a detailed description of their subjective experience at the beginning of their seizures (aura), even though they may be amnesic for this after the attack. Specific somatosensory and visual auras at the beginning of a seizure typically have a higher localising value than the scalp EEG pattern.

Seizure history, ictal behaviour and EEG thus provide complementary information that help to localise the seizure onset zone. How many seizures need to be recorded varies depending on aetiology and results of neuroimaging. If there are doubts about laterality or localisation then more seizures will need to be recorded. It is also important to ensure that the attacks recorded during long-term monitoring are representative of the patient's habitual attacks.

Protocols for electrode placement and drug reduction vary from unit to unit. In all patients being investigated for TLE, additional EEG electrodes covering the sphenoidal area are used (the authors use surface zygomatic electrodes and have found no significant advantage in using needle sphenoidal electrodes). In cases without an identifiable lesion, high density EEG with source localisation can be helpful.

Although most epilepsy surgery candidates can be adequately investigated by scalp interictal and ictal EEG, intracranial EEG monitoring over 1–2 weeks may be required in selected cases. Typical indications are dual or possible multiple potential epileptogenic pathologies, bilateral hippocampal sclerosis, focal lesions in eloquent cortex and individuals with negative neuroimaging in whom other investigations have suggested a likely location of the epileptogenic region. Invasive EEG uses a range of electrode types (depth, strip, grid) inserted neurosurgically. Electrode choice and placement is determined by where the epileptogenic region is sited: subdural grids are best for coverage of a relatively large cortical surface area, and they allow extensive cortical mapping of eloquent areas. They do require a craniotomy and carry a 3–5% risk of infection. Depth electrodes are more suited to deep foci, and can be used to sample from both hemispheres. They carry a risk of approximately 0.2% of hemorrhage per electrode. In any case, only a limited area of cortex can be sampled (usually there are 6–15 contacts in each electrode). Subdural grids do not broach the pial boundary, have a lesser chance of causing haemorrhage and can cover a much larger area. The disadvantage of subdural grid electrodes is that they require a craniotomy and carry a higher risk of infection (approximately 3–5%); over one-quarter of patients develop an aseptic meningitis – usually restricting recordings to 10 days or less. The placement of the electrodes is dependent on the hypothesis that is to be tested. Intracranial stimulation either during awake craniotomy or with chronic subdural electrodes may also be necessary to delineate eloquent cortex and so determine the safe margins of resection. Newer methods of analysing the intracranial EEG such as single pulse stimulation techniques and the identification of high frequency bursting activity are beginning to be used to localise the epileptogenic zone. The yield of an intracranial EEG investigation thus largely depends on an appropriately formulated implantation hypothesis. Intracranial electrocortical stimulation either during awake craniotomy or with chronic subdural electrodes may also be necessary to delineate eloquent cortex and to determine the safe margins of resection.

Acute electrocorticography at the time of resection is used in some units to define the extent of resection, but we usually use extra-operative recordings.

There is an increasing role of MEG in defining the epileptogenic zone in people without an identifiable lesion, and in addition MEG can be used to identify eloquent cortex such as speech areas. Measuring changes in the magnetic field has the advantage of detecting currents that run perpendicular to the brain surface (such currents are often undetectable by scalp EEG). MEG can also detect spikes that originate deeper in the cortex. Recordings are usually limited to 1 hour. Currently, it is useful only in patients with relatively frequent interictal epileptiform discharges, and is used mainly in patients who are considered for intracranial EEG, in order to refine the implantation plan.

Neuropsychology

Neuropsychological assessment has a role in localisation; discordant neuropsychological deficits implicating cortex distinct from the putative epileptogenic cortex indicate more widespread cortical pathology. Psychometric testing can also be used to estimate the psychological sequelae of epilepsy surgery, most commonly in the context of memory deterioration following temporal lobe resection.

Injection of sodium amytal into each hemisphere (the 'amytal test') is used to 'anesthetise' each hemisphere in turn. This test was originally devised to lateralise language in uncertain cases, but this function is now increasingly determined by fMRI. The amytal test is also extensively used to determine the possible neuropsychological sequelae of temporal lobe resection, and fMRI cannot substitute for this. However, because of variations of blood flow, access of the drug to relevant structures (e.g. the mesial temporal structures) and cross flow the amytal test can be misleading. More selective amytal tests can be performed by super-selective injections of amytal into specific cerebral vessels; however, these are more technically challenging and provide a greater risk for the patient. In some units, an intracarotid sodium amytal test is used in every patient undergoing temporal lobe resection. Other units restrict the use of this test to patients in whom there is discordance between neuropsychometric testing and neuroimaging. The authors now rarely use the amytal test and depend upon the information gleaned from standard neuropsychometric testing and neuroimaging. The amytal test has an approximately 0.5% risk of causing cerebral infaction because of the risk of arterial catherisation.

Counselling

All patients should be counselled prior to surgery. They should be given details of risks and benefits; the authors find it advantageous not only to record these discussions in the notes, but also to send a letter to the patient with all these details. An estimate of the odds of success along with associated risks including catastrophic risks (stroke/death), neuropsychological risks, neuropsychiatric risks and more specific risks (e.g. visual defect) is given to the patient. The counsellor will also describe in more detail the practicalities (e.g. the length of time off work). They will also ascertain the degree of postoperative social support.

Surgery

Surgery for epilepsy can be divided into resective curative surgery and palliative surgery, although some forms of palliative surgery can occasionally render patients seizure free, and on some occasions resective surgery is performed to palliate rather than to cure the epilepsy.

Curative resective surgery

Although resective surgery has been the mainstay of curative surgical techniques, other approaches such as stereotactic radiosugery using a gamma knife have grown in popularity. The gamma knife is ideal for lesions that are difficult to resect (e.g. hypothalamic hamartomas) or for patients who are unlikely to be able to tolerate resective surgery. Whether the technique has a place in other situations remains to be determined. The main disadvantages are a lack of long-term follow-up, the risk of delayed radionecrosis and a significant delay from the radiosurgery to obtaining maximum benefit (as long as 1 year).

Lesionectomy Patients with discrete lesions have a good outcome from resective surgery, provided that the lesion can be completely removed and that there is no concomitant pathology. Thus, patients with dysembryoplastic neuro-epithelial tumours or discrete vascular lesions have a 50–80% chance of seizure freedom following removal of the lesion. In situations where the lesion is less well defined or is associated with more widespread abnormalities, the chance of seizure freedom drops markedly. Thus, cortical dysplasia visualised on MRI may only be the 'tip of the iceberg' and resection margins invariably have to be delineated using intracranial recordings. Nevertheless, resections of focal cortical dysplasia have a 10–50% chance of rendering a patient seizure free. Temporal lobe lesions are frequently associated with hippocampal sclerosis, and experience dictates that removal of both the lesion and the hippocampus is usually necessary for a successful outcome. The complications of surgery depend upon the location of the lesion, and in particular its proximity to eloquent cortex.

Surgery in temporal lobe epilepsy Temporal lobe resection is the most common operation for seizure control. The most common pathology is hippocampal sclerosis although temporal lobe resection is also used to treat other lesions in the temporal lobes. There have been a variety of surgical approaches to temporal lobe resection, with variations aimed to minimise the temporal neocortex resection, while maintaining the hippocampal resection. The usual operations are either anterior temporal lobectomy or selective amygdalo-hippocampectomy. The relative advantages and disadvantages of each of these approaches are relatively minor. These operations result in approximately 50% of patients becoming seizure free in the long term (this figure may be higher in those with hippocampal sclerosis and concordant investigations) and 20% showing significant improvement. However, the chances of remaining seizure free diminish over time (probably by 3% per year for the first 5 years). The overall mortality of temporal lobectomy is less than 0.5%. A transient hemiparesis can occur in up to 5%, but the risk of permanent hemiparesis is less than 1%. The chance of significant memory decline depends upon baseline memory test, age and side of operation (dominant versus non-dominant). Significant visual field defects occur in 10%, and 5% of patients in the United Kingdom may be unable to drive because of these. Postoperative depression is not uncommon. Postoperative psychosis is less common and usually occurs in patients whose seizures are continuing. Other organic mental disorders can result, in a seemingly largely unpredicatable fashion. There is also a risk of a late decline in cognitive function some years later due, it is postulated, to reduction in cerebral reserve.

Extratemporal surgery Extratemporal surgery is performed less frequently and mainly consists of frontal lobe surgery. The presence of a lesion is the most important predictor of surgical success. Overall, approximately 30–50% become seizure free, depending on nature and extent of the pathological basis of the epilepsy, but a normal MRI reduces these odds. The risks of operation are related to the site of resection.

Hemispherectomy This is particularly effective in controlling seizures, with approximately 80% becoming seizure free. This operation is only suitable for people with a profound hemiparesis, and care needs to be taken if it is the dominant hemisphere. Early theories concerning language development suggested that resection of the dominant hemisphere should not occur after the age of 6 years, but recent experience suggests a cut-off of 9 years and indeed language recovery has been noted at even later ages. The operation is usually carried out in people with extensive abnormalities of one hemisphere or with a pathology affecting one hemisphere (e.g. Rasmussen's encephalitis). Mortality is approximately 1–2%. In the past, long-term outcome was poor because of problems resulting from hydrocephalus that is attributed to superficial haemosiderosis. These risks have diminished with modern refinements of the operation – most centres now carry out the safer functional hemispherectomy. In this operation, the temporal lobe is removed, a corpus callosotomy is performed and the frontal and occipital lobes are disconnected rather than resected.

Palliative procedures

These operations aim to reduce the frequency or severity of seizures but rarely render people seizure free.

Corpus callosotomy Callosotomy is considered in patients with frequent tonic or atonic seizures (and more controversially tonic–clonic seizures) and when resective surgery is not possible. The chances of long-term seizure freedom with this operation are slim, approximately 5%. The morbidity from this operation can be considerable. When language representation occurs in both hemispheres language problems can occur and disconnection syndromes with apraxia and 'alien' hand are the cause of considerable disability. These are more common in patients who undergo the operation after the age of 12 years. The operation is often performed as a two-stage procedure with first section of the anterior two-thirds and then, if seizure control is inadequate, a further procedure to section the posterior one-third can be considered. Because of the morbidity and disappointing long-term results, many centres have discontinued this operation and use vagal nerve stimulation in its place.

Multiple subpial transection This procedure is considered when eloquent areas of cortex form part of the epileptogenic zone. The procedure is based on the concept that functional cortical activity occurs in a radial plane, whereas seizures spread in a tangential plane. Thus, by making radial sections it should be possible to prevent seizure spread without interfering with physiological function. The cortex is exposed and acute corticography is used to determine the extent of the irritative zone. Radial cuts are made at intervals of less than 5 mm and the procedure is deemed successful once interictal discharges are abolished or minimised. Some groups report that 60–70% of patients experience a 95% reduction or more in seizure frequency, but in other centres the success rate is much lower. Some 20–30% of patients sustain focal deficits as the result of surgery and there is also a significant long-term relapse rate. The operation therefore is now usually performed only as an adjunct to and in combination with a cortical lesion resection with subpial transections made around the edge of the resection margin, or for the treatment of patients with Landau–Kleffner syndrome.

Neuro-stimulation The use of stimulation of various structures has a long and chequered history, but has recently been placed on a more scientific basis, with better trials and a better understanding of mechanisms of action.

Vagal nerve stimulation (VNS) for epilepsy has now been licensed throughout the world. This involves the placement of a stimulator under the skin with a wire to the left vagus nerve which is then intermittently stimulated. The stimulation parameters vary but are usually in the range: amplitude 0.25–3.5 mA; pulse width 250–500 μs; frequency 20–30 Hz; duty cycle 30 seconds on, 5 minutes off. In addition, patients or caregivers can activate a stimulation cycle with a magnet in an attempt to abort a seizure in its early stages. Long-term results are generally disappointing and <50% of patients can expect a 50% or greater reduction in seizures. The technique is considered worthwhile in patients with tonic or atonic seizures, and VNS is increasingly being used in preference to corpus callosotomy. Dyspnoea, throat pain and hoarse voice are the main adverse events. It has to be noted that some patients are unable to tolerate the stimulation even at very low intensity. Furthermore, VNS currently precludes MRI at field strengths >1.5 T.

More recently, trigeminal nerve stimulation (TNS) has been introduced. This has the advantage that it is carried out with external electrodes and stimulator just at night, removing the need for an operation and not posing problems for MRI examination. How effective this procedure will prove to be is currently uncertain.

Stimulation of other targets such as the thalamus, subthalamic nuclei and the hippocampus are still in the early stages of development, but these methods are beginning to show promise not only as palliation, but also as potential cures. A recent trial of bilateral stimulation of the anterior thalamic nucleus (SANTE) and responsive cortical stimulation of one or two predetermined seizure foci (NEUROPACE) reported results similar to those of VNS, with approximately 50% of patients reporting a >50% reduction in seizure frequency at 2 years, and around 10% of patients reporting periods of seizure freedom of 3 months or more. Although these results are encouraging, the authors feel that they do not justify the routine use of deep brain or cortical stimulation yet.

Follow-up and prognosis

All patients undergoing epilepsy surgery need close follow-up in order to detect postoperative problems (e.g. depression, psychosis, organic mental disorders, seizure recurrence) to inform surgical practice and to counsel patients. The authors routinely repeat neuropsychological tests and MRI at 3–6 months following surgery, and then may repeat the neuropsychology again at a year.

If a patient becomes seizure free, then drug withdrawal will need to be considered. In the authors' series less than 30% of those who are seizure free following surgery choose to withdraw antiepileptic drugs completely. In those who do wish to reduce or withdraw medication, some recommend withdrawal at 1 year postoperatively and slowly taper over the subsequent year (drug withdrawal thereby usually occurs by 2 years post-operation). Others withdraw drugs more slowly, and the authors' practice is not to withdraw drugs in the first 5 years. The occurrence of early seizures, the inability to remove all the pathology, normal preoperative MRI, longer duration of epilepsy and older age all predict a less successful withdrawal from drugs.

Driving regulations in the UK

In the United Kingdom, it is the role of the Driving and Vehicle Licensing Agency (DVLA) to issue driving licences. Epilepsy is a condition in which special rules for licensing apply, and the patient must notify the DVLA of the occurrence of epilepsy or an isolated seizure. In other countries different rules apply. The DVLA applies the following rules.

Group 1 licensing

Driving rules for a group 1 licence (a normal driving licence for car and motorcycles) are as follows:

1. The occurrence of a single epileptic attack will result in the removal of a driving licence for 6 months from the date of the seizure. If there are clinical factors or investigation results that suggest an unacceptably high risk of a further seizure (i.e. 20% or greater per annum), driving will be prohibited for 12 months from the date of the seizure.
2. For some types of awake seizures, driving is permitted after 1 year after the first attack, even if seizures are continuing. This is only the case if consciousness is preserved in all seizures, the seizures do not affect the ability to react and control a vehicle normally during the seizure, and providing that no other seizure types have occurred.
3. If epilepsy has developed with sleep attacks, licensing will be prohibited for a period of 1 year from the date of the attack. However, if a pattern of sleep-only attacks has been established for 3 years or more, without any awake attacks occurring during this period, licensing is allowed even if sleep attacks have occurred in the preceding year.

A provoked or acute symptomatic seizure may be dealt with on an individual basis by the DVLA if there is no previous seizure history. The decision to prohibit driving in this situation will be influenced by such aspects as:

1. Whether the provoking stimulus carries any risk of recurrence, and
2. Whether the stimulus had been successfully or appropriately treated or was unlikely to occur at the wheel.

Thus, for example, the following seizures are usually considered provoked: eclamptic seizures; reflex anoxic seizures; an immediate seizure at the time of a head injury; a seizure in first week following a head injury, which is not associated with any damage on CT scanning, nor with post-traumatic amnesia of longer than 30 minutes; a seizure at the time of a stroke/TIA or within the ensuing 24 hours; or a seizure occurring during intracranial surgery or in the ensuing 24 hours. Seizures associated with alcohol or drug misuse, sleep deprivation or a structural abnormality are not considered as 'provoked' for licensing purposes.

Driving during periods of change of medication is discretionary, and depends on the advice given by the doctor on the risks of a seizure. Special care needs to be exercised where complete withdrawal of medication is being carried out.

Group 2 licensing

Group 2 licences cover the driving of lorries, heavy goods vehicles and buses, and the rules are much stricter.

1. After a single seizure, driving is prohibited for a period of 5 years after the seizure, providing antiepileptic drugs have not been taken.
2. In patients with a diagnosis of epilepsy, a period of 10 years must pass without a seizure and without antiepileptic medication.

For taxis, many local authorities apply the regulations for Group 2 licences. However, each local authority has the ability to decide its own standards for driving.

For both types of licence

A person must have no other medical reason which may affect his/her ability to drive. The person must comply with advised treatment and check-ups for epilepsy, and the driving of a vehicle by such a person should not be likely to cause danger to the public.

Role of the doctor vis-à-vis the driving regulations

The following policy should be followed. The doctor must make it clear to a driving licence holder that they have a condition that may affect their safety as a driver, and therefore that the driver has a legal duty to inform the DVLA about the condition.

If the patient refuses to accept the diagnosis or the effect of the condition on their ability to drive, the doctor should advise the patient that a second opinion can be sought and appropriate arrangements should be made for this. It is important that the patient is advised not to drive until the second opinion has been obtained. If the patient continues to drive when not fit to do so, the doctor should make every reasonable effort to dissuade driving. If the patient continues to drive despite the above measures, the doctor should disclose relevant medical information immediately, in confidence, to the DVLA. Before giving information to the DVLA, the doctor should inform the patient of the decision to do so. Once the DVLA has been informed, the doctor should also write to the patient to say that a disclosure has been made.

Other types of vehicle

The DVLA regulations cover vehicles that are driven on public highways, not vehicles that are used on private land, and thus the driving for instance of forklift trucks, tractors and quad bikes, or sit-on lawnmowers is permitted providing this is on private land. However, employers need to take into account health and safety regulations.

Electric wheelchairs and mobility scooters also are not considered to be 'vehicles', so a driving licence is not needed to use them, on public or private land.

Acknowledgement

Dr Beate Diehl and Dr Tim Wehner wish to be acknowledged as co-authors of the EEG section only in this chapter (pp. 247–252).

References

Chadwick D, Taylor J, Johnson T. Outcomes after seizure recurrence in people with well-controlled epilepsy and the factors that influence it. The MRC Antiepileptic Drug Withdrawal Group. *Epilepsia* 1996; **37:** 1043–1050.

Hart YM, Sander JW, Johnson AL, Shorvon SD. National General Practice Study of Epilepsy: recurrence after a first seizure. *Lancet* 1990; **336:** 1271–1274.

ILAE Commission Report. Commission on Classification and Terminology of the International League Against Epilepsy. Proposal for revised clinical and electroencephalographic classification of epileptic seizures. *Epilepsia* 1981; **22:** 489–501.

Shorvon S. The biochemical, haematological and immunological and genetic investigation of epilepsy. In *The Oxford Textbook of Epilepsy and Epileptic Seizures.* Shorvon S, Guerrini R, Cook M, Lhatoo S. eds. Oxford: Oxford University Press, 2013: 127–135.

Shorvon S, Ferlisi M. The treatment of super-refractory status epilepticus: a critical review of available therapies and a clinical treatment protocol. *Brain* 2011; **134** (Pt 10): 2802–2818.

Winston GP, Daga P, Stretton J, Modat M, Symms MR, McEvoy AW, *et al.* Optic radiation tractography and vision in anterior temporal lobe resection. *Ann Neurol* 2012; **71:** 334–741.

Further reading

Useful websites with epilepsy information for patients

www.epilepsy.org Official portal of the International Bureau Against Epilepsy.

www.epilepsynse.org.uk Site of the National Society for Epilepsy, UK.

www.epilepsy.com Site of a US organisation providing support for epilepsy.

www.epilepsy.org.uk Site of Epilepsy Action, a UK-based charity providing support for epilepsy.

www.epilepsyfoundation.org Site of the Epilepsy Foundation for Epilepsy, a US based organisation providing support for epilepsy.

www.ninds.nih.gov/disorders/epilepsy/epilepsy.htm Patient information from the NINDS in the USA.

Books

Arzimanoglou A, Guerrini R, Aicardi J. *Aicardi's Epilepsy in Children*, 3rd edn. Philadelphia: Lippincott, Williams and Wilkins, 2003.

Engel J. (ed.) *Surgical Treatment of the Epilepsies*, 2nd edn. New York: Raven Press, 1993.

Engel J, Pedley T. (eds) *Epilepsy: A comprehensive Textbook*. Wolters Kluwer/Lippincott Williams & Wilkins, 2008.

Levy R, Mattson RH, Meldrum BS, Perucca E. *(eds) Antiepileptic Drugs, 5th edn.* Philadelphia: Lippincott, Williams and Wilkins, 2002.

Luders H. (ed.) *Textbook of Epilepsy Surgery*. London: Informa Healthcare, 2008.

Panayiotopoulos CP. *The Epilepsies: Seizures, Syndromes and Management*. London: Bladon Medical Publishing, 2004.

Panayiotopoulos CP. (ed.) *Atlas of Epilepsies*. Springer, 2010.

Schomer DL, Lopes da Silva FH. (eds) *Niedermeyer's Electroencephalography*, 6th edn. Philadelphia, Wolters Kluwer Health/Lippincott Williams & Wilkins, 2011.

Shorvon S, Guerrini R, Cook M, Lhatoo S. *Oxford Textbook of Epilepsy and Epileptic Seizures*. Oxford: Oxford University Press, 2012.

Shorvon SD. *Status Epilepticus: Its Clinical Features and Treatment in Children and Adults*, Cambridge: Cambridge University Press, 1994.

Shorvon SD. *Handbook of Epilepsy Treatment: Forms, Causes and Therapy in Children and Adults*. 3rd edn. Oxford: Blackwell Science, 2010.

Shorvon SD, Andermann F, Guerrini R. *The Causes of Epilepsy: Common and Uncommon Causes in Adults and Children*. Cambridge: Cambridge University Press, 2011.

Shorvon SD, Perucca E, Engel J. (eds) *The Treatment of Epilepsy*, 3rd edn. Oxford: Wiley-Blackwell, 2009.

Temkin O. *The Falling Sickness: A History of Epilepsy from the Greeks to the Beginnings of Modern Neurology*. Baltimore: Johns Hopkins Press, 1971.

Wyllie E. Cascino G. Gidal B, Goodkin HP. (eds) *Wyllie's Treatment of Epilepsy: Principles and Practice*, 5th edn. Lippincott Williams & Wilkins, 2012.

Journal articles

Adab N, Tudur SC, Vinten J, Williamson P, Winterbottom J. Common antiepileptic drugs in pregnancy in women with epilepsy. *Cochrane Database Syst Rev* 2004; **3**: CD004848.

Arts WF, Brouwer OF, Peters AC, Stroink H, Peeters EA, Schmitz PI, *et al.* Course and prognosis of childhood epilepsy: 5-year follow-up of the Dutch study of epilepsy in childhood. *Brain* 2004; **127**: 1774–1784.

Arroyo S, Anhut H, Kugler AR, Lee CM, Knapp LE, Garofalo EA, *et al.* Pregabalin add-on treatment: a randomized, double-blind, placebo-controlled, dose–response study in adults with partial seizures. *Epilepsia* 2004; **45**: 20–27.

Bang L, Goa K. Oxcarbazepine: a review of its use in children with epilepsy. *Paediatr Drugs* 2003; **5**: 557–573.

Barry JJ, Ettinger AB, Friel P, Gilliam FG, Harden CL, Hermann B, *et al.*; Advisory Group of the Epilepsy Foundation as part of its Mood Disorder. Consensus statement: the evaluation and treatment of people with epilepsy and affective disorders. *Epilepsy Behav* 2008; **13** (Suppl 1): S1–29.

Battino D, Tomson T, Bonizzoni E, Craig J, Lindhout D, Sabers A, *et al.*; EURAP Study Group. Seizure control and treatment changes in pregnancy:observations from the EURAP epilepsy pregnancy registry. *Epilepsia* 2013; **54:** 1621–1627.

Baxendale S, Thompson P, McEvoy A, Duncan J. Epilepsy surgery: how accurate are multidisciplinary teams in predicting outcome? *Seizure* 2012; **21**: 546–549.

Beghi E, Leone M, Solari A. Mortality in patients with a first unprovoked seizure. *Epilepsia* 2005; **46** (Suppl 11): 40–42.

Bell B, Lin JJ, Seidenberg M, Hermann B. The neurobiology of cognitive disorders in temporal lobe epilepsy. *Nat Rev Neurol* 2011; **7**: 154–164.

Benbadis SR, Tatum WO. Overinterpretation of EEGs and misdiagnosis of epilepsy. *J Clin Neurophysiol* 2003; **20**: 42–44.

Bough KJ, Rho JM. Anticonvulsant mechanisms of the ketogenic diet. *Epilepsia* 2007; **48**: 43–58.

Brenner RP. EEG in convulsive and nonconvulsive status epilepticus. *J Clin Neurophysiol* 2004; **21**: 319–331.

Camilo O, Goldstein LB. Seizures and epilepsy after ischemic stroke. *Stroke* 2004; **35**: 1769–1775.

Chan EM, Andrade DM, Franceschetti S, Minassian B. Progressive myoclonus epilepsies: EPM1, EPM2A, EPM2B. *Adv Neurol* 2005; **95**: 47–57.

Cendes F. Febrile seizures and mesial temporal sclerosis. *Curr Opin Neurol* 2004; **17**: 161–164.

Cramer JA, Mintzer S, Wheless J, Mattson RH. Adverse effects of antiepileptic drugs: a brief overview of important issues. *Expert Rev Neurother* 2010; **10:** 885–891.

Crino PB. Malformations of cortical development: molecular pathogenesis and experimental strategies. *Adv Exp Med Biol* 2004; **548**: 175–191.

de Tisi J, Bell GS, Peacock JL, McEvoy AW, Harkness WF, Sander JW, *et al.* The long-term outcome of adult epilepsy surgery, patterns of seizure remission, and relapse: a cohort study. *Lancet* 2011; **378:** 1388–1395.

Devlin AM, Cross JH, Harkness W, Chong WK, Harding B, Vargha-Khadem F, *et al.* Clinical outcomes of hemispherectomy for epilepsy in childhood and adolescence. *Brain* 2003; **126** (Pt 3): 556–566.

Drivers Medical Group, DVLA. *At a glance guide to the current medical standards of fitness to drive*. Swansea: DVLA, 2012.

Duncan JS. Imaging in the surgical treatment of epilepsy. *Nat Rev Neurol* 2010; **6:** 537–550.

Duncan JS, Winston GP, Koepp MJ, Ourselin S. Brain imaging in the assessment for epilepsy surgery. *Lancet Neurol.* 2016 Feb 23. doi: 10.1016/S1474-4422(15)00383-X.

Elger CE, Helmstaedter C, Kurthen M. Chronic epilepsy and cognition. *Lancet Neurol* 2004; **3**: 663–672.

Engel J Jr, Bragin A, Staba R, Mody I. High-frequency oscillations: what is normal and what is not? *Epilepsia* 2009; **50:** 598–604. doi:10.1111/j.1528-1167.2008.

Ferlisi M, Shorvon S. The outcome of therapies in refractory and super-refractory convulsive status epilepticus and recommendations for therapy. *Brain* 2012; **135** (Pt 8): 2314–2328.

Fisher RS, van Emde Boas W, Blume W, Elger C, Genton P, Lee P, *et al.* Epileptic seizures and epilepsy: definitions proposed by the International League Against Epilepsy (ILAE) and the International Bureau for Epilepsy (IBE). *Epilepsia* 2005; **46**: 470–472.

Foldvary N, Klem G, Hammel J, Bingaman W, Najm I, Lüders H. The localising value of ictal EEG in focal epilepsy. *Neurology* 2001; **57**: 2022–2028.

French JA, Kanner AM, Bautista J, Abou-Khalil B, Browne T, Harden CL, *et al.* Efficacy and tolerability of the new antiepileptic drugs I: treatment of new onset epilepsy: report of the Therapeutics and Technology Assessment Subcommittee and Quality Standards Subcommittee of the American Academy of Neurology and the American Epilepsy Society. *Neurology* 2004; **62**: 1252–1260.

French JA, Kanner AM, Bautista J, Abou-Khalil B, Browne T, Harden CL, *et al.* Efficacy and tolerability of the new antiepileptic drugs II: treatment of refractory epilepsy: report of the Therapeutics and Technology Assessment Subcommittee and Quality Standards Subcommittee of the American Academy of Neurology and the American Epilepsy Society. *Neurology* 2004; **62**: 1261–1273.

Genton P, Roger J, Guerrini R, Medina MT, Bureau M, Dravet C, *et al.* History and classification of 'myoclonic' epilepsies: from seizures to syndromes to diseases. *Adv Neurol* 2005; **95**: 1–14.

Glauser T, Ben-Menachem E, Bourgeois B, Cnaan A, Chadwick D, Guerreiro C, *et al.* ILAE treatment guidelines: evidence-based analysis of antiepileptic drug efficacy and effectiveness as initial monotherapy for epileptic seizures and syndromes. *Epilepsia* 2006; **47**: 1094–1120.

Glauser T, Ben-Menachem E, Bourgeois B, Cnaan A, Guerreiro C, Kälviäinen R, *et al.;* ILAE Subcommission on AED Guidelines. Updated ILAE evidence review of antiepileptic drug efficacy and effectiveness as initial monotherapy for epileptic seizures and syndromes. *Epilepsia* 2013; **54**: 551–563.

Gobbi G, Boni A, Filippini M. The spectrum of idiopathic rolandic epilepsy syndromes and idiopathic occipital epilepsies: from the benign to the disabling. *Epilepsia* 2006; **47** (Suppl 2): 62–66.

Gourfinkel-An I, Baulac S, Nabbout R, Ruberg M, Baulac M, Brice A, *et al.* Monogenic idiopathic epilepsies. *Lancet Neurol* 2004; **3**: 209–218.

Guerrini R, Aicardi J. Epileptic encephalopathies with myoclonic seizures in infants and children (severe myoclonic epilepsy and myoclonic-astatic epilepsy). *J Clin Neurophysiol* 2003; **20**: 449–461.

Guerrini R, Parrini E. Neuronal migration disorders. *Neurobiol Dis* 2010; **38**: 154–166.

Hitiris N, Brodie MJ. Evidence-based treatment of idiopathic generalized epilepsies with older antiepileptic drugs. *Epilepsia* 2005; **46** (Suppl 9): 149–153.

Hauser WA, Annegers JF, Kurland LT. Prevalence of epilepsy in Rochester, Minnesota: 1940–1980. *Epilepsia* 1991; **32**: 429–445.

Helmstaedter C, Kurthen M, Lux S, Reuber M, Elger CE. Chronic epilepsy and cognition: a longitudinal study in temporal lobe epilepsy. *Ann Neurol* 2003; **54**: 425–432.

Henry TR, Van Heertum RL. Positron emission tomography and single photon emission computed tomography in epilepsy care. *Semin Nucl Med* 2003; **33**: 88–104.

ILAE Commission Report. Commission on Classification and Terminology of the International League Against Epilepsy. Proposal for revised classification of epilepsies and epileptic syndromes. *Epilepsia* 1989; **30**: 389–399.

ILAE Commission Report. Commission on Diagnostic Strategies. Recommendations for Functional Neuroimaging of Persons with Epilepsy. Neuroimaging Subcommission of the International League Against Epilepsy. *Epilepsia* 2000; **41**: 1350–1356.

ILAE Commission Report. Guidelines for Neuroimaging Evaluation of Patients with Uncontrolled Epilepsy Considered for Surgery. Commission on Neuroimaging of the International League Against Epilepsy. *Epilepsia* 1998; **39**: 1375–1376.

ILAE Commission Report. Recommendations for Neuroimaging of Patients with Epilepsy. Commission on Neuroimaging of the International League Against Epilepsy. *Epilepsia* 1997; **38**: 1255–1256.

Jallon P. Mortality in patients with epilepsy. *Curr Opin Neurol* 2004; **17**: 141–146.

Kaplan PW. The EEG of status epilepticus. *J Clin Neurophysiol* 2006; **23**: 221–229.

Koutroumanidis M, Smith SJ. Use and abuse of EEG in the diagnosis of idiopathic generalized epilepsies. *Epilepsia* 2005; **46**: 96–107.

Leach JP, Stephen LJ, Salveta C, Brodie MJ. Which EEG for epilepsy? The relative usefulness of different EEG protocols in patients with possible epilepsy. *J Neurol Neurosurg Psychiatry* 2006; **77**: 1040–1042.

Löscher W, Potschka H. Drug resistance in brain diseases and the role of drug efflux transporters. *Nat Rev Neurosci* 2005; **6**: 591–602.

Logroscino G, Hesdorffer DC, Cascino G, Hauser WA, Coeytaux A, Galobardes B, *et al.* Mortality after a first episode of status epilepticus in the United States and Europe. *Epilepsia* 2005; **46** (Suppl 11): 46–48.

Luciano AL, Shorvon SD. Results of treatment changes in patients with apparently drug-resistant chronic epilepsy. *Ann Neurol* 2007; **62**: 375–381.

McIntosh AM, Kalnins RM, Mitchell LA, Fabinyi GC, Briellmann RS, Berkovic SF. Temporal lobectomy: long-term seizure outcome, late recurrence and risks for seizure recurrence. *Brain* 2004; **127**: 2018–2030.

Man CB, Kwan P, Baum L, Yu E, Lau KM, Cheng AS, *et al.* Association between HLA-B*1502 allele and antiepileptic drug-induced cutaneous reactions in Han Chinese. *Epilepsia* 2007; **48**: 1015–1018.

Mauguiere F, Ryvlin P. The role of PET in presurgical assessment of partial epilepsies. *Epileptic Disord* 2004; **6**: 193–215.

Marson AG, Al-Kharusi AM, Alwaidh M, Appleton R, Baker GA, Chadwick DW, *et al.*; SANAD Study group. The SANAD study of effectiveness of carbamazepine, gabapentin, lamotrigine, oxcarbazepine, or topiramate for treatment of partial epilepsy: an unblinded randomised controlled trial. *Lancet* 2007; **369**: 1000–1015.

Marson AG, Al-Kharusi AM, Alwaidh M, Appleton R, Baker GA, Chadwick DW, *et al.*; SANAD Study group. The SANAD study of effectiveness of valproate, lamotrigine, or topiramate for generalised and unclassifiable epilepsy: an unblinded randomised controlled trial. *Lancet* 2007; **369**: 1016–1026.

Moran NF, Poole K, Bell G, Solomon J, Kendall S, McCarthy M, *et al.* Epilepsy in the United Kingdom: seizure frequency and severity, anti-epileptic drug utilization and impact on life in 1652 people with epilepsy. *Seizure* 2004; **13**: 425–433.

Musicco M, Beghi E, Solari A, Viani F, for the First Seizure Trial Group (FIRST Group) Treatment of first tonic–clonic seizure does not improve the prognosis of epilepsy. *Neurology* 1997; **49**: 991–998.

Neligan A, Shorvon SD. Frequency and prognosis of convulsive status epilepticus of different causes: a systematic review. *Arch Neurol* 2010; **67**: 931–940.

Neligan A, Shorvon SD. Prognostic factors, morbidity and mortality in tonic–clonic status epilepticus: a review. *Epilepsy Res* 2011; **93**: 1–10.

Noachtar S, Borggraefe I. Epilepsy surgery: a critical review. *Epilepsy Behav* 2009; **15**: 66–72.

O'Brien MD, Guillebaud J. Contraception for women with epilepsy. *Epilepsia* 2006; **47**: 1419–1422.

Panayiotopoulos CP. Autonomic seizures and autonomic status epilepticus peculiar to childhood: diagnosis and management. *Epilepsy Behav* 2004; **5**: 286–295.

Panayiotopoulos CP. Syndromes of idiopathic generalized epilepsies not recognized by the International League Against Epilepsy. *Epilepsia* 2005; **46** (Suppl 9): 57–66.

Patsalos PN. Clinical pharmacokinetics of levetiracetam. *Clin Pharmacokinet* 2004; **43**: 707–724.

Patsalos PN. Properties of antiepileptic drugs in the treatment of idiopathic generalized epilepsies. *Epilepsia* 2005; **46** (Suppl 9): 140–148.

Patsalos PN, Berry DJ, Bourgeois BF, Cloyd JC, Glauser TA, Johannessen SI, *et al.* Antiepileptic drugs – best practice guidelines for therapeutic drug monitoring: a position paper by the subcommission on therapeutic drug monitoring, ILAE Commission on Therapeutic Strategies. *Epilepsia* 2008; **49**: 1239–1276.

Patsalos PN, Perucca E. Clinically important drug interactions in epilepsy: interactions between antiepileptic drugs and other drugs. *Lancet Neurol* 2003; **2**: 473–481.

Pitkänen A, Lukasiuk K. Molecular and cellular basis of epileptogenesis in symptomatic epilepsy. *Epilepsy Behav* 2009; **14** (Suppl 1): 16–25.

Pitkänen A, Lukasiuk K. Mechanisms of epileptogenesis and potential treatment targets. *Lancet Neurol* 2011; **10**: 173–186.

Polkey CE. Clinical outcome of epilepsy surgery. *Curr Opin Neurol* 2004; **17**: 173–178.

Potschka H. Transporter hypothesis of drug-resistant epilepsy: challenges for pharmacogenetic approaches. *Pharmacogenomics* 2010; **11**: 1427–1438.

Qureshi IA, Mehler MF. Epigenetic mechanisms underlying human epileptic disorders and the process of epileptogenesis. *Neurobiol Dis* 2010; **39**: 53–60.

Rakhade SN, Jensen FE. Epileptogenesis in the immature brain: emerging mechanisms. *Nat Rev Neurol* 2009; **5**: 380–391.

Rogawski MA, Löscher W. The neurobiology of antiepileptic drugs for the treatment of nonepileptic conditions. *Nat Med* 2004; **10**: 685–689.

Ryvlin P, Nashef L, Lhatoo SD, Bateman LM, Bird J, Bleasel A, *et al.* Incidence and mechanisms of cardiorespiratory arrests in epilepsy monitoring units (MORTEMUS): a retrospective study. *Lancet Neurol* 2013; **12**: 966–977.

Ryvlin P, Rheims S, Risse G. Nocturnal frontal lobe epilepsy. *Epilepsia* 2006; **47** (Suppl 2): 83–86.

Sackellares JC, Ramsay RE, Wilder BJ, Browne TR 3rd, Shellenberger MK. Randomized, controlled clinical trial of zonisamide as adjunctive treatment for refractory partial seizures. *Epilepsia* 2004; **45**: 610–617.

Schmidt D, Rogawski MA. New strategies for the identification of drugs to prevent the development or progression of epilepsy. *Epilepsy Res* 2002; **50**: 71–78.

Schuele SU, Lüders HO. Intractable epilepsy: management and therapeutic alternatives. *Lancet Neurol* 2008; **7**: 514–524.

Shorvon S. We live in the age of the clinical guideline. *Epilepsia* 2006; **47**: 1091–1093.

Shorvon S. The treatment of chronic epilepsy: a review of recent studies of clinical efficacy and side effects. *Curr Opin Neurol* 2007; **20**: 159–163.

Shorvon S, Luciano AL. Prognosis of chronic and newly diagnosed epilepsy: revisiting temporal aspects. *Curr Opin Neurol* 2007; **20**: 208–212.

Shorvon S, Tomson T. Sudden unexpected death in epilepsy. *Lancet* 2011; **378**: 2028–2038.

Siegel AM. Parietal lobe epilepsy. *Adv Neurol* 2003; **93**: 335–345.

Stephani U. The natural history of myoclonic astatic epilepsy (Doose syndrome) and Lennox–Gastaut syndrome. *Epilepsia* 2006; **47** (Suppl 2): 53–55.

Tan RY, Neligan A, Shorvon SD. The uncommon causes of status epilepticus: a systematic review. *Epilepsy Res* 2010; **91:** 111–122.

Taylor I, Scheffer IE, Berkovic SF. Occipital epilepsies: identification of specific and newly recognized syndromes. *Brain* 2003; **126**: 753–769.

Téllez-Zenteno JF, Dhar R, Wiebe S. Long-term seizure outcomes following epilepsy surgery: a systematic review and meta-analysis. *Brain* 2005; **128** (Pt 5): 1188–1198.

Téllez-Zenteno JF, Dhar R, Hernandez-Ronquillo L, Wiebe S. Long-term outcomes in epilepsy surgery: antiepileptic drugs, mortality, cognitive and psychosocial aspects. *Brain* 2007; **130** (Pt 2): 334–345.

Thiele EA. Managing epilepsy in tuberous sclerosis complex. *J Child Neurol* 2004; **19**: 680–686.

Tomson T, Battino D. Teratogenic effects of antiepileptic drugs. *Lancet Neurol* 2012; **11:** 803–813.

Tomson T, Beghi E, Sundqvist A, Johannessen SI. Medical risks in epilepsy: a review with focus on physical injuries, mortality, traffic accidents and their prevention. *Epilepsy Res* 2004; **60**: 1–16.

Urdinguio RG, Sanchez-Mut JV, Esteller M. Epigenetic mechanisms in neurological diseases: genes, syndromes, and therapies. *Lancet Neurol* 2009; **8:** 1056–1072.

Van Paesschen W, Dupont P, Sunaert S, Goffin K, Van Laere K. The use of SPECT and PET in routine clinical practice in epilepsy. *Curr Opin Neurol* 2007; **20:** 194–202.

Vecht CJ, Wagner GL, Wilms EB. Interactions between antiepileptic and chemotherapeutic drugs. *Lancet Neurol* 2003; **2**: 404–409.

Velis D, Plouin P, Gotman J, da Silva FL, ILAE DMC Subcommittee on Neurophysiology. Recommendations regarding the requirement and applications for long-term recordings in epilepsy. ILAE Commission report. *Epilepsia* 2007; **48**: 379–384.

Vezzani A, Granata T. Brain inflammation in epilepsy: experimental and clinical evidence. *Epilepsia* 2005; **46:** 1724–1743.

Walker M, Cross H, Smith S, Young C, Aicardi J, Appleton R, *et al.* Nonconvulsive status epilepticus: Epilepsy Research Foundation workshop reports. *Epileptic Disord* 2005; **7**: 253–296.

Wiebe S, Blume WT, Girvin JP, Eliasziw M. A randomized, controlled trial of surgery for temporal-lobe epilepsy. *New Engl J Med* 2001; **345**: 311–318.

Zaccara G, Franciotta D, Perucca E. Idiosyncratic adverse reactions to antiepileptic drugs. *Epilepsia* 2007; **48**: 1223–1244.

Zupanc ML. Neonatal seizures. *Pediatr Clin North Am* 2004; **51**: 961–978.

CHAPTER 8

Dementia and Cognitive Impairment

Martin Rossor[1], John Collinge[1], Nick Fox[1], Simon Mead[1], Catherine Mummery[2], Jonathan Rohrer[1], Jonathan Schott[1] and Jason Warren[1]

[1] UCL Institute of Neurology

[2] National Hospital for Neurology & Neurosurgery

Dementia and cognitive impairment are very common and accompany many neurological as well as systemic diseases. The array of syndromes arising from damage to the neural circuitry underlying cognition can be as bewildering as the terminology. Cognitive impairment is a useful umbrella term that encompasses the severe dementia of late stage degenerative diseases such as Alzheimer's disease (AD), the mild cognitive slowing of a patient on a sedative drug and the florid confusional state or delirium in the severely systemically ill. A useful distinction, easier in theory than in practice, is the distinction between delirium and dementia. Delirium, also referred to as an acute confusional state, is characterised by fluctuation, prominent impairment of attention and/or arousal, and accompanied often by agitation and autonomic features. Delirium is commonly seen in systemic diseases and as a side effect of a variety of drugs and toxins (see delirium tremens, Chapter 19). Dementia, by contrast, refers to widespread cognitive impairment in the setting of normal arousal. This distinction can be difficult especially because confusional states can supervene in patients with many forms of dementia, and dementia with Lewy bodies (DLB) can present with fluctuating arousal and attentional deficits.

Definitions of dementia vary. The key features of the International Classification of Diseases (ICD) and the Diagnostic and Statistical Manual of Mental Disorders (DSM) definitions are that the disruption of cortical function should involve more than one cognitive domain which should include memory, more specifically episodic memory. The requirement for a memory impairment has largely been determined by the prototypic dementia AD which normally has a major amnestic component. However, other dementias such as frontotemporal dementia may only develop memory impairment late in the disease. The cognitive deficits should be sufficiently severe to cause significant social and occupational impairment. It is often assumed that dementia is progressive but a dementia can be progressive, static or reversible, depending on the aetiology. There is an increasing need to identify patients early before they fulfil the criteria of dementia, which has led to the introduction of terms such as mild cognitive impairment (MCI) to describe those patients with early disease who have not progressed to fulfil the criteria for dementia. If memory is impaired (amnestic MCI) most patients are in the early stages of AD. The recent DSM revision DSM5 now refers to minor and major neurocognitive disorders.

A useful distinction has been drawn between patients with prominent cognitive deficits arising from pathology in the cerebral cortex (cortical dementia) and those with prominent basal ganglia, thalamic or brainstem pathology (subcortical dementia). The latter patients are often very slow but accurate and exemplified by progressive supranuclear palsy (PSP). Cortical and subcortical pathologies often overlap, but the clinical distinction is useful.

It is important to realise that:

- Dementia is a syndrome caused by many different diseases, and
- Dementia may be reversible if the correct diagnosis of the cause is made and treated.

Epidemiology: Delirium, dementia and cognitive impairment

Delirium is a problem of universal importance; it is encountered in all branches of medicine, and in both community and hospital practice. It has been estimated to occur in 5–15% of patients in general hospital wards, and a higher proportion in intensive care units. A plethora of systemic and intracranial disease processes may give rise to delirium (Table 8.1); the elderly and patients with any pre-existing cognitive impairment, and those with chronic systemic illness are especially vulnerable.

Dementia is an issue of enormous medical and socio-economic significance in societies with ageing populations. Prevalence rates in Europe, for people over the age of 65 years, are approximately 6% for all causes of dementia and approximately 4% for AD. Dementia in people under the age of 65 years (young onset dementia) is increasingly recognised as an important social problem, with UK prevalence rates estimated as 67–81/100 000 in people aged 45–65 years. Although data for individual diseases are limited by diagnostic accuracy, as a group degenerative diseases are numerically the most important causes of dementia in both older and younger adults in Western countries and probably worldwide. The young onset forms of these diseases are frequently familial. Some rarer degenerative dementias such as variant Creutzfeldt–Jakob disease (vCJD) occur typically in the young patient, while other disease processes, such as frontotemporal dementia (FTD) and alcohol-related dementia, are also common in younger age groups. In contrast, DLB, a common cause in patients over 65 years of age, accounts for only a small proportion of young onset cases. Vascular

Neurology: A Queen Square Textbook, Second Edition. Edited by Charles Clarke, Robin Howard, Martin Rossor and Simon Shorvon.

Table 8.1 Causes of delirium and dementia.

Category of disease	Delirium	Dementia
Acquired/sporadic		
Metabolic disturbance	Electrolyte disorders (especially hyponatraemia, hypercalcaemia), hypoglycaemia, respiratory failure/hypoxia (any cause), uraemia, liver failure, pancreatic encephalopathy, cardiac failure, dehydration, severe anaemia	Uraemia, dialysis dementia (now rare), liver failure, respiratory failure, cardiac failure, pancreatic encephalopathy, chronic/recurrent hypoglycaemia (e.g. insulinoma)
Intoxication/withdrawal syndromes	Alcohol, anticholinergics, antihistamines, anxiolytic-hypnotics, corticosteroids, anticonvulsants, cardiovascular drugs, opiates, levodopa, dopaminergic agonists, neuroleptic malignant syndrome, prescription of multiple drugs, illicit drugs, carbon monoxide, heavy metals, herbicides (organophosphates), industrial poisons	Alcohol, carbon monoxide, heroin (inhaled), heavy metals, organic solvents, organophosphates, lithium, methotrexate, alpha-interferon
Nutritional deficiency	Thiamine (Wernicke–Korsakoff syndrome), nicotinic acid	Thiamine, vitamin B_{12}, nicotinic acid, multiple vitamin deficiencies
Endocrinopathies	Thyroid, adrenal, parathyroid, pituitary	Thyroid, adrenal, parathyroid, pituitary
Infections	Systemic Urinary tract infection, viral exanthemas, pneumonia, endocarditis, septicaemia (all causes)	
	CNS Encephalitis (especially herpes simplex), meningitis, brain abscess, HIV, cerebral malaria, neurocysticercosis, Mycoplasma, post-infectious syndromes	CNS HIV, neurosyphilis, tuberculosis, Whipple's disease, Lyme disease, cryptococcal/fungal meningitis, neurocysticercosis, JC virus (PML), measles (SSPE), encephalitis lethargica (may be post-infectious-autoimmune)
Inflammation and autoimmune	ADEM, cerebral vasculitis (primary CNS or systemic), voltage-gated potassium channel antibody/other channelopathies	Multiple sclerosis (primary progressive), cerebral vasculitis (primary CNS or systemic), neurosarcoidosis, Behçet's disease, voltage-gated potassium channel antibody/other channelopathies, anti-basal ganglia antibody syndrome, Hashimoto's encephalopathy, coeliac disease
Epilepsy	Epileptic status (non-convulsive), post-ictal states	Non-convulsive status, transient epileptic amnesia, Rasmussen's encephalitis
Neoplastic	Raised intracranial pressure (including acute hydrocephalus), carcinomatous or lymphomatous meningitis, paraneoplastic limbic encephalitis, post-radiotherapy (acute radionecrosis, thrombo-angiopathy)	Brain tumours (especially frontal/callosal/midbrain), CNS lymphoma, carcinomatous/lymphomatous meningitis, limbic encephalitis and other paraneoplastic syndromes, post-radiotherapy (accelerated cerebral atherosclerosis, radiation leukodystrophy)
Vascular	Subarachnoid haemorrhage, venous sinus thrombosis, arterial stroke (esp posterior circulation, non-dominant parietal), hyperviscosity syndromes, polycythaemia	Multiple cortical or subcortical strokes, lacunar state, strategic infarct (esp thalamus, medial frontal), hyperviscosity syndromes, polycythaemia, sickle cell disease, steal syndromes (e.g. AVM), Susac's syndrome

Table 8.1 (continued)

Category of disease	Delirium	Dementia
Head injury	Post-concussional syndrome, diffuse axonal injury, subdural haematoma, focal cerebral trauma	Subdural haematoma, repeated head injury/dementia pugilistica, late deterioration post-head injury
Other treatable causes	Pain, sleep deprivation, sensory deprivation and distortion (as in ITU), hypothermia, heat stress, postoperative recovery (multifactorial), migraine	Obstructive sleep apnoea, normal pressure hydrocephalus, obstructive hydrocephalus/aqueduct stenosis
Degenerative	Rapid cognitive fluctuation in Lewy body/ Parkinson's disease dementia	Alzheimer's disease, Parkinson's disease/dementia with Lewy bodies, frontotemporal lobar degenerations, corticobasal degeneration, progressive supranuclear palsy, motor neurone disease dementia, neurofilament inclusion body disease, Creutzfeldt–Jakob/other prion diseases
Genetic		
Metabolic	Metabolic crises in porphyria, urea cycle disorders, others	Wilson's disease, acute intermittent porphyria, lysosomal and peroxisomal storage disorders, urea cycle disorders, leukodystrophies, others
Arteriopathies	Strokes and stroke-like episodes	CADASIL, cerebral amyloid angiopathies, British dementia, Fabry's disease, others
Degenerative	Rapid cognitive fluctuation in familial parkinsonism syndromes	Familial Alzheimer's disease, frontotemporal lobar degeneration (chromosome 17/chromosome 3/other), Huntington's disease, DRPLA, familial Parkinson's disease/Lewy body disease, mitochondrial encephalopathies, spinocerebellar ataxias, neuro-acanthocytosis, pantothenate kinase-associated neurodegeneration, neuro-ferritinopathy, neuro-serpinopathy, familial prion diseases, others

Ab, antibody; ADEM, acute demyelinating encephalomyelopathy; AVM, arteriovenous malformation; CADASIL, cerebral autosomal dominant arteriopathy with subcortical infarcts and leukoencephalopathy; DRPLA, dentato-rubro-pallido-luysian atrophy; HIV, human immunodeficiency virus; PML, progressive multifocal leukoencephalopathy; SSPE, subacute sclerosing panencephalitis.

disease is a common cause of dementia across all age groups. The epidemiology of dementia diseases in younger and older adults is presented graphically in Figure 8.1. It is important to recognise that data on the epidemiology of less common neurodegenerative diseases causing dementia, less well defined entities such as 'mild cognitive impairment', precursors or transitional states leading to established dementia, and dementia secondary to other neurological or systemic diseases remain very limited.

Cognitive functions and their clinical syndromes

Cognition, like other aspects of human brain function, has a modular organisation, and different cognitive functions have distinct anatomical substrates. While a global impairment of cognitive function is often observed in delirium, specific cognitive profiles in acute brain disease are potentially of great localising and diagnostic value. This is exemplified by the different subtypes of dysphasia in left hemisphere strokes, or the profound amnesia of Wernicke–Korsakoff syndrome. Our present understanding of the dementias has been transformed by the concept that different brain regions are affected in a characteristic and non-uniform manner as disease evolves (Table 8.2); the identification of an evolving rather than static pattern of cognitive deficits is often critical in establishing a clinical diagnosis of dementia.

Attention

Considered very broadly, attention is the ability to gate and focus sensory information and to direct awareness. The control mechanisms for attention are mediated by a hierarchy of brain structures: awareness and alertness are maintained by the ascending reticular activating system in the brainstem which projects to the thalamus and cortex; a bilateral frontal and parietal cortical network enables selective attention to particular events and types of stimuli, and divided attention to multiple events and stimuli. This cortical control system modulates activity in sensory cortices as well as the

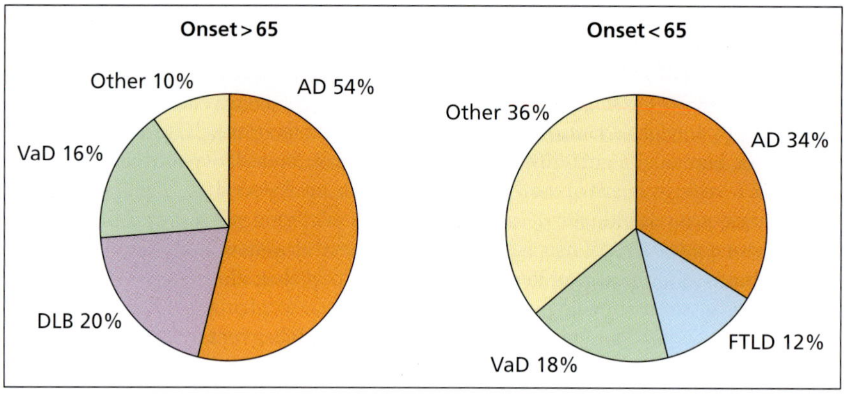

Figure 8.1 Epidemiology of dementia in older adults (onset age >65 years) and younger adults (onset age <65 years). Composite prevalence data derived from European series are displayed. The prevalence of dementia with Lewy bodies (DLB) shows wide variation between series. AD, Alzheimer's disease; DLB, dementia with Lewy bodies; FTLD, frontotemporal lobar degeneration; VaD, vascular dementia.

motor areas involved in response preparation. The distributed brain networks that regulate attention are vulnerable to many different disease processes. Deficits of attention are a cardinal feature of delirium, and impaired or inefficient attention is a feature of many dementias. However, the most striking deficits of attention, and those with greatest localising value, occur with focal lesions such as stroke involving the non-dominant parietal lobe. The syndrome of hemi-neglect manifests as unawareness of contralateral (most frequently left) space. The patient may not perceive contralateral stimuli, or contralateral stimuli may be perceived when presented alone, but extinguished on presentation of simultaneous bilateral stimuli (sensory extinction). The neglect syndrome is not simply attributable to sensory deficits such as hemianopia or hemianaesthesia. Failure to direct attention to the affected field is illustrated by constructional or cancellation tasks in which stimulus features on the affected side are systematically omitted or overlooked, and there may be associated neglect of contralateral auditory stimuli that have a bilateral cortical sensory representation. Breakdown in body schema is suggested by lack of awareness of deficits involving the contralateral side of the body (anosognosia) or failure of the patient to own their contralateral limbs. The deficit may also extend to mental imagery (Figure 8.2).

Memory

Impaired memory is a defining feature of acute disorders of cognition such as the discrete clinical syndrome of transient global amnesia, and a very common complaint in a variety of different dementias. In order to make an accurate diagnosis, it is important to determine the nature of the memory complaint. Memory is a multi-component process supported by anatomically and functionally distinct brain networks. There is a fundamental distinction between explicit memory, the contents of which can be consciously accessed, and implicit memory, the contents of which are accessed automatically and do not depend on conscious mediation (e.g. the sequence of procedural skills required when driving a car). Explicit memory has 'short-term' and 'long-term' components. In the neuropsychological sense, 'short-term' memory refers to the span for which information is retained for immediate repetition or reproduction, without rehearsal or other reinforcement (typically, less than a minute). Information that is retained for longer periods constitutes 'long-term' memory. Long-term memory can be further subclassified into memory for episodes or events from the individual's past experience, i.e. remembering what has happened (episodic, event or autobiographical memory), and conceptual knowledge about the world, i.e. remembering what something is (semantic memory). The selective breakdown of semantic memory is a cardinal feature of the semantic dementia phenotype of FTD.

Episodic memory can itself be further divided into operationally distinct processes: the encoding and subsequent retrieval of new events (anterograde memory); retrieval of events prior to the onset of the illness (retrograde memory); and memory for different types of material (e.g. verbal material, faces and topography).

A characteristic amnestic syndrome with severe deficits of anterograde and retrograde memory in the setting of a clear sensorium and with preserved immediate (short-term) recall was originally described in the setting of thiamine deficiency in chronic alcoholism (Wernicke–Korsakoff syndrome, Chapter 19), and subsequently in patients undergoing bilateral temporal lobe resection for intractable epilepsy (notably the much-studied patient known as H.M.) and in other conditions such as herpes simplex encephalitis (Chapter 9). Such patients are profoundly disabled, as they are effectively marooned in the immediate present with no capacity to lay down new memories, although it may be possible to demonstrate preserved implicit memory and procedural learning. Amnestic syndromes of varying severity are common after traumatic brain injury.

Less profound and incomplete deficits of verbal, visual and topographical memory are common early in the course of AD, DLB, vascular dementia (VaD) and other diseases. Patients frequently describe an inability to recall the details of conversations and messages, and the names of acquaintances. Impaired verbal episodic memory is the most sensitive cognitive marker of early AD, although it is not specific. Impaired topographical memory commonly presents as a difficulty with route finding, and a tendency to become lost in unfamiliar locations.

The medial temporal lobes (hippocampal formation, parahippocampal gyrus and entorhinal cortex, Chapter 2) are critical for episodic memory. The diencephalic system, comprising the thalamus and its limbic connections including the fornix and mamillary bodies, and the basal forebrain also have important roles. Postmortem findings in Wernicke–Korsakoff syndrome typically include petechial haemorrhages with astrocytic degeneration in the mammillary bodies and medial dorsal thalamic nuclei. Functional imaging studies during transient global amnesia have demonstrated

Table 8.2 Clinical and other features in selected dementias.

Disease	Episodic memory	Visuospatial perception	Halluc	Literacy skills	Praxis	Speech prod	Speech comp	Exec	Cogn slowing	Behav	Mood	Brain MRI	EEG	CSF	Other*
Alzheimer's disease	+	+	±	+	+		±	±			±	Disprop hippo atrophy	Abn alpha		Myoclonus
Posterior cortical atrophy	±	+		+	+										
Corticobasal degeneration		+		+	+	±		±	±						Asymmetry, alien limb, EPS
FTLD:															
Frontotemporal dementia	±					±		+		+	±				
Semantic dementia				+			+	±		±		L > R TL atrophy			
Progressive non-fluent aphasia						+		±		±		L > R peri-sylvian atrophy			
Vascular dementia	+	±		±	±		±	+	+	+	±	Vasc changes	Bitemp slowing		Strokes, brisk reflexes
Lewy body/ Parkinson	+	+	+	±	±			+	+	+	±		Abn alpha		EPS Fluctuation
Huntington's disease§		±						+	+	+	+	Caudate atrophy			Chorea/other EPS, genetics
Prion disease	+	+	±	±	±			+	±	+	+	Abn BG signal	Periodic compl		Myoclonus, ataxia, rapid

(continued)

Table 8.2 (continued)

Disease	Episodic memory	Visuospatial perception	Halluc	Literacy skills	Praxis	Speech prod	Speech comp	Exec	Cogn slowing	Behav	Mood	Brain MRI	EEG	CSF	Other*
Transient epileptic amnesia	+							±		±	±	Abn MTL signal/atrophy	Epilep changes		Fluctuation, seizures
Limbic encephalitis	+	±	+					±		+	+		Epilep changes	Cells, OCBs	Ca, ANAb VGKC, rapid
Cerebral vasculitis	±	±	±	±	±	±	±	±	±	±	±	Abn signal	Slowing	Cells, OCBs	Rapid
Multiple sclerosis	±							+	+	±	+	Abn wm signal		OCBs	VEPs, BAERs, abn MRI cord
Metabolic dieseases	±							+	+	+	±				Metabolic, other invest
Psychiatric disease	+		±			±		±		+	+				Fluctuation, inconsistency

+, Characteristic feature; ±, less prominent or inconsistent feature.

* Helpful but not invariable.

§ Similar 'subcortical' profile of cognitive impairment in many diseases with basal ganglia involvement.

Abn, abnormal; ANAb, antineuronal antibodies; BAERs, brainstem auditory evoked responses; behav, behaviour; bitemp, bitemporal; ca, cancer; cogn, cognitive; comp, comprehension; compl, complexes; disprop, disproportionate; epilep, epileptiform; EPS, extrapyramidal syndrome; exec, executive function; FTLD, frontoemporal lobar degeneration; halluc, hallucinations; hippo, hippocampal; invest, investigations; L, left; MTL, mesial temporal lobe; OCB, oligoclonal band (especially unmatched); prod, production; R, right; vasc, vascular; VEPs, visual evoked responses; VGKC, voltage-gated potassium channel antibodies; wm, white matter.

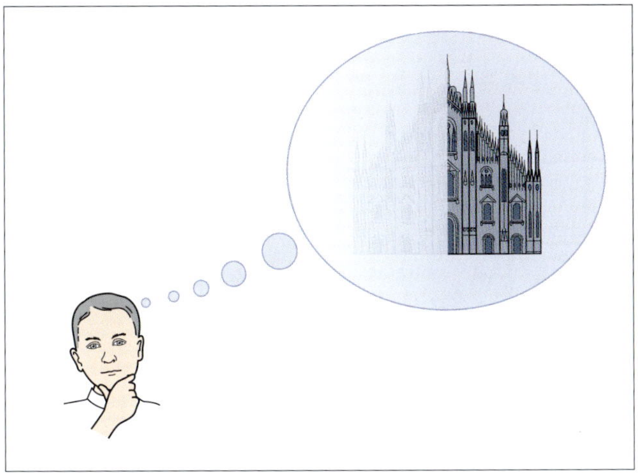

Figure 8.2 In their seminal paper, Bisiach and Luzzatti (1978) reported two left neglect patients who, when asked to imagine and describe from memory familiar surroundings (the Piazza del Duomo in Milan), omitted to mention left-sided details regardless of the imaginary vantage point that they assumed. Source: Bartolomeo *et al.* 2012. Reproduced under the terms of the Creative Commons Attribution Licence, CC-BY.

localised transient hypo- or hyperperfusion consistent with dysfunction of these structures and their connections. The ascending cholinergic projection pathways, which exert important modulatory and attentional influences on the medial temporal lobe and neocortex (Figure 8.3), are disrupted in cholinergic deficient disease states such as AD and DLB. Posterior cortical areas including the posterior cingulate, retrosplenial and temporoparietal association cortex are densely connected via the diencephalic system with the medial temporal lobes and have also been implicated in AD. Memory impairment in the setting of frontal lobe disease is likely to be heterogeneous and multifactorial: memory processes that may be affected include the editing of encoded material, organised search of memory stores, attribution of the source of particular memories, and possibly emotional valence or significance.

Short-term memory comprises separate systems for the temporary storage of auditory verbal, visual and spatial information. Rather than being passively stored, information in short-term memory generally undergoes some form of cognitive manipulation, for example when dialing a new telephone number, making sense of an ambiguous spoken message or visualising an unfamiliar route. These are active processes that are directed by executive systems (see later). The interaction of executive systems with short-term memory stores constitutes 'working memory'. This interaction is illustrated in the distinction between forward digit span (passive storage of information) and backward digit span (active manipulation of online material). Working memory deficits are common in acute conditions with impaired attention and have been documented in many degenerative disorders, including AD, DLB, VaD and FTD. It is likely that verbal short-term memory is supported by a fronto-parietal network in the left cerebral hemisphere, and visuo-spatial short-term memory by a corresponding network in the right cerebral hemisphere. These short-term storage mechanisms can be regarded as 'slave' systems under the executive control of fronto-subcortical networks.

Paramnesias

The paramnesias are characterised by false or distorted recall and may occur in acute or chronic settings. When prompted to fill a gap in the record of everyday experience the patient may describe events that never occurred, or may spontaneously supply detailed accounts of events that could not possibly have occurred (confabulation). Reduplicative paramnesias are characterised by the belief that particular places or persons have been transposed or duplicated: the patient may report that their house is an exact replica of the 'real' one (topographical paramnesia), or that their spouse has been replaced by an impostor with identical appearance (the Capgras delusion, Chapter 22). Confabulatory disturbances are most often observed in the setting of frontal lobe or frontolimbic damage.

Transient global amnesia

Transient global amnesia is a distinct and striking syndrome characterised by the sudden onset of severe anterograde amnesia generally lasting less than 24 hours. The patient often appears bewildered, repetitively asking the same questions. There is no disturbance of alertness and, in contrast to psychogenic fugue, personal identity is retained. Procedural and semantic memory are spared (e.g. the person may carry on driving or perform occupational tasks competently during the episode), other cognitive functions are intact and the neurological examination is normal. Complete recovery with amnesia for the period of the episode and a variable retrograde time-span is usual, although there may be persistent subtle memory deficits, and recurrence is rare. The condition generally occurs in later life. There are a number of associations, including physical exertion, exposure to cold, strong emotion, sexual activity and migraine; however, in the substantial majority, the aetiology remains unclear. Investigations are indicated to exclude mimics such as temporal lobe lesions, but are generally unrevealing. Recurrent attacks, especially on waking from sleep, suggest the syndrome of transient epileptic amnesia (Chapter 7), often accompanied by interictal memory impairment; this is an important differential diagnosis of dementia.

Perception

Perceptual analysis of the environment is a complex multi-stage process. Visual processing is the most widely studied modality and in general the most clinically relevant. The processing of visual objects involves dissociable stages of early sensory analysis, formation of structural representations and the association of those representations with meaning. Objects have locations in space, and the perception of space requires specific neural mechanisms. The mechanisms that process visual objects and visual space can be damaged selectively, supporting a broad anatomical and physiological distinction between ventral 'what is an object' and dorsal 'where is an object' cortical processing streams (Chapter 2). Selective impairments of visual functions such as motion detection (akinetopsia) and colour perception (achromatopsia) have been described with posterior circulation strokes and other focal lesions involving the cortical visual pathways in the posterior cerebral hemispheres. These syndromes may be transient or appear during the recovery phase of a more extensive visual deficit. Syndromes of progressive visual dysfunction are associated with relatively focal tissue loss and metabolic derangements involving the posterior cerebral hemispheres, and are often classified together on anatomical grounds as the posterior cortical atrophies (PCA). The most frequent tissue pathology is AD; however, a variety of others are

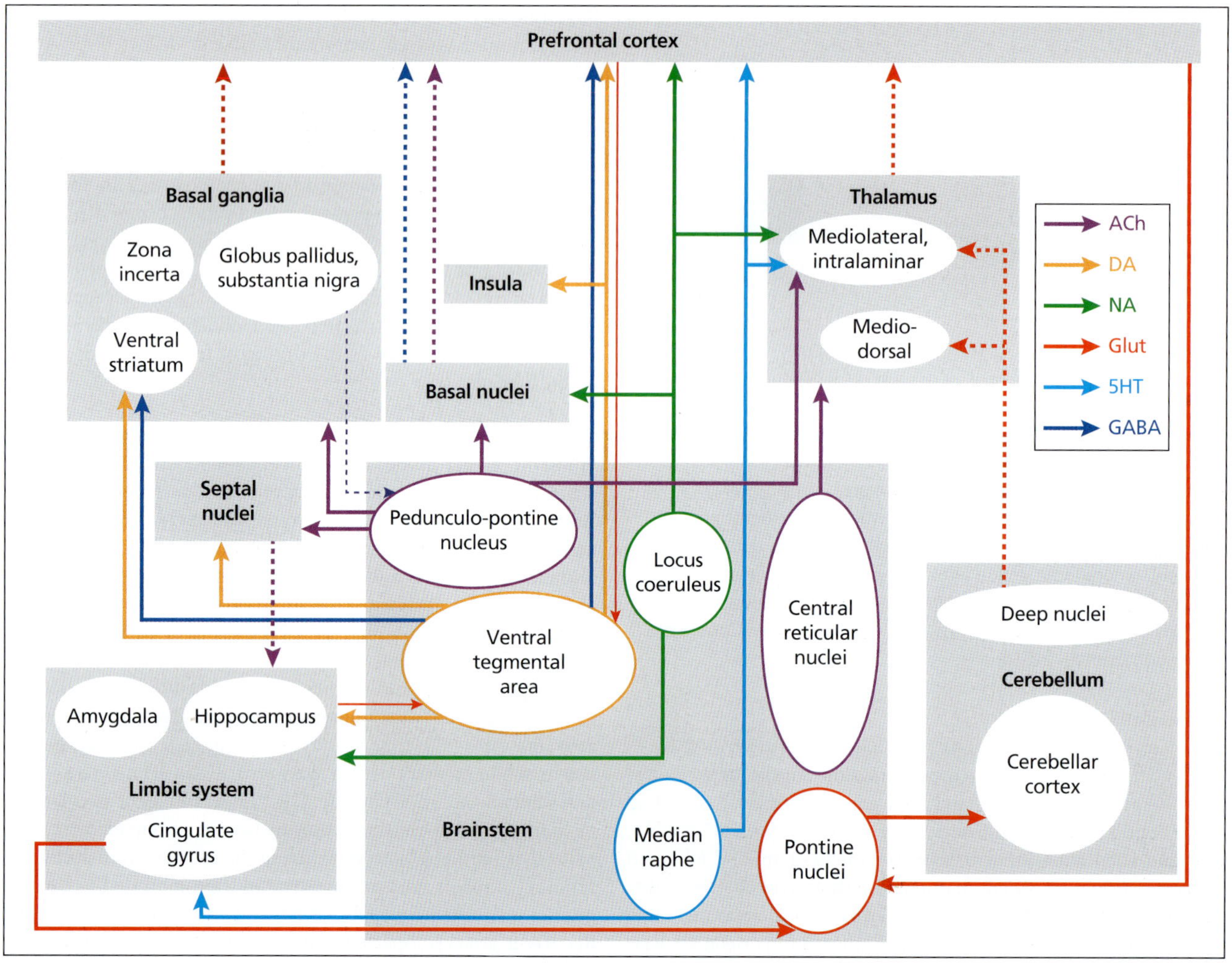

Figure 8.3 A schematic diagram of the major pathways linking the brainstem with other cortical and subcortical regions. The schema is based on evidence derived from both humans and non-human species. Pathways are colour-coded according to their major neurotransmitters. Direct efferent pathways from the brainstem are represented using heavy solid lines; other efferent pathways are represented using heavy dotted lines; afferent projections to the brainstem are represented using fine lines. It is likely that most of these pathways are functionally bi-directional. The pedunculo-pontine nucleus, locus coeruleus, median raphe and central reticular nuclei can be loosely grouped on anatomical grounds as the 'reticular formation'. 5-HT, 5-hydroxytryptamine; ACh, acetylcholine; DA, dopamine; GABA, γ-aminobutyric acid; Glut, glutamate; NA, noradrenaline. Source: Omar *et al.* 2007. Reproduced with permission of Taylor & Francis.

represented, including cortico-basal degeneration (CBD), DLB and prion disease.

Cortical blindness may result from bilateral occipital lobe damage and involvement of lateral occipito parietal areas may be associated with denial of blindness or visual anosognopia (Anton's syndrome). Partial forms of cortical blindness affecting visual acuity, stereopsis or the discrimination of elementary visual patterns (form, colour or motion) also occur in PCA. Clinically, such deficits may mimic peripheral visual loss: patients may complain of blurred vision, decreased acuity or desaturation of colours. Letters of similar shape may be confused. Difficulties may be particularly apparent under conditions of reduced contrast or changing illumination. Misperceptions of visual information may occur; patterns on fabric or wallpaper may seem to shift and change, objects in the environment or body parts (especially faces) may appear distorted (metamorphopsia), abnormally persistent or transposed (palinopsia) or multiply reduplicated (polyopia).

Identification of visual objects may be impaired despite intact early visual processing. The patient may fail to recognise common household items or familiar people. There may be difficulty in distinguishing coins, banknotes or playing cards, and on examination the patient may be unable to identify fragmented, distorted or overlapping pictures or letters, silhouettes or unusual views (Figure 8.4). Such patients have apperceptive visual agnosia: this means an inability to form structural representations of visual objects, the distinctive geometric and volumetric features that enable object identity to be abstracted despite changing contexts and viewpoints. The anatomical substrates of early visual processing and object representation are likely to involve a cortical pathway extending from early visual cortices into parieto-occipital association areas. This pathway is vulnerable to various disease processes, such as infarcts, hypoxic damage and focal degeneration in PCA. Processing of complex objects such as faces involves the ventral 'what' visual stream in the inferior temporal lobe, including the 'fusiform face area'.

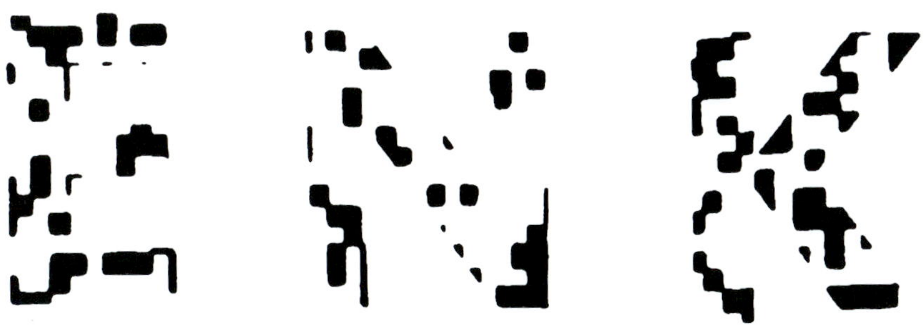

Figure 8.4 An example of a test of visual apperceptive function (fragmented letters) for use at the bedside. Patients with visual apperceptive agnosia have difficulty identifying the letters when presented in fragmented form but can read them easily when presented in unfragmented form and (unlike patients with reduced visual acuity) may find the letters easier to resolve at a distance. Source: Warrington and James 1967. Reproduced with permission of Elsevier.

Damage involving this region may lead to impaired face perception (prosopagnosia).

Deficits in the perception of visual space are more common than selective disorders of visual object processing. These deficits interact with mechanisms for spatial attention, which are generally more severely affected in focal brain lesions such as stroke involving the parietal lobes. However, visuo-spatial deficits are often prominent in dementias affecting the posterior cerebral hemispheres such as AD and DLB. Visuo-spatial disorders can be broadly classified as visual disorientation, the impaired perception of space relative to self (egocentric space), and visuo-spatial agnosia, the impaired perception of spatial configurations that are not referenced to one's own position (exocentric space). Patients with visual disorientation may be unable to locate objects such as cutlery immediately after they are put down or when the item is in front of them, and typically misreach for items. Threading a needle, reading lines of text, writing, using an index or even keeping within traffic lanes when driving may become impossible. Accidents when walking or driving are common, because of loss of the ability to judge distances or motion. Ultimately, such individuals become functionally blind. On examination, these patients have components of Balint's syndrome: fragmented perception of the visual field (simultanagnosia), inability to perform visually guided movements (optic ataxia) and/or inability to direct the eyes to a point in space (ocular apraxia). Because of the retinotopic encoding of egocentric space, these deficits frequently resemble hemi- or quadrantanopic field defects.

Patients with visuo-spatial agnosia may be unable to orient clothing when dressing, a camera when taking a photograph or an envelope when posting a letter. Loss of the ability to tell the time from a clock is characteristic. Patients are commonly unable to navigate familiar routes, and become lost in the neighbourhood or even within their own house (topographical disorientation). Skills such as reading text or maps, writing and calculation, which depend on accurate perception of spatial patterns, are often degraded. On examination, copying and constructional tasks are poorly performed and there may be specific deficits of spatial discrimination or spatial search (such as counting dots in an array). Anatomically, visuo-spatial deficits are associated with damage to the superior and posterior parietal lobes, within the dorsal cortical 'where' visual processing stream.

Perceptual defects in cognitive disorders are not confined to the visual domain. Cortical deafness is a rare accompaniment of bilateral damage involving auditory cortex and ascending auditory pathways, and auditory agnosia for complex sounds such as music and environmental noises may occur with diseases involving either temporal lobe. Loss or distortions of taste (dysgeusia) occurs with damage involving the gustatory pathways and cortex in the region of the insula. Olfactory identification deficits may occur early in the course of AD, Parkinson's disease and other degenerative dementias, and are likely to be at least partly central in origin. Disorders of cortical somatosensory function such as impaired perception of shape (astereognosis) and spatial configurations on the body surface (such as drawn numbers: agraphaesthesia) and impaired recognition of objects by touch (tactile agnosia) may occur with both acute damage involving the parietal lobes and in degenerative conditions such as CBD.

Hallucinations

Hallucinations are perceptual experiences in the absence of an external sensory stimulus. They may occur in normal individuals under conditions of fatigue or sensory deprivation, or at the onset of sleep (hypnagogic hallucinations). In organic brain disease, hallucinations occur most commonly in the visual modality, and are a frequent feature of delirium. However, hallucinations in other disease states and in non-visual modalities are well recognised (e.g. olfactory hallucinations in temporal lobe epilepsy). Complex verbal (auditory) hallucinations are typical of psychiatric disorders such as schizophrenia but distinctly unusual in organic disease. Visual hallucinations can arise from a variety of insults at different stages of the retino-calcarine and cortical ventral visual pathways. Hallucinations may arise from two general mechanisms: abnormal release of sensory cortex because of loss of sensory inputs from the periphery or other regulatory controls, or abnormal excitation or disinhibition of sensory cortex by irritative processes such as seizures or migraine. Deafferentation of early visual cortex in the setting of peripheral visual loss may be associated with isolated well-formed visual hallucinations in the absence of cognitive decline (Charles Bonnet syndrome). An analogous auditory mechanism may produce musical hallucinations in acquired deafness. Damage involving the ventral midbrain may produce vivid 'dream-like' peduncular hallucinations of cartoon-like images or complex scenes, resulting from dysfunction of the reticular activating system. Structural or functional lesions involving early visual cortices may produce elementary visual hallucinations (exemplified by 'fortification spectra' or teichopsia in migraine) while more complex or multimodal hallucinations, sometimes involving distortions of self-perception, may occur in the setting of temporal lobe disease.

Visual hallucinations are modulated by dysfunction of neurotransmitter pathways. Hallucinations are particularly striking and complex in diseases such as DLB in which there is a cortical deficiency of acetylcholine. Descriptions of hallucinations are often remarkably stereotyped: the patient typically sees unfamiliar people or animals (especially cats or other small creatures), mobile or stationary, often multiple, but generally silent. Hallucinations frequently appear in the evening or in darkness. They may be glimpsed transiently at the edge of view, or emerge from an environmental feature such as a piece of furniture or a garden scene. Extracampine hallucinations are associated with the sense of a presence beyond the field of view. The 'phantom boarder' delusion (the sense that there is another person in the house when there is not) may be a related phenomenon.

Knowledge

The brain mechanisms that mediate the storage and retrieval of knowledge constitute those of semantic memory. The most striking and selective deficits of knowledge are produced by focal lesions involving the ventral visual pathways in the inferior temporal lobes and by focal degeneration of the left temporal lobe in semantic dementia (SD). In SD, disintegration of word knowledge produces a progressive impairment of word-finding and word comprehension which is generally the presenting and most prominent feature of the syndrome. Naming deficits are characteristically early and prominent; a generic or superordinate term is often used in place of the more specific one (e.g. 'animal' in place of 'camel'). These patients do not grasp the meaning of words and typically have particular difficulty with definitions.

The selective inability to associate visual representations of objects with meaning constitutes an associative visual agnosia, which may occur as a relatively isolated deficit with temporo-occipital lesions or may develop in the course of SD. As is the case for verbal knowledge, semantic deficits can be relatively specific for the visual domain. Patients may be unable to identify everyday objects or describe their function despite accurate and detailed analysis of perceptual features. Patients with prosopagnosia lose the ability to recognise familiar faces, including acquaintances, famous people or even close family members. The recognition deficit may be selective for faces, dissociating from other types of person knowledge and from other categories of knowledge.

Neocortical regions in the anterolateral and inferior temporal lobes are likely to be critical for conceptual knowledge. Impaired word knowledge in SD is associated with atrophy involving the dominant (left) anterolateral temporal lobe. Person knowledge is likely to be asymmetrically distributed between the right and left anterior temporal lobes, the left anterior and inferolateral temporal lobe representing verbal information (such as personal names) and corresponding regions of the right temporal lobe representing familiar face information. Progressive prosopagnosia has been described much less frequently than SD. This is likely to be at least partly attributable to the clinical silence of the right temporal lobe relative to the eloquent left temporal lobe.

Voluntary action

Diseases that disturb the cognitive control processes involved in programming and guiding voluntary action produce apraxia: a disturbance of voluntary movement that cannot be explained by elementary motor or sensory deficits. The classification of apraxia poses conceptual and practical difficulties; however, a basic distinction can be drawn between disorders that affect unfamiliar, novel or meaningless actions (ideomotor apraxia), and disorders that affect previously learned actions (ideational apraxia). Apraxia generally occurs in association with more widespread deficits involving the dominant parietal or frontal lobes; however, cases of primary progressive apraxia have been described.

Apraxia for novel and meaningless actions is a prominent feature of dementias such as AD that involve the posterior hemispheres, and in this setting there is often additional evidence of impaired visuo-spatial perception. Novel tasks requiring mechanical problem-solving (such as assembling prefabricated furniture or models) and learning new motor skills pose particular difficulties. The patient has difficulties in imitating the examiner's meaningless hand positions. There may be particular difficulty when movements must be combined into a short sequence. Characteristically when attempting to imitate a gesture the patient will attempt to put their own hand into the space occupied by the examiner's (analogous to overlaying the drawing when attempting to copy a design): the 'closing-in' phenomenon.

Less commonly, apraxia leads to impaired production of actions previously learned. Manual occupations and hobbies may be abandoned, and the patient may be unable to use common household tools and utensils, or attempt to use them inappropriately (e.g. attempting to write with scissors). When instructed to perform a symbolic gesture (such as waving goodbye or saluting) or to pantomime the use of a tool (such as a screwdriver or hammer) an awkward or fragmentary approximation may be produced. Both the configuration of the fingers and the movements themselves are typically abnormal. Action production may be facilitated by holding the corresponding tool or other contextual cues. In addition, the patient may fail to recognise familiar gestures mimed by the examiner.

Apraxias affecting specific parts of the body are well recognised. Asymmetric limb apraxia is a cardinal presenting feature of CBD, where it is characteristically accompanied by asymmetric rigidity and other extrapyramidal or cortical sensory signs. Actions involving the affected limb comprise coarse, uncoordinated or mutilated constituent movements, sometimes termed limb-kinetic apraxia. Impairments affecting the voluntary control of orofacial movements often dissociate from disorders of limb praxis. Orofacial apraxia is frequently observed in association with impaired speech production. The patient may lose the ability to whistle and may complain of difficulty initiating chewing or swallowing. When instructed to cough, yawn or sigh the patient may produce an inadequate facsimile or simply repeat the instruction emphatically; however, these actions are typically normal when performed spontaneously and the examiner's orofacial gestures may be imitated competently.

So-called constructional apraxia, impaired ability to copy drawings of objects or designs, is observed both with focal lesions and degenerative diseases variously affecting visuo-spatial perception, spatial attention and executive processes. In the majority of cases it is likely to be multifactorial in origin rather than representing a specific disorder of voluntary action. Similar reservations apply to several other disorders, including dressing apraxia which is probably largely attributable to deficient visuo-spatial analysis, and apraxia of eyelid opening which in many cases has the features of a focal dystonia. The true status of gait apraxia, the selective impairment of walking (and often other axial motor programmes), remains somewhat controversial, as gait abnormalities may arise at various levels of the motor hierarchy. However, it is observed in association with focal lesions and degenerative processes affecting the frontal lobes and subcortical projections (as in hydrocephalus).

Patients with asymmetric limb apraxia may have difficulty in making cooperative movements using both hands because the more affected hand tends to mirror the other or otherwise interferes with the action: the alien limb phenomenon. The patient may complain that the affected arm is useless or seems not to belong to them, and the arm may tend to levitate or assume other odd postures (especially when attention is diverted or during walking). Forced grasping or reaching for objects in the immediate environment may occur, or there may be more organised purposeless actions such as repeatedly removing and replacing spectacles. Among the dementias, the most characteristic association is with CBD, although other pathologies have been described.

The neural control mechanisms for the control of voluntary action are distributed within a network of cortical and subcortical areas, and mixed forms of limb apraxia are common. Conceptual knowledge of gestures is likely to be mediated at least in part by the dominant temporal lobe, while the left parietal lobe is likely to have a key role in the integration of sensory information in the organisation of actions. An anterior system for the production of gestures may represent motor programmes for action in each hemisphere, and predominantly unilateral damage involving this system may lead to asymmetric limb-kinetic apraxia involving either side. Orofacial apraxia is associated with focal lesions or degenerative syndromes (such as progressive non-fluent aphasia) with asymmetric atrophy predominantly involving left inferior frontal and opercular regions.

Speech and language

The complex operations of human speech can be broadly classified as sensory decoding, comprehension, repetition, retrieval and production. Each of these operations can be considered at the level both of single words and sentences. These different operations are affected in a variety of acute and chronic cognitive disorders. Speech and language impairments (the dysphasias) are most commonly the result of focal lesions affecting the cortex of the dominant (left) cerebral hemisphere, but the recent recognition of focal 'language-based' dementias has revolutionised contemporary thinking about the degenerative brain diseases. Classic concepts of the human language system such as that of Lichtheim posited a cortical centre for word concepts connected by transcortical pathways with a posterior centre for processing word sounds and an anterior centre for programming speech output. This model has undergone considerable refinement in recent decades, influenced by functional imaging studies in healthy individuals as well as clinical observations in both stroke and focal cortical degenerations. The basic bedside distinction between fluent ('Wernicke's', 'sensory', 'posterior') and non-fluent ('Broca's', 'motor', 'anterior') dysphasia remains useful; however, it is not absolute clinically, anatomically or pathologically. Because of its quite different anatomical and clinical significance, it is important to distinguish fluent dysphasia from confusion (e.g. in the context of delirium); this can usually be accomplished by a careful analysis of the patient's spontaneous speech, in particular the presence of speech errors (paraphasias).

Comprehension of speech depends fundamentally on the accurate decoding of the acoustic signal at the level of its constituent sounds. In the setting of acute disease such as stroke, impaired speech comprehension or Wernicke aphasia is generally associated with damage involving Wernicke's area in the dominant posterior superior temporal lobe. However, the true functional and anatomical status of this area remains contentious. Selective impairments of speech perception manifesting as word deafness have been described rarely with acute bilateral or left-sided damage and degenerative disease affecting the posterior temporal lobe. Such patients have difficulty both in understanding and repeating spoken words despite normal comprehension of written material. Impaired comprehension of single words in the setting of intact acoustic analysis and repetition constitutes a transcortical sensory aphasia, originally described with posterior watershed infarcts. However, a similar syndrome is associated with breakdown in verbal knowledge systems in SD, suggesting an important role of the left anterior temporal lobe in normal language processing which is more difficult to reconcile with classic models of language organisation derived from the study of stroke and other acute lesions. Impaired sentence comprehension occurs in dementias such as progressive non-fluent aphasia (PNFA) in which there is disturbed processing of grammatical structure. Functional disconnection of posterior (input) from anterior (production) language areas produces a selective impairment of speech repetition or conduction aphasia, observed chiefly with focal damage involving the left parieto-temporal junction and the arcuate fasciculus.

Impaired word retrieval leads to word-finding pauses or circumlocutions in everyday conversation and a reduced ability to name (anomia). It is most often studied using confrontational naming tasks, in which nouns must be produced in response to pictures or other stimuli. Failure of retrieval in this situation is characteristic of anomic aphasia, which may be associated with a variety of focal lesions affecting the language system (e.g. during the recovery phase of stroke). Progressive anomia is a hallmark of SD; however, naming (and, more generally, word retrieval, often known loosely as nominal aphasia) deficits are also observed in AD and many other dementias. It is important to appreciate that confrontational naming depends on many distinct subprocesses, including intact perception and executive function, and intact connections between the cortical areas mediating these functions. This is illustrated by naming impairment resulting from visuo-perceptual deficits in PCA, and modality-specific impairments (e.g. optic and tactile anomia) with focal lesions interrupting transcortical and interhemispheric sensory pathways. Normal propositional speech involves not simply the retrieval of individual words, but the construction of a sentence that conveys an idea or message. Disruption of the process of message generation produces dynamic aphasia, with characteristics similar to transcortical motor aphasia: reduced spontaneous propositional speech despite the ability to produce speech relatively normally in specific contexts such as naming, repetition or reading. Dynamic aphasia has been documented with focal lesions and dementias that damage frontal or fronto-subcortical circuitry.

The spoken output of words and sentences in turn requires a number of distinct operations. The components of the verbal message must be combined according to morphological and syntactic rules. The breakdown of grammatical output (syntax) is a hallmark of Broca's aphasia, observed classically with focal lesions involving the inferior frontal gyrus of the dominant hemisphere. As is the case with Wernicke's area, however, the true functional role of Broca's area has not been fully clarified and should not be equated simply with language output. Broca's aphasia is characterised by effortful, dysfluent and agrammatic speech with a disjointed and telegraphic quality because of omission of verbs, prepositions and other function words. The production of single words involves both the selection and grouping of appropriate syllable codes (phonology) and the articulation of the corresponding motor programme. Progressive breakdown in either or both of these operations commonly occurs in PNFA, and in other disorders such as

CBD and motor neurone disease dementia. This syndrome includes relatively pure cases of cortical anarthria. Phonemic paraphasias (such as 'stirel' for 'squirrel') are often accompanied by articulatory errors. Prosody, the pattern of stress and timing that constitutes the melody of speech, is frequently abnormal. It is also important to distinguish dysfluency resulting from a primary disorder of speech production from interrupted output resulting from prolonged word-finding pauses ('logopenic' aphasia), which may occur in other conditions including AD. The spontaneous production of novel non-words (neologisms) and jargon may accompany fluent aphasia in acute disorders but rarely in degenerative disease.

Disorders that produce selective impairments of speech processing are associated with focal lesions or asymmetric atrophy predominantly involving the left peri-sylvian region. Deficits of speech perception are associated with damage involving the left posterior superior temporal gyrus, a region that includes early auditory areas. Impaired syntactic comprehension has been correlated with involvement of the left posterior temporo-parietal region. Impaired word retrieval occurs with interruption of a distributed asymmetric (predominantly left-sided) brain network including left lateral temporal cortex, left inferior and lateral frontal areas. Partially overlapping regions including the left inferior frontal gyrus, frontal operculum and anterior insula have been identified in group and single-case studies of speech production breakdown in stroke, PNFA and other disorders, implicating these dominant anterior regions in the motor programming of speech. The basal ganglia, thalamus and subcortical pathways in the dominant hemisphere participate in distributed cortico-subcortical networks mediating language and speech, and focal lesions involving these structures may closely resemble the corresponding cortical functional deficit.

Literacy and numeracy

An individual's premorbid level of literacy and numeracy is heavily influenced by educational attainment and potentially by specific long-standing limitations such as developmental dyslexia or dyscalculia. Such factors must be taken into account when interpreting the effects of disease.

A basic distinction is often made between reading disorders that occur without writing impairment (alexia without agraphia) and those that are accompanied by writing impairment (alexia with agraphia), originally described with acute lesions such as stroke affecting the posterior cerebral hemispheres. Alexia without agraphia is classically produced by the conjunction of a right homonymous hemianopia and damage involving the posterior corpus callosum, precluding the transfer of information from the left hemi-field (right occipital lobe) to the verbal left hemisphere; alexia with agraphia results from more extensive lesions involving the posterior left hemisphere. An alternative classification of the dyslexias is based on the cognitive operations involved, whereby disturbed visual analysis of written words produces a peripheral dyslexia (often with preserved writing ability) and disturbed analysis of written words for sound or meaning produces a central dyslexia (often with associated deficits of written output). Impaired visual analysis of written words or peripheral dyslexia is often a prominent feature of PCA, in which associated visuo-perceptual and visuo-spatial impairments are common. These individuals typically read letter by letter. Central deficits of written word processing beyond the stage of visual analysis fall into two general categories, which may dissociate: these correspond to two parallel routes to reading, based on analysis for sound (the phonological encoding of print-to-sound correspondences) and analysis of meaning (sight vocabulary). If reading by sound is damaged, there is a failure to use the general rules of phonological encoding (phonological dyslexia). These patients have particular difficulty reading meaningless words, grammatical function words (e.g. 'and', 'if', 'for') and morphological features such as tense or plurals. If reading by sight vocabulary is damaged (surface dyslexia), there is reliance on reading by sound. Irregular words are incorrectly regularised according to surface orthographic features (e.g. 'yacht' may be pronounced 'yached'), while regular words are read correctly. Impaired reading by sight vocabulary is a frequent and characteristic feature of SD.

Visually based (peripheral) dyslexia is associated with bilateral or predominantly left-sided occipito-temporo-parietal damage or specific involvement of the ventral visual pathway. In central dyslexia, impaired reading by sight vocabulary is associated chiefly with degeneration of the left anterior and inferior temporal lobe, in common with other components of the SD syndrome, while impaired reading by sound is associated with pathology in left peri-sylvian language regions.

Impairments of writing and spelling (the dysgraphias) can be broadly classified according to whether the core defect lies with spelling processes (central dysgraphias) or the motor programming and execution of writing (peripheral dysgraphias). As is the case for the dyslexias, mixed forms are common. Spelling can proceed via sound-based (phonological) and vocabulary-based routes, and central dysgraphias affecting each route have been described in patients with dementia. Impaired spelling by sound (phonological dysgraphia) is associated with particular difficulty writing grammatical function words and word endings. The breakdown of vocabulary-based spelling (surface dysgraphia) manifests as regularisation errors in rendering exception words (e.g. 'juice' may be spelled 'juse') while phonologically regular words are spelled correctly. Impaired spelling vocabulary is a characteristic feature of the SD syndrome, but also occurs commonly in AD and in other dementias. The various stages of letter shape selection, formation, placement and sequencing that underpin the motor output process of writing may be deranged in disease processes that disrupt visuospatial analysis or voluntary action. Dysgraphia is generally a feature of diseases involving the left parietal lobe; however, surface dysgraphia is associated with surface dyslexia and other features of SD in the setting of left temporal lobe atrophy.

Disorders of calculation can be classified according to whether the core defect lies with computation proper or with the procedures required to process written and spoken numbers. Patients typically complain of a loss of facility in handling change or household accounts, and may have relinquished these responsibilities to others. There may be specific difficulties in adding scores and calculating totals in games, in using measuring instruments, or in reading and writing numerals and number words (e.g. when issuing a cheque). Like dysgraphia, dyscalculia is often a prominent feature of diseases affecting the dominant parietal lobe. The association of dysgraphia and dyscalculia with finger agnosia and right–left disorientation is known as Gerstmann's syndrome (Chapter 4), although it is unlikely this particular constellation has special significance other than implicating the dominant angular gyrus.

Executive function

The generation of complex behaviour demands that many cognitive operations are combined, coordinated, adapted to different contexts and directed to relevant goals. The regulatory and supervisory brain mechanisms that achieve this together constitute the cognitive executive. These mechanisms reside chiefly in frontal lobe cortex and its subcortical connections, and indeed the recognition that frontal lobe damage may produce profound alterations in conduct and personality (as in the celebrated case of Phineas Gage) was one of the cornerstones of modern behavioural neurology. However, it is important to recognise that executive dysfunction and frontal lobe impairment are not equivalent concepts. The cognitive and anatomical organisation of the executive remains poorly understood: while it is possible to identify broad syndromes of executive dysfunction, in clinical practice these almost invariably overlap. Executive impairments are produced by a very wide range of acute and chronic diseases.

Perhaps the most striking frontal lobe syndrome is characterised by loss of capacity to gate or modulate the effects of cognitive inputs according to the overall context. Patients with impaired response modulation have particular difficulty in taking account of feedback or assessing the consequences of their own behaviour. Affected individuals almost invariably lack insight into their difficulties, but a change in the patient's personality is all too evident to others, and is accompanied by poor social judgement and inappropriate behaviour or insensitive remarks. Disinhibition and impulsivity may disrupt personal and occupational relationships. There is a reduced capacity for abstract thought, and patients typically display an inflexible and concrete approach to occupational and daily life tasks. Defective processing of social signals may contribute to impaired understanding of the mental states of self and others ('theory of mind'). Checking or counting routines, ritualised daily routes and schedules, clock-watching and hoarding are common. Analogies and similarities may not be recognised, and proverbs interpreted literally (e.g. 'People in glass houses shouldn't throw stones' meaning 'that the glass will break'). The ability to formulate a strategy for searching cognitive or sensory inputs is often compromised: this commonly manifests as reduced verbal fluency (the number of words generated in 1 minute according to a specified criterion, usually semantic category or initial letter).

An impaired ability to generate behavioural outputs leads to a loss of autonomy and increasing dependency on environmental cues and events to initiate behavioural subroutines. Apathy (abulia), inertia, passivity, perseveration, and motor and verbal stereotypies are common features of this syndrome. Left undisturbed, patients may contentedly spend all day watching television or absorbed in jigsaw puzzles or word games, and they may be disengaged from these activities only with difficulty. Loss of initiative commonly extends to household tasks and personal hygiene. There may be utilisation behaviour (e.g. the patient may don spectacles or peel a piece of fruit automatically when the item is placed before them), hyperorality (sometimes including mouthing of inedible items) or mimicry of others' speech (echolalia) or actions (echopraxia).

Slowness of thought (bradyphrenia) and difficulty in switching between behavioural subroutines or 'sets' spontaneously or according to context are hallmarks of fronto-subcortical damage. There may be perseverative errors on attempting to draw a sequence of alternating shapes or produce a sequence of alternating hand movements. Palilalia (repetition of the patient's own words or terminal phrases) also occurs.

Executive difficulties are exposed by tasks that demand planning, abstract thought, flexibility and consideration of alternative solutions. There is often little consistency between tests or even between testing sessions in the individual patient. Characteristic features include implausible but over-precise estimates (distance from London to New York is '266 miles'), impaired performance on dual tasks (such as tracking a visual target while reciting a list of numbers), and difficulty grasping simple rules (sorting multidimensional items by size, shape or colour) or in devising a problem-solving strategy (such as the 'Tower of London' puzzle). More complex behaviours that underpin social cognition including the understanding of social signals (such as sarcasm) and other people's mental states can be assessed quantitatively using widely available tests such as the Awareness of Social Inference Test (TASIT) and the Reading the Mind in the Eyes test, though these are time-consuming to perform.

The anatomy and pathophysiology of executive dysfunction remains poorly understood, and there is little consensus regarding the neural correlates of core executive functions. A similar pattern of cognitive and behavioural impairments may be associated with variable findings on structural and metabolic brain imaging. Disinhibition, sociopathic behaviour and altered physiological drives broadly correlate with predominantly right-sided anterior temporal and inferior frontal lobe damage and hypometabolism, and abulia with dorsolateral frontal and anterior cingulate involvement. Disinhibition, impaired theory of mind and disturbed modulation of sensory inputs are associated particularly with orbitofrontal and ventromedial frontal damage.

Emotion

Although they have traditionally been regarded as the domain of the psychiatrist, disturbances of emotion comprehension and expression are integral to many neurological disorders and are often closely allied with other behavioural and executive impairments, particularly those around social cognition and the understanding of others' mental states. Defective processing of emotions often has major social consequences. Poor understanding of the emotional states of people and animals, lack of empathy and reduced expressivity are often interpreted as coldness and lack of affection. Other patients display fatuous and puerile emotional responses. Paradoxically, there may be increased engagement with religious, philosophical or artistic pursuits. A dramatic illustration of the breakdown of normal emotion processing is the Klüver–Bucy syndrome, originally described in monkeys following bilateral temporal lobe ablation. The syndrome has been reported rarely in humans, but does occur in the context of acute destructive processes such as herpes simplex encephalitis, and is characterised by loss of normal emotional reactivity, abulia, altered sexual responses and hyperorality.

Disturbances of mood (in particular, depression and dysphoria) are commonly associated with stroke, temporal lobe epilepsy and head injury, and with AD and other degenerative disorders (Chapter 22). These affective changes are likely to be caused, at least in part, by damage involving limbic circuits (Chapter 2) and their neocortical projections. Specific deficits of emotion comprehension have been documented in both acute and chronic disorders with mesolimbic damage, and are a hallmark of certain degenerative diseases, notably FTD and Huntington's disease. A distributed predominantly right-sided frontotemporal network including the amygdala and orbitofrontal cortex is likely to be critical for normal emotion processing: this network is a plausible interface between primitive emotional states linked to biological drives and the neocortical cognitive machinery of complex goal-directed behaviours.

Investigation of the patient with cognitive impairment

Basic principles

The differential diagnosis of delirium and dementia is very extensive (Table 8.1), and a structured approach to the investigation of cognitive impairment is therefore essential. This approach should be tailored to the clinical problem at hand, guided by an accurate and complete history and examination (Tables 8.1 and 8.2). However, the first priority of investigation in every patient is to exclude a reversible condition. Most causes of delirium and a number of causes of dementia fall into this category, and delirium frequently supervenes on a background of more insidious cognitive decline in elderly patients and those with limited cognitive reserve. Accurate diagnosis, particularly in dementia, may have important implications for prognosis and possibly genetic counselling of other family members.

Initial investigation

Initial investigations should be minimally invasive and directed toward the identification of reversible metabolic, infective, inflammatory and other systemic processes. A number of investigations are relevant in the initial approach to both acute and chronic impairment, especially where the precise time course is difficult to establish or more than one process is likely (Tables 8.3 and 8.4). A basic initial battery includes full blood count and differential, biochemistry including serum calcium, renal, liver and thyroid function tests, coagulation profile, serum B_{12} and folate, inflammatory markers (erythrocyte sedimentation rate and C-reactive protein), an autoimmune screen (antinuclear factor), a chest radiograph, ECG and urinalysis. Clinical judgement is required in interpreting the significance of such screening results e.g. a low serum B_{12} is common in the elderly, but it is rarely the sole cause of cognitive decline.

Neuropsychometry

Neuropsychometry is an extension of the bedside cognitive examination and can be very valuable in characterising the cognitive profile in more detail (in particular, the identification of subclinical deficits that might not be volunteered in the history). It is most useful and relevant for the detection of change in cognitive function, either in assessing the effect of static insults, where ongoing deterioration is a diagnostic issue (typically, in the identification of dementia) or in assessing response to therapy. Many neuropsychometric tests provide quantitative and normative data that allow the individual's premorbid cognitive attainment to be estimated and their current cognitive performance to be measured in relation to a healthy age-matched population. Documentation of performance in particular cognitive domains allows the likely origin of the cognitive problem to be specified, because particular patterns of deficit have localising value (Table 8.2). A plethora of neuropsychological tests is available. These require a trained neuropsychologist to administer and interpret, ideally informed by a clinical summary that identifies the purpose of the referral and areas of chief concern. The timing of test administration should be considered carefully: it is rarely informative to perform neuropsychometry during a delirium or the acute phase of a stroke or head injury (because further alteration in cognitive state can be anticipated), or repeatedly within a short timeframe (because practice effects are likely to make interpretation difficult). The patient's age and level of education must always be taken into account and, as with any investigation, results should be interpreted in the context of the specific clinical scenario.

Brief mental state schedules such as the 30-point Mini Mental State Examination (MMSE; the Folstein test) are simple to administer at the bedside and give an overall snapshot of cognitive performance, but lack sensitivity for the detection of subtle or isolated cognitive deficits while depending heavily on particular domains, notably verbal processing. Such schedules may be of most value in charting change in cognitive function over time, although they remain crude indices. Frequently used standardised tests include the National Adult Reading Test (NART), which provides an index

Table 8.3 An approach to investigation of the patient with rapid onset cognitive impairment.

Associated features	Investigations
	Screening investigations
May have systemic symptoms and signs	Blood: full blood count, renal function, electrolytes, liver function, coagulation, glucose, thyroid function, ammonia, amylase, ESR/CRP, ANF urinalysis ECG, chest X-ray
	Additional investigations
Head injury, signs of raised ICP, focal cognitive deficit, neurological symptoms and signs, no systemic explanation, neurological assessment unreliable, headache, meningism, fever	Brain imaging: CT, MRI, MRI venography, angiography CSF examination, including cultures and viral PCR, septic screens, serology vasculitis screens, neoplasia screens
Recurrent attacks suspicion inherited disease	EEG, echocardiogram autoimmune, thrombotic screens, urinary catecholamines, serotonin metabolites, porphyrins, consider specialised metabolic screens
Drug use/possible toxic exposure	Rationalise medications Drug/toxicological screens
Poor nutrition	Nutritional screens
Pain sensory/sleep deprivation environmental factors	Identify source
Major affective disorder, psychosis not attributable to above; fugue state, factitious disorder	Psychiatric evaluation

ANF, antinuclear factor; CRP, C-reactive protein; CSF, cerebrospinal fluid; CT, computed tomography; EEG, electroencephalography; ESR, erythrocyte sedimentation rate; ICP, intracranial pressure; MRI, magnetic resonance imaging; PCR, polymerase chain reaction.

Table 8.4 An approach to investigation of the patient with dementia.

Associated features	Investigations
	Screening investigations – all patients
May have systemic symptoms and signs	Blood: full blood count, renal function, electrolytes, liver function, coagulation, glucose, thyroid function, ESR/CRP, ANF, syphilis serology, B_{12}, folate, urinalysis ECG, chest X-ray, brain imaging: CT, MRI if available EEG
	Additional investigations – selected patients
Young onset, non-cognitive neurological features, family history	HIV serology, copper studies, slit lamp examination, consider specialised metabolic and genetic screens, muscle/axillary skin, marrow, liver biopsy
Rapid course, headache, meningism, fever other features atypical for common degenerations (including age <65, systemic features, neurological signs)	Vasculitis, auto-antibody screens (incl ANCA, APL, VGKC Ab, coeliac screens) antineuronal antibodies, other neoplasia screens (incl whole-body PET, CT) CSF examination (including cells, protein, glucose, oligoclonal bands, cytology, cultures; may include 14-3-3, S100, Whipple PCR, JC/other viral PCR, cryptococcal Ag, measles Ab, syphilis serology, TB and other special cultures) MRI FLAIR sequences, prion genotyping if suspect prion disease, tonsillar biopsy if suspect vCJD
Clinical seizures prominent fluctuation (not in context of DLB)	Prolonged EEG (if routine EEG not diagnostic) autoimmune, thrombotic screens echocardiogram, other vascular screens urinary porphyrins
Sleep disorder	Sleep study
Drug use/possible toxic exposure	Rationalise medications drug/toxicological screens
Poor nutrition, suspicion of deficiency	Nutritional screens
Major affective disorder, psychosis not attributable to above; fugue state, factitious disorder	Psychiatric evaluation
Suspicion of treatable (inflammatory) process when diagnosis not established by non-invasive means	Brain biopsy

Ab, antibody; Ag, antigen; ANCA, antineutrophil cytoplasmic antibody; ANF, antinuclear factor; APL, antiphospholipid antibody; DLB, dementia with Lewy bodies; FLAIR, fluid-attenuated inversion recovery; PCR, polymerase chain reaction; PET, positron emission tomography; vCJD, variant Creutzfeldt–Jakob disease; VGKC, voltage-gated potassium channel antibody.

of premorbid intellectual attainment, and the Wechsler Adult Intelligence Scale (WAIS; revised, WAIS-R), which provides a profile of a range of verbal and non-verbal abilities. A variety of quantitative memory tests are in use, including the Recognition Memory Test for words and faces, which provides measures of verbal and non-verbal material-specific memory. Automated tests such as the Cambridge Neuropsychological Test Automated Battery (CANTAB) are in widespread use, incorporating specific subtests (e.g. paired associative learning) with demonstrated sensitivity for detecting the early stages of AD. Many tests have been used to assess executive function, including the Wisconsin Card Sorting Test (which requires the classification of stimuli according to various implicit rules) and Raven's Progressive Matrices (a test of abstract pattern continuation that does not depend on verbal mediation); however, this is a notoriously difficult domain to quantify and results are heavily affected by deficits in other domains (e.g. visual perception). Batteries to assess other functions such as visual object and space perception, praxis, naming and semantic knowledge are widely available.

Brain imaging

Structural brain imaging is indicated in all patients with dementia, and in patients with delirium where no systemic cause is identified, or where focal cognitive or neurological signs, headache, evidence of raised intracranial pressure or head trauma are present. This may be particularly critical in situations where neurological status cannot be reliably assessed, for example in acute alcohol or drug intoxication, or where an acute process may have supervened on pre-existing cognitive impairment. Computed tomography (CT) is widely available, and is adequate for detection of hydrocephalus and focal intracranial lesions such as subdural haematoma, brain abscess and tumours. CT is specifically indicated for detection of subarachnoid haemorrhage or intracranial calcification. However, magnetic resonance imaging (MRI) is distinctly superior for examination of the brainstem and posterior fossa structures, the basal ganglia and detail of cerebral white matter and the cortical mantle. In patients with dementia, T1 MRI sequences can be particularly valuable in detecting pathological atrophy: volumetric MRI employing thin slices can be used to delineate patterns of regional atrophy that may have diagnostic significance, while serial MRI has an increasing role in the assessment of progressive atrophy (both generalised and regional) for diagnosis and prognosis. T2-weighted sequences are used to assess white matter signal change and tissue oedema. Additional sequences may be useful for certain indications, for example fluid attenuated inversion recovery (FLAIR) sequences to assess basal ganglia and thalamic signal in suspected prion disease, and diffusion-weighted imaging (DWI) to detect acute ischaemic damage and prion disease with cortical diffusion signal change, reflecting spongiform histology.

Functional brain imaging techniques have a limited role in clinical practice. Metabolic imaging using single photon emission tomography (SPECT) or positron emission tomography (PET) may occasionally be useful in identifying regional functional changes in patients with frontal lobe syndromes and normal structural imaging; however, these techniques are not widely available and interpretation is difficult. The use of ligands to image amyloid is likely to become a useful adjunct in the investigation of AD.

Electroencephalography

The EEG is generally of limited diagnostic usefulness in delirium, which is frequently accompanied by generalised slowing of cerebral rhythms indicating diffuse cortical dysfunction. As a tool for the detection of local pathology it has been largely supplanted by brain imaging techniques; however, it remains essential for the detection and localisation of seizure discharges (particularly in non-convulsive status epilepticus). In dementia, the EEG is often helpful in the differential diagnosis. Conditions such as AD with diffuse cortical dysfunction are frequently accompanied by degeneration or loss of the normal alpha rhythm, while in focal dementias such as FTD alpha rhythm is generally preserved at presentation. The EEG may also detect covert epileptiform changes in amnestic syndromes resulting from partial seizures, or periodic complexes in classic CJD, subacute sclerosing panencephalitis (SSPE) and other conditions with severe cortical derangement. Prolonged ambulatory or video-EEG may be indicated where there is strong suspicion of covert or unrecognised partial seizures.

Cerebrospinal fluid examination

Examination of the cerebrospinal fluid (CSF) is indicated where CNS infection is suspected, provided no contraindications exist (Chapter 9). Lumbar puncture is also recommended for younger patients with dementia and in cases where there is an unusual presentation or rapid course, to exclude an inflammatory process. Suspicious features include a raised CSF cell count (pleocytosis), and/or unmatched oligoclonal bands (indicating local synthesis of immunoglobulin in the CNS). Polymerase chain reaction (PCR) can be used to amplify and detect viral and other infectious agent DNA. Cytological examination may reveal atypical or malignant cells. Elevated total CSF protein is a non-specific finding in isolation. Elevated protein 14-3-3 is associated with rapid neuronal destruction in classic CJD, while elevated S-100 is associated with gliosis. AD is associated with a reduction in CSF Aβ 1–42 and an increase in tau, and diagnostically specific CSF protein biomarkers are increasingly entering routine clinical practice.

Additional investigations

Additional investigations are dictated by clinical features in conjunction with the results of the initial battery (Tables 8.3 and 8.4). These may include vasculitic, infectious, autoimmune, neoplastic and toxicological investigations, and in younger patients, copper studies, white cell enzymes and genetic testing. HIV serology, although not routine, should always be considered, especially where risk factors exist. The more common familial dementias have autosomal dominant inheritance, and the diagnostic yield of genetic analysis is therefore likely to be higher in the younger patient with a positive family history (see Table 8.8); however, late onset cases of genetically mediated dementia do occur (e.g. in Huntington's disease) and the family history may be censored, incomplete or inaccurate.

Tissue biopsy may be required to establish the diagnosis in a minority of patients with dementia, especially in younger individuals, as directed by clinical features (Tables 8.2 and 8.8). Skin biopsy (including apocrine sweat glands) may detect abnormal accumulations in Lafora, Kufs or other storage diseases and in CADASIL (cerebral autosomal dominant arteriopathy with subcortical infarcts and leukoencephalopathy). Nerve biopsy may be diagnostic in rare dementias with peripheral nerve involvement. Muscle biopsy including histochemistry and respiratory enzyme analysis may confirm a mitochondrial disorder. Marrow biopsy may identify the 'sea-blue histiocyte syndrome' of Niemann–Pick disease type C and other storage diseases, and may also be indicated in the diagnosis of haematological and other malignancies in suspected paraneoplastic syndromes. Small bowel biopsy may be indicated to exclude Whipple's disease, and liver biopsy is occasionally indicated to exclude Wilson's disease. In exceptional cases, brain biopsy may be necessary where there is unresolved suspicion of a treatable (inflammatory or infectious) process where the diagnosis cannot be made by other means and potentially toxic treatment is contemplated. In some cases this is directed to a focal lesion; however, in most patients it is necessarily a 'blind' biopsy from the non-dominant frontal lobe. A full-thickness open biopsy including cortex, white matter and meninges should be performed by a neurosurgical team experienced in the technique. Disposable instruments should be used in cases where the risk of prion disease is considered clinically significant. Brain biopsy in patients with dementia carries an approximately 10% combined risk of significant morbidity or mortality, and should always be a carefully weighed decision.

The dementias

Alzheimer's disease

AD is the most common cause of cognitive decline with AD pathology, in part or in whole, underlying at least 50% of all cases of dementia. AD is the prototypical cortical dementia against which other dementias are compared in a differential diagnosis. An understanding of the clinical features and diagnostic approach to AD is central to being able to distinguish the different dementias.

The prevalence of dementia due to AD is strongly age-dependent – doubling every 5 years after the age of 60 years with around 1% of those aged 65–69 years affected rising to almost 20% in those aged 85 years or over. It is therefore important to have a low threshold of suspicion for cognitive decline in elderly patients who may not necessarily have cognitive problems as the presenting complaint;

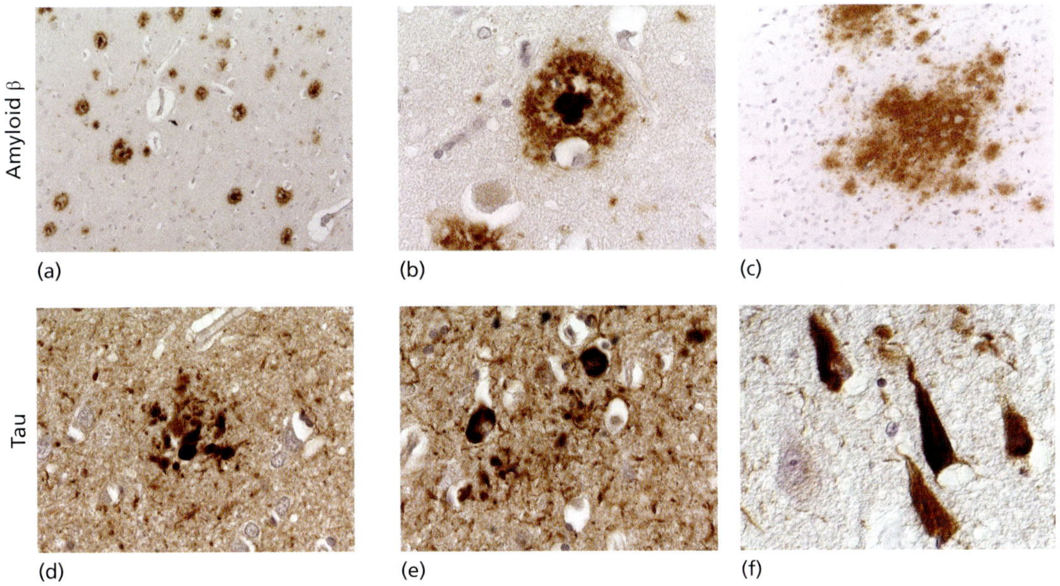

Figure 8.5 Alzheimer's disease: amyloid-β (a, b, c) and tau deposits (d, e, f). Autopsy specimen with abundant amyloid plaques in the neocortex seen at low power magnification (a), which are predominantly mature (neuritic) plaques which are characterised by a dense core and a peripheral halo seen at high power magnification (b). Diffuse plaques or large protein deposits (c) are probably a precursor of core plaques and can also be found in the ageing brain without being necessarily associated with dementia ('pathological ageing'). Neurites crossing the plaque become dystrophic and contain hyperphosphorylated tau protein, as shown in (d). Tau immunohistochemistry also shows multiple intraneuronal inclusions, neurofibrillary tangles, which may assume various shapes: small globose perikaryal (e) band shaped, or flame shaped (f), all at high power magnification.

however, these (undeclared) impairments can complicate management of other neurological or medical conditions.

AD is also the most common cause of early onset dementia, arbitrarily defined as symptom onset before the age of 65 years. However, sporadic AD starting before the age of 50 years is very rare, and in these cases a genetic cause should, even in the absence of a family history, be suspected.

A definitive diagnosis of AD requires histopathological examination of brain tissue usually only confirmed at postmortem demonstrating excess accumulation of extracellular amyloid plaques and intracellular neurofibrillary tangles (Figure 8.5). In established AD, amyloid plaques are found widely distributed throughout the cortex with heaviest deposition in the cortical association areas. Amyloid may also be laid down in cerebral blood vessels leading to amyloid angiopathy. The key building block of the amyloid plaque is beta-amyloid (Aβ), a 40–42 amino acid long peptide, formed following the cleavage of a much larger precursor polypeptide called amyloid precursor protein (APP) encoded by the *APP* gene on chromosome 21.

The relative proportions of parenchymal amyloid (plaques) and vascular amyloid (angiopathy) varies considerably between patients. In transgenic mouse models of AD, the relative proportions of these two forms of amyloid deposition seem to be related to the length of peptide generated by the pathogenic mutation, with a higher proportion of Aβ1-42 promoting parenchymal deposition whereas relatively greater amounts of Aβ1-40 leads to more vascular amyloid.

Neurofibrillary tangles result from the breakdown of the microtubule component of the neuronal cytoskeleton. Tau, a protein whose normal function is to promote and stabilise microtubule assembly, becomes hyperphosphorylated in AD and aggregates into an insoluble tangle of paired helical filaments (PHF) within the neurone. Autopsy studies suggest that neurofibrillary tangles first appear in the entorhinal cortex before progressively involving the hippocampus and other limbic structures and then becoming widely distributed in neocortical association areas. Primary motor and sensory cortices are relatively spared.

The vast majority of AD is 'sporadic'; however, in a small number of cases there is a strong family history usually with an early age at onset. Mutations in three genes (*APP, PSEN1* and *PSEN2*) cause autosomal dominant AD with a high level of penetrance. Together these mutations account for only 1% of all cases of AD. They have contributed greatly to the understanding of AD and underpin the amyloid cascade hypothesis for AD pathogenesis and also led to transgenic models of disease (Figure 8.6).

APP mutations cause single peptide substitutions largely clustered around either end of the Aβ peptide – at sites of enzymatic cleavage from APP – and result in either greater amounts of Aβ or a greater proportion of longer Aβ peptide. This longer peptide has a greater propensity to aggregate into dimers, oligomers and then fibrils and ultimately amyloid plaques. Presenilin is a key component of the gamma secretase complex that cleaves the Aβ peptide, at its C terminus end, from APP – with pathogenic mutations also causing a higher proportion of longer and more amyloidogenic forms of Aβ.

Point mutations in the *APP* gene on chromosome 21 were the first genetic causes of AD to be discovered. These account for approximately 15% of autosomal dominant familial AD and produce symptom onset typically between 45 and 60 years of age. Trisomy 21 and *APP* gene duplications also cause early onset AD with a similar age at onset. Mutations in the presenilin-1 gene (*PS-1*) on chromosome 14 account for over 50% of all familial AD and overall have the youngest age at onset: typically between 35 and 50 years of age but some manifest as early as 30 years of age and may

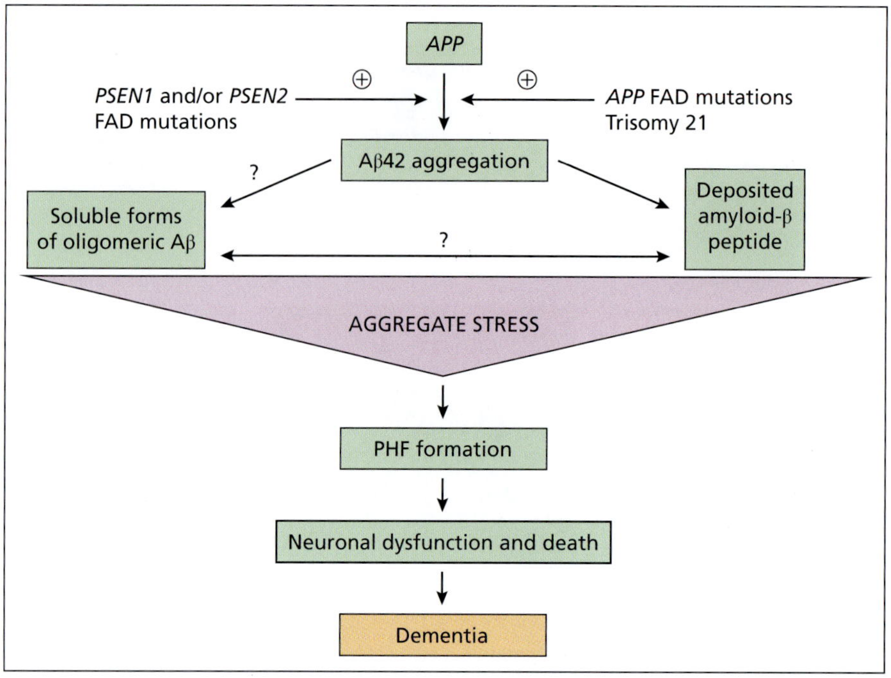

Figure 8.6 The amyloid cascade hypothesis posits that the deposition of the amyloid-β peptide in the brain parenchyma is a crucial step that ultimately leads to Alzheimer's disease. Autosomal dominant mutations that cause early onset familial Alzheimer's disease (FAD) occur in three genes: presenilin 1 (*PSEN1*), *PSEN2* and amyloid precursor protein (*APP*). This hypothesis has been modified over the years as it has become clear that the correlation between dementia or other cognitive alterations and amyloid-β accumulation in the brain in the form of amyloid plaques is not linear, either in humans or in mice. The concept of amyloid-β-derived diffusible ligands or soluble toxic oligomers has been proposed to account for the neurotoxicity of the amyloid-β peptide. These intermediary forms lie somewhere between free, soluble amyloid-β monomers and insoluble amyloid fibrils, but the exact molecular composition of these oligomers remains elusive. Toxic, soluble amyloid-β in different forms has been isolated from transfected Chinese hamster ovary cells transgenic mouse brains the human brain or it has been reconstituted *in vitro* under various experimental conditions. The amyloid cascade hypothesis now suggests that synaptotoxicity and neurotoxicity may be mediated by such soluble forms of multimeric amyloid-β peptide species. The dynamic nature of these species and the poorly defined mechanism (or mechanisms) of toxicity make this topic particularly controversial in the field. Given this uncertainty, we prefer to use the term 'aggregate stress' to describe the potential mechanisms that may lead to amyloid-β aggregation, the formation of paired helical filaments (PHFs) of tau aggregates and, ultimately, result in neuronal loss. Aβ42, the 42-amino acid form of amyloid-β. Source: Karran *et al.* 2011. Reproduced with permission of Macmillan.

occasionally present after the age of 65 years. Mutations in presenilin-2 (*PSEN2*) on chromosome 1 are relatively rare as causes of AD; cases have a young, although variable age at onset.

The clinical features of familial AD are similar to each other and to sporadic AD although there are rare atypical presentations such as a spastic paraparesis in *PSEN1*. Therefore, in a patient presenting with cognitive decline suggestive of AD with a family history of early onset dementia, testing for mutations in all three genes is appropriate. Presymptomatic testing of 'at-risk' individuals from known pedigrees is also possible, with appropriate counselling. In a number of countries, pre-implanation genetic diagnosis is now available and relevant to mutations carriers or at-risk individuals thinking about starting a family.

Overall, a family history of AD in a first degree relative occurring at any age confers an approximately twofold increase in an individual's lifetime risk. This is largely because of the risk-modifying effect of the apolipoprotein E gene (*ApoE*). ApoE exists in three isoforms: e2, e3 and e4. The most common isoform is e3, with e4 being less common and e2 relatively rare. Inheriting a single e4 allele increases the risk of AD approximately two- to threefold and is associated with an earlier age at onset. This risk is dose dependent, with e4 homozygosity being associated with a four- to eightfold relative risk, and a mean age at onset 5–10 years earlier than average. The e2 allele is relatively protective. However, the e4 allele is neither sufficient (in contrast to *APP* and *PSEN*) nor necessary to produce AD: approximately 20–30% of the general population carries one or more e4 alleles, and only 60–70% of all cases of AD have one or more e4 alleles. As a result, current consensus guidelines do not recommend testing for ApoE as part of the diagnostic work-up of a patient with possible AD. Recent genome-wide association studies have identified a number of genetic associations each with much lower relative risk than ApoE. With increasing longevity more and more people will have a family history of late onset AD; in most cases (e.g. a parent with onset in their seventies or eighties) it will be possible to reassure individuals that this confers very little additional risk and that genetic testing is not indicated.

Clinical features and assessment

The regional distribution and progression of the pathology of AD largely accords with the march of clinical symptoms, which start insidiously, and gradually and inexorably progress. Obtaining a reliable history is key to the diagnosis. Patients often lack insight and it is essential to obtain a collateral history from a close informant. Partners or family members may not want to embarrass or contradict the patient and therefore, with the patient's consent, it is helpful to speak in part without the patient present in order to understand the extent of an individual's problems.

The most common complaint, often made by a carer, spouse or other family member rather than by the patient, is of problems with memory. Patients become repetitive in questioning, forgetting that they asked the same question recently, be it minutes, hours or days ago. Messages or errands are forgotten, there is progressive difficulty often with misplacing items (e.g. keys, glasses) and errors may be made in route finding. A particular early feature of the memory deficit is the inability to place memories correctly; thus, patients may remember that someone visited but be unsure of the context (when the visit happened or who else was there). While many of these symptoms may be reported during normal ageing or by patients later determined to be 'worried well', what distinguishes AD is the severity of the deficit and its inevitably progressive nature.

In neuropsychological terms, these early symptoms reflect impairment of episodic memory. Recall is usually worse than recognition memory and although patients commonly lack insight into the severity of their problems they are often aware that memory is a problem. This memory deficit is a harbinger of the progressive impairment of other higher cortical functions. However, an isolated memory deficit is not sufficient for a clinical diagnosis of AD. Historically diagnostic criteria for AD required dementia to be present before a diagnosis of AD could be made. Dementia by definition involves deficits in multiple cognitive domains of sufficient severity to impair activities of daily living. Recent advances in biomarkers have led to new criteria being proposed that allow a diagnosis of AD to be made prior to dementia if there is biomarker support. In particular, these criteria recognise that AD is very likely if memory deficits are accompanied by evidence of cerebral amyloid deposition, from CSF measurement showing low $A\beta_{1-42}$ or from PET amyloid imaging; or a typical pattern of AD atrophy or hypometabolism (see Investigations). In the earliest stages, patients may have objective deficits of episodic memory without any other cognitive impairments and may have little problem continuing their activities of daily living. Amnestic MCI describes such individuals with objective impairment of memory (scoring 1.5 standard deviations below the age-related mean for healthy controls) but without dementia. Longitudinal studies have shown that patients fulfilling criteria for MCI develop AD at a rate of about 10–15% per year. However, MCI represents a heterogeneous group and includes individuals who score badly on tests of memory because of anxiety or depression and also individuals who have static deficits (e.g. resulting from vascular damage).

How best to identify those patients who will go on to develop AD is a major topic of research. Some factors in the history may provide clues: if the carer is more aware of the problems than the patient, the probability of the symptoms being caused by AD is more likely. Conversely, if it is the patient who is complaining more of their problems than the informant, an alternative non-neurodegenerative cause is more likely. Asking the patient and informant to provide detailed examples of memory problems is often helpful. It is clearly less significant if someone occasionally forgets a message or cannot remember where they have placed an item when they have been distracted, multi-tasking or simply not been giving it their full attention. However, it is of more concern if the carer reports salient information being forgotten (a conversation the day before) or more frequently repeating questions (e.g. the timing of hospital appointments). It is also characteristic for problems to be apparently 'brought on' by a change in environment (e.g. hospitalisation) or illness – reflecting a reduced cognitive reserve that makes acute confusional states more likely.

There are a number of associated features that may accompany these early deficits. In particular, carers often report that the patient has become less confident, less spontaneous and more apathetic, and may seem depressed. Depression and AD commonly coexist and depressive symptomatology may mimic AD. It is sensible to have a low threshold for suspecting and treating depression, ideally avoiding antidepressants with anticholinergic activity. However, the presence, proportion and progression of cognitive deficits are the key to determining that depression is related to the onset of AD rather than an alternative explanation. A common complaint of relatives of patients with AD is that initial problems were attributed to depression, and the cognitive decline was overlooked because the informant's history was not properly considered.

As the pathological process progresses beyond the medial temporal lobes, so too do the cognitive deficits. Patients with AD typically develop cortical deficits that are symmetrical, left and right hemisphere involved simultaneously, and generalised, posterior cognitive functions affected at least as much as frontal. The clinical assessment therefore should aim to assess the pattern of cognitive decline from the history, from bedside testing and, ideally, with formal neuropsychometry. In addition to memory and orientation problems there are often early subtle impairments of planning, decision-making and working out complex sequences, and learning new tasks (e.g. failures to master new equipment either at home or at work). The presence of posterior dysfunction (i.e. parietal and/or occipital problems – such as calculation, spelling, praxis or visual processing problems) should be sought, as this makes an alternative diagnosis of FTD less likely.

Unlike FTD or the frontal subcortical deficits of VaD, AD is not usually associated with marked behavioural and personality change in the early stages apart from a loss of confidence and some apathy. Thus, a useful contrast to FTD is that spouses of those with AD usually feel that the patient has essentially the same personality albeit less outgoing. While individuals with AD are less confident in a number of cognitive areas (especially memory), maintenance of a remarkably preserved social façade is a common feature whereas insight may be poor.

As the disease progresses, all these initially subtle cognitive deficits become more marked and generalised and behavioural problems become more common. More severe language problems develop, including naming difficulties. Carers often report that patients no longer read as much as they have before, often because of a combination of impaired memory for what they have read and difficulties following the plot. With time, problems with speech and naming become increasingly marked, eventually leading to significant impairment of communication.

There may also be a history of increasing difficulty in using tools or implements that had previously not been a problem. Problems with praxis, which may sometimes be picked up in the early stages as subtle difficulty in copying complex hand movements, become more obvious with time.

Visuo-spatial difficulties may manifest as a deterioration in an individual's ability to drive, more often reported by their passengers. Minor accidents may occur, as a consequence of misjudging distances or delayed decisions. This is compounded by a greater tendency to get lost in unfamiliar circumstances, and errors of

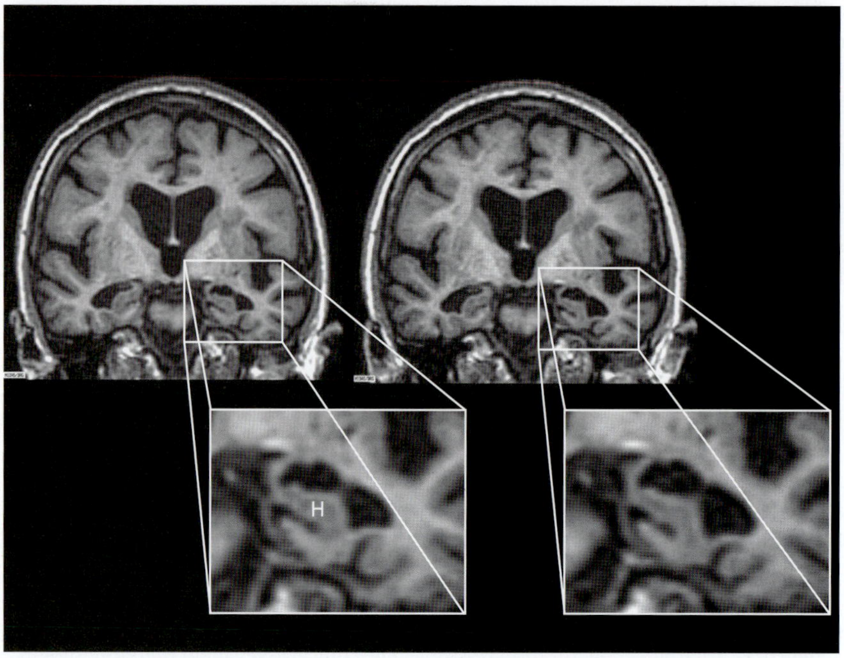

Figure 8.7 Hippocampal atrophy. Two coronal T1-weighted MRI scans of a patient with probable AD: baseline on the left; follow-up 1 year later registered to baseline. The inset shows a magnified view of the left hippocampus (H) with progressive atrophy over the year.

judgement. Therefore, patients with a diagnosis of AD and their carers must be reminded of their legal obligation to inform licensing authorities (DVLA in the United Kingdom) and depending on severity may need to be advised to stop driving. In the later stages, agitation is relatively common and occasionally aggression often associated with frustration may be a major problem. Delusions are common and can be particularly distressing for patient and carer. The kernel of the delusions can often be understood in the context of failing memory and reasoning abilities (e.g. delusions of theft are common as an inpatient).

In the early stages, there are generally no focal neurological signs and apart from the praxis problems mentioned earlier, the examination may be normal. Myoclonus (often most noticeable in the fingers) may occur later in the disease, although patients with autosomal dominant AD tend to have early and prominent myoclonus, often a harbinger of seizures later on. In the late stages, there may be a generalised increase in tone in a *Gegenhalten* fashion.

Brainstem and motor function are typically preserved when many higher cognitive abilities have been significantly degraded. Patients ultimately become unable to self-care but may still be capable of wandering, often with marked sleep–wake cycle reversal. In the later stages, problems with continence develop. Relentless progression leads to increasing dependency and institutional care. Diminishing capacity means that it is important for the person with AD to plan for the end of their life at an early stage. Symptomatic treatments may give a period of some months of apparent stabilisation of symptoms (see Management) but there is no evidence that current treatments alter the underlying disease progression. Seizures, when present, are usually a late feature. Swallowing difficulties can also develop and contribute to pneumonia, one of the most common causes of death. Survival is age-related (lower with older patients) but is typically 4–8 years from diagnosis of AD although may be up to 15 years in a minority; survival from first symptoms is 2–3 years longer because of delays in diagnosis.

Investigations

Apart from familial cases where demonstration of a pathogenic mutation in *APP*, *PSEN1* or *PSEN2* is diagnostic, there are no definitive laboratory tests for AD. It is therefore important to exclude, as detailed elsewhere in this chapter, alternative causes for cognitive decline.

A number of investigations have positive predictive value for AD. Neuropsychometry is important in establishing the extent and pattern of cognitive deficits, and in established cases typically demonstrating deficits in a broad range of cognitive domains, prominent problems with episodic memory and posterior dysfunction at least as significant as anterior without a marked left–right asymmetry.

Current (e.g. National Institute for Health and Care Excellence; NICE) guidelines suggest that all patients with dementia should undergo structural imaging (preferably MRI) as part of their diagnostic work-up. As with neuropsychometry, structural imaging, in addition to excluding a space-occupying lesion, can help in making a diagnosis of AD by identifying the pattern of atrophy. AD is associated with marked and disproportionate medial temporal lobe atrophy, which is most easily assessed by looking for evidence of bilateral hippocampal atrophy (Figure 8.7). AD is also associated with ventricular enlargement and generalised cortical atrophy symmetrically involving both parietal and frontal lobes. These findings are best seen with MRI using a coronal T1-weighted volumetric sequence.

Imaging, and in particular MRI (T2-weighted or FLAIR), can be used to assess the extent of cerebrovascular disease. Functional imaging, PET and SPECT, show symmetrical temporo-parietal hypometabolism and hypoperfusion. Nonetheless, the wide range

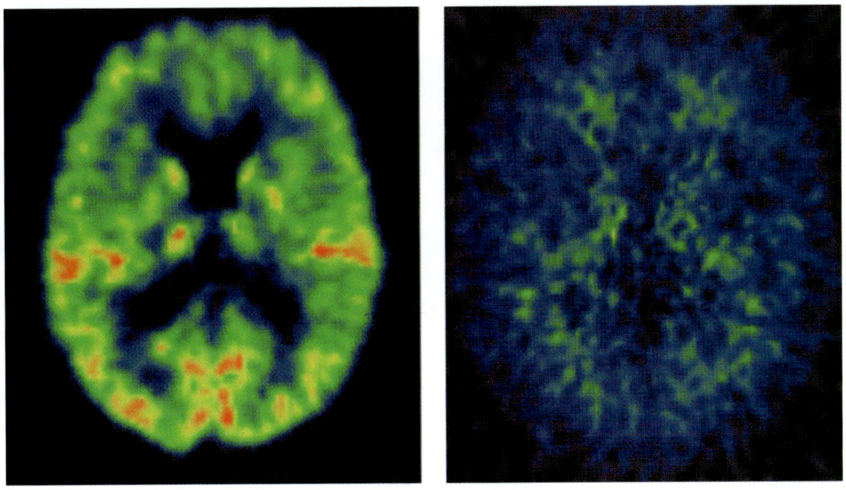

Figure 8.8 The left image shows a positive amyloid (11C-PIB) scan with the cortical amyloid binding shown in red and yellow; this is typical of Alzheimer's disease (AD). On the right is a negative scan with only non-specific white matter binding. Both subjects had mild cognitive impairment and were of a similar age. The individual on the left progressed to AD dementia in the following year whereas the subject on the right has remained well with stable memory complaints.

of normality means structural or functional scans may be reported as normal in the early stages of AD. NICE guidelines recommend functional imaging (SPECT or PET) to be used to help differentiate AD, vascular dementia and frontotemporal dementia if the diagnosis is in doubt.

Amyloid imaging (with C^{11} or F^{18} PET ligands) has high sensitivity for the presence of cerebral amyloid. Asymptomatic amyloid deposition may precede dementia by up to a decade; 25% of healthy elderly individuals aged about 75 years have positive amyloid scans. Although currently mainly research tools they are likely to be used increasingly in clinical practice but may find most utility in younger patients; in older patients they may be most useful in ruling out AD if the scan is negative (Figure 8.8).

EEG may be important to exclude seizure activity as a relatively uncommon cause of memory impairment and, if this is suspected, prolonged recordings may be required. In AD the EEG typically shows generalised slowing and loss of alpha rhythm, although in mild cases may appear normal.

There is increasing interest in using CSF markers to differentiate AD from other neurodegenerative dementias. In AD the CSF is usually acellular with normal protein. CSF tau (total levels and specific phosphorylated forms) are increased in AD while CSF Aβ 1-42 is reduced. The combination of these markers appears to differentiate AD from controls with sensitivity and specificity of approximately 90% but rather lower discriminatory ability to separate AD from other dementias such as FTD or DLB.

Management

It is important that both patient and carer are considered in management. A holistic approach that covers social support, prognostic information and advice on legal, benefit and support issues is essential. Treatment of depression must not be missed. Specific symptomatic pharmacological treatments for AD are discussed later; these include the cholinesterase inhibitors and memantine, an NMDA antagonist.

AD continues to be the subject of intensive research. Drugs aimed at modifying the disease process are under development. Aβ immunotherapy has so far failed to show efficacy in Phase III clinical trials. In mice such therapy has been shown to clear amyloid plaques from the brain and be neuroprotective if given before the onset of significant pathology. Other strategies include beta or gamma APP secretase inhibitors which aim to reduce Aβ production; or targeting tau or ApoE4.

Cholinesterase inhibitors The cholinesterase inhibitors (AChEIs) have been specifically developed as symptomatic treatment for AD. The rationale for their use is based on neurochemical findings in the cerebral cortex of patients with AD, in whom there is reduced activity of the enzyme choline acetyltransferase, with subsequent reduction in cortical levels of the neurotransmitter acetylcholine (ACh). By inhibiting the breakdown of ACh, AChEIs enhance the levels of ACh in cerebral cortex. There are currently three AChEIs licensed for the treatment of mild to moderate AD: donepezil (Aricept), galantamine (Reminyl) and rivastigmine (Exelon). Donepezil is a specific and reversible inhibitor of acetylcholinesterase (AChE); galantamine is a selective, competitive and reversible inhibitor of AChE, which additionally enhances the intrinsic action of ACh on nicotinic receptors; and rivastigmine inhibits both AChE and butyrylcholinesterase. They have similar symptomatic efficacy and there is no evidence of any disease slowing benefit. Once daily modified release formulations, oral solutions and patches are available.

The clinical efficacy of AChEIs has been measured using the Alzheimer's Disease Assessment Scale (ADAS-Cog), which assesses cognitive function, and the Clinician Based Impression of Change plus carer input (CIBIC-plus), which takes a more holistic view of the patient. A number of large randomised controlled trials have shown statistically significant, if clinically modest, symptomatic benefits of AChEIs on both ADAS-Cog effects and CIBIC over their 6-month duration, equivalent to a delay in symptomatic cognitive decline and temporary stabilisation of the patient's clinical and functional state. Further, in open label extensions of these trials effects have been reported to last up to 5 years, and Cochrane reviews report significant improvements on rating scales for activities of daily living and neuropsychiatric symptoms. Current NICE guidelines (www.nice.org.uk) for treatment with AChEIs (Table 8.5)

Table 8.5 Summary of NICE Guidelines for treatment of Alzheimer's disease (November 2006).

NICE recommend donepezil, galantamine and rivastigmine as options for managing mild to moderate Alzheimer's disease (typically, but not exclusively MMSE >10/30) under the following conditions:

- Treatment should be initiated by specialists but may be continued by general practitioners using a shared care protocol
- The carer's views should be sought before and during treatment
- Patients should be reviewed regularly and treatment should be continued only when it is considered to be having a worthwhile effect on cognitive, global, functional or behavioural symptoms
- It is recommended that therapy should be initiated with a drug with the lowest acquisition cost (since there is insufficient evidence to differentiate between the AChE inhibitors in terms of cost effectiveness)
- Memantine is recommended as an option for managing Alzheimer's disease for people with: moderate Alzheimer's disease who are intolerant of or have a contraindication to AChE inhibitors; or severe Alzheimers disease

Source: http://www.nice.org.uk/page.aspx?o=288826. Reproduced with permission of NICE.

suggest that cholinesterase inhibitors should be used in mild to moderate AD and can be continued into the more severe stages of the disease as long as it is felt they are still providing benefit. Treatment should be stopped when benefit is no longer evident. This is often a subjective and difficult decision made by the clinician after discussion with the patient and carer, based on either a global impression or deterioration on a rating scale such as the MMSE. As AChEIs can provide other benefits, particularly on behavioural and neuropsychiatric symptoms, their effectiveness in all areas should be considered. If in doubt, the drug should be withdrawn for a few weeks and if there is rapid decline in behaviour and/or cognition, the drug should be restarted.

Memantine Memantine has an entirely different mode of action from the AChEIs, potentially preventing glutamate-mediated neurotoxicity. It is a voltage-dependent, moderate affinity, non-competitive *N*-methyl-D-aspartate (NMDA) receptor antagonist and blocks the effects of pathologically elevated tonic levels of glutamate by preventing calcium influx into the neurone. It has beneficial effects in slowing cognitive decline in mild to moderate AD, but also in vascular dementia and is generally well tolerated. It was previously licensed for use in moderately severe AD. It is currently used when AChEIs are thought to have lost efficacy, in AD patients intolerant of AChEIs or in whom these are contraindicated. There is some evidence that a combination of donepezil and memantine gives greater improvement in cognition, activities of daily living and neuropsychiatric symptoms than donepezil combined with placebo; however, combination therapy is not currently recommended by NICE. Side effects are uncommon; they include hallucinations, confusion, dizziness, headaches and tiredness.

Frontotemporal dementia

Frontotemporal dementia (FTD) is an umbrella term used to describe a clinically and pathologically heterogeneous group of non-Alzheimer's neurodegenerative disorders, characterised by relatively focal frontal and temporal cerebral atrophy. The nosology

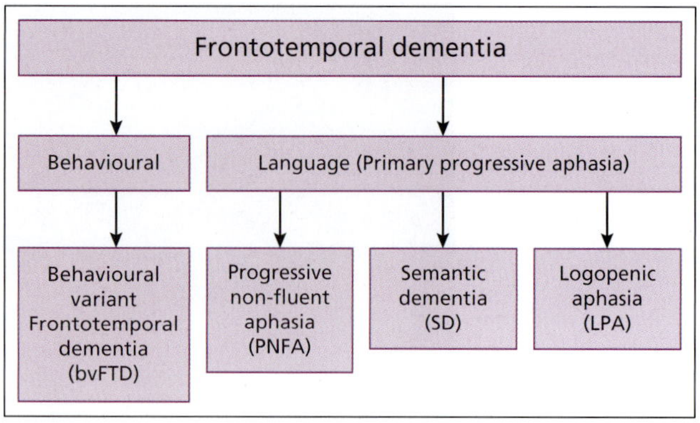

Figure 8.9 Syndromic variants of frontotemporal dementia.

for this group of disorders is complex. Cases have been recognised since the nineteenth century, when Pick first described a case of dysphasia with focal temporal atrophy and historically his name was used to describe the entire group of disorders. Recognition of the different clinical syndromes led to a proliferation of descriptive names although for this chapter we use the descriptions as outlined in Figure 8.9.

FTD is less common than AD, with prevalence estimates of 4–15/100 000 under 65 years. In general, onset occurs between 50 and 70 years, with most patients surviving 6–12 years. However, onset can be much earlier (twenties) or much later (eighties) and is likely to be under-recognised.

In recent decades, the clinical and pathological complexity of these disorders has been better understood. There are three broad syndromic variants, each of which is associated with a distinct set of presenting symptoms. Over half of the patients present with behavioural change (behavioural variant FTD) and the remainder present with language decline often referred to as primary progressive aphasia (PPA). Traditionally, two subtypes of PPA have been described, those with impaired comprehension, naming and semantic impairment (semantic dementia), and those with impaired speech production (progressive non-fluent aphasia). However, more recently further subtypes have been described.

Behavioural variant frontotemporal dementia

Patients with behavioural variant frontotemporal dementia (bvFTD) typically present with personality change and breakdown in behaviour, including apathy, disinhibition, loss of empathy and abnormal eating behaviour such as the development of a sweet tooth. Repetitive, obsessive or compulsive behaviours may also be seen. Early changes can be very subtle, and recognition of minor changes in social behaviour is important in detection of the problem, for example switching jobs, 'forgetting the rules' of social engagement or becoming more childlike. It is vital that the caregiver is interviewed as well as the patient, as frequently the patient lacks insight into the problem. Often, carers have recognised a change but have not realised why, for example in taste in clothes, in politeness with others or in developing obsessions about certain things.

As the disease progresses, disruptive behavioural symptoms usually worsen. Disinhibited patients often develop inappropriate antisocial behaviours, and may even be arrested for stealing or disorderly behaviour. Angry outbursts are common, and conversation can be punctuated by tactless remarks. When apathy is dominant, patients become progressively inert, robotic and emotionally detached. Such issues are distressing for the family, and greatly increase the caregiver burden. Drug treatments or other mechanisms for dealing with these problems are unfortunately limited.

Often observation of the patient's behaviour during the consultation is more revealing than formal neuropsychology. They can show impulsivity, be easily distracted (e.g. by the computer screen saver in the office), they may be disinhibited towards the examiner, picking up things on their desk or show suggestive behaviour towards them. Neuropsychological testing early on can be remarkably normal. It may reveal executive dysfunction as the sole or most prominent finding, particularly within the first couple of years of disease onset. Specific deficits (and the neuropsychological instruments with which they may be detected) include a tendency to perseverate (verbal fluency), impaired planning (Wisconsin card sorting test), loss of inhibition (go-no-go task), sequencing (Luria's test), failure of recall with improvement on cueing (Wechsler Memory Scale), limited problem-solving (Raven's progressive matrices) and concreteness of thought (Cognitive Estimates test). In contrast to executive dysfunction, memory and posterior functions tend to be relatively spared. Social cognition (including theory of mind) is commonly impaired early in the disease process but is rarely tested in formal neuropsychometric batteries.

Imaging (MRI) may normal in the early stages, but usually reveals focal atrophy of the frontal and/or temporal lobes, often asymmetrical. Fluoro-deoxyglucose positron emission tomography imaging (FDG-PET) can be useful in patients where structural imaging is normal to reveal frontal hypometabolism.

A subgroup of patients with bvFTD present with behavioural symptoms consistent with the diagnostic criteria and yet do not seem to progress over many years. These patients are often men and commonly are in their fifties or sixties. They have been called FTD 'phenocopies' and have normal structural and functional imaging. The underlying cause is uncertain but may represent decompensation of a previous personality or autistic spectrum disorder.

Semantic dementia

The onset of semantic dementia (SD) is insidious with a characteristic presentation of progressive deterioration in semantic memory. Patients may complain of 'memory' problems with words; the presenting feature is typically word-finding difficulty, especially problems with producing common nouns. During a typical consultation, if asked for example where they went on holiday, a patient might say 'what's a holiday?' – this loss of understanding of what a word means is pathognomonic of SD. Spontaneous speech is fluent and grammatically correct but empty of content, with word-finding difficulties, circumlocution, impaired confrontation naming and reduced verbal fluency, especially for conceptual categories (e.g. types of animal or vehicle). Typical responses when asked to name might be superordinate; for example, 'owl' becomes 'bird' or a description of the item is given that is autobiographical; for example, when asked to name a dog 'oh, you know, I see that every day next door; I like him'. Although verbal semantic impairment is usually predominant, with progression, semantic impairment of other modalities occurs, for example recognition of faces (prosopagnosia) or of visual objects (visual agnosia).

In contrast to the severe semantic deficit, phonology, prosody and grammar remain relatively intact. Other aspects of language become affected to a degree. Patients typically show surface dyslexia such that irregularly spelt words (such as 'sew' or 'pint') are read according to typical spelling-sound mappings (in this example, to rhyme with 'few' and 'mint'). Behavioural changes similar to those seen in bvFTD will develop as the disease progresses.

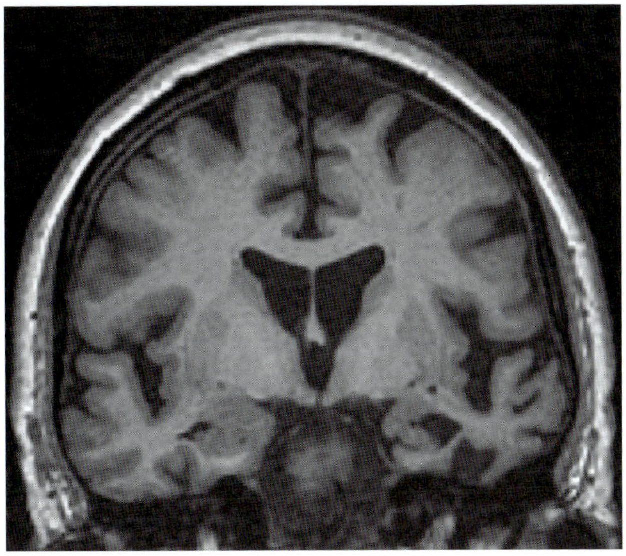

Figure 8.10 Coronal section of T1-weighted brain MRI showing focal atrophy predominantly involving the antero-inferior left temporal lobe, a pattern typical of semantic dementia.

Other cognitive domains such as episodic memory, perceptual and visuo-spatial abilities are relatively preserved until late in the course of the disease.

Imaging is particularly characteristic in SD. MRI of brain reveals severe asymmetrical antero-inferior temporal lobe atrophy, in particular affecting the fusiform gyrus (Figure 8.10). The temporal poles often appear as 'knife-blade'. Left temporal atrophy is dominant when the earliest symptom is one of verbal semantic loss, but when there is initial non-verbal semantic loss right temporal atrophy is present. In these right temporal cases, there may also be more evident behavioural change.

Progressive non-fluent aphasia

Patients with progressive non-fluent aphasia (PNFA) have a non-fluent language disorder, a deficit that may remain circumscribed for many years. Patients produce hesitant, effortful speech (often called 'apraxia of speech') and/or agrammatism with the presence of phonemic errors. With agrammatism, phrases become telegraphic, sentences short and disjointed, and comprehension is often impaired at the sentence level. However, there is a strikingly preserved ability to understand individual words in the early phases of the disease. Writing is similarly affected in many cases. Insight is usually retained, often with extreme distress.

In addition to the language-specific features there may be an associated orofacial apraxia, which can be tested by asking the patient to cough or yawn. This can sometimes lead to difficulty swallowing. It is not until late in the course of the disease that overt behavioural features such as rigidity and loss of concern for others arise; however, there may be evidence of executive dysfunction on formal psychometric testing. MRI of the brain often shows dominant left peri-sylvian atrophy involving the inferior frontal and anterior insular cortex; however, findings vary widely.

Other PPA syndromes Logopenic aphasia (LPA, or the logopenic variant of PPA) is a recently described further clinical subtype of primary progressive aphasia and is worth differentiating as it is usually associated with underlying AD pathology. The presentation is

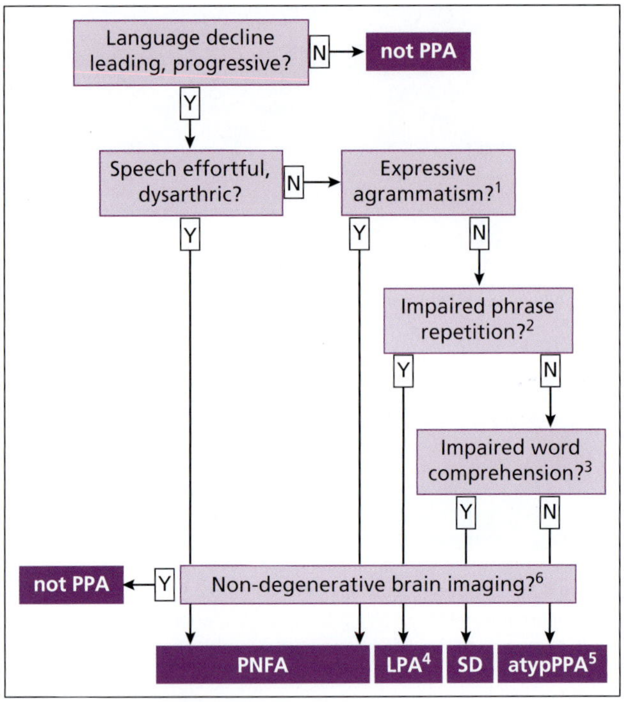

Figure 8.11 Bedside clinical assessment of the progressive aphasias: a simple algorithm (informed by current consensus criteria for progressive aphasia) for syndromic diagnosis of patients presenting with progressive language decline. The clinical syndromic diagnosis should be supplemented by neuropsychological assessment, brain magnetic resonance imaging (MRI), and ancillary investigations including cerebrospinal fluid examination. atyp, atypical; LPA, logopenic aphasia; PNFA, progressive non-fluent aphasia; PPA, primary progressive aphasia; SD, semantic dementia.
1 Terse, telegraphic phrasing with errors of tense or function words.
2 Disproportionate to repetition of single (polysyllabic) words.
3 This can be probed by having the patient select a nominated item from an array or supply a definition. Associated semantic deficits should also be sought: in other language channels (surface dyslexia and dysgraphia; a tendency when reading aloud or writing to 'regularise' words according to superficial rules of phonemic correspondence rather than learnt vocabulary, such as sounding 'sew' as soo) and other semantic domains (such as by asking the patient to list visual attributes of an object or to indicate the purpose of a familiar household item from sight.
4 Third major subtype of progressive aphasia, in most cases a result of Alzheimer's pathohody.
5 Atypical PPA variants represent a substantial minority of cases, including patients presenting with 'pure anomia' deficits primarily affecting language channels other than speech or relatively pure dysprosody.
6 Non-degenerative pathologies (such as brain tumours) should always be excluded on brain imaging.
Adapted from Warren *et al.* 2013 with permission of BMJ.

one of word-finding difficulties, anomia and poor working memory leading to difficulty repeating phrases rather than single words (Figure 8.11).

Recent studies have suggested that there may be other subtypes of PPA, with up to 20% of patients not fitting diagnostic criteria for SD, PNFA or LPA. In particular, there is some evidence that familial PPA syndromes are phenotypically distinct.

Overlap with other syndromes Neurological examination in FTD is usually normal, although there is overlap with other clinical syndromes including motor neurone disease and atypical parkinsonism, particularly PSP and cortico-basal syndrome. In FTD-MND, behavioural symptoms (or more rarely language problems) are present in conjunction with weakness and wasting in limb and/or bulbar muscles, although in the early stages the only sign of MND may be fasciculations. Around 10–15% of patients with FTD develop MND and, vice versa, 10–15% of patients with MND develop FTD (although up to 50% will develop cognitive impairment not meeting criteria for FTD).

Investigations

These syndromes must be distinguished from non-degenerative processes such as primary psychiatric illness, tumours, vascular disease and from atypical forms of AD. Neuropsychological assessment can help define the phenotype and reinforce the clinical impression, especially detecting subclinical cognitive involvement and for documenting progression. Structural imaging with MRI can be helpful, commonly showing the characteristic imaging pattern of asymmetrical frontal and/or temporal lobe atrophy. Distinct patterns are seen in the PPA syndromes with asymmetrical (usually left predominant) anterior and inferior temporal lobe atrophy in SD, left inferior frontal, insula and peri-sylvian atrophy in PNFA, and left posterior temporal and inferior parietal atrophy in LPA. Increasingly, CSF Aβ1–42 and tau assays are used to diagnose underlying AD pathology in those cases where differentiation from FTD is difficult.

Genetic pathological correlations

Recent advances in the genetic field have accelerated our understanding of molecular genetics, biochemistry and neuropathology of FTD. Some 35–50% of patients with FTD have a family history of dementia with an autosomal dominant inheritance pattern or an identified genetic mutation in around 20%. Most cases have mutations in the *MAPT* (microtubule associated protein tau), *GRN* (progranulin) or *C9orf72* genes. These three genes account for the majority of cases of genetic FTD but rarely mutations in other genes can also be causes, for example mutations in the valosin containing protein (*VCP*) gene cause FTD in association with inclusion body myositis and Paget's disease of bone.

The term frontotemporal lobar degeneration (FTLD) is a collective term sometimes used to denote the three major pathological forms that cause FTD, characterised by the abnormally aggregated proteins found in the neuronal inclusions:

1 *Tauopathies* In tau-positive FTLD (around 40–50% of cases), histology shows cellular inclusions containing phosphorylated protein tau. Subtypes of the tauopathies include Pick's disease, PSP, CBD and the pathology seen in patients with *MAPT* mutations (often called FTLD with parkinsonism linked to chromosome 17 or FTDP-17).
2 *TDP-43 proteinopathies* (around 40–50% of cases) Four subtypes of TDP-43 positive FTLD are described, named A to D. Patients with mutations in the *GRN* (type A), *C9orf72* (type A or B) and *VCP* (type D) genes fall into this group
3 *FUS proteinopathies* A minority of cases (5–10% of cases) have inclusions containing fused-in-sarcoma (FUS) protein.

For most cases there is poor clinico-pathological correlation (e.g. bvFTD can be associated with tau, TDP-43 or FUS inclusions). However, FTD-MND is reliably associated with TDP-43 pathology as is semantic dementia. Very young onset sporadic FTD (age of onset <40) is commonly associated with FUS pathology (Figure 8.12).

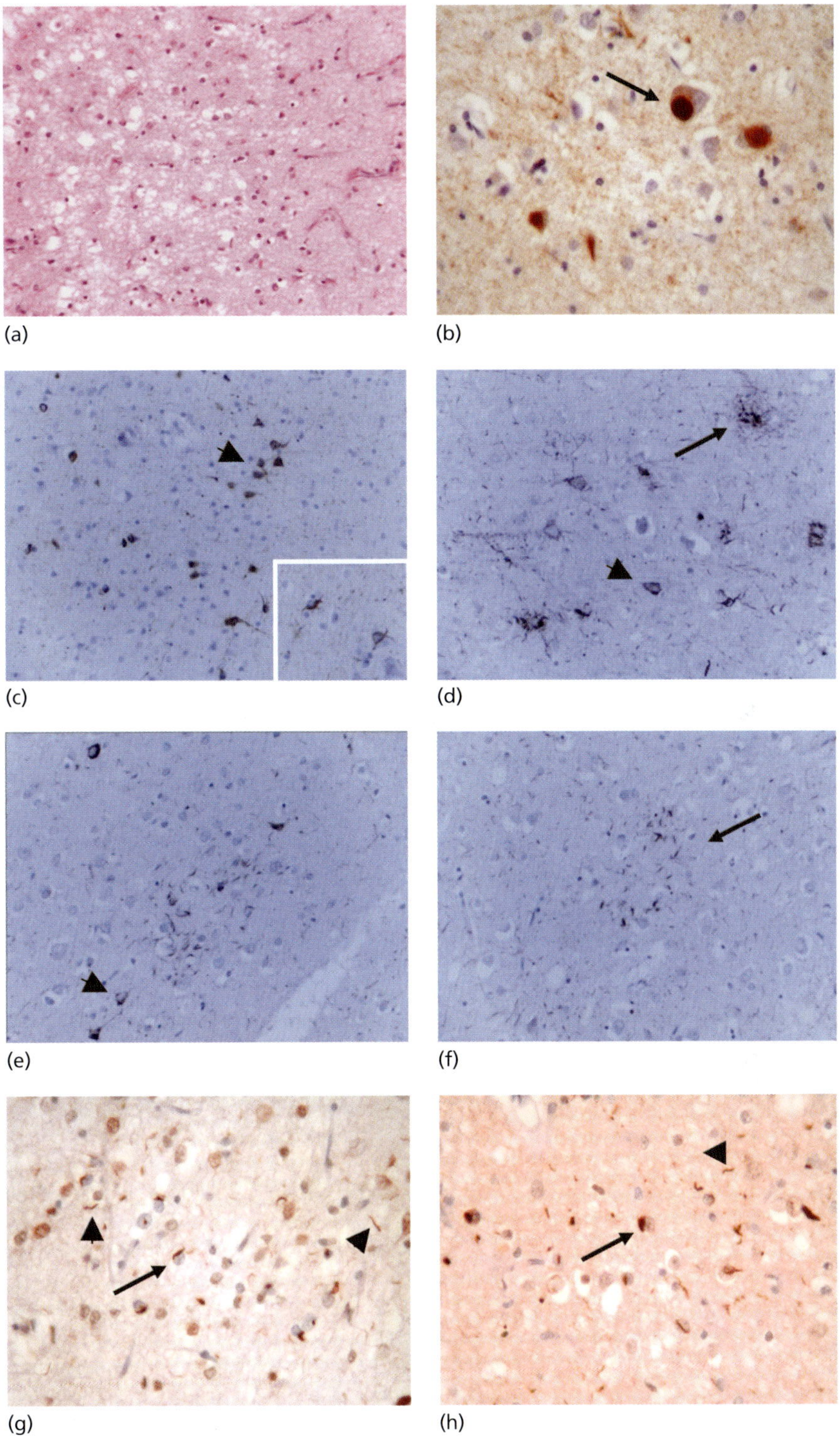

Figure 8.12 (a) Neurophil spongiosis occurring in superficial cortical laminae is seen in FTLDs (haematoxylin and eosin preparation, frontal cortex). (b) Tau-positive Pick body is a characteristic feature of Pick's disease (AT8 immunohistochemistry, temporal cortex). (c) A combination of tau-positive neuronal (arrowhead) and glial pathology is found in frontotemporal lobar degeneration (FTLD) due to intronic mutations located close to the alternatively spliced exon 10 (this case: exon 10 +16 mutation). Insert showing tau-positive oligodendroglial coiled bodies (AT8 immunohistochemistry, temporal cortex). Tau-positive neurofibrillary tangles and pretangles (arrowhead) occur both in progressive supranuclear palsy and cortico-basal degeneration (d and e arrowhead). However, tufted astrocytes are the characteristic glial pathology in progressive supranuclear palsy (d arrow) and the so-called astrocytic plaques are found in cortico-basal degeneration (f arrow) (AT8 immunohistochemistry, frontal cortex). Neuronal intracytoplasmic inclusions (arrow) and neurites (arrowhead) are ubiquitin-positive (g) and are immunoreactive for TDP-43 (h) in FTLD-U (g: ubiquitin immunohistochemistry; (h) TDP-43 immunohistochemistry, temporal cortex). Courtesy of Professor Tamas Revesz, Queen Square Brain Bank, Department of Molecular Neuroscience, UCL Institute of Neurology.

Prognosis

All syndromes slowly progress over time leading to dependency and institutional care. The most aggressive course is found in FTD-MND, with death within 3–5 years of onset. For the other syndromes many patients survive for well over a decade.

Management

The carer burden for this group of patients is significant and distinct in quality both comparing syndromes such as bvFTD and PNFA and from the more typical issues in AD. Often carer burden in this group is particularly severe because of behavioural issues and lack of insight from patients. Respite and counselling are vital for the carer and family – they often feel they have lost their loved one and this can lead to significant distress. There are difficult decisions to be made to balance independence and safety. For example, improving wandering behaviour by changing the environment, alerting local community police or shopkeepers about forensic behaviour, removing bank cards to avoid indiscriminate spending. For the language variants, speech and language therapy can be very helpful in providing strategies to improve communication, such as use of tablet programs to 'speak for' the patient if significant word-finding difficulties. In addition, it may be necessary to assess swallow, especially where there is orofacial apraxia in PNFA. Management is primarily symptom control and supporting patients and their carer cope with the disease burden. This includes signposting to local services in the mental health and social services teams, and disease-specific support networks such as the FTD Support Group and the Association for Frontotemporal Degeneration.

There are currently no disease-modifying treatments for FTD. There is limited evidence that selective serotonin re-uptake inhibitors may modulate abnormal behaviours in some patients. New generation neuroleptics are reserved for when agitation cannot be controlled by other means and are used very cautiously at low dosage.

Dementia with Lewy bodies and Parkinson's disease dementia

Dementia with Lewy bodies (DLB; also known as 'Lewy body dementia' or 'diffuse Lewy body disease') and dementia associated with Parkinson's disease (Parkinson's disease dementia; PDD) together constitute the second or third most common cause of dementia in later life in most series. These disorders appear to lie on a neuropathological and clinical continuum. Although estimates vary, in cross-sectional studies approximately 30% of patients with idiopathic Parkinson's disease have dementia; and in longitudinal studies individuals with idiopathic Parkinson's disease have a three- to sixfold higher risk of developing dementia than age-matched controls. Risk factors for development of PDD include older age, duration of disease and motor disability (especially symmetric, non-tremor dominant disease with postural instability and gait disturbance), diminished response to levodopa and levodopa-induced confusion, early visual hallucinations, olfactory dysfunction and mood and sleep disturbance.

Pathologically, both DLB and PDD are characterised by the formation of Lewy bodies (the hallmark of Parkinson's disease, Chapter 6): intracytoplasmic eosinophilic neuronal inclusions with a central core and pale halo, containing the protein α-synuclein aggregated with abnormally phosphorylated neurofilaments and ubiquitin. Lewy bodies are found in the neocortex, limbic cortices and subcortical nuclei and there is associated neuronal loss. Pathological subtypes of DLB have been categorised as brainstem predominant, limbic (transitional) or diffuse neocortical based on the predominant distribution of pathological changes. No neuropathological features that reliably separate DLB, PDD and Parkinson's disease without dementia have been identified, and the particular clinical phenotype is likely to depend on the pattern of spread of pathological changes in the brain. In individuals developing DLB in later life, pathological features of AD (senile plaques and neurofibrillary tangles) and vascular disease commonly coexist at postmortem.

The pathological determinants of cognitive dysfunction in association with DLB and PDD are complex. Although it is not a universal finding, a number of studies have found a correlation between the regional density of cortical Lewy bodies and cognitive dysfunction (in particular visual hallucinations), while conversely, dementia is uncommon in patients with *parkin* mutations that lack cortical Lewy body involvement. Lewy bodies have also been correlated with cortical Alzheimer's changes, and it has been suggested that the interaction of these factors predisposes to the development of dementia and modifies the clinical phenotype. However, the development of dementia in some patients with *SNCA* mutations that lack significant associated Alzheimer pathology suggests that this is not a critical factor in all cases. Disruption of ascending dopaminergic and cholinergic pathways gives rise to clinically significant deficiencies of these neurotransmitter systems that interact with intrinsic cortical pathology.

Unresolved issues of pathological classification notwithstanding, DLB and PDD remain clinically defined syndromes and together these diseases present characteristic clinical problems that justify their status as a distinct dementia category. According to the current revised DLB consortium guidelines, and Movement Disorders Society Task Force clinical criteria for PDD DLB should be diagnosed when dementia occurs before or coincides within 1 year of parkinsonism, and PDD when dementia develops in established Parkinson's disease (criteria for probable PDD and DLB are shown in Table 8.6). DLB is typically a sporadic disease of later life with an overall survival similar to AD; however, young adult, familial and rapidly progressive forms, although rare, are well described. As with AD, there is an increasing move to diagnose the cognitive impairments associated with PD earlier, leading to the concept of PD-mild cognitive impairment (Table 8.6).

Core features of DLB are progressive cognitive decline with fluctuating cognition, recurrent visual hallucinations and spontaneous parkinsonism. The cognitive profile is often dominated by executive, attentional and visuo-spatial disturbances. A history of some variation in cognitive function from day to day is common in many dementias; however, the fluctuations in DLB are more marked and often paroxysmal within a 24-hour period. They may manifest as drowsiness, decreased responsiveness or disorganisation of speech or behaviour. Fluctuations may be profound and prolonged, and frank delirium with protracted confusion and hallucinosis may supervene. Visual hallucinations should be enquired about specifically: in DLB, they are generally animate, vivid, stereotyped and silent, and often emerge from background visual features or patterns under low-light conditions. Although it is a core diagnostic feature of DLB, parkinsonism is not recorded in a significant proportion of autopsy-proven cases, implying that the absence of extrapyramidal features does not exclude the diagnosis. Other characteristic features of DLB are marked neuroleptic sensitivity and REM sleep behaviour disorder, the occurrence of complex and bizarre (often violent) sleep-related behaviour because of acting of dream content (the result of abnormal restoration of muscle tone resulting from synuclein pathology in the region of the pontine tegmentum). Additional supportive features include recurrent

Table 8.6 (a) Criteria for probable Parkinson's disease dementia (PDD).

1 Diagnosis of Parkinson's disease according to Queen Square Brain Bank criteria
and

2 A dementia syndrome with insidious onset and slow progression, developing within the context of established Parkinson's disease and diagnosed by history, clinical and mental examination, defined as impairment in more than one cognitive domain; representing a decline from premorbid level. Deficits severe enough to impair daily life (social, occupational, or personal care), independent of the impairment ascribable to motor or autonomic symptoms
and

3 Typical profile of cognitive deficits including impairment in at least two of the four core cognitive domains (impaired attention which may fluctuate, impaired executive functions, impairment in visuo-spatial functions, and impaired free recall memory which usually improves with cueing). The presence of at least one behavioural symptom (apathy, depressed or anxious mood, hallucinations, delusions, excessive daytime sleepiness) supports the diagnosis of probable PDD, lack of behavioural symptoms, however, does not exclude the diagnosis

Exclusion criteria

- Coexistence of any other abnormality which may by itself cause cognitive impairment, but judged not to be the cause of dementia (e.g. presence of relevant vascular disease in imaging)
- Time interval between the development of motor and cognitive symptoms not known
- Features suggesting other conditions or diseases as cause of mental impairment, which, when present, make it impossible to reliably diagnose PDD
- Cognitive and behavioural symptoms appearing solely in the context of other conditions such as acute confusion caused by systemic diseases or abnormalities; drug intoxication; 'major depression' according to DSM-IV; features compatible with 'probable vascular dementia'

Source: Emre *et al.* 2007. Reproduced with permission from John Wiley & Sons.

Table 8.6 (b) Criteria for probable dementia with Lewy bodies (DLB).

1 Dementia defined as progressive cognitive decline of sufficient magnitude to interfere with normal social or occupational function. Prominent or persistent memory impairment may not necessarily occur in the early stages but is usually evident with progression. Deficits on tests of attention, executive function and visuo-spatial ability may be especially prominent

2 Core features (two required for a diagnosis of probable DLB, one for possible DLB):
- Fluctuating cognition with pronounced variations in attention and alertness
- Recurrent visual hallucinations that are typically well formed and detailed
- Spontaneous features of parkinsonism

3 Suggestive features (probably DLB can be diagnosed with ≥1 core + ≥1 suggestive feature)
- REM sleep behaviour disorder
- Severe neuroleptic sensitivity
- Low dopamine transporter uptake in basal ganglia demonstrated by SPECT or PET imaging

4 Supportive features (commonly present but not proven to have diagnostic specificity): repeated falls and syncope; transient, unexplained loss of consciousness; severe autonomic dysfunction (e.g. orthostatic hypotension), urinary incontinence; hallucinations in other modalities; systematised delusions; depression; relative preservation of medial temporal lobe structures on CT/MRI scan; generalised low uptake on SPECT/PET perfusion scan with reduced occipital activity; abnormal (low uptake) MIBG myocardial scintigraphy; prominent slow wave activity on EEG with temporal lobe transient sharp waves

5 A diagnosis of DLB is less likely: in the presence of clinical or imaging evidence of cerebrovascular disease; in the presence of any other physical illness or brain disorder sufficient to account in part or in total for the clinical picture; if parkinsonism only appears for the first time at a stage of severe dementia

6 Temporal sequence of symptoms. DLB should be diagnosed when dementia occurs before or concurrently with parkinsonism (if it is present). In research studies in which distinction needs to be made between DLB and PDD, the existing 1-year rule between the onset of dementia and parkinsonism DLB continues to be recommended

Adapted from McKeith *et al.* 2005 with permission of AAN/LWW.

syncope and falls, significant autonomic dysfunction, hallucinations in non-visual modalities and early prominent delusions (including misidentification delusions such as the Capgras phenomenon and topographical and other reduplicative paramnesias), apathy and depression.

PDD has a very similar neuropsychological profile to DLB and shares many other clinical characteristics. Visual hallucinations are common in PDD even after medication effects are taken into account. In contrast to spontaneously occurring visual hallucinations, drug-induced hallucinations in treated Parkinson's disease are

Table 8.6 (c) Criteria for mild cognitive impairment–Parkinson's disease dementia (MCI-PDD).

1	Diagnosis of Parkinson's disease (PD) as based on the UK PD Brain Bank Criteria
2	Gradual decline, in the context of established PD, in cognitive ability reported by either the patient or informant, *or* observed by the clinician
3	Cognitive deficits on either formal neuropsychological testing or a scale of global cognitive abilities*
4	Cognitive deficits are not sufficient to interfere significantly with functional independence, although subtle difficulties on complex functional tasks may be present
Exclusion criteria	
1	Diagnosis of PD dementia based on MDS Task Force proposed criteria
2	Other primary explanations for cognitive impairment (e.g. delirium, stroke, major depression, metabolic abnormalities, adverse effects of medication or head trauma)
3	Other PD-associated co-morbid conditions (e.g. motor impairment or severe anxiety, depression, excessive daytime sleepiness, or psychosis) that, in the opinion of the clinician, significantly influence cognitive testing

* Depending on the scales used and how comprehensive the neuropsychological battery, PD-MCI can be classified as level 1 (lesser diagnostic certainty) or level 2 (higher diagnostic certainty); and for classifications within level 2 as single or multiple domain PD-MCI.
Source: Litvan *et al.* 2011.

often perceived as frightening or threatening and accompanied by paranoid delusions. REM sleep behaviour disorder is also a feature of PDD. Parkinsonism in both PDD and DLB may closely mimic that of uncomplicated idiopathic Parkinson's disease, although predominant axial involvement with postural instability, absence of tremor and limited response to levodopa are more common.

Certain investigations in DLB and PDD can help to support the clinical impression, although no diagnostic or disease-specific biomarkers have been identified. On structural brain MRI, mesial temporal structures tend to be relatively better preserved than in AD. Metabolic brain imaging typically shows reduced striatal dopamine transporter uptake, and cortical perfusion and metabolism are globally reduced, often with a posterior emphasis. Degradation of alpha rhythm in the EEG occurs as a non-specific marker of cortical degeneration.

No specific or disease-modifying therapies are currently available for DLB or PDD. Cholinesterase inhibitors (AchEIs) modestly improve cognitive function, attention, alertness and behaviour in a substantial proportion of patients, and indeed may be more effective than in AD at a comparable disease stage. More particularly, these agents may help in the management of fluctuations, sleep disturbance, confusion and hallucinations. The side effect profile of the AChEIs in DLB and PDD is broadly similar to that in AD. The impact on extrapyramidal symptoms is variable: modest benefit is seen in some patients, but significant worsening of parkinsonism or dystonia does occasionally occur and patients should be monitored for this possibility. The evidence base in favour of particular AChEIs remains limited and the choice of agent should be tailored to the individual patient (e.g. the convenience of once-daily dosing with donepezil set against the shorter half-life and more flexible regimen of rivastigmine, which can also be given as a transdermal patch). Neuroleptic drugs should in general be avoided in DLB and PDD, in view of the potential to cause severe, prolonged and sometimes life-threatening extrapyramidal reactions. However, these drugs may sometimes be necessary for the management of agitation or hallucinations where behavioural strategies or cholinesterase inhibitors have failed. In this situation, a new generation agent such as quetiapine or aripiprazole should be introduced cautiously and titrated slowly to the smallest effective dose. Clozapine is probably the most effective neuroleptic and least likely to cause extrapyramidal side effects, but its use is limited by the requirement for close supervision and blood monitoring because of the risk of agranulocytosis.

Management of parkinsonism in both DLB and PDD follows principles similar to those in idiopathic Parkinson's disease, although dopamine agonists are generally avoided because of their higher incidence of psychiatric side effects. Levodopa may benefit motor symptoms less than in uncomplicated Parkinson's disease, and dopaminergic effects on cognition are variable. Special care is needed to avoid exacerbating hallucinations and psychotic symptoms; in practice, the balance between immobility and confusion is often very finely poised and difficult to strike.

Dementia with other movement disorders

Cognitive decline is a feature of a number of other extrapyramidal disorders (described in more detail in Chapter 6), and most commonly manifests as a subcortical dementia resulting from involvement of fronto-subcortical circuitry. Although diagnosis generally rests on non-cognitive features, the type and relative prominence of cognitive deficits may assist in the clinical differentiation of atypical parkinsonism and 'Parkinson's-plus' syndromes. Progressive supranuclear palsy (Steele–Richardson–Olszewski syndrome) is frequently accompanied by profound bradyphrenia and executive deficits, which may include perseverative responses, environmental dependency and utilisation behaviours. The 'applause sign', when a patient asked to clap three times as fast as possible after the examiner, makes additional handclaps or may initiate applause, is suggestive of PSP. In contrast to other 'Parkinson's-plus' disorders, cortico-basal degeneration can present as a purely motor, purely cognitive, or more commonly mixed disorder. As cortico-basal degeneration is strictly a pathological diagnosis, the term 'cortico-basal syndrome' is increasingly preferred to describe the clinical syndrome, which can comprise early prominent cortical deficits such as limb and orofacial apraxia, parietal signs and impaired speech production, which may be relatively focal or asymmetric, and which overlap with disorders in the FTD spectrum. The presence of alien limb phenomena of variable complexity is said to be characteristic, but can occur in other pathologies. Although severe cognitive decline is an exclusion criterion for multiple system atrophy, many patients do have mild executive deficits and cognitive slowing.

Cognitive impairment is a core feature of Huntington's disease. Attentional deficits and behavioural disturbances often dominate early in the disease course, and patients frequently present via psychiatric services, especially where the family history is concealed or not recognised. Visuo-spatial deficits are also well documented. Deficits of emotion recognition may be present, even in presymptomatic carriers. Cognitive decline in Huntington's disease has been shown to correlate with caudate atrophy and frontal hypometabolism, consistent with a primary disruption of fronto-subcortical circuitry.

Cognitive dysfunction is common in the expanding group of inherited spinocerebellar ataxias (Chapter 17), and executive and verbal memory deficits, affective disturbances and personality change have all been described. The severity of cognitive decline varies with the underlying genetic abnormality and may be particularly evident in *SCA2* and *SCA17*. There is much interest in defining a cognitive and behavioural signature of cerebellar damage, but this is difficult because of the frequent co-occurrence of damage involving other neuronal systems.

Prion disease

Introduction and disease biology

The prion diseases, or transmissible spongiform encephalopathies, affect both humans and animals. The human prion diseases have been traditionally classified into CJD, Gerstmann–Sträussler–Scheinker (GSS) disease, fatal familial insomnia and kuru. Animal prion diseases include scrapie of sheep and goats, transmissible mink encephalopathy, chronic wasting disease of mule deer and elk, and bovine spongiform encephalopathy (BSE) which first appeared in the United Kingdom from the mid-1980s and rapidly evolved to a major epizootic estimated to have infected over 2 million UK cattle. The recognition of a novel human prion disease, vCJD, from the mid-1990s onwards and experimental confirmation that it was caused by the same prion strain as BSE raised major public health concerns. While the number of human cases to date has been relatively modest, key uncertainties, notably with respect to major genetic effects on incubation period, allied with the widespread population exposure, suggest the need for caution.

Prions are transmissible agents with unique composition and properties, being apparently devoid of significant nucleic acid. Prion diseases are associated with the accumulation in the brain of an abnormal, partially protease-resistant, isoform of a normal cell surface glycoprotein found in healthy people known as prion protein (PrP). The disease-related isoform, PrP^{Sc}, is derived from its normal cellular precursor, PrP^{C}, by a post-translational process that involves conformational change and aggregation. According to the 'protein-only' hypothesis, an abnormal PrP isoform is the principal, and possibly the sole, constituent of the transmissible agent or prion. PrP^{Sc} is hypothesised to act as a conformational template, promoting the conversion of PrP^{C} to further PrP^{Sc} by an autocatalytic process. In addition to public health concerns, prions have assumed much wider relevance in understanding neurodegenerative and other diseases involving accumulation of misfolded host proteins (protein-folding diseases).

Aetiological categories and classification of human prion disease

The human prion diseases are unique in having three distinct aetiologies (Table 8.7). They may occur sporadically, be acquired by dietary or iatrogenic exposure to prions, or inherited in an autosomal dominant fashion as a result of coding mutations in the prion protein gene (*PRNP*). Remarkably, Mendelian inherited forms of prion disease are also experimentally transmissible by inoculation of laboratory animals. The majority of recognised human prion disease occurs as sporadic CJD. The aetiology of sporadic CJD is unclear but may arise from somatic mutation of *PRNP* or spontaneous conversion of PrP^{C} to PrP^{Sc} as a rare stochastic event. The alternative hypothesis, exposure to an environmental source of either human or animal prions, is not supported by epidemiological evidence.

Prion diseases show marked phenotypic variability. A major factor in explaining this diversity is the existence of distinct prion strains. Prion strains can be distinguished by differences in the biochemical properties of PrP^{Sc}. Prion strain diversity appears to be encoded by differences in PrP^{Sc} conformation and pattern of glycosylation. Four main types are seen amongst CJD cases, sporadic and iatrogenic CJD being of PrP^{Sc} types 1–3, while all vCJD cases are associated with a distinctive PrP^{Sc} known as type 4 (London classification). A similar type 4 PrP^{Sc} is seen in BSE and in BSE when transmitted to several other species.

A common *PRNP* polymorphism at codon 129, where either methionine or valine can be encoded, is a key determinant of genetic susceptibility to acquired and sporadic prion diseases, the large majority of which occur in homozygous individuals. Heterozygosity is protective against developing sporadic and acquired prion disease and leads to increased age at onset in some forms of inherited prion disease. Codon 129 genotype also has a key role in determining clinicopathological phenotypes, in part via an effect on selection of particular prion strain types.

Sporadic prion disease

Creutzfeldt–Jakob disease The core clinical syndrome of classic sporadic CJD is of a rapidly progressive multifocal dementia usually with myoclonus. The onset is usually in the 45–75 year age group with peak onset between 60 and 65 years. The clinical progression is typically over weeks progressing to akinetic mutism and death often in 2–3 months; most die in under 6 months. Prodromal features include fatigue, insomnia, depression, weight loss, headaches, general malaise and ill-defined pain sensations. Frequent additional neurological features include extrapyramidal signs, cerebellar ataxia, pyramidal signs and cortical blindness. About 10% of patients present initially with cerebellar ataxia.

Routine haematological and biochemical investigations are normal. Routine CSF examination is normal but 14-3-3 protein is usually elevated. However, it is also positive in recent cerebral infarction or haemorrhage and in viral encephalitis, and may also be elevated in rapidly progressive AD which may be difficult to clinically distinguish from CJD. New CSF tests such as the real-time Quaking Induced Conversion (rtQUIC) assay may be more specific. CT or MRI is crucial to exclude other causes of subacute neurological illness but MRI has become increasingly useful in diagnosis of sporadic CJD, showing high signal in the striatum and/or cerebral cortex in FLAIR or DW images (Figure 8.13). Cerebral and cerebellar atrophy may be present in cases of longer duration. The EEG may show characteristic pseudoperiodic sharp wave activity. Brain biopsy may be considered in highly selected cases to exclude treatable alternative diagnoses using appropriate CJD infection control precautions.

Neuropathological confirmation of CJD is by demonstration of spongiform change, neuronal loss and astrocytosis together with positive PrP immunohistochemistry. PrP amyloid plaques are usually not present in CJD. PrP^{Sc} can be demonstrated by immunoblotting of brain homogenates and is diagnostic of prion disease. PrP^{Sc} types 1–3 are demonstrated, distinct from type 4 which is exclusively seen in variant CJD. *PRNP* analysis is important to exclude pathogenic mutations even in the absence of a family history because several mutations are not fully penetrant. Most cases of classic CJD are homozygous with respect to the common 129

Table 8.7 Classification of human prion disease.

Aetiology	Phenotype	Frequency
Sporadic		
Unknown: random distribution worldwide; incidence of 1–2 per million per annum	Sporadic CJD: subacute myoclonic form and range of atypical forms; multiple distinct prion strains associated with distinct clinico-pathological phenotypes which includes sporadic fatal insomnia	~85%
Inherited		
Autosomal dominantly inherited conditions with high penetrance; all forms have germline PRNP coding mutations	Extremely variable: readily mimics familial Alzheimer's disease and other neurodegenerative conditions; over 30 mutations identified; includes Gerstmann–Sträussler–Scheinker disease, familial CJD and fatal familial insomnia	~10–15%
Acquired		
Iatrogenic infection with human prions via medical or surgical procedures: human cadaveric-derived pituitary hormones, tissue grafts and contaminated neurosurgical instruments	Iatrogenic CJD: typical CJD when direct CNS exposure; ataxic onset when peripheral infection	<5% (most from USA, UK, France and Japan)
Exposure to human prions via endocannibalism	Kuru	Unique to small area Papua New Guinea; major epidemic in 1950s with gradual decline since cessation of cannibalism
Environmental exposure (presumed dietary) to BSE prion strain	Variant CJD	Total to date ~200. Mainly in UK but now reported from a number of countries
Iatrogenic infection via blood transfusion from healthy donor infected with vCJD prions	Secondary vCJD	UK only to date

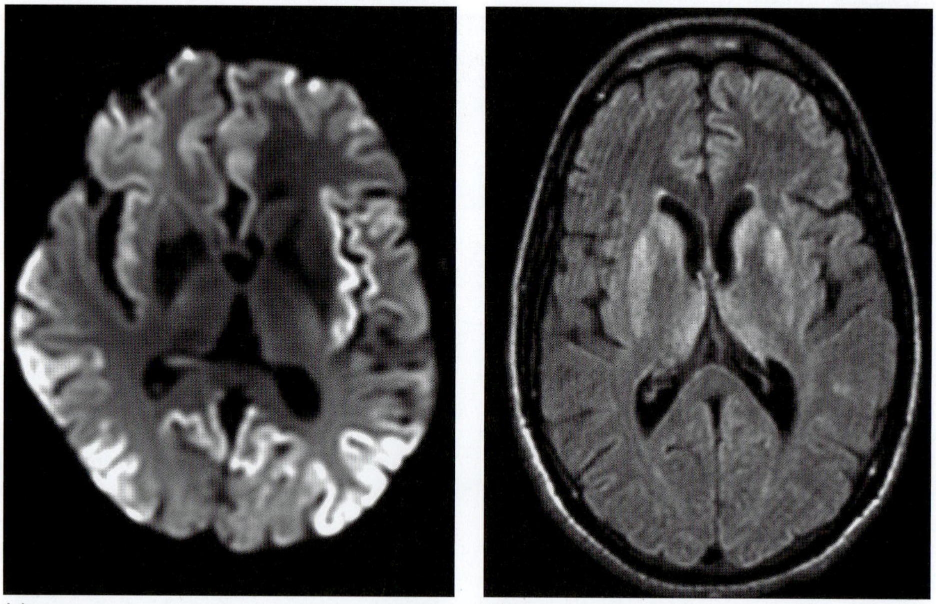

Figure 8.13 Sporadic Creutzfeldt–Jakob disease (CJD). MRI demonstrates typical increased signal intensity in the caudate and putamen bilaterally and widespread increased cortical signal intensity involving the occipital, frontal, temporal and insula cortex on (a) fluid attenuated inversion recovery (FLAIR) and (b) diffusion-weighted imaging (DWI) (b = 1000 s/mm^2) sequences. The cortical signal changes are more apparent on the DWI sequence.

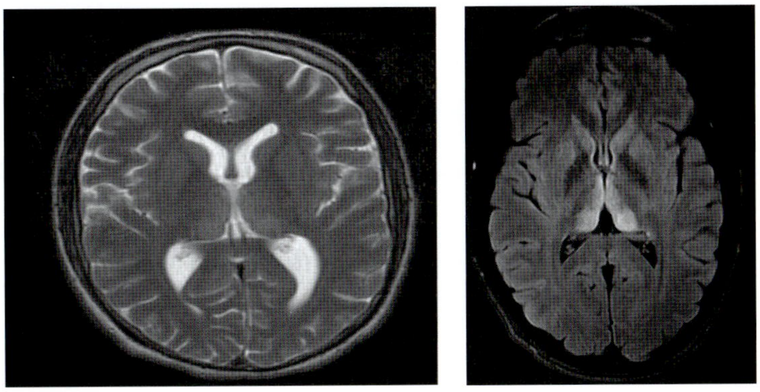

(a) (b)

Figure 8.14 Variant CJD. MRI demonstrates symmetrical increased signal intensity in the pulvinar nuclei bilaterally ('pulvinar sign') and dorsomedial thalami on (a) T2 weighted and (b) FLAIR sequences.

polymorphism of PrP and MM is by far the most common genotype in classical subacute CJD.

Atypical forms of CJD are well recognised. Around 10% of cases of CJD have a much more prolonged clinical course of over 2 years. *PRNP* codon 129 genotype is often VV or MV, rather than the MM type usually seen in subacute myoclonic CJD. Around 10% of patients with CJD present with cerebellar ataxia rather than cognitive impairment, so-called ataxic CJD, although this presentation should lead to a consideration of acquired prion disease. Heidenhain's variant of CJD refers to cases in which cortical blindness predominates with severe involvement of the occipital lobes.

Acquired prion diseases

Kuru Kuru is now largely of historical interest. It reached epidemic proportions amongst a defined population living in the Eastern Highlands of Papua New Guinea and was the major cause of death amongst adult women and children in the affected region when first described by Western medicine in the 1950s. It was the practice in these communities to engage in consumption of dead relatives as a mark of respect and mourning. Males over the age of 6–8 years participated little in mortuary feasts, which is thought to explain the differential age and sex incidence. Its gradual disappearance since the cessation of cannibalism in the late 1950s has allowed estimation of the range of incubation periods possible in human prion infection which may exceed 50 years. The mean clinical duration of illness is 12 months with a range of 3 months to 3 years. The dominant clinical feature is progressive cerebellar ataxia. In contrast to CJD, dementia is much less marked.

Iatrogenic Creutzfeldt–Jakob disease Iatrogenic transmission of CJD has occurred by accidental inoculation with human prions as a result of medical procedures. Such iatrogenic routes include contaminated neurosurgical instruments, dura mater and corneal grafting, and human cadaveric pituitary-derived growth hormone or gonadotrophin. The diagnosis is usually based on a progressive cerebellar syndrome and behavioural disturbance or a classic CJD-like syndrome together with a history of iatrogenic exposure to human prions, and may occur in any age group. The incubation period in intracerebral cases is short (2–4 years for dura mater grafts) compared with peripheral cases (typically 15 years or more). EEG, CSF and MRI are generally less diagnostically helpful than in sporadic CJD. *PRNP* analysis is important to exclude pathogenic mutations. Diagnosis is confirmed by PrP immunocytochemistry or Western blot of brain tissue for PrP^{Sc} types 1–3.

Variant CJD vCJD was first described in 1996. Its occurrence initially in teenagers and young adults and distinctive neuropathology differentiated it from sporadic CJD. A link with BSE was confirmed by molecular and biological strain typing of prions.

The early features of vCJD are non-specific, often with behavioural and psychiatric disturbances and in some cases with sensory disturbance. Initial referral has frequently been to a psychiatrist and the most prominent feature is depression but anxiety, social withdrawal and behavioural change are frequent. Delusions, which are complex and unsustained, are common. Other features include emotional lability, aggression, insomnia and auditory and visual hallucinations. A prominent early feature in some is dysaesthesiae or pain in the limbs or face which is persistent rather than intermittent and unrelated to anxiety levels. In most patients a progressive cerebellar syndrome develops with gait and limb ataxia. Cognitive impairment then occurs with inevitable progression to akinetic mutism. Myoclonus is seen in most patients, and chorea is often present which may be severe in some. Cortical blindness develops in a minority in the late stages of disease. Upgaze paresis has been noted in some patients. Age at onset ranges from 12 to 74 (mean 28) years and the clinical course to death is relatively prolonged (median 14 months).

The EEG is abnormal, most frequently showing generalised slow wave activity, but without the pseudoperiodic pattern seen in most sporadic CJD cases. MRI, particularly FLAIR sequence, demonstrates bilateral increased signal in the posterior thalamus (the pulvinar sign) in the large majority of cases (Figure 8.14). However, this sign appears as a late feature of the disease process and is not specific for vCJD.

Tonsillar biopsy is a sensitive and specific diagnostic procedure for vCJD. CSF 14-3-3 protein may be elevated or normal. *PRNP* analysis is essential to rule out pathogenic mutations, as the inherited prion diseases present in younger patients and may clinically mimic vCJD, and should be performed prior to tonsil biopsy. To date all clinically probable cases of vCJD have been of the *PRNP* codon 129 MM genotype; a single patient has been reported who possibly died from vCJD with a codon 129 MV genotype, but no autopsy was conducted.

The neuropathological appearances of vCJD are striking and relatively consistent, generally allowing differentiation from other forms of prion disease. While there is widespread spongiform change, gliosis and neuronal loss, most severe in the basal ganglia and thalamus, the most remarkable feature is abundant PrP amyloid plaques in cerebral and cerebellar cortex. These consist of kuru-like, 'florid' (surrounded by spongiform vacuoles) and multicentric plaque types. Western blot analysis (molecular strain typing) of brain tissue demonstrates PrP^{Sc} type 4 which is pathognomonic of vCJD.

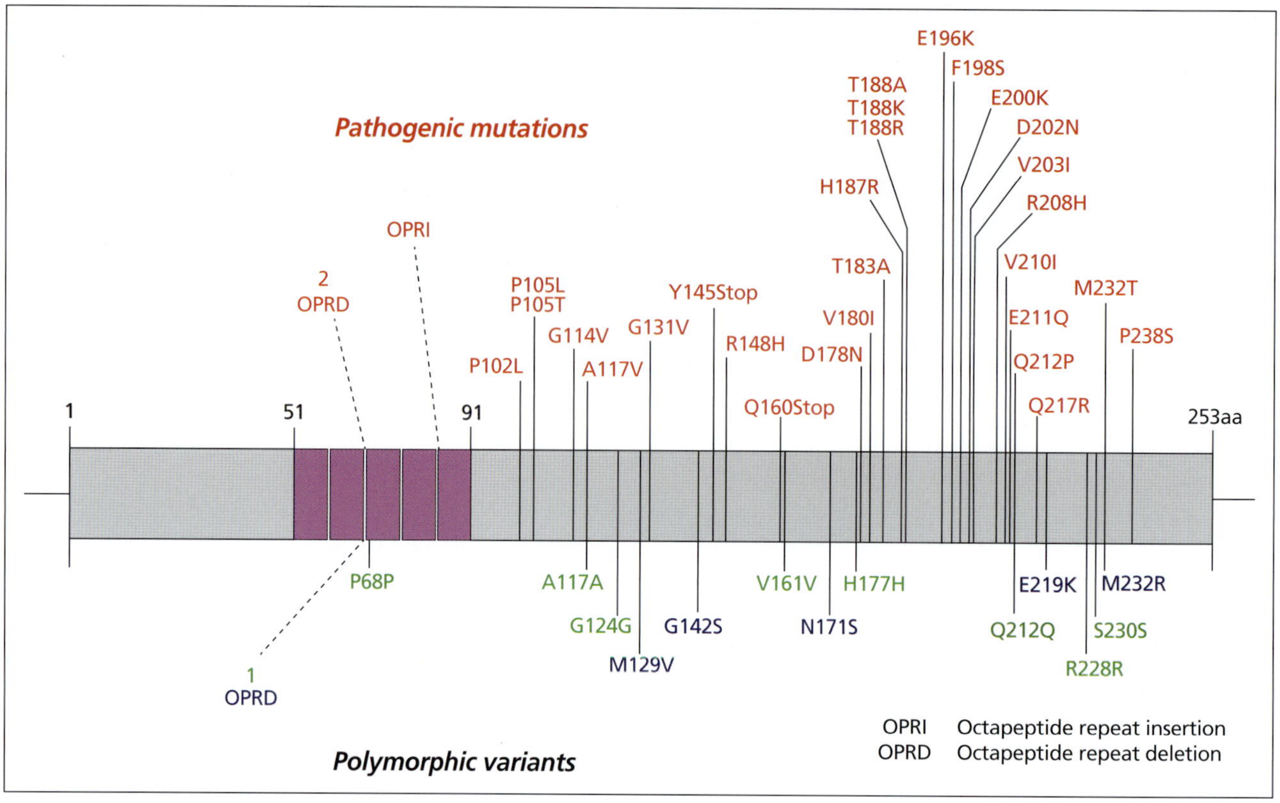

Figure 8.15 Pathogenic mutations and polymorphic variants in the prion protein gene.

Secondary (iatrogenic) vCJD The prominent lymphoreticular involvement prompted speculative concerns that vCJD may be transmissible by blood transfusion. Since 2004, four transfusion-associated cases of vCJD prion infection have been recognised amongst a small cohort of 23 surviving patients identified as having received blood from a donor who subsequently developed vCJD. The three clinical cases had the *PRNP* codon 129 MM genotype, while one patient, who died of an unrelated condition, was found to have prion infection at autopsy. This patient had the *PRNP* codon 129 MV genotype associated with relative resistance to prion disease. In each case transfusion was with a single unit of implicated red cells. Clinical features and investigations are as for primary vCJD.

Inherited prion diseases

These are adult onset autosomal dominantly inherited conditions associated with *PRNP* coding mutations (Figure 8.15). They were first classified as familial CJD and GSS. Classic GSS is a chronic cerebellar ataxia with pyramidal features, with dementia occurring later in a much more prolonged clinical course than that seen in CJD. The onset of GSS is usually in either the third or fourth decades and characterised histologically by the presence of multicentric PrP-amyloid plaques. However, inherited prion disease kindreds show remarkable phenotypic variability, which can encompass both CJD-like and GSS-like cases as well as atypical cases which readily mimic other neurodegenerative conditions. Inherited prion diseases are a frequent cause of presenile dementia and a family history is not always apparent: *PRNP* should be analysed in all suspected cases of CJD, and certainly considered in all early onset dementia and in ataxias. Cases diagnosed by *PRNP* analysis have been reported that are not only clinically atypical, but also lack the classic histological features.

The identification of a pathogenic *PRNP* mutation allows not only molecular diagnosis of an inherited prion disease but also its subclassification according to mutation. Over 30 pathogenic mutations are reported in the human PrP gene and consist of two groups:

1. Point mutations within the coding sequence resulting in aminoacid substitutions in PrP or production of a stop codon resulting in expression of a truncated PrP, and
2. Insertions encoding additional integral copies of an octapeptide repeat present in a tandem array of five copies in the normal protein (octapeptide repeat insertion; OPRI).

The key clinical features in inherited prion disease are progressive dementia, cerebellar ataxia, pyramidal signs, chorea, myoclonus, extrapyramidal features, pseudobulbar signs, seizures and amyotrophic features, which are seen in variable combinations. The most frequent forms include PrP E200K, which may mimic subacute sporadic CJD (and, in contrast to other inherited prion diseases, often has a typical EEG), PrP P102L which may present as a progressive cerebellar ataxia or dementia, and insertional mutations which have a particularly variable clinical presentation, often with a long duration mimicking AD. Fatal familial insomnia, usually associated with the D178N mutation, is characterised clinically by untreatable insomnia, dysautonomia and motor signs, and neuropathologically by selective atrophy of the anterior-ventral and mediodorsal thalamic nuclei. One variant, PrP P105L, presents as a progressive spastic paraparesis. Parkinsonism may be prominent in A117V and peripheral neuropathy occurs in E200K. Age at onset varies from the early twenties (seen often with insert mutations) to the seventies. The duration varies from less than a year to over 20 years.

Direct gene testing allows unequivocal diagnosis in patients with inherited forms of the disease and presymptomatic testing of unaffected but at-risk family members, as well as antenatal testing. Most of the mutations appear to be fully penetrant; however, experience with some is extremely limited. Exceptions include E200K and D178N (fatal familial insomnia) where there are examples of elderly unaffected gene carriers. Genetic counselling is essential prior to presymptomatic testing and follows a protocol similar to that established for Huntington's disease. It is vital to advise both those testing positive for mutations and those untested but at-risk that they should not be blood or organ donors and that they should inform surgeons, including dentists, of their risk status prior to significant procedures, as precautions may be necessary to minimise risk of iatrogenic transmission. Some truncation mutations are associated with PrP-systemic amyloidosis which presents with diarrhoea, autonomic failure and a mixed predominantly sensory neuropathy. Cognitive involvement is late in these pedigrees.

Prevention and treatment

While prion diseases can be transmitted to experimental animals by inoculation, it is important to appreciate that they are not contagious in humans. Documented case-to-case spread has only occurred by cannibalism (kuru) or following accidental iatrogenic inoculation with prions. As already discussed, there is now evidence that vCJD prion infection is transmissible by blood transfusion. UK policy for some time has been to leukodeplete all whole blood and to source plasma for plasma products from outside the United Kingdom. A further possible route of transmission of vCJD is via contaminated surgical and medical instruments. Prions resist conventional sterilisation methods and neurosurgical instruments are known to be able to act as a vector for prion transmission: several cases of iatrogenic transmission of sporadic CJD prions via neurosurgical instruments are documented.

Certain occupational groups are at risk of exposure to human prions: neurosurgeons and other operating theatre staff, pathologists and morticians, histology technicians, as well as an increasing number of laboratory workers. Because of the prolonged incubation periods for prions following administration to sites other than the CNS, associated with clinically silent prion replication in the lymphoreticular tissue, treatments inhibiting prion replication in lymphoid organs may represent a viable strategy for rational secondary prophylaxis after accidental exposure. A short course of immunosuppression with high-dose oral corticosteroids in individuals with significant accidental exposure to human prions has been advocated.

All patients with or at-risk of developing prion disease should be counselled on infection control as described for gene carriers. New diagnoses should be notified to the local consultant in communicable disease control who can assess if public health measures are necessary, notably if a patient has had recent surgery or donated blood prior to diagnosis.

All recognised prion diseases are invariably fatal following a progressive course. A variety of drugs have been tried in individual or small numbers of patients but there is no clear evidence of efficacy of any agent.

Vascular dementia and vascular cognitive impairment

Cerebrovascular disease (Chapter 5) is a major cause of cognitive impairment and dementia both in its own right and in association with AD ('mixed dementia'). In the acute phase, stroke may be associated with delirium and this in turn is associated with increased mortality and a worse functional outcome in survivors. Dementia has been estimated to occur in up to one-third of individuals within a year of stroke. Despite its frequency and importance, there is little consensus as to how 'vascular dementia' should be defined, whether in clinical or research settings. 'Vascular cognitive impairment' (VCI) may be a more appropriate catch-all term, because it reflects the broad range of clinical presentations including (in addition to clearly progressive cognitive decline) static or indolent cognitive syndromes and mild cognitive impairment on a vascular basis. In contrast to AD and other primary neurodegenerative disorders, VCI has been relatively little studied. The status of 'mixed' dementia is a particularly vexed issue. The frequent coexistence of vascular and Alzheimer changes presents serious practical challenges to the development and interpretation of treatment trials in both diseases, as well as complicating the interpretation of epidemiological studies suggesting common factors that may predispose to both AD and VCI.

Pathologically, there are no absolute criteria for a diagnosis of VCI. A spectrum of changes of variable severity occurs. Atheromatous involvement of large vessels may be found, although small vessel disease is typically prominent. Vascular changes are accompanied by lacunar and sometimes larger infarcts, typically in watershed regions between large arterial territories. Microscopically, there is lipohyalinosis of small arteries and arterioles, rarefaction and cavitation of white matter (leukoaraiosis) resulting from the conjunction of nerve fibre degeneration, gliosis and demyelination, and scattered cortical microinfarcts. Foci of old haemorrhage and amyloid angiopathy may also be observed. Pathophysiologically, lacunes are the result of completed infarction, whereas incomplete ischaemia resulting from partial vessel occlusion or hypotension can give rise to white matter lesions. There is evidence that autoregulatory perfusion reserve is decreased in zones of white matter damage, which is probably compounded by labile blood pressure control and raised plasma viscosity in vascular disease. The blood–brain barrier breaks down in these areas, and extravasated plasma proteins and other factors may contribute to neurotoxicity. Metabolic brain imaging and diffusion tensor MRI can demonstrate white matter abnormalities extending beyond the zone of damage on conventional structural brain imaging, underlining the dynamic nature of the vascular lesion and helping to explain why the relation between structural damage and cognitive impairment is not straightforward.

The clinical picture of VCI is diverse, and a given cognitive phenotype can result from a spectrum of pathogenetic mechanisms, including atherosclerosis, thromboembolism, thrombophilia, haemodynamic insufficiency, haemorrhage, and specific metabolic and genetic arteriopathies. Executive and attentional impairments, behavioural changes (disinhibition or abulia) and cognitive slowing with relative sparing of memory are clinical features common to many forms of vascular damage. This reflects the relative vulnerability of cognitive processes that depend on distributed neural networks and subcortical structures and pathways: an essential theme in our current understanding of VCI. Traditionally, emphasis was placed on the cognitive effects of acute stroke affecting a single large arterial territory or the stepwise accumulation of cognitive deficits accompanying recurrent cortical strokes: 'multi-infarct dementia'. However, it is increasingly recognised that VCI comprises a number of other clinico-anatomical syndromes, defined according to distinct patterns of clinical and brain imaging findings. Vascular changes are very common on brain imaging of

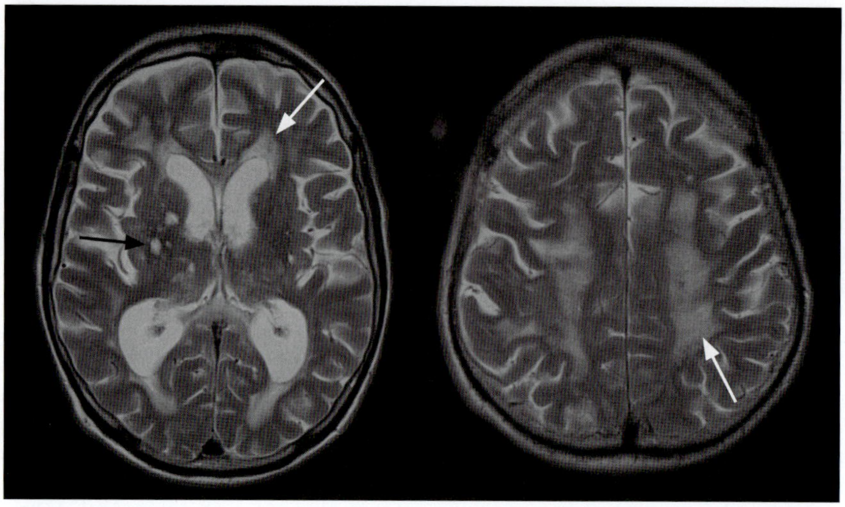

Figure 8.16 Small vessel disease. T2-weighted axial MR images showing confluent abnormal signal around the ventrical margins and throughout the centrum semiovale (white arrow) and multiple lacunes in the basal ganglia (black arrow) typical of severe small vessel disease.

healthy elderly individuals, and determining that a particular cognitively impaired individual has VCI, rather than an alternative cause such as AD, may be difficult. Diagnostic instruments such as the Hachinski Ischaemia Score are available but are of limited value in clinical practice.

Discrete strategically located cortical infarcts that implicate the medial frontal lobe (anterior cerebral artery) or mesial temporal lobe (posterior cerebral artery) can have a disproportionate effect on executive function and memory respectively: such lesions may simulate the cognitive effects of more diffuse brain damage. Single strategic subcortical infarcts can lead to impairment of multiple cognitive functions by damaging functional circuitry linking the cortex with subcortical structures or by interrupting projection pathways to the cortex. Critical sites include the thalamus, basal ganglia, internal capsule, limbic circuit and upper brainstem. Because of the distributed cortical connections of these sites, infarcts here may give rise to a surprising diversity of clinical presentations: for example, thalamic lesions may present with varying combinations of diencephalic amnesia (in which the patient may become mentally 'marooned' in a remote place or time), semantic deficits, perceptual disorders, apraxia or other sensori-motor disturbances.

More commonly, VCI results from diffuse involvement of cerebral white matter and subcortical nuclei caused by small vessel disease. This is the clinical entity known as Binswanger's disease, a somewhat controversial term that has also been applied to the neuropathological substrate. These patients typically present with an indolent cognitive decline and lack a history of clinical vascular episodes; the syndrome may closely mimic primary degenerative dementias such as AD. Clinical clues include fluctuating deficits, bradyphrenia and prominent dysexecutive features. Memory impairment is frequent, although it is more variable, more dependent on attentional factors and more responsive to cueing than in AD. On neurological examination there may be brisk facial and limb reflexes and a short-stepped wide-based apraxic gait or *marche à petit pas*. Other features include parkinsonism and other extrapyramidal syndromes, urinary incontinence or pseudobulbar palsy. A history of vascular risk factors (especially hypertension) should be sought but is of limited discriminating value. Patients undergoing major surgery (especially cardiac bypass) and those with congestive cardiac failure and orthostatic hypotension are especially vulnerable. However, an identical picture can occur even with a paucity of conventional vascular risk factors, suggesting that as yet undefined genetic and other factors also influence the development of cerebral small vessel disease.

The diagnosis rests on brain imaging findings of extensive, typical peri-ventricular white matter changes which predominantly spare subcortical U fibres and the corpus callosum and lacunes in the deep grey matter (Figure 8.16). MRI is the preferred modality because of its greater sensitivity; however, white matter changes may arise from a variety of different mechanisms and care is needed not to misclassify prominent peri-vascular spaces, which have no pathological significance. Existing brain imaging criteria for subcortical ischaemic vascular dementia have not been prospectively evaluated and do not reliably distinguish cases of 'mixed' dementia: although diffuse atrophy accompanies white matter damage, disproportionate atrophy of mesial temporal structures is a marker of AD. The relationships between cerebrovascular disease, neurodegeneration and atrophy as captured on brain imaging are complex and still poorly understood: cerebrovasuclar disease can itself lead to cortical atrophy, particularly in association with small vessel (lacunar) disease, which in turn is the clinical VCI syndrome most likely to produce insidious cognitive decline. Promising approaches for identifying concurrent Alzheimer pathology include MRI (in particular T2* and susceptibility-weighted) sequences with sensitivity for detection of microhaemorrhages associated with amyloid angiopathy, functional brain imaging based on amyloid-binding ligands, and assays of neurodegeneration-associated protein markers (tau and Aβ1-42) in CSF: these techniques are becoming increasingly widely available. Although cognitive dysfunction (and more specifically, executive and attentional deficits) correlates with cerebral atrophy and with more severe white matter involvement, there is no agreement regarding the threshold, extent or distribution of the vascular lesion load required to produce cognitive impairment. Also uncertain is the relationship to the rate of accumulation of vascular lesions on serial imaging, although the rapid appearance of new lesions raises concern regarding an atypical aggressive process such as vasculitis or an active embolic source.

While MCI on a vascular basis is well-recognised clinically, consensus diagnostic criteria that could form the basis of large-scale observational studies or therapeutic trials have yet to be agreed. However, it is likely that conventional definitions of MCI that emphasise memory impairment will need to be modified to incorporate the early attentional and executive deficits that are clinical hallmarks of small vessel disease. Depression is an important consideration in such patients (as it is in all forms of VCI) because it is strongly associated with cerebral white matter disease and may amplify any cognitive deficit.

Although less common than ischaemic cerebrovascular disease, cerebral haemorrhage presents distinct diagnostic and management challenges, and multiple haemorrhages may simulate multi-infarct dementia. Hypertension is the key risk factor for most clinically significant cerebral haemorrhages; however, recurrent lobar haemorrhages are a marker for cerebral amyloid angiopathy. Pathologically, there is deposition of congophilic material (beta-amyloid peptide) in vessels of the cortex and leptomeninges, and there is a strong association with cerebral leukoaraiosis and cortical and subcortical microhaemorrhages. The origin of the vascular beta-amyloid is presently unclear. The extent of associated Alzheimer changes is variable, although these commonly coexist. Genetic factors influence the development of cerebral amyloid angiopathy: it is associated with *ApoE* e4 and e2, while the risk of cerebral haemorrhage is increased in association with the e2 allele. Rarely, cerebral amyoid angiopathy occurs on a familial basis with autosomal dominant inheritance, and various mutations leading to the deposition of specific amyloid proteins have been identified (Table 8.8).

A variety of other haematological, autoimmune, metabolic and genetic processes can cause VCI (Chapters 5 and 19). Clues to a process in one of these categories often lie in associated non-cognitive features, and they should be suspected in younger patients with a vascular phenotype but a paucity of conventional risk factors. The antiphospholipid antibody syndrome may produce dementia via ischaemic mechanisms and there may also be additional direct effects of the antibody on neural tissue. Cognitive impairment in sickle cell disease may reflect chronic hypoxia in addition to focal infarction. Of the genetic vasculopathies, CADASIL has attracted much interest recently as the culprit protein (a transmembrane receptor in smooth muscle cells coded by the *Notch3* gene) appears to have a fundamental role in cell signalling, suggesting that this entity may be part of a broader spectrum of related disorders. Various presentations are possible, including psychiatric disturbance and acute encephalopathies, and a history of adult onset migraine is common. Brain MRI (T2 or FLAIR) characteristically shows involvement of white matter in the temporal pole and external capsule (see Figure 5.30), unusual sites for conventional small vessel disease, and skin or muscle biopsy shows periodic acid–Schiff (PAS) staining of vessels and on electron microscopy granular osmophilic deposits adjacent to the basement membrane of arteriolar smooth muscle cells. The diagnosis is confirmed by screening the *Notch3* gene for known mutations; however, this is not straightforward as the gene is large and over 50 different mutations have been described.

The differential diagnosis of VCI is potentially very extensive, because it overlaps with the spectrum of diseases causing subcortical dementia with cerebral white matter change. These include multiple sclerosis, progressive multifocal leukoencephalopathy, HIV dementia, lymphoma, post-irradiation, post-traumatic and post-hypoxic states, hereditary leukodystrophies and rare familial forms of AD with presenilin mutations. This list can usually be rationalised based on the clinical context. On imaging grounds, associated cortical infarction and involvement of the deep grey matter and brainstem are pointers to a primary vascular aetiology. Investigation of the patient with suspected VCI should include, in addition to the standard investigations listed in Table 8.4, an assessment of other end-organ damage (especially ischaemic heart disease) which may dictate overall prognosis. Brain imaging is essential and MRI is generally more informative than CT. Assessment of the carotid circulation is indicated where there is large-territory ischaemia or other suspicion of a symptomatic stenosis. Thrombophilia or other haematological or metabolic screens may be indicated, especially in younger patients. EEG often shows non-specific bitemporal slowing but preserved alpha rhythm, unless AD or another cortical degenerative process has supervened. CSF examination is indicated in younger patients or where an inflammatory or infective process is suspected and brain biopsy may be required in exceptional cases where cerebral vasculitis cannot be excluded by other means.

The management of VCI rests on primary and secondary prevention of further vascular damage, based on principles similar to those that hold for cerebrovascular disease in general (Chapter 5), and symptomatic treatment of cognitive deficits. Limited experience with the use of neuroprotective agents after stroke has been disappointing. Control of hypertension and other vascular risk factors remains the core management priority to prevent recurrent stroke. Antihypertensive treatment should be introduced cautiously in light of the evidence for impaired autoregulation in patients with subcortical ischaemic damage together with antiplatelet therapy. Although clear guidance is currently lacking, antiplatelet agents should probably be avoided in the presence of microhaemorrhages as these may signify associated amyloid angiopathy and a propensity to lobar cerebral haemorrhage. The benefit of statins on VCI is not clear, probably reflecting a weaker contribution of cholesterol to cerebrovascular disease. Randomised controlled trials suggests that the cholinesterase inhibitors are likely to be of symptomatic benefit in vascular dementia, although this is a difficult issue to resolve partly because of the problem of associated AD and also to the relative lack of suitable outcome measures (which tend to emphasise memory rather than the executive or attentional functions that are more relevant to VCI).

Dementia in young adults

Dementia is very rare before the fifth decade: in young adults and adolescents, inherited errors of metabolism and other genetic disorders are over-represented and many of these present as a 'dementia-plus' syndrome. The cognitive profile frequently takes the form of a subcortical dementia with prominent behavioural and affective features, or even frank psychosis, which may be misinterpreted as a pseudodementia. As cognitive impairment in young adult life is often constitutional or the result of congenital brain damage or static insults in early life, it is always important to establish whether cognitive dysfunction is progressive: this depends on a detailed history of pregnancy, birth and early milestones, and physical, social and scholastic development in later childhood. Cognitive decline often occurs in the setting of more widespread neurological and systemic disturbance and diagnosis generally depends on additional clinical and laboratory findings.

Effective treatments with the potential for prevention or reversal of deficits are available for some inborn errors of metabolism, such as Wilson's disease (Chapter 6) and the porphyrias (Chapter 19), which although rare should always therefore be considered in the correct clinical context. The large and diverse group of metabolic conditions also includes the mitochondrial cytopathies (Chapter 10) and a bewildering array of storage disorders (Chapter 19), in which the absence or partial inactivity of an affected enzyme leads to accumulation of abnormal material. The storage diseases can be subclassified in various ways: for example, according to the type of material deposited (e.g. glycolipid, glycosaminoglycan, lipopigment, cholesterol metabolites, polyglycosans), the primary site of cellular deposition (white matter in leukodystrophies, cell bodies in neuronal storage diseases), or the subcellular organelle affected (lysosomes, peroxisomes).

Clinicians may find it more useful to adopt a pragmatic approach based jointly on the availability of a family history and cardinal clinical features. This is the approach outlined in Tables 8.4 and 8.8. Many of these disorders have autosomal recessive inheritance, and family history is therefore often unrevealing; a history of parental consanguinity may therefore be crucial. Other diseases show variable inheritance (e.g. the mitochondrial diseases, as components of the respiratory chain are encoded both by nuclear DNA and maternally inherited mitochondrial DNA; Chapter 10). The presence of pyramidal, extrapyramidal, cerebellar or peripheral nerve signs are key diagnostic clues and help to direct investigations. Additional features such as seizures, retinopathy or deafness further restrict the differential diagnosis while certain features (such as corneal Kayser–Fleischer rings in Wilson's disease, or tendon xanthomas in cerebrotendinous xanthomatosis), if present, are pathognomonic of particular conditions.

Despite recent progress in elucidating the genetic and molecular basis of many inborn errors of metabolism, diagnosis remains challenging. This is compounded by the protean nature of the diseases themselves. Genetic diagnosis is not practical in many cases (e.g. Wilson's disease and Niemann–Pick disease), both because of the limited availability of the relevant tests and the intrinsic heterogeneity of the causative mutations, although this may change with the advent of next generation genetic sequencing techniques. Specialised processing of tissue samples is often required (e.g. muscle for respiratory enzyme analysis in mitochondrial disease; axillary skin for storage bodies in Kufs or Lafora body disease; fibroblast cultures in Niemann–Pick disease; Table 8.8). Despite much recent interest in disease-modifying therapies such as enzyme replacement or bone marrow transplantation in certain diseases (e.g. Gaucher's disease), the availability of such therapies remains limited, and cognitive deficits are unfortunately generally refractory to their effects. Accurate diagnosis is nevertheless of paramount importance in this group both for prognosis and genetic counselling.

In addition to genetically based disorders, non-degenerative acquired causes of dementia are also relatively more common in younger patients. The importance of this group lies in the potential for reversibility in many infective, inflammatory and acquired metabolic conditions. Advances in genetic sequencing techniques are also revealing links between hitherto unrelated conditions. Thus, while certain homozygous mutations in the *TREM2* gene cause a very rare dementia associated with leukoencaphalopathy and bone cysts (Nasu–Hakola disease), other heterozygous *TREM2* mutations have recently been shown to be risk factors for sporadic AD.

Potentially reversible causes of dementia

Although they are individually rare, many causes of dementia are potentially reversible and this group includes many diverse disease processes. A syndrome-based approach to the diagnosis of reversible dementias is presented in Table 8.9. Patients presenting with these syndromes demand particular vigilance to ensure that a treatable process is not overlooked. Rapid clinical evolution is a feature common to a number of diseases in this category. However, it is important to emphasise that many cases of dementia resulting from a reversible process do not present with such clinical clues: all patients with dementia should therefore be screened for treatable contributions to their cognitive decline.

Neoplasms and other space-occupying lesions

A variety of intracranial space-occupying lesions may present with insidious cognitive or behavioural decline. Potential causes include tumours, infectious lesions, chronic subdural haematoma and hydrocephalus. Cognitive and behavioural presentations are particularly associated with lesions in the frontal lobes, corpus callosum and midbrain. There may be associated features such as papilloedema or focal neurological signs, seizures, or systemic evidence of infection or primary tumour; however, such clues are often lacking and the detection of a process that may be amenable to surgical intervention is the single most important justification for brain imaging in all patients presenting with dementia. Biopsy or resection of the lesion is usually required for a definitive pathological diagnosis.

There are a number of other mechanisms besides focal cerebral damage by which neoplasms may produce cognitive dysfunction: metabolic disturbances associated with systemic cancers, paraneoplastic syndromes and meningeal infiltration. Cerebral lymphoma is notoriously protean, especially the intravascular variant which can closely mimic cerebral vasculitis and requires brain biopsy for diagnosis. Antineoplastic therapies may also be implicated in both acute and chronic cognitive decline, including cytotoxic drugs (especially methotrexate, or where multiple agents have been used) and cranial irradiation; these different modalities interact and show a dosage effect, and their delayed effects may be difficult to distinguish from tumour recurrence. Leukoencephalopathy and cerebral atrophy may manifest as a late decline in cognitive function up to several years post therapy. Cranial radiotherapy also predisposes to accelerated cerebral atherosclerosis and secondary tumours.

Epilepsy and dementia

There are a number of mechanisms by which seizures can be associated with cognitive decline and dementia. Seizures themselves may cause cognitive decline, and it is particularly important to identify covert temporal lobe seizures that may cause an amnestic syndrome similar to degenerative dementias such as AD. The syndrome of transient epileptic amnesia is characterised by fluctuations in cognitive function associated with episodes of anterograde amnesia and retrograde amnesia incorporating time periods for which the patient has essentially no recollection. Exacerbation of deficits following sleep is characteristic. Other clinical features of temporal lobe seizures often coexist but these are variable and indeed pure 'amnestic seizures' may occur. Temporal lobe spikes may be evident in the surface EEG; however, a prolonged recording may be required. There may be evidence of hippocampal damage on MRI. Although the pathophysiology is not understood in detail, ictal hippocampal paresis with inability to transfer events into long-term storage is a plausible mechanism.

Cognitive dysfunction (in particular, impaired attention and bradyphrenia) may develop in association with a number of anticonvulsant agents, including phenytoin, phenobarbital, topiramate and valproate (the last may also cause a hyperammonaemic encephalopathy, which in its more severe state can mimic CJD).

Table 8.8 A clinical classification of young onset and inherited dementias.

Family history	EPS	PYR	Atax	PN	Other features	Useful investigations	Gene	Diagnosis
a.d.	**Primary neurodegenerations**							
	–	+**	–	–	Myoclonus	MRI: symmetric hippocampal atrophy EEG: absent alpha	*APP, PSEN1, PSEN2*	Alzheimer's disease
	–	–	–	–	Epilepsy in neuroserpinopathy; inclusion body myopathy and Paget's disease with valosin mutations Language output problems with progranulin mutation	MRI: frontotemporal atrophy	ESCRT-III/ Neuroserpin/ Valosin/ Progranulin	Frontotemporal dementia
	+	–	–	–	May have amyotrophy	MRI: asymmetric frontotemporal atrophy	Tau exon10	FTDP-17
	+	–	–	–	Gaze apraxia	MRI: caudate atrophy	Huntingtin CAG repeat[§§]	Huntington's disease
	–	+	–	–	Dysfluency, fasciculations	MRI: asymmetric frontotemporal atrophy		Motor neurone disease dementia
	+	–	+	–	Seizures		Atrophin1 CAG repeat	DRPLA
	+	+	+	+	Abn saccades	MRI: cerebellar atrophy	SCA1–17	Spinocerebellar ataxias
a.d.	**Prion diseases**							
	+	+	+	–	Florid myoclonus, cortical blindness, rapid course	MRI: signal change in basal ganglia EEG: periodic complexes in CJD	PRNP20: codon 178 (codon 129 val)	Creutzfeldt–Jakob disease
	+	+	+	–	Gaze palsy, pseudobulbar palsy, cortical blindness		Codon 102/others	Gerstmann–Sträussler–Scheinker
	+	+	+	–	Sleep disorder, dysautonomia		Codon 178 (codon 129 met)	Fatal familial insomnia
a.d.	**Vasculopathies**							
	–	–	–	–	Migraine, strokes	MRI: w.m. change anterior temporal lobe, external capsule Skin bx: osmophilic perivascular material	Notch3	CADASIL

(continued)

Table 8.8 (continued)

Family history	EPS	PYR	Atax	PN	Other features	Useful investigations	Gene	Diagnosis
	–	–	–	–	Strokes	MRI: lobar haemorrhages	APP, cystatin	Cerebral amyloid angiopathies
	–	+	+	–		MRI: w.m. changes	BRI	British dementia
a.d.	**Metabolic disorders**							
	–	–	–	+	Acute attacks, abdo pain, dysautonomia, seizures, urine discoloration in light	Urinary porphyrin screens		Porphyria* (acute intermittent)
	+	+	+	–	Palatal tremor	MRI: iron in basal ganglia Dec plasma ferritin	Ferritin light chain	Neuroferritinopathy
	Other disorders							
§	–	+	+	–	May have relapsing:remitting course	MRI: abn w.m. signal esp frontal, sparing U fibres	GFAP	Alexander's disease
X-L	–	–	–	+	Strokes, renal disease, angiokeratoma corporis diffusum, extremity pain	WBC enz: dec alpha-galactosidase		Fabry's disease*
	–	+	+	–	Episodes of vomiting, stupor, hyperammonaemia	Urinary organic acids		Ornithine transcarbamylase deficiency
	–	+	+	+	Adrenal insufficiency	MRI: diffuse w.m. change Inc plasma VLCFAs		Adrenoleukodystrophy
mat	+	+	+	+	Seizures, strokes, CPEO, myopathy, deafness, abn fundi, DM, LA, short stature	MRI: w.m. disease Muscle bx: may have ragged red fibres	mtDNA	Mitochondrial encephalopathies
a.r. (neg)	**Storage diseases**							
	+	–	+	–	Supranuclear vertical gaze palsy, seizures, organomegaly	Marrow bx: sea-blue histiocytes Fibroblast cultures: abn cholesterol esters		Niemann–Pick type C
	+	–	+	–	PME, facial dyskinesias	Skin, muscle bx: inclusion bodies		Ceroid lipofuscinosis (Kufs)
	–	+	+	–	PME	Skin bx: Lafora bodies	Laforin	Lafora body disease

	–	+	+	–	Facial coarsening, recurrent infections, dysostosis, deafness, organomegaly	WBC enz: dec alpha-mannosidase		Alpha-mannosidosis
	–	+	+	–	PME, supranuclear horizontal gaze palsy, organomegaly	WBC enz: dec glucocerebrosidase Marrow bx: Gaucher cells		Gaucher's disease (subacute neuronopathic form)
	–	–	+	+	PME, visual loss with retinal cherry red spot, deafness, dysostosis	Inc urinary sialyloligosaccharides WBC enz: dec alpha-*N*-acetylneuraminidase		Sialidosis (mucolipidosis I)
	–	+	+	+	Optic atrophy	Fibroblast cultures: dec galactosylceramide beta-galactosidase		Globoid cell leukodystrophy (Krabbe's)
	–	+	+	+	Tendon xanthomas, cataracts, diarrhoea, seizures	MRI: abn signal, esp cerebellar Inc cholestanol (bile acid intermediate) in serum, nervous tissue, tendons	Mitochondrial sterol 27-hydroxylase	Cerebrotendinous xanthomatosis*
	+	+	+	+	Seizures	WBC enz: dec hexosaminidase A		GM2 gangliosidosis
	+	+	+	+		MRI: w.m. changes Urinary and peripheral nerve metachromatic deposits WBC enz: dec arylsulphatase-A		Metachromatic leukodystrophy
	+	+	+	+	Urinary incontinence	Skin bx: polyglucosan bodies	Glycogen brancher enzyme	Adult polyglucosan body disease
a.r.	**Other metabolic disorders**							
	+	–	+	–	Corneal Kayser–Fleischer rings, cirrhosis, haemolytic anaemia	MRI: 'face of the giant panda' sign Dec serum copper and caeruloplasmin, inc urinary copper excretion		Wilson's disease*
	+	+	–	–	Seizures, visual loss	MRI: iron in globus pallidus ('eye of the tiger')	PANK2	PKAN (Hallervorden–Spatz)

(continued)

Table 8.8 (continued)

Family history	EPS	PYR	Atax	PN	Other features	Useful investigations	Gene	Diagnosis
a.r.	**Other disorders**							
	+	+	–	–	Bone cysts, seizures, postural dyspraxia	MRI: basal ganglia calcification, inc w.m. signal	DAP12 TREM2	PLOSL: Nasu–Hakola disease
	–	+	+	–	Optic atrophy; may have onset with febrile illness or trauma	MRI: very extensive w.m. signal change	Eukaryotic initiation factor 2B	Vanishing white matter disease
Var								
	+	–	+	+	Orofacial dyskinesiae, seizures haemolysis in McLeod syndrome (X-L)	Acanthocytes on wet smears Inc serum CK Kell blood typing (McLeod)	VPS13A chorein/XK protein	Neuro-acanthocytosis

Pathognomonic features in italics.

* Specific treatment available.

§ Many cases represent new mutations.

§§ Mutations in SCA17 and Junctophilin-3 genes can cause a Huntington disease-like phenotype.

** Spastic paraparesis associated with some Presenilin 1 mutations.

abn, abnormal; a.d., autosomal dominant; APP, amyloid precursor protein; a.r., autosomal recessive; Atax, ataxia; bx, biopsy; CADASIL, cerebral autosomal dominant arteriopathy with subcortical infarcts and leukoencephalopathy-; CK, creatinine kinase; CPEO, chronic progressive external ophthalmoplegia; dec, decreased; DM, diabetes mellitus; DRPLA, dentato-rubro-pallido-luyesian atrophy; enz, enzymes; EPS, extrapyramidal syndrome; esp, especially; FTD, frontotemporal dementia; FTDP-17, frontotemporal dementia–parkinsonism linked to chromosome 17; GFAP, glial fibrillary acidic protein; HD, Huntington's disease; inc, increased; LA, lactic acidosis; mat, maternal; neg, negative; PKAN, pantothenate-kinase-associated neurodegeneration; PLOSL, polycystic lipomembranous osteodysplasia with sclerosing leukoencephalopathy; PME, progressive myoclonic epilepsy; PN, peripheral neuropathy; PS, presenilin; PYR, pyramidal signs; SCA, spinocerebellar ataxia; var, variable; VLCFAs, very long-chain fatty acids; WBC, white blood cell; w.m., white matter; X-L, X-linked.

Table 8.9 Diagnosis of some reversible dementia syndromes.

Syndrome/clinical features§	Candidate diagnoses	Relevant investigations
Intracranial space-occupying lesions		
Insidious behavioural change, frontal-executive dysfunction, may have papilloedema, focal neurological signs, seizures Constitutional disturbance, fever, other systemic evidence of infection, immunosuppression (esp HIV)	Intracranial tumour (primary, CNS lymphoma, metastasis), esp frontal lobe, corpus callosum, midbrain* Brain abscess, cysts, other infectious lesions	CT/MRI: focal or multifocal space-occupying lesions Biopsy or resection of lesion May have serological, CXR or other findings; may require biopsy or resection of lesion
History of head trauma (often absent), coagulopathy, altered alertness	Chronic subdural haematoma	CT: subdural haematoma (may be isodense depending on age; may be bilateral)
History of meningitis, subarachnoid haemorrhage; gait apraxia, urinary incontinence, subcortical dementia	Hydrocephalus (any cause)	CT/MRI: findings of hydrocephalus (disproportionate ventricular enlargement) ± causative lesion
CNS vasculitis (various syndromes may occur)		
Rapid course, headache, fluctuation	Primary angiitis of CNS CNS lymphoma, esp intravascular	EEG: slowing of rhythms (non-specific) MRI: ischaemic lesions, signal abnormalities CSF: >3 cells, OCBs Brain biopsy
Systemic features of autoimmune/connective tissue disease (esp lupus, polyarteritis, Wegener's granulomatosis) Fever, other evidence of chronic infection (e.g. varicella zoster)	Vasculitis associated with systemic disorders Vasculitis associated with infection	Inflammatory markers, serological and other investigations, tissue diagnosis (e.g. skin, kidney, lung) CSF: positive PCR May require brain biopsy
Limbic encephalitis		
Memory and behavioural disturbances, fluctuating alertness, confusion, temporal lobe seizures	VGKC Ab syndrome	MRI: abnormal mesial temporal signal EEG: temporal lobe spikes Serum: hyponatraemia (non-specific); VGKC titre CSF: OCBs
May have peripheral neuropathy, ataxia, hypothalamic dysfunction, brainstem signs	Paraneoplastic syndrome*	CSF: pleocytosis, OCBs Antineuronal antibodies (anti-Hu, anti-Ma2), systemic screens for malignancy incl whole body PET, CT
May have systemic features of autoimmune/connective tissue disease	CNS vasculitis (isolated or associated with systemic disorders)	CSF: pleocytosis May require brain biopsy Systemic serological and other investigations, other tissue biopsy (e.g. skin, kidney, lung) if indicated
Acute onset, may have fever, immunosuppression	Infectious encephalitis	CSF: pleocytosis; HSV, HHV6/7 PCR
Epilepsy		
Discrete episodes, fluctuating course, patchy retrograde amnesia	Temporal lobe epilepsy – Transient epileptic amnesia	EEG: epileptiform discharges (esp temporal lobe) MRI: abn mesial temporal signal, hippocampal damage
Refractory seizures increasing in frequency (may be epilepsia partialis continua), lateralised signs	Rasmussen encephalitis*	EEG: lateralised epileptiform discharges MRI: progressive atrophy and abnormal signal involving one cerebral hemisphere

(continued)

Table 8.9 (continued)

Syndrome/clinical features§	Candidate diagnoses	Relevant investigations
Extrapyramidal syndromes		
Tics – motor stereotypies, psychiatric disturbances, may have precipitating factor (e.g. respiratory infection)	ABGA syndrome	MRI: basal ganglia signal change Serum: ABGA titre
Encephalitis lethargica: sleep disturbance, psychiatric disturbances, ocular abnormalities, parkinsonism, dyskinesias; may have precipitating factor (e.g. upper respiratory tract infection)	Encephalitis lethargica* (?post-infectious)	MRI: basal ganglia, thalamic, midbrain signal change CSF: OCBs Serum: ABGA may be positive
Chronic meningitis		
Uveitis, hypothalamic dysfunction, cranial nerve signs or polyradiculopathy, systemic features; often recurrent episodes	Neurosarcoidosis	CXR: various patterns MRI: w.m. lesions ± meningeal enhancement CSF: lymphocytic meningitis
Oral and genital ulcers, uveitis, rash, posterior circulation strokes, racial predilection (especially Turkish/Japanese)	Behçet disease	MRI: brainstem, basal ganglia lesions CSF: lymphocytic meningitis
May have evidence of primary tumour; headache, confusion, cranial nerve and radicular signs	Carcinomatous/lymphomatous/ leukaemic	CT/MRI: may have mass lesions CSF: cytology, immunophenotyping (may need several)
Immunosuppression (incl HIV), systemic features, may have cranial nerve signs, strokes; travel, occupational exposures	TB/fungal/'atypical' infectious agents	CXR: frequently abnormal CT/MRI: meningeal enhancement, may have hydrocephalus, mass lesions (tuberculoma) CSF: lymphocytic meningitis, AFB and fungal cultures, cryptococcal Ag
Tick bite/travel to endemic area, skin lesion, arthritis, may have radiculopathies/ mononeuropathies/encephalomyelitis	Lyme disease (neuroborreliosis)	Serum: Lyme serology (may be negative) CSF: pleocytosis (may be absent), Lyme serology
Argyll Robertson pupils (light-near dissociation), strokes, dorsal column signs (tabes dorsalis), HIV infection	Neurosyphilis	Serum: treponemal serology CSF: pleocytosis, treponemal serology
Infectious syndromes with posterior hemisphere signs		
Adolescent or young adult, history of measles, rapid course, florid myoclonus and seizures	SSPE*	EEG: periodic burst-suppression CSF: OCBs (measles-specific Ab)
Immunosuppression/haematological malignancies, often hemiparesis, ataxia	PML*	MRI: confluent posterior w.m. changes CSF: JC virus PCR
Other infectious syndromes		
HIV risk factors, AIDS-related illnesses, advanced immunosuppression, gait disorder, seizures	HIV (AIDS–dementia complex)	MRI: confluent w.m. changes Serum: HIV serology, low CD4 count
Arthralgia, gut symptoms, facial movement disorder (oculomasticatory myorrhythmia), supranuclear gaze palsy, myoclonus	Whipple's disease of CNS	CSF: Whipple PCR Duodenal biopsy
Acquired metabolic disturbances		
History of poor nutrition, food faddism, vegan, features of malabsorption; specific features (e.g. Wernicke–Korsakoff, pellagra)	Nutritional deficiency states	Dietary assessment, nutritional and malabsorption (incl coeliac) screens, empirical therapy (e.g. thiamine)

Table 8.9 (continued)

Syndrome/clinical features§	Candidate diagnoses	Relevant investigations
Clinical features of endocrine dysfunction	Endocrinopathies	
Clinical features of organ failure; organ transplantation	Uraemia Hepatic encephalopathy Pancreatic encephalopathy Cardiorespiratory failure	Biochemical and metabolic screens, organ-specific imaging findings
Obesity, morning headaches, daytime somnolence, snoring	Obstructive sleep apnoea	Sleep study
Toxicological exposures		
Alcohol dependence, may have cerebellar ataxia, peripheral neuropathy, features of Wernicke–Korsakoff encephalopathy	Alcoholic dementia*	Co-morbidities: nutritional screens, liver function tests, brain imaging (exclude SDH)
History of heroin inhalation ('chasing the dragon'), parkinsonism, ataxia, cortico-spinal signs, subacute encephalopathy	Pyrolysate encephalopathy	MRI: diffuse w.m. increased signal sparing U fibres (esp posteriorly)
Polypharmacy, recent changes in therapy, culprit agents	Iatrogenic	Medication review
Suspicion of overt or covert poisoning (e.g. occupational/environmental, recreational drugs, self-harm), specific systemic features; specific neurological syndromes may occur (e.g. vasculitis with cocaine, amphetamines)	Environmental poisons (e.g. carbon monoxide, heavy metals, solvents, herbicides), illicit drugs	Specific urine and blood screens if available, other specific findings (e.g. blood picture, EMG)

* Limited potential for reversibility.

§ Rapid course in many.

Ab, antibody; ABGA, antibasal ganglia syndrome; abn, abnormal; Ag, antigen; CXR, chest X-ray; esp, especially; HHV, human herpes virus; HSV, herpes simplex virus; incl, including; OCB, oligoclonal band; PCR, polymerase chain reaction; PML, progressive multifocal leukoencephalopathy; SDH, subdural haematoma; SSPE, subacute sclerosing panencephalitis; VGKC, voltage-gated potassium channel antibodies; w.m., white matter.

The potential for cognitive deficits following surgical resections for intractable epilepsy (chiefly, temporal lobectomy) has long been recognised and must be taken into account during surgical planning and preoperative studies of the lateralisation of cognitive functions (especially language and memory).

A number of disorders predispose to the development of both cognitive dysfunction and seizures: examples include intoxications and drug withdrawal (notably alcohol), intracranial infections, head trauma, stroke, intracranial space-occupying lesions, cerebral vasculitis and degenerative dementias including AD (generally later in their course). In such disorders, care is needed to distinguish the cognitive effects of seizures from the underlying disease process. Complex partial seizures frequently accompany limbic encephalitis, whether infectious, paraneoplastic or autoimmune. Certain epilepsy syndromes are integral to primary disease processes that also produce progressive cognitive decline: these include epilepsia partialis continua in Rasmussen's encephalitis and progressive myoclonic epilepsy in neuronal storage diseases associated with inborn errors of metabolism (Table 8.8).

Limbic encephalitis

Limbic encephalitis (LE) is typically considered to be a subacute encephalopathy characterised by short-term memory impairment, confusion, alteration of consciousness, complex partial temporal lobe seizures and psychiatric syndromes. While it is mandatory always to consider, exclude and where doubt remains treat for infectious causes, including herpes simplex encephalitis (Chapter 9), classically LE is considered in the context of autoimmunity. LE was initially described as a paraneoplastic phenomenon associated with small cell bronchial (50%), testicular (>20%) and breast tumours (>13%). Several specific autoantibodies are recognised in this context, including *ANNA1 (anti-Hu)* in bronchial small cell carcinoma; *Anti-Ma2 (anti-Ta)* in testicular tumour; *CRMP5/(anti-CV2)* in lymphoma, thymoma, bronchial small cell carcinoma; *ANNA3* in bronchial small cell carcinoma; and *N type VGCC* in bronchial small cell carcinoma and breast tumours. Paraneoplastic LE is usually associated with the subacute (weeks to months) onset of anterograde memory impairment, temporal lobe seizures and psychiatric symptoms (particularly depression, aggressive psychosis, hallucinations and personality change). There may be other associated constitutional symptoms resulting from the underlying cancer, and other specific neurological features depending on the particular antibody (e.g. brainstem and eye movement abnormalities are common with *Ma2*). The MRI in paraneoplastic LE typically shows non-enhancing increased signal in the mesial temporal lobes, which can undergo prominent atrophy as the disease progresses. The EEG shows diffuse slowing with epileptiform discharges and there is a CSF pleocytosis and elevated protein in the majority. Serum antineuronal antibodies are not detected in approximately 40% of cases of histologically proven paraneoplastic LE, and it is important therefore that the diagnosis should not rely on their identification. In the majority (approximately 60%) of cases, the neurological presentation antedates the diagnosis of cancer and usually occurs in the absence of local or distant spread, emphasising the importance of early diagnosis. While a neoplasm may be identifiable on examination – underscoring the importance of a thorough physical examination including the breasts and testes in rapid and unusual dementia syndromes – occult tumours may be very difficult to detect. CT scanning, mammography or ultrasound of testicles/ovaries may detect tumours, supplemented where available by whole body FDG-PET which is very sensitive at detecting occult glucose-avid malignancy. The mechanism of paraneoplastic LE is unclear but is probably related to cell-mediated immunity developing against cancer cells. Paraneoplastic LE may improve following removal of the primary tumour usually with immunosuppression but there is often a considerable residual cognitive impairment and seizures may persist.

While classic antibody mediated syndromes including CNS vasculitis, Susac's syndrome, lupus cerebritis, Sjögren's syndrome and antiphospholipid syndrome may cause cognitive syndromes, over the last decade or so a number of novel antibodies directed against cell-surface antigens have been specifically associated with autoimmune encephalitis. Antibodies against the voltage-gated potassium channel complex are associated with a variety of peripheral hyperexcitability syndromes including cramp fasciculation syndrome and autoimmune neuromyotonia. In Morvan's syndrome, as well as these peripheral features, there is additional CNS involvement, with severe insomnia, seizures, hyperhidrosis, autonomic instability and subacute encephalopathy, often in association with thymoma. Recently it has emerged that antibodies directed against the VGKC complex are more frequently associated with limbic encephalitis, without peripheral manifestations and usually without an underlying tumour. Patients with significantly elevated (e.g. >400 pM, NR <100 pM) VGKC complex antibodies typically present in middle age, males more affected than females, with a subacute onset of behavioural changes, seizures and amnesia. MRI scanning typically but not always shows high signal change in medial temporal lobe structures, there is often significant and treatment resistant hyponatraemia, with normal CSF. Untreated, a significant proportion of patients will develop irreversible cognitive impairment, including an unusual, temporally ungraded dense retrograde amnesia, which may be prevented by prompt recognition and treatment with immune suppression (typically plasma exchange/IVIg followed by steroids). However, some patients may present with *formes frustes*, including REM behaviour disorder and unusual seizures, which may resolve spontaneously. Recent work has demonstrated a number of specific antigenic targets within the VGKC complex which begin to explain the phenotypic diversity: thus, patients with antibodies against the Lgi1 subunits of the channel are most likely to have 'classic' LE with signal change and hyponatraemia, and importantly may present with brief, frequent jerks of the face and hand (so-called faciobrachial dystonic jerks) preceding the development of cognitive impairment. Conversely, individuals with CASPR2 antibodies are more likely to have peripheral manifestations, although they can also have LE.

A distinct neuropsychiatric syndrome with antibodies directed against the NMDA receptor was first described in 2007 in young women with ovarian teratomas presenting with behavioural change, amnesia, movement disorders including choreoathetoid movements and orofacial dyskinesia, and autonomic disturbance including hypoventilation. The phenotype of this syndrome has since expanded to include women with teratomas or other tumours, men and children; and to include a variety of different cognitive and neuropsychiatric phenotypes including late onset psychosis. As with VGKC complex antibody encephalitis, recognition of this syndrome should prompt a hunt for an occult neoplasm, as resection (with immunosuppression) can result in dramatic improvements. Non-paraneoplastic cases can respond very well to treatment with immunosuppression, although there is a risk of relapse. A number of other antibodies including GAD, glycine and GABA-B antibodies have rarely been associated with autoimmune encephalitis.

Infective, metabolic, toxic and other causes of dementia

Cognitive dysfunction is a frequent accompaniment of infective, metabolic and toxic disorders, whether systemic or restricted to the CNS. The primary disorders are dealt with at greater length in Chapters 9 and 19: here, basic principles relating to their effects on cognition are summarised. In the majority of cases, cognitive decline is acute and manifests as a delirium; however, in a smaller proportion an insidious deterioration ensues which may be difficult to distinguish from more common degenerative causes of dementia. The exact pathophysiology of cognitive decline is poorly understood in many cases and is probably multifactorial. The cognitive profile itself is rarely diagnostic, and indeed remains poorly characterised for many of the disorders in this large and diverse group. Posterior hemisphere signs may be prominent in some conditions, such as progressive multifocal leukoencephalopathy and subacute sclerosing panencephalitis. However, most diseases in this group can produce a variable combination of behavioural and executive deficits, often with bradyphrenia: the pattern of a subcortical dementia. General clues that one may be dealing with a disease process in one of these categories include an aggressive course, evidence of active systemic disease and younger age. Risk factor profiles based on ethnic or geographical origin (many of these diseases are more common in poorer populations), occupational, travel or sexual habits, clinical infection or infectious contacts, immunosuppression or toxic exposures may raise suspicion of a particular cause. Impairment of cognition in patients with HIV is common and is known as HIV-associated neurocognitive disorder (HAND). In the early days of the HIV epidemic, prior to the introduction of combination antiretroviral therapy (cART), a subcortical dementia (AIDS dementia complex) would often develop, characterised by cognitive slowing and impaired attention and concentration in the early stages. Despite the introduction of cART, the overall prevalence of cognitive impairment has been relatively unchanged, seen in around a half of all patients, but in the cART era the majority of patients have mild cognitive impairment rather than dementia. Current criteria separate asymptomatic neurocognitive impairment from mild neurocognitive disorder (both defined as scoring one standard deviation below the mean in two cognitive domains but with no impairment in activities of daily living in the former). HIV-associated dementia (HAD) (defined as scoring two standard deviations below the mean in two cognitive domains with impairment of ADLs) is much less common and generally has a different cognitive profile now than in the pre-cART era, with more cortical (rather than subcortical) impairment, often with memory problems predominating. Characteristic and discriminating clinical features and investigations for some of these diseases are summarised in Table 8.3.

Controversial entities

A number of conditions often listed as causes of dementia continue to arouse controversy, because of uncertainty regarding the pathogenetic mechanism or the validity of the association with cognitive decline.

In addition to its well-recognised acute effects on cognition and behaviour, alcohol has an established association with dementia and forms a high proportion of young onset cases in community-based series. However, it is often unclear to what extent cognitive decline in an individual patient is attributable to the toxic effects of ethanol *per se* rather than associated factors such as malnutrition (in particular, thiamine deficiency and Wernicke–Korsakoff syndrome), concomitant drug use, hepatic encephalopathy and other associated medical conditions, head trauma or the interaction of multiple factors. Marchiafava–Bignami disease, a rare degeneration of the corpus callosum, was described initially in male Italian red wine drinkers but is likely to be the result of an uncharacterised nutritional deficiency or osmotic dysmyelination. On balance, it is likely that chronic heavy alcohol intake can itself produce a dementia that includes frontal deficits and difficulty with complex learning and which is accompanied by generalised cerebral atrophy. Improvement in cognitive function may occur with prolonged abstinence, although little information is available concerning the time course or extent of this. A variety of neuropathological changes have been described in alcoholics, including cortical neuronal loss and gliosis, cerebellar degeneration, and atherosclerosis; however, none could be considered pathognomonic. In some cases, alcoholism can be the result of behavioural change caused by an alternate cause of dementia.

Head trauma is linked with 'dementia pugilistica', a syndrome of cognitive deterioration, behavioural change and parkinsonism of variable severity that is observed in boxers and other individuals who have sustained significant repeated head injuries. Pathologically, dementia pugilistica shares many features with AD, and indeed head injury is a risk factor for later development of AD in epidemiological studies. The level of risk is influenced by the severity and tempo of the injury (greater with loss of consciousness and with repeated insults) and possibly *ApoE* status (greater in those with the e4 allele).

The association between dementia and common autoimmune disorders such as Hashimoto's thyroidopathy and coeliac disease is not straightforward. Such diseases may lead to cognitive deterioration secondary to a systemic disturbance such as hypothyroidism or malabsorption. The key issue concerns the potential pathogenetic role of autoantibodies in causing cognitive decline in such disorders. Despite a growing literature on 'Hashimoto encephalopathy' its nosological status remains to be defined, although there is growing consensus that thyroid antibodies are not causative. While the aetiology remains unclear, it is important to exclude other treatable processes (e.g. cerebral vasculitis or VGKC complex or NMDA-antibody associated syndromes) in all suspected cases of Hashimoto's encephalopathy.

Normal pressure hydrocephalus (NPH) is considered here insofar as it has been overdiagnosed in patients presenting with cognitive impairment. It is traditionally listed as a cause of reversible dementia, heralded by a clinical triad of gait apraxia, urinary incontinence and cognitive decline. However, the validity of the term has been criticised. NPH appears to be an idiopathic communicating hydrocephalus in a high proportion of cases, although it may follow arachnoiditis, subarachnoid haemorrhage or head trauma. Impaired CSF resorption at the arachnoid granulations is most often proposed as the pathogenetic mechanism. Supportive radiological features include ventricular enlargement that is disproportionate to the degree of gyral atrophy, occluded cortical sulci, prominence of the third and fourth ventricles with no macroscopic evidence of ventricular obstruction, and (on MRI) an aqueductal CSF flow void. The demonstration of normal CSF pressure and clinical improvement following removal of a diagnostic aliquot of CSF are put forward as additional criteria for the diagnosis. This can be supplemented by prolonged monitoring to document phasic increases in CSF pressure, CSF conductance studies or cisternography. Although the potential for improvement following surgical insertion of a CSF shunt has often been emphasised, the relationship between NPH and cognitive decline, as opposed to gait impairment, remains unclear. 'Pure' NPH is uncommon. Many patients diagnosed with NPH have changes of small vessel disease and/or AD at postmortem, and it has been shown that patients with AD may improve transiently following ventricular drainage (the mechanism is not clear). Patients with 'idiopathic' NPH, long-standing symptoms, established dementia, or radiological evidence of significant cerebral atrophy or cerebrovascular disease generally fail to improve cognitively following CSF shunting. The shunt procedure itself carries a significant risk of complications such as subdural haematoma in this population. It may be helpful to use molecular means (CSF or amyloid PET) to determine the extent of Alzheimer-related pathology in such patients, as there is evidence that individuals with AD pathology have a poor prognosis following shunting.

Management of dementia

Risk factor management

The greatest risk factor for development of dementia is age. However, there are several modifiable risk factors. Moderate exercise reduces the risk of dementia as does modification of vascular risk factors: obesity, hypercholesterolaemia, diabetes, hypertension and smoking.

Co-morbidity

Delirium is often a harbinger of dementia and patients with dementia have a lower threshold for developing delirium and will take longer to recover than those who are cognitively normal. The usual causes apply, such as infection (usually involving the urinary or respiratory tract), metabolic/biochemical derangement, hypoxic/ischaemic damage or medication. These should all be excluded as a cause and treated actively if identified. Multiple drugs can have a significant adverse effect on cognition.

Depression is both an important treatable cause and compounding feature of dementia, occurring in up to 20% of individuals with AD, vascular dementia and DLB. Over 50% of patients with dementia experience depressive symptoms at some stage. Symptoms should be actively sought and treated in any patient at presentation and during the course of their illness. Tricyclics should be avoided because of their anticholinergic effects. Selective serotonin reuptake inhibitors (SSRIs) are also preferable in FTD, as they may be effective in modifying the behavioural symptoms, in addition to any depressive symptoms. As in all patients, side effects should be looked for and response monitored.

Epileptic seizures occur in patients with dementia more frequently than among healthy elderly individuals. The incidence of seizures among patients with dementia varies with the aetiology of the dementing illness. In patients with AD, approximately 10–20%

have at least one seizure. Seizures usually occur several years post diagnosis, in moderate to severe AD. There is an increased incidence in early onset AD, especially with *PSEN1* mutations. The incidence of seizures in other dementing diseases is less clear. Diagnosis can be delayed by difficulty in description as a result of cognitive impairment. The potential cognitive adverse effects of some antiepileptic drugs must be taken into consideration, and the lowest effective dosage should be used.

The majority of patients with dementia are cared for in the community, at home or in nursing homes. Up to 30% of patients in UK nursing homes have received antipsychotic drugs, usually neuroleptics, although their use is steadily declining. In dementia, particularly DLB, these drugs can have catastrophic consequences; atypical antipsychotics should be used in preference. Even these are not free of the risk of increasing side effects and confusion, therefore treatment titration must be cautious. It is also important to remember the reported increase in stroke risk with risperidone and olanzapine.

Behavioural management

Coping on a daily basis with challenging behaviour is a major burden for the carer of a patient with dementia. In the early stages, the major behavioural changes are seen in FTD, but other disorders may also produce significant behavioural problems at some stage. The loss of insight seen in some diseases, combined with the change in personality and disinhibition, have a huge impact on the carer, causing strain on the relationship and loss of sense of control. Another problem apparent in mild dementia is significant anxiety, which also may exacerbate behavioural problems.

In more severe dementia, a multidisciplinary assessment is required for behavioural modification. This approach tends to be most successful in patients in nursing homes. Behavioural modification may be achieved by altering the environment, if there is an external precipitant, or by conditioning techniques with positive reinforcement. Strategies may improve performance, for example scheduled toileting or prompted voiding can reduce urinary incontinence. Playing music during meals and bathing can reduce disruptive behaviour. Exercise, massage and pet therapy have all been used to reduce abnormal behaviours.

Hallucinations often occur at home in dimly lit surroundings ('sundowning') and improved lighting may help; as always, intercurrent infections and drugs should be considered as possible exacerbating factors.

Patients may become irritable or angry at being disturbed at times of washing, dressing or eating. A considered response is needed, with maintenance of a respectful friendly approach, removal of exacerbating factors and consideration of behavioural measures such as distraction or 'time out'.

Sleep cycle is often very disturbed – patients may be up all night and sleep all day. This can be extremely distressing for carers. It is important to exclude delirium, and to ensure structure and rewarding activities during the day. A routine should be established with a fixed bedtime, no stimulants and meal before sleep. If these fail, it is reasonable to provide a trial of medication, such as an anxiolytic.

Urinary and faecal incontinence may become a problem for multiple reasons: medical causes such as diabetes mellitus, or cortical loss of bladder control, reduced mobility; or cognitive causes such as poor recognition, disorientation or impaired planning. In addition to prompt treatment of medical problems such as urinary tract infections, simple physical measures can make a significant difference. Regular visits can reduce the likelihood of accidents; avoidance of bedtime drinks, labelling of the toilet to provide cues and the use of incontinence pads all help. Pharmacological therapies (Chapter 25) may help, but have the potential for worsening confusion and need to be monitored closely.

Safety

Patients with mild to moderate dementia usually function best in familiar surroundings. It is important to create an appropriate, safe and supportive environment to encourage optimal function. A home safety evaluation and appropriate modifications should be organised. For example, signs may be placed around the house to orientate patients.

Patients may become increasingly unstable on walking, yet be unaware of this because of their cognitive impairment. Wandering is a frequent problem, often associated with lack of stimulation and ensuing frustration. Behavioural measures such as increasing interaction, providing stimulation at day centres, encouraging exercise and increasing the structure of the day may help. At times, locking doors is the only solution.

In patients with significant orobuccal apraxia (e.g. in progressive non-fluent aphasia), a feeding nasogastric tube, or even a percutaneous endoscopic gastrostomy, may be required. Patients and family may opt not to have this, but discussion is important. Broaching the subject early in the course of the illness, if swallow is involved, will enable the patient and carers to make an informed decision.

As dementia progresses, increasing supervision is necessary, eventually becoming continuous. This curtails the carer's ability to continue working, and progressively reduces their independence. Day care centres can provide release for the carers during the week and give structure to the patient.

The issue of fitness to drive creates enormous anxiety for the patient diagnosed with dementia, who perceives removal of a licence as a loss of independence. Driving for patients with frontal impairment can be particularly difficult because of their lack of insight and poor judgement, and families often have difficulty in persuading patients to stop. In contrast, patients with AD often progressively curtail their driving activities as they realise they or their relatives feel unsafe. It is difficult to determine at what point an individual becomes sufficiently impaired to cease driving, and the relationship between the severity of dementia and driving abilities is complex. The UK driving licence law states that if at any time the licence holder becomes aware that he/she has a disability he/she must inform the driver and vehicle licensing authority (DVLA). The guidelines state that in general a patient able to attend to day-to-day needs, with adequate insight and judgement, and not disorientated in time or place may be fit to drive. A licence may be issued on a yearly basis with reassessment on each renewal. If in doubt, assessment at a mobility centre may be required; if serious doubt exists a medical adviser at the DVLA may require a test to be taken.

In practical terms, the issue must be discussed with the patient and family once a diagnosis of dementia is made. The patient should be reminded of their legal obligation to inform the DVLA. If the patient and family do not inform the DVLA, and the physician is concerned, then he/she can inform the DVLA directly. Each case is individual, and the discussion should include carers and the patient.

Caring for the carer

In the United Kingdom and the United States, 33–60% of carers of patients with dementia are spouses over 75 years, of whom 75% are women. This profile, and the perception of the role of a carer, varies across cultures and socio-economic groups. In most of the Western world, where the extended family is small or may not exist, the burden of caring can be very high, often focusing almost entirely on a single, often elderly individual.

Compared with age-matched non-carer controls, carers have problems in several areas:

- Depression, stress, low self-esteem and poorer sense of well-being are common and are more severe in young onset dementia and if the premorbid relationship was ambivalent.
- Carers experience poorer physical health, with higher levels of chronic conditions, more drug prescriptions and GP attendances and poorer self-perception of health.
- Social isolation is frequent as carers have less time for themselves for hobbies and going out, and may have difficulty coping with social embarrassment caused by the patient's behaviour.
- The cost of nursing, respite care and lost earnings should not be underestimated, and often has a huge impact on quality of life, compounding the above factors.

This complex relationship requires both formal support from professionals and informal support from friends and relatives. The carer's needs change through the evolution of the illness and often continue after the death of the patient. Local support groups and national associations are extremely important in this regard.

Planning for the future and end of life issues

If no will is in existence, this should be discussed amongst the family. In order to make a will the patient needs to understand what they are doing and the effect it will have: what they have to leave, and who might make claims on it. Advanced directives concerning treatment should also be considered when patients are competent.

In the later stages of dementia the individual becomes totally dependent in activities of daily living, needing continuous nursing care. Profound loss of memory may lead to inability to recognise familiar surroundings or family and friends. Almost all comprehensible speech may be lost. There are particular issues that emerge at this stage, many with ethical implications, including whether to place the patient in institutional care. Important issues in any setting include:

- *Feeding* Swallowing may be difficult and good nutrition becomes a priority. Individuals at this stage need speech therapist assessment of swallowing, dietitian advice on nutrition and consultation with family as to when and if to institute feeding devices.
- *Medical treatment* Weight loss and immobility contribute to vulnerability to pressure sores and infection. Issues of withholding life-prolonging curative treatment, including cardiorespiratory resuscitation, need to be discussed with the family.
- *Postmortem diagnosis and brain donation* Clinical diagnostic accuracy in patients with dementia is at best 70–80%. Postmortem neuropathological examination can provide an accurate diagnosis with potentially important aetiological information for familial diseases. Families often gain benefit from contributing to research from tissue donation. Examination of the brain and use of tissue, however, can only be performed with written informed consent from the next of kin, even in the case of a coroner's postmortem.

References

Bartolomeo P, Thiebaut de Schotten M, Chica AB. Brain networks of visuospatial attention and their disruption in visual neglect. *Front Hum Neurosci* 2012; **6:** 110. doi:10.3389/fnhum.2012.00110.

Emre M, Aarsland D, Brown R, Burn DJ, Duyckaerts C, Mizuno Y, *et al.* Clinical diagnostic criteria for dementia associated with Parkinson's disease. *Mov Disord* 2007; **22:** 1689–1707. doi: 10.1002/mds.21507.

Karran E, Mercken M, De Strooper B, The amyloid cascade hypothesis for Alzheimer's disease: an appraisal for the development of therapeutics. *Nat Rev Drug Discov* 2011; **10:** 698–712.

Litvan I, Aarsland D, Adler CH. MDS task force on mild cognitive impairment in Parkinson's disease: Critical review of PD-MCI. *Mov Disord* 2011; **26:** 1814–1824. doi: 10.1002/mds.23823.

McKeith IG, Dickson DW, Lowe J, Emre M, O'Brien JT, Feldman H, *et al.* Consortium on DLB. Diagnosis and management of dementia with Lewy bodies - Third report of the DLB consortium. *Neurology* 2005; **65:** 1863–1872.

Omar R, Warren JD, Ron MA, Lees Aj, Rossor MN, Kartsounis LD. The neurobehavioural syndrome of brainstem disease. *Neurocase* 2007; **13:** 452–465.

Warren JD, Rohrer JD, Rossor MN. Frontotemporal dementia. *BMJ* 2013; **347:** f4827.

Warrington EK, James M. Disorders of visual perception in patients with localised cerebral lesions. *Neuropsychologia* 1967; **5:** 253–266.

Further reading

Epidemiology

Lambert MA, Bickel H, Prince M, Fratiglioni L, Von Strauss E, Frydecka D, *et al.* Estimating the burden of early onset dementia; systematic review of disease prevalence. *Eur J Neurol* 2014; **21:** 563–569. doi: 10.1111/ene.12325. Epub 2014 Jan 13. Review.

Matthews FE, Arthur A, Barnes LE, Bond J, Jagger C, Robinson L, *et al.* Medical Research Council Cognitive Function and Ageing Collaboration. A two-decade comparison of prevalence of dementia in individuals aged 65 years and older from three geographical areas of England: results of the Cognitive Function and Ageing Study I and II. *Lancet* 2013; **382:** 1405–1412. doi: 10.1016/S0140-6736(13)61570-6. Epub 2013 Jul 17.

Prince M, Bryce R, Albanese E, Wimo A, Ribeiro W, Ferri CP. The global prevalence of dementia: a systematic review and metaanalysis. *Alzheimers Dement* 2013; **9:** 63–75. e2. doi: 10.1016/j.jalz.2012.11.007. Review.

Qiu C, De Ronchi D, Fratiglioni L. The epidemiology of the dementias: an update. *Curr Opin Psychiatry* 2007; **20:** 380–385.

Cognitive function and clinical syndromes

Inouye SK, Marcantonio ER. Delirium. In: Blue Books of Neurology: The Dementias II. Growdon JH, Rossor MN, eds. Philadelphia: Butterworth Heinemann, 2007: 329–380.

Omar R, Warren JD, Ron MA, Lees Aj, Rossor MN, Kartsounis LD. The neuro-behavioural syndrome of brainstem disease. *Neurocase* 2007; **13:** 452–465.

Warrington EK, James M. Disorders of visual perception in patients with localised cerebral lesions. *Neuropsychologia* 1967; **5:** 253–266.

Warren JD, Warrington EK. Cognitive neuropsychology of dementia syndromes. In: *Blue Books of Neurology: The Dementias II.* Growdon JH, Rossor MN, eds. Philadelphia: Butterworth Heinemann, 2007: 329–380.

Investigations

Ahmed RM, Paterson RW, Warren JD, Zetterberg H, O'Brien JT, Fox NC, Halliday GM, Schott JM. Biomarkers in dementia: clinical utility and new directions. *J Neurol Neurosurg Psychiatry* 2014; **85:** 1426–1434. doi: 10.1136/jnnp-2014-307662

Blackwell AD, Sahakian BJ, Vesey R, Semple JM, Robbins TW, Hodges JR. Detecting dementia: novel neuropsychological markers of preclinical Alzheimer's disease. *Dement Geriatr Cogn Disord* 2004; **17:** 42–48.

Harper L, Barkhof F, Scheltens P, Schott JM, Fox NC. An algorithmic approach to structural imaging in dementia. *J Neurol Neurosurg Psychiatry* 2014; **85**: 69208. doi:10.1136/jnnp-2013-306285.

Mattsson N, Zetterberg H, Hansson O, Andreasen N, Parnetti L, Jonsson M, *et al.* CSF biomarkers and incipient Alzheimer disease in patients with mild cognitive impairment. *JAMA* 2009; **302:** 385–393.

Nordberg A. Dementia in 2014: Towards early diagnosis in Alzheimer disease. *Nat Rev Neurol* 2015; **11:** 69–70. doi:10.1038/nrneurol.2014.257

Waldemar G, Dubois B, Emre M, Georges J, McKeith IG, Rossor M, *et al.* Recommendations for the diagnosis and management of Alzheimer's disease and other disorders associated with dementia: EFNS guideline. *Eur J Neurol* 2007; **14:** 1–26.

Alzheimer's disease

Albert MS, DeKosky ST, Dickson D, Dubois B, Feldman HH, Fox NC, *et al.* The diagnosis of mild cognitive impairment due to Alzheimer's disease: recommendations from the National Institute on Ageing – Alzheimer's Association workgroups on diagnostic guideines for Alzheimer's diease. *Alzheimers Dement* 2011; **7:** 270–279.

Dubois B, Feldman HH, Jacova C, Hampel H, Molinuevo JL, Blennow K, *et al.* Advancing research diagnostic criteria for Alzheimer's disease: the IWG-2 criteria. *Lancet Neurol* 2014; **13**: 614–629. doi: 10.1016/S1474-4422(14)70090-0. Erratum in: *Lancet Neurol* 2014; **13:** 757.

Hannson O, Zetterberg H, Buchhave P, Londos E, Blennow K, Minthon L. Association between CSF biomarkers and incipient Alzheimer's disease in patients with mild cognitive impairment: a follow-up study. *Lancet Neurol* 2006; **5**: 228–234.

Knopman DS, DeKosky ST, Cummings JL, Chui H, Corey-Bloom J, Relkin N, *et al.* Practice parameter: diagnosis of dementia. *Neurology* 2001; **56**: 1143–1153.

Schott JM, Kennedy J, Fox NC. New developments in mild cognitive impairment and Alzheimer's disease. *Curr Opin Neurol* 2006; **19**: 552–558.

Frontotemporal lobar degeneration

Baker M, Mackenzie IR, Pickering-Brown SM, Gass J, Rademakers R, Lindholm C, *et al.* Mutations in progranulin cause tau-negative frontotemporal dementia linked to chromosome 17. *Nature* 2006; **442:** 916–919.

Chan D, Walters RJ, Sampson EL, Schott JM, Smith SJ, Rossor MN. EEG abnormalities in frontotemporal lobar degeneration. *Neurology* 2004; **62:** 1628–1630.

Gorno-Tempini ML, Hillis AE, Weintraub S, Kertesz A, Mendez M, Cappa SF, *et al.* Classification of primary progressive aphasia and its variants. *Neurology* 2011; **76:** 1006–1014.

Hodges JR, Davies R, Xuereb J, Kril J, Halliday G. Survival in frontotemporal dementia. *Neurology* 2003; **61:** 349–354.

Rascovsky K, Hodges JR, Knopman D, Mendez MF, Kramer JH, Neuhaus J, *et al.* Sensitivity of revised diagnostic criteria for the behavioural variant of frontotemporal dementia. *Brain* 2011; **134** (Pt 9): 2456–2477.

Renton AE, Majounie E, Waite A, Simón-Sánchez J, Rollinson S, Gibbs JR, *et al.* A hexanucleotide repeat expansion in C9ORF72 is the cause of chromosome 9p21-linked ALS-FTD. *Neuron* 2011; **72:** 257–268.

Rohrer JD, Lashley T, Schott JM, Warren JE, Mead S, Isaacs AM, *et al.* Clinical and neuroanatomical signatures of tissue pathology in frontotemporal lobar degeneration. *Brain* 2011; **134** (Pt 9): 2565–2581.

Rohrer JD, Guerreiro R, Vandrovcova J, Uphill J, Reiman D, Beck J, *et al.* The heritability and genetics of frontotemporal lobar degeneration. *Neurology* 2009; **73:** 1451–1456.

Warren JD, Rohrer JD, Rossor MN. Frontotemporal dementia. *BMJ* 2013; **347:** f4827. doi: 10.1136/bmj.f4827 PMID 23920254.

Vascular cognitive impairment

Gorelick PB, Pantoni L Advances in vascular cognitive impairment. *Stroke* 2013; **44:** 307–308. doi: 10.1161/STROKEAHA.111.000219. Epub 2013 Jan 15.

Markus HS, Martin RJ, Simpson MA, Dong YB, Ali N, Crosby AH, *et al.* Diagnostic strategies in CADASIL. *Neurology* 2002; **59**: 1134–1138.

O'Brien JT, Erkinjuntti T, Reisberg B, Roman G, Sawada T, Pantoni L, *et al.* Vascular cognitive impairment. *Lancet Neurol* 2003; **2**: 89–98.

O'Sullivan M. *Leukoaraiosis. Pract Neurol* 2008; **8**: 26–38.

Revesz T, Ghiso J, Lashley T, Plant G, Rostagno A, Frangione B, *et al.* Cerebral amyloid angiopathies: a pathologic, biochemical, and genetic view. *J Neuropathol Exp Neurol* 2003; **62**: 885–898.

Selnes OA, Vinters HV. Vascular cognitive impairment. *Nat Clin Pract Neurol* 2006; **2**: 538–547.

Warren JD, Thompson PD. Diencephalic amnesia and apraxia after left thalamic infarction. *J Neurol Neurosurg Psychiatry* 2000; **68**: 248.

Parkinson's disease dementia and dementia with Lewy bodies

Burn DJ. Cortical Lewy body disease and Parkinson's disease dementia. *Curr Opin Neurol* 2006; **19**: 572–579.

Emre M, Aarsland D, Brown R, Burn DJ, Duyckaerts C, Mizuno Y, *et al.* Clinical diagnostic criteria for dementia associated with Parkinson's disease. *Mov Disord* 2007; **22:** 1689–1707.

Litvan I, Aarsland D, Adler CH, Goldman JG, Kulisevsky J, Mollenhauer B, *et al.* MDS Task Force on mild cognitive impairment in Parkinson's disease: critical review of PD-MCI. *Mov Disord* 2011; **26:** 1814–1824.

McKeith I, Mintzer J, Aarsland D, Burn D, Cohen-Mansfield J, Dickson D, *et al.* Dementia with Lewy bodies. *Lancet Neurol* 2004; **3**: 19–28.

McKeith IG, Dickson DW, Lowe J, Emre M, O'Brien JT, Feldman H, *et al.* Diagnosis and management of dementia with Lewy bodies: third report of the DLB Consortium. *Neurology* 2005; **65**: 1863–1872.

Poewe W. When a Parkinson's disease patient starts to hallucinate. *Pract Neurol* 2008; **8:** 238–241.

Svenninsson P, Westman E, Ballard C, Aarsland D. Cognitive impairment in patients with Parkinson's disease: diagnosis, biomarkers and treatment. *Lancet Neurol* 2012; **11:** 697–707.

Dementia in young adults: general

Guerreiro R, Wojtas A, Bras J, Carrasquillo M, Rogaeva E, Majounie E, *et al.* TREM2 variants in Alzheimer's disease. *N Engl J Med* 2013; **368:** 117–127.

Rossor MN, Fox NC, Mummery CJ, Schott JM, Warren JD. The diagnosis of young onset dementia. *Lancet Neurology* 2010; **9**:793–806

Others

Armstrong CL, Gyato K, Awadalla AW, Lustig R, Tochner ZA. A critical review of the clinical effects of therapeutic irradiation damage to the brain. *Neuropsychol Rev* 2004; **14**: 65–86.

Buckley C, Vincent A. Autoimmune channelopathies. *Nat Clin Pract Neurol* 2005; **1**: 22–33.

Chan D, Henley SM, Rossor MN, Warrington EK. Extensive and temporally ungraded retrograde amnesia in encephalitis associated with antibodies to voltage-gated potassium channels. *Arch Neurol* 2007; **64:** 404–410.

Chong JY, Rowland LP, Utiger RD. Hashimoto encephalopathy: syndrome or myth? *Arch Neurol* 2003; **60**: 164–171.

Dale RC, Church AJ, Surtees RA, Lees AJ, Adcock JE, Harding B, *et al.* Encephalitis lethargica syndrome: 20 new cases and evidence of basal ganglia autoimmunity. *Brain* 2004; **127**: 21–33.

Dalmau J, Gleichman AJ, Hughes EG, Rossi JE, Peng X, Lai M, *et al.* Anti-NMDA-receptor encephalitis: case series and analysis of the effects of antibodies. *Lancet Neurol* 2008; **7:** 1091–1098.

Gallia GL, Rigamonti D, Williams MA. The diagnosis and treatment of idiopathic normal pressure hydrocephalus. *Nat Clin Pract Neurol* 2006; **2**: 375–381.

Hamilton R, Patel S, Lee EB, Jackson EM, Lopinto J, Arnold SE, *et al.* Lack of shunt response in suspected idiopathic normal pressure hy7drocephalus with Alzheimer disease pathology. *Ann Neurol* 2010; **68:** 535–540.

Høgh P, Smith SJ, Scahill RI, Chan D, Harvey RJ, Fox NC, *et al.* Epilepsy presenting as AD: neuroimaging, electroclinical features, and response to treatment. *Neurology* 2002; **58**: 298–301.

Jellinger KA. Head injury and dementia. *Curr Opin Neurol* 2004; **17**: 719–723.

Oslin D, Atkinson RM, Smith DM, Hendrie H. Alcohol related dementia: proposed clinical criteria. *Int J Geriatr Psychiatry* 1998; **13**: 203–212.

Rees JH, Hain SF, Johnson MR, Hughes RA, Costa DC, Ell PJ, *et al.* The role of [18F] fluoro-2-deoxyglucose-PET scanning in the diagnosis of paraneoplastic neurological disorders. *Brain* 2001; **124** (Pt 11): 2223–2231.

Schott JM. Limbic encephalitis: a clinician's guide. *Pract Neurol* 2006; **6**: 143–153.

Vernine S, Geschwind M, Boeve B. Autoimmune encephalopathies. *Neurologist* 2007; **13**: 140–147.

Vincent A, Bien CG, Irani SR, Waters P. Autoantibodies associated with diseases of the CNS: new developments and future challenges. *Lancet Neurol* 2011; **10:** 759–772.

Vincent A, Buckley C, Schott JM, Baker I, Dewar BK, Detert N, *et al.* Potassium channel antibody-associated encephalopathy: a potentially immunotherapy-responsive form of limbic encephalitis. *Brain* 2004; **127** (Pt 3): 701–712.

Zeman A, Butler C. Transient epileptic amnesia. *Curr Opin Neurol* 2010; **23:** 610–616. doi: 10.1097/WCO.0b013e32834027db.

Management

Treatment of Alzheimer's disease

Hort J, O'Brien JT, Gainotti G, Pirttila T, Popescu BO, Rektorova I, *et al.* EFNS Scientist Panel on Dementia. EFNS guidelines for the diagnosis and management of Alzheimer's disease. *Eur J Neurol* 2010; **17:** 1236–1248. doi:10.1111/j.1468-1331.2010.03040.

Howard R, McShane R, Lindesay J, Ritchie C, Baldwin A, Barber R, *et al.* Donepezil and memantine for moderate-to-severe Alzheimer's disease. *N Engl J Med* 2012; **366:** 893–903. doi: 10.1056/NEJMoa1106668.

Karran E, Hardy J. A critique of the drug discovery and phase 3 clinical programs targeting the amyloid hypothesis for Alzheimer disease. *Ann Neurol* 2014; **76:** 185–205. doi: 10.1002/ana.24188. Epub 2014 Jul 2.

Lanctôt KL, Herrmann N, Yau KK, Khan LR, Liu BA, LouLou MM, *et al.* Efficacy and safety of cholinesterase inhibitors in Alzheimer's disease: a meta-analysis. *CMAJ* 2003; **169**: 557–564.

Trinh NH, Hoblyn J, Mohanty S, Yaffe K. Efficacy of cholinesterase inhibitors in the treatment of neuropsychiatric symptoms and functional impairment in Alzheimer disease: a meta-analysis. *JAMA* 2003; **289**: 210–216.

CHAPTER 9

Infection in the Nervous System

Robin Howard, Carmel Curtis and Hadi Manji
National Hospital for Neurology & Neurosurgery

Infections that involve the nervous system carry a high morbidity and mortality, particularly in developing countries where the burden of disease is great, diagnosis is difficult and limited resources mean that availability and access to treatment is poor. In the developed world, neurological infection is less frequent but continues to cause significant problems of diagnosis and management. Acute bacterial meningitis and viral encephalitis remain significant causes of morbidity and mortality in all ages everywhere. Increasing global travel means that unfamiliar organisms are encountered unexpectedly. There is also increasing recognition that familiar pathogens may manifest disease in unexpected patterns and settings and emergent pathogens have become important, particularly in the immunosuppressed patient because of HIV and post transplant. The increasing burden of AIDS continues to present worldwide social and economic concern.

Infections of the nervous system can be caused by viruses, bacteria, fungi or protozoa. They may affect the meninges, cerebrospinal fluid (CSF), brain parenchyma, spinal cord, nerve roots, peripheral nerve or muscle. Infections of the central nervous system (CNS) may be divided into meningitis, encephalitis and focal suppuration or inflammation. In meningitis there is inflammation involving the pia and arachnoid mater and the subarachnoid space. Encephalitis is infection and inflammation within the brain parenchyma. Focal infection causes abscess formation within or immediately adjacent to the brain or spinal cord. These patterns may overlap and when infection involves the meninges, brain, spinal cord and nerve roots descriptive compound terms are used: meningoencephalitis, meningomyelitis, encephalomyelitis, meningoradiculitis and meningoencephalomyelitis. Neurological disturbances may also arise as a consequence of direct infection or from a secondary para-infectious immune-mediated mechanism.

The presentation of infections of the nervous system can be highly variable, ranging from acute fulminating meningitis or encephalitis leading to death within hours, to the development of disease many years after the initial infection. The spectrum of neurological manifestation is also highly variable, ranging from meningism and impaired consciousness, to signs of cortical and subcortical dysfunction, or involvement of the spinal cord, nerve roots, peripheral nerve or muscle.

The understanding of neurological infection has been advanced by new techniques of molecular diagnosis, in particular wider availability of polymerase chain reaction (PCR) assay to detect bacterial and viral nucleic acid in CSF, and improved imaging of brain and spinal cord. There have also been many important recent advances in the development of therapies targeted towards specific pathogens, such as antiretroviral therapy, and in facing the challenges presented by increased antibiotic resistance of pathogens such as pneumococci, tuberculosis and malaria. Even more importantly, the global burden of infections of the nervous system has been greatly reduced by the development of effective strategies of prevention for conditions such as poliomyelitis, leprosy and malaria.

Bacterial meningitis

Bacterial meningitis is caused by a primary infection within the subarachnoid space that leads to acute inflammation of the meninges (pia and arachnoid mater). It can be caused by a variety of organisms which vary in frequency according to the age of the host and other risk factors.

Epidemiology

The incidence of bacterial meningitis is 2–6/100 000 per annum, with peaks in infancy, adolescence and the elderly. Common causes of meningitis by age and risk factors are shown in Table 9.1. The incidence of *Haemophilus influenzae* type b, group C meningococcal (*Neisseria meningitidis*) and pneumococcal (*Streptococcus pneumoniae*) meningitis have declined dramatically with the introduction of vaccination, particularly in young children. The burden of bacterial meningitis is now borne by the older population. The most common infective species in adults in the United States are now *S. pneumoniae* (58.0%) followed by group B streptococcus (18.1%), *N. meningitidis* (13.9%), *H. influenzae* (6.7%) and *Listeria monocytogenes* (3.4%). The overall case fatality rate is 14.3% and has not changed significantly over the last decade.

Pathogenesis

Bacterial infection reaches the CNS either by direct invasion, haematogenous spread or embolisation of infected thrombi. In addition, there may be direct extension from contiguous structures via the diploic veins or erosion of an osteomyelitic focus and infection may be iatrogenic (e.g. following external ventricular drainage, ventriculoperitoneal shunt, intracranial pressure monitor or surgery).

Neurology: A Queen Square Textbook, Second Edition. Edited by Charles Clarke, Robin Howard, Martin Rossor and Simon Shorvon.

Table 9.1 Common causes of bacterial meningitis by age and risk factors.

Neonates (<3 months)	Group B streptococcus *Escherichia coli* *Listeria monocytogenes*
Infant and child (>3 months)	*Streptococcus pneumoniae* (pneumococcus) *Neisseria meningitidis* (meningococcus) *Haemophilus influenzae* type b
Adults <50 (healthy and immunocompetent)	*S. pneumoniae* *N. meningitidis*
Adult >50	*S. pneumoniae* *N. meningitidis* *L. monocytogenes* Aerobic Gram-negative organisms
Pregnancy	*L. monocytogenes*
Immunosuppressed (e.g. malignancy, alcohol, diabetes mellitus, septicaemia)	*S. pneumoniae* *N. meningitidis* Gram-negative bacilli *L. monocytogenes* Group B streptococcus *Staphylococcus aureus*
Impaired T-cell immunity (HIV, immunosuppressant medication, e.g. corticosteroids, post-transplant, TNF-alpha inhibitors, myeloproliferative disorders)	*S. pneumoniae* *N. meningitidis* Gram-negative bacilli *L. monocytogenes* Group B streptococcus *S. aureus*
Rarer causes	Non-typhoidal salmonellae *Shigella* spp. *Clostridium* spp. *N. gonorrhoeae*
Foreign bodies within the CNS (e.g. CSF shunts)	Coagulase-negative staphylococci *Propionibacterium* spp.
Splenectomy or splenic dysfunction, as in sickle cell disease	*S. pneumoniae* *H. influenzae* type b Non-typhoidal *Salmonellae*
Postoperative meningitis	Gram-negative bacilli including *Pseudomonas aeruginosa*, *S. aureus*

CSF, cerebrospinal fluid.

In community-acquired meningitis, the transmission of pathogenic bacteria occurs by respiratory droplet spread or close contact with a carrier. The process by which these bacteria gain access to the CNS is complex. Bacteria initially colonise the nasopharynx by attaching to epithelial cells using outer adhesive pili and membrane proteins. The risk of colonisation of the respiratory epithelium is increased by damage caused by irritants such as a preceding viral illness or cigarette smoke. Their capsular polysaccharides help to overcome host defence mechanisms including impairment of mucosal immunoglobulin A (IgA). The bacteria are carried across the epithelial cell into the intravascular space where they are relatively protected from the complement-mediated humoral response because of their polysaccharide capsule.

Bacteria that survive in the bloodstream gain access to the CSF via the choroid plexus epithelium or cerebral capillaries. They cross between endothelial cells by disrupting intercellular tight junctions or causing endothelial cell injuries. Once the bacteria reach the CSF they are in an immunologically privileged site where there is minimal complement-mediated humoral response. Bacteria multiply rapidly within the CSF and bacterial wall components released by lysis induce an inflammatory process involving the meninges and brain substance. This, in turn, leads to increased permeability of the blood–brain barrier allowing further leakage of plasma proteins into the CSF which contributes to the inflammatory and purulent exudates within the subarachnoid space (an immunologically priviledged site). There is initially a temporary increase in cerebral blood flow leading to disruption of cerebral autoregulation and an increase in intracranial pressure. Worsening exudates infiltrate the arterial walls leading to intimal thickening and large vessel constriction, together with an inflammatory vasculopathy eventually culminating in cerebral ischaemia. The development of systemic shock leads to a reduction in systemic arterial blood pressure and, because of the impairment in cerebral autoregulation, a consequent reduction in cerebral blood flow which exacerbates the cerebral ischaemia or infarction. There may also be secondary thrombosis of the major venous sinuses and thrombophlebitis of the cortical cerebral veins. Finally, the purulent exudate can obstruct the resorption of CSF by the arachnoid villi or the flow through the ventricular system leading to obstructive or communicating hydrocephalus with interstitial cerebral oedema.

Clinical presentation

Meningitis is characterised by the presence of fever, headache, altered mental state and neck stiffness. There is usually associated nausea, vomiting, photophobia and progressive lethargy, stupor or coma; seizures may occur. Meningitis may evolve as a fulminating illness over a few hours, particularly in children, but progression is variable and less commonly can be a progressive (subacute) infection worsening over several days, particularly in the elderly and the immunosuppressed. Meningism is characterised by the presence of neck stiffness on passive flexion and Kernig's sign is positive when the thigh is flexed at the hip and knee at 90° and subsequent extension of the knee is painful (leading to resistance). Brudzinski's sign is positive when flexion of the neck results in spontaneous flexion of the hips and knees when the patient is in a supine position. Seizures may be focal or generalised and may occur either at presentation or at any time during the course of bacterial meningitis in 40% of patients. They may arise from focal arterial or venous infarction, haemorrhage, localised cerebral oedema or as a consequence of systemic features including pyrexia, septicaemic shock, toxicity or other metabolic derangement. Meningitis may lead to vascular occlusion and subsequent infarction of the brain or spinal cord, progressive cranial nerve lesions and hydrocephalus secondary to impaired CSF absorption and obstruction. Organ failure, hearing loss and limb infarction may also occur.

Table 9.2 Possible imaging findings in CNS infection.

Imaging appearance	Possible infective cause	Differential diagnosis
Mass lesion	Abscess Subdural empyema Cerebritis	Tumour MS Acute disseminated encephalomyelitis Lymphoma
Temporal lobe signal change	HSV-1 or 2	Autoimmune limbic encephalitis (VGKC antibody) Paraneoplastic
Extensive white matter signal change	HSV HHV6	PML PRES ADEM
Brainstem	*Listeria* infection Bickerstaff encephalitis Viral encephalitis (VZV, HSV-2,WNV)	CPM Wernicke PRES Autoimmune encephalitis Whipple's disease CLIPPERS
Basal ganglia	*Toxoplasma gondii*, encephalitis (WNV, EEE, WEE, Jap B)	
Infarction	Infective endocarditis VZV Fungal (aspergillus, mucormycosis)	Vasculitis
Multiple enhancing lesions	Abscess *T. gondii* Tuberculomas *Cryptococcus* Neurocysticercosis	Multiple metastases Vasculitis

ADEM, acute disseminated encephalomyelitis; CLIPPERS, chronic lymphocytic inflammation with pontine perivascular enhancement responsive to steroids; CPM, central pointine myelinolysis; EEE, Eastern equine encephalitis; HHV, human herpes virus; HSV, herpes simpex virus; Jap B, Japanese B encephalitis; PML, progressive multifocal leukoencephalopathy; PRES, posterior reversible encephalopathy syndrome; VGKC, voltage-gated potassium channel; VZV, varicella zoster virus; WEE, Western equine encephalitis; WNV, West Nile virus.

Investigation

Bacterial meningitis is usually accompanied by an elevated peripheral white cell count and raised inflammatory markers. In the presence of septicaemia, platelet consumption may occur with loss of clotting factors. There may be associated hypocalcaemia, hyponatraemia and impaired renal function with metabolic acidosis. Imaging should be undertaken urgently to exclude mass lesions, hydrocephalus or cerebral oedema which are contraindications to lumbar puncture. The cornerstone of the diagnosis of meningitis remains a positive CSF Gram stain and culture, additional support for the diagnosis can be made by positive blood cultures (50% cases), a positive throat swab (in cases of *N. meningitidis*), CSF biochemical analysis, and PCR of blood or CSF. However, there is a considerable risk that lumbar puncture may cause coning in the presence of cerebral oedema. Lumbar puncture should be avoided if the patient has:

- Impaired consciousness (Glasgow Coma Scale [GCS] <12, or fall in GCS of ≥2)
- Signs of raised intracranial pressure or incipient herniation
- Focal neurological signs
- Papilloedema
- Prolonged focal seizures within 2 weeks of presentation
- Signs of shock or bleeding diathesis
- Purpuric or petechial rash
- Known immunocompromised state
- Evidence of obstructive hydrocephalus, cerebral oedema or herniation on computed tomography (CT) or magnetic resonance image (MRI) scan of brain.

Imaging may also provide important clues to the aetiology of the infective process (Table 9.2).

Gram staining of the CSF is positive for meningococcus in approximately 50% of patients with acute meningococcal meningitis. Blood cultures may be helpful but are not sensitive. CSF tests may directly identify an organism and its nucleic acid or surface constituents by staining, culture or capsular antigen detection (less helpful in adults). PCR is particularly sensitive in CSF for *S. pneumoniae* and *N. meningitidis*. The CSF findings in different forms of meningitis are summarised in Table 9.3.

Table 9.3 Comparison of CSF findings in different forms of meningitis.

	Normal	Acute bacterial	Viral meningitis	TB meningitis	Fungal meningitis
Appearance	Clear colourless	Turbid	Clear / opalescent	Clear / opalescent	Clear
Pressure (mm H_2O)	Normal (<180)	Increased	Normal or increased	Increased	Normal or increased
White cell count (cells/mm^3)	0–5	100–50 000	5–500	5–500	20–500
Neutrophils (%)	None	>80%	<50%	<50%	<50%
Glucose	>3.5 mmol/L (75% blood glucose)	Low (<50% blood glucose)	Normal	Low (<50% blood glucose)	Low (usually between 50% and 75% blood glucose)
Protein (g/L)	<0.4	>0.9	0.6–0.9	0.6–5	0.6–5
Others		Gram stain positive <90% Culture positive <80% Blood culture positive <60% PCR	Culture positive <50% PCR, if cellular	ZN stain positive <90% Culture positive 50–80%	Gram stain negative Culture positive 25–50% India ink

Previous or partial antibiotic treatment of bacterial meningitis usually leads to reduction in CSF cell count and protein level, shift from polymorphonuclear to lymphocytic CSF and marked reduction in the yield on Gram stain and culture. PCR, polymerase chain reaction.

Management

In patients with severe meningitis, the first priority is to commence empirical antibiotic treatment, usually immediately after sending a blood culture. Empirical therapy in the absence of staining and culture depends on the age and immune status of the patient and any other underlying risk factors:

- In any child or adult with suspected meningococcal meningitis, primary care physicians are recommended to commence benzylpenicillin before transfer to hospital. If the situation is less urgent it is preferable to undertake a lumbar puncture, if safe, and send CSF for staining and culture before antibiotics are commenced.
- In healthy immunocompetent adults with suspected bacterial meningitis, hospital treatment should be initiated with a third generation cephalosporin (2 g ceftriaxone 12-hourly IV) and not penicillin (because of potential pneumococcal resistance) and in those older than 50 years amoxicillin and gentamicin to cover *Listeria* infection (2 g amoxicillin 4-hourly, 7 mg/kg gentamicin once daily)
- When there is the possibility of nosocomial infection (i.e. acquired in hospital, such as following surgery, trauma or in the presence of a shunt), ceftazidime (2 g 8-hourly) is preferred because it is more active against *Pseudomonas aeruginosa* than other third generation cephalosporins. Vancomycin (15 mg/kg 8-hourly) is added to cover highly resistant staphylococcus.
- If the patient has penicillin or cephalosporin allergy, chloramphenicol (12.5 mg/kg 6-hourly) should be given with vancomycin (add co-trimoxazole if *Listeria* is suspected).
- Dexamethasone (10 mg every 6 hours) should be given concurrently with the antibiotics and continued for 4 days in all cases. This is primarily effective if Gram stain or culture is positive for pneumococcus but may be beneficial for other causes of bacterial meningitis.
- Aciclovir (10 mg/kg IV 8-hourly) should be commenced if viral encephalitis resulting from herpes simplex virus (HSV) is considered possible.

Specific antibiotic treatment for acute bacterial meningitis is summarised in Table 9.4 but therapy depends on demonstration of appropriate microbiological sensitivities.

Specific causes of bacterial meningitis

Neisseria meningitidis (meningococcal meningitis)

This is a Gram-negative diplococcus. It is the most common identified cause of meningitis in children and young adults, with an incidence of 1–1.5/100 000/year. In the United Kingdom, meningococcal disease remains the leading infectious cause of death in childhood with a mortality of approximately 10%. It occurs throughout the year but the majority of cases are in the winter and early spring. Transmission occurs by droplet spread, particularly with close contact, and 5–10% of all adults are asymptomatic nasopharyngeal carriers of these pathogenic bacteria.

Meningococcus is classified into subgroups according to the immunoreactivity of the capsular polysaccharide. While there are at least 13 serogroups, most cases of meningococcal disease are caused by subgroups A and C (geographically dependent) for which a polysaccharide vaccine is effective. In November 1999 the United Kingdom established a programme for vaccinating all infants with conjugate sero-group C vaccine. In 2014, two subgroup B meningococcal vaccines were approved for use and from 2015 quadrivalent conjugate vaccine against meningococcal subgroups A, C, W135

Table 9.4 Treatment of bacterial meningitis.

	First line treatment	Alternative treatment
Neisseria meningitidis (meningococcus)	Ceftriaxone 2 g (IV) 12-hrly for 7 days or Cefotaxime 2 g (IV) 6-hrly for 7 days	Benzylpenicillin (penicillin G) 2.4 g (IV) 4-hrly for 7 days or Chloramphenicol 12.5 mg/kg 6-hrly or Amoxicillin 2 g (IV) 4-hrly for 7 days
Streptococcus pneumoniae (pneumococcus)	Ceftriaxone 2 g (IV) 12-hrly for 14 days or Cefotaxime 2 g (IV) 6-hrly for 14 days	Benzylpenicillin <2.4 g (IV) 4-hrly for 14 days
Haemophilus influenzae type b	Ceftriaxone 2 g (IV) 12 hrly for 14 days or Cefotaxime 2 g (IV) 6-hrly for 14 days	Chloramphenicol 12.5 mg/kg 6-hrly or Meropenem 2 g (IV) 8-hrly for 14 days
Streptococcus Group B or *milleri* group	Ceftriaxone 2 g (IV) 12-hrly for 14 days or Cefotaxime 2 g (IV) 6-hrly for 14 days	Benzylpenicillin 2.4 g (IV) 4-hrly for 14 days and Gentamicin 8-hrly for 7 days
Listeria monocytogenes	Amoxillin 2 g (IV) 4-hrly for 3 weeks and gentamicin for 7 days	Co-trimoxazole 3 mg/kg (IV) 6-hrly for 21 days
Staphylococcus aureus – non-MRSA	Flucloxacillin 2 g (IV) 6-hrly for 4 weeks	Ceftriaxone 2 g (IV) 12-hrly for 4 weeks
Methicillin-resistant *Staphylococcus aureus* – MRSA	Vancomycin 1 g (IV) 12-hrly for 4 weeks	Linezolid 600 mg (IV) for 28 days maximum (limited clinical experience)
Gram negatives (excluding *Pseudomonas)* i.e. *E. coli, Klebsiella* spp. *and Proteus* spp.	Ceftriaxone 2 g (IV) 12-hrly for 3–4 weeks or Cefotaxime 2 g (IV) 4-hrly for 3–4 weeks	Meropenem 2 g (IV) 8-hrly for 14 days (for more resistant isolates)
Pseudomonas aeruginosa	Ceftazidime 2 g (IV) 8-hrly for 3 weeks	Meropenem 2 g (IV) 8-hrly for 3 weeks

and Y will be undertaken routinely in all infants. Risk factors for meningococcal infection include close contact with carriers or infected individuals, low socio-economic status, poor housing and impairments of both humoral and cell-mediated immunity.

Clinical manifestations of meningococcal infection may develop within minutes or hours. In approximately 40% of patients there is isolated meningitis; 10% have septicaemia alone and the remainder a mixed pattern. Isolated meningococcal meningitis carries a better prognosis than meningococcal septicaemia or a mixed picture. Clinically, fulminant meningitis is characterised by pyrexia, headache and meningism associated with nausea and vomiting, photophobia and progressive lethargy. In early meningococcal meningitis there is a diffuse erythematous macular papular rash which eventually develops into the characteristic non-blanching petechiae found across the trunk and lower extremities in the mucous membranes, conjunctiva and occasionally on the palms and soles. These lesions should be distinguished from other infective disorders that cause a purpuric rash, including enterovirus meningitis and bacterial endocarditis. The development of meningococcal septicaemia is associated with progressive vasomotor disturbance culminating in profound hypotension, tachycardia and a rising respiratory rate indicating pulmonary oedema or raised intracranial pressure resulting from cerebral oedema.

Waterhouse–Friderichsen syndrome is a form of fulminant meningococcal disease, in which severe septicaemia is complicated by the development of bilateral haemorrhage into the adrenal glands and disseminated intravascular coagulation leading severe sudden febrile illness associated with septic shock, petechiae, purpura and coma.

Management Patients with probable fulminant meningococcal meningitis should be treated immediately in primary care settings with parenteral benzylpenicillin (2.4 g) given intramuscularly or preferably intravenously because of uncertain absorption in patients with shock (Table 9.4). They should be transferred immediately to an accident and emergency department. In secondary care settings first line treatment is 2 g ceftriaxone IV stat; alternatively cefotaxime can be used. Antibiotics should be given prior to any diagnostic procedure if there is a petechial or purpuric rash or shock.

Septicaemic shock should be treated with appropriate volume replacement, elective intubation and ventilation. Patients may require inotropic support and metabolic abnormalities, coagulopathy and anaemia should be promptly treated. In the presence of raised intracranial pressure it may be necessary to administer mannitol, muscle relaxation and appropriate intensive care nursing.

Contacts Meningococcal meningitis is a notifiable disease in the United Kingdom and there is a high risk of family members developing the disease. All household close contacts should therefore be treated to eradicate nasopharyngeal carriage. It is recommended that 600 mg rifampicin 12-hourly should be given as prophylaxis for 2 days. Ciprofloxacin (750 mg as a single dose) is also effective.

Immunisation Meningococcal vaccination is currently available and contains polysaccharides to monovalent subgroup B and quadrivalent conjugate serogroups A, C, Y and W135.

Outcome Complications of the acute infection are common and occur in more than 35% of patients, they include cerebral oedema, hydrocephalus, vasculitis, venous thrombosis, ventriculitis, labyrinthitis and spinal cord involvement. The mortality rate is approximately 25% although this rises to 40% in those with meningococcal septicaemia coexisting with meningitis. Of survivors, 20% have neurological sequelae such as hearing loss, loss of limbs secondary to large vessel vasculitis and neurological disability resulting from cerebral ischaemia.

Streptococcus pneumoniae (pneumococcal meningitis)

This is the most common cause of meningitis in adults over the age of 18 years and carries a case fatality rate of approximately 20%. The organism is a Gram-positive coccus and spread occurs by respiratory droplet infection. The primary site of colonisation is the nasopharynx and the carrier state is common. *S. pneumoniae* meningitis can have a more insidious onset and is commonly caused by local extension from otitis media, or a paranasal source of infection, following a skull base fracture or sinus injury with dural tear. Other predisposing features include pneumonia, alcoholism, diabetes, immunodeficiency states (e.g. splenectomy, hypogammaglobulinaemia, HIV). Clinical presentation is similar to other forms of pyogenic meningitis but a coexisting pneumococcal pneumonia may be present. The course may be aggressive with rapid progression to coma and respiratory arrest. Neurological complications are similar to those described for mengococcal meningitis and include cerebral oedema, hydrocephalus, vasculitis, venous thrombosis, ventriculitis, labyrinthitis and spinal cord involvement. Residual sequelae occur in more than 30% of patiients and include seizures, focal neurological deficits (cranial nerve palsies, hemiparesis), sensorineural hearing loss, stroke and intellectual impairment.

Management Conventional treatment is with penicillin, ampicillin and ceftriaxone or cefotaxime but this treatment has been complicated by the development of penicillin and cephalosporin resistant strains. If penicillin-resistance is suspected then vancomycin should be added. However, vancomycin itself only crosses the blood–brain barrier poorly and therefore should not be used in isolation. Adjuvant dexamethasone (10 mg 6-hourly IV for 4 days) improves the outcome and should be commenced before or with the first dose of antibiotics. Failure to improve despite antibiotic treatment implies either the development of cerebral complications, a persistent primary focus or an inadequate or inappropriate regimen of antibiotics. In the United Kingdom, pneumococcal vaccine is recommended for all infants as part of the routine childhood immunisation programme, for those over the age of 65 and for children and adults at clinical risk (asplenia or splenic dysfunction, chronic respiratory, cardiac, renal or liver disease, diabetes, immunosuppressive or individuals with CSF leaks). Primary immunisation with conjugate vaccine (PCV 13) is recommended in childhood but polysaccharide vaccine (PPV 23) is used in those over 65 years or in the at risk group over 2 years.

Haemophilus influenzae type b

This is a small Gram-negative coccobacillus. Prior to the introduction of *Haemophilus influenzae* type b (Hib) vaccination this was the most common cause of meningitis in children with a fatality rate of approximately 5% and permanent neurological damage in some 30% of cases. Meningitis occurs as a consequence of respiratory droplet spread and adults remain vulnerable to the non-encapsulated strains. Risk factors include otitis media, splenectomy, head trauma, previous neurosurgery or a CSF leak. Presentation may be with acute meningitis but an associated vasculitis may occur, leading to focal signs.

Management The primary treatment of *H. influenzae* is ceftriaxone or cefotaxime because of the significant incidence of penicillin resistant strains in up to 40%. Chemoprophylaxis is recommended for non-immune household contacts, 600 mg rifampicin once daily for 4 days. Vaccination is recommended for all children with the first dose being given at 2 months.

Listeria monocytogenes

This is a beta-haemolytic Gram-positive rod with 12 subtypes based on antigenic properties. It is an intracellular pathogen that lyses phagocytic cells before entering the bloodstream. The overall case fatality rate is around 15%. Outbreaks are associated with contaminated food including soft cheese, unpasteurised milk and occasionally raw meat. Predisposing factors include pregnancy, advanced age, the neonatal period or immunosuppression, and listeria is more common in patients with malignancy, renal failure or following organ transplantation or steroid treatment. Listeria may cause a meningitis or meningoencephalitis but seizures, disturbances of consciousness and movement disorders may also occur. A brainstem meningoencephalitis develops in <10%, this presents with a prodromal phase followed by progressive ponto-medullary involvement with cranial neuropathy, pyramidal and sensory signs. The differential diagnoses of brainstem meningoencephalitis are listed in Table 9.5.

Management Treatment is with amoxicillin for 21 days; however, gentamicin for 7 days is recommended in addition to enhance bacteriocidal activity. If there is a penicillin allergy then co-trimoxazole (Septrin) is recommended but chloramphenicol should be avoided because of the high risk of relapse.

Group B streptococcus

Group B streptococcus (*Streptococcus agalactiae*) is an important cause of neonatal sepsis and meningitis. It also causes purulent meningitis in adults with a case fatality rate of approximately 5%. Risk factors in neonates include premature birth or low birth weight, prolonged rupture of membranes, intrapartum fever or maternal group B streptococcus infection during pregnancy. In non-pregnant adults, group B streptococcal meningitis is associated with advanced stage diabetes, cirrhosis and systemic malignancy; it can be acquired nosocomially. The treatment is with benzylpenicillin.

Table 9.5 Differential diagnosis of brainstem meningo-encephalitis.

Virus	Enterovirus EBV/CMV Tick-borne encephalitis, *Coxiella*
Bacterial	*Listeria, Mycoplasma* *Legionella, Brucella* *Borrelia*
Non-infectious	Multiple sclerosis Sarcoid Behçet's Acute disseminated encephalomyelitis Vasculitis Carcinomatous meningitis Bickerstaff's encephalitis Fisher's syndrome CLIPPERS

CMV, cytomegalovirus; CLIPPERS, chronic lymphocytic inflammation with pontine perivascular enhancement responsive to steroids; EBV, Epstein–Barr virus.

Gram-negative meningitis

Gram-negative meningitis (excluding *N. meningitidis*) may arise spontaneously, when the onset is often acute, and the condition follows an aggressive course. More commonly, Gram-negative meningitis may follow neurosurgical intervention when the onset and progression is insidious and gradual. Nosocomial infection is usually caused by *Klebsiella* spp. (approximately 40%), *Escherichia coli* (<30%) or *Pseudomonas aeruginosa* (<20%) with *Serratia* spp., *Proteus* spp. and *Salmonella* spp. meningitis occurring less commonly. Meningitis may be associated with seizures, confusion and focal signs including cranial nerve palsies. The diagnosis is made on CSF Gram stain and culture but this is only helpful in <50% of untreated patients. The limulus lysate assay can detect endotoxin but is limited in sensitivity and has little clinical role. Treatment of organisms with minimal resistance is with a third generation cephalosporin (Table 9.4).

Gram-positive meningitis (non-pneumococcal, non-group B)

Gram-positive meningitis usually results from a CNS shunt infection. Nosocomial shunt infections are usually caused by coagulase-negative staphylococci or *Propionibacterium acnes*. Spontaneously occurring *Staphylococcus aureus* meningitis may be predisposed by coexisting disease including diabetes mellitus, carcinomatosis, alcohol and intravenous drug abuse. It is usually associated with a focus of infection outside the CNS (e.g. endocarditis or osteomyelitis). The diagnosis is made on the basis of CSF staining and culture. Treatment depends on drug resistance. For fully sensitive staphylococci, treatment with high dose flucloxacillin or ceftriaxone is appropriate, with vancomycin or linezolid being used for methicillin resistant *S. aureus* (MRSA). There is a high mortality rate of approximately 50% with a further >10% experiencing neurological sequelae. *Streptococcus suis* is the second most common cause of community-acquired meningitis in South-East Asia and is associated with contact with pigs or raw pork. Treatment is with benzylpenicillin or ceftriaxone for 14 days. Other streptococci implicated in meningitis include group D streptococci (including *S. milleri* group) as a result of local invasion or haematogenous spread. Treatment with ceftriaxone is recommended.

Nosocomial meningitis

Nosocomial bacterial meningitis results from invasive procedures, such as craniotomy (0.8–1.5%), placement of internal (4–17%) or external (8%) ventricular catheters, lumbar puncture, intrathecal infusion or spinal anaesthesia, complicated head trauma or metastatic infection in patients with hospital acquired Gram-negative sepsis.

The initial choice of antibiotic treatment depends on the age of the patient and any underlying risk factors. In the neonate in whom there is a possibility of group B streptococcal infection or *Listeria*, then ampicillin and cefotaxime should be used. For anyone over the age of 3 months, ceftriaxone is the preferred treatment; cefotaxime is an alternative. Vancomycin should be added if there is a significant risk of *S. pneumoniae* with penicillin resistance and in those over 50 years.

Meningitis may occur as a complication of closed head trauma, particularly if there is a basal skull fracture causing the subarachnoid space to be in communication with a paranasal sinus cavity. The onset may be delayed for several days after the initial injury. Leakage of CSF is a further risk factor and is often unrecognised. Head trauma is the most common cause of recurrent meningitis and, in those over 50 years, the incidence of meningitis after moderate or severe head trauma is approximately 1.4%, usually resulting from a persistent dural tear and CSF leak. Open compound cranial fractures occur in 5% of head injuries and have been associated with rates of meningitis of 2–11% but prophylactic antibiotics are not indicated.

The specific bacteria causing nosocomial meningitis vary according to the pathogenesis and timing of the infection after the predisposing event. In the early stages after neurosurgical or ENT procedures the causative organism is generally pneumococcus but following prolonged hospitalisation after neurosurgery, penetrating trauma or skull base fracture infection meningitis is usually caused by staphylococci or aerobic Gram-negative bacilli. In those with a foreign body (e.g. external ventricular drain), infection is often caused by cutaneous organisms such as coagulase negative staphylococcus. CSF examination may be misleading and cell count may be normal even in culture positive meningitis. The choice of antibiotics depends on the pathogenesis of the infection. Following basilar skull fracture or ENT surgery a third generation cephalosporin and vancomycin are recommended but if there has been prolonged hospitalisation ceftazidime and vancomycin or meropenem are indicated.

Focal CNS infection

Cerebral abscess

Cerebral abscess is a focal suppurative (pus forming) infection occurring within the cerebral parenchyma. It develops as a result of contiguous spread of infection from paranasal sinuses, mastoiditis, otitis media, osteomyelitis, following postoperative and post-traumatic infections or, rarely, as a consequence of penetrating craniocerebral injuries. Less commonly, it may arise as a result of haematogenous spread from distant sites including teeth and lungs. No cause is found in around one-fifth of cases. The causative agents depend on the underlying abnormality, and the age and immunological status of the patient but 80–90% of all bacterial abscesses are polymicrobial. These are summarised in Table 9.6.

Table 9.6 Microbiological pathogens in brain abscesses.

Source/predisposition	Pathogens
Paranasal sinuses, otitic, mastoiditis or dental infection	Streptococci (esp. Group D strep including *Strep. milleri*) 60–70%, Enterobacteriaceae 20–40%, anaerobes, fusobacteria. More rarely *Actinomyces* spp., *Listeria monocytogenes*
Post-neurosurgery and penetrating head injury	*Staphylococcus aureus*, aerobic Streptococci, Enterobacteriaceae *Pseudomonas aeruginosa*
Pulmonary	Streptococci, Nocardia spp., Actinomycosis, Prevotella spp.
Infants	*S. aureus*, Enterobacteriaceae, *Pseudomonas aeruginosa*
Endocarditis	*Strep. viridians, S. aureus,* Enterococci spp.
Immunocompromised (immunosuppressant medication, post transplant, HIV, diabetes mellitus, IV drug user)	*Pseudomonas aeruginosa*, *Mycobacterium tuberculosis,* Enterobacteriaceae, Nocardia, Listeria, fungi (Cryptococcus, Candida, Aspergillus) and *Toxoplasma gondii*
HIV	*Toxoplasma gondii, Cryptococcus neoformans, Mycobacterium tuberculosis*

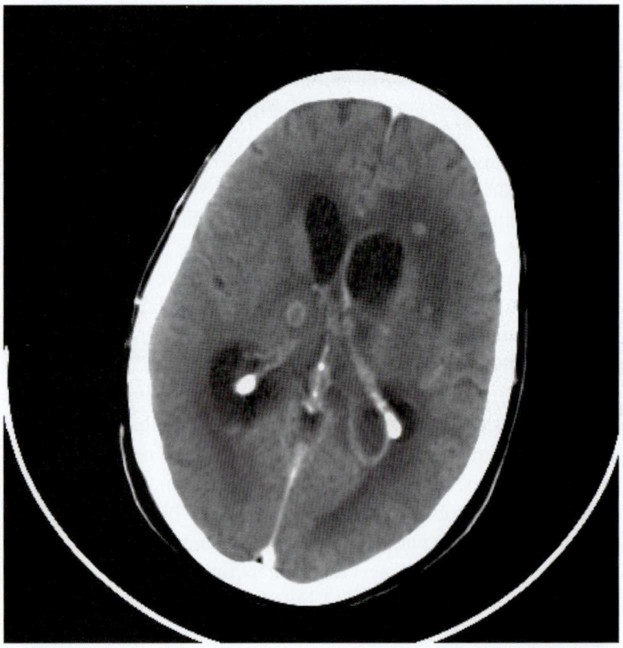

Figure 9.1 CT scan showing multiple bacterial abscesses and ventriculitis in a 53-year-old woman with Gram-negative septicaemia.

Most commonly, cerebral abscesses that arise from dental, frontal or ethmoid sinuses tend to involve the frontal lobe while those arising from the sphenoid sinuses or otitic infection particularly involve the temporal lobes. Cerebral abscesses resulting from haematogenous spread tend to occur as multiple rather than single abscesses (Figure 9.1), often in the region of greatest blood flow, within the basal ganglia.

Clinical features

The peak frequency is 35–45 years but abscesses can occur at any age. Although the characteristic onset is subacute and indolent with fever, headache, nausea, vomiting, seizures or focal neurological signs, there may be a rapid course of neurological symptoms suggesting a tumour or cerebral infarction. Fever is variable and may be absent in around half of cases, and usually those who are older; fever tends to resolve rapidly with steroids. Rupture of an abscess into the ventricles may cause a dramatic severe headache and emerging signs of meningism. Cerebellar abscess may cause obstruction to CSF flow and acute hydrocephalus.

Investigations

Following imaging, the gold standard investigation is aspiration of the abscess, urgent Gram stain, microscopy and culture. Depending on the age and immune status of the patient, analysis of the pus may include auramine stain for acid-fast bacilli, toxoplasma microscopy, fungal culture or PCR if culture fails to grow an organism. All specimens should have histopathology reporting. Routine haematology usually shows a raised ESR and white cell count. Blood cultures are positive but only in about 10%. CT scan may show a thin enhancing ring of uniform thickness with smooth margins which tends to be thicker nearer the cortex and thinner near the ventricles. MRI with enhancement is more sensitive and will show the extent of surrounding oedema more accurately than CT. Pyogenic abscesses exhibit restricted diffusion within the central pus (Figure 9.2). This is an important finding which allows distinction from other cystic lesions such as metastases. Lumbar puncture is contraindicated in patients with mass lesions and yield is usually low because of the focal nature of the abscess.

Treatment

Treatment is urgent, with surgical drainage being most effective but also necessitating administration of appropriate antibiotics and control of cerebral oedema (Table 9.7).

Surgical intervention

Pus evacuation using image guidance techniques usually utilising a mini-craniotomy is the optimum method and it carries a low risk, and should provide a microbiological diagnosis. Simple pus aspiration is easier than attempts at abscess excision and carries a smaller risk of subsequent seizures. Despite appropriate antibiotic therapy, recurrent abscesses are common. Cerebral oedema should be treated with dexamethasone, hyperventilation and/or mannitol.

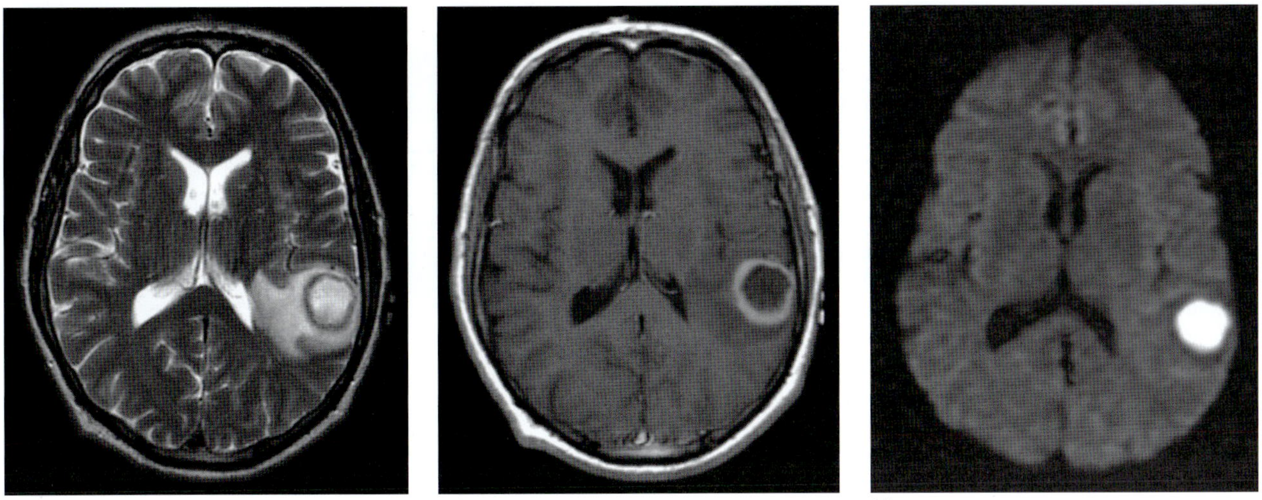

Figure 9.2 Left temporal abscess MRI: (a) T2-weighted, (b) T1 weighted post-contrast and (c) diffusion weighted images. Note the central T2 hyperintensity, relatively T2 hypointense, enhancing margin and central restricted diffusion.

Table 9.7 Antibiotic treatment of cerebral abscess.

Unknown source (covers sensitive steptoccocci, sensitive staphylococci, minimally resistant Gram-negatives and anaerobes)	Ceftriaxone/cefotaxime plus metronidazole
Streptococcus (resistant)	Add vancomycin or linezolid (limited clinical experience)
MRSA risk	Add vancomycin or linezolid (limited clinical experience)
Highly resistant Gram-negative organisms risk	Meropenem
Pseudomonas aeruginosa risk	Ceftazidime or meropenem

Prognosis

The prognosis depends on the clinical state of the patient and the organism isolated or suspected. Survival is excellent for those fully alert and conscious who receive appropriate treatment but declines to 40% if a patient is unrousable at initial assessment. Intraventricular rupture carries a mortality of up to 80%.

Subdural empyema

Subdural empyema occurs when intracranial suppuration develops between the dura and the arachnoid (Figure 9.3). This is usually a consequence of ear or paranasal sinus infection, particularly involving the frontal ethmoid sinuses. Empyemas also follow skull osteomyelitis, penetrating head trauma, neurosurgery and infection of a subdural effusion following childhood meningitis. Empyema from haematogenous spread does occur, but is rare.

Pathophysiology

Infection gains entry to the subdural space by direct extension through the bone and dura (e.g. ear and sinus infection, cranial osteomyelitis, penetrating head trauma) or by spread from septic thrombosis of the venous sinus particularly the superior sagittal sinus. Rarely, subdural empyema may result from metastases from infected lungs by haematogenous spread.

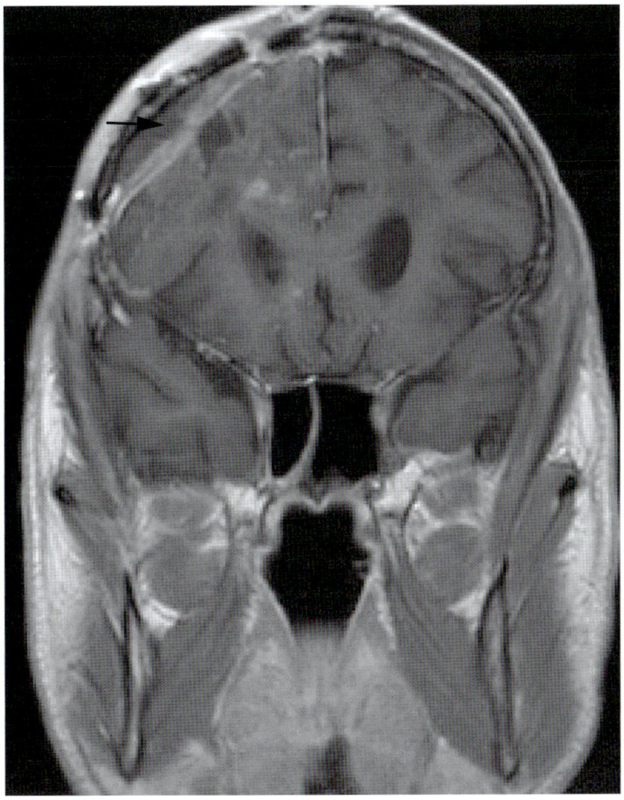

Figure 9.3 Large subdural empyema in a patient with a previous craniotomy for grade 2 glioma (coronal T1 MRI) (arrow).

Causative agents

Infection is usually secondary to paranasal sinus disease from viridans streptococci, aerobic streptococci (including *Strep. milleri* group [now called *Strep. anginosus* group]) and anaerobes. Less often subdural empyema may be caused by *S. aureus, Pseudomonas aeruginosa* or Enterobacteriaceae including Proteus, Klebsiella and *E. coli.* However, no organism is isolated in 20–50% of patients.

Clinically, there is an acute onset with rapid progression to extensive hemispheric involvement or mass effect with tentorial herniation; occasionally a more gradual meningitis-like conditions may evolve over several weeks. The onset is with pyrexia in >80%, localised cranial pain, focal or generalised headache, but meningism may develop and focal neurological deficits evolve into hemiparesis. Seizures occur in <50% of patients and there may be progressive obtundation. Venous extension of the infection may lead to the development of meningitis, brain abscess or septic intracranial venous thrombosis. The diagnosis is made by CT or MRI with enhancement. The management is immediate surgical decompression with antibiotic cover. There is debate about whether to undertake craniotomy drainage or multiple burr holes. Because many patients with empyema have a mixed culture of organisms, two or more antibiotic agents are required. For initial therapy where no information exists on the source of infection, ceftriaxone and metronidazole are recommended; if Gram-positive resistance is a concern then vancomycin should be added and treatment should be continued for at least 4 weeks. The outcome of surgically treated subdural empyema and intracerebral abscess has been transformed by image-guidance surgical techniques and antibiotics.

Intracranial epidural abscess

Intracranial epidural abscess develops as a result of infection between the outer most layer of the meninges (dura) and the overlying skull. These abscesses are associated with cranial osteomyelitis complicating ear, sinus or orbital infection or neurosurgical intervention. Infection is rarely metastatic. Epidural abscesses are commonly caused by streptococci (including *Strep. anginosus* group). The diagnosis and management are similar to subdural empyema. The onset is generally insidious with localised cranial pain following generalised headache. The abscess may be accompanied by superficial subcutaneous infection and oedema. Patients develop focal or generalised seizures, focal neurological deficit or alterations in their mental state. Epidural abscess near the petrous bone affecting the V and VI cranial nerve may cause Gradenigo's syndrome characterised by unilateral facial pain and lateral rectus weakness. Extension inwards across the dura, along the emissary veins leads to subdural empyema, meningitis, brain abscess or venous sinus thrombosis. CT imaging may be normal, but usually these abscesses will be seen on MRI. Small epidural abscesses can be managed by antibiotics alone, following the guidelines indicated earlier but larger abscesses require surgical drainage.

Spinal epidural abscess

Spinal epidural abscess is an infection of the epidural space of the spinal cord (Figure 9.4). It is usually caused by osteomyelitis or metastatic spread of infection from injuries to the back associated with skin wounds, bacteraemia or septicaemia. It may rarely occur following spinal surgery, lumbar puncture or epidural/spinal anaesthetic. Patients present with fever and back pain which may be severe and localised or radicular. Typically, the patient develops a fever and signs of progressive spinal cord compression leading to paraparesis, sensory loss and sphincter involvement, with localised spinal tenderness. Rarely, there may be a more chronic and indolent onset with a history suggesting a spinal cord neoplasm or a tuberculous abscess.

S. aureus is the most common cause of spinal epidural abscess, found in 50–90% of patients, although a few may be caused by aerobic streptococci, Gram-negative bacilli and, more rarely, anaerobic organisms. CSF shows a clear pleocytosis but this is usually modest with <100 white cells/mm^3 and these may be both polymorphonuclear and lymphocytes. The protein is usually high. Surgical treatment with laminectomy and drainage with prolonged antibiotic cover is indicated. There is a danger of vascular compromise to the cord causing infarction and permanent cord injury. Recovery may be slow with residual incomplete cord compression caused by formation of a fibrous and granulomatous reaction at the operative site.

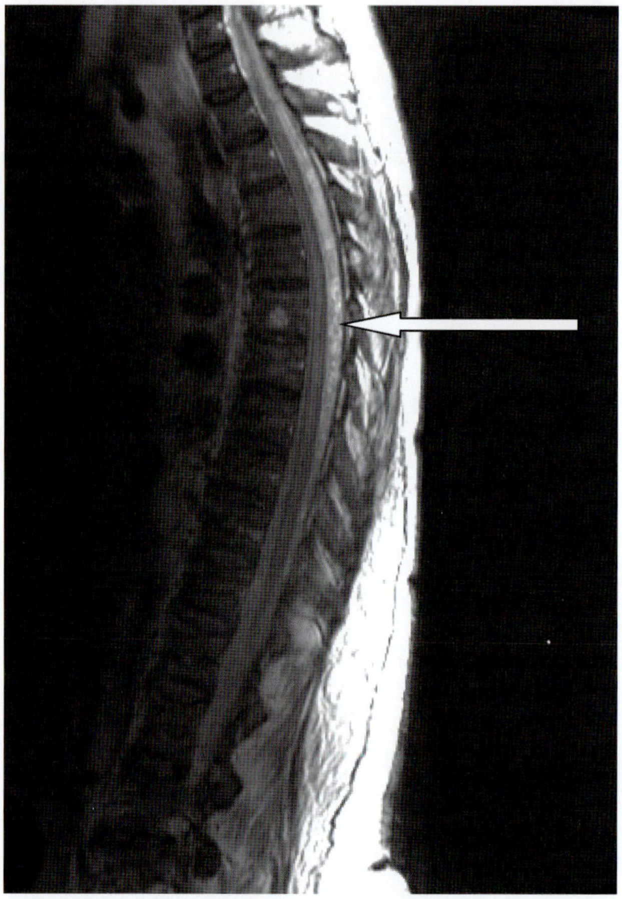

Figure 9.4 Extensive posterior epidural abscess on T2-weighted sagittal MRI.

Spinal subdural abscess

Subdural spinal abscess may be acute or chronic and caused by osteomyelitis or metastatic spread of infection and may be impossible to distinguish from the more common epidural infection. Presentation is similarly with fever, back and neck pain and rapidly developing signs of spinal cord compression. The onset is variable and may be over days or weeks. The causative agent is *S. aureus* in >50% of patients. A clue to the presence of subdural empyema comes from imaging, which tends to show that these lesions have a less sharp margin and a greater vertical extent than epidural abscess.

Spinal cord intramedullary abscess

Spinal cord intramedullary abscess is rare. It may present with a syringomyelia-like picture. The spinal cord is usually involved by direct spread from a contiguous abscess in the skin or if there is spinal dysraphism leading to an open track. Surgical drainage may be necessary.

Infective endocarditis

Infective endocarditis is caused by direct bacterial colonisation of the endothelial surface of the heart, usually on the valves. Endocarditis affecting a native valve is usually associated with congenital, rheumatic or degenerative valve disease but occurs on previously normal valves in intravenous drug users. Endocarditis develops on around 6% of prosthetic valves over 5 years. Approximately 30% of patients with endocarditis have neurological complications and often these are the presenting features. Most cases of native valve endocarditis are caused by *Streptococcus viridans* group, Enterococci or *Staphylococcus aureus;* the latter is common in endocarditis amongst intravenous drug users. Native valve endocarditis typically affects left heart valves, except in intravenous drug users, where right heart valves tend to be infected; the reasons are unclear.

Clinical presentation is characterised by fever, systemic symptoms including weight loss and anorexia, new or changing heart murmurs or peripheral vasculitic signs including petechiae, splinter haemorrhages or Osler nodes. Neurological complications are common and brought about either by bacteraemia leading to meningitis, cerebritis or a parameningeal focus or by recurrent emboli which may be infective. Cerebral emboli commonly involve the anterior cerebral circulation and are frequently multiple with up to 10% becoming haemorrhagic. There is often a preceding transient ischaemic attack and concurrent systemic emboli are common. Septic emboli may cause cerebral infarction, meningitis or parenchymal abscess but they also lead to the development of mycotic aneurysms which occur when an infected arterial wall becomes weakened (Figure 9.5). Mycotic aneurysms usually develop at arterial bifurcation or in distal arterial vessels and carry a high risk of rupture into the parenchyma and subarachnoid space leading to stroke, causing focal neurological deficits, meningism, declining consciousness and coma. Cerebral abscesses may be multiple and also lead to severe focal or generalised neurological deficits. Bacterial meningitis is common in endocarditis and carries a poor prognosis. Meningitis may lead to cerebral vasculitis, a condition seen particularly in staphylococcal infection. Ocular involvement may occur with vasculitis involving the retina, optic nerve, oculomotor nerves or brainstem. Central retinal artery occlusion, ophthalmoplegia or field loss may follow.

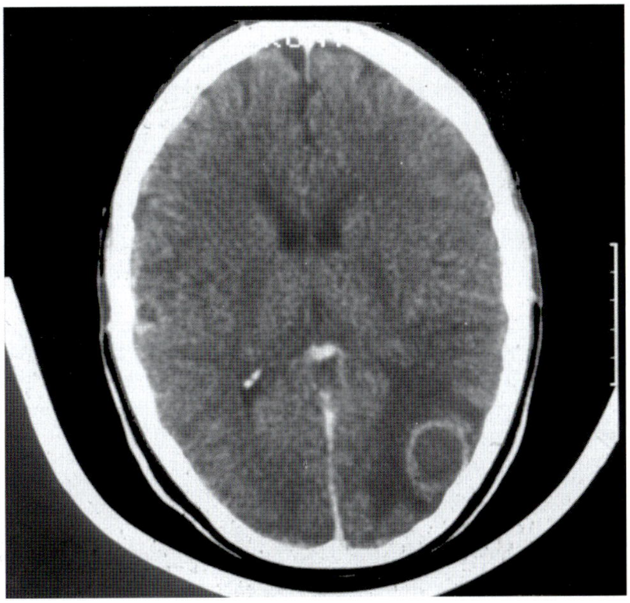

Figure 9.5 CT scan showing mycotic aneurym in *Streptococcus viridans* endocarditis.

Endocarditis should be carefully considered in any patient with a focal or generalised neurological deficit and unexplained pyrexia. The diagnosis depends on appropriate cardiac imaging including transthoracic and transoesophageal echocardiography, serial blood cultures and urine microscopy for red cells. Neurological investigation includes imaging of the brain and intracranial vessels with CT and/or MRI, and CSF examination; catheter angiography may be needed in cases of parenchymal or subarachnoid haemorrhage.

Treatment involves the urgent initiation of organism-specific antibiotics and depends on bacterial sensitivities and underlying risk factors. There should be close liaison with a bacteriologist. The 2012 British Society of Antimicrobial Chemotherapy guidelines recommend the following.

- Native valve *S. viridans* endocarditis should be treated with benzylpenicillin (or ceftriaxone) and gentamicin in regimens varying between 2 and 6 weeks depending on penicillin resistance. Longer courses are given for prosthetic valve *S. viridans* endocarditis. Vancomycin is used if there is penicillin allergy.
- Native valve staphylococcal endocarditis requires a 6-week course of flucloxacillin; if there is MRSA, vancomycin and rifampicin are used.
- Prosthetic valve staphylococcal endocarditis requires the addition of gentamicin and rifampicin to flucloxacillin or vancomycin.

The management of cerebral emboli and mycotic aneurysms is difficult. Longer courses of endocarditis treatments are recommended in cases of cerebral complications. Anticoagulation should be avoided because of the high risk of haemorrhagic transformation. Neurosurgical intervention is rarely indicated, endovascular procedures are occasionally undertaken. However, a conservative approach is usually justified depending on the size and location of the aneurysm. Despite advances in antibiotic management and supportive care, the prognosis of endocarditis once there is CNS infection is poor, with mortality of <20%.

Granulomatous infections of the nervous system

CNS tuberculosis

Tuberculous meningitis

Mycobacterium tuberculosis infection occurs by person-to-person droplet spread. The organism is inhaled into the lower portion of the lungs and there multiplies locally before disseminating through lymphatic and haematological spread into other organs. The general decline of tuberculosis in Europe has led to a marked reduction in the incidence of tuberculous meningitis (TBM) but the condition is still frequent in developing countries and in patients who are immunosuppressed, particularly because of HIV. However, there has been a recent increase in TB in the United Kingdom and other nations in the European Union. TBM develops secondary to a small caseating subpial and subependymal foci in the brain and spinal cord adjacent to the CSF (Rich foci). In some individuals, foci rupture and release bacteria into the subarachnoid space causing meningitis. In others, foci enlarge to form tuberculomas without meningitis. Both tuberculomas and parenchymal tuberculosis occur as a result of haematogenous spread. They may develop in the absence of pulmonary tuberculosis.

TBM is characterised by inflammatory meningeal adhesive exudates leading to a florid small and medium vessel vasculitis which culminates in occlusion of cerebral arteries and infarction. There is also a disturbance of CSF flow because of impairment of absorption

Table 9.8 Poor prognostic factors in tuberculous meningitis.

Disease severity
Impairment of consciousness
Presence of neurological deficits, seizures or abnormal movements
Extremes of age
Co-existing miliary disease
CSF protein with spinal block
Very low CSF glucose
CT scan showing abnormalities
HIV positive, low CD4 (below 50/mm^3)
Illness longer than 14 days

CSF, cerebrospinal fluid; CT, computed tomography.

at the arachnoid villi and blockage at the aqueduct and 4th ventricular outlet. In tuberculous meningitis, vasculitis particularly affects the vessels at the base of the brain – the internal carotid and proximal middle cerebral arteries – and perforating arteries to the basal ganglia and internal capsule. TBM was almost invariably fatal before the development of antituberculous chemotherapy. Tuberculosis in immunosuppressed adults, especially those with HIV infection, is likely to be disseminated and involve the CNS. Other risk factors for TBM include alcoholism, diabetes mellitus, malignancy, corticosteroid treatment and tumour necrosis factor (TNF) blocking drugs. Table 9.8 summarises factors of prognostic significance in the outcome of CNS tuberculosis.

Clinical manifestations TBM is often preceded by a prolonged prodrome (>6 days) of non-specific malaise, anorexia, low grade fever, myalgia, photophobia and headache. Neck stiffness is usually absent. The development of meningitis may be insidious, with worsening headache, nausea, vomiting, focal or generalised seizures and progressive impairment of consciousness. Cranial nerve palsies are common and often initially involve eye movements resulting from IIIrd, IVth or VIth nerve palsy. There may be facial weakness (VII), optic neuropathy (II), progressive hearing loss (VIII) and eventual bulbar involvement (X–XII). Fundal examination may show papilloedema, optic atrophy or the presence of choroidal tubercles. Visual impairment may also develop because of involvement of the optic chiasm, tuberculomas compressing the optic pathways or optic nerve toxicity resulting from treatment with ethambutol. Other neurological signs include hemiparesis and hemiplegia as a consequence of vasculitic infarction or space-occupying tuberculomas. Movement disorders may be manifest as tremor, myoclonus, chorea, hemiballismus or dystonia and cerebellar ataxia may occur from direct involvement or vasculitic infarction. Vasculitis usually occurs in the distribution of the anterior circulation, particularly affecting the deep structures, but occasionally involves the posterior territory. The major complications of TBM are:

- Hydrocephalus
- Stroke
- Tuberculoma formation.

Diagnosis The diagnosis of TBM or focal parenchymatous involvement can be difficult clinically. Tuberculin skin test is variable in its response and unreliable as there may be an anergy even in the presence of miliary tuberculosis. Interferon gamma release assays are increasingly used but cannot differentiate active from latent disease and are negative in 25% of cases. CSF examination is characterised by the presence of an elevated opening pressure in 50%, lymphocytic pleocytosis with a high protein and low glucose. The white cell count is usually 5–500 /mm^3 and should not generally exceed 1000/mm^3 but there may be a significant proportion of polymorphonuclear cells in the initial stages. The protein is generally elevated up to 1 g/L but may be greater than this particularly if there is a spinal block. The glucose concentration is low (often <2.2 mmol/L) and this is usually below 50% of the serum glucose.

A tissue diagnosis (by histopathology and culture) should be attempted whenever possible, either by meningeal biopsy or through diagnostic sampling from extraneural sites of disease (e.g. lung, gastric fluid, lymph nodes, liver or bone marrow). PCR can be performed directly on clinical specimens in untreated patients but is less sensitive than culture, particularly in extrapulmonary specimens. All patients with suspected or proven tuberculosis should be offered HIV testing.

CSF bacteriology No specific test has high sensitivity. Direct examination of the CSF for acid–alcohol fast bacilli (AFB) using Ziehl–Neelsen or auramine staining requires large volumes of CSF (minimum 10 mL) and is dependent on the experience of the microscopist. AFB are only seen in approximately 10% of cases with appropriate staining. CSF culture is the diagnostic investigation but requires up to 6 weeks, has a yield of 10–60% and is therefore of only limited value in clinical practice. CSF culture has the advantage of indicating drug sensitivities if the samples are taken before treatment has commenced.

Nucleic acid amplification techniques (NAATs) for the diagnosis of TBM are 98% specific but only 56% sensitive. Therefore, NAATs can confirm the diagnosis but cannot exclude it. The use of real-time PCR can improve the sensitivity but is expensive. The only way to diagnose drug resistant TBM is through CSF NAATs and the detection of genetic mutations that confer drug resistance. However, at present, this approach is limited by the low sensitivity of CSF NAATs and uncertainty about which mutations best predict resistance for some drugs.

Radiology Approximately 50% of patients with TBM show evidence of previous tuberculosis on chest X-ray, with up to 10% having miliary tuberculosis. CT brain scanning is commonly abnormal with marked enhancing exudate in the basal cisterns. There may also be hydrocephalus, parenchymal enhancement, evidence of cerebral infarction or cerebral oedema or focal tuberculoma. MRI is sensitive in showing meningeal enhancement, focal parenchymal abnormalities or the development of communicating or obstructive hydrocephalus (Figure 9.6).

Management of tuberculous meningitis TBM, like all bacterial meningitides, is a medical emergency. Treatment delay is strongly associated with death and empirical antituberculous treatment should be started promptly in all patients in whom the diagnosis of TBM is suspected without awaiting microbial or molecular confirmation. Chemotherapy for CNS tuberculosis consists of an intensive phase of treatment followed by a continuation phase. This is aimed at eradicating the causative organisms and management of the complications caused by the inflammatory response including hydrocephalus, vasculitis and raised intracranial pressure. The standard treatment of TBM is with an intensive primary phase of treatment followed by a continuation phase as summarised in Table 9.9 and

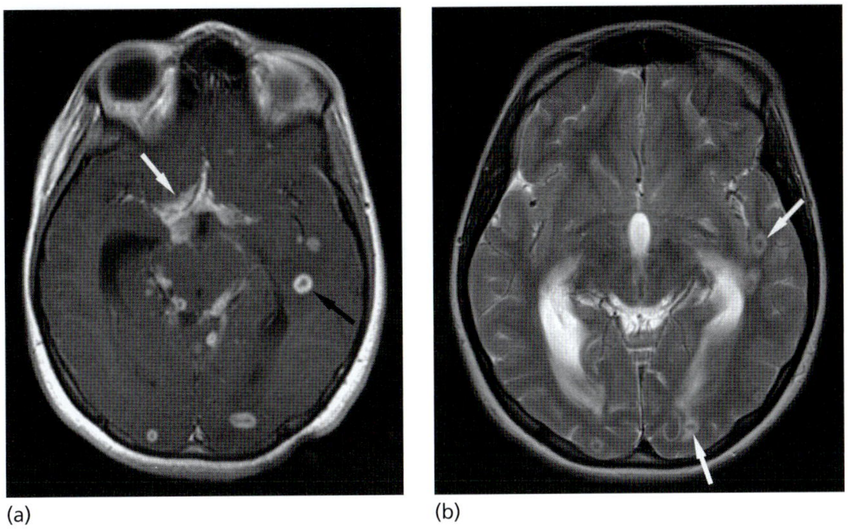

Figure 9.6 TB: basal meningitis and multiple tuberculomas. (a) T1-weighted post-contrast MRI showing extensive enhancing material within the basal cisterns encasing the vessels of the circle of Willis (white arrow) and multiple ring enhancing tuberculomas typified by the left temporal lesion (black arrow). (b) T2-weighted MRI showing hydrocephalus and multiple tubercluomas with characteristic hypointense centre and hyperintense rim (white arrows).

Table 9.9 Treatment of tuberculous meningitis – initial phase using four drugs for 2 months.

	Adult daily dose	Comment	Side effects
Isoniazid	300 mg	Essential drug Penetrates CSF freely and has potent early bacteriocidal activity Add pyridoxine to avoid peripheral neuropathy	Hepatitis, haemolytic anaemia, aplastic anaemia, peripheral neuropathy, optic neuritis, mania, fits
Rifampicin	450 mg (wt <50 kg) 600 mg (wt >50 kg)	Essential drug Bacteriocidal but poor CSF penetration (10%)	Hepatitis, thrombocytopenia, headache, confusion, drowsiness
Pyrazinamide	1.5 g (wt <50 kg) 2.0 g (wt >50 kg)	Bacteriocidal with good penetration	Hepatitis, anorexia, flushing
Fourth drug: use one of			
Streptomycin	20–40 mg/kg	Neither penetrates CSF well in absence of inflammation (10–50%)	Avoid in pregnancy and renal impairment Neuromuscular blockade
Ethambutol	15 mg/kg		Retrobulbar neuritis, peripheral neuropathy, confusion
Ethionamide	500–750 mg	Penetrate healthy and inflamed meninges but no evidence of advantage over other drugs	

Table 9.10. Treatment should commence with isoniazid, rifampicin, pyrazinamide and ethambutol for 2 months and this should be followed by a 9–12 month continuation phase of treatment with isoniazid and rifampicin or pyrazinamide. There remains some debate about the duration of treatment. Expert opinion should be sought where possible: TBM has a poor prognosis.

Isoniazid and pyrazinamide are bacteriocidal and show good penetration through inflamed meninges, easily achieving therapeutic concentrations. Rifampicin, ethambutol and streptomycin have poorer penetration and achieve lower CSF concentrations (maximum concentration around 30% of plasma) but the high mortality from rifampicin resistant tuberculosis confirms its role. The fourth drug (ethambutol) is added to cover the possibility of isoniazid resistant bacteria. All antituberculous treatment carries significant risks of toxicity. Treatment with a fourth drug during the initial phase remains indicated despite the poor ability of streptomycin and ethambutol to cross the blood–brain barrier. Ethambutol-induced optic neuropathy is a concern but is infrequent. The dose conventionally follows those used in pulmonary TB but remains controversial.

There is an increasing incidence of tuberculosis caused by organisms resistant to conventional treatment. The risk of drug resisitance must be assessed individually for all patients with CNS

Table 9.10 Treatment of tuberculous meningitis– continuation phase using two drugs for 9–12 months.

Isoniazid	
Rifampicin	
Pyrazinamide	
Suspected or proven multidrug resistance:	
Aminoglycoside	Kanamycin, amikacin, capreomycin
Ethionamide	
Protionamide	
Fluoroquinolones	Moxifloxacin, levofloxacin
Linezolid	

tuberculosis. Suspected isoniazid resistant disease should be treated with conventional four-drug first line therapy followed by 12 months treatment with rifampicin, isoniazid and pyrazinamide. If high level isonizid resistance is proven the isoniazid should be exchanged for levofloxacin or moxifloxacin for 12 months treatment. With suspected or proven multi-drug resistance initial therapy should be with a fluoroquinone (levofloxacin or moxifloxacin), pyrazinamide, ethionamide or prothionamide and an injectable agent (kanamycin, amikacin or capreomycin) followed by a maintenance course for 9–18 months.

Corticosteroids Adjunctive corticosteroids reduce death and disability from TBM by about 30% and are recommended for all patients with the disease. Treatment should be with 0.4 mg/kg dexamethasone, intravenously initially, gradually reducing and switching to oral, stopping after 6–8 weeks. Alternative treatment is with 2–5 mg/kg prednisolone intravenously initially and then reducing and switching to oral over 4 weeks. More prolonged courses may be considered if there is cerebral oedema, spinal block, severe tuberculous meningitis, spinal arachnoiditis or cerebral vasculitis.

Surgical intervention Surgical intervention may be required in the presence of obstructive hydrocephalus that has not responded to medical treatment. This usually consists of an external ventricular drain initially but may eventually necessitate a ventriculo-peritoneal shunt. Shunt complications are common (<30%) thus endoscopic 3rd ventriculostomy has become an alternative surgical treatment option. Success rates for this procedure are approximately 65%, with failure being caused by distorted anatomy of the 3rd ventricular floor in the acute phase of the disease.

Outcome The outcome of TBM has remained poor and the mortality is still >20%, with severe neurological sequelae occurring in up to 30% of survivors. Early drug treatment is essential, particularly before the development of impaired consciousness and coma. Late neurological disability is predicted by the presence of extrameningeal tuberculosis, cranial nerve palsies, limb weakness and multiple neurological abnormalities including hydrocephalus, cerebral infarction, expanding tuberculomas and hyponatraemia.

Parenchymal CNS tuberculosis

Tuberculous granuloma (tuberculoma) Tuberculous granulomas can be found in the cerebrum, brainstem, cerebellum, spinal cord, subarachnoid or epidural space but are generally supratentorial; they may be multiple in up to two-thirds of patients and may coexist with TBM in about 10% of patients. They present as space-occupying lesions with headache, intracranial hypertension, seizures and papilloedema. There may be motor, cerbellar or brainstem signs. Imaging confirms the presence of an enhancing space-occupying lesion, occasionally with central calcification. They usually resolve with conventional antituberculous treatment but there may be an initial phase of paradoxical expansion even with appropriate therapy. Occasionally, surgical intervention is indicated.

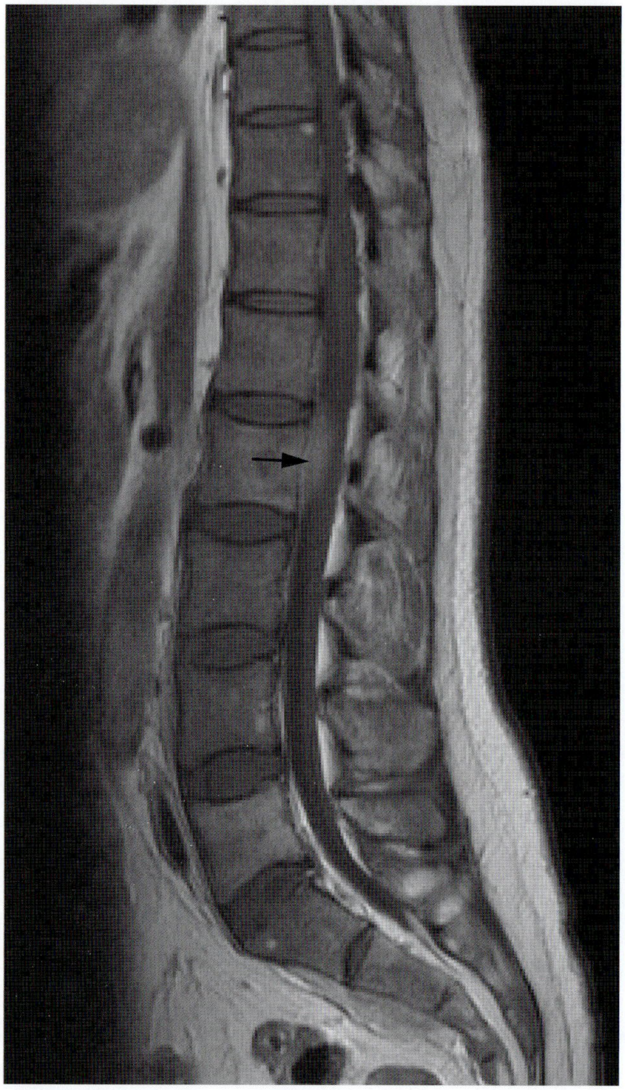

Figure 9.7 Anteriorly placed tuberculous spinal abscess (arrow).

Tuberculous abscess

Tuberculous abscess results from liquifaction of the central core of the tuberculoma. The lesions often enlarge and become multilocular and have mass effect associated with oedema. They tend to resemble pyogenic abscesses rather than tuberculomas and are difficult to distinguish clinically. They do not always respond well to antituberculous chemotherapy; surgical excision may be necessary.

Spinal tuberculosis (tuberculous spondylitis)

Tuberculosis may involve the spinal vertebral bodies, with a predilection for the anterior elements (Figure 9.7). In adults, at least two contiguous levels and their intervening disc space are involved, particularly in thoracic and lumbar regions. Paraspinal soft tissue involvement is common and a paravertebral tuberculous abscess (Pott's abscess) may occur in up to 30% of patients with tuberculous spondylitis. Spinal collapse is also frequent and leads to gibbus, extrinsic cord compression and paraparesis.

Tuberculous spinal meningitis may be localised to the spinal cord. In this condition there is a gross granulomatous exudate in the subarachnoid space, which causes a vasculitic response in the spinal vessels, particularly the anterior spinal artery, culminating in ischaemia or infarction of the spinal cord. There may also be a progressive radiculopathy, myelopathy or transverse myelitis. Intramedullary spinal cord tuberculous abscess or, rarely, tuberculoma may occur within the substance of the spinal cord mimicking a tumour. Tuberculous radiculomyelopathy or transverse myelitis often present acutely but may be slower in onset. They may be characterised by radicular pain, bladder disturbance or progressive paraparesis. CSF shows a high protein content with lymphocytic pleocytosis and a low glucose. MRI scan shows contrast enhancements surrounding the spinal cord and roots and often a diffusely increased intramedullary signal. Spinal cord disease is treated with prolonged standard antituberculous treatment and systemic steroids. If there is significant bone destruction, bracing and/or surgical decompression may be necessary.

Leprosy (Hansen's disease)

Leprosy is a common condition worldwide, but occurs predominantly in Africa (particularly Sudan and Nigeria), South America (particularly Brazil), South-East Asia, Nepal, India, Pakistan, Bangladesh and China. The prevalence is difficult to establish because of incomplete reporting. The disease remains widely feared and poorly understood but it is not highly contagious and curative treatment is available. However, early diagnosis and appropriate management are necessary to minimise the risk of irreversible neuropathy, deformity and disability. Leprosy is due to *Mycobacterium leprae* which causes granulomas to form in the peripheral nerves and skin. The organism is an intracellular AFB that resembles the tubercle bacillus. It multiplies at a cool temperature (27°C and 33°C) and therefore favours distal parts of the human body. There is a prolonged incubation period of 2–5 years but this may be as long as 20 years. The organism has a predilection for Schwann cells associated with thinly myelinated axons. The infective risk of leprosy is relatively low, even after exposure, and the means of transmission are not fully understood. The disease is probably transmitted from person to person by aerosol with a high subclinical rate of infection. Household and prolonged close contact seem important. There is anecdotal evidence that it may be transmitted by inoculation, such as by contaminated tattoo. Primary infection is followed by haematogeneous spread to preferential sites including skin, peripheral nerves, upper respiratory tract, anterior chamber of the eye and the testes.

The pattern of illness is determined by the host's immune response to the mycobacterial antigen. When there is an active cell-mediated immune reaction directed against *M. leprae*, tuberculoid leprosy develops which is restricted to a few peripheral nerves. However, a poor immune response leads to lepromatous leprosy in which there is an extensive proliferation of bacilli. Some patients have borderline patterns with features of both tuberculoid and lepromatous. The World Health Organization (WHO) now uses a simplified classification scheme that relies on clinical examination and skin scrapings, dividing cases into paucibacillary and multibacillary leprosy. Paucibacillary leprosy is defined as five or fewer skin lesions without detectable bacilli on skin smears while in multibacillary leprosy there are six or more lesions and skin smear may be positive. The risk of transmission from close contact is much greater in the multibacillary form.

Clinical features

Leprosy is characterised by hypoaesthetic skin lesions, thickened peripheral nerves and positive skin smear showing AFB.

In tuberculoid leprosy, the earliest skin lesions are single or few with clearly demarcated asymmetrical hypopigmented or erythematous skin lesions which are hypoaesthetic and are scattered across the body with no obvious preferential areas. They have a sharp edge but vary in size. Patients may complain of a numb patch or patches and/or minor and typically painless skin lumps.

In lepromatous leprosy, there is a more diffuse involvement of the skin with extensive hypopigmented, nodular or maculopapular infiltration affecting the body, the skin of the face and the earlobes, with progressive loss of the eyebrows and eyelashes. Over the course of years, there may develop coarse thickening of the features, particularly the earlobes, nose and cheeks, giving rise to the characteristic leonine facies. The larynx may also be involved. The testes become atrophic; gynaecomastia and sterility may follow. Visual impairment occurs because facial weakness and anaesthesia of the conjunctiva and cornea lead to corneal ulceration and scarring culminating in exposure keratitis. There also may be an iridocyclitis and cataracts secondary to intraocular involvement by the bacilli.

Peripheral nerve involvement

In tuberculoid leprosy, there is involvement of the small superficial nerves in the cooler part of the body and at points where they are exposed, leading to pain and temperature, touch and pressure impairment over affected skin areas but nerve thickening is less common than in lepromatous disease.

The most frequently affected peripheral nerves (nerves of predilection) are:

- Ulnar nerve
- Posterior tibial nerve and sural (at the medial malleolus of the tibia)
- Common peroneal nerve (at the knee where it winds around the neck of the fibula)
- Median (at the wrist)
- Facial (crossing zygomatic arch)
- Trigeminal nerve involvement of ophthalmic division of the trigeminal nerve leading to corneal and conjunctival sensory loss, ulceration and blindness
- Greater auricular (posterior triangle of the neck)
- Supraorbital
- Superficial radial (cutaneous at the wrist).

Lepromatous involvement of the peripheral nerves is insidious over many years. Peripheral nerve thickening affects sensori-motor and autonomic nerves to a varying extent and may cause either a focal or diffuse mononeuritis multiplex or a progressive symmetrical distal peripheral neuropathy. Sensory impairment is more common than motor but there may be atrophy and weakness leading to claw hands or bilateral foot drop.

Immunological reactions are systemic inflammatory complications that occur either before, during or after treatment and affect 30–50% of patients. There are two types of reaction: type I occurs in patients with borderline disease and seems to be caused by an intensification of the cellular immune response to *M. leprae*. It is manifest as a worsening erythema or swelling of an existing lesion; inflammation leading to severe nerve injury with pain and tenderness in a peripheral nerve distribution with subsequent paralysis and deformity; peripheral oedema and ulcerated skin lesions. Type 2 reaction (erythema nodosum leprosum) occurs in lepromatous disease. It is characterised by the acute eruption of numerous painful nodules which can form pustules or ulcerate. There may also be pyrexia, headache, generalised pain, tender lymphadenopathy, iridocyclitis, muscle tenderness and swollen joints. The mechanism of type 2 reactions is uncertain but has previously been thought of as an immune complex disorder.

Borderline leprosy

In borderline leprosy there are features of both tuberculoid and lepromatous forms. Hypoaesthetic skin lesions occur but they differ slightly in appearance from lepromatous leprosy. Borderline patients are particularly vulnerable to nerve damage and may develop severe deformities including trophic ulceration. The affected nerve trunk is often swollen and painful.

Primary neuritic leprosy

This is seen in India and Nepal and presents as peripheral nerve involvement without the characteristic skin lesions. Skin smears are negative for AFB. Neurological manifestations are caused by asymmetrical involvement of one or several peripheral nerve trunks and sensory changes develop before motor features. Isolated nerve thickening may occur. Skin lesions may develop later in the course of the illness.

Diagnosis

This is difficult and primarily clinical. Nerve conduction studies show axonal loss and demyelination with focal slowing across thickened nerve segments suggesting segmental demyelination. There is loss of the sensory action potentials. A skin smear is used to assess the density of AFBs – they are always found in the multi-bacillary form but only in 30% of borderline disease. Skin biopsy is essential for correct classification and diagnosis when skin smears are negative. Nerve biopsy of a thickened sensory nerve (usually sural or radial cutaneous nerve) may also yield a diagnosis. The Lepromin skin test assesses the patient's cell-mediated immunity against *M. leprae* and is strongly positive in tuberculoid leprosy but is negative in lepromatous leprosy. This test is of no value in patients who have received bacille Calmette–Guérin (BCG) vaccination or who have had previous subclinical disease. Serology tests use radioimmune assay and ELISA based on the detection of antibodies to *M. leprae* antigen. The *M. leprae* genome has now been entirely sequenced and it is possible to detect the organism using PCR amplification in skin and nerve biopsies.

Management

Accurate classification is essential to establish the correct treatment. Multi-drug therapy with a combination of rifampicin, dapsone and clofazimine is effective in both multibacillary and paucibacillary leprosy and nerve function appears to improve with early treatment. The skin lesions in paucibacillary leprosy resolve within a year but in patients with multibacillary leprosy they persist for much longer. However, with prolonged treatment relapse rates are low. Dapsone, the original drug treatment, is only slowly bactericidal and needs to be given daily. It is limited in its effectiveness and there is a high incidence of resistance if the drug is used alone. Side effects are rare but malaise, haemolytic anaemia and leukopenia can occur. Rifampicin is a strongly bactericidal drug which is rapidly effective. Because of the slow rate of replication of *M. leprae* the drug need be given only once a month but resistance may occur on monotherapy. Clofazimine is weakly bactericidal but is highly effective in controlling lepromatous leprosy, particularly in suppressing the inflammation of erythema nodosum.

Patients with paucibacillary leprosy are generally treated with two drugs. The WHO recommends rifampicin 600 mg once a month (supervised) and dapsone 100 mg/day (unsupervised) for 6 months. This regimen should be followed by treatment with dapsone as monotherapy for 3 years in patients with tuberculoid leprosy or 5 years in patients with borderline lepromatous leprosy. The National Hansen's Disease Program (NHDP) recommends rifampicin 600 mg/day and dapsone 100 mg/day for 12 months. Patients with multibacillary leprosy receive three drugs. The WHO recommends dapsone 100 mg/day (unsupervised), clofazimine 50 mg/day (unsupervised) and rifampicin 600 mg once a month plus clofazimine 300 mg once a month (unsupervised) for 12 months. The NHDP recommends dapsone 100 mg/day, rifampicin 600 mg/day and clofazimine 50 mg/day for 24 months. All treated patients should be followed up for reactions or relapses for many years after completing treatment. There is a small but increasing incidence of resistance to dapsone, notably in Vietnam. The neuropathy is often treated with oral steroids; 60% of patients usually regain some nerve function but this can take many months.

Mild immunological reactions can be managed with supportive care and antimicrobial treatment should be continued. Severe reactions with neuritis or erythema nodosum, cropping of facial lesions and ocular involvement require corticosteroids (prednisolone 40–60 mg/day tapered when the reaction is controlled – this may be up to 3 months in borderline disease and up to 9 months for lepromatous forms). Second line treatment includes ciclosporin for severe type 1 reactions and thalidomide (300–400 mg/day) for type 2 leprosy reactions, although teratogenicity limits its use in women of child-bearing age.

The social stigmata associated with deformity and scarring from leprosy remain a considerable worldwide problem despite extensive health education programmes run by WHO and other community projects. Leprosy control has been integrated into general health services in endemic areas, increasing access to diagnostic and treatment facilities. Despite these advances leprosy remains feared – difficulty in achieving diagnosis and poor compliance with treatment remain a major concern.

Brucellosis (undulant fever)

Brucellosis is a zoonotic infection caused by Gram-negative coccobacilli, *Brucella melitensis*, *B. abortis* and *B. suis*, harboured in sheep, cattle and pigs, respectively. Camels' milk can also become infected. Transmission of brucellosis to humans occurs through consumption of infected and unpasturised milk, through direct contact with animals, living or dead, and through direct inhalation of aerosol particles. It is a granulomatous disease, either acute or indolent in character. There is a non-specific prodrome with a variable and irregular (undulant) fever and flu-like symptoms of malaise, night sweats, malodorous perspiration, arthralgia and myalgia. Lymphadenopathy and hepatosplenomegaly follows; this either resolves or is followed by localised single organ infection. Osteoarticular disease is the most common and this can manifest as polyarthritis, sacroileitis or spondylitis.

The nervous system is affected in about 5% of patients; meningitis and meningo-encephalitis are the most common presentation with meningism, confusion and impaired level of consciousness. Cranial nerve deficits occur as a consequence of granulomatous involvement at the skull base, with facial weakness, sensorineural hearing loss and ocular symptoms from retrobulbar neuritis, papilloedema, optic neuropathy and ophthalmoplegia, all of which may occur. Brucella meningitis can lead to hydrocephalus and raised intracranial pressure. Brain and spinal cord abscesses can develop. There may be a granulomatous endarteritis or focal vasculitis causing stroke, myelitis or a radiculopathy. Polyneuropathy may also develop. Endocarditis is the principal cause of death. This organism is regarded as a biohazard and the laboratory should be warned of the possibility of a case of brucellosis. The diagnosis is often made serologically but culture is the gold standard. However, blood cultures are positive in only 40% of acute cases, with bone marrow cultures offering an additional 20% yield. CSF is positive 25% on culture or serological tests include tube agglutination and enzyme linked immunosorbent assay. There is no standardised PCR test yet available. CSF shows an elevated protein with a lymphocytic pleocytosis and a low glucose; occasionally oligoclonal bands are present. MRI may show contrast enhanced inflammatory changes in the spinal cord or brain.

Brucellosis is treated by various combinations of antibiotics: there is a high relapse rate with a single drug. WHO guidelines recommend doxycycline for 6 weeks (though not in pregnancy) with either streptomycin for 2-3 weeks or rifampicin for 6 weeks. Alternative drug combinations are co-trimoxazole with a quinolone, such as ciprofloxacin or moxifloxacin. Brucella meningitis should be treated with three drugs for 2–6 months. Regimens include doxycycline, rifampin and either ceftriaxone or co-trimoxazole. Ceftriaxone-based regimens may be more successful and allow shorter duration of therapy but therapy is generally prolonged (months) and needs to be individualised according to clinical signs and symptoms; in general, it should be continued until CSF parameters have returned to normal. The role of corticosteroids is uncertain and they are not part of routine therapy. Steroids may be appropriate in the setting of neurobrucellosis complicated by iritis, papilloedema, myelopathy, polyneuropathy and/or cranial nerve palsies.

Surgical drainage of brucella abscesses may be necessary.

Spirochete CNS infections

Syphilis

Syphilis is increasing in prevalence in the United Kingdom, in particular amongst homosexual men with HIV. It is a chronic systemic infection caused by the spirochete *Treponema pallidum* subsp. *pallidum*. It is transmitted through contact with an infected lesion (usually sexual contact), from mother to fetus during pregnancy (congenital syphilis) and through contaminated blood products. It readily penetrates intact mucus membranes and abraded skin, rapidly reaching the bloodstream and lymphatics.

Syphilis is characterised by four stages:

1. *Primary* Local primary chancre with regional lymphadenopathy
2. *Secondary* Multisystem involvement with generalised mucocutaneous lesions
3. *Latent* Previous infection with positive serological tests but no symptoms or signs
4. *Late (tertiary)* Involvement of the heart, bone, skin and CNS, many years after primary infection. The most common manifestations of late syphilis are cardiovascular (especially aortitis), CNS (general paralysis and tabes dorsalis) and gummatous (granulomatous, nodular lesions affecting a variety of organs, particularly skin and bones.)

Primary syphilis usually develops within a few days of exposure but may be delayed up to 90 days. It is characterised by a painless ulcer known as a chancre at the site of inoculation, with local lymphadenopathy. A chancre is highly infectious, but heals spontaneously over the course of some weeks.

Secondary syphilis usually develops 6–12 weeks after the chancre heals and consists of a characteristic generalised maculopapular rash involving the palms, soles and mucosal surfaces, with diffuse generalised lymphadenopathy, fever, weight loss and malaise. The patient is highly infectious during secondary disease. Secondary syphilis also causes meningitis. There may also be proctitis, hepatitis, gastritis, nephrotic syndrome and iridocyclitis.

The secondary infection resolves spontaneously, to become latent with a prolonged quiescent phase for a decade or more. About one-third of patients with latent syphilis who remain untreated develop tertiary disease and one-third of these develop symptomatic neurosyphilis. In a study of patients with untreated syphilis, 10% developed cardiovascular syphilis, 16% gummatous and 6.5% symptomatic neurosyphilis. With HIV infection, all stages of syphilis tend to be accelerated.

Syphilitic meningitis usually develops within the first year after infection but the onset may be delayed. The onset is with progressive headache, confusion and meningism. There may be progressive cranial nerve (particularly VII and VIII) involvement and focal signs such as aphasia, hemiparesis and focal epilepsy. Ocular involvement includes uveitis, vitritis, retinitis and optic neuritis. Focal meningeal inflammation may give rise to syphilitic gummas (see Intracerebral gumma) or a diffuse hyperplastic pachymeningitis affecting the cortex or spinal cord. Spinal involvement leads to back pain, muscle wasting and weakness (occasionally resembling motor neurone disease), urinary incontinence and sensory impairment.

Pachymeningitis refers to a localised, inflammatory thickening of the dura which has a number of causes:

- Infective
  - neurosyphilis
  - CNS tuberculosis: tuberculous pachymeningitis
  - CNS cryptococcosis
  - bacterial meningitis
- Inflammatory
  - Wegener's granulomatosis
  - polyarteritis nodosa
  - rheumatoid arthritis
- Neurosarcoidosis
- IgG4 disease
- Haemodialysis
- Mucopolysaccharidoses
- Idiopathic hypertrophic pachymeningitis.

Meningo-vascular syphilis is a form of early symptomatic neurosyphilis. It develops within 10 years of infection and is caused by syphilitic meningitis causing an infectious obliterative endarteritis and periarteritis with meningitis and spinal arachnoiditis (Figure 9.8). Impairment of CSF absorption may lead to hydrocephalus, with headache or confusion; there may be signs of focal cortical involvement brought about by ischaemic stroke including aphasia, hemiplegia, hemisensory disturbance or multiple cranial nerve palsies leading to diplopia, vertigo and dysarthria. Spinal cord involvement caused by meningo-myelitis is characterised by the slow evolution of a spastic paraparesis with bowel and bladder involvement and lower limb sensory loss. There may also be a more acute transverse myelitis caused by infarction caused by anterior spinal artery occlusion. Meningo-vascular syphilis should be considered in the differential diagnosis of ischaemic stroke in a young person. The CSF changes in meningo-vascular neurosyphilis are generally less severe than those in acute meningitis with a lymphocytic pleocytosis of 10–100 cells/mm^3 and a protein of 1–2 g/L.

Late neurosyphilis

Tabes dorsalis Tabes dorsalis has the longest latent period between primary infection and the onset of symptoms of late neurosyphilis with an average duration of 20 years although the time to onset can be much shorter. There is involvement of the posterior columns and root entry zones with diffuse inflammatory infiltration and atrophic change. Symptoms include characteristic lightning pains in the legs – intensely painful, sharp shooting paraesthesiae and pain – often associated with episodic acute abdominal pain, known as tabetic crises. The proprioceptive loss leads to a severely ataxic gait

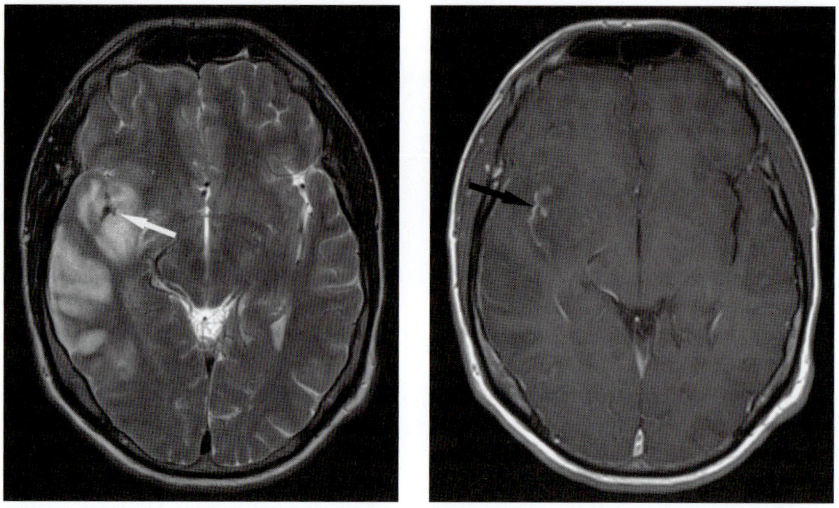

(a) (b)

Figure 9.8 Meningovascular syphilis: T2-weighted and post-contrast T1-weighted images (a and b, respectively) showing right temporal lobe infarction. A thrombosed right middle cerebral artery branch can be seen (white arrow) with enhancement of the vessel and adjacent leptomeninges (black arrow).

with characteristic stamping. There is also impaired deep pain sensation in the limbs and the development of bladder, bowel and sexual dysfunction. Progressive posterior column impairment leads to neuropathic (Charcot) joints, a severe destructive arthropathy caused by repeated trauma, ulcers may develop around these joints. Cranial nerve abnormalities are associated with tabes including optic atrophy and pupillary abnormalities.

General paralysis General paralysis is a recrudescence of infection (GPI) caused by direct invasion of the brain by spirochetes leading to frontal and temporal atrophy. GPI develops >15 years after the initial infection. There is a progressive cognitive impairment with memory loss and disintegration of personality and behaviour leading to severe dementia. Psychiatric problems include emotional lability, paranoia, delusions of grandeur and hallucinations. There may be a coarse tremor of the tongue and similar tremor of the extremities with pyramidal signs including hyper-reflexia. Pupillary abnormalities are characterised by the Argyll Robertson pupil, a tiny irregular pupil, fixed to light but with a preserved accommodation reflex.

Intracerebral gumma

Gummas are granulomatous masses formed by a chronic cellular hypersensitivity reaction resulting from late benign syphilis. Gummas form in skin, bone, abdominal viscera and the brain. Intracerebral gummas may act as mass lesions causing compression of adjacent structures, raised intracranial pressure or epilepsy. Cutaneous and intracerebral gummas usually heal rapidly after penicillin therapy with little scarring.

Diagnosis

The diagnosis of neurosyphilis is initially clinical but if neurosyphilis is suspected on the basis of positive serology CSF examination is mandatory. *T. pallidum* cannot be cultured. Diagnosis depends on identifying the spirochete by direct visualisation or by serology. In primary and secondary syphilis, direct visualisation is achieved by dark field microscopy of tissue samples from skin and mucous membranes. The diagnosis of latent syphilis and neurosyphilis relies on serological tests. These are either non-specific antigen tests such as the Venereal Disease Research Laboratory (VDRL) and rapid plasma reagin (RPR) or specific tests based on the detection of IgG and IgM directed against treponemal antibodies such as the fluorescent treponemal antibody absorption test (FTA-AbS), *Treponema pallidum* particle agglutination assay (TPPA) and the syphilis enzyme-linked immunosorbent assay (ELISA). The non-specific tests such as VDRL and RPR may be non-reactive in late syphilis, particularly in tabes dorsalis. It is thus essential to undertake specific treponemal tests to establish a diagnosis. The specific tests (TPPA, FTA, ELISA) remain reactive for life regardless of treatment.

The definitive diagnosis of neurosyphilis depends on the presence of a positive serum treponemal test and a reactive CSF with pleocytosis, increased protein and IgG and possibly also oligoclonal bands. In asymptomatic early neurosyphilis, the CSF shows a lymphocytic pleocytosis (typically 5–100 cells/mm^3), an elevated protein concentration (<1 g/dL) and a reactive CSF-VDRL. The CSF changes in symptomatic meningitis are more severe with CSF lymphocyte counts of 200–400 cells/mm^3 and protein of 1–2 g/dL with a reactive CSF-VDRL. In paretic neurosyphilis, the lymphocytic pleocytosis persists (25–75 cells/mm^3) with a raised protein (0.5–1 g/dL). In tabes, the CSF may be entirely normal or show only a mild elevation in protein concentration (0.5–0.75 g/dL).

Positive VDRL/RPR in CSF may indicate neurosyphilis but there is a high incidence of false positive findings, particularly because of previous infection with yaws, caused by the spirochete *T. pallidum pertenue*). The CSF-FTA Ab test is sensitive but not specific, particularly in asymptomatic neurosyphilis but a non-reactive CSF VDRL and FTA-Abs largely excludes the diagnosis of neurosyphilis.

In early neurosyphilis, the CSF findings may be difficult to interpret if there is coexisting HIV infection because HIV itself causes mild CSF pleocytosis and mild elevation of CSF protein levels.

Treatment

Standard treatment for early syphilis is intramuscular benzathine penicillin G 2.4 megaunits (MU) given in a single dose. Alternatives are procaine benzylpenicillin 0.6 MU intramuscularly daily for 10 days, or doxycycline 100 mg orally 12-hourly for 14 days for patients who are allergic to penicillin or who refuse parentral therapy. Late latent, cardiovascular or gummatous syphilis requires intramuscular benzathine benzylpenicillin in three doses of 2.4 MU at weekly intervals. Alternatives are procaine benzylpenicillin 0.6 MU intramuscularly daily for 17 days or doxycycline 100 mg orally 12-hourly for 28 days for patients who are allergic to penicillin or who refuse parenteral therapy.

Treatment of neurosyphilis (including neurological and ophthalmological involvement in early syphilis) is with with intramuscular procaine benzylpenicillin 1.8–2.4 MU given intramuscularly once daily and probenecid 500 mg 6-hourly for 17 days. Alternatives are benzylpenicillin 18–24 MU daily given as 3–4 MU intramuscularly every 4 hours for 17 days. These regimens can be used following desensitisation to beta-lactams for patients who have serious penicillin allergy. Limited data suggest that ceftriaxone (2 g intramuscularly or IV for 10–14 days) or high dose doxycycline (200 mg orally 12-hourly for 28 days) could be used as alternatives. HIV positive patients should be given the same treatment regime.

Treatment of early syphilis may be associated with a Jarisch–Herxheimer systemic reaction – the sudden onset of severe systemic features including fever, chills, headache and tachycardia – due to rapid destruction of treponemes. All patients being treated for syphilis should be pretreated with prednisolone 60 mg for 24 hours.

Antibiotics do not reverse the cardiovascular and neurological manifestations of late non-cutaneous gummatous syphilis but may prevent further progression.

The CSF should be re-examined after treatment has been completed to show a fall in the pleocytosis and then at 6-monthly to 1-year intervals until the cell count and protein levels have returned to normal although this is rarely undertaken in practice.

Zoonoses

Lyme neuroborreliosis

Lyme disease is caused by *Borrelia burgdorferi* which is a helical motile spirochaete. Neuroborreliosis is the most common complication of Lyme disease in the United Kingdom. The infection is a zoonosis; the spirochaete is maintained in populations of large and small mammals, such as deer, field mice and birds and transmitted by the tick bite of the hard-bodied *Ixodes* tick. Bites are small and easily overlooked. Within Europe, Lyme disease is a significant problem in Germany, Austria, France, Switzerland and Sweden where the annual incidence has been as high as 69/100 000. In the United Kingdom, the south-west regions are endemic areas. In North America, most cases occur in the north-east and mid-Atlantic regions, with 15 000 cases reported each year. Lyme also occurs widely in Asia.

Lyme disease affects all ages, with time outdoors being the most significant risk factor (e.g. forest workers). An occupational and travel history with a focus on hobbies such as shooting and rambling is therefore crucial. The infection occurs between May and September in Europe when the tick feeds, as they become inactive in cold weather. The substantial clinical differences between infections in the United States and Europe arise as a result of the differing strains – *B. burgdorferi sensu stricto* in North America and *B. garinii* and *B. afzelii* in Europe and Asia. Lyme disease also occurs in the southern hemisphere.

Clinical features of early neuroborreliosis

Local infection After a tick bite, 50–90% of patients develop the pathognomic skin lesion erythema migrans, 3–30 days later. Typically, the lesion is not painful or pruritic and enlarges centrifugally over the ensuing days. The rash may be accompanied by malaise, fever, headache, meningism, arthritis and lymphadenopathy (Table 9.11).

Early disseminated infection

Haematogenous dissemination within a few days or weeks after the initial inoculation results in:

- Cardiac involvement in 5–10% with conduction abnormalities such as complete heart block requiring temporary pacing.
- Neurological complications which include an aseptic lymphocytic meningo-encephalitis, cranial neuropathy and a painful radiculoneuropathy, singly or in combination.

Although some of these early disseminated syndromes may resolve without therapy, 10% will go on to develop late chronic disease that is less responsive to antibiotic therapy, hence the necessity for early diagnosis and treatment.

Table 9.11 Clinical spectrum of Lyme disease.

Infection stage	Incubation period	Clinical features
Early local infection	<1 month	EM Lymphocytoma cutis Flu-like illness Headache
Early disseminated infection	<3 months	Multifocal EM, arthritis, myalgia, myositis, Cardiac (conduction block, pericarditis, myocarditis) Conjunctivitis Meningitis, meningoencephalitis Cranial neuropathy (VII) Acute painful radiculoneuropathy
Late stage	>3 months	Acrodermatitis chronica atrophicans Arthritis Keratitis, uveitis Chronic encephalomyelitis Chronic polyneuropathy Possible motor neurone disease like syndrome

EM, erythema migrans.

Cranial neuropathy

A facial palsy occurs in 50–75% of patients with early disseminated disease. Clues that may lead to the suspicion of Lyme disease are a facial palsy during the summer months in endemic areas with systemic symptoms such as headache, meningism and arthritis. In one-third, the facial palsy is bilateral – highly unusual in Bell's palsy (Chapter 13). This narrows the differential diagnosis to a limited number of conditions:

- Guillain–Barré syndrome (GBS)
- Meningitis (e.g. due to HIV)
- Chronic meningitic disorders such as sarcoidosis
- Malignant meningeal infiltration
- Amyloidosis

Involvement of the IIIrd, Vth, VIth and VIIIth cranial nerves has also been described.

Acute radiculoneuropathy

This complication is more common in European Lyme disease than in North America. Patients present with severe radicular pain, which may affect the limbs or trunk, resembling mechanical root pain. Weakness, sensory loss and areflexia develop over the next few days, preferentially affecting the lower limbs. When acute and severe, the clinical picture may resemble GBS although demyelination on neurophysiological studies is unusual in neuroborreliosis and the CSF pleocytosis seen typically in Lyme disease should raise doubts about the diagnosis of GBS, in which cells are typically absent in CSF. The differential diagnosis of such a painful radiculoneuropathy with a pleocytic CSF includes:

- Herpes zoster with or without a rash (zoster sine herpete)
- Cytomegalovirus infection, in the context of immunosuppression
- Malignant infiltration
- Sarcoidosis
- Vasculitis
- Proximal diabetic radiculoplexo-neuropathy (diabetic amyotrophy)
- Diabetic truncal radiculopathy.

Other syndromes

Anecdotal reports have described brachial and lumbosacral plexopathies similar to neuralgic amyotrophy (Parsonage–Turner syndrome; see Acute brachial neuritis, Chapter 10) associated with borrelia. A few cases of a motor neurone disease-like phenotype have been described with exclusively lower motor neurone signs; however, these patients usually have a cranial or polyradiculopathy due to borrelia which is associated with clear serological evidence of acute infection. While borreliosis is often considered in the differential diagnosis of motor neurone disease, the serology is generally equivocal and the condition does not respond to appropriate treatment.

Clinical features of late neuroborreliosis

A few patients with early untreated Lyme disease go on to develop a chronic disorder and, occasionally, this may be the first presentation of neuroborreliosis. Problems include:

- Acrodermatitis chronica atrophicans.
- Chronic axonal neuropathy: distal sensory symptoms, radicular involvement and/or restless legs. Neurological examination is either unremarkable or minor sensory abnormalities are found. Neurophysiological abnormalities are consistent with a patchy sensori-motor axonal neuropathy. The CSF is normal. Nerve biopsies are unhelpful but can reveal minimal changes of an axonal neuropathy.
- Chronic meningitis, progressive myeloradiculopathy or encephalomyelitis.
- Subacute chronic progressive encephalomyelitis which may mimic multiple sclerosis.

Table 9.12 American Academy of Neurology guidelines for the diagnosis of nervous system Lyme borreliosis.

Diagnosis of definite nervous system Lyme disease requires:
1 Possible exposure (in wooded, brushy or grassy areas) to appropriate ticks in an area where Lyme disease occurs. A history of tick bite is not necessary
2 One or more of the following:
i Erythema migrans, the pathognomonic rash, or histopathologically proven borrelia lymphocytoma or acrodermatitis
ii Immunologic evidence of exposure to *Borrelia burgdorferi* (e.g. positive serology)
iii Culture, histologic or PCR proof of the presence of *B. burgdorferi*
3 Occurence of one or more of the following neurologic disorders after exclusion of other potential aetiologies. If CNS disease is suspected, CSF should be examined for intrathecal antibody production, culture or PCR
Causally related neurologic disease:
i Lymphocytic meningitis, with or without cranial neuritis or painful radiculoneuritis
ii Encephalomyelitis
iii Peripheral neuropathy

Source: Halperin *et al.* 1996. Reproduced with permission of AAN/LWW.

Post Lyme syndrome

Despite effective antibiotic treatment, some patients complain of persistent fatigue, myalgia, paraesthesias, memory difficulties and depression. Post Lyme syndrome remains contentious. In any event, serological tests continue to remain positive after treatment so there is no diagnostic test.

Diagnosis

The diagnosis of neuroborreliosis can be difficult for several reasons. The diagnosis remains clinical with laboratory support provided by serological tests and CSF examination. Features worth noting in the history are exposure in an endemic area, and associated systemic symptoms. The American Academy of Neurology has produced practice parameters for the diagnosis of patients with nervous system Lyme disease (Table 9.12).

Culture is the gold standard but is difficult to achieve and is a reference laboratory service. Punch biopsy or aspiration of the erythema migrans lesion has the highest positive rates of 40–80%. Less than 10% of CSF cultures are positive, reflecting the low density of organisms. Serology provides the basis for the laboratory support of the clinical diagnosis with a number of caveats:

1 The demonstration of positive antibody is evidence of exposure rather than active disease. Furthermore, these will remain positive even after adequate treatment regimens and cannot be used to assess treatment response.
2 Serology may be negative, especially in early disease because IgM antibodies take 2 weeks to develop and IgG antibodies 4–6 weeks after inoculation. Patients prescribed inadequate doses of antibiotics

early in the course of the illness may remain antibody negative despite persistence of viable organisms.

3 False positive results may occur because of cross reactions with infections such as EBV, syphilis, ricketsial and bacterial infections and autoimmune disorders.

The current recommendation is to use a two-tier system for serodiagnosis – screening with an ELISA or immunofluorescence assay (IFA) which is rapid and sensitive. Positive tests are followed up by a more specific Western blot analysis. Western blots are considered positive in acute disease if two of three selected bands are positive. In disease of longer duration five out of ten positive bands are required. A follow-up serology test may be required 2–4 weeks later to confirm seroconversion.

CSF examination is abnormal in most cases of neuroborreliosis – the exception being the chronic axonal neuropathy described earlier. There is usually a lymphocytic pleocytosis of up to a few hundred cells with an elevated protein level. The glucose is usually normal or slightly reduced. Intrathecal antibody production against *B. burgdorferi* is a useful indicator of infection; however, like blood serology, it may be a marker of past infection and remains positive after treatment. It is therefore necessary to assess CSF cytochemical parameters for evidence of active infection or a treatment response. PCR has proved disappointing with less than 50% of patients with meningitis demonstrating a positive response. As with serology, a positive PCR can be a marker of prior infection without viable organisms being present in the CSF.

Treatment

Although early disseminated neurological syndromes may resolve spontaneously, 10% go on to develop late complications. The current recommendation is that early and late neurological and cardiological borreliosis be treated with intravenous third generation cephalosporins such as ceftriaxone 2 g once daily for 2–4 weeks. Because it has not yet been determined whether a 2-week course is as effective as a 4-week course it seems reasonable to err on the side of caution. The alternative is another third generation cephalosporin, cefotaxime 2 g 8-hourly, which is less convenient. Intravenous penicillin G 3–4 mU six times daily (18–24 mU/day), provided renal function is normal, is another alternative. Oral doxycycline 100 mg 12-hourly was found to be effective for neuroborreliosis including meningitis in one European study and is an alternative. It may be argued that facial palsy is a peripheral disorder and oral antibiotics will suffice. However, many patients have symptoms of meningism and the CSF is abnormal. It is therefore reasonable to consider lumbar puncture in patients presenting with facial palsy in endemic areas before deciding on the most appropriate treatment regimen.

Leptospirosis

Leptospirosis is a widespread and prevalent zoonosis caused by the spirochete *Leptospira interrogans* carried in domestic animal and rodent urine. Risk factors for infection include occupational exposure – (farmers, abattoir workers, vets and sewer workers), recreational activities (freshwater swimming, canoeing) and household exposure (pet dogs, domesticated livestock). Although clinical manifestations vary in severity, presentation is gradual and nonspecific with a flu-like illness, pyrexia, nausea, vomiting and myalgia. Systemic involvement may rapidly develop with chest and abdominal pain. Aseptic meningitis is characterised by headache, photophobia and meningism progressing to encephalopathy with seizures. Ocular features include conjunctival injection, optic neuritis and uveitis. In the most severe form of the condition (Weil disease) there is hepatic and renal impairment with a bleeding diathesis. Less commonly, leptospirosis may result in acute disseminated encephalomyelitis or cerebrovascular disease manifest as vasulitic ischaemia or haemorrhagic complications. Cranial neuropathy, peripheral nerve involvement including radiculopathy, mononeuritis multiplex and an axonal or demyelinating peripheral neuropathy may occur.

CSF in the meningitic state shows a mononuclear pleocytosis usually around 100/mm^3 but may rise to >10 000/mm^3. The protein concentration may also be elevated. The diagnosis depends on culture requiring special media and growth is very slow. Diagnosis can also be made by serology with rising titres and specific agglutination tests.

The meningitic illness is usually self-limiting. *Leptospira* are sensitive to antibiotics during the initial febrile phase and treatment is with intravenous benzylpenicillin 6 mU/day or ceftriaxone or doxycycline but there is a risk of Jarisch–Herxheimer reaction.

Anthrax

Anthrax is caused by *Bacillus anthracis*, a Gram-positive rod that can exist for prolonged periods as a dormant spore in the soil. When introduced subcutaneously spores become vegetative organisms and multiply with the production of exotoxins which lead to extensive tissue necrosis and brawny oedema. Spores may be disseminated into the alveoli where they are phagocytosed into alveolar macrophages and transported to mediastinal lymph nodes. Following secondary haematological spread, they cause a haemorrhagic mediastinitis and overwhelming toxaemia with hypotension and hypoxaemia.

Haemorrhagic meningitis develops in about half of the cases of inhaled anthrax. Some patients develop severe parenchymal brain haemorrhage; coma rapidly supervenes and the prognosis is grave. The diagnosis is established by isolation of *B. anthracis* using culture, PCR or immunohistochemistry.

Treatment of localised cutaneous anthrax is with ciprofloxacin or doxycycline. Meningitis caused by anthrax is treated with IV ciprofloxacin and two additional antibiotics with good CNS penetration (e.g. rifampicin, vancomycin, ampicillin or meropenem).

Psittacosis

Psittacosis is infection with *Chlamydophila psittaci* transmitted from birds to humans, usually following inhalation of organisms in dried faeces, for example during cage cleaning. It generally presents with a pyrexial pneumonic illness. Neurological involvement is uncommon but there may be a brainstem encephalitis, cerebellar disturbance or uveomeningitic syndrome or it may be associated with the development of Guillain–Barré syndrome. Diagnosis is established by serology. First line treatment is with doxycycline (100 mg 12-hourly), tetracycline or erythromycin.

Cat scratch disease

Cat scratch disease is a zoonosis spread by exposure to cat bites or scratches or flea bites. It is caused by *Bartonella henselae* and is characterised by regional lymphadenopathy. Ocular manifestations include a form of conjunctivitis with granuloma formation (Parinaud's oculoglandular syndrome), neuroretinitis with visual loss from optic nerve oedema and macular exudates. Neurological involvement includes encephalopathy, transverse myelitis or radiculitis and occasionally cerebellar ataxia. Treatment is with azithromycin, clarithromycin or rifampicin.

Infections of the nervous system associated with toxin production

Diphtheria

Diphtheria is now extremely uncommon in developed countries as a consequence of immunity induced by mass immunisation with diphtheria toxoid. However, sporadic cases still occur and there is a risk that a decline in population immunity may render the individual at greater risk given that immunisation does not necessarily confer life-long immunity.

Diphtheria is caused by the toxin of *Corynebacterium diphtheriae (*and less often *C. ulcerans)*, an aerobic Gram-positive bacteria which most commonly causes local mucosal necrosis with the formation of a thick 'pseudomembrane' of fibrin, epithelial cells, bacteria and neutrophils affecting the skin and the throat. The toxin may disseminate leading to myocarditis and neurological complications. The incubation period is 1–7 days (usually 2–4 days) and infection is generally manifest as inflammation or pseudomembrane formation over the pharynx or skin.

Systemic involvement caused by dissemination of the toxin leads to neurological complications characterised by cranial nerve involvement and peripheral neuropathy. Palatal and posterior pharyngeal wall paralysis commonly follows pseudomembrane formation and is associated with progressive cranial neuropathy leading to bulbar weakness, with dysarthria, dyphagia and aspiration; ocular involvement may also occur. A mixed sensorimotor demyelinating peripheral neuropathy develops later in the course of the disease, often many months after the onset. There is usually proximal weakness extending distally with severe paralysis and areflexia. Diaphragm and respiratory muscle weakness may develop requiring tracheal intubation and prolonged ventilation. Distal sensory impairment affects all modalities. Autonomic involvement is common, with sinus tachycardia, postural hypotension and urinary retention.

The diagnosis is initially clinical and confirmed by nose or throat swabs, membrane sampling for *C. diphtheriae* and toxin detection. Serological testing for antibody to the toxin can also help support the diagnosis in cases where culture is negative but does not stand alone as a definitive test.

Management

Treatment involves the immediate administration of diphtheria antitoxin to neutralise circulating toxin, antibiotic treatment against *C. diphtheriae* (penicillin or erythromycin) and supportive management of cardiac, respiratory, bulbar and secondary infective complications. It is essential to recognise that immunity can wane and booster immunisation should be offered every 10 years. Public health notification is essential: diphtheria is contagious. Contacts are at considerable risk and throat swabs should be collected and antibiotic prophylaxis offered.

Botulism

Botulism is caused by a highly potent neurotoxin elaborated by *Clostridium botulinum*, an anaerobic Gram-positive rod which survives in the soil by forming spores. There are eight antigenically distinct strains of toxin (A–G) but each strain of *C. botulinum* produces only a single toxin. In food-borne botulism, the toxin is absorbed from the gastrointestinal tract and haematogenously disseminated. Toxin binds irreversibly to the presynaptic membrane of peripheral neuromuscular and/or autonomic nerve junctions to inhibit acetylcholine release. Recovery depends on the sprouting of new nerve terminals. Wound botulism has a longer incubation period but the symptoms and signs are similar to food-borne botulism. This condition also follows subcutaneous or intramuscular injection (skin or muscle popping) of black tar heroin contaminated with *C. botulinum* spores when being cut or diluted prior to street sale.

Forms of botulism

- Infantile
- Food-borne
- Wound
- Iatrogenic
- Inhalation (possible bioterrorism).

The mean incubation period of food-borne botulism (where the food is contaminated with the toxin) is 12–36 hours. Classically, patients develop non-specific gastrointestinal symptoms, a descending flaccid paralysis, cranial nerve symptoms, autonomic disturbance and ventilatory failure. They remain afebrile and have normal sensation.

Local botulinum toxin injected therapeutically or for cosmetic reasons is generally safe but weakness of muscles adjacent to injection site can be significant (e.g. worsening of dyspahagia in motor neurone disease following injection of the salivary glands). Life-threatening toxicity can also occur with paralytic symptoms resulting from spread of toxin. Patients may complain of dysphagia, ptosis, difficulty holding up the head and leg weakness. Occasionally, respiratory difficulties may occur.

Clinical presentation

Patients are apyrexial but may have nausea, vomiting, anorexia and abdominal pain. Cranial nerve deficits develop early including blurred vision, diplopia, dysarthria, dysphagia, dysphonia, facial weakness, ptosis and external ophthalmoplegia with mydriasis occurring because of accommodation paresis. There is flaccid limb weakness affecting the arms more than the legs and progressive respiratory impairment and arrest. Autonomic involvement is characterised by a dry mouth, unreactive pupils, paralytic ileus, gastric dilatation, bladder distension, orthostatic hypotension and constipation. Respiratory muscle weakness may be severe and prolonged. There is an important differential diagnosis which is summarised in Table 9.13.

Diagnosis

Botulism is a clinical diagnosis which may or may not be supported by laboratory findings. CSF and blood examination are normal. *C. botulinum* may be isolated from the wound site, stool or food.

Table 9.13 Differential diagnosis of botulism.

Guillain–Barré syndrome and Fisher variant
Myasthenia gravis and myasthenic syndrome
Borrelia (neuroborreliosis)
Diphtheritic polyneuropathy
Tick bites
Curare poisoning
Poliomyelitis
Organophosphate poisoning
Nerve gases (Chapter 19)

Table 9.14 Management of botulism.

Early administration of antitoxin	Antitoxin should not be delayed pending laboratory results Monitor for signs of allergic reaction to the antitoxin Antitoxin will not reverse established paralysis but should prevent progression Repeated doses can be considered after consultation with an expert if symptoms progress
Wound debridement	Search for and debride any wound no matter how small Examine carefully to ensure that small abscesses or sinuses have not been missed
Give antibiotics if wound present	Benzylpenicillin and metronidazole should be continued until the wound has healed completely
Supportive care	Patients should be admitted to ITU with close bulbar and respiratory monitoring Intubation and ventilation should be undertaken as necessary
Notify public health authorities immediately	Food-borne botulism is a public health emergency

The toxin is detected in serum, stool and food by bioassay using mice, but detection rates are less than 70% in food-borne cases and less than 50% in wound botulism. Immunoassays to detect toxins in the stool and food are being developed but have not been validated.

Neurophysiology
Nerve conduction studies are normal but repetitive stimulation shows a decremental response at low rates but an incremental response occurs at higher rates. Needle electromyography confirms small polyphasic motor units and single fibre studies show jitter and block.

Management
The management of botulism is summarised in Table 9.14. The mortality of patients with food-borne botulism is approximately 10%, wound botulism 15% and infant botulism 5%.

Tetanus
Tetanus is a disease preventable by immunisation. It is rare in the United Kingdom but common worldwide and probably kills 500 000 adults per year. Tetanus is caused by the neurotoxin tetanospasmin, elaborated by the anaerobic Gram-positive rod *Clostridium tetani*. This is a ubiquitous organism found in soil and faeces which persists as resilient spores capable of surviving many years and resistant to most disinfectants and boiling for 20 minutes. The spores germinate under appropriate anaerobic conditions. The toxin is produced in the wound and binds to peripheral motor nerve terminals before being transported via retrograde axonal transport into the spinal cord and/or brainstem. The toxin ultimately migrates to the presynaptic terminals. It inhibits release of gamma-aminobutyric acid (GABA) and glycine, important inhibitory neurotransmitters. In the absence of the inhibitory influence of GABA and glycine, alpha motor neurones fire rapidly, producing muscle spasms and rigidity. Preganglionic sympathetic neurones are also affected, resulting in increased catecholamine levels and sympathetic over-activity. Tetanospasmin can also produce weakness through blockade of acetylcholine release in a manner analogous to that of botulinum toxin.

Epidemiology
Tetanus occurs in neonates because of contamination of the umbilical stump. Children and adults may develop tetanus as a consequence of infected wounds, skin lacerations, as a consequence of intramuscular injections or drug abuse and occasionally after abdominal surgery. In adults incidence is greatest at ages >65 years, usually as a result of inadequate reimmunisation and waning immunity.

Clinical features
The incubation period varies from a few days to several weeks depending on the site of spore inoculation. There may be localised spasm and rigidity in the region of the wound. The onset may be with back pain, increased muscle tone and rigidity of the masseter muscles leading to trismus (lockjaw) and a similar rigidity of the facial muscles (risus sardonicus). There is a localised stiffness near to the injury with sustained rigidity of the axial muscles with involvement of the neck, back and abdomen and, in severe cases, reflex spasms and opisthotonus. Paroxysmal contractions of muscles appear in response to slight stimuli, and in severe cases are bad enough to cause limb fractures, tendon avulsion and rhabdomyolysis. Spasms of respiratory muscles lead to asphyxia, vocal cord obstruction and aspiration associated with increased bronchial secretions, hypersalivation and dysphagia.

Autonomic manifestations are common in severe tetanus with profuse sweating, hypersalivation and extreme hyperpyrexia. Fluctuations of blood pressure and heart rate are cardinal features and these may be followed by arrhythmias and circulatory failure. There may be transient glycosuria. There is also excessive bronchial secretion, gastric stasis, diarrhoea, acute renal failure and volume depletion.

Diagnosis
The diagnosis is predominantly clinical, from the history of the spasms and examination findings. Culture of *C. tetani* from a wound is confirmatory. Serology can also have a supportive role in diagnosis, with serum tests for tetanus toxin and tetanus toxin antibody.

Differential diagnosis
- Strychnine poisoning: strychnine is a competitive antagonist for glycine and poisoning causing spasms and rigidity, typically in the abdominal muscles.
- Dystonic drug reactions cause stiffness and involuntary muscle spasms.
- Autoimmune limbic encephalitis (particularly anti-*N*-methyl-D-aspartate [NMDA] receptor encephalitis) can cause severe involuntary spasms of the face and limbs.
- Non-organic spasms and rigidity may also be mistaken for tetanus.

Table 9.15 Management of tetanus.

Neutralise any unbound toxin	TIG intramuscular in multiple sites at 5000–10 000 IU. In the event of reduced availability of TIG, intravenous human normal immunoglobulin can also be used
Debridement of the wound	This encourages eradication of tetanus bacteria and arrest of toxin release
Antibiotics	Metronidazole 500 mg 4 times daily for 7–10 days
Supportive therapy during the acute phase	Nursing in a calm, quiet environment with cardiorespiratory monitoring Fluid balance, nutrition and the control of muscle spasms with diazepam, midazolam Tracheal intubation, ventilation and neuromuscular blockade with vecuronium
Immunisation	Immunisation is recommended following recovery from tetanus Primary childhood immunisation programmes as five doses of combined DPT in the UK given at 2 months, 4 months, 6 months, 3–5 years and 13–18 years Boosters are recommended every 10 years

DPT, diphtheria, pertussis and tetanus; TIG, tetanus immunoglobulin.

Treatment

Treatment in the ICU has resulted in a marked improvement in prognosis for patients with tetanus but the mortality is still approximately 10%. Severe muscular rigidity may last for weeks and assisted ventilation may be required for several weeks. Complete recovery is typical, although mild painful spasms can persist for months. Management is summarised in Table 9.15.

Miscellaneous infections of the nervous system

Mycoplasma

Mycoplasma are among the smallest free living organisms; they have no cell wall and grow in both aerobic and anaerobic conditions. They are difficult to identify and isolate. Pathogenic mechanisms are immune-mediated rather than caused by direct infection. Antibodies produced against the glycolipid antigens of *Mycoplasma pneumoniae* probably act as autoantibodies as they cross-react with human brain cells and erythrocytes.

The most common manifestations of mycoplasma infection include atypical pneumonia, skin rashes, gastrointestinal involvement, arthritis, glomerulonephritis, uveitis and cardiac disease. Neurological involvement is unusual and occurs most commonly in children as encephalitis. Other manifestations include aseptic meningitis, peripheral neuropathy, brainstem encephalitis, cranial nerve palsies and cerebellar ataxia. Acute transverse myelitis, although rare, can be severe (often affecting the high cervical cord); some patients suffer permanent sequelae, including tetraplegia.

There may be a haemolytic anaemia with positive Coombs test and an elevated reticulocyte count. The CSF typically shows a lymphocytic pleocytosis with elevated protein but normal glucose. Isolation of *M. pneumoniae* from the CSF is exceptional, antigen detection is occasionally positive but unreliable, PCR is more sensitive and specific but has a low diagnostic yield. Treatment is often empirical for atypical pneumonia. Specific anti-mycoplasma treatment includes doxycycline, erythromycin, azithromycin or a fluoroquinolone such as levofloxacin or moxifloxacin. Prolonged treatment may be necessary because of the organism's ability to reside intracellularly.

Whipple's disease

Whipple's disease is a multi-system disorder that usually presents with systemic and gastrointestinal features before neurological involvement. However, the condition may occasionally present with neurological features or these may be the only manifestation. Whipple's is caused by a Gram-positive bacillus *Tropheryma whippeli* which is ubiquitous and slow-growing.

Patients usually develop weight loss with abdominal pain, diarrhoea and steatorrhoea. Joint pain occurs, a consequence of a seronegative migratory arthropathy. There may be a low grade chronic pyrexia with lymphadenopathy, splenomegaly and hyperpigmentation. Cardiac involvement includes culture negative endocarditis and constrictive pericarditis.

CNS involvement occurs in 40% of patients, often late in the disease, after many months or years. The most common manifestation is slowly progressive cognitive change with memory loss, behaviour and personality change, evolving into frank dementia. Ocular involvement is also frequently seen with inflammatory changes causing retinitis or uveitis but there may also be papilloedema and progressive optic atrophy. Supranuclear vertical gaze palsy may occur with a characteristic movement disorder of oculomasticatory myorhythmia in which there is an associated repetitive movement of the masticatory muscles that persists during sleep or oculofacial skeletal myorhythmia that involves the facial and neck muscles. Seizures and myoclonus occur about 25% of cases in whom there is neurological involvement. There may also be a progressive ataxia. Rarely, the level of consciousness may be affected with progressive obtundation and even coma. Thalamic involvement causing polydipsia, hyperphagia, insomnia or hypersomnia have been described.

Tropheryma whippeli can be identified on biopsy of the jejunal mucosa which shows macrophages filled with periodic acid–Schiff (PAS +) staining intracellular inclusions that contain the organism. Similar staining may be seen in biopsies of lymph nodes, heart valves and cerebral tissue and in the CSF. Diagnostic PCR assay for *T. whippeli* is used widely to establish and confirm the diagnosis of Whipple's disease. CSF is characterised by pleocytosis with an elevated protein. MRI may show diffuse high signal on T2-weighted (T2W) images particularly affecting the frontal cortex, basal ganglia and periventricular white matter but the hypothalamus and cortex may also be involved. Occasionally, mass lesions may develop with ring enhancement. There may also be diffuse atrophy or focal abnormalities and, occasionally, hydrocephalus.

Management remains unsatisfactory. Conventionally, patients have been treated with parenteral penicillin and streptomycin followed by long-term tetracycline. Relapses occur and the outlook for recovery with neurological involvement is particularly poor. Newer recommendations suggest that more intense and vigorous treatment is indicated in the presence of neurological involvement because of the likelihood of clinical relapses. The initial phase should be treated with intravenous antibiotics that are active against *T. whipplei* and penetrate the blood brain barrier (Ceftriaxone 2g daily or Penicllin G 4mu 4 hrly) for 4 weeks followed by maintenance with co-trimoxazole or doxycycline and hydroxychloroquine. Meropenem is also considered an alternative to ceftriaxone. Although antibiotics are usually given for 1 year it has been argued that with neurological involvement treatment should be given indefinitely because of the high likelihood of relapse when therapy is stopped.

Melioidosis

Melioidosis is an infection caused by a facultative Gram-negative bacteria *Burkholderia pseudomallei* which occurs in South Asia (particularly Thailand), China and Australia. Transmission is by percutaneous inoculation during exposure to contaminated water or wet season soil. The predominant manifestation is a cavitating, nodular and fibrotic pneumonia but it may cause an encephalomyelitis often affecting the brainstem, occasionally with abscess formation. Treatment is with ceftazidime or meropenem.

Tick-borne disease

Ticks are small arachnids which are external parasites feeding on the blood of hosts including mammals and amphibians. They harbour disease-causing agents and act as vectors transmitting diseases including:

- *Bacteria*
  - Lyme disease *(B. burgdorfei)*
  - Relapsing fever (other species of borrelia)
  - Ehrlichiosis
  - Tularemia
- *Rickettsiae or rickettsiae-like*
  - Rocky Mountain spotted fever
  - Q fever
- *Viruses*
  - Tick-borne meningoencephalitis
  - Colorado tick fever
  - Crimean–Congo haemorrhagic fever
- *Protozoa*
  - Babesosis
- *Toxins*
  - Tick paralysis.

Ehrlichiosis

Ehrlichiae are obligate intracellular bacteria that grow within membrane-lined vacuoles in leukocytes (affecting either monocytes or granulocytes). In adults, the condition may present with malaise, myalgia and headache with a characteristic rash. Leukopenia and thrombocytopenia are common. Neurological manifestations include mental state changes, meningitis, seizures and coma. Diagnosis is established by a fluorescent antibody test. Treatment is with doxycycline.

Tularaemia

Tularaemia is a tick-borne infection caused by *Francisella tularensis*. It may cause severe typhoid-like or pneumonic disease. Neurological manifestations include meningitis and rhabdomyolysis. Treatment is with aminoglycosides or ciprofloxacin.

Rickettsial disease

Rocky Mountain spotted fever (RMSF) occurs in North, Central and South America and is caused by a minute polar staining Gram-negative bacillus *(Rickettsia rickettsii)* that occurs in freshly laid eggs of infected ticks. Attachment by the tick to the skin for more than 6 hours is required before rickettsiae are transmitted. There is subsequent invasion and multiplication within endothelial smooth muscle cells leading to the development of a vasculitis. The onset is with a maculopapular rash. Severe RSMF is associated with encephalitis and systemic signs including purpura, hypovolaemia, hypotension, prerenal failure and cerebral and pulmonary oedema. There may be non-specific muscular weakness which can progress to rhabdomyolysis.

Other rickettsial-like infections including *Coxiella burnetii* (Q fever) develop over 10–14 days and tend to be slightly less severe but are also associated with a purpuric rash, seizures, aseptic meningitis and encephalitis. There is also a chronic form characterised by endocarditis. Treatment with doxycycline is given until the patient has been afebrile for >2 days. Tetracycline and chloramphenicol are alternatives.

Viral infections of the nervous system

Viruses can cause a variety of diseases in the CNS. The most important are viral meningitis, encephalitis and encephalomyelitis.

Viral meningitis

Viruses cause an isolated aseptic meningitis characterised by symptoms and signs of meningeal irritation with a CSF pleocytosis in the absence of bacterial, fungal or parasitic infection – hence the term aseptic. There is no parenchymatous brain or spinal cord inflammation. However, in most cases there is mixed meningo-encephalitic or encephalomyelitic involvement.

Aetiology

Non-polio enteroviruses are by far the most common cause of viral meningitis, these include coxsackie and echovirus strains (Table 9.16).

Viral meningitis is a relatively uncommon complication of systemic viral infection. Most viruses gain access to the body from the oropharynx. They are amplified (multiply) in lymphatic tissue, spread to the bloodstream (viraemia) and cross the choroid plexus or capillary endothelial cells to reach the CNS. Rarely, viruses may enter the CNS by direct transmission through axons.

Table 9.16 Main causes of viral meningitis.

Enterovirus: • Echovirus • Coxsackie A, B • Enterovirus 70, 71
Mumps
Measles
Parvovirus B19
Herpes viruses • Herpes simple virus 2 (HSV-2) • Varicella zoster virus (VZV) • Epstein–Barr virus (EBV) • Cytomegalovirus (CMV) • Human herpes virus 6 (HHV-6)
Arboviruses (e.g. West Nile virus)
Influenza
Parainfluenza
Acute HIV infection
Adenovirus

Table 9.17 Differential diagnosis of aseptic meningitis.

Infections
Viruses
Viral meningitis
Bacterial
Partially treated bacterial meningitis
Bacterial endocarditis
Brucellosis, Listeriosis, Mycoplasma pneumoniae
Spirochete infection (syphilis, leptospirosis, *Borrelia*)
Mycobacterium (TBM)
Whipple's disease
Parameningeal infection – abscess, empyema, osteomyelitis, sinusitis, subdural empyema
Rickettsial infection
Fungi
Parasites – malaria
Vasculitis
Inflammation – sarcoid, Behçet's
Collagen vascular – SLE, RA, polyarteritis nodosa, mixed connective tissue disease, Sjögren's, Wegener's, lymphomatoid granulomatosis
Uveo-meningitic syndromes – Vogt–Koyanagi–Harada syndrome
Meningeal carcinomatosis
Leukaemia/lymphoma
Vascular
Previous subarachnoid haemorrhage
Chemical meningitis
Contrast materials
Drugs
Non-steroidal anti-inflammatory drugs
Antineoplastic drugs
Immunosuppressants – azathioprine
Antibiotics – septrin, sulfasalazine, ciprofloxacin, amoxicillin
Intravenous immunoglobulin G

RA, rheumatoid arthritis; SLE, systemic lupus erythematosus; TBM, tuberculous meningitis.

Clinical features

In viral meningitis there may be a flu-like prodrome followed by the sudden onset of intense frontal headache, fever and neck stiffness associated with photophobia, malaise, myalgia and severe nausea and vomiting. Although there is pyrexia, neck stiffness and meningeal signs, patients are generally less unwell than those with bacterial meningitis. A pruritic rash, pleurodynia or myocarditis may be present. There is a wide differential diagnosis of aseptic meningitis which is summarised in Table 9.17.

Diagnosis

The peripheral white cell count is usually normal but may be increased or decreased. Liver function tests may be abnormal. The CSF is clear and colourless with a normal to moderately elevated pressure; the cell count is usually <300 cells/mm^3 but may be up to 1000 cells/mm^3; mononuclear lymphocytes predominate, although polymorpholeukocytes may be present particularly in the early stages. CSF glucose is usually normal but may be slightly depressed. CSF protein is normal or mildly elevated.

Viral isolation

Viral isolation is undertaken from the throat, urine or stool and antibody studies are possible in serum or CSF. The detection of viral RNA or DNA is now undertaken using PCR in the serum or CSF. Not infrequently no virus is isolated in presumed viral meningitis.

Management and prognosis

Treatment is supportive but it is usual to admit a patient to exclude bacterial meningitis. A clinical diagniosis of viral meningitis is not secure; substantial errors have occurred by presuming a viral infection, when the underlying infection has been pyogenic or tuberculous.

Herpes virus meningitis should be treated with aciclovir (famciclovir, valaciclovir, ganciclovir and foscarnet are alternatives). The only therapy of clinical use for enterovirus meningitis is immune serum globulin. The prognosis in viral meningitis is good, with spontaneous recovery usually occurring within 1–2 weeks. However, there may be residual deficits in up to 5% including malaise, fatigue, mild intellectual and language difficulties, seizures, isolated cranial nerve lesions and optic neuritis.

Chronic and recurrent meningitis

Meningitis may be recurrent either because the patient is predisposed to repeated bacterial infection, recurrent non-purulent infection or because of a non-infective aetiology. Chronic meningitis may be defined as meningitis that persists for 4 weeks or more without showing any recovery. The condition often presents with a more encephalitic-like picture of progressive impairment of cognition and consciousness following a fluctuating course. Any of the conditions listed in Table 9.18 may cause a chronic meningitis or recurrent meningitis.

Mollaret's meningitis

This is a rare condition in which recurrent self-limiting episodes of pyrexia and lymphocytic meningism occur but may be separated by asymptomatic periods lasting weeks or months. The attacks resolve spontaneously in days with no residual deficit and they usually cease within a few years. During attacks the CSF shows a mild elevation in the protein and pleocytosis (200-several thousand cells/mm^3 which are predominantly monocytes with aggregated 'giant cells' (Mollaret's cells) with a background of polymorpholeukocytes and plasma cells). The cause of the condition is HSV-2, although HSV-1 has been implicated in some cases, presumably related to a viral resevoir in dorsal root ganglia.

Encephalitis

Encephalitis is acute inflammation of the parenchyma of the brain which is usually diffuse and may involve the meninges. Most common viral infections can, if rarely, lead to viral encephalitis. Encephalitis may also be caused by a parainfectious or autoimmune process. Encephalitis causes focal or multi-focal neurological deficits or seizure activity. Acute disseminated encephalomyelitis (Chapter 11) may occur as an immunologically mediated parainfectious phenomenon following a variety of infections or after vaccination. Encephalopathy refers to disruption of brain activity in the absence of a direct inflammatory process in the brain parenchyma.

Table 9.18 Causes of chronic or recurrent meningitis.

Continuing sepsis, potential access to CNS (e.g. skull base or middle ear defect) or immunosuppression (e.g. hypogammaglobulinaemia)
Chronic meningeal infection *Brucella*, syphilis, *Borrelia*
Fungi – cryptococcus, coccidioidomycosis, histoplasmosis, blastomycosis
HIV
Para-meningeal infection
Periodic reactivation of latent infection HSV, VZV, EBV, CMV
Toxoplasmosis
Immunosuppression Antibody deficiency
Complement deficiency
Splenic dysfunction
Inflammatory disorders Vasculitis
Collagen vascular disease
Uveo-meningitic syndromes Sarcoidosis, Behçets, Vogt–Koyanagi–Harada syndrome
Medication Non-steroidal anti-inflammatory drugs
Antineoplastic drugs
Immunosuppressants – azathioprine
Antibiotics – septrin, sulfasalazine, ciprofloxacin, amoxicillin
IVIg
Valacyclovir
Antiepileptic medication – lamotrigine, carbamazepine
Lymphoma
Immune reconstitution in highly active retroviral treatment in AIDS
Chemical meningitis
Mollaret's meningitis

Within the United Kingdom and North America, after the neonatal period, the most common severe forms of infectious encephalitis are shown in Table 9.19. Worldwide, the most common causes of encephalitis are arboviruses (e.g. Japanese encephalitis and West Nile virus). Table 9.20 summarises the more characteristic patterns of neurological involvement in encephalitis. Table 9.21 summarises viruses that can affect the CNS.

Pathophysiology

There are several mechanisms by which viruses can cause encephalitis. Organisms that cause encephalitis require the ability to infect brain tissue (neurotropism) but not necessarily the ability to infect neurones (neuronotropism). They usually enter the CNS via direct haematogenous dissemination but may infect the brain via retrograde neuronal spread.

Table 9.19 Most common causes of viral encephalitis.

HSV-1
VZV
EBV
CMV
HHV 6
Enteroviruses
Adenovirus
Influenza virus A and B
Arbovirus
HIV related

CMV, cytomegalovirus; EBV, Epstein–Barr virus; HHV, human herpes virus; HSV-1, herpes simplex virus type 1; VZV, varicella zoster virus.

Table 9.20 Features of encephalitis with specific organisms.

Cerebellar ataxia	VZV EBV Mumps Whipple's disease St Louis encephalitis *Trypanosoma brucei gambiense* *Mycoplasma pneumoniae*
Cranial nerve abnormalities	HSV (often HSV-2) EBV *Cryptococcus neoformans*
Cognitive impairment	HIV HSV Measles
Myorrhythmia	*Tropheryma whipplei*
Parkinsonism	Japanese encephalitis St Louis encephalitis West Nile virus

Arbovirus encephalitides are zoonoses in which the virus life cycle takes place both in the biting arthropod and an invertebrate host. The virus is then transmitted by an insect bite and undergoes local replication in the skin before spreading to the brain and causing human encephalitis. Pathological examination shows involvement of the grey matter with perivascular inflammation, neural destruction, neuronophagia and tissue necrosis.

Parainfectious and autoimmune encephalitides are discussed in Chapters 11 and 20.

Incidence

In the United States, the annual incidence of viral encephalitis is between 3.5 and 7.4/100 000 of the population. In the United Kingdom, the reported incidence is lower. HSV-1 is the most frequent cause but varicella zoster virus (VZV), enterovirus and influenza A are also common. There remains considerable geographical variation and arbovirus encephalitis is common in the Americas and Asia, and rare in Europe.

Clinical features

The clinical manifestations of encephalitis are often most severe in infants and those over the age of 65. Fever is present in >90% of patients, seizures are common and help to distinguish acute infective encephalitis from acute disseminated encephalomyelitis. The presence of headache, pyrexia and meningism suggest leptomeningeal irritation while parenchymatous involvement leads to focal neurological signs, seizures and alteration of consciousness progressing to stupor and coma. Behavioural and speech disturbances may develop and abnormal movements are associated with lesions in the basal ganglia and pituitary, involvement of the hypothalamus may cause hypothermia. Common patterns of encephalitis related to individual viruses are summarised in Table 9.21.

Diagnosis

In assessing a patient with suspected viral encephalitis it is essential to take a detailed history of travel and to note the season of onset, geographical location, recreational activities, occupation and vaccination history or any contact with animals and any evidence of immunosuppression. CSF examination should be undertaken if possible and HSV PCR should be performed on all CSF samples. MRI appearances may be characteristic in herpes simplex encephalitis (see Herpes simplex virus) but are non-specific in other causes. Immunological studies (e.g. voltage-gated potassium channel and NMDA antibodies) may provide a definitive diagnosis in autoimmune encephalitides.

Herpes simplex encephalitis

Herpes simplex encephalitis (HSE) is the most common cause of sporadic fatal viral encephalitis. There is a bimodal age distribution with most patients being below 20 or above 50 years. Ninety per cent are caused by HSV-1 and up to 10% by HSV-2, the later often associated with immuno-compromise or occurring in the neonate. Primary infection usually develops in the oropharyngeal mucosa before the virus is transported by retrograde transneuronal spread via the trigeminal nerve to establish latency in the olfactory bulb or trigeminal ganglion. Molecular analysis of paired oral and brain sites have indicated HSE can occur as the result of a primary infection, a reactivation of latent HSV in the trigeminal ganglion or reinfection by a second HSV. The reason for reactivation is unknown. The presence of labial herpes has no diagnostic specificity to HSE. The herpes virus leads to inflammation, infection and necrotising lesions particularly in the inferior and mesial temporal lobes which may also involve the orbital frontal cortex and limbic structures.

The onset of HSE is with symptoms of meningo-encephalitis including fever, headache and alteration of consciousness which may develop gradually or rapidly over a matter of hours, occasionally associated with neck stiffness. The most common manifestations are personality change, dysphasia with progressive behavioural disturbance and occasional psychotic features. Less typical features include the development of hemiparesis or a visual field defect (particularly superior quadrantic). Focal or generalised seizures are often associated with olfactory or gustatory hallucinations. HSE only develops in an immunocompromised patient following bone marrow transplant or in AIDS.

Investigation CT scanning is usually normal within the first 4–6 days. EEG is non-specific but may allow early localisation. MRI is more sensitive, demonstrating high signal intensity lesions on T2W diffusion-weighted and FLAIR images early in the course.

The MRI characteristically shows high signal areas of focal oedema on T2 images in the medial and inferior temporal lobes, extending into the insular cortex and frontal lobe; the changes may be unilateral or bilateral and extensive. Midline shift may be present if there is significant vasogenic oedema (Figure 9.9).

The EEG is characterised by periodic stereotyped, lateralised sharp and slow wave complexes occurring at regular intervals between 2 and 3 seconds.

The CSF is abnormal in >95% of patients. CSF is generally under an increased opening pressure and may show a mild to moderate lymphocytic pleocytosis of 5–500/mm^3; there may be a mild to moderate elevation in the protein (0.6–0.9 g/L) and a normal or mildly decreased glucose. In approximately 5% of patients CSF examination is normal.

Demonstration of intrathecal production of anti-HSV antibodies, has been replaced by PCR for HSV-1 DNA that is very sensitive (98%) and specific (94%), when compared to the gold standard of brain biopsy which was commonly undertaken in the past.

False negative PCR results can occur during the first days of the disease and, in cases of doubt, a repeat LP after 1–2 days is indicated. The optimal chance of obtaining positive PCR is 2–10 days after onset of illness. It should be positive after about 5 days of infection but clears again after 14 days of illness. PCR may also be used to guide the duration of treatment with aciclovir. PCR has also become increasingly valuable in the diagnosis of virus encephalitides from other causes such as cytomegalovirus CMV, VZV, influenza and enterovirus. Brain biopsy is now rarely undertaken but may be considered if diagnostic uncertainty remains.

Treatment HSE remains a serious infection of the CNS. Aciclovir has reduced the mortality of HSE from 70% to <25%. Despite early and appropriate treatment two thirds of patients may be left with significant residual deficits. Empirical therapy with IV acyclovir (10 mg/kg 8-hourly for 14–21 days) should be commenced as soon as the diagnosis is considered with dose adjustments for renal insufficiency.

Other causes of encephalitis

Varicella zoster virus VZV is a large herpes virus. Primary infection causes chickenpox and secondary reactivation leads to dermatomal shingles or disseminated herpes zoster. Chickenpox (varicella) is usually a self-limiting exanthematous disorder characterised by a diffuse vesicular rash in different stages of development on the face, trunk and extremities. It may be associated with pneumonitis or secondary bacterial infection. Neurological complications include severe encephalitis, meningitis, myelitis and cerebellar ataxia. Rarely, an acute toxic encephalopathy or Reye's syndrome may occur.

VZV encephalitis is treated with aciclovir (10–15 mg/kg 8-hourly for 10–14 days) although ganciclovir is also effective.

Shingles The most common acute peripheral nervous system infection in the United Kingdom is herpes zoster or shingles, caused by reactivation of VZV. VZV becomes latent in the ganglia of sensory and autonomic peripheral and cranial nerves following primary infection in chickenpox. Shingles is associated with reduced cell-mediated immunity through ageing, drugs, malignancy and HIV, but there may be no underlying risk factors. Patients typically experience tingling pain in one or more dermatomes a few days before the development of a vesicular rash. The thoracic dermatomes are most commonly affected. The rash of shingles starts as erythematous papules which rapidly evolve into grouped vesicles or bullae. The vesicles become pustular or haemorrhagic after 3–4 days. Zoster is generally limited to one dermatome but can spread to neighbouring dermatomes and occasionally scattered lesions occur in immunocompetent patients. Shingles most commonly affects the thoracic or lumbar dermatomes. The most common feature of shingles is pain which occurs in approximately 75% and may precede

Table 9.21 Viruses that may infect the CNS (excluding arboviruses).

Family of virus	Virus		
Herpes virus	HSV-1 HSV-2 VZV CMV EBV		See text
	HHV-6, HHV-7		Linked with meningoencephalitis, GBS and retinitis Occasionally found in CSF of patients with AIDS but significance unknown Treatment is with ganciclovir, foscarnet is an alternative
Orthomyxovirus	Influenza		May present as a frontal lobe or limbic syndrome without disturbance of consciousness Guillain–Barré like neuropathy, myelitis, ADEM Treatment – oseltamivir
	Avian flu A (H5N1)		Characterised by diarrhoea, seizures and progression to severe encephalopathy leading to coma and death CSF protein is elevated
Picornavirus	Enterovirus (non-polio) Coxsackie Echo Polio		Enterovirus infection is usually asymptomatic or manifest as an erythematous or maculopapular rash. Aseptic meningitis may occur Usually associated with a good prognosis but enterovirus 71 may present with herpangina, hand, foot and mouth disease, myoclonus, tremor and cranial nerve involvement May be complicated by acute flaccid paralysis or long-standing chronic meningo-encephalitis particularly in the young or patients who are immunosuppressed Enterovirus can be isolated from CSF faecal, throat and serum specimens
Paramyxoviruses	Mumps	Worldwide (winter and spring)	Usually starts several days after parotitis and usually resolves without sequelae except for occasional hydrocephalus due to ependymal cell involvement
	Measles	Worldwide (winter and spring)	Rash, myelitis, encephalitis Treatment – ribavirin (particularly in SSPE)
	Nipah virus	Asia (all year)	Rare. Contracted from infected pigs Presents with encephalitis and focal cerebellar or brainstem signs Segmental myoclonus and systemic involvement is characterised by hypertension and tachycardia Encephalitis may be delayed for several months after exposure to the virus MRI shows increased signal in cortical white matter
Arenavirus	Lassa fever	Africa	
	LCMV	Europe, Americas, Australia, Japan (usually winter)	
	Rabies		See text
Filovirus	Marburg Ebola	2014 outbreak – West Africa (Guinea, Liberia, Sierra Leone)	Person to person contact with virus containg body fluids Non-specific influenza which can progress to multi-organ failure and shock. Haemorrhagic involvement of multiple organs Headache, confusion, seizures and cerebral oedema reflecting systemic involvement Recurrent infections due to residual virus in privileged sites (e.g. eye) can lead to recurrent viral meningitis
Polyomavirus	JC BK		PML in immunosuppressed (e.g. HIV) Encephalitis in immunodeficiency

ADEM, acute disseminated encephalomyelitis; GBS, Guillain–Barré syndrome; LCMV, lymphocytic choriomeningitis; SSPE, subacute sclerosing panencephalitis; PML, progressive multifocal leukoencephalopathy.

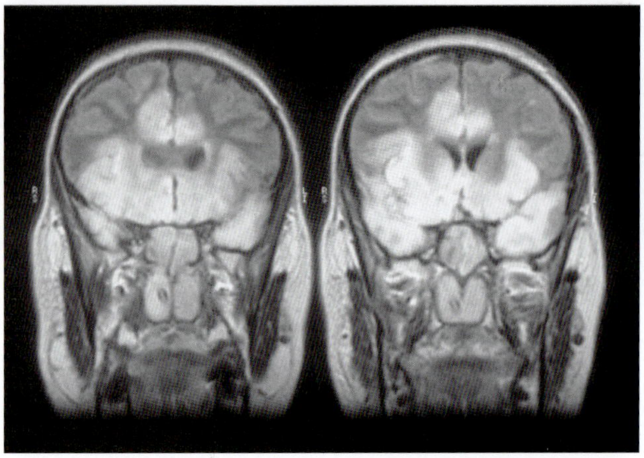

Figure 9.9 Fulminant herpes simplex encephalitis: extensive temporal lobe and diffuse parenchymal inflammation (coronal FLAIR MRI).

the rash. It is often severe and allodynia may develop. Occasionally, shingles may occur with pain but no rash (herpes zoster sine herpete). Zoster may be associated with a number of complications. Post-herpetic neuralgia increases in frequency with age and occurs in 20% of patients over 80 years. Herpes zoster ophthalmicus (HZO) affects the ophthalmic division of the trigeminal nerve and may be associated with conjunctivitis, episcleritis, iritis and most patients also develop corneal involvement (keratitis). Vesicular lesions on the nose (Hutchinson's sign) are associated with HZO and indicate involvement of the nasociliary branch of the trigeminal nerve which also innervates the globe. VZV has also been associated with the development of acute retinal necrosis which may lead to rapid loss of vision caused by iridocyclitis, vitritis, necrotising retinitis and occlusive retinal vasculitis.

Herpes zoster oticus (Ramsey-Hunt syndrome) is caused by VZV reactivation in the geniculate ganglion with subsequent spread of the inflammatory process to involve the auditory cranial nerve. The condition is characterised by its ipsilateral facial paralysis, ocular pain and vesicles in the auditory canal and auricle. Taste perception, hearing and lacrimation may be affected. Multiple cranial nerves may be involved, especially V, IX and X. Facial paralysis is more severe than in Bell's palsy and carries a worse prognosis for recovery. Other complications of zoster include the development of aseptic meningitis, peripheral motor neuropathy and Guillain–Barré syndrome. Transverse myelitis and radiculopathy may be caused by zoster but they may develop may be more than 6 months after the onset of zoster. Zoster associated encephalitis may occur months after acute shingles or in the absence of a clinically evident infection. However, it is often associated with extensive zoster particularly in the immunocompromised and in patients with HIV.

VZV can cause stroke resulting from a granulomatous vasculitis of large and small arteries. It is thought to occur by direct viral invasion of the media of cerebral arteries by VZV with extension along the intracranial branches of the trigeminal nerve. Extensive stroke may occur as a result of multifocal occlusion of the anterior and middle cerebral arteries. Immunocompromised patients are at particular risk of infection by VZV, particularly those with HIV, bone marrow and solid organ transplants recipients or patients receiving chemotherapy.

Antiviral therapy is indicated to promote more rapid healing of skin lesions, to lessen the severity and pain associated with acute neuritis and to reduce the incidence and severity of post-herpetic neuralgia. Antiviral drugs should be given to all patients within 72 hours of treatment using valaciclovir (1000 mg 8-hourly) or famciclovir (500 mg 8-hourly) for 7 days. Aciclovir (800 mg five times daily) needs to be given more frequently. Steroids are indicated if there is vasculitis but there is no evidence to support their routine use in shingles to improving quality of life or reducing the incidence of post-herpetic neuralgia. The management of post-herpetic neuralgia is discussed in Chapter 23 and includes the use of tricyclic antidepressants, gabapentin, pregabalin, opioids and topical treatments but side effects are common.

Cytomegalovirus CMV is a ubiquitous herpes virus that only affects humans. The virus often persists in the throat following infection and may become latent for many years. Infection is usually transient and asymptomatic but it may cause cytomegalic inclusion disease in the newborn infant and neurological disease in the immunocompromised adult, particularly following organ transplant or in patients who are HIV-positive in whom the most common complications are lumbo-sacral polyradiculopathy and retinopathy. Peripheral nerve vasculitis, encephalitis and myelitis are also described in the context of HIV infection. Treatment is with ganciclovir (5 mg/kg 12-hourly) and foscarnet (60 mg/kg 8-hourly).

Epstein–Barr virus EBV is a lymphotropic herpes virus which, like all herpes viruses, may establish latency before being reactivated. It replicates in B cells, causes infectious mononucleosis and is associated with lymphoproliferative disorders – Burkitt's and Hodgkin's lymphomas, hairy cell leukaemia, lymphocytic lymphoma and nasopharyngeal carcinoma. In patients with HIV, primary CNS lymphoma is associated with EBV infection. Neurological complications include aseptic meningitis, encephalitis, acute cerebellar ataxia, cerebritis, transverse myelitis, polyneuropathy (including Guillain–Barré), mononeuropathy (including brachial plexopathy) and cranial nerve palsies (especially facial nerve). These may occur as a consequence of direct viral infection or as a parainfectious phenomenon. EBV causes <5% of viral encephalitis and is associated with impaired level of consciousness, seizures and focal deficits. Although recovery is usual, permanent deficit may occur with residual chorea and cognitive impairment. Management is supportive; there is no evidence of benefit from aciclovir.

Arboviruses (arthropod-borne viruses)

Arthropod-borne viruses are adapted to particular reservoir hosts and are spread from animal to animal via the bite of an infected arthropod, usually a mosquito or tick (Table 9.22). Specific arboviruses can be predicted on the basis of geographical location and the demographic pattern of infection. Subacute inoculation by mosquito or tick vector is followed by local tissue and lymph node replication, viraemia and finally invasion of deep soft tissues, organs and CNS. Arbovirus encephalitis predominantly affects cortical grey matter but it may also involve the brainstem and thalamic nuclei. Arboviruses can occasionally cause meningitis or meningo-encephalitis.

Japanese encephalitis Japanese encephalitis is caused by the mosquito-borne Japanese encephalitis arbovirus. The disease is most prevalent in South-East Asia and the Far East. Japanese encephalitis is the most common arbovirus worldwide, particularly affecting children and young adults. Most infections are asymptomatic. The prodrome is non-specific with fever, headache and malaise. There may be an acute, severe fulminant encephalitic presentation with fever, vomiting, convulsion and impaired consciousness leading to coma. Mortality is high, up to 50%, with a high incidence of residual

Table 9.22 Arboviruses that may infect the CNS.

Togavirus (Alphavirus)	Eastern Equine	Eastern and Gulf USA (summer)	Severe, rapidly progressive, virulent encephalitis that affects children High mortality (<35%)
	Western Equine	Western USA (summer)	Encephalitis, predominantly affects children Mortality <10%
	Venezuelan	South and Central America (rainy season)	Occurs in large outbreaks but usually self-limiting and encephalitis is rare but neurological sequelae in <20%
Flavivirus	St Louis	USA (Summer)	Most common vector transmitted cause of aseptic meningitis in the USA Aseptic meningitis accounts for approximately 15% of all symptomatic cases Often asymptomatic and characterised by a mild febrile illness but severe encephalitic illness (characterised by tremor, seizures, headache, vomiting and stupor) can occur in the older age group when mortality may rise to 20% Urinary symptoms common (dysuria, urgency, incontinence) Sequelae occur in 10% including memory loss chronic fatigue, sleep disturbance, headaches and occasional seizures SIADH
	Japanese	See below	
	West Nile	See below	
	Far East	Eastern Russia (summer)	Associated with partal epilepsy and high mortality (<20%)
	Central European	Central Europe (tick-borne)	Flaccid proximal weakness
	Powessan	Canada (summer and autumn, tick-borne)	Severe encephalitis Residual cognitive impairment common High fatality rate
	Dengue	Tropics (SE Asia and Indian subcontinent) (transmitted by mosquito)	Presents with severe influenza like illness or haemorrhagic fever Headaches, arthralgia and myalgia Less commonly this can give rise to encephalitis or encephalopathy and rarely transverse myelitis or polyneuropathy resembling Guillain–Barré syndrome Haemorrhagic form also causes intracerebral haemorrhage, hepatic failure and Reye syndrome-like illness Low risk of sequaelae and low mortality with appropriate supportive management.
	Zika	Americas (Brazil) Africa SE Asia	Transmitted by mosquito (*Aedes aegyptus*) Acute low grade fever with maculopapular rash Associated with Guillain–Barré syndrome Microcephaly and foetal loss when acquired during pregnancy
	Yellow Fever	West & Central Afriuca, South America	Mosquito-borne viral haemorrhagic fever, hepatic dysfunction, renal failure, coagulopathy, shock, metabolic encephalopathy and coma. No direct neuroinvasion or encephalitis (high mortality rate)
	Murray Valley	Australia (mosquito-borne)	Mostly in children Rapid progression in infants
	Kunijin	Australia	
	Rocio	Brazil	
	Russia	Russia (tick-borne)	In cooler northern climates, flaviviruses transmitted by ticks rather than mosquito
Bunyavirus	La Crosse	Central USA	Predominantly a viral encephalitis of children which tends to be mild and self-limiting with a low mortality Occasionally fulminant onset with seizures and focal weakness

CSF, cerebrospinal fluid; ELISA, enzyme-linked immunosorbent assay; JE, Japanese encephalitis virus; PCR, polymerase chain reaction; SIADH, syndrome of inappropriate antidiuretic hormone.

neurological sequelae including deafness, focal deficits and cognitive impairment.

In adults, extrapyramidal involvement may occur with a transient parkinsonian-like syndrome, tremor, choreo-athetotic head nodding or axial rigidity. A flaccid paralysis can occur because of damage of anterior horn cells.

The diagnosis is established by IgM capture ELISA of serum or CSF. Japanese encephalitis virus may be isolated or the genetic viral sequence may be identified in tissue, blood or CSF. Imaging may show bilateral lesions in the basal ganglia, putamen and thalamus. The pons, cerebellum and spinal cord may also be involved. There is no specific antiviral treatment. Vaccination is recommended with three doses of inactivated Japanese encephalitis virus.

West Nile virus West Nile virus (WNV) is related to Japanese encephalitis. It is the most widely distributed arbovirus occurring in North and Central America, Africa, the Middle East, Europe and Australasia. It is transmitted by mosquito bites of the genus Culex.

Infection may be asymptomatic in <40%. Presentation is usually with a self-limiting pyrexia, malaise, myalgia and anorexia. A maculopapular rash is associated with dysasthesiae and systemic involvement may also include arthralgia, hepatosplenomegaly and pancreatitis. Neurological involvement occurs in <15% and is characterised by encephalitis, encephalomyelitis, aseptic meningitis, flaccid paralysis, tremor, myoclonus and parkinsonism. Flaccid weakness is generally caused by anterior horn cells involvement and this may lead to bulbar and respiratory muscle weakness. Guillain–Barré syndrome and axonal neuropathy may occur. WNV has been associated with a wide range of systemic and other neurological complications. Imaging changes are non-specific with signal intensity abnormalities in the brain (particularly the basal ganglia and thalamus), brainstem and spinal cord.

The diagnosis is established by demonstrating either specific IgM antibodies by ELISA or viral nucleic acid by PCR in sera, tissue or CSF. The treatment of WNV infection is supportive and no human vaccine is available.

Serious adverse outcome is limited to neurological involvement with a mortality rate of 2% with meningitis and 12% with encephalitis. Long-term residual weakness commonly follows WNV poliomyelitis.

Viral haemorrhagic fevers

Viral haemorrhagic fevers (VHF) are characterised by coagulation deficits, a capillary leak and shock. The condition is caused by heterogeneous group of viruses discussed earlier: Rift Valley fever; Crimean–Congo haemorrhagic fever; Lassa fever; yellow fever; dengue; ebola and marburg virus infection.

Polio and the post-polio syndrome

Despite a global policy aimed at eradication, pockets of wild polio still exist and there is a low reported incidence of vaccine-induced polio in infants and adults. Present policies are directed towards mopping up residual sources with the eventual discontinuation of routine immunisation. Acute poliomyelitis is rarely encountered in the United Kingdom following its successful eradication; however, imported poliomyelitis still occurs and it is necessary to distinguish acute poliomyelitis from other causes of acute flaccid paralysis (Table 9.23).

Poliomyelitis is caused by an enterovirus of high infectivity whose main route of infection is via the human gastrointestinal tract. There are three subtypes but, before the introduction of polio vaccine, type I accounted for 85% of paralytic disease. Epidemics of polio occurred, most commonly during the summer months, in the temperate climates of the northern hemisphere and the incidence was greatest where children bathed together.

The incubation period is 7–14 days. The acute illness is characterised by minor flu-like symptoms, followed by a meningitic phase as the virus reaches the CNS. The onset of spinal poliomyelitis is associated with myalgia and severe muscle spasms and the subsequent development of an asymmetrical, predominantly lower limb, flaccid weakness which becomes maximal after 48 hours. A purely bulbar form, with minimal limb involvement, also occurs carrying a particularly high mortality rate because of vasomotor disturbances such as hypertension, hypotension and circulatory collapse, autonomic dysfunction, dysphagia, dysphonia and respiratory failure. Polio may also cause an acute encephalitis. Recovery from the acute infection can be slow and prolonged periods of rehabilitation are necessary for recovery of limb function, severe permanent impairment is common.

The virus is commonly isolated from the nasopharynx or the stool. In the absence of a viral isolate, serological diagnosis can be established by neutralisation of sera against paired antigens of the three serotypes. PCR is now the technique of choice for serotypic identification of poliovirus and for differentiation of wild and vaccine-strain poliomyelitis.

Table 9.23 Causes of acute flaccid paralysis.

Infection
Viral
Enterovirus – poliomyelitis (wild and vaccine associated), enterovirus 71, Coxsackie A
Flavivirus – Japanese, West Nile encephalitis
Herpes virus – CMV, EBV, VZV
Tick-borne encephalitis
HIV related (associated with opportunistic infections, particularly CMV)
Other neurotropic viruses – rabies
Bacterial
Borrelia, mycoplasma, diphtheria, botulism
Neuropathy
Acute inflammatory polyneuropathy (AIDP)
Acute motor axonal neuropathy (AMAN)
Critical illness neuropathy
Lead poisoning, other heavy metals, porphyria, hyperkalaemia
Spinal cord
Acute transverse myelitis, acute spinal cord compression, trauma, infarction
Neuromuscular junction
Myasthenia gravis
Muscle
Polymyositis
Viral myositis
Post infectious myositis
Critical illness myopathy
Non-organic

Differential diagnosis

Acute flaccid paralysis is associated with infection by other enteroviruses including coxsackie virus A7 and enterovirus 71, tick-borne encephalitis and by flaviviruses including Japanese encephalitis and, more recently, West Nile virus (Table 9.23). The differential diagnosis of asymmetric motor flaccid paralysis includes Guillain–Barré syndrome, acute intermittent porphyria, HIV neuropathy, diphtheria and *B. burgdorferi* (Lyme disease) infections.

Prevention

Sabin trivalent oral live attenuated polio vaccine (OPV) is composed of live attenuated strains of polioviruses I, II and III grown in cell culture. The advantages over the older inactivated polio (IPV) (Salk) vaccine are that it can be administered orally, and causes an active attenuated infection of the oropharynx and intestinal endothelium, stimulating local secretary IgA in addition to serum antibody production. It is also cheap. Furthermore, the attenuated virus is excreted in the faeces leading to herd immunity. Complete immunisation with OPV has, conventionally, included four doses routinely given at 2, 4 and 6–18 months, with a booster at 4–6 years. Despite the success of the global eradication campaign difficulties remain and new outbreaks continue to occur. It is difficult to provide adequate heat-stable OPV, to ensure adequate sero-conversion in tropical populations and this has led to a suggestion that OPV should be abandoned in favour of IPV. OPV derived poliomyelitis is attenuated but can mutate and acquire properties similar to the wild type resulting in vaccine associated paralytic poliomyelitis. Vaccine derived poliomyelitis may occur in unimmunized direct contacts (particularly those changing the nappies of infants who have recently received OPV).

Post-polio syndrome

Many patients with residual impairments following previous paralytic poliomyelitis develop new disabilities after a period of prolonged stability. These late changes include progressive muscular atrophy, weakness, pain and fatigue but most patients are aware of late functional deterioration giving rise to impairment of activities of daily living, mobility, upper limb function and respiratory capacity. The new wasting and weakness is probably caused by distal degeneration of post-poliomyelitis motor units associated with age, overuse or disuse. New impairments often occur as a consequence of prolonged stresses on skeletal deformity and previously weakened muscles. The extent of the original limb, trunk, respiratory and bulbar weakness is an important factor in predisposing to the development of late functional deterioration. Although there are no adequate longitudinal studies, experience suggests that post-polio functional deterioration is not necessarily an ongoing process. Fatigue and reduced mobility, often may progress slowly or stabilise. The prognosis also depends on the nature of any underlying cause for the functional deterioration.

Subacute sclerosing panencephalitis

Subacute sclerosing panencephalitis (SSPE) is a progressive neurological condition associated with measles occurring at a young age (usually <2 years). The onset is usually in childhood at an average of 6–8 years, with a male : female ratio of 3 : 1. SSPE can also occur in adults and can be triggered during pregnancy. The clinical course is highly variable but the onset is usually with behavioural and intellectual change developing over weeks or months. There is frequently a decline in school performance with withdrawal, hyperactivity, aggressive behaviour and emotional lability. Motor signs progressively develop with dysarthria, incoordination and tremor. There is usually a progressive decline with periodic stereotyped attacks of myoclonic jerks and seizures. Higher functions deteriorate with worsening apraxia, visuo-spatial abnormalities and progressive language impairment. Profound disability is associated with choreoathetosis, dystonia, persistent myoclonic jerking and autonomic instability with hyperpyrexia, tachycardia and an abnormal respiratory pattern. There may be an associated choroidoretinitis pigmentosa and optic atrophy. The condition usually progresses to become fatal in 1–3 years. Ten per cent survive for up to 10 years. A more rapidly progressive course with death in 3 months occurs in about 10% of patients. The condition is associated with infection by measles virus at a young age. The virus is an enveloped RNA virus and can be recovered from the CSF and brain in most patients. The diagnosis is based on the clinical pattern and on EEG findings. There are characteristic bilateral synchronous and symmetrical periodic discharges occurring every 4–12 seconds. There is also associated slower background EEG activity which becomes disorganised. An elevated measles virus antibody is found in serum and CSF. MRI shows focal or generalised high white matter lesions in frontal, temporal and occipital regions. There is no effective treatment – inosoplex and intrathecal ribavirin have been used but evidence is lacking.

Rabies

Rabies is a zoonosis of certain mammals endemic in all continents; it is caused by a lyssavirus which is inoculated into the tissue of a wound usually caused by a canine or bat bite. The virus may replicate locally in muscle cells or attach directly to nerve endings. It then enters the presynaptic nerve terminal and is carried in a retrograde direction. On reaching the CNS there is massive viral replication in neurones before transynaptic transmission of the virus occurs from cell to cell. Viral proteins accumulate in the cytoplasm appearing as inclusions (Negri bodies).

Clinical features

Clinical features develop 1–3 months after the bite although longer incubation periods are known. The onset is with a prodrome of fever, nausea, vomiting, chills, malaise, fatigue and insomnia together with the development of pain, pruritus, paraesthesiae and fasciculation close to the bite site. This is followed by the development of progressive encephalopathy. The disease is described as either furious rabies (80%) or paralytic rabies (20%).

Furious rabies is characterised by fluctuating episodes of excitement and hyper-excitability with periods of lucidity. Aggressive behaviour, confusion and hallucinations develop. Autonomic dysfunction is manifest as hypersalivation, sweating and pilo-erection. Patients develop severe muscle spasms of the throat, trunk and respiratory muscles triggered either by the sight or sound of water or attempts to drink (hydrophobia) or even by a draft of air (aerophobia). The spasms cause generalised extension, convulsions and opisthotonus with death usually occurring within a week of the onset of furious rabies as a consequence of cardiac arrhythmias, myocarditis and respiratory arrest.

Paralytic rabies is less common; it may occur following vampire bat transmission, in patients who have been infected by an attenuated virus or following post-exposure vaccination. It is associated with an ascending paralysis leading to constipation, urinary retention, respiratory failure and an inability to swallow. Flaccid muscle weakness develops early in the course of the disease. Hydrophobic spasms may also occur. Patients may go on to develop bulbar and respiratory muscle involvement but tend to survive longer than those with furious rabies.

The differential diagnosis includes:
- Viral encephalitis
- Tetanus
- Post-vaccinal encephalomyelitis
- Guillain–Barré syndrome.

Diagnosis
The clinical features may be obvious. A CSF mononuclear pleocytosis develops, usually within the first week, but serum neutralising antibodies are not present until the tenth day of the illness. Viral isolation is occasionally possible from saliva, throat, trachea, CSF or brain biopsy and skin biopsy and immunofluorescent antibody techniques will demonstrate an antigen in the small nerves of the skin taken from the nape of the neck, often in a hair follicle. PCR detection of rabies virus RNA has also been demonstrated from the brain, saliva and CSF. Postmortem virus isolation and brain cultures should be taken if possible.

Management
Management is supportive. Rabies is almost invariably fatal. Patients with rabies need heavy sedation and adequate analgesia to relieve terror or pain. Acute interventional care may be necessary to manage cardiac arrhythmias, cardiac and respiratory failure, raised intracranial pressure, convulsions and fluid and electrolyte disturbances. Only very occasional survival has been documented, usually in patients who had received rabies vaccine before the onset of symptoms. Immunisation before possible exposure is strongly recommended to travellers who plan to visit regions where rabies is endemic, as it provides protection after unrecognised exposure and may simplify treatment. Post-exposure treatment is summarised in Table 9.24.

Table 9.24 Post-exposure treatment of rabies.

Post-exposure prophylaxis	If there is any doubt about the possibility of rabies then post-exposure prophylaxis should begin immediately • *Local wound care* – washed thoroughly with soap and water, debridement as necessary and tetanus prophylaxis • *Active immunisation* – using either human diploid cell vaccine or alternatively purified chick embryo cell culture vaccine in five doses given over 28 days. If a bite occurs in a previously immunised individual only two booster doses are necessary • *Passive immunisation* – human rabies immunoglobulin should be given immediately before the vaccine. The wound should be infiltrated with the immunoglobulin and then a dose given intramuscularly
Examination of the biting animal	Ideally, the animal should be captured confined and observed for 10 days If there is any clinical suspicion of rabies, the animal should be killed and the brain examined for virus
Antigen detection in animals	Using fluorescent antibody techniques or cell culture of mouse inoculation

Prevention is achieved with careful attempts to eradicate rabies from dogs by immunisation, careful border control and preventing contact of domestic pets with wild animals. Pre-exposure immunisation results in highly effective prevention and should be considered in individuals who are considered at high risk (e.g. vets, laboratory workers or those who handle imported animals) or those travelling to, living or working in endemic areas.

HTLV-1
Human T-lymphotropic virus type 1 (HTLV-1) is a double-stranded RNA retrovirus that causes adult T-cell lymphoma/leukaemia and also neurological involvement manifest as tropical spastic paraparesis and, less commonly, myositis. Only a small proportion of seropositive people infected go on to develop neurological manifestations.

The virus is endemic in southern Japan, the Caribbean, South America and sub-Saharan Africa. Risk factors for transmission of HTLV-1 include sexual contact, exchange of blood products and vertical transmission from mother to child (see also Chapter 16).

HTLV-1 associated myelopathy (tropical spastic paraparesis)
Tropical spastic paraparesis (TSP) is a progressive inflammatory myelopathy evolving over many decades. The incubation period may be many years. Females are more commonly affected than males. Onset tends to be in the fourth or fifth decades; symptoms develop insidiously with a slowly progressive paraparesis predominantly affecting proximal muscles with brisk reflexes and extensor plantar responses. Upper limb involvement develops as the condition progresses but the bulbar muscles are not involved. Bladder dysfunction becomes evident as urgency and incontinence; chronic retention and overflow may also occur leading to recurrent urinary tract infections; sexual dysfunction is common. There may be burning low back pain and painful dysaesthesiae in the legs. The myelopathy is occasionally associated with cerebellar ataxia. Examination shows mild to moderate progressive spastic pyramidal weakness more marked proximally. In TSP the brunt of pathological change is seen within the thoracic cord. There is occasionally mild distal vibration sense impairment to the ankles.

The major differential diagnosis is:
- Primary progressive multiple sclerosis
- Hereditary spastic paraparesis (HSP)
- Primary lateral sclerosis.

The diagnosis may be suspected on clinical grounds. HTLV-1 antibodies can be detected in serum and CSF using Western blot techniques. CSF shows a mild lymphocytosis with elevated protein and local IgG synthesis. Oligoclonal bands are found that are specific for HTLV-1 core and envelope antigen. PCR is available in some centres. MRI may show atrophy of the cervical or thoracic cord and brain MRI often shows subcortical, periventricular white matter high signal.

Antiviral agents have been used in an attempt to inhibit replication of the HTLV-1 proviral load. Immunosuppression is now increasingly used to suppress the immune response to the virus. There is no clearly effective treatment although transient benefit may be gained from steroids. The condition is progressive, although the rate of evolution is variable and generally slow.

Other neurological manifestions of HTLV-1 infection

Rarely, muscle inflammation is the only manifestation of HTLV-1 although muscle disease may accompany the myelopathy. Myalgia and progressive proximal muscle weakness develop over many months, occasionally associated with a dermatomyositis-like rash. The myositis is relentlessly progressive and does not respond to steroids. There have been no consistent reports of benefit from intravenous immunoglobulin (IVIG) or immunosuppression. Pathologically there is an inflammatory response with myofibre necrosis, regenerating fibres and mononuclear cell infiltrate.

HTLV-1 also causes both axonal and demyelinating neuropathies. Anterior and posterior uveitis have been described in association with HTLV-1. In these conditions the visual prognosis is good but there is a high relapse rate. A variety of other associations have been suggested, in particular between HTLV-1 and cognitive impairment or other autoallergic conditions, but these are unproven.

HTLV-2

HTLV-2 is closely related to HTLV-1, sharing 70% genomic homology. It is found in intravenous drug abusers and Native Americans but has not been clearly linked to any disease. HTLV-III was previously the term used for HIV-1 and HTLV-IV for HIV-2, but these terms have fallen out of use. HTLV-III and HTLV-IV have recently been used to denote two newly characterised viruses of uncertain significance.

Fungal infections

Fungi differ from bacteria by having a nucleus bounded by an organised membrane and a chitinous cell wall. They divide by mitosis, lack chlorophyll and are non-motile. Fungi exist in two forms: yeast and filamentous (hyphae and pseudohyphae). Yeasts are unicellular, multiply by budding and infections generally involve the CSF or meninges (Table 9.25). Filamentous fungi grow by extension of their hyphae, liberate spores and usually lead to parenchymous cerebral involvement. Fungal infections have increased because of the increased numbers of patients who are immunocompromised as a result of HIV/AIDS, an immunodeficiency state or immunosuppression.

Fungi produce neurological disease by direct invasion, allergic phenomena and liberating toxins. Fungal meningitis generally develops insidiously over several days or weeks and is secondary to systemic mycosis elsewhere in the body. The CNS is seeded haematogenously either from a pulmonary or cardiac focus or secondary to direct spread from the sinuses or skull involving the subarachnoid space and leading to a basal meningitis. Fungal meningitis is characterised by meningism with subacute involvement of cranial nerves and an arteritis with thrombosis and cortical or subcortical infarction and micro-abscess formation.

Primary fungal pathogens include *Cryptococcus neoformans*, *Coccidioides immitis*, histoplasmosis, blastomycoses and *Paracoccidioides*. Secondary opportunistic pathogens are more common and occur with immune dysfunction, these include *Candida*, *Aspergillus* and mucormycosis. *Cryptococcus*, *Aspergillus*, *Candida* and *Mucor* occur worldwide but histoplasmosis and blastomyces are generally confined to the Americas. *Cryptococcus*, histoplasmosis and *Coccidioides* are true yeasts, *Candida* mainly exists as pseudohyphae while *Aspergillus* and mucormycosis are filamentous.

Risk factors

Cancer, chemotherapy and resulting neutropenia predispose particularly to *Candida* and *Aspergillus* meningitis and HIV to *Cryptococcus*, *Histoplasmosis* and *Coccidioides*. Fungal infection can also occur as a consequence of direct inoculation of fungi followed penetrating trauma or neurosurgery. Other risk factors include:

- Pregnancy
- Lymphoreticular malignancy including leukaemia and lymphoma
- Diabetes

Table 9.25 Main fungal infections of the nervous system.

	Geography	Risk factors	Clinical features	Treatment
Cryptococcus neoformans	Worldwide	HIV, cytotoxic drugs, RE malignancy	Granulomatous meningitis, hydrocephalus, raised intracranial pressure	Amphotericin B and flucytosine (induction) and fluconazole maintenance
Histoplasmosis	USA, Central America, Asia, Africa	HIV, steroids, organ transplant	Chronic basal meningitis or cerebritis Rarely, encephalitis or abscess	Amphotericin B then itraconazole maintenance
Coccidiocoides	USA, Central and South America	HIV, pregnancy, immunosuppression	Diffuse parenchymatous meningitis Meningoencephalitis Mass lesions	Amphotericin B or Fluconazole followed by prolonged Fluconazole maintenance
Candida	Worldwide	See text	Meningitis, vascular infiltration	Amphotericin B
Aspergillus	Worldwide	Neutropenia, immunosuppression	Cerebral abscess, diffuse granulomatous meningitis, ascular infiltration	Voriconazole or amphotericin B Debulking
Mucormycosis	Worldwide	DM, malignancy, steroids	Rhinocerebral invasion	Amphotericin B and surgical debridement. Posaconazole can be used as salvage

- Organ transplantation
- Severe burns
- Connective and vascular disease
- Malignancy.

There is an extensive differential diagnosis of fungal meningitis summarised in Tables 9.17 and 9.18. The most important differential diagnoses are:

- Tuberculous meningitis
- Granulomatous cerebral vasculitis (Churg–Strauss, Wegener's granulomatosis)
- Viral meningoencephalitis
- Acute disseminated encephalomyelitis
- Sarcoidosis
- Lymphoma
- Carcinomatous meningitis
- Partially treated bacterial meningitis
- Other forms of chronic meningitis – lupus and idiopathic chronic meningitis.

The diagnosis of fungal meningitis is made on the basis of CSF examination which usually shows a mononuclear pleocytosis (20–500 cells/mm^3) with occasional predominance of polymorphonuclear cells especially in aspergillosis. The cell count may be reduced if the patient is immunosuppressed. CSF India ink staining and agglutinin testing is important in the diagnosis of *Cryptococcus* infection. In culture, *Candida* is identified in 2–3 days but dimorphic fungi such as *Histoplasma* may take several weeks to grow. Serology is occasionally helpful.

CT and MRI may show meningeal enhancement and accompanying parenchymatous mass lesions, possibly with hydrocephalus. Meningeal biopsy is only occasionally of value.

True yeasts

Cryptococcus neoformans

Cryptococcus neoformans is an encapsulated yeast which is the most common pathogen causing fungal meningitis. It occurs in bird excreta and has a worldwide distribution. *Cryptococcus* characteristically occurs in patients with impaired cell-mediated immunity in HIV, or those who have received cytotoxic drugs or steroids and it is also associated with sarcoid and reticulo-endothelial malignancy. *Cryptococcus* occurs as a result of inhalation of small yeast forms into the respiratory tract. Infection may remain dormant for many years or lead to immediate local pulmonary or disseminated infection.

There is an acute or subacute granulomatous meningo-encephalitis with meningism, headache and pyrexia, culminating in the progressive development of raised intracranial pressure with or without hydrocephalus. There may be multiple cranial nerve palsies or focal neurological features including paraparesis, hemiparesis and ataxia. Visual impairment and cerebral infarction also occur. The onset may be subacute over many weeks with cognitive impairment and dementia. The diagnosis is based on culture, direct observation with India ink staining, CSF fungal culture or crytococcal antigen (CrAg) testing which is both specific and sensitive. The CSF shows a variable lymphocytic pleocytosis.

The outcome of cryptococcal disease is variable. Untreated it can become disseminated and fatal within a few weeks but more often infection leads to persistently raised intracranial pressure with repeated lumbar puncture or a ventriculo-peritoneal shunt being necessary. It accounts for about 20% of all AIDS-related deaths.

Cryptococcus is treated with an induction phase of intravenous amphotericin B and flucytosine followed by fluconazole or itraconazole for 8–10 weeks. Because of the high relapse rate in patients with AIDS, the third level of treatment using fluconazole 200 mg/day as a lifetime suppressive agent is recommended.

Histoplasmosis

Histoplasmosis usually manifests as a respiratory illness that resembles miliary TB of the lung. It is associated with AIDS, steroids and organ transplantation. Histoplasmosis can also become disseminated; CNS involvement occurs in up to 20% of patients with a chronic basal meningitis or cerebritis. Less often there may be hydrocephalus, encephalitis, cerebral or spinal cord abscess. The diagnosis is made by CSF culture, which is positive in only about 30%; microscopy is usually negative. CSF antigen detection is also possible but there is a high incidence of false positives. Treatment is with amphotericin B but relapses are common and maintenance with itraconazole is indicated. Similar chronic basal meningitis occurs with blastomycosis and actinomycosis.

Coccidiomycosis

Coccidiomycosis occurs particularly in the south-west United States, Mexico and South America and is caused by air-borne spores. The onset is usually with a self-limiting flu-like illness and pulmonary infiltrates but the *Coccidioides* may disseminate to cause a chronic diffuse parenchymatous basal meningitis or meningoencephalitis. This causes lethargy, confusion and memory loss. Lytic skull and vertebral lesions occur and intracranial mass lesions may lead to communicating hydrocephalus.

The diagnosis is made by CSF culture and positivity to complement fixation tests. Treatment is with intravenous amphotericin B given over a prolonged period followed by prolonged or even lifelong treatment with fluconazole. Itraconozole and voriconozole are alternatives.

Pseudohyphae

Candida species

Candida albicans is a normal commensal but is the most common cause of fungal meningitis in neonates and young children.

Risk factors

- Neutropenia
- Immunodeficiency (acquired in congenital shunt infection)
- Immunocompromised hosts
- HIV
- Organ transplants
- Diabetes
- Severe burns
- Total parenteral nutrition
- Malignancy
- Debility
- Steroids and broad-spectrum antibiotics
- Following neurosurgery.

Candidiasis typically involves the lungs, heart, urogenital system, skin and mucous membranes. There can be an acute meningitis; diffuse infiltration occasionally leads to small vessel thrombosis with microinfarcts particularly in the middle cerebral artery territory. There may also be haemorrhage from rupture of mycotic aneurysms. Rarely, there is a subacute onset where invasion of the subarachnoid space occurs. Patients may have a ventriculoperitoneal shunt or ventriculostomy in place for other reasons and be receiving prophylactic antibiotics.

The diagnosis is made on the basis of clinical features together with the CSF showing a mild pleocytosis and low glucose. CSF staining has a low yield (<20%) but in nearly half of *Candida* cases the diagnosis can be confirmed by culture. While a very serious disease, mortality has been reduced by 10–20% by combined amphotericin B and flucytosine which act synergistically. Treatment should be continued for 6–8 weeks. Shunt replacement may be necessary. The mortality rate is still up to 30% in patients with HIV.

True hyphae (moulds)

Aspergillus fumigatus

Aspergillus fumigatus accounts for about 5% of CNS fungal infections and carries a poor prognosis. It develops in association with prolonged neutropenia, immunosuppression and parenteral drug abuse. It can also occur as a complication of sinusitis, otitis or mastoiditis. Manifestations include cerebral abscess (Figure 9.10), diffuse and granulomatous meningitis. Direct hyphal invasion of the cerebral blood vessels causes thrombosis, necrosis and haemorrhage, particularly involving the posterior circulation. Intracranial mass lesions also occur which may be solitary or, less commonly, multiple. Progressive vascular infiltration may lead to multiple mycotic intracranial aneurysms clinically manifest as encephalopathy, seizures and focal neurological deficit. Haematogenous spread occurs. Diagnosis is difficult as cultures are rarely positive. Products of metabolism may show evidence of *Aspergillus*. Treatment is both medical and surgical involving debulking and amphotericin B (0.7–1.0 mg/kg/day) but higher doses may be used. Treatment is less effective than in cryptococcosis. In many centres voriconazole has replaced amphotericin B. The prognosis remains poor often because of the impaired status of the host.

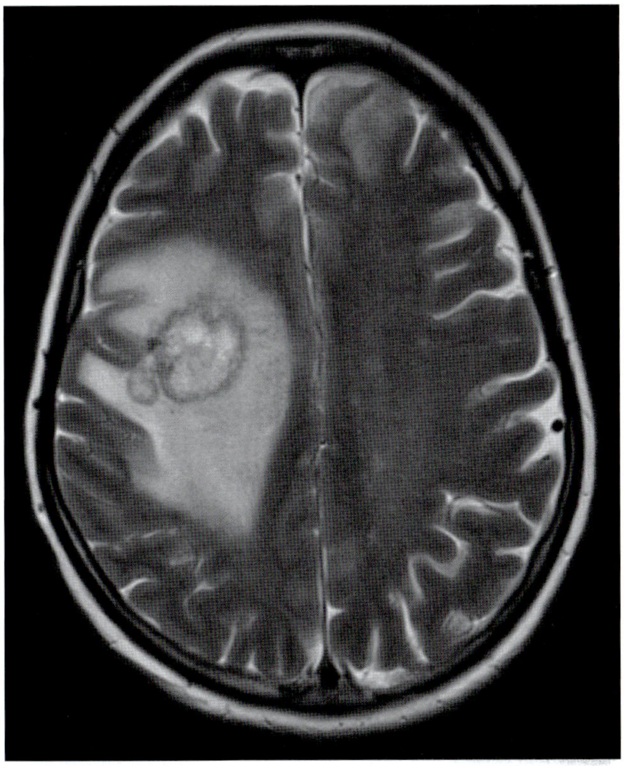

Figure 9.10 Aspergillosis: T2-weighted image showing a heterogeneous, irregular intraparenchymal aspergillus abscess with a hypointense rim.

Mucormycosis

Mucormycosis is a rare fungal infection associated with diabetes, steroids, malignancy, pregnancy or drug addiction. There may be malignant infiltration of cerebral vessels with hyphae commencing in the nasal turbinates and paranasal sinuses and spreading along infected vessels to retro-orbital tissue. Cavernous sinus or internal carotid artery thrombosis and involvement of the adjacent brain contribute to haemorrhagic infarction. Ocular involvement is manifest as central retinal and ophthalmic artery occlusion or optic nerve compression. Treatment is with rapid correction of any hyperglycaemia and acidosis from diabetes, surgical debridement and amphotericin B but the prognosis is poor. Posaconazole can be used as salvage treatment.

Parasitic disease of the nervous system

The parasitic causes of CNS lesions are summarised in Table 9.26, Table 9.27 and Table 9.28. Parasitic infection should be considered if the absolute number of eosinophils in blood is $>0.4 \times 10^9$ cells/L or if any eosinophils are found in the CSF. These infections are rare in the United Kingdom with the exception of toxoplasmosis in the immunosuppressed patient and *Toxocara canis* in children.

Neurocysticercosis

Neurocysticercosis is caused by infection of the human CNS by the larval form of *Taenia solium,* the pork tapeworm. It is the most common cause of acquired epilepsy in most low income countries and of major importance worldwide.

Adult *T. solium* tapeworms reside only in the small intestine of humans, who are the definitive host. Humans only develop cysticercosis if they ingest viable *T. solium* ova which are the larval forms of the *T. solium* tapeworm. These eggs or ova are only shed in the faeces of humans who are infected by the tapeworm. Humans ingest tapeworm eggs from contaminated water, food or from food handlers or others who harbour the adult tapeworms in their small intestines. Human carriers of *T. solium* tapeworm are at very

Table 9.26 Parasitic causes of CNS lesions.

Nematodes (Roundworms)
Trichinosis
Angiostrongylodiasis (*Angiostrongylus cantonensis*)
Strongylodiasis (*Strongyloides stercoralis*)
Visceral larva migrans (*Toxocara canis*)
Cestodes (Tapeworms)
Cysticercosis (*Taenia solium*)
Hydatid disease (Echinococcus)
Coenuriasis (Multiceps)
Sparganosis (Spirometra)
Trematodes (Flukes)
Schistosomiasis (*Schistosoma japonicum, S. mansoni, S. haematobium*)
Paragonimiasis
Protozoa
American trypanosomiasis (Chagas' disease)
African trypanosomiasis (sleeping sickness)

Table 9.27 Nematodes (roundworms).

Angiostrongyloidiasis	Ingestion of raw or inadequately cooked shellfish or snails which are the intermediate host	Asymptomatic or associated with pruritus, abdominal pain Neurological involvement is rare – may be chonic meningitis with headache, progressive cranial neuropathy, spinal cord involvement or retinal detachment CSF eosinophilic pleocytosis and raised protein. Larvae may be found in biopsy or the CSF Imaging shows meningeal enhancement with oedema and high signal in the basal ganglia Treatment is supportive as the illness is self-limiting
Strongyloides	Human intestinal infection. Associated with poor sanitation Occurs on contact with the parasite in contaminated water or by direct penetration of the skin	Migrates via the venous circulation to the lungs and small intestine where it remains dormant for many years May subsequently reinfect the host and render them liable to secondary bacterial infection Affects the lungs and gastrointestinal tract but rarely may involve the CNS leading to encephalopathy, meningism and, rarely, vascular involvement including mycotic aneurysms, intracerebral haemorrhage or vasculitis Serum eosinophilia Larvae can be identified in stool, serum, CSF or peritoneal fluid Antibodies can be detected with immuno assay MRI scan shows atrophy and may show the presence of mycotic aneurysms or abscesses Treatment is with ivermectin (alternatives includes thiabendazole, albendazole or mebendazole)
Toxocara canis	Ingestion of parasites after contact with infected cats or dogs in whom the excreted eggs survive for many years	Endemic throughout the world The eggs hatch into larvae, which migrate to the liver and then to the viscera leading to an inflammatory response and granuloma formation Infection is usually mild and self-limiting but visceral larva migrans may migrate to the lungs, liver, kidney, heart muscle, brain or eyes and ocular involvement can cause optic ocular neuritis and blindness. Cognitive impairment occasionally occurs with CNS involvement The diagnosis is difficult because the eggs are not excreted in the faeces Serum and CSF eosinophilia. Antibody testing on CSF confirms the diagnosis Imaging may show subcortical and white matter disease suggesting a vasculitis Treatment is with diethylcarbamazine or alternatively mebendazole and albendazole

CSF, cerebrospinal fluid; MRI, magnetic resonance imaging.

high risk of auto-infection with cysticercosis through faeco-oral transmission and family members are at particular risk. Poor sanitation can cause contamination of food and water leading to widespread low level exposure. Pigs acquire infection through ingestion of food or water contaminated with human faeces containing ova. In the pig, the ova hatch and invade the intestinal wall. Larval cysts (onchospheres) are carried in the bloodstream throughout the body. Cysticercosisis is not caused by eating raw or uncooked pork, which only causes adult tapeworm infestation (taeniasis) because infected pork contains the (onchospheres) which develop into adult worms in the human intestine but does not contain the eggs that cause cysticercosis.

Neurocysticercosis develops when ingested eggs (ova) hatch in the human intestine and the resulting embryos (onchospheres) become larvae that cross the intestinal wall and are carried by the bloodstream to various organs, including the nervous system, where they lodge in small blood vessels and develop into viable cysts (cysticerci) after 2–3 months. Cysticerci are vesicles consisting of a wall and scolex. The main target organs of the cysticerci are the eye, skeletal muscle and the nervous system, where cysticerci form in the brain parenchyma often following blood flow or they become localised in the subarachnoid space, ventricular system or spinal cord.

Parenchymatous cysts are common in patients with heavy infections and are frequently located at the grey–white interface. They develop in the cerebral cortex or the basal ganglia because of the relatively high blood flow to these areas.

Other extraparenchymatous cysts affect the basal subarachnoid region or pass into the ventricles becoming lodged in the choroid plexus or 4th ventricle and lead to hydrocephalus. They may become massive and lodge within the cortical sulci or the basal CSF

Table 9.28 Cestodes (tapeworms).

Echinococcus (Hydatid disease)	Humans and sheep are infected by ingesting eggs excreted by infected animals and the source is usually water or vegetables contaminated by canine faeces After ingestion the parasite rapidly disseminates to the liver, lungs and vertebrae	CNS involvement is characterised by cyst formation causing compression of the brain or intracerebral blood vessels which may manifest as raised intracranial pressure with headache, nausea, vomiting and seizures and is generally difficult to distinguish from cysticercosis. The cysts may also cause compressive spinal cord lesions *Investigations* Elevated ESR, serum eosinophilia and positive immunophoresis testing Imaging confirms the presence of cysts (often multiple) of various sizes *Management* Surgical intervention is necessary to remove enlarged cysts with mass effect. Medical treatment is with albendazole
Sparganosis	A form of the tapeworm – contracted from contaminated water or eating undercooked fish	Invasion of the CNS occurs occasionally and there may be focal neurological features including seizures and hemiparesis *Investigations* Peripheral eosinophilia Parasite may be demonstrated in human tissue specimens. Immunofluorescent antibody techniques are sensitive and specific. Imaging will show calcified lesions *Treatment* Praziquantel – only moderately successful and surgical excision of the parasite may be necessary

ESR, erythrocyte sedimentation rate.

cisterns and they may also involve the subdural space, the sellar and parasellar regions, the eye and the spinal cord.

Cysticerci elicit a mild inflammatory response when they enter the CNS. Cysts either remain viable for many years or enter a process of degeneration that ends with their death and calcification. Viable cysts are not associated with inflammation and remain static until they are eventually recognised by the host and undergo an intense inflammatory response which then leads to granuloma formation and degenerative change associated with varying amounts of enhancements on MRI and oedema. Eventually, the granuloma decreases in size and becomes nodular. Cysts can resolve entirely but most degenerating cysts hyalinize and calcify although intermittent flares of inflammation and oedema can still occur.

Following death, cysticerci undergo progressive involution in which the cyst becomes surrounded by a thick collagen capsule. Brain parenchyma develops astrocytic gliosis and diffuse oedema, progressing to granuloma formation and then calcification and astrocytic change as the oedema subsides. Cysticerci in the meninges induce an intense inflammatory response in the subarachnoid space with formation of a dense exudate leading to leptomeningeal thickening which may cause hydrocephalus or occlusion of the vessel lumen and cerebral infarction.

Clinical features

CNS infection is often asymptomatic. Epilepsy is the most common presentation – the seizures are usually generalized tonic–clonic or simple partial but can be complex partial. Cognitive function may be impaired. Intrasellar cysticerci present with visual field loss and endocrine disturbances from pituitary involvement while ocular cysticerci cause decreased visual acuity or visual field loss. Spinal cord involvement is characterized by root pain or motor and sensory deficits that vary according to the level of the lesion. Massive infection of striated muscle may lead to generalised weakness with progressive muscle enlargement.

Extraparenchymal neurocysticercosis generally has a worse prognosis. It can be divided into ventricular and subarachnoid locations.

Cysts lodging in the ventricles (usually 4th but may involve a 3rd and lateral ventricles) may cause mechanical obstruction to CSF flow leading to hydrocephalus, often associated with headache, nausea, vomiting and vertigo. Focal signs may develop.

Subarachnoid cysts may affect the brain convexity causing surface compression and leading to epilepsy or the effects of a space occupying lesion. Involvement of the Sylvian fissure by multiple cysts or a single giant cyst may result in a mass effect or calcification and infarction of the middle cerebral artery. Basal subarachnoid neurocysticercosis often causes and extensive inflammatory response affecting the arachnoid space, meninges, foramina and brain tissue leading to arachnoiditis, pachymeningitis and mass effect. Spread may occur throughout the subarachnoid space and in the spinal cord and may lead to arachnoiditis or cord compression.

Diagnosis

Plain films may show small <1 cm cigar-shaped soft tissue calcification in brain or cysticerci in the anterior chamber of the eye and in muscles. In countries where neurocysticercosis is prevalent, small <1 cm brain lesions are often regarded as neurocysticercosis cysts unless proved otherwise, and are common incidental findings.

Imaging appearances depend on the stage of the cysticercus. On MRI, the initial vesicular stage appears as a CSF-like cyst with the scolex as a dot at its centre. Oedema and rim-enhancement develop

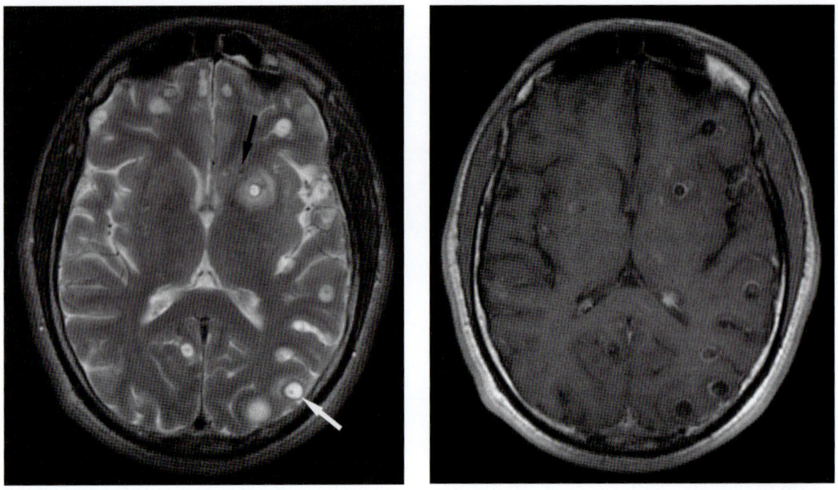

(a) (b)

Figure 9.11 Cysticercosis: (a) T2-weighted and (b) T1-weighted post contrast images showing multiple lesions in varying states of maturity. The scolex can be seen as a central hypointense dot in several of the vesicular lesions (white arrow). Old calcified lesions are visible as punctate hypointense foci (black arrow).

as the scolex degenerates, eventually contracting to a small calcified nodule. CT shows the viable cystercerci as hypodense lesions, occasionally with a central hyperdense scolex, and is particularly sensitive for detection of the mature calcified nodular stage (Figure 9.11). Degenerating cysts appear as contrast enhancing rings on FLAIR MRI sequences. There may be hydrocephalus. Cysticerci should be distinguished from lesions of tuberculosis which tend to be larger and to have mass effect. The differential diagnosis also includes tumours, particularly glioma.

Serological tests – enzyme-linked immunoelectro-transfer blot with purified glycoprotein antigens (Western blot) – can be undertaken on serum or CSF but may be negative. Cysticerci may be noted on muscle biopsy. Stool examination may reveal *T. solium* ova in those who carry gut tapeworms, which typically cause no symptoms.

Management

Acute treatment includes in immediate measures to manage raised intracranial pressure or mass effect (mannitol or high dose steroids). Surgical procedures are necessary to remove the cyst or to relieve the blockages or hydrocephalus. Antiepileptic drugs are used to control seizures. Corticosteroids reduce the acute inflammatory response and antihelminthic medication will kill the cysts.

There remains uncertainty about the value of medication in neurocysticercosis because many clinical manifestations are caused by calcified cysts rather than active lesions. In most patients a single enhancing lesion will disappear spontaneously. There is evidence to support the use of antihelminthic medication, usually accompanied by corticosteroids, to treat patients with viable cysts. The purpose is to kill the parasites and to alleviate symptoms.

There is debate about treatment of the patient with a single enhancing lesion. The two most used antihelminthic drugs are albendazole and praziquantel. Both are cysticidal and result in either cyst degeneration followed by clearance and eventual calcification of the cyst. However, many patients develop treatment-related exacerbations of disease.

The treatment of patients with cystic disease decreases generalised and partial seizures but the efficacy for single enhancing lesions remains unproven. Uncomplicated parenchymal disease is commonly treated with 15 mg/kg albendazole in two divided doses for 8 days to 2 weeks. Praziquantel at 50 mg/kg/day is taken for 1–2 weeks with cimetidine to prevent metabolism of the active drug in the liver. The commonly used antihelminthic treatment regimens provide relatively low cure rates and repeated courses of treatment are often necessary. Combined therapy is increasingly used. In patients with numerous or large areas of cysts there may be an extensive inflammatory response and this can be exacerbated by treatment. These patients require corticosteroids. A single course of albendazole or praziquantel kills 60–85% of viable brain cysts leading to rapid radiological resolution of the cysts. Corticosteroids are indicated in the presence of encephalitis angiitis or chronic meningitis causing progressive entrapment of cranial nerves. Antiepileptic medication may need to be life-long. Ventricular shunting to resolve hydrocephalus may be necessary but is associated with a high level of shunt malfunction.

Antihelminthic treatment is not indicated in patients with calcified neurocysticercosis because calcified lesions are non-viable and consist only of encapsulated cyst remnants.

Trematodes

Paragonimus is the only mammalian lung fluke that can infect humans. CNS involvement is extremely rare although chronic meningo-encephalitis, focal lesions including transverse myelitis, myelopathy and seizures may occur. There is often a marked serum and CSF eosinophilia. The eggs may be demonstrated in the CSF or on brain biopsy material. Serum antibody tests are positive and imaging showing multiple clusters of calcified density in the right frontal and temporal region. Treatment is with praziquantel and steroids.

Schistosomiasis (bilharzia)

Schistosomiasis occurs in up to 200 million people worldwide. There are five forms but CNS involvement occurs particularly with *Schistosoma mansoni*, *S. haematobium* and *S. japonicum*. Infection is acquired in areas where the water supply or sanitation is poor. The larva invades the skin and migrates into the venous system.

Subsequent spread depends on the species involved. Schistosomiasis commonly causes hepatointestinal and urinary tract disease. The eggs of *S. japonicum* cause 60% of all schistosomal brain infections while *S. mansoni* tends to be confined to the spinal cord. *S. haematobium* can involve brain or cord. Eggs enter the CNS and cause a granulomatous response which walls off the invading parasite. The granulomas expand, become exudative and necrotic, involving vascular walls as well as local tissue.

The onset is with an acute pyrexia, urticarial swelling, myalgia, bloody diarrhea and eosinophilia. Neurological involvement occurs in <5% of patients and develops after weeks or months when the eggs migrate through the vascular system to the brain or spinal cord. Mass lesions may be produced by expanding granulomas leading to raised intracranial pressure or erosion of vessel walls culminating in intracranial haemorrhage. Spinal cord involvement may be caused by granuloma formation and transverse myelitis (usually below T6) is the most common manifestation although cauda equina and conus syndromes are also characteristic.

There is usually a CSF eosinophilia. Diagnosis is made by detection of the eggs in stool, urine or tissue biopsy. Antibody detection, using ELISA, is possible but this is not reliable as seroconversion takes 4–12 weeks. CT scan shows single or multiple small, hyperdense enhancing lesions caused by granuloma formation, which is inflammatory and surrounded by oedema with variable contrast enhancement. They are usually seen in the frontal, parietal and occipital lobes and the brainstem. The diagnosis depends on a high level of suspicion in those exposed to fresh water in endemic areas.

Treatment Treatment is conventionally with praziquantel, which is effective against all schistosome species and curative for >90% of patients. If patients continue to excrete the eggs then it is necessary to have a further course of treatment. Alternative treatments include niridazole or artemether, which kills immature migrating larvae and is synergistic with praziquantel. Steroids are used for lesions if there is extensive surrounding oedema and large granulomas may need to be excised surgically. Most patients make a full recovery if diagnosis and treatment are prompt.

Protozoa

American trypanosomiasis (Chagas disease)

American trypanosomiasis (Chagas disease) is caused by *Trypanosoma cruzi*, which is endemic in South and Central America. Infection occurs secondary to contact with reduviid bug, ingesting guinea pig excretia, blood transfusion or organ transplantation. Larval eggs are taken through the site of pruritic skin lesions. The larvae then mature and are transported by the bloodstream to distant sites. They divide intracellularly before rupture of the cell releases the infectious parasite and inflammatory substances.

Chagas disease has an onset with malaise, myalgia, headache and anorexia. There is unilateral or bilateral periorbital oedema (Romana's sign). Cardiac failure and intestinal involvements are common. Meningo-encephalitis may occur in a minority of patients depending on the severity of infection and extent of host immune response. The diagnosis is made by CSF demonstration of trypanosomes. Serum antibody detection tests are sensitive and specific for acute and chronic forms. MRI scanning may show one or more ring enhancing lesions involving the grey and white matter. Acute Chagas disease can be eradicated by benznidazole or nifurtimox but chronic infection remains symptomatic and is difficult to clear.

African trypanosomiasis (sleeping sickness)

African trypanosomiasis (sleeping sickness) occurs in humans in two forms: *Trypanosoma brucei gambiense* (West African) and *Trypanosoma brucei rhodensiense* (East African). The condition is widespread throughout sub-Saharan Africa. The vector of both species is the tsetse fly which feeds from infected animals. A superficial chancre forms at the site of the bite and the parasite larvae migrate, via the bloodstream, to the lymphatic vessels before maturing and reproducing. There is then a secondary spread of mature forms to the lymph nodes, spleen, liver, heart, endocrine system, eye and CNS leading to a host immune response and meningo-encephalitis.

West African trypanosomiasis is slow or indolent in onset and characterised by rash, intermittent fever and lymphadenopathy. The symptoms are episodic. The East African form is more aggressive with behavioural disturbance, psychiatric manifestations including anxiety and agitation with manic and uncontrolled behaviours. Sleep disruption occurs with day–night reversal and uncontrolled urges to sleep. The condition progresses to motor disturbances including ataxia, rigidity, akinesis and progressive pyramidal signs but meningism is rare. Visual involvement includes optic neuritis, optic atrophy and papilloedema. Death occurs as a result of coma, secondary infection or cardiac involvement but chronic forms occur. The diagnosis of trypanosomiasis can be made by direct observation in wet preparations of stained blood, CSF or biopsy. However, antibody and PCR tests are unreliable. MRI may demonstrate abnormal signal within the deep white matter and basal ganglia (Figure 9.12). The treatment is with suramin and pentamidine but this is not suitable if there is CNS involvement when melarsoprol or eflornithine are recommended. Some of the

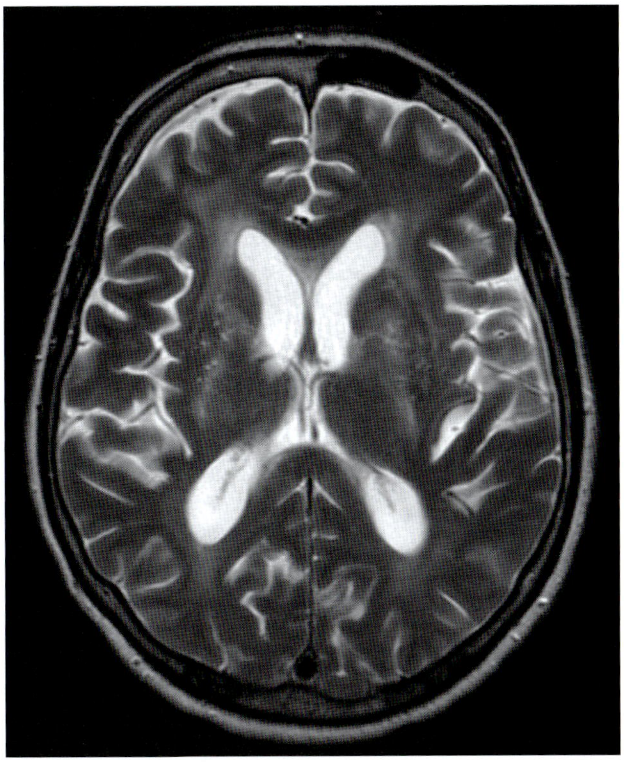

Figure 9.12 African typanosomiasis: T2-weighted axial image showing abnormal signal within the basal ganglia, internal and external capsules and peri-ventricular white matter.

agents are toxic and should be used at specialist centres with experience of the condition and its management.

Toxoplasma gondii

Toxoplasma gondii is an intracellular protozoan which is widely distributed. Invasion occurs as a result of ingestion of uncooked meat and exposure to cat faeces. *Toxoplasma* may invade multiple organs but in immunocompetent individuals infection is generally asymptomatic or associated with a mild mononucleosis-like illness with lymphadenopathy and a non-specific systemic illness. However, severe disease may occur in the immunocompromised patient, particularly in association with HIV, and this is discussed below.

Malaria

Malaria is the most important parasitic disease of humans and it is estimated that >5% of the world population has been infected. Each year >500 million new cases of malaria occur worldwide, 90% of these are in Africa or South-East Asia. The condition accounts for 200 million deaths per year.

Malaria is caused by five parasitic protozoa of the genus *Plasmodium*: *P. vivax*, *P. falciparum*, *P. ovale*, *P. malariae* and *P. knowlesi*. It is predominantly *P. falciparum* that can cause severe generalised disease and in particular cerebral malaria. The protozoa is transmitted by the female *Anopheles* mosquito which feeds at night-time although, rarely, transmission may also be transplacental or from contaminated needles. Infection is initiated by sporozoites injected in the bite of the mosquito. The protozoa undergoes a complex life cycle in the human host in which the sporozoites multiply within hepatocytes, producing thousands of multinucleated merozoites which enter the red blood cells and become mature forms (trophozoites and schizonts) before rupturing and releasing further merozoites. In falciparum malaria the red blood cells become distorted and excessively adherent binding to endothelial cells and causing sequestration, clumping and eventually vascular obstruction within the cerebral vessels. There is also an associated suppression of haemopoiesis leading to anaemia, thrombocytopenia and hepatosplenomegaly. *P. vivax*, *P. ovale* and *P. malariae* are either asymptomatic or cause recurrent episodic fever of varying severity. *P. knowlesi* is a primate malaria which causes non-relapsing disease that can also rarely lead to a rapidly severe and generalised malaria in parts of South-East Asia. In *P. falciparum* malaria, clinical manifestations depend on the load of parasite and the immune state of the host. Onset is with a flu-like illness, headache, fever and muscle aches. There are often paroxysms of rigor and shivering in between the pyrexia with extensive diaphoresis and hypothermia. Cerebral malaria is manifest by the onset of coma often heralded by focal or generalised seizures. Raised intracranial pressure develops rapidly, leading to possible brainstem herniation; in addition, vascular engorgement leads to the development of cerebral arterial occlusion, aneurysms or intracranial haemorrhage. A subacute syndrome or diffuse symmetrical encephalopathy may also occur associated with brainstem signs, eye movement abnormalities, pyramidal signs or extrapyramidal movements including choreoathetosis and myoclonus. Retinal haemorrhages are characteristic. Severe malaria is an acute form of the condition, generally but not exclusively due to *P. falciparum* (90%), and associated with organ dysfunction and a high level of parastaemia (>5%). In endemic areas children, pregnant women and travellers with no previous exposure are at particular risk of severe infection. Severe malaria may be associated with respiratory distress syndrome, pulmonary oedema, acidosis, circulatory collapse, pulmonary oedema, renal failure with haemoglobinuria (Blackwater fever), jaundice, disseminated intravascular coagulation, anaemia and hypoglycaemia. Neurological involvement is manifest as seizures and altered consciousness culminating in coma.

Diagnosis

The diagnosis of cerebral malaria is made on thick blood films and light microscopy ensuring that large amounts of blood are available and a minimum of 100 fields are observed. Thin film assessment allows species recognition. Newer antigen tests are now available based on recognition of the HRP-2 antigen of falciparum. PCR techniques are specific and sensitive to *Plasmodium*, but do not give an estimate of the parasite load.

Coma occurring in patients with cerebral malaria carries a fatality rate of up to 20% when appropriately treated and is invariably fatal if untreated. Complications include cerebral or dural venous thrombosis and cortical infarction. The management of acute malaria depends on the infecting species, the severity of parasitaemia, the pattern of clinical involvement and potential drug resistence.

Acute management

Acute management of cerebral malaria involves supportive care with appropriate attention to ventilation, fluid balance, renal function and seizures. *P. malariae*, *P. ovale*, *P. vivax* and *P. knowlesi* should be treated with a standard course of chloroquine over 48 hours. In severe cases it may be necessary to treat with an intravenous infusion of chloroquine. Primaquine may be added to eradicate the exerythrocytic forms and prevent relapses (Table 9.29).

Because chloroquine resistant *P. falciparum* is widespread, treatment of mild infections is with oral quinine sulfate followed by doxycycline or clindamycin to eradicate remaining asexual forms. Alternatives include mefloquine or co-artemether.

The management of acute malaria requires the provision of intensive care with ventilatory and haemodynamic support as well as treatment of hypoglycaemia, fluids, pyrexia, anaemia, sepsis and thrombotic risk.

Table 9.29 Antimicrobial treatment for malaria.

Plasmodium *P. malariae* *P. ovale* *P. vivax* *P. knowlesi* Chloroquine sensitive *P. falciparum*	Chloroquine and primaquine
Chloroquine resistant *P. falciparum*	Quinine sulfate and tetracycline (alternative to tetracycline is sulfadoxine and pyrimethamine or amiodaquine or doxycycline)
Multi-drug resistant *P. falciparum*	Mefloquine or artesunate or sulfadoxine and pyrimethamine or proguanil and atovaquone
Severe complex multi-drug resistant *P. falciparum* (particularly if mefloquine resistant)	Quinine dihydrochloride or artesunate

There are two major classes of drugs available for parental treatment of severe malaria: the cinchona alkaloids (quinine and quinidine) and the artemisinin derivatives (artesunate, artemether, artemotil). Artesunate, administered intravenously, is the preferred therapy for acute severe falciparum in children and adults. It is given as a high doses of 2.4 mg/kg over 3 days. However, the emergence of artemisinin resistance in South-East Asia is an important concern and monotherapy is now strongly discouraged. An important contribution to the recent success in malaria control has been the widespread use of highly effective artemisinin-based combination therapy. Intravenous quinine or quinidine remains the treatment of choice that areas where artesunate is an available or unreliable. Quinine can also be given by intramuscular injection.

In rural environments, if intravenous treatment cannot be commenced immediately, the patient should be treated with intramuscular quinine or artesunate or rectal artesunate.

The total duration of therapy with quinine/quinidine of the severe malaria is 7 days and for artemisinin-based therapy is 3 days.

Prevention

Although the complete genome of the *Anopheles* mosquito and *P. falciparum* has been sequenced, this has not yet led to new therapy and therefore traditional prophylaxis is still mandatory. Recommendations concerning appropriate prophylaxis vary depending on the characteristics of malaria and drug resistance in particular areas. There is considerable variation in the advice given when travellers are to visit a malarial zone. Meticulous attention to physical prevention with appropriate clothing, mosquito-repellants and nets at night are the most important.

Neurological disorders resulting from HIV

It is now more than 30 years years since the onset of the HIV/AIDS pandemic. Although it was soon apparent that the CNS was frequently involved with opportunistic infections and tumours, it was subsequently recognised that patients developed complications from HIV itself such as dementia, myelopathy, neuropathy and myopathy. With the introduction of HAART (highly active anti-retroviral therapy) in 1997, the incidence of opportunistic infections and tumours, as well as HIV-related complications, have drastically reduced, with a fall in the incidence of opportunistic infections from 13.1 per 1000 in 1996 to 1.0 per 1000 in 2006. This group of patients now present with problems resulting from drug side effects such as neuropathy and a metabolic syndrome that may predispose to cerebrovascular and cardiovascular disease. Newer clinical syndromes now encountered include the phenomena of immune reconstituition inflammatory syndrome (IRIS) and CNS compartmentalisation (with a viraemia in the blood but independent replication of the virus in the CSF which acts as a sanctuary site). There is also concern regarding effective CSF penetration of antiretroviral drugs, CNS drug neurotoxicity and much current research is focused on patients who may continue to decline cognitively despite adequate HIV treatment. In addition, because of greater longevity, patients with HIV are now prone to the same disorders associated with ageing found in the non-infected population.

HIV-1 is a retrovirus (lentivirus) which is single-stranded with a positive sense RNA. It contains reverse transcriptase, which transcribes viral RNA into DNA that is integrated into the host genome. It targets CD4 receptors and infects CD4+ lymphocytes as well as monocytes and macrophages. HIV is neuroinvasive (with invasion occurring early in the course of the infection), neurovirulent (causing a neuropathy, myopathy, myelopathy and encephalopathy) but not particularly neurotropic (capable of infecting nerve cells). The virus is rarely isolated from the neurones of the peripheral or central nervous systems and productive infection is usually found within the associated inflammatory infiltrate, predominantly in macrophages and microglia.

HIV infection can be divided into the following stages:

- Primary acute HIV infection
- Seroconversion
- Chronic latent infection (often associated with generalised lymphadenopathy)
- Early symptomatic HIV infection
- AIDS (CD4 count below 200/mm^3)
- Advanced AIDS infection (CD4 cell count below 50/mm^3).

HIV infection is generally acquired through sexual intercourse, exposure to contaminated blood or perinatal transmission.

Primary acute HIV infection is usually associated with fever, lymphadenopathy, rash, myalgia, arthralgia, headache and mucocutaneous ulceration. In the absence of treatment with HAART, disease progression is highly variable and the mean time to the development of AIDS is 10–11 years with the mean survival after the development of AIDS of 1.3–3.7 years. Up to 25% of patients with symptomatic primary acute HIV infection may develop symptoms or signs of aseptic meningitis or a self-limiting encephalopathy. Acute encephalitis due to HIV-1 and HIV-2 has rarely been reported in seronegative patients as a form of primary infection.

Most patients seroconvert to positive HIV serology 4–10 weeks after exposure but 95% have converted by 6 months. At seroconversion, a glandular fever-like illness occurs in 70% of cases. Seroconversion may be associated with neurological symptoms and signs in 10% – syndromes described include aseptic meningo-encephalitis, acute disseminated encephalomyelitis (ADEM), transverse myelitis, polymyositis, brachial neuritis or a cauda equina syndrome. Guillain–Barré syndrome has also been described at seroconversion and during the asymptomatic phase of HIV infection although the CSF shows a significant pleocytosis in contrast to the findings in HIV-negative patients where CSF examination is usually acellular with a high protein.

During the asymptomatic phase of HIV infection, when there is no evidence of immunosuppression clinically and the CD4 count is above at least 350 cells/mm^3, there are no neurological symptoms or signs. This has been ascertained by a number of large cohort serial studies using clinical, neurophysiological, neuroradiological and neuropsychological methods of assessment. During the clinically latent phase the only abnormal finding may be a persistent generalised lymphadenopathy.

Early symptomatic HIV infection (AIDS related complex, ARC) is associated with a variety of systemic manifestations that are not AIDS defining but occur more frequently and severely in association with HIV infection: thrush, leukoplakia, herpes zoster, peripheral neuropathy, cervical dysplasia, persistent pyrexia and diarrhoea.

Neurological conditions defining AIDS generally occur when the CD4 count falls below 200/mm^3 and include:

- HIV-associated dementia (HAD)
- Opportunistic infection (toxoplasmosis, *Cryptococcus*, CMV or mycobacterium)
- HIV-associated wasting
- Cerebral lymphoma
- Progressive multifocal leukoencephalopathy (PML).

Other AIDS defining conditions include pneumocystitis pneumonia, oesophageal candidiasis, cervical carcinoma, Kaposi's sarcoma, mycobacterial infection, CMV, toxoplasmosis, histoplasmosis and lymphoma. Advanced AIDS is considered to be present if the CD4 count falls below 50/mm^3.

Some patients exhibit remarkable clinical stability and remain asymptomatic over many years without antiretroviral therapy (long-term non-progressors). Elite controllers are HIV seropositive individuals who have no evidence of viraemia and maintain a high CD4 count.

Prior to the introduction of HAART, in up to 5% of cases HAD was the AIDS defining diagnosis. HIV infection should therefore be considered in the differential diagnosis in any young patient presenting with cognitive impairment. HIV-associated psychosis develops suddenly without a prodrome. There may be delusions, hallucinations and mood swings. When psychosis occurs in patients with HAD, it is characterised by prominent agitation, irritability and delusions (AIDS mania). HIV infection may be associated with a vasculitis or a thrombophilic state with anticardiolipin antibody and lupus anticoagulant and therefore enters the differential diagnosis of young stroke.

The timing of initiating HAART may be critical to the management of opportunistic infection for which no effective treatment is available (e.g. PML). HAART carries a significant risk of complications including drug intolerance, toxic effects and immune reconstitution inflammatory syndrome. Failure of HAART may be because of viral resistance, drug toxicity or poor compliance (which may be a result of cognitive impairment).

Basic principles of neuroAIDS

- As a result of immunosuppression, the clinical presentations may be atypical. For example, only one-third of patients with cryptococcal meningitis develop classic features of meningism. A low threshold for investigation with CT and/or MRI and lumbar puncture is necessary.
- Each area of the neuro-axis in an HIV infected individual may be affected by multiple different aetiological agents. For example, a patient may have a mass lesion in the brain resulting from toxoplasmosis, a concurrent HIV-related myelopathy and a drug-induced neuropathy.
- Dual infections are relatively common and this possibility must be borne in mind when assessing a treatment response. For example, patients may have meningitis resulting from *C. neoformans* and *M. tuberculosis*.
- CSF examination may be abnormal as a consequence of HIV infection alone even in the asymptomatic immunocompetent stages. These include a mild lymphocytic pleocytosis, an elevated CSF protein and oligoclonal bands. Conversely, as a result of HIV-induced immunosuppression, patients with meningitis or encephalitis may have normal CSF indices. The diagnosis of neurological disorders therefore relies on specific tests on the CSF such as the detection of cryptococcal antigen (by latex agglutination – CRAG), culture or using PCR techniques.
- Serological studies (e.g. in toxoplasmosis) are unhelpful in making a diagnosis as used in immunocompetent cases as there is no diagnostic fourfold rise in IgM and IgG titres.
- In patients who have not received HAART, the CD4 count is a useful guide in attempting to determine the specific aetiologies of opportunistic infections and tumours:
  - CD4 >500 cells/mm^3 – seroconversion manifestations include Guillain–Barré syndrome, myopathy and aseptic meningitis
  - CD4 <350 cells/mm^3 – complications resulting from *M. tuberculosis*
  - CD4 <200 cells/mm^3 – opportunistic infections (toxoplamosis, cryptococcal meningitis, HSV and *Mycobacterium*) PML, peripheral neuropathy, vacuolar myopathy, cerebral lymphoma and HAD
  - CD4 <50 cells/mm^3 – disseminated CMV retinitis, encephalitis and polyradiculopathy and cerebral lymphoma.

In HAART exposed patients, these guidelines are less robust because even if there is a rise in the CD4 count, these lymphocytes may not be fully competent as some antigen-specific clones will have been lost.

The major neurological complications of HIV-1 infection are summarised in Table 9.30.

Table 9.30 Major neurological complications in HIV-1 infection.

Opportunistic infections	*Toxoplasma gondii* – abscesses, encephalitis *Cryptococcus neoformans* – meningitis, cryptococcoma *Mycobacterium tuberculosis* – meningitis, abscesses, tuberculoma, myeloradiculopathy *Mycobacterium avium, M. kansasii* *CMV* – encephalitis, retinitis, lumbosacral polyradiculopathy, vasculitic neuropathy *JC virus* – PML *Varicella zoster virus* – encephalitis, CNS vasculitis, myelitis *Herpes simplex virus* – encephalitis, myelitis
Tumours	Primary CNS lymphoma (EBV-related) Metastatic systemic lymphoma
Caused by HIV	Peripheral neuropathy Distal sensory peripheral neuropathy Inflammatory demyelinating neuropathy (GBS and CIDP) Vasculitic neuropathy Diffuse inflammatory lymphocytosis syndrome HIV associated dementia Vacuolar myelopathy HIV polymyositis
Cerebrovascular disease	HIV associated thrombophilia Cardioembolic – endocarditis, infectious and marantic Vasculitis – HIV associated, infectious (varicella zoster)
Drug-related complications	Peripheral neuropathy Drugs (ddC, ddI, d4T) Other drugs (thalidomide, isoniazid, dapsone) Myopathy (AZT)
Immune reconstitution	Immune reconstitution inflammatory syndrome – related to JC virus (PML), MTb, cryptococcus, CMV, HIV

CIDP, chronic inflammatory demyelinating polyradiculoneuropathy; CMV, cytomegalovirus; EBV, Epstein–Barr virus; GBS, Guillain–Barré syndrome; JC, Japanese encephalitis; MTb, *Mycobacterium tuberculosis*; PML, progressive multifocal leukoencephalopathy.

Opportunistic infections in HIV

Toxoplasma gondii

Toxoplasmosis is the most common opportunistic infection but there has been a decline in the incidence. It occurs as a consequence of reactivation of the disease after prior infection. Human infection occurs as a result of ingestion of oocytes in cat faeces and the ingestion of tissue cysts in undercooked meat. Variations in dietary habits explain the differing seroprevalence rates worldwide – 90% in French adults compared with 50% in the United Kingdom. Symptomatic toxoplasmosis is usually caused by reactivation of latent infection which persists in the brain and muscle in immunosuppressed individuals. The risk of an HIV-infected patient who is seropositive for IgG *T. gondii* antibody developing toxoplasmosis is around 25%.

Toxoplasmosis is the most common cause of mass lesions in the CNS of HIV patients even in developing countries where tuberculosis is rife. Reactivation occurs when the CD4 count drops to 100–200 cells/mm^3 and the CD4 T cells are unable to suppress the latent infection. The clinical presentation is with headache, fever, confusion and/or seizures in association with hemiplegia, dysphasia and visual field defects. Other clinical features include a variety of movement disorders (choreoathetosis, dystonia and hemiparkinsonism); psychiatric illness such as depression and personality change resulting from frontal lobe pathology; brainstem syndromes and, rarely, a rapidly progressive diffuse encephalitis. Rarely, the spinal cord may be involved with a myelitis or a cauda equina syndrome.

On imaging studies, preferably MRI, *Toxoplasma* lesions have a predeliction for the grey–white interface of the frontal or parietal lobes and the basal ganglia and thalamus (Figure 9.13). There is normally mass effect with surrounding oedema with patchy ring enhancement. A single lesion or peri-ventricular lesions are more likely to be caused by primary CNS lymphoma, the main differential diagnosis that occurs with a similar clinical presentation and at similar low CD4 counts.

Although negative blood serology makes the diagnosis less likely, this may still occur in up to 17% of cases. These cases are a result of impaired antibody synthesis with increasing immunosuppression and only occasionally caused by primary infection. It is useful therefore to document *Toxoplasma* serology at the time of HIV diagnosis. IgG antibodies to *T. gondii* may be present in the serum and PCR can be undertaken on the CSF although the sensitivity is only 50%. A definitive diagnosis of *Toxoplasma* encephalitis can only be made by brain biopsy. With increasing experience and pragmatism, it is now standard practice to treat any HIV-infected individual with a low CD4 count and mass lesions on imaging with anti-*Toxoplasma* therapy. A response, clinically and radiologically, confirms the diagnosis.

The treatment is with combined pyrimethamine, folinic acid and sulfadiazine or co-trimoxazole for 6 weeks' induction and then maintenance treatment until the CD4 count is above 200 for at least 6 months (Table 9.31).

Response to treatment is seen in 90% of patients by the second week of treatment. It is important to re-image even if there is clinical improvement because it is not rare for some lesions to improve and others, such as those due to *M. tuberculosis*, to enlarge making it necessary to consider biopsy. The radiological improvement generally lags behind the clinical improvement.

Patients who are HIV infected and who are seropositive for IgG against *T. gondii* should be offered primary prophylaxis with 980 mg co-trimoxazole (trimethoprim and sulfamethoxazole) when the CD4 count drops below 200 cells/mm^3. This also offers protection against *Pneumocystis jirovecii*.

Table 9.31 Treatment of toxoplasmosis in HIV positive patients.

Acute phase (for 6 weeks)
First line therapy
Pyrimethamine (100 mg po for 3 days, then 75 mg/day) and sulfadiazine 6–8 g/day po/IV (or clindamycin 600–900 mg/day po/IV) and folinic acid 15 mg/day
(Side effects: pyrimethamine – marrow suppression; sulfadiazine – rash, nephrotoxicity, marrow suppression; clindamycin – rash, diarrhoea)
Maintenance treatment
Pyrimethamine 25–50 mg/day and sulfadiazine 2– g/day or clindamycin 600 mg/day and folinic acid 10 mg/day

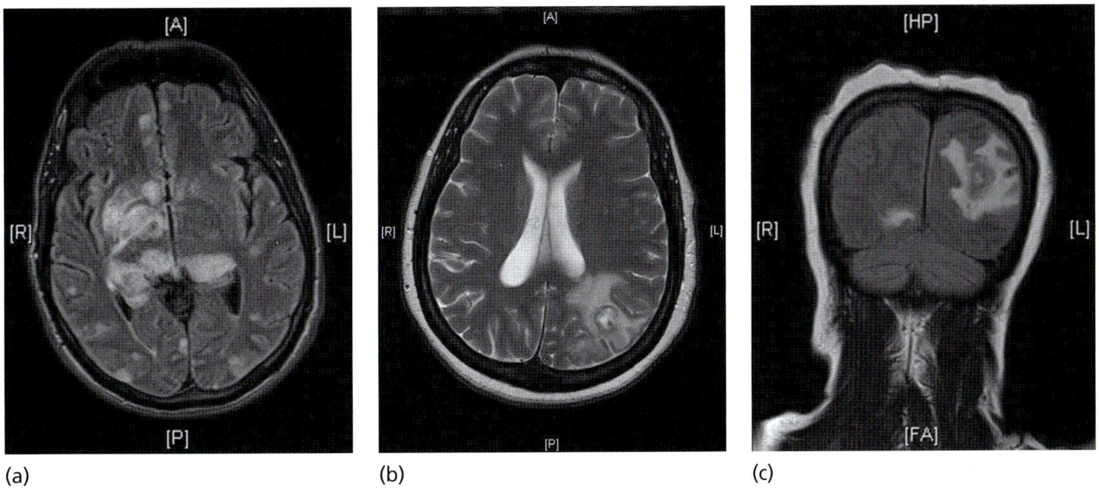

Figure 9.13 Cerebral toxoplasmosis in HIV: (a) FLAIR axial, (b) T2 axial and (c) FLAIR coronal MRI.

Tuberculous meningitis and brain abscess

The issues relating to tuberculous infection of the CNS in AIDS are a similar to those in that non-AIDS patients considered earlier in the chapter. The WHO estimate that one-third of the world population has latent *M. tuberculosis* and co-infection with HIV increases the risk of dissemination and tuberculous meningitis.

Clinical presentation of TBM is with fever, change in mental state, headache, seizures, cranial nerve or focal limb deficit. The CT may show hydrocephalus, tuberculomas, abscess or haemorrhage and in approximately 50% there is basilar enhancement. MRI may confirm the presence of a mass lesion and define exudates and vasculitis (with or without infarction) particularly affecting infratentorial regions and the basal ganglia. There may be infarcts secondary to vasculitis. The CSF shows a lymphocytosis with elevated protein levels and reduced glucose. AFB may be seen and *M. tuberculosis* may be cultured. The CSF TB PCR increases total sensitivity to 80% but as a stand alone test is less sensitive than culture. It is important to ensure that large volumes of CSF (at least 10 mL) are taken at repeated lumber puncture.

The diagnosis may be difficult because the sensitivity of standard detection of AFB, culture and even PCR is only approximately 50% although it may be higher in HIV because of the higher infective load and incomplete immune response. Other investigations including tuberculin skin test and interferon gamma release assays (e.g. Quantiferon, TB Gold) may increase sensitivity although they do not discriminate between latent and active infection. Occasionally, it may be necessary to resort to a brain biopsy to confirm the diagnosis.

The treatment is as previously described but the mortality rate is >50% which is double the rate occurring in non-HIV patients. Multi-resistant TB is seen in approximately 3% of cases worldwide and this may include resistance to isoniazid, rifampicin and fluoroquinolones.

Mycobacterium avium complex refers to infections caused by non-tuberculous *Mycobacterium* species. They may cause localised lymphadenopathy or disseminated infection involving the respiratory or gastrointestinal tract and occasionally cause localised abscess.

Cryptococcal meningitis

C. neoformans is ubiquitous in the environment and is commonly found in the soil and in the excreta of pigeons. Exposure occurs by inhalation of spores leading to primary pulmonary infection followed by secondary dissemination following reactivation of latent infection in an immune-compromised host with haematogenous spread to the meninges.

In patients infected with HIV, meningitis caused by *C. neoformans* occurs in 10% of patients with advanced HIV disease, usually when the CD4 count falls below 50 cells/mm^3. The incidence has fallen significantly since the introduction of HAART.

The clinical presentation is usually with headache which initially may be mild, fever and drowsiness. Only 30% of individuals present with features of meningism: photophobia, neck stiffness and a positive Kernig's sign. There may be communicating hydrocephalus in 15% because of impaired resorption of CSF by arachnoid villi leading to headache, vomiting, visual impairment and VIth nerve palsy. Multiple cranial nerve palsies may occur secondary to basal meningitis.

In 20% of cases there may be extraneurological involvement with diffuse pulmonary infiltrates, lobar consolidation or cavitating lesions on chest X-ray, skin lesions (small papules which resemble molluscum contagiosum) and infection of the urinary tract.

Table 9.32 Treatment of cryptococcal infection in HIV positive patient.

Acute phase therapy for 4–6 weeks or until CSF culture negative
Amphotericin B 0.7–1.0 mg/kg/day (via central line) and flucytosine 100–150 mg/kg/day p.o.
In milder cases Fluconazole 400 mg IV/p.o. for 8 weeks
Maintenance treatment
Fluconazole 200–400 mg/day p.o.
(Side effects: amphotericin B – nephrotoxicity, anaemia, hepatitis; flucytosine – marrow suppression; fluconazole – rash, hepatitis). Liposomal amphotericin B is associated with a lower risk of renal toxic effects but is more expensive

Brain imaging may be normal or may reveal hydrocephalus, cryptococcomas which are dilated Virchow–Robin spaces filled with the fungal organisms, and basal meningeal enhancement. Measurement of the serum cryptococcal antigen is a useful screening test in those with mild symptoms and, if positive, necessitates imaging and CSF examination. At lumbar puncture, CSF pressure is frequently elevated. In most cases there is a moderate mononuclear pleocytosis, elevated protein and a low glucose; however, in 25%, the CSF maybe normal. The diagnosis is established by the identification of India ink positive hypae in 75% and the detection of cryptococcal antigen in 95% of cases. A number of poor prognostic markers have been identified:

- CSF opening pressure >25 cm CSF
- Altered mental status
- CSF cryptococcal antigen titre >1 : 1024
- CSF white cell count <20 cells/mm^3
- Hyponatraemia.

Amphotericin B with or without flucytosine is the treatment of choice, but in patients with mild disease without any of the poor prognostic markers fluconazole maybe considered (as long a *C. gattii* has been excluded). Acute treatment should be continued until the CSF culture is sterile which may take 4–6 weeks, following this, secondary prophylaxis should continue with fluconazole (Table 9.32). HAART should be commenced on complete recovery if the patient was not already receiving this. However, if HAART is started too soon there is a risk of developing IRIS.

Raised intracranial pressure, unrelated to hydrocephalus, should be managed aggressively, as it may result in visual loss, by repeated lumbar puncture with high volume CSF removal and, if required, by the placement of a lumbar or ventricular drain. Acetazolamide may also be used as an adjunct.

Cytomegalovirus infection

CMV infections of the nervous system occur when the CD4 counts are very low (usually below 50 cells/mm^3). It is due to reactivation and is usually associated with CMV disease elsewhere in the body.

- CMV encephalitis presents with a rapidly evolving encephalopathy with headache, fever, seizures, change in mental state or cranial neuropathy. There may be hyponatraemia due to adrenal involvement and a brainstem syndrome (retinitis often coexists). Imaging studies have shown a range of abnormalities including a periventriculitis with progressive ventricular enlargement, periventricular enhancement and increased peri-ventricular signal or widely distributed multi-focal, non-enhancing hypodense lesions

Table 9.33 Treatment of CNS CMV infection in HIV.

Acute phase therapy	
Ganciclovir 5 mg/kg every 12 hours for 14–21 days	
or	
Foscarnet 60 mg/kg 8-hourly for 14–21 days	
Maintenance treatment*	
Ganciclovir 5 mg/kg every 24 hours	
or	
Foscarnet 90–120 mg/kg/day	
(Side effects: ganciclovir – anaemia, leukopenia, thrombocytopenia; foscarnet – renal failure, leukopenia)	

* Consider stopping maintenance treatment if after HAART is started the CD4 remains >200 cells/mm^3 for >6 months.

in the cortex, brainstem and basal ganglia, resembling PML and, rarely, single or multiple ring-enhancing mass lesions with oedema and mass effect.

- CMV retinitis presents with floaters, loss of peripheral vision and central scotoma leading to haemorrhagic infarction, vascular sheathing and retinal opacification. Visual loss is a result of retinal necrosis which may be associated with macular oedema or retinal detachment. Prior to HAART, CMV retinitis was the most common cause of blindness in this group of patients. Typically, patients present with painless visual loss. Fundoscopy shows extensive haemorrhage and necrosis described as a 'ketchup and cheese' appearance.
- CMV lumbosacral polyradiculopathy presents subacutely with back pain and progressive weakness of the legs with sphincter involvement. Radiculomyelitis affecting the lumbosacral area can present with rapidly progressive cauda equina syndrome. The differential diagnosis includes Guillain–Barré syndrome. Imaging studies may be normal or show thickened nerve roots. CSF examination, which is essential to exclude other causes of a polyradiculopathy such as syphilis and lymphomatous infiltration, shows a polymorphonuclear pleocytosis which is unusual in a viral infection, an elevated protein and low glucose. CMV DNA can be isolated from the CSF by PCR. CMV has also been associated with a mononeuritis multiplex, usually in the context of CMV elsewhere such as a retinitis. The diagnosis is confirmed by sural or superficial peroneal nerve biopsy.
- The preferred treatment for CMV is either ganciclovir (or oral valganciclovir, the prodrug) or foscarnet. Cidofovir has also been used (Table 9.33).

Herpes simplex virus

Herpes simplex virus type 1 (HSV-1) is generally acquired in early life and remains latent in sensory ganglia while HSV type 2 is acquired via contact with infected mucosal surfaces. HSV-1 causes necrotising encephalitis which is usually acute but may evolve over weeks. Onset is with fever, headache, vomiting and seizures. There may be disorientation, memory loss, confusion and personality change. Herpes simplex type 2 (HSV-2) is associated with a diffuse meningo-encephalitis often affecting the brainstem and rarely causes a rapidly progressive myelitis in those presenting with back pain, progressive leg weakness and sphincter disturbance.

CSF PCR is both sensitive and specific for viral DNA but may be negative in the first 72 hours. MRI shows high signal change on T2W imaging in the inferior temporal lobe but this may spread to involve the parenchyma, cerebellum and diencephalon. In HSV-2 myelitis, MRI shows an oedematous cord.

Treatment is with aciclovir 10 mg/kg three times daily IV over 21 days. If there is a failure to respond or aciclovir resistance ganciclovir or foscarnet are alternatives.

Varicella-zoster virus

Although dermatomal zoster (shingles) is common in the HIV population, occasionally patients may progress to a severe myeloradiculopathy. Following zoster involving the trigeminal nerves, VZV involvement of the small cerebral vessels can cause granulomatous angiitis. The clinical presentation is with headache, progressive focal neurological deficits and seizures. MRI shows multiple abnormalities on T2W images. The CSF is diagnostic with the identification of viral DNA by PCR. Treatment is with high-dose aciclovir and corticosteroids.

Progressive multifocal leukoencephalopathy

Progressive multifocal leukoencephalopathy (PML) is caused by the reactivation of the JC virus (JC; the initials of the patient from whom the virus was first isolated), a common polyoma DNA virus, which infects 75% of the general population. As the virus is frequently excreted in the urine of healthy individuals, primary infection is postulated to occur via the urine–oral route. Primary JC virus infection is asymptomatic and the virus remains permanently in the kidneys, bone marrow and lymphoid tissue.

Because impaired cell-mediated immunity is the major predisposing factor for the development of PML, prior to the AIDS epidemic, the condition was occasionally encountered in patients with lymphoproliferative disorders, sarcoidosis and those treated with immunosuppressive drugs (e.g. after transplant operations and systemic lupus erythematosus, SLE). A marked increase in the incidence of PML is reported in patients treated with monoclonal antibodies (natalazumab, rituximab, efalizumab, alemtuzumab). HIV-induced immunosuppression currently accounts for 85% of cases of PML. Prior to HAART, 5% of AIDS patients developed PML with CD4 counts usually below 100/mm^3. However, after the introduction of HAART, PML has remained more prevalent than expected and this may be related to increased activation of JC virus by the HIV proteins. The underlying pathology results from replication of the virus within the oligodendrocytes and astrocytes causing lysis and demyelination. It is unclear whether PML results from reactivation of the virus in the CNS following immunosuppression or if it is a result of invasion of the CNS by infected lymphocytes from the peripheral circulation (30% shed the virus in the urine).

The clinical presentation is with a progressive subacute focal deficit which includes hemiparesis, hemianopia or ataxia. Cognitive dysfunction is usually associated with focal neurological signs. Lesions adjacent to the cortex may occasionally result in dysphasia and seizures. Optic nerve involvement occurs rarely but spinal cord involvement does not seem to occur. In contrast to other more common causes of focal lesions found in HIV infected patients such as toxoplasmosis, there are usually no symptoms or signs of systemic infection or raised intracranial pressure. A cerebellar syndrome with isolated cerebellar atrophy on MRI scans may occur, pathological studies show JC virus infection of the granular cells (JC virus granule cell neuronopathy).

Cranial CT shows low attenuation lesions. MRI shows large single or multiple lesions involving white matter, with scalloping at the grey–white interface; the parieto-occipital and frontal lobes are most commonly affected. The affected areas are low signal on

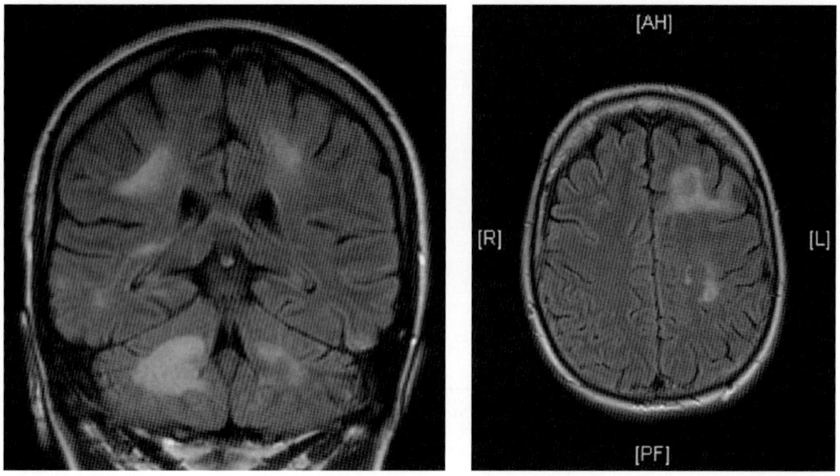

(a) (b)

Figure 9.14 Progressive multifocal leukoencephalopathy: FLAIR coronal and axial images demonstrating multiple regions of white matter hyperintensity both supratentorially and within the posterior fossa.

T1-weighted images and hyperintense on T2-weighted sequences. This may help distinguish PML from HIV dementia. There is no mass effect but contrast enhancement may be seen and has been identified as a good prognostic marker (Figure 19.14).

Early in the AIDS epidemic the diagnosis was only possible by brain biopsy showing the histological demonstration of demyelination, enlarged oligodendrocyte nuclei with JC virus inclusion particles and bizarre enlarged astrocytes. Prior to the HAART era, JC virus DNA could be isolated from the CSF by PCR with a sensitivity of 75% and a specificity of 99%. Since HAART, the sensitivity seems to have dropped to 58% perhaps because of decreased viral replication. The yield can be increased to 85% with repeated CSF examination in PCR negative cases but stereotactic brain biopsy may be necessary.

The treatment of PML in patients with HIV is two-pronged: reversing the underlying immunosuppression with HAART and specific anti-JC virus therapy. Institution of the former has resulted in fourfold improvement in survival, with some patients' neurological status stabilising or improving. A number of drugs such as cytosine arabinoside (araC) given intravenously or intrathecally, alpha interferon and cidofivir have anti-JC virus activity but have not been shown to be of clear benefit. Anecdotal reports have suggested benefit with mirtazipine and mefloquine but more data are required.

Primary CNS lymphoma

Primary CNS lymphoma (PCNSL) is the second most common cause of mass lesions in adults and the most common in children with AIDS although the incidence has fallen with the introduction of HAART. The incidence of PCNSL in HIV-infected patients is approximately 5%, compared to 1% of the general population, and it accounts for approximately 15% of all non-Hodgkin lymphoma (NHL). Histologically, PCNSL is a high grade, NHL diffuse, large B-cell lymphoma (Chapter 21), less commonly Burkitt's lymphoma may occur and also, rarely, T-cell lymphoma is seen. The Epstein–Barr virus is causally linked to PCNSL, with the identification of the viral DNA incorporated into that of the neoplastic cells. It usually occurs in patients with more advanced HIV infection and a CD4 count usually <100/mm^3 and a high viral load with plasma HIV RNA levels >100 000 copies/mL.

The common presenting symptoms are non-specific with headache, focal neurological deficits, cognitive change, altered level of consciousness and seizures. PCNSL remains confined to the central nervous system, but within this space leptomeningeal spread to all compartments including the spinal cord and the anterior chamber of the eye may occur.

Imaging shows single or multifocal enhancing mass lesions, with surrounding oedema, which are predominantly supratentorial and may spread into the white-matter tracts (Figure 9.15). It characteristically involves the corpus callosum, periventricular and periependymal areas. PCNSL is more likely to present with a single lesion than toxoplasmosis and is also more likely to invade the ventricular walls and exert mass effect. Whole body imaging is indicated to exclude systemic lymphoma. Studies using thallium-201 single photon emission computed tomography (SPECT) suggest that it may be possible to differentiate between an abscess and a tumour with the former having little uptake compared with high uptake of the mitotically active lymphoma. CSF analysis is usually not performed because of raised intracranial pressure but when possible the identification of EBV by PCR is useful diagnostically with a sensitivity of 50–100% and a specificity of 94%.

The diagnosis often depends on the exclusion of other causes of mass lesions (toxoplasmosis, PML, other infective lesions or tumours). There is no effective therapy for PCNSL and most patients succumb within 2–3 months. Radiotherapy may increase survival times by a few months. However, recent data suggest that treatment with HAART can also improve survival times.

A scheme for the diagnosis and management of HIV presenting with focal neurology and CD4 <200 cells/mm^3 is presented in Figure 9.16.

Neurological complications resulting directly from HIV

HIV enters the CNS early in the course of infection. The evidence for this includes the neurological seroconversion illness, the presence of CSF abnormalities in asymptomatic immunocompetent individuals and the presence of HIV DNA in brain pathological studies of asymptomatic HIV-infected patients who died from other causes. In one case of iatrogenic HIV transmission caused by a blood product given intravenously, the patient died 15 days after

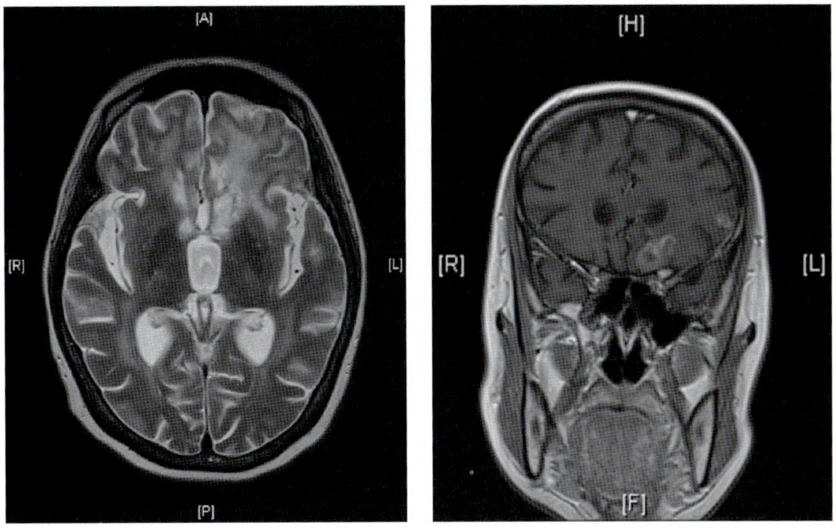

(a) (b)

Figure 9.15 High grade primary CNS lymphoma in a patient with HIV: (a) T2 axial; (b) T1 enhanced coronal MRI.

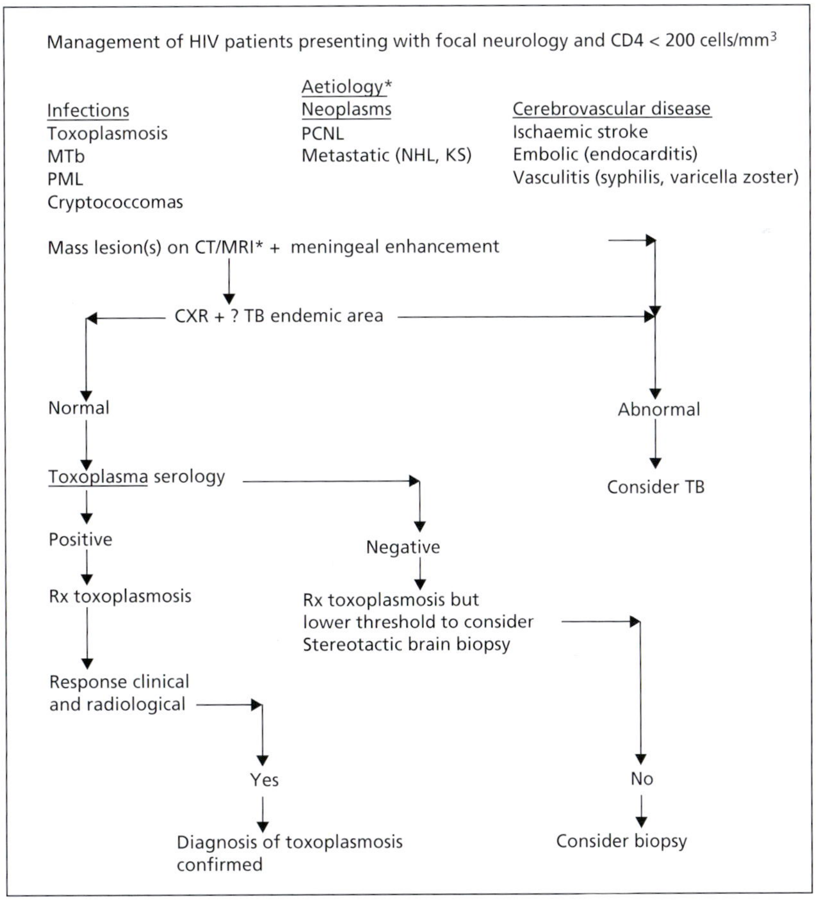

Figure 9.16 Management of HIV patients presenting with focal neurology and CD4 <200 cells/mm^3. CT, computed tomography; CXR, chest X-ray; KS, Kaposi's sarcoma; MRI, magnetic resonance imaging; MTb, *Mycobacterium tuberculosis*; NHL, non-Hodgkin's lymphoma; PCNL, primary CNS lymphoma; PML, progressive multifocal leukoencephalopathy.

the accident from an unrelated cause. HIV DNA was identified in the brain on day 14.

The mechanism of viral entry into the CNS remains controversial because the blood–brain barrier is an effective physical and metabolic barrier. The most accepted current theory is the Trojan horse mechanism, which proposes that HIV viral entry through the blood–brain barrier occurs via infected macrophages from the peripheral circulation. The choroid plexus, which resides outside the blood–brain barrier, is another potential site of viral entry because the choroid capillary endothelial cells are freely permeable with the stromal cells containing monocytes and macrophages.

Within the brain, neurones and oligodendrocytes are resistant to direct invasion by HIV and infection is localised primarily within the microglial cells and macrophages which are derived from peripheral blood monocytes. HIV does not infect neuronal cells even though neuronal cell death is an important aspect of the neuropathology of HIV dementia. There is some evidence suggesting a low level of astrocyte infection; this may be important because the astrocytic foot processes are an integral part of the blood–brain barrier and a low level of infection may be enough to disrupt functioning of the tight junctions between the endothelial cells. Neuronal damage is usually caused by viral proteins or as a result of chronic inflammation. Although demyelination is also a feature of HIV brain disease, infection of the oligodendrocytes has rarely been reported.

The neurovirulence of HIV occurs later in the course of the disease when immunosuppression develops and HIV acts like an opportunistic infection. It remains uncertain if this is a result of activation of the virus seeded in the nervous system early in the course of disease or trafficking of new HIV viral species from the peripheral circulation, or both. There is no doubt that since the introduction of HAART the incidence of HIV dementia has reduced, suggesting that suppression of HIV in the peripheral circulation has a crucial role.

HIV-associated neurocognitive disorders

HIV infection is associated with a hierarchy of progressively more severe cognitive dysfunction (HAND). It may be classified as:

- Asymptomatic neurocognitive impairment (ANI)
- HIV-1 associated mild neurocognitive disorder (MND)
- HAD, also called AIDS dementia complex (ADC) or HIV encephalopathy (HIVE).

Because neuronal cells are rarely infected, HAND probably results from the release of inflammatory cytokines such as tumour necrosis factor, quinolinic acid and platelet-activating factor by activated macrophages and microglia as well as toxic viral proteins such as Gp41 and Tat. These neurotoxins affect developing and mature nervous tissue leading to degeneration of synaptic function and contributing to neuronal cell death.

The pathological feature HIVE usually occurs at the grey–white interface, suggesting haematogenous dissemination. The hallmark for HIVE is the presence of microglial nodules which are a fusion of HIV infected and non-infected macrophages. Most infection is demonstrated in the basal ganglia, the brainstem and the deep white matter areas. Other pathological features include a leukoencephalopathy and areas of neuronal cell loss, especially in the hippocampal areas and the frontal and temporal lobes.

In the early stages the clinical features of HAND may be mild, with symptoms of poor concentration, mental slowing and apathy, which may mimic a depressive disorder. Later, as the syndrome progresses, more specific cognitive changes with memory loss and personality change develop. These occur in association with motor changes such as impaired dexterity and gait problems which result from the associated vacuolar myelopathy and peripheral neuropathy. Examination may show impaired pursuit and saccadic eye movements, generalised hyperreflexia, cerebellar and frontal release signs. HIV-associated psychosis develops suddenly without a prodrome. There may be delusions, hallucinations and mood swings. When psychosis occurs in patients with HAD, it is characterised by prominent agitation, irritability and delusions (AIDS mania).

HAD is a subcortical dementia which occurred in 15% of AIDS patients prior to the introduction of HAART but the incidence has now been reduced by 50%, although the incidence of ANI and MND are probably unchanged or may have increased slightly. Risk factors for the development of HAD include:

- Nadir CD4 count
- Increasing age
- Systemic symptoms, anaemia, low body mass index
- Substance abuse
- Co-infection with other viruses (e.g. hepatitis C)
- Host genetic factors (e.g E4 isoform of apolipoprotein E, polymorphisms in the TNF alpha promoter and *CCR2* genes)
- Viral clade subtypes.

Investigations are indicated to exclude other causes – MRI typically shows evidence of atrophy with diffuse white matter changes on T2-weighted images. The CSF shows non-specific cytochemical abnormalities but must be examined to exclude conditions such as neurosyphilis, CMV and PML. The CSF viral load correlates with severity of dementia but is not sensitive enough for diagnostic purposes. Formal neuropsychological assessments typically reveal abnormalities in the following cognitive domains: psychomotor speed, attention, frontal lobe function and verbal and non-verbal memory.

In patients with cognitive impairment, especially if progressive, it is prudent to first optimise the antiretroviral therapy to render the blood aviraemic. In patients who have an undetectable viral load in the blood, a CSF viral load should be checked in case of the compartmentalisation syndrome and changes made to the antiretroviral treatment using more CSF penetrating drugs.

Pre-HAART, the mean survival rate for patients with HAD was 12 months. With the introduction of HAART, some patients may improve implying some degree of reversibility, some remain static (perhaps because of burnt out brain damage) and some with virological failure may continue to deteriorate. A minority of patients with evidence of viral suppression in the peripheral circulation may continue to deteriorate as a result of 'compartmentalisation' with a high viral load in the CSF which will necessitate a change in HAART regimen. There is concern regarding the ability of the currently available antiretroviral drugs to penetrate the blood–brain barrier. The CNS penetration effectiveness (CPE) score has been proposed as a numeric tool to evaluate CNS penetration. The system is arbitrary in that scoring is based upon publications incorporating available pharmacokinetic data, results of clinical studies and drug properties. Although the CPE has been criticised it nevertheless represents an attempt at rationalisation of drug regimens in patients with HAND.

HIV-related vacuolar myelopathy

Clinically significant vacuolar myelopathy affects up to 10% of patients with AIDS, usually in patients who also have HAD. The condition is characterised by a slowly progressive spastic paraparesis, sphincter disturbance and a sensory ataxia resulting from posterior column involvement. There is no sensory level. Pathological specimens demonstrate a vacuolar degeneration of the white matter within the thoracic spinal cord similar to that seen in subacute degeneration of the cord resulting from vitamin B_{12} deficency. Although B_{12} levels are usually normal, it is possible that a methylation defect is responsible because *S*-adenosylmethionine is reduced in the CSF of patients with vacuolar myelopathy. This degeneration is not specific to AIDS and has been described in other immunodeficient states and malignancy. As with the other complications of HIV, significant productive HIV infection is not found. However, there is evidence of macrophage activation and increased levels of cytokines. MRI shows increased signal in the white matter tracts on T2 images or may be normal. CSF examination is necessary to exclude viral myelitis resulting from herpes zoster, herpes simplex and CMV although these myelitides tend to be much more acute. Co-infection with HTLV-1, which has a similar mode of transmission to HIV, merits consideration. There is no specific treatment apart from HAART. A small study using 3 g methionine showed some limited benefit but results of larger studies are awaited.

HIV-related neuropathy

The most common peripheral nerve disorder encountered in association with HIV is distal sensory peripheral neuropathy (DSPN) (Table 9.34). The prevalence rate pre-HAART was estimated at 35% and at necropsy 95% of patients had sural nerve pathological abnormalities. The underlying pathology in DSPN is one of a dying back axonopathy with secondary demyelination. Increased numbers of macrophages are found in the dorsal root ganglia and within the peripheral nerves. HIV RNA is rarely detected in the peripheral nerves and the pathophysiological mechanisms for the development of DSPN are the same as those for HAD (i.e. neurotoxicity of viral proteins such as Gp 120 and tat) as well as a bystander effect of neurotoxic cytokines released by activated macrophages.

Risk factors for the development of DSPN include age, higher viral load and lower CD4 counts. Patients with other risk factors for neuropathy such as diabetes, excess alcohol intake and genetic neuropathies are more vulnerable. The presentation is with 'painful, burning, numb feet'. Patients also complain of paraesthesiae, dysaesthesiae and allodynia but the upper limbs are rarely involved. Examination may reveal limited weakness, often confined to the intrinsic foot muscles. The reflexes may be normal, depressed or absent. There is characteristically impaired sensation to pain and temperature but subsequently other modalities are involved. Nerve conduction tests (NCTs) may be normal or show mild axonal abnormalities. Thermal thresholds are abnormal indicating small fibre involvement. Punch skin biopsies with the assessment of epidermal nerve fibre densities are increasingly being utilised in diagnosis and treatment trials of DSPN. In atypical cases where, for example, there is more extensive weakness with foot drop or significant upper limb involvement clinically or on NCTs, CSF examination and nerve biopsy should be considered to exclude vasculitis, demyelinating neuropathies and lymphomatous infiltration.

Table 9.34 Peripheral nerve complications in HIV infection.

HIV related	Axonal neuropathy (DSPN) Demyelinating neuropathy (GBS and CIDP) Vasculitic neuropathy Diffuse inflammatory lymphocytic syndrome Mononeuritis multiplex Lower motor neurone syndrome (resembling MND)
CMV related	Lumbosacral polyradiculopathy Vasculitic neuropathy
Drugs	Antiretroviral drugs (ddI, ddC, D4T) Isoniazid (treatment of TB) Thalidomide (treatment of mouth ulcers) Dapsone (treatment and prophylaxis of toxoplasmosis and *Pneumocyctis jirovecii*) Vincristine and vinblastine (treatment of KS and lymphoma) Paclitaxel (Taxol) (treatment of KS)
Others	Syphilis (polyradiculopathy) Metastatic NHL Dorsal root ganglionitis Autonomic neuropathy

CIDP, chronic inflammatory demyelinating polyradiculoneuropathy; DSPN, distal sensory peripheral neuropathy; GBS, Guillain–Barré syndrome; KS, Kaposi's sarcoma; MND, motor neurone disease; NHL, non-Hodgkin's lymphoma; TB, tuberculosis.

The treatment of DSPN is symptomatic – only lamotrigine and recombinant human nerve growth factor have been shown to be effective in relieving the pain of DSPN in randomised placebo controlled trials. Gabapentin, although often used, has only been shown to be effective in small trials. Amitriptyline, although not proven to be effective in placebo controlled trials, has a role in individual patients starting at low doses. Mexiletine, acupuncture and topical capsaicin have not shown benefit.

A form of mononeuritis multiplex may occur either as an early and mild self-limiting condition with CD4>200 cells/mm^3 or in association with severe immunosuppression and CMV infection. There may be multifocal cranial nerve or limb involvement. Neurophysiology studies confirm a patchy axonal neuropathy and nerve biopsy shows an endoneurial or epineurial perivascular inflammatory infiltrate with axonal degeneration. The neuropathy may respond to treatment with corticosteroids.

Diffuse inflammatory lymphocytosis syndrome

Some patients respond to HIV infection by developing diffuse inflammatory lymphocytosis syndrome (DILS), a syndrome characterised by a persistent circulating CD8 lymphocytosis with visceral lymphocytic infiltration particularly affecting the salivary glands. This multisystem disorder resembles Sjögren's syndrome, although anti-Ro/SS-A and anti-La/SS-B antibodies are absent. Patients present with salivary gland enlargement, xerostomia, keratoconjunctivitis sicca, uveitis and lymphocytic pulmonary, gastrointestinal and renal involvement. An uncommon form of HIV-associated neuropathy is seen in DILS which is eminently treatable with antiretroviral drugs and corticosteroids. The peripheral nerve complications present with a painful sensorimotor neuropathy which may be symmetrical or asymmetrical. Neurophysiological studies show an axonal neuropathy although rare cases of demyelination are reported. The CD4 counts are variable but the CD8 counts are consistently high, resulting in a low CD4 : CD8 ratio. The diagnosis is confirmed at nerve biopsy which shows angiocentric CD8 T-cell infiltration in endoneurium and epineurium.

Toxic neuropathy for antiretroviral drugs

The nucleoside reverse transcriptase inhibitors (NRTIs) didanosine (ddI), zalcitabine (ddC) and stavudine (d4T) have all been shown to cause a dose-dependent peripheral neuropathy but an association with lamivudine (3TC) is not well documented. Although their use in industrialised countries is now infrequent, in view of their low cost they are increasingly used in resource-poor settings. Mitochondrial toxicity from inhibition of the DNA polymerase enzyme may be the underlying mechanism for the neuropathy and the same mechanism may also account for the other side effects of this class of drug – pancreatitis, fulminant hepatic failure, lactic acidosis and lipodystrophy. The clinical presentation of toxic neuropathy for antiretroviral drugs (TNA) is similar to that seen with DSPN. The drug-related neuropathies are, however, more likely to be painful, have an abrupt onset and progress rapidly. After stopping the appropriate drug, there may be a paradoxical worsening of neuropathic symptoms over a period of 4–8 weeks (coasting). An improvement of symptoms may occur in some patients but a number may be left with underlying DSPN which has been unmasked by the TNA.

As with DSPN, the management of this group of patients can be difficult. The development of this painful sensory neuropathy is a significant cause of morbidity and poor drug compliance. If the patient is on a neurotoxic drug, the issue of stopping it needs to be discussed with their HIV physician. In practice, this maybe a difficult decision if there has been a good virological response and the CD4 count has risen significantly as lowering the drug dosage risks the possibility of viral drug resistance. Treatment is otherwise symptomatic. One small study has shown acetylcarnitine improves neuropathic pain scores and epidermal skin nerve fibre densities.

HIV-associated myopathy

An immunologically mediated polymyositis may occur at seroconversion or during the asymptomatic phases of the disease. As with non-HIV patients, the subacute illness manifests with proximal weakness, myalgia, and myopathic changes on EMG studies but the patients tend to be younger and the CK levels are lower. The disorder is usually steroid responsive. The inflammatory infiltrates found on muscle biopsy are similar to HIV – negative polymyositis with endomysial infiltrates of cytotoxic CD8+ T cells and MHC-I expression but there is a reduction of CD4-positive T cells. Zidovudine (AZT), an NRTI introduced in 1986, causes a mitochondrial myopathy. Muscle biopsies show ragged red fibres and muscle mitochondrial DNA levels are significantly depleted. Patients improve when the drug is stopped. This complication is now rare since the drug doses have been reduced from 1000–1500 to 600 mg/day.

Motor neurone disease

Anecdotal case series have described an association between motor neurone disease (MND) and HIV infection. Motor neurone loss is caused by viral proteins or by immune activation but the relationship to HIV remains uncertain. The clinical pattern may be similar to non-HIV MND but some patients have a more indolent course and an exclusively lower motor neurone pattern of disease often in a segmental distribution (e.g. flail upper limbs). The incidence and progression are not related to the CD4 counts or viral load and the response to HAART is often poor.

Immune reconstitution inflammatory syndrome

IRIS is a paradoxical worsening of pre-existing infectious processes following the initiation of HAART in HIV-infected individuals. It has been defined as the paradoxical deterioration of clinical or laboratory parameters including imaging studies, despite a favourable response of the HIV surrogate markers (i.e. viral load and CD4 count) to HAART. Some 10–25% of patients on HAART may develop IRIS, which usually occurs within the first 2 months although more chronic forms of IRIS with a long duration between the initiation of antiretroviral therapy and the development of the first symptoms may occur. IRIS develops in the setting of treatment of HIV with immune restoration leading to the recovery of CD4 T lymphocytes and memory T cells. After initiation of HAART, plasma HIV RNA levels fall to less than 10% of pre-therapy levels within 2 weeks. In parallel a biphasic increase in CD4 T lymphocyte count occurs. When this process of immune reconstitution develops in the presence of an antigenic stimulus (either a foreign or self-antigen), the immune reaction to the antigen may be excessive and pathological leading to IRIS. Risk factors in the development of CNS – IRIS include:

- Low CD4 nadir (<50 cells/mm^3)
- Rapid fall in viral load following initiation of HAART
- Underlying opportunistic infection
- Genetic factors.

In the presence of an existing opportunistic infection IRIS may either occur because the underlying opportunistic infection becomes 'unmasked' after immune restoration or because immune restoration leads to a devastating T-cell mediated encephalitis with infiltration of the brain by activated T cells in an attempt to control the underlying CNS infection. The inflammatory cell infiltrate is composed predominantly of CD3 and CD8 T cells with scattered CD68 macrophages. No CD20 B cells are seen. CD3 and CD8 T cells are also seen in increased numbers in the white matter, away from the blood vessels. Both forms of IRIS are associated with enhancing MRI lesions due to breakdown of the blood–brain barrier.

Several different pathogens have been associated with the development of IRIS, the most serious being *Mycobacterium*, *Cryptococcus*, *Pneumocystis* or viruses (HSV, VZV, CMV, EBV, hepatitis B and C and JC virus).

In neurological IRIS with co-existing *M. tuberculosis* there may be meningitis and abcesses in addition to systemic manifestations. IRIS resulting from reactivation of *M. avium* may cause paravertebral and brain abscesses. Following previous cryptococcus infection, IRIS may cause a recurrence of meningo-encephalitis or cavitating lung lesions leading to respiratory failure. IRIS due to prior cytomegalovirus infection leads to the development of vitritis, uveitis and cystoid macular oedema with visual loss. Unmasked PML IRIS resulting from pre-existing infection with JC virus is is the most devastating form of the disease as no antiviral agent is available to treat JC virus. It is associated with CD4 counts <200/mm^3. IRIS-induced cases of PML demonstrate gadolinium enhancement on MRI and biopsy shows extensive inflammatory infiltrates and demyelination. Occasionally, IRIS occurs without a clear pathogen; it may then be associated with sarcoid-like granulomatous lesions in the lungs or an autoimmune diathesis with patients developing disorders such as thyroiditis, SLE, polymyositis and rheumatoid arthritis.

Systemic IRIS is usually mild and self-limiting with the majority of cases occurring within 3 months after the initiation of HAART. Neurological presentation of IRIS is much less common than systemic IRIS, with an estimated incidence of <1%.

The management of neurological IRIS consists of treating any identified opportunistic infection and corticosteroids for the inflammatory component. HAART should be initiated early in the course of AIDS, despite the risk of IRIS, because it reduces mortality and it should also be initiated within 2 weeks of commencing therapy for opportunistic infections. If IRIS develops after commencing HAART the question of whether to stop or continue treatment is controversial. In most cases it is reasonable to continue HAART providing the IRIS is not serious or there is little risk of permanent sequelae. However, if there is a life-threatening complication such as a mass lesion within the brain, HAART should be discontinued for a period of time. Corticosteroids (prednisolone 1 mg/kg/day; maximum dose 60–80 mg) or other non-steroidal anti-inflammatory agents may decrease the inflammatory response. Prevention of IRIS may be possible by identifying potential opportunistic infections 1 or 2 months prior to commencing HAART.

Conclusions

Since the onset of the AIDS epidemic, tremendous strides have been made in unravelling the immunobiology of HIV; the development of the antiretroviral drugs which have made HIV a chronic medical disorder rather than an inexorably fatal one; identifying and treating the opportunistic complications with better diagnostic and therapeutic options. However, these benefits have not to date reached the areas of the world most affected by the epidemic. From the neurology point of view, toxic neuropathy continues to pose problems although less so since the use of d-drugs has declined at least in resource-rich settings. Although the incidence of HAD has declined, as a result of increased longevity, the prevalence has increased. There is concern regarding effective CSF penetration of drugs, which is currently being addressed as is the issue of ongoing cognitive decline despite undetectable virus in the blood. This could be a result of drug neurotoxicity, a low grade inflammation that is triggered when immunosupression supervenes (HAND legacy) and continues despite adequate antiviral treatment or to a persistent low grade IRIS phenomenon. Neurological IRIS mainly associated with PML and HIV itself has also proved difficult to diagnose and manage.

Acknowledgement

The authors are very grateful to Dr Frank Mattes, Consultant Virologist at UCLH, for reviewing the chapter and for his helpful comments and advice.

References

Halperin JJ, Logigian EL, Finkel MF, Pearl RA. Practice parameters for the diagnosis of patients with borreliosis (Lyme disease). Quality Standards Subcommittee of American Academy of Neurology. *Neurology* 1996; **46:** 619–627.

Further reading

Bacterial meningitis

Davis LE, Greenlee JE. Pneumococcal meningitis: antibiotics essential but insufficient. *Brain* 2003; **126**: 1013–1101.
Harden A, Ninis N, Thompson M, *et al.* Parentral penicillin for children with meningococcal disease before hospital admission: case–control study. *BMJ* 2006; **332**: 1295–1297.
Lee W-K, Mossop WP, Little AF, *et al.* Infected (mycotic) aneurysms; spectrum of imaging appearances and management. *RadioGraphics* 2008; **28**: 1853–1868.
Rosenstein NE, Perkins BA, Stephens DS, Popvic T, Hughes JM. Meningococcal disease. *N Engl J Med* 2001; **344**: 800–806.
Tan LKK, Carlone GM, Borrow R. Advances in the development of vaccines against *Neisseria meningitides*. *N Engl J Med* 2010; **362:** 1511–1520.
Van de Beek D, Drake JM, Tunkel AR. Nosocomial bacterial meningitis. *N Engl J Med* 2010; **362:** 146–154.
Van de Beek D, de Gans J, Tunkel AR, Wijdicks EFM. Community-acquired bacterial meningitis in adults. *N Engl J Med* 2006; **354**: 44–53.
Whitfield P. The management of intracranial abscesses. *ACNR* 2005; **5:** 12–15.

Tuberculosis

British Thoracic Society. Chemotherapy and management of tuberculosis in the United Kingdom: recommendations 1998: Joint Tuberculosis Committee of the British Thoracic Society. *Thorax* 1998; **53**: 536–548.
Nathanson E, Nunn P, Uplekar M, *et al.* MDR Tuberculosis – critical steps for prevention and control. *N Engl J Med* 2010; **362:** 1511–1520.
Thwaites GE. The diagnosis and management of tuberculous meningitis. *Pract Neurol* 2002; **5**: 250–261.
Thwaites GE, van Toorn R, Schoeman J. Tuberculous meningitis: more questions, still too few answers. *Lancet Neurol* 2013; **12:** 999–1010.
Zumla A, Raviglione M, Hafner R, *et al.* Tuberculosis. *N Engl J Med* 2013; **368:** 745–755.

Syphilis and leprosy

Britton WJ, Lockwood DN. Leprosy. *Lancet* 2004; **363**: 1209–1219.
Carr J. Neurosyphilis. *Pract Neurol* 2003; **3:** 329–341.
Guatilake SB, Settinayake S. Leprosy. *Pract Neurol* 2004; **4:** 194–203.
Kingston M, French P, Goh B, *et al.* UK National Guidelines on the management of syphilis 2008. *Int J STD AIDS* 2008; **14:** 729–740.
Lockwood DN, Reid AJ. Treatment of leprosy. *Q J Med* 2001; **94**: 207–212.
Ooi WW, Srinvasan J. Leprosy and the peripheral nervous system: basic and clinical aspects. *Muscle Nerve* 2004; **30**: 393–409.

Toxins

Cherington M. Clinical spectrum of botulism. *Muscle Nerve* 1998; **21**: 701–710.
Thwaites GE. Tetanus. *Pract Neurol* 2002; **5**: 130–137.

Zoonoses

Wokke J, Vanneste J. Neuroborreliosis. *Pract Neurol* 2004; **4**: 152–161.

Viral infections

Association of British Neurologists and British Infection Association. National Guidelines: Management of suspected viral encephalitis in adults. *J Infections* 2012; **64**: 449–477.
Davies NW, Brown LJ, Gonde J, Irish D, Robinson RO, Swan AV, *et al.* Factors influencing PCR detection of viruses in cerebrospinal fluid of patients with suspected CNS infections. *J Neurol Neurosurg Psychiatry* 2005; **76**: 82–87.
Davison KL, Crowcroft NS, Ramsay ME, *et al.* Viral encephalitis in England 1989–1998: What did we miss? *Emerg Infect Dis* 2003; **9**: 234–240.
Kennedy PGE, Chaudhuri A. Herpes simplex encephalitis. *J Neurol Neurosurg Psychiatry* 2002; **73**: 237–238.
Tunkel AR, Glaser CA, Bloch KC, *et al.* The management of encephalitis: clinical practice guidelines by the Infectious Diseases Society of America. *Clin Infect Dis* 2008; **47:** 303–327.

Tropical diseases

Akinosoglou K-A, Pasvol G. The management of malaria in adults. *Clin Med* 2011; **11:** 497–501.
Amlie-Lefond C, Kleinschmidt-DeMasters BK, Mahlingam R, Davis LE, Gilden DH. The vasculopathy of varicella-zoster encephalitis. *Ann Neurol* 1995; **37**: 784–790.
Davies NWS, Sharief MK, Howard RS. Infection-associated encephalopathies: their investigation, diagnosis, and treatment. *J Neurol* 1996; **253**: 833–845.
Ferrari TCA, Moreira PR. Neuroschistosomiasis: clinical symptoms and pathogenesis. *Lancet Neurol* 2011; **10:** 853–864.
Garcia HH, Del Brutto OH. Neurocysticercosis: update concepts about an old disease. *Lancet Neurol* 2005; **4**: 653–661.
Garcia HH, Evans CAW, Nash TE, *et al.* Current consensus guidelines for treatment of neurocysticercosis. *Clin Microbiol Rev* 2002; **15:** 747–756.
Greenwood B. Treatment of malaria: a continuing challenge. *N Engl J Med* 2014; **371:** 474–475.
Hotez PJ, Molyneux DH, Fenwick A, *et al.* Control of neglected tropical diseases. *N Engl J Med* 2007; **357:** 1018–1027.
Howard RS. Poliomyelitis and the postpolio syndrome. *BMJ* 2005; **330**: 1314–1318.
Nash TE, Garcia HH. Diagnosis and treatment of neurocysticercosis. *Nat Rev Neurol* 2011; **7:** 584–594.
Neary D, Snowden JS. Schistosomiasis and the nervous system. *Pract Neurol* 2003; **3**: 12–21.
Newton CR, Hien TT, White N. Cerebral malaria. *J Neurol Neurosurg Psychiatry* 2000; **69**: 433–441.
Saag MS, Graybill RJ, Larsen RA, *et al.* Practice guidelines for the management of cryptococcal disease. Infectious Diseases Society of America. *Clin Infect Dis* 2000; **30**: 710–718.
Walker MD, Zunt JR. Neuroparasitic infections: cestodes, trematodes and protozoans. *Semin Neurol* 2005; **25**: 262–271.
Walker MD, Zunt JR. Neuroparasitic infections: nematodes. *Semin Neurol* 2005; **25**: 252–261.
White NJ. Cerebral malaria. *Pract Neurol* 2004; **4**: 20–29.
White NJ. The treatment of malaria. *N Engl J Med* 1996; **335**: 800–806.
Willoughby RE, Tieves KS, Hoffman GM, *et al.* Survival after treatment of rabies with induction of coma. *N Engl J Med* 2005; **352**: 2508–2514.

HIV-related

Benjamin LA, Bryer A, Emsley HCA, Soloman T, Connor MD. HIV infection and stroke: current perspectives and future directions. *Lancet Neurol* 2012; **11:** 878–890.
Havlir DV, Kendall MA, Ive P, *et al.* Timing of antiretroviral therapy for HIV-1 infection and tuberculosis. *N Engl J Med* 2011; **365:** 1482–1491.
Huang L, Quartin A, Jones D, Havlir DV. Intensive care of patients with HIV infection. *N Engl J Med* 2006; **355:** 173–181.
Tan IL, Smith BR, von Geldern G, *et al.* HIV-associated infections of the CNS. *Lancet Neurol* 2012; **11:** 605–617.

CHAPTER 10

Nerve and Muscle Disease

Michael Lunn[1], Michael Hanna[2], Robin Howard[1], Matthew Parton[1], Shamima Rahman[1], Mary Reilly[2], Katie Sidle[1] and Christopher Turner[1]

[1] National Hospital for Neurology & Neurosurgery

[2] UCL Institute of Neurology

Neuromuscular diseases have traditionally been overlooked, underdiagnosed and poorly treated when compared with neurological diseases with greater visibility (e.g. Parkinson's disease or epilepsy), social impact (such as the dementias) or which pose a threat for survival (e.g. brain tumours or meningitis). However, neuromuscular disorders are diverse and extremely common, possibly accounting for up to 40% of neurological diagnoses. They may lead to significant disability or death. The accurate and early diagnosis of a cause may lead to effective treatment, reduction in disability and improved quality of life.

This chapter provides a comprehensive summary of disorders of peripheral nerve, neuromuscular junction, muscle and the anterior horn cell.

Peripheral nerve disorders

An understanding of the many peripheral nerve disorders relies upon a comprehension of the complexities of the macro- and micro-anatomy of peripheral nerves, their molecular biology, immunology and pathophysiology. Much of this is beyond the scope of this chapter but a short synopsis is provided here.

Macro-anatomy of the peripheral nerve

Peripheral nerves are bundles of axons, Schwann cells, elaborated myelin and the supporting cellular tissues whose primary purpose is to communicate neural information between the central nervous system (CNS) and peripheral sensory or effector structures (e.g. muscles, sweat glands, blood vessels). In very simplified terms, the peripheral nervous system (PNS) functions via a series of reflex arc circuits with efferent and afferent arms controlled from above by the CNS (Figure 10.1).

The anatomy of the major nerve trunks and their connections has been known for more than 500 years, even if there was little understanding of their function (Figure 10.2). The PNS consists of 10 of the 12 cranial nerves and the spinal roots, becoming the peripheral nerves, exiting from the spinal cord. Knowledge of basic peripheral neuroanatomy, physiology and immunology is the key to understanding the pathophysiology of diseases affecting peripheral nerves.

Upper limbs

The brachial plexus is formed from the anterior rami of the spinal roots from C5 to T1 (Figure 10.3). Within the course of the brachial plexus, axons originating from these cervical roots are rearranged and exit in major and minor nerve branches to supply sensory, motor and autonomic inputs and outputs to the upper limb and shoulder girdle (Table 10.1a; Figure 10.4). Many find the localisation of processes affecting the brachial plexus or cervical roots difficult but it is simplified by an understanding of the anatomy. The identification of affected muscle groups and sensory territories assist.

The major nerves leaving the brachial plexus are the musculocutaneous, median, ulnar and radial nerves (Figure 10.4). Each nerve has its innervated muscles, although there are occasional anatomical variations.

Lower limbs

The lumbosacral plexus is formed from the ventral rami of L1–S4 nerve roots (Figure 10.5). The upper (or lumbar) part of the plexus gives rise to the obturator and femoral nerves. The lower part of the plexus gives rise to the sciatic nerve, which is regionally organised in its cross-section, and this later divides into the tibial and common peroneal nerves at the knee. As with the brachial plexus, some smaller nerves exit the plexus directly (e.g. the genitofemoral and lateral cutaneous nerve of the thigh). The major nerves of the lumbosacral plexus innervate individual muscles as indicated in Figure 10.5 (see also Table 10.1b). An ability to identify which muscles or areas of skin innervation are affected on clinical and neurophysiological examination and to correlate this to the anatomical innervation is central to being able to make successful peripheral nerve diagnoses (Figures 10.6 and 10.7).

Micro-anatomy of the peripheral nerve

Each peripheral nerve comprises a collection of neurones and their bundles of axonal processes, supporting cells, blood vessels, connective tissue and other elements including cells of the immune system (e.g. macrophages and mast cells). An axon and its supporting cells (an axon–Schwann cell unit) are often referred to as nerve fibre. A fascicle is a group of nerve fibres with associated endoneurial elements enclosed in ensheathing perineurium. A nerve is a collection

Neurology: A Queen Square Textbook, Second Edition. Edited by Charles Clarke, Robin Howard, Martin Rossor and Simon Shorvon.

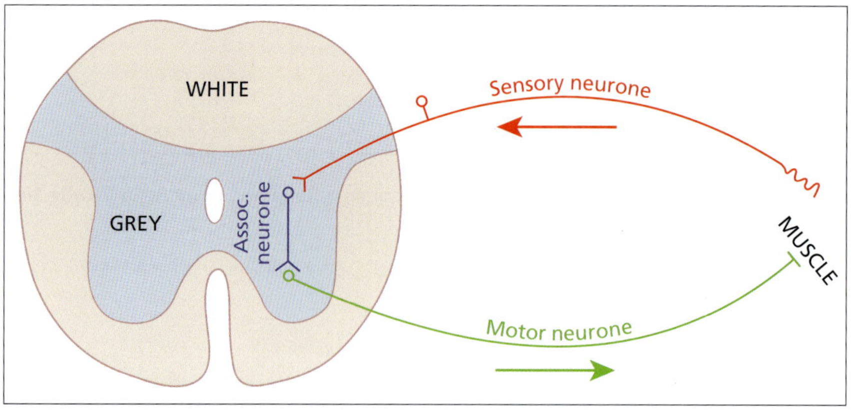

Figure 10.1 The reflex arc is the foundation of peripheral nerve function. Although highly stylised, peripheral stimuli enter the arc along the afferent limb and exit to effector organs along the efferent limb. Responses may be modified by synaptic connections along this pathway.

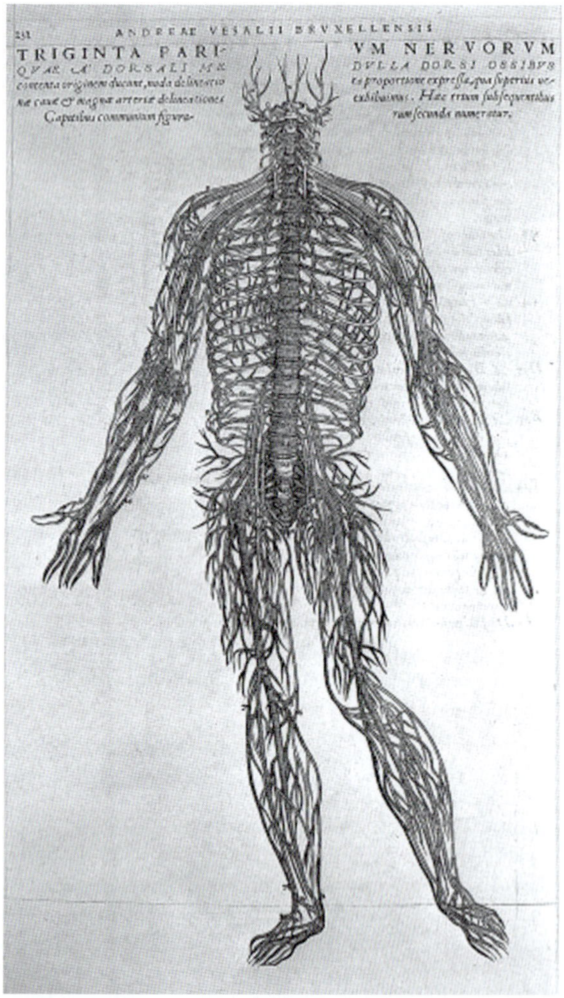

Figure 10.2 Vesalius, 1543. Source: Wellcome Library, London.

of fascicles surrounded by supportive and protective epineurium. Apart from post-ganglionic neurones of the autonomic nervous system, all PNS axons have a CNS extension or origin where the axonal and support matrix characteristics are different.

Peripheral nerve compartments

The peripheral nerve is divided into distinct compartments easily visible when cross-sectioned nerves are examined under the light microscope (Figure 10.8). The compartmentalisation of the peripheral nerve provides several layers of protection able to resist physical and immunological attack. Axons are protected from most immune reactions that might otherwise interfere with effective electrical impulse transmission.

The outer layer of epineurium is composed of loosely packed collagenous connective tissue containing adipocytes, fibroblasts, collagen and mast cells and serves to provide tensile strength and resist impact and trauma. The perineurium is a tight sleeve of flattened cells separated by collagen within the epineurium, and surrounds each individual nerve fascicle. The specialised flattened fibroblasts, connected by occlusive tight junctions, form an effective barrier to diffusion of macromolecules between the epineurium and endoneurium.

The endoneurium is a tissue space containing connective tissue, axon–Schwann cell units, pericytes, fibroblasts, macrophages and mast cells. The blood vessels in the endoneurium have a specialised endothelium which forms tight junctions and is also impermeable to macromolecules. There is no endoneurial lymphatic drainage. The endoneurial space is bathed in endoneurial fluid, the composition of which betrays the specialised protection afforded to this space. The electrolyte composition is that of extracellular fluid to enable electrical nerve conduction but the protein and immunoglobulin content is some 250 times less than that found extracellularly. The fluid is under positive pressure. This unique set of characteristics is possible because the perineurium and the specialised endoneurial endothelium form a blood–nerve barrier (BNB) that is relatively impenetrable to cells and macromolecules under normal conditions. Any active transcellular traffic of essential substances through the perineurium and into the endoneurium probably occurs in pinocytotic vesicles.

Immunology

The peripheral nerves are isolated behind the BNB which provides relative protection from circulating immune factors and perturbations of homeostasis. Not only is the endoneurium physically protected from outside attack, but it is also relatively deficient in the immunological machinery with which to make an internal immunological response. A few macrophages constitutively displaying major histocompatibility complex (MHC) Class II are found within

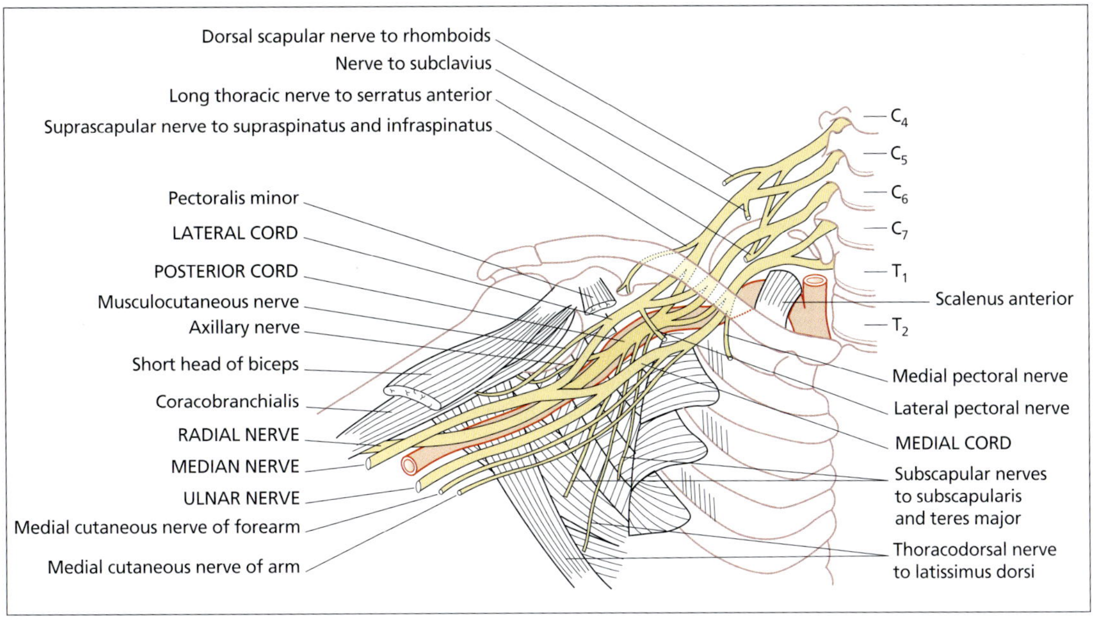

Figure 10.3 Diagram of the brachial plexus, its branches and the muscles which they supply. Source: O'Brien 2000. Reproduced with permission of The Guarantors of Brain.

Tabe 10.1 (a) Innervations. Upper limb. The bold type indicates the predominant innervation of the muscle where that exist.

	Muscles innervated	Spinal roots
Spinal accessory nerve	Trapezius	C3, C4
Brachial plexus	Rhomboids	C4, C5
	Serratus anterior	C5, C6, C7
	Pectoralis major – clavicular head	**C5**, C6
	Pectoralis major – sternal head	C6, **C7**, C8
	Supraspinatus	**C5**, C6
	Infraspinatus	**C5**, C6
	Latissimus dorsi	C6, **C7**, C8
	Teres major	C5, C6, C7
Axillary nerve	Deltoid	C5, C6
Musculocutaneous nerve	Biceps	C5, C6
	Brachialis	C5, C6
Radial nerve	Triceps (long, lateral and medial head)	C6, C7, C8
	Brachioradialis	C5, C6
	Extensor carpi radialis longus	C5, C6
Posterior interosseous nerve	Supinator	C6, C7
	Extensor carpi ulnaris	**C7**, C8
	Extensor digitorum	**C7**, C8
	Abductor pollicis longus	**C7**, C8
	Extensor pollicis longus	**C7**, C8
	Extensor pollicis brevis	**C7**, C8
	Extensor indicis	**C7**, C8
Median nerve	Pronator teres	C6, C7
	Flexor carpi radialis	C6, C7
	Flexor digitorum superficialis	C7, **C8**, T1
	Abductor pollicis brevis	C8, **T1**
	Flexor pollicis brevis	C8, **T1**
	Opponens pollicis	C8, **T1**
	Lumbricals I and II	C8, **T1**

(continued)

Table 10.1 (continued)

	Muscles innervated	Spinal roots
Anterior interosseous nerve	Pronator quadratus	C7, **C8**
	Flexor digitorum profundus I and II	C7, **C8**
	Flexor pollicis longus	C7, **C8**
Ulnar nerve	Flexor carpi ulnaris	C7, **C8**, T1
	Flexor digitorum profundus III and IV	C7, **C8**
	Hypothenar muscles	C8, **T1**
	Adductor pollicis	C8, **T1**
	Flexor pollicis brevis	C8, **T1**
	Palmar interossei	C8, **T1**
	Dorsal interossei	C8, **T1**
	Lumbricals III and IV	C8, **T1**

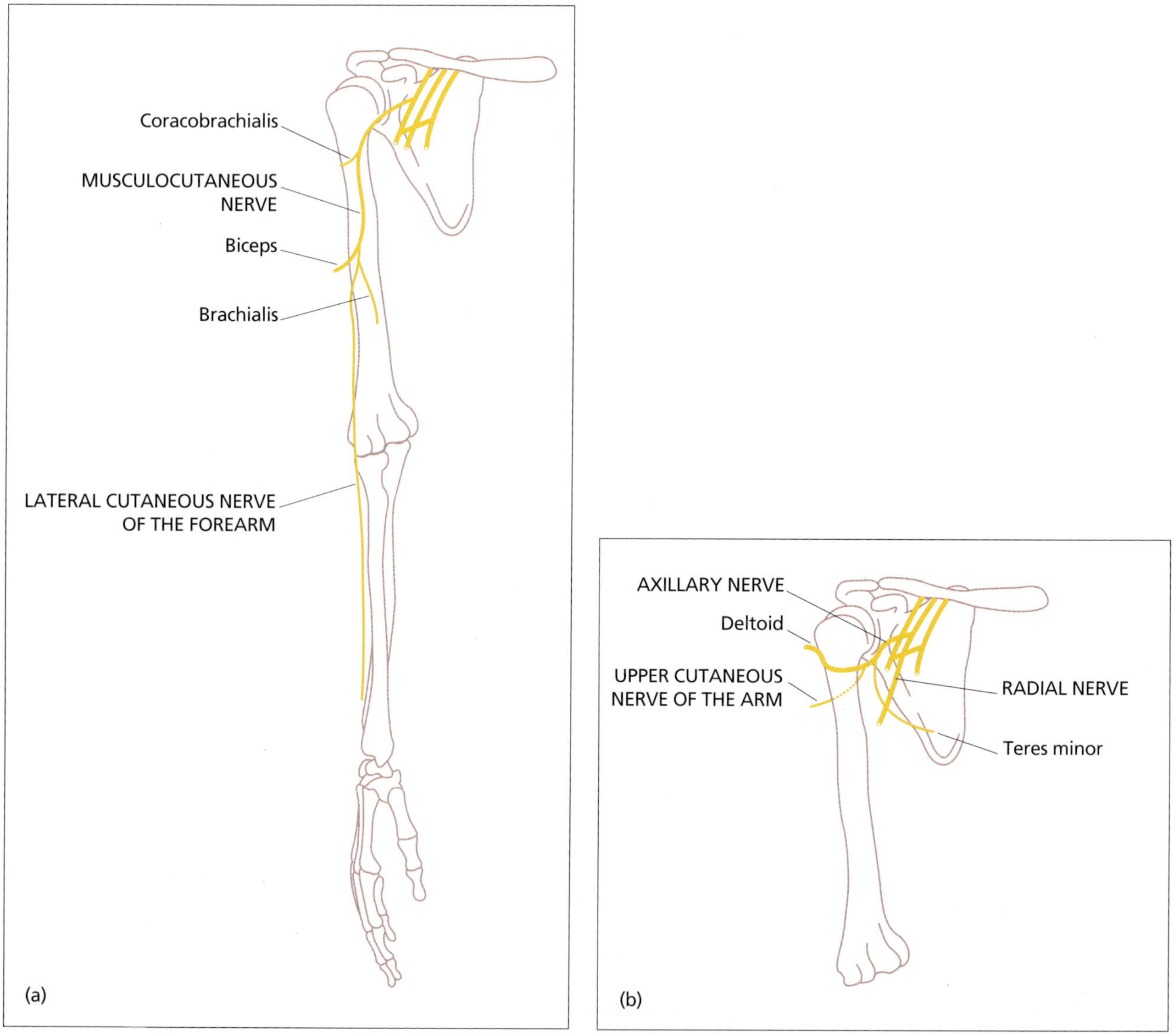

Figure 10.4 Nerves of the upper limb: (a) musculocutaneous nerve, (b) axillary nerve, (c) radial nerve, (d) median nerve, (e) ulnar nerve, their major cutaneous branches and the muscles which they supplies. Source: O'Brien 2000. Reproduced with permission of The Guarantors of Brain.

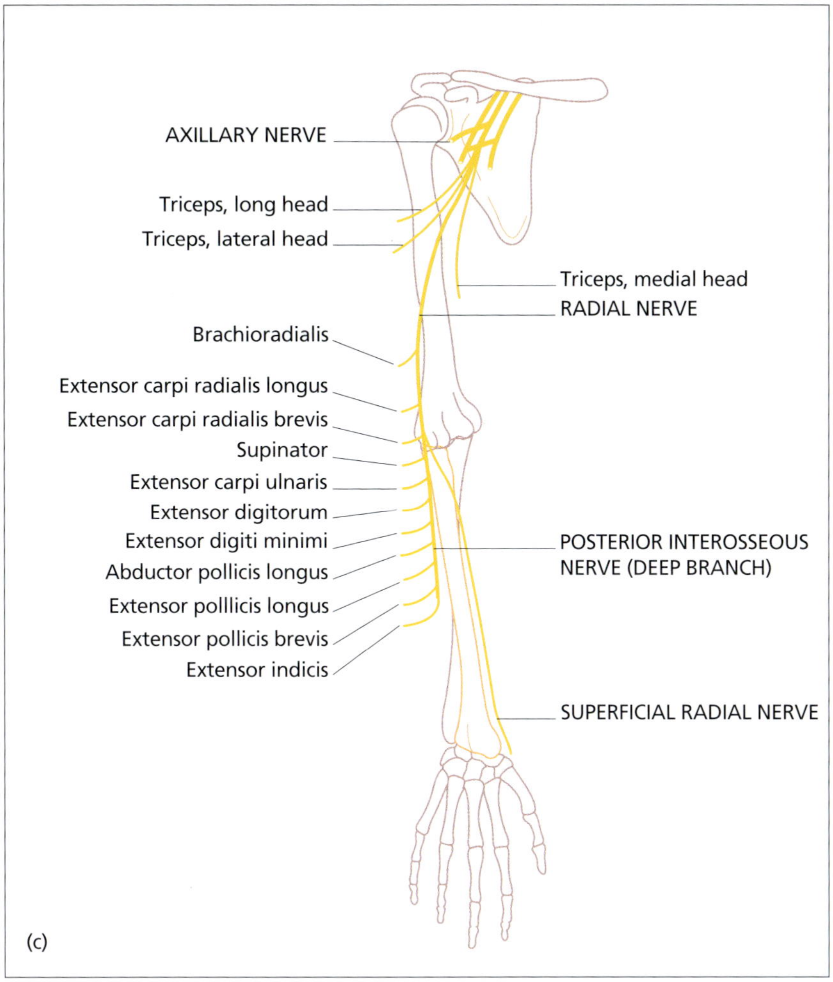
AXILLARY NERVE
Triceps, long head
Triceps, lateral head
Triceps, medial head
RADIAL NERVE
Brachioradialis
Extensor carpi radialis longus
Extensor carpi radialis brevis
Supinator
Extensor carpi ulnaris
Extensor digitorum
Extensor digiti minimi
Abductor pollicis longus
Extensor polllicis longus
Extensor pollicis brevis
Extensor indicis
POSTERIOR INTEROSSEOUS NERVE (DEEP BRANCH)
SUPERFICIAL RADIAL NERVE
(c)

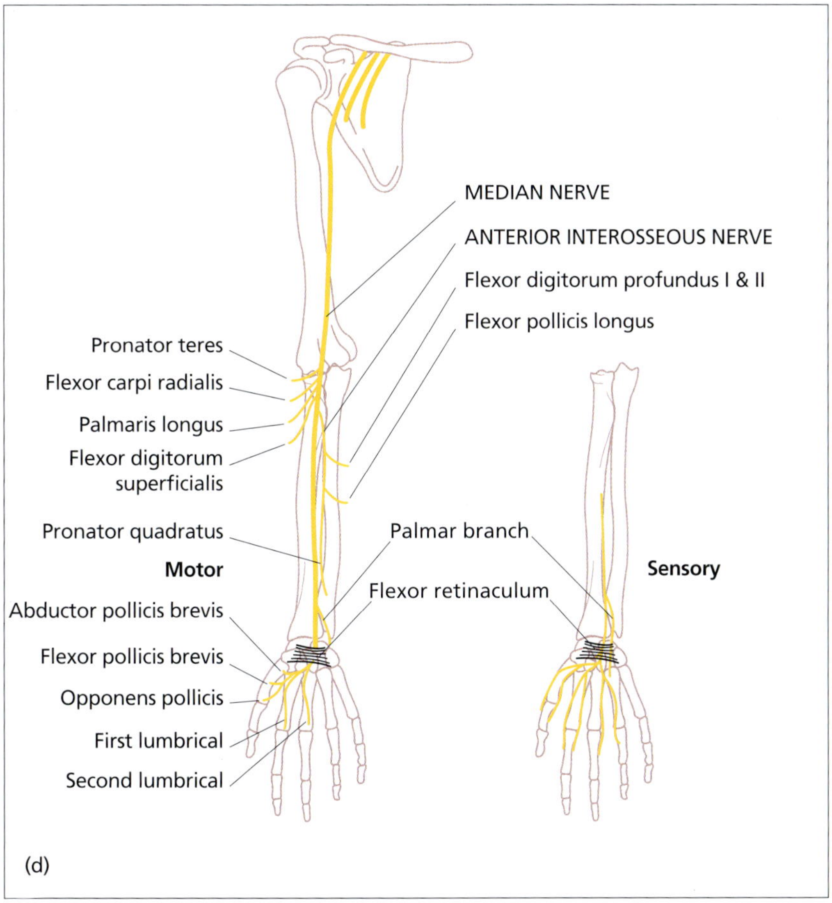
MEDIAN NERVE
ANTERIOR INTEROSSEOUS NERVE
Flexor digitorum profundus I & II
Flexor pollicis longus
Pronator teres
Flexor carpi radialis
Palmaris longus
Flexor digitorum superficialis
Pronator quadratus
Motor
Abductor pollicis brevis
Flexor pollicis brevis
Opponens pollicis
First lumbrical
Second lumbrical
Palmar branch
Flexor retinaculum
Sensory
(d)

Figure 10.4 *(continued)*

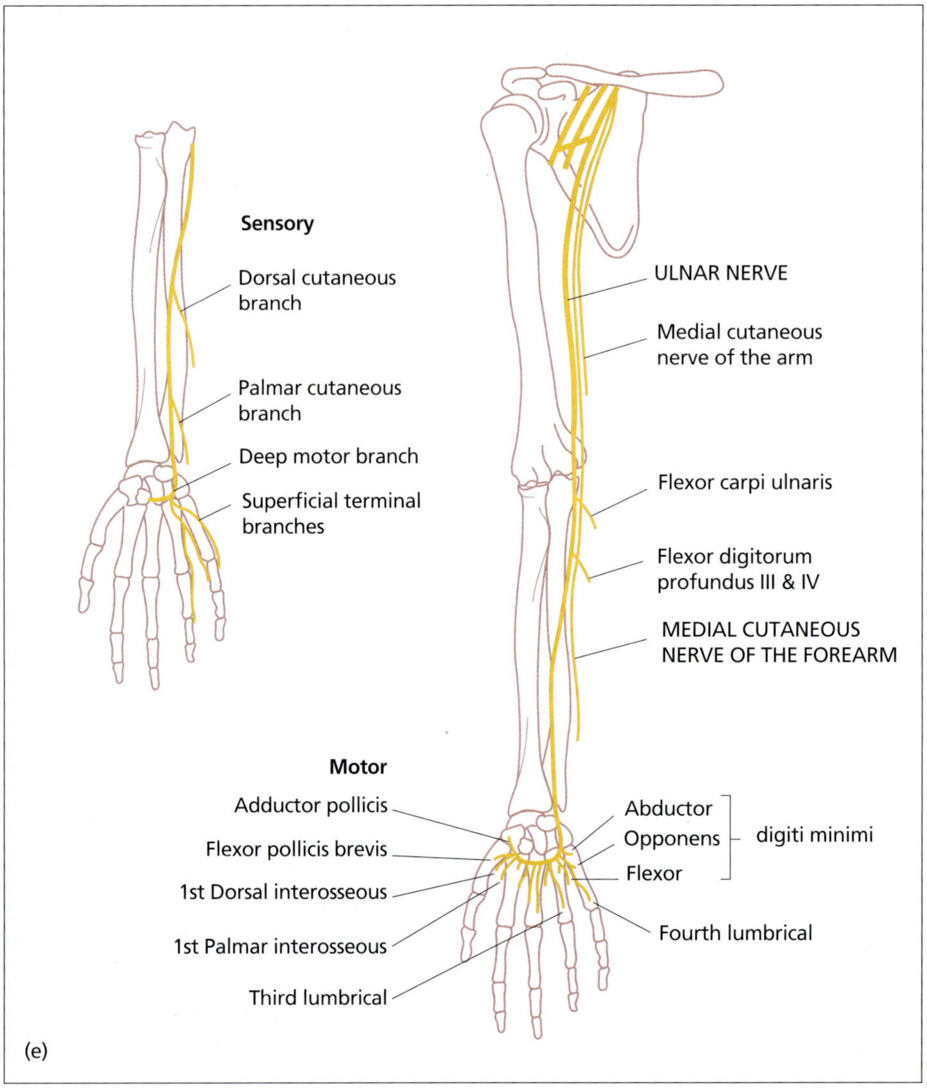

Figure 10.4 *(continued)*

the endoneurium and Schwann cells do not usually express MHC markers. Only very limited T-cell traffic occurs into and out of the endoneurium under normal conditions. Restricted access and egress of cells and molecules, raised endoneurial pressure, low constitutive MHC expression and limited patrol by cells of the immune system all contribute to antigen sequestration in the PNS and the relative BNB.

The physical characteristics of the BNB are not the same throughout the PNS. The barrier is relatively deficient at the trigeminal and dorsal root ganglia (DRG), the motor nerve terminals and the sensory endings. MHC Class II expression is up-regulated at the DRG as a result of continuous immune stimulation because of the physical deficiency and the need to patrol more effectively for invading pathogens. In some neuropathies these are the preferred sites for immune attack and development of pathology.

Pathophysiology of the peripheral nerve

All PNS axons are ensheathed by Schwann cells and the Schwann cells are, in turn, invested by a continuous layer of basal lamina. Schwann cells surrounding smaller axons (0.5–1.5 μm) do not elaborate myelin and one Schwann cell may surround several unmyelinated fibres (a Remak bundle). Those surrounding axons of larger calibre (1–20 μm) wrap a single axon only and form a tightly compacted multi-lamellar myelin sheath. Myelin is a lipid-rich specialised extension of the Schwann cell membrane in the PNS (and of oligodendrocytes in the CNS). Although broadly similar in structure, PNS differs from CNS myelin in its molecular composition (Chapter 2).

The pathophysiological mechanisms that result in peripheral neuropathies are almost as diverse as the number of peripheral nerve diagnoses. However, the patterns of damage at a microscopic level are few. Axonal degeneration occurs distal to a site of nerve transection (which may be physical, inflammatory or vascular; and focal, multi-focal or diffuse). Axonal degeneration can also occur as a distal dying back phenomenon especially in toxic, metabolic and hereditary neuropathies. The primary pathology in the most common hereditary neuropathies is demyelination which classically is uniform. In many inflammatory neuropathies segmental demyelination occurs which may result in conduction failure but not necessarily subsequent axonal degeneration. Remyelination

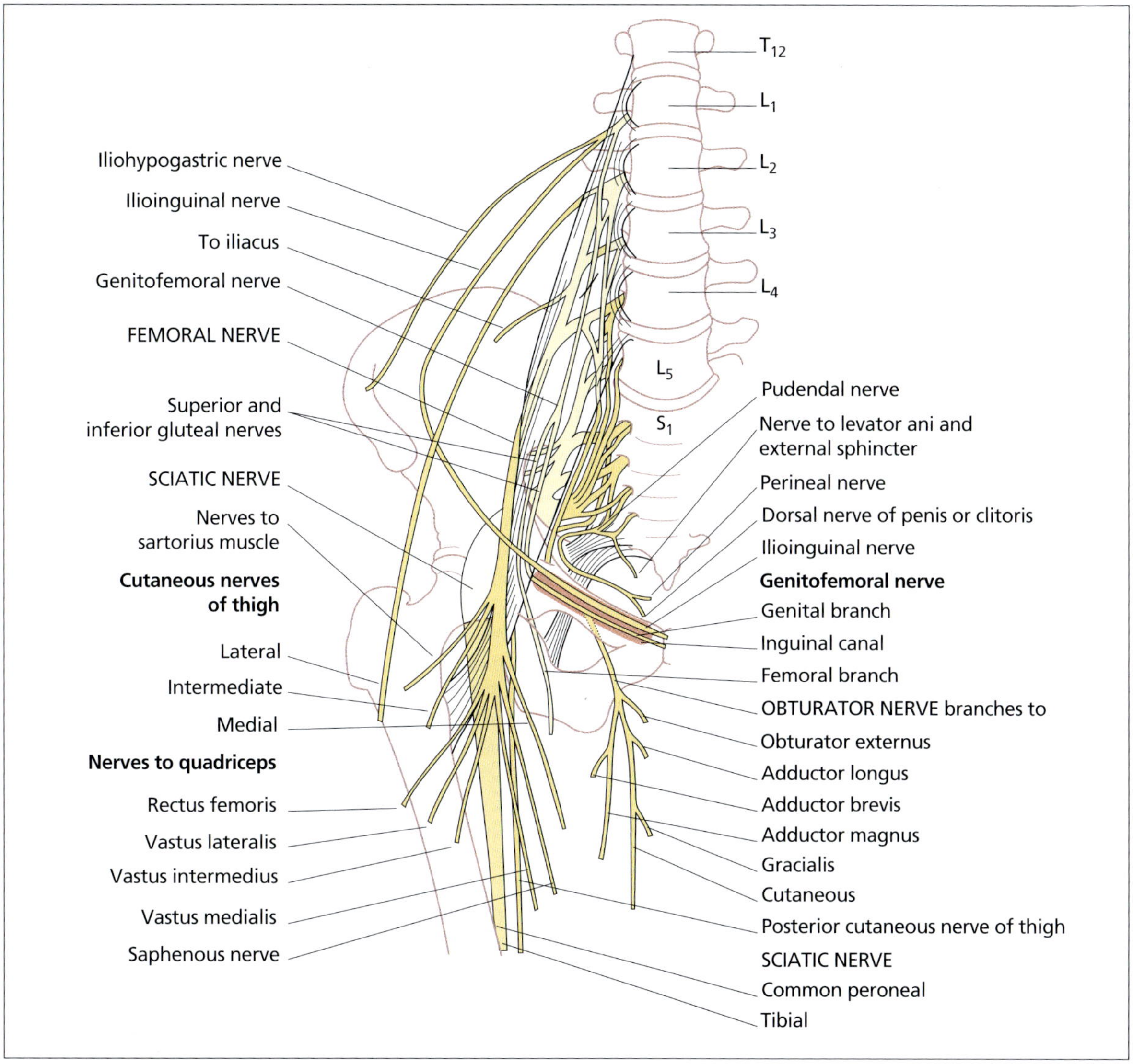

Figure 10.5 Diagram of the lumbosacral plexus, its branches and the muscles that they supply. Source: O'Brien 2000. Reproduced with permission of The Guarantors of Brain.

(with thin myelin, short internodes and onion bulbs) may occur, restoring adequate clinical nerve function. Axonal regeneration occurs less consistently and over distances of centimetres only.

Diseases of the peripheral nerve

Diseases of the peripheral nerve can be genetic or acquired. The acquired neuropathies may be primary or secondary to other conditions. The initial clinical approach is similar in all peripheral nerve disorders.

General approach to peripheral nerve disease

History

Patients with peripheral nerve disease complain of sensory disturbances, muscle weakness or wasting, sometimes fasciculation and cramping and/or symptoms referable to the autonomic nervous system.

Sensory disturbance may be numbness or hypoaesthesia (a term that does not have a correlate in many languages), pain, pins and needles (paraesthesiae), heightened sensation (hyperaesthesia), prolonged painful responses (hyperpathia) or abnormal unpleasant sensations perceived from innocuous stimuli (allodynia) or combinations (e.g. a 'painful numbness'). Abnormal sensations are often described in colourful terminology such as 'like walking on shards of broken glass' or sponges or as if limbs 'were wrapped in cotton wool', '…hot boots' or '…gripped in a vice'. Pain may have a number of qualities that can help the physician. For example, lancinating or shooting pain often associates with large fibre involvement and in the context of an apparent inherited neuropathy may suggest an abnormality in the *SPTLC-1* or *SPTLC-2* genes (see Autosomal dominant CMT2). Burning or stinging pain associates with small fibre involvement. The site of onset and subsequent progression help to differentiate the length dependent sensory neuropathy from the patchy multiple mononeuropathy or dermatomal radiculopathy.

Table 10.1 (b) Innervations. Lower limb. The bold type indicates the predominant innervation of the muscle where that exists.

	Muscles innervated	Spinal roots
Femoral nerve	Iliopsoas	**L1, L2**, L3
	Rectus femoris	L2, **L3, L4**
	Vastus lateralis	L2, **L3, L4**
	Vastus intermedius	L2, **L3, L4**
	Vastus medialis	L2, **L3, L4**
Obturator nerve	Adductor longus	**L2, L3**, L4
	Adductor magnus	**L2, L3**, L4
Superior gluteal nerve	Gluteus medius and minimus	**L4, L5**, S1
	Tensor fasciae latae	**L4, L5**, S1
Inferior gluteal nerve	Gluteus maximus	**L5, S1**, S2
Sciatic and tibial nerves	Semi-tendinosus	**L5, S1**, S2
	Biceps	L5, **S1**, S2
	Semi-membranosus	L5, **S1**, S2
	Gastrocnemius	S1, S2
	Soleus	S1, S2
	Tibialis posterior	L4, L5
	Flexor digitorum longus	L5, **S1, S2**
	Abductor hallucis	S1, S2
	Abductor digiti minimi	S1, S2
	Interossei	S1, S2
Sciatic and common peroneal nerves	Tibialis anterior	**L4**, L5
	Extensor digitorum brevis	**L5**, S1
	Extensor hallucis longus	**L5**, S1
	Extensor digitorum brevis	L5, S1
	Peroneus longus	L5, S1
	Peroneus brevis	L5, S1

Weakness may be described in terms of handicaps ('I can no longer run for a bus' or 'I can no longer do up my zip fastener') or disability ('My foot flaps' or 'I cannot lift my arms'). The pattern of such deficits helps to point to polyneuropathy, multiple mononeuropathies or radicular involvement. Weakness should always be differentiated from fatigue.

Autonomic disturbances may be missed through lack of recognition of their importance (diarrhoea or bladder dysfunction) or social embarrassment (impotence) by the patient, often compounded by a doctor's unwillingness to enquire. More than infrequent postural hypotension with presyncope or syncope is seldom innocuous. Nocturnal diarrhoea, urinary hesitancy or urgency, impotence and reduced sweating or tearing often require a proactive line of questioning and should be taken seriously if answered in the affirmative.

The tempo of symptom onset is definitive in some conditions and highly useful in the diagnosis of others. In the inflammatory neuropathies accurate determination of the time to the nadir of a first episode distinguishes between Guillain–Barré syndrome (GBS), subacute and chronic inflammatory demyelinating polyradiculoneuropathy (CIDP) and subsequently determines the selection of treatment. Likewise, a progressive sensory neuropathy with autonomic involvement that has evolved over 7 years is unlikely to be amyloid or paraneoplasia. Furthermore, relapses and remissions (whether spontaneous or following treatment) may favour one diagnosis over another (e.g. CIDP over GBS or an inflammatory neuropathy over a metabolic cause).

The pattern of weakness or sensory loss is a clue to the site of pathology and often to a pathogenic mechanism. It is important to establish the pattern of involvement as symmetrical, asymmetrical, focal, multi-focal, monomelic or upper or lower limb predominant and any transition from one to another (e.g. multi-focal to symmetrical in vasculitides).

Cranial nerve involvement is important to identify as some conditions have a predilection for one or more cranial nerves (e.g. sarcoidosis and Sjögren's syndrome). Phrenic nerve and diaphragmatic involvement may be disclosed with a history of orthopnoea, early morning headaches or daytime somnolence. A failure to recognise this may lead to a silent and unnecessary death.

Parts of the history, which at first sight may not seem relevant either to the patient or the doctor, are sometimes more important than the reported symptom complex. Other concurrent or previous diseases should not necessarily be assumed at face value and should be chased down and checked. For example, a diagnosis of 'asthma', so often reported, when established as relatively recent in an older person may give the clue to Churg–Strauss syndrome or if misattributed to lung disease may give the clue to cardiac involvement in amyloidosis.

An extensive multi-generational family history including details such as consanguinity, non-paternity, early infant death or adoption is crucial to identifying reduced penetrance or recessive disorders. In genetic disorders, careful probing of early and developmental history will often establish a relevant history of symptoms pre-dating the apparent onset of the condition (lack of interest in sport or numbness of the feet after wearing high heels) by a decade or more.

In all situations, exposures to other agents through sex, travel, insect, animal, toxin or drug exposures, should be sought. A systematic and thorough search for other systemic clues should be made, enquiring about skin and nails, joints, sicca symptoms, weight loss and appetite, masses, eyes and other body systems not covered by previous enquiry.

Examination

On inspection the examiner is looking for classic deformities such as pes cavus (Figure 10.9) or other indicators of diagnosis such as amputations, ulceration, wasting (or prominent lack of wasting in conditions with conduction block), trophic skin changes and fasciculations. Tremor usually occurs in demyelinating disease. Thickened nerves (Figure 10.10; Table 10.2) may be visible, but should be sought and palpated for. Common sites are the ulnar, superficial radial, greater auricular, sural and peroneal nerves.

Examination of the gait can identify both subtle abnormalities of the PNS such as mild distal weakness, or associated features (e.g. ataxia or dystonias). Romberg's sign is of limited use but may be illuminating in sensory neuronopathies. Tone is usually normal or apparently 'reduced'. A careful and correctly performed quantitative motor examination (O'Brien 2010) is crucial to identify the pattern of root, plexus, nerve or muscle and CNS involvement. Some neuropathies are predominantly or entirely motor (Table 10.3) but most will involve both motor and sensory modalities. Reflex loss may be variable and may evolve (e.g. GBS). Careful documentation of sensory loss in each modality using vibration, proprioception, pain, temperature or tickle and light touch may again illuminate disease patterns and pathogenesis. These may be the only findings in some purely sensory neuropathies (Table 10.4).

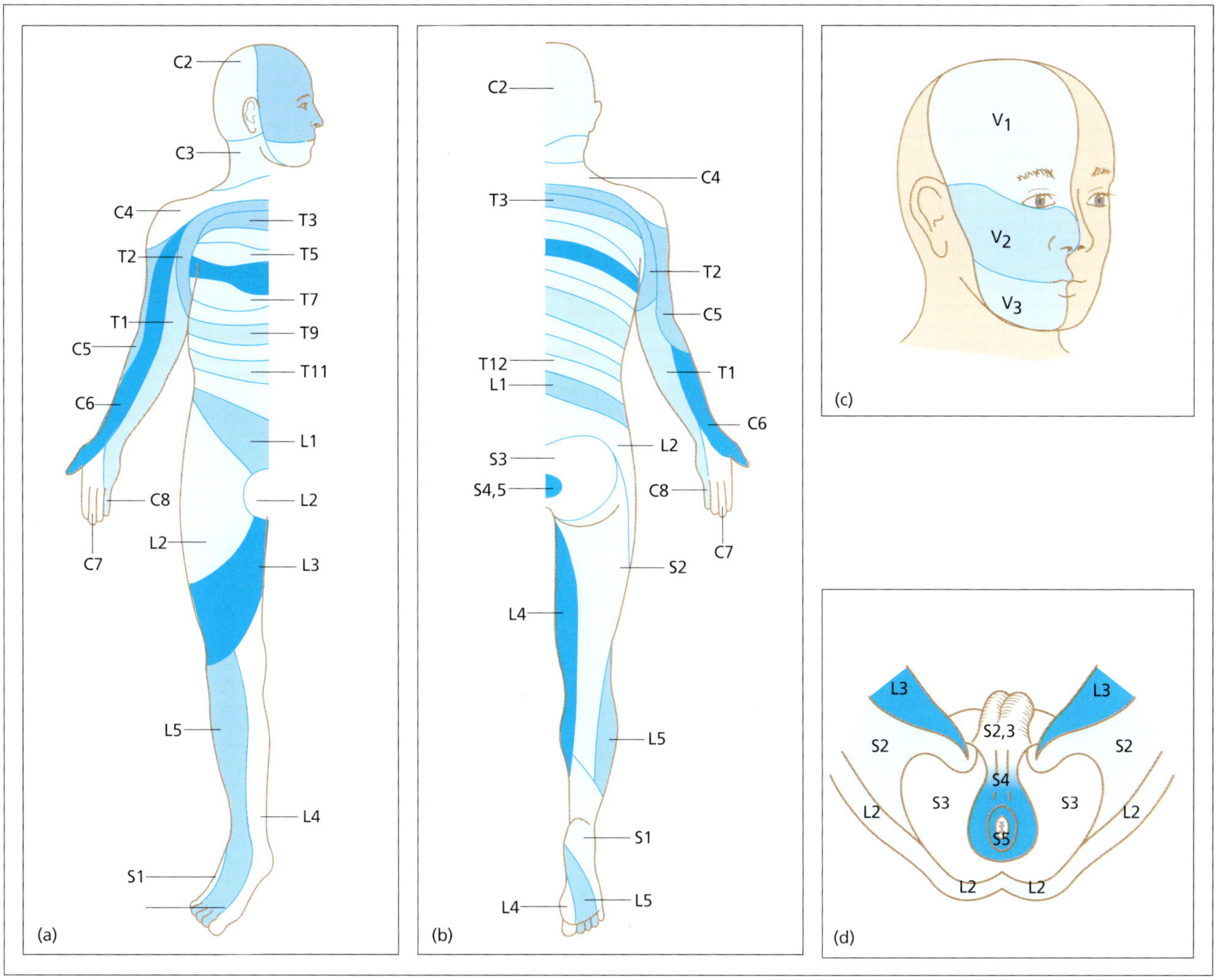

Figure 10.6 Dermatomes. (a) Anterior dermatomes, (b) Posterior dermatomes, (c) Trigeminal divisions, and (d) perineal dermatome. Source: O'Brien 2000. Reproduced with permission of The Guarantors of Brain.

A subsequent general examination should be thorough but tailored and include close inspection of fundi, skin, nails, joints, testes, breasts and a search for palpable nodes or organomegaly as well as a structured systems examination.

Scores

The quantification of the examination findings by their incorporation or translation into one of the many available scoring systems is useful for documenting levels of impairment, disability and handicap at a point in time and following patients over the course of their disease or treatment. The use of standardised and validated scales is also useful in combining and comparing data in clinical trials. Commonly used scales are the MRC Scale (for assessment of power; Chapter 4), the Overall Neuropathy Limitation Score, the new Rasch-Built Overall Disabilty Score (R-ODS), the Modified Rankin Scale, the 10-metre walk time, the Walk-12 and the SF36.

Neurophysiology

A neurophysiological examination should be regarded as an extension of the clinical examination (Chapter 4). If it is not performed by the examining physician then it should be performed with detailed communication between the neurologist and neurophysiologist to ensure that problems and specific issues can be addressed and clarified. Conduction block may be particularly difficult to identify.

Nerve biopsy

A nerve biopsy should be requested and performed only after careful consideration of the other options available to achieve a diagnosis. Biopsies are generally of sensory nerves, and usually a sensory nerve identifiably and recently affected; a neurophysiologically normal nerve should not be biopsied. The biopsy should be performed with informed patient consent; complications, especially of biopsy site pain, are not infrequent. The nerve biopsy should be performed by someone competent and experienced, as crush or diathermy artefact is easily caused and may render the biopsy uninterpretable. At least 4 cm should be excised for examination.

Staining and examination should again be carried out in consultation with a trained neurohistopathologist, preferably with specialist interest in peripheral nerve disease. Generic and specific tincturic and immunohistochemical stains can be used to identify or exclude suspected pathologies and special preparation of parts of the specimen for electron microscopy or teased fibre studies should be requested and discussed beforehand.

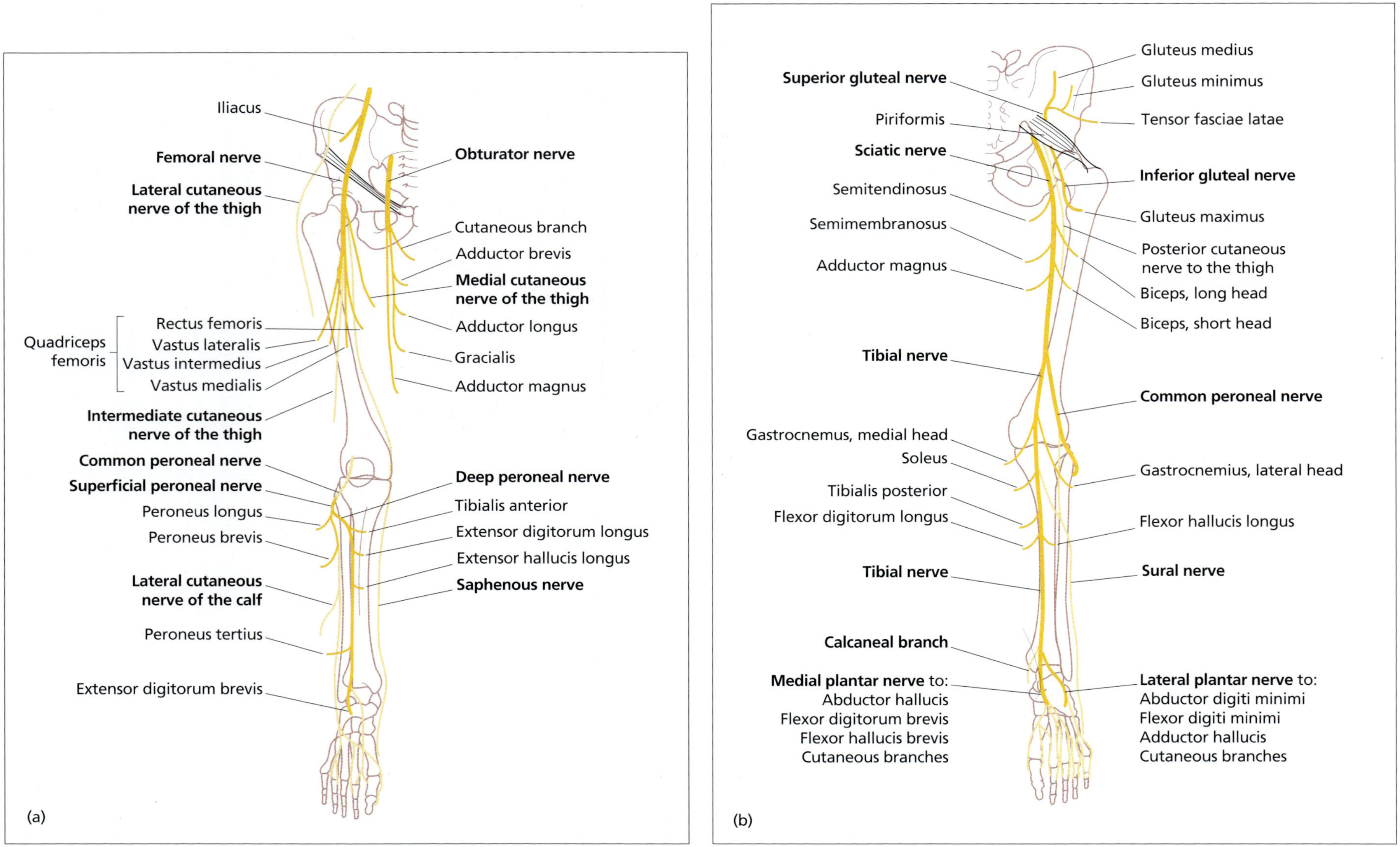

Figure 10.7 Nerves of the lower limb: (a) anterior aspect and (b) posterior aspect of the lower limb, their cutaneous branches and the muscles that they supply. Source: O'Brien 2000. Reproduced with permission of The Guarantors of Brain.

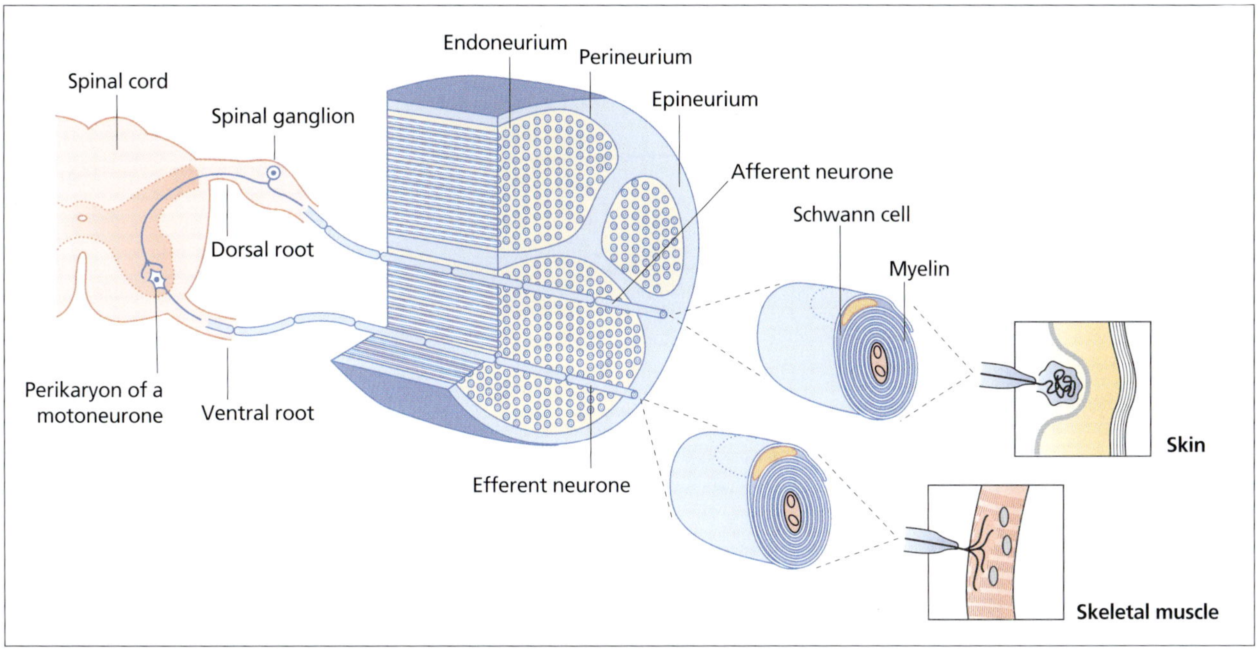

Figure 10.8 Cross-section of nerve diagram. Axons are associated with Schwann cells which in some cases elaborate myelin. Neurones are gathered in fascicles limited by a perineurial sheath. The endoneurium also contains supporting stromal cells endoneurial vessels and, in health, low numbers of immune cells including resident macrophages and mast cells. Fascicles are grouped into nerves limited by the epineurium.

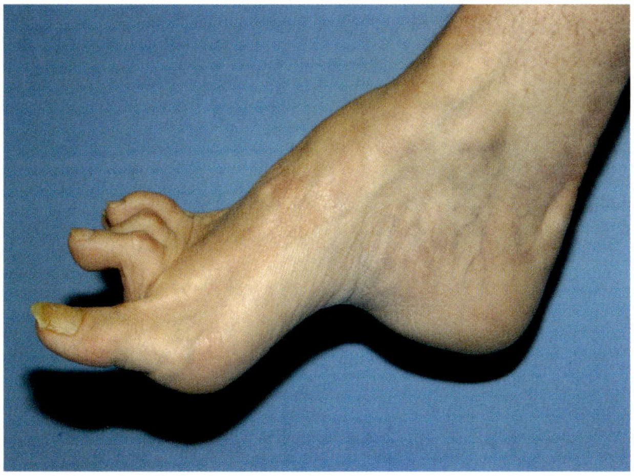

Figure 10.9 The typical lower limb appearances of CMT1A with distal wasting, pes cavus and clawed toes.

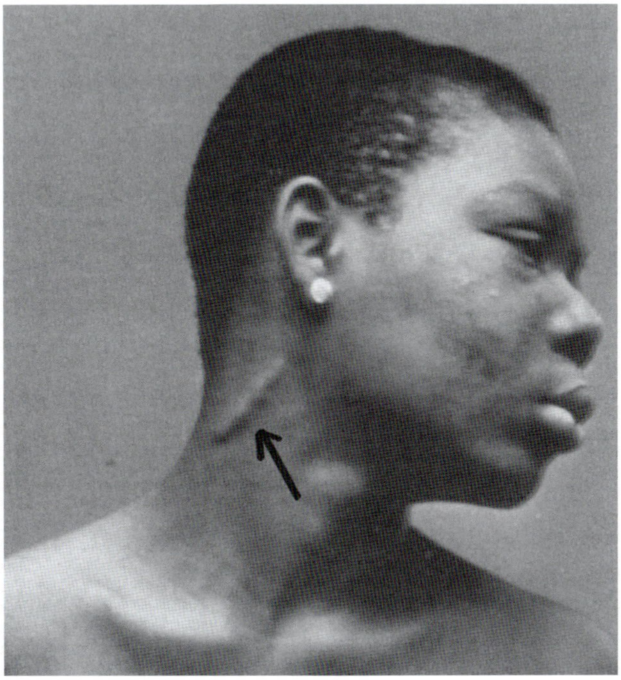

Figure 10.10 Thickened nerves. Source: Forbes 1993. Reproduced with permission of Elsevier.

Inherited neuropathies

The inherited neuropathies can be divided into those in which the neuropathy is the sole or primary part of the disease and those in which the neuropathy is part of a more widespread neurological or multi-system disorder (Table 10.5). The first group includes Charcot–Marie–Tooth disease (CMT). CMT is the most common inherited neuropathy affecting approximately 1/2500 in the Caucasian population, and usually presents with a length dependent motor and sensory neuropathy. Most of the other neuropathies in this group are either genetically related to CMT (e.g. hereditary neuropathy with liability to pressure palsies) or can present in a similar fashion (e.g. hereditary sensory neuropathy [HSN] and distal hereditary motor neuropathy [HMN]). This group also includes hereditary neuralgic amyotrophy (HNA) which presents with recurrent brachial plexus lesions and familial

Table 10.2 Causes of thickened nerves.

Hypertrophic Charcot–Marie–Tooth diseases (especially CMT1A and HNPP)
CIDP
Neurofibromatosis
Refsum's disease
Leprosy
Infiltration (lymphoma/secondary deposits)
Amyloidosis
Acromegaly
Perineuroma and other rare primary tumours

CIDP, chronic inflammatory demyelinating polyradiculoneuropathy; CMT1A, Charcot–Marie–Tooth disease type 1A; HNPP, hereditary neuropathy with liability to pressure palsies.

Table 10.3 Motor neuropathies.

Inherited
Distal hereditary motor neuropathies
Spinal muscular atrophy
SMN: chromosome 5q; recessive
Bulbo-spinal muscular atrophies (Kennedy X-linked, recessive, dominant)
Tay–Sachs (hexosaminidase A deficiency): chromosome 15; recessive
Acquired
Motor neurone disease (progressive muscular atrophy)
Monomelic atrophy (Hirayama) and other idiopathic focal motor neurone disorders
Inflammatory
Acute motor axonal neuropathy
Multifocal motor neuropathy with conduction block
Distal lower motor neuropathy associated with anti-GM1 IgM paraprotein
Paraneoplastic motor neuropathy (breast/lymphoma)
Brachial amyotrophy
Metabolic and medical
Diabetic amyotrophy
Porphyria
Post-asthmatic amyotrophy (Hopkins' syndrome)
Infective
Poliomyelitis, West Nile virus, Central European encephalitis
Toxins
Lead, dapsone, botulism, tick paralysis
Compressive neuropathies (motor branches)
Differential diagnoses
Neuromuscular junction disorders: myasthenia gravis, Lambert–Eaton myasthenic syndrome
Myopathies: distal myopathies; myotonic dystrophy; inclusion body myositis

Table 10.4 Sensory predominant neuropathies.

Inherited
Hereditary sensory and autonomic neuropathies
Acute intermittent porphyria
Fabry disease
Acquired
Neuronopathies
Paraneoplastic (anti-Hu)
Sjögren's syndrome
Toxic (pyridoxine, cis-platinum)
HIV
Idiopathic inflammatory
Copper deficiency
Metabolic and deficiency states
Diabetic
Renal failure
Thiamine deficiency, pellagra, Cuban neuropathy (Strachan's syndrome)
Toxins
Alcohol, chemotherapy agents (especially platinums), metronidazole, nitrofurantoin, thalidomide, thallium, mercury, phenytoin
Infectious agents
Herpes zoster
HIV
Leprosy
Focal compressive (e.g. meralgia paraesthetica, plantar nerves)
Small fibre neuropathies
Idiopathic distal sensory axonal neuropathy
Others: myelopathies, tabes dorsalis, B_{12} deficiency

Table 10.5 Classification of the inherited neuropathies.

Neuropathies in which the neuropathy is the sole or primary part of the disease
Charcot–Marie–Tooth disease
Hereditary neuropathy with liability to pressure palsies
Hereditary sensory neuropathy (hereditary sensory and autonomic neuropathy)
Distal hereditary motor neuropathy
Hereditary neuralgic amyotrophy
Familial amyloid polyneuropathy
Neuropathies in which the neuropathy is part of a more widespread neurological or multi-system disorder
Disturbances of lipid metabolism, for example
Leukodystrophies
Lipoprotein deficiencies
Phytanic acid storage diseases

Table 10.5 (continued)

α-Galactosidase deficiency
Cerebrotendinous xanthomatosis
Porphyrias, for example
Acute intermittent
Hereditary coproporphyria
Variegate
Amino lavulinic acid dehydrase deficiency
Disorders with defective DNA, for example
Ataxia telangiectasia
Xeroderma pigmentosum
Cockayne's syndrome
Neuropathies associated with mitochondrial diseases
Neuropathies associated with hereditary ataxias, for example
Friedreich's ataxia
Spinocerebellar ataxias
Miscellaneous

amyloid polyneuropathy (FAP), a disease in which neuropathy (often including autonomic neuropathy) is the cardinal feature although other systems can be involved (e.g. heart).

The second group is a very large varied group of disorders that usually also involve the CNS (e.g. leukodystrophies, spinocerebellar ataxias) or where systems other than the nervous system are significantly involved (e.g. mitochondrial disorders and porphyrias). Many of these disorders have been covered elsewhere in this book and will not be dealt with in this chapter which concentrates on the first group where the neuropathy is the sole or primary part of the disease.

Although this classification is still very useful, next generation sequencing (NGS) techniques has identified genes that normally cause a complex neurological syndrome which includes neuropathy such as some forms of spinocerebellar ataxia, hereditary spastic paraparesis and mitochondrial diseases, but which can occasionally present with just a neuropathy and be diagnosied as CMT. This needs to be kept in mind in the evaluation of these patients.

The autosomal spinal muscular atrophies (SMA) and hereditary motor neurone disease is covered elsewhere in this chapter.

Charcot–Marie–Tooth disease and related disorders

CMT disease is a group of neuropathies that are clinically and genetically heterogeneous (Table 10.6). They are also referred to as hereditary motor and sensory neuropathies (HMSN) although CMT is now the more commonly used term. CMT is characterised clinically by distal muscle wasting and weakness, reduced reflexes, impaired distal sensation and variable foot deformity, and neurophysiologically by a motor and sensory neuropathy. There is a wide variation in the age of onset and the severity of CMT, the variation depending to a large extent on the underlying genetic defect. CMT is a motor and sensory neuropathy that is closely related to two other rarer inherited neuropathies: the hereditary sensory neuropathies (HSN) also called the hereditary sensory and autonomic neuropathies, (HSAN; Table 10.7) that either only involve sensory nerves or where sensory involvement predominates, and the hereditary motor neuropathies HMN, (Table 10.8) in which there is only motor involvement. These three disorders (CMT, HSN and HMN), often collectively termed CMT, and related disorders represent a continuum from pure motor neuropathy (HMN) through to motor and sensory neuropathy (CMT) and to sensory predominant and pure sensory neuropathy (HSN). Some recently described causative genes for axonal CMT also cause forms of distal HMN. Certain forms of CMT and HSN are very difficult to distinguish clinically. Therefore, the same phenotypes may be caused by different genes and the same gene may cause different neuropathy phenotypes. Technology is now advanced enough using NGS techniques to allow the rapid screening in an individual patient of all genes identified so far. Therefore, classification systems (Table 10.6, Table 10.7 and Table 10.8) based on clinical features including neurophysiology and neuropathology as well as the genetic cause, when known, is the most useful current classification for the practising clinician. The rate of discovery of new causative genes for CMT and related disorders has increased dramatically with the advent of NGS techniques with over 75 causative genes now reported (Figure 10.11). The genes listed in Table 10.6, Table 10.7 and Table 10.8 although comprehensive currently will need constant updating as new genes are identified. Despite this long list of causative genes, multiple studies in the United Kingdom, United States and northern European countries have shown that mutations in four genes (*PMP22, GJB1, MPZ* and *MFN2*) account for over 90% of patients receiving a genetic diagnosis. It is beyond the scope of this chapter to discuss all types of CMT; a general overview and the phenotypes of most frequent types are given.

An approach to the diagnosis of CMT and related disorders

1 *Is the neuropathy hereditary?* When a patient attends with an obviously affected family member or there is a positive family history, a genetic neuropathy is likely. Unfortunately, many patients are from small sibships (especially in the United Kingdom, United States and northern Europe) and extensive family histories are often not available. Furthermore, rates of non-paternity in Western societies are reported to be approximately 10% and *de novo* dominant mutations are not uncommon in CMT. Factors that may help the clinician decide that the neuropathy in 'sporadic' patients is hereditary include:
   - A long, slowly progressive history.
   - The presence of foot deformity such as pes cavus in an adult patient (Figure 10.9).
   - The absence of positive sensory symptoms in patients with clear sensory signs.
   - In the dominant demyelinating forms of CMT (CMT1), neurophysiology can be very useful in distinguishing hereditary from acquired neuropathies, as the motor conduction velocities are usually uniformly slow in the common hereditary neuropathies.
2 *Classifying the neuropathy*. Is the neuropathy most compatible with CMT, hereditary neuropathy with liability to pressure palsies (HNPP), HSN or distal HMN?
   - CMT is numerically the most likely diagnosis.
   - CMT is a motor *and* sensory neuropathy although the patient may not have sensory symptoms and sometimes no sensory signs (the most sensitive sensory sign is a reduction in distal vibration sensation).
   - Because distal HMN (Table 10.8) can be indistinguishable clinically from CMT it is often necessary to perform a neurophysiological examination to differentiate between these two conditions. The sensory action potentials (SAPs) should

Table 10.6 Classification of Charcot–Marie–Tooth (CMT) disease.

Type	Gene / locus	Specific phenotype
Autosomal dominant CMT1 (AD CMT1)		
CMT1A	Dup 17p (PMP22) PMP22 (point mutation)	Classic CMT1 Classic CMT1 / DSD / CHN (rarely recessive)
CMT1B	MPZ	CMT1 / DSD / CHN / CMT2 (rarely recessive)
CMT1C	LITAF	Classic CMT1
CMT1D	EGR2	Classic CMT1 / DSD / CHN
CMT1F	NEFL	CMT2 but can have slow MCVs in CMT1 range ± early onset severe disease (rare AR CMT2 cases described)
CMT1 plus	FBLN5	CMT1 plus macular degeneration, cutis laxa / HMN
Hereditary neuropathy with liability to pressure palsies (HNPP)		
HNPP	Del 17p (PMP-22) PMP-22 (point mutation)	Typical HNPP Typical HNPP
Autosomal recessive CMT1 (CMT4 / AR CMT1)		
CMT4A	GDAP1	CMT1 or CMT2 usually early onset and severe / vocal cord and diaphragm paralysis described (rare AD CMT2 families described)
CMT4B1	MTMR2	Severe CMT1 / facial / bulbar / focally folded myelin
CMT4B2	SBF2	Severe CMT1 / glaucoma / focally folded myelin
CMT4B3	SBF1	CMT1 / focally folded myelin
CMT4C	SH3TC2	Severe CMT1 / scoliosis / cytoplasmic expansions
CMT4D (HMSNL)	NDRG1	Severe CMT1 / gypsy / deafness / tongue atrophy
CMT4E	EGR2	CMT1 / DSD / CHN phenotype
CMT4F	Periaxin	CMT1 / more sensory / focally folded myelin
CMT4G (HMSN Russe)	HK1	Severe early onset CMT1; gypsy
CMT4H	FGD4	Classic CMT1
CMT4J	FIG4	CMT1 / predominantly motor / progressive
CCFDN	CTDP1	CMT1 / gypsy / cataracts / dysmorphic features
CMT4	SURF1	CMT1 / lactic acidosis / abnormal brain MRI / cerebellar ataxia
AR CMT1	PMP22 (point mutation)	Classic CMT1 / DSD / CHN
AR CMT1	MPZ	CMT1 / DSD / CHN / CMT2
Autosomal dominant CMT2 (AD CMT 2)		
CMT2A	MFN2	Classic CMT2 / more progressive / optic atrophy (rarely recessive)
CMT2B	RAB7	CMT2 with predominant sensory involvement and sensory complications
CMT2C	TRPV4	CMT2 with vocal cord and respiratory involvement / congenital distal SMA
CMT2D	GARS	CMT2 with predominant hand wasting / weakness or distal HMN5
CMT2E	NEFL	CMT2 but can have slow MCVs in CMT1 range ± early onset severe disease (rarely recessive)
CMT2F	HSPB1	Motor predominant CMT2 or distal HMN2B

Table 10.6 (continued)

Type	Gene / locus	Specific phenotype
CMT2I	MPZ	Late onset CMT2
CMT2J	MPZ	CMT2 with hearing loss and pupillary abnormalities
CMT2K	GDAP1	Classic CMT2 (dominant); severe CMT2 (recessive)
CMT2L	HSPB8	Motor predominant CMT2 or distal HMN2A
CMT2M	DMN2	CMT2 or intermediate CMT / cataracts / ophthalmoplegia / ptosis
CMT2O	DYNC1H1	Motor predominant CMT2 / learning difficulties
CMT2P	LRSAM1	CMT2 (can be recessive)
CMT2Q	DHTKD1	CMT2
CMT2	MARS	Late onset CMT2
CMT2	HARS	CMT2
HMSNP	TFG	CMT2 with proximal involvement
SPG10	KIF5A	CMT2 / hereditary spastic paraparesis
CMT2	MT-ATP6	CMT2 / ptramidal signs / relapsing
Autosomal recessive CMT2 (AR CMT2)		
CMT2B1	LMNA	CMT2 proximal involvement and rapid progression described / also causes muscular dystrophy / cardiomyopathy / lipodystrophy
CMT2B2	MED25	Classic CMT2
CMT2H	GDAP1	CMT2 or CMT1 usually early onset and severe / vocal cord and diaphragm paralysis described (rare AD CMT2 families described)
AR CMT2	LRSAM1	Classic CMT2
AR CMT2	TRIM2	Early onset CMT2
AR CMT2	HADHB	Early onset CMT2
AR CMT2	C12 or f65	CMT2 plus optic atrophy / pyramidal signs
X-linked CMT		
CMTX1	GJB1	Males CMT1 (patchy NCV); females CMT2
CMTX4 (Cowchock syndrome)	AIFM1	CMT2; infantile onset, developmental delay, deafness, learning difficulties
CMTX5	PRPS1	CMT2; deafness, usually optic atrophy
CMTX6	PDK3	CMT2
Dominant intermediate CMT (DI-CMT)		
CMTD1B	DNM2	Intermediate CMT or CMT2; cataracts; ophthalmoplegia; ptosis
CMTDIC	YARS	Intermediate CMT
CMTDID	MPZ	Intermediate CMT
CMTDIE	INF2	Intermediate CMT; focal segmental glomerulosclerosis; end-stage renal failure
CMTDIF	GNB4	Intermediate CMT

(continued)

Table 10.6 (continued)

Type	Gene / locus	Specific phenotype
Recessive intermediate CMT (RI-CMT)		
CMTR1A	GDAP1	Intermediate CMT
CMTR1B	KARS	Intermediate CMT; learning difficulties; vestibular Schwannoma
PRI-CMT	PLEKHG5	Intermediate CMT; SMA
Hereditary neuralgic amytrophy		
	SEPT9	Recurrent neuralgic amyotrophy

AD, autosomal dominant; AR, autosomal recessive.

Table 10.7 Classification of the hereditary sensory neuropathies (HSN/HSAN).

Type	Inheritance	Gene/locus	Specific phenotype
HSN1A	AD	SPTLC-1	Mainly sensory, sensory complications Occasionally motor early, males more severe
HSN1C	AD	SPTLC-2	Mainly sensory, sensory complications Occasionally motor early
CMT2B	AD	RAB7	Sensorimotor, sensory complications
HSN1D	AD	ATL1	HSN with sensory complications/hereditary spastic paraparesis
HSN1E	AD	DNMT1	HSN; deafness; dementia
HSN2A	AR	WNK1	HSN with severe sensory complications, mutilations
HSN2B	AR	FAM134B	HSN with sensory complications
HSN2C	AR	KIF1A	HSN with sensory complications
HSN2D	AR	SCN9A	Congenital insensitivity to pain (dominant mutations paroxysmal extreme pain disorder; primary erythermalgia; small fibre neuropathy)
HSN3	AR	IKBKAP	Familial dysautonomia or Riley–Day syndrome Prominent autonomic, absence fungiform papillae of the tongue
HSN4	AR	NTRK1	Congenital insensitivity to pain with anhydrosis (CIPA) with severe sensory involvement, anhydrosis, mental retardation Unmyelinated fibres mainly affected
HSN5	AR	NGFB	Congenital insensitivity to pain, minimal autonomic No mental retardation Mainly unmyelinated fibres affected
HSN6	AR	DST	HSAN
HSN	AR	CCT5	HSN with spastic paraplegia
HSN	AD	PRNP	HSAN; autonomic dysfunction; dementia
HSAN	De novo dominant	SCN11A	HSAN

AD, autosomal dominant; AR, autosomal recessive.

Table 10.8 Classification of the distal hereditary motor neuropathies (distal HMN).

Type	Inheritance	Gene/locus	Specific phenotype
HMN 2A	AD	HSPB8	Classic distal HMN/CMT2F
HMN 2B	AD	HSPB1	Classic distal HMN/CMT2L
HMN2C	AD	HSPB3	Classic distal HMN
HMN	AD	SETX	Distal HMN with pyramidal features
HMN	AR	DNAJB2	Classic distal HMN
HMN5A	AD	BSCL2	Upper limb predominant; Silver syndrome; occasional mild sensory
HMN5A	AD	GARS	Upper limb predominant; occasional early onset
HMN5B	AD	REEP1	Predominant hand wasting; pyramidal signs
HMN6	AR	IGHMB2	Spinal muscle atrophy with respiratory distress (SMARD1), infantile onset respiratory distress
HMN7A	AD	SLC5A7	Adult onset, vocal cord paralysis
HMN7B	AD	DCTN1	Adult onset, vocal cord paralysis/facial weakness
SMAX3	X-linked	ATP7A	Classic distal HMN
SMALED	AD	DYNC1H1	Congenital; contractures; lower limb predominant; cortical migration defects; learning difficulties
SMALED	AD	BICD2	Congenital; contractures; lower limb predominant; late pyramidal signs
HMN	AD	TRPV4	HMN; scapular winging; vocal cord paralysis; can be congenital
HMN	AD	AARS	Classic distal HMN
HMN	AD	HINT1	Distal HMN; neuromyotonia
HMN	AD	FBOX38	Distal HMN with calf predominance

AD, autosomal dominant; AR, autosomal recessive.

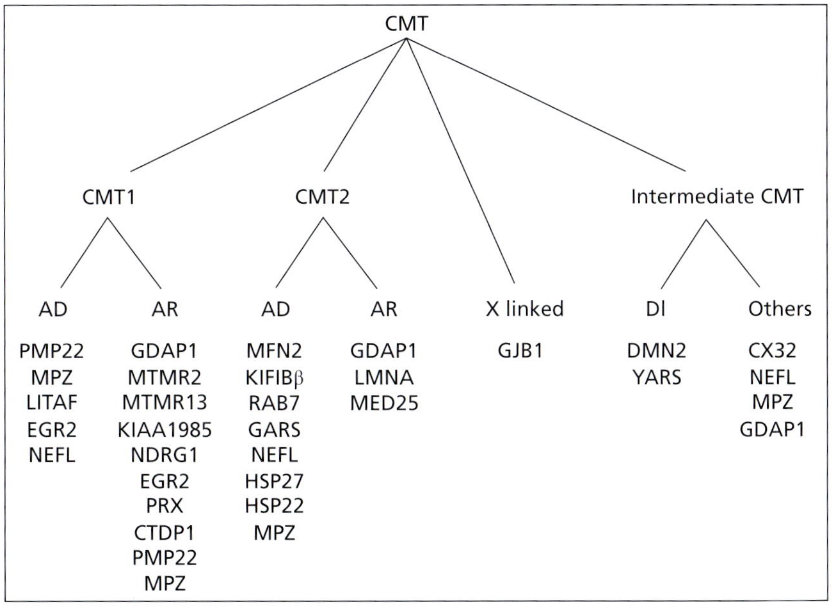

Figure 10.11 Causative genes for Charcot–Marie–Tooth disease (CMT). AD, autosomal dominant; AR, autosomal recessive; CTDP1, CTD phosphatase, subunit 1; DMN2, dynamin 2; EGR2, early growth response 2; GARS, glycyl-tRNA synthetase; GDAP1, ganglioside-induced differentiation-associated protein 1; GJB1, gap junction protein, beta 1; HSP 27, heat shock 27 kDa protein 1; HSP 22, heat shock 22 kDa protein 8; KIAA1985, K1AA1985 protein; KIF1Bß, kinesin family member 1B-ß; LITAF, lipopolysaccharide-induced tumour necrosis factor; LMNA, lamin A/C; MED25, mediator of RNA polymerase II, subunit 25; MFN2, mitofusin 2; MPZ, myelin protein zero; MTMR2, myotubularin-related protein 2; MTMR13, myotubularin-related protein 13; NDRG1, N-myc downstream-regulated gene 1; NEFL, neurofilament, light polypeptide 68 kDa; PMP-22, peripheral myelin protein 22; PRX, periaxin; RAB7, RAS-associated protein RAB7; YARS, tyrosyl-tRNA synthetase. Source: Forbes 1993. Reproduced with permission of Elsevier.

always be involved (reduced or absent) in CMT and normal in distal HMN.

- The neuropathy of HNPP is usually easily distinguished from CMT as the patient normally has a history of recurrent pressure palsies but may later accumulate neurological deficits. The neurophysiological findings are usually patchier in HNPP than in the common forms of CMT1.
- Most forms of HSN (Table 10.7) have more sensory and in some forms autonomic involvement and less motor involvement than CMT. The presence of neuropathic pain makes HSN1 secondary to *SPTLC* mutations more likely and is a useful differentiating feature.
- Additional features such as upper motor neurone signs can be found in certain forms of CMT, HSN and distal HMN.

Charcot–Marie–Tooth disease

CMT disease is the most common of the hereditary neuropathies. The classification of CMT is in a state of constant flux reflecting the rapid advances in the identification of the underlying causative genes. Despite the rapid genetic advances the most useful method of classification for clinicians is a combination of clinical presentation, neurophysiology and inheritance pattern combined with the causative gene when known (Table 10.6).

CMT is classified as either demyelinating (CMT1) if the median (or ulnar) nerve motor conduction velocity (MCV) is <38 m/s or axonal (CMT2) if the median MCV is >38 m/s (Table 10.6). The concept of an intermediate form of CMT with median MCVs in the intermediate range (25–45 m/s) has been around since the 1970s and although sometimes out of favour it can be helpful in directing genetic diagnosis.

The inheritance pattern may not be clinically obvious until a genetic diagnosis has been established as *de novo* dominant mutations, autosomal recessive (AR) mutations and other factors may obscure it. In most UK, north European and US populations where there are few consanguineous marriages, about 90% of cases of CMT are either autosomal dominant (AD) or X-linked; the ethnic background of the population should always be taken into account.

Autosomal dominant CMT1

Classic CMT1 The most common form of CMT in most populations is AD CMT1; patients usually present with a 'classic CMT' phenotype in the first two decades with motor symptoms in the lower limbs, for example difficulty walking or foot deformity. On examination, they have evidence of distal wasting and weakness and hyporeflexia affecting the lower limbs to a greater extent than the upper limbs. Distal sensory loss and foot deformity are frequent findings. Neurophysiologically, the median MCVs are <38 m/s and the SAPs are either reduced or absent. Nerve biopsies are no longer necessary to make the diagnosis but if performed show a demyelinating neuropathy with classic onion bulbs (Figure 10.12).

If there is a clear family history of AD inheritance, or if the patient is apparently 'sporadic', then the most likely diagnosis is CMT1A secondary to a duplication of the peripheral myelin protein 22 gene (*PMP22*). In a European population this duplication accounts for 70% of all CMT1 cases. Point mutations in the *PMP22* gene can also cause CMT1A but a wider spectrum of phenotypes is described with these.

CMT1B is less common and is caused by mutations in the myelin protein zero gene (*MPZ*). Patients may present with the classic CMT1 phenotype but are more likely to present with either a more severe, early onset form of CMT1 or a much milder, late onset form of CMT with median MCVs in the axonal range. As a result patients with *MPZ*-related CMT can be classified as CMT1, intermediate CMT or CMT2, depending on the MCVs.

Mutations in *EGR2* and *LITAF* are very rare and account for fewer than 1% of cases each and have no particular distinguishing features. Mutations in *NEFL* (neurofilament light polypeptide) were originally described as a cause of CMT2. Some patients with *NEFL* mutations have median MCVs in the demyelinating range and so patients with *NEFL*-related CMT can be classified as CMT1, intermediate CMT or CMT2, depending on the MCVs.

Severe CMT1 (HMSN III, Dejerine–Sottas disease, congenital hypomyelinating neuropathy) The severe cases of CMT1 used to be called HMSN III in older classifications and were subdivided into Dejerine–Sottas disease (DSD) and congenital hypomyelinating neuropathy (CHN) depending on the underlying pathology. They

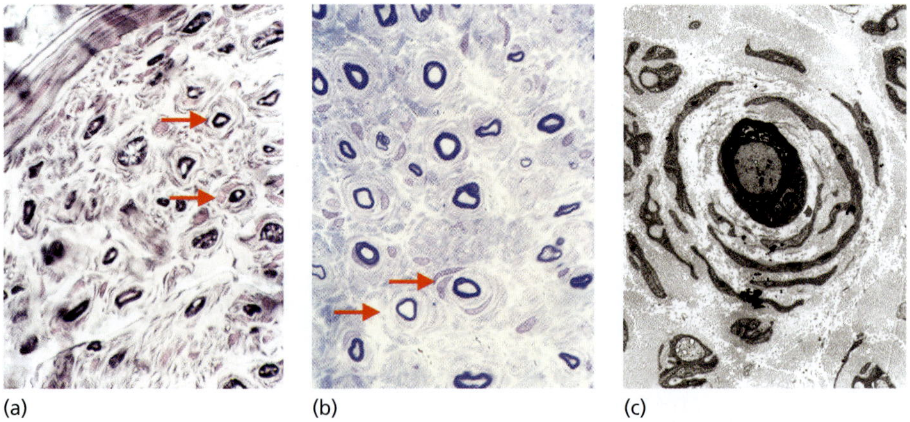

Figure 10.12 Charcot–Marie–Tooth type 1a with formation of onion bulbs. (a) Paraffin section (transverse) shows concentric formations (arrows) with a reduction of fibre density. The interstitial space is widened, indicating an oedema with a mucoid component. (b) Semithin resin section (tolouidin blue) confirms the abundant presence of onion bulbs (arrows). (c) Electron microscopy of the same nerve with concentric arrangement of Schwann cells around myelinated axons. The Schwann cells appear as plump, elongated and rounded stacks, separated by longitudinally oriented collagen fibres (light grey).

usually present in the first decade with very slow MCVs and a more severe neuropathy than classic CMT1. It was thought that most of these cases were recessive but we now know they are usually secondary to *de novo* dominant mutations in the three genes that commonly cause AD CMT1 (*PMP22, MPZ, EGR2*). Mutations in these three genes, which cause the DSD/CHN phenotype, can also occasionally be inherited in an AR fashion (Table *10.6*). Some of the other genes that cause recessive CMT1 can present with a similar phenotype (see Autosomal recessive CMT1 and Table *10.6*).

Hereditary neuropathy with liability to pressure palsies HNPP is an AD condition usually caused by a deletion of the same portion of chromosome 17 as is duplicated in CMT1A. Point mutations in *PMP22* can also rarely cause HNPP. Most patients with HNPP present with episodic recurrent pressure palsies, although atypical presentations have been described. Diagnostically, an important point is that although patients may present with only one nerve clinically involved at a particular time, there is always a more generalised patchy demyelinating neuropathy neurophysiologically. Screening for the chromosome 17 deletion is therefore not warranted in isolated pressure palsies that do not have electrophysiological abnormalities outside the clinically involved nerve.

X-linked CMT1 The X-linked form of CMT1 is caused by mutations in the gap junction β1 gene (*GJB1*) which codes for connexin 32. This is the second most common form of CMT. Over 300 mutations have been described in *GJB1*. Males are more severely affected than females. The MCVs in affected males are usually in the demyelinating range. Conversely, the MCVs in the females are usually in the axonal range but can be in the demyelinating range. Connexin 32 related CMT is therefore another form of intermediate CMT.

Patients (especially males) can have a rather patchy neuropathy both clinically and neurophysiologically with less uniform conduction slowing, differences in conduction velocities between nerves (e.g. ulnar and median) and more pronounced dispersion than that seen with AD CMT1. This can lead to difficulties in diagnosis in patients without a family history and occasionally to patients being diagnosed with CIDP, leading to unnecessary immunosuppressive therapy. CNS involvement is occasionally seen and is usually mild (extensor plantars, mild deafness, abnormal brainstem evoked potentials). A useful clue diagnostically is that abductor pollicis brevis is usually more wasted, weaker and has a lower compound muscle action potential (CMAP) that the first dorsal interosseous (the so-called split hand syndrome).

Autosomal recessive CMT1 In communities where consanguinity is high AR CMT may account for 30–50% of all CMT cases. There are now 15 genes described that can cause AR CMT1 (including the three genes *PMP22, MPZ* and *EGR2* that more commonly cause AD or *de novo* dominant CMT1). AR CMT1 is also commonly called CMT4 and the various forms are classified as CMT4A, CMT4B, etc.

Unfortunately, there is no one gene that is a major cause of AR CMT1/CMT4 which makes the diagnosis difficult for the clinician presented with a patient with presumed AR CMT1/CMT4.

Although no one algorithm is suitable for the diagnosis of AR CMT1/CMT4, there are some clinical indicators that can be used to aid diagnosis. These indicators are still pertinent in the era of NGS as often more than one variant is identified in multiple candidate genes in a patient and clinical features are invaluable is helping decide the most likely causative gene.

1 As a general rule, AR forms of CMT have an earlier onset and are more severe than AD cases. They usually start as a length dependent neuropathy but are more likely to progress to involve the proximal muscles and to result in loss of ambulation than AD patients. Associated clinical features, the ethnic background of patients and specific neuropathological features can aid the diagnosis (Table 10.6).
2 Neurophysiology may be difficult, as in severe cases all the nerves may be inexcitable although proximal nerves such as the axillary and facial nerves can sometimes be studied. In the cases where neurophysiology is not useful, nerve biopsies can be particularly helpful. Biopsy is also more useful in AR CMT1/CMT4 in general than in AD CMT1 as specific features in nerve biopsies may make a particular genetic diagnosis more likely (e.g. cytoplasmic processes in CMT4C). This is the major diagnostic use for nerve biopsy in genetic neuropathies.
3 Specific phenotypes in AR CMT1 (CMT4) are recognised:
   - CMT4A secondary to mutations in *GDAP1* is usually an early onset progressive neuropathy and can be associated with diaphragmatic and vocal cord involvement. Mutations in *GDAP1* can also cause AR CMT2 and even more rarely AD CMT2, making *GDAP1*-related CMT another intermediate form of CMT.
   - Nerve biopsies showing focally folded myelin are characteristic of CMT4B1 (*MTMR2* mutations), CMT4B2 (*SBF2* mutations) and CMT4B3 (*SBF1* mutations) although this finding has also been described with *MPZ* mutations and in CMT4F secondary to periaxin mutations.
   - Severe and early scoliosis is seen with CMT4C secondary to mutations in the *SH3TC2* gene. Patients with mutations in this gene also have characteristic nerve biopsy features including basal membrane onion bulbs and multiple cytoplasmic processes of the Schwann cells of unmyelinated axons.
   - Three forms of AR CMT1 are largely confined to patients of Balkan Romany origin. CMT4D secondary to *NDRG1* mutations is characterised by a demyelinating neuropathy with a high incidence of deafness. Tongue atrophy has also been described in this form of CMT. Another form of AR CMT1 seen in this Romany population is CCFDN (congenital cataract, facial dysmorphism and neuropathy syndrome) secondary to *CTDP1* mutations. The third form of CMT in this population, HMSN Russe, is caused HK1 mutations.
   - A phenotype ranging from a severe DSD type phenotype to a milder neuropathy with mainly sensory involvement is seen in CMT4F secondary to periaxin mutations.
   - *FIG4* mutations (CMT4J) cause a severe and progressive demyelinating phenotype; patients can develop a rapid increase in weakness with acute denervation in one or more limbs mimicking an acquired inflammatory neuropathy. Although the acute denervation and rapidity of the evolution of weakness in these cases has also been described to mimic motor neurone disease, the slow conduction velocities and accompanying sensory involvement help to distinguish between these two diseases.

To summarise, although there are many different genes identified as causing AR CMT1 careful phenotyping of the patients together with consideration of the ethnic background can help guide the genetic diagnosis.

Autosomal dominant CMT2 The true prevalence of CMT2 is not known. However, any adult presenting with a long-standing mild axonal neuropathy without an obvious family history and where an acquired cause has not been identified may have CMT2 but this is difficult to prove. Nineteen causative genes for AD CMT2 have been described (Table 10.6). These still account for less than 50% of the total cases of AD CMT2 and, until all the causative genes for CMT2 are identified, we will not know the true prevalence of this condition.

Autosomal dominant CMT2 can broadly be divided into three different groups by phenotype which can be helpful in establishing the causative gene.

1 Most patients with AD CMT2 present with the 'classic CMT' phenotype, clinically indistinguishable from AD CMT1. The neurophysiology revealing an axonal sensorimotor neuropathy distinguishes between the two. Nerve biopsies are rarely performed in patients with AD CMT2 as a non-diagnostic axonal neuropathy is usually described. Many patients with the classic CMT2 phenotype do not have a genetic diagnosis although some have mutations in Mitofusin 2 (*MFN2*), the gene that accounts for approximately 20% of all cases of AD CMT2 in all populations tested so far. Patients with mutations in *MFN2* often present early and with a more severe phenotype with fairly rapid progression to proximal muscle involvement and loss of ambulation. Occasionally, patients may have brisk reflexes. Furthermore, approximately 20% of the mutations are *de novo*, explaining why so many of these patients have normal parents. Mutations in *MFN2* also cause axonal CMT with optic atrophy (HMSN VI in previous classifications). In patients with classic AD CMT2 and no mutation in *MFN2*, both *MPZ* and *NEFL* should be screened as they can cause this phenotype. Other genes listed in Table 10.6 are rare causes of the classic CMT2 phenotype.
2 The second phenotype seen with AD CMT2 has much more sensory involvement than is usually seen with CMT. These patients have been described as having an 'autosomal dominant inherited neuropathy with prominent sensory loss and ulceromutilating features'. They were originally classified as CMT2B. Presentation is in the second or third decade with typical motor CMT features but also severe sensory complications including ulcerations, osteomyelitis and amputations. The causative gene for CMT2B is *RAB7*. The presentation of these patients is also very similar to patients with HSN1 secondary to mutations in the *SPTLC-1* or *SPTLC-2* genes (Table 10.7; i.e. different genes, same phenotypes). Patients with *SPTLC-1* or *SPTLC-2* mutations usually have less motor involvement at presentation and also lancinating pain, an unusual feature in hereditary neuropathies. Sometimes conduction velocities can be in the demyelinating range in patients with *SPTLC-1* or *SPTLC-2* mutations and males are often more severely affected than females. There remain other families with this phenotype who do not have mutations in either *SPTLC-1, SPTLC-2* or *RAB7*, suggesting other unidentified genes can also cause this phenotype.
3 The third phenotype seen with AD CMT2 is a motor predominant phenotype where there is very little sensory involvement,. Some patients with this phenotype have a typical length dependent motor predominant neuropathy with lower limbs more affected than upper limbs. Two genes, *HSPB1* and *HSPB8,* can cause this phenotype and these are of additional interest as they more commonly cause a purely motor phenotype, distal HMN type 2 (Table 10.8; i.e. same gene, different phenotype). A characteristic feature of the neuropathy associated with *HSPB1* and *HSPB8* is that ankle plantar flexion is usually affected early and is as severely affected as ankle dorsiflexion, unlike classic CMT where ankle dorsiflexion is involved much earlier and to a greater extent then ankle plantar flexion. Some patients with the motor predominant form of AD CMT2 have more more upper limb than lower limb involvement, classified as CMT2D. Patients were originally described presenting with wasting and weakness of the small muscles of the hand (onset can also be unilateral and misdiagnosed as thoracic outlet syndrome) with much later involvement of the distal lower limb muscles. Interestingly, as with mutations in *HSPB1* and *HSPB8*, some of these patients had no sensory involvement and were classified as distal HMN type 5 (Table 10.8). CMT2D and distal HMN 5 have now been shown to be allelic with two causative genes identified for this phenotype, *GARS* and *BSCL2* although there are patients with this phenotype without mutations in either of these genes. Mutations in the *BSCL2* gene can also cause Silver's syndrome (spastic legs and distal amyotrophy of the upper limbs). Another interesting gene that cause either CMT2 or a hereditary motor neuropathy (which can be associated with scapular winging or congenital onset) is *TRPV4*. Vocal cord palsy is common with *TRPV4* mutations.

Autosomal recessive CMT2 There are 10 causative genes known for AR CMT including AR CMT2 due to homozgous or compound heterozygous mutations in *MFN2* and *NEFL*, which more commonly cause AD CMT2. All forms of AR CMT2 are rare and the causative genes are listed in Table 10.6 but a few warrant further mention as they have interesting phenotypes.

Mutations in lamin A/C (*LMNA*) cause AR CMT2A. Moroccan and Algerian families were reported with this phenotype. Most patients present in the second decade with a severe CMT phenotype including proximal muscle involvement although some patients have been reported with a milder phenotype. Lamin A/C mutations have been associated with a wide spectrum of phenotypes including Emery–Dreyfuss muscular dystrophy, cardiomyopathy, Dunniugan-type familial partial lipodystrophy and many others.

The second form of AR CMT2, AR CMT2B, was described in a Costa Rican family and the gene for this type is *MED25*. The phenotype of AR CMT2B is milder than seen with the other AR CMT2 genes and is more like classic CMT2. Another rare AR cause of the classic CMT2 phenotype are mutations in *LRSAM1*. As shown in Table 10.6, *LRSAM1* mutations can also cause AD CMT2.

Mutations in *GDAP1* have been described above as a cause of AR CMT1 (CMT4A) but they can also cause AR CMT2 with a similar severe early onset phenotype which can include vocal cord paresis.

A characteristic feature of AR CMT2 secondary to mutations in *HINT1*, which has been described as an important cause of AR CMT2 in a number of Euroepan countries, is a high incidence of neuromyotonia. Some patients have no sensory involvement and are classified as having distal HMN.

X-linked CMT2 X-linked CMT2 is very rare and can be caused by mutations in *AIFM1*, *PRPS1* and *PDK3*. As seen in Table 10.6, there are commonly associated clinical features such as deafness.

Dominant intermediate CMT It is increasingly recognised that many forms of CMT can present with MCVs in the intermediate range as discussed earlier. These include patients with X-linked CMT resulting from *GJB1* mutations, patients with AD CMT caused by *MPZ* or *NEFL* mutations and patients with AR CMT caused by *GDAP1* mutations. In addition to these forms of intermediate CMT, a number of genes have recently been described including *DNM2, YARS, GNB4* and *IFN2* that cause CMT with intermediate MCVs and these have been classified as dominant intermediate CMT (Table 10.6). Mutations in *IFN2* cause an unusual form of CMT associated with renal failure resulting from focal segmental glomerulosclerosis.

Hereditary sensory neuropathy

HSN is much rarer than CMT but a number of causative genes for these disorders have been identified (Table 10.7). Generally, these disorders are characterised by prominent sensory and in some cases autonomic involvement and less motor involvement than CMT. The sensory involvement can be severe and result in mutilating injuries. Education of the patients to try to prevent these complications is crucial. Many patients with HSN have not had a genetic cause identified but phenotypes associated with specifc genes include:

- HSN1A secondary to *SPTLC-1* and HSN1C secondary to *SPTLC-2* mutations have already been mentioned. This disease is more appropriately termed HSN than HSAN as there is usually no autonomic involvement. Mutations in *ATL1* which more commonly causes a spastic paraparesis can also cause HSN1.
- Mutations in *DNMT1* cause an unusual form of HSN1 (HSN1E) with associated deafness and dementia.
- Mutations in the prion protein, PRNP, have also been described to cause a sensory and autonomic neuropathy with dementia in two families.
- All other forms of HSN are rare. HSN2 is an early onset, AR, severe sensory neuropathy with prominent sensory complications and is caused by mutations in a number of genes including *WNK1*, *FAM13B4* and *KIF1A*.
- HSAN3 (Riley–Day syndrome) is a distinct autosomal recessive neuropathy seen in Ashkenazi Jews and characterised by mainly autonomic involvement but it also involves the PNS, particularly the sensory nerves. The causative gene is the *IKBKAP* gene. Presentation is often in infancy or childhood with poor feeding, swallowing difficulties and recurrent chest infections.
- HSAN4 and HSAN5 are both AR neuropathies characterised by congenital insensitivity to pain. HSN4 (also called congenital insensitivity to pain with anhydrosis [CIPA]) presents with a severe sensory neuropathy, anhydrosis and mental retardation and is caused by mutations in the *NTRK1* gene, a receptor for nerve growth factor. HSN5 is similar but without the mental retardation or significant anhydrosis. This phenotype has been described with both *NTRK1* mutations and also with *NGFB* mutations. A recent development in the hereditary sensory neuropathies has been the identification of homozygous mutations in the gene (*SCN9A*) for the voltage-gated sodium 1.7 channel ($NA_v1.7$) in a form of HSAN resembling type V and termed HSN2D or channelopathy-associated insensitivity to pain.

Distal hereditary motor neuropathy

The distal hereditary motor neuropathies (dHMNs) are a complex group of disorders (Table 10.8) also referred to as distal spinal muscular atrophies (distal SMA). Forms that resemble CMT have been discussed earlier. Like HSN, many patients with HMN have not had a genetic cause identified but phenotypes associated with specifc genes include the following.

- Distal HMN2 is the classic form of AD distal HMN and is caused by mutations in the *HSPB8 (HMN2A)* and *HSPB1 (HMN2B)* genes. These patients present with classic CMT (but as described above with more ankle plantar flexion weakness) but without any sensory involvement.
- Mutations in *GARS* and *BSCL2* cause distal HMN5 as previously described and this phenotype can also be caused by mutations in *REEP1*, which usually causes a spastic paraparesis.
- Distal HMN6 is an unusually severe AR form of distal HMN that presents in infancy with respiratory and distal limb involvement (called spinal muscle atrophy with respiratory distress type 1 [SMARD1]) and is caused by mutations in the *IGHMBP2* gene.
- Mutations in dynactin (*DCTN1*) or *SLC5A7* cause distal HMN7, which is characterised by vocal cord paralysis and progressive weakness and atrophy of the face, hands and legs. Missense mutations in senataxin (*SETX*) can cause a form of distal HMN with pyramidal features. Nonsense mutations in the same gene cause autosomal recessive ataxia oculomotor apraxia type 2 (AOA2).
- A rare X-linked form of HMN due to mutations in the *ATP7A* gene (which also causes the severe infantile onset developmental disorder, Menkes disease and its milder variant, occipital horn syndrome) has been described.
- A form of hereditary motor neuropathy which has been called spinal muscle atrophy with lower extremity predominance (SMALED) is due to mutations in two genes, *DYNC1H1* and *BICD2*, which give a distinct phenotype of almost exclusive involvement of the distal and proximal lower limb muscles which is usually congenital and non-progressive. Some patients with mutations in *DYNC1H1* also have learnng difficulities and some with mutations in *BICD2* develop mild spasticity in later life.

Hereditary neuralgic amyotrophy

HNA is an autosomal dominant condition caused by mutations in the SEPT9 gene and characterised by recurrent episodes of typical brachial neuritis. The attacks are characterised by pain, weakness and sensory disturbance in the brachial plexus distribution. These attacks are indistinguishable from sporadic brachial neuritis but are recurrent, often starting in childhood.

Importance of a genetic diagnosis in CMT and related disorders

Our ability to identify the genetic causes of CMT and its related disorders in patients has been revolutionised by the advent of NGS which allows large number of genes to be screened simultaneously either by disease-specific panels, whole exome or whole genome sequencing. In inherited neuropathies, the major challenge is validating identified mutations as pathogenic as multiple variants are usually identified, most causative genes for inherited neuropathies are ubiquitously expressed and there are very few functional tests available in inherited neurpapthies to prove a particular mutation in a specific gene is the cause of the neuropathy. Careful phenotyping remains a crucial step in validating identified mutations.

An accurate genetic diagnosis is extremely important for these patients. There are obvious benefits including diagnostic testing for other family members, accurate genetic counselling and prognosis, predictive and antenatal testing but an accurate diagnosis also prevents patients from having unnecessary and invasive diagnostic tests, for example nerve biopsies and lumbar punctures. In certain situations where inflammatory neuropathies are being considered a genetic diagnosis can prevent a trial of potentially dangerous immunosuppressive therapy.

The era of treatment for genetic neuropathies is here. The first therapeutic trials in CMT have been completed (ascorbic acid for CMT1A, which were unfortunately negative) and more are planned. Drug discovery programmes are actively hunting for new therapeutics and although some of these may be mechanism driven, it seems likely that other developments (at least at the trial stage) could now be gene-specific, making the case for an accurate genetic diagnosis even more convincing.

Familial amyloid polyneuropathy

Familial amyloid polyneuropathy (FAP) is an AD condition first described in Portugal in 1952. The amyloidoses are characterised by deposition of a fibrillar β-pleated protein in the extracellular space of many organs. Only AL (light chain) amyloidosis and FAP cause a generalised neuropathy with autonomic involvement. AL amyloid is discussed later. Within the familial amyloidoses there are more than 30 proteins that can form amyloid deposits but there are only four different forms of FAP classified by the constituent amyloid-forming protein: transthyretin (TTR), apolipoprotein A-1 (Apo A-1), gelsolin and beta-2 microglobulin (one family).

Transthyretin-related familial amyloid polyneuropathy

Clinical features The cardinal clinical features of TTR-related FAP are a sensory motor peripheral neuropathy usually with autonomic involvement, a cardiomyopathy and to a lesser extent vitreous involvement. Other systems can be involved. Over 100 mutations in TTR have been described, the most common of which is the index Met30 point mutation. Clinical features do not always correlate well with a specific mutation.

Patients with TTR Met30 usually present with painful dysaesthesia in the lower limbs progressing to a severe mixed polyneuropathy. Early there is greater small fibre susceptibility giving rise to lack of pain and temperature sensation, but eventually all sensory modalities are involved. Mutilating injuries can occur. Later motor involvement is universal, with upper limb involvement occurring months to years after lower limb manifestations. Carpal tunnel syndrome (CTS) as a presenting feature is rare in TTR Met30. Autonomic involvement occurs frequently and can be severe and early.

Neurophysiological studies confirm an axonal neuropathy although SAPs may be normal early in the course of the disease, reflecting the mainly small fibre involvement. Cardiac involvement is common, presenting as an arrhythmia, heart block or heart failure, and amyloid deposition results in abnormal echocardiographic appearances. Vitreous involvement is more common in Swedish than Portuguese TTR Met30 patients and may be the presenting feature. Kidneys and, more rarely, pulmonary or bone involvement also occur.

Other common mutations include TTR Tyr 77 and TTR Ala 60. FAP TTR Tyr 77 has a high incidence of CTS but absent vitreous involvement. FAP TTR Ala 60 is mainly seen in patients of Irish descent and typically presents in the sixth decade with more prominent small and large fibre sensory loss than TTR Met30. Cardiomyopathy is a major and commonly a presenting feature.

CNS involvement in FAP TTR is very rare and, although postmortem studies have shown leptomeningeal amyloid deposition, this is usually asymptomatic. Oculoleptomeningeal amyloidosis (OLMA) is associated with TTR point mutations. The clinical features vary even within a kindred and include vitreous opacities, progressive dementia, stroke, subarachnoid haemorrhage, ataxia, hydrocephalus, seizures, spasticity and episodes of fluctuating consciousness often with focal neurological signs. The hallmarks of the CNS disease are meningeal enhancement of the brain and spinal cord on magnetic resonance imaging (MRI) and a raised cerebrospinal fluid (CSF) protein.

Pathology The pathological changes in the PNS are similar in FAP and AL amyloidosis. The amyloid in the PNS appears as extracellular, amorphous, eosinophilic deposits, which are found both diffusely in the endoneurium and epineurium and surrounding endoneurial and epineurial blood vessels. They are also present in sensory and autonomic ganglia. In milder cases there is predominant loss of small myelinated and unmyelinated axons; at later stages larger myelinated fibres are also lost. The pathology is predominantly one of axonal degeneration with some regenerative activity. Segmental demyelination has also been described. Congo red staining has apple green birefringence under polarised light and under electron microscopy (EM) rigid 10–15 nm fibrils are seen (Figure 10.13).

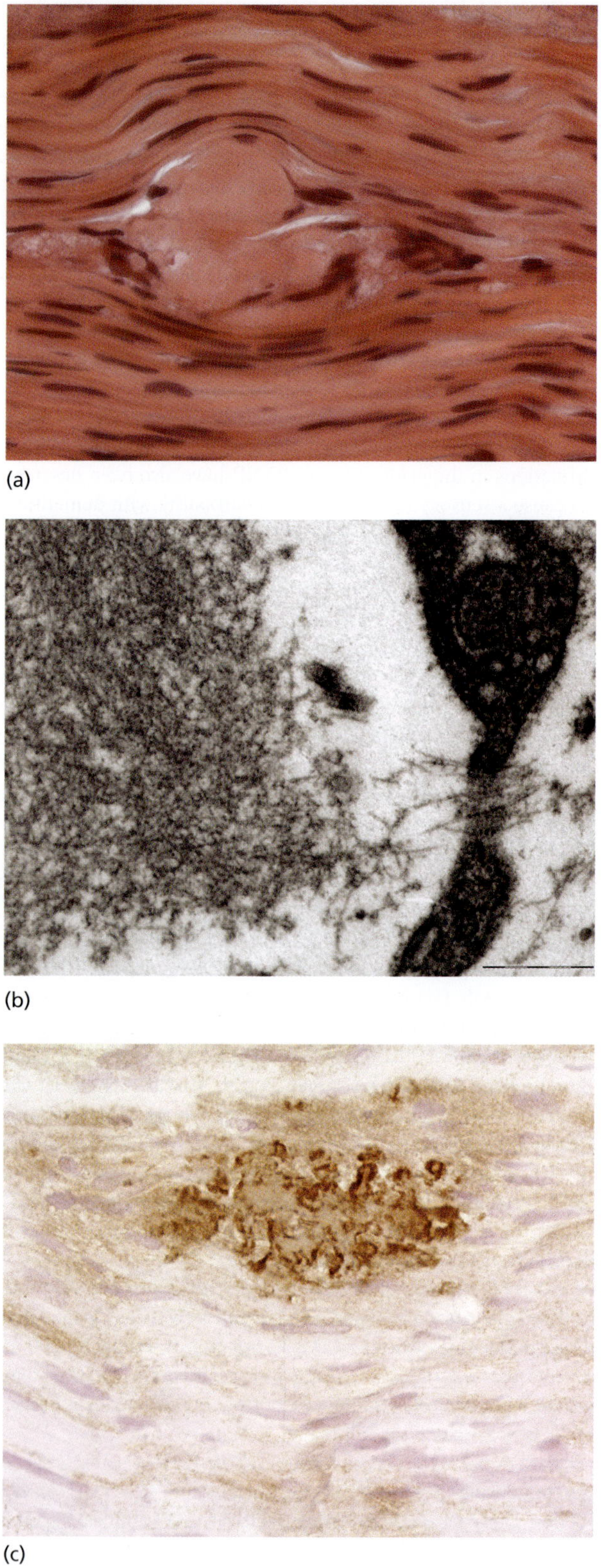

Figure 10.13 Amyloid neuropathy. (a) Haematoxylin and eosin stained paraffin section with a large amyloid deposition in the endoneurium, displacing normal structures. The nerve is severely depleted of large myelinated axons. (b) Electron microscopy of the same nerve, visualising amyloid fibrils. (c) The amyloid is composed of transthyretin (determined by immunohistochemistry).

Diagnosis The most important step in the diagnosis of TTR-related FAP is having a clinical suspicion. It should always be considered in patients with a family history and a neuropathy and/or cardiomyopathy, CTS or vitreous deposits. The diagnosis should also be considered in patients with an unexplained small fibre neuropathy especially with autonomic involvement or a cardiomyopathy regardless of family history. Neurophysiologically, the neuropathy is an axonopathy and has no specific features.

The diagnosis of amyloid can be made by direct examination of biopsy material from rectum, peripheral nerve, heart, subcutaneous fat or other tissue depending on the presentation. Congo red staining with apple green birefringence under polarised light is the primary examination. A number of methods for Congo red staining are available, some more effective in some tissues than others. Immunohistochemistry with monoclonal antibodies against TTR or the λ or κ light chains differentiates TTR amyloid from light chain amyloid but the method is neither 100% sensitive nor specific. Light chains should be sought by immunofixation in urine and serum if AL amyloid is suspected and the antibodies to TTR are negative. The use of mass spectrometry to identify the constituent amyoid protein looks promising and is more sensitive than immunohistochemistry but is not yet widely available.

Sequencing of the TTR gene is widely available for genetic testing and confirmation of a histopathological diagnosis. Predictive testing remains difficult because of uncertainties about the penetrance of certain mutations.

Once the diagnosis is made the extent and stage of the disease must be assessed and iodine-123 labelled serum amyloid protein scan is a useful tool to help with this, especially if liver transplantation (see Treatment) is being considered.

Treatment Ninety per cent of TTR is produced in the liver. Until the early 1990s the treatment of TTR-related FAP was limited to symptomatic treatments and rehabilitative measures. Since then liver transplantation has been used in the treatment of TTR-related FAP. More than 2000 liver transplants have been performed for patients with TTR-related FAP worldwide. The consensus is that liver transplantation halts or slows the progression of TTR-related FAP in most Met30 patients. The 5-year survival is now 82%. There is concern that patients with mutations other than Met30 do not do as well.

Although liver transplantation has been a major advance in the treatment of TTR amyloidosis, it is associated with a significant mortality and other safer and more effective treatments are being developed:

- Drugs that stabilise TTR in the tetrameric state and prevent its dissociation into amyloidogenic monomers. Two drugs, tafamadis and diflunisal, with this action have been introduced in clinical use in some countries although both are still undergoing further efficacy evaluation studies.
- TTR gene silencing strategies to inhibit the production of wild type and mutant TTR. Trials are currently ongoing for both antisense oligonucleotides and small interfering RNA strategies.
- Monoclonocal antibodies against serum amyloid protein (SAP) to increase the clearance of amyloid deposits are also in development.

Prognosis The average life expectancy for patients with untreated TTR-related FAP is about 10 years but varies with ethnicity, mutation and treatment. This figure is likely to improve further as newer genetic and chemotherapeutic treatments are developed.

Apolipoprotein A-1 related FAP

One type of FAP, originally described in an Iowa kindred, has been shown to be associated with deposition of a variant apolipoprotein A-1. The phenotype is similar to that of FAP TTR Met30 except for a higher incidence of renal amyloidosis and severe gastric ulcer disease.

Gelsolin-related FAP

Gelsolin amyloidosis was first described in a Finnish kindred. This usually presents in the thirties with corneal lattice dystrophy caused by amyloid deposition in the corneal branches of the trigeminal nerve. This is followed by a progressive cranial neuropathy. The facial nerve is the most common cranial nerve involved with the upper fibres as manifested by forehead muscle weakness initially being affected. Other cranial nerves may also be affected including the vestibulocochlear, hypoglossal and trigeminal with varying clinical manifestations. Peripheral nerve and autonomic involvement is usually mild.

The fibril protein in this type of amyloidosis is an abnormal fragment of a plasma protein, gelsolin, a calcium-binding protein that fragments actin filaments.

Beta-2 microglobulin FAP

A single family is described with an Asp76Asn mutation in beta-2 microglobulin and an otherwise classic presentation of FAP. More commonly, beta-2 microglobulin causes a dialysis related amyloid manifesting as carpel tunnel syndrome.

Acquired neuropathies

The acquired peripheral nerve diseases are a diverse group of conditions with a variety of pathogenic mechanisms. Some are primary peripheral nerve disorders affecting a single system. Many are disorders with multi-system dysfunction such as the neuropathies associated with diabetes, autoimmune diseases or toxic exposures. The inflammatory neuropathies, in their various guises, constitute the largest group of peripheral nerve disorders.

Inflammatory neuropathies

The inflammatory neuropathies (Table 10.9) are a diverse group of peripheral nerve disorders linked by their presumed immune-mediated pathogenesis. They are characterised pathologically by inflammatory infiltration of the peripheral nerves associated with destruction of myelin and/or axons. The inflammatory neuropathies are typified by the idiopathic demyelinating neuropathies, both acute and chronic, and the closely related neuropathies associated with paraproteinaemia. However, vasculitic, infectious and parainfectious, paraneoplastic and, more recently, diabetic plexopathy are included. Some of these may be thought of as primary disorders of the PNS (e.g. GBS and CIDP) and others secondary to a systemic immune process with subsequent involvement of the peripheral nerves (e.g. the neuropathy associated with vasculitis and the connective tissue diseases).

Acute neuromuscular weakness and the inflammatory neuropathies

Acute neuromuscular weakness can be caused by disease of muscle, neuromuscular junction, peripheral nerve, roots or the CNS. The distinction between these sites of pathology can largely be made on clinical grounds, with supportive investigations where necessary (Chapters 4 and 20).

Table 10.9 Inflammatory neuropathies.

ACUTE
Guillain-Barré (GBS) variants
Acute inflammatory demyelinating polyradiculoneuropathy
Acute motor axonal neuropathy
Acute motor sensory axonalneuropathy
Fisher syndrome and other regional variants
Pharyngeal-cervical-brachial
Paraparetic
Facial palsies
Pure oculomotor
Functional variants of GBS
Pure dysautonomia
Pure sensory GBS
Ataxic GBS
INTERMEDIATE
Subacute inflammatory demyelinating polyradiculoneuropathy
Vasculitic neuropathies (may present acutely, subacutely or chronically)
Primary vasculitis
Polyarteritis nodosa
Churg–Strauss syndrome
Microscopic polyangiitis
Wegener's vasculitis
Non-systemic vasculitic neuropathy
Giant cell arteritis
Systemic autoimmune diseases with associated vasculitis
Rheumatoid arthritis
Systemic lupus erythematosus
Sjögren's syndrome
Mixed connective tissue disease
Other vasculitis
Diabetic and non-diabetic lumbosacral plexopathy
Other inflammatory neuropathies
Serum sickness
Infections (hepatitis B and C, HIV, Lyme disease), leprosy
Malignancy (small cell lung cancer, lymphoma, leukaemia, renal and adenocarcinomas)
Chemotherapy
Paraneoplastic
Subacute sensory neuropathy/neuronopathy – small cell lung carcinoma and anti-Hu Abs
Other paraneoplastic tumour–antibody syndromes
CHRONIC
Chronic inflammatory demyelinating polyradiculoneuropathy
Multifocal motor neuropathy with conduction block
Multifocal acquired demyelinating sensory and motor neuropathy
Chronic relapsing axonal neuropathy
Chronic ataxic sensory neuronopathy
CHRONIC, WITH PARAPROTEINAEMIAS
Monoclonal gammopathy of undetermined significance
Multiple myeloma
Solitary plasmacytoma
Lymphoma or chronic lymphocytic leukaemia
Waldenström's macroglobulinaemia
POEMS syndrome
Cryoglobulinaemia
Cold agglutinin disease

Table 10.10 Infections predisposing to Guillain–Barré syndrome.

Campylobacter jejuni
Cytomegalovirus
Mycoplasma pneumoniae
Epstein–Barr virus
HIV
Haemophilus influenzae
Zika virus

A differential diagnosis of acute inflammatory neuropathies exists (Table 10.9). By far the most common of these is GBS. The acute infectious neuropathies (poliomyelitis, diphtheria, HIV, tick paralysis) are dealt with in Chapter 9 and paraneoplastic neuropathies in Chapter 21.

Guillain–Barré syndrome and its variants

GBS is the most common cause of acute neuromuscular weakness in the developed world following the near eradication of polio, but certainly occurs worldwide. The incidence is about 1–2/100 000 population. There is no sex difference. It affects all ages including children and infants but is more frequent in older age groups. In some populations a seasonal variation in the incidence is reported coinciding with the seasonal incidence of predisposing infections (Table 10.10). In Europe and the United States, GBS is synonymous with acute inflammatory demyelinating polyradiculoneuropathy (AIDP) as axonal variants only occur in 3–5% of cases. However, axonal forms are far more common in China, Japan and Mexico (see Variants of GBS).

Symptoms and signs The diagnosis of GBS remains a clinical one, supported by investigations which may be normal in the early stages of disease. Patients present with a progressive ascending sensorimotor paralysis with areflexia, affecting one or more limbs and reaching a nadir in less than 4 weeks. Patients who progress beyond this time or present with 'recurrent GBS' are reclassified into subacute or chronic inflammatory demyelinating neuropathies (SIDP/CIDP, see Chronic inflammatory demyelinating polyradiculoneuropathy). Pain, cranial nerve involvement and autonomic disturbances with arrhythmias and labile blood pressure are often features. Papilloedema may occur, which if unrecognised and untreated may lead to blindness. A clinical diagnosis of GBS should be questioned if there is persistent asymmetrical weakness, bladder or bowel involvement or a sensory level suggestive of spinal cord pathology. Furthermore, the presence of a known toxin, HIV, diphtheria, tick exposure or neoplasia broadens the differential. In the first few days the examination may be normal and reflexes retained. However, some patients may progress to tetraparesis and require ventilation in as little as 48 hours and vigilance for either scenario is important. Functional variants exist with acute pure autonomic failure, pure sensory neuropathy and pure ataxic neuropathy described. Recognised regional variants (Table 10.9) are associated with particular serum antiganglioside antibodies (see Antiganglioside antibodies). The differential diagnosis of acute GBS is summarised in Chapter 20.

Investigations

Cerebrospinal fluid In GBS the CSF is acellular or should contain <10 cells/mm^3. Ten per cent of patients have cell counts of 10–50 cells/mm^3 but these do not persist for more than a few days. Cell counts >50 cells/mm^3 should stimulate a search for an alternative diagnosis. Note that intravenous immunoglobulin (IVIG) can stimulate an aseptic meningitis and may provoke increased cell counts (as well as falsely raised CSF protein levels). CSF protein is usually raised for 4–6 weeks but may be normal in the first 7 days of illness and may also remain normal in a greater proportion of the regional variants (e.g. Fisher syndrome) than typical GBS. CSF pressure is typically normal but raised levels of CSF pressure and protein contribute to papilloedema.

Nerve conduction studies In the correct clinical context, abnormalities of nerve conduction studies suggestive of patchy proximal and distal demyelination are highly suggestive of GBS. Nerve conduction tests may be normal in the first few days of illness. Typical changes of slowed motor nerve conduction velocities, with prolonged F-wave and distal motor latencies with largely preserved amplitudes are typical. Conduction block may be demonstrated. Early on the lower limb sensory nerve action potentials are relatively preserved but they are later lost and electromyographic (EMG) evidence of denervation may emerge. Inexcitable nerves are common in severe cases and are unhelpful in diagnosis. Axonal changes without evidence of slowing are found in acute motor axonal and acute motor and sensory axonal neuropathies (AMAN and AMSAN) and these may indicate a worse prognosis.

Blood tests Blood tests are unhelpful in the context of the diagnosis of GBS. However, they importantly serve to exclude major biochemical disturbances that may mimic GBS, identify coexistent disorders that may complicate treatment (e.g. renal failure and IVIG), and point to conditions that may cause a GBS-like illness (systemic lupus erythematosus [SLE], HIV, malignancy). All patients should have urea and electrolytes, calcium, magnesium, liver and thyroid function, full blood count, erythrocyte sedimentation rate (ESR), vitamin B_{12} and folate and antinuclear antibodies (ANA) checked.

Ten per cent of patients will have abnormal liver function tests, possibly the result of viral (Epstein–Barr virus [EBV] or cytomegalovirus [CMV]) hepatitis. Hyponatraemia occurs in a proportion of patients caused both by syndrome of inappropriate antidiuretic hormone (SIADH) or an excess of atrial natriuretic factor.

Antiganglioside antibodies Antiganglioside antibodies are frequently requested but seldom help in diagnosis. They are sometimes found more commonly associated with one or other of the regional GBS variants. In the acute neuropathies only IgG antibodies are of relevance. IgG anti-GQ1b antibodies are found in 90–95% of cases of Fisher syndrome and also a substantial proportion of cases of GBS with ophthalmoplegia. Anti-GD1a and anti-GalNAcGD1a antibodies are associated with AMAN. IgG anti-GM1 antibodies associate with more severe disease. Anti-GM2 antibodies sometimes follow CMV infection and seem to be associated with a predominantly sensory neuropathy. Ganglioside species share epitopes and therefore more than one antiganglioside activity is commonly found.

Campylobacter stool testing and serology Serological testing with acute and convalescent serum may confirm seroconversion following infection with any of the infectious agents implicated in GBS causation. Stool should also be cultured for *Campylobacter* species. Its identification also has public health implications.

Lung function testing and monitoring Forced vital capacity (FVC) should be measured and recorded immediately on presentation and at least every 4 hours thereafter (more frequently if necessary) until the patient has begun to recover. Elective intubation should be considered if the FVC falls below 15 mL/kg. A fall in FVC of one-third between erect and supine indicates diaphragm weakness.

Cardiac monitoring A 12-lead ECG should be recorded and the patient monitored for arrhythmia and blood pressure fluctuations until clinically stabilised and improving.

Nerve biopsy Sural nerve biopsy is seldom helpful as much of the pathology in GBS is proximal to any intended biopsy site and changes may take days to weeks to develop. In severe, unusual cases or cases unresponsive to treatment sural nerve biopsy may be helpful to exclude alternative diagnoses.

Variants of GBS AMAN and AMSAN form a spectrum of axonal GBS. Although responsible for only 3–5% of cases of GBS in the western hemisphere, axonal variants may constitute up to 50% or more of GBS cases in China and Latin America. Here GBS occurs in seasonal summer outbreaks and is closely associated with *Campylobacter jejuni* infection. Anti-GD1a, GalNAcGD1a and GM1 antibodies occur frequently. The pathology involves direct macrophage attack on the axolemma resulting in profound axonal degeneration.

Limited and regional variants of GBS are shown in Table 10.9. Individual variants are rare but the combined incidence rate of all variants is about 7–13% of the incidence of GBS. Fisher syndrome, the triad of ataxia, areflexia and ophthalmoplegia, is the most common variant accounting for between one-third and half of variant cases. There is a frequent association with *C. jejuni* infection and up to 95% of cases are associated with anti-GQ1b antibodies. Fisher syndrome seldom progresses to require supportive or therapeutic treatment. Occasionally, a Fisher/GBS overlap syndrome or GBS with ophthalmoplegia may progress to full-blown weakness and thus it should be monitored and treated like GBS.

Other limited and regional variants are rare. The pharyngo-cervico-brachial variant involves predominantly the bulbar and upper limb musculature with weakness and areflexia but sparing the lower limbs. Anti-GT1a antibodies (sometimes cross-reacting with GQ1b) are often found. The pathophysiology is predominantly axonal. Paraparetic lower limb variants have been described as having pure motor and pure sensory or sensory ataxic forms. Acute dysautonomia has more recently been recognised in this group of conditions. It presents with profound postural hypotension and impaired sweating, impotence and bladder and bowel dysfunction. Antibodies to the nicotinic, preganglionic acetylcholine receptor have been described associated with this condition which improves with immunotherapy.

Pathogenesis The infectious agents associated with GBS probably all display ganglioside-like epitopes on their surface. Humoral and cellular immune responses to these epitopes cross-react with gangliosides displayed on nerve cells, resulting in an immunological attack.

The pathogenic hallmark of typical GBS is macrophage-mediated attack of either the Schwann cell or the axolemma resulting in demyelination or axonal degeneration. The BNB becomes inflamed and leaky allowing for the ingress of activated T cells, IgG and complement. IgG and activated complement is found on actively degenerating cells. The inflammatory milieu stimulates up-regulation of MHC Class II receptors and antigen presentation by endoneurial cells including Schwann cells, promoting endoneurial damage.

Treatment

General treatment (Chapter 20)

1 Respiratory monitoring is essential. Elective endotracheal intubation may be life-saving with early conversion to tracheostomy for comfort and prevention of complications.
2 Cardiac monitoring in a high dependency unit setting should be performed in all patients while the diagnosis is being confirmed and until recovery begins. Arrhythmias and blood pressure fluctuations should be treated appropriately. Persistent or severe bradyarrhythmias may require the insertion of a pacemaker.
3 Anticoagulation (low molecular weight heparin), pressure stockings and calf massage devices as prevention against deep venous thrombosis (DVT) should be used routinely.
4 Fluid balance, nutrition and electrolyte monitoring should be carried out. A nasogastric tube may be necessary for feeding, which may need to be supplemented. Hyponatraemia is more often brought about by excess atrial naturetic factor (ANF) (with loss of salt *and* water) than SIADH (dilutional through retention of water).
5 Physiotherapy should start immediately with hand and foot splints to prevent contractures.
6 Excellent nursing care of the paralysed patient prevents many complications associated with immobility and recumbency (pneumonia, pressure sores, DVT) and should be the central point of all care. Detection and treatment of issues related to pain, emotion, continence, nutrition and mouth care are crucial.

Specific treatment Plasma exchange was the first GBS treatment shown to have substantial benefit. It halves the time on ventilation, hastens recovery and improves outcome at 1 year if administered within 4 weeks of onset. Usually four to five 3-L exchanges are given over the course of 5–10 days. More practically, IVIG 2 g/kg over 5 days is as effective as plasma exchange and more likely to be completed as it has fewer complications. No additional benefit has been shown for following plasma exchange with IVIG. No trial has been performed to examine the benefit of a second dose of IVIG 14 days after the first in cases of minimal or delayed response, but an international study is ongoing. Patients who make an IgG increment of more than 7.5 g/L after a standard dose of 2 g/kg IVIG have a better outcome than those who have a lower increment. Steroids are not indicated in the treatment of GBS.

Pain may be severe. Treat with combinations of high-dose anticonvulsants (gabapentin, pregabalin, carbamazepine) and tricyclic antidepressants or selective serotonin re-uptake inhibitors (SSRIs), in conjunction with opiates (e.g. fentanyl). Epidural anaesthesia is sometimes helpful.

Outcome Despite many advances in therapeutics and intensive care, GBS remains a severe illness. Poor prognostic factors include advanced age, axonal degeneration in the context of AIDP and if the patient is ventilator-dependent or bed-bound at the nadir of the illness. Predictions of the need for ventilation and of the eventual mobility outcome can be based on scores evaluable at admission or shortly afterwards, known as mEGOS (modified Erasmus GBS Outcome Score) and EGRIS (Erasmus GBS Respiratory Insufficiency Score). Even with the best medical care 5–8% of patients die and about one-third are left with significant disability. The remainder make a good recovery and have few residual symptoms. Fatigue is an under-recognised and poorly treated residual outcome.

Chronic inflammatory neuropathies

The chronic inflammatory neuropathies include the idiopathic and those associated with other diseases, for example the paraproteinaemias and the vasculitides (Table 10.9). Although the latter group, especially the vasculitides and paraneoplastic disorders, may present more acutely and progress more rapidly, they are included here for convenience.

Chronic inflammatory demyelinating polyradiculoneuropathy

CIDP is an acquired, treatable, demyelinating PNS disease characterised by progressive or relapsing proximal and distal weakness of the limbs with sensory loss and/or cranial nerve involvement reaching a nadir in more than 8 weeks with absent or reduced reflexes in all limbs. Prevalence estimates vary at 1.2–7/100 000 population. Unlike GBS there are no known predisposing infections.

Symptoms and signs The diagnosis of CIDP is clinical, supported by electrophysiological, CSF and other tests (see Investigations) and the exclusion of other causative pathologies.

Patients with CIDP present with a progressive or relapsing limb weakness or numbness which may have an asymmetrical onset. Parasthesiae are common. Limb and back pain occurs but if prominent should stimulate a search for alternative causes especially vasculitis, lymphoma or infection. As with all demyelinating conditions a tremor may be prominent. Autonomic and bladder or bowel involvement is distinctly unusual. 'Recurrent GBS' can sometimes be classified as CIDP. Unusual forms can occur including monomelic paralysis, lower limb variants and sensory ataxic forms.

The clinical signs mirror the presentation. Proximal and distal weakness with areflexia and a distal sensory loss are normal and tremor occurs frequently. Wasting is not evident until late in untreated disease. Bulbar weakness and progression to respiratory involvement with ventilation are rare.

A careful general examination is crucial to identify systemic causes or contributing factors (e.g. malignancy, pre-existing CMT, SLE and other connective tissue diseases, diabetes or alcohol).

Investigations The European Federation of Neurological Sciences and the Peripheral Nerve Society have published criteria (2010) for essential and supportive investigations.

1 *Nerve conduction studies* Clear demonstration of demyelination in at least two nerves is mandatory for a definite diagnosis of CIDP if no other supportive criteria are employed. Demyelinating features include reduced motor conduction velocity, prolonged distal motor latencies, proximal F-waves reduction or conduction block or dispersion, all in the presence of relatively preserved compound muscle action potentials are acceptable. Later in the condition axonal degeneration may supervene.
2 *CSF* The CSF protein is raised in 90% of cases. A CSF white cell count of >10 mm^3 should prompt a search for alternative causes.
3 *MRI* Nerve root enlargement and/or enhancement with gadolinium is often seen. Most commonly imaged areas include the cervical and lumbosacral regions. MRI findings are now included in the supportive criteria for the diagnosis.
4 *Nerve biopsy* A diagnosis of CIDP does not usually require a nerve biopsy as the clinical presentation, neurophysiology and other less invasive paraclinical investigations are usually sufficient to make a diagnosis. Furthermore, complications include a 10–30% risk of permanent dysaesthesia at the biopsy site and other routine surgical complications of wound healing and infection. Although the sural nerve is the most commonly biopsied, a suitable nerve should be selected on the basis of symptoms and electrophysiological findings; only very rarely should an electrically 'normal' nerve be biopsied.

   Biopsies contain reduced numbers of myelinated nerve fibres with evidence of active demyelination or previous onion bulb formation (Figure 10.14). Endoneurial macrophage activity is usually increased and endoneurial T cells are present in increased numbers. Unequivocal diagnostic findings in the correct clinical context are macrophage-associated demyelination on electron microscopy (EM), evidence of demyelination or remyelination in five fibres by EMG or demyelinated segments of at least 20 fibres in teased preparations.
5 *Blood tests* There are no diagnostic blood tests for CIDP. Full blood count, ESR, B_{12} and folate, urea and electrolytes, glucose, liver and thyroid function tests, immunoglobulins, protein electrophoresis and immunofixation and ANA are normal or negative but should be requested as an initial screen to rule out other conditions.
6 *Exclusion of other conditions* Exclusion of other causative or contributing conditions is essential. Coexistent CMT disease should be considered and genetic tests requested as necessary.

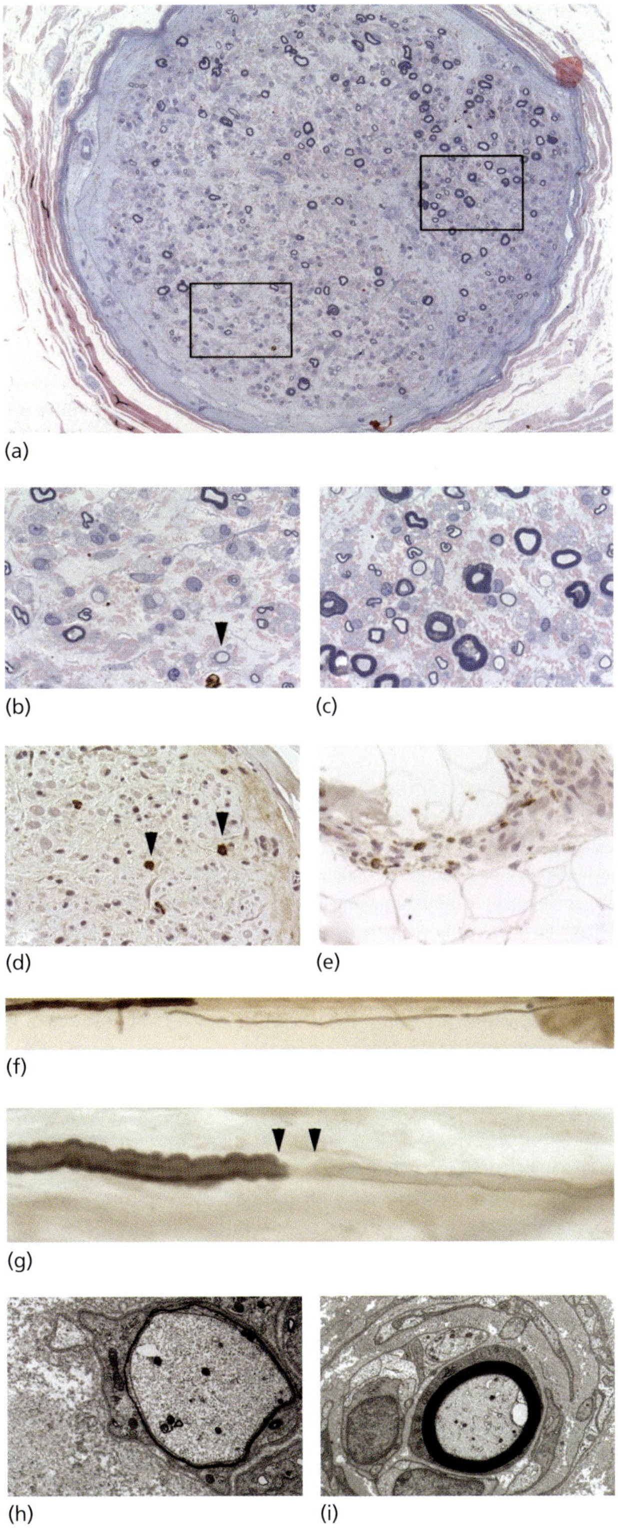

Figure 10.14 Chronic inflammatory neuropathy. (a) Patchy loss of myelinated fibres in a fascicle of the sural nerve (semi-thin resin section, toluidine blue). The left lower rectangle is shown in higher magnification in (b). (b) Close-up of the area with a significant loss of large myelinated fibres (arrowhead indicates a thinly myelinated fibre). There are several other thinly myelinated and entirely demyelinated fibres. (c) More densely populated area corresponding to the right upper rectangle in (a). (d) Endoneurial T-cells (CD8 immunohistochemical staining). (e) Most CIDPs are also characterised by a variable perivascular infiltrate as shown here (CD8 Immunohistochemistry). (f) Teased fibre preparation which shows a segmental demyelination. To unequivocally identify segmental demyelination, myelinated fibres have to be identified on either end of the demyelinated stretch. (g) Close-up of demyelination, which shows a myelinated segment on the left, the end of which is indicated by the left arrowhead. This is followed by an expanded internode length, the end of which is indicated by the right arrowhead. The subsequent stretch of the axon is very thinly myelinated. (h) Electron microscopy of a demyelinated and thinly remyelinated axon. (i) Axon with almost regular myelin thickness, surrounded by concentric formations of Schwann cell laminae, also designated onion bulbs.

CIDP variants

Multi-focal motor neuropathy with conduction block Multi-focal motor neuropathy with conduction block (MMNCB) is a progressive immune-mediated demyelinating motor neuropathy which often begins asymmetrically in the upper limbs. Weakness in the distribution of individual nerves, often with prominent cramps but without wasting or fasciculation, and patchy reduced reflexes are the most usual signs. Wasting and fasciculation can occur later which causes confusion with motor neurone disease. Subjective sensory symptoms can occur but no more than minor disturbance of vibration sense at the ankle is acceptable on examination. Cranial nerve or respiratory involvement are extremely rare and upper motor neurone, sphincter or marked bulbar involvement exclude the diagnosis. The prevalence of MMNCB is about 10% of that of CIDP. Men are more often affected than women.

Both IgG and IgM antibodies to ganglioside GM1 are described in the serum from 30–80% of patients, rarely as a paraprotein. CSF protein should not be raised to >1 g/L. The hallmark of the condition is the demonstration of multi-focal conduction blocks at sites other than common sites of compression. Extremely thorough neurophysiological assessment may be necessary to identify them.

MMNCB was originally described in 1988 as a subtype of CIDP but it may be a distinct entity as illustrated by its dramatically different response to immunosuppressive therapy including worsening with steroids (see Treatment of typical CIDP).

Multi-focal acquired demyelinating sensory and motor neuropathy Multi-focal acquired demyelinating sensory and motor neuropathy (MADSAM), previously called Lewis–Sumner syndrome, has similarities to CIDP and MMNCB. It may respond to treatment with IVIG.

Sensory ataxic CIDP This rare inflammatory disorder presents with profound sensory ataxia and may be caused by inflammatory involvement of the dorsal root ganglia. HIV, paraneoplasia, Sjögren's syndrome, copper deficiency and pyridoxine toxicity should be excluded.

Distal acquired demyelinating sensory neuropathy Many cases of distal acquired demyelinating sensory neuropathy (DADS) are associated with an IgM paraprotein.

Chronic relapsing axonal neuropathy Chronic relapsing axonal neuropathy (CRAN) is a rare entity that has an uncertain position in the nosology of CIDP.

Treatment of typical CIDP Treatment should be commenced as soon as possible in patients who warrant it after discussion of the risks and potential benefits with the patient. The first line treatments for CIDP are either oral steroids (although various regimens are used, 1 mg/kg given for 2 months and then slowly tapered is common) or IVIG (0.4 g/kg for 5 days repeated at 4–6 weeks and then as necessary according to the response). Both steroids and IVIG have been shown to be better than placebo and there is no clear difference between IVIG and steroids. Recent studies have shown that, if tolerated, steroids may produce a longer lasting remission than IVIG. Steroids should be co-prescribed with a bisphosphonate to protect against bone loss (unless contraindicated), and gastric pharmacoprotection should be considered. IVIG is a blood product and patients should be made aware of and consented for the risks. If IVIG or steroids are contraindicated or ineffectual then plasma exchange should be considered.

Other immunosuppressants have been tried in CIDP but cyclophosphamide is the only one to have shown promise. MMNCB, MADSAM and possibly motor-predominant CIDP may deteriorate with steroids and plasma exchange and therefore steroids should be avoided in these conditions.

Outcome CIDP is a chronic progressive or relapsing disease. About 80% of patients will respond to treatment. Where patients fail to respond to treatment an occult paraprotein should be sought annually.

Over half (54%) of patients require assistance to walk or are bed-bound at some stage of their illness; 13% of patients require assistance to mobilise or are bed-bound at any one time. Over 50% require continuous treatment to maintain stability.

Paraproteinaemic neuropathies

Neuropathies associated with a paraprotein occur more often than by chance alone. The prevalence of a paraprotein in the serum at the age of 50 is approximately 1%, rising to 3% aged 70. Some 30–70% of patients with a paraprotein have a demonstrable peripheral neuropathy. Conversely, of a group of patients with no other identifiable cause for their neuropathy, 10% have a paraprotein. Most neuropathies are associated with 'benign' paraproteinaemias (monoclonal gammopathies of undetermined significance [MGUS]). Although IgG paraproteins account for 61% of all paraproteins, IgM MGUSs are over-represented in association with neuropathies and in many the MGUS is thought to be implicated in causation. Neuropathies associated with malignant gammopathies are more often caused by compressive lesions, direct infiltration or amyloidosis.

If a paraprotein is discovered in the serum it should be fully investigated with a full clinical examination, search for urine light chains, a skeletal survey and a bone marrow aspirate and trephine to establish whether it is benign or malignant. The differential diagnosis of gammopathies associated with neuropathy is shown in Table 10.9.

Neuropathies associated with IgM paraproteins The neuropathy associated with IgM paraproteins is most frequently demyelinating. About 50–70% of the paraproteins react with the peripheral nerve epitope displayed by myelin-associated glycoprotein (MAG). A κ light chain is most frequent although IgMλ anti-MAG paraproteins do occur. The clinical picture associated with anti-MAG antibodies is relatively homogeneous. A slowly progressive distal sensorimotor neuropathy with a variable degree of ataxia and prominent tremor is typical. Men are affected more than women, with a mean age of onset of 59 years. The neurophysiological features are demyelination with characteristic prominent distal slowing. Nerve biopsy (not required for diagnosis) shows characteristic widening of the myelin lamellae (Figure 10.15).

There is good evidence to indicate that anti-MAG IgM paraproteins are pathogenic, although it is likely that the current assays are highly sensitive and pick up a subgroup of non-pathogenic antibodies. The evidence for the pathogenesis of other IgM paraproteins is less robust even though other serum activities to specific epitopes are reported. Thus, when IgM paraproteins occur in conjunction with otherwise CIDP-like or axonal neuropathies the neuropathies are treated according to their non-gammopathy related features (see Treatment of paraproteinaemic neuropathies).

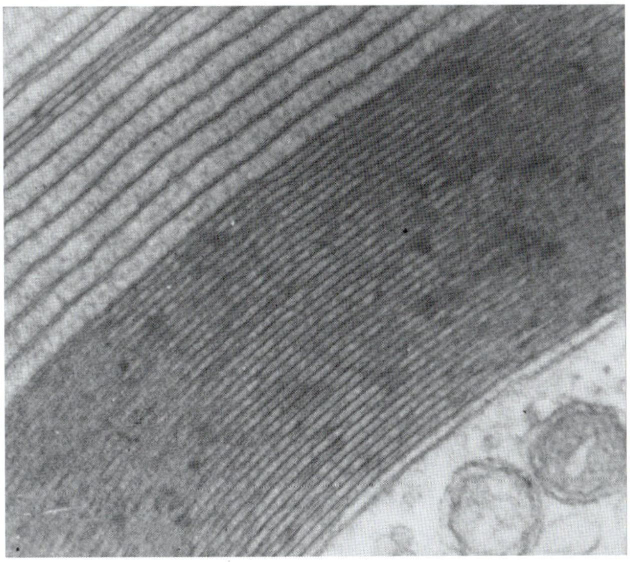

Figure 10.15 Widely spaced myelin. The normal myelin lamellae are tightly compacted and have a periodicity in electron microscope preparations of 12–15 nm. In the demyelinating neuropathy associated with IgM paraprotein that has activity against MAG (anti-MAG PDPN) the intraperiod line becomes split giving an overall periodicity of 30–40 nm. There is a suggestion of material within the widened spaces, possibly immunoglobulin M.

Neuropathies associated with IgG and IgA paraproteins The neuropathy associated with an IgG or IgA paraprotein is most often a chronic symmetrical predominantly sensory neuropathy similar to CIDP, but the presentations are much more heterogeneous than for IgM. People with IgG and IgA MGUS neuropathy often have less weakness and relatively more sensory involvement, both clinically and neurophysiologically, than do people with idiopathic CIDP. Electrophysiologically the neuropathies are either demyelinating or axonal/mixed neuropathies in approximately equal numbers. Debate continues about whether a patient with an IgG MGUS and otherwise typical CIDP justifies a separate diagnosis.

Neuropathies associated with lymphoma/CLL/Waldenström's macroglobulinaemia Neuropathy may be the presenting feature of a malignant gammopathy. A progressive painful neuropathy is common. Axonal and demyelinating large fibre and small fibre involvement occur. Several pathogenic mechanisms have been described including direct antibody attack on the nerves, immunoglobulin deposition, cryoglobulinaemic vasculitis, cold agglutinin activity, amyloid deposition, increased serum viscosity and ischaemia and direct infiltration by malignant cells (neurolymphomatosis).

POEMS syndrome Polyneuropathy, organomegaly, endocrinopathy, M-protein and skin changes constitute the POEMS syndrome, a rare haematological paraneoplastic disorder in which the cytokine vascular endothelial growth factor (VEGF) is strongly implicated in the pathogenesis. All five clinical features are not always present at presentation. The minimal criteria to establish the diagnosis are the presence of a demyelinating and axonal polyneuropathy associated with an IgA or IgG monoclonal gammopathy, the light chain being almost always λ, as well as one other major criterion (Castleman's disease, osteosclerotic bone lesion(s) or a raised plasma VEGF) and at least one secondary minor criterion; endocrinopathy (excluding diabetes), skin change (glomeruloid haemangiomas are specific to POEMS), organomegaly, generalised oedema, papilloedema or thrombocytosis/polycythaemia. A number of associated features are also recognised including (but not limited to POEMS) weight loss, low B_{12}, diarrhea, clubbing, restrictive lung disease. Ultrastructural identification of uncompacted myelin lamellae on the peripheral nerve biopsy is also a strong argument in favour of the diagnosis.

Cryoglobulinaemic neuropathy See Vasculitic neuropathies.

Neuropathies associated with multiple myeloma, solitary myeloma and other malignant plasma cell dyscrasias The neuropathies associated with a malignant plasma cell dyscrasia are heterogeneous. They should be managed in conjunction with a haematologist.

Treatment of paraproteinaemic neuropathies Because the neuropathy associated with paraproteinaemia is often mild and only slowly progressive treatment may not be required. The level of paraprotein and the neuropathy should be monitored as there is a risk of approximately 1% per year of malignant transformation of the B-cell clone which is greater in the first few years after identification. Treatments are aimed at reducing the amount or activity of antibody in the serum. IVIG has short-term benefit in IgM paraproteinaemic neuropathies. Rituximab is showing promise as an effective treatment. Plasma exchange, steroids, chlorambucil, azathioprine, cyclophosphamide, α-interferon, fludarabine and cladribine have all been used with variable success. For IgG and IgA paraproteinaemic neuropathies those with a slowly progressive distal axonal polyneuropathy tended to show a poor response to immunotherapy. Patients with a sensorimotor demyelinating neuropathy tend to respond better. In POEMS syndrome, specific treatment of osteosclerotic bone lesions may improve the other features of the syndrome, especially the neuropathy. Autologous bone marrow transplantation has been effective in some.

Acquired amyloid neuropathy In AL (light chain) amyloidosis the constituent amyloid protein is derived from monoclonal immunoglobulin light chains secondary to multiple myeloma, malignant lymphoma or Waldenström's macroglobulinaemia, or to a non-malignant immunocyte dyscrasia. Amyloid develops in approximately 15% of patients with myeloma and less frequently in other malignant B-cell disorders.

The amyloid is more commonly derived from λ than κ light chains.

Clinical features The incidence of AL amyloidosis is 5.1–12.8 per million. Light-chain amyloidosis occurs predominantly in later life, two-thirds between the ages of 50 and 70. It may present with non-specific symptoms such as malaise, fatigue and weight loss or with system specific symptoms, the most common being nephrotic syndrome, congestive cardiomyopathy, peripheral neuropathy (sometimes with autonomic involvement) and hepatomegaly. Associated features include purpura, oedema, hepatosplenomegaly and macroglossia.

Patients with neuropathy present with an acquired length dependent sensory loss with prominent small fibre involvement. Pain is often burning, especially nocturnally, or lancinating stabs. Autonomic involvement including distal limb anhydrosis, orthostatic hypotension, difficulty in voiding urine, and erectile and ejaculatory difficulty tends to be an early manifestation. Diarrhoea and gastroparesis may be prominent but whether this is related to direct gut wall or autonomic infiltration is uncertain.

On examination, nerves may be thickened, pain and temperature are selectively involved and autonomic involvement is often evident (including pupillary involvement).

Pathology The pathological features of AL amyloidosis are similar to those already described in the section above on pathology of transthyretin-related FAP.

Diagnosis Histological confirmation of amyloid deposition in nerve, rectum, abdominal fat or other tissue with Congo red is described above. Immunohistochemical staining for λ or κ light chains has a sensitivity of only 50%.

Once the diagnosis of AL amyloidosis is made it is necessary to screen for a paraprotein. Protein electrophoresis will detect a paraprotein in serum or urine in about 50% of patients where it is present. Immunofixation of serum and urine should be routinely performed and quantification of free light chains detects abnormality in 92% of patients. If all of the above techniques are used the sensitivity is 99%.

Bone marrow aspirate with a trephine biopsy and detailed systemic investigation should then be undertaken to assess the degree of other organ involvement, especially renal, cardiac and gastrointestinal. A serum amyloid protein scan identifies and quantifies tissue deposits in many tissues but not peripheral nerve.

Treatment of amyloid neuropathy Symptomatic treatments for pain, autonomic symptoms and the neuropathy can be tried as outlined above for TTR-related FAP. Extensive cardiac or renal involvement may merit organ transplantation. Chemotherapeutic regimens of different intensity are available to treat patients diagnosed at different stages of their disease. It is very important that patients are treated by centres with expertise in amyloidosis as regimes are continually being researched and updated.

Prognosis Prior to recent advances in treatment a median survival time of 35 months for patients with acquired amyloid peripheral neuropathy compared to 16 months for those without neuropathy was typical although longer survival is reported. Death was usually because of involvement of systems other than the peripheral nerves.

With treatment the outcome is better; a recent review reported that 22% of patients survived more than 10 years.

Vasculitic neuropathies

The vasculitic neuropathies are uncommon but are some of the most devastating but treatable peripheral neuropathies. The principal pathology is vascular inflammation in the vessels of the vasa nervorum with fibrinoid necrosis and occlusion of the vessel leading to nerve infarction. The early recognition, diagnosis and appropriate treatment can prevent considerable morbidity. They can be classified into systemic or non-systemic and then into primary or secondary causes (Table 10.9).

Symptoms and signs Sequential progressive painful sensorimotor mononeuropathies presenting over days or weeks is typical of the presentation of vasculitis. Lower limb nerves tend to be affected first. Progression to confluence occurs, especially in polyarteritis nodosa (PAN) and Wegener's granulomatosis, and more slowly in some of the secondary vasculitides. Systemic involvement may present as fever, weight loss, myalgia, fatigue and night sweats or as organ-specific symptoms of rash, wheeze or shortness of breath, haematuria and arthritis or arthralgias.

Primary vasculitides

1 Eosinophic granulomatosis with polyangiitits *(Churg-Strauss syndrome)* Up to 80% of patients with Churg–Strauss syndrome present with a neuropathy. Fever, pulmonary infiltrates, late onset asthma, skin rash and eosinophilia are often all present. Antineutrophil cytoplasmic antibody (ANCA) is positive in up to 70%.
2 Granulomatosis with polyangiitis *(Wegener's granulomatosis)* This is a midline necrotising vasculitis associated with a positive c-ANCA in 90% of patients. A neuropathy occurs in up to 40% of patients and may be confluent.
3 *Polyarteritis nodosa* True PAN is rare. It affects muscular arteries and arterioles only and is ANCA negative. Neuropathy occurs in 75% of cases and presents quite frequently as a painful symmetrical picture. Hepatitis B infection is often associated and implicated in the genesis.
4 *Microscopic polyangiitis* This is an overlap syndrome in which neuropathy occurs in 50–60% of cases. p-ANCA is often positive.

Secondary vasculitides

1 *Rheumatoid arthritis* (RA) The most common neuropathy associated with RA is a slowly progressive distal symmetric sensory neuropathy, many of which are asymptomatic. This is not vasculitic. Vasculitic neuropathies occur more often in late seropositive disease.
2 *SLE* This may present with a multiple mononeuropathy with vasculitis on nerve biopsy. However, a CIDP or GBS-like illness also occurs.
3 *Infection* Hepatitis C is strongly associated with the presence of type II (mixed) cryoglobulinaemia. This may cause a painful asymmetric multiple mononeuritis. The treatment is that of hepatitis C with ribavarin and interferon, although there are a number of case reports of vasculitis occurring in association with treatment per se. Vasculitis is directly attributable to HIV in <1% of cases. More frequent is a vasculitis secondary to coexistent hepatitis B, CMV or lymphoma.

Non-systemic vasculitides

1 Non-systemic vasculitic neuropathy usually has a more subacute or chronic course, but again with multiple mononeuropathies. Systemic symptomatic features are absent, except occasionally weight loss or fevers. No other organ involvement is identified on investigation. The prognosis and response to treatment are more favourable than with systemic forms.
2 Diabetic lumbosacral plexopathy (diabetic femoral neuropathy, Bruns–Garland syndrome, diabetic amyotrophy). There remains controversy about the classification of this entity but it seems to be a form of monophasic vasculitis.

Investigation of vasculitic neuropathies

1 *Haematological and biochemical investigation* Routine investigations should include full blood count, ESR, urea and electrolytes, C-reactive protein (CRP), liver and thyroid function, glucose (+/− HbA1c), ANA, ANCA, rheumatoid factor and RA latex, complement, serum protein electrophoresis and immunofixation, cryoglobulins (transfer to the laboratory at 37°C), hepatitis B and C. Consider requesting anti-ENA (extractable nuclear antigen), anti-CCP (cyclic citrullinated peptide), serum ACE (angiotensin converting enzyme), HIV testing and Lyme serology. The urine should be examined for red cell casts and Bence-Jones proteinuria.
2 *Radiology* A chest X-ray should be performed.

3 *CSF* is not usually helpful in vasculitic neuropathies. It could be performed to rule out differentials including HIV, carcinomatosis, lymphoma and Lyme disease if these are relevant.
4 *Neurophysiology* Patchy asymmetric sensorimotor axonal damage is typically found with evidence of acute or subacute denervation on EMG. Demyelinating neuropathies are sometimes found but should point to alternative or additional pathologies.
5 *Nerve biopsy* Patients with vasculitis are likely to need treatment with high dose, potentially toxic immunotherapies for a considerable time. A biopsy-proven diagnosis can usually only be made before treatment commences and it will reassure both physician and patient about their treatment. A biopsy of skin, liver, kidney or lung might be an alternative. If a nerve biopsy is performed, a recently affected sensory nerve should be selected. Biopsy of the superficial peroneal nerve and the underlying peroneus brevis muscle increases the chances of diagnosis over biopsy of the superficial peroneal nerve alone.

Patchy axonal fibre loss with active axonal degeneration is frequently seen in vasculitides. The diagnostic hallmarks of T-cell infiltration into vessel walls with destruction of the elastic lamina and fibrinoid necrosis with vessel occlusion (Figure 10.16) are seen less frequently. Biopsies should be carried out by an experienced surgeon and interpreted by a histopathologist with specific experience in peripheral nerve disease.

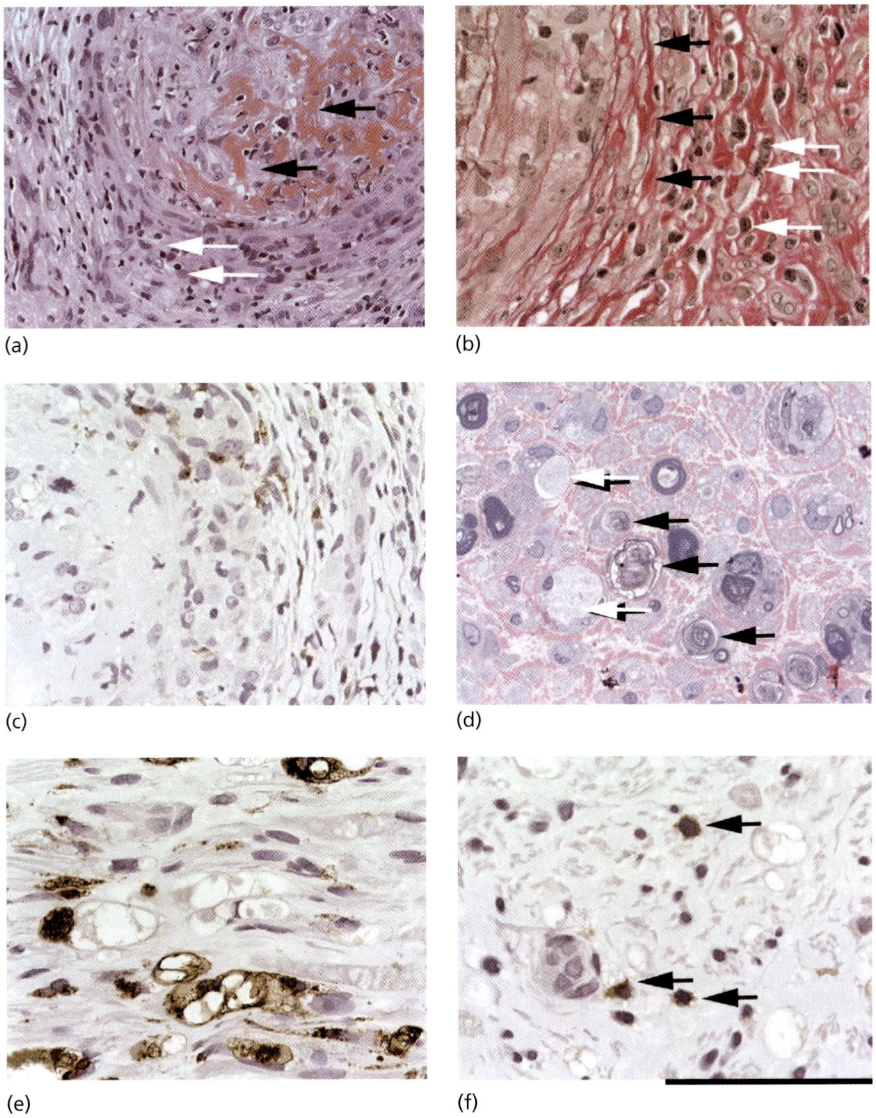

Figure 10.16 Vasculitis and severe axonal neuropathy in a peripheral nerve. (a) Fibrinoid necrosis (black arrow) of a medium-sized vessel. The vessel wall is densely infiltrated by inflammatory cells (white arrows). (b) Van Gieson elastica staining to visualise the distended and infiltrated vessel walls (red, black arrows) and interdispersed lymphocytes (white arrows). (c) CD8 immunohistochemical staining to visualise T-cells in the vessel walls. (d) Semi-thin resin sections on a transverse section of the adjacent nerve. Black arrows show acutely degenerating axons. White arrows indicate macrophages with the characteristic fine granular bright cytoplasm and peripheral small dark nucleus. (e) CD68 immunohistochemical staining to visualise digestion chambers and macrophage in the acutely degenerating nerve. (f) Accompanying occasional T-cell infiltrates in the affected nerve. This is regarded as a bystander effect to the overall inflammatory disease and should not be regarded as primary inflammation. Scale bar: A = 160 μm; b, e = 90 μm; c = 110 μm; d, f = 50 μm.

Treatment The vasculitides are a treatable group of disorders. Because of the ischaemic pathology, missing the opportunity to treat early may result in permanent irrecoverable peripheral nerve lesions. Randomised controlled trial evidence for specific therapeutic regimens in vasculitic neuropathy does not exist.

Non-virus-associated vasculitis Treatment is usually required, except in mild or non-progressive cases (usually non-systemic vasculitic neuropathy) and usually urgently. The key to treatment is the initial induction of remission followed by a maintenance phase. Oral steroids at a dose of 1–2 mg/kg or pulsed methylprednisolone (monthly courses 1 g/day for 3–5 days with 1 mg/kg oral prednisolone between) are usual. Wegener's granulomatosis and microscopic polyangiitis often require a more aggressive treatment course than Churg–Strauss or the non-systemic vasculitides. However, each case should be judged on its merits. Furthermore, there is good retrospective evidence that the addition of additional agents to the remission regimen improves the rate of remission, disability at 1 year and the rate of relapse even in non-systemic vasculitis. Cyclophosphamide is the most commonly used agent. Oral cyclophosphamide (2 mg/kg/day) was traditionally used; however, many clinicians now prefer to use monthly pulsed intravenous cyclophosphamide (10–15 mg/kg, maximum 1 g per dose and modified by age and renal function) with prehydration and MESNA cover for 6 months because of its reduced side effect profile (CYCLOPS regimen).

Many agents have been used for maintenance which usually covers the tail of oral steroids and continues to 2 years depending upon outcomes and patient tolerance. Methotrexate, azathioprine, mycophenolate and leflunomide have all been shown to be beneficial in case reports. Rituximab is useful in cryoglobulinaemic and lymphoma-associated vasculitis and demonstrated to be effective in other primary vasculitides (Rituxvas trial).

Virus-associated vasculitis Hepatitis B associated PAN responds to a short (2-week) induction course of steroids followed by 6 months of antiviral treatment, either interferon-2α or lamivudine. Hepatitis C cryoglobulin associated vasculitis is treated with pegylated interferon-2α with ribavarin, although neuropathy has on occasion been induced when this regimen is used to treat hepatitis C alone. Plasma exchange is traditionally used alongside the treatment for both viruses to clear circulating immune complexes but is of no demonstrable benefit.

Outcome Untreated vasculitis has a very poor outcome. In most types of vasculitis induction and maintenance treatment is associated with partial or complete recovery in about 50% of patients over months to years. Non-systemic vasculitis has much the best prognosis in terms of remission and low rates of recurrence.

Other acquired peripheral nerve disorders

Endocrine disorders

Diabetes Neuropathies occur extremely frequently in association with diabetes and, after leprosy, diabetes is the most common cause of neuropathy worldwide. Many neuropathies are asymptomatic or minor. Most occur later in the course of the disease; the prevalence of neuropathy is 50% after 25 years. The risk of neuropathy increases with duration of disease, poor control, height, male sex and with other cardiovascular risk factors constituting the 'metabolic syndrome'. Diabetic neuropathies can be classified as in Table 10.11.

Table 10.11 Classification of diabetic neuropathies.

Distal symmetric sensory neuropathy (DSSN)
Autonomic neuropathies
Vasculitic plexopathies and thoracolumbar radiculopathies (amyotrophies)
Focal and multifocal mononeuropathies
Small fibre neuropathy
Acute reversible hyperglycaemic neuropathy
Insulin neuritis and hypoglycaemic neuropathies
Neuropathies associated with diabetes (e.g. CIDP)

CIDP, chronic inflammatory demyelinating polyradiculoneuropathy.

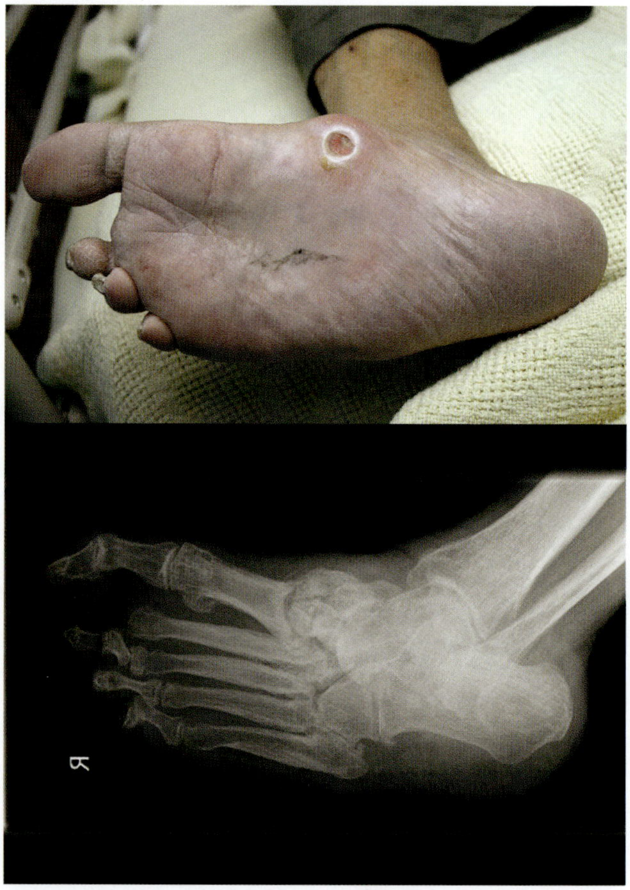

Figure 10.17 Charcot joint in a foot secondary to recurrent severe vasculitic neuropathy. The second phalanx has been amputated and a new vasculitic ulcer is present on the sole of the foot.

Distal symmetric sensory neuropathy Distal symmetric sensory neuropathy (DSSN) is the most common of the diabetic neuropathies. It presents with a slowly progressive 'glove and stocking' sensory loss which may be painful. Small fibre symptoms may also be present. With severe neuropathy, neuropathic Charcot joints may be present (Figure 10.17).

It is rarely necessary to perform a sural nerve biopsy on someone with apparently uncomplicated DSSN. Many of the biopsy features are non-specific but reduplication of basement membranes (Figure 10.18) and other endothelial alterations are commonly found.

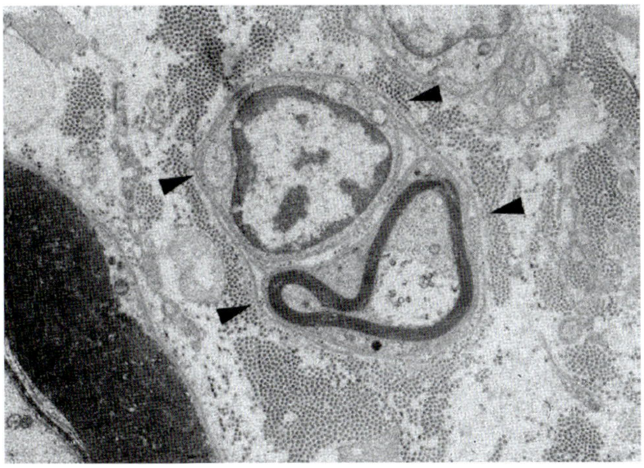

Figure 10.18 A diabetic nerve demonstating reduplication of the basal lamina (arrows) around a Schwann cell and myelinated nerve fibre.

The pathophysiology is poorly understood but relates to prolonged periods of hyperglycaemia increasing flux through the polyol pathway. Increased metabolic and oxidative stresses result in advanced glycated end-products in nerve.

There is no effective treatment but progress of the neuropathy can be largely arrested with aggressive diabetic control, although this is only achieved in about 25% of patients. Pain can be treated with antiepileptic and antidepressant medication.

Autonomic neuropathies These occur in both type 1 and 2 diabetes but are often most severe in type 1. Diabetes is the most common cause of autonomic neuropathy in the West. Up to 75% of men have impotence. Gastrointestinal motility disorders are common with constipation and nocturnal diarrhoea. Subclinical cardiovascular autonomic involvement is common with sympathetic and parasympathetic cardiac denervation demonstrated by fixed high heart rates. Postural hypotension is demonstrable in more than 40% of patients but is seldom symptomatic.

Vasculitic plexopathies The most common plexopathy is the diabetic lumbosacral plexopathy (also known as diabetic femoral neuropathy, diabetic amyotrophy, lower limb asymmetric motor neuropathy or Bruns–Garland syndrome). Patients present with asymmetric aching pain in the buttock, hip or thigh followed by progressive weakness and wasting affecting the hip flexors and quadriceps. The knee jerks are lost but sensory loss is unusual unless there is a coexistent DSSN. Patients describe a progressive history of asymmetric leg ache or pain followed by weakness and wasting, mostly in the femoral compartment. Usually, dramatic weight loss and the appearance of diabetes or worsening of its control are prominent. Cervical plexopathies and thoracolumbar radiculopathies have also been described. These probably have the same pathogenesis.

Nerve conduction studies show radicular neurogenic changes in the quadriceps muscles. Pathological studies have suggested that this is a microvasculitis.

Regaining tight control of the diabetes is the basis of treatment. Both IVIG and pulsed intravenous and oral steroids have been anecdotally been said to be of benefit. However, spontaneous recovery (which is sometimes complete) may occur over 18–24 months without any treatment.

Focal and multi-focal mononeuropathies Individual mononeuropathies including CTS and peroneal neuropathies are more common in diabetes than in the healthy population because nerves are more susceptible to the mechanical effects of compression.

Cranial nerve palsies, most commonly pupil-sparing 'microvascular' IIIrd nerve palsies, are not uncommon. The VIIth and VIth nerves may also be affected.

Small fibre neuropathy See Small fibre neuropathies.

Acute reversible hyperglycaemic neuropathy In patients with uncontrolled hyperglycaemia, an uncomfortable mainly lower limb sensory neuropathy can develop acutely. Nerve conduction is slowed. The symptoms resolve with reversal of the hyperglycaemia.

Insulin neuritis Rarely, an acute painful neuropathy may develop after the introduction of insulin, leading to rapid normalisation of glycaemic control. There is scant evidence to support a pathology but a pre-existing diabetic neuropathy may be unmasked with sudden relative hypoglycaemia. Prognosis is good if insulin therapy is continued.

Neuropathies associated with diabetes (e.g. CIDP) CIDP, but not GBS, was thought to occur more commonly in diabetics than the otherwise healthy population although this epidemiological association may not be correct from more recent studies. Severe proximal and distal diabetic neuropathy should be investigated for supra-added CIDP.

Hypoglycaemia Recurrent and severe hypoglycaemia, as occurs in insulinoma, results in a distal symmetric sensorimotor neuropathy. Distal painful parasthesiae are usually prominent. Correction of the hypoglycaemia by treatment of the insulinoma results in improvement of the sensory symptoms but not the motor.

Hypothyroidism Frank hypothyroidism is associated with a sensory axonal neuropathy in a substantial number of cases. CTS occurs frequently as a presenting feature.

Acromegaly Unrecognised and untreated acromegaly is now unusual. Most commonly weakness is caused by myopathy. Carpal tunnel syndrome is common as are other entrapment neuropathies partly through hypertrophy of nerves. A distal predominantly sensory axonal neuropathy also occurs.

Toxic, nutritional and metabolic peripheral neuropathies

Toxic neuropathies Peripheral nerve is relatively sensitive to the effects of systemic toxins (Chapter 19). The number of implicated drugs, chemicals and neurotoxins are too numerous to discuss each individually (Table 10.12). The reader is referred to http://neuromuscular.wustl.edu for a discussion of individual toxins.

If toxin exposure is suspected a full history and examination should be performed and a sample of the toxin should be retrieved if possible. Serum and urine specimens should be collected and, for acute poisoning, an acute poisons unit consulted.

Most toxins cause axonal neuropathies, some of which have either a motor or sensory predominance. Far fewer toxins cause demyelination (e.g. amiodarone or bortezomib). Frequently, the severity of the neuropathy is dose related. Removal of the source of the toxin may result in recovery which may be complete. Some agents, for example taxol, 'coast' (i.e. the neuropathy tends to

Table 10.12 Toxic neuropathies. After http://www.neuro.wustl.edu/neuromuscular.

Axonal				
Sensory	**Sensory and motor**	**Motor**	**Demyelinating**	**Mixed**
Bortezomib	Acrylamide	β-bungarotoxin	Buckthorn	Amiodarone
Chloramphenicol	Alcohol (ethanol)	Botulism	Chloroquine	Ethylene glycol
Dioxin	Allyl chloride	Dimethylamine borane	Diphtheria	1,1′-Ethylidinebis
Doxorubicin	Arsenic	Gangliosides	FK506 (tacrolimus)	[tryptophan]
Ethambutol	Cadmium	Latrotoxin (Black widow spider venom)	Hexachlorophene	Gold
Ethionamide	Carbon disulphide	Lead	Muzolimine	Hexacarbons
Etoposide	Ciguatoxin	Mercury	Perhexiline	n-Hexane
Gemcitabine	Colchicine	Misoprostol	Procainamide	Na^+ cyanate
Glutethimide	Cyanide	Tetanus	Tellurium	Suramin
Hydralazine	Dapsone	Tick paralysis	Zimeldine	
Ifosfamide	Dichloroacetate			
Interferon-α	Disulfiram			
Isoniazid	DMAPN (foams)			
Lead	Ethylene oxide			
Leflunomide	Heroin			
Metronidazole	Lithium			
Misonidazole	Methyl bromide			
Nitrous oxide	Nitrofurantoin			
Nucleosides	Organophosphates			
ddC; ddI;	Podophyllin			
d4T; 3TC	Polychlorinated biphenyls			
Phenytoin	Saxitoxin			
Platinum analogues	Spanish toxic oil			
Propafenone	Taxol			
Pyridoxine	Tetrodotoxin			
Statins	Thallium			
Thalidomide	Trichloroethylene			
	Tri-ortho-cresyl phosphate			
	Vacor (PNU, a rat poison)			
	Vinca alkaloids			

continue to worsen) for several weeks or months after removal of the toxin. Heavy metal poisoning may require specific treatment (e.g. lead, mercury and thallium) and toxins (e.g. α-latrotoxin, botulinum toxin) may benefit from antitoxin therapy. Prolonged supportive therapy in ITU may be required (e.g. botulism, tick paralysis).

Nutritional Vitamin deficiencies occur through inborn errors of metabolism (e.g. vitamin E deficiency, methylcobalamin deficiency; Chapter 19), limited dietary intake (vegan/vegetarian diet, alcoholism) or failure of absorption (post-ileal resection, pancreatic failure, coeliac disease). Deficiencies may therefore be isolated or combined. Neuropathies are invariably axonal, some associated with pain or ataxia and many with CNS involvement. Replacement of deficient vitamins by supplementation or providing an alternative metabolite can halt and sometimes improve the neuropathy.

Multi-vitamin malabsorption syndromes

1. *Coeliac disease* Coeliac disease is associated with a typical length-dependent sensory neuropathy, sometimes with pain. As well as the systemic disease features, coeliac has also been associated with seizures, ataxia, myopathy, headaches and vitamin A deficient night-blindness. Causation is difficult to prove except in the latter.
2. *Inflammatory bowel disease* Occasionally, a neuropathy occurs proportionate to the severity of the illness. Vitamin B_{12} deficiency through terminal ileal malabsorption is common.
3. *Cuban epidemic neuropathy* (Strachan's syndrome) Strachan's syndrome was described in prisoners of war. Cuban epidemic neuropathy occurs in patients of Afro-Caribbean origin and is very similar. It is thought to be caused by deficiencies in B vitamin and sulphur compounds. It typically occurs between 25 and 65 years of age with no sex predominance. Risk factors include tobacco and cassava consumption. The neuropathy is distal, axonal, sensory and often painful and occurs with an optic neuropathy presenting as central scotomata. Early treatment with B and multi-vitamin preparations can lead to resolution of the neuropathy although visual field defects may persist.
4. *Post gastroplasty/gastrectomy* Patients may become malnourished through severely reduced dietary intake, diversion, bypass or resective procedures and sometimes vomiting. Copper and selenium deficiency may occur. Polyneuropathy, mononeuropathies (especially CTS), radiculopathies and myelopathies are all described.

Vitamin deficiencies (Chapter 19)

1. *Vitamin B_1* (beri-beri) presents with an acute or chronic length dependent sensorimotor axonal neuropathy primarily affecting the legs. Burning feet with lancinating pains are common as is autonomic involvement in severe disease. Wernicke–Korsakoff syndrome, cerebellar degeneration and cranial nerve palsies also occur as well as the systemic features of beri-beri (heart failure, oedema and weight loss).
2. *Pyridoxine* (vitamin B_6) In excess, pyridoxine typically causes a neuropathy/neuronopathy syndrome. Deficiency causes a length-dependent polyneuropathy. Users of isoniazid, penicillamine and hydralazine as well as alcoholics, the elderly and the malnourished are all at risk and should receive appropriate supplements.
3. *Vitamin B_{12}* The causes of B_{12} deficiency are legion and all neuropathy blood profiles could include the measurement of B_{12} and folate. Symptoms are compounded by central and peripheral involvement. Deficiency may be long-standing and chronic. Nitrous oxide dental anaesthesia may unmask it. Typically, large fibre modality distal sensory loss begins first and motor involvement occurs later. Corticospinal tract involvement may lead to pyramidal weakness and extensor plantar responses. Treatment with vitamin B_{12} may stabilise or improve the neuropathy but seldom improves the central involvement.
4. *Vitamin E* Deficiency states cause a distal axonal neuropathy associated with cerebellar and posterior column involvement. Plantar responses may be extensor.

Metabolic neuropathies

Porphyrias Acute intermittent porphyria (AIP), coproporphyria, variegate porphyria and δ-amino-levulinate dehydratase porphyria cause neurological syndromes (Chapter 19). The most common is AIP.

AIP typically occurs in attacks, affecting women more than men. Abdominal pain and constipation reflect the sympathetic and parasympathetic involvement which can cause great management difficulties with additional cardiovascular instability. The neuropathy is motor and sensory and may be severe enough to result in respiratory failure and require ventilation.

Nerve conduction studies typically show axonal degeneration with denervation and small sensory potentials.

Treatment of attacks is with haem arginate or haematin and supportive measures to treat pain, constipation and weakness (including ventilation).

Uraemic neuropathy Renal failure, uraemia and dialysis are all associated with a multi-factorial neuropathy. Up to 60% of patients have a subclinical neuropathy. Symptoms and signs are of a length dependent sensory axonal neuropathy occasionally with pain and prominent itching. Recovery from renal failure or renal transplantation may improve or reverse the symptoms.

Critical illness neuromyopathy

The existence of a severe critical illness neuropathy in the absence of a myopathy is controversial (Chapter 20). Most patients who have a period of intensive care will develop a mild distal sensory neuropathy and some limb weakness of unknown cause. However, some patients have a severe proximal and distal weakness, sometimes affecting ventilation and weaning because of a myosin loss myopathy. This is most common in sepsis, dialysis-dependent renal failure and as a consequence of severe and prolonged ITU admission. On examination patients may be profoundly weak (including neck flexors), have absent reflexes and they often have distal sensory loss. Small compound muscle action potentials (CMAPs) are found on electrophysiology because of muscle inexcitability rather than axonal loss. Myosin is depleted in muscle biopsy specimens. Treatment is supportive.

Small fibre neuropathies

Small fibre neuropathies (SFN) are an increasingly recognised and symptomatically troublesome group of disorders with diverse causation. There are no studies of the epidemiology of SFN. This is largely because of the lack of a satisfactory definition for SFN and standardised methods of investigation and detection. A reasonable definition is a neuropathy characterised by positive (spontaneous or stimulus-induced) or negative sensory symptoms caused by dysfunction of Aδ or C fibres with or without autonomic abnormalities as assessed by specific neuropathological or electrophysiological tests. Asymptomatic small fibre involvement also occurs.

Table 10.13 Small fibre neuropathies.

Idiopathic
Idiopathic small fibre neuropathy
Recognised syndromes (e.g. burning mouth, burning feet, Ross syndrome, rectal hypersensitivity, vulvodynia)
Metabolic
Diabetes mellitus
Impaired glucose tolerance
Hyperlipidaemia
Toxic
Alcohol
Metronidazole
HAART
Statins
Environmental and marine toxins
Infective
HIV
EBV
Leprosy
Chagas disease
Botulism
Immune
Associated with MGUS
Paraneoplastic
Sjögren's syndrome
Sarcoidosis
SLE
Inflammatory bowel disease
Hereditary
Fabry disease
Tangier disease
Hereditary sensory and autonomic neuropathies (especially HSAN I, IV and V)
Familial amyloid polyneuropathy
Familial burning beet
Systemic amyloidosis

EBV, Epstein–Barr virus; HAART, highly active antiretroviral therapy; MGUS, monoclonal gammopathies of undetermined significance; SLE, systemic lupus erythematosus.

The list of causes of SFN is increasing (Table 10.13). Unfortunately, perhaps 50% or more small fibre neuropathies have no identifiable cause. Recently up to one-quarter of patients with idiopathic small fibre neuropathy have been shown to have mutations in the *SCN9A* gene encoding the voltage gated sodium channel $NaV_{1.7}$.

Symptoms SFN most often presents with positive sensory symptoms of pain (often burning, pricking or aching) in the feet. Sometimes the symptoms also affect the upper limbs. Pain may be spontaneous or stimulus evoked. It is often worse at night, may interfere substantially with sleep and can be relieved temporarily by walking or immersing the feet in cold water. Lancinating pain and paraesthesiae are usually indicative of additional large fibre involvement.

An association with restless legs syndrome is not uncommon. Significant autonomic disturbances are uncommon in idiopathic small fibre neuropathy and most often mild. Prominent orthostatic hypotension, faecal urgency, diarrhoea (especially nocturnal) and incontinence, urinary difficulties, impotence and sweating abnormalities should all prompt a search for diabetes, amyloid, vasculitis or a hereditary cause.

Signs The allowable clinical signs in SFN vary between experts in the field. Usually there is reduced temperature and pain sensation in the feet. Otherwise there should be no muscle wasting or weakness, deep tendon reflexes should be present and bedside vibration and proprioception should be normal.

Investigation Causation should be sought with appropriate blood tests and chest X-ray. Genetic testing for mutations in *SCN9A* should be considered (many polymorphisms exist). Standard nerve conduction tests are normal. Thermal threshold testing (especially warm thresholds which correlate well with intra-epidermal nerve fibre densities) is an effective method to confirm the diagnosis. Other tests are being developed (contact heat evoked potentials, laser evoked potentials, measurement of cutaneous silent periods and axon reflex flare responses) but are yet to be fully validated or widely used. Skin biopsy is a useful, largely painless, site specific and minimally morbid procedure to quantify intraepidermal nerve fibre density with high diagnostic efficiency and predictive value. Sural nerve biopsy does not form part of the investigation of SFN.

Treatment No treatments are yet available to treat or reverse SFN. Treatment is largely symptomatic and trials of gabapentin, pregabalin, sodium valproate, topiramate and opiates all demonstrate some benefit. Tricyclic antidepressants, duloxetine, oxcarbazepine and others are often tried. Enzyme replacement is helpful for the SFN in Fabry disease. Erythropoietin has shown promise in limited *in vitro* studies.

Idiopathic axonal neuropathy

Despite best practice the cause of at least 25% of neuropathies remain undiagnosed. These are largely a group of slowly progressive but usually non-disabling axonal and SFN. Careful history-taking, examination and sometimes the ability to examine 'unaffected' relatives improves diagnosis. It is to be hoped that over the coming years many of these conditions will be diagnosed more successfully.

Focal and compressive neuropathies

Focal neuropathies are the result of local damage to individual nerve trunks. They may be single or multiple; the occurrence of more than one pressure palsy should stimulate a search for a predisposing cause. Damage occurs most frequently because of compression, usually as the nerve passes through a tissue tunnel (bone, ligament, aponeurosis, muscle), or against an underlying surface at an exposed site (e.g. the peroneal nerve as it passes around the head of the fibula). Compression may also occur with prolonged abnormal postures (e.g. radial paralysis in the 'Saturday night palsy'). Diabetes, HNPP and alcohol overuse render nerves susceptible to the effects of otherwise non-damaging pressure.

The pathogenesis of focal compressive nerve dysfunction is probably multi-factorial and in experimental studies the mechanisms of acute and chronic compression have been shown to differ. At sites of acute compression endoneurial fluid, axonal contents and subsequently myelin are squeezed down the pressure gradient at the edge of the compression, resulting in nerve intussusception and subsequently Wallerian degeneration. In chronic compression, focal demyelination is found with alterations in nodal structure suggestive of a 'myelin slippage' secondary to stretching. In addition, endoneurial ischaemia may occur and contribute to focal pathology. The transperineurial venous plexus may be easily compressed as it obliquely exits the perineurium resulting in increased endoneurial tissue pressures, reduced blood flow and alteration in the endoneurial metabolic microenvironment. Over the longer term, impaired axonal transport may result in reduced distal trophic support. Furthermore, a nerve that becomes tethered at a site of inflammation can become further damaged; the inability of the nerve to glide during limb movement results in more nerve stretching.

Compression palsies cause signs in the motor and sensory distribution distal to the site of compression. Symptoms may occur both proximal and distal to the site. The reader is referred to diagrams of neuromuscular innervation at the beginning of this chapter (Figure 10.3, Figure 10.4, Figure 10.5 and Figure 10.6). The most common focal neuropathies affect the median (CTS), ulnar and common peroneal nerves. Many other nerves may be affected producing a variety of syndromes, many with colloquial names; e.g. orator's [anterior interosseous] and claw [ulnar] hand, waiter's tip and Saturday night [radial] palsies in the upper limb and toilet seat [sciatic], strawberry and turnip picker's and hoeing [peroneal] palsies in the lower limb). These are not always entirely 'typical' as anatomical variations may vary muscle and cutaneous innervation (e.g. Martin–Gruber anastomoses between median and ulnar nerves). Lesions of any other individual nerve trunk are possible and result in motor and/or sensory signs in the distribution of their innervation. The most common are the lateral cutaneous nerve of the thigh (resulting in meralgia paraesthetica), sciatic, radial, long thoracic, 'tarsal tunnel' (distal tibial [posterior] and peroneal [anterior] neuropathies) and femoral neuropathies.

History, examination and investigation follow similar principles to those already described. These are outlined with their colloquial terminology in Table 10.14. For more detailed descriptions the reader is referred to specialised texts.

Median nerve compression and carpal tunnel syndrome

Median nerve compression between the flexor retinaculum of the wrist and the bones of the carpus is referred to as carpal tunnel syndrome (CTS) and is the most common of the median compression palsies. The prevalence has been estimated at more than 6% of the population.

Table 10.14 Other focal neuropathies.

Colloquial terminology	Sites of compression	Weakness	Sensory loss
UPPER LIMB			
Median nerve			
Carpal tunnel syndrome (CTS)	Wrist (carpal tunnel)	Opponens pollicis, abductor pollicis brevis, flexor pollicis brevis, lumbricals	Palmar skin of thumb, digits II, III (and lateral IV)
Circle sign	Anterior interosseous nerve (below elbow)	Flexor pollicis longus and flexor digitorum profundus (median) – the circle sign	None
Orator's hand	Bicipital aponeurosis (elbow), or ligament of Struthers (above elbow)	Median innervated flexors (profundus/superficialis) and pollicis + pronators quadratus and teres	Palmar + CTS loss
Ulnar nerve			
Guyon canal syndrome	Guyon canal at wrist	Interossei and abductor digiti minimi (variable)	Distal superficial ulnar (variable)
'Claw hand'/tardy ulnar palsy/cubital tunnel syndrome	Elbow	As above + flexor carpi ulnaris, flexor digitorum profundus (ulnar)	Medial surface of palm and digits V and IV
Radial nerve			
Waiter's tip palsy	Upper arm/axilla	Triceps (strong in proximal lesions), brachioradialis, wrist and finger extensors	Superficial radial territory of hand (snuff box)
Tourniquet palsy			
Saturday night palsy			
Crutch palsy (sometimes with ulnar and median = triad neuropathy)			

(continued)

Table 10.14 (continued)

Colloquial terminology	Sites of compression	Weakness	Sensory loss
Wartenberg syndrome	Wrist	None	
Cheiralgia paraesthetica			
Axillary nerve	Axilla or humeral head	Deltoid	Skin over deltoid
Suprascapular nerve			
Pitcher's neuropathy	Suprascapular notch or ligament	Supra- and infraspinatus weakness (often painful)	None
Long thoracic nerve			
Rucksack palsy Long thoracic neuropathy	Shoulder or lateral thoracic wall	Serratus anterior	None
Brachial plexus			
Neurogenic thoracic outlet syndrome	C7 transverse process, anterior scalene muscle, fibrous band	C8 root > T1 root hence thenar > hypothenar muscles	Ulnar border of hand, forearm and arm
LOWER LIMB			
Sciatic nerve			
Toilet seat palsy	Gluteal compression	Hamstrings and all muscles below knee	Tibial and common peroneal territories (latter more common if partial)
Yoga paralysis	Sciatic notch	May also involve superior/inferior gluteal nerve	? + posterior cutaneous nerve of thigh
Catamenial sciatica (with endometriosis)			
Peroneal nerve			
Strawberry picker's, (olive) harvester's, turnip picker's, hoeing or clergyman's palsy	Popliteal fossa, lateral fibular head and fibular tunnel	Tibialis anterior, extensor hallucis longus, extensor digitorum and peronei	Lateral lower leg and dorsum of foot
Anterior (tibial) compartment syndrome	Tibial compartment	Tibialis anterior, extensor hallucis longus, extensor digitorum	Interspace and dorsum of digit I and II
Anterior tarsal tunnel syndrome	Ankle	None	Interspace and dorsum of digit I and II
Tibial nerve			
Tibial neuropathy	Posterior knee	Gastrocnemius, soleus, tibialis posterior, flexor digitorum longus and intrinsic foot muscles	Sole of foot ± sural
(Posterior) tarsal tunnel syndrome	Tarsal tunnel	Intrinsic foot muscles	
Femoral nerve	Pelvis, thigh	Psoas, quadriceps	Anterior thigh and medial aspect of calf
Lateral cutaneous nerve of the thigh			
Meralgia paraesthetica	Inguinal ligament	None	Lateral thigh

Table 10.15 Causes of median neuropathy at the elbow.

Fractured humerus
Elbow dislocation
Direct trauma
Anatomical compression
Supracondylar ligament/spur
Biceps aponeurosis
Pronator teres
Tumours and masses
Angiography/venepuncture

Compression in the more proximal upper limb occurs more rarely. Median nerve compression in the axilla usually co-occurs with radial and ulnar nerve compressions and is most commonly caused by traumatic or surgical injury, or unusual compressive forces (e.g. crutches or heavy sleep through intoxication). In the upper arm trauma is the most common insult and the median nerve may be affected in isolation. At the elbow the median nerve is susceptible to numerous injuries (Table 10.15). Compression at the elbow or more proximally is easily clinically identifiable as it leads to inability to pronate the forearm and flex the distal phalanx of thumb and index finger (orator's hand). Numbness affects the palm as well as the distal fingers.

Carpal tunnel syndrome

CTS is 3–8 times more common in women than men. It most commonly affects both hands, usually the dominant hand first. There are many recognised causes of CTS (Table 10.16). Numbness, paraesthesiae and pain in the hand and sometimes in the more proximal arm, often occurring at night, are the most common presenting complaints. When the pain is intermittent, shaking the hand or wrist relieves the symptoms and is a relatively reliable sign of compression at the wrist. The provactive tests of median nerve compression include Tinel's sign in which a light tapping over the nerve elicits tingling in the sensory distribution of the nerve or Phalen's test when the patient holds their wrists in complete and forced flexion to reproduce the symptoms. If not treated, these sensory symptoms become permanent and weakness and wasting of the thenar eminence may become apparent.

Examination Compression of the median nerve at the wrist typically results in sensory disturbance on the palmar skin of the thumb, second, third and half the fourth digit and weakness of abductor pollicis brevis, opponens pollicis, first and second lumbricals and sometimes flexor pollicis brevis. There are many anatomical variations. The palmar cutaneous branch arises proximal to the flexor retinaculum and does not pass through the carpal tunnel. Occasionally, the motor branch may pierce the retinaculum and may escape compression but be damaged during surgery.

Investigation Nerve conduction studies are required to confirm the diagnosis as demonstration of the clinical symptoms and signs is not 100% reliable. About 5% of studies are falsely negative, but a negative study should provoke a search for an alternative diagnosis (C6/7 radiculopathy, thoracic outlet syndrome or thalamic infarction). Severely affected patients are unlikely to benefit from surgical decompression as there is no remaining nerve to save. Where anatomical variants or structural abnormalities of the wrist are considered MRI can be most helpful in assisting both diagnostician and surgeon. The yield from haematological and biochemical testing where no pathology is detected on thorough clinical examination is low.

Table 10.16 Causes of carpal tunnel syndrome.

Rheumatoid arthritis
Bony osteophytes, degenerative wrist disease, wrist fractures
Gouty tophi
Congenitally narrow tunnel
Intracanalicular ganglia
Work-related repetitive strain
Pregnancy
Hypothyroidism/hyperthyroidism
Diabetes
Acromegaly
Amyloidosis
Vasculitides
Multiple myeloma
Chronic renalailure, renal failure, uraemia and dialysis
Mucopolysaccharidosis
Infections (e.g. leprosy)
Predisposing conditions: diabetes, HNNP, inflammatory neuropathy (e.g. CIDP, MMNCB)
Idiopathic

CIDP, chronic inflammatory demyelinating polyradiculoneuropathy; HNNP, hereditary neuropathy with liability to pressure palsies; MMNCB, multi-focal motor neuropathy with conduction block.

Treatment There is evidence of variable quality that non-surgical interventions including oral steroids, ultrasound, yoga and carpal bone mobilisation are effective in the short term for symptom relief. There is no benefit from the use of non-steroidal anti-inflammatory drugs or diuretics. Nocturnal splinting can relieve the symptoms in mild disease. Local steroid injections into the carpal tunnel seems to provide short-term relief, and while this procedure is carried out widely, a needle can cause median nerve injury. Surgical decompression gives the most satisfactory relief (90–95% success) in both the short and long term (3% recurrence rate) and is associated with minimal risks. Results are better if symptoms have been present for less than 3 years. Endoscopic release has few advantages over open procedures and is more often associated with failure.

Ulnar nerve compression

The ulnar nerve can also be damaged anywhere along its course from the brachial plexus to the hand. The most common site of damage is at the elbow. Here the nerve is exposed to trauma, pressure and stretching as it passes the medial epicondyle through the ulnar groove and then deep to the flexor aponeurosis under flexor carpi ulnaris. Other causes reflect the causes – similar to median neuropathy (Table 10.17). An extensive differential diagnosis of conditions mimicking ulnar neuropathy exists (Table 10.18).

Table 10.17 Causes of ulnar neuropathy.

Bony deformity at elbow
Fractures
Rheumatoid arthritis
Osteophytes
Paget's disease
Congenitally shallow condylar canal
Pressure
Bony
Prolonged elbow flexion
Peri-operative/ITU compression
Soft tissue/neural/bony masses
Variable anatomy (muscles/fibrous bands)
Supracondylar spur
Diabetes
Vasculitides
Leprosy
Predisposing conditions – diabetes, HNNP, inflammatory neuropathy (e.g. CIDP, MMNCB)
Idiopathic

CIDP, chronic inflammatory demyelinating polyradiculoneuropathy; MMNCB, multi-focal motor neuropathy with conduction block.

Table 10.18 Conditions mimicking ulnar neuropathy.

Cord lesions/myeloradiculopathy
Syringomyelia
Hirayama monomelic atrophy
Amyotrophic lateral sclerosis
C8/T1 radiculopathy
Thoracic outlet syndrome
Lower brachial plexus lesions (trauma/infiltration/radiation/post sternotomy)
Brachial neuritis (neuralgic amyotrophy)
Multi-focal motor neuropathy with conduction block

Symptoms Numbness and tingling affecting the fourth and fifth digits of the hand are the most frequent presenting complaints. Deep pain may be felt proximal to the nerve. Weakness of hand grip appears later but may be the only symptom in some. The elbow may be identified as a site of previous damage, trauma or pressure and occasionally sensitivity of the ulnar nerve at the elbow is reported.

Signs Accurate clinical localisation of ulnar neuropathies is essential to guide exploration and treatment. Weakness of first dorsal interosseous and abductor digiti minimi in the hand is most common. Motor branches and the distal superficial cutaneous branches all pass through Guyon's canal; signs confined only to this territory could result from compression at the wrist or more proximally. Sensory loss should not extend above the wrist; the medial cutaneous nerve of the forearm emerges from the brachial plexus. Weakness of the flexor digitorum profundus to the fourth and fifth digits or flexor carpi ulnaris puts the lesion at the elbow or above. Involvement of the palmar skin of the medial border of the hand or the dorsal skin of the affected fingers excludes compression in Guyon's canal at the wrist. Additional weakness of median nerve innervated muscles (see Median nerve compression and carpal tunnel syndrome) suggests alternative diagnoses. The presence of a thickened nerve at the elbow suggests inflammatory, hereditary, tumour or lepromatous involvement.

Treatment Effective treatment of ulnar neuropathies usually involves surgical intervention. Conservative measures aimed at educating the patient to avoid leaning on the elbow, nocturnal splinting and diffusing pressure with sheepskin elbow pads may all assist. Surgery should be offered to patients who have sensory and motor signs consistent with the diagnosis, especially if there is clear worsening. Patients with sensory signs only should be closely reviewed to detect signs of progression – most will remit. In late severe cases with weakness, wasting and sensory loss surgical intervention may not be beneficial but tendon transfer procedures may help hand function. Surgical approaches involve removing compressing structures (e.g. masses) if appropriate, and thereafter releasing and mobilising the nerve to a greater or lesser extent. Transposition of the nerve is associated with greater risks of peri-operative damage and thus extensive exploration and release may often be the most appropriate intervention.

Other ulnar neuropathies Ulnar neuropathies at other sites are identified by careful history-taking, examination directed at ulnar nerve innervation and more widely in the neck, chest and upper limb and neurophysiological 'inching studies' (inch by inch). Imaging (both MRI and ultrasound) are more widely used to identify abnormalities in sites other than the elbow.

Common peroneal neuropathies

Isolated lesions of the peroneal nerve are the third most common of the mononeuropathies. The common peroneal nerve is most liable to damage as it winds laterally around the knee and fibula head. It then passes through the fibular tunnel (a fibrous arch derived from peroneus longus) before dividing into superficial and deep peroneal nerves (Figure 10.7).

Symptoms Complete common peroneal lesions cause a foot drop with inability to evert the foot or extend the toes and a characteristic high-stepping and audibly slapping gait. The sensory loss covers the lower half of the lateral part of the leg and dorsum of the foot, sparing the sural nerve territory. The history may or may not reveal an obvious cause (Table 10.19). A history of focal pain elsewhere in the leg or other systemic symptoms should prompt a search for a local or systemic cause.

Signs The site of the lesion may be clear from the history or obvious site of damage from examination. However, the variability of innervations in the leg, and common occurrence of partial nerve lesions of the sciatic, lumbosacral trunk or multiple radiculopathies, means that an electrical study is often crucial for localising the site of damage and directing further investigation and treatment.

Investigation Nerve conduction and EMG studies enable localisation of any lesion from root (often L5) through the lumbosacral trunk and sciatic nerve to the more distal branches of the superficial and deep peroneal nerves. Although plain radiographs, CT and

Table 10.19 Causes of common peroneal nerve palsy.

Pressure
Leg crossing
Prolonged crouching (for example childbirth, 'strawberry pickers' palsy, yoga)
Lithotomy stirrups
Plaster casts
Peri-operative/ITU
Anterior (fibial) compartment syndrome
Nerve entrapment
Fibula tunnel
Post fracture fibrosis
Trauma
Direct penetrating or blunt trauma
Fibula fracture
Knee dislocation
Popliteal fossa lesions
Baker's cyst, haematoma, DVT
Nerve tumours
Neuroma, schwannoma, lymphoma
Diabetes
Leprosy
Vasculitis
Idiopathic

DVT, deep venous thrombosis.

arteriography have diagnostic use in specific scenarios, MRI scanning has greatest utility in demonstrating intrinsic and extrinsic mass lesions (both tumours and inflammatory) of the nerve.

Treatment Acute trauma with nerve transection or compartment syndromes are surgical emergencies and intervention to explore and relieve pressure and/or repair the nerve is indicated. Where an episode of prolonged nerve compression is identified avoidance of further injury and watchful waiting are appropriate. Most lesions recover. Lesions that progress or fail to recover, or lesions associated with other structural abnormalities should be surgically explored.

Plexopathies

The two major nerve plexuses are the brachial and lumbosacral. Lesions of a plexus cause complex post-ganglionic motor and sensory deficits in the distribution of part or all of the plexus. The reader is referred to the anatomical diagrams (Figures 10.3 and 10.6) to assist with identifying and localising involvement. Causes are shown in Table 10.20. Many of these are common to both plexuses. Some, for example neuralgic (brachial) amyotrophy and diabetic lumbosacral plexopathy, have a predilection for one or the other.

Table 10.20 Plexopathies (brachial or lumbosacral, except where indicated).

Trauma (mostly brachial plexus)
Shoulder injury – upward or downward
Peri-operative
Arm manoeuvres during pharmacological neuromuscular paralysis
Median sternotomy
Jugular/subclavian cannulation and thrombosis
Shoulder supports in head-down procedures
Fracture dislocation
Traction in newborns (Klumpke palsy)
Compression
Back pack
Haematomas and aneurysms
Thoracic outlet syndrome
Pregnancy and prolonged labour (lumbosacral plexus)
Retroperitoneal masses (lumbosacral plexus)
Abscess
Haematoma
Abdominal aortic aneurysms (lumbosacral plexus)
Malignancy
Invasive (e.g. metastases)
Brachial – lung (Pancoast), breast, lymphoma, melanoma
Lumbosacral – cervix, ovary, colon, prostate, bladder
Primary – neurofibroma and malignant nerve sheath tumour
Radiotherapy
Acute brachial neuritis (e.g. neuralgic amyotrophy/ Parsonage–Turner syndrome/acute brachial plexus neuropathy)
Diabetes (most commonly lumbosacral plexopathy)
Vasculitis
Inflammatory
CIDP
MMNCB
Hereditary
Hereditary brachial plexopathy (SEPT9)
Hereditary neuropathy with liability to pressure palsies (chromosome 17p11.2 deletion)

CIDP, chronic inflammatory demyelinating polyradiculoneuropathy; MMNCB, multi-focal motor neuropathy with conduction block.

Acute brachial neuritis

Parsonage and Turner described this entity also known as neuralgic amyotrophy in 1948. Typically, acute deep aching pain occurs spontaneously and affects the neck, shoulder and upper arm in a diffuse pattern. This may last from hours to 2 weeks or more; it is sometimes exceedingly painful. This is followed by focal wasting and weakness, most commonly in the distribution of nerves originating from the upper plexus (deltoid, serratus anterior, supraspinatus and infraspinatus and biceps). Muscles in the distributions of the lower brachial plexus may also less commonly be affected. Sensory symptoms occur in about one-third of patients and sensory signs in about two-thirds, most often sensory loss in the territory of the axillary nerve. Prolonged pain, bilateral involvement, structural or mass lesions on examination should prompt a search for an alternative cause.

The cause of brachial neuritis remains uncertain. Occasional rapid recovery and the finding of conduction block point to demyelination as an initial mechanism but clearly axonal degeneration swiftly follows. Rare pathological reports of inflammatory nerve lesions exist. Associations with immunisation, infection, trauma, surgery, pregnancy and childbirth, intravenous heroin and vasculitides point to an immune mechanism. Steroids, although sometimes useful for pain, usually fail to alter the outcome. Other analgesics (including opioids) are usually necessary. About 90% of patients with a typical brachial neuritis will recover in 3 years. Rarely, a similar condition affects the lumbosacral plexus.

Anterior horn cell diseases

Many motor nerve diseases principally affect the anterior horn cell body; these are usually neurodegenerative (e.g. motor neurone disease) or hereditary (e.g. spinal muscular atrophy). However, there is a broad differential diagnosis (Table 10.21).

Table 10.21 Differential diagnosis of motor neurone disease.

Bulbar weakness	
Brainstem	
	(tumour, infarction, infection, demyelination)
	Syringobulbia
Neuromuscular junction	
	Myasthenia gravis
Muscle	
	Oculopharyngeal dystrophy
Others	
	Allgrove's (AAA) syndrome (achalasia, adrenal deficiency, alacrima)
	Neuro-acanthocytosis
	Superficial siderosis
	Neuro-degenerative conditions
Upper motor neurone	
Compressive	
	Cervical spondylosis/radiculopathy
Intrinsic	
	Multiple sclerosis
	Soliliary sclerosis
	Spinal cord tumour
Degenerative	
	Hereditary spastic paraparesis
Infective	
	HTLV1-related myelopathy
Metabolic	
	Subacute combined degeneration
	Adrenomyeloleukodystrophy
Vascular	
	Cord infarction/haemorrhage
Lower motor neurone	
Unknown cause	
	Benign fasciculation/cramps
Hereditary	
	Spinal muscular atrophy
	X-linked bulbospinal neuronopathy (Kennedy's disease)
	Benign monomelic amyotrophy (Hirayama syndrome)
	Charcot–Marie–Tooth diseases
	Distal hereditary motor neuropathies
	Muscular dystrophy – fascio-scapulohumoral
Autoimmune	
	VGKC Ab mediated disease (neuromyotonia, Isaac's syndrome, Morvan's syndrome)
	SLE, Sjögren's syndrome
Infective	
	Postpolio syndrome
	Borrelia
	Syphilitic pachymeningitis
	HIV related
Inflammatory	
	CIDP
	Inflammatory muscle disease (polymyositis, inclusion body myositis)
	Multifocal motor neuropathy with conduction block
Metabolic/endocrine	
	Hexosaminidase A deficiency
	Metabolic muscle disease (acid maltase deficiency)
	Thyrotoxicosis
	Hyperparathyroidism
Toxins	
	Heavy metal toxicity – lead, thallium, arsenic toxicity
	Konzo, lathyrism
	Radiation
	Organophosphate toxicity
Compressive	
	Multiple radiculopathies
Paraneoplastic syndromes	
Neurodegenerative	
Corticobasal degeneration	
Progressive supranuclear palsy	
Multiple system atrophy	
Parkinson's disease	
Huntington's disease	

Motor neurone disease

Motor neurone disease (MND) is a progressive neuronal degenerative disease involving the corticospinal tract, brainstem and anterior horn cells of the spinal cord that leads to severe disability and death. There is considerable variability in presentation, clinical course and prognosis. The condition is divided into several different clinical subtypes. Amyotrophic lateral sclerosis (ALS) is the most common and is characterised by upper and lower motor neurone involvement of the bulbar, upper and lower limb territories; presentation with predominantly or exclusive bulbar weakness (lower and/or upper motor neurone) is referred to as progressive bulbar palsy (PBP). In primary lateral sclerosis (PLS) there is exclusively upper motor neurone involvement and progressive muscular atrophy (PMA) involves only lower motor neurones although there is a considerable overlap between these patterns.

Amyotrophic lateral sclerosis

The onset of ALS is usually with asymmetrical focal wasting and weakness affecting contiguous limb muscles more commonly in the upper limbs. Occasionally, there may be severe isolated wasting and weakness of individual limbs (e.g. flail arms). Other patients may present with bulbar dysfunction, progressive dysarthria and, less commonly, dysphagia. Rarely, there may be selective involvement of respiratory muscles leading to respiratory failure. ALS is characterised by the progressive development of wasting, fasciculation, cramp, weakness, spasticity, brisk reflexes and extensor plantar responses. Limb involvement is more often distal than proximal leading to weakness of the hands or bilateral foot drop. Patients may complain of clumsiness or impaired mobility. Bulbar involvement is characterised by weight loss, dysarthria, wasting, fasciculation and slow movement of the tongue, sialorrhoea and dysphagia. Patients complain of difficulty speaking or occasionally hoarseness which usually precedes swallowing difficulties. Clear fluids tend to aspirate causing the patient to cough after drinking. Hypersalivation becomes difficult to clear and leads to the development of drooling and dribbling. Pseudobulbar involvement is also associated with pathological emotional lability in which there is excessive uncontrolled laughter or crying and a brisk jaw jerk.

Fasciculation is variable but may be prominent after exercise. It is well seen in the tongue and across the back. Head droop may be an early feature because of weakness of the neck extensors and paraspinal muscles. Progressive respiratory muscle weakness may lead to exertional dyspnoea and selective diaphragm weakness will cause breathlessness on lying flat and progressive hypoventilation; examination shows paradoxical movements of the abdomen on inspiration. Increasing limb and truncal weakness causes worsening immobility and self-care. Bulbar weakness leads to increasing difficulty with communication and eventual anarthria with worsening dysphagia. Sleep disturbance is common and multi-factorial related to difficulty turning in bed, periodic limb movements, hypersalivation and inability to clear secretions, difficulty with communication, emotional lability and depression. Sensory, ocular and bladder symptoms are unusual.

Progressive bulbar palsy

PBP is restricted to bulbar musculature at presentation and during the initial progression. The clinical pattern is usually predominantly upper motor neurone but wasting, fasciculation and palatal weakness may also be present. Subsequent spread to the cervical regions and then more generally is usual, but not inevitable, after several months. Occasionally, bulbar weakness remains isolated or the predominant manifestation for many years, although generalised involvement usually develops eventually. PBP constitutes about 15–20% of cases of MND.

Flail arm/leg syndrome

Progressive isolated wasting and flaccid weakness of an arm or leg may be the presenting feature in up to 10%. Upper motor neurone features develop later. This form of the condition is considerably more common in males, often below the age of 50, and carries a better prognosis than ALS.

Primary lateral sclerosis

This is an exclusively upper motor neurone form of MND which occurs in about 10% of patients. Lower motor neurone features may develop in a minority after 5–10 years. The condition develops at an older age and may be slow in its progression. Survival for 20 years is not uncommon. Bladder symptoms are frequent but bulbar involvement often occurs later and is less severe.

Progressive muscular atrophy

This is a heterogeneous syndrome in which there is exclusively lower motor neurone involvement. However, at least 30% of patients with PMA develop upper motor neurone signs within 18 months and progress to ALS. Patients with an exclusively lower motor neurone syndrome and disease duration of 4 years or more have a more favourable prognosis, particularly if muscle involvement is predominantly segmental.

Cognitive involvement

Frontotemporal dementia occurs in <15% of patients with MND. It is characterised by personality change, irritability, poor insight and persuasive deficits on frontal executive tests. A milder form of executive impairment occurs in up to 20% of patients with ALS. It is associated with impaired judgement, behavioural disturbance, impulsivity and is a poor prognostic indicator.

Other forms

The hemiplegic variant of Mills is a rare presentation with mixed upper and lower motor neurone signs occurring on one side of the body. Overlap of MND occurring with features of other neurodegenerative disease including parkinsonism and progressive supranuclear gaze palsy may occur. Facial onset sensory motor neuronopathy (FOSMN) has recently been described. Although there are marked similarities to classic bulbar onset MND, FOSMN is set apart clinically by the striking facial-onset sensory deficits with subsequent development of motor deficits, slow evolution in a rostral–caudal direction and a much better prognosis. The different forms of MND are summarised in Table 10.22.

Aetiology

Sporadic MND is a complex disease and both genetic and environmental factors contribute to the development of the disease.

Genetics Between 5% and 10% of cases of ALS are familial (FALS) and most have an autosomal dominant pattern of inheritance. This is likely to be an underestimate because of incomplete recording or knowledge of family history and the possibility that some cases of sporadic MND represent familial forms with reduced penetrance.

Table 10.22 Forms of motor neurone disease.

Genetic
Familial ALS
Brown–Vialetto–van Laere syndrome
Fazio–Londe
Hexosaminidase A deficiency
HSP
SMA
X-linked bulbo-spinal atrophy (Kennedy's disease)
Multisystem (spino-cerebellar)
Sporadic
Sporadic MND (PBP, ALS, PMA)
PLS
Distal focal SMA
Madras form
Western Pacific form
MND and frontotemporal dementia
Multi-system atrophy
Progressive supranuclear palsy
Corticobasal degeneration
Focal onset sensory motor neuropathy
Acquired
HTLV1-associated myelopathy
HIV-associated MND
Creutzfeldt–Jakob disease
Acute poliomyelitis and post polio syndrome

ALS, amyotrophic lateral sclerosis; HSP, hereditary spastic paraparesis; HTLV, human T-lymphocyte virus; MND, motor neurone disease; PBP, progressive bulbar palsy; PLS, primary lateral sclerosis; PMA, progressive muscular atrophy; SMA, spinal muscular atrophy.

Mutations in more than 15 genes have been found to cause familial MND (Table 10.23). In approximately 20% of patients with FALS the genetic defect is a mutation on chromosome 21 in the gene for copper/zinc superoxide dismutase (*SOD1*). More than 100 mutations of the *SOD1* gene are now known. There is a small incidence of *SOD1* mutation occurring in sporadic MND. *SOD1* mutation screening is available, but counselling is essential before predictive testing can be undertaken. At present genetic screening for predictive testing is not performed routinely. Mutations in several other chromosomal loci have now been described in patients with autosomal recessive inheritance.

Patients with ALS and the C9orf72 repeat expansion are characterised by an earlier age of disease onset, cognitive and behavioural impairment, specific neuroimaging changes (i.e. non-motor cortex change on high resolution [3T] MRI and reduced grey matter volume), a family history of neurodegeneration with autosomal dominant inheritance and reduced survival. Identification of the transactive response DNA-binding protein 43 (TDP 43) as the major inclusion protein, common both to patients with ALS and frontotemporal dementia (FTD-TDP) suggests these conditions are closely related.

Environmental factors There is a 50–150 fold increase in the incidence of MND in the Western Pacific and other geographical clusters are described. The condition differs pathologically from sporadic ALS because dementia and parkinsonism frequently coexist. The pathological findings in these patients differ from sporadic ALS and are characterised by the presence of neurofibrillary tangles. It seems likely this form of the condition is related to a toxin, possibly from the cycad seed.

Lymphoproliferative disease An association between MND and lymphoproliferative disorders has been reported. PLS may rarely occur as a paraneoplastic disease associated with antineuronal antibodies.

Diagnosis of MND

Routine haematology and biochemical screening is usually normal. Creatine kinase (CK) may be mildly or moderately elevated. Underlying lymphoproliferative, infective, endocrine, vasculitic or toxic causes should be excluded. Hexosaminidase A should be checked in the young. Genetic analysis may include *SOD1* and *SMN* in the predominantly lower motor neurone presentation.

Investigations

Neurophysiology is essential in establishing the diagnosis and severity of MND and excluding the differential diagnoses (Tables 10.21 and 10.22). Sensory nerve action potentials (SNAPs) are normal and motor conduction velocities should be >70% of normal. There must be no conduction block. Needle EMG shows neurogenic changes of denervation and reinnervation. There is considerable variability in EMG findings and extensive sampling of bulbar, cervical, thoracic and lumbosacral muscles may be necessary. MRI is important to exclude structural or inflammatory conditions that may mimic MND. MRI may show high signal in the pyramidal tracts indicating Wallerian degeneration in patients with upper motor neurone involvement. Positron emission tomography (PET) imaging has shown cortical changes, particularly in patients with cognitive impairment.

Incidence and prognosis

The annual incidence is 2–3/100 000 and the prevalence approximately 4–8/100 000. Males are more commonly affected than females (1.5 : 1). The incidence increases with age, with a mean age of onset of 63 years and peaks at 50 and 75 years.

The natural history of MND is variable and occasional prolonged periods of stability may occur. Patients with PBP have the worst prognosis because of the risk of aspiration with a median survival of 2–2.5 years. In ALS the mean disease duration is 3–4 years. Over 50% of patients die within 3 years but <10% survive for more than 8 years. In PLS a survival of 20 years is relatively common. In general, rapid rate of progression, early respiratory or bulbar symptoms and increasing age are adverse prognostic indicators, while exclusively upper or lower motor neurone syndromes and young age are associated with a better prognosis.

Management

Telling the patient the diagnosis Diagnostic uncertainty is common during the early stages of the disease. Thus, the diagnosis is usually established 9–15 months after the first symptoms and usually two or three specialists will have been consulted, often resulting in profound anxiety and uncertainty. The communication of the diagnosis is a major and potentially devastating life event which must be handled with great sensitivity. All too often patients complain that the diagnosis has been given in a hurried, off-hand

Table 10.23 The genetic associations of motor neurone disease.

Genetic subtype	Chromosome locus	Gene	Inheritance	Phenotype
Oxidative stress				
ALS 1	21q22	SOD1	Adult/AD	ALS/PMA/(PBP, BFA rarely) Cerebellar ataxia FTD/cognitive impairment
mRNA processing				
ALS 4	9q34	SETX	Juvenile/AD	ALS Oculomotor apraxia Cerebellar ataxia Motor neuropathy
ALS 6	16p11.2	FUS	Adult/AD	ALS–FTD (Parkinsonism)
ALS 9	14q11.2	ANG	Adult/AD	ALS–Parkinsonism
ALS 10	1p36.2	TARDBP	Adult/AD	ALS ALS–FTD Parkinsonism–FTD
ALS-FTD	9q21-q22	C9orf72	Adult/AD	See below
Endosomal trafficking and cell signalling				
ALS 2	2q33	ALS2	Juvenile/AR	Juvenile PLS/ALS
ALS 11	6q21	FIG 4	Adult/AD	CMT/cognitive
ALS 8	20q13.3	VAPB	Adult/AD	
ALS 12	10p13	OPTN	Adult/AD and AR	
Glutamate excitotoxicity				
ND	12q24	DAO	Adult/AD	
Ubiquitin/protein degredation				
ND	9p13-p12	VCP	Adult/AD	
ALSX	Xp11	UBQLN2	Adult/X-linked	
Cytoskeleton				
ALS–dementia–PD	17q21	MAPT	Adult/AD	
Other genes				
ALS 5	15q15-q21	SPG11	Juvenile/AR	Juvenile ALS
ALS–FTD	9p13.3	SIGMAR 1	Adult/AD Juvenile/AR	
Unknown genes 1				
ALS 3	18q21		Adult/AD	
ALS 7	20ptel-p13		Adult/AD	

ALS, amyotrophic lateral sclerosis; ALS-2, alsin; ANG, angiogenin; C9ORF72, chromosome 9 open reading frame 72; DAO, D-amino-acid oxidase; FTD, frontotemporal dementia; FUS, fused in sarcoma; MAPT, microtubule-associated protein tau; OPTN, optineurin; PBP, progressive bulbar palsy; PD, Parkinson's disease; PMA, progressive muscular atrophy; SETX, senataxin; SIGMAR 1, sigma non-opiod intracellular receptor 1; SOD1, superoxidase dismutase 1; SPG11, spatacsin; TARDBP, TAR DNA-binding protein; UBQLN2, ubiquilin 2; VAPB, vesicle-associated membrane protein; VCP, valosin containing protein.

Table 10.24 Important websites related to motor neurone disease.

www.wfnals.org	World Federation of Neurology, Amyotrophic Lateral Sclerosis site
www.mndassociation.org	Motor Neurone Disease Association (England, Wales and Northern Ireland)
www.alsmndalliance.org	International Alliance of ALS/MND Associations
www.cochrane.org	The Cochrane collaboration (includes report on riluzole)
www.theabn.org/downloads/mnddoc.pdp	Guidelines for the management of motor neurone disease, endorsed by the Association of British Neurologists
www.alsa.org	ALS Association (USA)
www.mndscotland.org.uk	Scottish Motor Neurone Disease Association
www.nice.org.uk	National Institute for Clinical Excellence – includes review and recommendations for the use of riluzole

and inappropriate manner. The diagnosis should be explained by a senior physician, in a quiet and private room, with a nurse specialist and a carer present. The patient should be provided written comprehensible information, contact telephone number or e-mail address and a follow-up appointment within a few weeks. Ongoing follow-up should be supervised by a single named doctor, in close liaison with the nurse specialist, GP and community services. The diagnosis and details of the information given to the patient and the management plan must be communicated to the GP without delay.

Principles of management The management of MND involves the coordination of multi-disciplinary care with a team that includes the patient's GP and primary care team, occupational and physiotherapists, clinical nurse specialists, support and social workers and the palliative care team. The supervising neurologist or physician should coordinate a continuum of care for each patient from diagnosis to the terminal phase of the disease. Each member of the team has an individual role. In the United Kingdom, the Motor Neurone Disease Association (MNDA) employs a network of regional care advisors. These individuals act as a point of contact for people with MND and their carers, and help to point to the provision of pieces of equipment such as splints and communication aids. They also provide a telephone helpline and are able to contribute to the support of relatives and carers following the death of the patient. Important websites are listed in Table 10.24.

Pharmacotherapy Riluzole has multiple actions which includes inhibition of glutamate release. It is the only drug that has been shown to increase survival in MND. Riluzole prolonged survival by 3 months after 18 months administration with little or no effect on functional deterioration in two clinical trials. It is usually well tolerated with occasional nausea and fatigue. The drug should be discontinued if liver function tests exceed five times the upper limit of normal. Many patients look to other possible treatments and antioxidants (vitamins C and E) and creatine are in common use despite the absence of evidence from randomised clinical trials. Acupuncture, reflexology, chiropractic manipulation and massage may contribute to the individual's personal feeling of well-being.

Respiratory management Respiratory impairment is common and may develop because of respiratory muscle weakness, impaired bulbar function and obstructive sleep apnoea (OSA) or defects in central control. It should be anticipated in all patients with a diagnosis of MND. Dyspnoea is caused by infection, pulmonary embolus or airway obstruction from mucus plug or inhaled pharyngeal contents. Prompt use of antibiotics should be supplemented with physiotherapy. Annual influenza vaccination should be undertaken. Nocturnal hypoventilation and OSA present as daytime hypersomnolence, lethargy, morning headaches, poor concentration, depression, anxiety and irritability with or without snoring and restless sleep with abnormal movements.

FVC reflects respiratory muscle strength, and serial measurements may be useful in predicting the onset of respiratory failure. Non-invasive ventilation is often initiated when FVC is <50% of predicted. Isolated or selective diaphragm weakness is a particular concern and FVC should be monitored, both standing and lying – a fall of >30% indicates diaphragm weakness. Other markers of impending respiratory failure include maximal inspiratory and expiratory mouth pressures and maximum sniff nasal pressure. Nocturnal oximetry, polysomnography, diaphragmatic EMG and phrenic nerve conduction studies may provide useful additional information.

Respiratory support can provide symptomatic relief and increase life expectancy. These benefits must be balanced against the demands on carers, practical problems of administration, the risk of iatrogenic problems and distressing and unwanted prolongation of life in the terminal stages of MND. Many of these difficulties can be avoided by early and careful discussion with patients and their carers. Elective ventilatory support is usually administered non-invasively (NIV), initially during sleep. NIV allows speech, oral feeding and leads to fewer respiratory infections, extends survival and improves quality of life. However, it may not be desirable in patients with severe bulbar weakness, facial abnormalities or where aspiration has already occurred. Some patients require ventilatory support for increasing periods and may choose to undergo tracheostomy. Tracheostomy carries a significant risk of complications and considerable difficulties in domiciliary management. There remains a concern that tracheostomy may lead to prolonged survival in the face of severe disability. Many patients will decide to use NIV support if their respiratory function deteriorates and is symptomatic. There has been recent interest in pacing the phrenic nerve but this technique is expensive and unproven. The provision and supervision of respiratory support should be through a specialist MND centre.

Management of bulbar weakness Bulbar palsy is one of the most distressing features of MND. Weakness of tongue, pharynx and facial muscles results in slow eating, choking, drooling, dysarthria and dysphonia. Sialorrhoea is generally managed with anticholinergic agents including atropine or amitriptyline taken orally, hyoscine (scopolamine) transdermally or glycopyrronium bromide subcutaneously. Side effects are common in the elderly. Antimuscarinic agents or mucolytic agents render secretions viscid whereas β-blockers have been reported to reduce secretions without increasing tenacity and a saline nebuliser may also be helpful. Portable home suction devices and cough enhancement techniques are also valuable in some patients. Unilateral parotid gland irradiation and botulinum toxin injection into the duct or directly into the parotid gland have also been used although the later may exacerbate any bulbar weakness.

Dysphagia The management of dysphagia requires detailed clinical assessment with videofluoroscopy or fibreoptic techniques. This must be followed by speech and language therapy advice on techniques to ease mastication and prevent aspiration (e.g. tucking chin and flexing neck forward to protect the airway).

Nutrition Patients with dysphagia may have inadequate calorific and fluid intake, leading to accelerated weight loss and dehydration. The initial management of dysphagia in ALS includes modification of food and fluid consistencies while ensuring maximal calorific intake. Percutaneous endoscopic gastrostomy (PEG) should be considered as an alternative or supplementary route for nutrition, hydration and medication. PEG should be undertaken before FVC falls below 50% of predicted as it is more successful, improves survival and is less complicated at this early stage. Radiologically inserted gastrostomy tubes do not require sedation or endoscopy and are preferable in patients with respiratory compromise.

Communication Progressive dysarthria is common and speech may become severely impaired or lost within a short time. Simple techniques for improving the intelligibility of speech include reducing background noise and facing the speaker. Writing is often an excellent alternative to speech if limb function is preserved. There are a variety of other aids ranging from pointing boards to computerised speech synthesisers, particularly using ipad applications.

Limb dysfunction Musculoskeletal pain is common and may respond to antispasticity agents, NSAIDs and stronger analgesics including opiates. Skin pressure pain caused by immobility may also occur. Cramps are usually nocturnal and may respond to quinine sulfate, diazepam, carbamazepine or phenytoin. Stiffness may be caused by spasticity or muscle or joint contracture. Tizanidine and baclofen may help with the pain of spasticity.

Cognitive impairment in ALS MND is associated with both mild frontal lobe impairment and also a more severe form of frontotemporal dementia. Cognitive impairment occurs most often in patients with pseudobulbar palsy who may show changes in character, personality and behaviour. However, this is difficult to assess because of the speech disturbance and motor retardation associated with pseudobulbar palsy, these may be exacerbated by distress, anxiety and depression. Frontotemporal dementia is characterised by disinhibition, loss of insight and social awareness, impulsivity, reduced speech output with echolalia and eventual mutism. In the late stages there may also be anxiety, agitation, apathy and even delusions. There are characteristic pathological changes including frontotemporal neuronal loss, gliosis and spongiform change.

Psychological factors Depression and anxiety often follow the diagnosis of MND. The drugs of choice are SSRIs. Anxiety may require specific drug therapy. This may be short-term treatment with benzodiazepines or amitriptyline. If aggression and disinhibition occur with cognitive impairment, phenothiazines may be necessary and psychiatric support is often helpful. Emotional lability may be distressing for patient and carers and may be eased by amitriptyline or an SSRI.

Other symptoms Insomnia is common in MND. If sleep remains disturbed after relief of pain then amitriptyline is preferable to hypnotics for sedation. Constipation is treated by dietary modification, ample fluid intake and aperients. With severe pyramidal involvement bladder frequency and urgency may occur requiring oxybutinin.

Terminal care Palliative care (Chapter 26) should be introduced before the terminal stages of MND. Home care teams and day centres offer respite care in parallel with home carers. Close liaison between GP, community health care and hospice teams and palliative care physicians is essential. In the later stages of the patient's illness, regular respite and psychological support should also be available for the primary carer.

Terminal care often involves alleviating psychological distress and the symptoms of bulbar weakness and respiratory failure. Patients may experience a frightening sensation of choking because of episodes of laryngospasm. Benzodiazepines and agents to dry secretions may be helpful but laryngospasm usually resolves spontaneously. Oral, subcutaneous or intravenous morphine may be indicated to relieve dyspnoea, anxiety, pain or other distress. The effectiveness of sedatives such as diazepam, midazolam or chlorpromazine in reducing anxiety in the terminal stages outweighs any depressive action of the drugs on respiratory function.

The 'Breathing Space Kit', provided by the Motor Neurone Disease Association in the United Kingdom, contains medication that can be used by the carer, nurse or GP for the emergency treatment of acute episode of respiratory distress which often occurs in the terminal stages. These include diazepam, diamorphine, chlorpromazine and hyoscine.

Some patients wish to consider an advanced directive to record their end-of-life decisions. For the large majority who decide against life-prolonging measures including tracheostomy and invasive ventilation it is important to reassure the patient and their carers that palliative care can control symptoms in the terminal phase of the illness.

Carers Following the death of a patient with MND the family and carers will require bereavement support. This can be provided by the palliative care team but continuing domiciliary support may also be necessary.

Spinal muscular atrophy

Spinal muscular atrophy (SMA) represents a group of predominantly autosomal recessive disorders characterised by degeneration of anterior horn cells and bulbar nuclei without corticospinal or sensory neurone involvement. After cystic fibrosis, SMA is the second most common autosomal recessive disease of childhood (1/6000–10 000 live births). There are four clinically distinct types (Table 10.25):

1 *SMA type I:* infantile SMA (Werdnig–Hoffmann disease)
2 *SMA type II:* intermediate SMA
3 *SMA type III:* juvenile SMA (Kugelberg–Welander disease)
4 *SMA type IV:* adult onset SMA.

Table 10.25 Summary of spinal muscular atrophy (SMA).

Condition	Genetic association	Clinical features
SMA type I (infantile, Werdnig–Hoffman)	5q13 (SMN gene)	See text
SMA type II (intermediate)	5q13 (SMN gene)	See text
SMA type III (juvenile, Kugelberg–Welander)	5q13 (SMN gene)	See text
SMA type IV Adult onset	Variable (AR or AD)	See text
X-linked arthrogryposis multiplex (X-linked infantile SMA)	Xp11.3–q11.2	Hypotonia, areflexia, multiple congenital contractures. Death in infancy
Diaphragmatic SMA (HMN III, IV)	11q13	Distal limb weakness
SMARD (HMN VI)	1GHMB2	Diaphragm weakness, death in infancy
Distal SMA (HMN V)	7p15 (GARS)	Often sporadic, predominantly upper limb

GARS, glycyl-tRNA synthetase; HMN, hereditary motor neuropathy; SMARD, SMA with respiratory distress type 1; SMN gene, survival motor neurone gene.

Genetics and aetiology

The most common types of SMA are associated with defects in ribonucleic acid (RNA) processing. Spinal muscular atrophy types I–III and some of type IV (95% of the total SMA cases) are associated with reductions in the product of the survival motor neurone (*SMNI*) gene (chromosome 5q11.2–5q13.3). The *SMNI* gene encodes a protein involved in RNA metabolism and the severity of the phenotype correlates with the level of SMNI protein. In the majority of patients it is functionally absent and survival depends on the expression of the *SMNII* gene.

Clinical features

SMA type I (infantile, Werdnig–Hoffmann) This develops in infancy with failure to achieve a sitting posture and death by 2 years. There may be loss of fetal movements *in utero* and the baby is born floppy with a weak cry and failure to suck, swallow and achieve head control or sitting posture. Contractures develop after immobilisation and death usually occurs by 2 years as a result of respiratory failure.

SMA type II (intermediate) In SMA type II (intermediate SMA) muscle weakness develops after 6 months and manifests as motor development delay. Independent sitting is achieved but not walking. Kyphoscoliosis, severe contractures, skeletal deformity and respiratory muscle weakness may lead to death in early adulthood but prolonged survival is possible if respiratory involvement is limited or with appropriate ventilatory support.

SMA type III (juvenile, Kugelberg–Welander) SMA type III (juvenile SMA) becomes symptomatic in early childhood (<18 months) and patients achieve mobility. Fasciculation, cramps and a fine tremor are common and there is proximal limb weakness and wasting more prominent in the lower limbs. SMA III is highly variable and often stabilises. Prognosis can often be predicted by the age of onset and severity. SMA III may be compatible with normal life expectancy.

SMA type IV (adult onset) Adult SMA represents a heterogeneous group. The pattern of weakness symmetrical with proximal muscles more affected than distal muscles, legs more than arms with little involvement of facial or bulbar muscles. The truncal muscles or often severely affected with involvement of the intercostals but relative sparing of the diaphragm. The distal SMAs or HMNs present with distal limb weakness. Many of these disorders are allelic with subtypes of CMT2 disease with the principal distinction being mild to moderate sensory nerve involvement in CMT2. The autosomal dominant HMN 2A-C present with distal leg followed by distal arm weakness. In contrast, patients with HMN5A present with weakness beginning in the hand muscles and subsequently spreading to the legs.

An autosomal dominant pattern of inheritance accounts for up to 30% of cases and is not associated with chromosome 5 abnormalities or known dHMN mutations. The clinical pattern is variable with onset between the third and sixth decades. There may be slowly progressive limb girdle or scapulo-peroneal weakness with difficulty climbing stairs, arising from chairs or walking which resembles limb girdle dystrophy. Respiratory muscle involvement and scoliosis are rare but there may be vocal cord impairment.

Other forms of SMA Severe forms of SMA associated with death in infancy include X-linked arthrogryphosis multiplex (X-linked infantile SMA) characterised by hypotonia, areflexia and multiple congenital contractures and diaphragmatic SMA (SMARD-1) in which there is gynaecomastia, congenital fractures and sensory neuropathy. Fazio–Londe disease is a form of MND limited to the lower cranial nerves starting in the second decade of life and progressing to death over 1–5 years. Brown–Vialetto–Van Laere syndrome presents largely in females in the second decade with bulbar palsy and deafness. The differential diagnosis of SMA is summarised in Table 10.26.

Kennedy's disease (X-linked spinobulbar muscular atrophy) Kennedy's disease is of particular importance because the clinical pattern resembles MND. With a frequency of 1/50 000 per year it is not uncommon. Kennedy's disease affects males with onset in the third decade or later. It is an X-linked disorder caused by a CAG trinucleotide repeat expansion in exon 1 of the androgen receptor gene on Xp11-12. The condition is characterised by prominent oral and

Table 10.26 The differential diagnosis of spinal muscular atrophy.

Limb girdle muscular dystrophy
Dystrophinopathy (Duchenne's and Becker's)
Acid maltase deficiency
Hexosaminidase deficiency
Congenital myopathy – nemaline, central core
Myasthenia gravis
Polymyositis
CIDP
CMT2
Kennedy's disease
MND
Paraneoplastic syndromes

CIDP, chronic inflammatory demyelinating polyradiculoneuropathy; CMT, Charcot–Marie–Tooth disease; MND, motor neurone disease.

peri-oral fasciculation, muscle cramps, progressive dysarthria and dysphagia and slowly progressive lower motor neurone bulbar, shoulder girdle, axial and limb weakness. Upper motor neurone signs are not seen. Sensory involvement occurs. Other features of Kennedy's disease include gynaecomastia, diabetes mellitus, testicular atrophy and infertility. Kennedy's disease progresses more slowly than conventional MND and respiratory muscle involvement is less common; patients have an almost normal life expectancy. Serum CK may be elevated and nerve conduction studies may show reduced amplitude of both motor and sensory action potentials with diffuse, predominantly chronic denervation changes on EMG. The diagnosis is confirmed by genotyping.

Hexosaminidase-A deficiency The most severe form of hexosaminidase-A deficiency is Tay–Sachs syndrome (Chapter 19). However, a milder form may develop in children or adults characterised by a form of SMA associated with prominent muscle cramps, tremor, dementia, cerebellar atrophy and sensory involvement.

Monomelic amyotrophy (Hiryama's disease) Monomelic amyotrophy is a form of non-progressive wasting and weakness affecting the upper limbs. It is usually unilateral and occurs predominantly in men (4 : 1) with onset typically between 15 and 25. There is focal involvement of the C7, C8 and T1 myotomes often sparing brachioradialis. There is no fasciculation or sensory involvement. The condition must be distinguished from the monomelic onset of motor neurone disease, chronic asymmetrical spinal muscular atrophy, brachial neuritis, multi-focal motor neuropathy and intrinsic cervical cord lesion.

The aetiology remains uncertain. The occurrence is sporadic and insidious in onset which had led to the suggestion that it is caused by focal compression of the cervical spinal cord possibly causing focal venous ischaemia. In support, typical MRI findings with the neck flexed include flattening of the spinal cord against the C5–6 vertebral bodies, lower cervical cord atrophy, reduction in the size of the posterior cervical subarachnoid space and hyperintensity in the anterior horn cell region on T2-weighted imaging.

Allgrove's syndrome Allgrove's syndrome is a rare multi-system disorder characterised by achalasia, adrenal insufficiency and alacrima. Presentation is often with severe dysphagia caused by delayed passage of food into the stomach. There may be a more generalised autonomic disturbance characterised by abnormal pupillary reflexes, reduced heart rate variability and postural hypotension. There may also be a peripheral neuropathy, pyramidal syndrome, cerebellar and cognitive impairment. Allgrove's syndrome is caused by a mutation in the *ALADIN* gene on chromosome 12q13.

Investigation

Serum CK is often normal in SMA I–IV but elevated in Kennedy's disease, SMARD-1 and other rare forms of SMA. Neurophysiological studies show reduced CMAPs but normal conduction velocities and SAPs, except in Kennedy's disease where sensory involvement is identified in 80% of cases. EMG shows acute denervation and chronic reinnervation. Muscle biopsy is not especially helpful and shows features of acute denervation and secondary myopathic change. Genetic confirmation of mutations in the *SMN1* or androgen receptor genes is diagnostic. Mutations may not be found in some rare forms of childhood SMA and in many patients with adult onset SMA.

Management

There is no specific treatment available for SMA. The management largely involves the treatment of musculoskeletal complications which vary with age of onset and severity.

Ventilatory support may be necessary in SMA II. Invasive respiratory support leads to improved survival in some patients. Non-invasive ventilation may be necessary if nocturnal hypoventilation develops. In HMN7B or SPSMA, particular attention must be paid to vocal cord paresis which causes stridor and eventual airway obstruction. Vocal fold tie back procedures or tracheostomy may be indicated.

Scoliosis develops if there has been paraspinal weakness prior to the growth spurt and spinal correction may be necessary to preserve mobility and ventilatory function. The provision of walking aids including braces and callipers may allow younger patients to remain ambulant for many years.

It is important to ensure early access to an experienced paediatric palliative care support team. Ventilatory support is increasingly available for infants with SMA but most families opt to withdraw support when tracheostomy and invasive ventilation are indicated.

Treatment and management for SMA has improved to such an extent that many patients are surviving into adulthood. Clinics often need to be multi-disciplinary with input from neurology, respiratory, gastrointestinal, orthotic and nursing services. Independent mobility may be lost in teenage years and appropriate wheelchair and even driving provision must be considered. Planning for further education, work, pregnancy, independent living and genetic counselling is often necessary.

Disorders of the neuromuscular junction

Functional or structural abnormalities of the neuromuscular junction (NMJ) interfere with the transmission of neural impulses from motor nerves to muscles. In myasthenia gravis, antibodies mediate damage to the post-synaptic acetylcholine receptor. In Lambert–Eaton myasthenic syndrome, antibody-mediated block of the pre-synaptic calcium channels results in a deficit of quantal release. Congenital myasthenia is caused by defects affecting presynaptic, synaptic and post-synaptic mechanisms leading to NMJ impairment.

Myasthenia gravis

Myasthenia gravis (MG) is an autoimmune disorder caused by antibodies directed against the acetylcholine receptor (AChR) in the muscle membrane (Figure 10.19 and Figure 10.20). The serum antibody to the AChR and its interaction with the target antigen are well characterised.

The nicotinic AChR is a transmembrane glycoprotein with five subunits arranged around a central ion channel. These subunits are designated α,β,γ,δ and ε, each of the two α units has an extracellular acetylcholine binding site. The fetal AChR has a γ subunit in place of the ε. The AChR ion channel is closed in the resting state and when the binding sites of both α-subunits are occupied the channel opens transiently. There is a continuous process of turnover and renewal of AChR at the NMJ; impaired transmission induces increased transcription of AChR genes, which eventually allows full recovery of the NMJ.

IgG anti-acetylcholine receptor antibodies (AChRAb) of the IgG1 and IgG3 subtypes are detectable in 75% of patients with MG. These antibodies:

- Bind complement leading to destruction of the muscle end-plate.
- Bind to the receptor leading to blockade
- Cross-link muscle surface AChR increasing their rate of internalisation

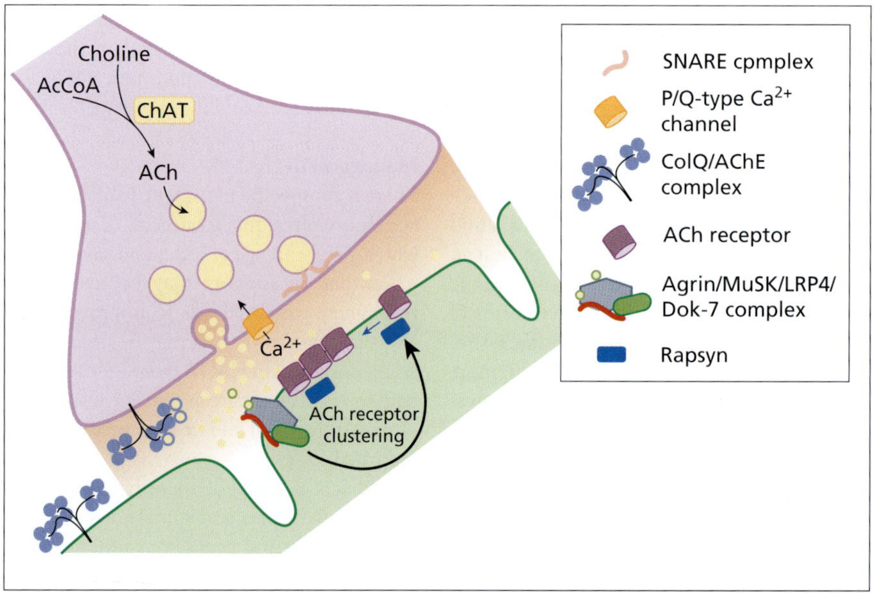

Figure 10.19 Key steps in acetylcholine (ACh) synthesis and release at the neuromuscular junction and the core pathway responsible for ACh receptor clustering. AChE, acetylcholinesterase; AcCoA, acetyl coenzyme A; ChAT, choline acetyltransferase; ColQ, AChE collagen-like tail subunit; Dok-7, downstream of tyrosine kinase 7; LRP4, low-density lipoprotein receptor-related protein 4; MuSK, muscle-specific kinase; SNARE, soluble NSF attachment protein receptor. Source: Spillane et al. 2010. Reproduced with permission of BMJ.

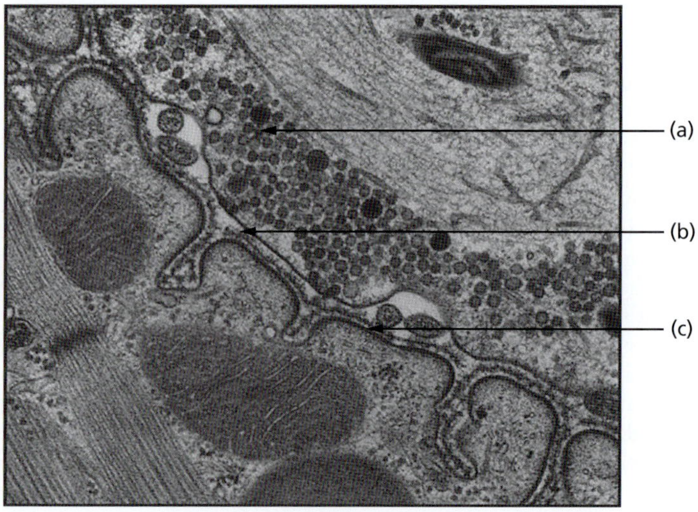

Figure 10.20 Electron micrograph of a normal neuromuscular junction showing presynaptic vesicle (a), synaptic cleft (b); post synaptic membrane (c).

Loss of voltage-gated Na^+ channels at the end-plate leads to reduced muscle membrane depolarisation and an increase in the threshold necessary to initiate a muscle action potential.

'Antibody negative' myasthenia gravis – Anti MuSK antibodies

Some 20–25% of patients with MG are AChRAb negative. IgG autoantibodies to muscle-specific kinase (MuSK) can be found in >50% of these patients with either ocular or generalised MG. MuSK is a receptor tyrosine kinase expressed selectively in the NMJ of mature skeletal muscle. MuSK has a critical role in the clustering of post-synaptic proteins, including AChR during NMJ development. Anti-MuSK do not activate complement but reduce the postsynaptic density of AChRs and impair their alignment. The remaining patients, negative for both AChRAb and MuSKAb, are referred to as 'seronegative' although there is a conversion rate of <15%. Recently some of these patients have been shown to have 'low-affinity' AChRAb.

Clinical features

MG has a bimodal pattern of onset; it occurs most commonly in women in the second and third decade but there is a second peak of incidence in the sixth and seventh decades with men being predominantly affected. The approximate incidence is 1.5 and prevalence 15/100 000. Presentation is characterised by fatigable weakness in the ocular, cranial nerve, limb, truncal or respiratory musculature.

A number of drugs impair neuromuscular transmission and therefore precipitate or exacerbate myasthenic weakness; these are summarised in Table 10.27. D-penicillamine MG is usually mild and may remit when the drug is withdrawn; however, in others it may precipitate severe MG which proves difficult to control.

The initial manifestation is often fatigable visual blurring, diplopia and/or unilateral or asymmetrical ptosis which worsens towards the end of the day. Weakness remains localised to the ocular muscles in 15% of patients. The jaw, facial muscles, speech and/or swallow, neck, respiratory muscles and proximal limbs are all commonly affected. Selective diaphragm weakness is rare.

On examination, fatigable weakness can be demonstrated in any affected muscle by repetitive or sustained activity. Cogan's lid twitch sign is pathognomic – when the patient rapidly refixates from downgaze to the primary position, there is overshoot of the eyelid before it settles down to the ptotic position. Cooling of the eye with an ice pack may lead to improvement in ptosis but its sensitivity and specificity in myasthenia remain uncertain. The ophthalmoplegia is fatigable and often does not fit the pattern of a single cranial nerve weakness. The medial and inferior rectus and superior oblique are most commonly affected but severe and occasionally total external ophthalmoplegia may occur. Up to 20% of patients with MG have prominent bulbar symptoms early in the course of their disease.

Respiratory muscle weakness is demonstrated by limited chest wall movement and excessive use of accessory muscles of respiration. Weakness of the truncal musculature leads to difficulty sitting from supine while limb weakness is characterised by fatigability in a limb girdle pattern. However, it may be markedly asymmetrical and occasionally distal musculature may be preferentially affected. The symptoms typically worsen at the end of the day and with extreme heat. They are also exacerbated by emotional stress, infection, pregnancy and menstruation.

The anti-MuSK phenotype often occurs in young women and is characterised by predominant facial, bulbar and respiratory muscle weakness. Myasthenic crisis is common, particularly at presentation, and many patients deteriorate rapidly early in the disease course and may require prolonged ventilatory support. Myasthenia can coexist with other autoimmune diseases such as diabetes rheumatoid arthritis, pernicious anaemia, SLE, vitiligo and thyroiditis. The differential diagnosis is summarised in Table 10.28.

Diagnostic tests

The diagnosis of MG can be supported by clinical, laboratory and electrophysiological investigations.

An intravenous bolus of edrophonium may transiently improve the symptoms and signs of myasthenia and is the basis of the Tensilon test. However, false negatives are common, false positives occur with many other neuromuscular diseases, and it is contraindicated in the elderly or patients with cardiac disease because of the risk of cholinergic haemodynamic side effects including bradycardia and ventricular fibrillation. It should not be undertaken in

Table 10.27 Drugs that impair neuromuscular transmission.

Antibiotics	Aminoglycosides (gentamicin, neomycin, streptomycin)
Antiarrhythmics	Quinine, quinidine, lidocaine and β-blockers
Antiepileptics	Phenytoin
Antirheumatoid drugs	D-penicillamine Chloroquine
Competitive neuromuscular junction blocking agents used during anaesthesia	D-tubocuarine Pancuronium Depolarising agents (e.g. succinylcholine)

Table 10.28 Differential diagnosis of myasthenia.

Ophthalmoplegia	Isolated cranial nerve palsies Thyroid eye disease Guillain–Barré syndrome Mitochondrial disease Oculopharyngeal muscular dystrophy Central causes (e.g. Internal carotid artery aneurysms, MS)
Bulbar and respiratory weakness	Botulism Acid maltase deficiency Motor neurone disease, Kennedy's disease Central causes (e.g. tumour, stroke and MS)
Proximal limb weakness	Myopathy including 'limb girdle', congenital myasthenia; inflammatory causes (e.g. polymyositis)
Myasthenic crisis	Guillain–Barré syndrome Botulism Myopathy (acid maltase deficiency) Motor neurone disease Brainstem stroke/inflammation LEMS Organophosphate poisoning Cholinergic crisis

LEMS, Lambert–Eaton myasthenic syndrome; MS, multiple sclerosis.

outpatients or without the availability of atropine to reverse the cholinergic side effects. Because neuroimmunological and electrical tests are now available the Tensilon test is often unnecessary.

Electrophysiological studies (Chapter 4) looking at repetitive stimulation and single fibre EMG (SFEMG) are abnormal in MG. Repetitive stimuli at a rate of 3 Hz lead to a decrement in the CMAP amplitude of >15% which should be reproducible. SFEMG is the most sensitive neurophysiological investigation of neuromuscular transmission. An increase in jitter (trial-to-trial variation in latency from stimulus to response) may be restricted to the ocular or facial muscles and blocking (intermittent failure of excitation of the muscle fibre) is also seen. However, SFEMG is not specific and jitter may be seen in other disorders of the NMJ, nerve or muscle.

The antibodies are measured mainly by immunoprecipitation of ^{125}I-α bungarotoxin labelled ACh receptors. AChRAb are detected in approximately 75% of patients with generalised myasthenia and 50% with pure ocular myasthenia. AChRAb are the most specific marker for MG but they may rarely be found in association with thymoma, SLE, autoimmune liver disease, inflammatory neuropathies and RA (especially when taking penicillamine) without any clinical evidence of myasthenia. Levels of AChRAb fluctuate with disease severity in an individual patient.

Anti-titin muscle antibodies are present in approximately 25% of patients with MG but in up to 90% with concurrent thymoma. Anti-MuSK antibodies occur in >50% of seronegative myasthenia gravis (SNMG) cases and are not found in ACRAb positive MG cases. Other autoantibodies that may be present in myasthenia include LRP4, titin, ryanodine receptor, anti-smooth muscle, antinuclear, antithyroid antibodies as well as rheumatoid factor and antibodies to gastric parietal cells and red blood cells.

Management

There are few randomised controlled trials in MG but treatment is based on clear principles which are determined by the age, sex, disease pattern and severity, the risk of side effects and the availability of close clinical and investigational monitoring. Treatment may be symptomatic (anticholinesterases), disease modifying (immunosuppression with steroids, immunosuppressant drugs, immunoglobulins or plasma exchange) and/or surgical (thymectomy).

Anticholinesterases are the first line of treatment. They are of value in the early symptomatic treatment of MG as a single therapy or later as an adjunct to immunotherapy. Pyridostigmine is the most widely used. Side effects of anticholinesterases include muscle fasciculation and weakness occurring as a result of excessive stimulation of the nicotinic acetylcholine receptors. The abdominal cramps, diarrhoea, increased bronchial and oral secretions can be mitigated by antimuscarinic medication. Persistence of myasthenic weakness despite increasing doses of pyridostigmine is an indication for immunosuppressant treatment. MuSKAb related myasthenia is less responsive to anticholinestarase medication than AChRAb positive myasthenia.

Corticosteroids can be extremely effective in improving myasthenic weakness and establishing remission. There is considerable variability in dosage, duration of treatment and clinical response to steroids. They should be commenced in hospital because of the significant risk of deterioration in proximal strength during the first 2 weeks of treatment. The risk is reduced if an incremental dosage is used. Marked improvement will occur in more than 50% of patients and remission in 25% with the time to maximum benefit approximately 6 months. Only 5% will show no significant improvement. While steroids are effective and inexpensive, their use is limited by considerable toxicity and they should be weaned to the lowest dosage possible to prevent glucocorticoid side effects. All patients likely to receive more than 7.5 mg/day steroid for more than 6 months should be treated to prevent iatrogenic osteoporosis, preferably with a bisphosphonate.

Azathioprine has been shown to reduce the dosage of prednisolone required to maintain remission and to reduce the number of treatment failures. The effects of azathioprine (<2.5 mg/kg) are extremely slow to develop and a therapeutic dosage may take up to 2 years for the full clinical effect to be seen. The risk of azathioprine toxicity is reduced by screening for the activity of the enzyme thiopurine methyltransferase (TPMT) which metabolises azathioprine. The risk of myelosuppression is increased in those with low activity.

Mycophenolate and methotrexate (MTX) have been used individually as alternative second line immunosuppressant agents if azathioprine has been ineffective or not been tolerated. They are both well tolerated with relatively few side effects although it is important to emphasise that MTX is administered weekly and carries a risk of hepatic toxicity.

Ciclosporin has also been shown to be effective in a randomised controlled trial. Ciclosporin has similar efficacy to azathioprine but works more rapidly. Its use is limited by significant side effects including nephrotoxicity and hypertension which contraindicate its use in pre-existing renal disease and necessitate the need for regular blood monitoring. Cyclophosphamide is now rarely used in MG because of its toxicity.

Rituximab is a monoclonal antibody to the B-cell marker CD20. It has been effective on an anecdotal basis in both ACRAb and MuSK Ab positive MG. Side effects include neutropenia and increased susceptibility to infection.

Plasma exchange reduces AChRAb titres significantly but is often ineffective in SNMG. It is valuable in producing short-term improvement of severe myasthenic weakness but difficulties and complications of venous access, biochemical derangements and high overhead costs limit its use. IVIG is similar in efficacy to plasma exchange and is valuable in producing short-term improvement in myasthenic crisis and also occasionally as a long-term maintenance therapy. There remains considerable uncertainty about the role of immunomodulation in MuSK myasthenia but a similar regimen of management is generally used.

Thymectomy has been used in the treatment of MG for 50 years. In most young patients with thymic enlargement the gland will show histological changes of thymic hyperplasia affecting the cortico-medullary junction and the germinal centres. Approximately 15% of patients with MG have a thymoma (Figure 10.21) while up to 50% of patients with thymoma will develop myasthenia which may occur even after thymectomy. CT or MRI of the mediastinum should be undertaken in all patients with MG to exclude thymoma. Most are benign and encapsulated; however, 10% show malignant features with invasion of the capsule, local spread, seeding or even distant metastasis. Postoperative radiotherapy is recommended for invasive thymoma in which the tumour capsule has been penetrated. If metastatic spread has occurred, chemotherapy may be highly effective with varying regimes including cyclophosphamide, vincristine, cisplatin and doxorubicin proving effective, not just in reducing the thymoma, but also in controlling the myasthenia. However late recurrence can occur.

Objective evidence of the efficacy and role of thymectomy has been elusive. Evidence from open studies indicates thymectomy for non-thymomatous autoimmune MG increases the probability of remission or improvement and a recent randomised control trial indicates a benefit of thymectomy over steroids alone. Up to 46% of

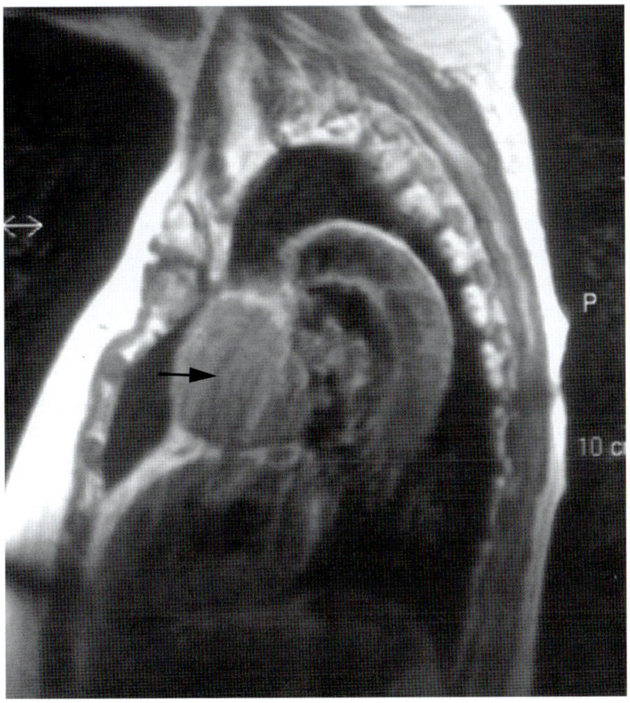

Figure 10.21 Large anterior mediastinal thymoma in an 80-year-old patient with mild generalised myasthenia gravis (black arrow).

patients with thymic hyperplasia may achieve full remission within 2–5 years of surgery and significant improvement and reduced treatment will be seen in up to 40%. Thymectomy is indicated for patients with seropositive MG from late childhood up to the age of 60 years. In those over 60 years, those with seronegative or ocular MG the role of thymectomy is less clear. The procedure is usually undertaken via the trans-sternal route but there is increasing use of video-assisted thoracoscopic surgery (VATS).

Ocular myasthenia gravis

In about 15% of MG the disease remains localised to the orbicularis oculi and extraocular muscles although EMG may show generalised NMJ abnormalities. Remission occurs in approximately to 20%. Response to anticholinesterases is often disappointing. Immunosuppression with steroids and azathioprine may be necessary if ptosis or diplopia are symptomatic.

Pregnancy and myasthenia

The effects of pregnancy on the patient and fetus should be considered separately. Myasthenia may worsen, improve or remain stable during pregnancy but there is a significant risk of deterioration in the puerperium. Pregnancy should ideally be planned when the patient is strong, steroids should be maintained at the lowest therapeutic dosage and, if possible, other immunosuppressants should be avoided. If pre-eclampsia occurs, magnesium sulfate should not be used because of the risk of further impairment of NMJ transmission.

The newborn infant is at risk of transient neonatal myasthenia which occurs in about 10% of myasthenic pregnancies. This condition is caused by transmission of AChRAb across the placenta. The neonate may require transient ventilator support but the weakness resolves over a few days.

Myasthenic crisis

Myasthenic crisis indicates the development of ventilatory failure. Approximately 20% of patients with MG will develop myasthenic crisis and in 10% there may be more than one episode. Respiratory failure in MG may be precipitated by bronchopneumonia, systemic sepsis, medication, surgery or inadequate treatment often related to a rapid tapering of the steroid dosage. Rarely, cholinergic crisis or the commencement of high-dose corticosteroids is to blame. In acute respiratory failure, urgent elective tracheal intubation and ventilation should be considered when the vital capacity falls below 15 mL/kg. The rate of progression, the presence of bulbar weakness and the state of the patient are also crucial to the decision (Chapter 20).

Cholinergic crisis

Cholinergic crisis is rare but should be suspected in patients taking high doses of anticholinesterase medication who have extensive cholinergic side effects including sweating, hypersalivation, excessive bronchial secretion and miosis. Eventually, flaccid weakness and respiratory failure develop. It may be necessary to admit the patient to ITU, intubate and ventilate and withdraw all anticholinergic medication.

Anaesthesia and peri-operative care

Elective surgery in patients with myasthenia should be undertaken with experienced anaesthetic support following pre-operative plasma exchange or IVIG if necessary. This is because myasthenic crisis may be precipitated by anaesthesia, the stress of surgery and non-depolarising neuromuscular blocking agents.

Other causes of abnormal neuromuscular transmission

Botulism is the most important condition which may mimic MG (Chapter 9). Snake venoms, tick paralysis and toxic agents including organophosphates may affect neuromuscular transmission. Organophosphates are used as nerve agents (Chapter 19) but are also widely employed as pesticides. Exposure may be occupational, food-borne or as a consequence of suicide attempts. Acute exposure results in cholinergic crisis. Respiratory muscle weakness is resistant to atropine and intubation is required. Longer term organophosphate exposure may lead to a myasthenic syndrome or an axonal sensory motor neuropathy. Rarely, organophosphate toxicity may also cause late onset of neuropsychiatric and cognitive impairment or a parkinsonian syndrome.

Lambert–Eaton myasthenic syndrome

Lambert–Eaton myasthenic syndrome (LEMS) is a rare disorder caused by impaired release of ACh by the presynaptic terminal of the NMJ. It is associated with underlying malignancy or autoimmune disease. The voltage-gated calcium channel (VGCC) at the NMJ is characterised by an $\alpha 1A$ subunit and antibodies to this P/Q type VGCC can be measured by immunoprecipitation using ^{125}I-conotoxin. VGCC antibodies cause aggregation and internalisation of the VGCC thereby reducing the number of functional P/Q type VGCCs on the presynaptic motor terminal of the NMJ. This, in turn, results in reduced action potential dependent ACh release from the motor nerve terminal.

Clinical features

The onset is often insidious with the gradual development of progressive weakness and fatigue. The condition may occur at any age but is more common after 40 years. Underlying malignancy may be present in about 50% of patients although this may not become apparent until more than 4 years after the onset of LEMS.

Fatigue is prominent at presentation. Weakness may affect the proximal muscles, particularly the legs, and is often associated with aching and stiffness. Autonomic features including dry mouth, constipation and impotence are also common. Ophthalmoplegia, ptosis, bulbar and respiratory muscle weakness can occur but are less common than in seropositive autoimmune MG. Examination findings are characterised by proximal weakness with a fatigable component. Reflexes are reduced or absent but after a short period of sustained effort they become brisker showing the phenomenon of post-tetanic potentiation.

The most common underlying tumour is small cell lung cancer (>80%) but LEMS also occurs with lymphoproliferative disorders, malignant thymoma and rarely with carcinoma of the breast, stomach, colon, prostate, kidney and bladder.

Aetiology

LEMS is an autoimmune disorder driven by antibodies to the VGCC (anti-VGCC Ab) of the presynaptic terminal. Serum from up to 90% of patients with paraneoplastic and autoimmune LEMS contain anti-VGCC Ab. In patients with small cell lung cancer it is likely that cancer cells contain antigen which mimics VGCC and induces the production of antibodies while the mechanism of production in the autoimmune condition is unclear.

Investigations

The diagnosis of LEMS is established by the presence of anti-VGCC Ab and by characteristic electrophysiological findings. A small CMAP, a decremental response to repetitive stimulation at low frequency (1–5 Hz) and an increment following sustained maximum voluntary contraction or 20–50 Hz repetitive stimulation are typical. SFEMG shows increased jitter and block.

A search for underlying malignancy and in particular small cell lung cancer must be conducted including FDG-PET if other tests are negative. Patients with malignancy negative LEMS should be closely followed up as an underlying tumour may become apparent after a long latent period.

Treatment

Any underlying carcinoma must be appropriately treated. Successful treatment often leads to improvement in LEMS.

Specific treatment is directed towards facilitation of neuromuscular transmission, removal of the antibody or suppression of its production. Pyridostigmine has a mild effect in enhancing neuromuscular transmission but most patients require 3,4 diaminopyridine (3,4 DAP) which blocks presynaptic Ca^{2+} channels, lengthens depolarisation of the nerve terminals and increases quantal ACh release. 3,4 DAP is associated with paraesthesiae, anxiety and insomnia and an increased risk of seizures. If severe weakness persists despite these treatments immunomodulation treatment is indicated. The response to plasma exchange and IVIG is less reliable than in MG. Prednisolone, azathioprine and ciclosporin are all effective in LEMS.

Congenital myasthenia

Congenital myasthenic syndromes (CMS) are a heterogeneous group of genetic disorders caused by abnormalities of the NMJ that interfere with normal synaptic transmission. They are generally autosomal recessive and are conventionally classified according to the site of defective neuromuscular transmission (presynaptic, synaptic and post-synaptic) although diagnosis increasingly depends on the identification of the specific gene defect. The conditions are rare but important to distinguish from SNMG because of the implications for management and genetic advice. In most patients there is a malformation in the structure or function of the pre- or post-synaptic NMJ. Presynaptic deficits are caused by reduced numbers of ACh molecules per synaptic vesicle, impaired quantal release mechanisms or reduced efficacy of individual quanta. The most common cause of post synaptic CMS is a mutation in the genes encoding the AChR subunits that can either impair ion channel gating or reduce the number of end plate receptors leading to slow channel, fast channel or AChR deficiency syndromes. Slow channel syndromes are dominantly inherited and are due to prolonged ion channel activation. Synaptic impairment is caused by end-plate acetylcholine esterase deficiency.

The classification of CMS is summarised in Table 10.29.

Clinical features

CMS may present in infancy with hypotonia, failure to thrive, delayed motor milestones and unexplained apnoeic episodes. In children and adults the conditions are manifest as fatigable or fluctuating, ocular, facial and bulbar weakness although limb and truncal wasting and weakness may also be prominent. The weakness tends to progress during adolescence but then often stabilises. There may be episodic worsening of the weakness, possibly triggered by intercurrent events such as pyrexia. On examination there is fatigable muscle weakness on exertion but a prominent myopathy and scoliosis may be present. Distal weakness, ocular and pupillary abnormalities are also occasionally present. There may be a positive family history. In infancy CMS may mimic muscular dystrophy, congenital and metabolic myopathy, spinal muscular atrophy or structural brainstem anomalies. In children and adults it is necessary to distinguish CMS from SNMG, forms of MND, LGMD and neuropathies. The differential diagnosis of CMS is summarised in Table 10.30.

Investigation

Standard MG investigations document an abnormality at the NMJ. Confirmatory diagnostic evidence comes from morphological and genetic NMJ studies. These include microelectrode recordings of miniature end-plate potentials to nerve stimulation, EM studies of intercostal muscle, AChR density studies using iodine-123 labelled bungarotoxin, patch clamp studies of individual channels at the NMJ and genetic studies of target genes in the AChR and post-synaptic structure.

Management

The management of CMS is summarised in Table 10.29.

Muscle diseases

The diagnosis of muscle disease has undergone groundbreaking transformation in the past 20 years, as a result of advances in immunohistochemistry, metabolic studies and genetics which enable accurate diagnosis of many inflammatory, genetic and metabolic muscle diseases. With the advent of new knowledge, many patients are now having their diagnoses revised and refined. This will inevitably lead to improved understanding of the natural history of muscle diseases and their treatment.

Table 10.29 Causes of congenital myasthenia.

Diagnosis	Defect in NMJ	Gene	Clinical features	Treatment
Pre-synaptic defect				
Choline acetyl transferase (ChAT) deficiency	Failure of ACh resynthesis or packaging	ChAT	Recurrent apnoeic spells Impaired pupillary responses	AChE inhibitors (variable response), 3,4 DAP
Synaptic				
End-plate acetylcholinesterase deficiency	Failure to anchor AChE in synaptic cleft	ColQ	Recurrent apnoeic episodes from infancy Variable myasthenic symptoms between attacks. Axial weakness.	Reduced active signal transmission No response to AChE inhibitors Ephedrine Ephedrine
Post-synaptic defect				
AChR deficiency				
AChR mutation	Reduce number of end-plate receptors. Non-functioning ε subunit replaced by fetal γ	CHRNE CHRNA CHRNB CHRND	Neonatal onset. Severe ophthalmoplegia, ptosis and feeding difficulties. Mild bulbar or respiratory involvement Generalised weakness	Reduced active signal transmission Cholinesterase inhibitors (partial response)
AChR kinetic abnormality				
Slow channel	Prolonged ion channel activation in response to ACh	CHRNE CHRNA CHRNB CHRND	Variable age of onset. Autosomal dominant Cervical weakness with mild bulbar or respiratory involvement. Weakness and wasting in extensor, distal muscles due to endplate myopathy caused by prolonged channel activation (depolarising block)	Drugs which block AChR ion channel when in an 'open state' Fluoxetine, quinidine, Salbutamol, AChE inhibitors
Fast channel	Abnormally brief ion channel activation in response to ACh	CHRNE CHRNA CHRNE	Respiratory insufficiency at birth. Recurrent respiratory crises. Severe ophthalmoplegia	Reduced active signal transmission AChE inhibitors or 3-4DAP
AChR clustering pathway				
Rapsyn mutation	Deficiency and instability of AChR at motor end-plate	RAPSN	Arthrogrypsis multiplex congenital. Early onset associated with hypotonia, bulbar and respiratory impairment Facial malformations, contracture of hands and ankles Episodes of respiratory failure Tendency to improve with time	Reduced active signal transmission AChE inhibitors or 3-4DAP
DOK 7	Binds to MuSK which controls the aggregation of AChR. Incomplete synaptogenesis results	DOK7	Highly variable Proximal > distal limb girdle weakness Childhood – waddling gait, falls. Ptosis, stridor, bulbar and respiratory impairment Benign forms may develop in adults	AChE inhibitors (variable response) – may worsen some patients 3-4 DAP Ephedrine, salbutamol

AChE inhibitors, Anticholinesterase inhibitors ACh, acetylcholine; ACR, acetylcholine receptor; CMS, congenital myasthenia syndrome.

Basic muscle biology

Muscle is a complex assembly of interacting proteins, outlined in Chapter 2. Its principal function is to respond to stimulus from a motor neurone by physically shortening its contractile apparatus with the conversion of electrical and chemical energy into mechanical energy.

The basic unit of a striated muscle is the myofibril. The myofibril is made up from many repeating functional multi-protein complexes of actin, myosin and titin called sarcomeres, the smallest functional unit of muscle. Thousands of sarcomeres are arranged end-to-end, giving muscle its striated microscopic appearance and form the contractile apparatus. 'Thin' filaments of actin and 'thick' myosin filaments are arranged such that they may slide over each other, retaining their own length but shortening the sarcomere as the thin filaments are pulled towards the centre. The myofibrils are enveloped in the mesh-like structure of the sarcoplasmic reticulum, which is central to excitation–contraction coupling. The electrical stimulation of the muscle cell causes a release of calcium ions from the intracellular sarcoplasmic reticulum. This in turn activates the contractile apparatus (Figure 10.22a) and an energy-dependent interaction occurs between the actin and myosin filaments of the sarcomere. As calcium levels fall, the interaction between actin and myosin ends, the sarcomere extends again and the muscle relaxes.

Together with the sarcomere is an array of other structures. First, a series of structural proteins anchor the contractile apparatus within the sarcomere (Figure 10.22a). A number of further proteins then link the sarcomere to the cell membrane (the sarcolemma) and extracellular matrix (Figure 10.22b). Dystrophin is attached at one end to actin and at the other to a complex of glycoproteins (including, amongst others, the dystroglycans, sarcoglycans and laminin) that are closely associated with the sarcolemma. In addition, various ion channels span the cell membrane, and their role in moderating the influx and efflux of potassium, sodium, calcium and chloride is crucial to proper muscle function.

Muscle is a complex structural and functional unit. Genetic or acquired abnormalities of any of the proteins or processes discussed earlier may result in disease. Muscle is also a highly metabolically active tissue and is therefore vulnerable to disturbances in energy including primary disorders of carbohydrate and lipid metabolism as well as mitochondrial oxidative phosphorylation.

Table 10.30 Differential diagnosis of congenital myasthenic syndromes (CMS).

Neonatal	Spinal muscular atrophy
	Congenital myopathies – central core, nemaline, myotubular
	Congenital muscular dystrophy
	Mitochondrial myopathy
	Brainstem anomaly
	Mobius syndrome
	Infantile botulism
	Autoimmune myasthenia gravis
Older patients	Motor neurone disease
	Peripheral neuropathy
	Congenital muscular dystrophy – fascioscapulohumoral, limb girdle
	Mitochondrial myopathy
	Myasthenia gravis (AChRAb, MuSKAb, SNMG)

Clinical assessment of the patient with muscle disease

A confident clinical diagnosis can often be made in disorders of muscle such as Duchenne muscular dystrophy, myotonic dystrophy type 1, fascioscapulohumoral dystrophy (FSHD) and inclusion body myositis. In other muscle diseases, the clinical assessment remains important in guiding genetic and metabolic testing as well as interpretation of the muscle biopsy.

History

There are a limited number of symptoms of muscle disease which are listed in Table 10.31. However, the interpretation of these symptoms is critical in guiding differential diagnosis and management. When patients describe 'weakness' they may be referring to 'stiffness', 'fatigue' or 'pain' as well as loss of power.

The onset and course of patients' symptoms is helpful in defining the aetiology of the muscle problem. Specific questions should be asked about the patient's antenatal history, birth, developmental milestones, sporting ability as well as academic and physical achievements in youth. The onset of a muscle problem can often be traced back many decades before the apparent onset and this can be helpful in formulating the differential diagnosis.

The history should document the current neuromuscular functional status of the patient. This would include a history of double

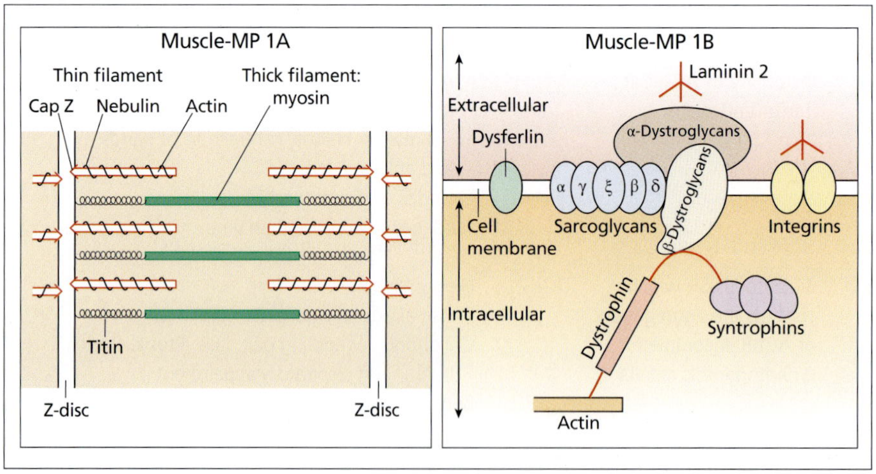

Figure 10.22 (a) Simplified schematic representation of the muscle contractile apparatus. Thin filaments are comprised of actin molecules as the core, wrapped in the template protein, nebulin, plus troponin and tropomyosin (latter two not shown). They are capped at the Z-disc with CapZ and at the other end with tropomodulin (not shown). Thick filaments of myosin are bound by titin to the Z-disc. One element of titin is elastic. Contraction involves interaction of the thick and thin filaments so the latter move towards the centre. (b) Simplified schematic representation of the muscle cell membrane and associated non-neuromuscular junction proteins (NB some components are omitted for clarity).

Table 10.31 Issues important in history-taking in muscle disease.

Symptom	Details
Weakness	Confirmation of reduced strength and function Onset, duration and progression Assessment of degree of weakness and subsequent disability (e.g. date of first use of walking aids) Pattern of muscle involvement – proximal limb (reaching objects from shelves, standing from sitting) versus distal limb (opening jars or bottles, tripping over) versus selective focal Variability and, if present, exacerbating or relieving factors (always consider the possibility of fatigability)
Pain	Confirmation of myalgia, rather than, for example, impaired sensation Localised versus generalised Severity Precipitating, exacerbating or relieving factors Association with any other symptom
Cramps	Localised versus generalised Precipitating, exacerbating or relieving factors Association with any other symptom
Stiffness	Identification of specific failure of relaxation (myotonia), e.g. difficulty releasing grip or opening eyes Localised versus generalised Exacerbating or relieving factors
Fatigue	Distinction from other symptoms Precipitating, exacerbating or relieving factors
Pigmenturia	Precipitating factors Association with any other symptom

vision, swallowing and speech difficulties, neck weakness, proximal and distal limb weakness and problems with mobility. It may be helpful to quantify this with clinical scales, such as the MRC grading system, to assess change over time. Clear documentation of functional abilities also aids completion of social care and driving assessment. Respiratory symptoms, especially those of neuromuscular respiratory failure, often first manifest as unrefreshing sleep, orthopnoea, morning headache or excessive daytime sleepiness. Recurrent chest infections and the use of non-invasive ventilation are also important in assessing the functional consequences of neuromuscular respiratory failure and dysphagia.

Pigmenturia ('coca-cola urine') should be specifically asked about, in conjunction with provocation factors such as exercise or fasting in patients who are felt to have had episodes of rhabdomyolysis. Some patients may have had solitary or only infrequent episodes.

Paroxysmal or variable symptoms (e.g. cramps, spasms, stiffness, weakness) require further questioning, seeking to identify provoking, exacerbating or relieving factors especially in defining the clinical features of a channelopathy.

Other organ systems are commonly involved in muscle diseases. Cardiac symptoms (palpitations, exertional dyspnoea, ankle swelling and paroxysmal nocturnal dyspnoea) may occur as cardiac disease often coexists with muscle disease. A suspected multisystem condition requires attention to other systems (e.g. the rash of dermatomyositis, cataracts in myotonic dystrophy type 1 and deafness in mitochondrial disease).

Table 10.32 Simple bedside functional motor tests.

Lifting head from lying down
Straight leg rising from lying down
Standing from lying down and/or squatting and/or sitting
Ability to walk on heels or on tiptoes
Ability to hop on one foot
Ability to run
Time to walk a specified distance
Time to climb a flight of stairs
Raising arms above head

Assessment of the past medical history is directed at identifying other conditions that may either cause muscle symptoms (e.g. rheumatological or endocrine disease), or make their management more difficult (e.g. orthopaedic conditions or a peripheral neuropathy). Specific questions should be asked about any difficulties with anaesthesia. Myotonic dystrophy may first be revealed by peri-operative cardiac arrhythmia or difficulty weaning from a ventilator, while certain myopathies, notably central core disease but also the dystrophinopathies, can lead to postoperative malignant hyperthermia. A thorough medication history is also required, particularly with regard to statin use, but also should include over-the-counter preparations, alternative remedies and recreational drugs. Any temporal association with symptoms should be explored.

Examination

A complete basic neurological examination is recommended and where appropriate further clinical tests performed, for example testing for myotonia. Inspection should be focused on assessment of muscle bulk, involuntary movements (fasciculation, myokymia, myotonia), skeletal abnormalities (e.g. kyphoscoliosis, dysmorphism), contractures and scars from previous muscle/nerve biopsies and orthopaedic surgery.

Power assessment may require additional examination techniques to those routinely employed. Subtle facial weakness can be revealed by formally testing eyelid and lip closure. Specific requests for buccal, palatal and lingual consonant production in addition to a demonstration of a cough and a sustained note can indicate more specific impairments. Neck extension and flexion should be tested with the patient both lying and upright. Experienced clinicians learn that muscle strength testing needs appreciation of the confounding effects of suboptimal effort ('give-way' weakness) or when pain is a limiting factor. Accordingly, bedside tests of disability rather than impairment can give a more useful guide, particularly on serial examinations, to assess disease progression or treatment effect when impairment testing is not reliable (Table 10.32).

Myotonia should be tested by sustained grip or eyelid closure, and/or by percussion of appropriate muscles (e.g. thenar eminence, forearm or tongue).

Respiratory function can be assessed by looking for abdominal paradox on deep inspiration and expiration (the abdomen normally distends on inspiration because the diaphragm descends as it contracts), as well as specific assessment of sniff and cough strength. Spirometry allows quantification of respiratory function, with the caveat that poor effort and air leak resulting from facial weakness must be taken into consideration.

Investigation of muscle diseases

Creatine kinase

This enzyme is continuously released at low level into the circulation. This process is increased by injury to the muscle including exercise. In addition, there is considerable variation in CK levels across a normal population. CK is proportional to the muscle bulk of an individual, and routine exercise and alcohol will increase levels. Furthermore, values in Afro-Caribbean are higher than in the Caucasian population. The CK result should be interpreted in light of an appropriate normal range and background exercise levels. Quantification of different isozymes (e.g. myocardial CK-MB) is usually unhelpful, and other enzymes may be released from skeletal muscle, such as ALT/AST. It is important to note that several muscle diseases may not be associated with a rise in CK in some patients.

Neurophysiology

Needle EMG can be helpful in distinguishing myopathy from neurogenic weakness. The classic findings in myopathy are spontaneous activity with fibrillations, positive sharp waves and complex repetitive discharges plus polyphasic, low amplitude, short duration units on voluntary contraction (Chapter 4). This pattern is common to several underlying processes and neurophysiological examination is less useful in refining the diagnosis of muscle disease than when used to investigate neuropathy. Other electrophysiological phenomena may be seen, such as myotonia, while specialised serial examination before and after cooling a limb, or after short or long periods of standardised exercise or 'exercise EMG' form a crucial element in assessing patients with possible muscle channelopathies.

Muscle biopsy

Muscle biopsy is often necessary to confirm a clinical diagnosis. It should be considered and, if possible, performed in all cases before any treatment is initiated. Close liaison with the pathologist and laboratory technician is essential because experience in both the preparation of biopsy material and its microscopic evaluation is critical. At a practical level, this will usually mean sending the patient to a specialist centre. The muscle selected for biopsy should ideally be moderately involved, and not fibrotic. Pathologists often have particular experience with interpreting changes in particular muscles and this information needs to be considered when planning a muscle biopsy.

Initial histological diagnosis is based on the presence or absence of inflammatory change, necrosis, fibrosis, fibre atrophy, fibre size and shape or other structural changes (vacuoles, inclusion bodies). Enzyme stains may identify certain conditions (e.g. absent acid phosphorylase in McArdle's disease, or reduced cytochrome oxidase staining in mitochondrial disorders). Immunostaining (e.g. dysferlin, dystrophin and the sarcoglycans) have greatly improved the diagnosis of dystrophies. Immunocytochemistry for MHC Class I and immune cell markers has greatly improved the diagnosis of primary inflammatory muscle disease as well as inflammatory dystrophies. If required, EM may detect more subtle abnormalities (e.g. features of mitochondrial disease).

Metabolic testing

Exercise testing (most safely performed non-ischaemically), with serial collection of blood samples for lactate and ammonia levels in normal subjects generates a three- to fivefold increase in both. In glycolytic or glycogenolytic disorders, the lactate rise is reduced (or absent) with excessive elevation of ammonia. Myoadenylate deaminase deficiency, by contrast, causes a normal rise in lactate but no change in ammonia. Exercise testing is increasingly not performed as more specialised metabolic and genetic testing has become available. Specialised centres can perform assays of enzyme function in muscle for the mitochondrial respiratory chain, carnitine metabolism, fatty acid flux studies, as well as the enzymes involved in glycogen metabolism.

Genetic testing

Specific DNA analysis has revolutionised diagnosis of muscle disease. Where a clinical diagnosis can often be accurately made, for example myotonic dystrophy type 1 or FSHD, genetic testing should be the first step in investigation. In other genetic disorders of muscle, such as the limb girdle dystrophies, genetic testing should be appropriately guided by other findings including the muscle biopsy although with the advent of improved genetic screening of several disorders at once as part of a 'panel', the need for a diagnostic muscle biopsy in these conditions will probably reduce.

Genetic muscle diseases

The clinical management and understanding of genetic muscle disease is changing rapidly as a direct result of the wealth of recent molecular genetic discoveries. Approximately 1/6000 of the UK population has one of many diverse genetically determined muscle diseases and the spectrum of clinical phenotypes is broad. Duchenne muscular dystrophy, caused by mutations in the dystrophin gene, is a young onset, severe, progressive muscle wasting disease which can be lethal in late teens without appropriate respiratory and cardiac support. In contrast, myopathies caused by mutations in mitochondrial DNA can develop in late adult life manifesting as external ophthalmoplegia or mild proximal myopathy with a relatively indolent course. The mortality in genetic muscles diseases is often determined by the degree of cardiac and/or respiratory muscle involvement and therefore cardiorespiratory screening is essential in the assessment of patients presenting with suspected genetic muscle disease. Careful clinical evaluation and attention to the family history can reduce the differential diagnosis sufficiently to rely on direct genetic testing alone and a muscle biopsy may not be required. The distinction between inflammatory and genetic myopathies can be difficult and genetic testing may be helpful in making a clear diagnosis. For example, a specialist muscle service may review patients where prominent inflammatory infiltrates on biopsy have led to the erroneous diagnosis of polymyositis in patients subsequently shown genetically to have dysferlinopathy or FSHD.

Where a precise DNA-based diagnosis is possible patients and families can be provided with accurate prognostic and genetic counselling information and entered into a rational screening programme for recognised complications. As national networks for DNA-based diagnosis become available more patients will have access to this diagnostic precision.

Genetic testing is now often the first investigation in myotonic dystrophy and FSHD and a muscle biopsy is usually not required. In other more clinically heterogeneous genetic muscle diseases, such as limb girdle muscular dystrophy (LGMD), muscle biopsy with careful immunohistochemical analysis is usually required to direct gene testing. However, as gene sequencing technologies become increasingly available even LGMD gene analysis may be selected at an earlier stage in the diagnostic process.

In this section we mention the more common genetic muscle diseases (Table 10.33) encountered by adult neurologists. The aim is to describe clinical features and to suggest efficient diagnostic strategies (Table 10.34). DNA-based diagnosis may accelerate and

Table 10.33 Genetic muscle diseases.

Muscular dystrophies
Dystrophinopathies
Emery–Dreifuss muscular dystrophy
Limb girdle muscular dystrophies
Facioscapulohumeral muscular dystrophy
Oculopharyngeal muscular dystrophy
Congenital muscular dystrophy
Myotonic dystrophy
Bethlem myopathy
Distal myopathies
Congenital myopathies
Myofibrillar myopathies
Skeletal muscle channelopathies
Metabolic myopathies
Mitochondrial myopathies
Glycogen storage myopathies
Lipid storage myopathies

simplify the diagnostic process, thereby providing the most accurate information for patients with these diseases.

Muscular dystrophies

The muscular dystrophies are a group of a genetic diseases that cause skeletal myodegeneration. Many genes causing muscular dystrophies have recently been described and the causative proteins have many cellular functions. Dystrophic muscle is possibly the non-specific end result of a number of different pathogenic pathways. The proteins identified include sarcolemmal structural proteins (e.g. dystrophin, sarcoglycans and dysferlin), nuclear envelope proteins (emerin, lamin A/C), enzymes (calpain, fukutin-related protein), sarcomeric proteins (e.g. myotilin, desmin) and extracellular matrix proteins (e.g. laminin, collagen type 6; Figure 10.22b). For some disorders, such as the myotonic dystrophies, two genes account for the majority of cases and their testing is readily available. In contrast, the LGMDs are genetically heterogeneous and require more complex assessment of clinical parameters with muscle biopsy testing to guide genetic analysis.

Xp21 dystrophies: the dystrophinopathies Dystrophin is a major muscle cell structural protein that lies just below the sarcolemma and helps to stabilise the sarcolemma during muscle contraction. It links intracellular actin to a complex set of transmembrane proteins which in turn link to elements of the extracellular matrix

Table 10.34 Diagnostic strategies for inherited myopathies.

Condition	DNA based diagnosis available?	Muscle biopsy needed?
Xp21 dystrophies (dystrophinopathies)	Yes, but negative gene test does not exclude diagnosis	Yes, if genetic test negative
Emery–Dreifuss muscular dystrophy	Yes, but usually only after immunohistochemistry for lamin a/c and emerin	Yes, muscle biopsy remains important
Limb girdle muscular dystrophies	Yes, check FKRP/calpain-3 genes initially. If negative muscle immunohistochemistry will reduce number of candidate proteins	Yes, muscle biopsy required in most cases
Facioscapulohumeral dystrophy	Yes, indirect genetic test available through regional genetics laboratory	Not usually unless genetic test for FSHD negative. Inflammatory muscle biopsy may cause difficulty distinguishing from polymyositis
Oculopharyngeal muscular dystrophy	Yes	Not usually
Myotonic dystrophy type 1 and 2	Yes	Not usually, unless gene tests for MD/PROMM negative
Bethlem myopathy	Consider skin and muscle biopsy. Exclude lamin a/c, emerin and SEPN1	May be helpful for exclusion. May not be definitive
Mitochondrial respiratory chain diseases	Yes (?age associated decline in MtDNA mutation load in blood). POLG gene analysis in CPEO	Yes (a) If blood MtDNA analysis negative (b) Muscle needed for mitochondrial enzyme analysis (c) Muscle MtDNA better for MtDNA analysis
Metabolic muscle disorders (glycogenoses, lipidoses)	Yes, but not usually first line	Yes. Also consider specialist metabolic testing, often first line, e.g. non-ischaemic lactate test (glycogenoses) or blood acylcarnitine/urinary organic acids (lipid disorders)

CPEO, chronic progressive external ophthalmoplegia; FKRP, fukutin-related protein; FSHD, facioscapulohumeral dystrophy; MD, mytonic dystrophy; POLG, polymerase gamma; PROMM, proximal myotonic myopathy; SEPN1, selenoprotein 1.

(particularly to an extracellular protein called laminin). Genetic defects in the dystrophin protein are associated with two major phenotypes: Duchenne and Becker muscular dystrophy.

Duchenne is a progressive and lethal dystrophy affecting boys in which there is a severe reduction in the amount of the dystrophin protein in muscle. There is no curative treatment, but improved ventilatory support, spinal surgery for kyphoscoliosis and the use of corticosteroids increase quality of life and life expectancy. Adult men with Duchenne are increasingly common and adult clinical practice needs to meet this new challenge with an active multidisciplinary approach.

Becker muscular dystrophy is commonly encountered in adult muscle practice. The severity of the phenotype correlates with the amount of dystrophin protein. Patients with Becker present with a limb girdle pattern of muscle weakness with pseudohypertrophy of calf muscles, which is often the clinical diagnostic clue. Cardiomyopathy is an important complication and occasionally severe dilated cardiomyopathy may be the presenting feature.

Diagnosis can be achieved by genetic testing through multiplex ligation-dependent probe amplification (MLPA) analysis, PCR and analysis of muscle dystrophin mRNA, although a 'negative' genetic test does not exclude the diagnosis of Becker's muscular dystrophy where reduced sarcolemmal dystrophin on muscle biopsy may be continue to support the diagnosis in spite of negative genetics.

Genetic counselling for families is important. One-third of cases of dystrophinopathy represent new mutations within a family. Female carrier status may be associated with a mild clinical phenotype but most female carriers are asymptomatic. The importance of the need for an effective treatment has provoked great interest in gene therapy approaches and clinical trials of genetic treatments, including exon skipping, are in progress.

Congenital muscular dystrophy The congenital muscular dystrophies are a genetically heterogeneous group of disorders which often present at birth with floppy infants and subsequently impaired motor and sometimes cognitive development. Skin, heart and bone can also be affected. Kyphoscoliosis is common. The degree of CNS involvement is often related to the overall severity of the condition. Patients at the mildest end of the spectrum may present later in life to the adult muscle clinic with an indolent myopathy and contractures.

Mutations in several genes may cause CMD and can be classified into five main subtypes, based on the underlying molecular defects. Several of these genes are allelic for other forms of muscular dystrophy such as lamin A (*LMNA*) (Emery–Dreifus muscular dystrophy (EDMD types 2/3) and limb girdle muscular dystrophy (*LGMD1B*)) and fukutin-related protein (FKRP) (*LGMD2I*).

1 Genes encoding for structural proteins of the basal membrane or extracellular matrix of the skeletal muscle fibres. This includes collagen 6 genes (Ulrich–Bethlem congenital muscular dystrophy); laminin α2 (merosin) and integrin α 7.
2 Genes encoding for putative or demonstrated glycosyltransferases, which affect the glycosylation of α dystroglycan, an external membrane protein of the basal membrane. Genes belonging to this category include *POMT1/2; POMGnT1*; fukutin; fukutin-related protein (FKRP);
3 Selenoprotein 1, which encodes an ER protein.
4 *LMNA*-related CMD.
5 Several CMD phenotypes have been described and linked but genetic clarification awaits.

Bethlem myopathy Bethlem myopathy is usually an autosomal dominant myopathy caused by mutations in one of three different genes for collagen type 6: *COL6A1* and *COLA6A2* on chromosome 21q22.3 and *COL6A3* on chromosome 2q37 and is allelic to the more severe form, Ulrich CMD. Onset of this so-called contractural phenotype is typically in the first or second decade. In childhood there are delayed motor milestones, waddling gait and tripping with falls. There is slow progression in the first decade although there may be stabilisation and even transient improvement of muscle strength in the second decade. There is subsequently slow progression. Life expectancy is usually normal and there is no evidence for cardiorespiratory involvement. Two-thirds of patients require a wheelchair by the age of 50 years. Physical examination shows generalised symmetrical muscle atrophy particularly in the shoulder girdle, upper arms and below the knees. Later there is forearm and neck flexor weakness. There is no ophthalmoplegia and facial weakness is rare. Prominent flexion contractures at the interphalangeal joints of the fingers, elbows and ankles are present in most patients and contractures at the metacarpophalangeal joints, shoulders (pectoralis major), tibialis anterior, hamstrings, quadriceps and erector spinae and jaw muscles frequently occur with no relationship between the severity of the weakness and the severity of the contractures. Treatment is supportive.

Muscle biopsy is non-specific. Immunofluorescence of patient fibroblast cultures sometimes shows a reduced expression of collagen type 6 but can be normal. Genetic testing is not widely available. The differential diagnosis includes other myopathies with prominent early contractures including EDMD, autosomal dominant LGMD and rigid spine syndrome with mutations in the selenoprotein N (*SEPN1*) gene.

Limb girdle muscular dystrophies The limb girdle muscular dystrophies (LGMD) share an association with progressive proximal limb girdle weakness but each form often has other particular clinical features, for example 'rippling muscles' in caveolin-3 and tongue hypertrophy in FKRP, although these features are not consistent. Several new genes have recently been described to cause LGMD and these code for proteins with many different functions (Table 10.35). Currently, patients often undergo a muscle biopsy with immunocytochemistry and immunoblotting being used to target genetic analysis. In the near future, a LGMD gene panel test will probably help in the diagnostic process and obviate the need for a muscle biopsy in some patients. The recessive LGMDs are far more common than the dominant forms. Three of the most common recessive forms for which gene testing is increasingly available are considered in detail.

Calpainopathy – LGMD2A LGMD caused by calpain mutations typically develops between 2 and 40 years with most patients presenting in their late teens to mid thirties. Early milestones are usually normal and pelvic girdle muscle weakness precedes later development of shoulder girdle weakness. Severe early onset forms with CNS involvement as well as more scapulohumeral upper limb variants have been described. On examination, there is typically a scapulohumeralpelvic distribution of weakness. The involvement of periscapular muscles is reminiscent of FSHD but facial involvement is minimal or absent. Muscle atrophy is usually a prominent feature, as opposed to hypertrophy in many other dystrophies (e.g. Becker dystrophy and LGMD2I). Particular atrophy of the posterior compartment of the thigh may be a distinguishing clinical feature compared to other LGMDs. Loss of ambulation usually occurs

Table 10.35 Genes/proteins causing limb girdle muscular dystrophies (LGMD).

Type	Chromosome	Protein	Clinical
Autosomal dominant			
LGMD 1A	5q22–q34	Myotilin	Rare, distal legs affected first; slow progression, late CMP in 50%; CK 2–10 × normal
LGMD 1B	1q	Lamin a/c	Rare; proximal legs affected first; slow progression; CMP in 60%; CK 1–2 × normal
LGMD 1C	3p25	Caveolin	Uncommon; variable phenotype: raised CK to progressive proximal weakness, no CMP, CK 3–40 × normal
LGMD 1D	7q	Unknown	Two families; proximal weakness, no CMP, CK 1–3 × normal
LGMD 1E	6q23	Unknown	Single family, proximal weakness, frequent sudden death from CMP; CK 2–4 × normal
LGMD 1F	7q32	Unknown	Single family, proximal weakness, no CMP CK often normal
Autosomal recessive			
LGMD 2A	15q15	Calpain	Uncommon but many different mutations found, very varied phenotype; no CMP, CK 3–80 × normal
LGMD 2B	2p13	Dysferlin	Uncommon with many different muations and variable phenotype (including within family); typically distal weakness; no CMP, CK 10–80 × normal
LGMD 2C	13q	γ-sarcoglycan	Rare, often early onset and loss of walking; respiratory weakness in some, CMP unusual, CK 5–20 × normal
LGMD 2D	17q21	α-sarcoglycan	Rare, variable phenotype but can be early onset, CMP unusual; CK 5–20 × normal
LGMD 2E	4q12	β-sarcoglycan	Rare; typically early onset with severe disability; CMP occasionally; CK 5–20 × normal
LGMD 2F	5q33	δ-sarcoglycan	Rare; early onset with severe disability; proximal weakness; CMP unusual; CK 10–50 × normal
LGMD 2G	17q11	Telethonin	Rare; teenage onset with proximal and distal leg weakness; CMP in 50%; CK 10–30 × normal
LGMD 2H	9q31	TRIM32	Very rare, slow progression; no CMP; CK 2–20 × normal
LGMD 2I	19q13	FKRP	Most common in UK; variable phenotype but respiratory involvement not uncommon and CMP in 30%; CK 4–30 × normal
LGMD 2J	2q31	Titin	Very rare; alleic to Finnish distal myopathy: causes proximal weakness but often relatives with distal weakness
LGMD 2K	9q34	POMT1	Rare; progressive proximal weakness with learning disability and ankle contractures; CK 8–40 × normal
LGMD 2L	11p13	None known	Very rare; CK very raised, no CMP. French–Canadian families, quadriceps and biceps weakness
LGMD 2M	9q31	Fukutin	Very rare; CK very high, infantile onset, proximal and distal weakness legs > arms. May improve with steroids

CK, creatine kinase; CMP, cardiomoyopathy; FKRP, fukutin-related protein; POMT, protein O-mannosyltransferase.

10–30 years after the onset. Cardiac involvement is not a feature and reduced vital capacity seems to occur only in severe very advanced cases. CK is elevated initially in the course of the disease but not as high as in LGMD2I, dystrophinopathies or LGMD2B.

Dysferlinopathy – LGMD2B There is a broad phenotypic range associated with mutations in the dysferlin gene and these include a proximal LGMD type presentation and a distal presentation (also known as Miyoshi myopathy; see Distal myopathies). In the LGMD presentation, weakness usually begins between in the late teens to early twenties and is associated with a pelvifemoral distribution, often with marked quadriceps involvement. The onset may be relatively abrupt with a very high CK leading to polymyositis as a differential diagnosis. Later, weakness in the arms develops with particular involvement of the biceps. Weakness usually spares the deltoids and also the periscapular muscles so scapula winging is not typical. The involvement of the posterior compartment of the leg is not uncommon and can be early. Imaging of gastrocnemius may show early changes and may be diagnostically helpful in an otherwise LGMD presentation. Facial and extraocular muscles are spared. Cardiac involvement is not reported, but may patients develop a reduced vital capacity with time.

In the lower limb posterior calf compartment presentation, weakness of ankle plantar flexors often prevents early walking on toes, and is called Miyoshi myopathy. The weakness often spreads to include the limb girdle muscles. A very high CK and sometimes marked inflammatory infiltrates in the muscle biopsy can cause confusion with myositis but immunohistochemistry using dysferlin antibodies in combination with genetic analysis of the dysferlin gene is usually diagnostic.

Fukutin-related protein (FKRP) dystrophy (LGMD2I) LGMD2I presents typically to adult clinics from late teens to early twenties with a mild phenotype but can present with a severe Duchenne-like pattern of weakness in infancy. The distribution of muscle involvement is similar, irrespective of the severity with a predilection for axial, neck flexor and the proximal pelvic and shoulder girdle muscles. Facial muscles are usually spared. Scapula winging is common. There may be striking hypertrophy of the tongue, brachioradialis, calves and sometimes the quadriceps. In contrast, there may be atrophy of pectoralis major and deltoid muscles. Prominent lumbar lordosis is common and exercise-induced cramping is a frequent symptom. Importantly, one-third of cases develop a dilated cardiomyopathy. Respiratory muscle involvement is also common, manifesting as nocturnal hypoventilation. In contrast to dystrophinopathies, respiratory failure may occur even while the patient remains ambulatory. LGMD2I is caused by mutations in the gene known as the fukutin-related protein (FKRP) which codes for a glycosylation enzyme.

Facioscapulohumeral muscular dystrophy FSHD is an important autosomal dominant disorder frequently encountered in adult specialist muscle practice. Patients commonly have facial muscle weakness as the initial symptom, which may be followed by periscapular and humeral muscle involvement. Later in the disease course lower limb weakness, particularly affecting the anterior tibial and abdominal wall, may occur. It is notable that the distribution of weakness is often asymmetric, with the right side often being more involved. Isolated periscapular weakness without facial involvement may occur. Prominent axial involvement often causes an exagerated lumbar lordosis and clavicular pectoral atrophy causes striking and typical appearances in the anterior chest wall. The severity is variable ranging from isolated asymmetrical scapular winging through to pronounced early onset weakness rendering the patient wheelchair-bound. Scoliosis, deafness and retinal vasculopathy are uncommon additional features and a severe infantile form with CNS involvement can occur.

FSHD is almost fully penetrant by the age of 30 years. FSHD is linked to chromosome 4q35, but identification of the causal gene remained elusive for many years. Recently, a mechanism has been proposed in the majority of cases, to involve the released expression of the gene DUX4 caused by contraction of a non-coding repeated DNA sequence or 'D4Z4'. The genetic test for FSHD currently still consists of examination for the D4Z4 contraction but this is likely to develop in the near future.

Oculopharyngeal muscular dystrophy Oculopharyngeal muscular dystrophy (OPMD) is an uncommon disorder characterised by late onset pharyngeal muscle weakness and ophthalmoplegia. It is usually autosomal dominant and highly penetrant although recessive inheritance may occur. OPMD may enter into the differential diagnosis in patients with late onset ophthalmoplegia and for those with bulbar weakness. The most common genetic defect is an expansion of a short (GCG) 7–13 triplet repeat in the poly-A binding protein 2 (*PAB2*) gene on chromosome 14q. Genetic testing for the expanded repeat sequence is available and usually obviates the need for muscle biopsy. Patients can develop a mild late onset limb girdle pattern of weakness although this is uncommonly severely disabling.

Myotonic dystrophies Myotonic dystrophy type 1 (dystrophia myotonica or DM1) is an autosomal dominant multi-system disorder ranging in severity from a severe congenital myopathy, which may be fatal, to late onset isolated cataracts. It is the single most common form of adult-onset muscular dystrophy. Neuromuscular symptoms include facial weakness, ptosis, neck flexion, long finger flexor and ankle dorsiflexion weakness with myotonia. Variable additional symptoms include cataracts, endocrine disturbance such as hypogonadism and impaired glucose tolerance, cardiac arrhythmias, frontal balding, cognitive impairment, primary daytime somnolence, bowel symptoms similar to IBS and respiratory muscle weakness. A clinical diagnosis can often be made with one or more of these additional features in combination with the typical muscle phenotype.

DM1 is caused by an expansion in an unstable trinucleotide repeat (CTG) in the 3′ untranslated region of a gene on chromosome 19 called myotonin protein kinase (*DMPK*). DM1 shows genetic anticipation and this correlates with expansion in the size of the repeat sequence. Recent evidence suggests that the expanded repeat may exert its toxic effect at the RNA level. The expanded untranslated repeat sequence in mRNA forms abnormal degradation resistant ribonuclear inclusions. The intranuclear inclusions impair the function of pre-mRNA splicing factors which in turn leads to mis-plicing of many pre-mRNA species. This may explain the diverse multi-system clinical involvement. For example, there is evidence that expression of the skeletal muscle voltage-gated chloride channel mRNA is altered in patients with myotonic dystrophy which would cause myotonia. Mutations in this chloride channel are also the basis of the pure myotonic disorder myotonia congenita.

The diagnosis of myotonic dystrophy is usually straightforward on clinical grounds but there is often a clinical delay of several years. DNA-based diagnosis is the initial investigation of choice. A detailed family history will usually reveal other affected members. Genetic counselling is a vital part of the consultation because of genetic anticipation. It is particularly important to identify females at risk of inheriting the gene in pedigrees because the severe, often lethal, congenital form is confined to the offspring of affected females. Women can be offered appropriate antenatal pre-implantation genetic diagnosis.

Patients with myotonic dystrophy should be followed up in a muscle clinic where they can be monitored for systemic complications. Premature mortality is high with an average life expectancy of 54 years which is mostly caused by cardiorespiratory complications. In most patients, myotonia is not symptomatic and does not require treatment. In those patients with symptomatic myotonia mexilitene can be effective. Excessive daytime sleepiness is a major problem and may respond to psychostimulants such as modafinil. Prominent imbalance causes falls, is a major cause of morbidity and is often multi-factorial in aetiology. Patients may require ankle foot orthoses which can improve imbalance.

In an appropriate clinical context, if the genetic test for DM1 is negative, then DM2 should be tested. This less common disorder is characterised by proximal rather than distal weakness, but in other respects may exhibit similar features to DM1. CNS involvement may occur. Muscle pain may be a prominent symptom. The genetic defect underlying DM2 is a CCTG repeat sequence expansion in intron 1 of a zinc finger protein gene on chromosome 3 (*ZNF9*). Similarly to DM1, there is evidence that this untranslated defect operates at the RNA level, causing ribonuclear inclusions. Both anticipation and a severe congenital form have not been described in DM2 (Figure 10.23).

Emery–Dreifuss muscular dystrophies The Emery–Dreifuss muscular dystrophies (EDMD) are often clinically characteristic and should be considered if contractures are a prominent early clinical feature. Patients present with a scapulo-humero-peroneal pattern of muscular weakness and often have strikingly thin muscles. Contractures of the cervical extensor muscles as well as the biceps and long finger flexor tendons are common. Cardiac conduction defects are also frequent and cardiac screening is important.

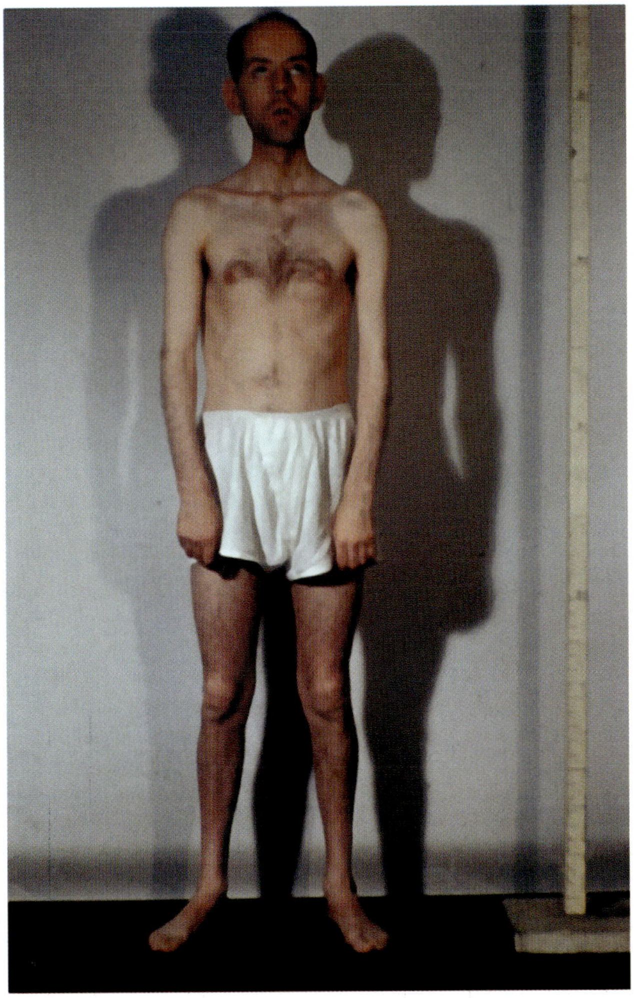

Figure 10.23 Typical clinical appearance of a patient with myotonic dystrophy. Note ptosis, frontal balding, typical facies and distal wasting.

EDMD is caused by mutations in several genes including those coding for nuclear envelope proteins emerin and lamin A/C whose function remains uncertain. Emerin mutations are associated with causing the X-linked form of EDMD and lamin A/C causes the less common dominant and recessive forms. Mutations in the lamin A/C gene have also been described other diseases including a form of LGMD (LGMD1B; Table 10.35), an autosomal recessive axonal neuropathy and partial lipodystrophy.

Myofibrillar myopathies The myofibrillar myopathies (MFM) are characterised by slowly progressive weakness with distal muscle involvement in 80% of patients and more prominent proximal than distal weakness in 25% cases. Facial involvement is uncommon. Some patients experience sensory symptoms, muscle stiffness, aching, or cramps. Peripheral neuropathy is present in about 20% of affected individuals. Clinically significant cardiomyopathy is present in 15–30% of patients and desminopathy may present with a pure cardiomyopathy. Respiratory muscle involvement may also occur.

Muscle histology often defines these conditions and consists of a combination of inclusions and vacuoles. The inclusions often stain immunocytochemically for myotilin and desmin. The CK is normal to modestly raised. Definitive diagnosis is made by genetic testing.

At the time of publication, the genetic basis of myofibrillar myopathies has been elucidated in approximately 50% of cases. Mutations have been identified in *DES*, the gene encoding desmin; *CRYAB*, encoding alpha-crystallin B chain; *MYOT*, encoding myotilin; *LDB3* (*ZASP*), encoding LIM domain-binding protein 3; *FLNC*, encoding filamin-C, and *BAG3*, encoding BAG family molecular chaperone regulator 3. More recently, mutations in *FHL1*, encoding four and a half LIM domains protein 1, and *DNAJB6*, encoding DnaJ homolog subfamily B member 6 have been described. These are all inherited in an autosomal dominant manner except for the X-linked *FHL-1* and the uncommon recessive form of *CRYAB*.

The differential diagnosis includes sporadic inclusion body myopathy (IBM) and IBM2 resulting from mutations in *GNE*. With the advent of genetic testing, some patients who were previously defined as having IBM have been found to have a form of MFM. Other differentials have been suggested to include DM1 and DM2 although these are often phenotypically very different from MFM. Other distal myopathies including dysferlinopathy are also included.

Distal myopathies

The distal myopathies are a heterogeneous group of genetic and acquired muscle disorders characterised by progressive muscle weakness and wasting predominantly affecting the feet and hands. Most genetic and acquired muscle diseases have a proximal presentation and distal myopathies may be confused with a primary neurogenic disorder. There are at least 17 genetically defined distal myopathies described in the literature and most of these are very rare (Table 10.36).

When a patient presents with a predominant distal myopathy, in addition to the disorders outlined in Table 10.36, other diagnostic possibilities to consider include IBM) myofibrillar myopathy, myotonic dystrophy and distal hereditary motor neuropathy. Usually, in each of these conditions there are associated clinical features which aid the diagnostic process. Exclusion of other conditions by careful clinical evaluation, genetic testing and often muscle biopsy. Often, biopsy of a distal lower limb muscle is more likely to reveal diagnostic pathology. Increasingly, MRI may be used to identify muscle involvement which may lead to the development of typical patterns associated with specific diseases and aid muscle selection for biopsy.

Table 10.36 Summary of the six well-characterised distal myopathies.

Disease	Onset	Weakness	Biopsy	Genes
Welander	>40	Hands	Dystrophic, rimmed vacuoles	AD, 2p13
Miyoshi	>15	Posterior calf	Dystrophic	AR, dysferlin
Nonaka	>15	Anterior calf	Myopathic, rimmed vacuoles	AR, GNE
Tibial MD	>35	Anterior calf	Dystrophic, rimmed vacuoles	AD, titin
LODM	>40	Anterior calf	Vacuoles	AD, 2q31
EODM	3–25	Anterior calf	Myopathic	AD, 14q

AD, autosomal dominant; AR, autosomal recessive; EODM, early onset distal myopathy; GNE, glucosamine (UDP-N-acetyl)-2-epimerase/N-acetylmannosamine kinase; LODM, late onset distal myopathy; MD, muscular dystrophy.

Congenital myopathies

The congenital myopathies are a group of uncommon muscle disorders that were defined on the basis of distinctive morphological muscle biopsy features and presentation at birth. They are a heterogeneous groups of disorders but, generally, patients present as floppy infants, with feeding and breathing difficulties, sometimes with congenitally dislocated hips, and then usually develop delayed motor milestones. The muscle weakness generally follows a fairly indolent course with a benign prognosis, at least when patients are younger. Some patients sometimes first come to attention in the adult muscle clinic. Central core myopathy, nemaline myopathy and centronuclear myopathy are of particular note and are described here.

Central core disease Central core disease (CCD) is an autosomal dominant disorder with onset often at birth or in early childhood with non-progressive limb and sometimes facial weakness with hypotonia. Patients usually live into adulthood. There may be a breech presentation, sometimes with dislocated hips, foot deformities or arthrogryposis. Motor milestones are delayed. There is mild proximal symmetrical muscle weakness and ambulation is usually achieved. Disability is usually mild. Significant cardiorespiratory problems are rare. CCD is associated with an increased risk of malignant hyperthermia (MH). However, the relationship between CCD and MH is complex and only around 30% of CCD patients have MH susceptibility. Most patients with pure MH have histologically normal muscle. Muscle biopsy in CCD typically shows central cores that are devoid of oxidative enzyme and phosphorylase activity. Both MH and CCD are often caused by mutations in the ryanodine receptor gene *RYR1*. MH susceptibility testing should be offered to patients with CCD. A more uncommon recessive form of central core disease is associated with CPEO and is often in the differential diagnosis of mitochondrial disease and congenital myasthenia gravis.

Nemaline myopathy Nemaline myopathy (NM) is characterised by the presence of rod-shaped structures (nemaline rods) in the muscle fibres. Inheritance can be autosomal dominant or recessive and to date mutations in seven genes have been described. Three clinical severities are seen: a severe congenital form, the typical congenital form and an adult onset form.

The severe congenital form presents with severe neonatal hypotonia and respiratory insufficiency. Reduced fetal movements are reported *in utero*. Occasionally there may be severe arthrogryposis and dilated cardiomyopathy. Early mortality because of respiratory complications is common. Occasional long-term survival with respiratory support has been described accompanied by major motor weakness and inability to ambulate. The typical congenital form presents with neonatal hypotonia with less respiratory difficulty. Weakness is milder and although motor milestones are delayed, independent ambulation is achieved and most patients have an independent life.

The adult onset form presents between the ages of 20 and 50 years. Myalgia may be predominant with moderate proximal weakness which is usually slowly progressive. Facial muscle weakness and neck flexion weakness are common in all forms. The face is often elongated with a tent-shaped mouth and a high arch palate. The degree of the facial abnormality correlates with the overall severity of the condition. Some adult cases have been described with more rapidly progressive weakness. Respiratory involvement, associated with diaphragm weakness, is rare but can occur; nemaline myopathy should always be considered in the adult presenting with unexplained respiratory muscle weakness. All the known NM genes identified encode components of the sarcomeric thin filaments. In AD NM mutations in α and β tropomyosin are described. In recessive NM, nebulin and troponin-1 mutations are described. Mutations in *ACTA1* may cause either dominant or recessive disease.

Centronuclear myopathy Three forms have been described. The severe X-linked form is associated with mutations in myotubularin. Bilateral ptosis, facial weakness, and ophthalmoplegia are common. Skeletal features include pectus carinatum, micrognathia, knee and hip contractures, elongated birth length, narrow face, slender/long digits, and macrocephaly. Patients often present *in utero* with reduced fetal movements and polyhydramnios. The prognosis is poor but those who survive the first year life, in spite of needing ventilatory support, will often survive in adulthood. The autosomal dominant form is often caused mutations in dynamin-2. Most patients have a mild phenotype with onset in adolescence or adulthood with axial/neck flexor as well as distal more than proximal limb weakness and slow progression. Other features include facial weakness, ptosis, ophthalmoplegia and contractures, especially of the ankles. The recessive form is often caused by mutations in amphiphysin-2 or RYR1. Presentation is often at birth but can be in childhood; approximately half of patients survive into adulthood.

Skeletal muscle channelopathies (Chapter 3)

Periodic paralyses and myotonias Periodic paralysis and inherited myotonia were the first human disorders in which genetic dysfunction of ion channel genes was identified. They are conditions in which there is a disturbance in skeletal muscle fibre membrane excitability. The periodic paralyses are autosomal dominant disorders in which patients experience focal or generalised episodes of muscle weakness of variable duration. They have been characterised on the basis of the change in serum potassium early in an attack. In hyperkalaemic periodic paralysis potassium triggers an attack which will be ameliorated by glucose ingestion. In contrast, patients with hypokalaemic paralysis will notice improvement with potassium ingestion but worsening with glucose. The classification based upon potassium is useful clinically although a genetic classification has now possible (Table 10.37). Mutations in one of four skeletal muscle ion channels genes associate with human periodic paralysis. These are the voltage-gated sodium and calcium channel genes *SCN4A* and *CACNA1S* and the voltage-independent potassium channel genes *KCNJ2* and *KCNJ18*. All forms of periodic paralysis share the common feature that during an attack the muscle fibre membrane becomes electrically inexcitable but the mechanisms leading to this state vary.

Myotonia is a clinical disorder in which patients experience muscle stiffness because of a failure of normal electrical inactivation of activated muscle. Myotonia may result from genetic mutations in either the muscle voltage-gated chloride channel *CLCN1* gene (dominant or recessive myotonia congenita) or the voltage-gated sodium channel *SCN4A* gene (dominant paramyotonia congenita).

Hyperkalaemic periodic paralysis and myotonias caused by skeletal muscle sodium channel dysfunction In hyperkalaemic periodic paralysis (hyperPP) patients typically experience recurrent attacks of muscle weakness starting in the first decade of life. Precipitants include rest following exercise, cold, potassium ingestion or stress. Attacks may vary in severity from mild weakness to total paralysis. The duration of attacks is usually less than 2 hours. Typically, the attack frequency declines with age but patients often develop a fixed myopathy of variable severity. Muscle biopsy in such cases often reveals tubular aggregates and or a vacuolar change. In humans, unlike equine forms, death is extremely rare in hyperPP or hypoPP. Cardiac arrhythmias are also uncommon except in Andersen's syndrome (see Periodic paralysis and cardiac arrhythmias).

HyperPP is caused by gain-of-function point mutations in the muscle sodium channel *SCN4A*. Sodium channel α-subunit mutations (*SCN4A*) lead to defective fast inactivation of the skeletal muscle Na^+ channel. The resulting persisting inward sodium current (a gain-of-function) impairs repolarisation and increases membrane excitability. Depending on the degree of increased membrane excitability, a patient may experience myotonia or paralysis. It is notable that similar gain-of-function mutations in a neuronal sodium channel gene *SCN1A* result in increased neuronal excitability and associate with a form of epilepsy, thus representing a direct pathophysiological parallel between muscle and brain sodium channel diseases.

Many attacks are brief and do not require treatment. If necessary, acute attacks can be terminated by ingestion of carbohydrate or inhaled salbutamol. Preventative treatment with acetazolamide or a thiazide diuretic may be required. It remains unproven if reducing attack frequency with such agents reduces the likelihood of the subsequent development of myopathy.

Paramyotonia congenita (PMC) is a form of myotonia that appears during exercise and worsens with continued activity. EMG at rest often shows some myotonia. Low temperature often precipitates symptoms in these patients and cooling produces repetitive

Table 10.37 Skeletal muscle channelopathies: a genetic classification.

Gene	Channel	Disease	Inheritance
CACNA1S*	Calcium channel	HypoPP1	AD
	L-type calcium α-subunit	MH	AD
SCN4A*	Sodium channel	HyperPP	AD
	Nav1.4 α-subunit	PMC	AD
		PAM	AD
		HypoPP2	AD
KCNJ2*	Potassium channel, $K_{ir}2.1$	Andersen's syndrome	AD
KCNJ18	Potassium channel K	Thyrotoxic Hypokalaemic Periodic paralysis	AD
	Kir 2.6		
CLCN1*	Chloride channel, ClC1	Myotonia congenita	AD/AR
		MD1, MD2†	AD
RYR1	Ryanodine receptor	MH	AD
	Calcium release channel	Central core disease	AD‡
			AR

AD, autosomal dominant; AR, autosomal recessive; ClC1, chloride channel 1 gene/channel; HyperPP, hyperkalaemic periodic paralysis; HypoPP, hypokalaemic periodic paralysis; $K_{ir}2.1$, potassium inward rectifier; MH, malignant hyperthermia; PAM, potassium aggravated myotonia; PMC, paramyotonia congenita.

* DNA-based diagnosis available in UK.

† Altered splicing of CLCN1 has been shown in both forms of myotonic dystrophy (MD) as the basis of the myotonia.

‡ Gain-of-function.

spontaneous motor unit discharges with a decrement in the muscle action potential amplitude. PMC is also caused by mutations in the voltage-gated skeletal muscle sodium channel α-subunit (*SCN4A*) and PMC is therefore allelic with hyperPP. PMC is inherited as a highly penetrant autosomal dominant trait. Mutations have been found throughout the gene, although exon 24 appears to be a hotspot for mutations. PMC associated point mutations confer a gain-of-function. However, the resulting impairment of fast inactivation is less than that associated with mutations associated with hyperPP. Mexiletene is an effective symptomatic treatment for PMC. Milder forms of myotonia without cold sensitivity are also described in association with different sodium channel point mutations, known as potassium aggravated myotonia.

Hypokalaemic periodic paralysis – a muscle calcium or sodium channel disorder Hypokalaemic periodic paralysis (hypoPP) is autosomal dominant with *de novo* dominant mutations accounting for one-third of cases. Attacks are precipitated by a period of exercise followed by rest or by carbohydrate loading. Attacks typically develop in the early hours of the morning and may last hours to days. Serum potassium is typically low at the onset but may normalise quickly. Attack frequency tends to decline with age but a fixed myopathy may develop. Myotonia does not occur in hypoPP.

Point mutations in two separate muscle channel genes may cause hypoPP. The majority of cases harbour one of three point mutations in the L-type calcium channel, *CACNA1S* (also known as hypoPP type 1). Far less frequent mutations have been described in the muscle sodium channel *SCN4A* (known as hypoPP-type 2).

Mutations in the L-type calcium channel α_1-subunit (dihydropyridine receptor; *CACNA1S*) account for about 70% of cases of hypoPP. All mutations are arginine substitutions in the voltage sensor (S4) of the channel protein. It remains unclear how mutations in *CACNA1S*, which does not have a major role in determining muscle membrane excitability, causes the symptoms; however, recent studies suggest that the S4 causative mutations result in a gating pore current that is important in causing episodic muscle membrane depolarisation.

HypoPP associated with *CACNA1S* mutations exhibits reduced penetrance in females (50%) compared to complete penetrance in males. Specific mutations appear to have discrete clinical features, for example R528H is common, with later onset and associated myalgias.

HypoPP can also be caused by missense loss-of-function mutations in the voltage sensor of domain 2 of *SCN4A* but these are uncommon in the United Kingdom. There is some evidence that such hypoPP cases may experience worsening of attacks with prominent myalgia when exposed to acetazolamide. In this setting an alternative carbonic anhydrase inhibitor dichlorphenamide seems to be effective.

In summary, current evidence indicates that hyperPP is a gain-of-function disorder caused by *SCN4A* point mutations. In contrast, hypoPP associates with S4 mutations that predict a gating pore current in either *CACNA1S* or *SCN4A*.

Thyrotoxic periodic paralysis This is a rare condition causing attacks indistinguishable from hypoPP but in the presence of thyrotoxicosis. The disorder is most common in young Asian and Latin American men in whom 10% of thyrotoxic males develop episodic weakness. Candidate gene sequencing has revealed mutations in *KCNJ18* which encodes Kir 2.6, an inwardly rectifying potassium channel that is expressed in skeletal muscle and transcriptionally regulated by thyroid hormones in one-third of patients.

Periodic paralysis and cardiac arrhythmias – a skeletal muscle potassium channel disorder Most cases of periodic paralysis do not associate with cardiac arrhythmias because the responsible channel (*CACNA1S, SCN4A*) is not expressed in cardiac muscle. Andersen–Tawil syndrome is a form of dyskalaemic periodic paralysis in which cardiac involvement is frequent (the resting ECG commonly shows bigeminy). In addition to periodic paralysis, patients may have atrial and/or ventricular arrhythmias and may also have characteristic facial and skeletal features (Figure 10.24). From a practical point of view, this disorder should be considered in any case of periodic paralysis with arrhythmia.

Andersen's syndrome is caused by mutations in a potassium channel termed Kir2.1. This inward rectifying potassium channel Kir2.1 is encoded by *KCNJ2* on chromosome 17q23. The functional channel is a homotetramer important for cardiac and skeletal muscle membrane hyperpolarisation and also has a role in skeletal bone precursor cell migration and fusion during development. There is intrafamilial variability and partial manifestation of the phenotype is common. During an attack, serum potassium is most commonly low but may be normal or high. In patients with hypokalaemia, oral potassium supplements may improve the weakness. In some families, increasing plasma potassium concentration with acetazolamide improves arrhythmias at the expense of exacerbating weakness. Once the diagnosis is made detailed cardiac assessment is needed. However, the optimum management to prevent malignant arrhythmias is not certain.

Myotonia congenita – a skeletal muscle chloride channel disorder Dominant (Thomsen's disease) and recessive (Becker's disease) forms of myotonia congenita are recognised. Patients experience differing degrees of muscle stiffness and muscle hypertrophy. The dominant form is less common and generally milder. Patients present with muscle stiffness because of impaired voluntary muscle relaxation. Patients describe marked muscle stiffness at the onset of activity, but the more they continue the less stiff the muscles become – the 'warm-up phenomenon'. While 90% show myotonia on EMG, only 50% have percussion myotonia on examination. There is usually normal power at rest, although a minority have proximal weakness. Muscle hypertrophy and myalgia may occur in both forms but are more prominent in the more common recessive form of the disease. Electrophysiologically, *in vivo* myotonia (and paramyotonia) is characterised by uncontrolled repetitive action potentials at the sarcolemma initiated by a voluntary activation. This persistent involuntary activation prevents the patient from relaxing the muscle, hence the complaint of muscle stiffness and limitation of free flowing movements.

Both forms of myotonia congenita are caused by mutations in a muscle voltage gated chloride channel (*CLCN1*) located on chromosome 7q35.10. There is evidence that, unlike all other voltage-gated ion channels, this channel has two separate ion pores through which chloride ion passage may occur. The resting membrane potential in skeletal muscle is mainly dependent upon the chloride channel conductance; *CLCN1* mutations result in impaired chloride conductance and so produce partial depolarisation of the membrane. This creates the electrophysiological condition of increased excitability and repetitive firing after muscle activation, necessary for myotonia to occur. In patients who require treatment there is randomised controlled trial evidence that mexiletine is effective.

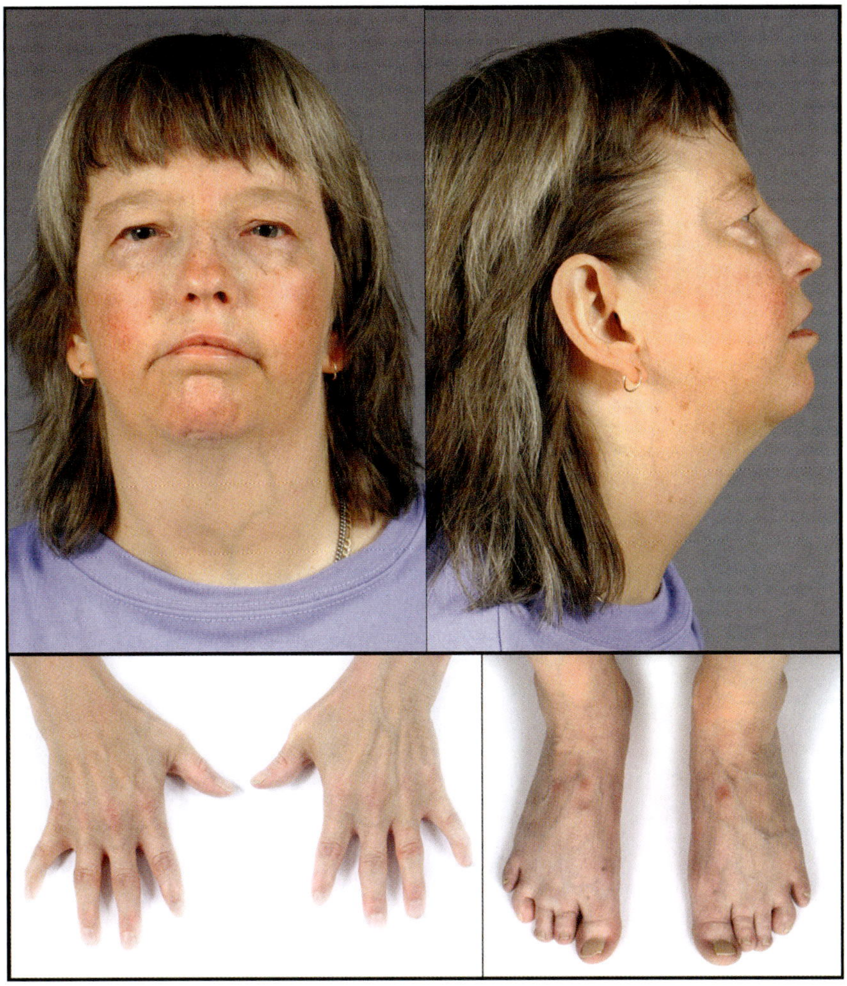

Figure 10.24 Typical facial and hand foot appearances in Anderson–Tawil syndrome. Note hypertelorism, micrognathism, low set ears, down-turned mouth, short digits, clinodactyly of the fifth digits and syndactyly of the toes.

Metabolic muscle disease

Mitochondrial respiratory chain diseases

Mitochondrial function and dysfunction Mitochondria are highly dynamic intracellular organelles with critical roles in numerous cell functions, including energy (ATP) generation via the respiratory chain and oxidative phosphorylation (OXPHOS) system (a series of enzyme complexes embedded in the inner mitochondrial membrane; Figure 10.25), calcium homeostasis, and cell-specific functions such as neurotransmitter biosynthesis. Mitochondria are unique among cellular organelles in possessing their own genetic material, a circular double-stranded 16.5 kb DNA molecule encoding 13 polypeptide components of OXPHOS enzymes and 24 RNA molecules needed for the intramitochondrial synthesis of these 13 polypeptides. Diseases related to mitochondrial dysfunction were first recognised more than 50 years ago, with the clinical description of Luft's disease (euthyroid hypermetabolism). However, the genetic basis of these disorders did not begin to be unravelled until 1988, when the first mitochondrial DNA (mtDNA) mutations were reported. Since then more than 150 pathogenic mtDNA mutations have been described (www.mitomap.org). Furthermore, it is now recognised that more than 1000 proteins make up the mitochondrial 'proteome' and that mutations in any of the nuclear genes encoding the vast majority of these proteins may, theoretically at least, cause mitochondrial disease. So far mutations in approximately 200 of these genes have been linked to human disease.

Clinical features of mitochondrial disorders Mitochondrial disorders are defined as inherited disorders affecting OXPHOS (directly or indirectly), and are estimated to have a birth prevalence of 1 in 5000. Presenting clinical features are extremely heterogeneous, particularly in childhood, but most affected adults have predominantly neuromuscular symptoms. Myopathic features include progressive external ophthalmoplegia (PEO), isolated proximal myopathy (or occasionally distal myopathy; Figure 10.26), exercise intolerance and rhabdomyolysis, which is an infrequent but recognised complication.

Although many adults have an isolated myopathic phenotype, complex multi-system disorders are increasingly recognised, including discrete constellations of symptoms forming specific clinical syndromes, as described later and summarised in Table 10.38.

Mitochondrial myopathies

Progressive external ophthalmoplegia The muscles most frequently involved by mitochondrial disease are the extraocular muscles, leading to PEO and bilateral symmetrical ptosis, usually without diplopia. Proximal limb musculature may also be involved by the

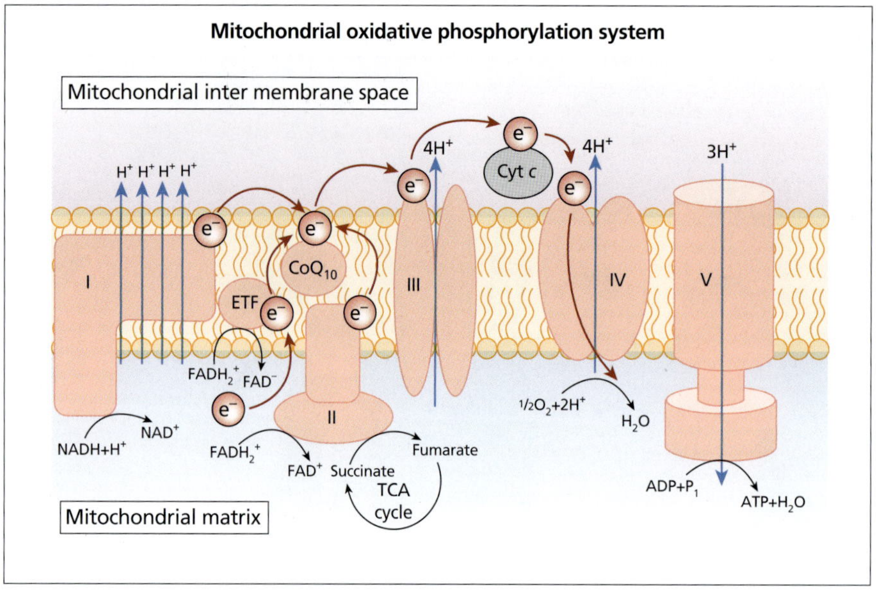

Figure 10.25 Mitochondrial oxidative phosphorylation system. I, NADH: ubiquinone oxidoreductase; II, succinate: ubiquinone oxidoreductase; III, ubiquinol: cytochrome oxidoreductase; IV, COX; V, ATP synthase. Source: Kanabus *et al.* 2014. Used under the terms of the Creative Commons licence. CC-BY.

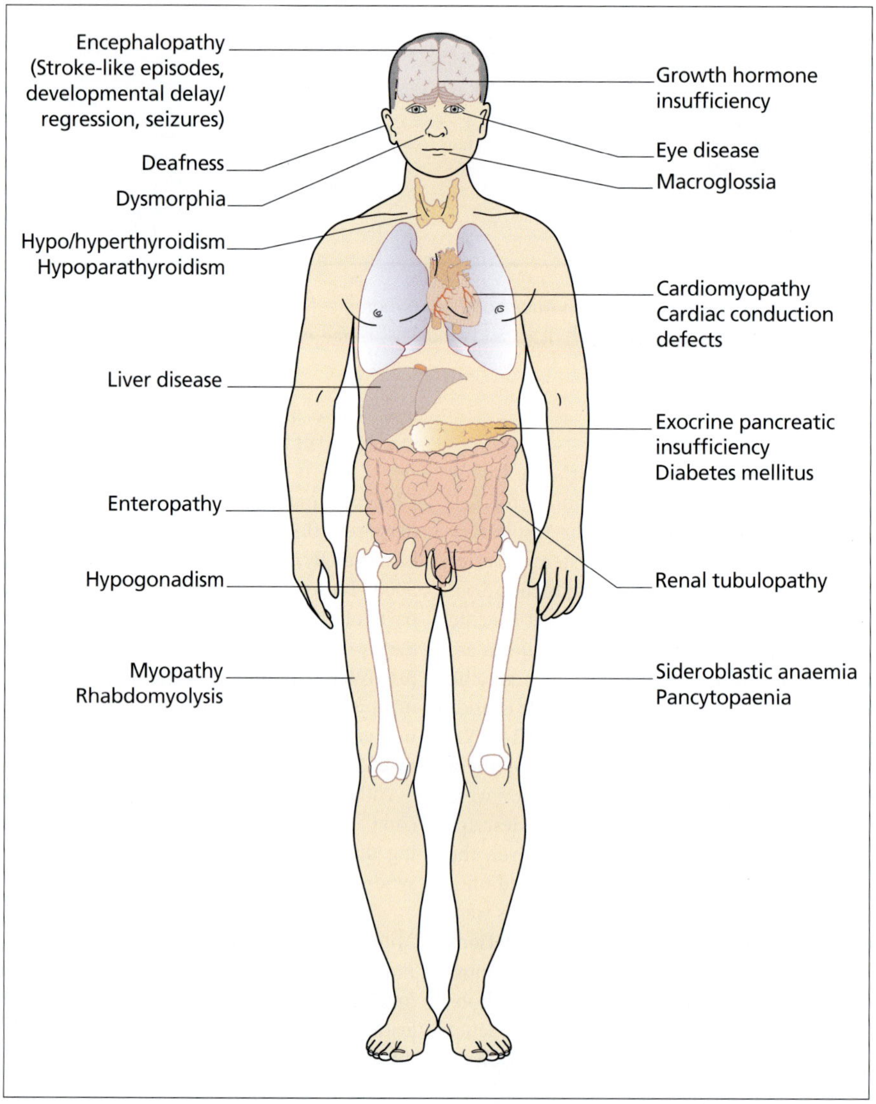

Figure 10.26 Clinical features of mitochondrial disease.

Table 10.38 Clinical mitochondrial syndromes presenting in adult life.

Acronym or eponym	Syndrome	Clinical features
MELAS	Mitochondrial encephalomyopathy, lactic acidosis, stroke-like episodes	Stroke-like episodes, migraines, dementia, ataxia, cardiomyopathy, deafness, gastrointestinal dysmotility
MIDD	Maternally inherited diabetes and deafness	Diabetes, deafness, maculopathy, cardiomyopathy, renal disease
MERRF	Myoclonus, epilepsy, ragged red fibres	Myoclonus, seizures, ataxia, deafness, dementia, lipomas
LHON	Leber's hereditary optic neuropathy	Subacute bilateral loss of vision
NARP	Neurogenic muscle weakness, ataxia, retinitis pigmentosa	Peripheral neuropathy, ataxia, pigmentary retinopathy
PEO	Progressive external ophthalmoplegia	Ptosis, limitation of eye movements
KSS	Kearns–Sayre syndrome	PEO (<20 years), pigmentary retinopathy, cerebellar ataxia, heart block
ADPEO	Autosomal dominant PEO	PEO, dysphagia
ARPEO	Autosomal recessive PEO	PEO, optic atrophy, cardiomyopathy
SANDO	Sensory ataxic neuropathy, dysarthria and ophthalmoparesis	Ataxia, neuropathy, dysarthria, PEO
MEMSA	Myoclonic epilepsy, myopathy, sensory ataxia	Epilepsy, ataxia, myopathy
MNGIE	Mitochondrial neurogastrointestinal encephalomyopathy	Gastrointestinal dysmotility, PEO, myopathy, demyelinating neuropathy
ADOA	Autosomal dominant optic atrophy	Optic atrophy, SNHL, SANDO-like disorder
CMT2A	Charcot–Marie–Tooth disease type 2A	Axonal sensorimotor neuropathy, optic atrophy
Alpers*	Progressive sclerosingpoliodystrophy	Intractable epilepsy, liver disease
Leigh's*	Subacute necrotising encephalomyelopathy	Progressive loss of neurological function, dystonia, ataxia, seizures, optic atrophy, respiratory failure

* Presentation in adult life is extremely rare.

disease process, manifesting as fatigue and exercise intolerance. Pain is an unusual feature. The most common cause of PEO is a sporadic single large-scale mtDNA deletion (SLMD). Several Mendelian PEO syndromes are now recognised, which may be inherited as autosomal dominant (ADPEO) or autosomal recessive (ARPEO) traits. These disorders are caused by mutations in nuclear-encoded genes needed for maintenance of the mitochondrial genome (Table 10.39) and may be suspected if multiple deletions are detected on long-range PCR of the mtDNA. ADPEO may also be suggested by the family history. Patients with ADPEO and ARPEO may present additional clinical problems, including ataxia, peripheral neuropathy, dysphagia and other bulbar symptoms, cataracts, depression, cardiac involvement and endocrine disturbance.

Kearns–Sayre syndrome Some patients with SLMDs have a more severe presentation, known as the Kearns–Sayre syndrome (KSS), which is defined as onset before 20 years of PEO with pigmentary retinopathy and one of: cardiac conduction defect, raised CSF protein (>1 g/L) or cerebellar ataxia. Eighty per cent of patients with KSS have a SLMD, but recently autosomal recessive KSS caused by *RRM2B* mutations has been reported.

Exercise intolerance and rhabdomyolysis Isolated myopathy with exercise intolerance and myoglobinuria may be associated with mtDNA point mutations affecting complex III and IV subunits, and are usually sporadic. Rhabdomyolysis is more usually a feature of mitochondrial fatty acid beta oxidation defects, but may also be seen in co-enzyme Q_{10} deficiency. Although proximal myopathy is typical in mitochondrial disease, recently distal myopathy caused by *POLG* mutations has been reported.

Mitochondrial neuropathies Peripheral neuropathy is an increasingly recognised feature of mitochondrial disease. In some cases it is mild or even subclinical, but in other individuals neuropathy may

Table 10.39 Classification of mitochondrial respiratory chain diseases.

Genetic defect	Inheritance	Phenotype
Defects of mitochondrial DNA		
Mutations affecting protein synthesis:		
SLMDs	Sporadic	PEO, myopathy, KSS
tRNA point mutations	Maternal	MELAS, MIDD, MERRF
rRNA point mutations	Maternal	Aminoglycoside-induced SNHL
Mutations of protein coding genes:		
Complex I subunits (*MTND1-6*)	Maternal	LHON, MELAS, LS
Complex III subunit (*MTCYTB*)	Maternal	Exercise intolerance
Complex IV subunits (*MTCO1-3*)	Maternal	Myopathy
Complex V subunits (*MTATP6/8*)	Maternal	LS, NARP, isolated neuropathy
Nuclear gene defects		
OXPHOS subunits, e.g.		
Complex I subunits	Recessive	LS
Complex II subunits(*SDHA-B*)	Recessive	LS
Complex II subunits (*SDHB-D*)	Dominant	Paraganglionoma, phaeochromocytoma
OXPHOS assembly factors, e.g.		
Complex I assembly factors (*NDUFAF…*)	Recessive	LS, cardiomyopathy, exercise intolerance
Complex IV assembly factors (*SURF1*)	Recessive	LS
mtDNA replication factors, e.g.		
POLG, PEO1	Dominant	ADPEO
POLG	Recessive	ARPEO, SANDO, MEMSA, Alpers' disease
Nucleoside metabolism, e.g.		
RRM2B, ANT1	Dominant	ADPEO
TK2, DGUOK, RRM2B	Recessive	ARPEO
TYMP	Recessive	MNGIE
Aminoacylt RNA synthetases, e.g.		
AARS2	Recessive	Leukodystrophy and ovarian failure
DARS2	Recessive	LBSL
HARS2, LARS2	Recessive	Perrault's syndrome (POF and SNHL)
MARS2	Recessive	ARSAL
YARS2	Recessive	MLASA
FeS cluster biogenesis, e.g.		
ISCU	Recessive	Myopathy with exercise intolerance
FXN	Recessive	Friedreich's ataxia
Co-enzyme Q_{10} biosynthesis, e.g.		
ADCK3	Recessive	Cerebellar ataxia ± seizures
Mitochondrial protein import, e.g.		
TIMM8A	X-linked	Deafness–dystonia syndrome
Mitochondrial dynamics, e.g.		
MFN2, GDAP1	Dominant	CMT2A, CMT4A
OPA1	Dominant	ADOA
Mitochondrial membrane lipid biosynthesis/remodelling, e.g.		
TAZ	X-linked	Barth's syndrome
SERAC1	Recessive	MEGDEL

This table has largely focussed on mitochondrial disorders presenting in or surviving into adult life.

ADOA, autosomal dominant optic atrophy; ADPEO, autosomal dominant PEO; ARPEO, autosomal recessive PEO; ARSAL, autosomal recessive spastic ataxia with leukoencephalopathy; CMT, Charcot–Marie–Tooth; KSS, Kearns–Sayre syndrome; LBSL, leukoencephalopathy with brainstem and spinal cord involvement and lactate elevation; LHON, Leber's hereditary optic neuropathy; LS, Leigh's syndrome; MEGDEL, methylglutaconicaciduria, deafness, encephalopathy, Leigh-like; MELAS, mitochondrial encephalomyopathy with lactic acidosis and stroke-like episodes; MEMSA, myoclonic epilepsy, myopathy, sensory ataxia; MERRF, myoclonic epilepsy with ragged red fibres; MIDD, maternally inherited diabetes and deafness; MLASA, myopathy, lactic acidosis, sideroblastic anaemia; MNGIE, mitochondrial neurogastrointestinal encephalopathy; NARP, neurogenic muscle weakness, ataxia and retinitis pigmentosa; PEO, progressive external ophthalmoplegia; POF, premature ovarian failure; SANDO, sensory ataxia, neuropathy, dysphagia and ophthalmoplegia; SLMDs, single large-scale mtDNA deletions; SNHL, sensorineural hearing loss.

be the predominant or only clinical manifestation of mitochondrial disease. Several multi-system disorders with a major neuropathy have been reported, most commonly a sensorimotor axonal neuropathy. Patients with moderate levels of maternally inherited point mutations (m.8993T > G/C) in the mitochondrial *MT-ATP6* gene, encoding a subunit of the ATP synthase, may have neurogenic muscle weakness, ataxia and retinitis pigmentosa (NARP) syndrome. The same mutations at very high mutant loads (>90%) are associated with Leigh's syndrome. However, other patients with point mutations in this gene have a much milder phenotype clinically indistinguishable from CMT disease. Patients with recessive *POLG* mutations may have a neuropathy syndrome known as sensory ataxia, neuropathy, dysphagia and ophthalmoplegia (SANDO) or ataxic neuropathy syndrome (ANS). These patients typically have multiple mtDNA deletions in skeletal muscle biopsies. In other patients neuropathy may be associated with DNA depletion (i.e. quantitative mutation of mtDNA), for example in patients with *MPV17* mutations. *MPV17* disease includes Navajo neurohepatopathy (a founder disease in the Navajo population in south-western United States) in which a severe sensorimotor neuropathy is associated with corneal ulceration, acral mutilation, liver disease, leukoencephalopathy and metabolic acidosis. Patients with mutations in the outer mitochondrial membrane GTPase mitofusin 2, which is critical for mitochondrial fusion, present with dominant CMT type 2A, and may additionally have optic atrophy, whereas mutations in another outer mitochondrial membrane protein GDAP1 are associated with recessive CMT4A. Finally, demyelinating peripheral neuropathy is a feature of mitochondrial neuro-gastrointestinal encephalopathy (MNGIE) syndrome (see Multi-system mitochondrial disorders), and rarely may be seen in MELAS, MERRF and Leigh's syndromes.

Mitochondrial optic neuropathies

LHON Leber's hereditary optic neuropathy (LHON) is a maternally inherited subacute optic neuropathy characterised by painless sequential loss of vision in both eyes. More than 90% of cases have one of three common mtDNA point mutations (m.11778G > A, m.3460G > A and m.14484T > C) in genes encoding subunits of complex I of the respiratory chain. These mutations are homoplasmic (i.e. present in 100% mutation load) but penetrance is extremely variable and differs between the sexes. Males have an approximately five times greater risk of loss of vision, possibly because of a protective effect of oestrogen in females. In most patients loss of vision is the only symptom, but occasional patients have additional problems, including cardiac arrhythmias, peripheral neuropathy and multiple sclerosis-like symptoms.

ADOA Autosomal dominant optic atrophy (ADOA, also known as Kjer's optic neuropathy) is the most common inherited optic neuropathy in Caucasian populations and is caused by mutations in *OPA1*, encoding an inner mitochondrial membrane GTPase with roles in mitochondrial morphology and dynamics and mtDNA maintenance. Optic atrophy beginsin childhood (typically by 6 years) and is slowly progressive, with vision loss varying from mild to severe. Intrafamilial variability is recognised. Individuals with the *R445H* mutation frequently have associated sensorineural hearing loss (SNHL) while up to 20% of patients may have a multi-system neurological disorder resembling SANDO (see Mitochondrial neuropathies).

Mitochondrial encephalomyopathies

MELAS Mitochondrial encephalomyopathy with lactic acidosis and stroke-like episodes (MELAS) syndrome is a multi-system disorder characterised by the occurrence of stroke-like episodes before the age of 40 years, frequently associated with seizures, migrainous headache, anorexia, vomiting and lactic acidosis. Transient hemiparesis, altered consciousness and cognitive blindness may occur during the stroke-like episodes, which are thought to be caused by microangiopathy and endothelial dysfunction, although the precise mechanisms are still debated. The disease course is usually relentlessly progressive, with recurrent stroke-like episodes leading to visual disturbance and motor and cognitive decline. Eighty per cent of cases have a common mtDNA point mutation, m.3243A > G. Nearly 30 different mtDNA point mutations have been implicated in the remaining 20% of cases, although similar symptoms may occasionally result from nuclear gene mutations such as *POLG* mutations. Other clinical features of MELAS syndrome include sensorineural hearing loss (SNHL), ataxia, diabetes mellitus, and cardiac, renal and gastrointestinal disturbance. Many of these features may occur in isolation in patients with the m.3243A > G mutation, with the full MELAS syndrome occurring in a minority (<10%) of individuals with this mutation.

MERRF In MERRF (myoclonic epilepsy with ragged red fibres) syndrome, onset is usually in late childhood with myoclonus, typically associated with ataxia. Other clinical features of this syndrome include generalised epilepsy, SNHL, optic atrophy, pigmentary retinopathy and lactic acidosis. Some individuals also have multiple symmetrical lipomatosis. Most patients with this syndrome have a mtDNA point mutation, m.8344A > G, although other mtDNA point mutations have also been associated with this phenotype, and patients with recessive *POLG* mutations (see Chapter 7) may have similar presentations. In practice, there is often considerable overlap between MERRF and MELAS, with stroke-like episodes sometimes occurring in the former. Moreover, recently it has become clear that the m.8344A > G mutation is associated with marked phenotypic heterogeneity.

Alpers' and other mitochondrial epilepsy syndromes Several epilepsy syndromes have been associated with recessive *POLG* mutations. Alpers–Huttenlocher syndrome (also known as progressive sclerosing poliodystrophy or progressive neuronal degeneration of childhood with liver disease) is one of the most severe presentations of recessive *POLG* mutations. Intractable seizures usually begin in infancy but may occur at any time during childhood. In some cases there is preceding developmental delay and hypotonia. Initial seizures are focal, often involving the right arm, evolving through epilepsia partialis continua to status epilepticus. Seizures are resistant to multiple antiepileptic drugs and death may follow status epilepticus or acute liver failure, which may be precipitated by sodium valproate. For this reason valproate therapy is generally avoided in the treatment of mitochondrial epilepsy, at least until *POLG* mutations have been excluded. Later onset *POLG* epilepsies are now considered under the umbrella term myoclonic epilepsy, myopathy, sensory ataxia (MEMSA) syndrome, which includes patients previously described as having spino-cerebellar ataxia with epilepsy (SCAE). The first symptom in MEMSA is often ataxia, together with recurrent seizures (usually myoclonic) and myopathy.

Leigh's syndrome Leigh's syndrome, or subacute necrotising encephalopathy, has a birth prevalence of at least 1/40 000. It usually presents in infancy with stepwise neurodevelopmental regression related to intercurrent illnesses and other metabolic stresses, and usually has a relentlessly progressive course leading to death in early childhood. However, occasional cases present in adult life and increasingly childhood-onset cases are surviving into adulthood (possibly related to improved supportive care), and so the adult neurologist should be familiar with this cause of severe neurodisability. Blood and/or CSF lactate levels are usually elevated, and characteristic neuro-imaging appearances are of bilateral symmetrical lesions in the basal ganglia and/or brainstem, which appear hyperintense in T2-weighted sequences. Leigh's syndrome is associated with remarkable genetic heterogeneity, with more than 50 genes (including both mitochondrial and nuclear genes) linked to this condition so far.

Multi-system mitochondrial disorders

MIDD Maternally inherited diabetes and deafness (MIDD) is one of the most common presentations of the m.3243A > G mutation which has been traditionally linked to MELAS (see Mitochondrial encephalomyopathies). Deafness usually precedes the onset of diabetes by several years. The diabetes is comparatively easy to manage although insulin may be needed. Other clinical features related to m.3243A > G may be observed in patients with MIDD, including hypertrophic cardiomyopathy, renal impairment (caused by focal segmental glomerulosclerosis), ataxia, myopathy and stroke-like episodes.

MNGIE Mitochondrial neurogastrointestinal encephalopathy (MNGIE) is caused by thymidine phosphorylase deficiency, leading to impaired mtDNA replication because of intramitochondrial nucleoside imbalance. This in turn leads to progressive mtDNA depletion and accumulation of mtDNA rearrangements and point mutations. Affected individuals may be healthy in childhood and typically present late in the second decade with intestinal pseudo-obstruction, which may be associated with demyelinating peripheral neuropathy, PEO and optic atrophy. MRI reveals a leukoencephalopathy, which is usually relatively asymptomatic.

Other multi-system disorders As mitochondria are present in all human cells with the exception of mature erythrocytes, mitochondrial dysfunction can potentially involve any organ system, as indicated by Figure 10.27, and these clinical features may present in any combination at any age.

Disorders associated with secondary mitochondrial dysfunction Space precludes the detailed discussion of these disorders, but secondary mitochondrial dysfunction has been reported in several neuro-degenerative disorders, including Parkinson's, Huntington's and Alzheimer's diseases, as well as in normal healthy ageing.

Diagnosis Investigation of mitochondrial disease needs to take a multi-modality approach, including some or all of the following investigations, depending on the clinical presentation.

Blood investigations Blood lactate may be elevated in mitochondrial disease, but is frequently normal in adult patients. CK may be mildly elevated but is not usually informative. In MNGIE syndrome, plasma and urine thymidine and deoxyuridine levels are elevated; the diagnosis is confirmed by demonstrating reduced activity of thymidine phosphorylase in platelets.

Neuro-imaging MRI of the brain is typically normal in patients with mitochondrial myopathies, neuropathies and optic neuropathies. However, acute stroke-like episodes, MRI of the brain in patients with MELAS usually reveals unilateral T2 hyperintensities in a parieto-occipital distribution (not confined to specific vascular territories), which subsequently resolve. Leigh's syndrome is characterised by bilateral symmetrical T2 hyperintensities involving the basal ganglia and/or brainstem. Leukoencephalopathy may be seen in MNGIE and other mitochondrial encephalopathies, such as the syndrome of leukoencephalopathy with brainstem and spinal cord involvement and lactate elevation (LBSL) caused by *DARS2* mutations.

Neurophysiology Approximately 50% of adult patients with mitochondrial disorders have electromyographic evidence of myopathy, while axonal sensorimotor polyneuropathy is observed in about 35% of cases. Demyelinating neuropathy is seen in MNGIE. The electroencephalogram has a characteristic appearance in the early stages of Alpers' syndrome (unilateral occipital rhythmic high-amplitude delta with superimposed [poly] spikes; RHADS), although later becomes non-specifically abnormal.

Muscle histology The histological hallmark of mitochondrial disease, the ragged-red fibre (RRF), is best visualised by the modified

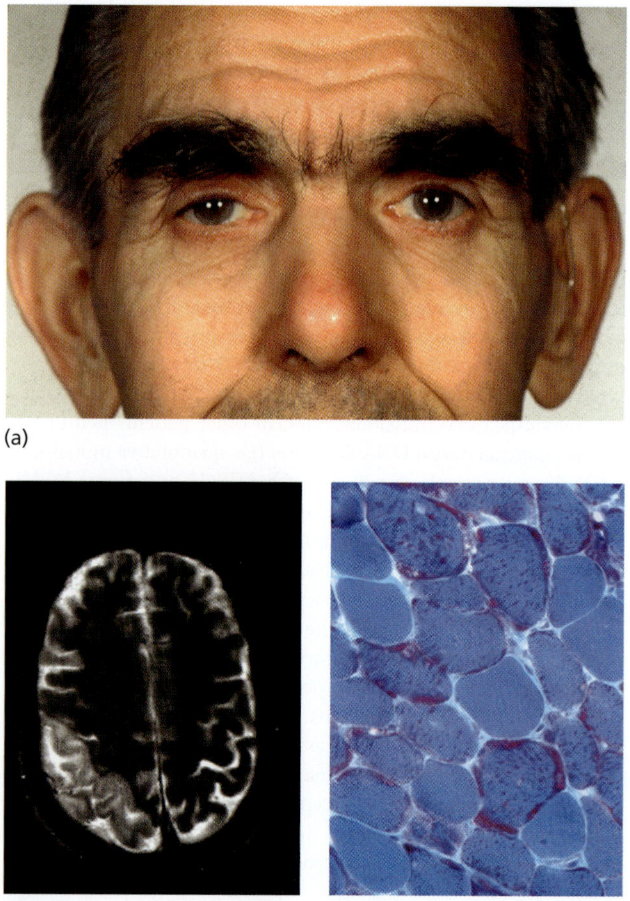

(a) (b) (c)

Figure 10.27 (a) Mitochondrial myopathy. Note not only the ptosis but hearing aid indicating deafness. (b) Typical stroke of a patient with mitochondrial disease, occipitoparietal and not respecting usual anatomical vascular territories. (c) Ragged red fibres stained with Gomori trichrome stain represent muscle fibres with peripheral accumulations of abnormal mitochondria.

Gomori trichrome stain, in which mitochondria appear red. The 'ragged' appearance results from subsarcolemmal accumulation of mitochondria. RRF frequently stain negatively for cytochrome oxidase (COX) and positively in the succinate dehydrogenase (SDH) stain, leading to 'ragged-blue' fibres in the sequential COX–SDH combined stain. Although a small number of RRF may be a normal feature of ageing muscle, the presence of any RRF below the age of 40 years is considered abnormal, as is the observation of greater than five RRF above the age of 60. Other non-specific histological features that may be observed in patients with mitochondrial disease include accumulation of lipid droplets within muscle fibres and type 2 fibre predominance.

Muscle biochemistry OXPHOS enzyme activities can be measured using spectrophotometric assays in skeletal muscle biopsies and may reveal isolated deficiency of a single enzyme or combined deficiencies of multiple enzymes, particularly in childhood-onset disease. However, OXPHOS enzyme activities are typically normal in most adults with mitochondrial disease, even those with confirmed genetic defects, reflecting the relatively milder disorders presenting in adults.

Mitochondrial genetics Point mutations of mtDNA were initially linked to LHON and later to a multitude of clinical presentations. To date >150 different mtDNA point mutations have been reported, and these have been catalogued in the Mitomap online database (www.mitomap.org). Many of these mutations have only been described in single families and so are considered provisionally pathogenic, until reported to cause a similar phenotype in a second unrelated family, at which time a confirmed pathogenicity status is assigned. The first genetic defects reported in mitochondrial disorders were large-scale rearrangements of the mtDNA in patients with PEO. Single mtDNA deletions arise sporadically, but some patients have multiple mtDNA deletions because they have a Mendelian disorder of mtDNA maintenance. Mutations in 11 different nuclear-encoded genes have so far been linked to defective mtDNA replication. With the recent widespread adoption of whole exome sequencing, a rapidly increasing number of nuclear genes have been associated with mitochondrial disease (Table 10.39).

A stepwise approach to the genetic diagnosis of mitochondrial disease in adults is illustrated by the flowchart (Figure 10.28).

Treatment Currently, very few curative therapies exist for mitochondrial disorders, with the following notable exceptions:

Disorders of coenzyme Q_{10} biosynthesis Primary CoQ_{10} deficiencies (i.e. disorders of CoQ_{10} biosynthesis) are usually diagnosed in childhood but may present in adult life, for example with ataxia, seizures or myopathy. Early CoQ_{10} supplementation has been associated with a good prognosis, but extremely high doses may be needed, up to 2.4 g/day.

MNGIE Allogeneic haematopoietic stem cell transplantation has been suggested as a potentially curative therapy for MNGIE, but mortality has been ~50% in reported cases to date, related to transplant-related complications or disease progression.

Symptomatic therapy For all other mitochondrial diseases, supportive treatment in a multi-disciplinary setting is the mainstay of management, as follows:

- *Seizures*: antiepileptic drugs, according to seizure type; valproic acid is contraindicated in patients with POLG mutations.
- *Dystonia*: baclofen, trihexphenidyl, botulinum toxin injections, consider deep brain stimulation.
- *Ptosis*: surgery (e.g. brow suspension) to improve the cosmetic appearance; problem frequently recurs, necessitating further surgery.
- *Hearing loss*: hearing aids and/or cochlear implants, according to severity.
- *Endocrine disturbance*: oral hypoglycaemics (avoid metformin as may precipitate lactic acidosis) or insulin, as clinically indicated, for diabetes mellitus; thyroxine for hypothyroidism; hydrocortisone for adrenal insufficiency.
- *Cardiac disease*: pacemaker or implantable cardiac defibrillator for conduction defects; medical therapy for cardiomyopathy; consider heart transplantation if isolated severe heart disease.
- *Renal disease*: electrolyte replacement in tubulopathy; consider renal transplantation in end-stage renal disease, depending on severity of neurological disease and other multi-system involvement.
- *Gastrointestinal disturbance*: formal dietetic evaluation and adequate nutritional support, including enteral feeding if unsafe swallow or unable to take sufficient calories orally; prokinetics and laxatives for constipation; antiemetics if persistent nausea/vomiting; pancreatic enzyme replacement if exocrine pancreatic insufficiency.
- *Psychological support*: this is extremely important for affected patients and their families, particularly as depression and psychiatric disturbance are increasingly recognised manifestations of mitochondrial disease.

Experimental approaches Many different agents have been proposed for the treatment of mitochondrial disorders, but it has proved extremely difficult to design and execute effective clinical trials for this group of clinically and genetically heterogeneous disorders, with unpredictable disease progression. Particular problems have been the selection of validated, objective and clinically relevant outcome measures. A recently updated Cochrane systematic review identified very few well-designed clinical trials for mitochondrial disease, and results were conflicting. Many treatments are still at the stage of preclinical evaluation and include novel antioxidants and agents designed to stimulate mitochondrial biogenesis (e.g. bezafibrate), manipulate mitochondrial dynamics and rescue defects of mitochondrial nucleoside metabolism. Gene therapy has been performed in mouse models of MNGIE using AAV vectors, while other gene therapy strategies (e.g. MitoTALENs) are at very early preclinical stages of development. Finally, techniques have been developed that have allowed exchange of nuclear genetic material between embryos in primates, and these are now being explored as potential methods to avoid transmission of mtDNA defects in humans.

Conclusions Mitochondrial disorders are clinically, biochemically and genetically heterogeneous conditions sharing the common feature of abnormal oxidative phosphorylation. Traditionally, syndromic neuromuscular (PEO) and CNS (MELAS, MERRF) diseases, characterised by RRF myopathy and underlying mtDNA mutations, were the most frequently recognised mitochondrial disorders in adults presenting to neurologists. However, multi-system disorders, often of childhood onset and caused by nuclear gene mutations, are increasingly being transitioned to the adult neurology clinic, leading to changing perceptions of these complex diseases. As the genetics of these disorders are resolved by next generation sequencing strategies, new therapeutic targets and modalities are likely to emerge.

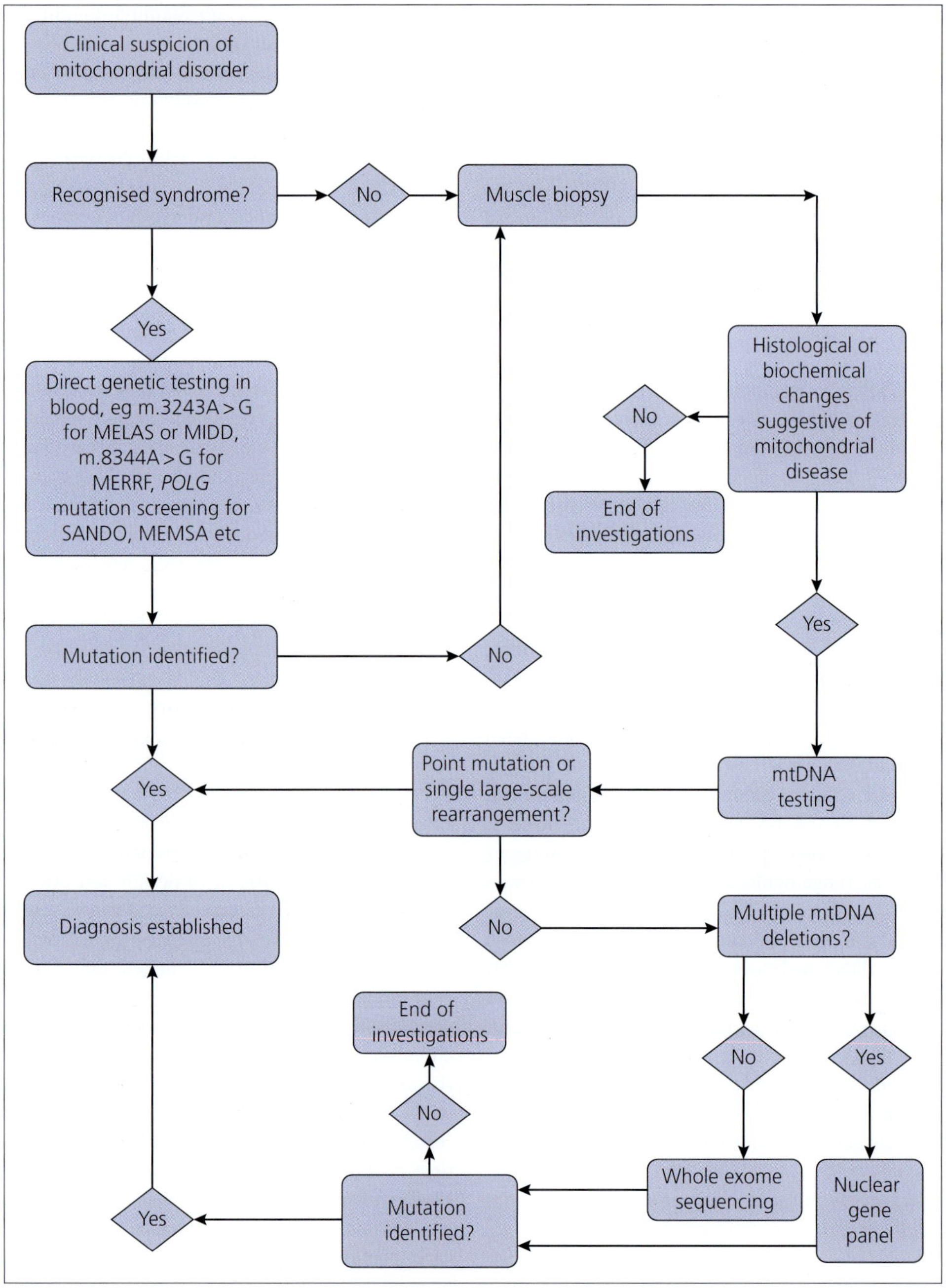

Figure 10.28 Flowchart for diagnosis of mitochondrial disorders in adults.

Glycogenoses and lipid storage disorders (Chapter 19)

In addition to mitochondrial respiratory chain disorders, the other metabolic disorders in muscle include defects in glucose metabolism (glycogen storage disorders) and defects in fat metabolism (lipid storage disorders). Patients with these autosomal recessive disorders generally develop muscle pain on exertion. Myoglobinuria and sometimes fulminant rhabdomyolysis may occur. Patients with McArdle's disease (the most common glycogenosis caused by myophosphorylase deficiency) present with muscle pain soon after commencing exercise. The pain can be severe and cramping, often causing the patient to stop. A second wind phenomenon is common. The forearm non-ischaemic lactate test will show a blunting of the expected rise in muscle lactate induced by repeated isometric exercise because of a failure to breakdown glycogen. Muscle biopsy will allow histioenzymatic staining for myophosphorylase, absent in McArdle's disease. Genetic testing is available but is usually performed after the metabolic defect has been confirmed.

Of the many disorders of lipid metabolism, the most common lipid storage disorder is carnitine palmitoyl transferase II (CPT-II) deficiency. Adults with CPT-II deficiency usually present with muscle pain induced by prolonged exercise, and often the pain may not develop until some time after exercise. Post-exercise myoglobinuria is frequent. Rhabdomyolysis is more likely to occur after fasting or if there is intercurrent infection or dehydration. Hypoketotic hypoglycaemia may occur. Occasionally, patients with CPT-II deficiency present with a painless proximal myopathy. Muscle biopsy light microscopy may reveal abnormal accumulations of lipid. Muscle tissue can be used for specific enzyme assays. The pattern of acylcarnitines in blood is particularly useful whenever a lipid storage disorder is being considered. Molecular genetic diagnosis is available.

Conclusions The diagnosis of patients with genetic muscle disorders has truly entered the molecular genetic era. DNA-based diagnosis is now available for many of these disorders and often removes the need for invasive tests such as muscle or nerve biopsy. Efficient selection of genetic tests is important and neurophysiology has a particularly important role in this regard for genetic muscle channelopathies. Muscle biopsy remains essential in certain situations, for example in the comprehensive investigation of patients with LGMD and in some metabolic myopathies. It is worth noting that while a blood sample is all that is required for testing in nuclear gene disorders, muscle tissue remains most useful for mitochondrial DNA analysis. In our view, all clinical neurologists need to be aware that a wealth of genetic diagnostic possibilities exists for these patients, and that achieving such diagnostic precision on a routine basis is important. Often, this will involve referral to a specialist muscle service.

Acquired muscle diseases

Inflammatory myopathies

The inflammatory myopathies are diseases whose primary pathology is inflammation within muscle. This definition thus excludes those genetic muscle disorders discussed earlier in which inflammatory change may occur (e.g. dystrophinopathy, FSHD or dysferlinopathy), and also diseases in which inflammation affects associated structures rather than muscle itself, as in polymyalgia rheumatica. The inflammatory myopathies can be divided into four principal classes on the basis of their aetiology (Table 10.40). Their diagnosis can be further refined by distinctive clinical and pathological features that reflect differing fundamental causes and processes, although at present the latter are incompletely understood.

Idiopathic inflammatory myopathies

These are the most commonly encountered acquired muscle diseases and discussion of them forms the framework for the remaining conditions. The three subtypes are:

1 *Dermatomyositis* (DM) in which the inflammatory process may also involve the skin.
2 *Polymyositis* (PM): isolated inflammation of the muscles (but similar findings may occur in association with several rheumatological diseases; see Polymyositis).
3 *Inclusion body myositis* (IBM) has a distinctive clinical pattern with less, if any, inflammatory change on biopsy.

All three share the key features of proximal lower limb wasting and weakness as the main clinical findings. However, they may be distinguished by specific features of both their clinical presentation and the findings of investigations. All are caused by separate pathological mechanisms. However, distinguishing one from another, or indeed from other conditions, can be difficult. There remains both incomplete understanding of their aetiology and a dearth of evidence on which to base decisions about their treatment.

Table 10.40 The inflammatory myopathies.

Idiopathic
Dermatomyositis, polymyositis, inclusion body myositis
Associated with connective tissue disease
SLE, rheumatoid arthritis, mixed connective tissue disease, Sjögren's disease
Infective/post-infective
Viral (HIV, EBV, CMV, HTLV-1), bacterial (staphylococcal, Lyme, tuberculosis), parasitic (nematodes, cestodes, protozoa)
Miscellaneous
Vasculitic, non-infective granulomatous (e.g. sarcoid), eosinophilic syndromes

CMV, cytomegalovirus; EBV, Epstein–Barr virus; HTLV, human T-lymphocyte virus; SLE, systemic lupus erythematosus.

Dermatomyositis

DM causes inflammation of muscle and typically, the skin. Epidemiological data are imprecise, but DM is uncommon, with an incidence of approximately 1/100 000. Unlike the other idiopathic inflammatory myopathies, cases in children are well recognised and it is by far the most common such condition in that age group. DM is more common in non-Caucasians and in women.

DM is a humorally mediated autoimmune disorder, in which the pathology is that of a microvasculopathy (Figure 10.29). Activated complement is found deposited in muscle capillaries and other tissues, which directs subsequent cellular inflammation. The trigger to this is unknown but postulated mechanisms include deposition of circulating immune complexes, or a response to an as yet unknown endothelial antigen.

Clinically, DM typically produces a subacute, progressive, proximal and symmetrical weakness, affecting the lower limbs more than the arms. Rarely does the condition lead to pronounced distal weakness. CK is usually raised. There is often some myalgia, but not severe pain. The extraocular and facial muscles are typically spared, but dysphagia may be a problem in severe or advanced cases, while neuromuscular respiratory compromise may also develop. Rarely, a more explosive presentation can occur, even leading to overt myoglobinuria.

The skin manifestations of DM usually precede the myopathy, but they may be difficult to detect if they are not specifically looked for, particularly in people with dark skin. The classic dermatological presentations are the 'heliotrope' erythematous rash of the face (especially the eyelids) and upper trunk. This rash is photosensitive, and often occurs with some oedema and telangiectasia. The hands can typically demonstrate Gottron papules, thickening over the surfaces of the knuckles, but may also show either a more subtle general coarseness of the skin ('mechanic's hands') or nail bed capillary change.

Occasionally, patients have only the skin changes, without clinical weakness or any elevation of CK, leading to the diagnostic term dermatomyositis sine myositis. However, muscle biopsy in these cases can demonstrate, even if only subtly, the abnormalities seen in DM. In such amyopathic patients, the condition may even resolve without need for immunosuppressive treatment, although recent work identified a high incidence of interstitial lung complications. Finally, typical DM over time may lead to calcinosis within affected tissues. This can be quite marked and produces striking changes on imaging. Early treatment is thought beneficial to minimise this last complication.

Other systems may also be involved in DM, notably the lungs and the heart. Approximately 20% of patients demonstrate evidence of an interstitial lung disease which can rarely be the first symptom.

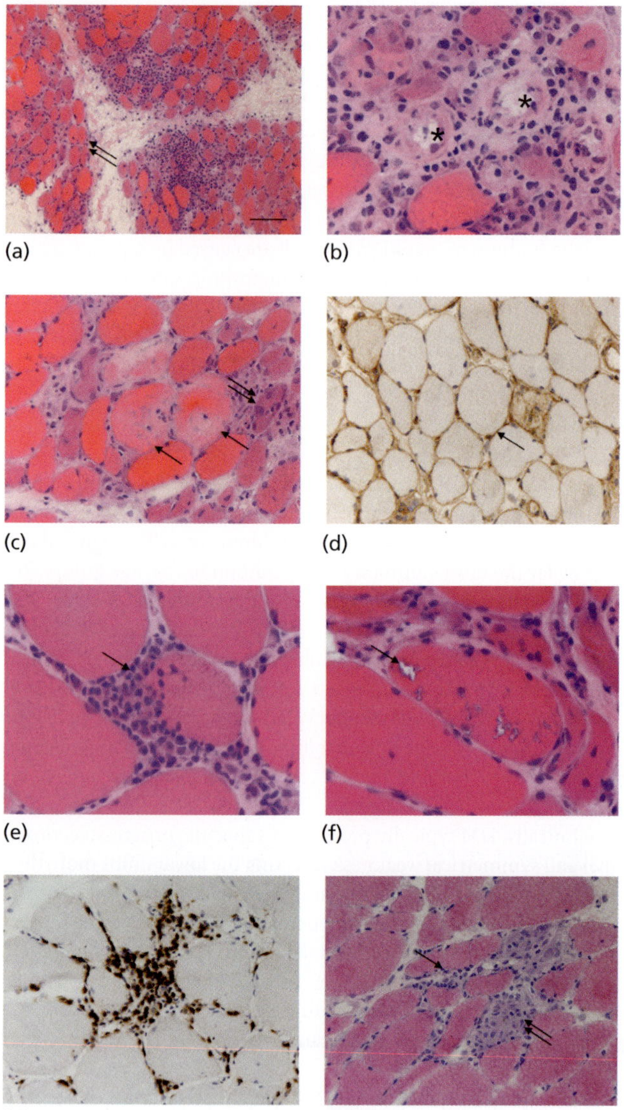

(a) (b) (c) (d) (e) (f) (g) (h)

Figure 10.29 In dermatomyositis atrophic fibres often display a perifascicular arrangement (a, double arrow). Lymphocytic infiltrates are frequently perivascular (b, *indicate small arterioles) and perimysial but may extend into the endomysium. There is fibre necrosis (c, arrows) and regeneration (c, double arrow). MHC Class I is expressed at the sarcolemma (d, arrow). The features of inclusion body myositis include endomysial lymphocytic infiltration with infiltration into intact muscle fibres (e, arrow) and rimmed vacuoles that occur in fibres without lymphocytic infiltration (f, arrow). The inflammatory infiltrate is composed predominantly of CD8-positive T lymphoctes (g). In polymyositis the inflammation is largely endomysial in location (h, arrow). In this example necrotic fibres infiltrated by macrophages are prominent (h, double arrow). a–c, e, f, h: haematoxylin and eosin; d: immunohistochemical staining for MHC Class I; g: immunohistochemical staining for CD8. Bar in (a) represents 100 μm in (a); 50 μm in (c), (d), (g) and H and 25 μm in (b), (e) and (f).

The most common symptoms are of cough and dyspnoea, typically with bibasal crepitations on auscultation of the chest. Lung complications are most commonly slowly progressive but symptoms can develop acutely. Twenty five per cent of those patients with abnormal pulmonary investigations remain asymptomatic. Pulmonary complications are associated with Jo-1 (anti-tRNA synthetase) IgG antibodies. These are present in 20% of patients with DM and of whom 70% have evidence of interstitial lung disease. The lung pathology is variable, but only bronchiolitis obliterans is likely to respond to immunosuppression. Early treatment, aiming to prevent permanent pathological muscle change, also prevents severe long-term pulmonary disease.

The exact incidence of cardiac involvement in idiopathic myositis is uncertain but several studies found congestive heart failure and ischaemia to be more common than in controls. Up to 50% of cases in some series have ECG evidence of dysrrhythmias, conduction block or ischaemic change pointing to a high incidence of subclinical cardiac involvement. Case reports have identified similar inflammatory changes in both the myocardium and conducting system to that found in skeletal muscle.

Large series of cases of DM find an approximate 20% association with malignancy, most commonly with adenocarcinoma and gynaecological tumours. Those most at risk are older, female and non-Caucasian patients. A thorough clinically directed approach to detecting an underlying malignancy is therefore indicated, with careful history-taking and examination for undisclosed symptoms or signs (e.g. weight loss, post-menopausal bleeding, breast lump or rectal mass). Appropriate further examination with imaging and/or specialist review is indicated to identify any occult cancer. Guidelines exist (see References) but these recognise the absence of clear evidence for how to investigate some conditions and which techniques to utilise. Our practice is to perform whole body FDG-PET-CT in all cases, together with mammography and pelvic imaging (ultrasound/MRI) in women, and testicular ultrasound in men, plus to consider older patients for colonoscopy.

The prognosis of DM is worse in those with pulmonary or cardiac complications, underlying malignancy, arthritis, hypergammaglobulinaemia or in acute or febrile presentations.

Polymyositis

Polymyositis is characterised by a progressive, proximal and symmetrical weakness without the skin lesions seen in DM. It is probably of similar or slightly lower incidence and prevalence to DM. It is very rare in those under 20 years, and is typically a disease of middle or later life. The course of PM is variable but is somewhat slower to evolve than DM. Although it can be rapidly progressive, the most frequent presentation is a slowly worsening proximal weakness over several months, in which the exact onset is difficult to pinpoint. Myalgia is typical but rarely severe. As with DM, the legs are typically more affected than the arms, distal and facial weakness is rare but respiratory muscle involvement can occur and can be life-threatening; the latter is most often seen when the disease is rapidly worsening.

Polymyositis differs fundamentally from DM in being a cell-mediated disease. CD8-positive T lymphocytes respond to an unknown muscle antigen by invading and destroying non-necrotic muscle fibres that express major histocompatibility complex protein (MHC-1; Figure 10.29). Unlike DM, blood vessels are spared. Respiratory and cardiac complications can develop at similar rates as occur in DM. Polymyositis also shares with DM the particular association of interstitial lung disease with antisynthetase antibodies.

Because PM presents with an absence of helpful associated clinical signs such as the skin involvement of DM or the particular pattern of weakness of typical IBM, 'pure' PM can be diagnosed in error. At the clinically milder end of the spectrum, care must be taken not to over-interpret pain or submaximal effort on examination. At the other, PM must be distinguished from other conditions that can provoke a raised CK and inflammatory changes on biopsy. All the clinical and investigation findings must be considered together and an open mind kept to the need to review or revise a diagnosis over time. In particular, 'failure' to respond to immunosuppressants should raise the possibility that a dystrophic process is, in fact, the cause.

There is a less established association of PM with neoplasia than with DM and guidelines for assessment of the latter do not extend to include PM. We recommend considering the possibility of an occult cancer and undertaking clinical review and investigation as per DM.

Inclusion body myositis

Sporadic inclusion body myositis occurs somewhat more frequently than DM or PM and is probably the most prevalent acquired myopathy. Unlike either PM or DM it appears to be most commonly a disease of Caucasian men. Other racial groups seem less frequently affected and the male to female ratio is 3 : 2. Typically, IBM occurs late in life and onset before age 30 years is highly unusual. Very rare familial forms of 'IBM' (either autosomal recessive or dominant) are increasingly recognised as instead being cases of myofibrillar myopathies, or caused by extremely rarely identified mutations in the gene encoding either valosin-containing protein (VCP): an overlapping but variable syndrome of a myopathy with inclusions on biopsy, Paget's disease of bone and frontotemporal dementia, or UDP-*N*-acetylglucosamine 2-epimerase (GNE), which causes a distal myopathy with rimmed vacuoles but which spares the quadriceps.

The onset of IBM is insidious and usually slower than seen with PM or DM. Classically, IBM causes a distinctive pattern of wasting and weakness most involving the quadriceps and deep finger flexors (Figure 10.30). This compromises the most crucial functions of the upper and lower limbs, hand grip and maintaining upright posture. Consequently, falls may occur relatively early, because of buckling of the knees. Dysphagia occurs in 10–30% but respiratory muscle weakness is unusual. Ankle dorsiflexion weakness can also occur, and taken together these distal signs, plus occasional mild facial involvement and a usually asymmetrical pattern of weakness, allow clinical distinction to be made from other conditions, including the other idiopathic inflammatory myopathies.

The aetiology of IBM is uncertain. Whether it is a degenerative process and whether any endomysial inflammatory component (which may be substantial) is merely a secondary process is still debated. Support for it being degenerative rests principally on both the finding of amyloid material in the almost pathognomic cellular inclusions and rimmed vacuoles seen on biopsy (Figure 10.30), and the failure of IBM to respond to all immunosuppressant medications in controlled trials. However, against this comes recent identification of antibodies to cytosolic 5′-nucleotidase 1A (CN1A) with reported high specificity (up to 98%) and sensitivity (up to 79%) for IBM, though with both false positives and false negatives. C1NA is of uncertain function, but may have a role in DNA repair. It is expressed in muscle and antibodies to it label the rimmed vacuoles of IBM patients' muscle biopsies. Antibody testing is not available as a diagnostic tool, but may prove useful as part of overall assessment and, if securely established, would point to immune system dysfunction underlying IBM.

There appears to be no link to malignancy and pulmonary or cardiac complications are not to be expected.

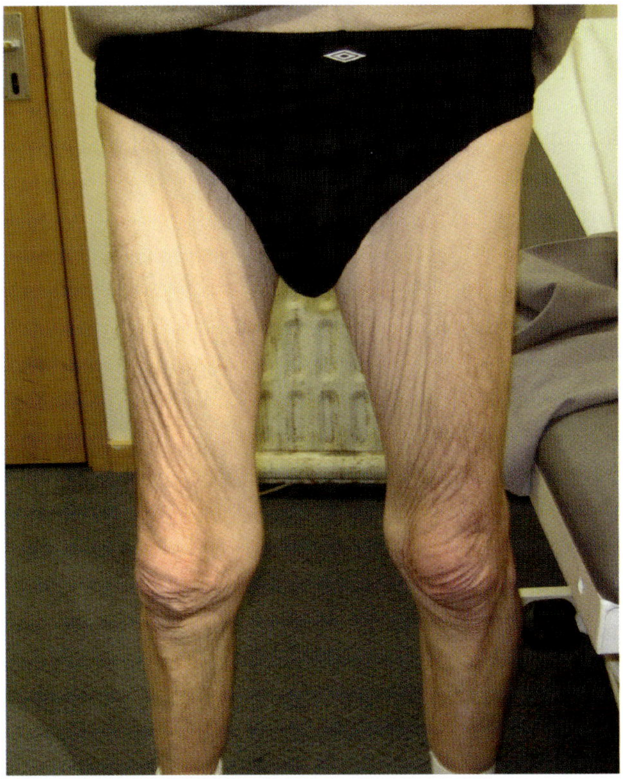

Figure 10.30 Inclusion body myositis may present with focal weakness of the quadriceps muscles, in this case easily identified by the focal wasting seen in comparison to the lower leg compartments.

Investigation of inflammatory myopathy

Serum creatine kinase levels The level of serum CK is raised in all three conditions and offers some guide to the degree of inflammation. It may be raised up to 50 times normal in severe PM and DM; the typical rise in IBM is, however, typically less than 10-fold. It is very important to note that definite deterioration can occur without an accompanying rise in CK, especially of DM. It is crucial to bear in mind that quoted 'normal' values of CK can be misleadingly low, as there is considerable variation in CK levels across a normal population. CK values are in rough proportion to muscle mass and also correlate with ethnic origin: people of African heritage show higher CK. Furthermore, exercise, muscle injury and alcohol intake will all raise measured CK. As such, diagnosis of 'pure PM' should never be made solely on a borderline elevation in CK levels.

Neurophysiology Typical myopathic features are common in myositis, while frequent fibrillation and spontaneous repetitive discharges can be indicative of active inflammation. A useful rule of thumb from highly experienced practitioners is that when EMG is performed to confirm myopathy, seemingly normal findings frequently turn out to be IBM.

Muscle biopsy Muscle biopsy is the keystone of diagnosis. It should be considered and if at all possible performed in every case before treatment is initiated. The idiopathic inflammatory myopathies share some pathological features but aspects of the pathology of each may be diagnostic (Table 10.41; Figure 10.29). Typical changes are not always present, however, and thus interpretation can be difficult. The clinical and pathological findings need to be interpreted in conjunction to make the correct diagnosis.

Table 10.41 Characteristic pathological findings of the idiopathic inflammatory myopathies.

Condition	Muscle fibres	Blood vessels
DM	Focal infarctions; perifascicular atrophy	Capillary necrosis and undulating tubules or other endothelial abnormalities; deposition of immunoglobulin and activated complement membrane attack complex
PM	Partial invasion of non-necrotic fibres by activated CD8 lymphocytes and macrophages (seen less in IBM and not in DM). Uniform expression of class I MHC products on surface of all fibres	Rarely involved: possible secondary capillary necrosis
IBM	Rimmed vacuoles; inclusions staining for ubiquitin and amyloid; 15–18 nm tubular filaments in nucleus or cytoplasm (may require extensive EM)	Can be normal; possible increased capillarity

DM, dermatomyositis; EM: electron microscopy; IBM, inclusion body myositis; MHC: major histocompatibility complex; PM, polymyositis.

Muscle MRI Imaging of muscle disease is increasingly undertaken but not yet established as a standard part of the diagnostic process for inflammatory myopathy. Serial imaging of cases undergoing treatment can be used as an indicator of response, but this should be undertaken only as part of a wider assessment, most crucially that of clinical change.

Extended investigation of inflammatory myopathies

- *Lung:* a chest radiograph may identify bibasal shadowing. Chest radiography is insensitive, being normal in 10% of those with proven lung involvement. High-resolution CT scanning is more sensitive, characteristically revealing linear opacities and a 'ground glass' appearance of the lung bases. Pulmonary function tests are also indicated; a restrictive pattern with reduced lung volumes and decreased diffusing capacity for carbon monoxide is typical.
- *Heart:* an ECG is indicated in all patients. Clinical evidence of cardiac involvement necessitates further assessment with 24-hour Holter recording, echocardiography and review by a cardiologist.

Treatment of idiopathic inflammatory myopathies

The treatment of idiopathic inflammatory myopathies is based largely on expert opinion rather than evidence. Indeed, the Cochrane collaboration's systematic review on the treatment of DM and PM concluded that, 'the small number of randomised controlled trials of immunosuppressants and immunomodulatory therapies are inadequate to decide whether these agents are beneficial'. Guidelines for management remain open to the influences of personal practice, but one suggested approach is given in Table 10.42.

For IBM no beneficial effect has been demonstrated for any agent tested. Despite this, individual cases may show a response to medication, essentially when a significant degree of inflammatory change is shown on biopsy. Under such circumstances, a trial of steroid (30–40 mg/day oral prednisolone for 3–4 months) should be considered, and if successful, the dose slowly reduced, introducing steroid-sparing drugs if appropriate.

In all cases, non-pharmacological measures to support the patient are also crucial. Multi-disciplinary assessment from physiotherapists, occupational therapists and, if indicated, speech therapists, dietitians and colleagues from other medical disciplines, is recommended. Regular follow-up to assess progress and identify and treat potential complications is essential.

Table 10.42 Treatment of the idiopathic inflammatory myopathies, in the absence of evidence.

Steroids, aiming for rapid stabilisation
Prednisolone 1 mg/kg/day by mouth until CK normal, then reduce (e.g. 5–10 mg monthly, with slower reduction for the last 20–30 mg)
If very acute resolution required: IV methylprednisolone 500mg / day for 5 days to initiate steroid course
Osteoporosis and gastric ulcer prophylaxis
Steroid-sparing agents (aiming to reduce side effects and maintain disease control)
First line
1 Azathioprine, starting at 1 mg/kg or below, and increasing by 25 mg every 1–2 months to a maximum of 2.5 mg/kg, as tolerated and guided by the degree of lymphocyte suppression and clinical response Thiopurine methyltransferase checked beforehand Blood monitoring of FBC and LFT necessary.
2 Methotrexate, increasing to 20–25 mg/day maximum once weekly with folic acid on other days, blood monitoring required; watch for pulmonary fibrosis and cirrhosis. NPSA guidelines available in UK
Second line
1 Ciclosporin: of use if first line drugs ineffective; blood monitoring required
2 IVIG: for refractory cases, particularly if deteriorating and rapid response sought
3 Cyclophosphamide, consider if poor response to other drugs (may be given as cycles of IV preparation in combination with other drugs; see peripheral nerve vasculitis)

CK, creatine kinase; FBC, full blood count; IV, intravenous; IVIG, intravenous immunoglobulin; LFT, liver function test; NPSA, National Patient Safety Agency.

Inflammatory myopathies associated with connective tissue disease Although rheumatological diseases can lead to weakness through either musculoskeletal deformity, neuropathy, muscle ischaemia or medication side effects, certain patterns of inflammatory myopathy are recognised, albeit infrequently. Systemic sclerosis occurs in conjunction with a DM-like picture in approximately 5–10% of cases, and a similar proportion of people with SLE have a condition that resembles PM. Sjögren's syndrome can rarely be seen with features similar to either DM or IBM. Myositis is very rare with either rheumatoid arthritis or polyarteritis nodosa. Muscle biopsy should be considered in any patient with a confirmed rheumatological illness who develops otherwise unexplained weakness, in particular if the CK is raised and EMG identifies myopathic features.

Inflammatory and other myopathies associated with infection A number of viruses cause myositis. Common infections (Coxsackie, EBV, CMV, influenza) have all been associated with acute and chronic muscle inflammation, although such complications are rare and the underlying mechanism is unclear. A definite causative link has been established for the retroviruses HIV and human T-lymphocyte virus (HTLV-1) and myositis.

At seroconversion, HIV can lead to a polymyositis that can be explosive enough to provoke myoglobulinuria, and which is steroid-responsive. A nemaline rod myopathy may also develop at this stage of infection, with a raised CK and specific findings on biopsy. With the onset of AIDS, a necrotising myopathy with proximal weakness, typically a normal CK and necrotic fibres on biopsy occurs. HIV wasting disease or 'slim' is frequently encountered in sub-Saharan Africa, but rarely in industrialised populations. 'Slim' is defined as more than 10% weight loss, weakness and fever or diarrhoea for at least 1 month, without any other causative condition. It appears to be caused by a combination of increased metabolic demand, anorexia, possible endocrine derangement and altered lipid metabolism. It leads to muscle wasting without myalgia, and when biopsied most typically shows type II fibre atrophy. Treatment is with improved nutrition and antiretrovirals. People with HIV are also at greater risk of infectious pyomyositis, which is typically multi-focal and slower to evolve than the non-HIV-associated form. The range of causative organisms also differs with cryptococcus, toxoplasma, CMV and atypical mycobacteria implicated.

HTLV-1 is endemic in the Caribbean and Japan and most commonly leads to a slowly evolving myelopathy. However, it can alternatively provoke a polymyositis, which seems to follow expression of HTLV-1's tax-1 protein in muscle cells, rather than any sustained viral replication. HTLV-1 induced PM may respond to immunosuppression.

Non-viral infective myopathies occur with bacteria or parasites. Suppurative pyomyositis is typically a tropically acquired illness in which a staphylococcal abscess forms at the site of injury. In industrialised populations, immunosuppression from medication or conditions such as diabetes, liver disease or malignancy are more commonly associated than HIV. Staphylococci account for the great majority of infections but others including TB and fungi also occur. The diagnosis is largely clinical and treatment includes aspiration (which aids identification of the infective organism) and drainage if required and appropriate antibiotics.

Lyme disease, in addition to its more frequent CNS and nerve involvement, can unusually lead to myositis; this may be either a localised painful swelling or a rarer generalised dermatomyositis-like picture. Treatment is of the underlying spirochaete with appropriate antibiotics.

Some parasites cause focal or multi-focal muscle inflammation. Cestodes (cysticerci), nematodes (trichinella) and protozoa (toxoplasma, trypanosomes), all typically ingested in undercooked meat, can infect muscle. Muscle symptoms are often mild and self-limiting and it is involvement of the CNS that prompts identification and medication.

Other rare inflammatory myopathies

Granulomatous myopathies Granulomatous myopathies present as a slowly evolving proximal weakness, which is often painful and possibly develops to include dysphagia. Over time, flexion contractures may develop in the forearms and muscle hypertrophy may become evident. The serum CK is typically elevated and muscle biopsy demonstrates focal non-caseating granulomas. The differential is wide, including sarcoidosis (which can rarely present in such a manner, and in which the CK may not rise), autoimmune conditions (rheumatoid arthritis, mixed connective tissue disease, granulomatosis with polyangiitis (Wegener's granulomatosis) or in association with myasthenia gravis and thymoma) plus some infections (fungal, mycobacterial, protozoal). Many, but not all, respond to treatment with steroids.

Eosinophilic myopathic syndromes Three forms of inflammatory myopathy are associated with eosinophilic infiltration of muscle, a systemic eosinophilia, or both. Eosinophilic polymyositis is similar to the classic PM described above, but occurs in conjunction with eosinophils, which are elevated in the circulation and prominently present on muscle biopsy. In eosinophilic fasciitis, pathological inflammation is limited to the fascia, and the fascia lata is the best site for confirmatory biopsy. Finally, dietary L-tryptophan, apparently contaminated by an acetaldehyde ditryptophan derivative, led to the eosinophilia myalgia syndrome. A marked eosinophilia developed with muscle pain and weakness with a scleroderma-like skin reaction and a peripheral neuropathy. Symptoms resolved after the medication was ended, although steroids were required to speed improvement in some cases.

Macrophagic myofasciitis This is a very rarely identified but pathologically distinctive focal reaction at the site of vaccination, possibly directed against the aluminium hydroxide adjuvant of the vaccines. Originally described in France, after the adoption of hepatitis B vaccination, cases have now been reported from other countries. Many patients report systemic systems of fatigue, and CK can be significantly raised. Several years may elapse between the vaccination and the onset of the syndrome. Periodic acid–Schiff (PAS) positive macrophage infiltration of connective tissue is seen on biopsy. Steroid treatment has been reported as beneficial.

Myopathies associated with malignancy Weakness may simply accompany tumour-induced cachexia, but cancers can cause a number of other muscle disorders. Dermatomyositis and (less so) polymyositis can be associated with a range of malignancies (ovary, lung, gastrointestinal, non-Hodgkin's lymphoma) and, if so, have a worse prognosis.

An aggressive necrotising myopathy is rarely seen in older patients with cancer (lung, gastrointestinal adenocarcinoma and breast). A rapidly progressive proximal weakness is typically accompanied by an elevated CK, while muscle biopsy demonstrates foci of necrosis. Steroids and treatment of the underlying tumour may help arrest symptoms.

Rare paraneoplastic antibody-driven myopathies have also been reported. Waldenström's macroglobulinaemia can generate IgM against the muscle proteoglycan decorin. Myasthenia gravis, with or without underlying thymoma, can generate antibodies against skeletal muscle that cause rippling muscle disease: painful cramps with visible ripples of the muscle that often worsen with pyridostigmine but improve with immunosuppression.

Endocrine myopathies

Thyroid Hypothyroidism frequently causes non-specific fatigue, myalgia and cramps and may also raise the CK level. Untreated and over time a proximal symmetrical weakness can develop. The CK is not related to the level of weakness. Typically, the EMG shows myopathic changes and the histopathological findings are non-specific. Less commonly, myokymia may be seen and rarely severe muscle oedema may develop with subsequent rhabdomyolysis. The myopathy responds to thyroid replacement but is slow to do so.

Hyperthyroidism when severe is often associated with muscle weakness. Unlike hypothyroidism, distal muscles can be affected, sometimes in isolation. CK is not elevated. Symptoms are worse with severe and acute hyperthyroidism ('thyroid storm'). There is a rare inflammatory myopathy associated with hyperthyroidism, clinically similar to the idiopathic condition, and also causing a raised CK.

Adrenal Cushing's syndrome leads to steroid myopathy as described later, while Addison's disease (whether primary or iatrogenic) typically causes myalgia, cramps and fatigue. Inadequate circulating levels of corticosteroids may lead to proximal weakness, which can lead to respiratory difficulty. Adequate steroid replacement is curative.

Parathyroid Both inadequate and excessive levels of parathyroid hormone may lead to a mild progressive proximal myopathy. CK is more frequently raised in the former case, but normal in the latter.

Acromegaly Untreated, excess growth hormone will cause a proximal weakness, sometimes with muscle hypertrophy and with an elevated CK. Some 50% of acromegalics show myopathic changes on EMG. Correction of the underlying condition leads to resolution of the myopathy.

Necrotising autoimmune myopathy

Necrotising autoimmune myopathy (NAM) is a form of acquired myopathy characterised by subacute onset of symmetrical, proximal, predominantly lower limb weakness associated with dysphagia, respiratory muscle weakness, abnormal echocardiogram, markedly elevated CK level and EMG showing fibrillation potentials and myotonic dyscharges. It is idiopathic in 50% but other cases are related to statin treatment, connective tissue disorders (e.g. scleroderma, mixed connective tissue disease) and malignancy. NAM is associated with autoantibodies specific for signal recognition particle (SRP) or 3-hydroxy-3-methylglutaryl-coenzyme A reductase (HMGCR). Muscle biopsy shows necrotic muscle fibres with regeneration but little or no inflammatory change. It is usually treated with IVIG and prednisolone but is refractory and often requires long-term immunosuppression with multiple agents.

Drugs and myopathy

A variety of drugs have been identified as causing a myopathy (Table 10.43). Some, such as steroids, will eventually cause a deleterious effect on all those who receive them. Others, such as statins, will do so to only some. The spectrum of drug-induced myopathy varies from an asymptomatic raised CK to profound weakness with rhabdomyolysis. Drugs may also worsen an existing muscle disease or, alternatively, unmask one that was previously hidden.

Statin myopathy Statins inhibit the enzyme HMG CoA reductase, reducing the formation of cholesterol and also ubiquinone (co-enzyme Q10). Series identify an eightfold risk of myopathy in those taking statins, raised to 42-fold if a fibrate is taken concurrently. This equates to about 1–6/10 000 treated. Large-scale studies of those who take statins find the most common problem is of an asymptomatic elevation of CK, and the most frequent symptoms are of myalgia and cramps. Together such mild to trivial findings affect up to 10% of patients. By contrast, side effects requiring hospitalisation (incapacatating pain, overt weakness or rhabdomyolysis) occur at less than 1/10 000 patient years. The increasing prescription of statins to prevent vascular disease (over 4 million people in the United Kingdom were taking a statin in 2014), has not been mirrored in specialist practice dealing with more cases of severe muscle side effects. Minor problems appear anticipated and managed in primary care, and the wider publicity and awareness of statin-associated myopathy appears effectively 'protective', with patients abandoning medication as soon as any mild symptom develops (perversely so, in terms of wider public health). Overall, it appears that the risk of statin-induced myopathy is dose-dependent and varies between individual drugs (one form, cerivastatin, was withdrawn from the market because of its higher risk of myopathy). Problems are also more likely in the elderly or those with diabetes, hypothyroidism or concurrent renal or liver disease. Also at greater risk are those taking fibrates, or inhibitors of the hepatic enzyme CYP3A4 (including ciclosporin, proton pump inhibitors, various antifungals, calcium-channel blockers, SSRIs, grapefruit juice).

The classic pathological finding of severe statin-induced myopathy is of muscle necrosis. Alternatively, statins can induce inflammatory or mitochondrial change (the latter with normal CK), or unmask an underlying metabolic condition.

A suggested management strategy for statin myopathy is given in Table 10.44. Stopping the statin usually leads to improvement within a few weeks, so allowing trial re-administration of either a lower dose or an alternative statin, but myalgia and raised CK may persist and severe myopathy can leave permanent sequelae.

Table 10.43 Drugs associated with myopathy.

Lipid-lowering: statins, fibrates, nicotinic acid, ezetimibe
Steroids
Abuse: alcohol, heroin, cocaine
Cardiac: amiodarone, perhexiline
Rheumatological treatments: colchicines, chloroquine, hydroxychloroquine
Other: ipecac (anorexics), streptokinase, zidovudine, α-interferon, d-penicillamine

Table 10.44 Management of statin myopathy.

Prevention	Start those at higher risk on lowest dose statin (e.g. simvastatin, pravastatin 10 mg/day)
CK raised without symptoms	Check CK again after 2 weeks; discontinue statin if CK rises further or symptoms develop
CK raised with symptoms	Stop statin. Consider co-enzyme Q10. Then: If symptoms resolve and the CK falls to normal, reinitiate statin at lowest dose If symptoms or elevated CK persist for 6 months off treatment, then perform muscle biopsy (to look for exposed inflammatory/mitochondrial myopathy) If the symptoms worsen or CK rises further, then proceed to urgent muscle biopsy

CK, creatine kinase.

Zidovudine and other antiretrovirals A toxic mitochondrial myopathy may follow the use of zidovudine (AZT), because of its inhibition of mitochondrial DNA replication. Those affected develop myalgia, exercise intolerance, proximal or generalised weakness and raised CK, usually after some time on the drug. A muscle biopsy is indicated, looking for cytochrome oxidase-negative fibres, not least to differentiate the diagnosis from that of HIV myositis. The myopathy usually resolves when zidovudine is stopped, although 3–4 months may be required. Zidovudine is also well recognised for its potential to expose a pre-existing carnitine deficiency.

Recently, the syndrome of nucleoside-associated lactic acidosis was been reported. Multiple symptoms including abdominal pain, vomiting, cough, shortness of breath, weight loss, together with myopathy and a painful axonal neuropathy develop subacutely in the first months of treatment. Cases have been reported up to 3 years after treatment began. Serum lactate is raised and muscle biopsy reveals necrosis plus mitochondrial abnormalities. Treatment is supportive, with fluids and bicarbonate to neutralise the acidosis, and the retroviral drug should be stopped. However, mortality is high at up to 50% and recovery is slow.

Steroid myopathy Chronic administration of steroids reduces muscle protein synthesis, leading to insidious proximal weakness, especially of the quadriceps muscles. CK is not elevated and so any such rise necessitates separate investigation. Myopathy can occur at any dose but the incidence is highest with dexamethasone, betamethasone and triamcinolone, while for prednisolone daily doses in excess of 40 mg appear to confer the highest risk.

The pathological change is of selective type II (particularly IIB) fibre atrophy. The condition is usually reversible and so if possible steroids should be withdrawn. If withdrawal is not possible, the dosage should be reduced to the minimum and/or switched to an alternate-day regimen.

Rhabdomyolysis

Rhabdomyolysis is the breakdown of striated muscle fibres that leads to the release of muscle enzymes into the circulation. It is the final common pathoway for varying aetiologies. Myoglobinuria occurs when the haem-binding protein, myoglobulin, appears in the urine leading to a brownish discoloration with concentrations >250 μg/mL. The severity of rhabdomyolysis can vary from an asymptomatic elevation of muscle enzymes to severe electrolyte imbalance with acute renal failure. Rhabdomyolysis usually results from muscle injury because of trauma or other external causes (e.g. medication or intoxication) but may also develop if there is an underlying muscle disorder (Table 10.45). Therapeutic medication, substance abuse and toxins can cause rhabdomyolysis through a

Table 10.45 Causes of rhabdomyolysis.

Acquired muscle disease	
Exertion	Extreme exertion, status epilepticus, status asthmaticus, prolonged involuntary movement
Crush	Multiple trauma, prolonged immobility (e.g. pre-operative, coma, torture)
Temperature	Pyrexia, exposure to extreme heat, burns
Ischaemia	Arterial occlusion, compartment syndrome, DIC, sickle cell disease
Metabolic	Hyper-/hyponatraemia, hypophosphataemia, hyperosmolar state
Endocrine	Hypothyroidism, diabetic ketoacidosis, non-ketotic hyperosmolar coma
Alcohol	
Inflammatory	Polymyositis, dermatomyositis, vasculitis, paraneoplastic necrotising myopathy
Drugs (Chapter 19)	Coma induced by alcohol, opioids or CNS depressants Agitation (e.g. following amphetamines). Possibly associated with serotonin syndrome or neuroleptic malignant syndrome Prolonged involuntary movements (e.g. drug-induced dystonic states) Metabolic effects – statins, antidepressants, carbon monoxide, colchicines
Toxins	Snake bites
Infections	Viral – HSV, enterovirus, influenza A + B, CMV, EBV, adenovirus, HIV Bacterial – acute pyomyositis, staphylococcal/streptococcal Others – plasmodium, trichinella, toxoplasma
Inherited muscle disease	
Metabolic	Disorders of glycolytic – glycogenolytic pathway Disorders of fatty acid oxidation Disorders of purine cycle Mitochondrial respiratory chain Malignant hypothermia
Other hereditary muscle disease	e.g. congenital myopathy, dystrophinopathy, myotonic dystrophy

CMV, cytomegalovirus; DIC, disseminated intravascular coagulopathy; EBV, Epstein–Barr virus; HSV, herpes simplex virus.

wide variety of mechanisms including prolonged coma, seizures, agitation, hypothermia, metabolic effects or direct myotoxicity.

Presentation depends on the cause of rhabdomyolysis. Onset may be subclinical or with mild muscle pain, cramps and swelling. However, there is usually severe myalgia, muscle swelling and pigmenturia in association with greatly elevated CK (often >100 000). Compartment syndrome is characterised by severe muscle swelling in a limited anatomical space which may cause extreme pain and secondary vascular and neural compromise. The onset of renal failure may be manifest as oliguria and hypotension with haem pigmented casts. Electrolyte derangement arises from muscle lysis and renal failure and may include severe hyperkalaemia and hyperphosphotaemia with hypocalcaemia resulting from deposition of calcium salts within injured muscles. A secondary hypoalbuminaemia with hypotension, shock and cardiac arrhythmias may develop.

Management is treatment of the underlying disorder, correction of fluid and electrolyte abnormalities and prevention of renal failure. This usually involves plasma volume expansion with forced diuresis. The development of compartment syndrome may require fasciotomy.

References

O'Brien MD (for the Guarantors of Brain). *Aids to the Examination of the Peripheral Nervous System*, 5th edn. London: W.B. Saunders, 2010.

Forbes CD, Jackson WF. *A Color Atlas and Text of Clinical Medicine.* Aylesbury: Wolfe Publishing, 1993: 49–50.

Further reading

Hereditary neuropathy

Auer-Grumbach M, De Jonghe P, Verhoeven K, *et al.* Autosomal dominant inherited neuropathies with prominent sensory loss and mutilations: a review. *Arch Neurol* 2003; **60**: 329–334.

Auer-Grumbach M, Mauko B, Auer-Grumbach P *et al.* Molecular genetics of hereditary sensory neuropathies. *Neuromol Med* 2006; **8**: 147–158.

Cox JJ, Sheynin J, Reimann F, *et al.* An SCN9A channelopathy causes congenital inability to experience pain. *Nature* 2006; **444**: 894–897.

Kleopa KA, Scherer SS. Molecular genetics of X-linked Charcot–Marie–Tooth disease. *Neuromolecular Med* 2006; **8**: 107–122.

Murphy SM, Laura M, Fawcett K, *et al.* Charcot–Marie–Tooth disease: frequency of genetic subtypes and guideliens for genetic testing. *J Neurol Neurosurg Psychiatry* 2012; **83**: 706–710.

Nelis E, Van Broeckhoven C, De Jonghe P, *et al.* Estimation of the mutation frequencies in Charcot–Marie–Tooth disease type 1A and hereditary neuropathy with liability to pressure palsies: a European collaborative study. *Eur J Hum Genet* 1996; **4**: 25–33.

Rossor A, Polke J, Houlden H, Reilly MM. Clinical implications of genetic advances in Charcot–Marie–Tooth disease. *Nat Rev* 2013; **9**: 562–571.

Saporta M, Sottile SL, Miller LJ, *et al.* Charcot–Marie–Tooth disease subtypes and genetic testing strategies. *Ann Neurol* 2011; **9**: 22–33.

Zuchner S, Mersiyanova IV, Muglia M, *et al.* Mutations in the mitochondrial GTPase mitofusin 2 cause Charcot–Marie–Tooth neuropathy type 2A. *Nat Genet* 2004; **36**: 449–451.

Amyloidosis

Adams D Theudin M, Cauquil C, *et al.* FAP neuropathy and emerging treatments. *Curr Neurol Neurosci Rep* 2014; **14**: 435.

Andrade C. A peculiar form of periphral neuropathy: familial atypical generalized amyloidosis with special involvement of the peripheral nervous system. *Brain* 1952; **75**: 408–427.

Gertz MA, Merlini G, Treon SP. Amyloidosis and Waldenström's macroglobulinaemia. *Hematology Am Soc Hematol Educ Program* 2004; 257–282.

Guidelines Working Group of UK Myeloma Forum. Guidelines on the diagnosis and management of AL amyloidosis. *Br J Haematol* 2004; **125**: 681–700.

Holmgren G, Steen L, Ekstedt J, *et al.* Biochemical effect of liver transplantation in two Swedish patients with familial amyloidotic polyneuropathy (FAP-met[30]). *Clin Genet* 1991; **40**: 242–246.

Meretoja J. Familial systemic paramyloidosis with lattice dystrophy of the cornea, progressive cranial neuropathy, skin changes and various internal symptoms. *Ann Clin Res* 1969; **1**: 314–324.

Nichols WC, Gregg RE, Bryan Brewer H, Benson MD. A mutation in apolipoprotein A-1 in the Iowa type of familial amyloidotic polyneuropathy. *Genomics* 1990; **8**: 318–323.

Acquired neuropathies

Allen D, Lunn M, Niermeijer J, Nobile-Orazio E. Treatment for IgG and IgA paraproteinaemic neuropathy. *Cochrane Database Syst Rev* 2007; **1**: CD005376.

Dyck PJ, Norell JE, Dyck PJ. Microvasculitis and ischemia in diabetic lumbosacral radiculoplexus neuropathy. *Neurology* 1999; **53**: 2113–2121.

Dyck PJ, Oviatt KF, Lambert EH. Intensive evaluation of referred unclassified neuropathies yields improved diagnosis. *Ann Neurol* 1981; **10**: 222–226.

European Federation of Neurological Societies/Peripheral Nerve Society. Guideline on management of chronic inflammatory demyelinating polyradiculoneuropathy. Report of a joint task force of the European Federation of Neurological Societies and the Peripheral Nerve Society – first revision. *J Peripher Nerv Syst* 2010; **15**: 185–195.

Fisher M. Syndrome of ophthalmoplegia, ataxia and areflexia. *N Engl J Med* 1956; **255**: 57–65.

Hughes RA. Immunobiology of the peripheral nervous system. In: Swash M, ed. *Guillain–Barré Syndrome.* London: Springer-Verlag, 1990: 19–48.

Hartung H-P, Willison HJ, Jung S, Pette M, Toyka KV, Giegerich G. Autoimmune responses in peripheral nerve. *Springer Semin Immunopathol* 1996; **18**: 97–123.

Lauria G. Small fibre neuropathies. *Curr Opin Neurol* 2005; **18**: 591–597.

Lunn MP, Nobile-Orazio E. Immunotherapy for IgM anti-myelin-associated glycoprotein paraprotein-associated peripheral neuropathies. *Cochrane Database Syst Rev* 2012; **5**: CD002827.

Patten J. *Neurological Differential Diagnosis*, 2nd edn. London, New York: Springer, 1996.

Schaublin GA, Michet J, Dyck PJ, Burns TM. An update on the classification and treatment of vasculitic neuropathy. *Lancet Neurol* 2005; **4**: 853–865.

Stewart JD. *Focal Peripheral Neuropathies*, 4th edn. Vancouver: JBJ Publishing, 2009.

Motor neurone disease and spinal muscular atrophy

Anderson K, Talbot K. Spinal muscular atrophies reveal motor neuron vulnerability to defects in ribonucleoprotein handling. *Curr Opin Neurol* 2003; **16**: 595–599.

Anderson PH, Al-Chalabi A. Clinical genetics of amyotrophic lateral sclerosis. *Nat Rev Neurol* 2011; **7**: 603–615.

Bedlack RS Amyotrophic lateral sclerosis: current practice and future treatments. *Curr Opin Neurol* 2010; **23**: 524–529.

Borasio GD, Volz R, Miller RG. Palliative care in amyotrophic lateral sclerosis. *Neurol Clin* 2001; **19**: 829–848.

Bourke SC, Bullock RE, Williams TL, *et al.* Non-invasive ventilation in ALS: indications and effect on quality of life. *Neurology* 2003; **61**: 171–177.

Bourke SC, Tomlinson M, Williams TL, Bullock RE, Shaw PJ, Gibson GJ. Effects of non-invasive ventilation on survival and quality of life in patients with amyotrophic lateral sclerosis: a randomised controlled trial. *Lancet Neurol* 2006; **5**: 140–147.

Bradley MD, Orrell RW, Clarke J, *et al.* Outcome of ventilatory support for acute respiratory failure in motor neurone disease. *J Neurol Neurosurg Psychiatry* 2002; **72**: 752–756.

Ferraluolo L, Kirby J, Gierson AJ, Sendtner M, Shaw PJ. Molecular pathways of motor neuron injury in amyotrophic lateral sclerosis. *Nat Rev Neurol* 2011; **7**: 616–630.

Hardiman O, van den Berg LH, Kiernan MC. Clinical diagnosis and management of amyotrophic lateral sclerosis. *Nat Rev Neurol* 2011; **7**: 639–649.

Howard RS, Orrell RW. Management of motor neurone disease. *Postgrad Med J* 2002; **78**: 736–741.

Leigh PN, Abrahams S, Al-Chalabi A, *et al.* The management of motor neurone disease. *J Neurol Neurosurg Psychiatry* 2003; **74** (Suppl IV): 32–47.

Lyall RA, Donaldson N, Polkey MI, Leigh PN, Moxham J. Respiratory muscle strength and ventilatory failure in amyotrophic lateral sclerosis. *Brain* 2001; **124**: 2000–2013.

Mercuri E, Bertini E, Iannaccone ST. Childhood spinal muscular atrophy: Controversies and challenges. *Lancet Neurol* 2012; **11**: 443–452.

Miller RG, Rosenberg JA, Gelinas DF, *et al.* Practice parameters. The care of the patient with amyotrophic lateral sclerosis (an evidence-based review): Report of the Quality Standards Subcommittee of the American Academy of Neurology: ALS Practice Parameters Task Force. *Neurology* 1999; **52**: 1311–1323.

Mitchell JD, Borasio GD. Amyotrophic lateral sclerosis. *Lancet* 2007; **369**: 2031–2041.

Motor Neurone Disease Association. Standards of Care. http://www.mndassociation.org/forprofessionals/mndmanagement/best-practice-guidelines-and-pathways (accessed 10 February 2016).

Sumner CJ. Therapeutics development for spinal muscular atrophy. *NeuroRx* 2006; **3**: 235–245.

Sykes N. End of life care in ALS. In: Oliver D, Borasio GD, Sykes N, eds. *Palliative Care in Amyotrophic Lateral Sclerosis*. Oxford: Oxford University Press, 2000: 159–168.

Traynor BJ, Alexander M, Corr B, *et al*. Effect of multidisciplinary amyotrophic lateral sclerosis clinic on ALS survival. *J Neurol Neurosurg Psychiatry* 2003; **74**: 1258–1261.

Wirth B, Brichta L, Hahnen E. Spinal muscular atrophy: from gene to therapy. *Semin Pediatr Neurol* 2006; **13**: 121–131.

Wokke J. Riluzole. *Lancet* 1996; **348**: 795–799.

Myasthenia gravis

Chen G, Marx A, Wen-Hu C, *et al*. New WHO histologic classification predicts prognosis of thymic epithelial tumours: a clinicopathologic study of 200 thymoma cases from China. *Cancer* 2002; **95**: 420–429.

Gronseth GS, Barohn RJ. Practice parameter: thymectomy for autoimmune myasthenia gravis (an evidence-based review): report of the Quality Standards Subcommittee of the American Acadamy of Neurology. *Neurology* 2000; **55**: 7–15.

McConville J, Forrugia ME, Beeson D, *et al*. Detection and characterization of MuSK antibodies in seronegative myasthenia gravis. *Ann Neurol* 2004; **55**: 580–584.

Newsom-Davis J, Beeson D. Myasthenia gravis and myasthenic syndromes, autoimmune and genetic disorders. In: *Disorders of Voluntary Muscles*, 7th edition. Karpati G, Hilton-Jones D, Griggs R, eds. Cambridge: Cambridge University Press, 2001: 660–675.

Palace J, Newsom-Davis J, Lecky BA. Randomised double-blind trial of prednisolone alone or with azathiuoprine in myasthenia gravis. *Neurology* 1998; **50**: 1778–1783.

Spillane J, Beeson DJ, Kullmann DM. Myasthenia and related disorders of the neuromuscular junction. *J Neurol Neurosurg Psychiatry* 2010; **81**: 850–857.

Muscular dystrophy and congenital myopathies

Bonilla E, Samiit CE, Miranda F. Duchenne muscular dystrophy deficiency of dystrophin at the muscle cell surface. *Cell* 1988; **54**: 447–452.

Engel AG, Franzini-Armstrong C, eds. *Myology*, 3rd edn. New York: McGraw Hill, 2004.

Maggi L, Scoto M, Cirak S, *et al*. Congenital myopathies: clinical features and frequency of individual subtypes diagnosed over a 5-year period in the United Kingdom. *Neuromuscul Disord*. 2013; **23**: 195–205.

Mercuri E, Muntoni F. Muscular dystrophies. *Lancet* 2013; **381**: 845–860.

Myotonic dystrophy

Brook JD, McCurrch ME, Harley HG, *et al*. Molecular basis of myotonic dystrophy; expansion of a trinucleotide repeat CTG at the 3′ end of a transcript encoding a protein kinase family member. *Cell* 1992; **68**: 799–808.

Liquori CL, Ricker K, Mosley ML, *et al*. Myotonic dystrophy type 2 caused by a CCTG expansion I intron 1 of ZNF9. *Science* 2001; **293**: 864–867.

Turner, C, Hilton-Jones, D. The myotonic dystrophies: diagnosis and management. *J Neurol Neurosurg Psychiatry* 2010; **81**: 358–367.

Muscle channelopathies

Beker PE. *Myotonia Congenita and Syndromes Associated with Myotonia*. Stuggart: Thieme Press, 1977.

Burge JA, Hanna MG. Novel insights into the pathomechanisms of skeletal muscle channelopathies. *Curr Neurol Neurosci Rep* 2012; **12**: 62–9.

Koch MC, Steinmyer K, Lorenz C, *et al*. The skeletal muscle chloride channel in dominant and recessive human myotonia. *Science* 1992; **257**: 797–800.

Kullmann DM, Waxman SG. Neurological channelopathies: new insights into disease mechanisms and ion channel function. *J Physiol* 2010; **588**: 1823–1827.

Russell JF, Fu YH, Ptáček LJ. Episodic neurologic disorders: syndromes, genes and mechanisms. *Annu Rev Neurosci* 2013; **36**: 25–50.

Spillane J, Fialho D, Hanna MG. Diagnosis of skeletal muscle channelopathies. *Expert Opin Med Diagn* 2013; **7**: 517–529.

Venance SL, Cannon SC, Fialho D, *et al*. The primary periodic paralyses: diagnosis, pathogenesis and treatment. *Brain* 2006; **129**: 8–17.

Mitochondrial disease

Archer SL. Mitochondrial dynamics: mitochondrial fission and fusion in human diseases. *N Engl J Med* 2013; **369**: 2236–2251.

Kanabus M, Heales SJ, Rahman S. Development of pharmacological strategies for mitochondrial disorders. *Br J Pharmacol* 2014; **171**: 1798–1817.

Koopman WJ, Willems PH, Smeitink JA. Monogenic mitochondrial disorders. *N Engl J Med* 2012; **366**: 1132–1141.

Pareyson D, Piscosquito G, Moroni I, Salsano E, Zeviani M. Peripheral neuropathy in mitochondrial disorders. *Lancet Neurol* 2013; **12**: 1011–1024.

Pfeffer G, Majamaa K, Turnbull DM, Thorburn D, Chinnery PF. Treatment for mitochondrial disorders. *Cochrane Database Syst Rev* 2012; **4**: CD004426.

Rahman S, Hanna MG. Diagnosis and therapy in neuromuscular disorders: diagnosis and new treatments in mitochondrial diseases. *J Neurol Neurosurg Psychiatry* 2009; **80**: 943–953.

Schapira AH. Mitochondrial diseases. *Lancet* 2012; **379**: 1825–1834.

Vafai SB, Mootha VK. Mitochondrial disorders as windows into an ancient organelle. *Nature* 2012; **491**: 374–383.

Metabolic muscle disease

Engel AG, Franzini-Armstrong C, eds. *Myology*, 3rd edn. New York: McGraw Hill, 2004: 1535–1677.

Rahman S, Hanna MG. Diagnosis and therapy in neuromuscular disorders: diagnosis and new treatments in mitochondrial diseases. *J Neurol Neurosurg Psychiatry* 2009; **80**: 943–953.

Turner C, Schapira AHV. Mitochondrial disorders. In: *Bradley's Neurology in Clinical Practice*, 6th edition. Daroff RB, Fenichel GM, Jankovic J, Mazziotta JC, eds. Saunders, 2012: 1473–1487.

Inflammatory myopathy

Fathi M, Lundberg IE. Interstitial lung disease in polymyositis and dermatomyositis. *Curr Opin Rheumatol* 2005; **17**: 701–706.

Gordon PA, Winer JB, Hoogendijk JE, *et al*. Immunosuppressant and immunomodulatory treatment for dermatomyositis and polymyositis. *Cochrane Database Syst Rev* 2012; **8**: CD003643. DOI: 10.1002/14651858.CD003643.pub4.

Greenberg SA. Biomarkers of inclusion body myositis. *Curr Opin Rheumatol* 2013; **25**: 753–762.

Karparti G, Hilton-Jones D, Bushby K, *et al*. *Disorders of Voluntary Muscle*. Cambridge: Cambridge University Press, 2010.

Lev EI, Tur-Kaspa I, Ashkenazy I, *et al*. Distribution of serum creatine kinase activity in young healthy persons. *Clin Chim Acta* 1999; **279**: 107–115.

Machado P, Brady S, Hanna MG. Update in inclusion body myositis. *Curr Opin Rheumatol* 2013; **25**: 763–771.

Mastaglia FL. Drug induced myopathies. *Pract Neurol* 2006; **6**: 4–13.

Titulaer MJ, Soffietti R, Dalmau J, *et al* European Federation of Neurological Societies. Screening for tumours in paraneoplastic syndromes: report of an EFNS task force. *Eur J Neurol* 2011; **18**: 19–e3.

Van Gelder H, Charles-Schoeman C. The heart in inflammatory myopathies. *Rheum Dis Clin North Am* 2014; **40**: 1–10.

CHAPTER 11

Multiple Sclerosis and Demyelinating Diseases

Siobhan Leary[1], Gavin Giovannoni[2], Robin Howard[1], David Miller[2] and Alan Thompson[1,2]

[1] National Hospital for Neurology & Neurosurgery

[2] UCL Institute of Neurology

Multiple sclerosis is an inflammatory demyelinating disorder of the central nervous system (CNS). Although the characteristic pathological lesions were first described over 150 years ago, its aetiology and pathophysiology remain to be fully elucidated. However, advances in pathological, immunological and genetic techniques have provided a greater understanding of the disease mechanisms involved. The application of magnetic resonance imaging (MRI) over the last three decades has also provided important insights into the dynamics of the disease which have subsequently been used in diagnosis and monitoring. Multiple sclerosis is a complex disease with an unpredictable prognosis which can cause numerous and diverse symptoms and accumulating disability. Major advances in disease modification have been made in the last two decades and multiple sclerosis is no longer an 'untreatable' condition. However, the efficacy of current therapeutic agents is limited to the earlier relapsing remitting phase of the disease. Management requires a responsive and comprehensive approach involving multiple health disciplines. This chapter outlines the features of multiple sclerosis as we understand them today and reviews current practice in diagnosis and management. Other demyelinating diseases are also reviewed.

Epidemiology

It is estimated that there may be 100 000 people living with multiple sclerosis in the United Kingdom (population ~ 63 million). The prevalence probably lies between 125 and 175/100 000 population, with an annual incidence of new cases between 3.1 and 7.2/100 000. The estimated lifetime risk from birth of receiving a multiple sclerosis diagnosis is 5.3/1000 in women and 2.3/1000 in men. The incidence of multiple sclerosis worldwide tends to increase with increasing latitude, although there are clear, and important, exceptions. It is more common in temperate regions, such as northern Europe, northern America and southern Australasia, but much rarer in the tropics. Geographical variations are seen over relatively small distances and, for example, it is more common in Scotland than in south-east England.

Multiple sclerosis typically presents between 20 and 40 years of age. Females are more susceptible than males by a factor of approximately 2.3 : 1. The incidence of multiple sclerosis in females has been disproportionately increasing, with a steady increase in the sex ratio of over 3 : 1 in several countries.

Migration studies

Migration studies have demonstrated that people who migrate from one geographical area to another before adolescence are essentially subject to the same level of risk of the area to which they migrate. Subjects who migrate after adolescence carry with them the risk, and hence incidence, of multiple sclerosis from the area from which they migrated. However, although the risk of multiple sclerosis consistently declines in migrants from high-risk to low-risk areas, the converse is not seen consistently in migrants from low-risk to high-risk areas. For example, an increase is not initially seen in Caribbean and Asian immigrants to the United Kingdom, although the risk can increase over time and the benefit is not passed on to the next generation. Migration may explain the higher incidence of multiple sclerosis than expected for latitude in countries like Israel and South Africa.

Health economics

Multiple sclerosis is the most common cause of neurological disability in young adults and health care costs result in considerable financial burden to society. Many people are in education or employment at the time of diagnosis but, over time, reduced capacity to work and unemployment is common, which results in further indirect costs to society. In 2010, the cost of multiple sclerosis in Europe was estimated at €27 000 per person with multiple sclerosis per year. The total annual cost across Europe was estimated at €14.6 billion, with just over one-third arising from direct health care costs and the remainder from non-medical and indirect costs.

Aetiology

The aetiology of multiple sclerosis is complex and cannot be ascribed to a single genetic or environmental factor. There is wide acceptance that interactions between genes and environmental factors lead to tissue injury by autoimmune mechanisms, implicated by immunological and pathological observations in people with multiple sclerosis and by extensive studies in the animal model experimental allergic encephalomyelitis (EAE). Multiple sclerosis is associated with other putative autoimmune disorders, including Hashimoto thyroiditis, psoriasis, inflammatory bowel disease and possibly type 1 diabetes mellitus, but not rheumatoid arthritis or systemic lupus erythematosus (SLE). This suggests that people with multiple sclerosis can be predisposed to autoimmunity in general.

Neurology: A Queen Square Textbook, Second Edition. Edited by Charles Clarke, Robin Howard, Martin Rossor and Simon Shorvon.

Genetic susceptibility

It is well recognised that genetic factors contribute to the occurrence of multiple sclerosis. Twin studies have demonstrated much higher concordance rates in monozygotic twins (~30%) than dizygotic twins (~5%), which also varies with latitude, but nowhere near the 100% rate which would be expected if it was solely a genetic disease. Family studies have demonstrated that relatives of people with multiple sclerosis have a greater risk for the disease than the general population, ~3–5% in first degree relatives. No increased risk is seen in adopted relatives, indicating that the risk is related to genetic rather than microenvironmental factors.

Numerous genes that contribute to multiple sclerosis susceptibility have been identified, but they exert a relatively modest effect on disease risk. The strongest genetic linkage identified is with alleles of the human lymphocyte antigen (HLA) region, part of the major histocompatibility complex (MHC). In the most recent international genome-wide association study, five alleles at three different loci in the HLA region influence multiple sclerosis susceptibility: the HLA-DRB1*1501, *0301 and *1303 alleles, the HLA-A*0201 allele and the HLADPB1*0301 allele. There are likely to be multiple epistatic interactions at the HLA class I and II loci with susceptibility and resistance alleles interacting to determine overall multiple sclerosis risk. Multiple sclerosis has been associated with over 100 single nucleotide polymorphisms in the human genome; the vast majority of these polymorphisms are linked to genes involved in the immune system. This strongly supports multiple sclerosis being an autoimmune disease.

Environmental factors

Geographical gradients, migration studies and high discordant rates in monozygotic twins indicate that the environment has a significant influence on the development of multiple sclerosis. Migration studies suggest that exposure to environmental factor(s) in early adolescence is associated with the development of multiple sclerosis. As multiple sclerosis may be uncommon in areas where sanitation is poor and the prevalence of parasitic infections is high, and as there is an increased incidence of autoimmune diseases in developed counties, the 'hygiene hypothesis' has been evoked. This suggests that exposure to infections in early childhood can protect against multiple sclerosis. However, the hygiene hypothesis has been largely discredited by conjugal pair, adopted children and sibship studies, which show no attributable risk to the familial microenvironment. Family-based genetic epidemiological approaches have found no evidence of non-genetic transmissibility within the familial micro-environment, which implies that the environment appears to influence the risk of multiple sclerosis at a population level. Several environmental factors have been proposed as aetiologically significant in multiple sclerosis, including transmissible agents and non-infectious factors.

Transmissible agents

Numerous transmissible agents have been implicated as the possible cause of multiple sclerosis. Suggested candidates include Epstein–Barr virus (EBV), human herpes virus type 6 (HHV-6) and human endogenous retroviruses (HERV). The epidemiological data associating EBV infection with multiple sclerosis is the strongest. A consistent finding is that almost all subjects with multiple sclerosis, >99%, are infected with EBV compared with only ~94% of control subjects. People who have had infectious mononucleosis or who have high titres of anti-EBV antibodies have a higher risk of developing multiple sclerosis than subjects who have not had infectious mononucleosis or who have low titres of anti-EBV antibodies.

The association of EBV infection with multiple sclerosis can simply be a ubiquitous epiphenomenon that is required at the onset of the disease. There are several theories to explain how infection causes multiple sclerosis but definitive evidence to suggest causation has been lacking. Pathological studies have found evidence of EBV infection in B cells and plasma cells in the brain, with viral reactivation in acute lesions and ectopic B-cell follicles, in multiple sclerosis and to a lesser extent in other neuro-inflammatory diseases. This still does not establish causation, but it suggests that EBV persistence and reactivation can have an important role in pathogenesis.

Vitamin D and sunlight exposure

Two associated factors that have been recognised as a potential explanation for the link between geography, in particular latitude, and the incidence of multiple sclerosis is sunlight exposure and vitamin D status. Experimental and epidemiological data suggest that high levels of vitamin D decrease the risk of multiple sclerosis. Taking vitamin supplementation, which includes vitamin D, has been associated with a reduction in the risk of developing multiple sclerosis. Small uncontrolled studies suggest vitamin D supplementation can decrease the incidence of relapses, but the results are inconsistent. A lower risk of multiple sclerosis is associated with high serum 25-hydroxy vitamin D levels in subjects of European extraction. In the Northern hemisphere it has been reported that significantly fewer people with multiple sclerosis are born in November and significantly more are born in May, with a reversal of this ratio in the Southern hemisphere, although these observations may be susceptible to confounding factors. For month of birth and risk of multiple sclerosis to be associated, there could be an interaction with the environment that acts during gestation or shortly after birth. This month of birth effect may be linked to the vitamin D status of the mother but this has not been confirmed. It has been proposed that immune system maturation *in utero* can be affected by vitamin D levels, with low levels predisposing to the development of autoimmunity later in life.

Smoking

Smoking prior to the onset of multiple sclerosis has emerged as a significant, albeit moderate, risk factor for the subsequent development of multiple sclerosis. Smoking can increase the risk of developing progressive disease. It has been suggested that smoking can explain the increase in incidence of multiple sclerosis in females, but this is unlikely as this increase predates the increase in incidence of female smokers.

Other environmental factors such as diet, alcohol consumption, recreational drug use, oral contraceptive pill exposure and vaccination have not been shown to increase the risk of multiple sclerosis.

Pathophysiology

The characteristic pathological feature of multiple sclerosis is the focal plaque or lesion. The lesions of multiple sclerosis were first depicted by Carswell in 1838 and the principal elements were described by Charcot in 1868 – demyelination, relative preservation of axons, gliosis and a variable amount of inflammation. This histological overview remains just as accurate today but the precise roles and inter-relationships of these elements in the pathogenesis of multiple sclerosis are still not fully elucidated. Furthermore, it is evident that the pathology of multiple sclerosis is not just confined to white matter lesions but involves the grey matter and macroscopically normal-appearing white matter (NAWM) and axonal loss can be marked in white matter lesions.

Pathology

Lesions occur throughout the CNS but particularly in the optic nerves, peri-ventricular white matter and corpus callosum, brainstem and cerebellar white matter, and cervical cord. Macroscopically, lesions are generally round or oval and, in broad terms, can be pink and soft, representing acute or active lesions, or grey and firm, representing chronic lesions (Figure 11.1). Brain atrophy and ventricular enlargement and atrophy of the spinal cord and optic nerves may be evident. Microscopically, acute lesions are characterised by active demyelination with marked inflammatory infiltrates, predominantly T lymphocytes and macrophages, associated with a variable degree of axonal damage and loss (Figure 11.1). In chronic lesions there is extensive loss of myelin, abundant astrocytic gliosis and axonal loss.

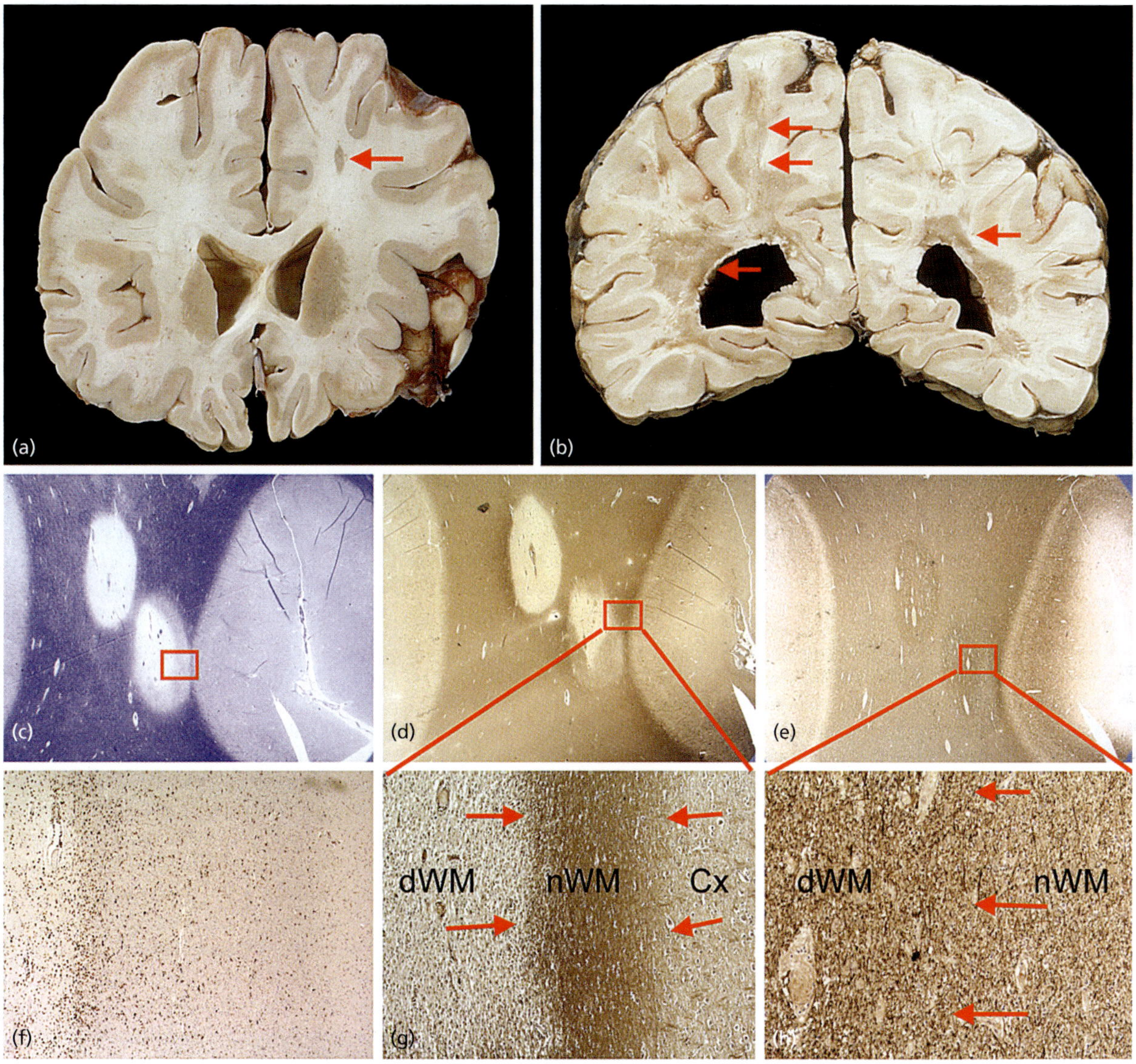

Figure 11.1 Macroscopic and microscopic findings in multiple sclerosis. (a,b) Macroscopic pathology of demyelination (coronal sections of formalin fixed brains). (a) Arrow pointing at a small circumscribed demyelination in the frontal white matter. Loss of myelin appears grey, similar to cerebral cortex. (b) Coronal section of the occipital lobe with extensive multifocal and confluent demyelinations (arrowhead). (c-e) Two foci of demyelination, one with partial remyelination (red box) stained for myelin or axons. (c) Luxol fast blue stains myelinated structures dark blue and the punched-out well-demarcated defects indicates loss of myelin. (d) Myelin basic product (MBP) immunohistochemistry labels myelinated fibres, and shows the same punched-out demyelination with a smaller rim of remyelination fibres in the lowest lesion. (e) Immunohistochemical staining of phosphorylated neurofilament demonstrates the presence of axons within the demyelinating lesions, which appear of slightly increased density than the surrounding intact white matter. (f) CD68 immunohistochemistry labels microglia and macrophage activity. The area corresponds to the red rectangle in (c-e), it clearly shows a demarcation between demyelinated and remyelinated regions. (g) High power magnification of the boxed area in (d) (MBP) on the left with loss of the myelin (demyelinated white matter [dWM]), a myelinated area in the centre (WM) and normal cortex (Cx) with myelinated on the right, all indicated by arrows. (h) High magnification of the labelled area in (e) shows the axons in the lesion on the left (dWM) and outside the lesion (nWM), the border is indicated by arrows. Source: Images and macroscopic specimens courtesy of Sebastian Brandner, UCL Institute of Neurology; histological specimens courtesy of Klaus Schmierer, Queen Mary, University of London.

Table 11.1 Pathological classification of active multiple sclerosis lesions.

I	T-cell/macrophage associated
II	Antibody/complement associated
III	Distal oligodendrogliopathy
IV	Oligodendrocyte degeneration in the peri-plaque white matter

Source: Adapted from Lucchinetti *et al.* 2000.

Different patterns of demyelination in active lesions have been described. Lucchinetti *et al.* (2000) studied actively demyelinating lesions in a large sample of multiple sclerosis biopsy and post-mortem samples and proposed four different patterns (Table 11.1). Inflammatory infiltrates, dominated by T lymphocytes and macrophages, were seen in all lesions. Patterns I and II were similar and lesions were typically sharply demarcated and centred on small veins and venules. High numbers of oligodendrocytes were seen. Pattern II was distinguished from Pattern I by prominent deposition of immunoglobulins and complement. Patterns III and IV were associated with signs of oligodendrocyte dystrophy. Pattern III lesions were diffuse with ill-defined borders. They were not centred on vessels and there was a preserved rim of myelin around vessels in some lesions. Unlike other patterns, where loss of myelin proteins was evenly distributed, there was a preferential loss of myelin-associated glycoprotein. There was pronounced loss of oligodendrocytes and oligodendrocyte apoptosis was seen. Pattern IV lesions were sharply demarcated. There was loss of oligodendrocytes and oligodendrocyte death was seen in a small rim of peri-lesional white matter. All active lesions within an individual patient exhibited the same pattern and there was no intra-individual heterogeneity. Patterns I and II were found in all clinical subtypes of multiple sclerosis. Pattern III was mainly found in people with disease duration of less than 2 months. Pattern IV lesions were least common and only found in a variant of primary progressive disease. Therefore it was suggested that mechanisms of demyelination can be different in different subtypes and stages of the disease. However, this concept has not been universally accepted and there is a potential bias associated with the inevitable limitations in access to tissue containing acute lesions. Since the original observation was made, other studies have reported different types of active lesions within the same individual, and it has been suggested that the Pattern III lesions represent a very early stage in the development of acute lesions.

The role of inflammation in the pathogenesis of lesions also remains unclear. Axonal damage, which is sometimes abundant, is seen in the presence of active inflammation, but is also evident in chronic demyelinated lesions. Lesions in people who have died shortly after a relapse have been shown to have zones of extensive oligodendrocyte apoptosis and microglial activation in myelinated tissue (Pattern III) containing few or no lymphocytes or myelin phagocytes suggesting that lesion formation can be related to a process other than inflammation.

Active lesions are predominantly seen in acute relapsing disease and are rare in secondary and primary progressive disease, in which chronic lesions predominate. However, slow expansion of chronic lesions can occur in progressive disease. These lesions are characterised by a rim of activated microglia, at the edge of the lesion, which are associated with active demyelination.

Remyelination is seen in a large proportion of lesions, often at the edges of lesions, although it can be present throughout the lesion. Remyelination can be extensive and result in remyelination of the complete lesion, described pathologically as a shadow plaque. Although historically remyelination has been felt to occur predominantly in early relapsing disease, it is now apparent that extensive remyelination can also occur in progressive disease. It is not known why remyelination occurs in some lesions and not others.

Pathological abnormalities are also seen in NAWM. In contrast to the extensive inflammation seen in focal lesions, there can be a mild but diffuse inflammatory reaction in NAWM. Peri-vascular cuffing and diffuse inflammatory infiltrates and microglia activation are seen. Diffuse axonal injury is also evident. This does not correlate with the extent of lesions and so is not explained by Wallerian degeneration arising from focal lesions alone. Therefore, there appears to be a mechanism of axonal injury that is independent of focal lesions. Pathological changes are also not just confined to the white matter, and striking cortical demyelination can be seen. Subcortical lesions can extend into the cortex or small focal lesions can be present within the cortex, but extensive subpial demyelination can also occur. Both cortical demyelination and the diffuse changes seen in the NAWM are present far more extensively in progressive than in relapsing disease. Subpial demyelination is especially marked in secondary progressive multiple sclerosis.

It has been previously suggested that relapses and disease progression can occur through distinct mechanisms, with relapses resulting from inflammatory demyelination and progression resulting from neurodegeneration. The recent advances in the elucidation of the immunopathology of multiple sclerosis provide support for a more unifying hypothesis. Multiple sclerosis typically starts with acute inflammation, arising from specific immune mechanisms, which are discussed later, resulting in focal inflammatory demyelinating lesions. Over time, inflammation becomes sequestered within the CNS. This inflammation can be non-specific and low grade but it drives the slow expansion of chronic lesions and the diffuse injury in the NAWM and cortex.

Autoimmune pathogenesis

The first step in the autoimmune pathogenesis of multiple sclerosis is believed to be that an environmental agent(s) combined with a genetic predisposition results in the production of pathological auto-reactive T cells. After a latent period of 10–20 years a breakdown in immunological tolerance, possibly by a systemic trigger such as a non-specific viral infection or exposure to a superantigen, activates these autoreactive T cells.

During the normal process of immunosurveillance, memory $CD4^+$ T-helper (Th) cells or a T-helper subset producing IL-17 (Th-17) cells, selectively cross the blood–brain barrier, through a process involving the interaction of their cell surface adhesion molecules with those expressed on CNS endothelium. Once within the peri-vascular space, these cells are presumably activated by professional antigen-presenting cells (probably macrophages or microglia) to proliferate and produce pro-inflammatory cytokines. Antigen recognition occurs via the trimolecular complex, consisting of HLA, T-cell receptor and CD3 molecules. This requires additional co-stimulatory signals, for example interactions between HLA MHC I and II molecules and their respective CD8 and CD4 molecules, and CD28/B7-2/1 pairs.

Humoral immunity appears to have an important role in multiple sclerosis, and intrathecal antibody synthesis is characteristic of the disease. The presence of B-cell clonal expansion in cerebrospinal fluid (CSF) and in lesions indicates an antigen-driven response within the CNS. Ectopic B-cell follicles have also been found in the meninges and are anatomically associated with sub-pial cortical demyelinating lesions, providing further evidence that B cells are involved in immunopathogenesis. Meningeal inflammation occurs in the brain and spinal cord and in both regions has been associated with neuroaxonal loss in the adjacent parenchyma, suggesting that it can be a significant mechanism contributing to the neurodegeneration and cortical grey matter demyelination that is prominent in progressive multiple sclerosis.

Potential autoantigens implicated in the pathogenesis of multiple sclerosis have included myelin basic protein (MBP), proteolipid protein (PLP), myelin-associated glycoprotein (MAG), myelin oligodendrocyte glycoprotein (MOG) and alpha-B crystallin. The presence of specific cytokines, like transforming growth factor β (TGF-β), IL-6, IL-12, IL-17, IL-21 and IL-23, govern the type of T-helper response. Th1-like cytokines (IL-2, IFNγ and TNF-α) or Th23-like cytokines (IL-17) initiate a cell-mediated inflammatory cascade which activates macrophages, microglia, astrocytes and endothelial cells. This results in further cytokine production and recruitment of inflammatory cells by the up-regulation of adhesion molecule expression on endothelial cells and by the production of chemo-attractants, such as chemokines. Astrocytes and macrophages produce mutually stimulating cytokines (IL-1 and TNF-α). These and other pro-inflammatory T-cell cytokines up-regulate the production of numerous mediators of inflammation, which are toxic to oligodendrocytes, axons and neurons. These substances include tumour necrosis factor α (TNF-α), free oxygen and nitrogen radicals, complement, proteases and eicosanoids.

Autoantibodies, particularly to surface myelin antigens, can be crucial to the development of demyelination. Autoantibodies to axonal elements (e.g. gangliosides and neurofilaments) can have functional consequences and can contribute to conduction abnormalities and axonal loss. In addition to myelin damage, programmed cell death or apoptosis of the oligodendrocyte can occur as a result of oxidative stress and death signalling induced by TNF-α. Antibodies and complement assist Fc-receptor mediated phagocytosis by opsonisation. Phagocytosis also occurs via the macrophage scavenger and low-density lipoprotein receptors. T-regulatory cells and immunomodulatory cytokines produced by these cells are important in down-regulating and controlling the focal inflammation. Elimination of autoreactive T cells by apoptosis can be important in controlling inflammation.

The combination of both cell and humorally mediated inflammatory cascades causes oligodendrocyte, axonal and neuronal toxicity, which in turn is believed to release sequestered CNS antigens which are hypothesised to initiate further cycles of autoimmune-induced inflammation via intra- or intermolecular antigen determinant spreading.

Inflammatory demyelination results in a reduction in the safety factor of conduction, with complete or intermittent conduction block, which produces clinical symptoms and signs, some of which can be intermittent. Resolution of inflammation and oedema initially can result in clinical improvement. Over a longer time, remyelination and/or axonal plasticity (synthesis of new sodium channels along demyelinated axonal segments) restores axonal conduction, albeit with a reduced safety factor of conduction, which results in remission. There is evidence that growth factors produced as part of the inflammatory response stimulate the process of remyelination. Synaptic plasticity can also compensate for defective conduction. Transient neurological symptoms can occur secondary to the residual reversible conduction block, typically in relation to fatigue, changes in body temperature and systemic inflammation. Ephaptic transmission can cause paroxysmal positive neurological symptoms. Axonal loss, as a consequence of acute or diffuse injury, causes permanent neurological impairment and disability.

In summary, the hypothetical autoimmune pathogenesis for multiple sclerosis has an initial phase of multi-focal inflammatory demyelination in white matter that is mediated through a systemic adaptive immune response (activated T cells) and accounts for a relapsing remitting clinical course. There is a subsequent phase characterised by a more widespread low grade inflammatory process – involving white and grey matter lesions and NAWM – which is mediated through an innate immune response within the CNS (activated microglia, meningeal and peri-vascular inflammation), leading to widespread neuroaxonal loss and a progressive clinical course. This sequential process would explain the evolution from a relapsing remitting to secondary progressive course and a primary progressive course could be because of a milder initial adaptive immune response phase that is not expressed clinically.

Clinical course

Multiple sclerosis is characterised by lesions disseminated throughout the CNS, which can appear, disappear or gradually worsen over time, and this is reflected in its clinical presentation and course. Its presentation is variable and its course and prognosis are unpredictable, although broad clinical categories of the disease are well recognised.

Types of multiple sclerosis

Clinical disease activity in multiple sclerosis can manifest as relapses or insidious progression. According to the occurrence and timing of these features, four main categories of multiple sclerosis were outlined in 1996 in the widely accepted classification of Lublin and Reingold (Figure 11.2).

Relapsing remitting multiple sclerosis

Approximately 85% of individuals present with relapses and remissions. A relapse is defined as an episode of acute or subacute neurological dysfunction lasting a minimum of 24 hours. A relapse usually evolves over days or weeks, plateaus and then remits to a variable degree, from minimal resolution to complete recovery. Further relapses can then occur at irregular intervals. The average relapse frequency in the relapsing remitting phase of the disease (without disease modifying treatment) is approximately one relapse per year.

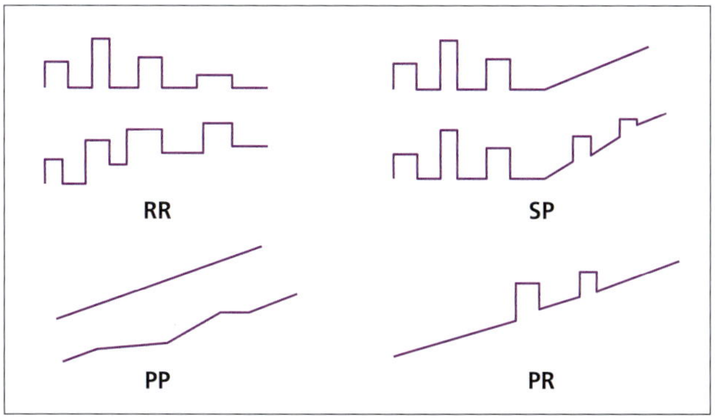

Figure 11.2 Clinical course of multiple sclerosis: illustration of the relationship between increasing disability and time in the different types of multiple sclerosis (PP, primary progressive; PR, progressive relapsing; RR, relapsing remitting; SP, secondary progressive). (After Lublin and Reingold 1996.)

Secondary progressive multiple sclerosis

Relapsing remitting multiple sclerosis can evolve into a gradually progressive course with accumulating irreversible neurological deficit and disability, classified as secondary progressive multiple sclerosis. The proportion of people developing secondary progressive disease increases with length of follow-up. In a large Canadian natural history study, 41% of people with relapsing remitting multiple sclerosis entered the secondary progressive phase within 6–10 years of disease onset increasing to 58% between 11 and 15 years after onset. After 20 years, approximately 80% had developed secondary progressive multiple sclerosis. Superimposed relapses can continue to occur in the secondary progressive phase, although less frequently as the disease progresses.

Primary progressive multiple sclerosis

In primary progressive multiple sclerosis there is insidious disease progression from onset, resulting in gradual accumulation of neurological deficit or disability, without relapse or remission. It accounts for approximately 10–15% of multiple sclerosis. Males and females are affected with equal frequency. The average age of onset is older in primary progressive multiple sclerosis, approximately 40 years compared to 30 years in relapsing remitting multiple sclerosis.

Progressive relapsing multiple sclerosis

Progressive relapsing multiple sclerosis refers to the small number of people who have progressive disease from onset with superimposed relapses, but the term is now rarely used. Insidious progression is the predominant feature and relapses are usually mild. Progressive relapsing multiple sclerosis is considered to be largely similar to primary progressive multiple sclerosis. Approximately one-quarter of people initially diagnosed with primary progressive multiple sclerosis will later have relapses, and a relapse can occur decades after disease onset.

The classification of clinical course was revised in 2013. Clinically isolated syndrome was added and progressive relapsing multiple sclerosis eliminated. It was recommended that all forms of multiple sclerosis should be subcategorised as either active or non-active. Active multiple sclerosis is defined as the occurrence of clinical relapse or new T2 or gadolinium-enhancing lesions over a specified period of time. Progressive multiple sclerosis should be subcategorised into those who have shown signs of disability progression over a given time period and those who have remained stable. It was also recommended that the patients whose disease is advancing through relapses should be described as 'worsening', and that the term 'disease progression' should be reserved for those with truly progressive disease.

Natural history and prognosis

The natural history of multiple sclerosis is extremely variable. The spectrum of disease activity ranges from clinically asymptomatic demyelinating lesions, detected incidentally on imaging (radiologically isolated syndrome) or at postmortem, to an aggressive course with rapidly accumulating disability. It is not possible to predict prognosis in an individual, but natural history studies have provided data on disease progression in different multiple sclerosis populations.

Clinically isolated syndrome

A clinically isolated syndrome refers to a first acute episode suggestive of CNS demyelination, and it can be the first presentation of multiple sclerosis. The average risk of developing multiple sclerosis following a clinically isolated syndrome has been reported as between 30% and 70%, although the risk increases with the length of follow-up. People presenting with unilateral optic neuritis may have a lower risk of converting to multiple sclerosis than other clinical presentations, although high conversion rates have been seen in the United Kingdom, where the prevalence of multiple sclerosis is also high. Abnormal MRI at first presentation has been consistently shown to confer a higher risk of conversion to multiple sclerosis than if MRI is normal. Long-term follow-up studies, ranging from 7 to 20 years, have reported the development of multiple sclerosis to occur in 56–88% of people with lesions on MRI and in 8–22% of those with a normal scan. The lesion number and load at first presentation can also have prognostic relevance, with higher lesion loads modestly predictive of the likelihood of developing disability in the long term.

Established multiple sclerosis

Natural history studies have conventionally assessed disease progression in multiple sclerosis by measuring the time taken to reach disability milestones. Such studies have shown that the median time to reach a level of disability requiring assistance for walking is between 15 and 30 years.

There has been debate as to the effect of the disease type on long-term prognosis. Relapsing remitting multiple sclerosis has been felt to carry a better prognosis, but a French natural history study from a single large centre reported that disease progression in the long term is largely independent of disease type once a person has acquired a moderate level of disability (level 4 on the Kurtzke expanded disability status scale). However, this requires replication in other studies. Although accumulation of irreversible disability is slower in the relapsing and remitting phase, once the secondary progressive phase is entered the initial course does not seem to significantly influence long-term prognosis.

The influence of residual disability from relapses on long-term accumulation of disability has been similarly debated. Residual neurological deficit following a relapse is common. For example, an increase in disability was demonstrated in one study in up to 42% of people at 2 months following a relapse. However, further recovery can take place over a longer time. Analysis of the placebo arms of treatment trials in relapsing remitting multiple sclerosis has suggested that relapses, although resulting in confirmed disability over 6 months, do not seem to have a consistent effect on the development of sustained disability over the course of a typical study (mean 2.66 years). Further study is required to understand the effect of relapses on long-term disability.

The age of onset does not seem to significantly influence long-term prognosis. Younger age of onset has previously been considered a good prognostic marker but this is not really the case as, although the time to develop permanent disability can take longer, disability still occurs at a younger age. The older age of onset associated with primary progressive multiple sclerosis has also previously been felt to be a poorer prognostic marker. However, the average age of onset in primary progressive multiple sclerosis is similar to that of the progressive phase in secondary progressive multiple sclerosis. The rate of progression is also similar in the primary and secondary progressive groups, with disability milestones being reached at similar ages.

Male sex has been suggested to be associated with a poorer prognosis, but recent studies suggest that this may not be clear-cut. Factors reported to be associated with a more favourable prognosis include monosymptomatic onset, afferent symptoms (sensory, optic neuritis) at onset, complete recovery from first attack, a long interval between first and second relapses, a low relapse frequency in early disease and minimal disability after 5 years from the onset of first symptoms. However, such associations are weak and it is not possible to reliably predict individual prognosis.

Benign multiple sclerosis

Benign multiple sclerosis refers to a disease course with accumulation of minimal or no disability. There is no consensus definition, but it is often taken as an Expanded Disability Status Scale (EDSS) score ≤3 (Table 11.2) at 10–15 years after disease onset. A systematic review of published studies has reported the frequency of benign multiple sclerosis as 26.7%, but the proportion of people with benign disease decreases with length of follow-up. In a large British Columbian cohort only half of those with benign disease at 10 years still fulfilled the criteria at 20 years, with the remainder having developed secondary progression. There are no reliable indicators of a benign course, although follow-up over 20 years in a US cohort found that the longer the disease duration and the lesser the disability, the more likely an individual was to remain stable. It is well recognised that even long-standing benign disease can progress with the development of severe disability.

Aggressive multiple sclerosis

An aggressive or malignant disease course can result from severe or frequent relapses with little or no neurological recovery or from rapid disease progression. However, aggressive disease is uncommon and early death in multiple sclerosis is rare.

The Marburg variant of multiple sclerosis refers to an acute fulminant disease course, usually monophasic, which can result in death within a few months. Its clinical presentation relates to its site, which can be cerebral, brainstem or spinal cord. In cerebral presentations, confusion and seizures can occur. MRI shows large tumefactive lesions, correlating with destructive hypercellular demyelinating lesions on neuropathological examination, which typically enhance and can have associated oedema and mass effect. The condition must also be distinguished from acute disseminated encephalomyelitis, acute haemorrhagic leukoencephalitis and vasculitis.

Baló concentric sclerosis refers to a particular neuropathological lesion variant, which can also be evident on MRI, characterised by alternating concentric layers of myelin loss and relative preservation of myelin. It can be seen in association with a fulminant course, although it can also occur in more benign disease.

Early onset multiple sclerosis

Although rare, the onset of multiple sclerosis can be in childhood. Early onset, before the age of 16 years, occurs in approximately 2–5% of individuals. A relapsing remitting disease onset is typical, and a primary progressive course is much rarer than in adult onset disease. Prognosis can be considered better in that the time to develop disability is longer than in adult onset multiple sclerosis, but overall individuals develop disability at a younger age. Over half are likely to develop secondary progressive multiple sclerosis by the age of 30 years. The paediatric multiple sclerosis population can be an ideal group in which to study aetiological factors, and there has been a recent upsurge of interest in this group. A large international collaboration has reported that paediatric multiple sclerosis can be associated with exposure to EBV, but not with other common childhood viral infections. A Canadian nationwide study has followed children who presented with a clinically isolated syndrome and found that the risk for developing multiple sclerosis was increased in the next 3 years by

Table 11.2 Expanded Disability Status Scale (EDSS). Functional systems (FS) are: pyramidal, cerebellar, brainstem, sensory, bowel and bladder, visual and cerebral.

0.0	Normal neurological examination
1.0	No disability, minimal signs in one FS
1.5	No disability, minimal signs in more than one FS
2.0	Minimal disability in one FS
2.5	Minimal disability in two FS
3.0	Moderate disability in one FS or mild disability in three or four FS, although fully ambulatory
3.5	Fully ambulatory but with moderate disability in one FS and mild disability in one or two FS; or moderate disability in two FS; or mild disability in five FS
4.0	Fully ambulatory without aid, self-sufficient up and about some 12 hours a day despite relatively severe disability in one FS or combinations exceeding limits of previous steps; able to walk without aid or rest some 500 m
4.5	Fully ambulatory without aid, up and about much of the day, able to work a full day, may otherwise have some limitation of full activity or require minimal assistance; able to walk without aid or rest some 300 m
5.0	Ambulatory without aid or rest for about 200 m; disability severe enough to impair full daily activities (e.g. to work a full day without special provisions)
5.5	Ambulatory without aid or rest for about 100 m, disability severe enough to preclude full daily activities
6.0	Intermittent or unilateral constant assistance (cane, crutch, brace) required to walk about 100 m with or without resting
6.5	Constant bilateral assistance (canes, crutches, braces) required to walk about 20 m with or without resting
7.0	Unable to walk beyond approximately 5 m even with aid, essentially restricted to wheelchair; wheels self in standard wheelchair and transfers alone, up and about in wheelchair some 12 hours a day
7.5	Unable to take more than a few steps; restricted to wheelchair; may need aid in transfer, wheels self but cannot carry on in standard wheelchair a full day; may require motorized wheelchair
8.0	Essentially restricted to bed or chair or perambulated in wheelchair, but may be out of bed itself much of the day; retains many self-care functions; generally has effective use of arms
8.5	Essentially restricted to bed much of day; has some effective use of arm(s); retains some self-care functions
9.0	Helpless bed patient; can communicate and eat
9.5	Totally helpless bed patient; unable to communicate effectively or eat/swallow
10.0	Death due to multiple sclerosis

Source: Kurtzke 1983. Reproduced with permission of AAN/LWW.

the presence of MRI brain lesions, CSF oligoclonal bands, the HLA DRB1*15 allele, previous EBV infection and low vitamin D levels.

Mortality

Mortality rates are increased compared to the general population. The average life expectancy in multiple sclerosis has been reported to be reduced by between 7 and 14 years. The proportion of deaths attributed to complications of multiple sclerosis is at least half. The risk of suicide in the multiple sclerosis population is increased and can be more than twice the rate of the general population. Although the long-term effects of disease-modifying therapy on the course of multiple sclerosis are not yet clear, their potential to increase survival is supported by a 21-year follow-up report from the pivotal interferon β-1b trial.

Factors affecting relapse activity

Various health and lifestyle factors have been proposed to affect relapse activity in multiple sclerosis. It is important that people with multiple sclerosis are aware of these factors to facilitate informed decisions regarding their lifestyle.

Infections

Systemic infections can trigger a relapse or exacerbate existing symptoms of multiple sclerosis. An association between common viral and bacterial infections and risk of relapse has been documented, but such infections are difficult to avoid. Infections can occur as a complication of multiple sclerosis (e.g. urinary tract infections resulting from retention and chest infections resulting from aspiration). Therefore, addressing the underlying cause of infections can be preventative and, where possible, infections should be anticipated and treated early. Cigarette smoking, aside from its well-known health risks, can increase the occurrence of respiratory tract infections and should be discouraged.

Pregnancy

The effect of pregnancy on disease activity is an important concern among women of childbearing age. A large prospective study of pregnancy in multiple sclerosis confirmed that relapse rate declines during pregnancy, especially in the third trimester, increases during the first 3 months postpartum and then returns to pre-pregnancy rate. The incidence of postpartum relapse was 28%. An increased relapse rate in the pre-pregnancy year and during pregnancy, and higher disability at pregnancy onset, were associated with a higher risk of postpartum relapse. Epidural analgesia and breastfeeding were not found to increase the risk of relapse. There is no evidence for an adverse effect of pregnancy on the long-term course of multiple sclerosis and some studies have identified a better long-term course in multiparous than nulliparous women.

Stress

Prospective studies have reported stressful life events to be associated with an increased risk of relapse. A meta-analysis also supported an association between stressful life events and subsequent relapses although did not link relapse to specific stressors. Physical trauma has been proposed to trigger relapses but a systematic review of the evidence has not supported this link.

Diet Despite popular interest in the effect of diet on multiple sclerosis there is currently little evidence to support an association between dietary factors and disease activity. A systematic review concluded that no dietary intervention has been shown to significantly affect disease progression. Linoleic acid, an omega-6 fatty acid, was associated with slight decreases in relapse rate and severity, but the studies were small and of limited design. Vitamin D supplementation has been reported to reduce relapse rates, but the available data are not conclusive; larger studies are ongoing.

Vaccines

The question of whether vaccination can immunologically trigger a relapse has been investigated and there is no clear evidence to support this hypothesis. Most vaccines have not been investigated prospectively, but a double-blind, placebo controlled study of influenza vaccine showed no effect on relapse rate or disease progression. There has been particular concern regarding hepatitis B vaccination but a large case cross-over study found no increased risk of relapse following either hepatitis B or indeed any vaccination. Current expert opinion is that vaccinations are not contraindicated in multiple sclerosis, and national guidelines recommend that people with multiple sclerosis can be offered vaccination against influenza according to the individual's needs. However, it must not be forgotten that live vaccines can be contraindicated in individuals on immunosuppressant therapy (i.e. BCG, oral polio vaccine, MMR [measles–mumps–rubella], rotavirus, yellow fever, varicella zoster).

Clinical features

Multiple sclerosis can cause a wide variety of symptoms mirroring involvement of any part of the CNS. The spinal cord, optic nerves and brainstem are commonly involved sites. In a European database of clinically isolated syndromes, 46% of individuals presented with a spinal cord syndrome, 21% with optic neuritis and 10% with a brainstem syndrome. The presentation was polysymptomatic in 23% of cases. Differences in presenting symptoms are seen between disease types. In relapsing remitting multiple sclerosis, the most common symptoms are sensory and visual, whereas in primary progressive disease the most usual presentation is locomotor. During the course of the disease a multitude of symptoms can occur: weakness, spasticity, numbness, paraesthesia, pain, visual loss, diplopia, ataxia, tremor, vertigo, sphincter and sexual dysfunction, dysphagia, dysarthria, respiratory dysfunction, temperature sensitivity, fatigue, cognitive and psychiatric disturbance.

There are no symptoms or signs that are pathognomonic for multiple sclerosis, although characteristic clinical features are seen. Optic neuritis is a common manifestation. It presents with eye pain, which is exacerbated by eye movement, and blurring of vision. The visual impairment can progress over a few days, but not usually longer than 1–2 weeks. Continued progressive visual failure or loss of perception to light should alert to the possibility of alternative diagnoses. On examination, colour vision and visual acuity are impaired and a scotoma, classically central, can be detected. The optic disc can be normal but swelling can be present, and pallor of the optic disc can develop later. A relative afferent pupillary defect is usually present.

Diplopia can be a presenting symptom and usually is symptomatic of a VIth nerve palsy or an internuclear ophthalmoplegia. As the disease advances, unilateral or bilateral internuclear ophthalmoplegia, identified on conjugate lateral gaze as impaired adduction on the side of the lesion and nystagmus of the abducting eye, is commonly seen but can often be asymptomatic.

A partial spinal cord syndrome is a frequent presentation. Typically, altered sensation starts in one foot and spreads to involve both legs and, to a varying extent, ascends to the trunk and arms. Variable degrees of numbness and tingling can occur but complete loss of sensation is unusual. On examination, all sensory modalities can be impaired and a sensory level can be discerned although, as the relapse recovers, a persistent bilateral sensory level is uncommon. Oppenheim hand, a functionally impaired hand caused by loss of position sense, can be a characteristic presentation of a lesion in the posterior columns of the cervical cord.

Motor involvement becomes more common as the disease advances and weakness is a prominent symptom. Weakness is usually greater in the legs than the arms, and paraparesis is frequently asymmetrical. Spasticity can manifest as stiffness, clonus or spasms. On examination, signs usually reflect upper motor neurone involvement with hypertonia, hyper-reflexia and positive Babinski responses. However, focal wasting, flaccidity and loss of tendon reflexes can be seen, and can result from denervation in the spinal cord.

Spinal cord involvement also commonly results in bladder and bowel disturbance. Bladder disturbance can result from a combination of detrusor hyper-reflexia, manifesting as urgency, frequency and incontinence, and incomplete emptying because of sphincter dyssynergia and poorly sustained detrusor contractions, resulting in hesitancy and incomplete emptying. Constipation is the most common bowel symptom, although urgency and incontinence are not infrequent. Sexual function in males and females is frequently affected, because of central neurological dysfunction, although psychological and other factors can also contribute.

An initial cerebellar presentation is uncommon but cerebellar involvement is frequent during the course of the disease, evidenced by nystagmus, dysarthria, limb ataxia, intention tremor and truncal ataxia. Gait ataxia can contribute to the classic spastic ataxic gait, but it can also cause disabling gait disturbance in the absence of significant weakness and spasticity.

Fatigue can be one of the most disabling symptoms in multiple sclerosis, and can impact on all activities. An exercise-induced motor fatigue, with increasing leg weakness on walking, and an unprovoked but severe generalised exhaustion may be reported. Fatigue appears to be related to electrophysiological and immunological effects of multiple sclerosis, and is often worse during relapses, but disturbed sleep, medication and depression can also be contributory factors. Heat sensitivity is a common symptom, caused by the increased temperature inducing slowing of nerve conduction. Uhthoff's phenomenon refers to the transient blurring of vision on exercise or in hot environments brought about by underlying optic nerve disease.

Cognitive impairment is well documented to occur in multiple sclerosis and mild deficits can be apparent in early disease. Attention, information processing, memory and executive functions are predominantly affected. Severe dementia can occur but, particularly in early disease, can suggest an alternate diagnosis. Depression occurs more frequently than in the general population but is usually mild and is often reactive to the diagnosis and ensuing neurological deficits. Emotional lability, with involuntary crying or laughing in the absence of subjective mood disorder, can occur. Psychosis is an uncommon manifestation of multiple sclerosis, but may rarely be the presenting episode.

Pain is common in multiple sclerosis and is usually chronic. It is often myelopathic in origin, typically resulting in a burning pain in the legs and hands. Paroxysmal pain can occur, most notably trigeminal neuralgia. Pain can also result indirectly from other related problems such as spasms and musculoskeletal complications.

A characteristic feature of multiple sclerosis is the occurrence of paroxysmal symptoms, resulting from electrical instability within lesions. A typical episode is of acute onset with symptoms of short duration, less than 2 minutes, occurring up to 30 or more times a day. The whole episode usually resolves spontaneously within a few weeks to months. The nature of the symptoms reflects the underlying site of the lesion. Infratentorial lesions can result in trigeminal neuralgia and paroxysmal dysarthria and ataxia. Tonic spasms, painful tonic contractions usually involving one or two limbs unilaterally, can arise from sites in the cortico-spinal tract. Other paroxysmal sensory disturbances can occur and paroxysmal itching is described.

Other positive symptoms include Lhermitte's symptom, a brief electrical sensation radiating down the back into the legs or arms precipitated by neck flexion, caused by a lesion in the cervical cord, and phosphenes resulting from optic nerve demyelination. Lesions involving the facial nucleus or nerve can cause hemifacial spasm or facial myokymia. Epilepsy, originating from juxtacortical or cortical lesions, is seen 2–3 times more commonly than in the general population, and rarely may be the presenting symptom.

Diagnosis

Multiple sclerosis is a clinical diagnosis that requires appropriate expertise to confirm evidence of CNS lesions disseminated in time and space and to exclude other diseases. Investigations can be used to:

- Exclude other diseases
- Provide evidence of dissemination in time and space, and
- Provide evidence of immunological disturbance.

Diagnostic investigations

Magnetic resonance imaging

The plaques of white matter demyelination in multiple sclerosis are readily visualised on MRI by virtue of an increase in the amount and mobility of water protons in the lesions. The standard imaging sequence is a T2-weighted spin echo or fast spin echo, with an additional fast FLAIR (fluid attenuated inversion recovery) sequence that suppresses signal from CSF and increases the conspicuity of cerebral hemisphere lesions.

The value of MRI in diagnosis comes through its high sensitivity for detecting clinically silent lesions, and showing them in characteristic locations; the detection of blood–brain barrier breakdown in acute lesions using gadolinium-enhanced T1-weighted MRI is also a useful finding. MRI can be normal in clinically definite multiple sclerosis, but this is unusual: lesions are seen in the brain in approximately 95% and spinal cord lesions in approximately 70% with a clinically definite diagnosis. The characteristic locations for foci of demyelination are peri-ventricular, corpus callosum, juxtacortical, brainstem, cerebellar white matter and spinal cord (Figure 11.3). Lesions are usually small (3–10 mm diameter), can have an oval or rounded shape, and usually extend to the parenchymal surface in the brainstem and spinal cord. Cord lesions are most often seen in a posterior or lateral location, involve white and grey matter, and affect only part of the cord in cross-section (Figure 11.4). Gadolinium enhancement is invariable in new lesions in relapsing multiple sclerosis, can be homogeneous or ring-shaped, and lasts an average of 2–6 weeks (Figure 11.5).

In people with a clinically isolated syndrome (CIS), clinically silent cerebral white matter lesions are seen in 50–70%. The presence of MRI lesions confers a relatively high risk for future development of clinically definite multiple sclerosis as already discussed. Development of new T2 or gadolinium-enhancing lesions on

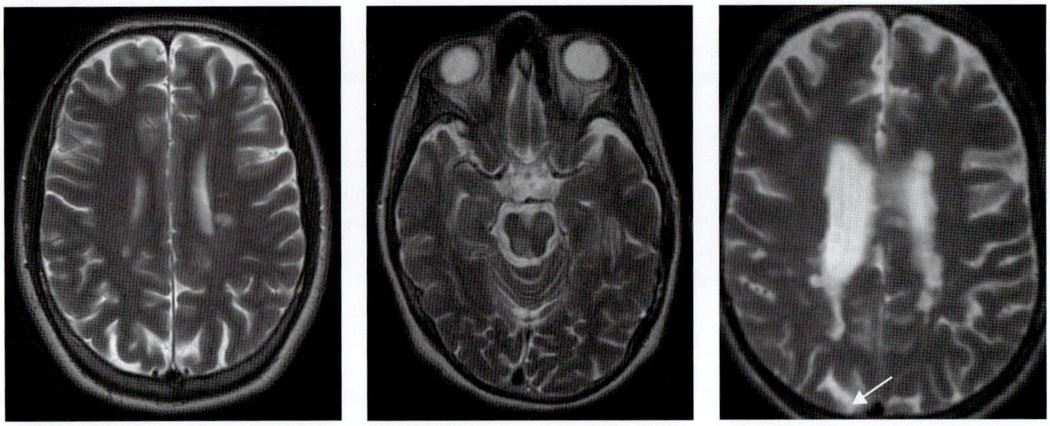

(a) (b) (c)

Figure 11.3 Typical lesions in multiple sclerosis: (a) periventricular; (b) infra-tentorial, (c) juxtacortical lesion (arrow) (MRI T2W axial).

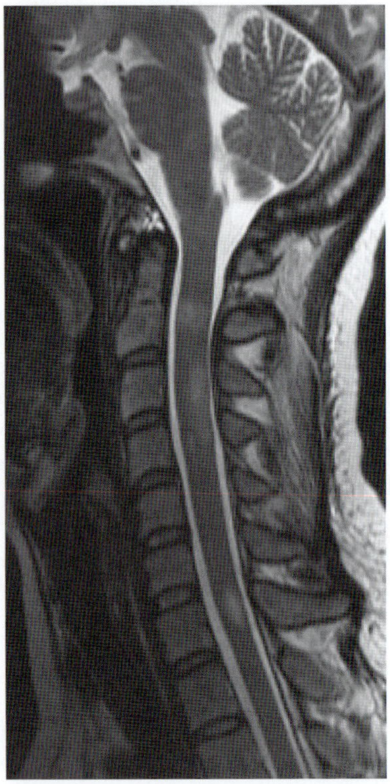

Figure 11.4 Typical lesions in the cervical cord in multiple sclerosis (MRI T2W sagittal).

follow-up MRI increases the likelihood of early clinical relapses and, accordingly, the development of clinically definite multiple sclerosis.

The major limitation of MRI is specificity: there are many other causes of cerebral white matter lesions (Table 11.3). Small vessel disease is an especially common cause of areas of T2 hyperintensity on white matter and over one-third of the general population aged over 50 years will exhibit areas of high signal. These are small, and mainly subcortical rather than peri-ventricular. Basal ganglia involvement is not uncommon and central pontine abnormalities are also seen (unlike multiple sclerosis, not extending to the surface). Cord lesions do not occur with ageing per se and their detection in older patients is a particularly useful pointer to demyelination.

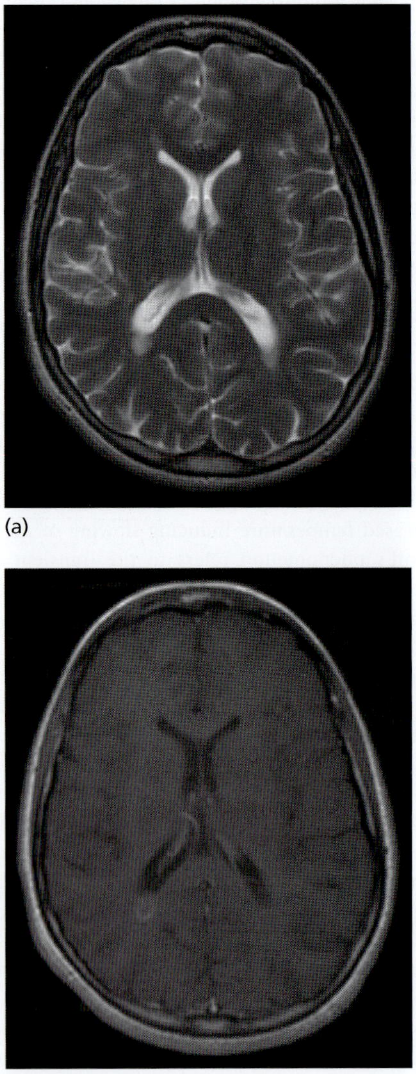

(a)

(b)

Figure 11.5 Typical lesions in multiple sclerosis: (a) an acute periventricular lesion (MRI T2W axial); (b) associated gadolinium enhancement (MRI T1W axial).

Table 11.3 Differential diagnosis of white matter lesions on magnetic resonance imaging (MRI).

Inflammatory
Multiple sclerosis
Acute disseminated encephalomyelitis
Neuromyelitis optica
Vasculitis (including SLE, Sjögren's syndrome)
Sarcoidosis
Behçet's disease
Primary angiitis of the CNS
Vascular
Small vessel disease
Antiphospholipid syndrome
CADASIL
Infectious
Progressive multifocal leukoencephalopathy
HIV encephalitis
Viral encephalitis
Lyme's disease
Whipple's disease
Syphilis
Subacute sclerosing panencephalitis
Intracerebral abscesses
Tuberculosis/fungal infections
Metabolic
Pontine/extra-pontine myelinolysis
Phenylketonuria
Vitamin B_{12} deficiency
Hyperhomocysteinaemia
Cerebrotendinous xanthomatosis
Leukodystrophies
Adrenoleukodystrophy/adrenomyeloneuropathy
Globoid cell leukodystrophy
Metachromatic leukodystrophy
Vanishing white matter disease
Alexander's disease
Canavan's disease
Other
Tumour (glioma, lymphoma, metastases)
Mitochondrial disease
Susac's syndrome

CADASIL, cerebral autosomal dominant arteriopathy with subcortical infarcts and leukoencephalopathy; SLE, systemic lupus erythematosus.

Other multi-focal and inflammatory disorders can at times be difficult to distinguish from multiple sclerosis on clinical and imaging grounds: sarcoidosis, SLE, Sjögren's syndrome, Behçet's disease, CNS vasculitis, acute disseminated encephalomyelitis (ADEM) and neuromyelitis optica (NMO). There are some distinctive imaging findings, for example meningeal enhancement in sarcoidosis; multifocal, punctate and peri-vascular enhancement in CNS vasculitis; extensive brainstem and diencephalic lesions in Behçet's disease; monophasic disease activity in ADEM, with partial and sometimes marked resolution at follow-up; extensive longitudinal cord lesions in ADEM and NMO. Numerous other non-inflammatory white matter disorders can also enter the differential diagnosis, for example progressive multifocal leukoencephalopathy, cerebral autosomal dominant arteriopathy with subcortical infarcts and leukoencephalopathy (CADASIL). In leukodystrophies (e.g. Krabbe's disease, adrenomyeloneuropathy) or metabolic disorders such as phenylketonuria, the white matter abnormalities are typically symmetrical. Rarely, demyelinating lesions can manifest as a single, large, atypical-appearing or tumefactive lesion within a cerebral hemisphere mimicking a cerebral tumour (Figure 11.6). Sometimes such lesions are accompanied by other smaller lesions that are typical for demyelination and thereby assist diagnosis. The tumefactive lesions tend to be extensive but circumscribed with little mass effect or vasogenic oedema and there may be pathological ring enhancement, although more atypical features can occur; ultimately, the lesions will become smaller, and sometimes appear to resolve rapidly with corticosteroid therapy.

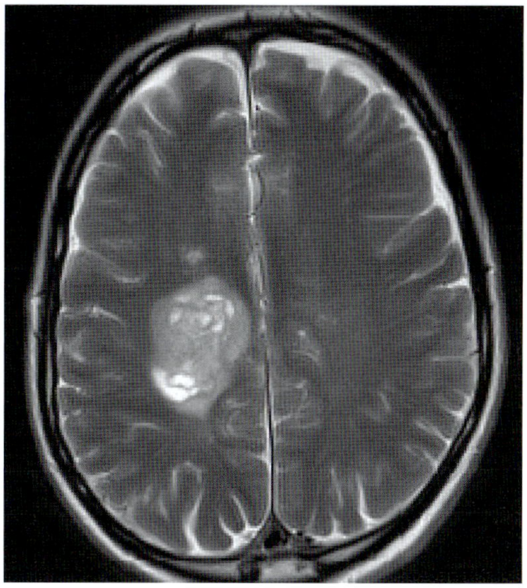

Figure 11.6 Atypical lesion in multiple sclerosis mimicking a cerebral tumour (MRI T2W axial).

Conventional T2-weighted MRI sequences are very insensitive to cortical grey matter lesions and abnormalities in NAWM that are nevertheless abundant in multiple sclerosis. Some cortical lesions are detected using more sophisticated imaging techniques, including double inversion recovery and phase sensitive inversion recovery sequences and higher resolution imaging on high field scanners, although an added diagnostic value of such approaches has not been shown. Quantitative MRI abnormalities have been demonstrated in NAWM and include decreased magnetisation transfer ratio, increased T1 relaxation time, increased mean diffusivity and decreased *N*-acetylaspartate on spectroscopy. While the development of techniques to better detect and quantify these more extensive abnormalities may have some diagnostic role in future, the greater importance seems likely to be in understanding pathogenic mechanisms and assigning prognosis.

Cerebrospinal fluid

When both clinical and imaging features are characteristic of multiple sclerosis, many neurologists will not feel that a lumbar puncture is required, although there are some geographical variations in practice. In those regions where Lyme disease is common (Chapter 9), exclusion of this treatable condition warrants a lumbar puncture in almost all suspected multiple sclerosis cases (however, it should be noted that the usual clinical features of neuroborreliosis – facial palsy and meningoradiculitis – are not a common presentation for multiple sclerosis). In clinically definite multiple sclerosis, intrathecally synthesised oligoclonal immunoglobulin G (IgG) bands are found in approximately 90% of patients. A parallel blood sample is required to demonstrate the intrathecal origin of bands as the passive transfer of bands from the systemic circulation has no diagnostic value. Isoelectric focusing and immunodetection of oligoclonal bands is the gold standard technique to provide evidence of intrathecal antibody synthesis (Figure 11.7). A raised IgG index can be informative but is not as sensitive or specific. About two-fifths of patients have a mildly raised CSF white cell count (5–50 mononuclear cells/mm^3) and protein.

Oligoclonal bands occur in other CNS inflammatory disorders including infections (e.g. neurosyphilis, subacute sclerosing panencephalitis [SSPE], neuroborreliosis, human T-lymphocyte virus type 1 [HTLV-1] associated myelopathy and CNS varicella zoster), vasculitis, collagen-vascular disorders and paraneoplastic disease but they are less common in neurosarcoidosis, Behçet's disease and NMO. Whereas in multiple sclerosis the antigenic specificity of the bands is largely unknown, in SSPE and varicella zoster they are largely directed against measles and herpes zoster antigens, respectively.

Laboratory procedures for optimal CSF examination in suspected multiple sclerosis have been defined recently by an expert international panel. Some new laboratory methods for detecting oligoclonal bands, including IgM bands, have been investigated and suggested as being more sensitive and specific in diagnosing and predicting the course of multiple sclerosis. More extensive studies are required to determine their clinical utility.

Evoked potentials

For 10–20 years prior to the widespread introduction of MRI, evoked potentials were important and frequently used diagnostic investigations. Their role was similar to MRI: detection of clinically silent CNS white matter lesions. Because they are less sensitive in this respect than MRI, they are not often requested as part of contemporary diagnostic work-up. The most useful of these investigations is the visual evoked potential; the demonstration of a markedly delayed P100 wave of normal amplitude provides strong evidence for optic nerve demyelination (Figure 11.8). It can still be useful in supporting the diagnosis, especially when the clinical syndrome is in the spinal cord or brainstem and MRI is normal or shows only minor non-specific abnormalities or is obtained in an older age group where the specificity of white matter abnormalities is less. Brainstem auditory evoked potentials and somato-sensory evoked potentials are generally less useful, although can sometimes have a role in establishing the nature of a lesion.

Autoantibodies

No autoantibody has been confirmed to be diagnostic for multiple sclerosis to date. A study of patients with CIS – who also had MRI abnormalities and CSF oligoclonal bands indicating a high likelihood for multiple sclerosis – reported that the presence of antimyelin antibodies in serum substantially increased the risk for developing clinically definite multiple sclerosis. However, several subsequent studies were consistently negative, reporting as high a frequency of such antibodies in healthy controls or in those with

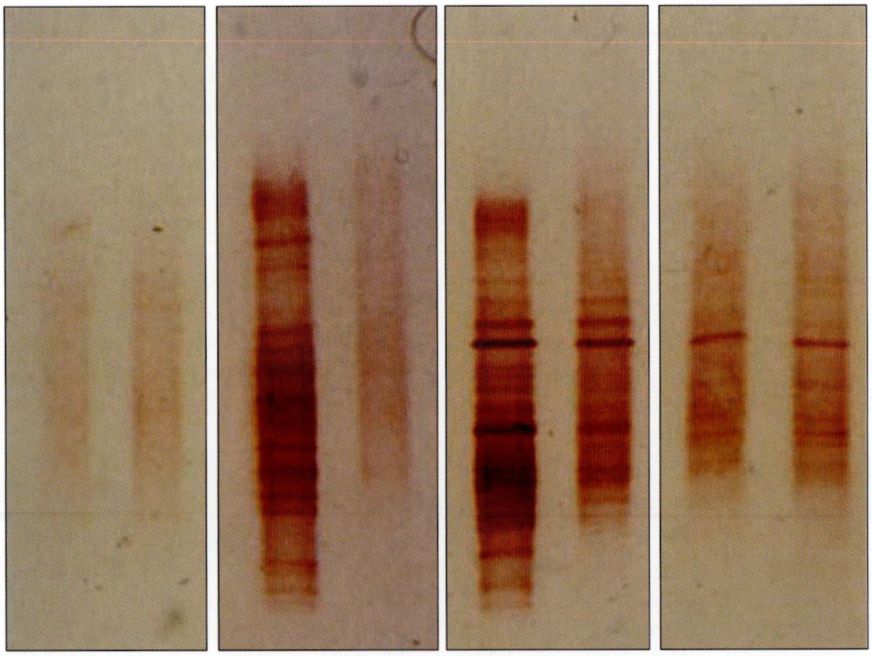

(a) (b) (c) (d)

Figure 11.7 Isoelectric focusing of paired cerebrospinal fluid (CSF) and serum. (a) CSF negative/serum negative; (b) CSF positive/serum negative; (c) CSF positive/serum positive but with fewer bands; (d) CSF positive/serum positive with the same bands. The oligoclonal band patterns in (b) and (c) indicate intrathecal antibody synthesis.

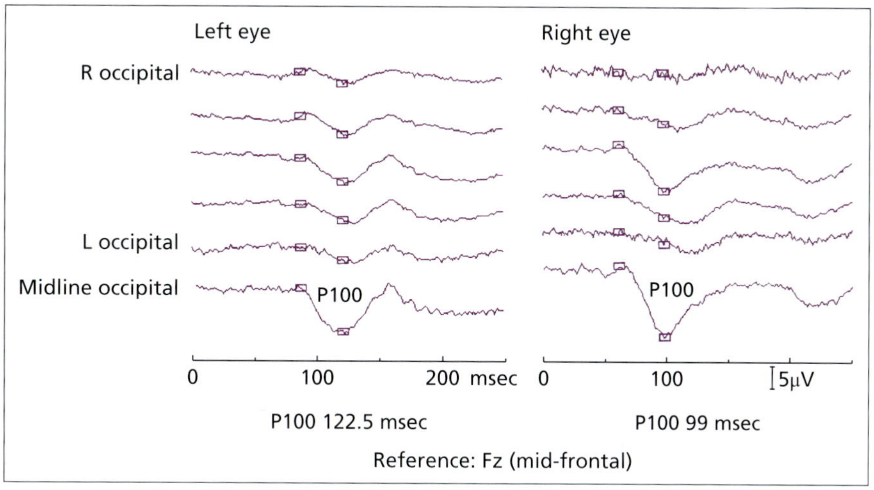

Figure 11.8 Visual evoked potential in left optic neuritis: delayed P100 waveform from left eye; normal response from right eye.

non-converting CIS as in those who develop multiple sclerosis. Anti KIR4.1 antibody (a potassium channel antibody) has been reported to be present in almost 50% of people with multiple sclerosis, but in only 1% with other neurological diseases and not at all in healthy controls, but this finding has not been reproduced in other studies.

Diagnostic criteria

Diagnostic criteria for multiple sclerosis have evolved over recent decades with the emergence and widespread availability of newer laboratory investigations that improve the accuracy of diagnosis, and allow it to be made earlier. However, an incontestable core requirement of all the criteria is objective clinical evidence for a disease affecting CNS white matter. Multiple sclerosis cannot be diagnosed in an asymptomatic individual based on MRI findings alone. The criteria also require evidence that the CNS white matter disorder is disseminated in space and time; where they vary is that the early criteria required clinical evidence for dissemination, whereas more recent criteria allow MRI evidence of dissemination. The evolution of diagnostic criteria over the last 50 years shows how experience of the use of new technology has changed the diagnostic process in patients with clinically suspected CNS demyelination.

Schumacher criteria

The diagnostic criteria of Schumacher *et al.* (1965) were an attempt to logically integrate dissemination in space and time based solely on clinical manifestations. Definite cases of multiple sclerosis were classed as having objective clinical evidence for disease affecting two or more regions of CNS white matter (dissemination in space), and occurring in episodes lasting at least 24 hours and separated by at least 1 month or with progression over 6 months (dissemination in time), in a person aged 10–50 years at onset and in whom no better explanation could be found by an experienced clinician. This clinically based description remains useful today, and while more detailed aspects of clinical, imaging and CSF findings should be appropriately focused on, one should always keep in mind the caveat 'there is no better explanation'.

Poser criteria

The Poser criteria (1983) retained the concept of at least two relapses with signs of a corresponding CNS white matter lesion in two or more locations as the basis for diagnosing clinically definite multiple sclerosis. They introduced laboratory features to strengthen the diagnostic classification in patients in whom clinical evidence suggested probable or possible multiple sclerosis but was insufficient to be certain, for example a patient with two relapses and clinical signs of one lesion could, with additional clinically silent evoked potential abnormalities (and silent MRI lesions when MRI became widely available subsequent to the criteria being published in 1983), be considered as definite multiple sclerosis. The Poser criteria gave particular weight to the evidence provided by CSF oligoclonal bands indicating an immunological disorder of the CNS. Thus, a patient with two relapses and signs of single CNS lesion plus unmatched CSF oligoclonal bands was classified as laboratory supported definite multiple sclerosis.

McDonald 2001 criteria

The major change in practice leading to further revisions of the Poser criteria was the widespread use of MRI and the emerging evidence that certain imaging features were suggestive of multiple sclerosis. In particular, Barkhof and Tintore had shown that in patients with CIS, three or four of the following brain MRI features had a high specificity for developing clinically definite multiple sclerosis:

- >9 T2 or ≥ 1 gadolinium-enhancing lesions
- >3 periventricular lesions
- >1 juxtacortical lesions, and
- >1 infratentorial lesions.

The International Panel that developed the McDonald 2001 diagnostic guidelines adopted the Barkhof–Tintore criteria as evidence for dissemination in space with the modification that one cord lesion could substitute for one brain lesion. The Panel also proposed an alternative, non-evidence based criterion for dissemination in space: two T2 lesions and the presence of CSF oligoclonal bands. They also had a complex MRI requirement for dissemination in time, erring on the side of caution, defined as either a gadolinium-enhancing lesion occurring at least 3 months after the clinical onset or a new T2 lesion shown to have developed more than 3 months after clinical onset. It was thus possible, for the first time, to use imaging evidence for dissemination in space and time to diagnose multiple sclerosis in patients with a single clinically manifest CNS lesion (CIS), but the MRI occurrence of new disease activity had to be at least 3 months following the CIS.

McDonald 2005 criteria

The 2001 criteria were criticised by some as being too liberal – the argument being that anything other than clinically definite mutiple sclerosis would run the risk of false positive diagnoses – and by others as being too conservative – the argument being that because patients with CIS with multiple MRI lesions have a high likelihood of developing clinically definite multiple sclerosis, they may as well be diagnosed as multiple sclerosis at presentation.

When the 2001 criteria were applied to two natural history cohorts that had been recruited with a CIS, from specialist centres, and were being followed up with serial clinical and MRI evaluation, they were found to have a high specificity and positive predictive value for development of clinically definite multiple sclerosis over the next 3 years. However, sensitivity of the early dissemination in time criterion – a gadolinium-enhancing lesion after 3 months – was low. One study reported that allowing a new T2 lesion at 3 months of follow-up (many of which must have occurred within 3 months of clinical onset) increased sensitivity without compromising specificity. The substitution of a single spinal cord lesion for a brain lesion had a negligible effect on performance of the criteria in patients with isolated optic neuritis, although substituting all visible cord lesions for an equivalent number of brain lesions considerably increased sensitivity of the Barkhof–Tintore criteria for dissemination in space in patients at the time of multiple sclerosis diagnosis.

A reconvened International Panel in 2005 made revisions to the MRI criteria for dissemination in space and time. These allowed any number of cord lesions to substitute for a brain lesion, and a gadolinium-enhancing cord lesion to substitute for an enhancing brain lesion. They also allowed for any new T2 lesion occurring more than 30 days after clinical onset to constitute evidence for dissemination in time. The criteria affirmed that there must be objective clinical evidence for a CNS lesion (i.e. an abnormality on neurological examination). A suggestive symptom alone (e.g. Lhermitte's symptom) was considered insufficient.

McDonald 2010 criteria

Application of the 2005 criteria to a multicentre European CIS cohort indicated that they retain a high overall specificity, and that dissemination in time is more specific than dissemination in space per se. However, the criteria were criticised for several reasons. First, the inclusion of a gadolinium-enhancing lesion as evidence for dissemination in space was illogical as it is actually a feature of lesion activity. Secondly, the counting of lesions (a total of nine brain lesions, or three in a periventricular location) was cumbersome in clinical practice. Thirdly, the dissemination in time criteria still imposed a delay to diagnosis, and there would often need to be three scans before a new T2 lesion qualified as evidence (i.e. the first at presentation with a CIS, a second 30 days or more later and a third scan at a still later time to show the qualifying new lesions). Through the work on the European (MAGNIMS) collaboration, simplified criteria for dissemination in space and time were developed and when implemented in a multi-center CIS cohort were found to have a high sensitivity and specificity for development of clinically definite multiple sclerosis. These criteria were adopted in the 2010 McDonald criteria and are as follows:

- *Dissemination in space:* one or more clinically silent T2 lesions involving at least two of four locations that are characteristic for multiple sclerosis: juxtacortical, periventricular, infratentorial and spinal cord.
- *Dissemination in time: either* a new T2 lesion seen on any follow-up scan regardless of the timing of the baseline scan in relation to CIS onset *or* both gadolinium-enhancing and non-enhancing lesions on a single scan.

The 2010 criteria continue to require clinical evidence of a process that involves CNS white matter. This will normally be confirmed by objective neurological examination although an historical episode that is highly suggestive of demyelination, but for which examination findings are not available, may qualify. The alternative dissemination on space criteria of two T2 lesions and oligoclonal bands are no longer included.

Diagnostic criteria for primary progressive multiple sclerosis

The diagnosis of primary progressive multiple sclerosis can be problematic. The differential diagnosis is different from relapse onset presentation: it is, most often, the differential diagnosis of a progressive spastic paraplegia or a progressive brainstem/cerebellar syndrome, in order the two most common presentations of primary progressive multiple sclerosis. Experience with the performance of MRI and/or CSF findings in two large cohorts with a diagnosis of primary progressive multiple sclerosis has helped to inform diagnostic guidelines. The McDonald 2010 criteria for primary progressive require that there has been a progressive CNS syndrome for at least 1 year, and two of three of the following.

- Evidence for dissemination in space in the brain based on one or more T2 lesions in at least one area characteristic for multiple sclerosis: juxtacortical, periventricular, infratentorial.
- Evidence for dissemination in space in the spinal cord based on two or more T2 lesions in the spinal cord.
- Positive CSF (isoelectric evidence of oligoclonal bands and/or elevated IgG index).

The MRI lesions should be asymptomatic in the case of a progressive brain stem or spinal cord syndrome, there should be no better explanation and in patients with a progressive myelopathy, an alternative structural disorder of the cord should always have been excluded by spinal MRI (Table 11.4).

Radiologically isolated syndrome

From time to time, patients with non-specific symptoms such as headache are found on MRI to have lesions that are typical for demyelination and that fulfill the MRI component of the McDonald criteria for multiple sclerosis. The term radiologically isolated syndrome has been used to describe such individuals. Radiologically isolated syndrome is not included in the McDonald diagnostic criteria as the requirement for having clinical evidence for demyelination is not satisfied. However, it is known from sequential autopsy series that clinically silent multiple sclerosis occurs: in series reported in Canada and Denmark in the 1980s, the frequency was about 1 in 500–1000, which approximates to the frequency of clinically manifest disease in these countries. Recent follow-up of cohorts with a radiologically isolated syndrome has reported the development of clinical manifestations of demyelination in about one-third after 5 years. It is prudent that such individuals are counselled about the association of such MRI findings with multiple sclerosis and offered follow-up.

Differential diagnosis

The differential diagnosis of multiple sclerosis is wide and a myriad of neurological disorders can mimic the varying manifestations of the condition. The differential diagnosis can be considered in terms of diseases that cause:

- A single episode of neurological disturbance which can be focal involving a single site (e.g. optic nerve or spinal cord), or multi-focal

Table 11.4 Differential diagnosis of a progressive spinal cord syndrome.

Tumour
Intramedullary – glioma, ependymoma
Intradural – meningioma, neurofibroma
Extradural – metastasis
Compression (non-tumour)
Vertebral spondylosis/disc prolapse/collapse
Arnold–Chiari malformation
Inflammatory
Multiple sclerosis
Vasculitis
Sarcoidosis
Infectious
HTLV-1
HIV
Syphilis
Schistosomiasis
Tuberculosis
Brucellosis
Metabolic
Vitamin B_{12} deficiency
Copper deficiency
Phenylketonuria
Vitamin E deficiency
Cerebrotendinous xanthomatosis
Degenerative
Amyotrophic lateral scelerosis
Primary lateral sclerosis
Vascular
Dural arteriovenous malformation
Cavernous haemangioma
Paraneoplastic
Hereditary
Hereditary spastic paraplegia
Adrenomyeloneuropathy
Friedreich's ataxia
Toxic
Nitrous oxide
Lathyrism

HTLV, human T-lymphotropic virus type 1.

- Relapsing neurological disturbance which can be focal or multi-focal, or
- Progressive neurological disturbance which can be focal or multi-focal.

The differential diagnoses of some of the most common presentations are given in Tables 11.4, 11.5, 11.6 and 11.7, although such lists are necessarily selective and incomplete.

Table 11.5 Differential diagnosis of optic neuritis.

Clinically isolated syndrome suggestive of multiple sclerosis
Anterior ischaemic optic neuropathy
Temporal arteritis
Vasculitis
Sarcoidosis
Neuromyelitis optica
Chronic relapsing inflammatory optic neuritis
Syphilis
Viral infection
Leber's hereditary optic atrophy
Compression/tumour
Raised intracranial pressure
Vitamin B_{12} deficiency
Tobacco-alcohol amblyopia
Susac's syndrome
Neuroretinitis
Eales' disease
Central serous retinopathy
Paraneoplastic optic nerve/retinal disease

Table 11.6 Differential diagnosis of an acute spinal cord syndrome.

Spinal cord compression
Transverse myelitis
Clinically isolated syndrome suggestive of multiple sclerosis
Acute disseminated encephalomyelitis
Neuromyelitis optica
Acute necrotizing myelitis
Infectious (viral, tuberculosis, syphilis, mycoplasma, fungal, parasitic) / post-infectious
Vasculitis
Sarcoidosis
Vascular
Spinal cord infarction
Spinal cord haemorrhage

The diagnostic process

It is important that the diagnostic process is centred on the needs of the individual with multiple sclerosis. The diagnostic phase is an anxious time, and delay in diagnosis and poor communication is a common cause for complaint. People want a clear and accurate diagnosis and access to appropriate support and information. National guidelines make recommendations for best practice during the diagnostic process. However, there is still wide variation in the services provided throughout the United Kingdom and diagnosis often occurs in a random and unsupported manner. This can be partly explained by the over-stretched medical services, but forward planning and reorganisation of

Table 11.7 Differential diagnosis of relapsing CNS neurological disturbance.

Inflammatory
Multiple sclerosis
Neuromyelitis optica
Recurrent optic neuritis/transverse myelitis
Systemic lupus erythematosus
Sjögren's syndrome
Behçet's disease
Sarcoidosis
Primary angiitis of the CNS
Susac's syndrome
Vascular
Recurrent transient ischaemic attack/stroke
CADASIL
Cerebral amyloid angiopathy
Fabry's disease
Antiphospholipid syndrome
Vasculitis
Primary angiitis of the CNS
Systemic lupus erythematosus
Sjögren's syndrome
Behçet's disease
Sarcoidosis
Susac's syndrome
Mitochondrial disease
MELAS
Chronic infections
Lyme disease
HIV encephalitis
Syphilis
HTLV-1
Subacute sclerosing panencephalitis
Whipple's disease
Brucellosis
Fungal/parasitic infections
Migraine
Migraine aura
Familial hemiplegic migraine
Epilepsy
Focal seizures
Todd's paresis

CADASIL, cerebral autosomal dominant arteriopathy with subcortical infarcts and leukoencephalopathy; HTLV-1, human T-lymphotropic virus type 1; MELAS, mitochondrial encephalopathy, lactic acidosis and stroke-like episodes.

services could address this problem. There is some evidence that a coordinated diagnostic clinic facilitates an efficient, supportive and cost-effective setting to manage the diagnostic phase. However, the diagnostic model will depend on the locally available expertise and resources. The clinical nurse specialist has been a key development in recent years and is well placed to facilitate the diagnostic process.

Management

In recent years, clinical guidelines have been published that aim to improve the standards of care provided to people with multiple sclerosis. Notably in the United Kingdom, the National Institute for Health and Care Excellence (NICE) published guidelines on the management of multiple sclerosis in 2003 and these were updated in 2014. Health and social care professionals involved in the care of people with multiple sclerosis should be aware of current evidence-based practice in order to optimise the standard of management. People with multiple sclerosis should be encouraged to participate fully in decisions on their management. Management requires a comprehensive and multidisciplinary approach addressing medical, functional, psychological and social aspects of the disease and interventions should be responsive and timely (Table 11.8). Management strategies are required to:

- Provide education and support
- Manage acute relapses
- Modify the course of the disease, and
- Treat symptoms and provide rehabilitation.

Education and support

Education and support are an integral part of management from the time of diagnosis and throughout the disease course (Table 11.9). Individuals should be provided with information regarding multiple sclerosis, and specific information relating to their disease type and its management. This will facilitate their active participation in their own management. Multiple sclerosis specialist nurses have an essential role in this in the United Kingdom, and can provide individualised educational and supportive sessions. Health care professionals work closely with voluntary organisations to provide educational materials such as information booklets, teaching manuals to explain the biology of multiple sclerosis and online decision-making aids for choosing disease-modifying therapies. The Multiple Sclerosis Society in the United Kingdom also coordinates educational programmes, such as Getting to Grips courses for newly diagnosed individuals.

Management of acute relapses

Management of acute relapses should be comprehensive, addressing all aspects of the relapse. Multi-disciplinary input may be required, particularly if recovery is less than complete. The first step is to assess whether new or increased symptoms are caused by a relapse of multiple sclerosis.

Assessment

In the event of new or increased symptoms, people with multiple sclerosis should be able to identify and contact a health care professional who can advise or direct them to the most appropriate local service. A formal assessment should be made to diagnose a relapse as early as possible. The possibility of another medical cause for the increase in symptoms must be considered. It is important that an infective cause such as a urinary tract infection, which can be otherwise clinically silent, is excluded. The possibility of dual neurological pathology (e.g. a compressive lesion mimicking a spinal cord relapse) should also be considered. If the new symptoms are thought to be unrelated to multiple sclerosis, access to the appropriate service and treatment should be facilitated.

It is essential that the service provided is flexible and responsive to the unpredictable and acute needs of people experiencing a

Table 11.8 Recommendations for comprehensive review (NICE 2014).

Ensure all people with MS have a comprehensive review of all aspects of their care at least once a year
Ensure the comprehensive review is carried out by healthcare professionals with expertise in MS and its complications. Involve different healthcare professionals with expertise in specific areas of the review if needed
Tailor the comprehensive review to the needs of the person with MS assessing: • MS symptoms ∘ mobility and balance including falls ∘ need for mobility aids including wheelchair assessment ∘ use of arms and hands ∘ muscle spasms and stiffness ∘ tremor ∘ bladder, bowel and sexual function ∘ sensory symptoms and pain ∘ speech and swallowing ∘ vision ∘ cognitive symptoms ∘ fatigue ∘ depression and anxiety ∘ sleep ∘ respiratory function • MS disease course ∘ relapses in last year. • General health ∘ weight ∘ smoking, alcohol and recreational drugs ∘ exercise ∘ access to routine health screening and contraception ∘ care of other chronic conditions • Social activity and participation ∘ family and social circumstances ∘ driving and access to transport ∘ employment ∘ access to daily activities and leisure. • Care and carers ∘ personal care needs ∘ social care needs ∘ access to adaptations and equipment at home
Refer any issues identified during the comprehensive review of the person with MS to members of the MS multidisciplinary team and other appropriate teams so that they can be managed
Ensure people with MS are offered a medication review
Ensure people with MS have their bone health regularly assessed and reviewed
Ensure people with MS and severely reduced mobility are regularly assessed and reviewed for risk of contractures
Check people with MS and severely reduced mobility at every contact for areas at risk of pressure ulcers
Discuss the care provided by carers and care workers as part of the person's care plan. Ensure carers know about their right to a local authority carer's assessment and how to apply for one
Refer people with MS to palliative care services for symptom control and for end of life care when appropriate

Table 11.9 Providing information and support for multiple sclerosis (MS) (NICE 2014).

Information at the time of diagnosis The consultant neurologist should ensure that people with MS and, with their agreement their family members or carers, are offered oral and written information at the time of diagnosis. This should include, but not be limited to, information about: • What MS is • Treatments, including disease-modifying therapies • Symptom management • How support groups, local services, social services and national charities are organised and how to get in touch with them • Legal requirements such as notifying the Driver and Vehicle Licensing Agency and legal rights including social care, employment rights and benefits
Discuss with the person with MS and their family members or carers whether they have social care needs and if so refer them to social services for assessment. Ensure the needs of people with MS are addressed
Offer the person with MS a face-to-face follow-up appointment with a healthcare professional with expertise in MS to take place within 6 weeks of diagnosis
Ongoing information and support Review information, support and social care needs regularly. Continue to offer information and support to people with MS or their family members or carers even if this has been declined previously
Ensure people with MS and their family members or carers have a management plan that includes who to contact if their symptoms change significantly
Explain to people with MS that the possible causes of symptom changes include: • Another illness such as an infection • Further relapse • Change of disease status (e.g. progression)
Talk to people with MS and their family members or carers about the possibility that the condition might lead to cognitive problems
When appropriate, explain to the person with MS (and their family members or carers if the person wishes) about advance care planning and power of attorney

relapse. The demands on general neurology and medical services often make this difficult. One model to address this issue is to set up a specialist relapse clinic to assess and manage acute episodes. A dedicated telephone line to the specialist service can also facilitate direct access.

Treatment

If a relapse has been diagnosed, treatment to hasten the recovery from the relapse should be considered. Steroid therapy is the only recommended drug treatment. NICE guidelines recommend that steroid therapy should be offered if the relapse affects ability to perform routine tasks.

Steroid therapy It has been established that steroid therapy can accelerate the recovery from a relapse, although a long-term benefit has not been proven. Its precise mode of action is uncertain but there are several potential mechanisms, including reduction of oedema, stabilisation of the blood–brain barrier, reduction of pro-inflammatory cytokines and induction of T-cell apoptosis. Efficacy was suggested in early studies with intramuscular adrenocorticotrophic hormone (ACTH), but this practice has been discontinued. Intravenous methylprednisolone, which is now widely used, has been proven to hasten recovery, and to be as effective as ACTH. The comparative efficacy of intravenous and oral steroid therapy has been more contentious. The largest study to address this issue, the Optic Neuritis Treatment Trial, was a randomised placebo controlled study in acute optic neuritis that compared intravenous methylprednisolone, followed by oral prednisone, with oral prednisone alone. Visual recovery was accelerated in the intravenous group, but not in the lower dose oral group. No benefit in long-term visual outcome was seen in either group. An increased rate of new attacks of optic neuritis was seen in the oral prednisone group, and a reduction in the rate of development of multiple sclerosis was reported in the intravenous group at 2 years. However, the beneficial effect of treatment on the development of multiple sclerosis was not sustained at follow-up of 3 years and longer. More recently, a large randomised controlled non-inferiority study showed that oral high dose methylprednisolone was not inferior in improving disability scores than intravenous methylprednisolone for acute relapses of multiple sclerosis and had a similar safety profile.

NICE guidelines recommend oral methylprednisolone 0.5 g/day for 5 days for the treatment of relapse of multiple sclerosis. Intravenous methylprednisolone 1 g/day for 3–5 days should be considered as an alternative for people in whom oral steroids have failed or not been tolerated, or who need hospital admission for a severe relapse or monitoring of conditions such as diabetes or depression.

Steroid therapy can have side effects and, although their incidence is low, the potential risks as well as benefits should be discussed with the individual. Adverse events from intravenous methylprednisolone in the short-term include taste disturbance, facial flushing, insomnia, psychiatric disturbance, exacerbation of acne and transient hypertension and hyperglycaemia. Steroid therapy can exacerbate infection, which should be excluded before treatment, and urinalysis to rule out urinary tract infection should be performed routinely. Urinary dipstick testing is a rapid screening technique with strong negative predictive value; if infection is suggested, co-treatment with antibiotics may be considered to avoid delay in steroid therapy while the result of urine culture is awaited. Gastrointestinal disturbance, such as peptic ulceration, can be exacerbated. Therefore it is prudent to screen for a history of any other risk factors and cover with a gastric acid inhibitor may be required. Long-term complications are rare with intermittent intravenous steroid therapy, but prolonged courses of oral steroids are more likely to assume the risks of long-term therapy. The relationship between pulsed steroids and osteoporosis has not been established, although osteoporosis can be seen as a result of impaired mobility. Serious complications, such as avascular necrosis, rarely occur.

Other therapies No other immunomodulating therapies are routinely recommended for the treatment of acute relapses. Placebo controlled trials of intravenous immunoglobulin (IVIG) in addition to intravenous methylprednisolone have demonstrated no significant benefit over methylprednisolone alone. A small randomised controlled trial of plasma exchange in patients with acute severe neurological deficits caused by demyelinating diseases, which had failed to respond to steroid therapy, showed improvement in some patients. Plasma exchange can be considered in the event of a catastrophic acute relapse that has not responded to steroid therapy.

Supportive measures Management of acute relapses should be comprehensive, addressing all consequences of the relapse and not just limited to steroid therapy. Practical supportive measures, such as the provision of care or equipment, may be required. Specific treatment for new symptoms is sometimes necessary, but if the relapse is responding to steroids or improving spontaneously the duration of symptoms may be too short to warrant treatment. Symptomatic treatment can be required for symptoms that persist, or that are distressing even for a short period such as trigeminal neuralgia.

Multi-disciplinary input from neurological rehabilitation services may facilitate the functional recovery from a relapse, and such input should run in parallel with any medical treatment. A randomised controlled trial showed that a multi-disciplinary rehabilitation approach was superior to a standard ward routine in people with multiple sclerosis receiving pulsed intravenous steroid therapy. Inpatient rehabilitation can also be beneficial, particularly in people with incomplete recovery from relapses with moderate to severe disability.

Disease-modifying therapy

Developing strategies to modify the course of multiple sclerosis requires an understanding of the underlying pathogenic mechanisms. Although these mechanisms are not fully understood, it is evident that inflammatory demyelination predominates in early disease and that neuroaxonal loss advances over time. Possible therapeutic strategies include:

- Immunomodulation to prevent or reduce inflammatory relapses
- Neuroprotection to prevent or slow disease progression
- Remyelination and repair to reverse neurological deficit and prevent disease progression.

Immunomodulation can be most useful in early disease. Neuroprotection and remyelination are plausible strategies for later disease, but can also be useful in early disease. The currently available therapies all seem to work through immunomodulation and the reduction of relapse activity. No therapies have been proven to be effective for relapse independent progression or to have a primary neuroprotective or reparative mechanism.

Currently available therapies

In the last two decades, a number of therapies have been shown to reduce relapse activity in multiple sclerosis. This is a major step forward in the management of multiple sclerosis but it is not without controversy as, although beneficial effects on relapses and disease progression can be seen in the short-term, the long-term effects on progression of disease and disability remain unproven. Furthermore, the treatments are expensive and their cost-effectiveness continues to be a cause for debate.

Interferon β and glatiramer acetate have been conventional first line disease-modifying therapy in relapsing remitting multiple sclerosis for more than a decade. There has also been a role for mitoxantrone as induction or rescue therapy in patients with rapidly progressive relapsing remitting or secondary progressive multiple sclerosis. However, alternative management strategies are now evolving as therapies with superior efficacy have become available. The licensing of the monoclonal antibody natalizumab marked a new development in disease modification of relapsing remitting multiple sclerosis. Natalizumab and the more recently licensed alemtuzumab are significantly more effective than conventional disease-modifying therapy, but this is tempered by life-threatening adverse events. Although this shift to more aggressive management of multiple sclerosis may be daunting, it is bringing the management approach in line with that of other immune-mediated diseases such as rheumatoid arthritis. The licensing of fingolimod has been another landmark development, being the first oral disease-modifying therapy, soon followed by teriflunomide and dimethyl fumarate.

Interferon β and glatiramer acetate

Natural interferon β is a glycosylated protein, synthesised by fibroblasts, that has antiviral, immunomodulatory and antineoplastic effects. The original rationale for its use in multiple sclerosis was based on the hypothesis that the condition is triggered by an underlying viral infection. Although this has not been established as the mechanism of benefit, interferon β was shown to be effective in reducing relapses in multiple sclerosis. The precise mechanism of action of interferon β in multiple sclerosis is unclear and it is likely to involve several different effects that modify the immune response. Relevant immunological effects include improvement of suppressor T-cell function, increased production of anti-inflammatory cytokines and neutrotrophic and gliotrophic factors, and antagonism of the effects of interferon γ. Interferon β reduces T-cell migration by inhibition of matrix metalloproteinases and down-regulation of adhesion molecules, which can inhibit T-cell migration across the blood–brain barrier. Interferon β also has a direct effect on plasma cells, modulating IgG synthesis, which can stimulate natural interferon production by lymphocytes and inhibit T-cell proliferation.

There are three recombinant preparations of interferon β available: interferon β-1b, which is non-glycosylated and differs slightly in amino acid sequence from natural interferon β, and two preparations of interferon β-1a, which are glycosylated and identical in sequence to interferon β. They have all been investigated in randomised placebo controlled Phase III trials in relapsing remitting and secondary progressive disease and in clinically isolated syndromes.

Interferon β-1b

A randomised controlled trial of subcutaneous interferon β-1b (250 μg on alternate days) in relapsing remitting multiple sclerosis was the first Phase III trial of interferon β to be completed. There was a 34% reduction in annual relapse rate over 2 years, a reduction in relapse severity and an increased proportion of subjects remaining relapse free on treatment. On MRI, there was an 80% reduction in disease activity, as measured by number of active scans and new lesions, and a reduction in lesion load. Interferon β-1b has also been shown to delay conversion to multiple sclerosis and development of disability in subjects with clinically isolated syndromes.

The effect of interferon β-1b in secondary progressive multiple sclerosis has been less clear. A European Phase III trial reported a delay in the progression of disability of 9–12 months over 2–3 years in treated subjects both with and without superimposed relapses. MRI showed a reduction in lesion load and new lesion activity. The clinical results were not reproduced in a North American trial which showed no effect on disease progression, although positive effects were seen on relapse rate and MRI activity. A post hoc analysis attributed this discrepancy to the North American cohort being less clinically active and having fewer relapses.

Intramuscular interferon β-1a

A Phase III trial of intramuscular interferon β-1a (30 μg once weekly) in relapsing remitting multiple sclerosis demonstrated a reduction of relapse rate by one-third in the treated group. The trial was terminated early and in the smaller group of patients who had completed the 2 years of follow-up the reduction in relapse rate was 18%. Time to sustained disability progression was significantly greater in treated subjects. A reduction in enhancing lesions was seen on MRI. Intramuscular interferon β-1a has also been shown to delay conversion to multiple sclerosis in clinically isolated syndromes.

Intramuscular interferon β-1a (60 μg once weekly) had limited clinical effect in secondary progressive multiple sclerosis in a Phase III trial. A favourable effect was seen on one measure of disability progression, the Multiple Sclerosis Functional Composite, but this was largely because of effects on upper limb rather than locomotor function, and no effect was seen on the EDSS. There was a reduction in relapse rate and MRI lesion activity in the treated group.

Subcutaneous interferon β-1a

A Phase III trial of subcutaneous interferon β-1a (22 μg or 44 μg three times weekly) in relapsing remitting multiple sclerosis demonstrated a reduction in relapse rate by 27% in the low-dose and 33% in the high-dose groups over 2 years. Progression of disability was delayed in both treatment arms, with greater delay in the higher dose group. A reduction in active lesions and in lesion load was seen on MRI. Subcutaneous interferon β-1a (22 μg once weekly) has also been shown to delay conversion to multiple sclerosis in subjects with clinically isolated syndromes.

In secondary progressive multiple sclerosis, a Phase III trial showed no effect of subcutaneous interferon β-1a on progression of disability, although positive effects were seen on relapses and MRI activity.

Side effects The most common systemic side effect of interferon β is a transient post-dose flu-like reaction with symptoms such as fever, myalgia and headache. These symptoms tend to improve over time and are ameliorated by symptomatic treatment. Injection site reactions are common with the subcutaneous preparations. Abnormalities of liver enzymes and the blood count sometimes occur; although not commonly clinically significant, and blood parameters should be monitored. Rarely, an autoimmune hepatitis or thyroid disease can develop and nephrotic syndrome has been reported. An association with depression has been reported, and interferon β can be contraindicated if there is a history of severe depression. Monoclonal gammopathy should be excluded prior to treatment as systemic capillary leak syndrome has been associated with the administration of interferon β.

Neutralising antibodies Treatment with interferon β is associated with the production of neutralising antibodies (NAbs), which can reduce or abolish the bioavailability and efficacy of interferon β. The incidence of NAbs in the pivotal relapsing remitting studies at 2 years was 42% with interferon β-1b, 24% (22 μg) and 13% (44 μg) with subcutaneous interferon β-1a and 22% with intramuscular interferon β-1a. Subsequent studies suggest a lower incidence of NAbs for intramuscular interferon β-1a. The presence of NAbs has been shown to correlate with reduced clinical, MRI and biological markers of therapeutic efficacy. NAbs cross-react with all preparations of interferon β and so the effects cannot be avoided by switching preparation. Guidelines for NAb testing have been suggested but they are not universally accepted and the role of NAb testing in routine clinical practice remains unclear. NAbs sometime disappear with follow-up, but a persistent and high titre is more likely to be associated with loss of efficacy.

PEGylated interferon β

Conjugation of polyethylene glycol (PEG) to interferon β is a possible approach to reduce the frequency of dosing and side effects and to optimise the efficacy of interferon β. Several PEGylated preparations of interferon β are in development. A Phase III trial of PEGylated interferon β-1a reported a 35% reduction in relapse rate with a 2-weekly dosing regimen, and this preparation has been licensed.

Glatiramer acetate

Glatiramer acetate is a synthetic mixture of polypeptides containing four amino acids. Its exact mechanism of action is not clear but can involve induction of regulatory T cells, MHC blocking and T-cell receptor antagonism. It has also been suggested that its effects can be mediated by brain-derived neurotrophic factor. A randomised placebo controlled Phase III trial of subcutaneous glatiramer acetate (20 mg/day) in relapsing remitting multiple sclerosis demonstrated a 29% reduction in relapse rate in the treated group. Subsequently, a randomised controlled MRI study reported a reduction in enhancing lesions and accumulation of lesion load as well as a reduction in relapse rate.

Glatiramer acetate has been shown to delay conversion to multiple sclerosis in subjects with CIS. No placebo controlled trials of glatiramer acetate in secondary progressive multiple sclerosis have been reported; a Phase III trial in primary progressive multiple sclerosis was negative. A randomised controlled study of oral glatiramer acetate in relapsing remitting multiple sclerosis was negative.

Glatiramer acetate has a favourable side effect profile. A transient acute post-dose reaction with shortness of breath and palpitations can occur. Erythema and lipoatrophy can occur at the injection site, and lymphadenopathy has been reported.

A placebo-controlled trial of glatiramer acetate 40 mg three times a week showed a 34% reduction in relapses. In an open label comparative study with the standard dose, glatiramer acetate 40 mg three times a week had a significantly lower rate of injection-related adverse events and was perceived to be more convenient.

Comparative studies Comparative studies of different interferon β preparations have been carried out. A prospective study of subcutaneous interferon β-1b and intramuscular interferon β-1a found interferon β-1b to have a superior effect on relapses, disease progression and the development of new lesions on MRI. Subcutaneous interferon β-1a (44 μg three times a week) has also been reported to have greater efficacy, as evidenced on relapses and MRI lesion activity, than intramuscular interferon β1a (30 μg once weekly). This seems to indicate that the effects of interferon β are dose-related. This is supported by a study of low-dose subcutaneous interferon β-1a (22 or 44 μg once weekly) in relapsing remitting multiple sclerosis which showed no significant clinical effect.

Prospective studies comparing high dose subcutaneous interferons β-1a and β-1b with glatiramer acetate showed no significant difference in relapse activity.

In summary, interferon β and glatiramer acetate have been proven to reduce relapse rate in relapsing remitting multiple sclerosis by approximately one-third over 2–3 years, and to delay conversion to clinically definite multiple sclerosis in clinically isolated syndromes. Interferon β can reduce accumulation of disability through prevention of relapses but the effect appears modest. Conflicting results have been found in secondary progressive multiple sclerosis, but interferon β does not seem to have a significant impact on progression unrelated to relapses. Open-label follow-up studies have suggested that the benefit from treatment may be sustained, but no controlled studies are available to answer the question of whether interferon β and glatiramer acetate improve prognosis in the long term. Axonal loss, the pathological correlate of disability, can occur from first presentation and so it is suggested that early treatment can have a long-term protective effect but this remains unproven. Currently, there is insufficient evidence to draw conclusions as to the long-term efficacy of interferon β and glatiramer acetate therapy.

Prescribing guidelines All the interferon β formulations and glatiramer acetate are licensed in the United Kingdom for ambulatory individuals with relapsing remitting multiple sclerosis. Interferon β-1b is also licensed for secondary progressive multiple sclerosis with superimposed relapses. Prescribing in the UK National Health Service (NHS) is subject to strict clinical guidelines, produced by the Association of British Neurologists (ABN), and funding of treatment is governed by the Department of Health's Risk Sharing Scheme. Treatment with interferon β and glatiramer acetate is recommended in subjects with active multiple sclerosis, which is normally indicated by two relapses in 2 years. Updated guidelines also allow for treatment of clinically isolated syndrome when MRI evidence predicts a high likelihood of recurrent episodes.

Natalizumab

Natalizumab is the first monoclonal antibody to be licensed for use in multiple sclerosis. Monoclonal antibodies are a new class of biological agent designed to interact with specific target antigens and thus have highly selective effects on the immune system. Natalizumab is a recombinant humanised monoclonal antibody directed against α4-integrin, an adhesion molecule that is primarily expressed on T cells. Natalizumab blocks the adhesion of activated T cells with the vascular cell adhesion molecule, expressed on the luminal surface of vascular epithelium, and so prevents activated cells crossing the blood–brain barrier.

In a randomised placebo controlled Phase III trial over 2 years, intravenous natalizumab (300 mg monthly) reduced relapse frequency by 68%, delayed disease progression by 42% and reduced enhancing lesions by 92%. Natalizumab was generally well tolerated, although 4% of subjects developed a hypersensitivity reaction. Other side effects included fatigue and headache. Persistent anti-natalizumab antibodies developed in 6% of subjects and were associated with a decrease in efficacy. A randomised controlled Phase III trial of combination therapy of natalizumab and intramuscular interferon β-1a found superior efficacy compared with interferon β-1a monotherapy. However, two subjects on combination therapy developed progressive multifocal leukoencepahalopathy (PML) and one subject died, and another fatal case of PML occurred during natalizumab treatment for Crohn's disease.

A recent randomised placebo-controlled study has shown no benefit from natalizumab in secondary progressive multiple sclerosis.

Natalizumab-related PML Post-marketing surveillance has revealed further cases of PML occurring on natalizumab monotherapy. As of September 2015, over 140 000 subjects have received natalizumab with 585 confirmed cases of treatment-related PML and an estimated overall risk of 4.03/1000 patients. The following risk factors have been identified to be associated with an increased risk of PML:

- *Presence of anti-JCV antibodies:* JC virus must be present in an individual for PML to develop. A reliable and validated assay to detect anti-JCV antibodies is now available and can be used to identify individuals carrying the JC virus. The risk of developing PML is significantly increased in patients who are anti-JCV antibody positive compared to antibody-negative patients, although the absolute risk is small. The risk in patients who are antibody negative is not zero as the assay has a false negative rate of approximately 2.5%, and seroconversion can occur. The rate of seroconversion appears to be higher in patients on natalizumab and has been reported as 16% over 18 months.
- *Duration of treatment:* the risk of PML is increased in patients treated for more than 2 years. There is limited experience in patients who have received more than 4 years of treatment and so the risk with longer duration of treatment is not yet clear.
- *Prior immunosuppressant use:* the risk of PML is increased in patients with a history of prior treatment with an immunosuppressant (excluding corticosteroids, interferon β and glatiramer acetate).

Analysis of these risk factors has led to the development of an algorithm to stratify risk (Figure 11.9). The risk of PML is lowest in patients who are anti-JCV antibody negative, with a currently estimated risk of 0.1/1000 patients. The risk is highest in patients who are anti-JCV antibody positive, have a history of prior immunosuppressant therapy and a treatment duration of >24 months, with an estimated risk of 11.2/1000 patients. The anti-JCV antibody index is a quantitative measure which can allow further stratification of an individual's risk of PML.

PML can be fatal (in ~23% of cases) or cause severe disability. Early diagnosis of PML appears to improve outcome, and so vigilance to the symptoms and signs of PML is vital. Management consists of discontinuation of natalizumab. Plasma exchange to accelerate the removal of natalizumab has been used in the majority of cases. Immune reconstitution inflammatory syndrome (IRIS) occurs frequently following the removal of natalizumab, within days to several weeks, and can also cause disability or be fatal. IRIS is usually treated empirically with high dose corticosteroids.

Other side effects Hypersensitivity reactions, including serious systemic reactions, can occur, usually during or up to 1 hour after the infusion and patients should be observed over this time. Reactions can occur with any infusion, but are greatest with early infusions and with re-exposure after an extended period without treatment. Hypersensitivity reaction is a permanent contraindication to further treatment. Cases of liver injury have been reported and liver function should be monitored. No increased incidence in malignancy has been seen to date, and reports of skin cancer appear to be in keeping with background incidence.

Prescribing guidelines In view of the risk of PML, the licence for natalizumab has been restricted. It is licensed in Europe for individuals who have failed to respond to interferon β or those with rapidly evolving severe relapsing remitting disease, defined as at least two disabling relapses in 1 year and evidence of active disease on MRI (Table 11.10). Prescribing in the United Kingdom is subject to NICE guidelines and natalizumab is only recommended for individuals with rapidly evolving severe relapsing remitting multiple sclerosis. Patients should be informed of the risk of PML (and IRIS)

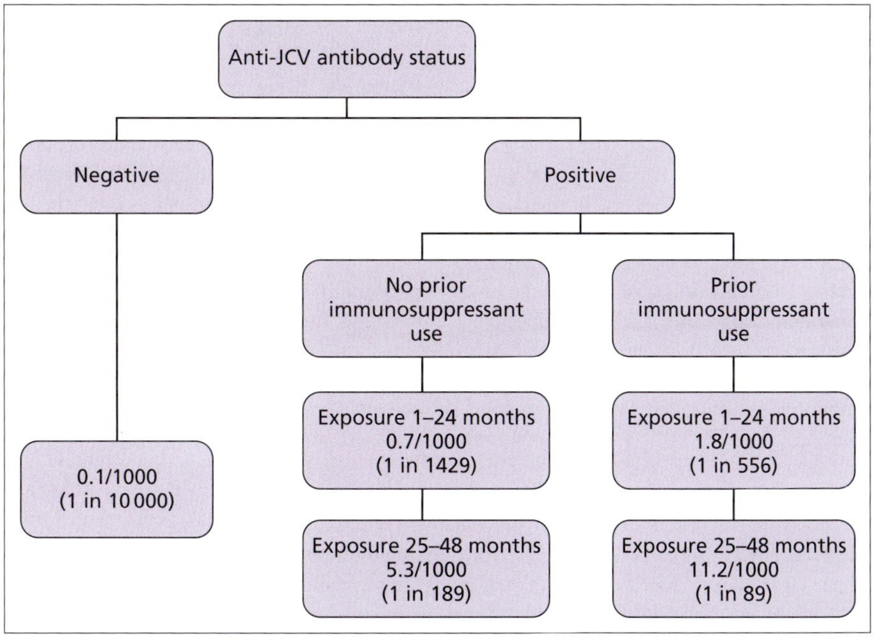

Figure 11.9 Risk stratification tool: risk of PML in patients exposed to natalizumab stratified according to presence of anti-JCV antibodies, prior immunosuppressant use and treatment duration. Source: Biogen Idec Medical Information Service 2014.

Table 11.10 Definition of rapidly evolving and severe relapsing remitting multiple sclerosis (NICE 2007).

Two or more disabling relapses in 1 year
and
One or more gadolinium-enhancing lesions on brain MRI
or
A significant increase in T2 lesion load compared with a previous recent MRI

with natalizumab, and that this risk increases after 2 years of treatment, and to be aware of the symptoms of PML and the need to report symptoms urgently. Informed consent to treatment should be obtained at initiation and if treatment is to be continued after 2 years. It is recommended that patients should be monitored with MRI within 3 months prior to starting natalizumab, annually during treatment, and if there any symptoms possibly indicative of PML. A wash-out period following previous immunosuppression is recommended.

Although there are currently no national guidelines incorporating risk stratification, this can be used to facilitate treatment decision-making in clinical practice. Testing for anti-JCV antibody should be offered prior to starting therapy, and re-testing of antibody negative patients every 6 months is suggested. It is also suggested that the frequency of MRI monitoring should be increased if anti-JCV antibody positive to a minimum of 6-monthly, and more frequently if the antibody index is high.

Fingolimod

Fingolimod is an oral immunodulatory agent derived from the fungal metabolite myriocin. It is phosphorylated *in vivo* and acts as an agonist of the sphingosine 1-phosphate receptor-1 on lymphocytes. This results in internalisation of the receptor, failure of lymphocyte egress and sequestration of lymphocytes in secondary lymphoid tissues, and so causes a reversible redistribution of lymphocytes. This reduces the infiltration of pathogenic lymphocytes into the CNS. Fingolimod crosses the blood–brain barrier and it has been suggested that it also can act via interaction with sphingosine 1-phosphate receptors on neural cells.

In a randomised placebo controlled Phase III trial of two doses of fingolimod (0.5 and 1.25 mg once daily) over 2 years, annualised relapse rate was significantly reduced by 54% with fingolimod 0.5 mg and 60% with 1.25 mg. Disability progression was reduced by 30% and 32% with fingolimod 0.5 and 1.25 mg, respectively. Significant effects were also seen on MRI activity with an approximately 75% reduction in new lesions and a 35% reduction in rate of brain volume loss. A randomised controlled Phase III trial over 1 year comparing fingolimod 0.5 and 1.25 mg with intramuscular interferon β-1a demonstrated a significantly reduced relapse rate on fingolimod, with the greatest reduction of 52% in the 0.5 mg group. Two fatal viral infections (disseminated primary varicella zoster and herpes simplex encephalitis) occurred in the 1.25 mg group. Other adverse events in the Phase III studies included transient bradyarrhythmias on initiation of treatment, non-fatal herpes virus infections, macula oedema, mild hypertension, elevated liver enzyme levels and lymphopenia. Skin cancers did occur, but the incidence of malignancies was not significantly raised. Post licensing, a few cases of serious viral infections, including PML, have been reported.

Prescribing guidelines Fingolimod (0.5 mg/day) is licensed in Europe for individuals with high disease activity despite treatment with interferon β or with rapidly evolving severe relapsing remitting multiple sclerosis. In the United Kingdom, NICE has recommended its use only for patients who have an unchanged or increased relapse rate or ongoing severe relapses compared with the previous year despite treatment with interferon β. The manufacturer also has to provide fingolimod with a discount as part of the UK NHS patient access scheme.

Since initial authorisation, an unexplained death in a patient within 24 hours of taking fingolimod has led to further regulatory advice on cardiovascular safety. Fingolimod is not recommended for patients with a history of cardiovascular or cerebrovascular disease or who take heart-rate lowering medication. On initiation of treatment, the electrocardiogram should be monitored before receiving the first dose and for at least 6 hours after. Vaccination against varicella zoster virus is recommended in antibody-negative patients prior to treatment. Monitoring of full blood count and liver function on treatment, and ophthalmological review for macula oedema are also recommended.

Teriflunomide

Teriflunomide is an oral agent that reversibly inhibits dihydroorotate dehydrogenase, an essential enzyme involved in pyrimidine synthesis, and decreases T and B-cell proliferation and function. Teriflunomide is the active metabolite of leflunomide which has been used in rheumatoid arthritis.

In a randomised placebo controlled Phase III trial of two doses of teriflunomide in relapsing multiple sclerosis with or without progression, annualised relapse rates were reduced by 31.2% in the 7 mg group and 31.5% in the 14 mg group. The risk of disability progression was reduced by 23.7% in the 7 mg group and 29.8% in the 14 mg group. An 80% reduction in enhancing lesions was seen on the higher dose, and a 25% reduction in brain atrophy was seen with both doses. The most common adverse events included diarrhoea, nausea, hair thinning and elevated liver enzyme levels. No serious opportunistic infections or increased incidence of malignancy were seen. In another placebo controlled Phase III trial, teriflunomide 14 mg reduced relapse rate by 36.3% and reduced disability progression by 31.5%, whereas teriflunomide 7 mg reduced relapse rate by 22.3% and showed no significant effect on disability. A randomised controlled Phase III trial of teriflunomide versus high-dose subcutaneous interferon β-1a showed no statistical superiority of either drug, but teriflunomide was better tolerated. The most common adverse events associated with teriflunomide in these studies included diarrhoea, nausea, hair thinning, headache, elevated liver enzyme levels and neutropenia. No serious opportunistic infections or increased incidence of malignancy were seen. Teriflunomide has also been shown to delay conversion to multiple sclerosis in clinically isolated syndrome.

Prescribing guidelines Teriflunomide is recommended for treating adults with active relapsing remitting multiple sclerosis, only if they do not have highly active or rapidly evolving severe relapsing remitting multiple sclerosis. The recommended dose is 14 mg once daily. Liver enzymes should be assessed before initiation of therapy, every 2 weeks during the first 6 months of treatment, and every 8 weeks thereafter or as clinically indicated. There is a serious risk of teratogenicity and a long washout period (2 years) or an accelerated elimination procedure is needed for women who wish to conceive having stopped treatment.

Alemtuzumab

Alemtuzumab is a humanised monoclonal antibody directed against CD52, a cell surface antigen expressed on >95% of T and B lymphocytes, as well as monocytes and macrophages, but not stem cells. Alemtuzumab causes prolonged lymphocyte depletion, including the autoreactive T cells that have a role in the pathogenesis of multiple sclerosis, while there is a reconstitution of B-cell numbers over several months. A small study in secondary progressive multiple sclerosis demonstrated a dramatic reduction in relapse rate and enhancing lesions but about half of the subjects still experienced progressive disability and increasing brain atrophy. Initial studies in relapsing remitting multiple sclerosis similarly showed a dramatic reduction in frequency of relapses and MRI activity, but there was also a favourable effect on disease progression. Therefore, it has been suggested that therapy may be most effective in early disease.

In a randomised controlled Phase III trial in subjects with previously untreated relapsing remitting multiple sclerosis over 2 years, intravenous alemtuzumab (12 mg/day for 5 days at baseline and 3 days at 12 months) was compared with high dose subcutaneous interferon β-1a. Alemtuzumab reduced relapse rate by 54.9% but, unlike the preliminary studies, no significant effect on disability progression was seen. A reduction in the proportion of subjects with enhancing and new lesions was seen, and alemtuzumab slowed brain volume loss by approximately 40%. In a Phase III trial over 2 years of alemtuzumab versus high dose subcutaneous interferon β-1a in subjects who had relapsed on interferon β or glatiramer acetate, alemtuzumab reduced relapse rate by 49.4% and reduced disease progression by 42%.

Infusion of alemtuzumab can cause an acute inflammatory response with pyrexia, malaise and rash, and can transiently exacerbate pre-existing neurological symptoms. Therefore, pretreatment with corticosteroids is recommended. Other adverse effects include infections and autoimmune complications. Infections have been predominantly of mild to moderate severity and include cutaneous herpes infections. Autoimmune thyroid disorders have been reported in one-third of subjects. There is an increased incidence of immune-mediated thrombocytopenia purpura, which can be life-threatening, and nephropathies, including antiglomerular basement membrane disease. An association with thyroid papillary carcinoma has been reported.

Prescribing guidelines Alemtuzumab is licensed in Europe for the treatment of adults with relapsing remitting multiple sclerosis with active disease defined by clinical or imaging features. The recommended dosage of alemtuzumab is 12 mg/day administered by intravenous infusion for two treatment courses. The initial treatment course lasts 5 consecutive days followed 12 months later by the second treatment course of 3 consecutive days. Patients should be pre-treated with corticosteroids immediately prior to administration, and given oral prophylaxis for herpes infection. Regular monitoring for early signs of autoimmune disease should be continued for 48 months following the last treatment course.

Dimethyl fumarate

Dimethyl fumarate is an oral fumaric acid ester. Fumaric acid esters have been used to treat psoriasis for several years and there has been evidence to suggest immunomodulatory effects. The mechanism of action of dimethyl fumarate has been proposed to be mediated through activation of the transcription factor Nrf2 antioxidant response pathway and experimental data have suggested anti-inflammatory and neuroprotective effects.

In a randomised placebo controlled Phase III trial of two doses of dimethyl fumarate (240 mg twice daily and 240 mg three times daily) in relapsing remitting multiple sclerosis over 2 years, a significant treatment effect was seen on the primary end-point of proportion of patients who had a relapse by 2 years. Annualised relapse rates were reduced by 53% in the twice daily dimethyl fumarate group and by 48% in the three times daily group, and the risk of disability progression was reduced by 38% and 34%, respectively. The number of new or enlarging lesions on MRI was reduced by 85% in the twice daily group and by 74% in the three times daily group. A randomised placebo controlled Phase III trial with an additional reference comparator group randomised to glatiramer acetate showed a similar treatment effect on relapses, with a 44% reduction in annualised relapse rate in the twice daily dimethyl fumarate group and 51% reduction in the three times daily group. However, no significant effect on disability progression was seen.

Previous experience of fumaric acid esters in the treatment of psoriasis has indicated a good safety profile with the main side effects being flushing and gastrointestinal symptoms, but PML has occurred rarely. In the Phase III trials, adverse events associated with dimethyl fumarate included flushing, gastrointestinal events and decreased lymphocyte counts. There were no opportunistic infections and no increased incidence of malignancy. Post licensing, a few cases of PML have been reported.

Prescribing guidelines Dimethyl fumarate is recommended for treating adults with active relapsing remitting multiple sclerosis, only if they do not have highly active or rapidly evolving severe relapsing remitting multiple sclerosis. The recommended dose is 120 mg twice daily in the first week of treatment and 240 mg twice daily thereafter. The frequency of flushing and gastrointestinal adverse reactions can be managed by temporarily (up to a month) reducing the dose to 120 mg twice daily.

To summarise the guidance for prescribing of the currently available disease modifying therapies for active relapsing remitting multiple sclerosis in the UK NHS:

- Interferon β, glatiramer acetate, teriflunomide, alemtuzumab and dimethyl fumarate are first line therapies.
- Natalizumab can be used first or second line in rapidly evolving severe disease.
- Fingolimod can be used second line following interferon β failure.

Initiation of treatment

It is widely accepted that treatment should be started as early as possible in eligible patients. Treatment should be initiated and supervised by a multiple sclerosis specialist neurologist, after careful and informed discussion with the individual and, where available, with nurse specialist support. The optimal strategy to approach treatment is not yet clear. One approach is to start with a less effective but less toxic therapy and, if there is continued disease activity, escalating to a more potent therapy. Alternatively, it may be decided to start the most effective therapy as early as possible. Treatment can now be aimed at not only suppressing clinical disease activity but also MRI activity, with a treatment goal of 'no evidence of disease activity'. The ABN has updated its guidelines for prescribing disease-modifying treatments in 2015 and its recommendations for starting treatment are summarised in Table 11.11. However, there remain considerable uncertainties concerning the appropriate indications for these new agents.

Table 11.11 ABN recommendations for starting disease-modifying treatment (after Scolding *et al.* 2015).

Eligible patients will normally be ambulant (maximum EDSS 6.5).
There are no treatments licensed for use during pregnancy

The currently licensed disease-modifying treatments divide broadly into two classes:

1 Drugs of moderate efficacy (Category 1)
- Interferon β
- Glatiramer acetate
- Teriflunomide
- Dimethyl fumarate
- Fingolimod

2 Drugs of high efficacy (Category 2)
- Alemtuzumab
- Natalizumab

Relapsing–remitting MS

Patients who have had two or more clinical relapses in the previous 2 years are considered to have 'active' disease that warrants consideration of disease-modifying treatments

Most are likely to start treatment with a Category 1 drug

Dimethyl fumarate and fingolimod are likely the more effective drugs in Category 1, with the advantage of being oral agents

More active relapsing–remitting MS

Patients can be classified as having more active MS by frequent clinical relapses and/or MRI activity either when untreated or while on a Category 1 drug

Recommend use a Category 2 drug

In individuals who are risk-averse or have infrequent minor relapses, it may be appropriate to change to another Category 1 drug

Clinically isolated syndrome

Consider treatment for individuals within 12 months of a significant clinically isolated syndrome, if MRI evidence establishes a diagnosis of MS or predicts a high likelihood of recurrent episodes, and perhaps particularly if CSF examination shows CNS-restricted oligoclonal immunoglobulin bands

Primary or secondary progressive MS

None of the current disease-modifying treatments is recommended in non-relapsing secondary progressive MS or in primary progressive MS

Some people with relapsing secondary progressive MS, whose relapses are their main cause of increasing disability, may benefit from disease-modifying treatment

Discontinuation of treatment

Deciding when to discontinue treatment is a difficult area in which evidence is lacking. The ABN recognises the importance of patient choice and that it is not feasible to have mandatory criteria which apply to all. It is recommended to consider stopping disease modifying therapy in the event of significant side effects (but to consider alternative treatment), the development of non-relapsing secondary progressive multiple sclerosis, and pregnancy.

Emerging therapies

The following therapies have demonstrated efficacy in Phase III trials but are not currently licensed.

Daclizumab Daclizumab is a monoclonal antibody targeted against the CD25 antigen, the IL-2 receptor alpha chain, and its effects can be mediated through blocking the expansion of autoreactive T cells or the expansion of regulatory natural killer cells. It is licensed for renal transplantation. In a randomised controlled Phase III trial, subcutaneous daclizumab 150 mg every 4 weeks reduced annualised relapse rate by 45%. The number of new or enlarging lesions was reduced by 54% and gadolinium-enhancing lesions by 65%. There was an increased risk of infection, rash, dermatitis and hepatic enzyme abnormalities.

Ocrelizumab Ocrelizumab is a humanised monoclonal antibody targeting CD20. It has previously been investigated in rheumatoid arthritis but study was discontinued because of opportunistic infections. In a placebo controlled Phase II trial of two doses of ocrelizumab (600 and 2000 mg), an 89% and 96% reduction in enhancing lesions and an 80% and 73% reduction in relapse rates were seen in the low and high dose groups, respectively. There was one death on high dose ocrelizumab as a result of systemic inflammatory response syndrome. Two Phase III studies of intravenous ocrelizumab (600 mg every 6 months) versus subcutaneous interferon β-1a in relapsing remitting multiple sclerosis have preliminarily been reported to reduce annualised relapse rates by up to 47%. A Phase III study of ocrelizumab in primary progressive multiple sclerosis has been preliminarily reported to reduce the risk of disability progression by 24%.

Other therapies

Mitoxantrone Mitoxantrone is a synthetic antineoplastic agent of the anthracendione family, with broad cytotoxic and immunomodulatory activity. It intercalates with DNA and inhibits DNA repair, and has immunosuppressive effects on proliferating cells, including T cells, B cells and macrophages. It also reduces pro-inflammatory cytokines and induces apoptosis and necrosis of B lymphocytes and monocytes. Two small trials initially suggested efficacy in relapsing remitting and secondary progressive subjects with very active disease, with a reduction in relapse rate and in enhancing lesions on MRI. A pivotal randomised placebo controlled trial of intravenous mitoxantrone (5 or 12 mg/m^2 3-monthly) for 2 years in worsening relapsing remitting and secondary progressive multiple sclerosis showed a significant effect of the higher dosage on a multivariate clinical measure, including a reduction in progression of disability and relapses.

Mitoxantrone is a potentially toxic agent. High cumulative doses impair ventricular function and can cause symptomatic cardiac failure. Treatment should not exceed a maximum cumulative dose of 140 mg/m^2 and monitoring of cardiac function is required throughout and following treatment. Mitoxantrone causes bone marrow suppression and leukopenia and the full blood count should be monitored. Treatment-related acute leukaemia occurs rarely; an incidence of 0.8% has been reported, but this may be higher with longer follow-up. Other side effects include nausea and vomiting, and alopecia, although usually mild. Amenorrhoea occurs in approximately one-quarter of women. It is usually transitory, but it is more likely to be permanent in older women, and women should be counselled regarding the possibility of infertility.

In view of the toxicity of mitoxantrone, its use should be restricted to subjects with aggressive and rapidly progressing disease. It is not licensed for multiple sclerosis in the United Kingdom, and there are no national prescribing guidelines. It is usually reserved for people who have failed or are not eligible for existing licensed disease-modifying therapies. In such circumstances it can be considered if there have been two relapses resulting in residual disability during the previous year, or documented substantial progression in disability over 1 year, and if there are new and enhancing lesions on MRI. However, its use in relapsing remitting multiple sclerosis is now largely superseded by natalizumab and other new agents.

The following non-licensed therapies have been investigated in multiple sclerosis, but are not routinely recommended because of insufficient evidence or side effects.

Azathioprine Azathioprine is a derivative of 6-mercaptopurine and acts as an antimetabolite to decrease DNA and RNA synthesis and therefore lymphocyte proliferation. Several randomised controlled trials of azathioprine have been carried out in multiple sclerosis. A meta-analysis confirmed a slight clinical benefit but debated whether this may be outweighed by side effects, which include hepatic and bone marrow toxicity.

Cladribine Cladribine (2-chlorodeoxyadenosine) is a purine nucleoside analogue. It acts as a prodrug and is activated through phosphorylation and its accumulation leads to apoptosis. It has a preferential effect on T and B lymphocytes and causes lymphocyte depletion. Initial exploratory study of subcutaneous cladribine had a favourable effect in relapsing remitting multiple sclerosis, but a randomised controlled trial of intravenous cladribine in progressive multiple sclerosis was negative. A placebo controlled Phase III trial of oral cladribine in relapsing remitting multiple sclerosis showed a significant reduction in annualised relapse rate and MRI activity. However, because of concerns about a small number of cancers and effects on the immune system, it has not been licensed in Europe or the United States and the manufacturer has withdrawn cladribine worldwide.

Cyclophosphamide Cyclophosphamide is a cytotoxic alkylating agent with immunosupppressant and immunomodulatory properties. It has been suggested that cyclophosphamide can suppress disease activity in patients with progressive disease, particularly with an active inflammatory component. Most studies have been uncontrolled and no benefit has been demonstrated on disability progression in small placebo controlled trials. The use of cyclophosphamide is also limited by side effects including leukopenia, bladder toxicity and increased risk of malignancy. A systematic review did not support its use in clinical practice.

Haematopoietic stem cell transplantation Autologous haematopoietic stem cell transplantation (HSCT) has been performed in people with progressive types of multiple sclerosis. No randomised controlled trials have been reported. In uncontrolled retrospective studies it is reported that about 60–70% of patients are progression-free, although study design precludes meaningful interpretation. Mortality was about 5–6% in early studies but in more recent years, as there has been a move away from high-intensity regimens, mortality rates have been about 1–2%.

HSCT is essentially a profoundly potent immunomodulatory therapy and so its use in progressive disease may be too late. A small uncontrolled study using a reduced-intensity regimen in patients with relapsing remitting disease reported at least stabilisation of progression in all patients. A larger multi-centre study is underway.

Intravenous immunoglobulin IVIG has been shown to have a beneficial effect on relapse rate and a significant reduction in enhancing lesions has been reported. IVIG is a blood product that is in scarce supply and so, with other agents of similar efficacy available, it is not widely used. A randomised controlled trial of IVIG in secondary progressive multiple sclerosis was negative.

Laquinimod Laquinimod is an oral formulation of quinoline-3-carboxamide. It appears to have immunomodulatory effects, reducing leukocyte infiltration into the CNS, and a neuroprotective effect has also been suggested. Two placebo controlled Phase III trials of laquinomod (0.6 mg once daily) in relapsing remitting multiple sclerosis showed only modest or non-significant reductions in annualised relapse rate. A positive effect on disability progression and significant reductions in brain atrophy were reported. Laquinimod has not been approved for use in relapsing remitting multiple sclerosis. Further studies of two doses of laquinimod (0.6 and 1.2 mg) in relapsing remitting multiple sclerosis and primary progressive multiple sclerosis are underway.

Methotrexate A small randomised controlled trial of low-dose oral methotrexate in progressive multiple sclerosis reported a favourable effect on progression on tests of upper limb function, but there is insufficient evidence to recommend its use.

Percutaneous venoplasty A small uncontrolled study suggested that chronic cerebrospinal venous insufficiency (CCSVI), caused by abnormalities in the internal jugular and azygous veins, is associated with multiple sclerosis, and proposed percutaneous venoplasty as a treatment for CCSVI. Findings from subsequent studies have been contradictory, and procedure-related deaths have occurred. NICE guidance has stated that the current evidence on efficacy is inadequate and the procedure should only be used in clinical trials. Multiple recent imaging studies that have included non-multiple sclerosis control subjects have found no significant association of CCSVI with multiple sclerosis.

Rituximab Rituximab is a chimeric monoclonal antibody directed against the CD20 antigen, which is expressed on B cells, and it causes depletion of B lymphocytes. It is already used in the treatment of B-cell lymphoma and rheumatoid arthritis. In a placebo controlled Phase II trial in relapsing remitting multiple sclerosis, rituximab halved relapse activity and significantly reduced gadolinium-enhancing lesions. The main adverse effects were infusion-associated events and about one-quarter of patients developed antibodies. Further investigation of rituximab in multiple sclerosis is not planned, but similar agents with less immunogenicity are being studied.

Negative studies Many other therapeutic trials have been carried out in multiple sclerosis and failed to show significant benefit. These include trials of hyperbaric oxygen, total lymphoid irradiation, sulfasalazine, oral myelin, anti-CD4 antibody, ustekinumab (a monoclonal antibody targeting interleukin-12/23) and dirucotide (a synthetic peptide analogue). There have also been therapies that have increased disease activity, including lenercept (a TNF neutralising agent) and atacicept (a B-cell targeted therapy), or caused unforeseen serious adverse events, such as cardiopulmonary toxicities with roquinimex.

Future immunomodulatory therapies

Monoclonal antibody therapies, directed at specific immune targets, remain among the most promising therapies for the future. Ofatumumab is a fully human monoclonal antibody which, like rituximab and ocrelizumab, targets CD20. Intravenous ofatumumab reduced MRI brain lesion activity by >99% in a Phase II study. A Phase II study of subcutaneous ofatumumab has been preliminarily reported to also significantly reduce MRI activity. Although monoclonal antibody therapies can be effective, in view of the associated immunological side effects, developing much smaller or more targeted agents is desirable. Firategrast is a small oral anti-α4β-integrin molecule and it has been shown to reduce gadolinium-enhancing lesions and to be well tolerated in a Phase II study.

Neuroprotection and remyelination

Most of the therapies investigated to date have primarily targeted the inflammatory response in multiple sclerosis. However, the role of acute inflammation mediated by a systemic adaptive immune response in the development of long-term axonal loss and permanent disability is not established and other potential mechanisms for chronic neuroaxonal loss exist. Therefore, it is also important to explore agents that can protect axons independently of acute inflammation and so prevent disease progression. Various neuroprotective agents have been suggested, including glutamate antagonists, sodium channel blockers, cannabinoids and statins. A protective effect of sodium channel blockers has been demonstrated in animal models, but a Phase II trial of lamotrigine in secondary progressive multiple sclerosis was negative. A Phase III trial investigating the neuroprotective effects of tetrahydrocannabinol in primary and secondary progressive multiple sclerosis has recently been reported to be negative. A significant beneficial effect of high dose simvastatin on brain atrophy, and small effects on measures of disability progression, has been preliminarily reported in a Phase II study.

Although it is hoped that the newer therapies, given in early disease, can have a beneficial effect on long-term outcome, therapeutic approaches are still required to address neuronal damage that has already occurred. Strategies to facilitate remyelination and axonal repair are being explored. Such therapeutic approaches include promotion of endogenous remyelination and stem cell replacement therapies. Various growth factors have been explored in animal models, but have not translated into clinical practice. Anti-LINGO-1 (leucine-rich repeat and Ig domain containing NOGO receptor interacting protein 1) antibody is a small domain-specific antibody which blocks inhibition of myelination and promotes remyelination in animal studies, and this is being evaluated further in clinical trials. Stem cell replacement therapies may be more promising, although there are a number of obstacles to overcome, not least how to replace cells in a disease that is disseminated throughout the CNS. Therapies can utilise embryonic stem cells or adult stem cells harvested from various sites. Clinical studies of autologous HSCT have been carried out, as discussed earlier, but have involved intensive immunosuppression which carries serious risks. Exploratory studies of autologous bone marrow derived mesenchymal stem cell therapy have been reported with no serious adverse events and evidence of neuroprotection has been suggested.

Disease-modifying therapy in primary progressive multiple sclerosis

Until recently, no treatment has been proven to modify the course of disease in primary progressive multiple sclerosis. Phase III trials of glatiramer acetate and rituximab found no significant clinical effect. Smaller trials of interferon β, mitoxantrone and riluzole have been negative or inconclusive. Ocrelizumab has preliminarily been reported to be the first drug to be beneficial in primary progressive multiple sclerosis, but peer-reviewed publication is still awaited.

Symptomatic treatment

Symptomatic treatment and rehabilitation remain essential elements of management and complement current disease-modifying therapies which have little impact on existing neurological impairment and disability. The evidence base for most symptomatic treatments is at best modest, although national management guidelines provide some limited direction. Symptomatic management can be challenging as people usually have multiple symptoms or functional deficits. Symptoms should not be considered in isolation, particularly as treatment of one problem can exacerbate or cause another, and management should take a holistic approach. This requires input from a wide range of health disciplines and draws on a variety of clinical resources, often best exemplified by specialised multidisciplinary clinics and inpatient or community-based rehabilitation. Education remains a fundamental component of management, and essential if successful self-management is the goal. The management of specific key symptoms is now discussed.

Fatigue

Fatigue is one of the most disabling symptoms of multiple sclerosis from the patients' perspective. Treatment is difficult and often unsatisfactory. Any treatable contributory factors such as disturbed sleep patterns because of nocturia, nocturnal spasms or pain and depression should be addressed. Fatigue can be worse as the day progresses. A fatigue management programme, addressing daily routine and conserving energy, is the mainstay of treatment. Graded aerobic exercise programmes can also be helpful. Symptoms may be worse in heat and humidity, which may need to be avoided, and some people can benefit from pre-cooling before undertaking activity.

Drug therapy can be considered, although the evidence for efficacy is limited. Amantadine, which has cholinergic, monoaminergic and glutaminergic effects on the CNS, has been reported to improve fatigue when compared with placebo, although the benefit is limited. Side effects include insomnia, hallucinations, gastrointestinal disturbance, dry mouth, livedo reticularis and peripheral oedema. Studies of modafinil, a central stimulating agent, have provided conflicting results and it is not recommended for use in Europe to treat conditions other than narcolepsy because of concerns about the risk of neuropsychiatric disorders, skin and hypersensitivity reactions, and cardiovascular side effects.

The potassium channel blocker 4-aminopyridine has been proposed to improve fatigue by potentiating synaptic transmission and improving nerve conduction. A beneficial effect on fatigue was initially suggested in small studies, but results were inconsistent. Other drug therapies, including pemoline and carnitine, have been suggested but there is little evidence to support their use.

Spasticity

Spasticity (Chapter 18) can cause stiffness, spasms, pain and contractures and as a result adversely affect mobility, seating, comfort, activities of daily living and care. Management should not primarily aim to abolish spasticity, but rather optimise function, alleviate pain and facilitate care. Management incorporates education, physical therapy, drug therapy and, very occasionally, surgery. A multi-disciplinary approach is essential. Exacerbating factors such as infection, constipation, pain and pressure ulcers must be identified and addressed, and it is important to educate the individual and carer to avoid such triggers. First line treatment is usually physiotherapy which can reduce tone without exacerbating weakness. Review of seating and bed positioning is often helpful. A home exercise or standing programme can be very valuable. Management should aim to prevent contractures but if they do occur, serial plaster casts, removable splints and standing programmes can all have a role in treatment.

Broadly speaking, spasticity is caused by disinhibition of spinal reflexes because of an upper motor neurone lesion and so drug therapies often target spinal pathways. Treatment should start with a small dose and be titrated up slowly until the desired effect is achieved or unacceptable side effects occur. Monotherapy is desirable. The most commonly used agent is baclofen, a chlorophenyl derivative of gamma aminobutyric acid (GABA) and a GABA β-agonist. It acts on pre- and post-synaptic receptors to potentiate spinal inhibition. The most common side effects are drowsiness and muscle weakness, which are particularly unwelcome in multiple sclerosis. Large doses can result in CNS and cardiorespiratory depression. Abrupt withdrawal should be avoided as it can cause rebound spasticity, hallucinations and epileptic seizures.

Gabapentin enhances GABA function and has been suggested to have a beneficial effect on spasticity in small placebo controlled studies. It is generally well tolerated, although side effects include sedation and dizziness. NICE guidelines recommend baclofen and gabapentin as first line drug agents for spasticity in multiple sclerosis.

Tizanidine acts through its α_2-adrenergic properties resulting in spinal inhibition. Placebo controlled trials have shown it to be effective in reducing spasticity. It has been reported that this is not associated with an increase in weakness, but there is little evidence for this in clinical practice. Side effects include dizziness, drowsiness, dry mouth, fatigue and hypotension. Hepatotoxicity can occur and liver function tests should be monitored during the first few months of treatment.

Dantrolene reduces muscle contraction via the inhibition of calcium release in muscle fibres. It acts peripherally and it can be used as an adjunct to a centrally acting drug. Side effects are common and include nausea, diarrhoea, weakness and fatigue. Irreversible hepatotoxicity can occasionally occur and liver function should be monitored closely. As less toxic drugs have become available, dantrolene is now rarely used.

Benzodiazepines, such as diazepam and clonazepam, reduce muscle tone through augmentation of the inhibitory effects of GABA. The use of benzodiazepines may be limited by their sedative effects but they can be useful as a short-term intervention or for treatment of nocturnal spasms.

Cannabinoids have generated much public interest and a beneficial effect on spasticity was initially reported in small studies. Their effect is mediated through cannabinoid receptors in the CNS. A large randomised placebo controlled trial of oral cannabis extract and the synthetic cannibinoid, delta-9-tetrahydrocannibinol, found no benefit on physician-based spasticity measures. There was an improvement in patient-reported spasticity measures, although they may have been affected by unmasking. Further randomised controlled trials of cannabis extract oromucosal spray have also reported a benefit on patient-reported measures of spasticity. Side effects include dizziness, disorientation and, rarely, psychiatric disturbance, gastrointestinal disturbance, increased appetite, dry mouth and oral ulceration. Cannabis extract oromucosal spray is licensed in the United Kingdom for people with multiple sclerosis with moderate to severe spasticity who have not responded

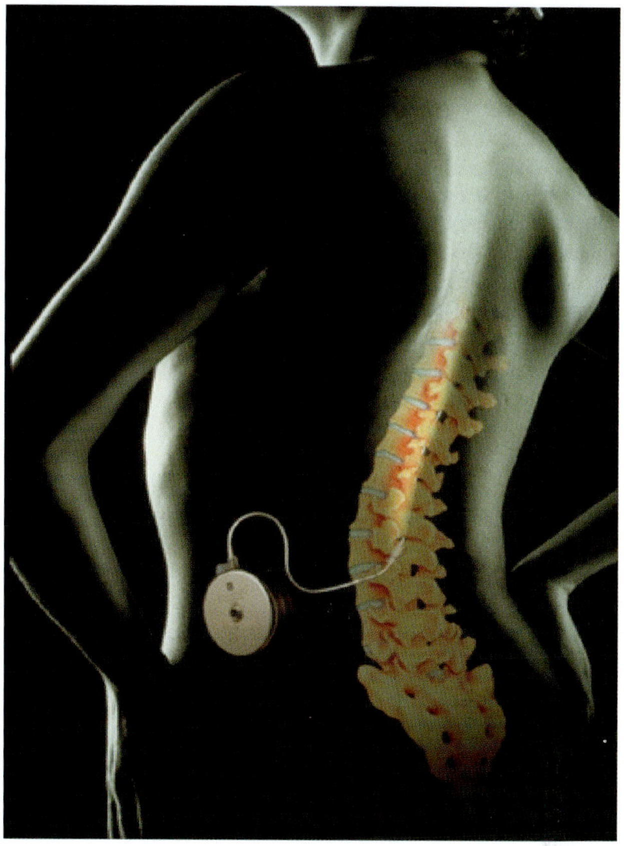

Figure 11.10 Abdominally placed baclofen pump and intrathecal catheter. Courtesy of Medtronic.

adequately to other antispasticity medication. An initial trial of therapy to demonstrate a significant response and a titration period to reach the optimal dose is required. It has proved useful in postponing more invasive management.

Oral spasticity agents can be limited by systemic side effects, particularly when high doses are required in severe spasticity. Locally administered agents, including intrathecal and intramuscular therapies, can therefore be helpful although they are more invasive. Such treatments should not be performed in isolation, and require a comprehensive approach with specialist multi-disciplinary input and monitoring.

For severe generalised spasticity, intrathecal therapies can be considered. Intrathecal baclofen directly targets the spinal receptors that mediate spasticity. Much smaller doses are required than orally and there is a reduction in systemic side effects. Baclofen is administered into the subarachnoid space via a catheter from an abdominally placed subcutaneous pump (Figure 11.10). The pump is externally programmable so that the regime of baclofen can be changed in response to clinical need; this flexibility is vital in a progressive disease such as multiple sclerosis. Long-term studies have indicated that intrathecal baclofen is an effective and well-tolerated treatment of spasticity. However, adverse effects, related to both the implanted device and the dosing, can occur and can rarely be life-threatening. Patients must be selected carefully and generally have severe spasticity resulting in severe functional disability or pain that has not responded to oral medication.

Intrathecal phenol can also be an effective treatment for spasticity in a small group of carefully selected patients. It causes indiscriminate nerve destruction, and damage to the sacral nerves can cause bladder, bowel and sexual dysfunction. However, it is a relatively simple procedure and is a useful option in severely disabled patients with existing loss of sphincter function and in whom the more complex treatment of intrathecal baclofen is not feasible.

For focal spasticity, intramuscular botulinum toxin can be useful. It reduces muscle activity through presynaptic neuromuscular blockade. Benefit has been reported in the treatment of distal limb spasticity. It is less helpful with spasticity in large muscles, although it can reduce leg adductor spasticity. It is maximally effective when used in combination with physiotherapy and a stretching exercise programme. Intraneural phenol injection is an alternative focal therapy but is now rarely used.

Surgery has a limited role in the current management of spasticity and techniques such as surgical rhizotomy are now little used. Surgical release of contractures can occasionally be required to improve comfort or function.

Weakness

Treatment for weakness should aim to optimise strength, endurance and function. Therapy-directed exercise programmes, including aerobic training, are the mainstay of treatment. Supportive measures, such as orthoses for focal weakness or specialist seating for postural weakness, should be provided as appropriate. Functional electrical stimulation can be of benefit for foot drop in selected individuals.

A recent large randomised controlled Phase III study of sustained-release 4-aminopyridine assessed its effect on walking ability. An improvement in walking speed was seen in 35% of subjects on active treatment, with an average improvement of 25%. Side effects include parasthesiae, dizziness, insomnia, anxiety, fatigue, nausea and seizures. Prescribing of 4-aminopyridine is not routinely funded in the United Kingdom, but can be considered for selected patients with severe walking disability who demonstrate a significant symptomatic improvement with a trial of therapy. It should not be used if there is a history of seizures or moderate to severe kidney problems.

Ataxia

Cerebellar ataxia is an extremely disabling symptom and is exceedingly difficult to treat. Truncal ataxia can adversely impact on walking, standing and even sitting, and limb tremor and dysmetria can restrict any limb function. Therapeutic options include physical therapy, drug therapy and surgery, although all have limited efficacy. Physiotherapy and occupational therapy are first line interventions and should address posture, seating and aids to improve function and safety. Drug therapy is usually unrewarding. Small studies or anecdotal reports of isoniazid, ondansetron, gabapentin, carbamazepine, propranolol, primidone, clonazepam and levetiracetam provide insufficient evidence to support their routine use in clinical practice. A small randomised controlled trial of targeted injection of botulinum toxin type A has reported a significant improvement in upper limb tremor.

Stereotactic thalamotomy and thalamic electrostimulation have been reported to be of benefit for tremor, particularly if proximal, although the evidence is limited and the interventions carry significant risks. Neurosurgery can be considered if tremor is severe and intractable. Gamma knife thalamotomy can be a less invasive alternative, and has been reported to induce functional improvement in tremor, but further study is required.

Bladder and bowel dysfunction

Bladder dysfunction in multiple sclerosis can result from detrusor hyper-reflexia and incomplete emptying. It is important to assess whether incomplete emptying is occurring before initiating treatment as this can be exacerbated by drugs for detrusor instability. This is carried out by measuring the post-micturition residual which can be measured simply by ultrasound. If the residual is >100 mL, clean intermittent self-catherisation should be considered. An external bladder stimulator can be tried in ambulatory individuals reluctant to self-catheterise.

If the residual is <100 mL, treatment should be directed at detrusor hyper-reflexia which can be treated successfully with antimuscarinic drugs. The most commonly used include oxybutynin, tolterodine and solifenacin. Side effects include dry mouth, which may be dose-limiting, constipation, blurred vision and fatigue. Desmopressin, usually administered intranasally, is an effective and well-tolerated treatment for nocturia and nocturnal enuresis; administered at bedtime it reduces diuresis overnight. It can also be used to reduce daytime urinary frequency (e.g. when travelling), but it must never be used more than once in 24 hours.

Detrusor injections of botulinum toxin type A have been shown to be highly effective for severe urgency and incontinence; its effect on bladder emptying usually requires clean intermittent self-catheterisation afterwards. Percutaneous and transcutaneous posterior tibial nerve stimulation have been reported to be beneficial for bladder overactivity, without compromising bladder emptying. Other nerve stimulation procedures, including sacral nerve root stimulation, can occasionally be considered.

If bladder symptoms are not controlled, despite the above measures, further assessment and advice from a specialist continence service should be sought. Supportive measures for urinary incontinence, such as reviewing toileting arrangements and considering a penile sheath or pads, should be offered. Pelvic floor exercises and encouraging regular bowel emptying can be beneficial. Education regarding the symptoms of urinary tract infections should be given, and infections should be treated with an appropriate antibiotic. If bladder dysfunction persists after other non-invasive measures have been tried, long-term indwelling catheterisation can be considered. Supra-pubic catheterisation is the preferred option, particularly if sexual function is active, and urethral catheterisation can cause long-term bladder neck and urethral damage. Surgical procedures such as urinary diversion or bladder augmentation may rarely have a role in refractory cases.

Bowel dysfunction may be less frequent than bladder dysfunction but is still common and can be difficult to treat. The most common symptoms are constipation, urgency and incontinence. Individuals with faecal incontinence should be assessed for constipation with overflow. It is important to establish a regular bowel regime. Maintaining an adequate fluid intake is advised, and increasing dietary fibre may be recommended although there is no specific evidence for this. Oral laxatives can be required. Bulking agents, such as ispaghula hulk, and osmotic laxatives, such as lactulose or polyethylene glycol, can be tried. Stimulant laxatives, such as senna and bisacodyl, can be used in more severe constipation. If constipation persists, the use of suppositories or enemas should be considered. Behavioural biofeedback therapy has been reported to be of benefit for constipation and faecal incontinence in small studies in multiple sclerosis. Transanal irrigation may be a potentially promising therapy. Surgical intervention such as stoma formation can be considered rarely in severe cases where other measures have failed.

Sexual dysfunction

Sexual dysfunction is a frequent but often neglected symptom. In males, the most common complaint is erectile dysfunction. Management has improved with the advent of phosphodiesterase inhibitors, such as sildenafil and tadalafil, which should be offered as a first line therapy. If ineffective, intracorporeal therapy with alprostadil (prostaglandin E1), administered as a urethral pellet, or papaverine can be used. In females, common symptoms include anorgasmia and decreased vaginal lubrication. Lubricants can be helpful, but drug therapy currently has little role. In both sexes any coexistent contributory factors such as depression, anxiety, diabetes, vascular disease and medications should be addressed. Counselling for individuals or couples should also be offered as appropriate.

Pain and paroxysmal symptoms

Pain occurs in the majority of people with multiple sclerosis. It can be neurogenic, as a consequence of direct involvement of central pain pathways, or it can be nociceptive, often musculoskeletal, caused by secondary complications of neurological impairment.

Chronic pain is common and includes dysaesthetic extremity pain, painful leg spasms and musculoskeletal back pain. Amitriptyline, gabapentin and pregabalin are often used for dysaesthetic extremity pain. Other anticonvulsants, including carbamazepine, lamotrigine and levetiracetam, opioid analgesics, mexilitene and intravenous ketamine and lidocaine can also be used. Painful leg spasms are best managed by treating the underlying spasticity. Musculoskeletal pain can result from abnormal posture and gait; physical therapy input is the first line of treatment, although anti-inflammatory drugs and other analgesics, electrical stimulation and tricyclic antidepressants all have a role in treatment. Cannabinoids have been reported to improve pain in multiple sclerosis. Although cannabis extract is not licensed for treatment of pain in the United Kingdom, it can be prescribed on a named patient basis. For intractable chronic pain, more invasive therapies such as intrathecal drug therapy, transcutaneous electrical nerve stimulation, spinal cord stimulation and deep brain stimulation can possibly be considered. Cognitive behavioural therapy can be helpful in selected individuals. Patients for whom pain is a major issue should be referred to a multidisciplinary pain clinic and not simply told they have to live with it.

A minority of people with multiple sclerosis experience acute and paroxysmal neurogenic pain. Lhermitte's symptom, tonic spasms and trigeminal neuralgia are the most common paroxysmal pains. Carbamazepine and gabapentin can be effective for trigeminal neuralgia and other anticonvulsants, baclofen and misoprostol have been used. Surgery can be considered for intractable trigeminal neuralgia but may be less successful than in idiopathic trigeminal neuralgia; percutaneous procedures may be preferred. Other painful, and non-painful, paroxysmal symptoms can also respond to carbamazepine, gabapentin and other anticonvulsants.

Cognitive and psychiatric dysfunction

Cognitive deficits are common in multiple sclerosis and can have a significant impact on all activities of daily living and quality of life. If symptomatic, a formal assessment of cognition should be offered and advice given regarding any implications of the results. In particular, cognitive dysfunction can affect employment and recognition of cognitive deficits allow adaptations to be made to enable the individual to maintain employment. Cognitive rehabilitation programmes can be of benefit, and techniques to assist memory, attention and executive function have been suggested, but are not widely available. Any other contributory factors such as medication or mood disturbance should also be addressed. Drug therapies are being investigated but are currently not recommended. Initial small studies of the anticholinesterase inhibitor donepezil in multiple sclerosis reported improvement in memory, but no significant benefit was seen in a larger randomised controlled trial. A recent small randomised controlled trial of the neurostimulant lisdexamfetamine dimesylate showed improvements in processing speed and memory in multiple sclerosis.

Psychiatric morbidity is increased in multiple sclerosis with depression and anxiety predominating. A lifetime prevalence of depression in multiple sclerosis of approximately 50% has been reported. People with low mood should be screened as to the severity of depression, and referred for specialist psychiatric input if depression is severe. There is a significant increased risk of suicide in multiple sclerosis, and it is important to be vigilant about suicidal ideation. Simple screening tools, such as the Beck Depression Inventory, can easily be incorporated into clinical practice. Contributory factors, such as pain or social isolation, should be reviewed. In mild to moderate depression and in anxiety disorders, counselling and cognitive behavioural therapy can be helpful. Antidepressant therapy can be effective in many patients but agents with anticholinergic effects can exacerbate bladder and bowel symptoms. Selective serotonin and noradrenaline re-uptake inhibitors appear to be effective for depression and anxiety and are well tolerated in patients with multiple sclerosis. There is an increased prevalence of bipolar affective disorder and psychotic disorders in multiple sclerosis; management is based on the treatment of these disorders in the general population. Emotional lability may be helped by tricyclic antidepressants and selective serotonin re-uptake inhibitors.

Visual dysfunction

Reduced visual function (Chapter 14) can occur as a result of optic neuritis, diplopia caused by ophthalmoplegia or oscillopsia from nystagmus. Drug therapy is of no help for permanent deficit from optic neuritis. Gabapentin and memantine have been reported to be of benefit in acquired nystagmus resulting from multiple sclerosis, but studies have been small. Prisms can be of some help in compensating for eye movement disorders. Visual function can also be improved by assessment in a low vision clinic and provision of adaptive equipment.

Vertigo

Vertigo can occur acutely as part of a brainstem relapse but may persist. In acute vertigo, which can be complicated by nausea and vomiting, vestibular sedatives such as prochlorperazine and cinnarizine are useful as well as supportive measures such as bed rest and rehydration. Vestibular sedatives should not be used in the long term as they may obstruct vestibular compensatory mechanisms. Vestibular rehabilitation physiotherapy, and supportive mobility aids as appropriate, have a role in the management of persistent symptoms.

Bulbar and respiratory dysfunction

Dysphagia is a common symptom and patients may most frequently describe coughing or choking on swallowing. Assessment by a speech therapist is at the core of management and advice on posture, eating patterns and diet is often helpful. In more severe cases, aspiration with the risk of chest infection can occur and individuals and carers should be alerted to this. Investigation with videofluoroscopy may be required. Further supportive measures such as the use of fluid thickening agents, provision of appropriate seating and chest physiotherapy are valuable. Percutaneous gastrostomy may be required if swallowing is unsafe or oral intake is insufficient.

Speech disturbance is usually caused by dysarthria. It may be helped by speech therapy. In severe disease, speech can become unintelligible or anarthric and communication aids are required.

Respiratory dysfunction resulting from respiratory muscle weakness is common, although often not symptomatic, in multiple sclerosis. More severe involvement can result from acute lesions in the medulla or high cervical cord, and respiratory insufficiency occurs in advanced disease. Respiratory muscle training can improve muscle strength and pulmonary function. Early recognition of respiratory complications is important and ventilatory support, including continuous positive airway pressure or non-invasive ventilation, is occasionally necessary.

Temperature sensitivity

Many people report a significant deterioration in function associated with an increase in temperature. Simple advice on heat avoidance, planning of activities around diurnal temperature variation and cooling should be given. Cooling garments can be of benefit for selected people. 4-Aminopyridine may improve function in patients with temperature sensitivity, but the evidence is very limited.

Neurological rehabilitation

Outpatient and inpatient neurological rehabilitation programmes can be an effective approach to the comprehensive management of many of the problems described above (Chapter 18). Although rehabilitation methods have not been evaluated as stringently as pharmacological therapies, there is now evidence to support their use. Randomised controlled studies have shown inpatient rehabilitation reduces disability and improves quality of life in multiple sclerosis. Benefits gained from inpatient rehabilitation may be maintained for several months, but carry-over of benefits declines over time, reinforcing the need for continuity of care into the community. However, in the only double-blind controlled trial of inpatient rehabilitation in multiple sclerosis no significant benefit was reported, although this perhaps reflects methodological issues and highlights the difficulties in evaluating rehabilitation methods. Outpatient multi-disciplinary rehabilitation has also been reported to reduce disability. Physiotherapy alone improves mobility and well-being in multiple sclerosis, with similar effects seen for outpatient and home physiotherapy, although the benefit may only last a few weeks. Exercise therapies have also been reported to have beneficial effects in multiple sclerosis including improvements in muscle strength and mobility.

In evaluating the efficacy of rehabilitation it is essential that the outcome measures used are valid, sensitive and reliable. Historically, outcome measures have been developed without the application of rigorous psychometric methods and have been disease-based. More recently, using standard psychometric methods, patient-based measures such as the Multiple Sclerosis Impact Scale (MSIS-29) and the 12-Item Multiple Sclerosis Walking Scale (MSWS-12) have been developed. Preliminary study has shown them to be reliable and responsive, and such measures should facilitate the assessment of rehabilitation in multiple sclerosis.

Symptomatic treatment and rehabilitation in multiple sclerosis is not just limited to addressing physical and cognitive impairments but should encompass the social and psychological needs. The different requirements of people with long-term neurological conditions, including multiple sclerosis, have been set out in the National Service Framework (NSF) for long-term conditions (Table 11.12). Among these requirements, vocational rehabilitation and palliative care are specifically highlighted.

Table 11.12 Quality requirements for the management of long-term neurological conditions (Department of Health 2005).

1	A person-centred service
2	Early recognition, prompt diagnosis and treatment
3	Emergency and acute management
4	Early and specialist rehabilitation
5	Community rehabilitation and support
6	Vocational rehabilitation
7	Providing equipment and accommodation
8	Providing personal care and support
9	Palliative care
10	Supporting family and carers
11	Caring for people with neurological conditions in hospital or other health and social care settings

Vocational rehabilitation

Work is a central activity for most adults and contributes to financial and social status. People with multiple sclerosis face restrictions in their ability to work leading to loss of employment. Factors relating to the disease and relating to the job and work environment affect the ability to work. Disease-related factors are not just confined to physical impairments but also include cognitive impairments and fatigue. The need for access to vocational rehabilitation has been highlighted, but specialist vocational rehabilitation services remain scarce. A focus group based study found that people with multiple sclerosis identified two key needs in the workplace: managing performance and managing expectations. It was suggested that people with multiple sclerosis required support to address the interaction of their impairments, workplace environment and demands of the work, and to provide expert knowledge about employment issues and legislation, and counselling and support to manage complex issues.

Palliative care

Palliative care (Chapter 26) services have traditionally addressed the needs of people with cancer and terminal illness. In recent years, there has been a shift within these services to also provide support for people with non-terminal long-term conditions. The NSF highlights the need for access to palliative care services for people in the later stages of long-term neurological conditions. Palliative care services have particular expertise in symptom control, provision of social, psychological and spiritual support, and end of life care. There should be multi-disciplinary working across neurology, rehabilitation and palliative care services and staff involved in the care of people with advanced disease should be trained in palliative care skills. A survey of consultants in neurology, rehabilitation and palliative care has found that there is a shortfall in provision of palliative care services, and a lack of coordination between services. A randomised controlled trial of delivering specialist palliative care to people severely affected by multiple sclerosis found positive effects on key symptoms and improvement in caregiver burden in the short term. Further work is required to develop palliative care services specific to the needs of people with multiple sclerosis.

Complementary and alternative medicine

Use of complementary and alternative medicine in multiple sclerosis is common, with at least one-third of people having tried at least one therapy. Although some therapies have been subject to controlled trials, the evidence base for most therapies is at best limited and insufficient to make definite recommendations. Cannabis has been one of the most extensively investigated therapies, as discussed, and there is limited evidence for dietary supplements such as linoleic acid. As many people will decide to use complementary and alternative medicine, access to accurate information should be available to assist decision making. It is particularly important that people are encouraged to evaluate any risks, both financial and health-related. Information is provided by voluntary organisations such as the MS Society and the MS International Federation.

Neuromyelitis optica

Neuromyelitis optica (NMO), also known as Devic's disease, is an inflammatory demyelinating disease of the CNS. Although historically there has been debate as to whether NMO is a variant of multiple sclerosis, recent advances have shown that NMO is immunologically and pathologically distinct from multiple sclerosis and requires different treatment.

Epidemiology

The median age of onset of NMO is in the late thirties, but there is a wide age range from childhood to late adulthood. Females are more commonly affected than males in a ratio of >3 : 1. The prevalence of NMO has been reported as 0.3–4.4/100 000, with an incidence of 0.05–0.4/100 000, in different populations worldwide. NMO is much rarer than multiple sclerosis in Europe and North America. It can affect all ethnic groups but it makes up a greater proportion of demyelinating diseases in non-Caucasian populations. The optico-spinal variant of multiple sclerosis, which is common in Japan, has been found to be associated with the NMO specific aquaporin-4 antibody suggesting that it is the same disease as NMO.

Familial occurrence of NMO occurs in about 3% of cases. Familial cases are clinically indistinct from sporadic cases. HLA associations with increased risk of NMO have been reported, including DRB1*0301 in Caucasian and DPB1*0501 in East Asian populations. NMO susceptibility is not significantly related to variations in the aquaporin-4 gene.

Pathophysiology

An autoimmune basis to NMO has long been suspected because of the association with autoimmune diseases such as SLE, Sjögren's syndrome and thyroid disease. In 2004, a new autoantibody, NMO-IgG, was reported to be highly specific for NMO and to distinguish it from multiple sclerosis. The target antigen of NMO-IgG is aquaporin-4 (AQP4), a cell membrane water channel which is important in maintaining water homeostasis and widely distributed in the CNS. AQP4 is highly expressed in astrocytic foot processes, particularly in direct contact with pia and capillaries. AQP4 antibody is approximately 75% sensitive for NMO and >90% specific.

The specificity of AQP4 antibody suggests a direct pathological role for the antibody. Experimental data indicate that AQP4 antibody binds to AQP4 in astrocytic foot processes and causes complement-dependent cytotoxicity. Astrocyte destruction appears to be the primary pathology and leads to secondary oligodendrocyte loss and demyelination and ultimately to axonal loss. Pathological data also provide support for this distinct pathophysiology. NMO lesions show peri-vascular inflammation with prominent complement and immunoglobulin deposition in keeping with a role for humoral immunity. Myelin may be preserved in early NMO lesions, whereas acute fragmentation and loss of glial fibrillary acid protein-positive astrocytes has been reported to be pathognomonic for NMO. *In vivo* magnetic resonance spectroscopy of the NMO lesions in the cervical cord has shown a reduction in the concentration of the glial cell marker myo-inositol, consistent with loss of astrocytes.

Clinical features

The hallmark features of NMO are episodes of optic neuritis and transverse myelitis. Concurrent optic neuritis and transverse myelitis occurs in a minority of patients. Optic neuritis is often rapidly evolving with severe visual loss, with recovery far less complete than in multiple sclerosis. Bilateral optic neuritis can occur, either simultaneously or sequentially over a few days. Transverse myelitis also develops rapidly and is often symmetrical and bilateral, with motor and sensory involvement. It often progresses to a severe paraparesis or quadriparesis with loss of bladder and bowel function. High cervical cord involvement can cause respiratory failure. Severe optic neuritis or transverse myelitis should alert to the possibility of NMO rather than multiple sclerosis. However, it is increasingly recognised that mild episodes of optic neuritis and transverse myelitis are also a presentation of NMO.

Other neurological features have previously been considered rare in NMO. However, with the availability of testing for AQP4 antibody as a biomarker of NMO, the spectrum of clinical phenotypes has expanded. Other characteristic clinical presentations include hiccups and vomiting caused by medullary involvement, and somnolence and endocrinopathies as a result of hypothalamic involvement. Presentations because of large cerebral hemisphere lesions and posterior reversible encephalopathy syndrome can also be seen.

Clinical differences have been reported between AQP4 seropositive and seronegative patients. The female predominance is not seen in seronegative disease. Seronegative patients are more likely to present with bilateral optic neuritis or simultaneous optic neuritis and transverse myelitis than seropositive patients, can have less severe attacks and are more likely to have a monophasic course.

Investigations

MRI has an important role in the investigation and diagnosis of NMO. In transverse myelitis, MRI of the spinal cord characteristically shows an intrinsic spinal cord lesion extending contiguously over three or more vertebral segments (Figure 11.11). Lesions typically occur in the cervical and thoracic cord, and there can be extension into the caudal medulla. Lesions are located centrally, and acute lesions can occupy most of the cross-sectional area and are often associated with cord swelling, T1 hypointensity and gadolinium enhancement. This appearance contrasts with multiple sclerosis where partial myelitis is usually associated with small, focal, asymmetrical and often superficial cord lesions that are T2 hyperintense but not T1 hypointense and that rarely extend over more than one segment. Following the acute phase, spinal cord atrophy may develop.

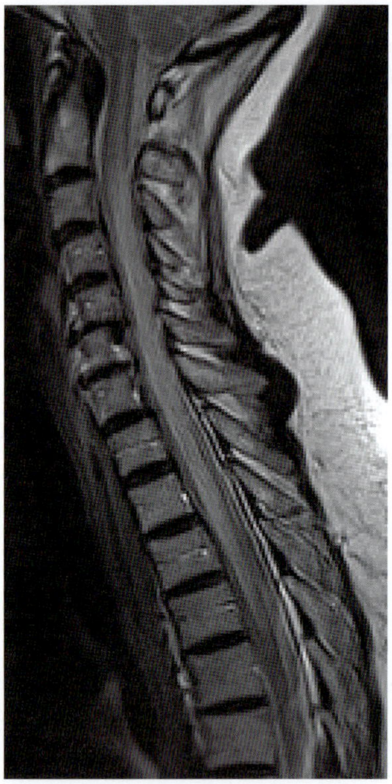

Figure 11.11 Longitudinally extensive spinal cord lesion in neuromyelitis optica (MRI T2W sagittal).

MRI of the brain can be normal, particularly at initial presentation, but brain lesions are seen in the majority of patients during the course of the disease. Lesions in the hypothalamus and peri-aqueductal brainstem region are considered typical for NMO. Non-specific white matter lesions can often be seen, but the brain lesions may fulfill radiological criteria for multiple sclerosis in a significant proportion of cases. However, thorough inspection of the morphology and distribution of brain lesions can distinguish multiple sclerosis from NMO and periventricular and juxtacortical lesions are more characteristic for multiple sclerosis. Large and extensive cerebral lesions can occasionally also occur in NMO.

MRI in optic neuritis shows an intrinsic lesion in the affected nerve and acute lesions are often associated with swelling and gadolinium enhancement. Optic nerve lesions can be more extensive than typically seen in multiple sclerosis, and posterior nerve and chiasmal involvement may be more common.

CSF examination is often abnormal particularly in the acute presentation. There can be a CSF pleocytosis, which is usually mononuclear, but neutrophils can be present and may predominate. A cell count of >50/mm^3 is not uncommon, and should alert that the diagnosis may not be multiple sclerosis. CSF protein is usually mildly elevated. Unmatched oligoclonal bands are present in less than one-third of cases and, unlike multiple sclerosis, their presence can be transient.

Testing for AQP4 antibody is now widely available and is an essential investigation in patients with suspected NMO. Second generation recombinant AQP4 antigen-based assays have been reported to yield the highest sensitivities (up to 87%). The role of testing for other putative biomarkers in seronegative NMO is not yet established, but myelin-oligodendrocyte glycoprotein antibodies have been reported in a few cases.

Table 11.13 Neuromyelitis Optica Spectrum Disorders (NMOSD) diagnostic criteria for adult patients.

Diagnostic criteria for NMOSD with AQP4-IgG:
- At least one core clinical characteristic
- Positive test for AQP4-IgG using best available detection method (cell-based assay strongly recommended)
- Exclusion of alternative diagnoses

Diagnostic criteria for NMOSD without AQP4-IgG or with unknown AQP4-IgG status
- At least two core clinical characteristics occurring as a result of one or more clinical attacks and meeting all of the following requirements:
  - at least one core clinical characteristic must be optic neuritis, acute myelitis with LETM, or area postrema syndrome
  - dissemination in space (two or more different core clinical characteristics)
  - fulfillment of additional MRI requirements, as applicable
- Negative tests for AQP4-IgG using best available detection method, or testing unavailable
- Exclusion of alternative diagnoses

Core clinical characteristics
- Optic neuritis
- Acute myelitis
- Area postrema syndrome: episode of otherwise unexplained hiccups or nausea and vomiting
- Acute brainstem syndrome
- Symptomatic narcolepsy or acute diencephalic clinical syndrome with NMOSD-typical diencephalic MRI lesions
- Symptomatic cerebral syndrome with NMOSD-typical brain lesions

Additional MRI requirements for NMOSD without AQP4-IgG or with unknown AQP4-IgG status
- Acute optic neuritis requires brain MRI showing
  - normal findings or only non-specific white matter lesions, *or*
  - optic nerve MRI with T2-hyperintense lesion or T1-weighted gadolinium-enhancing lesion extending over>½ optic nerve length or involving optic chiasm
- Acute myelitis requires associated intramedullary MRI lesion extending over
  - ≥3 contiguous segments (LETM), *or*
  - ≥3 contiguous segments of focal spinal cord atrophy in patients with history compatible with acute myelitis
- Area postrema syndrome requires associated dorsal medulla/area postrema lesions
- Acute brainstem syndrome requires associated periependymal brainstem lesions

LETM, longitudinally extensive transverse myelitis
Source: Wingerchuk *et al.* 2015. Reproduced with permission of AAN/LWW.

Diagnostic criteria

With the discovery of AQP4 antibody, diagnostic criteria have been revised to include seropositivity and have been widely adopted. The criteria have been updated in 2015 and no longer refer to NMO but use the unifying term NMO spectrum disorders (NMOSD; Table 11.13). NMOSD is stratified further by the presence or absence of AQP4 antibody. Core clinical characteristics are required for diagnosis, but the occurrence of both optic neuritis and transverse myelitis is not necessary for a diagnosis of NMOSD.

Course and natural history

Although initially described as a monophasic disorder, the clinical course of NMO is relapsing in about 80–90% of cases. AQP4 seropositivity predicts a high risk of relapse, and the majority of seropositive patients may relapse within the first year. Many patients acquire severe and permanent disability with the initial attack, and recurrent attacks result in accumulating disability. Before the current era of early diagnosis and treatment, over half of patients were functionally blind in at least one eye or were unable to walk without assistance within 5 years. Mortality rates of approximately 30% within 5 years were also reported, but recent data suggest that mortality rates with longer follow-up are now <10%. The development of a secondary progressive phase is, unlike multiple sclerosis, very uncommon.

Management

Acute attacks of NMO necessitate early and aggressive treatment. First line treatment is high-dose intravenous methylprednisolone followed by maintenance oral prednisolone. In patients with acute severe attacks unresponsive to high-dose steroids, the next step is plasma exchange. Efficacy of plasma exchange in acute attacks of demyelinating disease including NMO has been demonstrated in a small randomised controlled trial.

In patients with relapsing NMO and in those with a first attack who are AQP4 seropositive, long-term immunosuppression for relapse prevention is indicated. The evidence for immunosuppressive therapies for relapse prevention in NMO is limited to retrospective and open-label studies, but their use is widely accepted in clinical practice. First line therapies include azathioprine, mycophenolate and methotrexate, in combination with oral prednisolone. If patients relapse on a therapeutic dose of first line therapy, rituximab is often used, which causes depletion of B cells and so may be expected to be useful in an antibody-mediated disease. Other second and third line therapies include mitoxantrone (although this cannot be used in the long-term because of the risk of cumulative cardiotoxicity), cyclophosphamide, ciclosporin and maintenance pulsed plasma exchange or IVIG. The importance of correct diagnosis is emphasised by reports that the multiple sclerosis disease modifying therapies of interferon β, natalizumab and fingolimod can make NMO worse.

The nationally commissioned NMO UK service has proposed a treatment algorithm for management of NMO (Figure 11.12). For patients with a single episode of longitudinally extensive transverse myelitis and negative AQP4 antibody, long-term immunosuppression is not recommended unless there is a relapse, although it has been suggested to continue maintenance oral prednisolone for a few months.

Potentially more disease-specific therapies such as the monoclonal antibodies eculizumab, which neutralises complement C5, tocilizumab, which targets the IL-6 receptor, and aquaporumab, a protective AQP4 binding antibody, are being explored.

In view of the significant symptoms and disability that can develop in NMO, symptomatic treatment and rehabilitation are

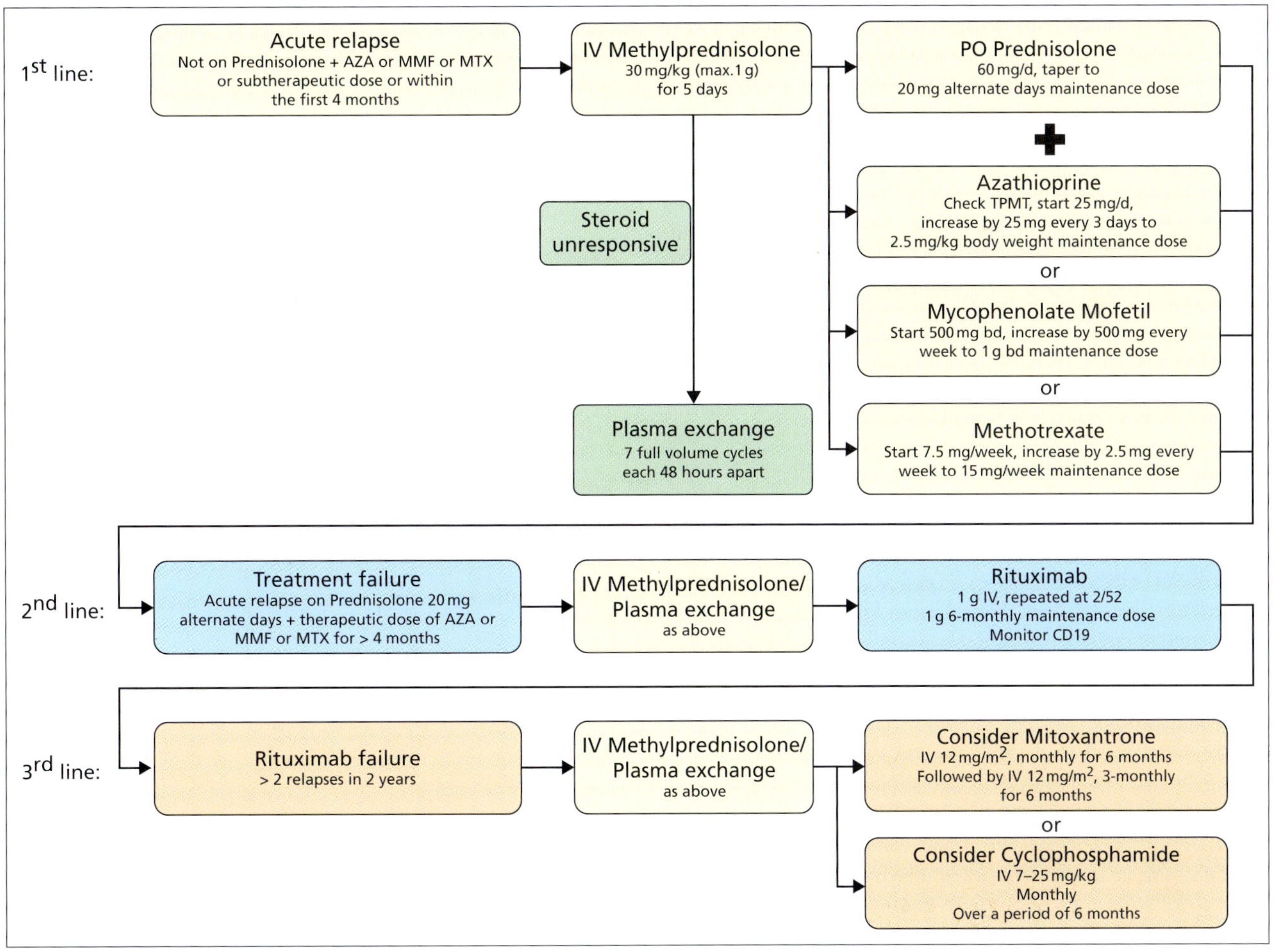

Figure 11.12 Neuromyelitis optica treatment algorithm. Source: Neuromyelitis Optica UK Service. (Courtesy of Dr J. Palace)

essential aspects of management. Management principles are the same as for multiple sclerosis, but it is important to be aware of and to treat symptoms that occur commonly such as hiccups, vomiting, tonic spasms and pain.

Acute para-infectious inflammatory encephalopathies

Acute para-infectious encephalopathies are typically monophasic encephalitides characterised by multifocal inflammatory lesions, principally affecting the white matter of the CNS. There are two consistently distinguishable pathological subdivisions: acute disseminated encephalomyelitis (ADEM) and acute haemorrhagic leukoencephalitis (AHL).

Acute disseminated encephalomyelitis

ADEM classically occurs in children and young adults. The mean age of onset in paediatric studies is reported as 5–8 years. It typically follows a febrile illness or vaccination by 1–4 weeks, often after the exanthem clears and the initial fever abates. ADEM is most frequently associated with childhood exanthemas particularly measles, rubella and varicella but other infections including mumps, enterovirus, EBV, herpes simplex virus, cytomegalovirus, HHV-6, HTLV-1, adenovirus, influenza A and B, *Mycoplasma*, *Chlamydia*, *Borrelia*, *Listeria*, *Leptospira* and beta-haemolytic streptococcus have all been implicated. Post-vaccination ADEM occurs less frequently. It has been particularly associated with rabies vaccine, notably the Semple neural vaccine, but has rarely been reported with the measles, pertussis, diphtheria, tetanus, rubella, Japanese B encephalitis, typhoid and hepatitis B vaccines.

Clinical features

The onset is usually with a low-grade fever, headache and meningism preceding the development of drowsiness and encephalopathy which can progress to stupor and coma. Neurological deficits are typically multi-focal and include seizures, hemiparesis, paraparesis, ataxia, visual loss, sensory disturbance, dysphasia, cranial nerve palsies, choreoathetosis, myoclonus and sphincter disturbance. ADEM evolves rapidly over hours to days. It is rarely fulminant, with acutely raised intracranial pressure leading to tentorial herniation and death within 72 hours. Respiratory failure resulting from brainstem involvement can also occur. In some patients there is an associated acute psychosis, depression and hypersomnolence. A number of characteristic patterns are seen. Following measles infection, myelitis with hemiparesis or paraparesis is common. Post-rubella ADEM can be associated with seizures, coma and moderate pyramidal signs. Varicella can lead to cerebellar ataxia with a mild pyramidal defect. Rabies vaccination is associated with radicular and peripheral nerve involvement.

Pathophysiology

It is generally accepted that the pathogenesis of ADEM is immune-mediated, rather than caused directly by infection. The exact mechanism of this is not clear. It has been proposed that the preceding infection or vaccine cross-activates an immune reaction to myelin through molecular mimicry. Alternatively, it has been suggested that the inflammatory response to the initial agent results in the activation of pre-existing encephalitogenic T cells.

Pathological examination of the brain in ADEM classically shows multiple peri-venous zones of demyelination in the cerebral white matter. The changes found in patients dying early in the disease affect the small blood vessels of both grey and white matter with hyperaemia, endothelial swelling, vessel wall invasion by inflammatory cells, peri-vascular oedema and haemorrhage all preceding the demyelination. Patients dying later in the disease process show zones of lymphocytic infiltration and demyelination, often with relative axonal-sparing lesions; these are discrete and surround small and medium sized vessels which have peri-vascular pallor. Advanced lesions can show astrocytic proliferation with gliosis and mild meningeal inflammation. The lesions are generally homogeneous in appearance and appear to be of the same age.

Differential diagnosis

ADEM can be difficult to distinguish from the first presentation of multiple sclerosis. A fulminant presentation may also be indistinguishable from AHL. In comparison with multiple sclerosis, ADEM tends to occur in younger patients (mainly children) and is more common in males. Encephalopathy, headache, fever and a multifocal presentation are more common, as is a history of a preceding infection or vaccination. Recently proposed diagnostic criteria for ADEM actually require there to be an encephalopathy and this is a particularly valuable point of distinction from clinically isolated syndromes associated with multiple sclerosis, which will not have clinical features of encephalopathy although there are sometimes extensive cerebral white matter lesions on MRI. Other CNS infections and inflammatory diseases must be excluded, and tumours are in the differential diagnosis of mass lesions (Table 11.14).

Distinguishing ADEM from multiple sclerosis can also be difficult if there are further episodes. In an attempt to distinguish ADEM and related disorders from multiple sclerosis, two international expert groups have proposed definitions for the major CNS

Table 11.14 Differential diagnosis of acute disseminated encephalomyelitis (ADEM).

Encephalitis
Herpes simplex encephalitis
Varicella zoster virus
HIV
Listeria monocytogenes
Mycobacterium tuberculosis
Inflammatory
Multiple sclerosis
Vasculitis – primary or secondary small vessel CNS vasculitis
Systemic lupus erythematosus
Behçet's disease
Sarcoidosis
Leukoencephalopathy
Toxic
Vascular
Metabolic
Genetic
Malignancy
Diffuse infiltration
Paraneoplastic

Table 11.15 Criteria for diagnosis of acute disseminated encephalomyelitis (ADEM).

Subacute encephalopathy (altered level of consciousness, behaviour or cognitive function)
Evolution over 1 week to 3 months; new symptoms, including focal/multifocal demyelinating syndromes, within the first 3 months from onset are allowed, as long as they are not separated by a period of complete remission from the initial symptoms (in which case the diagnosis is multiple sclerosis)
Accompanied by improvement or recovery although residual neurological deficits may be present
MRI shows predominantly symptomatic white matter lesions that • Are acute • Are multiple but rarely a single large lesion • Are supra- or infra-tentorial or both • Generally include at least one large (1–2 cm diameter) lesion • Variably enhance with gadolinium (gadolinium enhancement is not required) • May be accompanied by basal ganglia lesions, but their presence is not required

Source: Adapted from Miller *et al.* 2008. Reproduced with permission of Sage.

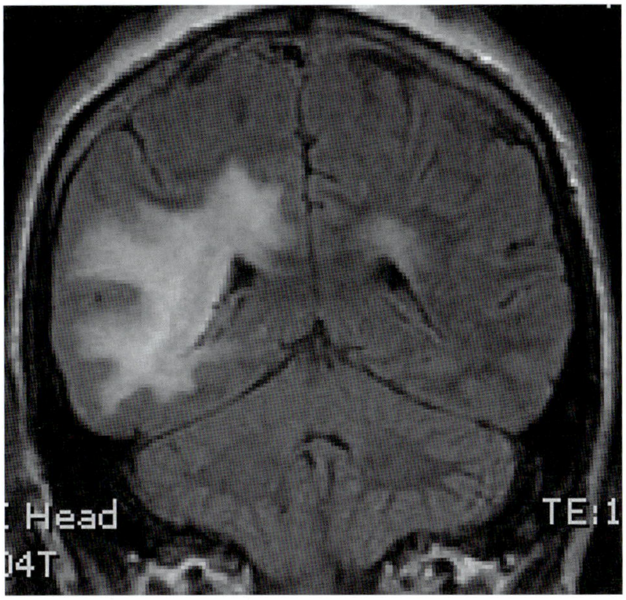

Figure 11.13 Extensive confluent demyelination in acute disseminated encephalomyelitis (MRI FLAIR coronal).

inflammatory demyelinating diseases including ADEM, although these are not yet validated. One group focused on the definitions for monophasic, recurrent and multiphasic ADEM in children. The other focused on adult presentation, when ADEM is uncommon, and rejected the category of multiphasic ADEM as it was felt to be indistinguishable from multiple sclerosis with an encephalopathic presentation (Table 11.15). This is an important distinction because there are specific disease-modifying treatments for such forms of relapsing multiple sclerosis.

Investigations

CSF can be normal in up to 50% of patients but can reveal an elevation in the opening pressure and a mild lymphocytosis (>50/mm^3), although occasionally there may be a polymorphonuclear leukocytosis. The protein is elevated in approximately 50%. Oligoclonal bands can be present acutely in up to 30% of patients but often disappear on repeat testing. CSF polymerase chain reaction (PCR) for viral infection can show the underlying precipitating agent. MRI is most useful in the diagnosis of ADEM, with abnormalities frequently evident on T2-weighted and FLAIR (Figure 11.13) imaging, although MRI can be normal early in the disease. The lesion load is often extensive with large and multi-focal lesions, which can be confluent and ill-defined. Lesions are not confined to the white matter but involve the cortical and deep grey matter. Mass lesions, mimicking tumours occur. 'Black holes', hypointense lesions on T1-weighted imaging, are typically absent. Lesions may enhance with gadolinium, reflecting their acute and synchronous development, but enhancement of the meninges is unusual. Spinal cord lesions are often large, extending over several levels, with swelling and mass effect, and have a predilection for the thoracic cord.

Although MRI appearances can be suggestive of ADEM, no features are specific to ADEM. It is not possible to distinguish ADEM from multiple sclerosis on the basis of MRI, although follow-up imaging can be helpful in the differential diagnosis. Brain MRI appearances can normalise in approximately 40% of patients with typical ADEM. The development of new lesions, after an interval of at least 3 months, is inconsistent with a diagnosis of monophasic ADEM.

Clinical course and prognosis

ADEM is usually a monophasic illness which is self-limiting. Recovery takes place over weeks to months, and full recovery can occur in about 50–75% of cases. However, major neurological sequelae can occur in up to one-third of patients and mortality is approximately 5%. There appears to be a worse prognosis if seizures and coma accompany the acute illness. Common residual deficits include hemiparesis, ataxia, blindness, cognitive dysfunction and epilepsy. Recurrent or multi-phasic ADEM has been reported in up to 20% of patients (mainly children) but in adults it would seem more likely to indicate the existence of multiple sclerosis.

Management

Management involves meticulous support and care, often in an intensive care unit, with adequate hydration and treatment of pyrexia, seizures and raised intracranial pressure. Patients can be given antibacterial and antiviral medication to treat the underlying infection. Empirically, first line treatment for ADEM is usually high dose intravenous methylprednisolone, for 3–5 days, followed by a tapering course of oral steroid over a few weeks. If unresponsive to steroids, plasmapheresis or IVIG can be considered, although the evidence for these is limited. Rarely, acute cerebral oedema, refractory to conventional management, may require decompressive hemicraniectomy.

Acute haemorrhagic leukoencephalitis

Acute haemorrhagic leukoencephalitis (Hurst's disease) is a rare, severe acute fulminant encephalopathy. There is generally an abrupt onset following an infection, usually respiratory tract, and the precipitating symptoms can be masked. Onset is usually between 20 and 40 years, and it is more common in males. It can occur in children, and has been reported to occur in 2% of a large cohort of children with ADEM. Pathologically it is characterised by peri-vascular inflammation with destruction of small vessels in association with haemorrhage and demyelination.

Clinical features

The course is generally brief and rapid, commonly leading to death. Patients present with acute pyrexia, headache, photophobia, meningism leading to progressive encephalopathy with confusion, lethargy and deepening coma over a few days. Focal neurological signs develop and seizures may occur. Cerebral oedema usually develops, frequently causing tentorial herniation resulting in death.

Investigations

There is marked elevation of the peripheral white cell count and erythrocyte sedimentation rate. The CSF pressure is raised with a moderately elevated protein level and a polymorphonuclear leukocytosis accompanied by an elevated red cell count and xanthochromia. Glucose levels are normal. Oligoclonal bands are rarely present. Computed tomography shows diffuse oedema and may show early haemorrhagic change, MRI shows numerous and large hyper-intense lesions on T2-weighted imaging. Haemorrhagic change can be seen with subsequent development of necrosis. Diffusion-weighted imaging can show restricted diffusion within lesions. Electroencephalography is abnormal in up to 90% of patients with diffuse slowing, although there may be lateralising features.

Prognosis

The prognosis of AHL is grave and most patients (up to 70%) die within 1 week of onset. Survivors may have severe residual deficits including seizures, cognitive and psychiatric disturbances. Complete recovery is exceptional.

Management

There is little evidence to guide management but, because of the acute inflammatory nature of the condition, high dose intravenous steroids are used. Surgical decompression can be necessary if severe cerebral oedema develops. Plasma exchange, IVIG and cyclophosphamide have also been tried, with a few reports of more favourable outcomes with early and aggressive treatment.

References

Kurtzke JF. Rating neurologic impairment in multiple sclerosis: an Expanded Disability Status Scale (EDSS). *Neurology* 1983; **33**: 1444–1452.

Lublin FD, Reingold SC. Defining the clinical course of multiple sclerosis: results of an international survey. National Multiple Sclerosis Society (USA) Advisory Committee on Clinical Trials of New Agents in Multiple Sclerosis. *Neurology* 1996; **46**: 907–911.

Lucchinetti C, Bruck W, Parisi J, Scheithauer B, Rodriguez M, Lassmann H. Heterogeneity of multiple sclerosis lesions: implications for the pathogenesis of demyelination. *Ann Neurol* 2000; **47**: 707–717.

Miller DH, Weinshenker BG, Filippi M, *et al.* Differential diagnosis of multiple sclerosis: a consensus approach. *Mult Scler* 2008; **14**: 1157–1174.

McDonald WI, Compston A, Edan G, Goodkin D, Hartung HP, Lublin FD, McFarland HF, Paty DW, Polman CH, Reingold SC, Sandberg-Wolheim M, Sibley W, Thompson A, van den Noort S, Weinshenker BY, Wolinsky JS. Recommended diagnostic criteria for multiple sclerosis: guidelines from the International Panel on the diagnosis of multiple sclerosis. *Ann Neurol* 2001; **50**: 121–127.

Poser CM, Paty DW, Scheinberg L, McDonald WI, Davis FA, Ebers GC, Johnson KP, Sibley WA, Silberberg DH, Tourtellotte WW. New diagnostic criteria for multiple sclerosis: guidelines for research protocols. *Ann Neurol* 1983; **13**: 227–231.

Schumacher GA, Beebe G, Kibler RF, Kurland LT, Kurtzke JF, McDowell F, Nagler B, Sibley WA, Tourtellotte WW, Wilmon TL. Problems of experimental trials of therapy in multiple sclerosis : a report by the panel on the evaluation of experimental trials of therapy in multiple sclerosis. *Ann N Y Acad Sci* 1965; **122**: 522–568.

Wingerchuk DM, Banwell B, Bennett JL, *et al.* International consensus diagnostic criteria for neuromyelitis optica spectrum disorders. *Neurology* 2015; **85:** 177–189.

Further reading

Epidemiology and aetiology

Ascherio A, Munger KL, Lunemann JD. The initiation and prevention of multiple sclerosis. *Nat Rev Neurol* 2012; **8**: 602–612.

Dyment, DA, Ebers GC, Sadovnick AD. Genetics of multiple sclerosis. *Lancet Neurol* 2004; **3**: 104–110.

International Multiple Sclerosis Genetics Consortium; Welcome Trust Case Control Consortium 2, *et al.* Genetic risk and a primary role for cell-mediated immune mechanisms in multiple sclerosis. *Nature* 2011; **476**: 214–219.

Trivedi P, Salvetti M, Faggioni A, Aloisi F. Dysregulated Epstein-Barr virus infection in the multiple sclerosis brain. *J Exp Med* 2007; **204**: 2899–2912.

Pathophysiology

Barnett MH, Prineas JW. Relapsing and remitting multiple sclerosis: pathology of the newly forming lesion. *Ann Neurol* 2004; **55**: 458–468.

Kutzelnigg A, Lucchinetti CF, Stadelmann C, Bruck W, Rauschka H, Bergmann M, *et al.* Cortical demyelination and diffuse white matter injury in multiple sclerosis. *Brain* 2005; **128**: 2705–2712.

Magliozzi R, Howell OW, Reeves C, *et al.* A Gradient of neuronal loss and meningeal inflammation in multiple sclerosis. *Ann Neurol* 2010; **68**: 477–493.

Clinical course

Banwell B, Ghezzi A, Bar-Or A, Mikaeloff Y, Tardieu M. Multiple sclerosis in children: clinical diagnosis, therapeutic strategies, and future directions. *Lancet Neurol* 2007; **6**: 887–902.

Confavreux C, Hutchinson M, Hours MM, *et al.* Rate of pregnancy-related relapse in multiple sclerosis. Pregnancy in Multiple Sclerosis Group. *N Engl J Med* 1998; **339**: 285–291.

Confavreux C, Vukusic S, Moreau T, Adeleine P. Relapses and progression of disability in multiple sclerosis. *N Engl J Med* 2000; **343**: 1430–1438.

D'hooghe MB, Nagels G, Bissay V, De Keyser J. Modifiable factors influencing relapses and disability in multiple sclerosis. *Mult Scler* 2010; **16**: 773–785.

Lublin FD, Reingold SC, Cohen JA, *et al.* Defining the course of multiple sclerosis: the 2013 revisions. *Neurol* 2014; **83**: 278–286.

Miller DH, Chard DT, Ciccarelli O. Clinically isolated syndromes. *Lancet Neurol* 2012; **11**: 157–169.

Diagnosis

McDonald WI, Compston A, Edan G, *et al.* Recommended diagnostic criteria for multiple sclerosis: guidelines from the International Panel on the diagnosis of multiple sclerosis. *Ann Neurol* 2001; **50**: 121–127.

Montalban X, Sastre-Garriga J, Filippi M, *et al.* Primary progressive multiple sclerosis diagnostic criteria: a reappraisal. *Mult Scler* 2009; **15**: 1459–1465.

Polman CH, Reingold SC, Banwell B, *et al.* Diagnostic criteria for multiple sclerosis: 2010 revisions to the McDonald criteria. *Ann Neurol* 2011; **69**: 292–302.

Polman CH, Reingold SC, Edan G, *et al.* Diagnostic criteria for multiple sclerosis: 2005 revisions to the 'McDonald Criteria'. *Ann Neurol* 2005; **58**: 840–846.

Management

Beck RW, Cleary PA, Anderson MM Jr, *et al.* A randomized, controlled trial of corticosteroids in the treatment of acute optic neuritis. The Optic Neuritis Study Group. *N Engl J Med* 1992; **326**: 581–588.

Department of Health. The National Service Framework for Long-Term Conditions. London: Department of Health, 2005.

LePage E, Veillard D, Laplaud DA, et al. Oral versus intravenous high-dose methylprednisolone for treatment of relapses in patients with multiple sclerosis (COPOUSEP): a randomised, controlled, double-blind, non-inferiority trial. *Lancet* 2015; **386**: 974–981.

National Institute for Clinical Excellence (NICE). *Management of multiple sclerosis in primary and secondary care.* NICE Guideline, 2014.

Disease-modifying therapy

Bloomgren G, Richman S, Hotermans C, *et al.* Risk of natalizumab-associated progressive multifocal leukoencephalopathy. *N Engl J Med* 2012; **366**: 1870–1880.

Cohen JA, Coles AJ, Arnold DL, *et al.* Alemtuzumab versus interferon beta 1a as first-line treatment for patients with relapsing-remitting multiple sclerosis: a randomized controlled phase 3 trial. *Lancet* 2012; **380**: 1819–1828.

Gold R, Kappos L, Arnold DL, *et al.* Placebo-controlled phase 3 study of oral BG-12 in relapsing multiple sclerosis. *N Engl J Med* 2012; **367**: 1098–1107.

IFNB Multiple Sclerosis Study Group. Interferon β-1b is effective in relapsing-remitting multiple sclerosis. I. Clinical results of a multicenter, randomized, double-blind, placebo-controlled trial. *Neurology* 1993; **43**: 655–661.

Jacobs LD, Cookfair DL, Rudick RA, *et al.* Intramuscular interferon β-1a for disease progression in relapsing multiple sclerosis. *Ann Neurol* 1996; **39**: 285–294.

Johnson KP, Brooks BR, Cohen JA, *et al.* Copolymer I reduces relapse rate and improves disability in relapsing-remitting multiple sclerosis: results of a phase III, multicenter, double-blind, placebo-controlled trial. *Neurology* 1995; **45**: 1268–1276.

Kappos L, Radue EW, O'Connor P, *et al.* A placebo-controlled trial of oral fingolimod in relapsing multiple sclerosis. *N Engl J Med* 2010; **362**: 387–401.

National Institute for Health and Clinical Excellence. *Natalizumab for the treatment of adults with highly active relapsing-remitting multiple sclerosis*. 2007.

National Institute for Health and Clinical Excellence. *Fingolimod for the treatment highly active relapsing-remitting multiple sclerosis*. 2012.

National Institute for Health and Clinical Excellence. *Alemtuzumab for treating relapsing-remitting multiple sclerosis*. 2014.

National Institute for Health and Clinical Excellence. *Dimethyl fumarate for treating relapsing-remitting multiple sclerosis*. 2014.

National Institute for Health and Clinical Excellence. *Teriflunomide for treating relapsing-remitting multiple sclerosis*. 2014.

O'Connor P, Wolinsky JS, Confavreux C, *et al.* Randomized trial of oral teriflunomide for relapsing multiple sclerosis. *N Engl J Med* 2011; **365**: 1293–1303.

Oh J, Calabresi PA. Emerging injectable therapies for multiple sclerosis. *Lancet Neurol* 2013; **12**: 1115–1126.

Polman CH, O'Connor PW, Havrdova E, *et al.* A randomized, placebo-controlled trial of natalizumab for relapsing multiple sclerosis. *N Engl J Med* 2006; **354**: 899–910.

Prevention of Relapses and Disability by Interferon β-1a Subcutaneously in Multiple Sclerosis (PRISMS) Study Group. Randomised, double-blind, placebo-controlled study of interferon β-1a in relapsing/remitting multiple sclerosis. *Lancet* 1998; **352**: 1498–1504.

Scolding N, Barnes D, Cader S, *et al.* Association of British Neurologists: revised (2015) guidelines for prescribing disease-modifying treatments in multiple sclerosis. *Pract Neurol* 2015; **15**: 273–279.

Symptomatic treatment and neurological rehabilitation

Beer S, Khan F, Kesselring J. Rehabilitation interventions in multiple sclerosis: an overview. *J Neurol* 2012; **259**: 1994-2008.

Bowling A. Complementary and Alternative Medicine and Multiple Sclerosis, 2nd edn. New York: Demos Medical Publishing, 2006.

Sweetland J, Riazi A, Cano SJ, Playford ED. Vocational rehabilitation services for people with multiple sclerosis: what patients want from clinicians and employers. *Mult Scler* 2007; **13**: 1183–1189.

Thompson AJ, Toosy AT, Ciccarelli O. Pharmacological management of symptoms in multiple sclerosis: current approaches and future directions. *Lancet Neurol* 2010: **9**: 1182–1199.

Turner-Stokes L, Sykes N, Silber E, Khatri A, Sutton L, Young E. From diagnosis to death: exploring the interface between neurology and palliative care in managing people with long-term neurological conditions. *Clin Med* 2007; **7**: 129–136.

Neuromyelitis optica

Jacob A, McKeon A, Nakashima I, *et al.* Current concept of neuromyelitis optica (NMO) and NMO spectrum disorders. *J Neurol Neurosurg Psychiatry* 2013; **84**: 922–930.

Lennon VA, Wingerchuk DM, Kryzer TJ, *et al.* A serum autoantibody marker of neuromyelitis optica: distinction from multiple sclerosis. *Lancet* 2004; **364**: 2106–2112.

Matthews L, Marasco R, Jenkinson M, *et al.* Distinction of seropositive NMO spectrum disorder and MS brain lesion distribution. *Neurology* 2013; **80**: 1330–1337.

Wingerchuk DM, Banwell B, Bennett JL, *et al.* International consensus diagnostic criteria for neuromyelitis optica spectrum disorders. *Neurology* 2015; **85**: 177–189.

Acute disseminated encephalomyelitis

Krupp LB, Tardieu M, Amato MP, *et al.* International Pediatric Multiple Sclerosis Study Group criteria for pediatric multiple sclerosis and immune-mediated central nervous system demyelinating disorders: revisions to the 2007 definitions. *Mult Scler* 2013; **19**: 1261–1267.

CHAPTER 12

Headache

Manjit Matharu[1], Paul Shanahan[2] and Tim Young[2]
[1] UCL Institute of Neurology
[2] National Hospital for Neurology & Neurosurgery

Headache is the most common neurological reason for new presentations to general practitioners and to neurologists, and has a lifetime prevalence of 93% in men and 99% in women. As such, it represents a significant part of many clinicians' workload. Despite this, headaches and migraine in particular are a commonly overlooked cause of disability. The World Health Organization ranks a day spent with severe migraine as being equivalent in disability to a day spent with dementia, quadriplegia or psychosis.

While it should go without saying that accurate diagnosis improves management, the Landmark study showed that 76% of patients who had been diagnosed with non-migraine primary headache in primary care had met the criteria for migraine and a further 18% met the criteria for probable migraine. This suggests that there is considerable scope to improve our diagnostic skills in headache, and this represents a significant opportunity for clinicians, given how treatable many of these conditions are.

Although primary headaches constitute the vast majority of what is seen in clinical practice, there is no doubt that the possibility of an underlying secondary aetiology can cause concern in both the patient and the treating clinician. An important part of the initial assessment, therefore, involves determining the likelihood of a secondary cause of headache and investigating as appropriate.

The clinical approach to headache should start with an appropriate assessment and diagnosis, assisted by investigations where necessary, before proceeding to treatment.

Evaluation of the headache patient

Headache history taking

Assessment of headache, as with much of neurology, relies primarily on an accurate and detailed history supplemented by clinical examination. As many patients find pain a difficult experience to describe, it is the job of the clinician to bring out the salient features through comprehensive and careful history taking. We recommend particular attention to the following points.

Onset and time course The abrupt (or 'thunderclap') onset of severe headache may indicate subarachnoid haemorrhage or other vascular events such as venous sinus thrombosis or arterial dissection and should always be taken seriously, whereas migraine generally evolves more slowly. Migraine also tends to resolve gradually, often with residual symptoms of lethargy and fatigue, whereas a trigeminal autonomic cephalalgia (TAC), such as cluster headache, may begin and end quite abruptly.

Frequency and pattern of pain As well as indicating the total burden of pain experienced, the frequency of attacks may provide a useful clue to diagnosis. For example, a patient experiencing several discrete attacks of pain per day (rather than a day-long headache with brief respites due to analgesia) is less likely to be describing migraine; other disorders such as a TAC or cranial neuralgia may need to be considered. Timing of the individual headaches may be informative: many patients with cluster headache experience attacks at fairly consistent times of day; patients with low cerebrospinal fluid (CSF) pressure may experience pain only on standing up.

Duration of pain Provided that the duration of the headache is not being influenced by analgesia, the duration of pain is one of the most helpful characteristics. Long-lasting headaches such as migraine, which typically lasts at least 4 hours without treatment, can be differentiated from shorter attacks such as cluster headache (typical duration 15–180 minutes), paroxysmal hemicrania (typical duration 5–30 minutes) or neuralgic pain (typically lasting seconds).

Severity and quality of pain While severity is clearly a subjective quality, it is an important component of overall headache disability and when combined with other attributes may suggest a diagnosis. The pain of tension-type headache, for example, is usually described as mild to moderate whereas that of cluster headache is generally severe or excruciating. The pain of migraine is often described as throbbing or pounding and trigeminal neuralgia is usually described as electric shock-like or stabbing, whereas tension-type headache may be described as pressing or tightening.

Variability and pattern of pain Predictable worsening or improvements in pain under certain conditions can be helpful. A consistent diurnal pattern of pain may raise the possibility of a secondary, pressure-related headache: pain caused by raised intracranial pressure may be worse in the morning after a night's recumbency, whereas that of low pressure headache (intracranial hypotension) is

Neurology: A Queen Square Textbook, Second Edition. Edited by Charles Clarke, Robin Howard, Martin Rossor and Simon Shorvon.

typically minimal on waking and worsens after getting up and as the day goes on. Other causes of a headache maximal on waking include analgesia rebound headache and obstructive sleep apnoea. Cluster headache in some individuals can occur with striking predictability at the same times of day.

Triggers A wide range of triggers for migraine attacks have been reported, with the most common including hunger, thirst, lack of sleep, or occasionally oversleeping, stress or occasionally the reverse – winding down following a stressful period, hormonal changes particularly premenstrually and alcohol. Dietary factors seem to be less consistent, and while the popular perception is that migraine has frequent dietary triggers, this can be confounded by food cravings which may occur as a premonitory symptom of migraine and create confusion as to cause and effect. In cluster headache, alcohol is a reliable trigger for the majority of patients when they are experiencing a bout of attacks but not while in remission. Triggering of pain by the Valsalva manoeuvre may occur in cases of raised intracranial pressure, though it may also be seen in cases of low intracranial pressure where there is significant cerebellar tonsillar descent, as well as in cases of Chiari malformation. The neuralgic pain of trigeminal neuralgia, and sometimes that of SUNCT (short-lasting, unilateral neuralgiform pain with conjunctival injection and tearing) may be triggered by having the affected site stimulated by touch, movement, such as speaking or chewing or by a cold breeze on the face.

Location of pain The pain of tension-type headache is generally bilateral or holocranial. Although migraine derives its name from the Greek *hemicrania*, its location is often inconstant and, while 60% of migraineurs will experience unilateral attacks, these may swap sides, and 40% will experience bilateral attacks. The TACs, on the other hand, are very rarely bilateral. The pain of trigeminal neuralgia affects the second (maxillary) and third (mandibular) divisions of the trigeminal nerve in approximately 95% of cases, whereas SUNCT more usually affects the first (ophthalmic) division.

Associated symptoms Whereas tension-type headache has a paucity of associated symptoms, migraine is a frequently 'feature-rich' headache. The most common associated symptoms of migraine are nausea, sensory hypersensitivities (photophobia, phonophobia, osmophobia and sensitivity to motion), fatigue, which may precede the pain and frequently outlasts it, and cognitive effects from impaired concentration to irritability and mood change. It should be noted that these so-called migrainous features, while common in migraine, can also be seen, albeit less frequently, in other headache disorders.

Cranial autonomic symptoms are seen in many primary headache types but are most obviously associated with the TACs. Symptoms such as ptosis, lacrimation, conjunctival injection, rhinorrhoea, nasal congestion, facial flushing or sweating and a sensation of aural fullness may occur singly or in combination. They are ipsilateral to the pain in cluster headache, SUNCT, SUNA (short-lasting unilateral neuralgiform headache with cranial autonomic symptoms), paroxysmal hemicrania and hemicrania continua. These symptoms can also be seen in migraine, but more commonly bilaterally.

Pulsatile tinnitus may be reported by patients with abnormal CSF pressure (either high or low) and is often described as a pulsating, 'whooshing' noise.

Aura While most commonly associated with migraine, and occurring in 30% of patients, aura has been reported in many of the primary headache syndromes. The time course of the evolution of symptoms often helps to distinguish it from other causes of transient neurological dysfunction such as transient ischaemic attacks. Typical migraine aura will develop gradually over minutes and may exhibit a somatotopic spread before settling. The most common form of aura is visual; indeed, as visual aura occurs in 99% of patients with aura, one should be wary of diagnosing aura in those who have never experienced visual symptoms. Typically, aura consists of a mixture of positive (e.g. scintillations, fortification spectra) and negative (e.g. scotomata) symptoms which evolves over several minutes and typically lasts from 5 minutes to an hour. Sensory aura (with spreading numbness and paraesthesiae) is the second most common form of aura, occurring in about 30% of patients with aura, with speech disturbance, motor aura and basilar-type aura (bilateral cortical or brainstem symptoms) occurring with decreasing frequency.

Evolution of symptoms While it is not unusual for primary headache syndromes to cause varying degrees of disability over time, a history of progressive worsening or evolving symptoms (e.g. the emergence of new aura in a patient with no prior history of aura), or abnormal findings on clinical examination may require further scrutiny or investigation to exclude the possibility of an emerging secondary headache.

Past medical history Any history of recent head or neck injury should be carefully sought. As well as being a significant cause of pain in its own right, trauma (occasionally minor trauma in those predisposed) may result in haemorrhage, arterial dissection, nerve injury, CSF leakage or infection, so it is helpful to note any relevant prior history such as anticoagulation or collagenopathy (Marfan's syndrome, Ehlers–Danlos syndrome) which may increase the risks of secondary headache. Patients with a new diagnosis of migraine may give a history of cyclical vomiting or possibly travel sickness in childhood or adolescence.

Co-morbidities that may exacerbate or contribute to migraine becoming chronic include obesity, sleep apnoea, head injury, stressful life events and overuse of acute relief medication or caffeine, and these factors should be explored in those with increasing headache frequency.

A patient's headache diary, recording carefully the frequency, severity and pattern of pain as well as any acute medication use, can be invaluable both in clarifying the diagnostic points above and in monitoring response to treatment.

Examination of the patient with headache

Examination should be directed at excluding any underlying cause and identifying signs that warrant further investigation. At first presentation, all patients should have a thorough examination with particular attention directed to the following points.

In the acute setting, temperature, pulse rate and blood pressure should be measured and the level of consciousness/orientation assessed. Neck stiffness and signs of meningeal irritation should be looked for, as should any evidence of purpuric rash to suggest meningococcal septicaemia.

Fundoscopy should be performed to look for any evidence of papilloedema, while bearing in mind that its absence does not exclude raised intracranial pressure. Subhyaloid haemorrhages may sometimes be seen in subarachnoid haemorrhage.

Examination of the head and neck should include auscultation for cervical or cranial bruits, and assessment of range of neck movement. Palpation of the temporal arteries in patients over 50 years of age may reveal the thickened, often tender arteries of giant cell arteritis (GCA).

Full neurological examination may reveal focal abnormalities including visual field defects (in cerebral or chiasmal lesions) or enlargement of the blind spot, oculomotor disturbance, particularly VIth nerve palsies in raised intracranial pressure or Horner's syndrome, for example in carotid dissection or any evidence of focal neurological dysfunction which requires further investigation.

Red flags for secondary headaches

In carrying out a full history and examination, the clinician should be alert to any symptoms or signs that raise the possibility of a secondary headache. In particular, the need for further investigations should be considered in the circumstances shown in Table 12.1.

Investigation of the patient with headache

In those patients where a secondary cause of headache is suspected, further investigation is essential. This includes consideration of the following.

Blood tests Erythrocyte sedimentation rate (ESR) and C-reactive protein (CRP) in cases of suspected GCA. Other investigation is directed at specific systemic diseases.

Neuroimaging Computed tomography (CT) imaging is capable of identifying subarachnoid haemorrhage with near 100% sensitivity when performed within 6 hours. Non-contrast magnetic resonance (MRI) enables high-quality structural imaging, including the posterior fossa, as well as highlighting arterial, venous and CSF circulation. Spinal imaging with heavily T2-weighted sequences may aid the detection of spinal CSF leaks in spontaneous intracranial hypotension. Imaging is of no diagnostic value in primary headache, and in patients with a history suggestive of migraine and normal clinical examination findings, the rate of any significant abnormality on imaging is low. Diagnostic imaging should therefore only be a consideration where a secondary headache is suspected. Any decision to perform imaging in headache patients must weigh the potential diagnostic yield, and the reassurance provided against cost, and a definite potential for identification of incidental abnormalities, unrelated to the presenting complaint but capable of causing diagnostic confusion and anxiety.

Table 12.1 Features that should prompt consideration of secondary headaches.

Worsening headache with fever
Sudden-onset headache reaching maximum intensity within five minutes ('thunderclap headache')
New-onset neurological deficit
New-onset cognitive dysfunction
Change in personality
Impaired level of consciousness
Recent (typically within the past 3 months) head trauma
Headache triggered by Valsalva manoeuvre, coughing or sneezing
Headache triggered by exercise
Orthostatic headache (headache that changes with posture)
Symptoms suggestive of giant cell arteritis
Symptoms and signs of acute narrow-angle glaucoma
A substantial change in the characteristics of their headache
New-onset headache in the presence of any of the following: • Compromised immunity, caused, for example, by HIV or immunosuppressive drugs • Age under 20 years and a history of malignancy • History of malignancy known to metastasise to the brain • Vomiting without other obvious cause

Source: National Institute for Health and Care Excellence Clinical Guideline 150: Diagnosis and management of headaches in young people and adults, September 2012.

Lumbar puncture In addition to its role in identifying inflammatory and infectious disorders, lumbar puncture, when not contraindicated, enables measurement of CSF pressure as well as its reduction by withdrawal of CSF, for example in cases of idiopathic intracranial hypertension.

Secondary headaches

The third edition of the International Classification of Headache Disorders (ICHD-III) classifies secondary headaches according to the underlying cause. It is a prerequisite for diagnosis of secondary headache that the underlying condition is recognised as being capable of producing the headache phenotype experienced, and that where possible that the headache can be demonstrated to resolve with successful treatment of the underlying condition.

Medication overuse headache

While for many clinicians the term secondary headache conjures images of intracranial catastrophes, it is important to remember that the most common cause of secondary headache is medication overuse. It has been estimated that 1.5% of the general population suffer from medication overuse headache (MOH). This entity develops most commonly in those patients with a pre-existing primary headache disorder, typically migraine or tension-type headache, and it is easy to see how a spiral of escalating headache frequency and escalating analgesia use can occur.

ICHD-III defines medication overuse as the use of simple analgesia (paracetamol, aspirin or non-steroidal anti-inflammatory drugs) on 15 or more days per month for at least 3 months. In contrast, triptan or opiate (including codeine) overuse is defined as use of these agents on 10 or more days per month for at least 3 months. It is important to note that frequency, not dosage, is the determinant of overuse; a small daily dosage is more likely to result in MOH than infrequent use of larger doses.

When occurring in the setting of a coexisting primary headache such as migraine, it may be very difficult to establish where migraine ends and MOH begins. Under such conditions, rationalisation of analgesia use is an important therapeutic as well as diagnostic step. Approximately half of patients with MOH who withdraw from analgesia for a 2-month period will experience an improvement in headaches; of the remainder, the majority will stay the same and only a minority (<10%) will worsen. The improvement with analgesia withdrawal is maximal in patients with migraine, in whom two-thirds will improve.

Regular caffeine use of >200 mg (about the equivalent of three espressos) per day, over a period of at least 2 weeks may be associated with withdrawal headaches when interrupted or discontinued. This headache typically resolves within 7 days.

Other medications may provoke headache in their own right, notably nitroglycerin, atropine, digitalis, disulfiram, hydralazine, imipramine, nicotine, nifedipine and nimodipine.

Headache caused by vascular disorders

Thunderclap headache is perhaps the most striking of the red flag symptoms suggesting secondary headache. It may arise from a number of vascular and non-vascular causes including arterial dissection, venous thrombosis, ischaemic stroke, pituitary apoplexy, reversible cerebral vasoconstriction syndrome and spontaneous intracranial hypotension, but the classic cause of thunderclap headache until proven otherwise is subarachnoid haemorrhage.

Subarachnoid haemorrhage

Approximately 12% of patients presenting with an acute 'worst headache of my life' and normal clinical examination will be found to have had a subarachnoid haemorrhage. As early recognition and treatment leads to improved outcomes a high index of suspicion in such cases is essential. Prompt non-contrast CT has a sensitivity approaching 100% within 6 hours, but in cases of delayed presentation a lumbar puncture looking for evidence of blood or blood degradation products may be necessary. Some 85% of subarachnoid haemorrhage is aneurysmal and endovascular or surgical occlusion of the aneurysm is necessary to reduce the risk of rebleeding.

Carotid and vertebral artery dissection

Arterial dissection may occur, particularly in susceptible individuals, in response to trauma of varying severity, though spontaneous cases are not uncommon. The presentation consists of pain in the neck and/or in the head and symptoms of ischaemia distal to the dissection, though 15% may present with headache alone, and ischaemia may be delayed. Neck pain with signs of posterior circulation ischaemia should raise the possibility of vertebral dissection, whereas an ipsilateral Horner's syndrome may be seen in carotid dissection, with or without carotid territory ischaemic symptoms.

Giant cell arteritis

GCA occurs virtually exclusively in those over 50 years, and incidence rises with age, occurring 10 times more commonly in those over 80 compared to those in the 50–60 age group. It is 2–3 times more common in women than men. Symptoms of scalp tenderness as well as ischaemic pain in the muscles of mastication (jaw claudication) or the tongue (tongue angina) should raise suspicion of the diagnosis. ESR and/or CRP will be elevated in over 95% of cases and definitive diagnosis is established on temporal artery biopsy. Prompt treatment with steroids, typically at least 1 mg/kg initially will rapidly alleviate symptoms and protect against the risk of anterior ischaemic optic neuropathy (AION).

Headache caused by disturbance of intracranial pressure

Intracranial hypertension

A history suggestive of raised intracranial pressure should prompt urgent imaging to look for a structural cause such as a space-occupying lesion (e.g. tumour, abscess, haematoma, hydrocephalus) or venous sinus thrombosis. Once a space-occupying lesion has been excluded, a lumbar puncture may be required to clarify the pressure and lower it if needed. A CSF opening pressure of >250 mm CSF (in the lateral decubitus position) should prompt removal of CSF and the patient should maintain a careful diary of symptoms to establish any improvement in headache post-lumbar puncture.

Idiopathic intracranial hypertension is most commonly seen in young women with a high body mass index (BMI). Papilloedema is usual though cases without papilloedema are recognised. Treatment is directed a lowering CSF pressure to prevent visual loss. Ultimately, reduction of BMI is usually curative but, as this is slow at best, pressure lowering strategies include drugs (e.g. acetazolamide, bendroflumethazide), repeated lumbar punctures and CSF shunting or optic nerve fenestration when necessary.

Other causes of raised CSF pressure include malignant meningeal infiltration and hypertrophic pachymeningitis and side effects of medications such as anabolic steroids, amiodarone, lithium carbonate, nalidixic acid, retinoids and tetracycline.

Low pressure headaches (intracranial hypotension)

The most common cause of intracranial hypotension is iatrogenic, following lumbar puncture or inadvertently after epidural anaesthesia. Low CSF pressure (defined as <60 mm CSF in ICHD-III) results in headache that is usually worsened on standing and relieved by lying, though in persistent cases the postural variability may diminish over time. There may be associated neck pain, photophobia, tinnitus (or even hearing loss) and nausea. Some relief may be obtained from caffeine intake. Spontaneous CSF leakage may occur, often as a result of a tear in a spinal nerve root sheath, and the initial trauma may not always be recalled. Spontaneous CSF leakage may be more common in those with a collagen disorders such as hypermobility or Marfan's syndrome.

In post-dural (post LP) headache, where the aetiology is clear, resolution is usually spontaneous within 2 weeks and further investigation may not be required. Cranial MRI in low CSF pressure states may show cerebellar tonsillar descent, sagging of the brainstem, post-contrast enhancement of the meninges and occasionally subdural fluid collections (Figure 12.1). In spontaneous intracranial hypotension the site of CSF leakage is usually spinal and careful imaging with heavily T2-weighted spinal MRI (such as constructive interference steady state [CISS] sequences) or even CT myelography may be required to identify the site of leakage.

Where leakage has been identified, or inferred in the case of persistent post-dural puncture headache, epidural blood patching with autologous blood is the treatment of choice. Effective closure of the leak should result in resolution of the headache, though in refractory cases repeated blood patching and (rarely) operative repair may be required.

ICHD-III lists a very extensive list of other causes of secondary headache, beyond the scope of this chapter, and the reader is encouraged to refer to this to appreciate the broad spectrum of causes of secondary headache.

When evaluating a patient for secondary headache, bear in mind that with the exception of MOH, secondary headaches are rare and the reassurance of excluding a secondary cause should not be a substitute for diagnosing and treating a primary headache.

Primary headaches

Primary headaches are disorders in which headache and associated features are seen in the absence of any exogenous cause. The common syndromes are tension-type headache, migraine and cluster headache.

Anatomy and physiology of headache

The disabling primary headaches, migraine and cluster headache, have been studied extensively and are now relatively well understood. The detailed anatomy of the neural substrate of head pain is now well described. Surrounding the largest cerebral vessels, meningeal vessels, large venous sinuses and dura mater is a plexus consisting largely of small-diameter myelinated and unmyelinated fibres which arise

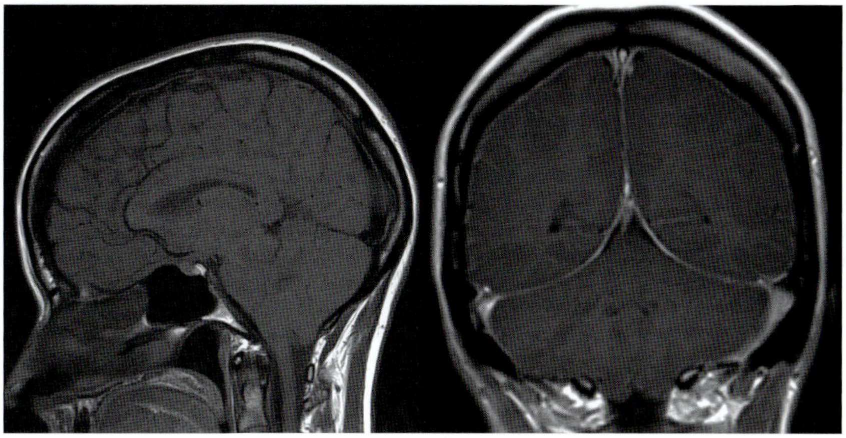

Figure 12.1 Low cerebrospinal fluid (CSF) pressure headache: magnetic resonance image (MRI) showing tonsillar descent and diffuse meningeal enhancement.

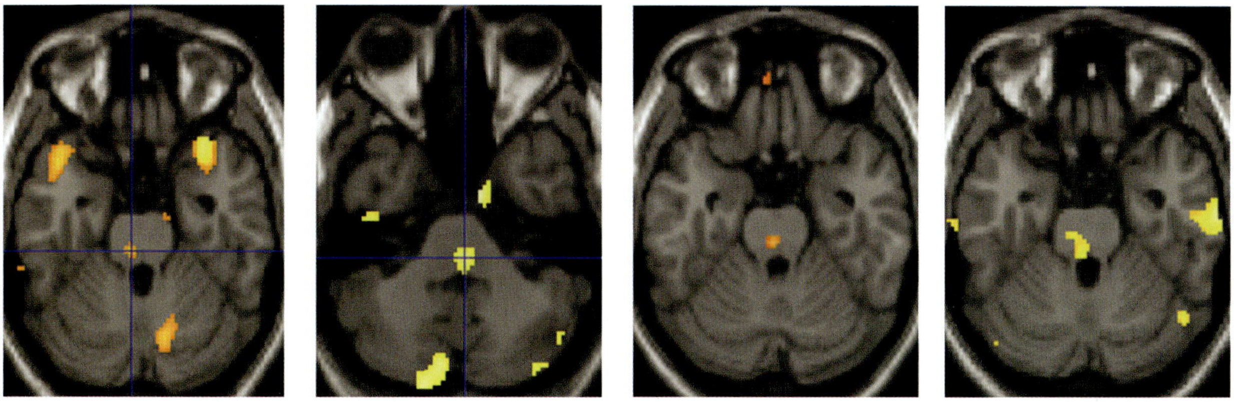

(a) (b) (c) (d)

Figure 12.2 Brainstem activation in migraine and hemicrania continua. (a) Spontaneous episodic migraine. Source: Afridi *et al.* 2005. Reproduced with permission of Oxford University Press and M.S. Matharu. (b) GTN-triggered episodic migraine. Source: Afridi *et al.* 2005. Reproduced with permission of Oxford University Press and M.S. Matharu. (c) Chronic migraine. Source: Matharu 2004. Reproduced with permission of Oxford University Press and M.S. Matharu. (d) Hemicrania continua. Source: Matharu *et al.* 2004. Reproduced with permission of John Wiley & Sons.

mainly from the trigeminal nerve and the upper cervical dorsal roots. These fibres project centrally to synapse on second order sensory neurones in the trigeminal brainstem nuclear complex, composed of the principal trigeminal sensory nucleus and the spinal trigeminal nucleus. Projections from this trigeminocervical complex cross the midline and ascend in the contralateral quinto-thalamic tract to connections in the brainstem (peri-aqueductal grey; PAG) and diencephalon (hypothalamus), and thence ultimately to thalamic nuclei and cerebral cortex (Chapter 2). Cortical areas associated with nociception include primary and secondary somatosensory cortices, cingulate cortex, insulae, visual and auditory areas, and frontal cortices. A reflex connection exists between neurones in the pons in the superior salivatory nucleus, which results in a cranial parasympathetic outflow that is mediated through the pterygopalatine ganglia; this provides the basis for symptoms, such as lacrimation and nasal stuffiness, which are prominent in trigeminal autonomic cephalalgias. Transmission of pain is modulated by a powerful descending antinociceptive neural network extending from the frontal cortex and the hypothalamus through the PAG to medulla.

Primary headaches such as migraine and cluster headache are neurovascular disorders. The central underlying abnormality is a disorder of the endogenous pain modulating antinociceptive systems. The structures of the antinociceptive system, besides participating in nociceptive control, modulate other sensory modalities and can alter brain blood flow. The abnormality underlying primary headaches is hypothesised to result in an alteration of function of these systems – either activation of descending systems that facilitate processing of pain signals by trigeminocervical neurones, or suppression of descending pathways that inhibit such processing of pain signals or a combination of systems dysfunctions. The result is central hyperalgesia and an augmentation of the central perception of pain.

Functional neuroimaging studies have provided evidence of a role for brainstem dysfunction in migraine and hemicrania continua (Figure 12.2) and a region near the posterior hypothalamic grey matter, the site of the human circadian pacemaker cells of the suprachiasmatic nucleus in the pathogenesis of the TACS, including cluster headache (Figure 12.3).

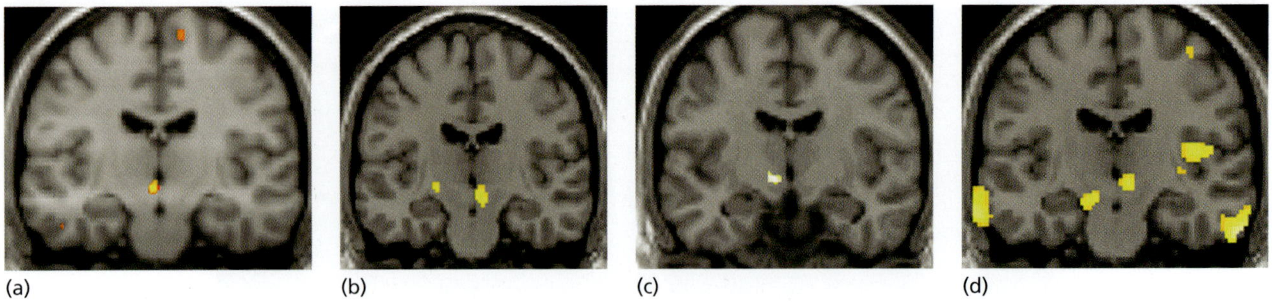

Figure 12.3 Posterior hypothalamic activation in trigeminal autonomic cephalalgias. (a) Cluster headache (PET study). Source: May et al. 1998. Reproduced with permission of Elsevier. (b) Peroxysmal hemicrania (PET study). Source: Matharu *et al.* 2006. Reproduced with permission of John Wiley & Sons. (c) SUNCT (fMRI study). Source: May *et al.* 1999. Reproduced with permission of John Wiley & Sons. (d) Hemicrania continua (PET study). Source: Matharu *et al.* 2004. Reproduced with permisison from John Wiley & Sons.

Migraine

Migraine is very common worldwide, affecting some 18% of the population, and is more frequent in women than men. It is a primary headache disorder which may be episodic or chronic. Migraine causes significant morbidity and lost productivity, and costs the United Kingdom over £2 billion a year in absenteeism alone. The Global Burden of Disease Survey recently estimated migraine to be the seventh greatest specific cause of disability globally. Despite this, it is frequently undiagnosed and undertreated. This section examines the features of migraine together with aspects of its management.

Epidemiology

In England the 1-year prevalence of migraine has been estimated at 7.6% for men and 18.3% for women. The 1-year prevalence of episodic migraine in the North American population has recently been estimated at 11.7% (17.1% in women and 5.6% in men) based on a large postal questionnaire survey. The incidence of episodic migraine is less clear. Based on a Danish 12-year follow-up population study the annual incidence of episodic migraine was 8.1/1000 person years.

The prevalence of chronic migraine has been widely studied with estimates between 0 and 5.1% for 1-year prevalence being described for the general population. The incidence for chronic migraine has not been well studied. A figure of 14% has been given as the annual incidence of transformation of episodic to chronic migraine but this was made in specialist headache clinics so may not be applicable to the general population. In the community an estimated 2.5% of episodic migraineurs transformed into chronic migraine over a 1-year period in the United States.

Clinical features

Migraine is usually episodic, with headaches occurring on less than 15 days per month. Chronic migraine involves headaches affecting the patient on 15 or more days a month for more than 3 months with features of migraine headaches on at least 8 days a month. It can be very helpful to ask patients how many headache *free* days they have had in the last month as well to pick up any additional lower level headaches, which are often described by patients as 'normal' headaches.

Migraineurs may have a warning that a headache is due to occur by premonitory symptoms up to 2 days before the headache, which can include yawning, increased micturition or fatigue. Estimates of the proportion of patients who experience premonitory symptoms vary widely, ranging from 7% to 87%. The migraine headache itself may have a variety of features and associated features. ICHD-III requires at least five separate attacks each lasting 4–72 hours if untreated. The headache should have at least two of the following characteristics: unilateral location, pulsating quality, at least moderately severe, and aggravated by routine physical movement such as walking or climbing stairs. In addition there should be at least one of the following associated features during the headache: nausea with or without vomiting, or both photophobia and phonophobia. Importantly, there are caveats to the above criteria. While useful to define migraine for research purposes many migraineurs will not exhibit all of the above features. On the other hand, a patient may exhibit all the clinical features of migraine and yet have a secondary headache disorder. No one characteristic is critical for the diagnosis though duration of the headache can be one of the most helpful characteristics in distinguishing migraine from other primary headaches.

Just over 30% of migraineurs will experience auras with some or all of their headaches. Auras are recurrent episodes of reversible focal neurological symptoms typically developing gradually over 5–30 minutes and lasting for less than 60 minutes. They usually occur before or at the start of the headache. The auras are most commonly visual with positive symptoms, such as flashing lights or zigzag lines and negative symptoms such as scotomata. Other relatively common types of auras include sensory and speech or language disturbance. Uncommon types of aura include motor (with hemiplegic symptoms) and brainstem (with dysarthria, vertigo, tinnitus, hyperacusis, diplopia, ataxia and decreased level of consciousness) disturbance for which careful exclusion of secondary causes is mandatory. The pathophysiology of the underlying auras is believed to involve a wave of cortical spreading depression in the relevant sensory area associated with initial hyperaemia followed by prolonged hypoperfusion. Less commonly, auras can occur with other primary headaches including cluster headaches, or even without headache at all, in which case it is especially important to exclude transient ischaemic attacks. Women who experience migraine with visual aura have an increased risk of stroke which is approximately trebled if they smoke and trebled if on the combined oral contraceptive pill.

Assessment and investigations

Where a clear phenotype of long-standing and stable migraine has been established from the history together with a normal examination, imaging should not routinely be requested. However, focal neurological signs, atypical aura or prolonged aura may well justify MRI. While unusual (except for MOH), secondary causes do need to be borne in mind in patients with migrainous sounding headaches that are rapidly worsening.

Potentially significant abnormalities on MRI in patients with headache without neurological signs are found in less than 1%. However, even in healthy young adults, incidental changes on MRI are seen in nearly 10% of cases and may then require follow-up before being cleared as harmless. This usually generates considerable anxiety.

Keeping a diary each day to record headaches is often a helpful step. Recording should include the pain severity, duration of attacks and medications used. In females, the time of menses can also be recorded. Diaries should document the numbers of days abortive treatments are used to try and identify or avoid medication overuse. Disability can be assessed using a scale such as the Migraine Disability Assessment Scale (MIDAS), which is well validated and easy to use in clinical practice (Figure 12.4).

Management

The management of migraine includes non-pharmacological strategies, pharmacological treatments (acute and preventive treatments) and, rarely, surgery.

Non-pharmacological strategies

Migraine triggers and predisposing factors Migraineurs are often more sensitive to sensory stimuli than non-migraineurs. Thus, factors such as sleep disruption, skipping meals, perceived changes in stress levels or menstrual cycle sometimes can be significant factors in triggering or worsening migraine attacks. Therefore, patients should be advised to lead as regulated a life as is possible and acceptable. Healthy diets with regular eating patterns, good hydration, regular sleep, regular exercise, avoiding excessive caffeine and alcohol, and modifying or minimising stress will benefit most patients.

Cognitive behavioural therapy (CBT) CBT typically involves face-to-face meetings with a clinical psychologist although group sessions are sometimes used. It may seem rational to have some negative thoughts and emotions about a painful situation, but it can be helpful to explore the exact thoughts and emotions the patient experiences. These may be irrational, even involving catastrophising, and these beliefs may be then targeted and the patient encouraged to substitute these with more logical alternatives. Successful CBT can allow the patient to shift the locus of control from external chance to internal control. Rather than being seen as alternative to pharmacological treatments, behavioural therapies can be used successfully in conjunction with drugs. When successful, CBT can not only help the headache experience, but may also help to lessen some of the associated anxiety which can be co-morbid with migraine. It is advisable to be as specific as possible if asking others to refer on for CBT; patients may mistakenly end up having alternative approaches such as psychoanalysis offered.

Acupuncture This is commonly tried by patients even before being seen in specialty clinics. There are different techniques but at least some evidence for effectiveness. A recent study claimed similar results in chronic migraine to topiramate, although physician–patient interaction time was very different between the groups. While the evidence for efficacy is not overwhelming, acupuncture from an accredited practitioner is generally seen as safe and is included as an accepted treatment in the recent National Institute for Health and Care Excellence (NICE) headache guidelines for migraine prophylaxis.

Acute attack treatments General approaches to acute pharmacological treatment in migraine include either stepped or stratified care. Stratified approaches develop a treatment plan for individual patients depending on the severity of the headaches while stepped approaches with treatment ladders provide a more generic approach starting at cheapest and safest options and build up as needed. Some pharmaco-economic evidence exists in favour of a stratified approach, which is more patient-centred.

Acute treatments are generally divided into non-specific (paracetamol, non-steroidal anti-inflammatory drugs, opioids), which may be effective for other pain types, or migraine specific (triptans or ergots) (Table 12.2). If an individual acute treatment is ineffective in at least two out of three trials, it is considered a treatment failure. While a useful rule of thumb, this 'three strikes and you're out' approach does not entirely exclude the possibility that a different formulation of the drug might sometimes work for that individual. Importantly, there may be different approaches to different types of headaches that the patient recognises.

While early treatment is important to success, some patients cannot predict early on which will be a severe headache and too frequent use of acute treatments may result in the dangers of medication overuse. Patients should be advised to limit the intake of paracetamol and NSAIDs to less than 15 days per month while triptans, ergots and any other combination of acute headache treatments should be limited to 10 days per month. The use of a headache diary is helpful to keep track of both the headaches and treatment days.

If an oral acute medicine is not effective a retrial with an antiemetic should be considered. In patients who have significant nausea or vomiting agents such as prochlorperazine 3–6 mg as buccal preparations, metoclopramide or domperidone can be used. Very importantly, however, antiemetics that have prokinetic action help counter the gastric stasis often seen in migraine which then aid absorption of the oral medication. These motility agents include metoclopramide 20 mg, or domperidone 10–20 mg. The use of motility agents with acute treatments can result in improved efficacy of the abortive treatment.

NSAIDs can be effective for migraine but high doses may be required, for example ibuprofen 400–800 mg or aspirin 600–1000 mg, ideally in a form to aid absorption such as effervescent tablets. Paracetamol can be added but opioids are generally discouraged for migraine, not least because of the dangers of developing medication overuse headaches. If nausea or vomiting is prominent, diclofenac suppositories (100 mg) have been used as well as antiemetics.

Migraine specific treatments are dominated by the triptans. Generally, they are fairly well tolerated although uncontrolled cardiovascular risk factors can be a contraindication. The recent NICE headache guideline has suggested that a triptan should be combined with an antiemetic and either paracetamol or an NSAID as an initial treatment if deemed appropriate. The response to one triptan does not predict the response to other triptans, hence they should be tried in turn until the patient can identify an effective agent. A common problem is the relapse of headaches in the first 24 hours after successful initial treatment. For this reason a second dose is often considered within 24 hours if there is relapse after at least 2 hours. Care again has to be taken to educate against the dangers of medication overuse. Triptans should be used for the headaches and not for any preceding aura.

Rather than randomly selecting triptans until all have been tried, an approach can be made to rationalise this by trying to opt first for those with better evidence of effectiveness, tolerability and price. The difficulty is that some triptans will be favourable for one or two of these criteria but not all. All prescription triptans have placebo-controlled evidence to suggest effectiveness in migraine.

The Migraine Disability Assessment Test

The **MIDAS** (Migraine Disability Assessment) questionnaire was put together to help you measure the impact your headaches have on your life. The information on this questionnaire is also helpful for your primary care provider to determine the level of pain and disability caused by your headaches and to find the best treatment for you.

INSTRUCTIONS

Please answer the following questions about ALL of the headaches you have had over the last 3 months. Select your answer in the box next to each question. Select zero if you did not have the activity in the last 3 months. Please take the completed form to your healthcare professional.

_____ 1. On how many days in the last 3 months did you miss work or school because of your headaches?

_____ 2. How many days in the last 3 months was your productivity at work or school reduced by half or more because of your headaches? (Do not include days you counted in question 1 where you missed work or school.)

_____ 3. On how many days in the last 3 months did you not do household work (such as housework, home repairs and maintenance, shopping, caring for children and relatives) because of your headaches?

_____ 4. How many days in the last 3 months was your productivity in household work reduced by half of more because of your headaches? (Do not include days you counted in question 3 where you did not do household work.)

_____ 5. On how many days in the last 3 months did you miss family, social or leisure activities because of your headaches?

_____ Total (Questions 1-5)

What your Physician will need to know about your headache:

_____ A. On how many days in the last 3 months did you have a headache? (If a headache lasted more than 1 day, count each day.)

_____ B. On a scale of 0 - 10, on average how painful were these headaches? (where 0=no pain at all, and 10= pain as bad as it can be.)

Scoring: After you have filled out this questionnaire, add the total number of days from questions 1-5 (ignore A and B).

MIDAS Grade	Definition	MIDAS Score
I	Little or No Disability	0-5
II	Mild Disability	6-10
III	Moderate Disability	11-20
IV	Severe Disability	21+

If Your MIDAS Score is 6 or more, please discuss this with your doctor.

Figure 12.4 MIDAS headache questionnaire. MIDAS score (add the total number of days from questions 1–5; ignore A and B) 0–5 little disability; 6–10 mild disability; 11–20 moderate disability; 21+ severe disability.

A meta-analysis has been performed to allow a comparison of triptans with results for sumatriptan 100 mg in terms of effectiveness and tolerability. While this acknowledged the greatest experience with sumatriptan, it suggested that rizatriptan 10 mg, eletriptan 80 mg and almotriptan12.5 mg gave the highest likelihood of consistent success. Zolmitriptan 2.5 or 5 mg tablets were comparable to sumatriptan 100 mg. Naratriptan 2.5 mg showed lower efficacy but better tolerability. Frovatriptan was not included in this study, but the available data suggests that it has a lower efficacy but better tolerability than sumatriptan 100 mg.

Non-oral triptans may be of use with early vomiting or rapid onset headaches:

- Buccal: 'melt' forms of rizatriptan and zolmitriptan exist with evidence for their efficacy and speed of onset.
- Intranasal forms of sumatriptan and zolmitriptan exist. Importantly though, intranasal sumatriptan is still mainly absorbed enterally therefore not by-passing the problem of gastric stasis. This is less of a problem with zolmitriptan spray with about 30% of absorption occurring via the nasopharyngeal route.
- A subcutaneous triptan option only exists for sumatriptan. Subcutaneous sumatriptan can be extremely effective and rapid in onset.

Ergotamine can be effective but tolerability is a concern and is poorly absorbed orally with significant contraindications and side effect profile. The recent NICE guidelines specifically advised against the use of ergot-derived treatments for acute treatment of migraine.

The use of migraine-specific treatments in some special circumstances is summarised in Table 12.3.

Table 12.2 Acute migraine treatments.

Non-specific treatments	Specific treatments
Simple analgesics	**Triptans**
Aspirin (600–1000 mg)	Sumatriptan (50–100 mg)
Paracetamol (1000 mg)	Almotriptan (12.5 mg)
	Rizatriptan (10 mg)
NSAIDs	
Ibuprofen (400–800 mg)	Zolmitriptan (2.5–5 mg)
Naproxen (500–1000 mg)	Eletriptan (40–80 mg)
Tolfenamic acid (200 mg)	Frovatriptan (2.5 mg)
	Naratriptan (2.5 mg)

Ergots and opiates should be avoided due to the risk of developing medication overuse headache.
Acute migraine treatments can be used with antiemetic/prokinetics such as domperidone, prochlorperazine or metoclopramide.
NSAIDs, non-steroidal anti-inflammatory drugs.

Table 12.3 Acute treatments for migraine in special circumstances.

Clinical situation	Treatment options	Comments
Early nausea or vomiting	Rizatriptan MLT wafer 10 mg Sumatriptan nasal spray 20 mg Zolmitriptan nasal spray 5 mg Subcutaneous sumatriptan 6 mg	
Rapidly developing symptoms	Subcutaneous sumatriptan 6 mg	
Headache recurrence	Frovatriptan 2.5 mg Naratriptan 2.5 mg Almotriptan 12.5 mg Eletriptan 40 mg Ergotamine 1–2 mg	Ergotamine should not be used within 12 hours of a triptan
Poor tolerance of side effects	Naratriptan 2.5 mg Frovatriptan 2.5 mg Eletriptan 20 mg	Efficacy may be slightly less with these drugs
Menstrually related migraine – acute treatment	Triptans Dihydroergotamine nasal spray	Mini-prophylaxis with frovatriptan 2.5 mg twice daily, zolmitriptan 2.5 mg three times daily or naproxen 500 mg twice daily can be considered for 5–7 days starting 2 days before the period
Pregnancy	Paracetamol NSAIDs such as ibuprofen may be considered but still can cause problems especially in the third trimester with risk of bleeding or premature closure of the ductus arteriosus Sumatriptan has the most available data for use in pregnancy. From the available pregnancy registers no significant associations with major fetal abnormalities have been established though the data available is limited	The majority of women will experience improvement in their migraines as their pregnancy progresses

Preventative treatments Preventative treatment may help not only to reduce the frequency of headaches, but also to reduce severity of attacks and improve the effectiveness of acute medication. While typically having more than four headache days per month could lead to consideration of preventatives for some, less frequent headaches, especially if not responsive to acute treatment, may also be an indication for the use of such measures.

MOH has been discussed earlier, with evidence to support withdrawal to improve the headache. Another difficulty that may arise from medication-overuse is that patients may become less susceptible to preventatives. For much of the last decade fairly standard practice would be either to withdraw the medications being overused first for 1–2 months and then introduce a preventative *or* introduce a preventative at the same time as withdrawing. Recent analysis of evidence from trials in which topiramate or onabotulinumtoxinA appeared to benefit some patients in whom medication overuse was present has led to some debate on this issue.

Most preventatives had been developed for conditions other than headache and many have some evidence to support their use. Commonly used agents can be grouped into antiepileptic drugs, beta-blockers and tricyclic antidepressants. Other groups of agents used include serotonergic antagonists (pizotifen, methysergide), calcium channel antagonists (flunarizine), angiotensin modulators (angiotensin-converting enzyme inhibitors and angiotensin receptor inhibitors), nutrients and vitamins (co-enzyme Q10, riboflavin, magnesium) and herbal products such as feverfew.

The co-morbidities of the patient should be factored into choice, for example asthma excludes beta-blockers, a history of kidney stones or depression may contraindicate topiramate while topiramate may promote weight loss and therefore be favoured in patients with high BMI. Most preventatives have teratogenic potential although this is likely to be greatest for valproate. This is an important point, especially as many patients may be of childbearing age and some agents such as topiramate may increase likelihood of oral contraceptive failure.

The currently available evidence base is best for propranolol or topiramate. Valproate also has evidence for efficacy but has a significant side effect profile and teratogenicity is a particular concern. All three medicines were deemed to be effective in a recent American Academy of Neurology and American Headache Society report and can be considered for migraine prevention. Tricyclic antidepressants have long been used in migraine though the available evidence is difficult to assess because a range of doses, durations and drugs have been used in studies. A recent meta-analysis of randomised clinical trials of tricyclic antidepressants in migraine included 13 studies between 1966 and 2010 and concluded that the overall evidence was favourable. The options available for preventive treatments are covered in Table 12.4.

Whichever preventative is chosen, starting low and gradually increasing the dose typically over 2–4 weeks until either unacceptable side effects develop, a clear improvement emerges or until a maximum dose is reached. There can be a lag of up to 2 months after the optimum dose is achieved and therefore it is important to ensure that patients remain on these agents for a suitable duration of time.

In selected cases, combinations of preventatives can be beneficial where monotherapy has failed. Specific evidence exists for beta-blockers with topiramate, beta-blockers with valproate and

Table 12.4 Preventive treatments in migraine.

Drug	Dose	Selected side effects
Beta-blockers		
Propranolol	40–120 mg twice daily	Reduced energy Tiredness
Metoprolol	100–200 mg/day	Postural symptoms Erectile dysfunction Contraindicated in asthma
Antiepileptic agents		
Topiramate	25–200 mg/day	Parasthaesiae Cognitive dysfunction Weight loss Glaucoma Renal stones
Valproate	400–600 mg twice daily	Drowsiness Weight gain Tremor Hair loss Fetal abnormalities Haematological and liver abnormalities
Tricyclic antidepressants		
Amitriptyline	10–75 mg nocte	Drowsiness
Dothiepin	25–75 mg nocte	Dry mouth
Nortriptyline	10–75 mg nocte	Some patients are very sensitive and may only need a total dose of 10 mg, although generally 1–1.5 mg/kg body weight is required for a response
Serotonergic modulators		
Pizotifen	0.5–3 mg/day	Drowsiness Weight gain
Methysergide	1–6 mg/day	Drowsiness Leg cramps Hair loss Retroperitoneal fibrosis (a 1-month drug holiday is required every 6 months)
Calcium channel antagonists		
Flunarizine	5–10 mg/day	Lethargy Weight gain Depression Parkinsonism
Angiotensin-based modulators		
Lisinopril	10–20 mg/day	Persistent dry cough
Candesartan	8–32 mg/day	Hypotension
Telmisartan	20–80 mg/day	

Table 12.4 (continued)

Drug	Dose	Selected side effects
Neutriceutical		
Riboflavin	400 mg/day	Diarrhoea
Coenzyme Q10	300–600 mg/day	
Magnesium	600 mg/day	
Controlled trials demonstrate no effect		
Selective serotonin reuptake inhibitors (e.g. fluoxetine)		
Gabapentin		
Nimodipine		
Clonidine		
No convincing controlled evidence		
Verapamil		

topiramate with nortriptyline. While chronic migraine is also treated with preventative agents, the evidence base for preventatives is mainly focused on patients with episodic migraine. Specifically for chronic migraine there is evidence for topiramate, and OnabotulinumtoxinA as well as some limited evidence for acupuncture.

The two key PREEMPT studies looked at the effect of onabotulinumtoxinA (Botox) on chronic migraine versus saline placebo. The studies used 155–195 units of onabotulinumtoxinA injected at 31–39 sites around the head and neck. The pooled results of the two PREEMPT studies showed that from a similar baseline of around 19 days a month, after 24 weeks those who received Botox experienced a mean of 8.4 fewer headache days compared with a drop of 6.6 days in the placebo arm ($P < 0.001$). A variety of other secondary end-points also favoured Botox over placebo.

For highly disabled chronic migraine patients who are intractable to medical treatments, there is emerging evidence that occipital nerve stimulation can be useful.

Tension-type headache

Tension-type headache (TTH) is a relatively featureless headache, unlike migraine. Like migraine, TTH can be divided into episodic or chronic forms depending on whether patients have headaches on less or more than 15 days per month.

Epidemiology

While TTH is more common in the community than migraine, affecting over 60% of the population in Europe, they are not often seen in isolation in specialist headache clinics unless coexisting with migraines. This reflects the lower severity of TTH compared with migraine. In secondary or tertiary care one should be careful before diagnosing TTH and carefully consider migraine first even if it does not have many migrainous characteristics.

Clinical features

The episodic forms tend not to be severe, although chronic TTH can be associated with significant disability. The duration range is typically wider than for migraine. The ICHD-III (beta) definition lists the range as between 30 minutes and 30 days. TTH are not typically associated with the migrainous features such as photophobia, phonophobia, nausea and motion sensitivity. They are usually pressing or tightening headaches rather than throbbing.

Investigations

Clear cases of episodic TTH with a normal examination do not require routine imaging. As with migraine, if there was rapid progression or abnormal signs on examination then imaging and even lumbar puncture may need considering.

Management

Education and reassurance is especially important for TTH. Medical treatment may not even be needed but there is a potential danger of exacerbating the situation with excessive analgesia use. For acute treatment there is some evidence to support the use of NSAIDs such as naproxen and aspirin as well as paracetamol for episodic TTH.

Amitriptyline is often used where prophylaxis is required for TTH. A recent meta-analysis of tricyclic antidepressants found 17 randomised published studies focusing on TTH. Overall, the outcome was found to be similar to that for tricyclic antidepressants in migraine. Topiramate has also been shown to be potentially helpful in TTH. For frequent episodic or chronic TTH a course of acupuncture up to 10 sessions over 5–8 weeks may be beneficial.

Trigeminal autonomic cephalalgias

The trigeminal autonomic cephalalgias (TACs) are a group of primary headache disorders characterised by unilateral head pain that occurs in association with ipsilateral cranial autonomic features. The TACs include cluster headache, paroxysmal hemicrania, short-lasting unilateral neuralgiform headache attacks with conjunctival injection and tearing (SUNCT) and its closely related variant short-lasting unilateral neuralgiform headache attacks with cranial autonomic symptoms (SUNA) as well as hemicrania continua. The TACs differ in attack duration and frequency as well as the response to therapy (Table 12.5). The importance of recognising these syndromes resides in their excellent but highly selective response to treatment.

Cluster headache

Cluster headache is an excruciating syndrome and is probably one of the most painful conditions known to mankind with female patients describing each attack as being worse than childbirth. The central feature of cluster headache is its striking circannual (cycles that recur each year) and circadian periodicity.

Epidemiology

Cluster headache is a rare primary headache with a prevalence of 0.2%. There is a male predominance of 3.5–7 : 1.

Clinical features

The headaches are strictly unilateral, though attacks of pain can switch sides. The pain is excruciatingly severe. It is located mainly around the orbital and temporal regions though any part of the head can be affected. The headache lasts between 15 minutes and 3 hours. The signature feature of cluster is the association with autonomic symptoms. ICHD-III (beta) require the cluster attacks to be accompanied by at least one of the following, which have to be present on the pain side: conjunctival injection, lacrimation, miosis, ptosis, eyelid oedema, rhinorrhoea, nasal blockage and forehead or facial sweating, or restlessness or agitation. The autonomic features are transient, lasting only for the duration of the attack, with the exception of partial Horner's syndrome; ptosis or miosis may rarely persist, especially after frequent attacks.

Table 12.5 Clinical features of trigeminal autonomic cephalalgias.

	Cluster headache	Paroxysmal hemicranias	SUNCT/SUNA	Hemicrania continua
Sex F : M	1 : 3.5–7	1 : 1	1 : 1.5	1.6 : 1
Pain:				
Type	Stabbing, boring	Throbbing, boring, stabbing	Stabbing, sharp, burning,	Background dull ache, throbbing/stabbing exacerbations
Severity	Excruciating	Excruciating	Moderate to severe	Moderate background pain; severe exacerbations
Site	Orbit, temple	Orbit, temple	Orbit, temple	Orbit, temple
Attack frequency	1/alternate day –8 daily	>5/day for more than half the time	1/day – 30/hour	Continuous
Duration of attack	15–180 mins	2–30 mins	1–600 s	Continuous background pain; exacerbations very variable lasting mins to days
Autonomic features	Yes	Yes	Yes	Yes
Migrainous features	Yes	Yes	No	Yes
Alcohol trigger	Yes	Occasional	No	Rare
Cutaneous trigger	No	No	Yes	No
Indometacin effect	–	++	–	++
Abortive treatment	Sumatriptan injection or nasal spray Oxygen	Nil	Nil	Nil
Prophylactic treatment	Verapamil Methysergide Lithium	Indometacin	Lamotrigine Oxcarbazepine Topiramate	Indometacin

There are several descriptions of the full range of typical migrainous symptoms in significant proportions of cluster patients. Migrainous symptoms such as nausea, vomiting, photophobia, phonophobia and even aura symptoms have all been described in relationship to cluster attacks. However, in contrast to migraine, cluster headache sufferers are usually restless and irritable, preferring to move about, and looking for a movement or posture that may relieve the pain.

The cluster attack frequency varies between one every alternate day to three daily, although some have up to eight daily. The condition can have a striking circadian rhythmicity, with some patients reporting that the attacks occur at the same time each day. Alcohol, the smell of volatile substances, exercise, and elevated environmental temperature are recognised precipitants of cluster attacks.

Cluster headache is classified according to the duration of the bout. About 80–90% of patients have episodic cluster headache (ECH), which is diagnosed when they experience recurrent bouts, each with a duration of more than a week and separated by remissions lasting more than 4 weeks. The remaining 10–20% of patients have chronic cluster headache (CCH) in which either no remission occurs within 1 year or the remissions last less than 1 month. Most patients with episodic cluster headache have one or two annual cluster periods, each lasting between 1 and 3 months. Often, a striking circannual periodicity is seen with the cluster periods, with the bouts occurring in the same month of the year.

Investigations

The diagnosis of cluster headache is made entirely on the basis of a clinical history and neurological examination. However, it is very difficult to clinically dissect the secondary causes from primary cluster headache. MRI of the brain is a reasonable screening investigation.

Management

The management of cluster includes using acute attack treatments, preventive agents and, rarely, surgical approaches.

Acute attack treatments The pain of cluster headache builds up very rapidly to such an excruciating intensity that most oral agents are too slowly absorbed to cure the pain within a reasonable period of time. The most efficacious abortive agents are those that involve parenteral or pulmonary administration (Table 12.6).

Table 12.6 Acute attack treatments for cluster headache.

Good efficacy	Oxygen 100% at 7–12 L/min for 15–30 minutes Sumatriptan subcutaneous injection 6 mg (maximum twice daily for the duration of the cluster bout)
Moderate efficacy	Sumatriptan nasal spray 20 mg (maximum thrice daily for the duration of the cluster bout) Zolmitriptan 5 or 10 mg (for episodic cluster headache only)
Poor efficacy or unproven	Ergotamine tablets or suppository Intranasal lidocaine

Inhalation of oxygen is highly effective in the majority of patients. Oxygen needs to be used at a high concentration (100%) and flow-rate (7–12 L/min) for 15–20 minutes. Injectable sumatriptan 6 mg is the agent of choice for the acute treatment of cluster attacks. It has a rapid effect and high response rate with no evidence of tachyphylaxis. Though sumatriptan 20 mg and zolmitriptan 5 mg nasal sprays are effective in acute treatment, they are considerably less efficacious than injectable sumatriptan. However, they offer a useful option for patients who do not wish to self-inject regularly. There is no controlled evidence to support the use of oral sumatriptan in cluster headache. Oral sumatriptan 100 mg three times daily taken prior to an anticipated onset of an attack or at regular times does not prevent the attack and therefore it should not be used. Oral zolmitriptan 5 mg provides meaningful pain relief in episodic but not chronic cluster headache. However, its efficacy is modest and does not approach the efficacy or speed of subcutaneous sumatriptan or oxygen.

Preventive treatments The aim of preventive therapy is to produce a rapid suppression of attacks and to maintain that remission with minimal side effects until the cluster bout is over, or for a longer period in patients with chronic cluster headache.

Verapamil is the preventive drug of choice in both ECH and CCH. Clinical experience has demonstrated that higher doses than those used in cardiological indications are needed. Dosages commonly employed range from 240–960 mg/day in divided doses. Verapamil can cause heart block by slowing conduction in the atrioventricular node. Observing for PR interval prolongation on ECG can monitor potential development of heart block. After performing a baseline ECG, patients are usually started on 80 mg three times daily and thereafter the total daily dose is increased in increments of 80 mg every 10–14 days. An ECG is performed prior to each increment. The dose is increased until the cluster attacks are suppressed, side effects intervene or the maximum dose of 960 mg/day is achieved. About 20% of patients with cluster headache on verapamil have cardiac conduction problems and these can develop after months of stable dosing and are not dose-dependent. Thus, an ECG needs to be performed every 6 months with long-term therapy.

Other preventive treatment options include lithium and methysergide. Though topiramate, sodium valproate, pizotifen and gabapentin are often used, they are of as yet unproven efficacy.

Transitional therapies As preventative medications can take a number of weeks to exert their full effect, patients with short bouts or patients in whom one wishes to quickly control attack frequency may benefit from a transitional or bridging treatment. These interventions are not suitable for long-term use and so may require concurrent use with traditional preventative agents. A short course of steroids is the most commonly used transitional agent but a greater occipital nerve block is another option.

Surgery This is a last-resort measure in treatment-resistant patients. Procedures may be destructive, such as pterygopalatine ganglion or trigeminal ganglion procedures, or even trigeminal nerve root section. Most recently, neurostimulation therapies with occipital nerve stimulation, sphenopalatine ganglion stimulation and deep brain stimulation of the posterior hypothalamic region have emerged. These approaches are very promising and especially occipital nerve stimulation and sphenopalatine ganglion stimulation offer a more acceptable side effect profile than destructive and invasive approaches.

Paroxysmal hemicrania

Paroxysmal hemicrania is a rare syndrome that responds in a dramatic and absolute fashion to indometacin, thereby underlining the importance of distinguishing it from cluster headache, SUNCT and SUNA, which are not responsive to indometacin.

Clinical features The clinical phenotype of paroxysmal hemicrania is highly characteristic. Patients typically have unilateral, relatively brief, severe attacks of pain associated with cranial autonomic features that recur several times per day. The attacks have an abrupt onset and cessation. The pain is strictly unilateral and centred around the orbital and temporal regions though any part of the head can be affected. It is excruciatingly severe. The headache usually lasts 2–30 minutes. Attacks of paroxysmal hemicrania invariably occur in association with ipsilateral cranial autonomic features. Up to 85% of patients report at least one migrainous feature of photophobia, nausea or vomiting during an attack. Similar to cluster headache, patients are often restless or agitated during an attack. The frequency of attacks in paroxysmal hemicrania is high, ranging from 1 to 40 daily. The attacks occur regularly throughout the 24-hour period without a preponderance of nocturnal attacks as in cluster headache. While the majority of attacks are spontaneous, approximately 10% of attacks may be precipitated mechanically, either by bending or by rotating the head. Attacks may also be provoked by external pressure against the transverse processes of C4–5, C2 root or the greater occipital nerve. Alcohol ingestion triggers headaches in only 7% of patients.

Investigations The diagnosis of paroxysmal hemicrania is made entirely on the basis of a good clinical history and a detailed neurological examination. As a relatively high number of symptomatic cases have been reported, MRI of the brain should be routinely performed in all patients with paroxysmal hemicrania.

Management Indometacin leads to complete resolution of the headache. This is usually prompt, occurring within 1–2 days of initiating the effective dose. The typical maintenance dose ranges from 25 to 100 mg/day but may vary inter-and intra-individually between 12.5 and 300 mg/day. Therapy with indometacin can lead to gastrointestinal side effects. For patients who cannot tolerate indometacin one faces a difficult challenge. No other drug is consistently effective in paroxysmal hemicrania. Some response is seen with a range of other NSAIDs, however, this is usually not helpful. Other therapies that have been reported to be effective in paroxysmal hemicrania include topiramate, verapamil, cyclooxygenase-2 inhibitors, and greater occipital nerve block blocks

Short-lasting unilateral neuralgiform headache attacks

Clinical features This syndrome is characterised by moderate to severe, strictly unilateral pain that is usually centered over the orbital, supra-orbital or temporal region but can occur in other trigeminal distribution. The attacks last for 1–600 seconds and occur as single stabs, series of stabs or in a saw-tooth pattern. The attack frequency during the symptomatic phase varies immensely between patients and within an individual patient. Attacks may be as infrequent as once a day or less to more than 60 per hour. The pain is accompanied by prominent ipsilateral cranial autonomic features. The majority of patients can precipitate attacks by touching certain trigger zones within trigeminal innervated distribution and, occasionally, even from an extra-trigeminal territory. Precipitants include touching the face or scalp, washing, shaving, eating, chewing, brushing teeth, talking and coughing. Unlike in trigeminal neuralgia, most patients have no refractory period. This syndrome is very rare, with a prevalence of 1/15 000 population.

The disorder is further sub-classified into SUNCT or SUNA depending on the cranial autonomic features. SUNCT is diagnosed if patients have both conjunctival injection and lacrimation, while SUNA is diagnosed if only one or neither of these two autonomic symptoms are present. SUNCT and SUNA are likely to represent the same disorder but have been kept separate in ICHD-III until definitive evidence emerges to support this notion. These syndromes are very similar to trigeminal neuralgia and may indeed turn out to be variants of trigeminal neuralgia rather than distinct disorders in their own right.

Investigations Secondary forms of SUNCT and SUNA are typically seen with either posterior fossa or pituitary tumours. This emphasises the absolute need for cranial MRI, including adequate imaging of the pituitary. These patients should also have a basal (as opposed to dynamic) pituitary hormone screen. Recent studies suggest that in a high proportion of subjects with SUNCT/SUNA, brain MRI shows an arterial loop contacting or deforming the trigeminal nerve. Given the potential benefit of surgical decompression of the trigeminal nerve in trigeminal neuralgia the diagnostic work-up of SUNCT and SUNA should also include dedicated MRI cuts of the trigeminal nerves.

Management As the attacks are short-lasting, abortive therapies are not generally useful. For patients with acute severe debilitating attacks of SUNCT or SUNA, short-term prevention with an intravenous lidocaine infusion can be tried, though the headaches usually recur when the infusion is stopped. The mainstay of therapy in SUNCT and SUNA is preventive treatment. The most effective treatment based on open-label experience is lamotrigine. Other effective treatments include carbamazepine, topiramate and gabapentin. For patients who are refractory to medical treatments, surgical approaches can be useful. Trigeminal microvascular decompression can be useful in two-thirds of patients who have trigeminovascular conflict. Occipital nerve stimulation and posterior hypothalamic region deep brain stimulation can be highly effective in selected medically intractable patients.

Hemicrania continua

Hemicrania continua, like paroxysmal hemicrania, is an indometacin-responsive headache. Unlike the other TACs, which are intermittent short-lasting headaches, hemicrania continua is a continuous headache.

Clinical features Hemicrania continua is a persistent headache that is exclusively unilateral without side-shifting though rare cases of side alternating attacks have been described. Patients describe a persistent background pain of mild-to-moderate intensity with superimposed exacerbations that can be very severe and are associated with cranial autonomic features, a sense of restlessness or agitation and aggravation of pain by movement. An absolute response to therapeutic doses of indometacin (at least 150 mg/day and increasing to 225 mg/day if necessary) is a prerequisite for diagnosis.

Investigations As with paroxysmal hemicrania, a relatively high number of symptomatic cases of hemicrania continua have been reported hence MRI should be routinely performed in all patients suspected to have hemicrania continua. Furthermore, systemic symptoms, atypical presentation or hemicrania continua which becomes unresponsive to indometacin over time should prompt careful search for a secondary cause.

Management Indometacin leads to complete resolution of symptoms but a significant minority are unable to tolerate the side effects. No other drug is consistently helpful in hemicrania continua. The treatment options in these cases include other NSAIDs, cyclooxygenase-2 inhibitors, topiramate, melatonin, verapamil, gabapentin, greater occipital nerve blocks and botulinum toxin type A injections. For patients who are intractable to medical treatments, occipital nerve stimulation can be considered.

Other primary headaches

Primary cough headache

In cough headache, the pain arises moments after performing a Valsalva manoeuvre such as coughing, sneezing, straining, laughing or stooping. The pain reaches its peak almost immediately, and then subsides over several seconds to a few minutes although some patients experience mild to moderate headache for 2 hours. It is usually bilateral and posterior. Associated symptoms such as vertigo, nausea and sleep abnormality have been reported by up to two-thirds of patients. There is a significant correlation between the frequency of cough and the severity of the headache. This headache predominantly affects patients older than 40 years of age. The lifetime prevalence of benign cough headache is 1%.

The syndrome of cough headache is symptomatic in about 40% of cases, and the majority of patients in whom this is so have Chiari malformation type 1. Other reported causes include CSF hypotension, carotid or vertebrobasilar disease, middle cranial fossa or posterior fossa tumours, midbrain cyst, basilar impression, platybasia, subdural haematoma, cerebral aneurysms and reversible cerebral vasoconstriction syndrome. Diagnostic neuroimaging has an important role in the search for possible intracranial lesions or abnormalities.

The most consistently reported effective treatment is indometacin used at between 25 and 250 mg/day. Treatment should be withdrawn periodically to ascertain whether the symptoms have remitted. Other treatments reported to be effective include acetazolamide, topiramate, naproxen, propranolol, methysergide and intravenous dihydroergotamine. In addition to medical therapy, there are several reports of high volume (40 mL) CSF removal by lumbar puncture. The response can be dramatic and long term. Any pulmonary disease causing coughing should be identified and treated if possible.

Primary exercise headache

Exercise or exertional headaches are triggered by physical exercise. They are characterised by bilateral, throbbing pain that persists from 5 minutes to 48 hours. Exertional headaches are not usually associated with migrainous features, though exercise is also a fairly common trigger in some migraineurs for their typical migrainous headaches. Exertional headaches can be prevented by avoidance of excessive physical exercise, particularly in hot weather or at high altitude.

Case series report the presence of structural intracranial lesions in 10–40% of patients. The underlying abnormalities associated with exertional headaches include supratentorial and posterior fossa space-occupying lesions (both metastatic and primary), vascular abnormalities such as cerebral aneurysm or arteriovenous malformation, intracranial haemorrhage, intermittent obstruction of cerebrospinal fluid flow caused by a third ventricular colloid cyst, lateral ventricular tumour, or Chiari type 1 malformation, and previous traumatic injury. Extracranial causes of exertional headache include pheochromocytoma and cardiac cephalgia, which is a rare exertional headache secondary to cardiac ischaemia. Patients with exercise-induced headache should have brain MRI, and a neurovascular evaluation with intracranial magnetic resonance angiography. These patients should usually have an evaluation for coronary heart disease, particularly if headache occurs exclusively with exercise, lacks features suggestive of migraine, or radiates to or from the neck or jaw.

In situations where exertion cannot be predicted, treatment is prophylactic. If exertion can be predicted then pre-emptive therapy 30–60 minutes before exercise can be used. Indometacin at daily doses varying from 25 to 250 mg is generally very effective. Propranolol, naproxen and ergotamine derivatives have also been reported to be beneficial in some patients.

Primary sex headache

Sex headache may be precipitated by both masturbation and coitus. Sex headache is of two types, preorgasmic and orgasmic, which have distinct clinical features. Preorgasmic headache is a bilateral occipital or generalised pressure headache that gradually intensifies with growing sexual excitement. Orgasmic headache has a sudden explosive onset followed by severe throbbing head pain that occurs just prior to or at the moment of orgasm. Sex headache tends to be short-lasting, with severe pain generally lasting between 10 minutes and 6 hours. Accompanying symptoms are uncommon. Some patients with preorgasmic headaches can terminate the attack by stopping sexual activity. In about 50% of patients benign sex headache will settle in 6 months. There is an association between sex headache and exercise headache as well as migraine.

Several symptomatic causes of sex headache have been reported including subarachnoid haemorrhage (underlining the importance of investigating for an underlying intracranial aneurysm), non-haemorrhagic stroke, phaeochromocytoma and drugs such as cannabis, oral contraceptives and pseudoephredine. Spontaneous low CSF pressure headache is another pressure-like positional type of headache that may arise during sexual activity. It is thus mandatory to exclude structural intracranial abnormalities in all cases of sex headaches with appropriate neuroimaging. Evaluation for phaeochromocytoma is warranted when symptoms such as prominent flushing, tachycardia and sweating are present remote from sexual activity.

Benign sex headaches are usually irregular and infrequent, hence management can often be limited to reassurance and advice about ceasing sexual activity if a milder warning headache develops. When sex headaches occur frequently, they can be prevented by propranolol (40–200 mg/day), diltiazem 60 mg three times daily or indometacin (25–250 mg/day). Triptans, ergotamine or indometacin (25–75 mg) taken 30–45minutes prior to sexual activity can be helpful.

Primary thunderclap headache

Thunderclap headache is characterised by the abrupt onset of a severe headache that reaches maximum intensity within 1 minute. Thunderclap headache is frequently associated with serious vascular intracranial disorders, particularly subarachnoid haemorrhage, as well as cerebral venous sinus thrombosis, arterial dissection, reversible cerebral vasoconstriction syndrome and acute cerebral ischaemia. It has also been reported with other pathologies including pituitary apoplexy, spontaneous intracranial hypotension, third ventricle colloid cysts, arterial hypertension and systemic or intracranial infections. Some longitudinal studies suggest that a benign form of recurrent thunderclap headache exists but the evidence for this is considered to be relatively poor.

It is not possible to differentiate between primary and secondary thunderclap headache on clinical grounds. Therefore all patient with thunderclap headache should be investigated. The first episode should be vigorously investigated with CT and CSF examination. For patients with thunderclap headache who have non-diagnostic head CT and lumbar puncture, we suggest obtaining brain MRI. Additional studies that may be indicated on a case-by-case basis include angiography and venography. Primary thunderclap headache should be a diagnosis of last resort, reached only when all organic causes have been demonstrably excluded.

Primary thunderclap headache is generally self-limiting, but can recur over months or years. For patients who have recurrent attacks nimodipine has been reported to be helpful.

Primary stabbing headache

Primary stabbing headache is characterised by transient, sharp jabbing pains that occur within a small, localised area of the scalp. The pain can be unifocal or multifocal in site, predominantly within the first division of the trigeminal nerve. The attacks appear suddenly either as single stabs or in volleys of intense stabbing pain. The stabs last from 1 to 10 seconds and occur at irregular intervals from rarely to many times each day. The pain is spontaneous and without any additional features. The main differential diagnosis are SUNCT, SUNA and trigeminal neuralgia; primary stabbing headache is relatively easily differentiated from these conditions on the basis of presence of autonomic symptoms, triggerability and site of pain. Primary stabbing headache responds to indometacin, melatonin or cyclooxygenase-2 inhibitors.

Nummular headache

Nummular headache is characterised by small circumscribed areas of pain on the head. The pain is generally of mild to moderate intensity and confined to a round or elliptical, sharp contoured, unchanging area 1–6 cm in diameter. The pain is continuous, although in a large minority of cases spontaneous remissions lasting weeks to

Table 12.7 Differential diagnosis of new daily persistent headache.

Primary	Secondary
Migrainous variant Featureless (tension-type variant)	CSF pressure disorders: • Low CSF pressure headache • Raised CSF pressure headache Infections: • Chronic meningitis • Sphenoidal sinusitis Vascular disorders: • Subarachnoid haemorrhage • Chronic subdural haematoma • Carotid or vertebral artery dissection • Dural arteriovenous fistula Post-traumatic headache Leptomeningeal metastasis

Table 12.8 Causes of chronic daily headache.

Long-lasting (>4 hours/day)	Short-lasting (<4 hours/day)*
Chronic migraine†	Chronic cluster headache
Chronic tension-type headache†	Chronic paroxysmal hemicrania
Hemicrania continua†	SUNCT/SUNA
New daily persistent headache†	Hypnic headache
Nummular headache	

SUNA, short-lasting unilateral neuralgiform headache with cranial autonomic symptoms; SUNCT, short-lasting unilateral neuralgiform headache with conjunctival injection and tearing.
* Patient with these disorders may have more than 4 hours/day of headache. This classification emphasises that the individual attacks last less than 4 hours.
† May be complicated by analgesia overuse, thereby resulting in concurrent medication overuse headache.

months may occur. Superimposed on the continuous pain, lancinating pain may occur that initially lasts seconds but may gradually increase in duration to minutes or hours. The affected area commonly shows variable combinations of hyperaesthesia, paraesthesiae or allodynia. Structural and dermatological lesions need to be excluded with appropriate investigations. Treatment with gabapentin (900–1800 mg/day) can be effective, but nummular headache often becomes refractory to standard headache therapies.

Hypnic headache

Hypnic headache, also known as 'alarm clock headache', is characterised by episodes of head pain that develop only during sleep and awaken the patient from sleep. The pain is usually mild to moderate in 80% of cases. It lasts from 15 minutes to 3 hours. The pain is bilateral in two-thirds of cases. The pain is usually featureless though nausea, photophobia, phonophobia and cranial autonomic features can rarely accompany the pain. Hypnic headache is one of the few headaches that occurs almost exclusively in later life, usually after the age of 50 years.

Other possible causes of headache developing during and causing wakening from sleep should be ruled out, with particular attention given to sleep apnoea and medication overuse; intracranial structural disorders must be excluded with neuroimaging.

Simple analgesics tend to be effective abortive treatments. Preventive treatments reported to be effective include lithium, caffeine, melatonin, indometacin and flunarizine.

New daily persistent headache

New daily persistent headache (NDPH) is a distinct headache that is daily and unremitting within 24 hours of onset, and lasts more than 3 months. Eighty per cent of patients can pinpoint the exact date their headache started. The pain lacks characteristic features, and in many cases the phenotype resembles migraine or, less often, tension-type headache.

NDPH can have both secondary and primary forms (Table 12.7). Diagnostically, it is important to first exclude secondary forms of NDPH. We recommend neuroimaging for all patients presenting with NDPH. Where available, we suggest brain MRI with gadolinium as the initial imaging study. For selected patients, additional studies such as venography and lumbar puncture may be warranted

There are no controlled trials of treatment in primary NDPH. As noted earlier, the phenotype of primary NDPH often resembles primary chronic tension-type headache or a chronic migraine. Although evidence is lacking, it is intuitive to treat NDPH based on the phenotype. Thus, our suggested approach is to first classify the phenotype of NDPH as most similar to either migraine or chronic tension-type headache, and then treat with appropriate preventive headache therapy accordingly. NDPH may take either of two subtypes: a self-limited one, or a persistent form that can last years or decades and is challenging to treat.

Chronic daily headache

The term chronic daily headache (CDH) remains in widespread usage, though it is not part of ICHD-III. It is defined as the presence of headache of any sort on at least 15 days per month for at least 3 consecutive months. As such, it is a heterogeneous entity which can indicate frequent or long-lasting headache of any cause; it may be a manifestation of primary headache, for example chronic migraine, tension type or cluster headache or secondary headache (notably MOH). A diagnosis of CDH is therefore not a substitute for a definite primary or secondary headache diagnosis. Secondary causes should be looked for where appropriate. Primary headaches that can result in CDH are listed in Table 12.8.

References

Afridi S, Giffin NJ, Kaube H, Friston KJ, Ward NS, Frackowiak RSJ, *et al.* A positron emission tomographic study in spontaneous migraine. *Arch Neurol* 2005; **62:** 1270–1275.

Matharu MS, Bartsch T, Ward N, Frackowiak RS, Weiner R, Goadsby PJ. Central neuromodulation in chronic migraine patients with suboccipital stimulators: a PET study. *Brain* 2004; **127** (Pt 1): 220–230.

Matharu MS, Cohen AS, Frackowiak RS, Goadsby PJ. Posterior hypothalamic activation in paroxysmal hemicrania. *Ann Neurol* 2006; **59:** 535–545.

Matharu MS, Cohen AS, McGonigle DJ, Ward N, Frackowiak RS, Goadsby PJ. Posterior hypothalamic and brainstem activation in hemicrania continua. *Headache.* 2004; **44:** 747–761.

May A, Bahra A, Buchel C, Frackowiak RS, Goadsby PJ. Hypothalamic activation in cluster headache attacks. *Lancet* 1998; **352:** 275–278.

May A, Bahra A, Buchel C, Turner R, Goadsby PJ. Functional magnetic resonance imaging in spontaneous attacks of SUNCT: short-lasting neuralgiform headache with conjunctival injection and tearing. *Ann Neurol* 1999; **46:** 791–794.

Further reading

Background reading

Lance JW, Goadsby PJ. *Mechanisms and Management of Headache*, 7th edition. Philadelphia: Elsevier Butterworth Heinemann, 2005.

Olesen J, Tfelt-Hansen V, Ramadan N, Goadsby P, Welch KMA. *The Headaches*, 3rd edition. Philadelphia: Lippincott, Williams & Wilkins, 2005.

Silberstein SD, Lipton RB, Dodick D. *Wolff's Headache and Other Head Pain*, 8th edition. Oxford: Oxford University Press, 2008.

Classification

Headache Classification Subcommittee of The International Headache Society. The International Classification of Headache Disorders, 3rd edition (beta version). *Cephalalgia* 2013; **33:** 629–808.

Epidemiology and clinical features

Li D, Rozen TD. The clinical characteristics of new daily persistent headache. *Cephalalgia* 2002; **22:** 66–69.

Markus HS. A prospective follow up of thunderclap headache mimicking subarachnoid haemorrhage. *J Neurol Neurosurg Psychiatry* 1991; **54:** 1117–1118.

Tepper SJ, Dahlof CG, Dowson A, Newman L, Mansbach H, Jones M, *et al.* Prevalence and diagnosis of migraine in patients consulting their physician with a complaint of headache: data from the LANDMARK Study. *Headache* 2004; **44:** 856–864.

Investigation

Afridi S, Matharu M, Lee L, Kaube H, Friston K, Frackowiak R, *et al.* A PET study exploring the laterality of brainstem activation in migraine using glyceryl trinitrate. *Cephalalgia* 2004; **9:** 775–776.

Bahra A, Matharu MS, Buchel C, Frackowiak RS, Goadsby PJ. Brainstem activation specific to migraine headache. *Lancet* 2001; **357:** 1016–1017.

Matharu MS, Cohen AS, McGonigle DJ, Ward N, Frackowiak RS, Goadsby PJ. Posterior hypothalamic and brainstem activation in hemicrania continua. *Headache* 2004; **44:** 747–761.

Specific and unusual headache syndromes

Boes CJ, Matharu MS, Goadsby PJ. Benign cough headache. *Cephalalgia* 2002; **22:** 772–779.

Cittadini E, Matharu MS. Symptomatic trigeminal autonomic cephalalgias. *Neurologist* 2009; **15:** 305–312.

Cittadini E, Matharu MS, Goadsby PJ. Paroxysmal hemicrania: a prospective clinical study of 31 cases. *Brain* 2008; **131** (Pt 4): 1142–1155.

Cohen AS, Matharu MS, Goadsby PJ. Short-lasting unilateral neuralgiform headache attacks with conjunctival injection and tearing (SUNCT) or cranial autonomic features (SUNA): a prospective clinical study of SUNCT and SUNA. *Brain* 2006; **129** (Pt 10): 2746–2760.

Dodick DW, Mosek AC, Campbell JK. The hypnic ("alarm clock") headache syndrome. *Cephalalgia* 1998; **18:** 152–156.

Evers S, Goadsby PJ. Hypnic headache: clinical features, pathophysiology, and treatment. *Neurology* 2003; **60:** 905–909.

Pareja JA, Pareja J, Barriga FJ, Baron M, Dobato JL, Pardo J, *et al.* Nummular headache: a prospective series of 14 new cases. *Headache* 2004; **44:** 611–614.

Pareja JA, Ruiz J, de Isla C, al-Sabbah H, Espejo J. Idiopathic stabbing headache (jabs and jolts syndrome). *Cephalalgia* 1996; **16:** 93–96.

Pascual J, Iglesias F, Oterino A, Vazquez-Barquero A, Berciano J. Cough, exertional, and sexual headaches: an analysis of 72 benign and symptomatic cases. *Neurology* 1996; **46:** 1520–1524.

Schwedt TJ, Matharu MS, Dodick DW. Thunderclap headache. *Lancet Neurol* 2006; **5:** 621–631.

Treatments

Cohen AS, Matharu MS, Goadsby PJ. Trigeminal autonomic cephalalgias: current and future treatments. *Headache* 2007; **47:** 969–980.

Diener HC. Detoxification for medication overuse headache is not necessary. *Cephalalgia* 2012; **32:** 423–427.

Dodick DW, Turkel CC, DeGryse RE, Aurora SK, Silberstein SD, Lipton RB, *et al.* OnabotulinumtoxinA for treatment of chronic migraine: pooled results from the double-blind, randomized, placebo-controlled phases of the PREEMPT clinical program. *Headache* 2010; **50:** 921–936.

Ferrari MD, Goadsby PJ, Roon KI, Lipton RB. Triptans (serotonin, 5-HT1B/1D agonists) in migraine: detailed results and methods of a meta-analysis of 53 trials. *Cephalalgia* 2002; **22:** 633–658.

Goadsby PJ. The pharmacology of headache. *Prog Neurobiol* 2000; **62:** 509–525.

Jackson JL, Shimeall W, Sessums L, Dezee KJ, Becher D, Diemer M, *et al.* Tricyclic antidepressants and headaches: systematic review and meta-analysis. *Br Med J* 2010; **341:** c5222.

Lambru G, Matharu M. Management of trigeminal autonomic cephalalgias in children and adolescents. *Curr Pain Headache Rep* 2013; **17:** 323.

Lambru G, Matharu MS. Occipital nerve stimulation in primary headache syndromes. *Ther Adv Neurol Disord* 2012; **5:** 57–67.

Lambru G, Matharu MS. Trigeminal autonomic cephalalgias: a review of recent diagnostic, therapeutic and pathophysiological developments. *Ann Indian Acad Neurol* 2012; **15** (Suppl 1): 51–61.

Linde K, Allais G, Brinkhaus B, Manheimer E, Vickers A, White AR. Acupuncture for tension-type headache. *Cochrane Database Syst Rev* 2009; **1:** CD007587.

Matharu MS, Zrinzo L. Deep brain stimulation in cluster headache. *Expert Rev Neurother* 2011; **11:** 473–475.

National Institute for Health and Clinical Excellence. Diagnosis and management of headaches in young people and adults 2012. Available from: http://guidance.nice.org.uk/CG150 (accessed 4 January 2016).

Olesen J. Detoxification for medication overuse headache is the primary task. *Cephalalgia* 2012; **32:** 420–422.

Silberstein SD, Dodick DW, Saper J, Huh B, Slavin KV, Sharan A, *et al.* Safety and efficacy of peripheral nerve stimulation of the occipital nerves for the management of chronic migraine: results from a randomized, multicenter, double-blinded, controlled study. *Cephalalgia* 2012; **32:** 1165–1179.

CHAPTER 13

Cranial Nerve Disorders

Jeremy Chataway, Charles Clarke, Robin Howard and Paul Jarman
National Hospital for Neurology & Neurosurgery

This chapter reviews typical features of lesions of individual cranial nerves and conditions affecting them, and some combinations of cranial nerve lesions. Conditions affecting the optic nerves and cranial nerves III, IV and VI are discussed in Chapter 13. Neuro-otological conditions are discussed in Chapter 15 and the anatomy of the cranial nerves, their nuclei and central connections in Chapter 2.

I. Olfactory nerve

Complaints about disorders of the sense of smell are relatively common; they are sometimes almost unnoticed by patients and tend to be downplayed by clinicians. Loss of olfaction is often an underestimated disability; it is of great importance in the professions where differentiation of complex odours is vital. Although seldom regarded as a major handicap, anosmia or hyposmia may be the first manifestation of a serious underlying disorder. Olfaction can be difficult to test in practice and is often not examined routinely.

Functional anatomy

Humans have two nasal chemosensory systems: the olfactory nerve system responsible for detecting odours, and trigeminal afferents that respond to irritants, high concentrations of odorants and the sensation of coolness (e.g. menthol vapour). Thus, in patients with anosmia resulting from lesions of the olfactory nerve, the response to nasal irritation from ammonia or menthol is still preserved. The olfactory pathways and the subtleties of the complex mechanisms of olfaction are described in Chapter 2.

Symptoms

Anosmia refers to complete loss of sense of smell and partial anosmia to loss of ability to detect certain smells. Hyposmia indicates generally diminished sense of smell. Dysosmia is distorted sense of smell (e.g. when pleasant odours smell unpleasant). Phantosmia refers to a sensation of smell that is constantly present, in the absence of objective odour.

Patients with impaired olfactory function also usually complain of loss of taste. This is because most of the perceived flavour of food is derived from smell rather than taste: try tasting food or drink with the nostrils occluded. The four basic tastes – sweet, sour, salty and bitter – are subserved by Vth, VIIth and IXth nerve afferents. *Umami*, the savoury, tomato-like taste recognised via glutamate-specific receptors is distinct from the four common basic tastes and is rarely tested in clinical practice. These remain intact in the patient with anosmia. Many people with gradual loss of smell over many years are unaware of the problem. Dysosmia and phantosmia, often with perception of a foul or medicinal odour, may occur during olfactory epithelium degeneration and regeneration; this may follow an upper respiratory infection or paranasal sinus infection, or head trauma. These complaints are also noted frequently after cancer chemotherapy and cranial radiotherapy; recovery is uncertain.

It is important to determine the tempo of onset and to distinguish clinically between total bilateral loss of sense of smell and unilateral loss, rarely noticed by patients; the latter can point to a lateralised lesion of the olfactory system. A history of local nasal symptoms indicative of nasal congestion, allergic rhinitis or sinusitis should be sought. A recent upper respiratory tract infection may be relevant. Past history of head injury, exposure to toxic fumes, drugs, chemotherapy or radiotherapy, excessive alcohol, smoking and cocaine use, systemic diseases, and features of Parkinson's disease or cognitive impairment may all provide clues to aetiology. Kallmann's syndrome is a rare cause of anosmia resulting from failure of the olfactory lobes to develop, with secondary hypogonadism caused by gonadotropic hormone deficiency.

Examination

Detailed smell testing is difficult in routine clinical practice. The usual assessment is to ask patients to sniff vials containing odours such as peppermint oil, cloves or coffee, using each nostril in turn with the other occluded. The examiner should be aware that even with a normal sense of smell it may be difficult for many people to identify these odours – the crux of the matter is to distinguish them. Non-organic anosmia may be suggested by the loss of ability to detect ammonia, which causes nasal irritation because of stimulation of trigeminal afferents within the nose; such testing with irritants should be carried out with particular care, if at all. However, all tests of this sort are relatively crude. More detailed testing of olfaction is possible using commercially available tests such as the University of Pennsylvania Smell Identification Test (UPSIT), a standardised panel of 40 microencapsulated 'scratch and sniff' odours with multiple choice identification of each. A percentile ranking, compared to age- and gender-matched controls is obtained

Neurology: A Queen Square Textbook, Second Edition. Edited by Charles Clarke, Robin Howard, Martin Rossor and Simon Shorvon.

and olfactory function may be classified into one of six categories from anosmia to normal, and includes malingering. Other shorter quantitative smell testing kits are also commercially available. There are no readily available objective neurophysiological tests, although evoked responses are used in some research protocols.

In addition to testing olfaction, taste should be tested in patients with olfactory disorders, and the mouth, nose and sinuses examined. Endoscopic examination by an ENT specialist is usually necessary.

Causes of anosmia

Olfactory disorders are caused either by transport disorders brought about by local obstruction of the nasal passages or sensori-neural impairment from damage to the olfactory neuro-epithelium, olfactory nerve or its central connections.

Ageing

Age-related reduction in sense of smell is the norm. About half of the population between the ages of 65 and 80 years have significant impairment, a figure that rises to almost three-quarters after the age of 80. This diminution of smell with age may contribute to the loss of appetite that sometimes occurs in the elderly. The number of olfactory receptors and neurones decreases with age and there may be cumulative damage from viruses and degenerative change. In some cases bone growth around the ethmoid, leading to compression of the olfactory fila, may be a cause.

Upper respiratory infections, nasal and paranasal sinus disease

Viral upper respiratory tract infections, including the common cold and influenza, are probably the most common cause of permanent loss of smell. Often the infection is more severe than usual and is remembered by the patient. Damage to the olfactory epithelium and receptors, including the basal cells from which receptor cells regenerate, is probably the cause. A wide variety of allergic and infective nasal disorders, including chronic rhinitis and sinusitis, as well as disorders causing nasal obstruction, may all be associated with anosmia.

Trauma and surgery

Acceleration–deceleration of the brain following injury can shear the delicate olfactory fila as they pass through the cribriform plate of the ethmoid, with or without fracture of the cribriform plate itself. A fall on to the occipital region can cause this, without loss of consciousness, sometimes with frontal lobe contracoup injury. Anosmia is also associated with more severe traumatic brain injury with evident damage to the olfactory bulb and frontal cortical and subcortical structures; nasal trauma may also be a contributing factor in some cases. Transient dysosmia can occur soon after injury; recovery of olfactory function occurs in 30–40% but is unlikely if symptoms persist for longer than a year. Anosmia, unilateral or bilateral, can follow surgery to the sub-frontal region, sometimes with a persistent cerebrospinal fluid (CSF) leak and risk of meningitis.

Neurodegenerative disorders

Impaired olfactory function has been well described in:

- Parkinson's disease
- Dementia with Lewy bodies
- Alzheimer's disease
- Huntington's disease
- Motor neurone disease
- Korsakoff's syndrome
- Multiple sclerosis (MS).

In Parkinson's disease, the anterior olfactory structures including the olfactory bulb and anterior olfactory nucleus have been shown to be involved, with Lewy body formation at an early stage of the disease. Similarly, in Alzheimer's disease, profound neuronal loss is seen in the olfactory bulb and limbic brain regions, areas that receive olfactory input become heavily laden with neurofibrillary tangles and plaques. In MS, olfactory loss is in direct proportion to the burden of demyelinating lesions in areas of the brain associated with olfactory processing (frontal and temporal regions).

In idiopathic Parkinson's disease, hyposmia predates the onset of motor symptoms, often by many years or even decades. Impaired olfactory function is found in up to 90% of patients with Parkinson's disease, irrespective of disease duration or severity. Perception of certain odours such as petrol, banana, smoke and cinnamon seem to be lost preferentially on detailed testing. Demonstration of hyposmia may be useful in the differential diagnosis of parkinsonian disorders, because other extrapyramidal disorders such as progressive supranuclear palsy, vascular parkinsonism and corticobasal degeneration are not associated with an increased prevalence of impaired olfaction compared to age-matched controls. However, hyposmia is sometimes seen in multiple system atrophy. There has been recent interest in olfactory testing as a biomarker of preclinical Parkinson's and Alzheimer's diseases.

Other causes of olfactory dysfunction

Olfactory groove meningiomas are an important, if rare, cause of unilateral anosmia; impairment of smell may be the only or principal symptom of this tumour. Eventually, unilateral visual loss resulting from posterior extension to involve the optic nerve and dementia because of frontal lobe involvement may follow. Other structural lesions such as pituitary tumours and aneurysms may also compress the olfactory tract below the frontal lobes. Toxic exposure to a wide variety of industrial agents including acids, acetone, solvents and benzene have been anecdotally related to impaired smell, possibly because of direct damage to the olfactory receptor cells in some cases. The highly metabolically active receptor cells are also vulnerable to exposure to a number of drugs including antibiotics, anti-inflammatory agents, antithyroid drugs, antimetabolites and chemotherapeutic agents or radiotherapy – the latter two can irreversibly damage the ability of olfactory receptor cells to proliferate. Similarly, cigarette smoking impairs olfactory ability, usually with recovery after abstinence.

A variety of medical disorders such as cirrhosis, renal failure, hypothyroidism and vitamin deficiency (vitamins A, B_6 and B_{12}) can cause impaired olfaction. Olfactory receptor cells may be congenitally absent in Kallmann's syndrome, Turner's syndrome and albinism.

Damage to cortical structures involved in olfactory processing can lead to impaired odour identification or impairment of recognition memory but rarely to total anosmia. Olfactory hallucinations are well-recognised as part of the aura preceding a temporal lobe seizure; such hallucinations rarely occur as the sole manifestation of a seizure (Chapter 7). An unpleasant but stereotyped smell is usually described but it is rarely an identifiable odour. Olfactory hallucinations may also occur in depression, schizophrenia and alcohol withdrawal. The complaint of a constant foul smell, or of a distortion of smell with everything smelling unpleasant, may sometimes be a result of suppurative paranasal sinus infection, but is more often of psychotic origin or associated with depressive illness.

V. Trigeminal nerve

The trigeminal is the largest cranial nerve. It contains sensory and motor components, the sensory territory includes the face and head anterior to the vertex, the mucous membranes of the oral and nasal cavities, paranasal sinuses, the teeth, intracranial vessels and the dura of the anterior and middle cranial fossae. The motor root supplies the muscles of mastication. Detailed anatomy is considered in Chapter 2. The distribution of the three peripheral divisions of the nerve is shown in Figure 13.1 and the arrangement of the distribution of the spinal Vth nucleus in Figure 13.2.

Examination

Motor and sensory functions of the trigeminal nerve need to be examined separately. Sensory examination should include examination of all three divisions of the nerve and comparison made with the other side. Cutaneous sensation including light touch, pin-prick and temperature should all be tested. In practice, temperature sensation is often quickly assessed with a cold metal tuning fork, asking if the patient can appreciate the cool temperature of the metal against the facial skin. Remember that the angle of the jaw is usually outside the trigeminal territory and that V_1, the ophthalmic division includes the side of the nose and extends back to the vertex. The back of the scalp and angle of the jaw are supplied by the C2/3 dermatomes. Non-organic patterns of sensory loss may include the angle of the jaw or stop at the hairline but it is essential to recognise that organic disease may occasionally result in atypical patterns of sensory loss (e.g. in syringobulbia).

The corneal reflex (Chapters 2, 4 and 20) is elicited with a wisp of cotton wool or sometimes by wafting air gently over the cornea while shielding the other eye. The afferent arc is mediated by V_1 for the upper cornea and V_2 for the lower portion of the cornea (Chapter 2); the efferent arc is via the facial nerve (blink) and nervus intermedius (lacrimation). In the normal corneal response, there is discomfort when the cornea is touched, accompanied by tearing and conjunctival injection. Abnormalities of the corneal reflex may be an early sensitive sign of trigeminal nerve sensory dysfunction; neurophysiological recording of the related blink reflex is a useful way of quantifying an abnormality.

Tactile sensory loss on the face in the absence of a reduced or absent corneal reflex should raise suspicion of a non-organic cause. Parietal lobe lesions (involving the peri-sylvian portion of the post-central gyrus) can cause depression of contralateral corneal sensation.

The muscles of mastication are tested, first by asking the patient to clench the jaw, palpating the muscles and looking for fasciculation. Strength of jaw opening and lateral deviation against resistance are also examined. Unilateral lesions causing jaw deviation towards the affected side (contralateral pterygoid contraction) and inability to deviate the jaw to the opposite side. The jaw jerk is elicited with the jaw relaxed and slightly open. The afferent arc is via stretch receptors in V_3 and the efferent arc via the trigeminal motor fibres. An absent jaw jerk is rarely helpful. An exaggerated jaw jerk indicates bilateral supranuclear lesions of the cortico-bulbar pathways rostral to the pons (i.e. pseudobulbar palsy).

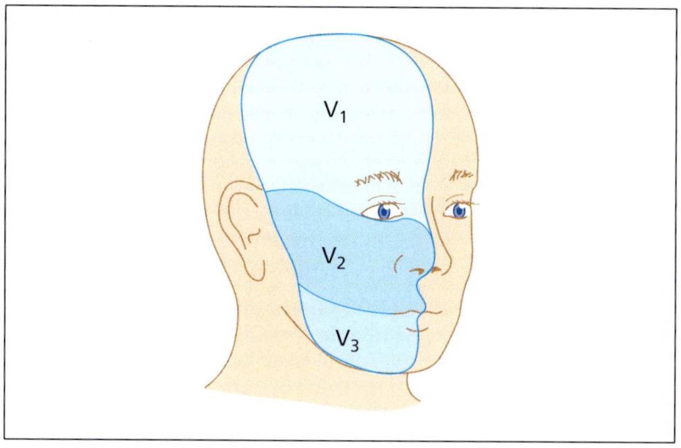

Figure 13.1 Cutaneous distribution of the three divisions of Vth nerve. Precise distribution varies amongst published sources. Source: Patten 1996. Reproduced with permission of Springer Science + Business Media.

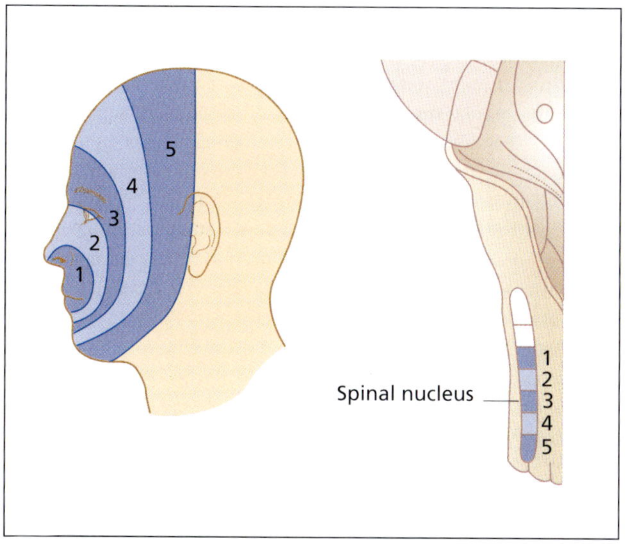

Figure 13.2 Distribution of spinal Vth nucleus. Source: FitzGerald 2010. © 2016 Elsevier. Reproduced with permission of Elsevier.

Peripheral Vth nerve lesions

Lesions of individual divisions and peripheral branches produce well-demarcated areas of sensory loss on the face and sometimes considerable pain. Trauma is a frequent cause; the supra-orbital and infra-orbital branches of V_1 are among the nerves most commonly affected. Numbness of half of the tongue accompanied by occipital and upper neck pain on head turning is a feature of the neck–tongue syndrome, believed to be caused by compression of the ventral ramus of C2 that carries sensory fibres from the tongue via the hypoglossal nerve. The ophthalmic, maxillary and mandibular divisions may be affected individually or in combination as they exit the skull base (through the superior orbital fissure, foramen rotundum and foramen ovale) by malignant meningeal infiltration, infective or granulomatous meningeal processes, or bony metastases in the skull. The Gasserian ganglion may be affected by similar processes at the petrous tip, causing ipsilateral sensory disturbance in the face; the abducens nerve may also be affected in this area (Gradenigo's syndrome). Trigeminal schwannomas may arise from the region of the trigeminal ganglion, either as an isolated tumour or as part of the spectrum of neurofibromatosis type 2. The trigeminal nerve may be involved in cerebellopontine angle syndromes (see Cerebellopontine angle syndrome).

Numb chin syndrome

Unilateral sensory disturbance affecting the chin and lower lip is a distinctive, important syndrome. It usually indicates a bony metastasis in the mandible involving the mental nerve. This can be a feature of a breast or prostate cancer recurrence, lymphoma or myeloma. Some cases are caused by more proximal infiltration of V_3. Non-malignant disorders affecting the mandible can also present in this way. A variant is the numb cheek syndrome, is caused by compromise of the infra-orbital nerve in the infra-orbital foramen, or proximal involvement of V_2.

Superior orbital fissure syndrome

The ophthalmic division V_1 within the superior orbital fossa (SOF) may be involved in various combinations with the IIIrd, IVth and VIth cranial nerves (Chapter 14). The typical presentation is with ophthalmoplegia accompanied by sensory disturbance and often pain in V_1 distribution, sometimes in combination with proptosis with large orbital lesions. Horner's syndrome and visual loss may also occur if the sympathetic supply to the eye or optic nerve become involved, the latter suggesting extension to the orbital apex. Tumours, such as nasopharyngeal cancers, trauma, infections, e.g. epidural abscesses (see Intracranial epidural abscess) and mucormycosis spreading from a paranasal sinus and inflammatory disorders (e.g. sarcoidosis and Wegener's granulomatosis; Chapter 26) are important causes of the SOF syndrome.

Cavernous sinus syndrome

This can be clinically indistinguishable from the SOF syndrome except that V_2 as well as V_1 may be involved in the cavernous sinus syndrome. Proptosis does not occur, except in the case of carotid cavernous fistulas (Chapter 14). Involvement of both the oculomotor nerve and the sympathetic supply to the eye may result in a mid position, non-reactive pupil, or the pupil may be dilated or miotic because of sympathetic or parasympathetic involvement in isolation. The causes are listed in Table 13.1. Cavernous sinus thrombosis is a serious condition that can follow infection of the face, paranasal sinuses (particularly the sphenoid sinus) or teeth. Spread to the opposite cavernous sinus usually occurs within a short time. The cavernous sinus syndrome is also discussed in Chapter 14.

Table 13.1 Causes of cavernous sinus syndrome (ophthalmoplegia, orbital congestion, chemosis, peri-orbital oedema, proptosis, facial sensory loss, Horner's syndrome).

Vascular	Carotid aneurysms (aneurysms of the intracavernous portion of the carotid artery)
	Carotico-cavernous fistula
	Thrombosis (secondary to paranasal sinus infection, orbital cellulitis, facial infection)
Neoplastic	Metastases
	Nasopharyngeal carcinoma
	Pituitary adenoma (lateral expansion)
	Craniopharyngioma
	Meningioma
	Lymphoma
Inflammatory	Any inflammatory granulomatous process
	Sarcoidosis
	Wegener's granulomatosis
	Polyarteritis nodosa
	Tolosa–Hunt syndrome

Nuclear Vth nerve lesions

As with other cranial nerves, trigeminal nuclear lesions resulting from intrinsic brainstem pathology, such as tumour, inflammatory or vascular lesions, frequently involve other brainstem structures. Because the lateral spinothalamic tract (which has already decussated) lies close to the trigeminal spinal tract and its nucleus, a common pattern is ipsilateral facial dissociated sensory loss (pain and temperature) with contralateral dissociated sensory loss in the limbs and trunk. Infarction of the lateral medulla (Wallenberg's lateral medullary syndrome; Chapter 5) is the most common cause.

The spinal trigeminal nucleus may be disrupted anywhere in the long course between the caudal pons and upper cervical cord. The somatotopic arrangement of the nucleus maps to an onion skin type distribution in the face, the nose and mouth being the centre of the onion, represented rostrally, with subsequent more posterior layers being more caudal in the nucleus (Figure 13.2). Thus, pontine nuclear lesions may result in intra-oral sensory loss with sparing of the face, while lesions of the lower part of nucleus (e.g. in syringobulbia) may be like a balaclava, sparing the muzzle area. The extension of the lower trigeminal spinal nucleus into the upper spinal cord means that lesions in this area may occasionally be a cause of facial pain and sensory disturbance.

Dorsal mid pons lesions involving the principal sensory nucleus and motor nucleus cause ipsilateral facial hemianaesthesia, usually to both light touch and pain/temperature, with paresis of muscles of mastication. There may be contralateral hemiplegia and spinothalamic sensory loss in the limbs. Ipsilateral tremor, internuclear ophthalmoplegia and Horner's syndrome can also occur with lesions in this area. Dorsal mid-pontine tumours can occasionally cause ipsilateral masticatory muscle spasm limiting jaw opening.

Trigeminal neuralgia

Trigeminal neuralgia (TN) is the most common disorder of the trigeminal nerve. Although not life-threatening, TN can be extraordinarily distressing. Prevalence is difficult to determine; incidence is approximately 4/100000/year. Women are more frequently affected than men. TN, often termed idiopathic but frequently caused by neurovascular compression, starts typically in the sixth and seventh decades; younger patients are more likely to have symptomatic TN (e.g. caused by MS) or occasionally a mass lesion.

Clinical features

The pain is usually quite characteristic, consisting of excruciating lancinating paroxysms in the face. This pain is severe, often described as shooting, stabbing, electric shock-like or as like a red hot needle. Paroxysms last for a few seconds or a minute at most; they tend to occur in bouts, sometimes with such frequency that paroxysms become indistinct. Often a refractory period of several minutes is seen after each attack, the duration being proportional to the severity and length of the paroxysm. The face may contort during an attack, hence the name tic douloureux. Patients are usually pain-free between attacks but in some a superimposed dull background pain may develop, often a sign of a poor response to treatment. Sensory triggering of pain by touching a specific affected part of the face (often no larger than a few millimetres), or by talking, chewing or even exposing the face to wind is very characteristic. Patients may be prevented from eating, drinking or brushing teeth; men may leave an area of the face unshaved. Weight loss can follow from pain triggered by eating. The mandibular and maxillary territories of the nerve are far more commonly affected than the ophthalmic division (only 5%); pain commencing in V_1 distribution should lead to consideration of an underlying cause for TN. Bilateral TN is rare (3%) and usually caused by intrinsic brainstem pathology such as demyelination.

Spontaneous remissions occur, lasting months or even years, but the pain almost always recurs. Successive bouts tend to be worse and more frequent, with shorter remissions and the pain may spread to affect a wider area of the face over time, typically commencing in V_3 distribution and moving to include V_2 and V_1. Patients may become fearful during a remission that the pain will return. Examination can be difficult as the patient may be hesitant to allow the face to be touched. Subtle areas of cutaneous sensory loss over the affected area are seen in a minority of patients if careful examination is performed, but examination is typically normal. The presence of other neurological signs points to an underlying cause for TN. Careful scrutiny of the teeth and oral cavity is important, to identify other causes of facial pain.

The diagnosis of TN is often made erroneously in patients with other causes of facial pain. The presence of characteristic paroxysms of lancinating pain is needed to make the diagnosis, supported by sensory trigger areas. The main differential diagnosis of TN is dental disease, particularly dental abscess and the cracked tooth syndrome, both of which can mimic localised forms of TN. Most patients consult a dentist initially, and many will have had dental work, with no improvement in pain, before the diagnosis of TN is suggested. Some will date onset of symptoms to a dental procedure. Acute glaucoma, sinusitis, giant cell arteritis and angina with referred jaw pain should all enter the differential diagnosis. Temporo-mandibular joint dysfunction causing facial pain is rarely like TN, it is usually associated with jaw movements and is probably over-diagnosed. Trigeminal autonomic cephalalgias such as cluster headache (Chapter 12) typically affect only the eye and surrounding area and usually easily differentiated from TN. Distinguishing V_1 TN from attacks of short-lasting unilateral neuralgiform headache with conjunctival injection and tearing (SUNCT) can be more difficult. The occasional occurrence of facial rather than eye pain in SUNCT may lead to particular problems. A useful distinguishing feature is the duration of attack. This is typically less than 5 seconds in TN and 5 seconds to 5 minutes in SUNCT. The younger age of patients with SUNCT with the presence of prominent autonomic features, or the finding on imaging of a vascular loop in patients with TN is helpful. Idiopathic stabbing headache may also enter the differential diagnosis of V_1 TN.

Atypical facial pain is frequently mistakenly labelled as TN initially. Unlike TN, atypical facial pain tends to be constant rather than paroxysmal, aching rather than lancinating, diffuse and poorly localised, often affecting the whole face and even areas outside the trigeminal territory. Trigger zones are usually absent. There is frequently associated depression or anxiety, although this does not necessarily imply a causal relationship.

Aetiology and pathogenesis

The main risk factors for apparently idiopathic TN are age and occasionally a history of hypertension. However, there is increasing evidence that in many cases TN is caused by compression of the trigeminal nerve root at or near the dorsal root entry zone by an ectatic vascular loop, often of the superior cerebellar artery. Abnormal ephaptic non-synaptic transmission between trigeminal axons, within areas of focal demyelination, caused by compression of the nerve has been proposed as the substrate of the pain, with increased excitability of the trigeminal–brainstem complex. High-resolution magnetic resonance imaging (MRI) studies demonstrate a distinct vascular loop in contact with the nerve in some cases. Other cerebellopontine angle masses including tumours (vestibular schwannomas, meningiomas, epidermoids) and aneurysms may sometimes compress the nerve.

Intrinsic brainstem pathology, particularly plaques of pontine demyelination in patients with MS, can cause symptomatic TN, which is occasionally bilateral. Patients with MS have a 20 times higher risk of developing TN. Up to 5% of patients with MS develop TN; occasionally TN is a presenting symptom of MS. Rarely, small infarcts in the dorsal root entry zone in the pons, or infiltration of the trigeminal nerve or ganglion by amyloid or tumour may lead to TN.

MRI is not essential in typical cases of TN, although increasingly carried out. Imaging is indicated where a symptomatic cause is suspected, for example in younger patients, in those with sudden onset of pain, abnormal examination findings or when surgical treatment such as microvascular decompression is contemplated.

Treatment

Until the advent of modern treatments patients were sometimes driven to suicide by the severity and distress of TN pain. A variety of effective medical and surgical treatments now exist, but evidence supporting their use is often observational rather than based on rigorous data.

Carbamazepine has been the first line drug for TN and it is effective or partially effective in 70% of cases (initially 100 mg every 12 hours, increasing gradually to 200 mg 6-hourly and occasionally to a total dose of 1.6 g/day in some patients). In practice, the problem is often achieving an effective therapeutic dosage quickly enough; side effects are often encountered in elderly patients when rapid titration regimes are used. Oxcarbazepine is used increasingly as a first or second line drug. It is as effective as carbamazepine and can be increased to an effective therapeutic dosage more rapidly and is often better tolerated (initially 300 mg 12-hourly increasing in increments to 2.4 g in divided doses). Other agents used alone or in combination include lamotrigine, baclofen, gabapentin and a variety of other anticonvulsant drugs. Conventional analgesics are not effective.

For patients with drug-resistant TN, or where drugs are not well tolerated, various surgical approaches are available. In general, surgery tends to be more effective than medical therapy. There is an increasing trend towards early surgical intervention, because sustained remission is the exception and natural history studies indicate TN often becomes gradually more severe and resistant to medical therapy. More than half of all patients with severe and intractable TN will require surgery.

Gasserian ganglion ablative techniques These techniques involve selective ablation of part of the trigeminal ganglion, using a percutaneous approach via the foramen ovale, by radio-frequency thermocoagulation, glycerol or balloon microcompression. These procedures, performed as day cases or with a short inpatient stay, have a low morbidity and immediate efficacy. However, some degree of postoperative facial sensory loss is almost inevitable and they may provide only temporary relief. Late recurrence is common. The extent of sensory loss is proportional to long-term efficacy; those with minor sensory loss tend to have recurrence of pain. Radio-frequency thermocoagulation is the most common modality used, destroying a selected part of the ganglion within Meckel's cave. Analgesia lasts on average 2 years and the procedure can be repeated. Glycerol injection is a simpler technique, usually associated with earlier recurrence of TN but it has fewer problems with postoperative numbness and pain than radio-frequency thermocoagulation.

Anaesthesia dolorosa, the distressing and sometimes very painful dysaesthesia in an anaesthetic area, occurs in around 1% of patients treated by ablation techniques; it is resistant to treatment.

Microvascular decompression This intracranial micro-neurosurgical procedure involves a general anaesthetic and the exposure of the trigeminal nerve at the brainstem. In some instances a vascular loop is seen to be compressing the nerve; the vessel is dissected away from the nerve and compression relieved, using Teflon felt or other material as a cushion. Decompression has a high long-term success rate, approximately 90% in published series, and has few frequent unwanted effects. Nevertheless, it is an intracranial procedure and carries a small risk of damage to other cranial nerves, especially unilateral deafness, as well as CSF leakage (2–5%) and, occasionally, cerebellar venous infarction.

Gamma knife radio-surgery High doses of focused irradiation are directed at either at the root exit zone or at the nerve itself within the pontine cistern, proximal to the Gasserian ganglion. Success rates for pain relief are reasonable, but the effects are usually delayed for several months. Long-term results and complications are not yet known.

Choice of surgical technique Ganglion ablation techniques are most appropriate for the elderly and infirm. For those able to undergo microvascular decompression, this is certainly the preferred option for TN affecting the ophthalmic division, where post-ablation corneal anaesthesia can lead to keratitis, and for patients with TN generally who prefer a more definitive procedure with a low risk of facial sensory loss. Symptomatic TN caused by MS is generally treated with medical therapy initially; ganglion ablation techniques are the preferred surgical technique, but decompression may be remarkably effective in some patients (40%) even in the absence of an identifiable vascular loop.

Trigeminal sensory neuropathy

Facial sensory loss in the absence of a defined lesion of the trigeminal nerve or its central connections is usually described as idiopathic trigeminal sensory neuropathy and is probably a heterogeneous disorder.

Patients develop gradually evolving facial numbness, often preceded by positive sensory symptoms such as tingling, but usually without significant pain. In many cases initial symptoms are localised, typically in a circumoral distribution, with disregard for the divisional boundaries of the nerve. Gradual spread to involve the rest of the face, and sometimes the opposite side, is usual over a period of months or years. Tactile, temperature and pain sensation are usually diminished and taste sensation becomes impaired in the anterior two-thirds of the tongue in many. The corneal reflex is usually diminished or absent in those with V_1 involvement; the blink reflex may be delayed or absent in neurophysiological recordings in some patients. The motor root is very rarely affected. A small subgroup have acute onset of sensory loss; this may represent a condition similar to Bell's palsy.

The association with autoimmune connective tissue diseases (CTDs) sometimes offers a clue to an underlying cause. Three conditions account for more than 90% of the CTDs associated with trigeminal neuropathy: undifferentiated connective tissue disease (47%), mixed connective tissue disease (26%) and scleroderma (19%). The condition is also seen in association with primary Sjögren's syndrome. Trigeminal neuropathy is seldom seen in the more common CTDs such as rheumatoid arthritis and systemic lupus erythematosus (SLE), and where it does occur in association with these disorders is more likely to be acute in onset with systemic and other neurological involvement because of vasculitis. In a minority of patients, facial numbness develops before other rheumatological or systemic symptoms. Vasculitic damage to the trigeminal ganglion may explain trigeminal neuropathy in some cases without evidence of a CTD and there is speculation that tissue-specific autoimmune damage may explain some idiopathic cases.

Neuroimaging is usually normal. There are few pathological studies but the available evidence indicates a destructive inflammatory process at or near the Gasserian ganglion.

Generally, symptoms do not improve with time but few patients are severely disturbed by their symptoms, particularly once more serious neurological disorders have been excluded.

Non-specific, often intermittent, facial sensory symptoms are common in neurological practice, sometimes accompanied by sensory symptoms elsewhere in the body, and may sometimes be a feature of somatisation (Chapter 22). Non-organic patterns of sensory loss are typical; examination is normal. Investigations are negative. Distinguishing such patients from patients with trigeminal sensory neuropathy is usually possible on clinical grounds.

Herpes zoster ophthalmicus

The lifetime risk of herpes zoster ophthalmicus (HZO) is about 1%. The other divisions of the trigeminal nerve are rarely affected. Elderly and immuno-compromised individuals are particularly at risk. Early ocular and later neurological complications are common and potentially serious.

As with shingles elsewhere, pain and sensory disturbance often precede appearance of vesicles. Vesicles over the side of the nose and medial to the eye indicate involvement of the nasociliary nerve and predict involvement of the eye itself (Hutchinson's sign). Most patients with HZO have conjunctivitis. Without antiviral therapy 50% of HZO patients will develop severe ocular complications, including keratopathy, episcleritis, corneal perforation and iritis, some of which result – potentially – in blindness. Corneal anaesthesia may lead to secondary damage to the eye. Retinal necrosis may occasionally occur in immuno-compromised patients.

All patients with HZO should receive oral antiviral therapy with aciclovir, valaciclovir or famciclovir as early as possible. The newer antiviral drugs may improve compliance, because dosing is three times daily rather than five times daily as with aciclovir. Treatment within 72 hours reduces the frequency of ocular complications from 50% to 20–30% and may reduce the duration of zoster-associated pain. Patients with eye involvement should be assessed by an ophthalmologist. Topical steroids may be indicated where there is anterior chamber inflammation. Taping of the lids is often helpful at night. There are some suggestions that steroids (oral and/or intravenous) in combination with antiviral drugs reduce the duration of pain and accelerate healing but there is no effect on the incidence of post-herpetic neuralgia (PHN). Steroids are not used routinely.

PHN is pain persisting more than 3 months after the rash (Chapter 23). This is the most common neurological complication of HZO. Overall, 7% of patients with shingles have PHN at 3 months and 3% at 1 year. PHN is much more common in the elderly, in whom HZO usually occurs, and 20% of HZO patients over the age of 60 years develop PHN, with 9% persisting at 1 year. However, after allowing for age, patients with HZO are no more likely to develop PHN than those with shingles affecting other dermatomes. Treatment of PHN is usually with tricyclic antidepressants (e.g. amitriptyline), or anticonvulsants, sometimes in combination. Topical capsaicin cream may also be helpful. PHN may be refractory to treatment and have a major impact on quality of life.

Rarer late neurological complications of HZO include cranial nerve palsies (optic neuropathy and III, IV and VI) and stroke as a result of granulomatous arteritis of the intracranial carotid artery or its branches, probably caused by direct viral invasion of the vessel. This usually develops 1–2 months after the rash.

Atypical facial pain

Atypical facial pain is a residual diagnostic category for otherwise unclassifiable facial pain without an apparent structural cause. The features are of chronic facial pain, lasting months to years, usually unilateral and within trigeminal distribution, but without signs of Vth nerve sensory loss. The pain is described as deep and burning in quality. Paroxysms and trigger areas are typically absent. There have often been incorrect diagnoses, and invasive diagnostic or therapeutic procedures, sometimes multiple. Patients are typically over 50 years of age, and predominantly female. Depressive features are prominent but patients with atypical facial pain appear to have little in the way of other unexplained pain. Investigation is negative. Treatment, with tricyclic antidepressants and other similar drugs, although sometimes helpful, is frequently distinctly unsatisfactory. Attempts at invasive treatment usually cause the pain to increase.

VII. Facial nerve

The facial nerve has a long and complex course and may be damaged at any point. Bell's palsy is seen commonly in primary care, at all ages, and worldwide.

Functional anatomy

The facial nerve has motor, sensory and autonomic components and a tortuous course from pons to extracranial innervation of facial muscles, lacrimal and salivary glands, and visceral and somatic sensory territories. The anatomy is described in more detail in Chapter 2.

The majority of the upper motor neurone corticobulbar fibres decussate in the pons but the upper third of the face is said traditionally to receive bilateral cortical innervation, resulting in sparing of the brow and frontalis muscles with supranuclear lesions (e.g. after a stroke). The situation is more complex; the upper part of the face probably receives relatively little direct cortical innervation. Separate supranuclear anatomical pathways subserve voluntary and emotional facial movements; as a result these movements may be dissociated. Thus, emotional movements such as smiling, which are separate from the internal capsule pathway, may be preserved when voluntary movements are affected following a stroke. The right cerebral hemisphere is dominant for expression of facial emotion.

The VIIth motor nucleus lies in the lower pons. The fascicle of efferent motor fibres travels backwards, before sweeping around in a U-turn around the VIth nerve nucleus, to emerge anteriorly from the lower border of the pons.

The nervus intermedius is the distinct sensory and autonomic component of the facial nerve that joins the motor fibres just after the internal genu (Chapter 2; Figure 13.3). After leaving the pons, the facial nerve traverses the cerebellopontine angle before entering the internal auditory meatus of the temporal bone with the nervus intermedius and VIIIth nerve. The facial nerve emerges from the skull via the stylomastoid foramen. After traversing the parotid gland the nerve divides into several branches that innervate the facial muscles, with the exception of the levator palpebrae superioris, supplied by the IIIrd nerve – which explains why facial palsy does not cause ptosis, but instead widens the palpebral fissure (Figure 13.4).

Examination

Facial symmetry should be inspected, particularly forehead creases and nasolabial folds, remembering that a proportion of the normal population have some degree of facial asymmetry. Facial myokymia, synkinesis or hemiatrophy may be observed on careful inspection at rest and during facial movements. When assessing power, test frontalis (eyebrow elevation), as well as eye closure, lip closure and emotional facial movements such as smiling. Platysma is tested by asking the patient to bare their teeth and open the mouth at the same time. Asking the patient to blow out the cheeks and whistle are also useful. For patients with facial weakness, Bell's phenomenon (Chapter 4) is assessed. The ability to close the eye to protect the cornea needs to be examined specifically, to

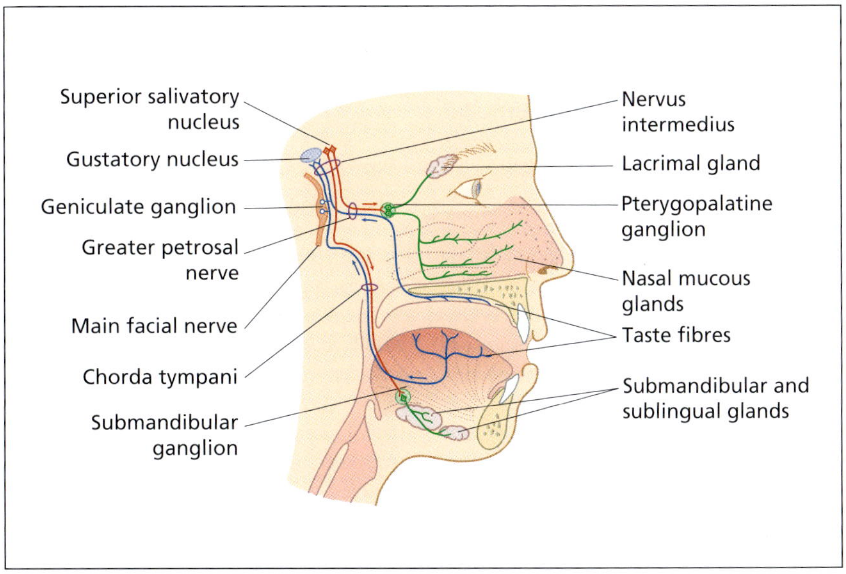

Figure 13.3 Nervus intermedius, greater petrosal nerve and chorda tympani. Source: FitzGerald 2010. © 2016 Elsevier. Reproduced with permission of Elsevier.

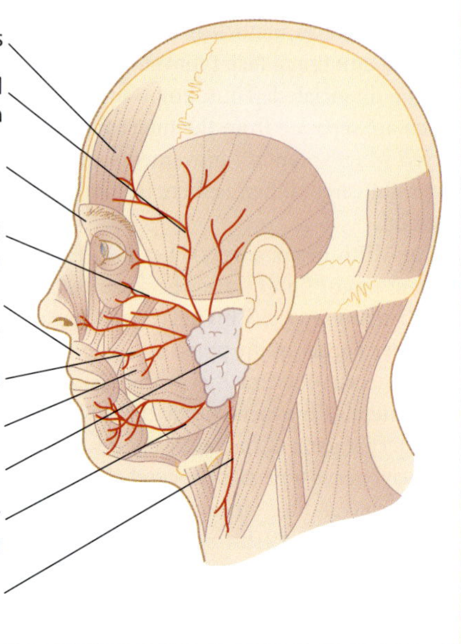

Figure 13.4 Principal facial branches of VIIth nerve. Source: FitzGerald 2010. © 2016 Elsevier. Reproduced with permission of Elsevier.

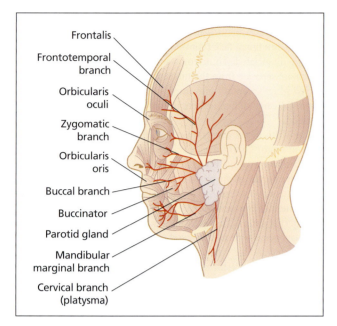

avoid exposure keratopathy. Upper motor neurone lesions produce relative sparing of the frontalis and orbicularis oculi muscles because of their bilateral innervation; voluntary and emotional movements may be affected differentially. Unilateral upper motor neurone facial weakness is often less evident to patients and relatives than lower motor neurone weakness. Gradual onset weakness or even bilateral facial weakness is less noticeable than sudden unilateral weakness.

The four common primary tastes – sweet, salt, sour and bitter – can be tested using sugar, salt, vinegar and quinine dabbed separately on to the tongue, rinsing the mouth between each test substance (*Umami*: see p. 531). In cases of facial weakness, examination should include inspection of the oral cavity, tongue and external auditory meatus for vesicles indicating zoster or for evidence of nasopharyngeal carcinoma or fissured tongue (lingua plicata). The parotid should be palpated for evidence of tumour, infection or inflammation. Otoscopic examination of the external auditory canal and tympanic membrane should be performed to look for evidence of infection or cholesteatoma. The causes of unilateral and bilateral facial weakness are summarised in Table 13.2.

Supranuclear facial weakness

Facial weakness caused by lesions of the upper motor neurones innervating the facial nucleus (e.g. following hemispheric stroke) are usually associated with ipsilateral limb weakness. In the face, the usual pattern is of relative sparing of the upper muscles because of their bilateral cortical representation and the fact that the cortical representation of the upper face is in the anterior cingulate gyrus rather than the motor cortex. Dissociation between voluntary and emotional facial movements may be seen; impairment of voluntary movement with relative sparing of emotional facial movements is more common than the converse.

In disorders such as progressive supranuclear palsy, disruption of supranuclear and brainstem mechanisms relating to facial movements may cause apraxia of eyelid opening; patients cannot voluntarily open eyes despite absence of overt facial weakness.

Table 13.2 (a) Causes of facial palsy.

Bell's palsy
Herpes zoster (Ramsay Hunt syndrome)
Otitis media/cholesteatoma
Borrelia (Lyme disease)
Guillain–Barré syndrome
Sarcoidosis
Sjögren's syndrome
IgG4-related disease (Melkersson–Rosenthal syndrome)
Stroke
Multiple sclerosis
Other infections – HIV (usually associated with seroconversion), TB, polio
Vasculitis – Granulomatosis with polyangitis (Wegener's), polyarteritis, Sjögren's syndrome
Tumour (usually involving temporal lobe, internal auditory canal, cerebellopontine angle, skull base or parotid gland): • Schwannoma VIIth nerve • Parotid gland tumour

Table 13.2 (b) Causes of bilateral facial palsy.

Bell's palsy
Guillain–Barré/Miller–Fisher syndrome
Brainstem encephalitis
Pontine tumour
Meningeal infection / inflammation / infiltration
Borrelia
Sarcoidosis
Amyloidosis
HIV seroconversion
Herpes simplex / herpes zoster
Poliomyelitis
Motor neurone disease
Moebius syndrome
Neuromuscular junction / myasthenia gravis
Muscle / e.g. FSH, OPMD, Myotonic dystrophy

FSH, Facioscapulohumeral muscular dystrophy; OPMD, oculopharyngeal muscular dystrophy

Nuclear VIIth lesions

Vascular, inflammatory and occasionally infiltrative brainstem lesions can affect the facial nerve nucleus within the pons or the intrapontine fascicle. This produces a lower motor neurone type facial palsy. This rarely occurs in isolation and like most brainstem lesions usually involves adjacent structures. The VIth nerve nucleus, around which the facial fasciculus sweeps, is often involved producing facial weakness and diplopia because of paralysis of lateral rectus on the same side. An associated contralateral hemiplegia (Millard–Gubler syndrome) is often caused by pontine vascular lesions; an ipsilateral gaze paresis reflects involvement of the paramedian pontine reticular formation.

Cerebellopontine angle syndrome

The petrous temporal bone, lying laterally, completes the triangular recess between the cerebellum and the lower border of the pons (Table 13.3). The Vth nerve lies at the upper corner of the cerebellopontine angle (CPA), the IXth and Xth nerves at the lower, and the VIIth and VIIIth nerves between them (Figure 13.5). Mass lesions in the CPA cause combinations of an VIIIth nerve lesion, a Vth nerve lesion and a VIIth. Additional features develop when the adjacent cerebellar lobe is damaged, and occasionally a IXth nerve lesion, upper motor neurone signs in the limbs and exceptionally hydrocephalus with papilloedema.

Table 13.3 Causes of cerebellopontine angle syndrome (invariably neoplasms; usually benign).

Vestibular schwannoma (most common)
Meningioma
Epidermoid
Cholesteatoma
Lipoma
Arachnoid cyst
Schwannoma of V, VII, IX, X or XI
Dermoid cyst
Hamartoma
Melanoma (primary or secondary)
Paraganglioma (glomus)
Choroid plexus papilloma
Primary CNS neoplasm
Lymphoma
Metastases (breast, prostate, lung and gynaecological)

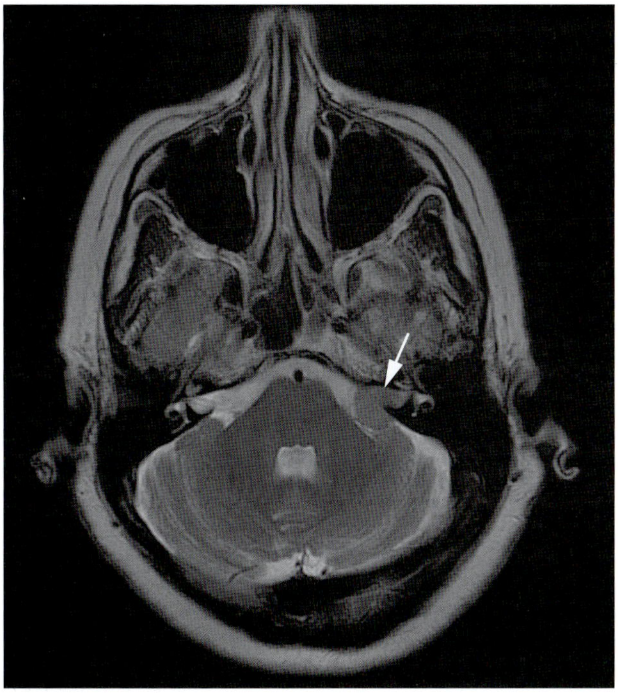

Figure 13.5 Vestibular schwannoma (MRI T2-weighted).

VIIIth nerve schwannoma (acoustic neuroma; Chapters 14 and 21) is the typical cause. Meningioma, cholesteatoma, metastasis or occasionally an aneurysm can also produce a CPA syndrome.

With an VIIIth nerve schwannoma there is a typical but not invariable sequence. High-pitched tinnitus, at first intermittent, is followed by progressive sensorineural deafness. Episodes of vertigo follow. Trigeminal facial sensory loss develops; initially this is symptomless – hence the importance of testing the corneal reflex. Facial weakness of lower motor neurone type follows. An IXth nerve lesion may be found. Later, as the tumour enlarges, cerebellar and other signs of brainstem involvement become apparent. In the elderly, when hearing loss has been neglected, hydrocephalus with raised pressure can be the presenting feature.

CPA lesions were sometimes hard to diagnose before the era of high-definition imaging but standard MRI sequences are now able to identify the great majority of CPA lesions.

Facial canal syndrome

At the internal auditory meatus the VIIth nerve lies close to the VIIIth, and may be affected with it. Damage to the nerve within the facial canal is common and it is here that the VIIth nerve is believed to be affected in Bell's palsy. The first (labyrinthine) portion of the facial canal is the narrowest and the only segment lacking anastomosing arterial arcades, making it vulnerable to ischaemia and compression at this point. The clinical picture will depend on where within the canal the lesion occurs:

- Damage proximal to the first branch of the VIIth nerve, the greater superficial petrosal nerve to the lacrimal gland, will result in facial palsy with loss of lacrimation, hyperacusis (nerve to stapedius) and loss of taste in the anterior two-thirds of the tongue (chorda tympani).
- Lesions distal to the origin of the nerve to stapedius will not cause hyperacusis.
- Lesions distal to the chorda tympani will spare taste.

Head injury may cause damage to the facial nerve within the facial canal, usually as a result of a transverse fracture of the temporal bone. After the olfactory nerve, the facial nerve is the cranial nerve most commonly involved in head trauma. Surgical decompression and use of steroids are sometimes advocated but there is little evidence to support their use. Malignant otitis externa in diabetic patients, usually caused by *Pseudomonas* infection, and suppurative middle ear infection may spread to adjacent tissue and the skull base resulting in facial palsy. Temporal bone metastases, nasopharangeal carcinoma and other tumours as well as disorders such as osteopetrosis and cholesteatoma may sometimes affect the facial nerve in this segment.

Lesions at and distal to the stylomastoid foramen

The facial nerve or its branches can be damaged at or distal to its exit from the skull at the stylomastoid foramen. Parotid tumours or inflammatory parotitis resulting from infection or granulomatous disease such as sarcoidosis may cause facial palsy. Individual branches of the nerve may be damaged by surgery to the parotid or face, carotid endarterectomy, facial trauma or carotid dissection. Misplaced botulinum toxin injections, for cosmetic purposes or for hemifacial spasm, may also result in localised, but temporary, facial weakness.

Bell's palsy

Bell's palsy is an acute peripheral facial palsy. A large retrospective study of almost 2500 cases presenting to UK GPs showed an incidence of 20/100 000 per year. Bell's palsy may occur in childhood; incidence increases steadily with age. There is no change in incidence with season, latitude or geography and no evidence for familial clustering. Weak associations may exist with diabetes and hypertension. A viral aetiology has been postulated on the basis that decompression of the nerve in the acute phase usually reveals swelling of the facial nerve proximal to the geniculate ganglion, a finding confirmed by MRI, and detection of herpes simplex virus type 1 (HSV-1) DNA in endoneurial fluid in most patients. Both primary HSV-1 infection and reactivation of latent infection have been implicated. Microvascular ischaemic mononeuropathy of the facial nerve may also be causal in older patients. Bell's palsy has also been reported after immunisation. Bell's palsy should no longer be considered idiopathic.

Clinical features The clinical picture is stereotyped and familiar to most clinicians. Rapid onset of facial weakness progressing over 48 hours (and occasionally up to 5 days) is preceded or accompanied by diffuse retro-auricular pain in the region of the mastoid. In some patients, mastoid pain may be severe and persist for a week or longer. Facial weakness and asymmetry with drooling of liquids from the corner of the mouth on the affected side often lead the patient to suspect a stroke; most patients present promptly to primary care physicians. Not infrequently, patients mistakenly report that the contralateral unaffected side is the weak side. All facial muscles are usually equally affected. The palpebral fissure is widened on the affected side, eye closure and blinking are reduced or absent (with a visible Bell's phenomenon on attempted eye closure). Ectropion formation may lead to overflow of tears on to the cheek. The angle of the mouth droops with reduction of the nasolabial fold, smoothing of skin wrinkles; the platysma muscle is also involved. The extent of maximal facial weakness is variable, but is severe in the majority, although occasionally patients present with very mild facial weakness. For example, this may be noticed only because the patient is unable to form an adequate embouchure to play a wind instrument. However, a mild, painless, progressive or patchy facial weakness developing over several weeks is distinctly unusual in Bell's palsy, and suggests an underlying cause.

A vague alteration of sensation on the affected side of the face is relatively common in Bell's palsy, although the corneal reflex is preserved. Loss of taste, often described as a muddy or metallic taste, and hyperacusis (because of paralysis of stapedius) indicate involvement of the chorda tympani and the branch to stapedius, respectively.

Other causes of acute facial paralysis should be considered:

- The Ramsay-Hunt syndrome caused by varicella-zoster reactivation in the geniculate ganglion may be diagnosed by careful inspection of the external auditory meatus and palate for vesicles in these small somatic sensory territories of the facial nerve. Vesicles may be absent in some patients – zoster *sine herpete*. Other symptoms are common in the Ramsay-Hunt syndrome including tinnitus, hearing loss and nystagmus, indicating involvement of the VIIIth nerve and occasionally involvement of other cranial nerves such as the IXth and Xth.
- The ear should be examined for evidence of local pathology such as cholesteatoma or malignant otitis externa, and parotid tumours excluded.
- Lyme disease may possibly account for one-quarter of cases of facial palsy in endemic areas.
- Acute VIIth nerve lesions are sometimes seen at HIV seroconversion.

When a possible Bell's palsy appears to be unusual, for example a minor persistent facial weakness or slowly progressive weakness without pain, an underlying cause should be considered. A skull base tumour, such as a breast cancer metastasis can cause an isolated VIIth nerve lesion. In some cases there is also post-auricular pain.

Investigation Investigations are not required in typical cases. MRI may show contrast enhancement of the distal intra-canalicular and labyrinthine portions of the facial nerve. Imaging is not routinely indicated, unless a brainstem or other cause is suspected. Gradual onset of facial weakness over weeks, the presence of other neurological signs or failure to recover within 6 months should prompt further investigation, including imaging. In areas of high HIV prevalence, acute facial weakness is more often because of HIV seroconversion than the typical Bell's palsy seen in largely HIV-negative populations. In areas of high Lyme disease prevalence, testing for *Borellia* serology is appropriate.

CSF examination is not indicated in Bell's palsy and the CSF constituents are normal.

Neurophysiological stimulation of the facial nerve with measurement of facial compound motor action potential 3–20 days after onset may identify those with severe Wallerian degeneration of the nerve and a correspondingly poor prognosis for recovery. In practice this is rarely required.

Management and outcome Complete or almost complete recovery, without recurrence, over 3–8 weeks is the norm in at least 85% of cases, even without any treatment. Reassurance about the good prognosis and absence of recurrence is important. Inability to blink in severe facial weakness may lead to exposure keratitis and early evaluation should include assessment of the eye. Lubricating eye drops are often required and patients should be shown how to tape the eye closed at night. Severe facial weakness with complete inability to close the eye requires urgent ophthalmological assessment; lateral tarsorrhaphy and/or temporary insertion of a gold weight into the upper lid may be necessary.

Early treatment with steroids and antiviral agents remains contentious although this is now near standard practice. Some studies indicate a better outcome with steroids but a rigorous analysis as part of a Cochrane review concluded that there was insufficient evidence to support the use of steroids. Nevertheless, many clinicians choose to treat patients with oral prednisolone (typically 1 mg/kg for 7 days) if they present within a week of onset. Evidence to support use of antiviral agents is even more limited. The two largest clinical trials failed to show additional benefit for antiviral therapy and its use is no longer routinely recommended. However, it remains possible that the addition of antivirals is beneficial in the subgroup of patients with severe facial palsy (total paralysis) and it has been suggested that these patients should be given valacyclovir (1000 mg three times daily) in addition to prednisolone for 1 week. Treatment with an aciclovir–steroid combination could also be justified on the basis that HSV reactivation may be a frequent cause of Bell's palsy, and that some cases of Ramsay-Hunt syndrome may occur *sine herpete*.

Surgical decompression of the labyrinthine portion of the facial nerve in the acute phase has had its proponents, but there is little evidence to support this practice – now rarely performed in the United Kingdom. Over 80% of UK patients with Bell's palsy are managed in primary care; most receive no medical treatment.

The extent of early weakness is an important prognostic sign, with incomplete facial weakness indicating a better prognosis than total paralysis. For the majority of patients where recovery occurs within several weeks, conduction block and segmental demyelination, with intact axonal integrity within the facial canal, is presumed to be the basis of facial weakness. Where axonal loss and Wallerian degeneration have occurred, recovery follows after axonal regrowth. This is delayed by 4–6 months, or even longer. In these cases, recovery is usually incomplete, particularly for the more distal branches supplying the brow and mouth, and often associated with contracture or tightness of facial muscles. Aberrant reinnervation of facial muscles and glands is common in late recovery, leading to synkinesis and the phenomenon of jaw-winking – involuntary eye closure with lip or mouth movement, known as the inverse Marcus Gunn phenomenon or Marin–Amat syndrome. Similarly, lip movement may occur on blinking. Aberrant parasympathetic reinervation may lead to watering of the eye when eating (crocodile tears), caused by misdirection to the lacrimal gland of fibres destined for the submandibular salivary glands. These complications may be successfully treated with botulinum toxin injections either into the active muscle or the lacrimal gland.

For the minority left with severe facial weakness after a year, reconstructive facial surgery can be helpful. A variety of procedures may be considered: botulinum toxin for synkinesis, and into the contralateral side of the face to rebalance the cosmetic appearance, and highly specialised surgical procedures such as reanimation. The latter involves sural nerve grafting of a branch of the contralateral facial nerve, the aim being to innervate the paretic side. After 6 months (to allow axonal growth along the sural graft), this is followed by insertion of a revascularised pectoralis muscle flap into the affected side to improve function. In some patients, particularly older people, a simple muscle sling procedure improves cosmetic appearance, without improving movement.

Recurrent facial palsy

Bell's palsy is rarely recurrent (<5% of cases) and should in any event prompt a search for an underlying cause, such as sarcoidosis.

Melkersson–Rosenthal syndrome This condition is a rare triad of intermittent VIIth nerve palsy, persistent or recurrent lip or facial swelling, and a fissured tongue (lingua plicata). The facial paralysis is identical to Bell's palsy, but has a distinct tendency to recur, and may be bilateral. These features are diagnostic clinically. Characteristic non-caseating granulomas are found on lip biopsy; the lip swelling is sometimes treated with local steroid injections. The aetiology was previously unknown, but now is thought to be associated with IgG4-related disease (Chapter 26).

Bilateral facial weakness

Bilateral facial palsy is rare, accounting for fewer than 1% of cases of facial palsy, and is much more likely to be a manifestation of a systemic disease than a unilateral palsy, isolated or recurrent. Paradoxically, patients with bilateral facial weakness are often slower to present than those with obvious facial asymmetry.

In one large case series, bilateral Bell's palsy was the most common cause of bilateral facial palsy. Infective diseases such as bilateral mastoiditis and diptheria have been replaced by HIV seroconversion, EBV infection and Lyme disease (Bannwarth's syndrome) as a cause of bilateral facial weakness. Lyme disease facial palsy is bilateral in one-quarter of cases and may be associated with a facial rash and CSF pleocytosis. Bilateral facial weakness may be a presenting feature of sarcoidosis. Other causes include trauma with skull base fracture, pontine glioma, tumours including bone metastases, leukaemic deposits within the skull base and malignant meningitis. These tend to cause gradually evolving facial weakness.

Bilateral facial weakness may be a feature of a more generalised neuromuscular disease. This occurs commonly in Guillain–Barré syndrome and the Miller Fisher variant, and is also a feature of disorders such as myotonic dystrophy, facioscapulohumeral dystrophy (sometimes presenting years before weakness of shoulder girdle muscles), myasthenia gravis, botulism, various congenital myopathies and motor neurone disease. Möbius syndrome is a congenital disorder characterised by bilateral facial weakness, usually in association with abducens palsy and other neurological deficits. A rare form of familial amyloid polyneuropathy caused by gelsolin gene mutations may cause bilateral facial palsy with corneal lattice dystrophy.

Hemifacial spasm

This is a benign, usually painless but often distressing condition, characterised by unilateral, involuntary, irregular tonic or clonic contractions of muscles supplied by the facial nerve. Prevalence is 14.5/100 000 and 7.4/100 000 in women and men, respectively. Onset is usually in the fifth and sixth decades.

In some patients the involuntary movements start in the orbicularis oculi muscle and gradually progresses over months or years to involve other facial muscles on the same side. In others, the problem begins with twitching around the mouth or the cheek. Movements are irregular in rhythm and degree but synchronous in all affected muscles. They may be spontaneous or triggered by voluntary facial movements including chewing and speaking, and they are made worse by stress or fatigue. Movements usually persist during sleep. Bilateral involvement is rare (3%), and when it occurs movements are never synchronous on the two sides. Examination is usually normal although subtle ipsilateral facial weakness is sometimes seen. It is now generally accepted that hemifacial spasm is usually caused by extrinsic compression of the root entry zone of the facial nerve, generally by vascular structures such as the vertebral or basilar arteries or their branches. Other mass lesions in the CPA, including tumours, are the cause in about 1% of cases. Secondary hemifacial spasm, following injury to the peripheral facial nerve or following Bell's palsy also occurs. High-resolution MRI with fine cuts through the region of the facial nerve root entry zone demonstrates a vascular structure in contact with the nerve in some cases. Imaging is not usually needed, except in atypical cases where onset is not around the eye, where there are abnormal findings on physical examination or when surgical treatment is being considered.

Botulinum toxin injection into affected muscles is now the first line for those patients who want treatment. Injections need to be repeated every 3–4 months and many patients eventually develop some degree of facial weakness and atrophy. Drug treatment with carbamazepine, gabapentin, clonazepam and baclofen are rarely very effective and seldom result in resolution of symptoms, certainly at tolerable doses. Microvascular decompression of the facial nerve in the posterior fossa involves interposing a non-resorbable sponge between the nerve and any adjacent vascular loop identified at operation. The procedure is sometimes claimed to give complete resolution of symptoms in some 60% of cases, but is associated with a risk of 3% facial weakness or 3% unilateral deafness.

Hemifacial spasm may occasionally occur with ipsilateral trigeminal neuralgia, one symptom usually preceding the other, a combination called *tic convulsif*. The paroxysms of pain and spasm occur independently. A compressive cause such as a vascular loop or other structural lesion is usually identified.

Other involuntary facial movements

- Myokymia of orbicularis oculi, an irritating twitch usually of the lower eyelid, is a normal phenomenon, but sometimes a cause of anxiety. More extensive facial myokymia, with persistent worm-like wriggling of the chin and other facial muscles is more sinister. This is typically caused by intrinsic brainstem pathology such as MS, or a pontine glioma, in both cases it is usually progressive. Facial myokymia is also a hallmark of some inherited ataxias, particularly spinocerebellar atrophy type 3 (SCA3).

- Tics and tardive dyskinesia frequently involve facial or perioral muscles.
- Neuro-acanthocytosis may cause prominent oro-facial dystonia, often including the tongue.
- Blepharospasm is a form of focal dystonia affecting orbicularis oculi (Chapter 6). Fasciculation of facial muscles can develop in motor neurone disease (particularly Kennedy's disease).
- Focal motor seizures may affect facial muscles alone in some cases; epilepsy partialis continua (Chapter 7) is a cause of persistent clonic–tonic facial movements, which can be localised and difficult to recognise.

Progressive hemifacial atrophy Also known as Parry–Romberg syndrome, this rare condition consists of progressive hemifacial atrophy of skin, soft tissue and bone, sometimes with pathological changes within the brain. This begins in childhood, with gradual progressive atrophy, typically in one or more trigeminal nerve dermatomes. Facial sensation remains normal. There is no denervation. The condition is believed in some cases to be related to linear scleroderma. Sometimes a vertical fissure, known as a coup de sabre, separates atrophic areas from normal facial structures. Brain imaging shows ipsilateral grey and white matter lesions in some cases. Epilepsy sometimes occurs. The cause is unknown. There are suggestions that a chronic inflammatory process underlies the condition.

Lower four cranial nerves: IX, X, XI and XII

An outline of the peripheral course of these four nerves is shown in Figure 13.6. Their complex central arrangement and nuclei are summarised in Chapter 2.

IX. Glossopharyngeal nerve

Functional anatomy

The IXth nerve (Chapter 2) is predominantly sensory but also contains motor and parasympathetic components. It arises from the lateral medulla as a series of small rootlets rostral to those of cranial nerves X and XI. All three nerves then pass through the jugular foramen. At this point or just beyond, the IXth nerve divides into the superior and petrous ganglia, before descending the pharynx between the internal jugular vein and internal carotid artery. The small motor root supplies pharyngeal constrictors and elevators. The principal sensory root supplies taste and tactile sensation from the posterior one-third of the tongue, the posterior pharyngeal wall, Eustachian tube and tympanic membrane, and other targets such as the chemo- and baro-receptors. The parasympathetic fibres, from the inferior salivatory nucleus, leave the glossopharngeal nerve at the petrous ganglion running in the tympanic and petrosal nerves. They terminate in the parotid gland, via the auriculo-temporal branch of the trigeminal nerve.

Examination

Pharyngeal sensation can be tested with the end of an orange stick. In a IXth nerve lesion, there is altered sensation of the soft palate and pharynx. This is frequently difficult to diagnose in isolation, and rarely of great importance because other neighbouring nerves are also often affected. Loss of taste over the ipsilateral posterior third of the tongue is rarely symptomatic and cannot be tested. Isolated weakness of stylopharyngeus (which elevates the palate) is difficult to detect, with only mild dysphagia or asymmetry of the palatal arch at rest. Because the nerve supplies the afferent limb of both the pharyngeal and palatal reflex arcs, as well as the motor component of the former, a IXth nerve lesion has the potential to interfere with both these reflexes. Stimulating the normal pharynx, base of tongue or tonsillar area, with an orange stick, will result in pharyngeal elevation and constriction, with a degree of tongue retraction. In an isolated IXth nerve lesion the muscles of the pharynx supplied by the vagus continue to contract, making it impossible to diagnose an isolated IXth nerve lesion by this method.

IXth nerve lesions, peripheral and central

An isolated peripheral glossopharyngeal nerve palsy is excessively rare and lesions can be generally identified by the additional structures involved. Unilateral supranuclear lesions cause no deficit because of the bilateral input to the nucleus ambiguous. It is only

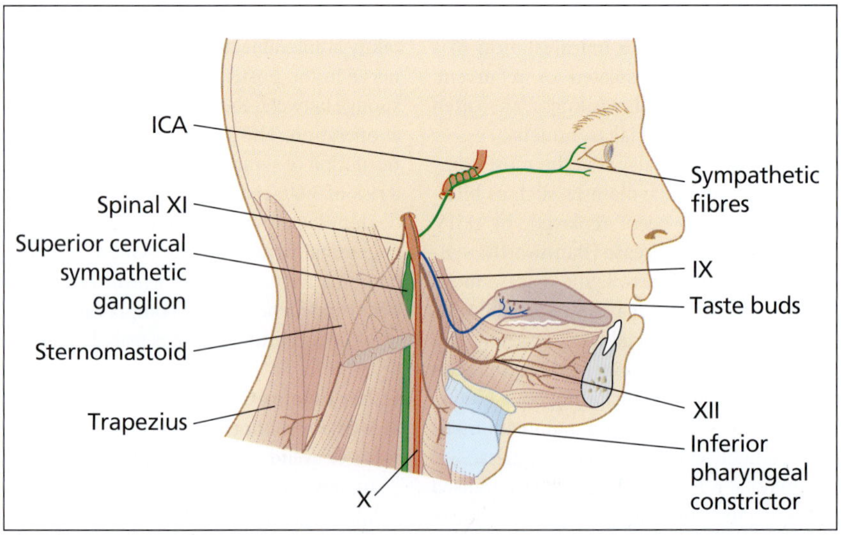

Figure 13.6 Distribution of IX, X, XI, XII and superior cervical ganglion. ICA, internal carotid artery. Source: FitzGerald 2010. © 2016 Elsevier. Reproduced with permission of Elsevier.

when there are bilateral corticobulbar lesions (as part of pseudobulbar palsy) that overt signs are seen which include tongue spasticity and dysarthria, with emotional lability.

Peripheral lesions usually occur as part of the jugular foramen and CPA syndromes. More distally the nerve can be injured in the retropharyngeal space by structural lesions (e.g. a primary tumour such as nasopharyngeal carcinoma or metastatic spread) and surgical complications (e.g. carotid endarterectomy).

Glossopharyngeal neuralgia

Glossopharyngeal neuralgia is a rare condition. There is unilateral sharp stabbing pain in the ear or throat, lasting for seconds or minutes. Like trigeminal neuralgia, pain is triggered by movement of neighbouring structures, such as yawning or chewing. The pain is intense and paroxysmal. Bradycardia or even asystole with hypotension and syncope have been described in an attack. The cause often remains obscure, although CPA structural lesions, demyelination and possibly vascular loop compression of the posterior inferior cerebellar artery have been found. As with trigeminal neuralgia, carbamazepine and gabapentin may be effective. Microvascular decompression is usually curative but nerve section is also sometimes carried out.

X. Vagus nerve

Functional anatomy

The central origins and connections of the vagus and its relations to IX, XI and XII are outlined in Chapter 2. The vagus exits at the jugular foramen with the spinal accessory nerve and glossopharyngeal nerve. Two ganglia are formed (jugulare and nodose), and from this region a number of rami project: auricular (external ear), meningeal (posterior fossa dura mater) and pharyngeal (soft palate and pharynx). There are two principal laryngeal nerves, the superior and recurrent laryngeal nerves (Figure 13.7), The vagus carries the parasympathetic supply to many thoraco-abdominal organs, with fibres from the nucleus ambiguus innervating the striated muscle of larynx, pharynx and soft palate, with the exception of stylopharyngeus (IXth) and tensor veli palati (Vth). Sensory input from the viscera and taste from the palate and epiglottis are carried back to the nucleus solitarius.

Clinical features

Vocalisation, swallowing and palatal movement are the major functions observable clinically. Bilateral lesions cause complete palatal, pharyngeal and laryngeal paralysis resulting in severe dysphagia, dysphonia and respiratory compromise with stridor, inability to cough and high risk of aspiration. Tracheostomy is usually required in acute bilateral nuclear or peripheral lesions, which may otherwise be life-threatening.

Unilateral vagus nerve palsy is characterised by dysphonia – the voice is hoarse and weak, with variable, usually mild, dysphagia. The vocal cords cannot be opposed, causing the cough to be weak and dependent upon forceful expiration; this is described as bovine. There is difficulty clearing the throat; the voice can often sound wet, because of pharyngeal pooling of secretions. Clinical examination demonstrates soft palate droop on the affected side; there is failure of elevation of the ipsilateral palate and the uvula may be pulled towards the unaffected side on phonation. Unilateral depression of the gag reflex occurs with a lesion of one vagus nerve. Autonomic dysfunction can occur and is discussed in Chapter 24.

With bilateral vagus involvement the palate cannot elevate on phonation and it may droop depending on the function of the tensor veli palatini. The palatal gag reflex is absent bilaterally. There is nasal speech and nasal regurgitation of liquids.

With pharyngeal weakness dysarthria is usually minimal unless there is also weakness of the soft palate or larynx. Spontaneous coughing and the cough reflex are impaired. Dysphagia may occur but without the tendency to greater difficulty with liquids and nasal regurgitation that occurs with palatal weakness. Examination of the

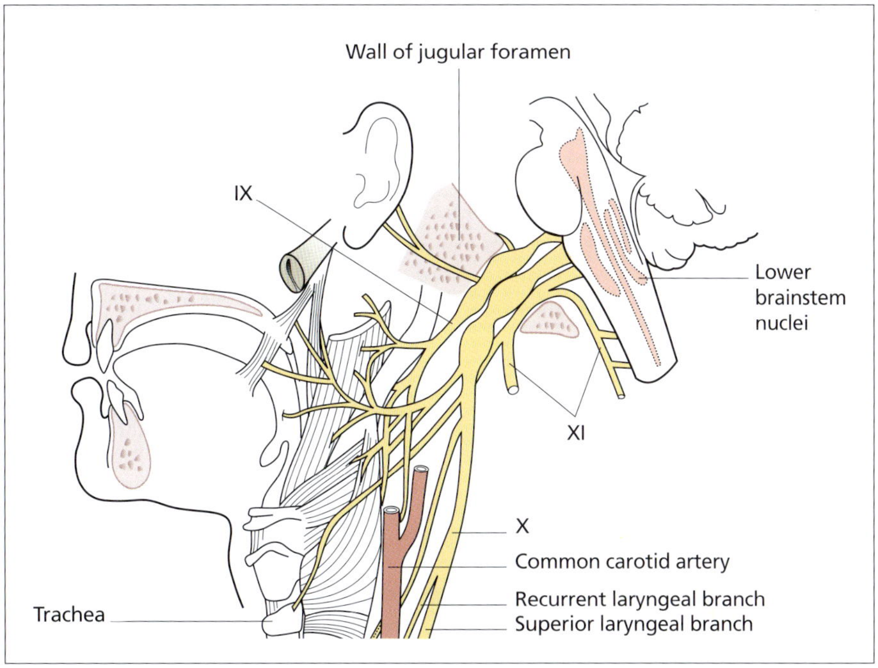

Figure 13.7 Scheme showing IXth, Xth, XIth nerves, skull base and brainstem.

pharynx includes observation of the contraction of the pharyngeal muscles on phonation, elevation of the larynx on swallowing and testing the pharyngeal gag reflex. Unilateral weakness of the superior pharyngeal constrictor may cause 'curtain movement' (Vernet's rideau phenomenon). With movement of the pharyngeal wall towards the non-paralysed side on testing the gag reflex or on phonation, the normal elevation of the larynx may be absent on one side unilateral lesions or on both sides in bilateral lesions.

Sensory examination is essentially impossible because of inaccessibility (meningeal structures) or co-innnervation (e.g. the pinna).

Causes and localisation of lesions

Major supranuclear lesions (e.g. acute hemispheric stroke), may cause transient swallowing difficulty, but the bilateral innervation of vagal brainstem nuclei means compensation usually occurs rapidly. Bilateral supranuclear lesions cause pseudobulbar palsy (see Pseudobular palsy). Nuclear lesions are usually accompanied by damage to adjacent structures within the medulla which may dominate the clinical picture. Brainstem stroke resulting from lesions of the vertebral artery or its branches may cause characteristic clinical syndromes of infarction, particularly affecting the lateral medulla (Wallenberg's lateral medullary syndrome; Chapter 5). Involvement of the nucleus ambiguus leads to dysphagia and dysphonia accompanied by vertigo, ipsilateral cerebellar signs, Horner's syndrome and spinothalamic sensory loss of the contralateral half of the body and the ipsilateral face. Other structural and inflammatory disorders in this region can also affect long motor and sensory tracts; there are a number of eponymous syndromes (Table 13.4).

- Syringobulbia, motor neurone disease and vascular lesions can cause bilateral nuclear lesions affecting the vagus, producing a complete or partial bulbar palsy. Multiple system atrophy may affect the vagal nuclei causing stridor because of partial vocal cord paralysis as well as the autonomic disturbances characteristic of this condition.
- Peripheral lesions in the extramedullary intracranial region and as the nerve exits the skull through the jugular foramen often involve the IXth, XIth and XIIth nerves.
- Primary tumours (e.g. chordoma, skull base or meningeal infiltration by metastatic tumour and inflammatory disorders) may all be responsible (see Jugular foramen syndrome). Extracranial lesions of the nerve trunk in the neck, where it runs in the carotid sheath, may result from carotid dissection, surgery or lymph node inflammation (e.g. tuberculous) at the skull base.

Table 13.4 Eponymous brainstem syndromes involving the cranial nerves.

Syndrome	Site	Artery	Neurology
Weber	Midbrain – base	PCA	i/l III, c/l pyramidal
Benedikt	Midbrain – tegmentum	PCA	i/l III, c/l pyramidal, ataxia, rubral tremor
Claude	Midbrain – tegmentum	PCA	i/l III, c/l ataxia, rubral tremor
Nothnagel	Midbrain – tectum	PCA	i/l III, ataxia
Millard–Gubler	Pons – basis and fascicles of VI and VII	Basilar (cicumferential and paramedian branches)	i/l VI, VII, c/l pyramidal
Foville	Pons – dorsal tegmentum in caudal third	Basilar (paramedian and short circumferential)	i/l VII, i/l PPRF (horizontal gaze impairment/ palsy), c/l pyramidal
Raymond	Pons – ventromedial	Basilar (paramedian)	i/l VI, c/l pyramidal
Wallenberg	Medulla – lateral	Vertebral (distal or superior lateral medullary) Posterior inferior cerebellar	i/l V (sensory loss and pain) i/l ataxia (limb and gait) i/l nystagmus, vertigo, hoarseness, dysphagia i/l Horner's c/l hemisensory loss Nausea, vomiting, hiccup
Dejerine	Medulla – medial	Vertebral/basilar/anterior spinal (anteromedial branches)	i/l XII, c/l pyramida, c/l hemisensory
Hughlings Jackson	Medulla – tegmentum	Vertebral/basilar/anterior spinal (anteromedial branches)	i/l X, XI, XII
Schmidt	Medulla – lower tegmentum	Vertebral/basilar/anterior spinal (anteromedial branches)	i/l X, XI

i/l, ipsilateral; c/l, contralateral; PCA, posterior cerebral artery; PPRF, parapontine reticular formation.

- More distally, beyond the point at which the pharyngeal nerve arises high in the cervical region, a complete isolated vagal palsy causes unilateral vocal cord palsy and laryngeal anaesthesia but spares pharyngeal and palatal muscles. The superior laryngeal nerve, which arises just distal to the pharyngeal nerve, is primarily sensory and lesions tend to be asymptomatic; classically, crico-thyroid dysfunction causes an inability to raise the vocal pitch, with a degree of hoarseness.

Lesions of the recurrent laryngeal nerve are more common than isolated vagus trunk lesions. These cause degrees of dysphonia, which may be transient if unilateral, or severe if bilateral. The left recurrent laryngeal nerve is more frequently involved than the right because of its longer intrathoracic course making it vulnerable to mediastinal lesions such as lung malignancy, left atrial enlargement and aortic arch aneurysm. A wide variety of pathological processes (e.g. thyroid masses, lymph node and oesophageal malignancy) can affect the recurrent laryngeal nerves as they ascend through the neck and they are vulnerable during thyroid and parathyroid surgery. In a significant proportion of cases, however, the cause of an isolated recurrent laryngeal nerve palsy often remains undetermined, even after extensive investigation; spontaneous recovery may occur.

Investigation

This is based around comprehensive ENT evaluation, with appropriate MRI and CT imaging of brainstem, skull base, neck and upper thorax. If no structural pathology is identified, CSF examination may be needed. The clinical picture will help to localise the lesion and guide targeted investigation. In practice, when confronted with a patient with a vocal cord palsy, the clinician needs to establish if there is evidence of other brainstem signs or involvement of other lower cranial nerves and to look for associated pharyngeal and palatal paralysis.

XI. Accessory nerve

Functional anatomy

The spinal accessory nerve is the motor nerve to the upper portion of the trapezius and sternocleidomastoid muscles. Unusually, the XIth nerve has twin origins: the caudal portion of the nucleus ambiguus forms the internal ramus (minority), and the accessory nucleus of the upper cervical spinal cord (C1–6), the spinal root and external ramus (majority). The pathway begins by ascent of the spinal root through the foramen magnum and the nerve then exits from the skull via the jugular foramen (Figure 13.8). From there, the

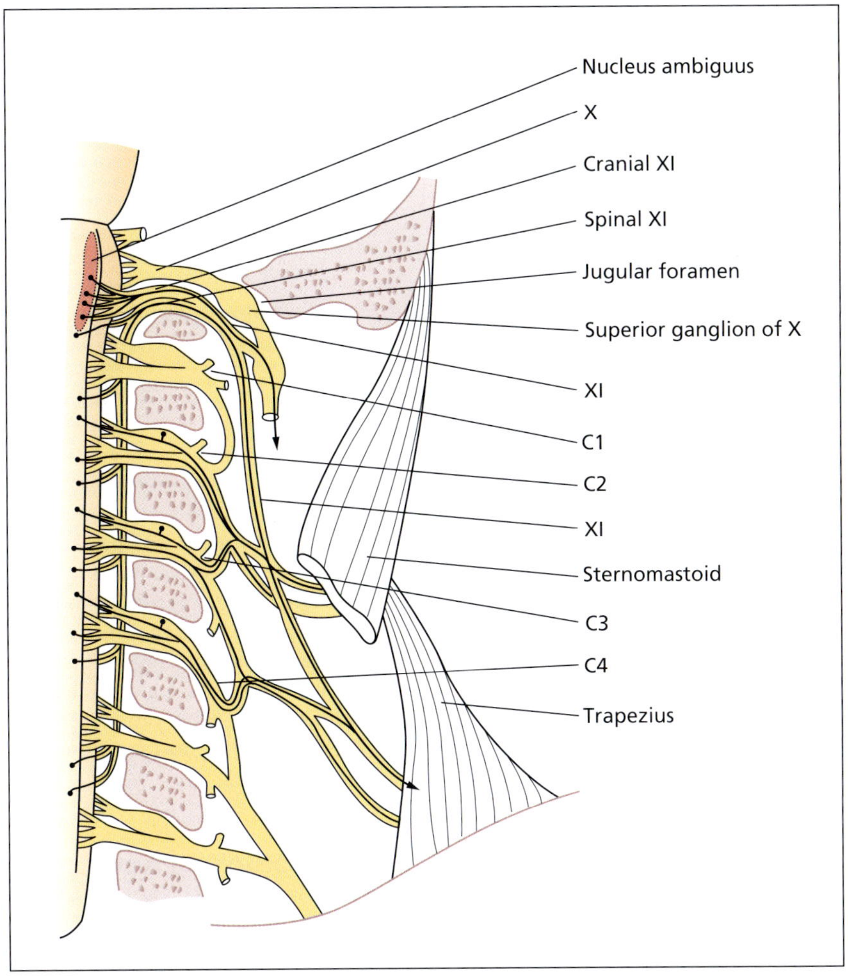

Figure 13.8 Jugular foramen (left), X and XI (AP view, cord and medulla).

internal ramus supplies the larynx and pharnynx with the Xth nerve; the external ramus supplies the sternocleidomastoid and trapezius muscles. Strictly speaking, the fibres of the cranial root of the nerve destined to form the internal ramus are functionally and anatomically part of the vagus nerve; thus, the accessory nerve is primarily a spinal nerve with an intracranial course rather than a true cranial nerve. Afferent twigs from the cervical and thoracic nerves combine with spinal XI as it pierces trapezius – an anomalous arrangement (Chapter 2). The spinal accessory nerve has an intimate relationship with the internal jugular vein (IJV): one surgical series of neck dissections for cancer found that in 96% it was lateral to the IJV at the level of the superior border of the posterior belly of digastric, in 3% medial and in 1% spinal XI travelled through the IJV.

Examination and localisation of lesions

The right sternomastoid is tested by asking the patient to turn the head to the left against resistance; both sternomastoids contracting together produce head flexion. The trapezius raises the abducted arm above horizontal, and is responsible for much of the scapular movement. This is tested by asking the subject to shrug their shoulders.

The clinical picture is relatively straightforward for unilateral peripheral lesions. The shoulder droops lower on the affected side, with wasting of the upper trapezius, accompanied by weakness of shoulder elevation and arm abduction above 90°. Winging of the scapular is seen, particularly when the arm is moved laterally, as opposed to damage of the long thoracic nerve when the winging is seen with forward movement of the arms against a flat surface, because of serratus anterior weakness. The so-called scapular flip sign is a cluster of shoulder girdle depression, trapezius atrophy, and active shoulder abduction limited to less than 90° with the postulated mechanism being the unopposed pull of the external humeral rotators by the inactive lower and middle trapezius.

Isolated bilateral sternocleidomastoid lesions are extremely rare but generalised neuromuscular processes such as myotonic dystrophy, inflammatory myopathies, some muscular dystrophies and myasthenia gravis also affect these and other neck muscles and are a more common cause of neck flexion weakness.

With central hemispheric lesions, the trapezius is weak on the side of the hemiparesis, while the sternomastoid is weak ipsilateral to the cortical lesion (so head turning is weak towards the side of the hemiparesis). Dissociated weakness has also been described, mainly indicating brainstem or upper cervical pathology.

Table 13.5 Lesions of the spinal accessory nerve.

Supranuclear (pseudobulbar palsy)	Cerebrovascular disease Extrapyramidal disorder (e.g. cervical dystonia, parkinsonism)
Nuclear	Motor neurone disease Syringobulbia
Infranuclear (intracranial)	Meningeal process (e.g. infective or malignant meningitis) Subarachnoid haemorrhage Tumours (e.g. schwannoma, neurofibroma, meningioma) Inflammation Trauma
Infranuclear (skull base)	Basal skull fracture
Infranuclear (jugular foramen)	Inflammatory Tumour Traumatic Metastatic
Infranuclear (extracranial – posterior triangle of neck)	Lymphadenopathy (deep cervical), biopsy Tumours – schwannoma, neurinoma Shoulder dislocation Infection – abscess Trauma – traction injury, hyperextension of cervical cord Surgery – sternotomy, carotid endarterectomy Jugular vein cannulation Carotid artery (e.g. aneurysm/ dissection) Neuropathy (e.g. neuralgic amyotrophy) Radiotherapy
Neuromuscular junction	Myasthenia, Lambert–Eaton
Muscle	FSH Myotonic disorders Inflammatory

FSH, facioscapulohumeral muscular dystrophy.

XIth nerve lesions

The leading cause of damage to the XIth nerve is iatrogenic trauma during operations such as lymph node biopsy in the posterior cervical triangle and other surgery in this region. Historically, tuberculosis of the neck was a major cause. Vascular procedures such as carotid artery endarterectomy and internal jugular vein cannulation are also well-recognised causes, especially with the intimate relationship to the IJV described earlier (Table 13.5).

These lesions cause weakness of trapezius but spare the sternomastoid. The trapezius weakness following XIth nerve lesions is sometimes associated with persisting severe local shoulder pain and/or deep pain in the trapezius, possibly caused by mechanical factors relating to shoulder droop and scapular winging, or to the anomalous afferents described earlier. Neurophysiology studies can confirm the site of the peripheral lesion, followed if needed by imaging. Surgical intervention has a distinct place in management, using direct grafting, end-to-end repair or neurolysis. There are also instances of spontaneous accessory neuropathy, perhaps allied to neuralgic amyotrophy with pain in the lateral neck or shoulder, which subsides over several weeks followed by weakness and wasting. Recovery is rare. A recurrent variant has been described, with one individual experiencing two episodes over 8 years.

The spinal nucleus of XI may be affected by local structural and inflammatory cord pathologies. In the posterior fossa, the intracranial portion of the nerve can be damaged, often in combination with the glossopharyngeal and vagus nerves (Table 13.4; see Jugular foramen syndrome).

XII. Hypoglossal nerve

Functional anatomy

Glossal muscles, both intrinsic and extrinsic, are supplied by the hypoglossal nerve; the peripheral route travelled is illustrated in Figure 13.9. The styloglossus elevates and retracts the tongue, the hypoglossus convexes and the genioglossus protudes the tongue. The nucleus is beneath the floor of the 4th ventricle, and the nerve

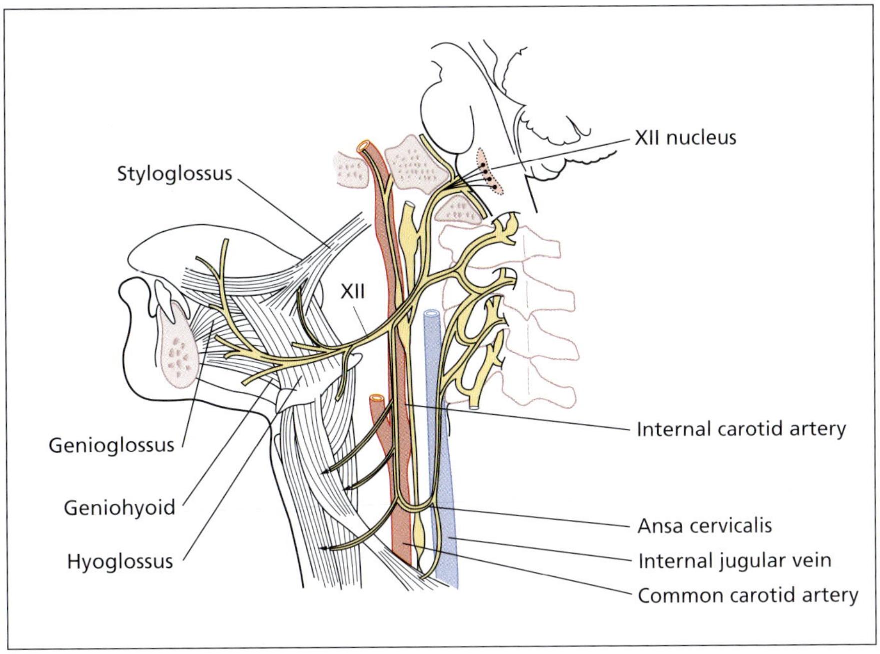

Figure 13.9 Peripheral distribution of XIIth nerve and other principal structures.

emerges as a series of rootlets between the olive and pyramid, in the ventrolateral sulcus. In the posterior cranial fossa, the XIIth nerve exits the skull through the hypoglossal foramen, close to the jugular foramen. Its proximity to both the internal carotid artery and internal jugular vein is important.

Localisation of lesions

Observation of the tongue in both resting and active states is essential, the latter including forward–backward and side–side movements. A variety of signs of unilateral or bilateral wasting can be seen: furrowing, atrophy, fissuring, discoloration and fibrillation. Tongue fibrillation, seen typically bilaterally in motor neurone disease, should only be diagnosed with the tongue at rest within the mouth; the normal tongue often has some flickering movements visible when protruded. The tongue can be spastic, with a small triangular appearance when protruded and slow clumsy movements (see Pseudobulbar palsy).

Peripheral pathology affecting one XIIth nerve causes the tongue to deviate to the side of the lesion on tongue protrusion. Subtle weakness is detected by asking the patient to press the tongue against the inside of each cheek (weakness is evident when the tongue is pressed against the cheek on the same side as the lesion). Typically, unilateral wasting and atrophy follow.

Unilateral upper motor neurone lesions can result in deviation of the tongue contralateral to the lesion, without evidence of wasting, although caused by the bilateral representation; this is uncommon (Chapter 2). Bilateral lower motor neurone lesions result in an inability to protrude the tongue, mild dysphagia and severe dysarthria (see Bulbar palsy).

Causes of XIIth nerve lesions

The causes of hypoglossal nerve lesions are summarised in Table 13.6. A variety of tumours account for half, mainly peripherally in the skull base or neck, with half of those being malignant (e.g. nasopharyngeal carcinoma, lymphoma and metastatic carcinoma). Nasopharyngeal carcinoma commonly involves the Vth and VIth nerves and can spread within the cavernous sinus to involve the IIIrd nerve. In a series of approximately 1000 patients with nasopharyngeal carcinoma, 22% presented with cranial nerve involvement, in which the XIIth nerve was involved in 19%, rising to nearly one-third at follow-up. Trauma is an important cause of XIIth nerve damage, in particular bullet, shrapnel and knife wounds. Damage from infection is rare but when there is evidence of sepsis, osteomyelitis of the clivus should be suspected, in particular in patients with diabetes who have *Pseudomonas* infection originating in the ear (malignant otitis externa). An isolated XIIth nerve lesion, usually associated with neck pain, is sometimes seen as part of carotid artery dissection (Chapter 5) or following carotid endarterectomy.

The proximity of the XIIth nerve to the other lower cranial nerves in the posterior fossa and neck has already been mentioned and combinations of cranial nerve palsies are frequently seen.

Investigation

Imaging of the skull base and neck is essential, predominantly using MRI and fine-cut CT, usually with contrast enhancement. If no cause is revealed, then CSF analysis looking for inflammatory and infiltrative causes may be needed. Electrophysiological studies can be useful (e.g. in motor neurone disease or Guillain–Barré syndrome).

Cranial nerve injury following carotid endarterectomy or carotid angioplasty with stenting

Cranial nerve injury is a common problem following carotid procedures and, in the authors' experience, often understated to patients prior to surgery (Table 13.7). In a recent Cochrane review of trials of carotid intervention, carotid endarterectomy compared to carotid artery stenting carried a higher risk of cranial nerve injury, 5.5% versus 0.3% (n = 7000 evaluated). The nerve most frequently affected is the hypoglossal.

Table 13.6 Causes of tongue weakness.

Supranuclear (pseudobulbar palsy)	Cerebrovascular disease Structural lesion (e.g. abscess, tumour) Extrapyramidal disorder (e.g. MSA) Inflammatory/demyelination (e.g ADEM, MS, CPM) Motor neurone disease
Nuclear	Motor neurone disease Tumour Structural (e.g. Chiari malformation) Vascular Syringobulbia Abscess Granuloma Infections (e.g. TB, syphilis, polio)
Infranuclear (intracranial)	Meningeal process (e.g. infective or malignant meningitis) Subarachnoid haemorrhage Tumours (e.g. schwannoma) Inflammation Trauma
Infranuclear (skull base)	Basal skull fracture Basilar invagination Platybasia Chiari malformation Clivus lesion (e.g. chordoma, epidermoid) Vascular (e.g. ICA dissection/aneurysm, dural AV fistula) Tumour (e.g. nasopharyngeal carcinoma, glomus, osteoma)
Infranuclear (hypoglossal canal)	Inflammatory Tumour Traumatic Metastatic
Infranuclear (extracranial)	Trauma Surgery Carotid artery (e.g. aneurysm/dissection) Tumours/infections of the retropharyngeal space Lymphadenopathy (deep cervical) Tumours (e.g. neck, tongue base, salivary gland) Neuropathy (e.g. GBS, CIDP, HLPP)
Neuromuscular junction	Myasthenia, LEMS
Muscle	Myotonic disorders Inflammatory

ADEM, acute disseminated encephalomyelitis; CIDP, chronic inflammatory demyelinating neuropathy; CPM, central pontine myelinolysis; GBS, Guillain–Barré syndrome; HLPP, hereditary liability to pressure palsy; ICA, internal carotid artery: LEMS, Lambert–Eaton myasthenic syndrome; MS, multiple sclerosis; MSA, multiple system atrophy; TB, tuberculosis.

Jugular foramen syndrome

This pattern of IXth, Xth and XIth nerve lesions is known as Vernet's syndrome but cranial nerve involvement may be more extensive (Table 13.8a). Figure 13.8 and Figure 13.9 demonstrate how structural disease at the jugular foramen can damage this trio of cranial nerves. As predicted, the presentation is dysphagia, dysphonia, sensory loss over the posterior third of the tongue, soft palate, pharynx and larynx (IXth and Xth) and ipsilateral sternomastoid/trapezius atrophy and weakness (XIth). The causes are listed in Table 13.8b.

An analysis of jugular foramen schwannomas found:

- Mean age at presentation was 40 years
- 2 : 1 left : right
- Common symptoms: hearing loss, tinnitus, hoarseness, dysphagia and ataxia, and
- Complete removal was possible in 80% but 7% recurred.

Schwannomas arose from the glossopharyngeal nerve in 24%, vagus in 13% and cranial XI in 6%. Postoperative complications included facial and lower cranial nerve palsies occurred in around 25%.

Table 13.7 Common nerve lesions following carotid endarterectomy and stenting.

Nerve involved	Effect	Usual outcome
Cervical sympathetic chain	Horner's syndrome	Permanent
Hypoglossal (XII)	Tongue deviation	Recovery
Recurrent laryngeal (X)	Hoarseness, dysphagia	Variable
Cutaneous cervical branches	Sensory loss around neck	Some numbness: common
Accessory (XI) – unusual	Weak sternomastoid; pain	Variable

Table 13.8 Causes of jugular foramen syndrome.

(a) Variants		
	Vernet	Ipsilateral involvement of CN IX, X, XI
	Collet–Sicard	Vernet + XII
	Villaret	Collet–Sicard + Horner's (due to carotid sympathetics)
(b) Causes		
	Tumours	Glomus tumour (paraganglioma, chemodactoma) Schwannoma Meningioma Ependymoma Glioma (ectopic) Chordoma Plasmacytoma Metastasis
	Infection	Malignant otitis externa Retropharyngeal abscess Herpes zoster
	Vascular	Thrombosis of the jugular bulb Giant cell arteritis
	Trauma	

Bulbar and pseudobular palsy

These terms refer to impairment of function of muscles supplied by lower cranial nerves (IX, X, XI and sometimes XII). The nuclei of these nerves lie in the medulla (the medullary bulb), within the brainstem. Lesions involving the descending corticobulbar pathways (from cortex to nucleus) cause pseudobulbar palsy and lesions of the nuclei, fasciculi, cranial nerves or muscles themselves produce bulbar palsy. In pseudobulbar weakness, there is no lateralisation. Bulbar weakness can be unilateral, though it is typically bilateral. The most obvious manifestation of diminished muscle movement is usually choking and neurogenic dysphagia, but both bulbar and pseudobulbar palsy include a constellation of characteristic associated clinical features. Patients with severe Parkinson's disease also have poverty of movement of bulbar muscles, and cerebellar disease causes disordered swallowing.

Normal swallowing

The normal swallow is a complex sequence of coordinated events requiring intact lower cranial nerve function. A pre-oral phase is associated with the sight, smell and taste of food that triggers saliva production and prepares for the food or liquid bolus. In the oral phase the lips close to form a seal (VII); the tongue and rotatory action of the jaw (XII, V) grind food, mixing it with saliva. The velum sits on the base of the tongue to seal off the nasal cavity. When the bolus has been formed the tongue raises against the hard palate, a central groove forms (XII) and the stripping motion of the tongue moves the bolus backwards. When the bolus reaches the faucial arches, the swallowing reflex is triggered. The pharyngeal stage is entirely involuntary. The soft palate rises to block off the nasal cavity (X). As the swallow is triggered the larynx rises and tilts forwards. The airway is protected by apposition of the true and false cords and of the arytenoids against the base of the epiglottis (the sphincteric action of the larynx). The epiglottis inhibits direct contact of the bolus with the laryngeal vestibule (all X). Upward and forward movement of the hyoid and larynx (V, VII, C1–3) enhance airway protection and pull open the relaxed upper oesophageal sphincter. The bolus moves over the closed airway and the cricopharyngeal sphincter relaxes. In the oesophageal stage the bolus passes through the cricopharyngeal oesophagus by peristalsis. Breathing is centrally inhibited during the swallow (deglutition apnoea); afterwards, structures return passively to their original positions, or with the aid of the infrahyoid muscles.

It is increasingly clear these swallowing reflexes are influenced by significant descending control to the medulla. Clinical observation in cerebrovascular disease and cortical mapping using transcranial magnetic stimulation and functional imaging indicate a role for the cerebral cortex (primary motor, inferior frontal gyrus and insula) with probable left hemispheric dominance. Dysphagia is also common in basal ganglia and cerebellar disorders – these systems are clearly also involved in descending control.

Table 13.9 Causes of bulbar palsy.

Lesions of medullary cranial nerve nuclei	
Cerebrovascular	Infarction Haemorrhage
Tumour	Glioma
Infection	Poliomyelitis
Inflammatory	Multiple sclerosis Acute haemorrhagic leuko-encephalitis Sarcoidosis Behçet's
Degenerative	Motor neurone disease Kennedy's disease
Structural	Syringobulbia
Rhomboencephalitis	Bickerstaff's encephalitis* Fisher's syndrome
Lesions of cranial nerves	
	Guillain–Barré syndrome Fisher's syndrome CIDP CMT type II
Neuromuscular junction lesions	
	Myasthenia gravis Lambert–Eaton myasthenic syndrome Congenital myasthenia gravis Botulism
Muscle diseases	
Inflammatory	Polymyositis Inclusion body myositis
Dystrophy	Myotonic Duchenne Oculopharyngeal

CIDP, chronic idiopathic demyelinating polyradiculoneuropathy; CMT, Charcot–Marie–Tooth.
* Bickerstaff's encephalitis: rare, sometimes with anti-GQ1b antibodies, cranial nerve palsies, cerebellar ataxia, coma.

Bulbar palsy

While bulbar palsy may be unilateral or bilateral, swallowing impairment usually only occurs with bilateral weakness (Table 13.9). Bulbar muscle weakness causes a nasal dysarthria, dysphagia with nasal regurgitation, a wasted atrophic tongue with fasciculation and slow tongue movement. There may also be associated facial weakness, dysphonia and limited jaw movement. There is consistent absence of both palatal and pharyngeal reflexes in bulbar palsy. Unilateral pharyngeal wall paresis causes the paralysed side to move towards the healthy side (Vernet's movement *de rideau*). It is not possible to distinguish reliably between IX and X nerve lesions, but lack of posterior pharyngeal sensation can have important implications in stroke. A unilateral XII nerve lesion causes tongue deviation – on retraction towards the healthy side (unopposed action of the styloglossus), and on protrusion towards the affected side (genioglossus). Impaired swallow can easily lead to poor dietary intake and dehydration, aspiration and bronchopneumonia – secretions pool in the pharynx.

Pseudobulbar palsy

Pseudobulbar palsy describes an upper motor neurone pattern of weakness affecting muscles innervated by the bulbar nuclei (Table 13.10). It is usually caused by bilateral involvement of the descending corticobulbar and/or cortico-pontine pathways anywhere from the insular cortex to the medulla. Pseudobulbar palsy is characterised by spastic dysarthria, slow and limited tongue movements with no wasting or fasciculation, an exaggerated jaw jerk and pharyngeal weakness. There may be complete anarthria with an

Table 13.10 Causes of pseudobulbar palsy.

Cerebrovascular disease	Infarction Haemorrhage Vasculitis
Inflammatory	Multiple sclerosis Acute disseminated encephalomyelitis Acute haemorrhagic leuko-encephalitis Sarcoidosis
Degenerative	Motor neurone disease – progressive bulbar palsy, amyotrophic lateral sclerosis or progressive lateral sclerosis Hereditary spastic paraplegia Progressive supranuclear palsy Corticobasal degeneration Multiple system atrophy
Inborn errors of metabolism	Friedreich's ataxia Mitochondrial disease Leigh's syndrome Adrenoleukodystrophy / adrenomyelodystrophy Alexander's disease GM2 gangliosidase deficiency Metachromatic leukodystrophy

inability to open the mouth, protrude the tongue, swallow or move the face at will or on command. Patients with pseudobulbar palsy show a striking incongruity with loss of voluntary movements of muscles innervated by the motor nuclei of the lower pons and medulla (inability to swallow, phonate, articulate, move the tongue forcefully, close the eyes) but preservation of reflex ponto-medullary actions: yawning, coughing, throat clearing, spasmodic laughter and crying. Pseudobulbar affect describes the combination of emotional lability and profound motor retardation. There may be associated frontal release signs and primitive reflexes; the jaw jerk, facial and pharyngeal reflexes can be particularly brisk, with clonic jaw movements or clamping down on a wooden tongue blade. Occasionally, these clinical features occur in isolation with no other manifestations of pseudobulbar palsy. In particular, isolated inappropriate spasmodic laughing or crying, unrelated to surrounding circumstances or stimulation and with no corresponding emotional feeling may be the first feature sign of pseudobulbar palsy. Movements of the palate and pharynx on phonation are variable but often reduced.

Pseudobulbar palsy may be divided into three forms:

1 *Cortical:* caused by lesions in the opercular region and characterised by isolated weakness of the face, pharynx and tongue with dissociation between automatic and voluntary function. This is associated with anarthria, a complete loss of swallow and hypotonic paralysed muscles. Emotional lability is unusual.
2 *Striatal:* caused by lesions in the descending corticobulbar tract in which the characteristic cortical features are associated with pyramidal signs, emotional lability and cognitive impairment.
3 *Pontine:* in which all these features occur with cerebellar signs and emotional lability but no cognitive impairment.

Dropped head syndrome

Certain clinical appearances narrow diagnostic possibilities. The dropped head syndrome (Figure 13.10) is one of these. A variety of neuromuscular diseases cause this syndrome (Table 13.11); motor neurone disease is one of the most common.

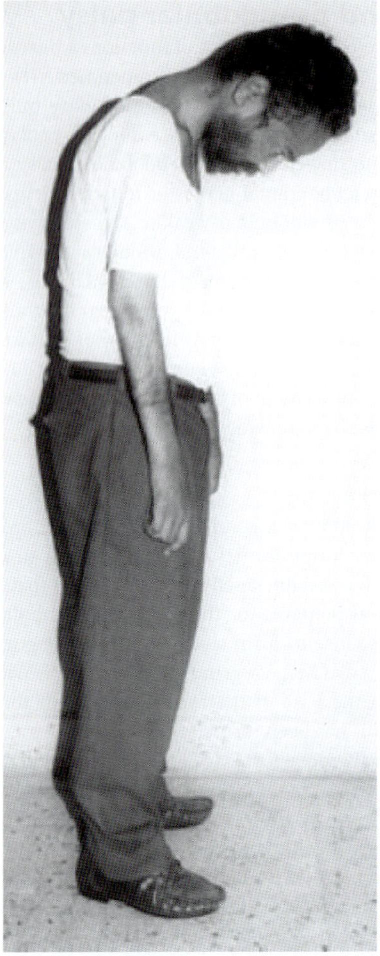

Figure 13.10 Dropped head syndrome in a patient with motor neurone disease. Source: Gourie-Devi 2003. Reproduced with permission of BMJ.

The condition is particularly distressing and difficult to help. Various supports and frames are sometimes suggested and some patients find a high-backed chair or a tailored U shaped cushion is more comfortable than a soft collar. Advice from an occupational therapist with experience of palliative care is helpful. Severe neck pain often accompanies the weak muscles.

Multiple cranial neuropathies

Multiple cranial neuropathies (MCNs) are either caused by local lesions such as tumours, vascular causes, trauma and infection, which affect clusters of neighbouring nerves, or by underlying systemic conditions. Some combinations of cranial nerve lesions have been mentioned already; others are described in Chapters 14 and 21. Some MCNs have a benign cause, such as a CPA tumour. However, when no such lesion is evident on initial imaging, MCNs should be regarded as ominous, because of the high chance of underlying malignancy (metastasis, primary tumour and malignant meningitis) or other serious systemic disease often affecting the clivus or the skull base (Table 13.12). Careful scrutiny, a review of detailed imaging and CSF analysis are needed, and may need to be repeated after an interval. Images of the skull base are sometimes particularly difficult to interpret; fine-cut CT, with bone windows is

Table 13.11 Causes of dropped head.

Inflammatory myopathy
Motor neurone disease
Myasthenia gravis
FSH
SMA
Isolated neck extensor myopathy
Rarely
Acid maltase deficiency
CIDP
Myofibrillary myopathy (e.g. desmin, lamin)
Nemaline myopathy
Mitochondrial myopathy
Hypothyroid myopathy
Hyperthyroidism
LEMS
Myotonic dystrophy

CIDP, chronic inflammatory demyelinating neuropathy; FSH, fascioscapulohumoral (dystrophy); LEMS, Lambert–Eaton myasthenic syndrome; SMA, spinal muscular atrophy.

Table 13.12 Clivus/skull base syndromes (commonly VI, II and V; XII sometimes).

Nasopharyngeal carcinoma
Chordoma
Meningioma
Pituitary adenoma, craniopharyngioma
Lymphoma, myeloma, leukaemia, histiocytosis
Dermoid, epidermoid
Exophytic glioma, ependymoma
Primary bone tumour, giant cell tumour
Schwannoma
Cholesteatoma
Glomus
Metastases – prostate, thyroid, kidney, lung, gastric
Radiotherapy
Paget's disease, osteopetrosis, fibrous dysplasia, hyperostosis

of particular value. The advice and expertise of an ENT surgeon and an ophthalmologist with experience of neurological conditions is invaluable.

One large series of over 1000 cases of MCNs found that tumours were responsible for 30%. Schwannomas, generally from the VIIIth nerve, followed by metastases were the most common neoplasms. The majority of vascular cases were lateral pontine or medullary infarcts. There were a small number of arteriovenous malformations and carotico-cavernous aneurysms. Infection made up 10% of the series, caused by meningitis (bacterial, tuberculous, cryptococcal). Other causes included botulism, mucormycosis, viral encephalitis and cysticercosis. The main causes of multiple cranial nerve palsies are summarised in Table 13.13.

Table 13.13 Other causes of multiple cranial nerve palsies (most common patterns are III and IV; V and VI; V and VII).

Meningitis	Infectious, carcinomatous, lymphomatous, pachymeningitis
Tumour	Clivus and skull base
Trauma	
Infection	Bacterial-*Borrelia*, TB, syphilis Viral – HZV, HSV, EBV, CMV, HIV, HTLV-1 Fungal – *Aspergillus, Cryptococcus, Mucormycosis, Histoplasmosis, Candida* Parasite – *Cysticercosis*
Neuropathy	Guillain–Barré, Miller–Fisher, idiopathic cranial polyneuropathy
Metabolic	Diabetes mellitus
Inflammatory	Sarcoidosis, Behçet's, amyloidosis
Vasculitis	Wegener, PAN, Churg–Strauss, lymphomatoid granulomatosis, giant cell arteritis, granulomatous angiitis
Connective tissue disease	Systemic lupus erythematosus, Sjögren's, scleroderma, mixed connective tissue disease
Pituitary	Apoplexy, lymphocytic hypophysitis
Vascular	Aneurysm, dissection, endarterectomy
Radiotherapy	
Bone disease	Osteopetrosis, Paget's disease, hyperostosis cranialis, fibrous dysplasia

CMV, cytomegalovirus; EBV, Epstein–Barr virus; HIV, human immunodeficiency virus; HSV, herpes simplex virus; HTLV-1, human T-cell lymphotrophic virus; HZV, herpes zoster virus; PAN, polyarteritis nodosa; TB, tuberculosis.

Other causes of MCNs

Other causes of MCNs are sarcoidosis, infection and vasculitides (Chapters 9 and 26). Nasopharyngeal carcinoma is also an important cause of MCN; usually branches of V are involved initially, but with tumour spread the VIIth, VIth and lower cranial nerves become affected.

Multiple recurrent cranial neuropathy of unknown cause

A recurrent multiple cranial neuropathy of unknown cause is seen particularly in South-East Asia. Clusters of MCNs, such as IIIrd, Vth and VIIth nerve lesions, develop, remit and recur over several years. Some of these cases are responsive to steroids.

Intracranial epidural abscess

Pyogenic intracranial epidural abscess is a rare cause of progressive sequential multiple cranial nerve lesions on one side. This occurs typically in the elderly, and in diabetic and cachectic patients. For example, deafness with a discharge from the external auditory meatus can be followed by a VIIth nerve palsy and progressively by lower cranial nerve palsies, to include the XIIth. The abscess, a thin sheet of pus, little more than 1 mm in thickness, can also track upwards to involve the Vth nerve, the three oculomotor nerves and even the optic nerve, the process taking weeks or months. In the early stages, these abscesses can be hard to visualise on imaging. Surgical exploration is usually required, and high doses of antibiotics, but the condition carries a high mortality.

Acknowledgement

Professor M.J. Turlough FitzGerald, Emeritus Professor, Department of Anatomy, National University of Ireland, Galway, kindly agreed that figures and information from the award-winning textbook *Clinical Neuroanatomy and Related Neuroscience* (FitzGerald MJT, Folan-Curran J. 4th edition, 2002; WB Saunders, Edinburgh) were made available for use in the first edition. This cooperation proved invaluable. Details from figures in the subsequent *Clinical Neuroanatomy and Neuroscience* (FitzGerald MJT, Gruener G, Mtui E. 6th edition, 2012; Elsevier Saunders) have been used here, again with permission from Professor FitzGerald. The *Queen Square Textbook* authors and editors are most grateful for this continuing cooperation.

References

Gourie-Devi M, Nalini A, Sandhya S. Early or late appearance of "dropped head syndrome" in amyotrophic lateral sclerosis. *J Neurol Neurosurg Psychiatry* 2003; **74**: 683–686.

Patten J. *Neurological Differential Diagnosis,* 2nd edition. London, New York: Springer, 1996.

Further reading

Trigeminal nerve (V)

Hagen NA, Stevens JC, Michet CJ. Trigeminal sensory neuropathy associated with connective tissue diseases. *Neurology* 1990; **40**: 891–896.

Lecky BRF, Hughes RAC, Murray NMF. Trigeminal sensory neuropathy a study of 22 cases. *Brain* 1987; **110**: 1463–1485.

Zakrzewska JM. *Trigeminal neuralgia. Major Problems in Neurology Series.* WB Saunders, 1995.

Zakrzewska JM, Lopez BC. Trigeminal neuralgia. *Clin Evid* 2006; **15**: 1827–1835.

Facial nerve (VII)

Adour KK, Ruboyianes JM, Van Doersten PG, Byl FM, Trent CS, Quesenberry CP, *et al.* Bell's palsy treatment with acyclovir and prednisone compared with prednisone alone: a double-blind, randomized, controlled trial. *Ann Otol Rhinol Laryngol* 1996; **105**: 371–378.

Auger RG, Whisnant JP. Hemifacial spasm in Rochester and Olmstead county, Minnesota, 1960 to 1984. *Arch Neurol* 1990; **47**: 1233–1234.

Burgess RC, Michaels L, Bale JF, Smith RJ. Polymerase chain reaction amplification of herpes simplex viral DNA from the geniculate ganglion of a patient with Bell's palsy. *Ann Otol Rhinol Laryngol* 1994; **103**: 775–779.

Hagelberg N, Forssell H, Aalto S, Rinne JO, Scheinin H, Taiminen T, *et al.* Altered dopamine D2 receptor binding in atypical facial pain. *Pain* 2003; **106**: 43–48.

Halperin JJ, Golightly M; Long Island Neuroborreliosis Collaborative Study Group. Lyme borreliosis in Bell's palsy. *Neurology* 1992; **42**: 1268–1270.

Harrison DH. Surgical correction of unilateral and bilateral facial palsy. *Postgrad Med J* 2005; **81**: 562–567.

Hato N, Yamada H, Kohno H *et al.* Valacyclovir and prednisolone treatment for Bell's palsy: a multicenter, randomized placebo-controlled study. *Otol Neurol* 2007; **28**: 408–413.

Helgason S, Petursson G, Gudmundsson S, Sigurdsson JA. Prevalence of postherpetic neuralgia after a first episode of herpes zoster: prospective study with long term follow up. *Br Med J* 2000; **321**: 1–4.

Holland NJ, Weiner GM. Recent developments in Bell's palsy. *BMJ* 2004; **329**: 553–557.

Keane JR. Bilateral seventh nerve palsy: analysis of 43 cases and review of the literature. *Neurology* 1994; **44**: 1198–1202.

Lascelles RG. Atypical facial pain and depression. *Br J Psychiatry* 1966; **112**: 165–169.

Murakami S, Honda N, Mizobuchi M, Nakashiro Y, Hato N, Gyo K. Rapid diagnosis of varicella zoster virus infection in acute facial palsy. *Neurology* 1998; **51**: 1202–1205.

Rowlands S, Hooper R, Hughes R, Burney P. The epidemiology and treatment of Bell's palsy in the UK. *Eur J Neurol* 2002; **9**: 63–67.

Sullivan FM, Swan IR, Donnan PT *et al.* Treatment with prednisolone or acyclovir in Bell's Palsy. *N Engl J Med* 2007; **357**: 1598–1607.

Sweeney CJ, Gilden DH. Ramsay-Hunt syndrome. *J Neurol Neurosurg Psychiatry* 2001; **71**: 149–154.

Wang A, Jankovic J. Hemifacial spasm: clinical findings and treatment. *Muscle Nerve* 1998; **21**: 1740–1747.

Bulbar and pseudobulbar palsy

Besson G, Bogousslavsky J, Regli F, Maeder P. Acute pseudobulbar or suprabulbar palsy. *Arch Neurol* 1991; **48**: 501–507.

Hughes TAT, Wiles CM. Neurogenic dysphagia: the role of the neurologist. *J Neurol Neurosurg Psychiatry* 1998; **64**: 569–572.

Wiles CM. Neurogenic dysphagia. *J Neurol Neurosurg Psychiatry* 1991; **54**: 1037–1039.

Glossopharyngeal nerve (IX)

Chalk C, Isaacs H. Recurrent spontaneous accessory neuropathy. *J Neurol Neurosurg Psychiatry* 1990; **53**: 621–625.

Pearce JMS. Glossopharyngeal neuralgia. *Eur Neurol* 2006; **55**: 49–52.

Accessory nerve (XI)

Bakar B. The jugular foramen schwannomas: review of the large surgical series. *J Korean Neurosurg Soc* 2008; **44**: 285–294.

Hinsley ML, Hartig GK, Hinsley ML, Hartig GK. Anatomic relationship between the spinal accessory nerve and internal jugular vein in the upper neck. *Otolaryngology Head Neck Surg* 2010; **143**: 239–241.

Kelley MJ, Kane TE, Leggin BG, Kelley MJ, Kane TE, Leggin BG. Spinal accessory nerve palsy: associated signs and symptoms. *J Orthop Sports Phys Ther* 2008; **38**: 78–86.

Kim DH, Cho Y-JC, Tiel RL, Kline DG. Surgical outcomes of 111 spinal accessory nerve injuries. *Neurosurgery* 2003; **53**: 1106–1112.

Makiese O, Chibbaro S, Marsella M, Tran Ba HP, George B, *et al.* Jugular foramen paragangliomas: management, outcome and avoidance of complications in a series of 75 cases. *Neurosurg Rev* 2012; **35**: 185–194.

Talacchi A, Biroli A, Soda C, Masotto B, Bricolo A, *et al.* Surgical management of ventral and ventrolateral foramen magnum meningiomas: report on a 64-case series and review of the literature. *Neurosurg Rev* 2012; **35**: 359–367.

Hypoglossal nerve (XII)

Bonati L, Lyrer P, Ederle J, Featherstone R, Brown M. Percutaneous transluminal balloon angioplasty and stenting for carotid artery stenosis. *Cochrane Database Syst Rev* 2012; **9**: CD000515.

Cunningham EJ, Bond R, Mayberg MR, Warlow CP, Rothwell PM. Risk of persistent cranial nerve injury after carotid endarterectomy. *J Neurosurg* 2004; **101**: 445–448.

Keane JR. Twelfth nerve palsy: analysis of 100 cases. *Arch Neurol* 1996; **53**: 561–566.

Multiple cranial nerve palsies

Campbell WW. In: *DeJong's The Neurological Examination*, 7th edition. Philadelphia: Wolters Kluwer Lippincott, Williams & Wilkins, 2013.

Carroll CG, Campbell WW. Multiple cranial neuropathies. *Semin Neurol* 2009; **29**: 53–65.

Keane JR. Multiple cranial nerve palsies. *Arch Neurol* 2005; **62**: 1714–1717.

CHAPTER 14

Neuro-Ophthalmology

James Acheson[1], Fion Bremner[1], Elizabeth Graham[1], Robin Howard[1], Alexander Leff[2], Gordon Plant[1], Simon Shorvon[2] and Ahmed Toosy[2]

[1] National Hospital for Neurology & Neurosurgery

[2] UCL Institute of Neurology

Patients generally relate visual disorders to the eye itself rather than recognising that the problem might be with the brain. In the United Kingdom, when a patient complains that he/she has impaired vision the first port of call is frequently an optometrist and if spectacles are not the answer a further referral is made to a hospital through the general practitioner. In many other countries without extensive service provision by optometrists and general practitioners the patient will seek the advice of an ophthalmologist directly.

A significant proportion of patients presenting with symptoms of visual abnormalities have primary neurological disorders or require neurological assessment. Therefore, ophthalmology and neurology should rightly be closely related disciplines; the eye is, after all, a part of the brain and many disorders of the brain have direct effects on vision.

The neuroanatomy of the visual pathway is outlined in Chapter 2. The basic examination of the visual and ocular motor system is dealt with in Chapter 4.

Unilateral visual failure

History

Mode of onset

In taking a history from a patient complaining of visual loss in one eye it is first essential to establish whether the onset was acute, subacute or gradual and whether, since the patient noticed the problem, the vision has deteriorated, improved or remained static. It is best to establish exactly how and in what circumstances he/she first became aware of the problem because the patient may suddenly become aware of vision loss that has been coming on for some time. Some people do not seem habitually to close one eye unless having a specific reason to do so – such as acquiring a foreign body in one eye or during a visit to the optometrist. Thus, a reported abrupt onset of unilateral visual loss, in contrast to when both eyes are affected, may be spurious and the precise circumstances need to be reviewed with an appropriate degree of scepticism. Once it is clear that the loss of vision was genuinely abrupt, painless and with no subsequent change, a vascular cause (e.g. central retinal artery occlusion or anterior ischaemic optic neuropathy) is almost certain but it is important to remember that some vascular syndromes can cause progressive or fluctuating loss of vision.

Subacute loss over days, with pain, is in keeping with an inflammatory cause (e.g. optic neuritis) but the differential diagnosis remains wide unless there has been spontaneous recovery of vision because a number of compressive lesions are capable of producing the same syndrome: notably, anterior communicating artery aneurysm, infections or mucocoele of the paranasal sinuses. The consequences of missing compressive optic neuropathy (e.g. pituitary tumour) can be disastrous as early intervention is required to prevent permanent visual loss. The general rule is that in demyelinating optic neuritis, associated with multiple sclerosis (MS), the pain precedes the loss of vision. Indeed, the pain often abates as the visual loss is noticed by the patient. Furthermore, the pain is not severe, rarely disturbing sleep and it may only be present on eye movement or even only on movement in a particular direction. Therefore an unusual degree of persistent pain would be a feature that should alert the clinician to possible compressive granulomatous or infective causes.

In many patients, the more typical history of gradually progressive loss of vision produced by a compressive lesion will be clear: in others, it may be necessary to acquire optometrist's records to confirm the tempo of the visual failure. Paradoxically, in some instances, loss of vision which would clearly have been abrupt at onset may not be noticed for some time – such as following a vascular occlusion that affected a part of the field only or following trauma. Again, any previous records of visual acuity or visual field testing will be invaluable. Another situation that causes confusion is when a patient is referred with asymptomatic unilateral visual field loss. Usually, visual acuity is normal in this situation and the patient presents with a visual field defect sparing central vision. It is first necessary to establish whether the patient had ever had a previous perimetric examination; if not, the loss could be congenital. If it is clear that the loss has been acquired at some time between two examinations it may require some detective work to decide the cause based on the examination findings and on occasion serial perimetry to determine whether or not the defect is static. Unilateral visual field defects that present in this way are commonly caused by focal retinal pathology, congenital optic nerve defects, glaucoma, optic disc drusen, previous trauma, compressive lesions and as chronic sequelae of subclinical branch retinal artery and vein occlusions or demyelinating optic neuritis.

Neurology: A Queen Square Textbook, Second Edition. Edited by Charles Clarke, Robin Howard, Martin Rossor and Simon Shorvon.

Positive symptoms

Positive symptoms are not commonly reported in optic nerve disease. Occasionally, patients with optic neuritis report that on eye movement a brief flash is perceived. Of interest, these flashes are not seen except in the dark, indicating that the perception is washed out by natural illumination. This is in contrast to positive stimuli generated in the occipital lobes which appear equally bright in the dark and in brightly lit surroundings. Patients who report continuous phosphenes (again appreciated more in low light levels) will have retinal disease and this is particularly true of cases of local retinitis such as the idiopathic big blind spot syndrome and acute zonal occult outer retinopathy. These two conditions are almost always unilateral and often referred as suspected optic nerve disease because the retina appears normal on fundus examination but there are discrete scotomas typical of retinal disease and within which the patient is aware of a more or less constant flickering.

Effect of light level

Humans have a duplex retina in which two independent systems of photoreceptors – the rods and cones – are specialised for low and high light levels, respectively. Indeed, in extreme low light levels the cone photoreceptors make no contribution to vision and at photopic levels the rods do not function. Hence, conditions that affect more or less independently the two classes of photoreceptor result in visual loss that is much more marked at low light levels (nyctalopia, e.g. rod dystrophies) or at high light levels (e.g. cone dystrophies); these disorders are rarely unilateral. However, post receptorally the rod and cone signals are shared (multiplexed) by the same pathways (bipolar cells and retinal ganglion cells). Hence, in optic nerve disease marked variation in visual performance at different light levels is not generally observed. There are exceptions to this and some patients with optic neuropathy may report seeing better in bright or dim light although it may be difficult to understand why. A more specific situation which occurs in demyelinating optic neuropathy is deterioration in bright light which patients describe as 'fading'. The pathophysiological basis of this is not known.

Direct questions

The following are a few direct questions worthwhile asking any patient with unilateral visual loss.

- *Subjective visual field changes* 'If you are viewing with that eye alone, is the entire field of vision affected, or only a part?' Central scotomas are frequently reported as appearing as if there is a cloud or other patch in front of the eye, saying: 'If only I could see around it my eyesight would be normal.' Patients with altitudinal field defects may have normal visual acuity but be aware that they cannot see above or below what they are looking at and this is highly suggestive of either anterior ischaemic optic neuropathy or a branch retinal artery occlusion.
- *Provoking factors* 'Does vision deteriorate after exertion or a hot bath?' In Uhthoff's symptom vision deteriorates with a rise in body temperature, returning to normal when the body cools down. This phenomenon is almost pathognomonic of demyelinating (MS-associated) optic neuritis. The loss of vision may be total or partial but recovery always occurs after a few minutes of resting. Most commonly, the symptom is noticed by patients who have recovered from acute optic neuritis but it may also occur in the acute phase or in patients who do not report an acute episode at all, that is to say as a result of subclinical demyelination.
- *Associated symptoms* 'Have you noticed any change in your sense of smell?' In cases of anterior cranial fossa masses (usually meningiomas) anosmia may precede loss of vision by several years and may well have passed without any neuroimaging being carried out.
- *Double vision* 'Have you had double vision?' The ocular motor nerves enter the orbit through the superior orbital fissure while the optic nerve enters through the optic canal and the combination of an optic neuropathy with a IIIrd, IVth or VIth cranial nerve lesion would indicate either an extensive lesion (and this can occur with meningiomas and granulomas) or the pathology must be within the orbit itself and on examination the neurologist should look particularly for orbital signs.
- *Distortion* 'Do you see distortion of anything that you are looking at, do straight lines appear crooked or do objects appear larger or smaller than they are?' Rarely, spatial distortion of images can occur with occipital lobe disease. This does not occur with optic nerve disease but is very commonly seen with retinal disease. A distorted photoreceptor layer will result in an equivalent geometric distortion of the perceived image. Thus, elevation of the retina will result in separation of the photoreceptors and the perceived image will be diminished in size. Central serous retinopathy in younger patients or age-related macular degeneration in older patients are the disorders that are most commonly confused with optic nerve disease and this simple question can provide an important clue.

Examination

Visual acuity

The first step for the neurologist is to decide whether unilateral visual loss is caused by refractive error, disorders of the lens and ocular media or retinal pathology and hence would require onward referral for appropriate management. Some knowledge of optometry is essential because the presence of emmetropia, myopia or hypermetropia and presbyopia has a marked effect on how patients respond to changes in vision resulting from neurological disease and also on the interpretation of findings on examination including the appearance of the fundus. Visual acuity examination for near and distance, with and without refractive correction, should be carried out under standardised conditions using correctly illuminated Snellen or equivalent charts at the correct distance.

Colour vision

The testing of colour vision can be performed simply by asking the patient to judge the saturation of a coloured target. 'Saturation' in chromatic terms refers to how far the colour is from white and it is generally the case in optic nerve disease that colours will appear less saturated – that is to say, closer to white. Quite simply, in unilateral optic nerve disease if a coloured target is held up to the affected eye and a comparison made with the unaffected eye this difference in colour will be reported. At the extreme the colour may be lost altogether and the object will appear white or grey depending upon its luminance/brightness. Tests are available in which patients are shown a series of discs of the same hue varying in saturation. The patient is asked to arrange them in order of increasing saturation which will indicate the least saturated disc that is perceived as being different from white. The degree of saturation can be quantified in this way.

Across the visual field this change can be observed regionally so that in a patient with a central scotoma which is relative the colour saturation of the target may be restored as it is moved from an abnormal to an unaffected region of the visual field. This is of particular importance when a hemianopic or altitudinal field defect is suspected as this change in colour saturation will appear abruptly as the target is moved across the vertical or horizontal meridian, respectively.

The Ishihara pseudoisochromatic plates are commonly utilised for the assessment of colour vision in ophthalmic and neurological practice. The term 'pseudoisochromatic' refers to the fact that the individual coloured dots which make up the figure are varied in brightness, thus making it impossible to use luminance differences to identify the figure. The advantage of this in the assessment of unilateral visual loss is that impairment of colour vision in optic nerve disease is much greater (for an equivalent loss of acuity) than in the case of retinal disease. The explanation for this is not known but it may in part be related to a selective effect of compressive and demyelinating optic pathology on the parvocellular pathway (these are the retinal ganglion cell axons that project to the parvocellular layers of the lateral geniculate nucleus and which subserve colour vision). In retinal disease the extent to which colour vision is affected can be predicted from the degree of involvement of the macular and paramacular regions of the retina. In other words, if acuity is reduced and there is a large enough central scotoma then colour vision will be affected. At the limit, patients with visual acuity of 6/60 cannot read even the control plate in the Ishihara test. This plate does not require any colour vision to read but indicates that the patient has adequate visual acuity to perform the test. In optic nerve disease, a patient with a visual acuity of 6/6 or 6/9 is likely to have significantly impaired colour vision and this would be very unusual in retinal disorders with the exception of the cone dystrophies.

The Ishihara plates were developed for the assessment of congenital colour anomalies (Daltonism) and so there is considerable detail in the testing that is not relevant to optic nerve disease where the losses do not follow the specific patterns seen in Daltonism but show instead largely global losses. Furthermore, specific illumination conditions are required for an accurate interpretation of errors. Therefore, loss of colour vision can be broadly quantified by recording the number of errors made on the charts but there is normally little to be gained from recording the individual errors. An exception to this is if the patient misses all of the numbers on the left or right-hand side of the double figure numbers as this may indicate a hemianopic defect on that side in that eye. It is also worth observing the speed with which the patient is able to read the numbers. This should be instantaneous and any reduction in the speed of reading in one eye is certainly significant. Some appreciation of the effect of Daltonism on performance on these plates is necessary so that results can be interpreted in the patients (female : male ratio 1 : 17) who are so affected.

Amsler's test

The Amsler grid is a very useful tool as patients may be able to visualise scotomas or report distortion (see Unilateral visual failure: direct questions). The findings can be recorded and used for serial monitoring of any defect. In fact, it is common practice to use the recording sheet (a black grid on a white background) for testing as well as recording rather than the test plates which are considerably more sensitive being a white or red grid on a black background.

Visual field testing

Confrontation perimetry remains an essential skill. A rapid assessment of the visual field can be obtained in any situation and any clinical environment. A normal confrontation test is usually an accurate assessment of a normal field. Monitoring of fixation is straightforward (even if the patient's cooperation may be problematic) because the patient is asked to fix on the tester's eye. In the case of unilateral visual loss not only should the visual loss in the affected eye be plotted, but the other eye should be tested carefully for any evidence of a contralateral temporal hemianopic visual field defect as this immediately gives the location of the lesion as involving the prechiasmal portion of the optic nerve and the chiasm itself. Such defects are best demonstrated looking for colour desaturation. There is considerable discussion in the literature regarding junctional visual field defects (i.e. defects affecting the junction of the optic nerve and chiasm) and readers may have heard of the 'junctional scotoma' and 'Wilbrand's knee' of optic nerve fibres which loop forward into the contralateral nerve before crossing in the chiasm. Suffice to say that the junctional scotoma (first described by Traquair, ophthalmologist in Edinburgh, 1875–1954) is a temporal hemianopic scotoma found in an eye that shows signs of optic neuropathy: an upper temporal hemianopic defect in the fellow eye was described by Wilbrand (ophthalmologist in Hamburg, 1851–1935). Whatever the anatomical explanation of these phenomena, the essential practical point is that a temporal hemianopic defect in either eye of a patient with unilateral visual loss immediately places the problem to the chiasm.

It is beyond the scope of this chapter to give detailed descriptions of other perimetric techniques such as Goldmann and Humphrey automated perimetry but it is helpful to appreciate their respective advantages and disadvantages. In a patient with unilateral visual loss either method can be used but in certain respects the information provided is complementary.

The Goldmann perimeter uses kinetic testing – the target is moved from an area where it is invisible to a seeing area and the patient is asked to report when he/she sees it, usually from the periphery towards the centre in plotting isopters (lines of equal sensitivity) for any particular size and brightness of target: thus, a scotoma can be plotted (including the physiological blind spot) by moving the target from within the scotoma to its borders. The Goldmann perimeter can also be used for static testing. The target spot is flashed on at a particular location in the visual field and the patient asked whether or not it was detected. The brightness of the target can then be adjusted to determine the *threshold* – the smallest increment of the target over the background that the subject can detect. To cover the entire visual field in this way can be extremely arduous and the method of plotting isopters to kinetic targets remains the most efficient way of screening the visual field; however, some static points should be tested within the central field to look for any evidence of central or paracentral scotomas.

The Humphrey and Octopus automated perimeters are in use in most ophthalmology departments and at the time of writing the manually operated Goldmann perimeter is no longer being manufactured. The automated perimeters are based on the Goldmann in that the target size employed is the same as one of the standard settings on the Goldmann (size III) and indeed the field plot produced for the Humphrey perimeter is the same scale as the Goldmann charts (they can be overlapped and held up to the light to compare them). The test is automated and the operator is needed to monitor fixation and encourage the patient to concentrate a task which they may find quite challenging. The most commonly used plot that the reader will come across is limited to the central 30° of the field and threshold sensitivity is measured along a grid of points covering the area. These automated machines are being modified to permit the kind of kinetic testing that is carried out on the Goldmann but this will be more time-consuming.

Interpretation of visual fields requires considerable knowledge. An understanding is required of refraction and it is necessary to be familiar with many potential artefacts and what happens when the subject is fatigued, and so on. For the general neurologist the most useful skill is to be able to carry out competent confrontation fields but for a detailed consideration of complex cases and strategies for monitoring it will be necessary to turn to colleagues with neuro-ophthalmic expertise.

Fundus examination

The primary interest is in the appearance of the optic disc and there are some important rules. The emphasis traditionally has been on the observation of a pale optic disc as evidence for optic neuropathy but there is considerably more detailed information to be obtained. First, it is important to observe the morphology of the optic disc and in particular the size of the cup. In the management of glaucoma the degree of cupping of the optic disc is of fundamental importance and it is essential to know the difference between normal cupping and pathological cupping in optic nerve disease including glaucoma. In hypermetropia there tends to be a small cup or none at all (crowded optic disc) while in myopia the disc can be very large so it is necessary to be familiar with identifying the neural elements within the disc circumference which is defined by the scleral opening.

Furthermore, we are interested not only in pallor of the disc but more directly with loss of the optic nerve fibres which is the primary pathology leading to the development of atrophy. The retinal nerve fibre layer is the closest layer to us as we examine the retina with the ophthalmoscope. The vessels, the arterioles and venules of the retina itself are in this same layer and it is the retinal nerve fibres (the retinal ganglion cell axons) that fill in the space between the vessels, altering in a subtle way the optical properties of the retinal surface. With some practice it is possible to observe thinning of this layer and the disappearance of sectors and slits associated with focal pathology at the disc.

Once familiar with the variations in morphology of the disc in health and disease and the changes that occur in the optic nerve fibre layer we can be confident in ascribing loss of vision to disc-related pathology (e.g. glaucoma, optic disc drusen, papilloedema) or to retrobulbar disease (optic neuritis or compressive optic neuropathy). It must be remembered also that severe retinal disease (especially retinal dystrophies) can lead to loss of retinal ganglion cells and thence to the appearance of optic atrophy. Another important fact is that it takes 4–6 weeks for the loss of retinal nerve fibres and optic atrophy to appear following an acute insult to the optic nerve. If a patient presents with a history of visual loss of less than a month but optic atrophy is already visible then the pathological process must predate the first symptom. This indicates that either the patient noticed the loss of vision sometime after the onset (as occurs in compressive optic neuropathy) or that there has been a previous subclinical event (as might occur in MS).

Swelling of the optic disc occurs in a number of pathological situations such as acute optic neuritis, acute ischaemia, retinal vein occlusion and in raised intracranial pressure. The disc may also appear swollen in hypermetropic crowded discs or with buried drusen (pseudopapilloedema).

The vessels are also of interest, not only in primarily vascular disease but also in compressive optic neuropathies because of the development of retinochoroidal collaterals (previously, and erroneously, known as optico-ciliary shunt vessels). In order to understand this phenomenon it is necessary to understand that there are two possible routes for venous blood to leave the retina:

- The ophthalmic vein, which is the continuation of the central retinal vein, and thence to the cavernous sinus, and
- The choroidal veins, which drain into the vortex veins and thence to the cavernous sinus indirectly.

Any pathology that gives rise to retinal venous hypertension will tend to lead to the opening up of collaterals between the retinal branch veins and the choroidal veins. Occlusion of the central retinal vein is a common cause of this but any pathology that compresses the central retinal vein within the optic nerve – typically, optic nerve sheath meningioma – will result in the formation of these collaterals. Papilloedema is another cause because the central retinal vein has a short course in the subarachnoid space of the optic nerve sheath and a rise in intracranial pressure will lead to retinal venous hypertension.

In inflammatory disorders of the optic nerve there may be evidence of periphlebitis or vitritis; these changes are more marked in sarcoidosis than in MS.

The macula is inspected primarily to look for any evidence of a maculopathy that could mimic optic nerve disease such as central serous retinopathy or a cone dystrophy. Exudates around the macula (a 'macular star') are seen in neuroretinitis. The clinical features resemble optic neuritis but the inflammation must be very anterior, possibly involving the ganglion cell layer, for sufficient retinal oedema to be generated for the macular star to result.

Associated features

Thorough general ophthalmological and neurological examinations must be undertaken but signs of orbital disease should also be sought, such as proptosis or motility defects. The sense of smell must be tested. Evidence of sinus disease should be sought and clues to any pre-existing central nervous system (CNS) dysfunction such as caused by MS.

The causes of transient unilateral visual loss are summarised in Table 14.1 and those of sudden fixed unilateral visual loss in Table 14.2.

Table 14.1 Causes and underlying conditions in transient monocular blindness.

Vascular*	Central retinal artery emboli Retinal or choroidal ischaemia Partial retinal vein occlusion Carotid artery stenosis or occlusion (e.g. atherosclerotic plaque, thromboembolism, dissection, radiation damage) Arterial vasospasm
Migraine	Uncertain whether monocular visual loss occurs in migraine
Hypoperfusion	Hypotension, hyperviscocity, hypercoagulability, carotid disease, giant cell arteritis
Ocular	Intermittent angle closure glaucoma Retinal detachment
Vasculitis	Giant cell arteritis
Others	Inflammatory – Uhthoff's phenomenon Idiopathic Psychogenic
Obscurations†	Papilloedema due to raised intracranial hypertension causes transient visual obscurations Optic nerve tumours (e.g. gaze-evoked amaurosis in optic sheath meningioma)

*Duration: several minutes.
†Duration: seconds only.

Table 14.2 Sudden onset fixed monocular visual loss.

Vascular
Non-arteritic anterior ischaemic optic neuropathy (posterior non-arteritic ischaemic optic neuropathy is rare)
Arteritic anterior and posterior ischaemic optic neuropathy
Branch or central retinal artery occlusion
Branch or central retinal vein occlusion
Inflammatory
Systemic inflammatory diease
Traumatic optic neuropathy
Retinal detachment
Vitreous haemorrhage
Functional visual loss

Table 14.3 Sudden onset fixed bilateral visual loss.

Occipital lobe infarction
Acute basilar artery occlusive disease
Posterior circulation hypoperfusion (posterior watershed (border-zone) infarction)
Sagittal sinus thrombosis
Pituitary apoplexy
Posterior reversible encephalopathy syndrome
Toxic encephalopathy (caused by drugs, e.g. ciclosporin, methotrexate, vincristine)
Head trauma
Functional visual loss

Bilateral visual failure

The diagnostic problem of progressive bilateral visual loss is usually solvable with a clear understanding of the knowledge of the visual pathways, patterns of visual symptoms and careful examination. Visual loss in both eyes may develop over months, weeks or days:

1 If visual loss > 6/9 develops on a background of previously normal visual acuity, this should be investigated initially by an optometrist and/or an ophthalmologist and, if visual loss remains unexplained, by a neurologist.

2 Progression of visual loss or progressive visual symptoms should always be investigated.

3 Accurate measurement and recording of visual acuity is essential. A 2 or 3 m hand-held Snellen chart is useful, even though these are less accurate than the standard 6 m wall chart. A pin-hole (this corrects up to 4 dioptres of refractive error) is essential.

4 As with uniocular visual loss, substantial diminished vision is sometimes an almost incidental finding in the context of vague visual complaints.

The principal issue is to distinguish between ocular disease and disease of the neural pathway, for example:

- Refractive errors, cataracts, uveitis, macular degeneration, bilateral retinal disease
- Optic nerve disease
- Conditions affecting the optic chiasm, and beyond, to the cortex.

Post-chiasmal conditions, such as optic tract lesions, are relatively rare. Others, such as optic radiation lesions, visual association area and bilateral occipital lobe infarction, tend to present acutely. Bilateral visual loss, with progression, which does not have an organic basis is relatively common. Its features are characteristic and need to be recognised. Non-organic visual impairment must be distinguished from cortical visual loss.

For the general neurologist, matters can be compounded by unfamiliarity with the fine detail of ophthalmology and relative inexperience of ocular and retinal conditions. Conversely, for the ophthalmologist, chiasmal compression and other neurological problems will be less familiar than the patterns of common ocular disease. The causes of progressive bilateral visual loss include the following:

1 *Ocular and retinal conditions*
Refractive errors and cataracts
Macular degeneration
Uveitis
Retinal disease:
Diabetes and other retinal vascular disease
Retinal dystrophies
Paraneoplastic degenerations.

2 *Bilateral optic nerve disease*
Leber's hereditary optic neuropathy
Other bilateral optic nerve lesions
Papilloedema as a cause of visual failure
Toxins, drugs and radiation.

3 *Chiasmal disease*
Chiasmal compression by mass lesions
Chiasmal (and optic nerve) glioma and meningioma.

4 *Post-chiasmal disease*
Optic tract and radiation lesions
Visual association area lesions
Cortical visual loss.

5 *Non-organic visual failure*

The causes of sudden onset fixed bilateral visual loss are summarised in Table 14.3 and progressive visual loss in Table 14.4.

Table 14.4 Neurological causes of bilateral progressive visual loss.

Anterior visual pathway inflammation	Optic neuritis Sarcoidosis Meningitis Neurosyphilis
Anterior visual pathway compression	Tumours Aneurysm Dysthyroid
Hereditary optic neuropathy	Leber's Dominant optic atrophy
Optic nerve drusen	
Low tension glaucoma	
Papilloedema	
Toxic and nutritional optic neuropathy	
Drugs (Table 14.5)	
Radiation damage	
Paraneoplastic retinopathy	

Special investigations in neuro-ophthalmology

Optical coherence tomography

Optical coherence tomography (OCT) permits non-cross-sectional imaging of internal structures in biological tissues using near infra-red light. All the layers of the retina can be studied in high magnification and consecutively. Quantitative analysis of retinal nerve fibre layer (RNFL) atrophy may serve as a biomarker for axonal loss in generalised neurological disease and has important applications in MS and neuromyelitis optica (NMO) (Figures 14.1, 14.2 and 14.3). This equipment has become widely adopted in general ophthalmology departments with facilities for the assessment and treatment of retinal disease.

Ultrasound

Real-time B-mode ultrasound can be used to study the optic nerve head; for example, it is very useful in demonstrating echogenic buried drusen in cases with elevated optic discs, giving the correct diagnosis without the need for more invasive investigations (Figure 14.4).

Clinical electrophysiology of the eye

The visual evoked potential (VEP) is a sensitive means of detecting optic nerve dysfunction. However, VEP abnormalities are not specific for optic nerve disease and can reflect dysfunction anterior to the optic nerve. Macular disease, in the presence or absence of fundus change, commonly causes VEP delay.

Full-field electroretinogram (ERG) will ascertain the nature of possible generalised retinal disease if the pattern ERG (PERG) suggests a macular abnormality (Figure 14.5).

Visual field testing

Visual field testing retains central importance in the localisation of defects in the visual system, and for monitoring natural history and responses to therapy. Qualititative confrontation testing with a red target remains useful, with quantitative recording provided by kinetic and static perimetry (Figures 14.6, 14.7, 14.8 and 14.9).

Fundus fluorescein angiography

Fundus fluorescein angiography (FFA) remains important in neuro-ophthalmology for certain specific situations (Figures 14.10, 14.11 and 14.12).

Optic nerve disease

Optic neuropathy

Optic nerve lesions generally lead to monocular visual loss and pain is a frequent accompanying features. The causes of optic nerve disease are listed in Table 14.5.

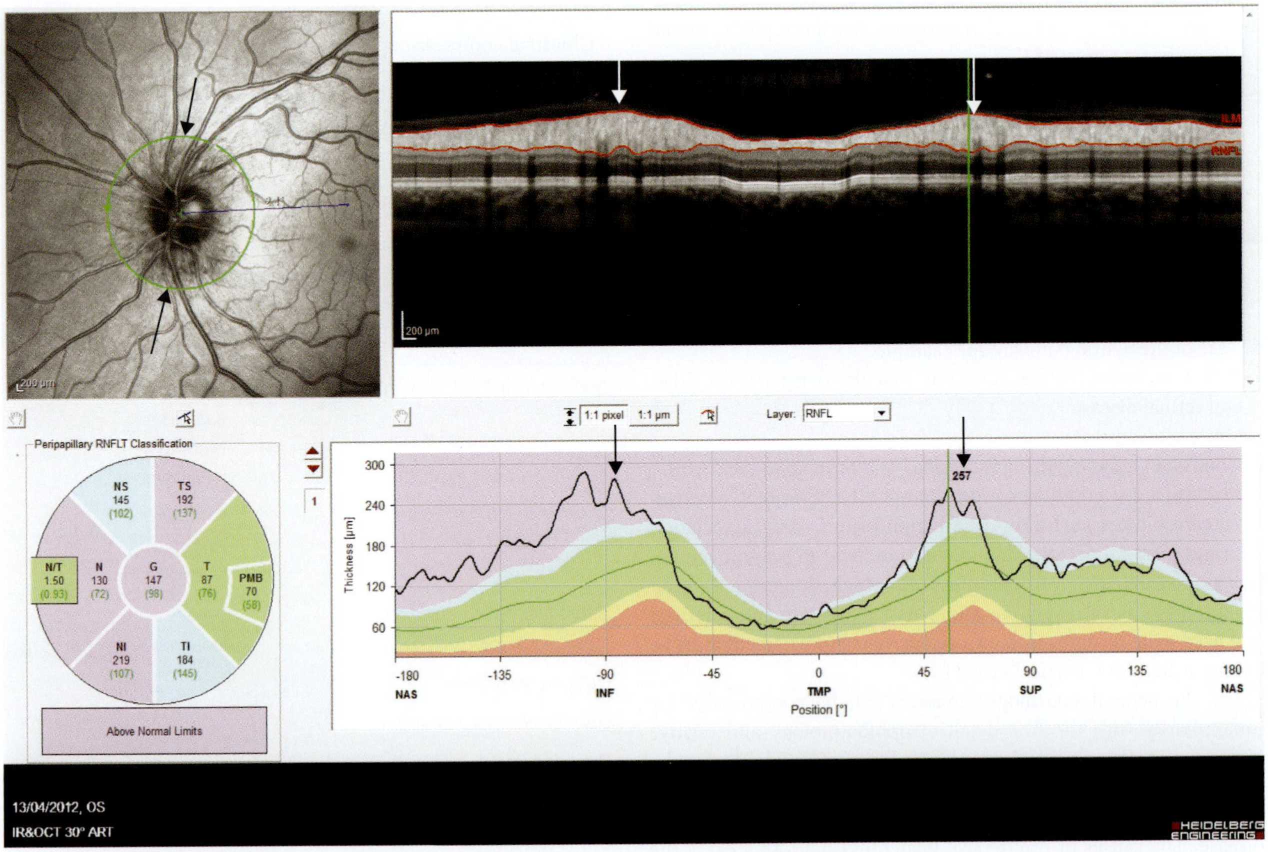

Figure 14.1 Fourier-domain optical coherence tomography (OCT) of the retina in a patient with acute optic neuritis showing mild retinal nerve fibre layer (RNFL) swelling around the optic disc which correlates with ophthalmoscopic disc swelling. This is most prominent at the superior and inferior poles (arrows).

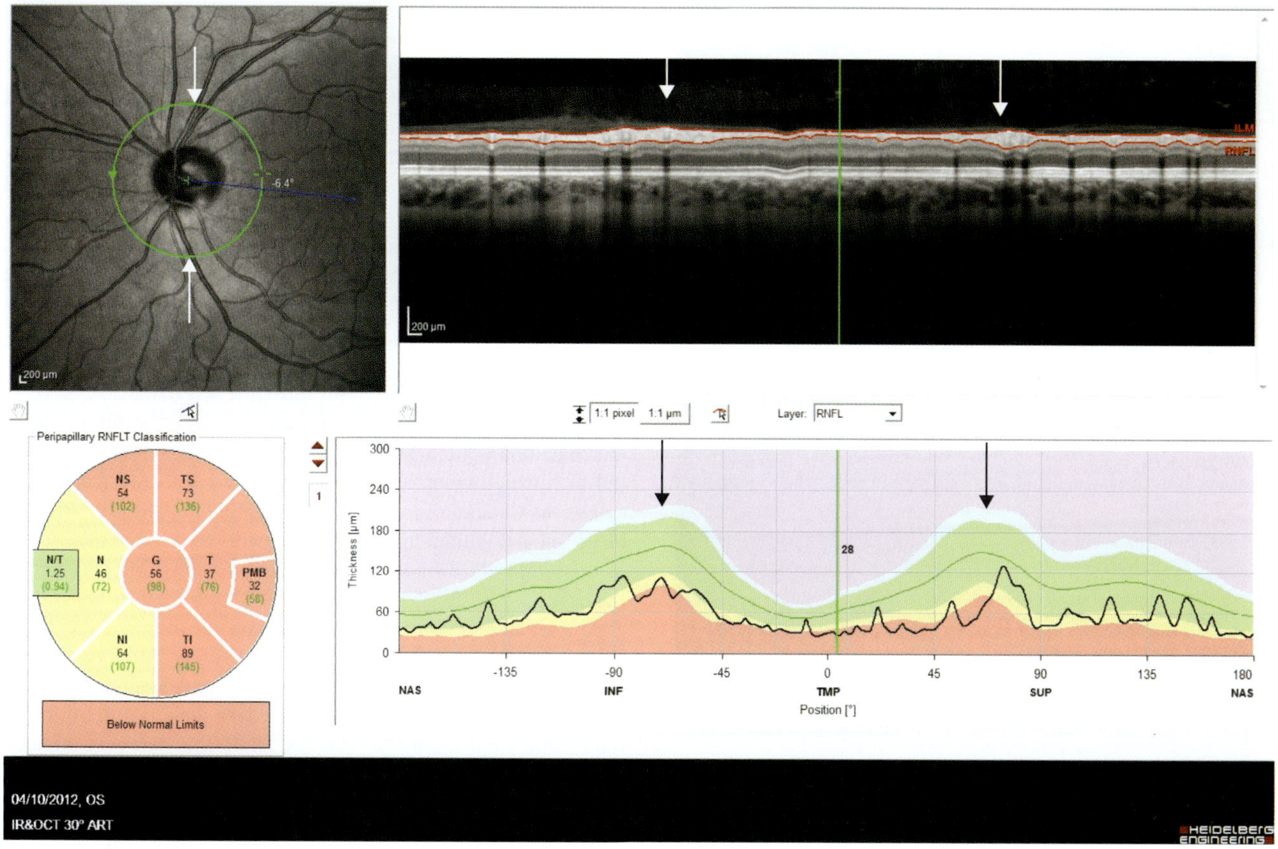

Figure 14.2 Repeat study on the same patient 4 months later shows that the peri-papillary RNFL swelling has resolved and is replaced by with measureable reduction of thickness of the peri-papillary RNFL on cross-sectional imaging (arrows).

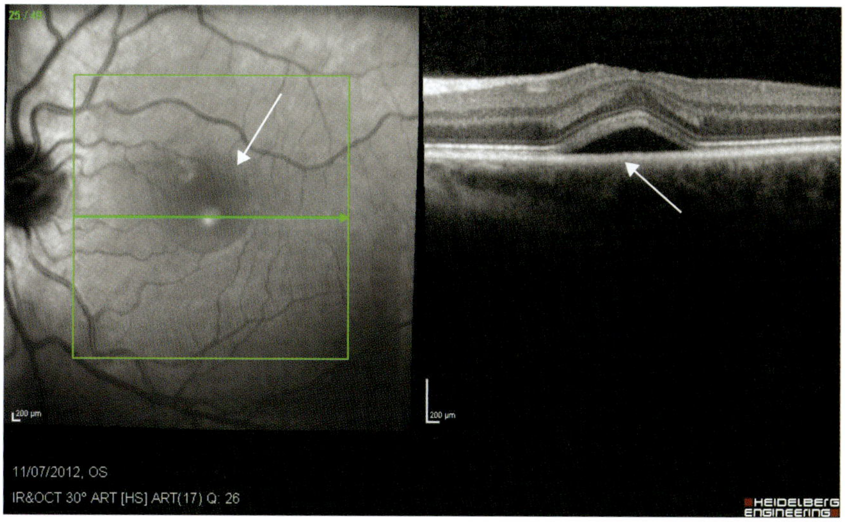

Figure 14.3 Not all patients with central visual acuity loss and an apparently normal fundus have retrobulbar neuritis. On closer examination this patient with systemic lupus erythematosus had a focal serous detachment of the neurosensory retina at the fovea, seen on biomicroscopy and demonstrated clearly on OCT (arrows).

Inflammatory optic neuropathies (optic neuritis)

Nosology of optic neuritis There is no consistent terminology in literature for describing optic neuritis. It is sometimes categorised by clinical presentation into typical and atypical forms, where typical indicates optic neuritis associated with multiple sclerosis in white populations. This has a characteristic tempo of recovery and visual loss tends not to be severe. An alternative classification describes optic neuritis by aetiology and this system is predominantly adopted in this chapter (Table 14.6). The most common form in white populations is

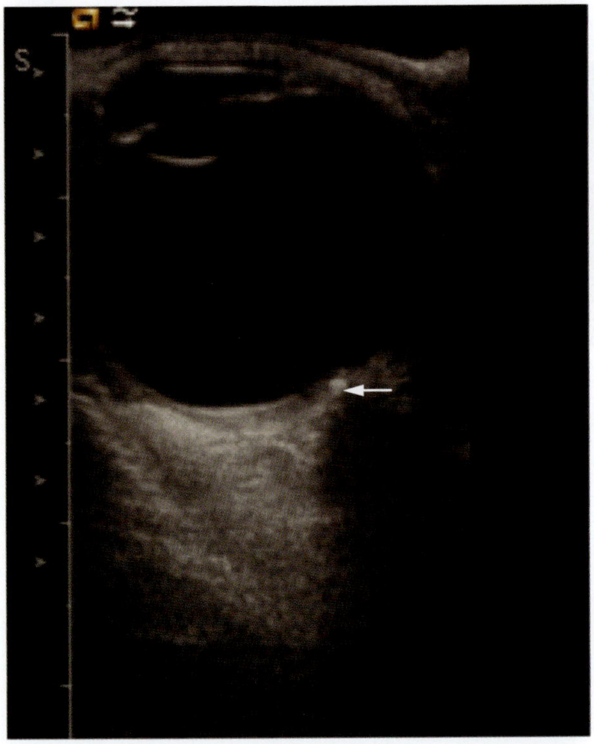

Figure 14.4 B-mode ultrasound: echogenic buried optic disc drusen (arrow).

multiple sclerosis associated optic neuritis (MS-ON) with the understanding that it can also occur as a demyelinating clinically isolated syndrome (CIS). Optic neuritis associated with neuromyelitis optica (NMO-ON) is an important cause of atypical optic neuritis, described later. These form part of a group of immune-mediated causes of optic neuritis, which can have no systemic features of inflammation (e.g. MS, NMO) or be related to certain systemic inflammatory disorders (e.g. sarcoid, lupus, vasculitis). Certain conditions closely related to optic neuritis, which do not fit neatly by aetiological classification, are described (neuroretinitis and optic perineuritis) at the end of this section.

Optic neuritis associated with multiple sclerosis

Clinical features Optic neuritis is one of the most common causes of subacute unilateral visual loss in young adults. It is first essential to distinguish optic neuritis associated with MS from other causes. In Caucasian populations in temperate latitudes, MS will be the most common form of optic neuritis seen but in other parts of the world and in non-Caucasian populations this may not be the case.

Almost all patients experience pain on eye movement prior to noticing loss of vision but this is rarely severe and as a general rule will not interfere with sleep. Severe or persistent pain should lead to a consideration of other disorders such as a granulomatous optic neuropathy or NMO-ON. If the nerve is affected entirely intracranially there will be no pain but this occurs

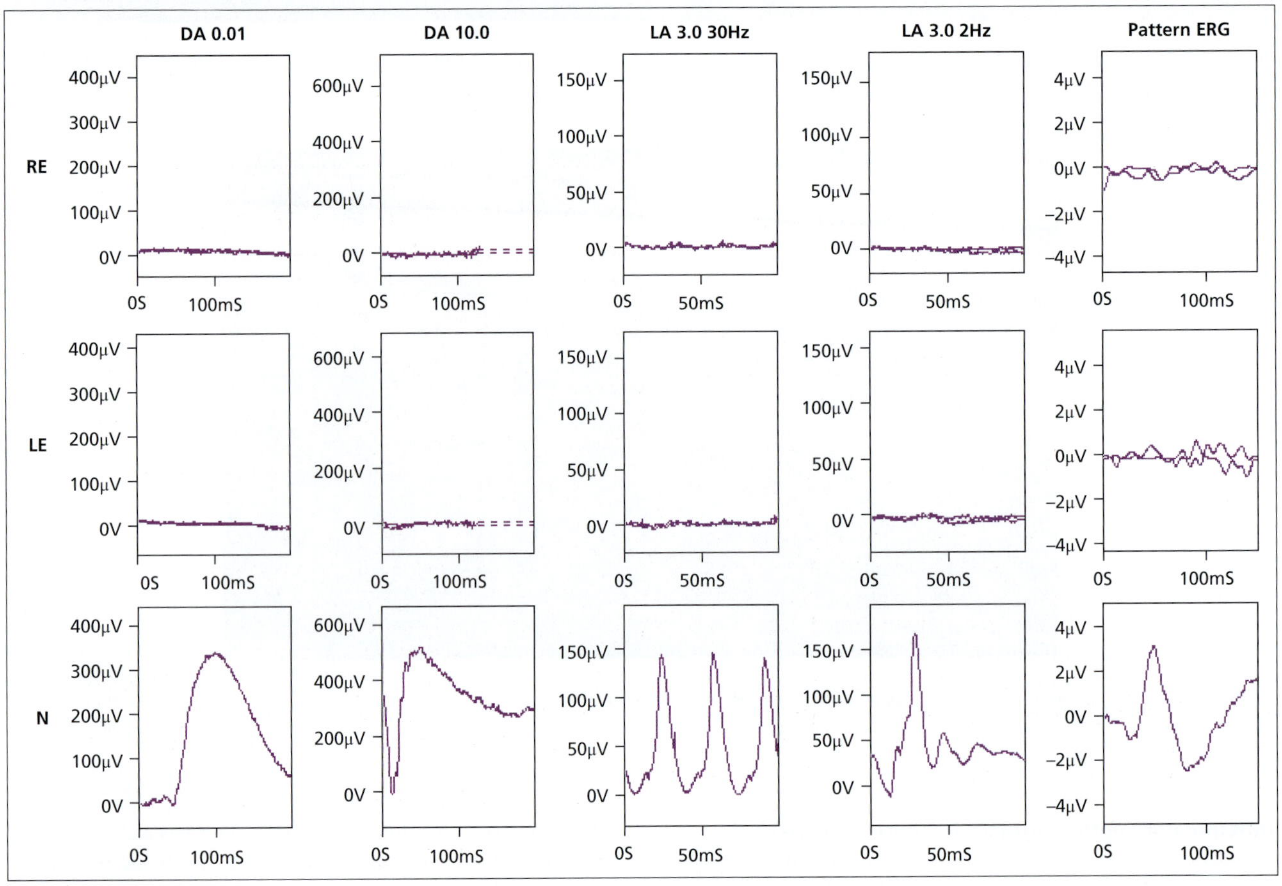

Figure 14.5 Flat electroretinogram (ERG) in left eye (LE) and right eye (RE) in both dark adapted (DA) and light adapted (LA) conditions, compared with normal (N) in a case of paraneoplastic retinopathy due to remote cancer.

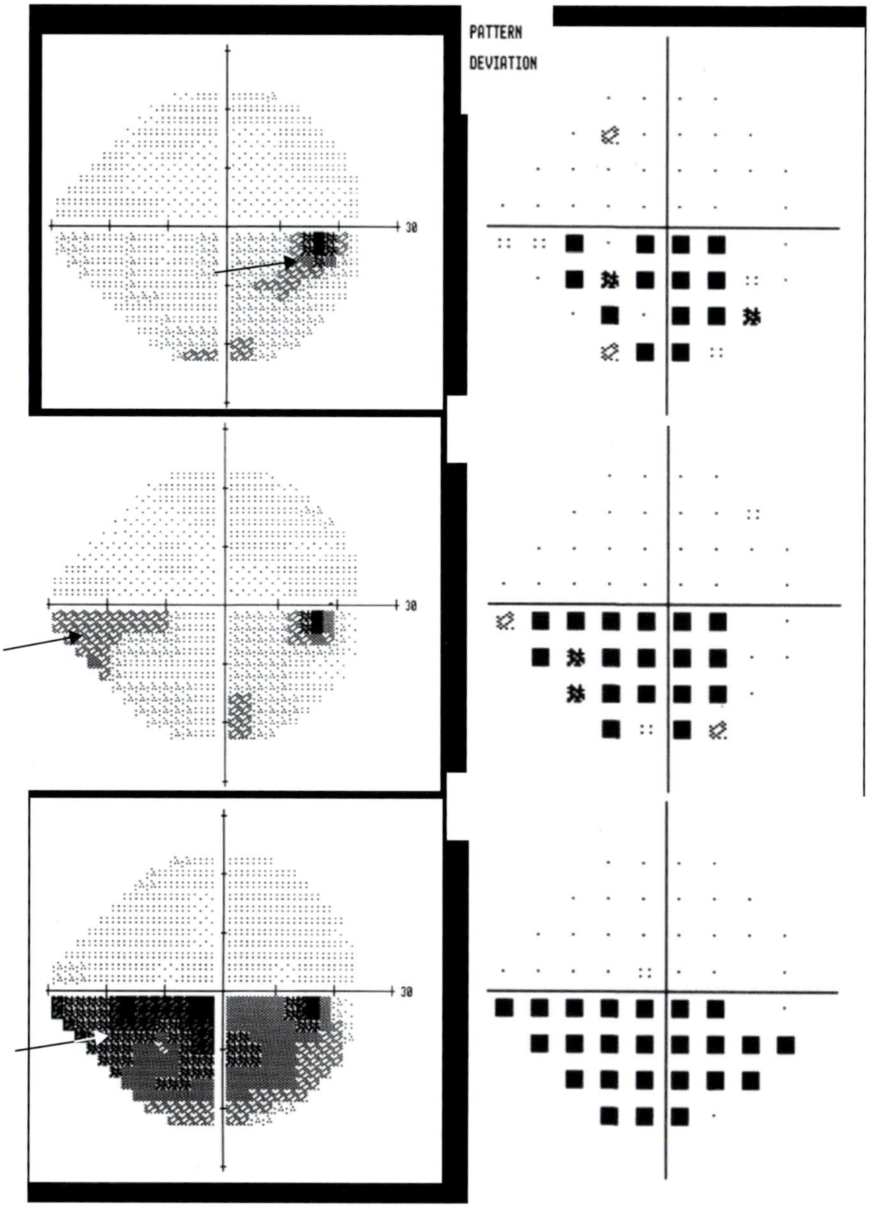

Figure 14.6 Progressive lower altitudinal scotoma evolving over 2 weeks in anterior ischaemic optic neuropathy: shown here on static automated perimetry equipment (arrows).

in only 10% of cases. Loss of vision typically progresses over days and can be minimal (indeed it may not be noticed by the patient) or, at the other extreme, lead to no light perception. Colour vision and the pupil light reflex are impaired disproportionately to the acuity loss. Central visual field defects are typical but not found universally. There is nearly always a degree of spontaneous recovery and 95% of cases will recover to a visual acuity of 6/9 or better. Disc swelling is seen acutely in one-third of cases, the disc appearing normal (retrobulbar neuritis) in two-thirds. After recovery, many patients exhibit some degree of disc pallor.

Investigations In patients where the clinical context and symptomatology point to a diagnosis of MS-ON, the diagnosis can usually be made on clinical grounds. However, there may be uncertainty and the investigations should follow the protocol given below for atypical forms of optic neuritis. It is customary to check the erythrocyte sedimentation rate (ESR) and C-reactive protein (CRP), and perform a chest X-ray and syphilis serology. MRI of the optic nerves will almost always show high signal in the affected optic nerve on T2-weighted (or STIR) orbital images (Figure 14.13) with gadolinium enhancement. In cases of diagnostic uncertainty, visual evoked potentials with pattern electroretinograms and optical coherence tomography can help to confirm optic nerve involvement or exclude maculopathy as a cause of the visual loss.

In CIS, the risk of future conversion to multiple sclerosis can be stratified with brain MRI and this should be routinely discussed with or offered to the patient (chapter 11). Abnormal brain MRI may show disseminated white matter lesions suggestive of

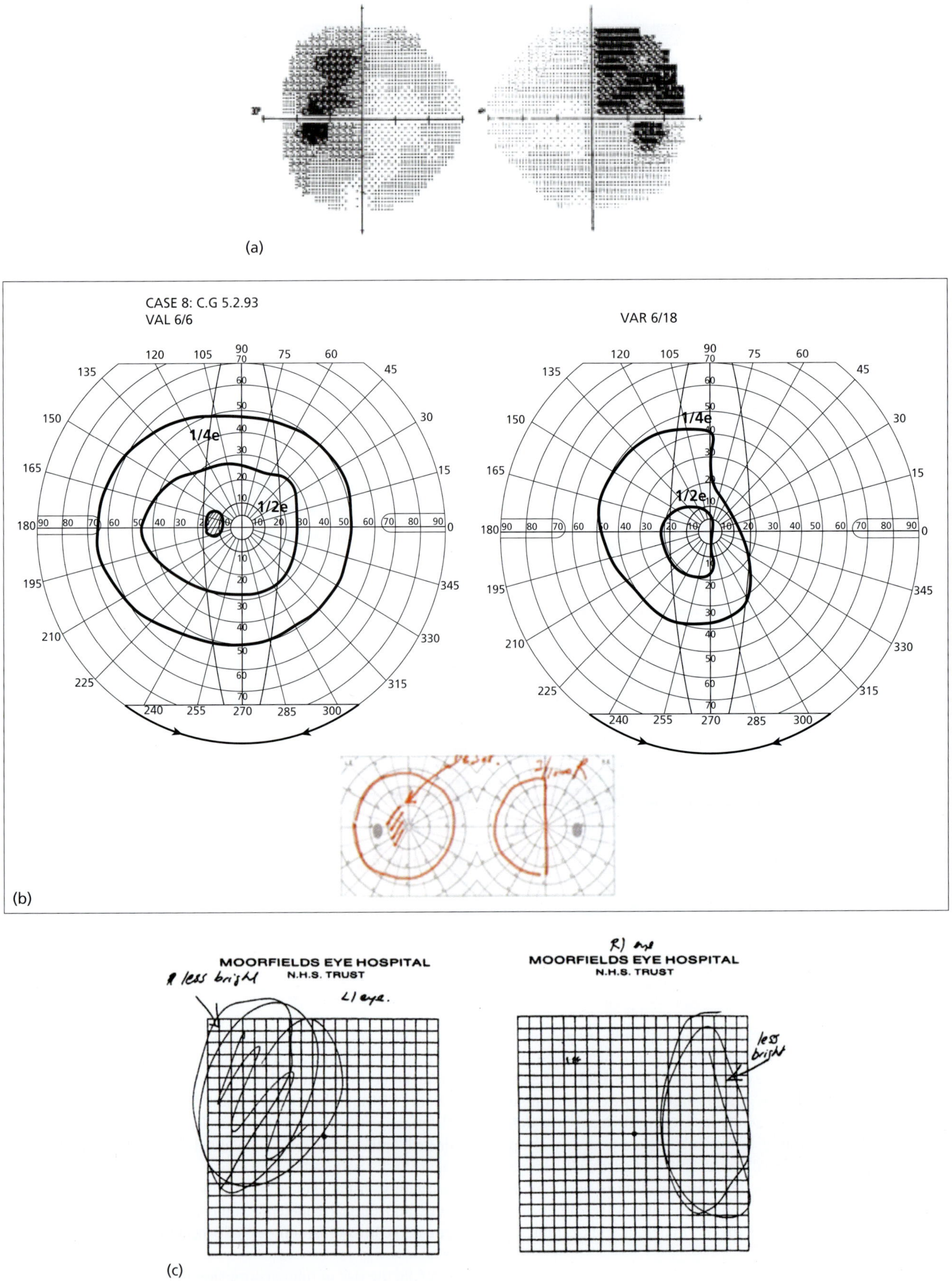

Figure 14.7 Bi-temporal hemianopia signifying chiasmal compression shown in different field testing formats. (a) Bilateral temporal defects on automated perimetry grey-scale. (b) Asymmetric temporal defects on Goldmann kinetic perimetry clarified on red target testing. (c) Amsler grid central visual field showing bi-temporal hemianopic scotomas due to chiasmal compression: as represented by the patient.

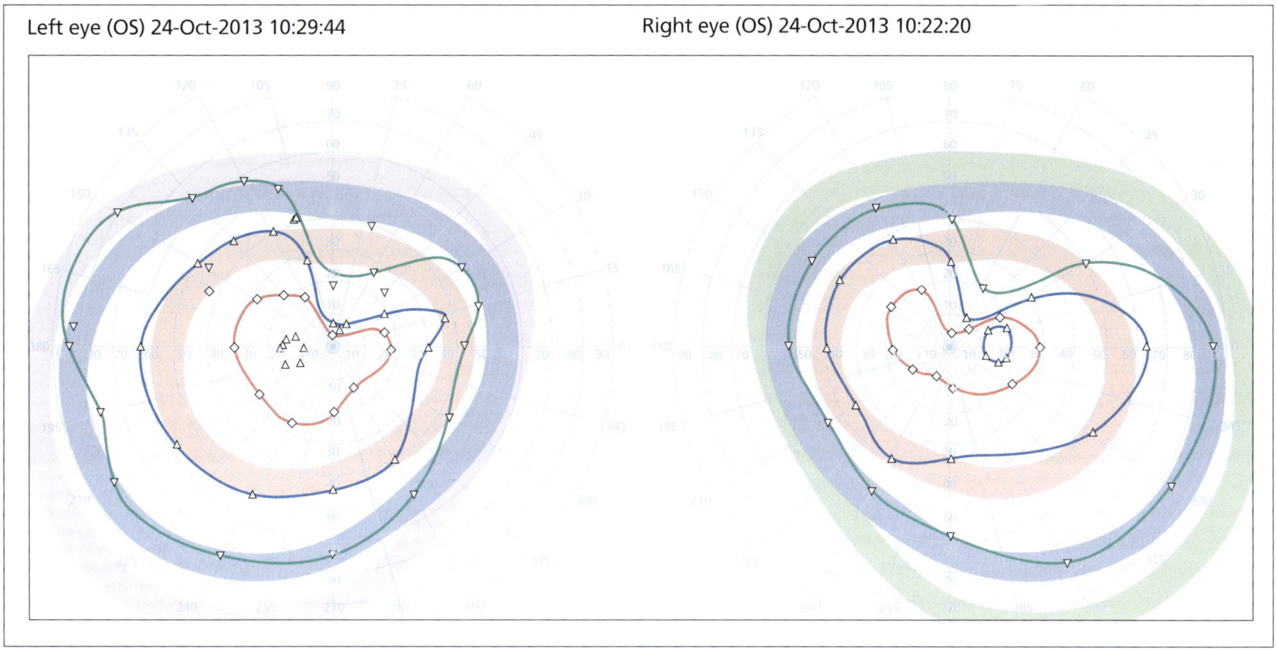

Figure 14.8 Upper quadrantic hemianopia after temporal lobectomy: automated full field kinetic perimetry.

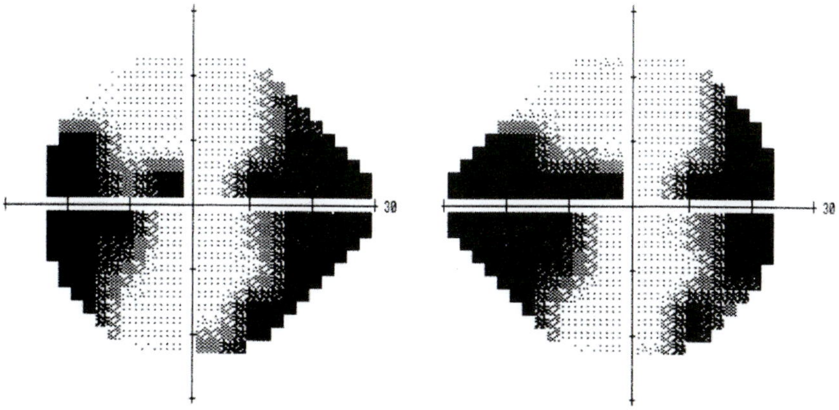

(a)

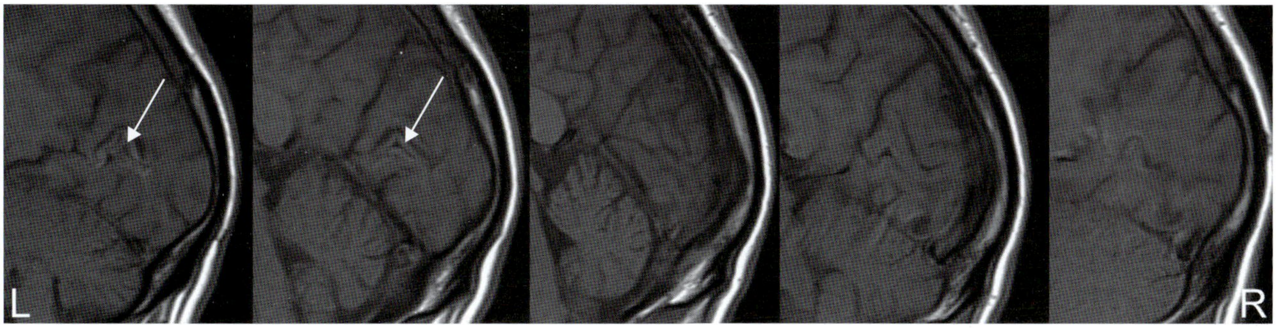

(b)

Figure 14.9 Bilateral macular sparing hemianopias: (a) automated visual fields; (b) MRI showing bilateral anterior calcarine fissure lesion (arrows).

demyelination. In the North American Optic Neuritis Treatment Trial (ONTT), 72% of patients with optic neuritis with abnormal baseline MRIs developed clinically definite MS after 15 years compared with 25% with normal baseline MRIs. Even the lower risk is not insignificant, hence patients should receive appropriate counselling. The longest prospective follow-up of CIS (ON, cord and brainstem) was for 20 years and reported a conversion rate to clinically definite MS of 82% for baseline abnormal MRIs compared

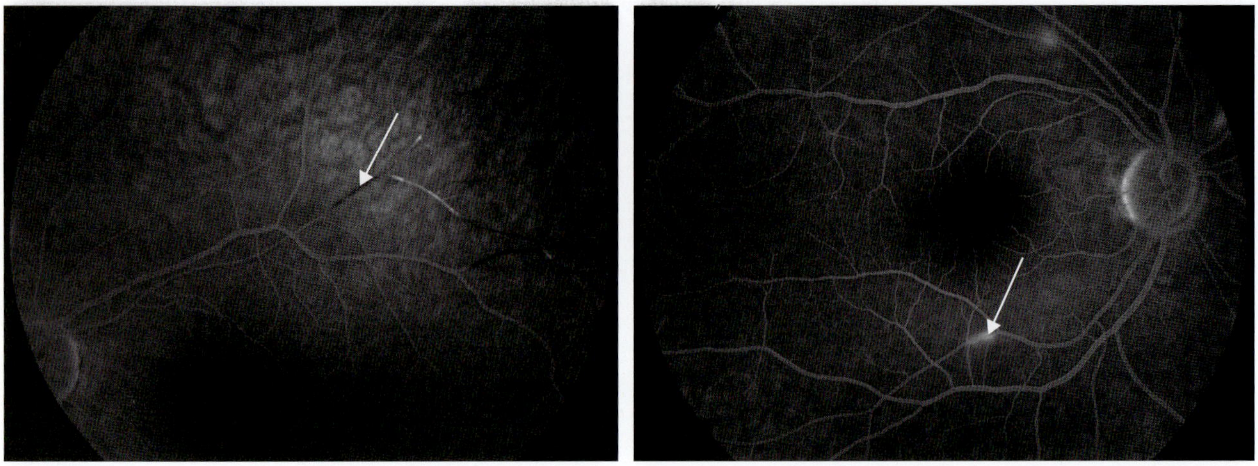

(a) (b)

Figure 14.10 Recurrent branch retinal artery occlusions with hyperfluorscence at remote artery bifurcation sites in Susac's micro-angiopathy of eye, brain and cochlea. (a) Fundus fluorescein angiography (FFA) showing occluded branch retinal artery (arrow). (b) FFA showing hyperfluorescence at a different branch artery bifurcation (arrow).

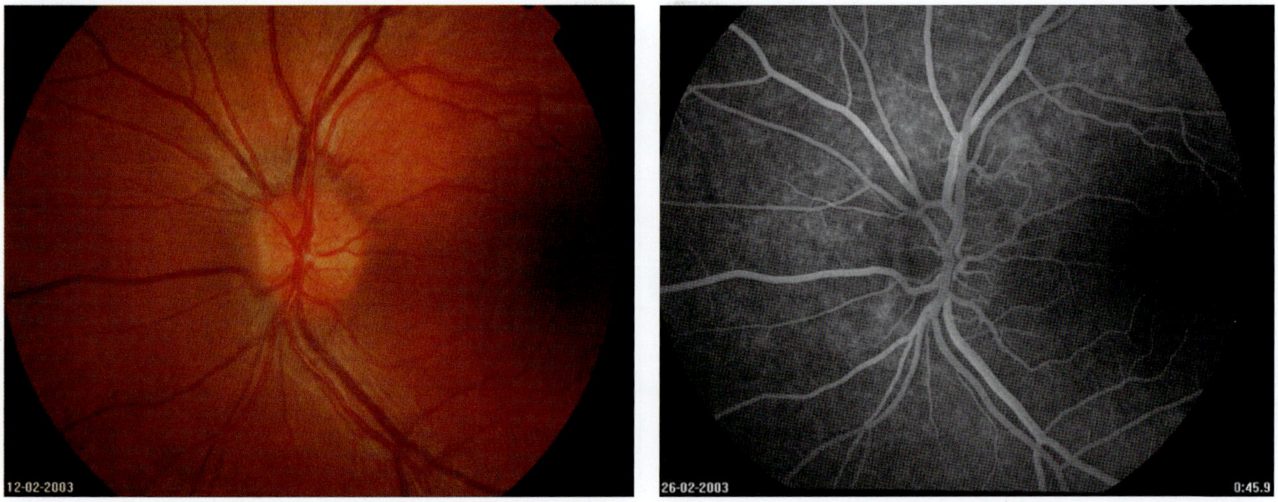

(a) (b)

Figure 14.11 Hyperaemia and likely optic disc swelling in a patient with subacute monocular visual loss. (a) Colour photograph of optic disc. (b) FFA showing absence of dye leakage supporting diagnosis of Leber's hereditary optic neuropathy and against diagnoses of ischaemic or inflammatory optic neuropathy.

with 21% for those with normal baseline MRIs. More recently, developments in MRI criteria can now allow the diagnosis of MS to be made after a single episode of MS-ON and after a single MRI brain with contrast in certain cases.

Treatment Many studies have confirmed that a short course of high-dose corticosteroids reduces the time taken for recovery in acute MS-ON but does not alter the eventual outcome. Methylprednisolone administered 1 g/day for 3 days intravenously or 500 mg/day orally for 5 days is usually recommended. However, approximately 10% of patients are left with acuities of 6/12 or worse. There is interest in developing neuroprotective or remyelinating therapies which potentially could improve visual outcome and several trials are in progress.

Optic neuritis associated with neuromyelitis optica (Devic's syndrome)

Clinical features (Chapters 11 and 16) NMO-ON can present with atypical ON features such as severe peri-ocular pain or severe visual loss, which are rarely seen in MS-ON. It is essential to recognise the possibility of NMO early, as prompt treatment can save vision. Spontaneous clinical recovery is less likely without treatment.

The disorder is more common in parts of the world where MS is less frequently the cause of optic neuritis and is likely to be related to the 'Asian optico-spinal form of multiple sclerosis' seen in East Asia. Although very few epidemiological studies have been performed, it is thought to be more common in non-Caucasians and has a greater female preponderance. Other autoimmune conditions (e.g. lupus, Sjögren's syndrome) may co-exist with

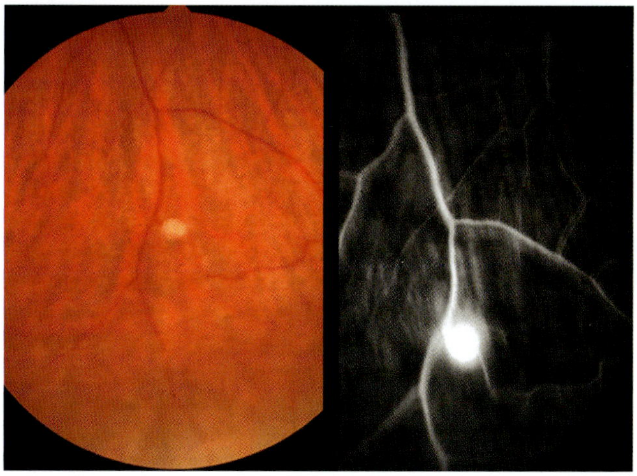

Figure 14.12 Fundus photograph and FFA in greater magnification: small peripheral retinal haemangioma in von Hippel–Lindau disease.

NMO-ON. Patients may have or develop other features of NMO (e.g. longitudinally extensive myelitis) or have an NMO spectrum disorder.

Investigations Aquaporin 4 (AQ4) antibody should be sought in any case of atypical optic neuritis. There are no absolute features of optic nerve imaging although the lesion is more likely to be posterior along the optic nerve and involve the chiasm. Patients with both optic neuritis and the typical spinal cord lesions of NMO are more likely to have AQ4 antibodies. There is also a small subgroup of patients who have recurrent optic neuritis alone without myelitis and who have the same antibody, about 5–10% of cases of optic neuritis for whom no specific cause (including MS) can be identified. However, the diagnosis is an important one to make because the management of NMO is quite different from the management of MS. Brain MRI may be normal or may show white matter lesions that look atypical for MS. Hypothalamic and peri-aqueductal grey matter lesions have also been seen. CSF may show a lymphocytic pleocytosis and oligoclonal bands are less likely to be found than in MS-ON. Post-acutely, OCT tends to show more severe retinal nerve fibre layer thinning than after MS-ON.

There is an emerging NMO phenotype found in a sub-group of AQ4 Ab-negative NMO patients who are positive for myelin oligodendrocyte glycoprotein (MOG) Ab. These patients are more likely to be male, have bilateral simultaneous optic neuritis, have spinal lesions lower down in the cord and tend to demonstrate better functional recovery.

Treatment Acute attacks are treated with high dose corticosteroids (intravenous methylprednisolone 1 g/day for 3–5 days) followed by a prolonged oral tail weaning over 4–6 months. Relapses during weaning can be treated by increasing the oral dose or providing a further intravenous course. Plasmapheresis should be considered for those patients who do not respond to steroids in the acute phase. Steroid sparing immunosuppressants should be commenced for long-term relapse prevention. No randomised controlled evidence exists but azathioprine and methotrexate are typically considered as first line agents. Rituximab is gaining favour as an alternative first line agent. Second line agents include mycophenolate. Future treatments may include toculizumab and eculizumab (Chapter 11).

Table 14.5 Causes and classification of optic neuropathy.

Anterior optic neuropathy with disc swelling
(Disorders causing visible axonal swelling at the optic nerve head: often monocular)
Anterior ischaemic optic neuropathy
Arteritic
Non-arteritic
Optic neuritis (papillitis)
Neuro-retinitis
Diabetic papillopathy
Papillophlebitis/venous papillopathy
Compressive optic neuropathy
Infiltrative optic neuropathy
Medication-associated (e.g. amiodarone, beta-interferon)
Raised intracranial pressure
Accelerated hypertension
Anterior optic neuropathy without disc swelling
(Disorders causing primary retinal ganglion cell failure: typically bilateral and symmetrical)
Toxic/nutritional optic neuropathy
Drugs (e.g. ethambutol, isoniazid, linezolid, chloramphenicol)
Toxins (e.g. methanol, ethylene glycol, toluene, heavy metals)
Nutritional (e.g. vitamin deficiency B_1, B_{12}, folate deficiency)
Endemic (Tanzanian, Jamaican)
Recreational (e.g. ethanol, tobacco)
Heredofamial optic neuropathy
Leber's hereditary optic neuropathy
Dominant optic atrophy
Syndromic (e.g. Friedreich's, Wolfram's, mitochondrial disease, storage diseases, hereditary motor sensory neuropathy)
Posterior (retrobulbar) optic neuropathy without disc swelling
Retrobulbar neuritis
Traumatic optic neuropathy
Radionecrosis
Compressive optic neuropathy
Obstructive hydrocephalus
Posterior ischaemic optic neuropathy
Pseudopapapilloedema
(Disorders mimicking acquired causes of optic neuropathy with disc swelling)
Optic disc drusen
Optic disc hamartomas
Optic disc dysplasia and dysversions
High refractive error
Myelinated nerve fibres

Optic neuritis: chronic relapsing inflammatory optic neuropathy

Chronic relapsing inflammatory optic neuropathy (CRION) is a condition that is not yet clearly defined and has an unknown aetiology. Presentation is with painful subacute visual loss but the pain is frequently more severe and prolonged than in MS-ON. In most cases the second eye is involved but not simultaneously.

Table 14.6 Causes of optic neuritis.

Immune-mediated	No systemic inflammation	MS-ON (if first episode then called clinically isolated syndrome) NMO-ON Solitary, isolated optic neuritis Recurrent isolated optic neuritis Chronic relapsing inflammatory optic neuropathy Post-viral/post-immunisation Acute disseminated encephalomyelitis
	Systemic inflammation	Sarcoidosis Connective tissue disease – lupus, Sjögren's syndrome Vasculitis – polyarteritis nodosa, Wegener's granulomatosis, Churg–Strauss
Infective	Bacterial Viral	Borrelia, syphilis, mycoplasma, tuberculosis, Whipple's disease Herpes simplex/zoster, EBV, CMV, Coxsackie, hepatitis A and B, measles, mumps, rubella
	Parasitic Fungal	Toxoplasmosis, cysticercosis, toxocara Cryptococcus, aspergillus, mucormycosis, candida
Other associated conditions	Perineuritis (contiguous sheath inflammation) Sinus disease (mucocoele, pyocoele) Neuroretinitis Extrinsic tumour (e.g. meningioma)	

CMV, cytomegalovirus; EBV, Epstein–Barr virus.

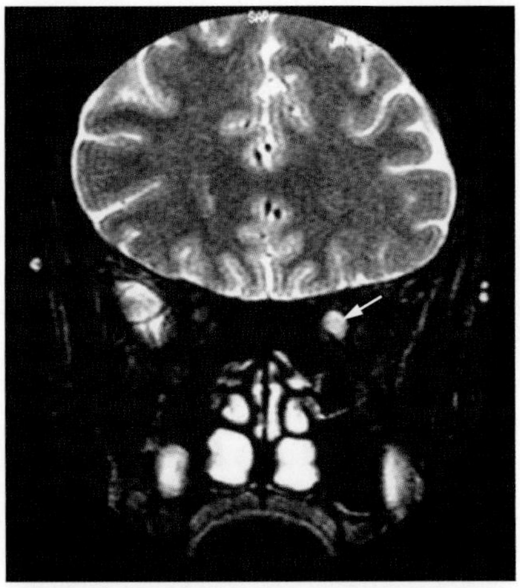

Figure 14.13 Coronal MRI showing high signal in the left optic nerve (arrow) in a case of demyelinating optic neuritis.

However, the essential point is that there is not only a response to corticosteroids but a relapse when these are withdrawn. This is in contrast to MS-ON where it is possible to give very short courses of high-dose steroids (even as short as 3 days) without fear of relapse when the course is completed. However, relapse is also common in sarcoid-related optic neuropathy and NMO-ON. Another feature often seen in CRION is late improvement (i.e. a long-standing optic neuropathy that appeared static can show recovery with corticosteroid therapy).

Investigations By definition, investigations are normal. Any evidence for an underlying systemic condition such as a vasculitis or granulomatous disorder must be excluded. There is no evidence of MS or NMO. A small number of patients with this phenotype do appear to have NMO antibodies.

Treatment The response to immunosuppression suggests that the essential difference between CRION and MS-ON is that in the former there is ongoing inflammation whereas in MS-ON there is a brief period of inflammation of acute onset which then subsides moving to a recovery phase. CRION is therefore appropriately treated with long-term immunosuppression and steroid-sparing agents. It is important to bear in mind that relapses can be associated with irreversible visual loss unless treated promptly.

Optic neuritis: infective disorders

Clinical features It is important to recognise these causes of optic neuritis because they require immediate and aggressive management. Viral infections can give rise to optic neuritis either by direct infection of the optic nerve or as a post-infectious syndrome. Bacterial infection of the optic nerve or sheath, such as in pneumococcal meningitis, can result in devastating visual loss as can fungal invasion (e.g. with *Aspergillus fumigatus*). Optic neuritis is one of many possible ophthalmic complications of neurosyphilis (Figure 14.14) and of another spirochaetal disease, Lyme disease, caused by *Borrelia burgdorferi*. In most cases there will be some clear evidence of the causative infective process for instance herpes zoster ophthalmicus, or bacterial meningitis. Vigilance is required for instances of underlying infection such as syphilis, tuberculosis, sinus disease or fungal disease. Atypical features of optic neuritis such as orbital signs or prolonged and severe pain should alert the physician to these possibilities. In many of these infective cases the optic nerve sheath is involved rather than the optic nerve itself and

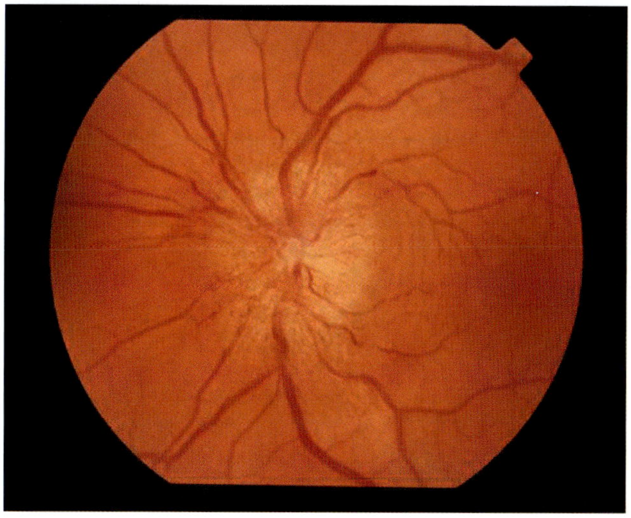

Figure 14.14 Optic neuritis in secondary syphilis.

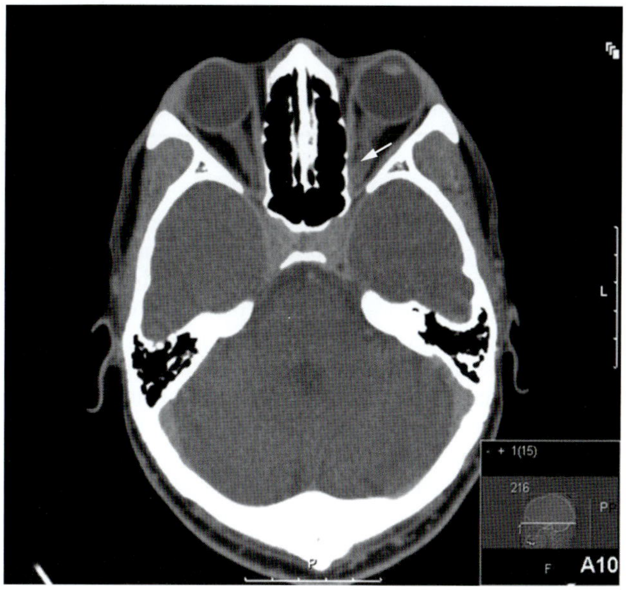

Figure 14.15 CT showing bilateral thickening of optic nerve sheaths (arrow) in sarcoid granulomatous optic neuritis.

the presenting syndrome is one of optic perineuritis (see Optic neuritis: optic perineuritis).

Investigations Serological testing for syphilis should be undertaken in every case of optic neuritis presenting as an isolated syndrome. Other serological tests will depend on the clinical presentation. Tuberculin testing may be required as may lumbar puncture, sinus biopsy and, occasionally, optic nerve biopsy. MRI of the optic nerve may give important clues in that the appearance may be of optic perineuritis rather than of swelling and inflammation affecting the intrinsic optic nerve and there may be evidence of infection elsewhere in the orbit, the paranasal sinuses or intracranially.

Treatment The management of these disorders is discussed in Chapter 9.

Optic neuritis: sarcoid-related optic neuropathy

Clinical features In neurosarcoidosis, optic neuropathy is not uncommon. Some patients have a syndrome indistinguishable from MS-ON with spontaneous recovery but more commonly the optic nerve is infiltrated with granulomata. This process may be visible at the optic disc and there is much greater likelihood of a vitritis and of peri-phlebitis than in MS-ON. The optic nerve may also be compressed extrinsically by a granulomatous mass causing contiguous involvement of nearby structures, for example leading to diabetes insipidus arising in sarcoid chiasmitis with associated orbital signs (Figure 14.15). Sarcoidosis is also a cause of optic perineuritis (see Optic neuritis: optic perineuritis).

Investigations On MRI, when there is intrinsic optic nerve disease the optic nerve is more likely to be enlarged than in MS-ON. There may be a granulomatous mass and features of optic perineuritis.

Treatment Corticosteroids are used in the acute phase. It is essential that steroid treatment is given over many weeks in slowly reducing doses. The treatment of neurosarcoidosis is reviewed in Chapter 26.

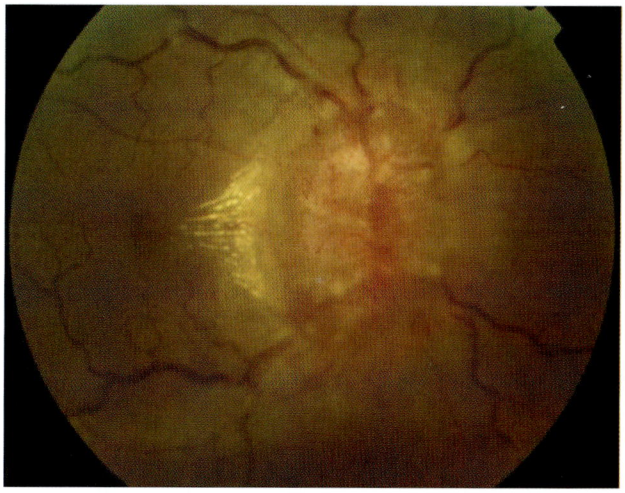

Figure 14.16 Swollen optic disc with hard exudates in retinal nerve fibre layer due to acute neuro-retinitis in a case of cat-scratch fever.

Optic neuritis: neuroretinitis

Clinical features This condition presents in similar fashion to MS-ON but the pathology is more anterior. The optic disc is swollen and within a few weeks a macular star develops. The macular star (exudates in a radial pattern around the macula) indicates that there has been oedema affecting the retina itself and it may be that this syndrome results from inflammation more of the retinal ganglion cell layer than of the optic nerve itself (Figure 14.16). It is an important diagnosis to make because it is not associated with MS.

Investigations This disorder commonly occurs after an infection and therefore appropriate serological tests may be revealing (e.g. *Bartonella* infection – cat scratch disease). In acute neuroretinitis the optic nerve does not show the features of demyelinating optic neuritis on MRI such as swelling, increased T2 hyperintensity or enhancement on gadolinium-enhanced MRI, and there are no CNS abnormalities (Figure 14.16).

Treatment Corticosteroids are usually given in more severe cases with vision reduced to 6/60 or worse.

Optic neuritis: optic perineuritis

Clinical features Optic perineuritis describes the situation in which the optic nerve is not directly involved in the inflammatory process, but rather the optic nerve sheath. Presentation can be much as any other form of optic neuritis but there may be considerable and sustained pain; in some cases the patient is reluctant to move the eye at all. There may be orbital signs of congestion or inflammation and disc swelling is almost universal. Peripheral visual field loss is more common than a central defect. The pathology is a meningeal-based process and is caused by infective disorders such as tuberculosis and syphilis or infiltration with a neoplastic process, particularly lymphoma or malignant meningitis. In some cases the condition is a component of orbital inflammatory disease with or without associated scleritis.

Investigations MRI shows a thickened and enhancing optic nerve sheath often with involvement of the orbital fat. Investigations are directed towards excluding a systemic condition. Rarely, a biopsy of the optic nerve sheath may be necessary. CSF examination should include careful cytology for neoplasia.

Treatment Treatment depends upon the exact cause, if this can be determined. All investigations should be carried out within 48 hours so that corticosteroid therapy can be instituted promptly if no other cause is found as any delay in treatment may result in a poor visual outcome.

Ischaemic ocular syndromes

Nosology of ischaemic syndromes

It is essential to have an understanding of the vascular supply to the intracranial and intraorbital portions of the optic nerve, to the optic nerve head and to the outer and inner layers of the retina. The ganglion cell layer of the retina is supplied in most individuals entirely by the central retinal artery which is a branch of the ophthalmic artery and is an end artery. Occlusion of this artery results in total visual loss and this is a common consequence of retinal embolism. In around 15% there is a branch of the choroidal circulation (cilioretinal artery) which is usually solitary and supplies the macula. Occlusion of this artery will give rise to a scotoma extending from the blind spot to the macula. This is a rare event in isolation but can occur in association with central retinal vein occlusion.

The prelaminar (most anterior) portion of the optic disc is supplied by the short posterior ciliary arteries which are several in number. These are also branches of the ophthalmic artery but these are not end arteries because there is an anastomosis (the circle of Zinn–Haller) around the optic nerve itself immediately behind the globe where the arterioles pierce the sclera to supply the optic nerve head and the choroid. Ischaemic events in posterior ciliary artery territory therefore are not related to embolic or arteriolar occlusive disease as is the case with the central retinal artery but to low perfusion. The optic disc is especially vulnerable in this respect because it is at a watershed between different branches of the short posterior ciliary vessels from the ophthalmic artery.

The anastomoses between the internal and external carotid artery in the orbit are extensive and for this reason occlusion of the ophthalmic artery in isolation does not result in any ischaemic consequence because the branches of the external carotid can take over the supply to all of the orbital structures. Similarly, occlusion of the internal carotid artery, in the presence of an adequate external carotid artery supply will not result in any ischaemic complications in the orbit and indeed the flow in the ophthalmic artery can be reversed.

The retrolaminar portion of the optic nerve and the remainder of the intraorbital nerve are supplied by pial vessels and by penetrating branches of the ophthalmic artery. The intracanalicular portion of the nerve is supplied by penetrating branches of the ophthalmic artery and the intracranial portion by pial vessels.

Central and branch retinal artery occlusion

Clinical features In central retinal artery occlusion (CRAO) abrupt loss of vision may be reported or loss of vision noticed on waking. Occasionally, the loss of vision may go unnoticed by the patient, more commonly in branch retinal artery occlusion (BRAO; Figure 14.17). There is no pain. In BRAO the field defects respect the fact that the branch arterioles of the central retinal artery do not cross the horizontal raphe of the retina so that altitudinal defects, or portions thereof, are the rule. Any portion of the retina supplied by a cilioretinal artery (most commonly the macula) will be spared. Acutely, there is retinal oedema (cloudy swelling; Figure 14.17) which is the hallmark of infarction of the inner layers of the retina which includes the ganglion cell layer. The 'cherry red spot' at the macula is in fact normal in colour; it is simply that this is a zone that is free of capillaries and ganglion cells, hence the red spot results from the intact choroidal supply, thrown into contrast by the surrounding pale and infarcted retina (Figure 14.18). If flow in the central retinal artery is restored within a matter of minutes following the occlusive event, then transient monocular blindness will result. If it is restored some time later, when infarction has occurred, then the appearance of the fundus can return remarkably to normal except that there is total loss of the retinal nerve fibre layer.

Of particular value is the search for the various types of embolus – calcific, cholesterol (Figure 14.19) or platelet/fibrin – as this can give some clue as to the source of the embolus. Not all retinal artery occlusions are caused by embolic disease, however, and CRAO can occur in giant cell arteritis and other causes of vasculitis. Some cases

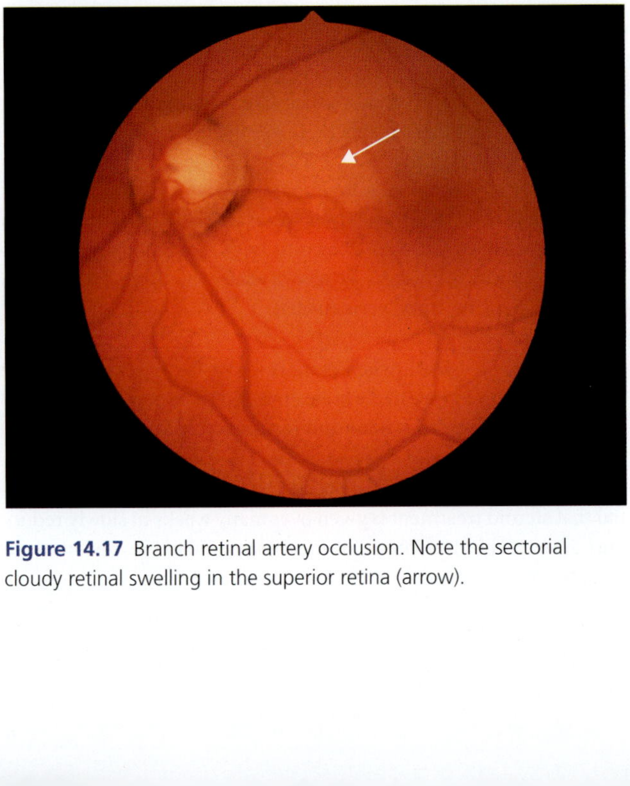

Figure 14.17 Branch retinal artery occlusion. Note the sectorial cloudy retinal swelling in the superior retina (arrow).

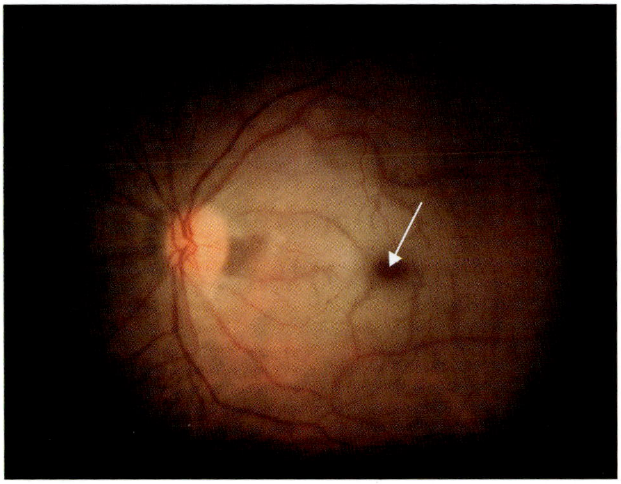

Figure 14.18 Central retinal artery occlusion with cherry red spot in Afro-Caribbean patient (arrow).

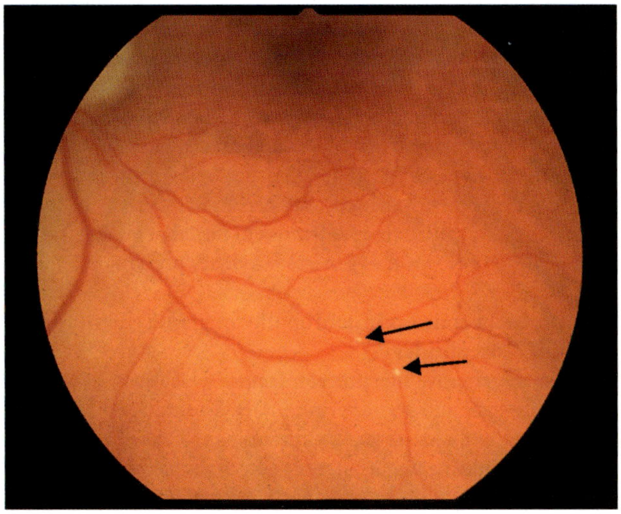

Figure 14.19 Cholesterol emboli (arrow).

are seen of recurrent BRAO and in this situation a more extensive vasculopathy should be suspected such as Susac's syndrome where recurrent arteriolar ischaemic events occur in the retina, the brain and the cochlea. Clearly, in these situations it is the systemic associated features that often give the clue (Chapter 26).

Investigations If a calcific embolus is seen as a cause of a CRAO then a cardiac source should be suspected, whereas platelet or fibrin embolus or cholesterol is more likely to have originated in atheromatous disease of the ipsilateral internal carotid or aortic arch.

Treatment Treatment of acute CRAO is attempted if seen early enough. Administering acetazolamide intravenously and performing ocular massage with or without paracentesis to lower intraocular pressure and improve perfusion is established practice but has no evidence base. Even cases with a blind eye for some hours can experience partial recovery spontaneously and it would be difficult to set up a controlled trial of such treatment. Local intra-arterial thrombolysis has not proved superior to conservative treatment and is associated with a risk of intracranial haemorrhage.

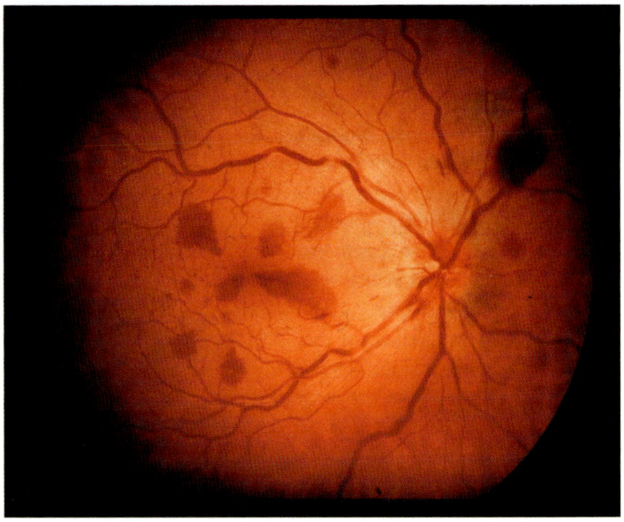

Figure 14.20 Central retinal vein occlusion showing scattered deep retinal haemorrhages.

Central and branch retinal vein occlusion

Clinical features Patients usually present complaining of painless abrupt onset of blurred vision or there may be no symptoms. The appearance of a central retinal vein occlusion (CRVO) is easily recognised – there is swelling of the optic disc and congestion of the retinal veins with extensive nerve fibre layer haemorrhages. Partial retinal vein occlusion (venous papillopathy or papillophlebitis) can cause diagnostic confusion because the patient may present with unilateral disc swelling with minimal haemorrhages and be investigated for raised intracranial pressure or an optic nerve tumour (Figure 14.20).

Investigations For the neurologist the task is usually to exclude any underlying prothrombotic disorder in the absence of obvious vascular risk factors such as hypertension or diabetes. CRVO can occur in young fit people and dehydration may have a part to play in some of these. Otherwise, most studies have shown an association between CRVO and various vascular risk factors particularly when recurrent. There is no need for imaging but it must be remembered that some optic nerve tumours (particularly malignant glioma of the optic nerve) can present with a picture resembling a CRVO but in these cases there is usually progression of visual loss and progression to arterial occlusion.

Treatment There is no treatment for the acute disorder but referral to the ophthalmologist is necessary because if there is significant retinal ischaemia new vessel formation can occur with all its attendant complications. Otherwise, management is limited to prevention of recurrence as with all occlusive vascular disease.

Non-arteritic anterior ischaemic optic neuropathy

Clinical features Ischaemia at the level of the posterior short ciliary artery supply to the prelaminar optic nerve head results in anterior ischaemic optic neuropathy (AION). By definition, the optic disc will be swollen acutely. Indeed, it should always be insisted that the diagnosis is not made unless the patient was seen acutely and the disc observed to be swollen. The common form of AION is non-arteritic. The pathogenesis of this condition is not understood but the condition may be caused by a drop in the perfusion pressure of the optic nerve head. It is almost never brought about by embolic disease, with the rare exception of atrial myxoma. Associations therefore include systemic hypotension, especially blood loss, during surgery and during renal haemodialysis, and obstructive sleep apnoea/hypopnoea syndrome. The other factor that influences perfusion of the optic disc is intraocular pressure and angle closure glaucoma may precipitate AION.

The morphology of the optic disc is of particular importance, the majority of cases have small 'crowded' optic discs, usually also hypermetropic (i.e. the scleral opening is small and the optic nerve has little or no cup; Figure 14.21). Therefore, if a minor degree of ischaemia leads to swelling of the optic nerve head, the ischaemia will be exacerbated and lead to infarction.

In non-arteritic AION the most common field defect is a lower altitudinal one – hence, the upper part of the optic disc is more vulnerable, a feature also in favour of the critical perfusion hypothesis. The optic disc will be swollen throughout initially but after 4–6 weeks the upper pole will become atrophic as the nerve fibres disappear while the lower pole remains swollen. A few weeks later sectoral optic atrophy is seen with loss of optic nerve fibre from the upper pole of the disc corresponding to the visual field defect (Figure 14.22).

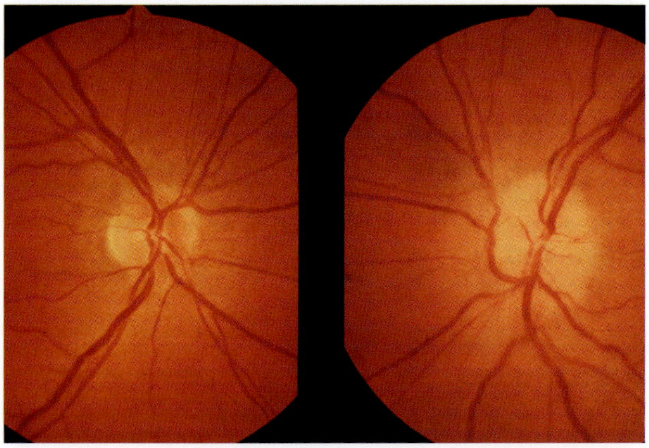

Figure 14.21 Left eye non-arteritic anterior ischaemic optic neuropathy with 'crowded disc at risk' in fellow right eye. The left disc is swollen and the right has an absent physiological cup.

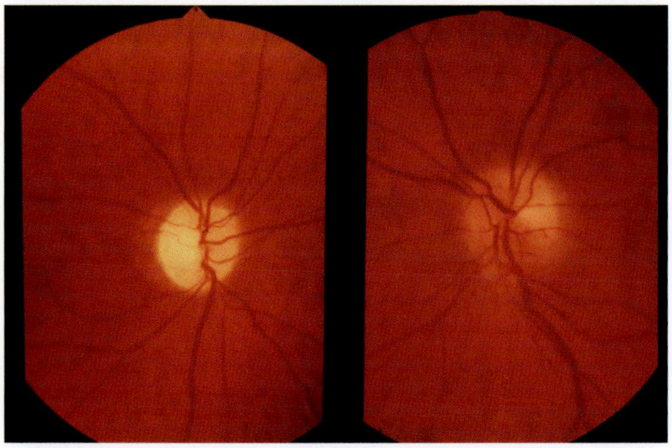

Figure 14.22 Pseudo-Foster Kennedy syndrome with swollen optic disc on left and optic atrophy on right.

Patients most commonly complain of sudden or subacute visual loss with some progression over hours to days, they may notice the loss on waking, or it may pass unnoticed until the visual field defect or optic atrophy is picked up some time later. AION rarely affects the same eye a second time but some cases show stepwise progression sometimes over many weeks. Unfortunately (and possibly related to the vulnerable optic disc morphology), there is a risk of the same process occurring in the other eye in about 20–40% of cases. Second eye involvement is usually within months to years, bilateral simultaneous involvement suggests systemic hypotension as the cause.

Investigations Non-arteritic AION is rarely associated with embolic disease and only exceptionally associated with disease of the ipsilateral carotid artery; in which case it is usually in the context of disease of both the internal and external carotid arteries and inadequate perfusion of the entire globe. Thrombophilic conditions, most of which cause venous rather than arterial occlusions, are rarely implicated. Investigations are limited to a general screen for vascular risk factors with consideration of nocturnal hypotension or obstructive sleep apnoea as cofactors.

Many patients with non-arteritic AION are relatively young and do not have extensive evidence of generalised vascular disease and in these patients the disc morphology may be the only predisposing factor.

Treatment Management is treatment of any underlying cause and of general vascular risk factors. There is no treatment known to influence the visual deficit although drugs to lower the intraocular pressure are sometimes used. Neither has it been shown that prophylactic aspirin can reduce the risk to the other eye but it seems reasonable to prescribe it as general secondary prevention.

Anterior ischaemic optic neuropathy in giant cell arteritis and other vasculitides

There is an extensive literature on factors which help distinguish between arteritic and non-arteritic AION. The argument is centred on the need to diagnose giant cell arteritis (GCA) and to prevent blindness. While the importance of this cannot be overemphasised, the arteritic versus non-arteritic AION dichotomy is only a part of the story. It is essential to realise that AION is not the only cause of visual symptoms and visual loss in GCA, furthermore there are other systemic inflammatory conditions that can lead to AION.

Clinical features By definition, all causes of AION will be associated with disc swelling but in GCA the loss of vision is more profound than in non-arteritic AION, indeed total blindness of the affected eye in a matter of hours is the rule. The swollen disc will look pale early – often within days – whereas in non-arteritic AION the disc only becomes pale as optic atrophy supervenes (Figure 14.23). Premonitory transient visual loss occurs in GCA but never in non-arteritic AION; this is not embolic but a result of poor perfusion. Usually, patients are aware that the loss of vision lasts seconds only and tends to come on with change of posture from sitting or lying to standing. This phenomenon is related to the pathological difference between the two conditions. Indeed, all of the distinctions between the two can be explained in these terms.

First in GCA, many arteries and arterioles are involved, hence there is more extensive ischaemia. The central retinal artery and the choroidal vessels may be involved, the entire globe or indeed entire orbit may be ischaemic because branches of both the internal and external carotid artery are affected. Secondly, GCA is a vascular occlusive disorder which accounts for the more profound visual loss

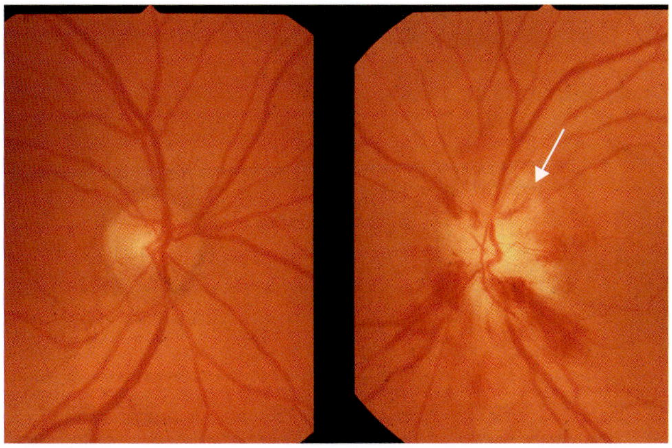

Figure 14.23 Vasculitic anterior ischaemic optic neuropathy (AION) showing haemorrhagic disc swelling.

as there is no collateral or anastomotic supply which may help to preserve vision. However, in GCA, the occlusion is generally not thrombotic and the lumen is occluded by the intimal hypertrophy which is the pathological hallmark of the disease.

Apart from the severity of the visual loss, for example, preceding symptoms – both visual and systemic – should be sought in any patient with visual loss that might be brought about by GCA. Headache and tenderness of the extracranial arteries, especially the superficial temporal and occipital arteries are important clues to the diagnosis as is other evidence of ischaemia in the territory of the branches of the external carotid artery (ischaemic jaw pain on chewing, scalp or tongue necrosis). Polymyalgia rheumatica often occurs in the same individuals and may precede or follow GCA by some years. The disease is rare below the age of 50 years.

An often neglected clinical sign is the palpation of the superficial temporal, occipital and facial arteries (Figure 14.24). In a severe case of GCA these arteries will be thickened, pulseless and tender. In the appropriate clinical context this confirms the diagnosis. In other cases they may be normal or thickened but still with a pulse. False positives are possible because arteriosclerosis alone can result in similar findings.

AION can occur in other true vasculitides where there is inflammation in the vessel wall especially where arterioles are affected (e.g. polyarteritis nodosa, Churg–Strauss syndrome and ANCA-positive vasculitis). It can also be seen where there is vascular occlusion because of antigen–antibody complex deposition in arterioles and capillaries such as in systemic lupus erythematosus. These conditions have characteristic systemic features but it is beyond the scope of this chapter to list them all. An important clinical point, however, is that these disorders lie somewhere between GCA and non-arteritic AION in their clinical features – visual loss may be intermediate in severity, for example. The importance in recognising these conditions is that, unlike non-arteritic AION and the vast majority of cases of GCA, there is some possibility of visual recovery if treatment is administered promptly.

Investigations A normal ESR and CRP do not exclude the diagnosis but in most cases these are reliable screening tests with all the usual concerns regarding false positive and false negative results. In clinically definite cases of GCA one needs to disregard blood tests, but they are usually helpful when monitoring the response to steroid therapy. A biopsy should be carried out if possible because it is always helpful to future management to have that result in the notes (Figure 14.25). The rapidity of the response of headache to steroids (usually measured in hours after the first dose) is also useful circumstantial evidence.

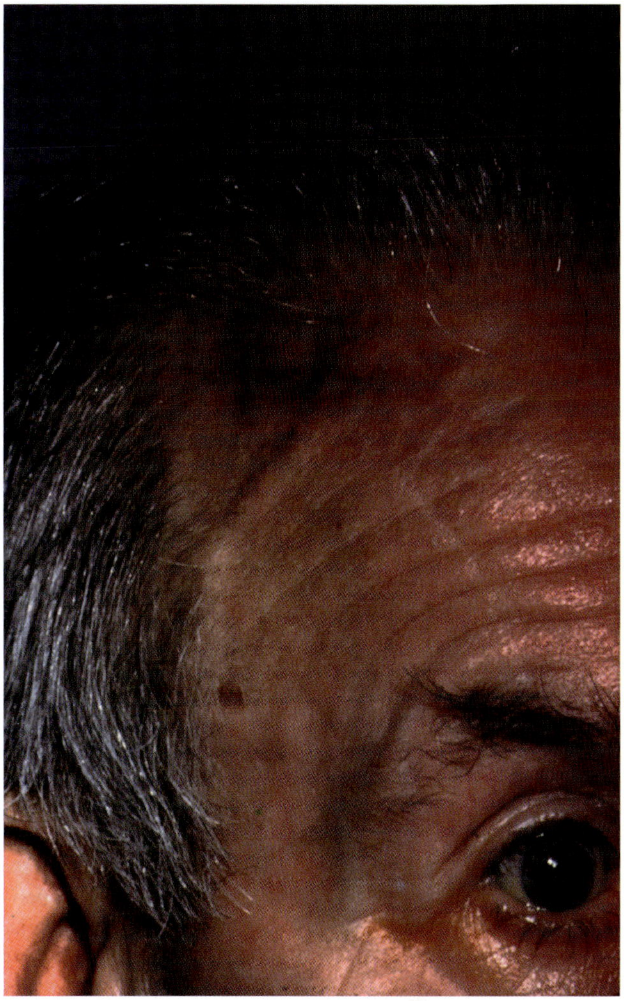

Figure 14.24 Giant cell arteritis with superficial scalp necrosis.

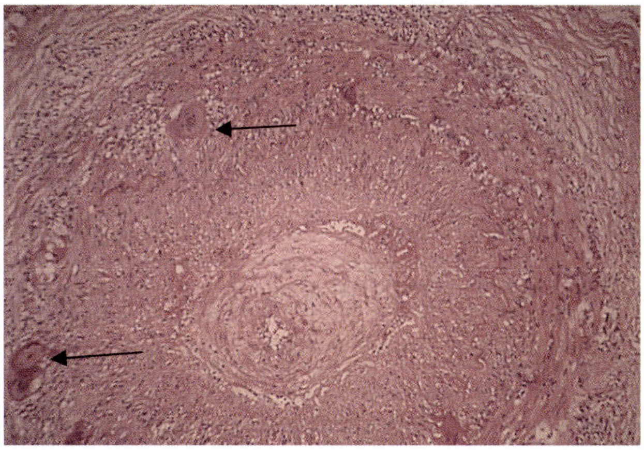

Figure 14.25 Giant cell arteritis histology. Granulomatous inflammation across vessel wall with fragmentation of the internal elastic lamina and occlusion of the lumen (arrows).

Treatment Therapy with oral prednisolone, at 1 mg/kg body weight, should be commenced urgently in any suspected case of GCA. Intravenous methylprednisolone to initiate therapy may have advantages if the second eye becomes involved. There is a time window of a few days in which visual loss can occur in the other eye even after treatment with steroids has been initiated. A delay of even hours can make a difference in preventing blindness. Unfortunately, the chances of recovery in an eye already showing signs of AION are low. It is possible to demonstrate that the lumen recanalises in affected arteries – simply by palpating the superficial temporal arteries again in a week or two when the pulse will be restored. In clinical practice the main problem is the need to minimise the adverse effects of corticosteroids and discontinue the treatment safely without risking relapse. In most cases it is possible to discontinue steroids after 18 months to 2 years.

Posterior ischaemic optic neuropathy

Posterior ischaemic optic neuropathy (PION) should only be diagnosed in the context of GCA or following severe hypotension, or for example following spinal surgery. A compressive disorder is erroneously diagnosed as PION more commonly than vice versa, a situation that has more serious potential consequences.

Clinical features There is acute or subacute painless loss of vision with variable patterns of visual field loss with, in the acute phase, a normal fundus although optic atrophy develops later. Where visual loss has occurred in the context of spinal surgery or blood loss the loss of vision is more likely to be bilateral (see Bilateral visual failure).

Investigations In the appropriate context, the investigations for arteritic AION are as those described earlier. In recovery from peri-operative visual loss little needs to be done except to exclude an unlikely compressive lesion by appropriate imaging. There is little information on the MRI appearances of the optic nerve in acute PION, there is no need to carry out this investigation in GCA and cases of spontaneous PION are very rare. There is often high signal and gadolinium enhancement of a segment of the nerve.

Treatment Treatment of GCA is discussed earlier. There is no treatment for PION in other contexts.

Chronic ocular ischaemic syndromes

Clinical features In a number of situations there may be chronic ischaemia of the retina, the optic disc or the entire globe. As far as the optic disc is concerned chronic ischaemia at the capillary level will lead to disc swelling with a variable degree of visual loss. The classic example is known as 'diabetic papillopathy' where a chronically swollen disc is seen in poorly controlled diabetes. Disc swelling in accelerated hypertension has a similar aetiology and can persist for some time without significant loss of vision. In both instances there is a risk of infarction of the optic nerve which will lead to permanent loss of vision. In the case of accelerated hypertension this may occur if the blood pressure is treated too aggressively.

'Slow flow retinopathy' is seen when there is poor perfusion of the retina. This situation occurs when there is severe impairment of both the internal and external carotid artery supply to the orbit.

Patients may complain of transient loss of vision, particularly associated with change from a sitting to a standing posture and on moving to bright illumination particularly sunlight. On examination, vision may be only mildly impaired but there is congestion of retinal veins, haemorrhages in the mid-periphery (characteristically petal-shaped) and macular oedema ('cattle-trucking') (Figure 14.26). The central retinal artery collapses with minimal digital pressure on the globe and indeed may show spontaneous pulsation because in diastole the pressure is lower than the intraocular pressure. In more severe cases the entire globe may be ischaemic, this leads to the formation of new vessels at the iris – rubeosis – which in turn leads to glaucoma.

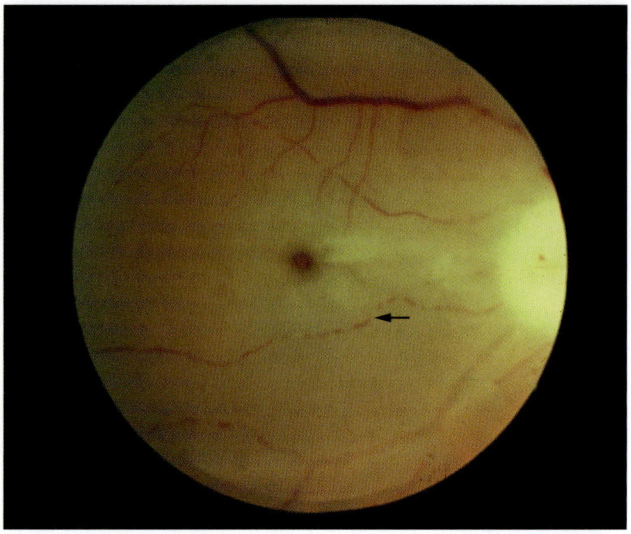

Figure 14.26 Arteritic AION + central retinal artery occlusion (CRAO) with cattle trucking in branch retinal artery (arrow) in a patient with GCA.

Investigations The task is to confirm that the problem is with occlusion of the ipsilateral carotid artery. The principal differential diagnosis is GCA which can also give rise to an ocular ischaemic syndrome.

Treatment The evidence that carotid endarterectomy is effective in these disorders is not compelling and many cases, if followed, will not deteriorate nor develop significant visual loss, except in the case of rubeotic glaucoma which should be treated by an ophthalmologist.

Tumours affecting the optic nerve

Compressive or infiltrative optic neuropathy

Visual loss may be unilateral or bilateral. In unilateral cases there will be a relative afferent pupillary defect, the disc may be normal, swollen or infiltrated. When the visual impairment is bilateral the lesion is almost always intracranial or in the paranasal sinuses and the optic discs appear normal at presentation although progressive loss of colour vision and an afferent pupillary defect may occur. The disc may develop collateral vessels to bypass the retinal circulation. Locally invasive tumours such as optic glioma and optic nerve sheath meningioma compress the optic nerve and directly cause axonal backflow. Systemic malignancies such as leukaemia, lymphoma and metastases can directly infiltrate the optic nerves usually via the dura and cause both compression and papilloedema leading to abrupt or rapidly progressive visual loss (Figure 14.27; Table 14.7).

Primary optic nerve sheath meningiomas Primary optic nerve sheath meningiomas arise from the arachnoid cells of the optic nerve sheath. Their origin is generally in the orbital portion of the nerve but intracranial extension may occur. Primary optic nerve

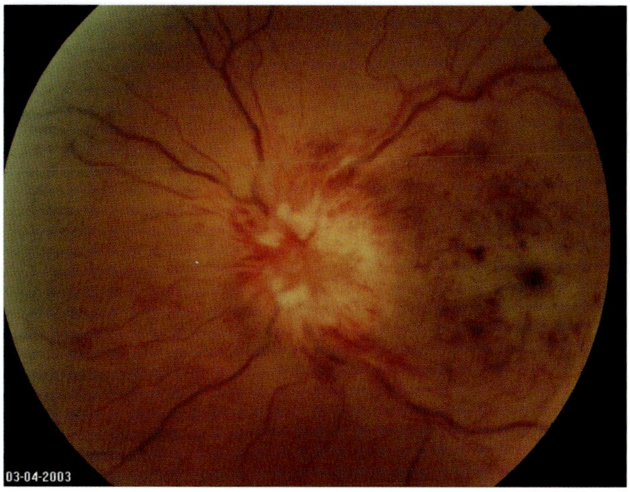

Figure 14.27 Neoplastic infiltration of the optic disc with associated central retinal artery occlusion (CRAO) causing a cherry red spot at the macula.

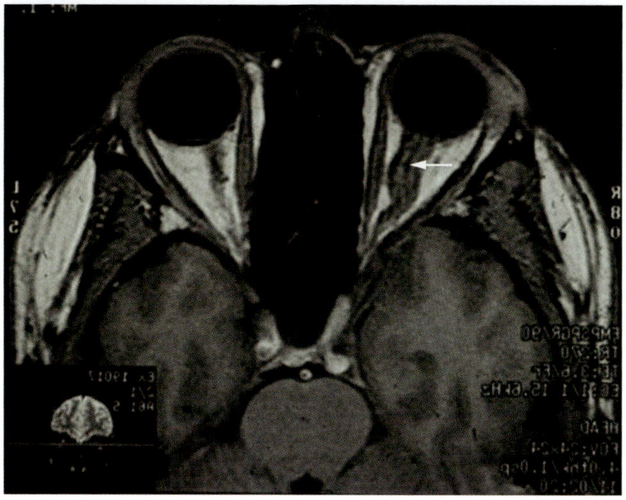

Figure 14.28 Peri-optic meningioma causing thickening of left optic nerve sheath (arrow).

Table 14.7 Causes of compressive and infiltrative optic neuropathies.

Compressive	
Tumour	Intraorbital tumours
	Optic nerve sheath meningioma
	Sphenoid wing meningioma
	Pituitary tumour
	Craniopharyngioma
Non-neoplastic	Thyroid eye disease
	Sphenoid mucocoele
	Orbital pseudotumour
	Orbital haemorrhage
	Paget's disease of bone
	Fibrous dysplasia of bone
Infiltrative	
Neoplastic	Optic nerve glioma
	Metastatic carcinoma
	Nasopharyngeal carcinoma
	Lymphoma
	Leukaemia
	Meningeal carcinomatosis and malignant meningitis
Non-neoplastic	Sarcoidosis

sheath meningiomas are more common in middle-aged females and are generally unilateral but may be bilateral or multifocal particularly in neurofibromatosis type 2. They may present with features of a slowly progressive optic neuropathy leading to loss of acuity, impairment of colour vision with a central scotoma and a relative afferent pupillary defect. Fundal examination shows unilateral optic atrophy but there may be chronic disc oedema with retinochoroidal venous collateral vessels indicating chronic retinal vein obstruction. Progressive visual loss is likely regardless of treatment but intracranial extension is rare (Figure 14.28). Stereotactic radiotherapy can slow progression in selected cases.

Other forms of meningiomas Meningiomas may also arise from the sphenoid wing, tuberculum sellae or olfactory groove. They cause visual failure by direct compression of the intracranial portion of the optic nerve or chiasm but they may invade the optic canal and orbit. Large olfactory groove or sphenoid wing meningiomas can cause optic atrophy in one eye due to compression and papilloedema in the other eye due to raised intracranial pressure (Foster Kennedy syndrome). Imaging of splenoid wing meningioma shows sphenoid hyperostosis and contrast enhancement on CT if there is orbital extension of the intracranial mass. Complete surgical excision is rarely possible but vision can be improved or stabilised by decompressing the optic canal and the posterior orbital segment of the optic nerve, sometime combined with adjuvant radiotherapy.

Optic and optochiasmal glioma

Primary glial tumours of the anterior visual pathway (optic glioma) occur either as benign gliomas of childhood or rarely as malignant glioblastoma in adults.

Benign optic gliomas of childhood arise in the chiasm more often than within the orbit or the canal. Patients present with proptosis and visual field loss which is generally bilateral and either scotomatous or bitemporal. There may be horizontal or rotatory nystagmus with head nodding. The optic disc is swollen or atrophic leading to fluctuations in visual function which may improve spontaneously in some patients. It is essential to exclude neurofibromatosis type 1. Optic glioma of childhood may be associated with hypothalamic or thalamic involvement and there may be hydrocephalus or signs of raised intracranial pressure and leptomeningeal spread may occur. The management is controversial as these tumours are slow-growing. Surgery is confined to palliative treatment for intraorbital tumours and chiasmal gliomas. Radiotherapy results in significant tumour shrinkage and improvement in visual function but carries a risk of radionecrosis of the optic nerve. However, surgical intervention may be required for hydrocephalus, decompression of intraneural cyst, in instances of significant exophytic extension, or biopsy.

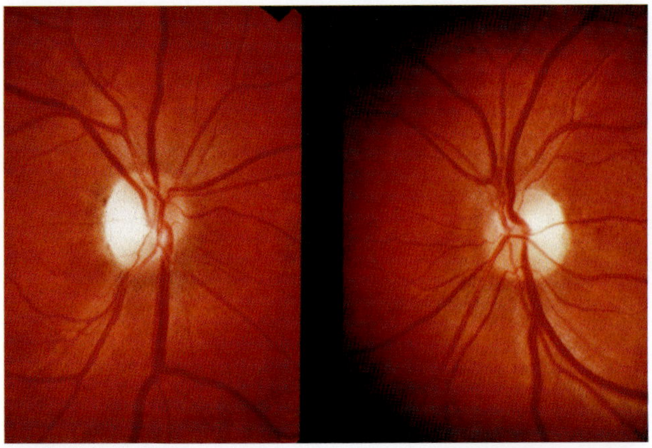

Figure 14.29 Autosomal dominant optic atrophy causing temporal optic disc pallor in both eyes.

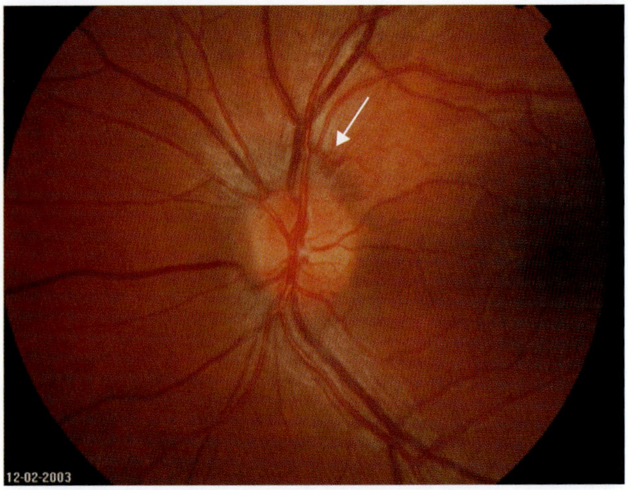

Figure 14.30 Acute Leber's hereditary optic neuropathy (LHON); optic disc shows hyperaemia and telangectatic vessels (arrow).

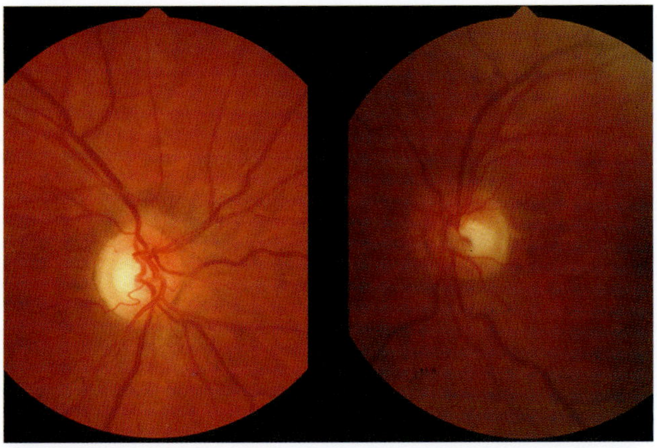

Figure 14.31 Bitemporal optic disc pallor in established LHON.

Primary malignant gliomas of the optic nerve generally arise in males aged 40–60 years and patients present with rapid monocular visual loss, retrobulbar pain and disc oedema with transient improvement on corticosteroids, signs mimicking optic neuritis. However, within several weeks of treatment visual function deteriorates again and contralateral visual loss develops. There may be an associated central retinal vein or artery occlusion as a result of vascular compression. Radiotherapy and adjunctive chemotherapy may slow progression somewhat but spread along the optic nerve sheath usually occurs within a few months with a uniformly poor prognosis.

Hereditary optic neuropathies

Autosomal dominant optic atrophy

Autosomal dominant optic atrophy typically commences in childhood or the teenage years and is characterised by insidious binocular visual loss which is highly variable. It commonly affects the papillo-macular nerve fibre bundle causing loss of central vision manifest as impaired visual acuity with a bilateral symmetrical central or centro-caecal scotoma and mild impairment of colour vision. Optic atrophy is often localised to the temporal portion of the optic nerve (Figure 14.29) and there may be associated sensorineural hearing loss. The condition is transmitted as an autosomal dominant with high penetrance although there is variability even within families. The gene responsible (*OPA1*) is located on the long arm of chromosome 3 although there is considerable genetic heterogeneity.

Leber's hereditary optic neuropathy

Leber's hereditary optic neuropathy (LHON) typically presents in young adults with subacute painless loss of central vision which develops over 3–6 months; however, there is considerable variability in the age of onset and rate of progression. While the onset may be bilateral and symmetrical, in up to 50% of patients one eye is affected initially followed by similar loss in the fellow eye developing within 4–6 weeks. The rate of visual loss is considerably quicker than in dominant hereditary optic atrophy and progressively worsens over several weeks although sudden and complete visual loss may occur.

On examination there is marked impairment of visual acuity and colour vision, with a central or centro-caecal scotoma with preservation of the peripheral field (Figure 14.30). The disc may appear normal but the condition is characterised by a triad of hyperaemia with swelling of the optic nerve fibre layer around the disc ('pseudopapilloedema'), telangiectatic vessels on the disc and in the circumpapillary region with the absence of leakage on fluorescein angiography. Optic nerve involvement progresses to optic atrophy with non-glaucomatous cupping, pallor and attenuation of the arterioles (Figure 14.31). The optic disc abnormalities may be present for many years prior to the onset of visual loss and may be seen in unaffected carriers of the mutation.

Some patients may have cardiac conduction defects or other neurological features including pyramidal signs with brisk reflexes, cerebellar ataxia and tremor, movement disorders, distal sensory neuropathy or encephalopathy and some patients have been reported to develop MS. It is therefore important to exclude LHON in patients with severe visual loss resulting from MS. The prognosis for restoration of vision is poor but some patients do recover vision spontaneously many years later.

LHON is a mitochondrial disorder that is maternally inherited. It is caused by point mutations within the mitochondrial genome at nucleotide positions 11778, 3460 and 14484 in genes that encode subunits of the respiratory chain. The 11778 mutation is the most common and has the worst visual prognosis with a 4% improvement rate. However, 25–40% of patients with mutations at sites 14484 and 3460 experience improvement in visual acuity and the field deficit.

It is important to consider the diagnosis in any patient with painless, relatively rapid visual loss particularly with an asymmetrical onset and to distinguish the condition from toxic nutritional optic neuropathy.

Toxic and nutritional optic neuropathies

Toxic and nutritional neuropathies are often considered together because it is difficult to distinguish the relative contribution, particularly in tobacco- or alcohol-related amblyopia. Clinically toxic and nutritional deficiencies present with subacute bilateral central visual loss with impaired acuity, centro-caecal scotomata and impaired colour vision. Toxic and deficiency optic neuropathies are almost always bilateral although one eye may be affected before the other. The optic disc appears hyperaemic at onset but temporal pallor develops as a later finding and there is selective vulnerability of the papillo-macular bundle. The loss of vision usually evolves slowly over months, with moderate to severe impairment of acuity although complete blindness may result from methanol toxicity.

Tobacco-alcohol amblyopia is usually associated with excessive tobacco consumption with or without alcoholism or poor nutritional intake. A similar syndrome is associated with vitamin B_{12} deficiency and may occur with vitamin B_{12} levels that remain in the low normal range. Nutritional optic neuropathy may occur in a number of settings including chronic alcohol abuse, starvation, malabsorption syndromes or depression.

Toxic amblyopia (Chapter 19) is particularly associated with amiodarone, ciclosporin and digoxin and may develop with other neurological manifestations including peripheral neuropathy, ataxia and tremor. In Cuban epidemic optic neuropathy there is an associated peripheral neuropathy, myelopathy and sensorineural hearing loss.

Traumatic optic neuropathy

Traumatic optic neuropathy typically results from damage to the optic nerve and its blood supply from pial vessels within the optic canal following an indirect blow to the boney orbital rim. Less commonly there is penetrating orbital trauma. Orbito-cranial fractures may be absent even when optic nerve function is significantly affected (Figure 14.32). Visual loss is variable but may be severe. There is no evidence for improvement following corticosteroids or decompression of the optic nerve.

Radiation-induced optic neuropathy (Chapters 19 and 21)

This can occur in up to 15% of patients who have received radiotherapy with doses up to 5000 cGy but may occur with smaller doses if there has been coexisting chemotherapy or diabetes mellitus. Visual loss occurs 4 months to 8 years after radiotherapy with a relatively rapid progression in one or both eyes. The optic disc is initially normal but pallor develops. There is no effective treatment but single case reports describe improvement in response to corticosteroids, anticoagulants and hyperbaric oxygen therapy. A transient and self-limiting form may occur which is usually treated with corticosteroids.

Swollen optic disc

Optic disc swelling (Figure 14.33) is the end result of many pathological processes (Table 14.8). A swollen disc implies axonal distension and elevation of the optic disc. Papilloedema is the term used when the cause is elevated intracranial pressure, but local disease of the optic nerve itself and intraocular processes may produce a similar ophthalmolscopic picture.

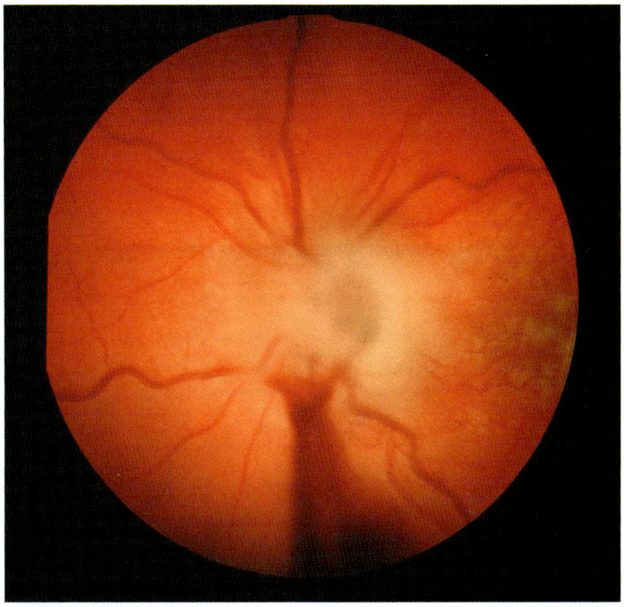

Figure 14.32 Traumatic optic nerve avulsion from scleral canal.

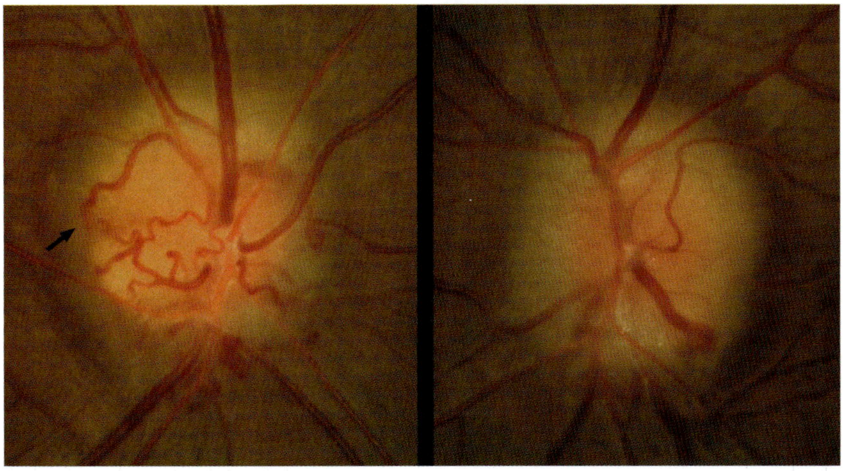

Figure 14.33 Florid chorio-retinal collateral vessels on right optic disc in chronic bilateral papilloedema due to raised intracranial pressure (arrow).

Table 14.8 Causes of optic disc swelling.

Raised intracranial pressure
Space-occupying lesions
Obstructive hydrocephalus
Idiopathic intracranial hypertension: associations with medications (e.g. vitamin A, retinoids, tetracyclines, doxycycline, nitrofurantoin, ciprofloxacin, corticosteroids) and with endocrine disorders (e.g. adrenal, thyroid, parathyroid dysfunction)
Cerebral venous sinus thrombosis
Venous outflow obstruction
Dural arteriovenous fistula
Local disease in eye or optic nerve
Anterior optic neuropathies (Table 14.5)
Intraocular disease
Uveitis
Hypotony
Retinal vein occlusion
Pseudopapilloedema (Table 14.5)

NB The term papilloedema should be reserved for cases of optic disc swelling caused by raised intracranial pressure.

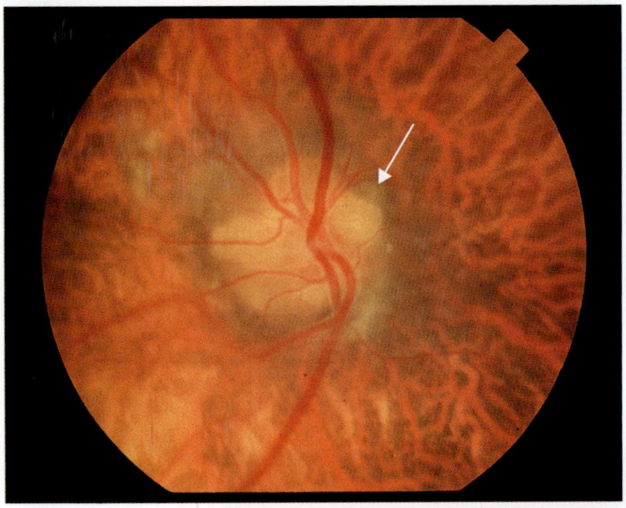

Figure 14.34 Optic disc drusen visible on disc surface (arrow).

The optic disc may also appear swollen because of bilateral anomalous disc appearances. Local causes for disc swelling (e.g. optic neuritis, ischaemic optic neuropathy and compressive lesions; Table 14.8) are frequently unilateral and often present with ipsilateral visual loss and a relative afferent pupillary defect.

Specific optic disc anomalies

Optic disc drusen These are small hyaline concretions on the surface or 'buried' beneath the optic nerve head causing elevation of the optic disc but no other features of true swelling. They are usually bilateral and drusen may be easily visible. Up to 70% of patients with this anomaly have a field defect including enlargement of the blind spot and arcuate or infero-nasal defects but central vision is preserved. Drusen may be associated with retinitis pigmentosa and are transmitted as an autosomal dominant trait (Figure 14.34).

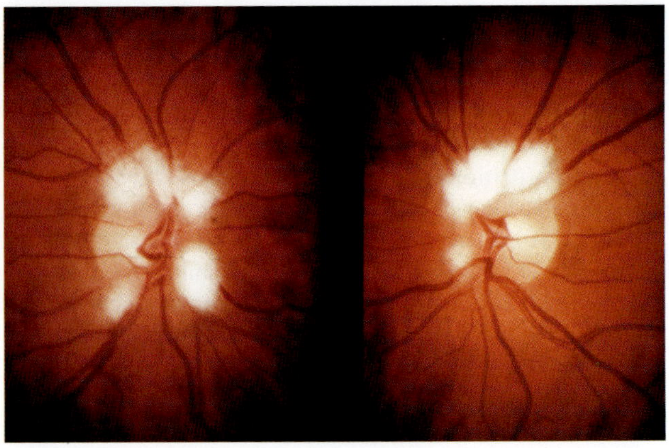

Figure 14.35 Myelinated retinal nerve fibres.

Tilted disc This is a non-hereditary condition characterised by bilateral elevation of the supero-temporal disc, posterior displacement of the infero-nasal disc, situs inversus of the retinal vessels and bitemporal visual field defects. The elevated superior disc may be mistaken for segmental swelling but there is no hyperaemia or obscuration of the peri-papillary vessels.

Myelinated nerve fibres These appear as white striated patches, often at the upper and lower poles of the optic disc, which typically spare the papillomacular bundle. They rarely affect acuity or visual field (Figure 14.35).

Papilloedema

Papilloedema is the most common cause of optic disc swelling without visual loss and is caused by raised intracranial pressure (Figure 14.36). This may occur as as a result of the following:

1 An intracranial mass (e.g. tumour, abscess or haemorrhage)
2 Excessive production of CSF (e.g. choroid plexus papilloma)
3 Blockage of arachnoid villi by blood or protein (e.g. infection, sarcoidosis, carcinomatous meningitis)
4 Obstruction of flow of CSF through the ventricles (e.g. aqueduct stenosis)
5 Decreased flow of venous blood through the dural sinuses (venous sinus thrombosis)
6 Idiopathic intracranial hypertension (see Idiopathic intracranial hypertension).

Patients with papilloedema may report transient binocular visual obscurations which occur occasionally or many times a day and are often related to changes in posture. There may be diplopia caused by unilateral or bilateral VIth nerve palsy. In the early stage, visual loss only occurs if haemorrhages, exudates and oedema develop over the macula or in the subretinal fluid or if there is a mass lesion involving the optic nerve or chiasm. On examination the visual field is initially normal but as disc swelling worsens, there is an enlarged blind spot. If intracranial pressure is severe enough to cause compression and axonal loss an arcuate scotomatous defect develops and with continued damage generalised field constriction occurs although visual acuity remains preserved unless the field loss is severe. It is unclear why the papillomacular bundle (i.e. the portion of the ganglion cell layer subserving central vision) is spared until late.

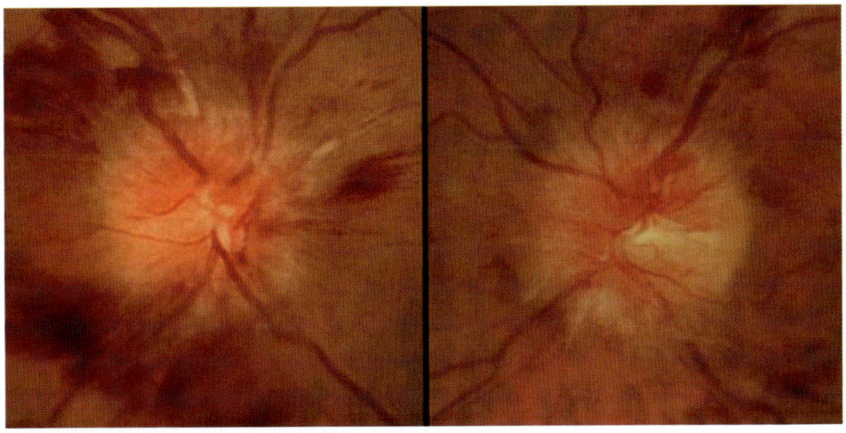

Figure 14.36 Acute haemorrhagic papilloedema.

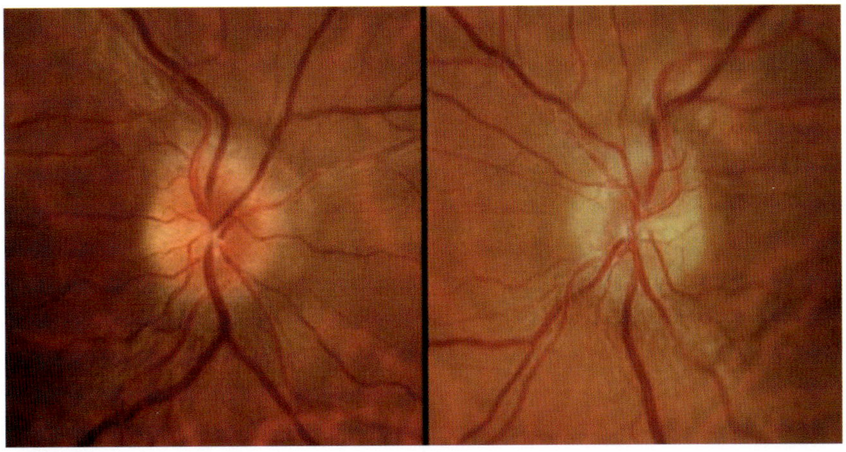

Figure 14.37 Early papilloedema.

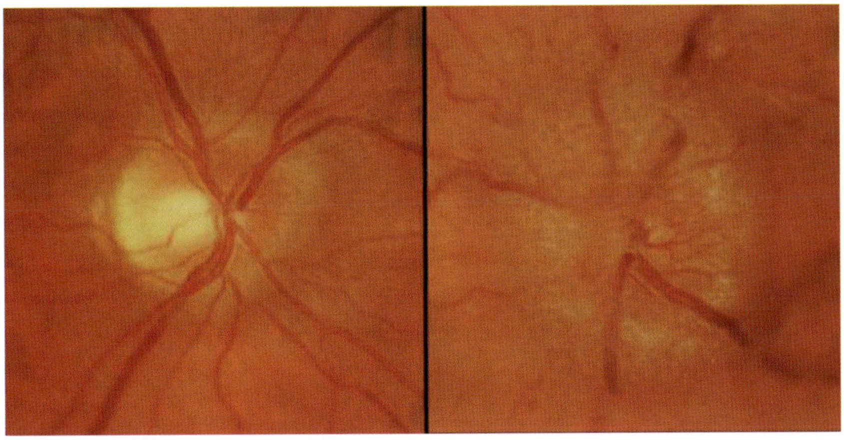

Figure 14.38 Asymmetric bilateral papilloedema.

The disc appearance varies with severity. In early papilloedema there may be only mild swelling of the optic disc with no evidence of haemorrhages or dilation of retinal veins (Figure 14.37). However, as papilloedema worsens the discs become increasingly swollen and hyperaemic and the vessels become obscured by swollen tissues and spontaneous venous pulsation is lost. Peri-papillary flame-shaped haemorrhages may appear with folds in the retina and/or macula which rarely compromise vision. When papilloedema is fully developed visual acuity and colour vision are normal but the blind spot is enlarged and severe field constriction is present. With chronic papilloedema the discs become pale and the margins clearer, haemorrhage resolves but the constricted visual field persists (Figures 14.38, 14.39 and 14.40). Eventually, atrophic papilloedema occurs when the swelling has resolved and led to the death of nerve

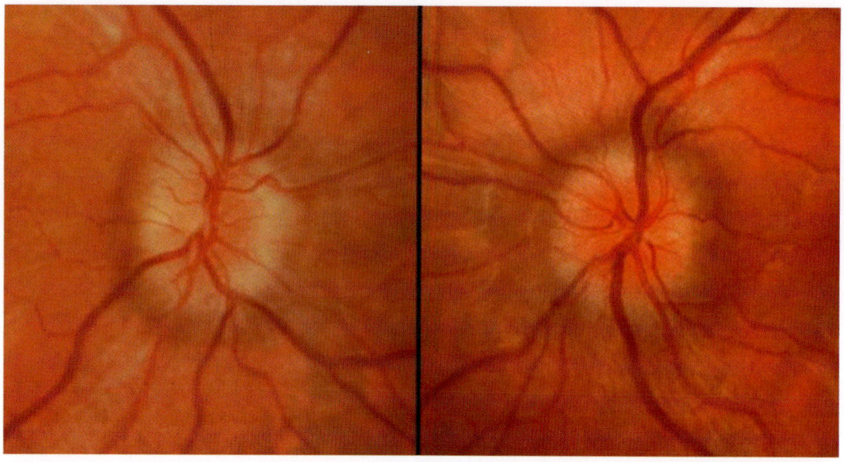

Figure 14.39 Chronic compensated papilloedema.

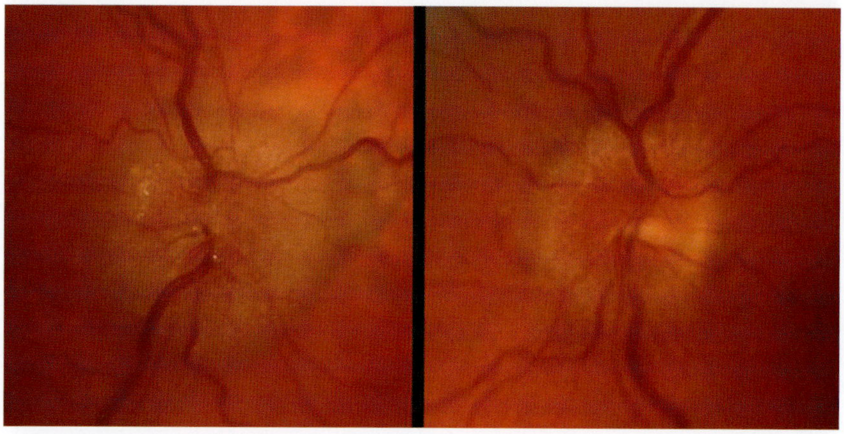

Figure 14.40 Vintage papilloedema with corpora amylacea.

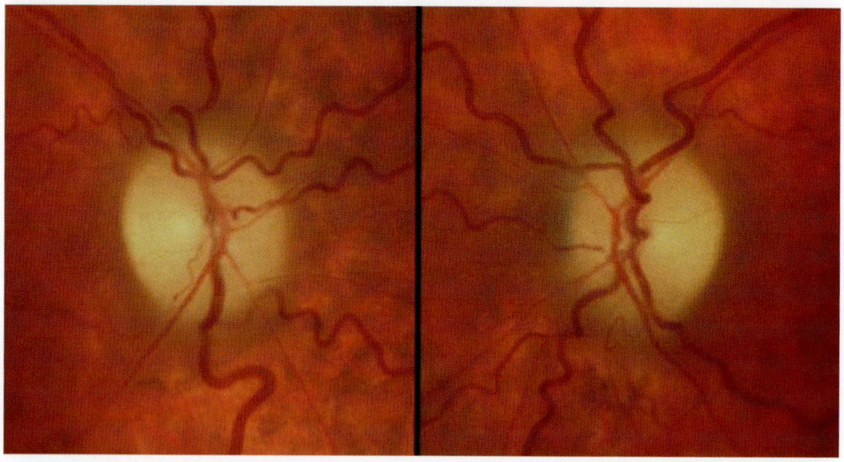

Figure 14.41 Atrophic papilloedema.

fibres (Figure 14.41). The optic discs are pale, visual acuity is reduced and the visual fields are severely constricted.

Papilloedema can only develop if there is patency of the subarachnoid space surrounding the optic nerve. If these spaces are blocked by adhesions, papilloedema does not occur. Loss of the nerve fibres in optic atrophy will also prevent the development of papilloedema. Development of papilloedema depends on increased pressure in the distal optic nerve sheath, decreased perfusion of the axons exiting through the lamina cribrosa and possibly elevated central retinal venous pressure. Disturbance of both slow and fast axoplasmic transport are a feature of papilloedema.

Idiopathic intracranial hypertension

Idiopathic intracranial hypertension (IIH) is a disorder of elevated intracranial pressure of unknown cause which may lead to visual loss due to papilloedema. The condition usually occurs in obese women of childbearing age.

The diagnosis depends on fulfilling the modified Dandy criteria:

1 Symptoms and signs of elevated intracranial pressure in an awake and alert patient.
2 No localising symptoms or signs other than a VIth nerve palsy.
3 Normal neuroimaging apart from changes due to the raised pressure itself.
4 Lumbar puncture showing elevated opening pressure (>250 mm/H_2O) but normal fluid analysis.

Intracranial hypertension may be idiopathic or may develop secondarily to a number of underlying conditions, particularly venous sinus thrombosis. The clinical features of idiopathic and secondary intracranial hypertension may be identical. However, the treatment of the secondary form depends on the underlying cause and it is therefore extremely important to exclude another underlying cause before making a final diagnosis of IIH.

Clinically, IIH presents with headache in >90% of patients, it is characteristically severe, daily and pulsatile; nausea and vomiting may be present. There may be retrobulbar pain with eye movements and radicular pain in the neck and shoulders radiating down the arms. Transient visual obscurations lasting for seconds or minutes and associated with postural changes are present in up to 70% of patients. Tinnitus is common and some patients develop hearing loss. Diplopia, usually horizontal is present in up to 40% of patients usually resulting from a VIth nerve palsy. Other symptoms include impaired coordination and sense of smell and numbness or motor weakness.

On examination only 15% of patients who present with IIH have impairment in visual acuity but significant visual field loss is common. An afferent pupillary defect suggests asymmetric visual loss and is present in the eye with the greatest amount of field loss. VIth nerve palsies are relatively common because of stretching of the nerve by intracranial hypertension. A IIIth nerve palsy may occur in IIH but other causes must be excluded. Signs of optic disc swelling include elevation and blurring of the disc margin, a peripapillary halo, venous congestion and tortuosity, retinal exudates and retinal infarcts (cotton wool spots). Significant visual loss is likely when there are nerve fibre layer haemorrhages, subretinal neovascularisation, cotton wool spots, choroidal folds or macular oedema. Papilloedema may be unilateral or asymmetrical, and optic nerve atrophy suggesting long-standing papilloedema may be present in up to 10% of patients. The appearances may be striking enough to mimic Foster Kennedy syndrome or AION.

Visual field abnormalities are frequent; enlargement of the blind spot and constriction of the fields are the most common manifestation. Other visual field defects include arcuate or centro-caecal scotomatous lesions, nasal visual field loss or loss of visual acuity alone. Visual field testing shows a greater sensitivity when compared with visual acuity and contrast sensitivity.

Venous sinus thrombosis leads to increased pressure within the dural sinuses which, in turn, causes poor absorption of CSF through the arachnoid granulations and this leads to papilloedema and headache. Venous sinus thrombosis is discussed in Chapter 5. The most important causes include:

- Hypercoagulable states
- Thrombocythaemia
- Behçet's disease
- Oral contraceptive use
- Pregnancy
- Local infection
- Iatrogenic trauma (e.g. subclavian vein thrombosis following catheter insertion)
- Mass lesions in the venous sinus (e.g. meningioma, metastases or cystic lesions).

IIH has been associated with a number of aetiological factors although clear evidence of a causal relationship is lacking. Endocrine disorders are likely to be important because of the strong female bias, association with obesity and the relationship of IIH to hypoparathyroidism and thyroid disorders, Addison's disease and Cushing's disease. IIH is also associated with obstructive sleep apnoea, medications including antibiotics (naladixic acid, ciprofloxacin, tetracyclines, minocycline and nitrofurantoin), hormonal medications including growth hormone and the oral contraceptive, and corticosteroids. The strongest link of IIH is with hypervitaminosis A or retinoid excess. Stopping the medication relieves the symptoms.

Investigations MRI shows that up to 70% of patients have an empty sella, presumably caused by long-standing effects of pulsatile high-pressure CSF causing downward herniation of the arachnoid through a defect in the diaphragm sellae. Other features include reversal of the optic nerve head, flattening of the posterior sclera, enhancement of the prelaminar optic nerve, distension of peri-optical subarachnoid space, vertical tortuosity of the orbital optic nerve and intraocular protrusion of the prelaminar optic nerve.

Poor prognostic features for visual loss include long-standing swelling of the optic disc with atrophy, visual field or acuity loss at first examination, delay in treatment, systemic hypertension, older age, male gender and increased intraocular pressure. Pre-existing disc anomalies such as drusen and an optic pit may also worsen the prognosis for visual outcome.

Management Medical treatment of the underlying condition includes weight loss with restriction of calorie, salt and fluid intake. Repeat lumbar punctures may be necessary and in self-limiting disease this approach may tide patients over until spontaneous remission.

Symptomatic therapy is routinely used. Acetazolomide is a strong carbonic anhydrase inhibitor that reduces CSF production and is highly effective in IIH. The dose is gradually increased to 0.5–1 g/day although higher doses are occasionally necessary. Many patients develop evidence of toxicity with digital or peri-orbital tingling, anorexia or a metallic taste. Other diuretics such as bendroflumethazide and can be used if acetazolomide is not tolerated. High-dose corticosteroids are normally only given in rare instances of severe visual failure in the short term, prior to CSF diversion surgery.

Surgical options, when required for intractable headache or progressive visual loss, include shunting and optic nerve sheath decompression (ONSD). The preferred shunt technique (normally either lumbar–peritoneal or ventricular–peritoneal) varies according to local expertise but effective shunting remains the best way of controlling headache and/or severe visual loss. ONSD is often used in instances when headache is minimal and visual loss is less severe, meaning that more invasive shunting procedures can be avoided.

Ocular involvement in other neurological disease

Uveomeningitic syndromes

Uveomeningitic syndromes are a group of disorders in which there is involvement of the uveal tract (either the iris, ciliary body or the choroid), the retina and the meninges. The causes are listed in Table 14.9.

Table 14.9 Causes of uveomeningitic syndromes.

Inflammatory	Vogt–Koyanagi–Harada Sarcoidosis Beçhet's syndrome SLE Wegener's granulomatosis
Infections	Borrelia, syphilis, TB, leprosy, *Neisseria meningitidis* Fungi – candida, coccidiodomycosis CMV, herpes simplex, HZV, HIV, hepatitis B SSPE
Neoplasia	Primary B-cell lymphoma Large cell or intravascular lymphoma Leukaemia Metastatic carcinoma, paraneoplastic
Primary ophthalmological	Acute posterior multifocal placoid pigment epitheliopathy Multiple evanescent white dot syndrome Posterior scleritis

CMV, cytomegalovirus; HZV, herpes zoster virus; SLE, systemic lupus erythematosus; SSPE, subacute sclerosing panencephalitis; TB, tuberculosis.

Sarcoidosis Up to 60% of patients with sarcoidosis may have ocular involvement and this may be the presenting feature (Chapter 26). Conjunctival nodules and uveitis are commonly associated conditions and posterior segment inflammation is particularly seen with neurological involvement. The optic nerve appears swollen because of the intraocular inflammation but may be directly involved by granulomas or meningeal change. Retinal abnormalities in sarcoidosis include periphlebitis with haemorrhages and choroidal granulomas.

Behçet's disease Inflammatory ocular disease can occur in 70% of patients and usually manifests itself as a bilateral panuveitis (Chapter 26). The pathognomonic features of the uveitis are a hypopyon in the anterior chamber and retinal infiltrates in the posterior segment. Recurrent attacks of retinal vein occlusion also occur and after sequential attacks optic atrophy and permanent visual loss ensue.

Inflammation of the optic nerve is unusual, but intracranial hypertension and papilloedema may develop in isolation or secondary to venous sinus thrombosis. Historically, visual prognosis has been poor as the ocular inflammation responds poorly to regular immunosuppressives but the introduction of biological agents such rituximab and infliximab is changing the outcomes.

Vogt–Koyanagi–Harada disease Vogt–Koyanagi–Harada disease (VKH) is a granulomatous multi-system inflammatory disorder that affects the eyes, the auditory system, meninges and the skin. The cause is unknown. There may be meningism, tinnitus and a CSF pleocytosis; skin involvement is characterised by alopecia, poliosis (whitening of the eyebrows) and vitiligo. Early ocular involvement is characterised by uveitis and serous retinal detachment. Late manifestations are usually bilateral and include choroidal and retinal depigmentation.

Table 14.10 Causes of retinal involvement in neurological disease.

Retinitis pigmentosa	Hereditary Neurodegenerative disorders – abetalipoproteinaemia (Bassen–Kornzweig syndrome), Refsum's disease, adrenoleukodystrophy
Salt and pepper retinopathy	Kearns–Sayre syndrome Hallervorden–Spatz disease
Cone–rod dystrophy	Multiple system atrophy Spinocerebellar atrophy type 7 Juvenile Batten's disease
Cherry red spot	Tay–Sachs disease Niemann–Pick disease Sialidosis
Paraneoplastic retinopathy	Cancer-associated retinopathy Melanoma-associated retinopathy
Viral retinitis	Acute retinal necrosis

Multiple sclerosis In MS (Chapter 11) the most common ocular manifestation is optic neuritis; however, symptomatic uveitis may occur in up to 3% of patients and asymptomatic changes in the retinal vessels including periphlebitis and sheathing or cuffing of the retinal veins with lymphocytes and plasma cells can be demonstrated on fluorescein angiography in a greater number. Visual loss in MS is therefore not always a result of optic neuritis but may, albeit rarely, be caused by uveitis with macular oedema, previous haemorrhage or retinal vascular change with neovascularisation.

Retinitis pigmentosa Retinitis pimentosa may occur as an isolated genetic defect or as part of a variety of other diseases in particular mitochondrial disorders (Table 14.10). Isolated hereditary forms of retinitis pigmentosa may be autosomal recessive (<60%), autosomal dominant (<25%) and, rarely, X-linked. The X-linked and recessive forms are typically more severe than the autosomal dominant form. More than 20 genes coding for this disorder have now been recognised but the most common abnormality lies in the genes for rhodopsin and peripherin.

The initial loss in the rod dystrophy form of retinitis pigmentosa occurs in the mid-peripheral visual field with an inability to see as clearly in dim light as in bright light (nyctalopsia). There is then a progressive loss of the peripheral visual field. The fundus initially shows a grey discoloration of the retinal pigment epithelium but with progression pigmented cells migrate into the retina leading to a characteristic bone spicule appearance with 'waxy' pallor of the optic nerve and attenuated retinal vessels.

In contrast, cone dystrophies are caused by involvement of the photoreceptors in the region of the macula. These cause blurred vision and an inability to see as clearly in bright light as in dim light. There is loss of the central field of vision manifest as a reduction in visual acuity or a central scotoma with loss of colour vision. Initially the fundus appears normal but as the condition progresses there is pigmentary degeneration of the macular ('bull's-eye maculopathy'). Eventually, optic disc pallor develops which mimics primary optic nerve disease.

Retinal pigmentary changes are associated with several forms of mitochondrial disease including neurogenic muscle weakness, ataxia and retinitis pigmentosa (NARP), myoclonic epilepsy, lactic acidosis, stroke-like episodes (MELAS) and Kearns–Sayre syndrome. In NARP, retinal involvement is manifest as a cone–rod dystrophy with variable involvement of each form of photoreceptors. The severity of the disease correlates with the extent of the mutation in mtDNA. Pigmentary change is noted in the first or second decade of life and associated with bilateral symmetrical ptosis. The macula is often affected initially followed by the peripheral retina with pigment clumping, atrophy and a 'salt and pepper' retinopathy. The visual acuity and fields are only mildly affected. There may be systemic and neurological involvement (Chapter 10). Retinal involvement has also occasionally been reported in subacute necrotising encephalopathy (Leigh's disease) which is also ascribed to a mitochondrial respiratory chain deficiency. Retinitis pigmentosa has also been associated with a variety of metabolic abnormalities affecting amino acid protein or lipoprotein metabolism (Chapter 19).

Neoplasia

Metastatic disease is the most common form of intraocular malignancy. Lesions may involve the choroid, retina or vitreous humor. The lung and breast are the most common primary sources. Primary intraocular lymphoma occurs in up to 25% of patients with primary CNS lymphoma but ocular involvement may occur in isolation. Ocular lesions are variable. There may be a posterior uveitis with vitreous cellular infiltration. The characteristic lesion is a subretinal infiltrate which appears creamy yellow and is associated with retinal pigment epithelial detachment. There may be discrete pale retinal lesions or vascular changes including vasculitis.

Paraneoplastic syndromes include carcinoma-associated retinopathy in which a progressive subacute bilateral visual loss is associated with pigmentary retinal change and arteriolar narrowing with sheathing. Patients who have the paraneoplastic disorder characterised by the IgG autoantibody CRMP-5 may present with progressive visual loss caused by a combination of vitritis, retinitis and optic neuritis. The optic disc becomes swollen, there is diffuse leakage from all retinal vessels and histologically lymphocytes are found throughout the retina, although on fundoscopy there is no frank area of white fluffy retinitis.

The phakomatoses in neuro-ophthalmology

The phakomatoses comprise a group of dominantly inherited diseases in which tumours both benign and malignant arise in different organ systems and in which tissues of ectodermal origin (CNS, skin and eye) are prominently involved.

Neurofibromatosis types 1 and 2 (Chapters 16 and 26)

Neurofibromatosis type 1 (NF1) is the most common with a frequency of about 1 in 3000. The gene has 100% penetrance but variable expression. NF1 is inherited as an autosomal dominant trait but about 50% of new cases are considered to be new mutations. The diagnostic criteria for NF1 are met if a person has two or more of the following:

- Six or more café au lait spots over 5 mm in greatest diameter in prepubertal individuals and 15 mm in post-pubertal individuals
- Two or more neurofibromas or one plexiform neuroma
- Axillary or inguinal freckles
- Optic glioma
- Two or more iris nodules

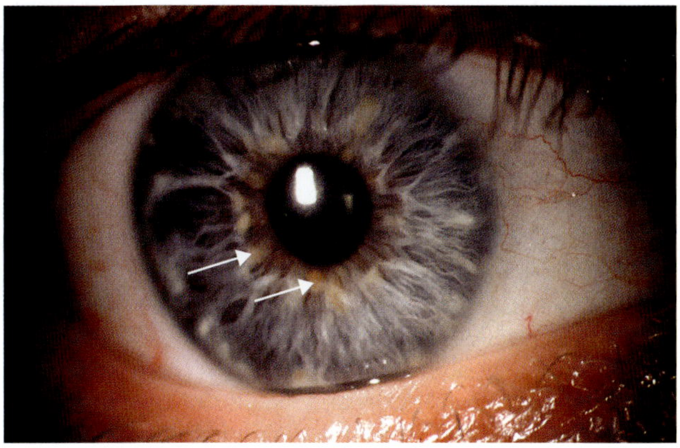

Figure 14.42 Iris hamartomas (Lisch nodules) in neurofibromatosis type 1 (NF1) (arrows).

- Distinctive osseous lesion (e.g. sphenoid dysplasia)
- A first degree relative with NF1.

Ocular features of NF1 include iris hamartomas, known as Lisch nodules (Figure 14.42) or melanocytic naevi which are detectable in about 50% of 5-year-olds, 75% of 15-year-olds and 95–100% of adults over 25 years. Individuals with NF1 may also have congenital glaucoma, anterior subcapsular cataract, posterior segment hamartomas, retinal vascular occlusions and pulsating exophthalmos due to sphenoid dysplasia. Retinal and choroidal hamartomas are occasionally seen, but these are a more typical feature of neurofibomatosis type 2 (NF2). Up to 70% of optic gliomas arise in patients with NF1 – typically these present in early childhood and have a benign histology and clinical course.

The gene for NF1 is located in the long arm of chromosome 17 – band q11.2. Within this gene is an area coding for a GAP-like protein which may act as a growth regulator interacting with an oncogene to produce benign and occasionally malignant tumours. The unpredictability of disease severity even in the same NF1 gene mutation makes genetic counselling difficult.

NF2 is a much rarer disease than NF1 with a population incidence of 1/33 000–40 000. At least 50% of new cases appear to be new mutations. Like NF1, NF2 has an extremely high penetrance. The hallmark of NF2 is the presence of bilateral vestibular nerve schwannomas: diagnostic criteria are met if a person has either of the following:

1. Bilateral VIIIth nerve masses seen with appropriate imaging
2. A first degree relative with NF2 and either unilateral VIIIth nerve mass or one of the following:
   - Neurofibromas
   - Meningioma
   - Glioma
   - Schwannoma
   - Juvenile posterior subcapsular lenticular opacity.

Patients with NF2 tend to develop tumours of neural converings and sheaths – meningiomas including optic nerve sheath meningiomas, schwannomas and ependymomas whereas those with NF1 tend to develop neural or astrocytic tumours – astrocytomas and gliomas. Although presentation in NF2 is typically the result of hearing loss, more than 75% of patients with NF2 have posterior subcapsular cataract, and occasionally optic nerve sheath meningioma. Other ocular findings include combined retinal pigment epithelial and retinal hamartomas, epiretinal membranes, optic disc gliomas, retinal haemangiomas, medullated nerve fibres, choroidal naevi, uveal melanoma and choroidal hamartoma. Lisch nodules are occasionally seen.

The NF2 gene is located on chromosome 22q band 11.2. In sporadic forms of the disease the vestibular schwannomas develop at a later age and may occur unilaterally.

Von Hippel–Lindau disease (Chapter 26)

Von Hippel–Lindau (VHL) disease is a pleiotrophic autosomal dominant inherited familial cancer syndrome characterised by a predisposition to develop haemangioblastomas of CNS and retina, renal cell carcinoma, phaeochromcytoma and renal, pancreatic and epididymal cysts. The minimum birth incidence in the United Kingdom is 1/36 000. The gene for VHL disease has been mapped to chromosome 3p25-p26, and the clinical importance lies in the fact that long-term morbidity and mortality can be reduced by presymptomatic diagnosis of ocular, CNS and renal involvement.

Although clinical heterogeneity is common, retinal angiomatosis is the most frequent initial manifestation and develops in more than 70% of patients by the age of 60 years. Retinal haemangiomas (or more correctly, haemangioblastomas) are most commonly seen in the peripheral retina but may also occur on the optic disc itself. Ophthalmological screening requires dilated direct and indirect fundoscopy together with fluorescein angioscopy for the detection of nascent, preclinical lesions.

Current criteria for diagnosis of VHL are as follows.

A. Without family history, two of the following:
- Retinal or CNS haemangioblastoma
- Phaeochromocytoma
- Renal cell carcinoma, or
- Renal/pancreatic/epididymal cysts.

B. Positive family history, one of the above.

Current screening recommendations in an affected individual are:
1. Annual physical examination and urinalysis including 24-hour vanillylmandelic acid levels (VMAs)
2. Annual ophthalmological examinations
3. Brain imaging 3-yearly to age 50, then 5-yearly
4. Annual renal ultrasound and 3-yearly abdominal CT scanning.

When screening of an at risk relative is required, this protocol is modified so that the eyes are examined from age of 5 years (with fluorescein angioscopy from age 10), brain imaging is undertaken 3-yearly from age 15 to 40 and then 5-yearly, and abdominal imaging is commenced from age 20.

Tuberous sclerosis

The triad of epilepsy, retinal tumours and adenoma sebaceum referred to as tuberous sclerosis or Bourneville's disease has now been widened and the term tuberous sclerosis complex (TSC) is applied. All tissues are involved, most typically brain and retina but also skin, heart, kidneys and lungs. TSC is inherited as an autosomal dominant trait showing marked genetic heterogeneity. It appears that different families may have different mutations: in some pedigrees the mutation location is at chromosome 9q34.1-q34.2 and in others it is at 11q14-q23. Diagnosis is based on the presence of:
1. Cortical tubers, or
2. Multiple hamartomas associated with cortical tubers:
   - Subependymal nodules
   - Facial angiofibromas
   - Renal angiomyofibroma

and three other associated lesions:
- Giant cell astrocytomas
- Retinal hamartoma
- Ungual fibroma
- Fibrous forehead plaque.

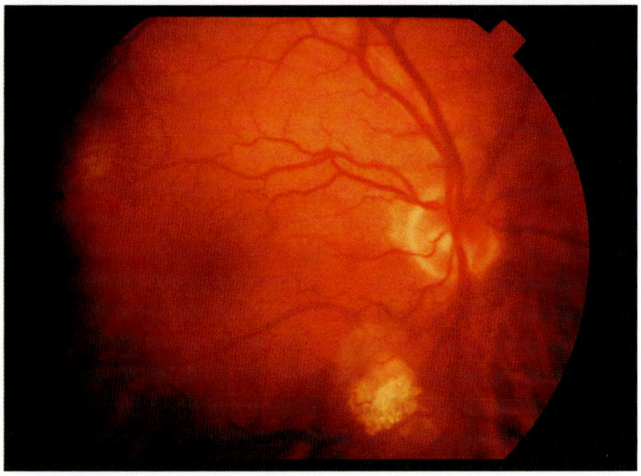

Figure 14.43 Retinal hamartomas in a patient with tuberous sclerosis.

Fifty per cent of patients have retinal or optic nerve hamartomas: other ocular abnormalities include adenoma sebaceum on the eyelids and colobomas. A wide range of neuro-ophthalmic features including retrochiasmal field defects, ocular motility abnormalities and papilloedema reflect intracranial involvement. The retinal hamartomas may be calcified or non-calcified lesions of both glioblastic and angioblastic origin – patches of focal congenital retinal pigment epithelial hypertrophy may also be seen (Figure 14.43). In contrast to VHL disease, retinal hamartomas in TSC are only rarely associated with visual loss. The differential diagnosis of non-calcified hamartomas includes retinoblastoma in infants, and calcified hamartomas on the optic nerve may resemble florid calcified peripapillary disc drusen seen in retinitis pigmentosa.

Sturge–Weber syndrome (encephalo-trigeminal angiomatosis)

Sturge–Weber syndrome (SWS) is a further vascular neuro-cutaneous syndrome often classed alongside the phakomatoses, but without a familial basis or associated tumours. Typically, angiomas involve the meninges and the skin of the face, typically the ophthalmic (V_1) and maxillary (V_2) distributions of the trigeminal nerve, giving rise to the cutaneous facial port-wine stain. Ipsilateral intracranial calcifying meningeal lesions affect the ipsilateral parietal and occipital regions leading to epilepsy, developmental delay, learning disability and homonymous visual field loss. Ocular involvement is characterised by glaucoma as well as haemangiomas of the choroid, conjunctiva and episclera. In type 1 SWS, both facial and leptomeningeal angiomata arise and patients may have glaucoma; in type 2, facial angiomata and glaucoma arise without leptomeningeal involvement, and in type 3 there is isolated leptomeningeal involvement without a facial angioma or glaucoma.

Abnormalities of eye movements

Diplopia

Disturbances of eye movements may occur as a consequence of either reduced or excessive ocular motility. Diplopia results from:
- Dysfunction of the extraocular muscles, caused by local factors
- Impairment of neuromuscular junction

- Disturbance of the cranial nerves at any point throughout their long course
- Lesions at a nuclear or supranuclear level within the brainstem or central pathways.

Oscillopsia (illusory movement of static objects) results from nystagmus or saccadic intrusion. Binocular diplopia is caused by ocular misalignment and therefore resolves if one eye is covered and is absent if there is severe monocular visual impairment. Monocular diplopia persists if one eye is closed and is generally caused by local eye disease, refractive error or functional disorders.

The character and pattern of diplopia should be established by history and examination. It is important to clarify whether the separation of images is maximal on vertical, horizontal or oblique gaze, whether any corrective head position is favoured and whether the diplopia is worse at a distance (typically in a VIth nerve palsy) or for near objects (e.g. medial rectus palsy). Diplopia is worse when looking in the field of action of a paretic muscle or in the opposite field to a restricted muscle (i.e. when it is being stretched). Diplopia may be absent, despite ocular misalignment, if there is impaired acuity in one eye, if the separation is particularly wide or narrow and the false image can be suppressed or if the ocular misalignment is long-standing or has been present from birth. The presence of pain on eye movement suggests a local orbital or myopathic process while orbital or peri-orbital pain is characteristic of vascular, neoplastic, inflammatory or infective disorders.

The principles of examination of the extraocular movements are outlined in Chapter 4. The presence of pupillary asymmetry or impaired reactions may be important (e.g. a fixed dilated pupil may indicate parasympathetic involvement in a compressive IIIrd nerve palsy). Involvement of other cranial nerves (e.g. II, V, VII and VIII) is important in localising lesions and a proptosis suggests thyroid ophthalmoparesis or a structural lesion of the orbit. Ocular alignment should be assessed by the corneal light reflex or cover test and the eye movement examination includes assessment of ocular motility in each eye in the nine positions of gaze. The presence of associated local factors (e.g. orbital swelling or dry eyes) or neurological features (e.g. other cranial nerve lesions) may be of localising importance.

Vertical diplopia is present when the patient sees two images displaced vertically or diagonally and suggests impairment of any or all of the superior or inferior recti or oblique muscles. Torsional diplopia from underaction of the oblique muscles is associated with an angular head tilt. Horizontal diplopia, in which the images appear side by side, is usually brought about by involvement of the medial or lateral rectus muscles.

Orbital disease

The principal causes of restrictive ophthalmopathy are summarised in Table 14.11.

Table 14.11 Causes of restrictive ophthalmoplegia (progressive infiltration and fibrosis of extraocular muscles).

Dysthyroid eye disease	
Orbital pseudotumour (myositis)	
Primary or metastatic orbital tumours	Lymphoma
Other orbital masses	Paranasal sinus mucocoele
Intracranial masses extending into orbit	Sphenoid wing meningioma
Infiltration of extraocular muscles	Sarcoidosis, amyloidosis, acromegaly, infection
Entrapment of extraocular muscle due to trauma	
Caroticocavernous fistula	

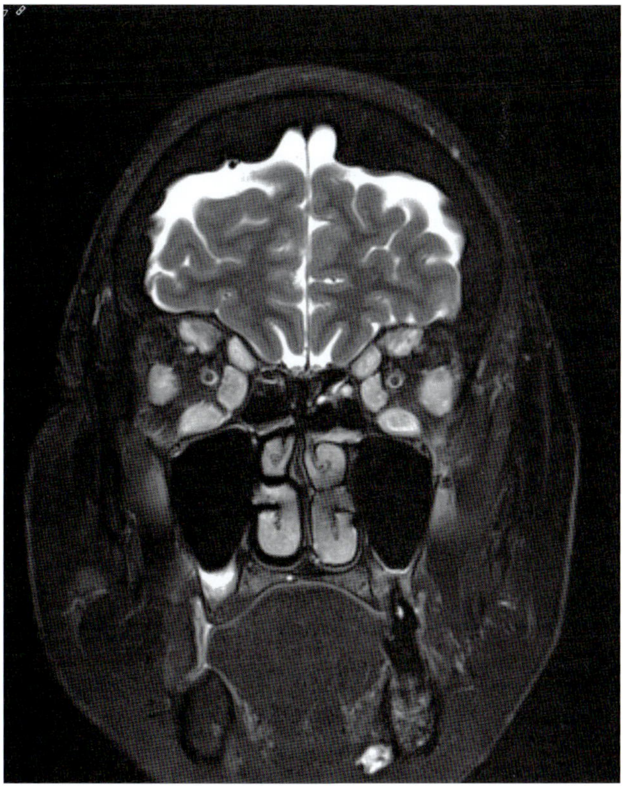

Figure 14.44 MRI scan (T2-weighted) showing extraocular muscle thickening in thyroid eye disease.

Thyroid ophthalmopathy

Thyroid ophthalmology is a common cause of proptosis with horizontal or vertical diplopia. It is associated with Graves' disease in >50% of patients and most of these patients are hyperthyroid at the time of diagnosis (Figure 14.44).

Two phases of the disease are recognised: active and fibrotic. In the active phase, the patient develops lid changes (upper lid retraction and lid lag, puffiness), conjunctival congestion (chemosis), orbital congestion (proptosis) and extraocular muscle swelling (ophthalmoplegia) in association with water and glycosaminoglycan deposition in the orbital structures together with an inflammatory infiltrate. Vision may be compromised either by such severe proptosis as to cause corneal exposure, or by optic nerve compression at the orbital apex leading to visual failure. Choroidal folds or optic nerve swelling may be seen although fundal examination may be normal.

In the fibrotic phase of the disease, evidence of inflammation (pain, conjunctival congestion, vascular engorgement at the site of tendon insertions into the globe) resolves leaving the patient with variable degrees of proptosis, lid lag and ophthalmoplegia. The limitation of eye movements in the fibrotic phase is principally caused by the healing with fibrosis of the inflammatory infiltrate of the acute phase leaving a restrictive myopathy. In some patients the acute phase is florid and readily diagnosed; in others it is limited and subclinical so that the patient presents later with a restrictive myopathy. The disease may be highly asymmetric or unilateral; extraocular muscle involvement may be selective or generalised. The inferior and medial recti are the two most commonly involved muscles. The diagnosis is made from the history and typical physical signs. Sometimes orbital signs are minimal or absent so that the patient may present with diplopia, most commonly vertical but lid retraction is still usually present.

Treatment of the endocrine disorder rarely affects the thyroid ophthalmology, and although ocular motility defects and lid problems may be treated by elective surgery, compressive optic neuropathy requires high-dose corticosteroids and sometimes urgent endoscopic surgical decompression.

Orbital inflammatory syndromes

Non-specific idiopathic inflammatory disorders cause double vision associated with marked local pain and may be classified according to their mode of onset, anatomical localisation and physical signs or histopathological subtype. In particular they may be divided into:

- *Orbital pseudotumour* when the inflammation primarily involves the structures in and around the orbit (sclera, ocular muscles and lids).
- *Tolosa–Hunt syndrome* when the inflammation primarily involves the cavernous sinus and superior orbital fissure.
- *Orbital inflammation:* the cellular component of the infiltrate is highly variable but includes mature T lymphocytes, plasma cells, macrophages, eosinophils and polymorpholeukocytes. Connective tissue may show oedema, fibrosis or sclerosis. Clinically, orbital inflammation is associated with localised ipsilateral pain, conjunctival injection, unilateral lid oedema and erythema, proptosis, ophthalmoplegia and a palpable orbital mass.

In Tolosa–Hunt syndrome, involvement of the superior orbital fissure is characterised by:

- Proptosis
- Ophthalmoplegia
- Trigeminal sensory loss
- Horner's syndrome.

Ophthalmoplegia without proptosis suggests cavernous sinus involvement.

Orbital myositis is often unilateral and occasionally only a single muscle is affected but any combination of extraocular muscles may be involved. Symptoms may be caused by paresis or restriction but conjunctival injection and pain on eye movements are characteristic.

Imaging is essential to assess possible orbital mass lesions and paranasal sinus disease: extraocular muscle enlargement in thyroid ophthalmology spares the tendon insertions into the globe in contrast to other inflammatory diseases. The course of orbital inflammatory pseudotumour, orbital myositis and Tolosa–Hunt syndrome is usually one of prompt response to systemic steroids but then relapse as the steroids are reduced which may prompt the use of additional steroid-sparing agents such as azathioprine, methotrexate or mycophenolate mofetil.

Lymphoid tumours are the most common orbital neoplasms and are the most important differential diagnosis of the inflammatory orbital syndromes. If prompt response to steroids does not occur then a biopsy should be considered. Other primary and systemic syndromes must be considered in the differential diagnosis of orbital inflammatory syndromes. Inflammatory disease of the orbit may be infective, particularly in children when it is a medical emergency. In orbital cellulitis, ophthalmoplegia is associated with fever and lid swelling. Proptosis occurs with paranasal sinus or metastatic infection.

Mucormycosis (Chapter 9) is an acute fungal infection which occurs in the immuno-compromised patient and is particularly associated with diabetic ketoacidosis, haematological malignancy and organ transplantation. Rhino-orbital cerebral mucormycosis develops by inhaling spores onto the oral and nasal mucosa following which direct invasion of the orbits occurs via the paranasal sinuses or the brain and via the sphenoid sinus, superior orbital fissure, cribriform plate or via the orbital vessels and nerves. The condition is characteristically unilateral with an acute onset of fever, headache, sinusitis, peri-orbital pain, cellulitis, rhinorrhoea and trigeminal anaesthesia. Ophthalmic involvement is a result of direct fungal infiltration or ischaemic infarction and this leads to acute ophthalmoplegia, proptosis, peri-orbital oedema and blindness from central retinal artery occlusion or an optic neuropathy. Mucormycosis may cause an orbital apex or cavernous sinus syndrome. Neurological involvement may lead to internal carotid artery occlusion, meningitis or cerebral abscess. Radiology shows mucosal thickening, orbital infiltration, bony destruction or ophthalmic vein thrombosis. However, tissue diagnosis is usually established by nasal biopsy demonstrating large branching hyphae that invade the vessels. Mucormycosis carries a high mortality rate and requires aggressive antifungal treatment and surgical debridement.

Inflammatory disease of the orbit may be caused by granulomatous disease (tuberculosis, sarcoidosis), systemic vasculitis (granulomatous polyangiitis) or neoplasm (lymphoma or metastasis). Metastatic cancer (particular breast) may spread to the orbit causing unilateral or bilateral inflammatory masses. Lymphoid neoplasm tends to develop at a later age, is often bilateral and is less characteristically associated with pain or ophthalmoplegia.

Cavernous sinus thrombosis

A number of conditions may lead to thrombosis within the cavernous sinus. Infection may spread from local structures either directly or via vascular pathways (e.g. facial and dental infections, sinusitis, otitis media or orbital cellulitis). Underlying medical conditions that may predispose to cavernous sinus thrombosis include diabetes mellitus, malignancy and collagen vascular disease. There is usually peri-orbital pain with proptosis, cheimosis, ptosis and ophthalmoplegia.

Patients may present with headache, nausea and vomiting, occasionally encephalopathy and early involvement of the VIth nerve occurs before total ophthalmoplegia develops. With increasing venous stasis optic disc swelling may develop leading to optic neuropathy or retinal ischaemia. Meningitis or cerebral abscess is associated with extension beyond the cavernous sinus. The CSF may show meningitis and imaging confirms involvement of the cavernous sinus and superior ophthalmic vein. Other causes of lesions of the cavernous sinus are considered later.

Carotico-cavernous fistula

Carotico-cavernous fistula (CCF) is an abnormal arteriovenous communication between the carotid artery and the cavernous sinus. The fistula is considered:

- *Direct:* if the arterial supply is derived from the internal carotid artery itself, or
- *Indirect:* if the supply is via the extradural meningeal branches of the internal or external carotid artery.

The fistula is indirect in >90% of cases and may be located anywhere along the course of the intracavernous carotid artery. It may project anteriorly or posteriorly.

The most common cause of CCF is head trauma which may be either penetrating or non-penetrating and not necessarily associated with a fracture of the skull base. Other causes include rupture of an intracavernous aneurysm, systemic vasculopathy, Ehlers–Danlos syndrome or fibromuscular dysplasia. Direct CCF may present within a few days of trauma but indirect CCF may be delayed and manifest with mild signs such as red eye and subtle orbital congestion. If the blood escapes posteriorly through the superior and inferior petrosal sinuses, ocular signs may be minimal although an expanded inferior petrosal sinus will cause direct compression of the VIth cranial nerve. However, anterior flow of high pressure arterial blood into the orbital veins leads to raised episcleral venous pressure, reduced arterial perfusion pressure and venous stasis. Although the signs are usually ipsilateral, the contralateral eye may be involved because of the variable connections between the two cavernous sinuses.

In an anterior direct CCF there is pulsatile proptosis associated with chemosis, arterialisation of the conjunctival vessels and an orbital bruit. Ophthalmoplegia may be a result of compression of the cranial nerves within the cavernous sinus or direct muscle involvement with orbital hypoxia and oedema due to venous stasis. Visual loss occurs as a result of retinal ischaemia, ischaemic optic neuropathy, intracranial optic nerve compression or corneal ulceration. These effects result from a reduction in retinal blood flow, because of a drop in effective ophthalmic artery perfusion pressure, together with venous stasis caused by arterialisation of the orbital venous circulation. Fundal examination shows features of a slow flow retinopathy with mild disc swelling, blot haemorrhages and micro-aneurysms, venous congestion and tortuosity. Central retinal vein occlusion, glaucoma, retinal detachment and vitreous haemorrhage may occur. The diagnosis is established on imaging by enlargement of the superior ophthalmic vein. Rapid diagnosis is essential because high intracranial venous pressure may cause venous haemorrhage. Transarterial balloon embolisation is the most effective treatment.

Indirect CCFs are low-flow dural-based arteriovenous malformations which are typically non-traumatic. Symptoms are often mild with conjunctival injection, mild ophthalmoplegia and elevated intraocular pressure or retinal vasculopathy which may threaten vision. Rarely, orbital congestion may become severe if there is thrombosis of the superior ophthalmic vein. MRI may show distension of the cavernous sinus, of the superior ophthalmic vein and enlargement of the extraocular muscles. Endovascular treatment is indicated if there is significant posterior venous hypertension with the risk of associated cortical venous thrombosis, or if there is significant intraocular pressure rise and risk of visual loss.

Myopathy

Myopathy involving the extraocular muscles leads to progressive ophthalmoparesis termed chronic progressive external ophthalmoplegia. This syndrome is brought about by a number of causes, each associated with limitation of eye movements and ptosis but normal pupillary function. Because of the slowly progressive and painless onset, patients are often asymptomatic. Oculocephalic and caloric stimulation do not increase the range of movements reflecting the infranuclear origin of the limitation and there is often symmetrical ptosis and moderate orbicularis oculi weakness.

Mitochondrial disease

Mitochondrial myopathy (Chapter 10) is an important cause of chronic progressive external ophthalmoplegia (CPEO) (Table 14.12) which may be an isolated finding in cases with mitochondrial or Mendelian autosomal recessive or dominant transmission. Sporadic mitochondrial DNA deletions or duplications are more common than maternally inherited cases. Dominant and recessive forms are associated with genetic mutations in *ANT1, POLG, POLG2* and *PEO* genes. There may be an associated 'salt and pepper' retinopathy or a symptomatic field constriction with bone spicules and disc pallor typical of retinitis pigmentosa.

In Kearns–Sayre syndrome, CPEO, ptosis and retinitis pigmentosa (developing before the age of 20) are associated with cardiac conduction deficit (heart block often requiring a pacemaker), cerebellar signs and a raised CSF protein. CPEO is also prominent in mitochondrial gastrointestinal encephalomyopathy. Muscle biopsy shows the presence of 'ragged red fibres' within a population of relatively normal fibres on modified Gomori trichrome staining representing degenerate mitochondria. Electron microscopy confirms abnormal morphology of the mitochondria. A deletion in the mitochondrial DNA can be detected in >90% of patients with Kearns–Sayre syndrome and in 50% with CPEO alone.

Oculopharyngeal dystrophy

This is an inherited dystrophy affecting extraocular and bulbar muscles which is usually transmitted in an autosomal dominant pattern but rarely may be recessive. Bulbar weakness, if prominent, leads to severe dysarthria and dysphagia, predominantly affecting liquids with marked nasal regurgitation. There is bilateral ptosis, progressive ophthalmoplegia and facial weakness with occasional involvement of the jaw muscles leading to difficulty chewing. Muscle biopsy shows characteristic vacuolar myopathy with tubules.

Table 14.12 Causes of progressive external ophthalmoplegia.

Mitochondrial myopathy – Kearns–Sayre
Myopathy
Congenital – central core, multicore, centronuclear, myotubular, nemaline
Congenital oculopharyngeal
Myotonic dystrophy
Neuromuscular junction – Myasthenia gravis, Botulism
Neurogenic disease
aBetalipoproteinaemia
Spinocerebellar ataxia

Other causes of myopathy affecting the extraocular muscles include abetalipoproteinaemia (Chapter 19) which is characterised by childhood onset of CPEO, retinopathy and chronic fatty diarrhoea. There is malabsorption, low serum cholesterol and complete absence of beta lipoprotein.

Neuromuscular junction abnormalities

Ocular myasthenia gravis is discussed in Chapter 10. The ophthalmoparesis is variable and may mimic any abnormal eye movement. It often fluctuates with prominent fatigability and variable ptosis. Nystagmus of an abducting eye mimicking internuclear ophthalmoplegia may occur and can develop rarely in the absence of extraocular muscle limitation. Weakness of orbicularis oculi is usually associated. In long-standing ocular myasthenia there may be a severe fixed ophthalmoplegia with ptosis which may be difficult to distinguish from myopathy or mitochondrial disorder. Extraocular muscle involvement may be found in congenital myasthenia but is not common in paraneoplastic Lambert–Eaton myasthenic syndrome.

Botulism (Chapters 9 and 20) is associated with external ophthalmoplegia and ptosis which may preceed the develop of dilated, poorly reactive pupils and paralysis of accommodation. The presence of associated gastrointestinal symptoms and muscarinic anticholinergic effects helps to distinguish botulism from myasthenia gravis.

Cranial nerve palsies

Oculomotor nerve (IIIrd nerve palsy)

The IIIrd nerve originates in several subnuclei in the dorsal midbrain (Table 14.13). The fascicles exit the brainstem ventrally in close relation to the red nucleus and cortico-spinal tract. The nerve traverses the subarachnoid space and passes through the lateral wall of the cavernous sinus (Table 14.14). Just before entering the orbit via the superior orbital fissure, it divides into a superior branch, which innervates the levator palpabrae superioris and the superior rectus, and an inferior branch which innervates the inferior and medial recti, the inferior oblique and the iris sphincter and ciliary muscle. In the subarachnoid space and cavernous sinus the pupillomotor fibres

Table 14.13 Causes of oculomotor (IIIrd) nerve palsy.

Location	Clinical features	Aetiology
Nucleus	III (i/l) but with c/l superior rectus involved. Ptosis either bilateral or absent	Infarction Haemorrhage Trauma Tumour Infection
Fascicular	Signs of midbrain impairment – c/l ataxia, cerebellar tremor, hemiparesis, choreiform movements	Infarction Haemorrhage Tumour Demyelination Syphilis Trauma
Subarachnoid space	Usually isolated May be headache or orbital pain	Aneurysm (PCommA, ICA, basilar, PCA) Ischaemic (microvascular) Tumour (meningioma, chordoma, pituitary, metastases, carcinomatous meningitis) Infectious (meningitis, syphilis, *Borrelia*, herpes zoster) Herniation Trauma
Tentorial edge	Uncal herniation	Raised intracranial pressure Idiopathic intracranial hypertension Hydrocephalus Trauma
Cavernous sinus and superior orbital fissure	IV, VI, VII, sympathetic fibres (Horner's); V_1 or its branches	(Table 14.14)
Orbital	Optic neuropathy, chemosis, conjunctival injection, proptosis	Trauma Tumour Inflammatory Infection (fungal) Dural arteriovenous malformation Sphenoid sinus mucocoele

i/l, ipsilateral; c/l, contralateral; ICA, internal carotid artery; i/l, ipsilateral; PCA, posterior cerebral artery; PcommA, posterior communicating artery.

Table 14.14 Causes of lesions of the oculomotor nerve in the cavernous sinus.

Tumours	Pituitary adenoma, meningioma, nasopharyngeal carcinoma, plasmacytoma, Hodgkin's disease and non-Hodgkin lymphoma, haemangioma, VIth nerve tumour, sphenoid sinus tumour, skull base tumour
Vascular	Cavernous sinus thrombosis, dural carotico-cavernous fistula, superior ophthalmologic vein thrombosis Internal carotid artery – aneurysm, dissection, occlusion Posteror communicating artery aneurysm Microvascular occlusion
Sphenoid sinus mucocoele	
Infection	Herpes zoster
Inflammatory	Tolosa–Hunt syndrome, vasculitis, Granulomatosis with polyangiitis (Wegener's granulomatosis)

of the IIIrd nerve lie superficially and dorsally and are vulnerable to compression from above. The IIIrd nerve supplies the medial rectus, inferior oblique, inferior rectus and superior rectus muscles, the lid levator and the parasympathetic innervation of the pupillary sphincter and ciliary body. Patients with a IIIrd nerve palsy complain of binocular diplopia. With a complete lesion there is ptosis, a fixed dilated pupil and the eye is deviated 'downward and outward' with residual function only in abduction (lateral rectus) and intorsion (superior oblique). Elevation, depression and adduction of the eye are impaired. With partial lesions involvement of extraocular muscles is incomplete and the pattern may resemble myopathic or restrictive disorders. In microvascular disease, the perforating vasae nervorum are primarily occluded affecting the central fibres and extraocular movements, and sparing the pupillomotor fibres.

Aberrant reinnervation (oculomotor synkinesis) is relatively common following oculomotor nerve injury or prolonged compression as with meningioma or aneurysm. A number of characteristic patterns are seen. These include co-contraction of the levator and medial rectus on attempted adduction or co-contraction of levator and inferior rectus on attempted down-gaze and pupillary constriction on medial or downward eye movement.

Abducens (V1th) nerve palsy

Abducens nerve palsy causes binocular horizontal diplopia due to ipsilateral rectus paresis with a primary position esotropia. The causes are summarised in Table 14.15.

The VIth nerve nucleus is located in the caudal paramedian pontine tegmentum beneath the floor of the IVth ventricle. The facial nerve loops around the nucleus and the medial longitudinal fasciculus (MLF) passes medially. The fascicle has a long intrapontine course and lesions are frequently associated with other neurological signs. It emerges from the brainstem ventrally and traverses the subarachnoid space in close relationship to the anterior inferior cerebellar artery. Within the cavernous sinus it lies free in the body unsupported by the sinus wall (unlike III and IV) before passing through the annular segment of the superior orbital fissure to innervate the lateral rectus muscle.

Trochlear (IVth) nerve palsy

Trochlear nerve palsy causes binocular vertical diplopia with tilting of objects (torsional diplopia) which is worse on looking down and is caused by ipsilateral superior oblique weakness (Table 14.16). There is elevation of the affected eye with vertical diplopia and head tilt away from the side of the lesion.

The trochlear nerve originates in the dorsal midbrain. The fascicle passes laterally to the aqueduct and exits the midbrain dorsally. The nerves cross in the superior medullary velum before passing around the midbrain tectum to reach the free end of the tentorium and then pass forward into the wall of the cavernous sinus. The nerve enters the orbit through the superior orbital fissure and innervates the contralateral superior oblique muscle.

Congenital trochlear palsy is relatively common and may be caused by aplasia of the nucleus or a developmental anomaly of the superior oblique tendon in the orbit. The trochlear nerve is rarely involved by intrinsic brainstem lesions because of the short intramedullary course of its fascicle. Isolated trochlear nuclear lesions cause a contralateral superior oblique palsy. There is usually also a Horner's syndrome ipsilateral to the lesion because of the proximity of sympathetic fibres. Bilateral IVth nerve palsy may be caused by a lesion in the superior medullary velum.

The most common cause of trochlear palsy is trauma, possibly because the tectum of the midbrain shifts as a result of contre-coup trauma and may compress the IVth nerve either in the superior medullary velum or against the tentorial notch. Microvascular ischaemic disease may also cause IVth nerve palsy. Other causes of IVth nerve palsy are summarised in Table 14.16.

Painful and combined ophthalmoplegia

Multiple ocular motor palsies are usually unilateral and result from lesions in the cavernous sinus or superior orbital fissure. The principal causes are summarised in Table 14.17.

Bilateral lesions suggest a diffuse disorder of muscle (see Myopathies), a neuromuscular abnormality (e.g. myasthenia gravis) or a neurogenic cause (e.g. Guillain–Barré syndrome, Miller Fisher syndrome), diffuse infiltrative brainstem lesions, infection or neoplastic disease affecting the meninges. Painful combined ophthalmoplegia is usually caused by inflammatory, neoplastic or vascular disease; other causes are summarised in Table 14.18.

Central disorders of eye movements

Normal vision requires the ability to shift gaze rapidly to bring an object of attention into foveal vision (saccadic system) and a system to stabilise the new image on this area even if there is movement of the object (smooth pursuit and vergence) or of the head and body (vestibulo-ocular and opto-kinetic reflexes). The anatomical and physiological basis of these systems is discussed in specialised texts.

Supranuclear eye movement abnormalities result when the cerebral, cerebellar and brainstem afferent inputs to the ocular motor nuclear are disrupted.

Saccadic eye movements

The assessment of saccadic eye movements is mentioned briefly in Chapter 4. They are best examined by telling the patient to fixate alternately between two targets: saccades in each direction can be examined in each field of gaze in both horizontal and vertical planes. The examiner notes whether the saccades are of normal velocity, promptly initiated, accurate and conjugate.

Table 14.15 Causes of abducens (VIth) nerve palsy.

Location	Clinical features	Aetiology
Nuclear	Horizontal gaze palsy (rostrolateral pons) c/l internuclear ophthalmoplegia	Möbius' syndrome Duane's syndrome Infection Tumour Demyelination Wernicke's encephalopathy Trauma
Fascicular	i/l dysmetria, i/l Horner's, c/l internuclear ophthalmoplegia	Infection Demyelination Tumour Inflammation Wernicke–Korsakoff syndrome
Subarachnoid	i/l dysmetria, c/l hemiparesis	Aneurysm – ICA Subarachnoid haemorrhage Trauma Infections – meningitis, syphilis, borrelia, TB, HIV Inflammatory – vasculitis, sarcoid, SLE, Wegener's granulomatosis Tumour – VI nerve, cerebellopontine angle, clivus, lymphoma, carcinomatous meningitis Raised intracranial pressure
Petrous apex	VI, VII, deafness. Facial pain	Infection of mastoid or tip of petrous bone Otitis media Gradenigo's syndrome Thrombosis of inferior petrous sinus or transverse/sigmoid sinus Trauma Downward displacement of brainstem by supratentorial mass Tumour – nasopharyngeal
Cavernous sinus and superior orbital fissure	III, IV, V_I, sympathetic	ICA aneurysm/dissection Cavernous sinus thrombosis Carotico-cavernous fistula Tumour (pituitary adenoma, nasopharyngeal carcinoma, meningioma) Sphenoid mucocoele Tolosa–Hunt syndrome Infection – VZV
Orbital	Ophthalmoplegia, proptosis, chemosis	Tumour Infiltration Infection Trauma

c/l, contralateral; i/l, ipsilateral; ICA, internal carotid artery; SLE, systemic lupus erythematosus; TB, tuberculosis; VZV, varicella zoster virus.

Disorders of saccadic eye movements consist of abnormalities of velocity, accuracy, initiation, premature termination of gaze during saccades and the presence of saccadic intrusions and oscillations.

Velocity Slow saccadic movements occur either in the direction of a paretic extraocular muscle or, if there is an internuclear ophthalmoplegia, in adduction. Slow saccades with a full range of movement occur in degenerative disorders affecting the parapontine reticular formation: spinocerebellar ataxia, Alzheimer's, Parkinson's and Huntington's diseases. Slowing of vertical saccades is characteristic of progressive supranuclear palsy (PSP) while prolonged latency of saccadic movements is seen in corticobasal degeneration. In myasthenia the initial velocity of the saccade may be abnormally fast with fatigue during the course of the movement.

Accuracy Dysmetric (inaccurate) saccades are seen in cerebellar disorders, neurodegenerative conditions or as a consequence of drug toxicity (particularly anticonvulsants). In lesions of the

Table 14.16 Causes of trochlear (IVth) nerve palsy.

Nuclear and fascicular	Aplasia Haemorrhage/infarction (mesencephalic) Tumour AVM Trauma Demyelination Neurosurgical complication
Subarachnoid	Trauma Tumour – pineal, tentorial meningioma, ependymoma, haemangioblastoma, metastases Aneurysm – superior cerebellar, PCA, PCommA Hydrocephalus Meningitis (infectious, neoplastic) Superficial siderosis Inflammatory – Wegener's granulomatosis
Cavernous sinus and superior orbital fissure	Tumour (pituitary adenoma, nasopharyngeal carcinoma, meningioma) Tolosa–Hunt syndrome Infection – VZV Carotid aneurysm/dissection Cavernous sinus thrombosis Carotico-cavernous fistula
Petrous	Infection of mastoid or tip of petrous bone Thrombosis of inferior petrous sinus Trauma Downward displacement of brainstem by supratentorial mass Aneurysm, AVM
Orbital	Trauma Tumour infiltration
Unknown	Microvascular infarction

AVM, arteriovenous malformation; PCA, posterior cerebral artery; PCommA, posterior communicating artery.

cerebellar vermis and brachium conjunctivum, saccades may have an abnormally large amplitude (hypermetric) away from the side of the lesion. Saccadic hypermetria leads to macro-saccadic oscillation around the target. These oscillations may also be associated with hypometric saccades.

Initiation Delayed initiation of saccadic movements and prolonged latency may be caused by lesions anywhere within the saccadic pathways, particularly frontal, collicular or pontine damage. Saccadic latency is increased in PSP and cortico-basal degeneration. Ocular motor apraxia is characterised by loss of voluntary control of saccadic and pursuit eye movements with preservation of reflex movements, especially slow and quick phases of the vestibulo-ocular reflex. Patients have difficulty in making horizontal and vertical saccades to command although reflex and random saccades are normal. Ocular motor apraxia may be congenital but when acquired indicates bilateral hemispheric disease and is particularly associated with Balint's syndrome and cortical visual loss (see Visual cortex). Abnormalities of saccadic initiation are also common in parkinsonian syndromes and progressive ataxia.

Table 14.17 Causes of unilateral multiple ocular motor nerve palsies.

Location	Clinical features	Aetiology
Brainstem	Supranuclear signs i/l limb ataxia c/l involuntary movements c/l hemiparesis i/l VII	Haemorrhage/infarction Tumour Infection – encephalitis
Subarachnoid		Meningitis (infectious, neoplastic) Trauma Tumour – clivus Aneurysm – superior cerebellar, PCA, PcommA
Cavernous sinus and superior orbital fissure	III, IV, V_I, VI, VII, sympathetic fibres	Tumour (pituitary adenoma, nasopharyngeal carcinoma, meningioma, cavernous angioma, lymphoma, myeloma, lymphoma, Waldenström's, metastases [breast, lung, prostate]) Carotid aneurysm, occlusion/dissection Cavernous sinus thrombosis Carotico-cavernous fistula Cavernous sinus sepsis Tolosa–Hunt syndrome Infection – VZV
Orbital		Infection – fungal (mucormycosis) Trauma Tumour Aneurysm of ophthalmic artery
Localisation uncertain		Guillain–Barré/Miller Fisher syndrome Sjögren's syndrome

c/l, contralateral; i/l, ipsilateral; PCA, posterior cerebral artery; PcommA, posterior communicating artery; VZV, varicella zoster virus.

Impersistence and gaze distractability Saccadic movements are often abnormal in neurodegenerative disease, particularly Alzheimer's, when large amplitude saccadic intrusions deviate the eyes away from the intended direction of gaze. There may also be a distractibility of gaze in which there is an inability to fix on a target while being distracted by an alternative peripheral target. On head turning there may be an ocular deviation with skew and the complete absence of saccadic movements. In neurodegenerative disorders period alternating gaze deviation with tonic deviation of the eyes and the head to one side may also occur followed by a slow deviation over 10–15 seconds to the other side.

Intrusions Saccadic intrusions may take several forms. Square wave jerks occur during fixation when there is a conjugate displacement of the eye followed by a refixation saccade. These are seen in

Table 14.18 Causes of painful ophthalmoplegia.

IIIrd nerve palsy due to aneurysmal compression	
Cavernous sinus disease	Thrombosis Intracavernous carotid aneurysm Inflammatory: Tolosa–Hunt Sarcoid Wegener's granulomatosis
ICA dissection	
Pituitary apoplexy	
Giant cell arteritis	
Nasopharyngeal carcinoma	
Basal meningitis	

ICA, internal carotid artery.

cerebellar disease and PSP but are also described in many other neurodegenerative disorders. High-amplitude macro-square wave jerks are seen in cerebellar disorders, multiple system atrophy and Chiari malformation. In ocular flutter, which occasionally occurs in MS, there are bursts of saccades with no intersaccadic interval. Opsoclonus (saccadomania) suggests brainstem (particularly pontine) disease. This is a multi-directional sequence of conjugate saccadic eye movements of large amplitude which persist during eye closure and sleep. It occurs as a paraneoplastic or post-infective phenomenon and may be associated with drug ingestion.

Horizontal gaze palsy

Horizontal gaze palsy refers to a restriction of conjugate eye movements that affect both eyes in a symmetrical manner. Unilateral restriction of horizontal voluntary gaze is usually caused by a contralateral frontal or ipsilateral pontine lesion.

Frontal lobe lesions occur acutely as the result of a cerebrovascular event affecting ipsilateral horizontal smooth pursuit and causing a sustained ipsilateral horizontal gaze deviation with head rotation – the patient is said to be looking towards the side of the lesion and away from the hemiparesis. The gaze palsy can be overcome by oculo-cephalic stimulation and usually resolves over several days although residual impairment of saccadic and smooth pursuit persists. Frontal horizontal gaze palsy is usually caused by an extensive vascular lesion often haemorrhagic involving the post-Rolandic cortex or subcortical fronto-parietal region and the internal capsule. Adversive eye deviation is associated with an epileptic focus but this often resolves rapidly.

Lesions of the posterior parietal cortex and temporo-occipital parietal region cause ipsilateral horizontal gaze preference and decrease the gain and maximum velocity of smooth pursuit eye movements towards the side of the lesion. Contralateral sensory and visual inattention may be associated.

Thalamic lesions cause abnormalities of horizontal and vertical gaze with conjugate deviation of the eyes away from the side of the lesion and towards the hemiparesis. Pontine lesions involving the paramedian pontine reticular formation (PPRF) or the VIth nerve nucleus lead to a horizontal gaze palsy with the eyes deviated away from the side of the lesion and an inability to move either eye beyond the midline towards the side of the lesion. The palsy may be incomplete. Oculo-cephalic stimulation by passive horizontal rotation of the head directly stimulates the VIth nerve but will not overcome the gaze palsy caused by pontine nuclear or infranuclear lesions. Horizontal gaze palsy in the pons may be a result of ischaemia, infarction, acute infection or inflammatory change, tumours or trauma.

Vertical gaze palsy

Vertical gaze palsy may be caused by lesions affecting the visual pathway from the cortex (frontal and parieto-occipital) to the vertical gaze centre in the rostral midbrain. Rarely, non-dominant hemispheric lesions may cause up-gaze palsies and thalamic lesions have also been associated with vertical gaze palsy.

Midbrain disorders most commonly result in disturbances of vertical eye movements that can be related to involvement of the posterior commissure, the rostral interstitial nucleus of the MLF (riMLF) or the interstitial nucleus of Cajal (iC). Lesions in the posterior commissure cause loss of up-gaze and Parinaud's syndrome (dorsal midbrain or pretectal syndrome) which includes lid retraction (Collier's sign) and occasionally ptosis, down-gaze preference, disturbance of vergence eye movements including convergence–retraction nystagmus, skew deviation and pupillary light near dissociation (see Convergence–retraction nystagmus in Parinaud's syndrome). The lesion is usually bilateral and Parinaud's syndrome is caused by tumours (pinealoma, glioma, metastases), obstructive hydrocephalus (dilation of the 3rd ventricle and aqueduct) and by vascular occlusion (perforating branches of posterior cerebral artery) or thalamic and midbrain haemorrhage.

Up-gaze palsy resulting from lesions of the rostral midbrain nuclei is associated with hypersomnolence and impaired consciousness because there is involvement of the reticular activating system. There may be behavioural disturbances, associated with thalamic impairment, including amnesia, apathy, slowness of thought and akinetic mutism. This clinical pattern is seen as part of the 'top of the basilar syndrome'.

Bilateral defects in the riMLF result either in paralysis of down-gaze or loss of downward saccades. This is seen in a number of neurodegenerative or metabolic storage diseases including PSP, Niemann–Pick disease type C, Whipple's disease, Wilson's disease and Wernicke's syndrome. Combined loss of up-gaze and down-gaze for all eye movements suggests extensive bilateral rostral midbrain impairment involving riMLF and interstitial nucleus of Cajal.

Oculogyric crises

Oculogyric crises are episodes of fixed conjugate upward (and occasionally lateral) deviation of the eyes first described in encephalitis lethargica. The crises are accompanied by behavioural disturbances including obsessive thoughts or depression and dystonic or dyskinetic limb movements. The episodes occur most commonly in association with metoclopramide or neuroleptic medication but are also described with other forms of brainstem encephalitis, parkinsonian syndromes or as a paraneoplastic phenomenon. The anatomical basis remains unknown.

Internuclear ophthalmoplegia

Internuclear ophthalmoplegia (INO) is caused by a lesion of the MLF which lies between the VIth nerve nucleus and the contralateral medial rectus oculomotor subnucleus. The abducens nerve and the MLF coordinate conjugate horizontal eye movements with co-contraction of the contralateral medial rectus and ipsilateral lateral rectus. If there is a lesion of the MLF the horizontal PPRF can communicate with the adjacent ipsilateral VIth but the other pathway to the contralateral IIIrd nerve nucleus is interrupted. This leads to impaired adduction (incomplete and decreased velocity) of the eye ipsilateral to the MLF lesion and ataxic nystagmus of the contralateral eye. The nystagmus may be the most prominent feature. Convergence is usually preserved because the IIIrd nerve and medial rectus continue to work normally if conjugate movements are not required. When INO is bilateral there is usually vertical nystagmus on up-gaze. INO is a characteristic sign of demyelination resulting from MS or other forms of inflammation but is also common in brainstem vascular disease. It is also seen in Wernicke's encephalopathy and can occur as a paraneoplastic sign.

One and a half syndrome

This is associated with a unilateral lesion of the dorsal pontine tegmentum affecting the ipsilateral PPRF, MLF and VIth nerve nucleus. There is dysconjugate horizontal gaze palsy and an internuclear ophthalmoplegia leading to complete impairment of horizontal gaze in the direction of the lesion and impaired adduction when looking in a contralateral direction. Vertical movements and convergence are spared. This condition is usually caused by a pontine infarct or MS although any structural lesion may be responsible.

Wall-eyed bilateral internuclear ophthalmoplegia

Wall-eyed bilateral internuclear ophthalmoplegia (WEBINO) occurs if, in the presence of bilateral internuclear ophthalmoplegia, both eyes deviate laterally rather than remaining aligned in the primary position, convergence is often absent. This is caused by extensive lesions involving each MLF.

Internuclear ophthalmoplegia of abduction

This describes paresis of ipsilateral abduction occasionally associated with adducting nystagmus in the contralateral eye. This has been associated with ipsilateral rostral pontine and mesencephalic lesions. The paresis of abduction may be prenuclear and suggests an ipsilateral inhibitory correction between the PPRF and oculomotor nucleus.

Disconjugate vertical gaze palsy

A number of disconjugate vertical gaze palsies have been described. These include mononuclear elevator paresis in which the eyes are straight in the primary position of gaze but the affected eye will not elevate. Full elevation on eye lid closure confirms the supranuclear origin of the defect. It is associated with a lesion immediately rostral to the oculomotor nucleus. A vertical one and a half syndrome may also occur in association with vertical up-gaze palsy and monocular paresis of down-gaze associated with thalamo-mesencephalic infarction.

Skew deviation and ocular tilt reaction

Skew deviation is a vertical misalignment caused by an acquired supranuclear or vestibulo-ocular dysfunction. Hypertropia may be the same (concomitant) in all positions of gaze or may vary with eye position or alternate in left and right gaze. Non-concomitant skew deviation can mimic a single extraocular muscle paresis but there are usually accompanying brainstem signs. Skew deviation represents an imbalance in the otolith input because of a peripheral or central lesion. There is generally a downward and outward rotation of the eye on the side of the lesion and upward and inward rotation of the opposite side. Skew deviation is often associated with an INO. In some patients, skew deviation may be associated with ocular torsion which can be sustained (tonic or paroxysmal) and give rise to a compensatory head tilt – the ocular tilt reaction. Skew deviations are seen commonly in disruptions of the otolith-ocular pathways as a result of acute peripheral disease, and lesions of the vestibular nerve and nuclei, intrinsic brainstem lesions affecting the MLF and cerebellar disorders.

Nystagmus

Horizontal nystagmus

Nystagmus is an involuntary rhythmic regular oscillatory movement in one or both eyes in any field of gaze. It usually consists of alternating phases of slow drift with a quick corrective fast 'jerk' saccade in the opposite direction (jerk nystagmus). In some cases the movements have the same speed in both phases which is usually slow and sinusoidal (pendular nystagmus). Nystagmus reflects a disorder in the mechanisms that maintain steady gaze. Nystagmus occurring in the comatose and critically ill patient is discussed in Chapter 20.

Nystagmus in normal subjects

Some normal subjects show endpoint gaze evoked nystagmus on extreme lateral or vertical gaze. This may be asymmetrical having a greater amplitude in the abducting eye but tends to wane after several seconds (Table 14.19). Optokinetic nystagmus (OKN) is a jerk nystagmus induced by moving repetitive visual stimuli across the visual field. It is composed of an initial slow pursuit eye movement and a compensatory fast saccadic movement that shifts the eyes back towards fixation. This is a physiological form of nystagmus and the amplitude in the two eyes is equal regardless of the direction in which the stimulus is moved. The optokinetic response is reduced in association with lesions of the deep parietal lobe. Reduced OKN amplitude of an affected eye in adduction is a valuable way of demonstrating an internuclear ophthalmoplegia. Normal OKN pattern is retained with functional visual loss.

Jerk nystagmus

Jerk nystagmus is characterised by an initial slow drift away from the fixation target followed by a fast correcting phase back towards the target. The abnormal slow phase is mediated by the smooth pursuit system and the fast phase by the saccadic system. It is the direction of the fast component that defines the direction of the nystagmus. The amplitude is normally increased on gaze in the direction of the fast component (Alexander's law). Nystagmus in the primary position is defined by its trajectory (i.e. horizontal, torsional, upbeat, downbeat or mixed) and by the direction of the fast phase.

Pendular nystagmus

In pendular nystagmus both phases of the oscillation are symmetrical. The movement is usually vertical with a torsional component superimposed but may be horizontal, oblique or rotatory.

Table 14.19 Nystagmus in normal subjects.

Endpoint nystagmus
Fatigue nystagmus
Optokinetic nystagmus
Voluntary nystagmus

It is usually present in the primary position and does not vary with gaze direction. The movements may fluctuate, be different in both eyes or may be monocular. Occasionally, saccadic or fast phases may be superimposed upon a pendular nystagmus. It may be congenital but in acquired cases typically causes severe oscillopsia which interferes with reading and is associated with impairment of visual acuity and visual blurring. Specific forms of pendular nystagmus include spasmus nutans, oculo-palatal myoclonus, see-saw nystagmus and oculo-masticatory myorhythmia (in Whipple's disease). Acquired pendular nystagmus arises as a late manifestation of MS and it may also be associated with lesions in the pontine tegmentum particularly with brainstem stroke and encephalitis.

Nystagmus in childhood

Latent nystagmus (fusional maldevelopment nystagmus syndrome) in childhood is a congenital jerk nystagmus that only appears when one eye is covered (Table 14.20). It is a conjugate jerk nystagmus beating with the fast phase towards the fixating eye. When the other eye is covered, the nystagmus reverses its direction. Latent nystagmus may become manifest as oscillopsia in patients with strabismus, amblyopia or acquired visual loss who are only able to fix monocularly (manifest latent nystagmus).

Congenital nystagmus (infantile nystagmus syndrome) is noted at birth or in early infancy but may rarely emerge in teenage years or adulthood. The oscillations are generally horizontal and conjugate in all directions of gaze and are either pendular or a mix of jerk and pendular wave forms. The movements diminish with vergence and increase on attempted fixation. The amplitude can vary in different gaze positions but the direction of the nystagmus does not fluctuate. Some patients adopt a compensatory head turn to use the position with the lowest amplitude of ocular movement. Patients with congenital nystagmus show an inversion of OKN in which the quick phase is directed in the same direction as the drum is rotating. Congenital nystagmus is absent during sleep. It is usually idiopathic but may be associated with structural ocular lesions, retinal dystrophies or optic neuropathies. The nystagmus block syndrome refers to a form of conjugate horizontal congenital nystagmus that is absent or minimal when the fixating eye is in adduction but becomes more marked when it is in abduction.

Pendular nystagmus from visual loss

Vertical pendular nystagmus can result from any condition that causes visual loss in early childhood (Table 14.20). In adults, vertical pendular nystagmus may develop many years after visual loss. Nystagmus is usually low amplitude and low velocity and may resolve if vision is restored.

Table 14.20 Types of nystagmus in children.

Congenital nystagmus	
Acquired nystagmus	Secondary to structural brain lesion
	Secondary to any condition causing reduced vision
	Monocular – optic glioma
	Spasmus nutans
	Nystagmus block syndrome

Spasmus nutans

This is a rare and benign syndrome that develops in infancy (<14 months) and resolves by 3 years. It is characterised by nystagmus, head nodding and abnormal head posture. The nystagmus is usually horizontal and pendular although it may be oblique. It is usually of low amplitude and high frequency and characteristically either monocular or markedly disconjugate. The head nodding usually appears first and disappears with sleep or changes in head position. The condition is often transient with good residual visual acuity although it can occasionally be associated with structural lesions causing impaired visual acuity.

Monocular nystagmus

This is often caused by spasmus nutans or uniocular visual loss from optic glioma. However, in practice it is more usually brought about by an asymmetrical congenital nystagmus.

Vestibular jerk nystagmus

This is caused by abnormalities in the peripheral or central vestibular system causing an imbalance in the mediation of the smooth pursuit eye movements. Diseases of the peripheral vestibular system involving the labyrinth or vestibular nerve result in a unidirectional horizontal or mixed horizontal jerk nystagmus with the fast phase directed away from the side of the lesion. The amplitude of the nystagmus increases as the eyes are turned in the direction of the fast phase. It is reduced by visual fixation and intensified by factors causing loss of visual fixation including the dark, wearing Frenzel goggles or by sudden changes in head position. Clinical correlates of peripheral labyrinthine disturbance include tinnitus, vertigo, deafness and falling in the direction of the lesion.

Gaze evoked or gaze paretic jerk nystagmus

Gaze evoked nystagmus is induced by holding gaze in an eccentric position. It is the most common form of nystagmus encountered in clinical practice. The eyes are unable to maintain the eye position and the orbital elastic tissue causes them to drift back into the primary position. This is followed by a corrective saccadic eye movement giving rise to the nystagmus. If an associated paresis of gaze is present, either because of a peripheral or central disturbance, the nystagmus is termed gaze paretic. Gaze evoked nystagmus is usually asymptomatic and is only rarely associated with oscillopsia or poor balance from gait ataxia. It is a relatively large amplitude nystagmus which beats in the direction of gaze and is associated with rebound nystagmus on return to primary position and impairment of horizontal smooth pursuit movements. An associated fatigue nystagmus may occur in normal subjects or in myasthenia gravis after extended maintenance of eccentric gaze. Gaze evoked nystagmus is associated with many medications including antiepileptic drugs, sedative and alcohol and may also be caused by structural lesions of the vestibulocerebellum or the brainstem.

Caloric nystagmus

Cold water instilled into the external auditory meatus results in a jerk nystagmus with the fast phase beating away from the irrigated side when the head is maintained at a 30° angle. Irrigation induces repetitive slow phases that are corrected by opposite directed saccadic quick phases. The presence of normal caloric nystagmus indicates that the brainstem vestibulo-ocular connections and the IIIrd and VIth cranial nerves are intact. Disturbances of caloric nystagmus have been discussed in more detail in Chapter 15.

Torsional nystagmus

This is usually caused by a brainstem lesion affecting the central projections from the anterior and posterior semicircular canals and the otolith, therefore interrupting the vestibular input to the ocular motor centres. Torsional nystagmus usually beats away from the side of a brainstem lesion and is a conjugate movement associated with oscillopsia. There is generally an associated skew deviation and impairment of smooth pursuit movements. There may also be an internuclear ophthalmoplegia and associated midbrain lesion affecting vertical gaze. Torsional nystagmus is usually caused by infarction of the brainstem but may be associated with MS, tumours or rhombencephalitis.

Central vestibular horizontal nystagmus

This is a low amplitude nystagmus in the primary position which is seen in patients with reduced pursuit movements because of large cerebral lesions. Lesions of the vestibular nuclei or cerebellar flocculus result in a variety of forms of nystagmus which may be bidirectional or purely vertical (upbeat or downbeat) but less commonly may be torsional or horizontal. Fixation does not reduce the amplitude and Frenzel goggles or darkness do not intensify the oscillations. Central vestibular nystagmus is usually associated with vascular lesions, MS or brainstem tumours. The fast phase of the nystagmus is directed towards the side of the lesion. Patients with cerebellopontine angle lesions may manifest both a gaze paretic nystagmus to the side of the lesion, as a result of a horizontal pontine gaze paresis, and a faster beating nystagmus in the opposite direction associated with vestibular involvement.

Vertical and other forms of nystagmus

Downbeat nystagmus

This is a jerk nystagmus in which there is a fast phase saccadic movement beating in a downward direction (Table 14.21). This occurs in the primary position and increases with downward and lateral gaze. It causes blurred vision, oscillopsia and gait imbalance. It is associated with lesions of the dorsal medulla leading to loss of tonic downward vestibular input causing the eyes to drift upwards or of the cerebellar flocculus which removes its tonic inhibition of upward vestibular eye movements. Downbeat nystagmus is therefore associated with gaze evoked and rebound nystagmus and abnormal smooth pursuit movements. Lower brainstem involvement may cause a coexisting internuclear ophthalmoplegia or skew deviation.

Downbeat nystagmus is particularly associated with lesions at the cervico-medullary junction (e.g. Arnold–Chiari malformation) but is also seen in spino-cerebellar degeneration and in association with drug toxicity in particular antiepileptic drugs, lithium and alcohol.

Upbeat nystagmus

Upbeat nystagmus is a jerk nystagmus characterised by a slow downward drift and a saccadic correcting fast phase beating upward (Table 14.22). It is associated with midline lesions of the ponto-medullary or ponto-mesencephalic junctions causing loss of vestibular upward eye movement input. Oscillopsia is less frequent than with downbeat nystagmus and patients are either asymptomatic or complain of blurred vision. Upbeat nystagmus occurs in the primary position and increases with up-gaze. Impaired upward pursuit is seen and the condition is often associated with poor horizontal pursuit, gaze evoked nystagmus and rebound nystagmus. If the cause is a low brainstem lesion there may also be a skew deviation and an internuclear ophthalmoplegia. Upbeat nystagmus is caused by cerebellar degeneration, brainstem or cerebellar strokes and demyelination but may also occur with toxicity and Wernicke's encephalopathy.

Other forms of vertical eye movement disorders may be seen in states of impaired consciousness and are discussed in Chapter 20.

Nystagmus in oculopalatal tremor

This may be associated with an asymptomatic palatal tremor. More commonly, palatal tremor is symptomatic and follows brainstem infarction or cerebellar degeneration. The nystagmus is usually a slow vertical regular pendular movement, synchronous with the palatal movement. Oculopalatal tremor is associated with brainstem involvement and is often seen with a horizontal gaze or lower cranial nerve palsy, cerebellar dysarthria or damage to the spinothalamic tract. It is associated with lesions of the dentato-rubro-olivary region (Mollaret's triangle) which lead to denervation of the inferior olive which appears hypertrophied on MRI.

Table 14.21 Causes of downbeat nystagmus.

Craniocervical abnormalities	Arnold–Chiari malformation, basilar invagination, syringobulbia, Paget's disease, platybasia
Toxic – metabolic	Antiepileptic drugs lithium, alcohol (Wernicke's encephalopathy)
Cerebellar degeneration	Spinocerebellar atrophy, paraneoplastic, familial episodic ataxia, multiple system atrophy
Raised intracranial pressure	
Infarction	
Infection	
Demyelination (rare)	
Cerebellar tumour	
Head trauma	
Heat stroke	

Table 14.22 Causes of upbeat nystagmus.

Infarction	Medulla, cerebellum or superior cerebellar peduncle
Posterior fossa tumour	
Demyelination (common)	
Wernicke encephalopathy	
Brainstem encephalitis	
Behçet's disease	
Meningitis	
Congenital	Leber's neuropathy
Toxins	Tobacco Antiepileptic drugs Ciclosporin
Paraneoplastic	

See-saw nystagmus

In see-saw nystagmus there is alternating elevation and intorsion of one eye while the opposite eye falls and extorts. Both components of the movements are pendular and they occur in rapidly alternating sequence. It is usually present in all positions of gaze but maximal in down-gaze. This form of nystagmus is associated with bitemporal hemianopia usually from a large suprasellar mass such as a craniopharyngioma or pituitary adenoma. The lesion often causes expansion of the 3rd ventricle. It is also associated with vascular disease, particularly affecting the rostral mesencephalon.

Oculomasticatory myorhythmia

Oculomasticatory myorhythmia is a continuous slow rhythmic convergent–divergent nystagmus (i.e. the eyes oscillate horizontally towards and away from each other). There are synchronous diffuse muscle contractions particularly involving masticatory or facial muscles and occasionally the palate and mouth. This form of nystagmus is associated with Whipple's disease and occurs in about 20% of patients. There is often also a supranuclear gaze palsy affecting vertical and then horizontal eye movements with eventual loss of all eye movements.

Periodic alternating nystagmus

Periodic alternating nystagmus may occur as a congenital or acquired manifestation; it is a spontaneous horizontal jerk nystagmus that is present in primary position of gaze. It is present in one direction for around 120 seconds, it then stops for 5–20 seconds before beating in the other direction for a similar duration. In the interval between direction change, there may be a vertical nystagmus or square wave jerks. The horizontal nystagmus is least when looking in the direction of the slow phase. A complete cycle takes approximately 4 minutes and therefore may be missed on routine clinical examination. Periodic alternating nystagmus may be congenital or acquired in association with impairment of the vestibular cerebellar pathways. It is particularly seen with Arnold–Chiari malformation or cerebellar degeneration but may also be associated with MS or brainstem tumours.

Convergence–retraction nystagmus in Parinaud's syndrome

This is characterised by rapid convergence movements of both eyes which also retract in the globe. It is best seen on attempted up-gaze or with a downward moving optokinetic drum and is caused by co-contraction of the horizontal recti on attempted convergence or up-gaze. Patients may have difficulty with upward saccadic movements but vertical pursuit is intact. It occurs with pupillary light near dissociation and bilateral lid retraction and is associated with lesions of the dorsal rostral midbrain which involve the posterior commissure (e.g. pineal tumours).

Voluntary nystagmus

Normal individuals may be able to perform high-frequency horizontal conjugate eye movements which appear to be pendular. Occasionally they are vertical or circumrotatory. The movements tend to fatigue after more than a few seconds.

Eye lid nystagmus

Eye lid twitches may occur in synchrony with vertical nystagmus and may also be provoked by convergence. Similar eye lid twitches are seen with the fast phase of horizontal nystagmus on lateral gaze.

Rarely, lid nystagmus may occur in isolation and it is particularly associated with medullary disorders. Irregular lid flutter may also be seen with weakness of up-gaze or in parkinsonism.

Medical treatment of nystagmus

A proportion of patients with neurological nystagmus develop visually disabling and intrusive oscillopsia which is sometimes responsive to medication. Examples of drugs that may help include gabapentin for particular acquired pendular nystagmus in multiple sclerosis, baclofen for acquired periodic alternating nystagmus and aminopyridine for downbeat jerk nystagmus.

Chiasmal and retrochiasmal visual pathways

Chiasmal disease

At the optic chiasm the nerve fibres from the temporal retina (nasal visual field) maintain their relative position in the lateral chiasm before passing into the ipsilateral optic tract while the nerve fibres from the nasal retina (temporal visual field) decussate in the chiasm and pass into the contralateral optic tract. The separation of the two hemifields occurs at the fovea so that the visual field is split at the point of fixation into the right and left halves, thus the macular fibres are both crossed and uncrossed in the optic chiasm. Bitemporal hemianopia is the characteristic clinical sign of chiasmal disease.

In some individuals the intracranial portion of the optic nerve is relatively long and the chiasm is formed in the posterior cistern (post-fixed) with the consequence that expanding sellar lesions may cause compression of the optic nerve and anterior aspect of the chiasm. Lesions of the anterior chiasm can result in a contralateral temporal hemianopic field defect with an ipsilateral central scotoma. This is referred to as a junctional field defect. A central scotoma with a temporal hemianopic scotoma in the same eye is also a junctional pattern but is less often identified.

Conversely, the chiasm may be pre-fixed so that mass lesions of the pituitary fossa may impinge on the posterior aspect of the chiasm or optic tract. Lesions of the posterior chiasmal notch may selectively involve only dorsal crossing fibres which predominantly serve central vision thus resulting in a bitemporal hemianopic scotoma. However, macular fibres, which form at least 30% of all fibres despite serving only 5° of field, are present throughout the chiasm and therefore any form of chiasmal lesion usually causes a defect in central vision (e.g. acuity or colour vision) in one or both eyes as part of the bitemporal field loss.

Patients with bi-temporal hemianopia may present with double vision despite normal eye movements. When there are dense temporal field defects, binocular fusion is not supported by overlapping temporal hemifields in the visual cortex. As a result, latent phorias may readily break down leading to variable vertical or horizontal diplopia. In other instances there may be difficulty in performing tasks requiring depth perception and judgement. The phenomenon of post-fixational blindness occurs when the subject with a bi-temporal hemianopia fixates on a near target, causing objects beyond the target to project on to both nasal hemiretina and therefore be invisible. In chiasmal disorders, diplopia may also be caused by direct cranial nerve involvement, either because of compression or direct invasion of the cavernous sinus or as a consequence of raised intracranial pressure.

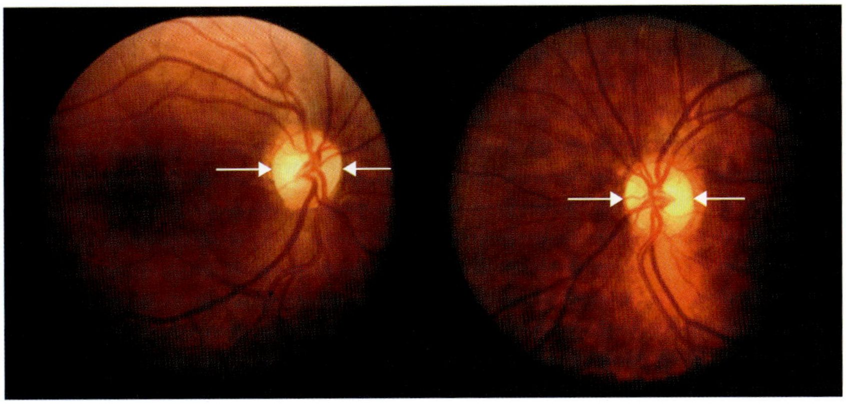

Figure 14.45 Bow tie or band atrophy in both discs with bi-temporal hemianopia caused by chiasmal transection (arrows).

The characteristic appearance of the optic disc in pure bi-temporal hemianopia is 'band' or 'bow-tie' atrophy. This occurs because exclusively crossing fibres enter the disc at the nasal and temporal poles. At all other locations there is a mixture of crossing and non-crossing fibres. Hence, if only crossing fibres are lost a 'band' of total atrophy results which is rarely seen in a complete form except in chiasmal transection caused by trauma (Figure 14.45).

Management of lesions in the pituitary region is described in Chapter 21.

Homonymous hemianopia

Homonymous hemianopia is caused by unilateral lesions of the visual pathway posterior to the optic chiasm (i.e. optic tract, lateral geniculate body [LGB], optic radiation and cerebral cortex). Clinically, these are often disabling causing difficulty with reading and visual scanning. Patients may fail to notice relevant objects or obstacles on the affected side causing collisions particularly in complex environments (e.g. with approaching people). Driving, reading, shopping, applying make-up and food preparation are the most commonly affected activities of daily living. Transient homonymous hemianopia may occur in migraine, transient ischaemic attacks or seizures. The most common cause is vascular but homonymous hemianopia may result from tumours, trauma or surgery.

Optic tract

Each optic tract contains crossed and uncrossed nerve fibres subserving the contralateral visual field, in particular nasal fibres subserving the temporal visual field of the contralateral eye and ipsilateral temporal fibres subserving the nasal visual field. Therefore, the left optic tract contains fibres carrying information for the right half of the visual field from both the right and left eyes. Lesions of the optic tract cause homonymous visual field defects of the contralateral visual field. The optic tract lies in close proximity to the internal capsule, cerebral peduncle and basal ganglia. Optic tract lesions are rare and are usually associated with other visual system abnormalities. Tract lesions typically occur with suprasellar lesions (craniopharyngiomas, aneurysm, optic chiasmal glioma and rarely, pituitary tumours) which extend posteriorly especially when there is a pre-fixed chiasm.

Involvement of the optic tract may lead to a homonymous hemianopia which may be complete or incomplete. When incomplete the visual field loss is often non-congruent. Optic atrophy occurs in a 'bow-tie' distribution (band atrophy) in the eye with the temporal hemianopia because the fibres at the temporal poles of the disc are exclusively crossing fibres, where fibres crossing from temporal hemifields to enter the disc at both lateral poles are preferentially lost. A contralateral relative afferent pupillary defect may be present because the temporal hemifield served by the nasal hemiretina carries a greater number of ganglion cells that drive the light reflex than does the nasal hemifield. Lesions of the optic tract may be associated with hypothalamic involvement and contralateral hemiparesis from internal capsular damage.

Lateral geniculate nucleus

Most of the nerve fibres of the optic tract (>80%) project to the ipsilateral lateral geniculate nucleus in the midbrain. Other optic tract fibres innervate the Edinger–Westphal nucleus in the pretectum, providing the afferent limb of the pupillary light reflex. The axons from the ipsilateral eye terminate in the second, third and fifth laminae of the lateral geniculate body while the axons from the contralateral eye terminate in the first, fourth and sixth laminae. The nerve fibres are believed to form a precise retinotopic map of the LGB.

Isolated lesions of the LGB are extremely uncommon and are caused by occlusive vascular disease involving the dual supply from the posterior cerebral and inferior choroidal arteries. Such lesions are often associated with contralateral hemiparesis from involvement of the adjacent posterior limb of the internal capsule or contralateral hemisensory loss from thalamic involvement.

Horizontal bands of the ganglion may be destroyed resulting in a specific hemianopic wedge field defect (known as geniculate hemianopia or sectoranopia) that straddles the horizontal meridian, although congruous or non-congruous hemianopia are more common. The wedge-shaped defects are located near the horizontal meridian either involving or sparing fixation. Pupillary reactions are normal. There may be associated signs resulting from involvement of the ipsilateral thalamus and/or pyramidal tract.

Optic radiation

The neurones originating from the LGB form the optic radiation or the geniculo-striate tract and end in the primary visual cortex in the occipital lobe. The first part of the optic radiation is associated with the posterior limb of the internal capsule and lies in close proximity to the cortico-spinal and cortico-bulbar tracts as well as the thalamus and cortical fibres. Lesions of the optic radiation in this region typically produce contralateral and usually complete homonymous hemianopia associated with contralateral hemianaesthesia and hemiplegia. Relative afferent pupillary defects may occur in lesions that are close to the lateral geniculate body.

The inferior fibres that subserve the superior visual field initially course anteriorly, superior to and around the temporal horn of the lateral ventricle. They then pass laterally and posterior to the striate cortex forming Meyer's loop. It is believed that as these fibres approach the occipital cortex their retinotopic order increases and the left and right eye fibres representing common visual loci separate into ocular dominance columns in the striate cortex. Lesions of the optic radiation in the temporal lobe usually result in a congruous homonymous hemianopia primarily affecting the superior quadrant with preserved visual acuity and pupillary light reflexes. The defect may be incomplete, incongruous and either confined to the superior quadrants ('pie in the sky') or more dense superiorly than inferiorly. This field defect is associated with aphasia, memory deficits and visual hallucinations. It is caused by intrinsic tumours such as gliomas, metastases or large demyelinating plaques rather more frequently than vascular occlusion.

More dorsal fibres pass through the parietal lobe. Lesions of the optic radiation in this region lead to incomplete or mildly incongruous homonymous hemianopia which is either limited to the inferior visual field or is more dense inferiorly than superiorly. However, more extensive lesions may produce a complete homonymous hemianopia with macular splitting, preservation of visual acuity and normal pupillary reflexes. There may be associated disruption of optokinetic nystagmus. Contralateral hemifield neglect is also seen in lesions of the non-dominant parietal lobe and should be distinguished from a visual field defect although sometimes both co-occur. There can be an associated sensory defect and lesions extending into the dominant angular gyrus produce Gerstmann's syndrome (finger agnosia, agraphia, acalculia, right–left disorientation).

Visual cortex

The anatomical structure of the visual cortex and the associated striate and extrastriate cortex is described in Chapter 2. The primary visual cortex (V1, calcarine cortex, striate cortex, Brodmann area 17) is believed to be retinotopically organised, based on visual information from the corresponding retinal loci from the two eyes. The posterior pole of the occipital lobe is concerned with the central visual field while the peripheral visual field is represented in the most anterior part of the striate cortex. The upper lip of the calcarine cortex receives projections from the inferior visual field. The striate cortex is surrounded by the visual association areas (V2–6, Brodmann areas 18 and 19). These areas are also believed to be retinotopically arranged with over-representation for the central visual field as in the primary visual cortex.

Various specific patterns of acquired field defect occur with lesions of the primary visual cortex. Occipital lobe lesions are the most common cause of homonymous hemianopia and are usually a result of infarction in the distribution of the posterior cerebral artery. Other aetiologies include venous infarction, haemorrhagic arteriovenous malformations and fistulas, tumours, abscess and trauma.

The most peripheral 30% of temporal field viewed by both eyes is not overlapped by corresponding nasal fields in the other eye (temporal crescent). This portion of the field therefore has a monocular representation in the anterior part of the contralateral visual cortex. Lesions of the anterior striate cortex cause a congruous homonymous scotoma with unilateral loss of the temporal crescent. This is the only example of a monocular visual field defect caused by a retrochiasmal lesion although a uniocular temporal scotoma is much more commonly caused by a peripheral retinal lesion. More commonly, when the anterior portion of the visual cortex is spared by an occipital lobe lesion, there is a complete homonymous hemianopia except for sparing of the temporal crescent in the contralateral eye.

Superior and inferior homonymous visual field defects respecting the vertical and sometimes the horizontal meridians occur with lesions of the occipital cortex selectively damaging either the inferior or superior banks (usually infarcts).

Macular sparing is rarer than macular splitting hemianopias. Mammals in general and humans in particular are foveo-centric, that is much of the occipital cortex (two-thirds) given over to central (0–5°) vision which is why macular sparing hemianopias are rarer than those that involve central vision. The mechanism of macular sparing has been debated with some arguing that the macula is bilaterally represented in the occipital cortex but the weight of evidence supports the theory that macula sparing is caused by incomplete damage to the striate cortex on the affected side, probably because of sparing of some of the four main branches of the posterior cerebral arteries (PCA) which supplies visual cortex. Conversely, homonymous visual field defects preferentially involving the macular may occur. These respect the vertical meridian and are limited to the central 30° and are usually enclosed within an area of normal peripheral visual field. The cause is most commonly occipital tip injury resulting from hypotension or ischaemic stroke. However, larger lesions involving the occipital radiations and optic tract have also been associated with this deficit.

Bilateral homonymous hemianopia

This may occur with bilateral lesions of the occipital cortex either simultaneously or consecutively. The extent of the visual field defect depends on the involvement of the striate cortex. Bilateral occipital cortex lesions are relatively frequent because the two posterior cerebral arteries are terminal branches of a single basilar artery and therefore basilar occlusion will cause occipital infarction and cortical blindness. This may also occur in metabolic, neurodegenerative or inflammatory disease. A variety of bilateral homonymous lesions may occur ranging from complete bilateral homonymous hemianopia (cortical blindness), to bilateral macular sparing hemianopia (ring scotoma), quadrantanopias or scotomatous and altitudinal defects.

Anton's syndrome is particularly associated with occipital cortex lesions extending to the calcarine cortex and including visual association cortices (Brodmann areas 18 and 19). Acute bilateral and extensive lesions of the occipital lobe lead to sudden visual loss. Patients with cortical blindness are sometimes unaware of their visual loss, deny any difficulty and confabulate about what they are able to see often being able to direct their gaze to auditory stimuli.

Blindsight and stato-kinetic dissociation

Blindsight or residual vision in an apparently blind hemifield (V1 scotoma) can be demonstrated in some patients. There is evidence that reflex motor responses may be generated in response to stimuli in the blind field. The underlying substrate for this is uncertain but is likely to involve subcortical visual pathway, the pulvinar of the thalamus and callosal connections. There is also a direct projection from the LGB to area 5, which may subserve preserved perception of movement. The Riddoch phenomenon of stato-kinetic dissociation may be demonstrated on Goldmann perimetry: a stimulus is perceived on movement in the periphery of a homonymous hemianopia despite failure to see colour or static forms.

Visual association areas (extrastriate cortex areas V2–6)

Lesions affecting the human area V1 often extend into underlying white matter in the prestriate area and adjacent parietal and temporal regions causing an inferior quadrantic field defect which respects the horizontal as well the vertical meridian. The pre-striate pathways or visual association areas can be considered as two separate systems: first, a ventro-mesial pathway which occupies the occipital lobe below the calcarine fissure and adjacent temporal lobes (the visual 'what' pathway) and, secondly, a dorsolateral area which is located in the occipital lobe above the calcarine fissue and in the adjacent parietal and temporo-parietal region (the 'where' pathway). The clinical significance of this is that there may be functional partitioning of the pre-striate cortex in such a way that focal lesions may result in selective impairment of aspects of higher visual function.

Lesions of the ventro-mesial pathway in the occipito-temporal cortex result in defects of object recognition colour vision and reading affecting the contralateral hemifield. These include cerebral dyschromatopsia, pure alexia and prosopagnosia (see Other disorders of visual perception). Hemianopic field defects are commonly found, often bilateral inferior quadrantanopia as a result of damage to the adjacent ventral portion of the optic radiation. Lesions of the dorso-lateral pathway may cause visuo-spatial neglect, Balint's syndrome, visual agnosia and, very rarely, cerebral akinetopsia (see Other disorders of visual perception).

Disorders of higher visual function

Visual hallucinations

Visual hallucinations are formed or unformed images perceived when in reality there is no stimulus present and are the result of endogenous neural activity. Illusions are the misperception or distortion of a stimulus present in the external environment.

Visual hallucinations may occur in medical, neurological or ocular disorders. In contrast to auditory hallucinations, they are not usually a result of psychiatric disorders. Simple visual hallucinations may consist of single discrete or flickering flashes of light (phosphenes or photopsia) which may result from lesions of the retina, choroid or optic nerve. There may be lines of different colours in the form of simple patterns (circles, fortification or zig-zag patterns) which may be associated with a defect in the field of vision and usually caused by migraine or occipital epilepsy. Simple visual hallucinations include brief vertical flashes of light (Moore's lightning streaks) which predominantly occur in the temporal field in association with eye movements and are associated with vitreous detachment. Spontaneous flashes precipitated by eye movement or loud unexpected sounds may be a manifestation of demyelination or other causes of optic neuropathy.

Migraine is the most common cause of visual hallucination and illusion. The disturbances may vary from elementary, predominantly black and white, visual disturbances, elementary positive (phosphenes or geometrical forms) or negative (scotomas) disturbances with more complex visual hallucinations and illusions. In particular, fortification spectra (teichopsia), scintillating lights and lines or zig-zag waves may occur and frank distortions including geometric forms, micropsia, macropsia and metamorphopsia. These may also occur in migraine without headache.

Visual hallucinations are particularly associated with simple and complex seizures arising in the occipital lobe with or without secondary generalisation (Figure 14.46). These seizures may be

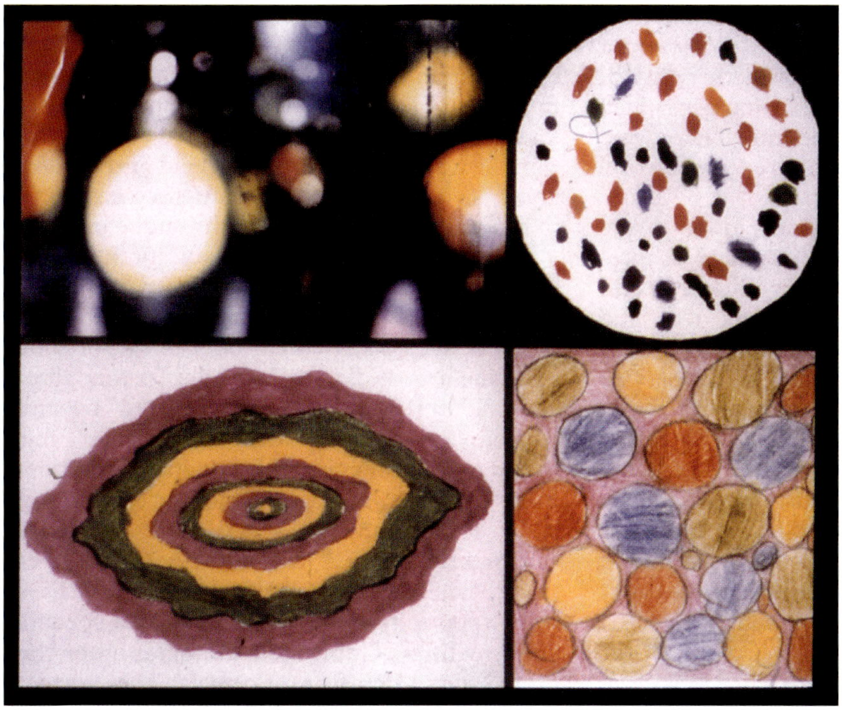

Figure 14.46 Visual phenomena recorded by four patients with occipital epilepsy. Source: Panayiotopoulos 1999. Reproduced with permission of John Libbey Eurotext.

associated with multiple types of hallucinations or illusions. In contrast to migraine, the hallucinations are usually brief, stereotyped and fragmentary and are usually multicoloured and occasionally complex with circular or spherical patterns. They are generally seen in the contralateral temporal field but may begin centrally. They may be prolonged in non-convulsive status and are sometimes perceived as unreal and associated with anxiety and an affective disturbance. It may be difficult to distinguish from migraine because a migraine-like headache may occur after an occipital lobe seizure, usually coming on several minutes after the hallucinations have stopped. Occipital and temporal lobe epilepsy may also be associated with distortions, particularly changes in size both micropsia and macropsia.

In transient visual loss caused by occipital ischaemia there may be coloured bright flashes (scintillations). Occipital lobe tumours may give rise to uniform visual hallucinations in one hemifield often associated with exercise, which are probably ictal in origin. Visual hallucinations may occur with posterior cerebral infarction involving the occipital lobe and thalamus (Figure 14.47).

Complex visual hallucinations are usually related to temporal lobe dysfunction. They may involve hallucinations of colour, face, texture and objects and correlate with cerebral activity in the ventral extrastriate visual cortex and their content reflects the functional specialisation of the particular region of occipital cortex affected.

Hallucinations and illusions occur in a variety of other neurological disorders (Chapter 8). They are frequently seen in delirium from any cause when they are associated with an alteration in attention, concentration and the level of consciousness with disrupted sleep–wake cycle and agitation. The symptoms characteristically fluctuate. In diffuse Lewy body disease there are characteristically vivid visual hallucinations and similar phenomena may also be seen in Parkinson's disease particularly in the older and more cognitively impaired patient taking dopamine agonists.

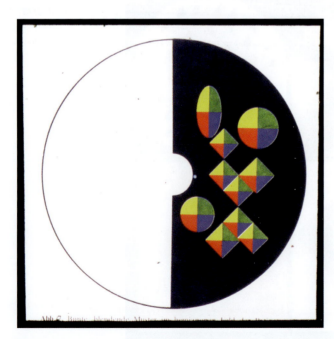

Figure 14.47 Geometric hallucinations within a hemianopic field defect recorded by the patient. Source: Kölmel 1985. Reproduced with permission of BMJ.

These hallucinations are often colourful, complex, involving scenes of people and animals. There may also be associated paranoid delusional disturbances. Visual hallucinations are less commonly seen in Alzheimer's disease, Pick's disease, Huntington's chorea and vascular dementia. Hypnogogic and hypnopompic hallucinations lasting several minutes are associated with narcolepsy. These are often colourful vivid images involving people, animals or landscape scenes and may be difficult to separate from reality.

Visual hallucinations associated with impaired vision (Charles Bonnet syndrome)

In patients with impaired visual acuity from a variety of primary ophthalmological disorders, particularly in the elderly, recurrent vivid hallucinations may occur despite normal cognition and insight. They may be more likely to occur in low light and are seen in the blind portion of the visual field. They are not stereotyped and often consist of vivid scenes which are predominantly coloured and often involve animals, flowers and people which are sometimes said to have a cartoon-like appearance. They may have normal proportion or be altered in size and may change shape when the subject reaches out to them. They can usually be stopped by opening and closing the eyes or by rapid eye movements. The patient invariably realises that the hallucinations are unreal.

This syndrome may result from lesions throughout the visual pathway but is particularly associated with age-related degenerative retinal or neurological disease and is considered to be a release phenomenon of the ventral occipito-temporal cortex.

Peduncular hallucinosis

This occurs with lesions of the thalamus and upper midbrain (usually bilateral). These are vivid and usually well-formed colourful hallucinations or people, animals or complex scenes. There may be illusionary micropsia and the scenes are often considered to be pleasant. The hallucinations can last for minutes to hours and usually occur in the evening. There may be associated auditory and tactile hallucinations but insight is well preserved.

Other visual illusions may be experienced by patients with partial visual loss (Table 14.23).

Table 14.23 Visual illusions in patients with partial visual loss.

Tessellopsia	Regular repeating patterns
Dendropsia	Branching patterns
Hyperchromatopsia	Hyperintense brilliant colours
Polyopia	Seeing a single target as multiple
Macropsia	Seeing objects enlarged
Micropsia	Seeing objects reduced in size
Metamorphopsia	Seeing distortion of perceived objects
Palinopsia	Persistence or recurrence of the visual image despite removal of the object
Allesthesia	Transportation of an object seen in a visual field to the contralateral visual field
Oscillopsia	Illusion of movement of the environment

Polyopia

Polyopia, in which a single target is seen as multiple, is a rare manifestation of lesions of the occipital cortex or central visual pathway and occurs with monocular viewing. The number of objects seen may vary from two to hundreds. The true image is seen and the false images are similar but tend to reduce in intensity, colour and size. Polyopia tends to develop several seconds after fixation and does not resolve with a pin-hole.

Palinopsia

Palinopsia is also associated with occipital or occipito-temporal disease and may occur as an ictal phenomenon. The image tends to recur immediately after the object has been removed or the gaze has been diverted, it is usually without colour and remains despite eye closure. Palinopsia may develop during recovery from cortical blindness and is particularly associated with non-dominant focal occipito-parietal lesions. It also occurs in association with a variety of medications, drug withdrawal and neurodegenerative disorders.

Other disorders of visual perception

Pulfrich's phenomenon

Pulfrich's phenomenon is loss of stereoscopic depth perception that causes objects to appear to cross the midline. It is caused by a difference in the latency of transmission in the optic nerve between the two eyes usually because of delay in conduction associated with demyelination or compression of the optic nerve.

Hemifield slide

Bi-temporal hemifield slide is caused by loss of overlapping regions of the binocular visual field. This may cause a disturbance to reading because there is a vertical break in horizontal lines of text. Similarly, a left homonymous hemianopia may impair the transition from the end of line of text to a new line on the left-hand side of the page.

Tilt

Environmental tilt is particularly seen following lateral medullary infarction. The tilt in the field of vision may be 90° or 180° and come on abruptly. Severe tilts tend to be brief in duration while smaller deviations may persist for longer periods.

Visual synaesthesia

Visual synaesthesia occurs when auditory, tactile or gustatory stimuli produce visual images and is associated with illusions throughout the visual pathway. Visual dysaesthesia occur when various unpleasant visual sensations are experienced when looking towards a blind field. They are often associated with lesions of the optic radiation.

Visual agnosia

Visual agnosia refers to an inability to recognise objects visually despite preservation of visual acuity, intellectual function, attention and language abilities. However, object recognition deficits may also occur as a result of visual form imperception despite normal acuity. These patients are unable to detect differences in object matching tasks. True visual object agnosia may occur at the level of perceptual analysis (apperceptive agnosia) or at the level of semantic analysis (associative agnosia). Apperceptive agnosia is observed in patients with lesions of the right dorsal posterior cortex and associative agnosia with left ventral lesions. Patients with apperceptive agnosia cannot copy a line drawing well; those with associative agnosia can copy the drawing but are unable to explain it. Both syndromes are seen most commonly in degenerative disorders, specifically Alzheimer's disease and a rare variant, posterior cortical atrophy.

Prosopagnosia

Prosopagnosia is a circumscribed form of visual agnosia in which there is failure to recognise previously familiar faces or to learn the appearance of new faces. In its severe form patients rely on individual facial features (e.g. glasses, beard or hairstyle) or non-visual clues (e.g. voice) to recognise others. However, some patients are able to judge age, gender and emotional expression. Prosopagnosia can be congenital or associated with bilateral lesions particularly affecting the ventral visual system, a milder form may occur with unilateral right hemisphere lesions.

Disorders of colour vision

Inability to recognise colours as a consequence of cortical deficits occurs in several different clinical patterns. In cerebral achromatopsia patients are not able to read Ishihara plates or sort colours according to hue. There is complete loss of colour vision with colours appearing as shades of grey. This is associated with bilateral lesions or involvement of the non-dominant occipito-temporal lobe and there is usually a superior quadrantic field loss with involvement of the inferior striate cortex or optic radiations. There is often accompanying visual agnosia.

Cerebral metamorphopsia

Patients notice distortion of images which may be caused by spatial remapping around homonymous scotomas in which case it can be mapped in a predictable fashion. In other instances the distortions are bizarre, often frightening and specific to faces and hands (Figure 14.48).

Visual simultanagnosia

This syndrome may occur in isolation or in association with cortical visual loss. There is an inability to understand the visual field as a whole while individual elemental parts are attended and recognised. If the patient is presented with several figures he/she is able to recognise them individually but sees only one when they are presented in a group. Formal testing is difficult because patients use only macular vision and fail to keep their eyes focused on the target. The syndrome appears to be associated with an inability to sustain visuo-spatial attention. It is particularly associated with the visual field defects involving unilateral or bilateral inferior quadrantic field and may occur as a sequelae of posterior circulation watershed infarction in Balint's syndrome. Dorsal (visuo-spatial) and ventral (visual agnosias) variants occur. Patients can be severely visually impaired despite a normal performance on tests of visual acuity.

Cortical visual impairment

Balint's syndrome is characterised by the following:

1. *Ocular motor apraxia*: an inability to shift gaze on command because of difficulty initiating voluntary saccades to redirect attention to visual targets despite an unrestricted range of eye movements.
2. *Optic ataxia*: the inability to benefit from visual guidance when reaching for a target under visual control; the inability to benefit from visual guidance when reaching. It is manifest as clumsiness of movement of the hand performed under visual guidance. This is present throughout the range of movement in contrast to cerebellar ataxia.

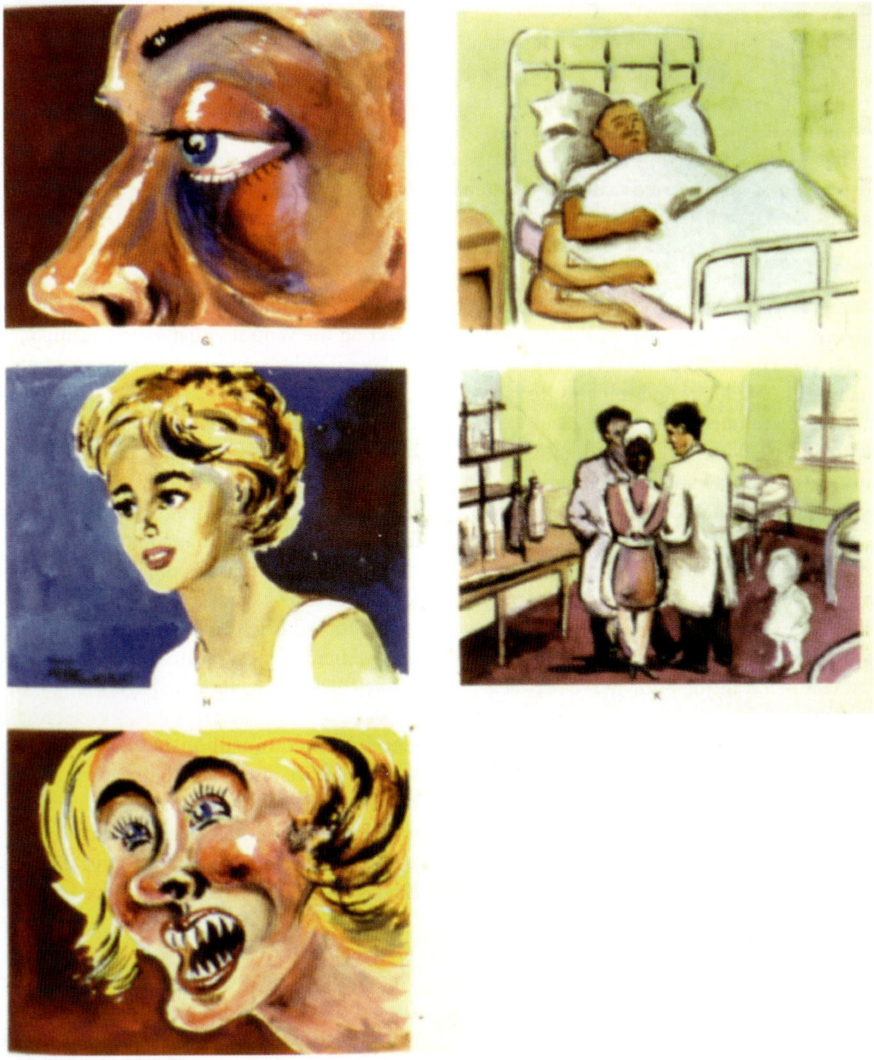

Figure 14.48 Metamorphopsia recorded by a patient following occipital lobe surgery. Source: Mooney et al. 1965. Reproduced with permission of Elsevier.

3 *Reduced visual attention manifest as simultanagnosia* (see Cortical visual impairment): there may also be a reduction in visual attention with functional constriction in the fields and altitudinal neglect.

Balint's syndrome is associated with bilateral posterior watershed lesions in the convexity of the hemispheres. It is also associated with Gerstmann's syndrome although the strength of associations with these defects as a syndrome remains open to question.

Occipital cortical visual disturbances may also occur as a consequence of posterior presentation of Alzheimer's disease which tends to come on at a young age with relatively preserved visual acuity and colour appreciation. There is often difficulty reading and marked visuo-spatial difficulties. MRI shows prominent occipito-parietal atrophy.

Neglect

This is different from hemianopia in the sense that it is not confined to one hemifield or the other, but rather is best considered as a disorder of attentional allocation over space, with a spatial gradient. Right parietal lesions are the most common cause with severe and persistent cases usually associated with widespread fronto-parietal damage. Patients preferentially respond to stimuli on the right leading to visual extinction. Cancellation tests are often used to diagnose the condition (patients with hemianopia alone will be slow but accurate in these tests); the more difficult the test that is, the more targets and distracters, the more a patient's tendency to only report stimuli to the right. Neglect can also affect interpersonal space with patients not recognising their own body parts in extreme cases.

Alexia

This is the loss of reading ability in previously literate subjects. When associated with other language disturbance (aphasia) it is known as central alexia, or as Dejerine called it 'alexia with agraphia' (patients with aphasia are usually agraphic). This is usually caused by a lesion affecting the dominant MCA territory. Peripheral alexia or 'alexia without agraphia' occurs in the face of otherwise normal language abilities (speaking, hearing speech, writing). The most common form is hemianopic alexia where a macular splitting hemianopia causes problems with text reading by robbing the reader of information about upcoming words. For texts, like this one, written and thus read from left-to-right, a right-sided hemianopia is more disabling. 'Pure' alexia is caused by lesions affecting the dominant fusiform gyrus and its connections. These patients have difficulty with single word reading and, in the more serve cases, resort to a letter-by-letter reading strategy. At the most severe end of the spectrum are patients who have problems at the single letter level: global alexia. Such patients retain their writing ability, at least to some degree, leading to the odd sign of a patient being able to write a sentence which, after a suitable gap to interfere with verbal recall of what they have just written, they cannot subsequently read.

Abnormalities of the pupil

The pupil is abnormal in a number of ocular as well as neurological disorders; only the latter is considered in this chapter. The importance of pupillary change is not so much the fact that they cause serious symptoms (they usually do not), but that they may indicate serious underlying neurological disease.

A knowledge of the anatomy of the direct and indirect light reflexes and of the sympathetic supply are important in understanding pupillary change (Chapter 2), and abnormalities of pupillary function can be very helpful in localising neurological disorders.

The size of the pupil is determined by the balance between parasympathetic drive (which determines the tone in the iris sphincter muscle) and sympathetic drive (which determines the tone in the iris dilator muscle). The size of the pupils is affected by the ambient lighting and many other factors including the level of alertness and emotional factors. Sometimes the pupils are naturally of slightly unequal size without any underlying pathology (physiological anisocoria). Physiological anisocoria describes clearly perceptible inequality of pupillary size and is present in 20% of the population. It varies from day to day and can even reverse in some people. Its physiological nature can be confirmed by the observations that the measured inequality is similar in light and dark, and by the fact that the direct and indirect light reflexes are quite normal.

The light reflex is mediated by afferent (optic nerve) and efferent (parasympathetic) fibres. The anatomy of these is also discussed in Chapter 2.

Pupillary abnormalities in neurological practice are best considered in two categories:

1 Disorders of the light reflex
2 Disorders of the sympathetic innervation to the eye.

Disorders of the light reflex

These can be divided into afferent, central and efferent disorders. The afferent limb of the light reflex is via the optic nerve where fibres pass to the pretectal region and thence to the Edinger–Westphal nucleus bilaterally. The parasympathetic efferent outflow, firing of which causes constriction of the pupil, originates in the Edinger–Westphal nucleus. The preganglionic fibres follow the course of the IIIrd nerve to the ciliary ganglion and then synapse with the post-ganglionic fibres which travel to the iris sphincter muscle in the short posterior ciliary nerves.

Complete afferent pupillary defect

When there is complete blindness in one eye because of pathology in the retina or optic nerve then a light shone in the blind eye produces no reaction in either pupil, whereas a light shone in the normally sighted fellow eye constricts both pupils. This situation is encountered in any complete optic nerve lesion, and the most common causes are tumour or trauma.

The light reflex tests the integrity of the anterior visual pathways. A preserved light reflex, in the presence of apparent total blindness in the eye, indicates either that the blindness is non-organic or that it arises from the posterior visual pathways.

Relative afferent pupillary defect

A pupil with a relative afferent defect (sometimes known as the Marcus Gunn pupil) is identified by the swinging light test. When light is directed into the affected eye this will cause only mild constriction of both pupils (because the afferent defect reduces the amount of light stimulus reaching the pretectum), and when directed into the unaffected eye it will cause a larger constriction of both pupils (because more of the light stimulus is reaching the pretectum to drive the pupils). When the light is rapidly alternated between the two eyes, the pretectum 'sees' the light stimulus as brighter when the stimulus is presented to the good eye and dimmer when the stimulus is presented to the affected eye; as a result, the pupils constrict when stimulating the good eye and dilate when stimulating the affected eye. This sign is called a relative afferent pupil defect (RAPD).

The presence of an RAPD indicates that there is unilateral (or markedly asymmetric) disease of the optic nerve (most commonly) or retina (less commonly). It is extremely rare for preretinal diseases (e.g. corneal pathology, cataract or vitreous haemorrhage) to cause this sign provided the torch light is bright enough, nor should an RAPD be attributed to a 'lazy eye' or maculopathy.

The most common optic nerve disorder causing an RAPD is optic neuritis associated with MS. Other causes include an ischaemic optic neuropathy, optic nerve tumour (optic nerve meningioma, glioma), orbital disease causing compression of the optic nerve (including thyroid orbitopathy), infection and inflammation (including sarcoidosis and Lyme disease), radiation damage or trauma. Other unilateral optic neuropathies including Leber's hereditary optic neuropathy will also result in this sign.

Extensive retinal disease will sometimes cause a 'Marcus Gunn' effect. This may be seen with retinal infarction, infection, tumours and detachment, but in these patients additional optic nerve disease must be excluded. Disease confined to the macula rarely gives rise to an RAPD.

Central (midbrain) lesions of the light reflex

When the pupil is affected by a midbrain lesion, there are two common patterns: the Argyll Robertson and Parinaud syndromes.

Argyll Robertson's syndrome This venerable sign is rarely encountered in clinical practice now. However, it used to be a common finding, characteristically in tertiary syphilis. The pupils typically are small and irregular and do not react to light but do react to accommodation (light near dissociation). The features are caused by damage of the central inhibitory fibres ventral to the aqueduct. Similar pupillary abnormalities are occasionally encountered in diabetes, MS or myotonic dystrophy. Occasionally, the 'inverse Argyll Robertson pupil' (no accommodation reflex but a preserved light reflex) is observed in cases of tertiary syphilis and was common in encephalitis lethargica.

Parinaud's syndrome Parinaud's syndrome (synonym: dorsal midbrain syndrome) is a term used to describe a cluster of five clinical signs:

- Dilated (or mid-dilated) pupils that do not react to light, but which do react to accommodation.

- Paralysis of voluntary up-gaze with preservation of down-gaze (a supranuclear gaze palsy where up-gaze can still be demonstrated using the doll's head manoeuvre, i.e. using the oculocephalic reflex).
- Convergence retraction nystagmus on attempted up-gaze. The eyes pull inward on up-gaze and the eyeballs retract.
- Eyelid retraction (Collier's sign).
- Convergence paralysis.

The syndrome is caused by damage to fibres in the dorsal midbrain, specifically to the posterior commissure. The syndrome can result from many pathologies in this anatomical location. It is a characteristic sign of a pineal gland tumour (usually a pinealoma) but is also commonly encountered with any extrinsic space-occupying lesions in this region including other brain tumours and hydrocephalus. Intrinsic mesencephalic pathologies such as MS, angiomas, infection (e.g. toxoplasmosis) and ischaemic or haemorrhagic stroke are uncommon causes. Transient Parinaud's syndrome may rarely result from a tonic–clonic seizure.

Treatment is primarily directed towards the aetiology of the dorsal midbrain damage. MRI is the common first choice investigation and will usually reveal the cause.

If the cause is alleviated, the eye findings of Parinaud's syndrome generally improve, either rapidly or over a period of months. If symptomatic therapy is needed (which is rare) up-gaze palsy and the retraction nystagmus can be improved by bilateral inferior rectus recession.

Efferent parasympathetic defects of the light reflex

Anatomically these can be divided into preganglionic and post-ganglionic parasympathetic lesions. In acute preganglionic block, there is a large unreactive pupil with absent light and accommodation reflexes. If in isolation, it is usually pharmacologic rather than neurogenic and caused by exposure of the eye to drugs or eye drops. Preganglionic lesions are usually associated with a IIIrd nerve palsy and may be caused by an acute compressive (neurosurgical) cause or basal meningitis. Other causes, and the clinical features, of IIIrd nerve palsy are considered above.

Holmes–Adie syndrome

The Holmes–Adie syndrome (HAS; named after William John Aidie, 1886–1935, and Gordon Morgan Holmes, 1876–1965, both from the National Hospital, Queen Square) is characterised by two key clinical signs: a tonic pupil and tendon areflexia. The tonic pupil shows little or no reaction to light, and when examined under magnification it is often observed that some meridians of the pupil margin respond to light whereas others do not ('sector palsy') causing the pupil to appear misshapen. In contrast, the pupil shows an exaggerated response to near but the constriction is markedly slowed (hence 'tonic'). The other cardinal feature of this syndrome is the absence of deep tendon reflexes (especially knee jerks), a clinical sign that is never associated with symptoms. HAS typically occurs in young adults (third to fifth decade), with a female preponderance. It often affects one pupil initially but the other eye usually becomes affected years or even decades later. Once present, the condition persists and the pupil changes are irreversible. Some individuals with HAS also develop sweating abnormalities, with patches of hyperhidrosis and hypohidrosis (Ross's syndrome).

HAS is most commonly noticed by chance, when the affected individual looks in a mirror and sees the pupil abnormality. Sometimes there is blurring of vision and photophobia (intolerance to bright light) because of the pupillary dilatation, or difficulty with near vision because of failure of accommodation of the lens. The clinical features of HAS are thought to be caused by damage to the ciliary ganglion and the dorsal root spinal ganglia, although the cause is unknown and the syndrome remains idiopathic. The diagnosis is made on clinical grounds. Treatment is not usually needed, but pilocarpine drops can be used, three times a day, to constrict the pupil if necessary. Thoracic sympathectomy or botulinum toxin injection is a definitive treatment for excessive sweating.

Tonic pupils are not always a result of HAS and may also be seen in a number of other ophthalmic (e.g. following eye or orbital surgery) and neurological conditions (e.g. in generalised dysautonomias and peripheral neuropathies), in which case there will always be other symptoms and signs indicating the underlying aetiology.

Disorders of the sympathetic nervous supply to the pupil

The sympathetic pathway originates in the posterior hypothalamus, travels through the brainstem (including the lateral medulla) and then descends in the cervical cord to the C8–T1 level. There the first order neurones synapse with the second order neurones which leave the cord and enter the paravertebral sympathetic chain to the superior cervical ganglion. They subsequently synapse with the third order (post-ganglionic fibres) which ascend around the internal carotid artery to the base of the skull. In the cavernous sinus they form a peri-arterial plexus in the adventitia of the artery. The oculosympathetic fibres pass through the superior orbital fissure in the long ciliary nerves while sudomotor and vasomotor fibres to the face travel with branches of the external carotid artery. Excitatory fibres supply the dilator pupillae, Müller's muscle and the blood vessels of the eye. Inhibitory fibres supply the ciliary muscle and the sphincter pupillae.

Horner's syndrome

Horner's syndrome is caused by dysfunction of the sympathetic nervous supply to the eye. It can be caused by damage anywhere along the lengthy three-neurone sympathetic pathway – and can be divided into 'central' (first-order), 'preganglionic' (second order) and 'post-ganglionic' (third order) lesions. It is an important syndrome, not because it affects vision itself (this is unusual) but because some of the common causes of the syndrome require urgent attention.

Clinical features The cardinal signs are ptosis (from loss of sympathetic tone in Müller muscle) and miosis (constricted pupil). Other signs include 'upside-down' ptosis (slight elevation of the lower lid) giving rise to narrowing of the palpebral aperture and apparent enophthalmos, conjunctival injection and anhidrosis (decreased sweating). If the syndrome develops around birth or in very early childhood, the iris on the affected side may become less pigmented (heterochromia iridis) because melanisation of the ocular tissues in early life requires an intact sympathetic nerve supply. An important clinical point is that the ptosis caused by Horner's syndrome occurs with a constricted pupil and the ptosis caused by a IIIrd nerve palsy is usually more severe and associated with a dilated pupil (from a loss of innervation to the sphincter pupillae).

Causes Horner's syndrome can be congenital but is usually acquired. A list of causes is shown in Table 14.24. Traumatic birth injury is one cause of a congenital Horner's (Klumpke paralysis) and the diagnosis is usually obvious. Most cases are isolated and idiopathic. Rare genetic causes also result in a congenital Horner's syndrome. Congenital cases show heterochromia (the affected iris is less pigmented).

The acquired causes are almost all unilateral if caused by a focal lesion, and can be caused by interference with the sympathetic nervous supply at any point in its long anatomical course (Chapter 2). Bilateral Horner's syndrome is characteristic of autonomic neuropathies (e.g. diabetes or amyloid). In children, the development of a Horner's syndrome requires urgent imaging to exclude a neuroblastoma. In adults, a characteristic presentation of dissection of the carotid artery is the development of a Horner's syndrome with ipsilateral neck or face pain. The Raeder syndrome (paratrigeminal syndrome) comprises oculo-sympathetic palsy and ipsilateral facial pain, often with some involvement of the trigeminal and oculomotor nerves. Pancoast tumour, carcinoma at the apex of the lung, also may present with a Horner's syndrome. Cluster headaches cause a transient Horner's syndrome, which is useful in diagnosis.

Table 14.24 Acquired causes of unilateral Horner's syndrome.

Type of lesion	Anatomical position	Common pathologies
Preganglionic		
First order neurone	Hypothalamus, midbrain, pons, medulla, cervical cord	Multiple sclerosis Tumour Vascular lesion (in medulla, as part of the lateral medullary syndrome; Wallenberg's syndrome) Syringomyelia
Second order neurone	T1 level of spinal cord/column, sympathetic chain, the superior cervical ganglion	Thoracic cord lesions Neck trauma Spinal column lesions and disc prolapse Cervical rib Aneurysm/dissection of aorta or subclavian artery Central venous catheteriisation Abscess or infection, lymphadenopathy Thyroid neoplasm Lesions in the apex of the lung (especially Pancoast's tumour)
Post-ganglionic		
Third order neurone	Internal carotid artery, base of the skull, ophthalmic nerve, cavernous sinus, superior orbital fissure, orbit	Aneurysms or dissection of the internal carotid artery Cavernous sinus lesion (fistula, aneurysm, granuloma) Skull base or orbital tumour Skull base malformation (e.g. Arnold–Chiari malformation) Infection Meningioma Trauma Nasopharyngeal carcinoma Orbital pathology (including trauma, tumour, granuloma, infection) Neuroblastoma (in children) Herpes zoster

Table 14.25 Summary of responses to topical agents in Horner's syndrome.

	0.5% apraclonidine	4% cocaine	1% hydroxyamphetamine
Normal	No response	Dilates	Dilates
Preganglionic Horner's syndrome (recent)	Dilates	No response	Dilates impressively
Preganglionic Horner's syndrome (long-standing)	Dilates	No response	May dilate if no transsynaptic degeration of third order neurones
Post-ganglionic Horner's syndrome	Dilates	No response	No response

Diagnosis The clinical features are so characteristic that no diagnostic tests are usually needed. However, the diagnosis of the underlying cause depends on the clinical situation and will often involve MRI and MR angiography.

Pharmacological tests can be used to confirm the diagnosis and to differentiate a preganglionic from a post-ganglionic Horner's syndrome. The most reliable test for confirmation of the diagnosis is instillation of topical 4% cocaine eye drops; this prevents re-uptake of noradrenaline in the sympathetic nerves to the iris dilator muscles and causes dilatation of the pupil in a normal eye but not in an eye with Horner's syndrome. Nowadays cocaine eye drops are often unavailable so an effective alternative drug to use is topical apraclonidine; this is a weak adrenergic agonist that has little or no effect on a normal pupil but causes dilation (and reversal of the anisocoria) in Horner's syndrome because of the denervation supersensitivity present in the dilator muscle fibres. Neither of these drugs can localise the lesion; for this it is necessary to use 1% hydroxyamphetamine, a drug that releases noradrenaline from intact sympathetic nerve endings – this drug dilates a normal pupil, has no effect on a patient with a post-ganglionic Horner and produces an exaggerated mydriasis in patients with a pre-ganglionic Horner (Table 14.25).

References

Kölmel HW. Complex visual hallucinations in the hemianopic field. *J Neurol Neurosurg Psychiatry* 1985; **48**: 29–38.

Mooney AJ, Carey P, Ryan M, Bofin P. Parasagittal parieto-occipital meningioma with visual hallucinations. *Am J Ophthalmol* 1965; **59**: 197–205.

Panayiotopoulos CP. Visual phenomena and headache in occipital epilepsy: a review, a systemic study and differentiation from migraine. *Epileptic Disord* 1999; **1**: 205–216.

Further reading

General texts

Acheson J, Riordan-Eva P. *Fundamentals of Clinical Ophthalmology: Neuro-ophthalmology.* London: BMJ Books, 1999.

Acheson JF, Sanders MD. *Common Problems in Neuro-ophthalmology*. London: WB Saunders, 1997.

Brazis PW, Masdeu JC, Biller J. *Localization in Clinical Neurology*, 4th edn. Philadelphia: Lippincott, Williams & Wilkins, 2001.

Miller NR, Newman NJ, Biousse V, Kerrison JB, eds. *Walsh & Hoyt's Clinical Neuro-Ophthalmology*, 6th edn. Philadelphia: Lippincott Williams & Wilkins, 2005.

Miller NR, Newman NJ. The eye in neurological disease. *Lancet* 2004; **364**: 2045–2054.

Purvin V, Kawasaki A. Neuro-ophthalmic emergencies for the neurologist. *Neurologist* 2005; **11**: 195–233.

Riordan-Eva P, Whitcher JP, eds. *Vaughan and Asbury's General Ophthalmology*. New York: McGraw-Hill, 2004.

Spalton DJ, Hitchings RA, Hunter P, eds. *Atlas of Clinical Ophthalmology*, 3rd edn. London: Elsevier, 2004.

Unilateral and bilateral visual failure

Holder GE, Gale RP, Acheson JF, Robson AG. Electrodiagnostic assessment in optic nerve disease. *Curr Opin Neurol* 2009; **23**: 3–10.

Jindhara P, Hedges T, Mendoza-Sebastian C, Plant GT. Optical coherence tomography of the retina: applications in neurology. *Curr Opin Neurol* 2010; **23**: 16–23.

Pandit RJ, Gales K, Griffiths PG. Effectiveness of testing visual fields by confrontation. *Lancet* 2001; **358**: 1339–1346.

Optic nerve disease

Arnold AC. Pathogenesis of nonarteritic anterior ischaemic optic neuropathy. *J Neuroophthalmol* 2003; **23**: 157–163.

Atkins EJ, Biousse V, Newman NJ. Optic neuritis. *Semin Neurol* 2007; **27**: 211–220.

Belcer LJ. Clinical practice: optic neuritis. *N Engl J Med* 2006; **354**: 1273–1280.

Bhatti MT. Orbital syndromes. *Semin Neurol* 2007; **27**: 269–287.

Digre KB, Corbett JJ. Idiopathic intracranial hypertension (pseudotumour cerebri): a reappraisal. *Neurologist* 2001; 7: 2–68

Frohman EM, Frohman TC, Zee DS, *et al.* The neuro-ophthalmology of multiple sclerosis. *Lancet Neurol* 2005; **4**: 111–121.

Guevara N, Roy D, Dutruc-Rosset C, Santini J, Hofman P, Castillo L. Mucormycosis: early diagnosis and treatment. *Rev Laryngol Otol Rhinol* 2004; **125**: 127–131.

Kerrison JB. Optic neuropathies caused by toxins and adverse drug reactions. *Ophthalmol Clin North Am* 2004; **17**: 481–488.

Klopstock T, Yu-Wai-Man P, Dimitriadis K, Rouleau J, Heck S, Bailie M, *et al.* A randomized placebo-controlled trial of idebenone in Leber's hereditary optic neuropathy. *Brain* 2011; **134** (Pt 9): 2677–2686.

Newman NJ. Hereditary optic neuropaties. In: *Walsh & Hoyt's Clinical Neuro-Ophthalmology*, 6th edn. Miller NR, Newman NJ, Biousse V, Kerrison JB, eds. Baltimore: Lippincott Williams & Wilkins, 2005: 293–348.

Optic Neuritis Study Group. Neurologic impairment 10 years after optic neuritis. *Arch Neurol* 2004; **61**: 1386–1389.

Purvin VA. Optic neuropathies for the neurologist. *Semin Neurol* 2000; **20**: 97–110.

Rucker JC, Biousse V, Newman NJ. Ischaemic optic neuropathies. *Curr Opin Neurol* 2004; **17**: 27–35.

Schumacher M, Schmidt D, Jurklies B, Gall C, Wanke I, Schmoor C, *et al*; EAGLE-Study Group. Central retinal artery occlusion: local intra-arterial fibrinolysis versus conservative treatment, a multicenter randomized trial. *Ophthalmology* 2010; **117**: 1367–1375.

Smith CH. Optic neuritis. In: *Walsh & Hoyt's Clinical Neuro-Ophthalmology*, 6th edn. Miller NR, Newman NJ, Biousse V, Kerrison JB, eds. Baltimore: Lippincott Williams & Wilkins, 2005: 293–348.

Tomsak RL. Giant cell arteritis. *Ophthalmology* 2002; **109**: 219–220.

Toosy A, Mason D, Miller DH. Optic neuritis. *Lancet Neurol* 2014; **13**: 83–99.

Van Stavern GP. Optic disc edema. *Semin Neurol* 2007; **27**: 233–243.

Ocular involvement in other neurological diseases

Brazis PW, Stewart M, Lee AG. The uveo-meningeal syndromes. *Neurologist* 2004; **10**: 171–185.

Diplopia

Keane JR. Cavernous sinus syndrome: analysis of 151 cases. *Arch Neurol* 1996; **53**: 967–971.

Keane JR. Bilateral involvement of a single cranial nerve: analysis of 578 cases. *Neurology* 2005; **65**: 950–952.

Kline LB, Hoyt WF. The Tolosa–Hunt syndrome. *J Neurol Neurosurg Psychiatry* 2001; **71**: 577–582.

Rucker JC. Oculomotor disorders. *Semin Neurol* 2007; **27**: 244–255.

Central disorders of eye movements

Caplan LR. 'Top of the basilar' syndrome. *Neurology* 1980; **30**: 72–79.

Leigh RJ, Zee DS. *The Neurology of Eye Movements*, 4th edn. Oxford: Oxford University Press, 2006.

Nystagmus

Dell'Osso LF, Daroff RB. Nystagmus and saccadic intrusions and oscillations. In: *Neuro-ophthalmology*, 3rd edn. Glaser JS, ed. Philadelphia: Lippincott Williams & Wilkins, 1999.

Chiasmal and retrochiasmal disorders

Barton JJ, Hefter R, Chang B, *et al.* The field defects of anteriotemporal lobectomy: a quantitative reassessment on Meyer's loop. *Brain* 2005; **128**: 2123–2132.

Fujino, T, Kigazawa K, Yamada R. Homonymous hemianopia: a retrospective study of 140 cases. *Neuroophthalmology* 1986; **6**: 17.

Levin LA. Topical diagnosis of chiasmal and retrochiasmal disorders. In: *Walsh & Hoyt's Clinical Neuro-Ophthalmology*, 6th edn. Miller NR, Newman NJ, Biousse V, Kerrison JB, eds. Baltimore: Lippincott Williams & Wilkins, 2005.

Miller Jacobson DM. The localizing value of a quadrantinopia. *Arch Neurol* 1997; **54**: 401–412.

Disorders of higher visual function

Zhang X, Keder S, Lynn MJ, Newman NJ, Biousse V. Homonymous hemianopias: clinical–anatomic correlations in 904 cases. *Neurology* 2006; **66**: 906–910.

Pupils

Bremner FD. In: *Fundamentals of Clinical Ophthalmology: Neuro-ophthalmology*. Acheson J, Riordan-Eva P, eds. London: BMJ Books, 1999.

Cooper-Knock J, Pepper I, Hodgson T, Sharrack B. Early diagnosis of Horner syndrome using topical apraclonidine. *J Neuroophthalmol* 2011; **31**: 214–216..

Thompson HS, Miller N. Disorders of pupillary function, accommodation and lacrimation. In: *Walsh & Hoyt's Clinical Neuro-Ophthalmology*, 5th edn. Miller NR, Newman NJ, eds. Baltimore: Lippincott Williams & Wilkins, 1998.

CHAPTER 15

Neuro-Otology: Problems of Dizziness, Balance and Hearing

Rosalyn Davies, Linda M. Luxon, Doris-Eva Bamiou and Adolfo Bronstein
National Hospital for Neurology & Neurosurgery

Dizziness and vertigo: introduction

Dizziness is an umbrella term describing symptoms varying from vague light-headedness and disorientation to imbalance and vertigo. Vertigo means the illusion of movement of either the body or the surroundings, typically spinning or sometimes tilting or rocking to and fro.

Vertigo is either of internal origin – a mismatch between sensory inputs – or it may be linked to retinal slip during the slow phase of nystagmus (i.e. the image moves across the retina); in each case the surroundings or the head seem to move. Much information can be gleaned from detailed descriptions of dizziness and especially vertigo, sometimes pointing to the specific semicircular canal involved. Any vestibular dysfunction can be accompanied by:

- Vertigo – rotary, swaying, tilting or postural imbalance
- Blurring of vision or slippage of the visual field with head movement, and
- Autonomic symptoms – nausea, vomiting, sweating, distress and anxiety.

Acute, severe vertigo causes prostration.

Epidemiology

Dizziness and vertigo are common. One UK community survey showed that one in four adults have had significant dizziness. Dizziness is a substantial cause of morbidity, loss of time from work, repeated medical attendances and costly investigation – one study showed that on average more than four physicians were visited before precise diagnosis of a vestibular problem. Dizziness is a frequent reason for consultation by those over 65 years and, like headache, is common worldwide.

Basic concepts

Three-dimensional spatial orientation

Balance is achieved and maintained by a complex sensorimotor system. Orienting sensory information is derived from the paired vestibular labyrinths, visual input and somato-sensory afferents (joint, tendon and muscle position sense, and superficial sensation). This information converges on the brainstem vestibular nuclei and is integrated with modulating influences from the reticular activating system and higher centres: cortex, cerebellum and extrapyramidal system. Effector pathways from the vestibular nuclei project to the oculomotor nuclei generating compensatory eye movements (i.e. the efferent limb of the vestibulo-ocular reflex, a three neurone reflex arc). Other efferents pass to the neck, trunk and limb muscles, the vestibulo-spinal tracts, which modulate spinal reflex arcs. Efferents also project to the vestibular cortex from the brainstem (Figure 15.1).

The vestibular system has three primary functions:

1. To stabilise gaze in space during head movement (e.g. reading a sign while walking)
2. To control posture when the head and body are static (e.g. while standing and during passive motion), and
3. To facilitate perception of orientation and motion.

Vestibulo-ocular reflexes

The parallel vestibular and oculomotor systems have evolved in such a way that they function in three similar planes. These planes of head movement are:

1. *Yaw*: head rotation about the vertical z-axis
2. *Pitch*: head flexion/extension about the horizontal y-axis, and
3. *Roll*: lateral head tilt about the horizontal x-axis.

This alignment, between spatial planes of the three semicircular canals and the planes of the three sets of extraocular muscles is such that when the two, paired labyrinths are excited, the two eyes move conjugately (i.e. they are yoked), producing an appropriately directed compensatory eye movement. This is the vestibulo-ocular reflex. For example, the paired horizontal semicircular canals function as a gauge of rotational acceleration in the yaw plane and are connected via the brainstem nuclei to the set of extraocular muscles whose primary direction of pull is also in the horizontal plane – the lateral and medial recti. The action of these muscles is to produce a compensatory eye movement in the horizontal plane in an equal and opposite direction to that of head movement, thus maintaining stable gaze.

The neuronal circuitry is similar for the vertical planes of pitch and roll: the anterior and posterior semicircular canals, sited diagonally to the sagittal plane (Figure 15.2) are connected to the paired extraocular muscles whose primary action is aligned to the spatial planes of each canal. Thus, the superior and inferior recti move the eye up or down when that eye is abducted; the inferior and superior oblique muscles move the eye up and down when it is adducted.

Neurology: A Queen Square Textbook, Second Edition. Edited by Charles Clarke, Robin Howard, Martin Rossor and Simon Shorvon.

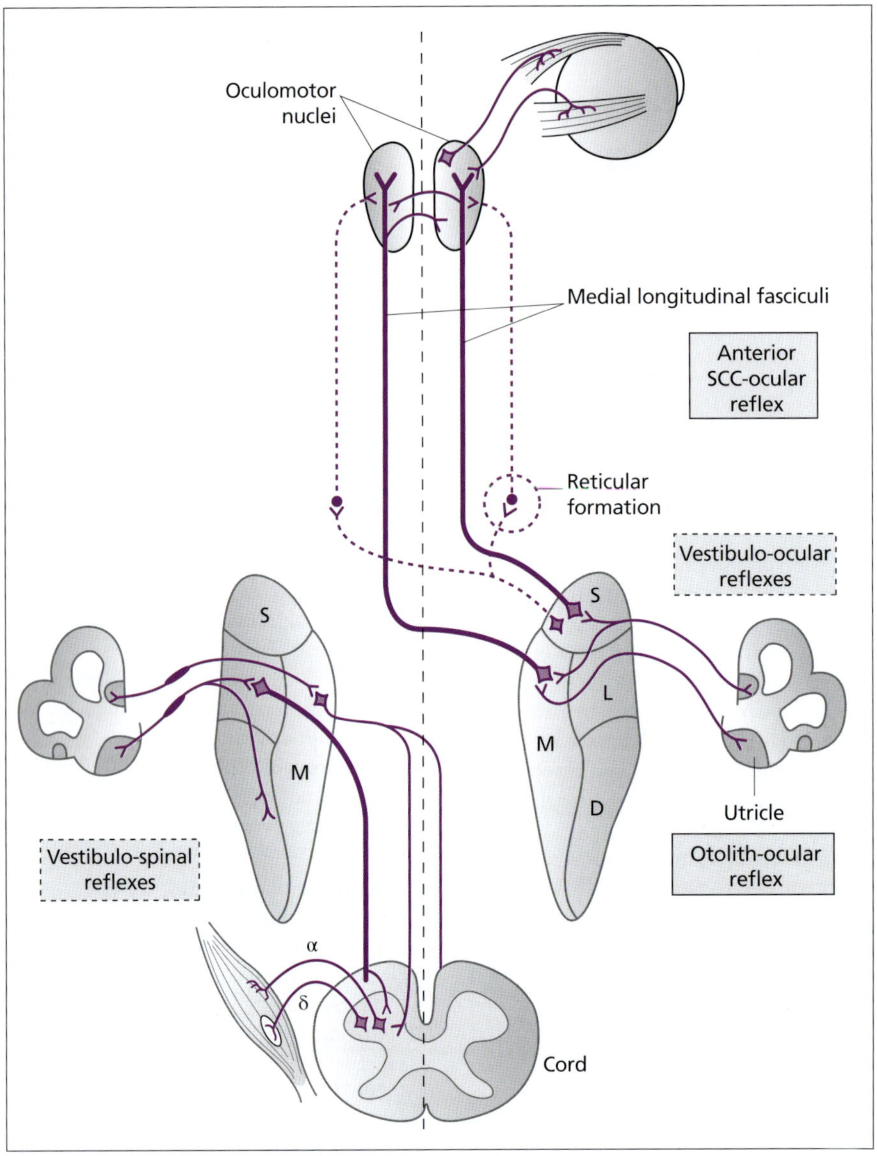

Figure 15.1 Vestibulo-ocular and vestibulo-spinal reflexes. S, L, M, D: superior, lateral, medial and descending vestibular nuclei.

The system is driven by the relationship between endolymph and cristae (Chapter 2). The relevant principles were described by Ewald in 1892:

1 Head and eye movements always take place in the plane of the canal that is stimulated and in the direction of endolymph flow.
2 In the horizontal canal, endolymph flow towards the ampulla (ampullo-petal) causes a greater response than endolymph flow away from the ampulla (ampullo-fugal).
3 In the vertical canals, endolymph flow away from the ampulla (ampullo-fugal) causes a greater response than endolymph flow towards the ampulla (ampullo-petal).

Encoding of head movements in space

Sensory epithelium of each vestibular end organ includes the maculae found in the utricle and saccule, and the cristae, found in the ampulla in each of the three semicircular canals. Both maculae and cristae contain sensory hair cells with projecting kinocilia. Linear acceleration and gravitational forces are transduced by the otolith organs of the utricle and saccule; angular acceleration is transduced by the cristae. As a result of the orientation of the semicircular canals and arrangement of hair cells, head movements in any plane are encoded by the pattern of deflection of kinocilia. Stabilising sensory information thus derived is relayed to the vestibular nuclei, integrated and stored in a data centre probably within the reticular formation. New sensory data are constantly compared with this data bank; under normal circumstances, there is a match between visual, proprioceptive and vestibular inputs, thus maintaining equilibrium (Figure 15.3). This matching up of sensory inputs is essential for spatial orientation and perception of motion. Vertigo results from a mismatch between sensory information from these inputs, leading to impaired perception of a stationary environment. Vestibular sensations can also occur as a response to a moving environment (e.g. motion sickness), or with pathology of any of the three sensory stabilising systems. Examples of the latter include

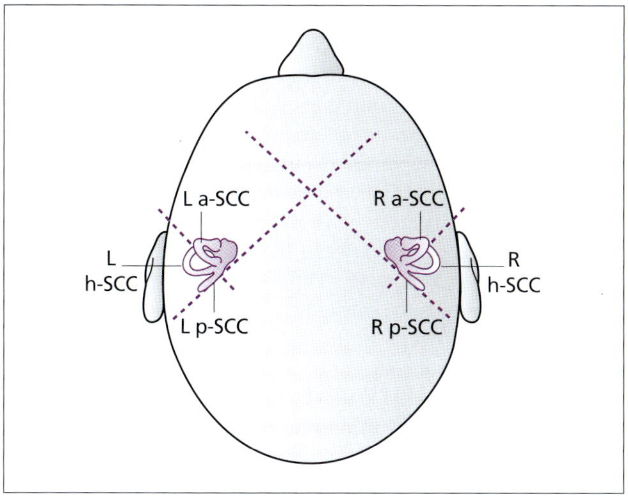

Figure 15.2 Topographical orientation of the anterior, horizontal and posterior semicircular canals. a-SCC, anterior semicircular canal; h-SCC: horizontal semicircular canal; p-SCC: posterior semicircular canal. Source: Rudge 1983. Reproduced with permission of Elsevier.

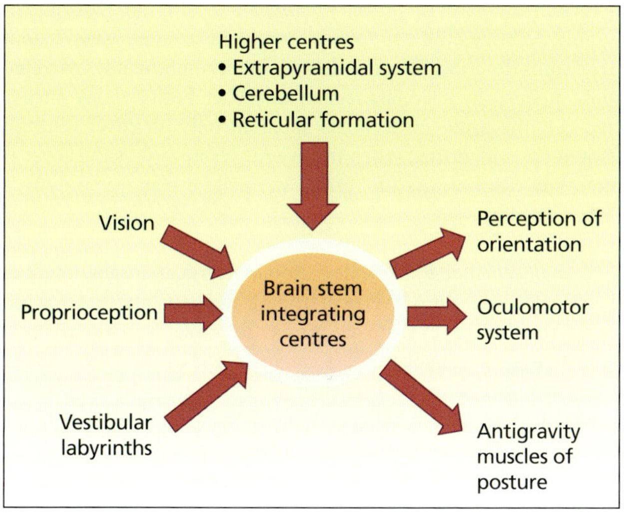

Figure 15.3 Sensori-motor physiology of the maintenance of equilibrium. Depicting the three sensory inputs required for maintenance of equilibrium, the central modulating influences and the efferent pathways. Source: Davies 2004. Reproduced with permission.

disturbed labyrinthine input during an attack of Ménière's disease; altered visual input with the first use of varifocal lenses; or with impaired proprioception following a knee joint replacement. The unpleasant autonomic sensations of nausea, vomiting and anxiety that often accompany vertigo are mediated by vestibulo-autonomic pathways.

Neuro-otological assessment

Clinical examination

What to examine

- Brief neurological examination
- Gait and posture
- Nystagmus, eye movements, positional testing
- Orthostatic blood pressure.

When to examine what – the clinical presentation of balance disorders

- Acute vertigo
- Recurrent vertigo and dizziness
- Chronic dizziness and imbalance.

As in any other clinical examination in medical practice, the physician is guided by the symptoms reported by the patient. A good physician would not spend too much time examining the vestibular-ocular reflex if his/her patient's dizzy spells are always preceded by chest pain and palpitations. If we focus on peripheral and central vestibular disorders, these can usually be diagnosed with a good history and examination. A summary of the clinical examination is first presented, followed by a strategy to apply the various components of the examination to the specific clinical presentations.

What to examine

Brief neurological examination

Neurological disease affecting the sensory input, strength, tone, coordination or praxis of the lower limbs will cause a degree of unsteadiness and sense of imbalance. As these sensations can be described by patients as 'dizziness', the clinician must be sure that the cause of his patient's dizziness or imbalance is not a lower limb neurological problem. Neuro-otologists of any background (ENT, audiovestibular medicine, audiology or neurology) should examine the patient neurologically, particularly the gait and postural reflexes, if explaining the patient's symptoms on the basis of a vestibular disorder prove elusive. Of note, patients may, during the early stages of a neurological gait disorder (small vessel white matter disease in particular) describe imbalance and yet formal examination of the lower limbs is normal. Slight unsteadiness during turning while walking or hypokinetic postural responses during pulls to the trunk may be the only objective abnormality during the examination, as is discussed later.

Gait and posture

Examination of gait with eyes open is very useful for detecting neurological disorders that compromise balance and gait and can therefore predispose to falls. It is indeed an important part of the general neurological examination and there are many specific gait types (e.g. parkinsonian, cerebellar, polyneuritic, tabetic and spastic gait). The clinician should observe the general speed of gait, size of the base of support, regularity of step production and turning. Difficulties in initiating gait can be seen in gait apraxias, small vessel disease and parkinsonism.

Increasing the base of support is an automatic reaction adopted when healthy people (walking on a boat, drunkenness) or patients perceive that their balance capabilities are reduced. Broad based gait is observed in any condition limiting balance, including acute vertigo (both peripheral and central), polyneuropathies, cerebellar disease and many pyramidal and extrapyramidal disorders. The relatively narrow gait present in patients with idiopathic Parkinson's disease may indicate reduced adaptability (to their objective imbalance) in their motor system. Unilateral vestibular disorders, except in the acute vertigo phase, do not cause significant abnormalities.

- *Gait test:* this is a 5 m walk, first with the eyes open and then with the eyes closed, with the examiner close alongside for safety. The patient should walk at normal speed towards a fixed target. As with Unterberger's test, patients with recent unilateral vestibular hypofunction tend to deviate towards the side of the lesion.

- *Tandem gait test:* this is useful for assessing vestibulo-spinal function. When performed with the eyes open, tandem walking is primarily a test of cerebellar function because vision compensates for chronic vestibular and proprioceptive deficits. Tandem walking with eyes closed is a good test of vestibular function as long as cerebellar and proprioceptive functions remain intact: ask the patient to take 10 heel–toe steps at a comfortable speed, starting with feet in the tandem (heel to toe) position and arms folded against the chest. Most normal subjects can manage 10 accurate tandem steps in three trials.
- *Romberg's test:* described in 1846 in patients with dorsal column loss following tabes dorsalis; the test is positive if there is increased body sway when the eyes are closed and the patient stands with feet close together. The principle behind the test is that balance is maintained with minimal physiological sway when all three sensory inputs are functioning (i.e. vision, vestibular input and proprioceptive input). With the loss of one or more of these inputs, there is increased physiological sway.
- *Unterberger's test:* In the 1930s, Unterberger described the tendency for vestibular imbalance to cause patients to turn when walking. The test identifies that the direction of turning in patients with unilateral vestibular deficits coincides with the direction of past-pointing and falling (i.e. in the direction of the slow component of nystagmus). The test is performed by asking the patient to stand with arms extended and thumbs raised, to close their eyes and asked to march on the spot for about 50 steps. However, there is often marked variability in the rotation angle in the same subject on repeated testing and non-organic problems frequently produce apparent abnormalities, thus Unterberger's test should be interpreted with care.

Nystagmus, eye movements, positional testing

Clinical examination of eye movements The vestibular system provides a powerful input to the oculomotor system so eye movements must be examined in detail. In a patient suspected to have a peripheral vestibular disorder (labyrinth and VIIIth nerve) one can consider that the examination has two broad aims:

1. To search for direct ocular signs indicative of a peripheral vestibular disorder, typically nystagmus, benign paroxysmal positional vertigo (BPPV) or a positive head thrust test (see Head impulse test)
2. To exclude a central nervous system (CNS) lesion by making sure that non-vestibularly mediated eye movements are normal.
   The oculomotor examination should include:
   - Cover test
   - Search for spontaneous and gaze-evoked nystagmus
   - Convergence
   - Smooth pursuit
   - Saccades
   - Vestibular-ocular reflexes
   - Positional manoeuvres.

If the patient reports diplopia, or if at any point during the examination the two eyes appear dysconjugate, examination of the individual cranial nerves III, IV and VI and a cover test is mandatory (Chapter 14). Beware of infantile strabismus as oculomotor findings become less reliable.

Cover test

Misalignment of the visual axes needs to be identified (i.e. manifest or latent strabismus). Either can lead to eye movement abnormalities as fixation switches from one eye to the other. If one eye has become amblyopic, the better eye should be assessed, both by clinical tests and oculography. Commonly, a patient with acquired strabismus will turn or tilt their head to minimise diplopia. Turning is seen typically with paresis of a horizontal extraocular muscle (e.g. following VIth nerve palsy), when the head is turned towards the weak lateral rectus. Following a IVth nerve palsy, the head tends to tilt, if slightly, towards the side of the weak superior oblique.

To perform the cover test, the patient is asked to fixate a distant target, with refractive correction in place. Each eye is covered in turn; this prevents foveal fixation by the covered eye. The cover test relies on the fact that foveation occurs in the eye forced to fixate; movement redress occurs if the retinal image was not directed to the fovea before the eye took up fixation. The patient is asked to fixate with the uncovered eye on a target; the covered eye is then observed as the cover is removed.

Horizontal misalignment A squint (manifest strabismus) is seen when the visual axes of the two eyes deviate with the eyes uncovered: an exotropion (divergent squint) means that the affected eye is turned outward in primary gaze; an esotropion (convergent squint) describes the eye turned inward in primary gaze. Latent strabismus describes the situation when misalignment is corrected spontaneously by fusional mechanisms when both eyes are uncovered (i.e. the problem becomes apparent only on cover testing). Exophoria is identified when the eye moves inward as the cover is removed; esophoria is identified when the eye moves outwards with refixation.

Vertical misalignment Skew deviation is a vertical misalignment of the visual axes (i.e. it is a vertical tropia), and may be either a hypotropia (uncovered eye moves up as the other is covered) or a hypertropia (the uncovered eye moves down as the other is covered). By convention, the higher of the eyes is referred to as hypertrophic/hyperphoric, regardless of which is at fault. The hypertropia may be the same in nearly all positions of gaze (concomitant) or vary with right or left gaze (non-concomitant) and is usually associated with the ocular tilt reaction (OTR). When non-concomitant, skew deviation can be distinguished from a superior oblique palsy by the direction of any torsion of the elevated eye (intorsion with a skew, extorsion with a IVth nerve palsy). Skew deviation can be either sustained or paroxysmal. Skew deviation is caused typically by brainstem or cerebellar lesions.

Latent nystagmus Nystagmus is seen in the uncovered eye during cover testing. Typically, the nystagmus beats away from the covered eye and is conjugate. Latent nystagmus can be unilateral or bilateral. Some cases are associated with congenital nystagmus (see Congenital nystagmus).

Spontaneous nystagmus

The search for spontaneous nystagmus begins in the primary (straight ahead position) of the eyes. In the presence of nystagmus, ascertain: (i) the waveform (e.g. saw-tooth, jerk or 'beating nystagmus'); or pendular nystagmus, and (ii) the direction of the beat (Figure 15.4a). As spontaneous nystagmus is often enhanced by convergence, it is convenient to examine convergence at the same time, by slowly moving an object in and out along the visual axis.

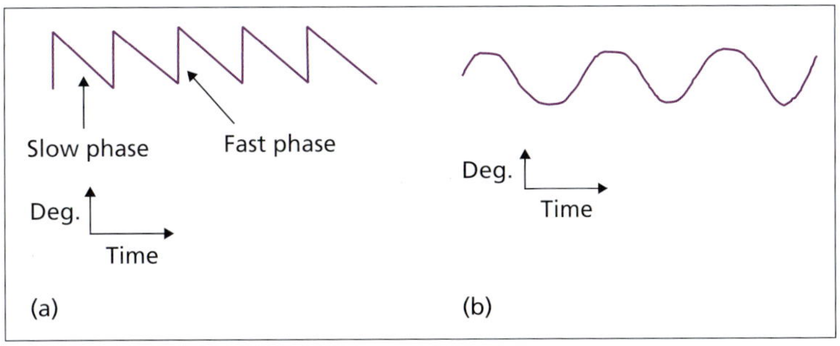

Figures 15.4 Oculographic recordings of types of nystagmus: (a) saw-tooth or 'beating' nystagmus (the direction of beat is defined as the direction of the fast phase with upwards deflection of the recording indicating movement to the right); (b) pendular nystagmus.

Absence of convergence occurs in midbrain lesions, but it must be remembered that reduced/absent convergence is very common in normal people above the age of 60 years.

Patients have to be clearly instructed to look at a pre-determined fixation object and the eyes should be well-illuminated. The presence of spontaneous nystagmus in primary gaze immediately raises the question, is this caused by a peripheral or central lesion? If the patient is in the midst of an acute vertigo attack, with severe unsteadiness and nausea, the nystagmus can be either peripheral or central, but if the patient comes as a routine ambulatory patient and does not look acutely ill, the nystagmus is more likely to be of central origin. A clinically visible nystagmus of peripheral vestibular origin can only be seen in the acute phase of the disorder (e.g. vestibular neuritis, Ménière's disorder). The nystagmus is essentially horizontal with a minor torsional (rotary) component. The fast phase beats contra-lesionally, but in the acute irritative phase of Ménière's attack, it can beat ipsi-lesionally.

Can a nystagmus like this result from a central lesion? Yes, in particular, lesions in the VIIIth nerve root entry zone or vestibular nuclei, but, almost invariably, there are additional brainstem symptoms and signs. Any other nystagmus is almost certainly of central origin. These differ from a peripheral vestibular nystagmus in waveform (e.g. pendular, a quasi-sinusoidal oscillation of the eye without distinction between the slow and fast phases; Figure 15.4b) or beat plane (e.g. vertical up or downbeat, or torsional nystagmus). A large horizontal nystagmus in a patient with no significant vestibular or neurological symptoms should always raise the possibility of congenital nystagmus.

Gaze evoked nystagmus

Soon after the acute stage of a peripheral vestibular lesion, the nystagmus is not visible in primary gaze but only on gaze deviation in the direction of the fast phase. A useful classification for the severity of nystagmus is Alexander's law:

- *First degree nystagmus:* only visible on gaze deviation in the direction of the fast phase
- *Second degree nystagmus:* when present in primary gaze as well as the direction of the fast phase, and
- *Third degree:* when it is also visible when the eyes are deviated in the opposite direction to that of the fast phase.

Alexander's law applies to most peripheral vestibular nystagmus. Downbeat nystagmus in primary gaze, which is always of central origin, often does not enhance on looking down but on looking sideways.

Nystagmus on gaze deviation can also indicate a central lesion. This is what is frequently called gaze paretic nystagmus, not to be confused with the broader term gaze evoked nystagmus. The term gaze paretic implies that the patient has difficulty in holding gaze in an eccentric position in the orbit. The eyes drift in centripetally with a slow phase which progressively decreases in velocity, until a new saccade re-fixates the eccentric target. This nystagmus, usually of larger amplitude than peripheral vestibular nystagmus, is caused by damage to the gaze holding mechanisms mediated by ipsilateral brainstem and cerebellar structures. An example of vestibular and gaze paretic nystagmus present in the same patient is Brun's nystagmus caused by a large, extracanalicular, acoustic neuroma. The vestibular nystagmus, as expected in any destructive vestibular lesion is in the opposite direction to the side of the tumour. The coarser nystagmus, evoked by looking in the same direction as the tumour, is gaze paretic because of brainstem–cerebellar compression (Figure 15.5). Gaze paretic nystagmus can be present in all directions of gaze in the same patient, typically in symmetrical processes such as cerebellar degenerations.

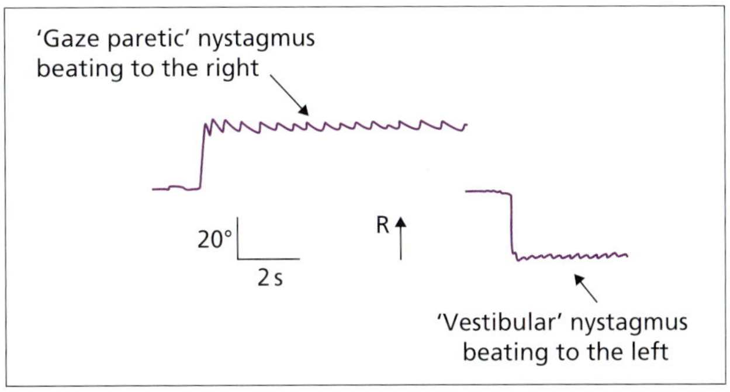

Figure 15.5 Oculographic recordings of Brun's nystagmus. Horizontal electro-oculography (EOG) in a patient with Brun's nystagmus caused by a large right-sided cerebello-pontine angle lesion. Note the larger amplitude 'gaze paretic' nystagmus beating to the right (top trace) and the smaller amplitude 'vestibular' nystagmus beating to the left (lower trace).

Congenital nystagmus

The patient with congenital nystagmus rarely complains of oscillopsia, but does have a central eye movement abnormality. The nystagmus is in the horizontal plane and may change direction. There is a null point, which is often the eye position the patient adopts for reading; the slow phase is dysmorphic with non-linear slow phases and may be exponential as can be demonstrated on the

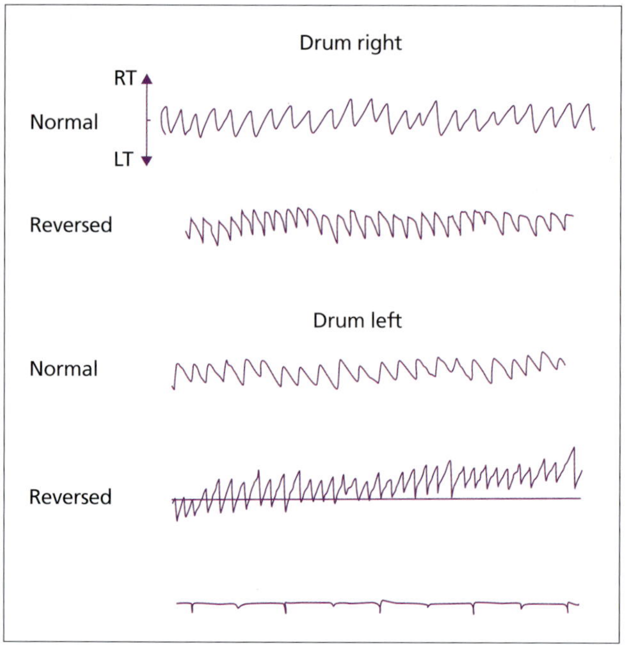

Figure 15.6 Congenital nystagmus. EOG showing the optokinetic response in a patient with congenital nystagmus (i.e. reversal of optokinetic nystagmus [OKN] direction with the slow phase of the patient's eyes in the opposite direction to the direction of the OKN drum). Source: Hood 1984. Reproduced with permission of John Wiley & Sons.

electro-nystagmogram (ENG). Characteristically, there is reversal of optokinetic nystagmus (OKN; i.e. the slow phase of OKN does not match the direction of drum rotation; Figure 15.6).

Smooth pursuit eye movements

When tracking an object with our eyes we use a combination of fast (saccadic) and slow phase eye movements. Strictly speaking, only the latter should be considered smooth pursuit. When the target moves slowly (<10–15°/s) the eye is capable of following it almost exclusively with smooth pursuit movements (i.e. with a gain of 1.0). When targets move at velocities >40°/s, the proportion of tracking carried out by saccades increases progressively and the gain decreases. Clinically speaking, smooth pursuit looks abnormal or 'broken up' when the observer detects too much saccadic tracking; this gives a cogwheel, jerky appearance to the pursuit movements.

In principle, the presence of normal pursuit rules out a central vestibular disorder. Similarly, a patient with balance symptoms and unequivocally broken pursuit movements almost certainly has a neurological rather than a labyrinthine disorder. In order for the clinician to reach these conclusions confidently, the examination has to be technically correct. To start with the patient should be able to see the target correctly. Any object can be a target, not only the examiner's finger or pen. In patients too young, too old or with attentional problems, a substantial, solid target such as a key, a toy, a mobile phone or a credit card can increase performance. Make sure that in elderly subjects, with presbyopia and age-related convergence insufficiency, the object is presented at comfortable viewing distance. Sometimes the examination must be conducted with the patient wearing his/her own glasses.

Also the target has to be moved slowly, taking 3–4 seconds to travel from right to left, and vice versa. One cycle is not usually enough because patients may not understand the task and jump their eyes ahead of target; the patient should be encouraged to 'glue' their eyes to the target. Pursuit should be assessed in both the horizontal and vertical planes.

It is easy to identify asymmetric pursuit with excessive 'catch up' saccades in one direction only. When pursuit is broken, say to the right, the lesion may be in the (right) cerebellum or (left) parietal lobe. Brainstem lesions can have more complex effects (e.g. if they involve the vestibular nuclei which can generate nystagmus), but often are ipsilateral too. Small asymmetries in the horizontal plane, if consistent, are significant whereas asymmetries in the vertical plane can occur in many normal subjects. Global or pan-directional abnormalities of smooth pursuit are more difficult to interpret because pursuit pathways are polysynaptic, including visual pathways, parietal and frontal cortices, vestibular nuclei and cerebellar flocculus. This makes them vulnerable to trivial sources of mild diffuse CNS dysfunction, including ageing, psychotropic drugs and alcohol. The influence of age on pursuit is considerable so one must be careful in diagnosing bilaterally abnormal smooth pursuit in an elderly patient.

Saccadic eye movements

Saccades are fast movements of the eyes (200–500°/s) which allow us to shift gaze from one object of interest to another. These refixations occur incessantly so that gross saccadic defects are often detected when simply speaking to the patient. It should be said at the outset that just saying that a patient has abnormal saccades is not sufficient to make a topographic diagnosis. There are at least three independent properties of saccades: (i) velocity (normal, slow or absent saccades, e.g. a gaze palsy); (ii) accuracy (normo-, hypo- or hypermetric) and (iii) binocular conjugacy (conjugate or dysconjugate, e.g. internuclear ophthalmoplegia). All these three aspects can be assessed clinically.

Saccadic velocity It is possible to gain some insight into saccadic velocity by simply asking the patient to look fully to the right, left, up and down. However, it is better to assess accuracy at the same time, in which a visible target should be provided, usually the examiner's finger placed at 20–30° to the right–left up–down of primary gaze. The patient is instructed to look at the target when, for instance, the right or left finger flick, or when the hand opens up. It is customary to reinforce the visual stimulus with a simultaneous verbal command such as 'right', 'left' (from the patient's point of view!) or 'pen', 'finger'. Subtypes of saccades (e.g. self-paced saccades, anti-saccades) can be elicited with more complex instructions and these can be selectively abnormal in fronto-basal ganglia disorders.

Saccadic accuracy Saccadic amplitude is normally smaller than target amplitude and the subject makes 1–2 additional, smaller, corrective saccades towards the target. The presence of 2–3 corrective saccades consistently is considered saccadic hypometria, and severely hypometric saccades look fragmented, often called 'multiple step' saccades. If the initial saccade is too large and travels past the target, the patient makes corrective saccades in the opposite direction of the initial saccade. This is saccadic hypermetria, a reliable cerebellar sign (Figure 15.7). The appearance is similar to abnormal past-pointing during a 'finger–nose' test in an ataxic patient. By contrast, saccadic hypometria is less specific and can be caused by lesions in the cortex, basal ganglia, brainstem, cerebellum and oculomotor nucleus, nerve and muscle. Combined slow and

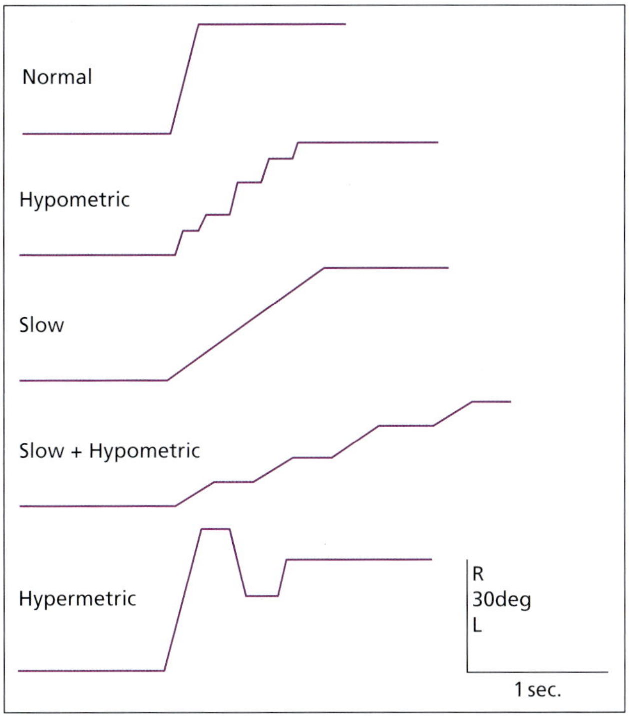

Figure 15.7 Examples of normal and abnormal saccades. Idealised examples of normal and abnormal saccades; apart from a small degree of symmetric hypometria, which can be normal, abnormalities of saccades suggest CNS (or neuromuscular) disorder.

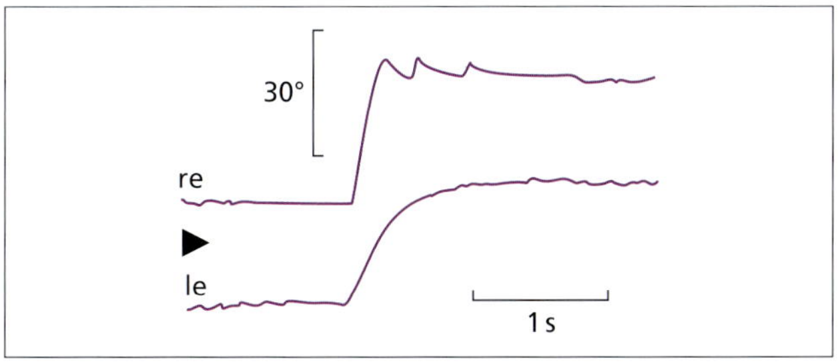

Figure 15.8 Left internuclear ophthalmplegia (INO). Right (re) and left eye (le) horizontal EOG in a patient with a left internuclear ophthalmoplegia (INO). Note the slower adduction velocity (slope) of the left eye, with respect to that of the right eye abduction velocity. The uniocular or 'ataxic' nystagmus of the abducting eye, as shown here in 're', is a frequent component of the INO.

hypometric saccades are not uncommon, an extreme case is progressive supranuclear palsy (PSP; Chapter 6).

Saccadic conjugacy When examining saccadic conjugacy (the two eyes should travel at the same speed) it is important to ensure there is no individual IIIrd, IVth or VIth nerve palsy. A common source of dysconjugacy in the horizontal plane is the internuclear ophthalmoplegia (INO) in which the abducting eye saccades are fast and large, whereas saccades in the adducting eye are slow and small. INOs are caused by lesions of the medial longitudinal fasciculus (MLF) which connects abducens interneurones of the VI nucleus with medial rectus motor neurones in the contralateral VI nucleus. Abducens interneurones cross the midline immediately to form the ascending MLF on the other side of the brainstem. Thus, a right INO means that right eye adduction during gaze to the left is slow, hypometric or incomplete because of a small right MLF lesion. As innervation to the eyes is yoked, the attempt of the CNS to overcome the limitation in adduction makes saccades in the abducting eye larger (hypermetric). This sequence of overshoots in the abducting eye leads to the characteristic monocular 'ataxic' nystagmus (Figure 15.8).

Optokinetic nystagmus

The OKN system in humans is not a truly separate oculomotor system. When OKN is elicited with a small hand-held drum or by moving a newspaper in front of a patient's eyes, the slow phase movement comes from the smooth pursuit system and the re-setting eye movements (fast phases of OKN) are saccades. For these reasons, if smooth pursuit and saccades have been properly examined what can be learnt additionally from observation of OKN is very little. Peripheral vestibular lesions, unless acute and massive with clinically visible spontaneous nystagmus, leave OKN unaffected. A slight directional preponderance, concordant with the peripheral vestibular nystagmus, may be observed in a peripheral vestibular disorder, but gross asymmetries indicate CNS lesions.

Vestibulo-ocular reflexes

The vestibulo-ocular reflex (VOR) stabilises gaze in space during head movements, thus allowing us to see clearly when for instance we walk, run or turn our head. It does so by generating slow phase eye movements of an almost equal velocity, but opposite in direction, to head movement. This is achieved by a three-neurone, short latency reflex: a Scarpa ganglion neurone, a vestibular nucleus neurone and an oculomotor neurone (III, IV or VI).

Thanks to our increased understanding of the physiological basis of the VOR and our improved skills in observing eye movements, we can assess the VOR in the clinic. Unilateral and bilateral loss of vestibular function can, in many cases, be identified clinically, but will be easier the more severe and the more acute the lesion is. In contrast, a unilateral, partial, long-standing, peripheral vestibular disorder cannot be detected clinically and a caloric test is required. The clinical manoeuvres available rely either on a slow doll's head manoeuvre assessed either by (i) direct observation of the eyes or ophthalmoscopy and (ii) measurement of visual acuity; or a fast version of the doll's head, the 'head impulse' or 'head thrust' test.

Doll's head eye manoeuvre

This manoeuvre requires the patient sitting in front of the examiner, close enough to be able to observe the patient's eyes carefully. The patient is instructed to fixate a feature of the examiner's face (nose or bridge of nose). The examiner then turns the patient's head from side to side, at a frequency of 0.5 to 1 Hz. In the complete absence of VOR, the patient's eye movements will not be smooth but will be interrupted by 'catch-up' saccades towards the fixation target. This occurs because at frequencies of 0.5–1 Hz, a head oscillation of +30°/s, will generate peak head velocities above 100°/s which are too high for the pursuit or cervico-ocular reflex to compensate. As slow phase eye movements are unable to keep up with the target, catch-up saccades are put in, and these can be easily observed if close enough. In patients with bilateral severe loss of vestibular function (e.g. gentamycin ototoxicity, meningitis or idiopathically), the manoeuvre is positive. A further procedure uses ophthalmoscopy for the assessment of vestibular disorders. The ophthalmoscope is a powerful magnifying glass and nystagmus of small amplitude or catch up saccades during head turns as described above can be detected easily.

Dynamic visual acuity

A similar movement of the head can be used to investigate the VOR while reading a visual acuity chart. A baseline, binocular visual acuity measurement is noted, say 6/6. Standing behind the patient, the examiner oscillates the patient's head at about 1 Hz while a new visual acuity measurement is taken. A normal subject's visual acuity does not change with respect to the baseline reading or it can deteriorate by one line, say 6/9. A loss of two lines in visual acuity must be treated as suspicious and when three lines or more are lost, the results are frankly abnormal, suggesting the patient's VOR is grossly reduced. False positives may occur if the patient has a spontaneous nystagmus (e.g. a down-beating nystagmus), which is exacerbated by head movement and/or lateral gaze. False negatives occur if the patients themselves oscillate the head, because they briefly stop the head motion and get a snapshot of the visual acuity chart. Although the examination of a patient's eyes during the doll's head manoeuvre can in some instances detect a unilateral lesion, this is detected more efficiently with the head impulse test.

Head impulse test

The value of VOR examination as described is limited by the fact that they are all carried out with relatively low head velocities. The VOR is only irreplaceable during high accelerations of the head. Neither pursuit, optokinetic nor cervical mechanisms can fully take over from the VOR during brisk head movements. For this reason, Halmagyi and Curthoys (1988) (Figure 15.9) have popularised the examination of the doll's head manoeuvre with discrete, brisk and unpredictable head turns. In essence, the patient is seated with the examiner at close range to observe the eyes carefully or with a video-camera if it is wished to document the findings. The patient is instructed to fixate a target such as the examiner's nose and the head is turned briskly in discrete steps of +10–15° across the midline by the examiner, thus producing head velocities of several hundred degrees per second. A fast right head (nose) turn will make a patient with a right-sided vestibular loss introduce one or more catch-up saccades towards the target (i.e. towards the left), in order to refixate. These catch-up saccades can easily be identified by a trained observer. The test is clearly useful for identifying an acute, unilateral, peripheral vestibular deficit, for instance in a patient with vestibular neuritis. In patients with chronic uncompensated, incomplete unilateral lesions, the test is often negative or inconclusive. A study comparing caloric testing with the head impulse test shows that the overall sensitivity

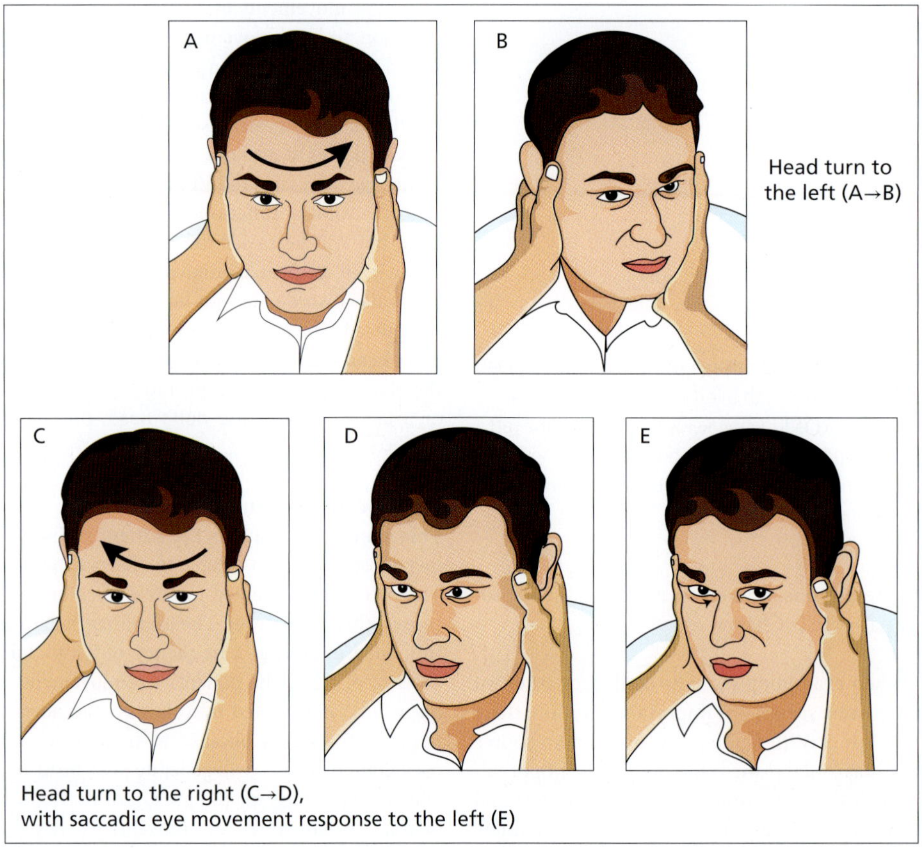

Figure 15.9 Halmagyi head thrust test. A fast right head turn will make a patient with a right-sided vestibular loss introduce one or more catch-up saccades towards the target (i.e. towards the left), in order to refixate.

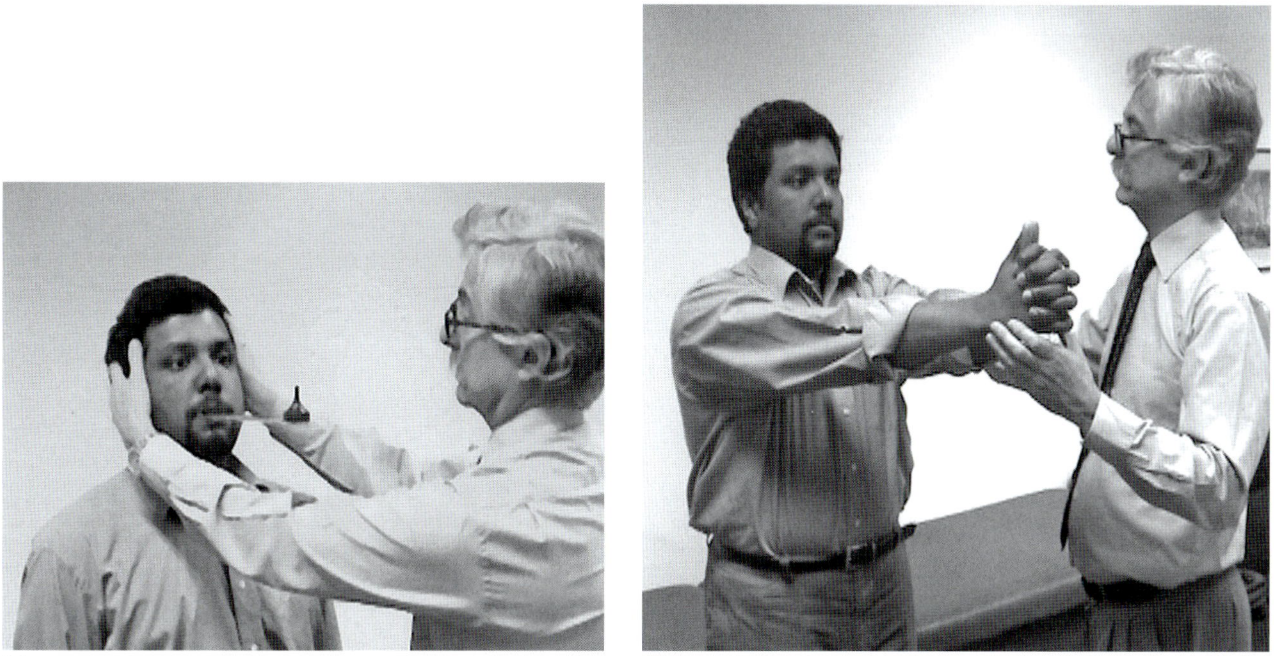

(a) (b)

Figure 15.10 Two ways of examining vestibulo-ocular reflex suppression (VORS). (a) The patient fixating an object carried in his bite and (b) his outstretched thumbs. The examiner helps the subject oscillate his head (a) or trunk (b) while carefully observing the patient's eyes, to see if vestibular nystagmus is suppressed (good VORS) or breaks through (poor VORS).

of the head impulse test is 34%. However, specificity is high (100%) and all patients with a canal paresis of >87% had a positive head impulse test.

Vestibulo-ocular reflex suppression

When a subject rotates the head in the environment, the eyes adopt a pattern of alternating slow and and fast phases, a physiological vestibular nystagmus. In a normally lit room, this is aided by OKN. The human brain can also suppress the vestibulo-ocular reflex suppression (VORS) with mechanisms closely related to pursuit mechanisms and pathways. Abnormalities in VOR are this indicative of central dysfunction, as discussed already for smooth pursuit.

Clinical examination of VORS is easy, both clinically and during oculography (Figure 15.10). The general principle is to oscillate the patient while s/he fixates a head-fixed target. Any obvious break-through nystagmus indicates poor suppression. In the clinic this can be achieved by asking the patient to clasp the hands together in front and put the thumbs up as a target; the patient can then oscillate side to side 'en bloc', by himself/herself if standing up, or the examiner can oscillate the patient's swivel chair if sitting down. Alternatively, the patient can bite and carry a ruler with his/her teeth and fixate on an object attached to the opposite end, while moving the head side to side. As with pursuit, the oscillation should be slow, say 2–5 s from left to right, and vice versa (0.1–0.25 Hz) and the examiner should have a good view of the patient's eyes.

Patients with peripheral vestibular lesions have a normal VORS (or even 'supra-normal' as they are trained to suppress their own nystagmus). In central lesions, the abnormality of pursuit and VORS go hand in hand (i.e. a patient with a right cerebellar lesion will have abnormal rightwards pursuit and abnormal VORS, with visible nystagmus breaking through, when turning the head rightwards).

Positional manoeuvres, Dix–Hallpike and roll manoeuvres

One of the most common causes of vertigo is BPPV. This accounts for one-quarter of all patients presenting with dizziness and vertigo. Positional manoeuvres are a vital component of the examination of the balance disordered patient, particularly in the light of effective treatments available for BPPV. This condition is usually diagnosed from the history and confirmed using the Dix–Hallpike and supine roll manoeuvres. With the pathological ear undermost, the Dix–Hallpike manoeuvre and roll manoeuvre produces characteristic nystagmus (Table 15.1).

The Dix–Hallpike manoeuvre is a valuable test in such patients and can distinguish between the peripheral nystagmus of BPPV, central positional nystagmus and atypical positional nystagmus (Figure 15.11):

- Seat the patient on a couch so that when supine, his/her head extends over the end of the couch.
- Ask the patient to remove spectacles (warn them they may feel intensely dizzy with the test) and to keep the eyes open and maintain gaze on the examiner's forehead (remove your stethoscope – it can fly around.)
- The patient's head is turned 30–45° towards the examiner and moved rapidly into the lying position with the head hanging 30° over the head of the couch. In this way the posterior semicircular canal of the undermost ear is moved directly through its plane of orientation. The patient's eyes are observed for nystagmus for up to 1 minute.
- The manoeuvre is carried out with one and then the other ear undermost.

Table 15.1 Characteristic features of different types of positional nystagmus.

	p-BPPV	h-BPPV geotropic	h-BPPV apogeotropic	a-BPPV	Central
History	Vertigo on turning over in bed, getting in or out of bed, looking up or down	Vertigo on rolling from side to side in bed	Same as for geotropic h-BPPV	Same as for p-BPPV	Often little in the way of positional vertigo
Diagnostic positional test	Hallpike or side-lying (on affected side)	Supine roll test	Supine roll test	Hallpike, or side-lying (on opposite side)	Hallpike
Latency	2–20 s	5 s	Nil	2–20 s	Nil
Nystagmus	Torsional (geotropic)/ vertical (upward) with head tilt in the plane of the posterior canal	Horizontal (geotropic) more marked towards affected ear	Horizontal (apogeotropic) more marked towards affected ear	Vertical (downbeat)/ small torsional component towards affected ear	Pure vertical or torsional not direction changing
Duration	40 s	<60 s	60 s	40 s	60 s
Reversibility	On sitting	On rolling to other side	On rolling to other side	On sitting	No
Fatiguability	Yes	Yes	No	Variable	No

a-BPPV, anterior canal benign paroxysmal positional vertigo; h-BPPV, horizontal canal benign paroxysmal positional vertigo; p-BPPV, posterior canal benign paroxysmal positional vertigo.

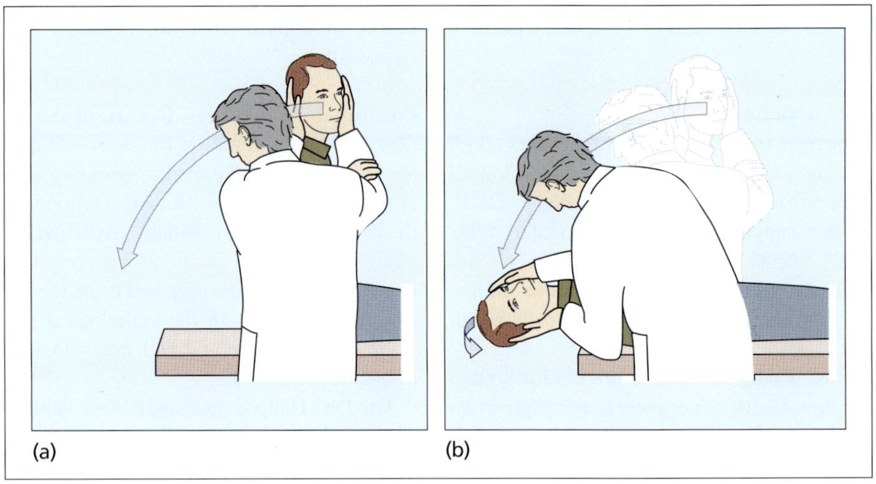

Figure 15.11 The Dix–Hallpike manoeuvre (see text).

In central positional nystagmus, sometimes seen in multiple sclerosis, Arnold–Chiari malformations, posterior fossa lesions or cerebellar vascular disease, typically there is no latency to the onset of nystagmus, frequently little vertigo and no adaptation or fatigability. The direction of nystagmus may be towards the uppermost ear, torsional or may be vertical. Positional nystagmus may be the only sign of posterior fossa pathology.

The supine roll manoevre is carried out by seating the patient on the couch with their legs outstretched (Figure 15.12). Holding their head, the examiner lays the patient straight back on the couch looking for horizontal nystagmus. Once supine, the patient's head is turned towards the right side through 90° around the longitudinal z-axis. Typically, the induced nystagmus of canalolithiasis of horizontal canal BPPV (h-BPPV) beats towards the undermost ear (geotropic), and is more prolonged than that of posterior canal BPPV (p-BPPV). The nystagmus and associated vertigo is allowed to settle. The patient's head is then turned 180° to the left around the same longitudinal z-axis. Any nystagmus

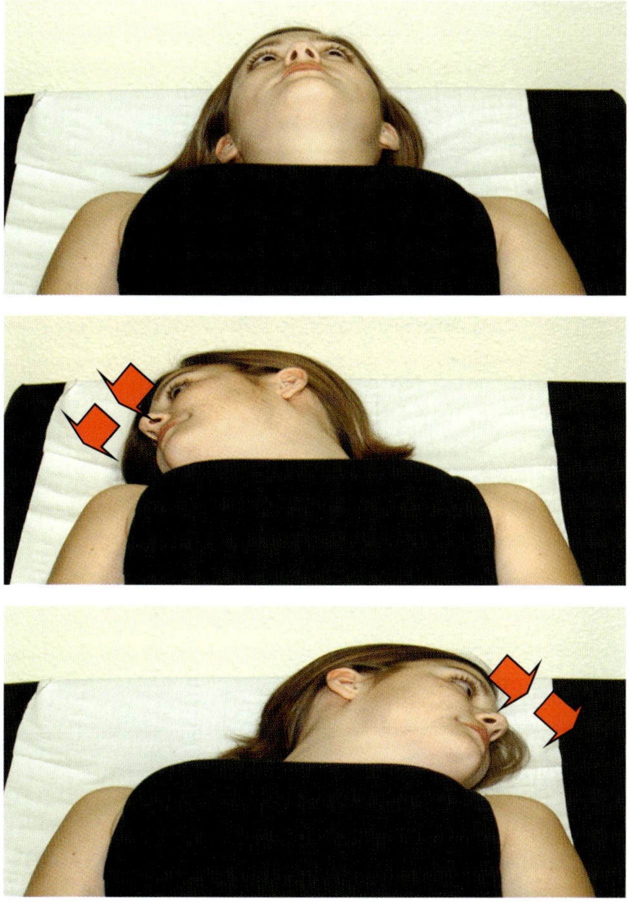

Figure 15.12 The roll test (see text). Source: Bertholon 2006. Reproduced with permission of Sage.

caused by horizontal canalolithiasis reverses (e.g. right-beating nystagmus becomes left-beating), in that it remains geotropic and is direction changing.

To check for h-BPPV in the opposite ear, repeat the manoeuvre, starting by moving the patient's head from the straight back position through 90° to the left side, waiting for the nystagmus to appear and disappear, and then rolling the head through 180° to the right. Laterality of h-BPPV is assigned to the side to which the more marked horizontal nystagmus occurs. Occasionally when the head is rolled there is apogeotropic horizontal nystagmus (i.e. beating away from the ground). This similarly reverses when the head is turned to the other ear and is a result of h-BPPV cupulolithiasis. In this instance the side of head turn resulting in weaker nystagmus indicates the affected ear.

Orthostatic blood pressure

Even in specialised neuro-otological clinics, many patient's symptoms turn out to be caused by orthostatic drop in blood pressure. The incidence is higher in non-specialised setting, often associated with old age, diabetes, antihypertensive medication and vaso-active medication (e.g. prostate alpha blocking drugs). In patients whose symptoms develop while standing or walking, the blood pressure should be measured when supine after 10 minutes lying, immediately on standing and again after a further 3 minutes standing. Heart rate should also be recorded as it can identify the postural orthostatic tachycardia syndrome (POTS;Chapter 24).

When to examine what – the clinical presentation of balance disorders

Acute vertigo

Here you need to establish if the vertigo is just bothersome but otherwise trivial, and if it is likely to be caused by a peripheral vestibular disorder or a CNS lesion, most commonly a stroke. Enquire directly about central symptoms and also about acute hearing loss or tinnitus. Look for general neurological signs (including oculomotor signs such as skew deviation, abnormal pursuit or saccades) and unilateral deafness. Establish if the nystagmus is compatible with a peripheral disorder (unilateral, mostly horizontal beating). If the above examination does not indicate CNS disease, a positive (abnormal) head impulse test in the opposite direction to that of the nystagmus would confirm the peripheral origin of the vertigo. Note that patients with BPPV present to A&E departments so be ready to do a positional manoeuvre. If you are in doubt organise a CT angiogram and/or MRI. Investigation suite audio-vestibular tests are rarely necessary in the acute situation and, except in specialised centres, not available as emergency investigations.

Recurrent vertigo

The common aetiologies in this group are BPPV and migraine. Thus, eliciting positional triggers and migrainous features in the history is paramount. Positional manoeuvres are essential for the diagnosis of BPPV but examination in patients with vestibular migraine is by and large normal. Diagnostic criteria for Ménière's disease require the presence of a sensori-neural hearing loss, so otoscopy plus clinical and instrumental hearing tests are mandatory. Postural blood pressure measurements are useful, particularly in the elderly. Audiological investigations can be helpful: normal in migraine and abnormal in Ménière's disease. Most patients with recurrent (and chronic) symptoms end up having MRI, but this is not strictly necessary if clinical and laboratory audio-vestibular examination is normal.

Chronic dizziness and/or unsteadiness

Most patients in this group will have a previous history of vestibular symptoms, followed by poor central vestibular compensation or secondary psychological symptoms. The examination is usually normal. Audio-vestibular investigations (if not performed already) may help to understand the underlying condition and quantify the overall level of residual vestibular function. The risk in the 'chronic dizzy patients' category is that a neurological gait disorder is missed – early or circumscribed (vestibulo-cerebellar) disorders are the most common. Patients need a general neurological examination, paying attention to sensory-motor function of the lower limbs and gait, and a detailed eye movement examination looking for CNS signs or bilaterally abnormal head impulse test (indicating bilateral vestibular failure). Eye movement recordings showing central-type nystagmus and abnormalities of saccades and/or pursuit will reinforce the diagnosis of a CNS disorder. MRI head scans are useful to document cerebellar disorder or white matter small vessel disease.

Table 15.2 lists the main causes of dizziness according to the generally recognised site of lesion, and Table 15.3 identifies the main medical causes of dizziness.

Table 15.2 Causes of peripheral and central vestibular problems.

Peripheral	Central
Middle ear pathology	***Mendelian heritability***
Peri-lymph fistula (trauma, cholesteatoma, surgery)	Friedreich's ataxia
Serous otitis media (glue ear)	Arnold–Chiari malformations
Chronic middle ear disease (e.g. suppurative otitis media)	Spino-cerebellar ataxias
Peripheral vestibular pathology	Episodic ataxias (types 1 and 2)
Vestibular neuritis	***Others***
Benign paroxysmal positional vertigo	Vestibular migraine
Bilateral vestibular failure	Multiple sclerosis
Anterior semicircular canal dehiscence	Posterior fossa mass lesions
Ménière's disease	Syringomyelia and syringobulbia
Vestibular paroxysmia	Posterior circulation ischaemia/infarction
VIIIth nerve lesion	Inflammatory disorders
Vestibular schwannoma	Malignant meningitis
Neurofibromatosis type 2	Multi-system atrophy
Other cerebellopontine angle tumour	Vestibular epilepsy
Basal meningitis (e.g. tuberculous meningitis)	Raised intracranial pressure
Neurosarcoidosis	Drugs
Lyme disease	

Table 15.3 General medical causes of dizziness.

Orthostatic hypotension	Causes:
i.e. reduction of 20 mmHg systolic blood pressure measured 0–3 min after assuming an upright posture after lying for 10 min	• Prolonged bed rest • Hypotensives, major tranquillisers, vasodilators, antidepressants, beta-blockers, levodopa • Autonomic neuropathy (e.g. diabetes, Shy–Drager syndrome) • Hyponatraemia, Addison's disease, chronic renal failure
Vasovagal episodes	Triggers:
Characterised by sense of hearing and vision receding, buzzing in the ears and sense of impending doom, light-headedness	• Standing at attention for too long • Noxious stimuli • Vertigo • Fear, emotional stress • Hot stuffy environments
Low cardiac output	• Cardiac dysrhythmia • Stokes–Adams attack • Carotid sinus hypersensitivity • Aortic stenosis • Hypertrophic cardiomyopathy
Hyperventilation	Clinical features include:
	• Muscle cramps, carpopedal spasm • Breathlessness, air hunger • Palpitation, chest tightness
Other	• Hypoglycaemia • Anaemia • Many acute illnesses (e.g. infections) • Chronic fatigue syndrome

Commonly used vestibular investigations

The three approaches to physiological investigation of the vestibular system are:

- Recording eye movements
- Measurements of postural changes, and
- Measurements of the caloric responses (to hot and cold thermal irrigations) of the semicircular canals.

Eye movements are well-suited to measurement. Ocular motility is restricted to the rotations of the globe, the eye muscles moving the globe against an unchanging resistance. Different types of eye movement can be distinguished by their physiological properties. Direct observation of eye movements is useful, while recording techniques such as electronystagmography, video-oculography (VOG) and spiral coil recordings allow detailed evaluation and provide a permanent record for comparative purposes.

Electronystagmograph

Electro-nystagmography (ENG; also known as electro-oculography, EOG) has traditionally been the simplest and most readily available system for recording eye movements. A recording electrode placed laterally to the eye becomes increasingly positive as the eye turns towards it and negative when the eye turns away. The voltage change represents the change in eye position. Only small angular movements are involved in nystagmus and thus the relationship between voltage change and eye movement is virtually linear within small degrees of arc. The polarity of the recording is arranged so that a deflection of the eye to the left causes a downward deflection of the pen and vice versa. The sensitivity of ENG is such that it can record consistently eye rotations of 0.5°. This sensitivity is actually less than that of direct visual inspection – approximately 0.1°.

The plane of the recording electrodes is in the plane of recorded eye movement; electrodes attached medially and laterally to the eye record horizontal components of eye movement, whereas those attached above and below record vertical components. A single-channel ENG machine summates horizontal movements of both eyes from bi-temporal recordings on to the same trace. A two-channel ENG records movement of each eye separately; four-channel ENG can record simultaneously vertical and horizontal movements. Paper speed at 10 mm/s is used, although when saccadic accuracy and velocity are measured, 100 mm/s or even faster speeds may be necessary. Calibration is such that a standard angle of eye deviation produces a defined amplitude of pen deflection – commonly 10 mm of pen deflection for each 10° of eye movement. A detailed standardised protocol is essential.

Clinical relevance of ENG

The main value of ENG recordings is that some patients have demonstrable nystagmus only when optic fixation is removed.

- *Peripheral vestibular disorders*: unless acute, these are unlikely to be associated with nystagmus in the presence of optic fixation but nystagmus can be revealed if fixation is removed, i.e. with the use of the Frenzel's glasses or video- or electro-nystagmoscopy, and is of increased amplitude in darkness (Figure 15.13). Nystagmus is unidirectional with the largest amplitude on horizontal gaze towards the direction of the fast component (see Gaze evoked nystagmus).
- *Vestibular nuclei lesions*: in darkness the amplitude of nystagmus may hardly alter but the velocity of the slow phase may be decreased. Often the nystagmus is bi-directional.
- *Cerebellar lesions*: these may be associated with pathological square waves with duration <200 ms. With direct current ENG recordings a characteristic abnormality of cerebellar pathology is the failure to maintain lateral gaze, with a slow drifting movement of the eyes towards the midline. Rebound nystagmus can also be seen, but when cerebellar, it is transient and persists for a maximum of 20 s. Patients with cerebellar disease may have difficulties in executing commands for saccadic movement. When asked to turn their gaze laterally quickly, they overshoot the target.

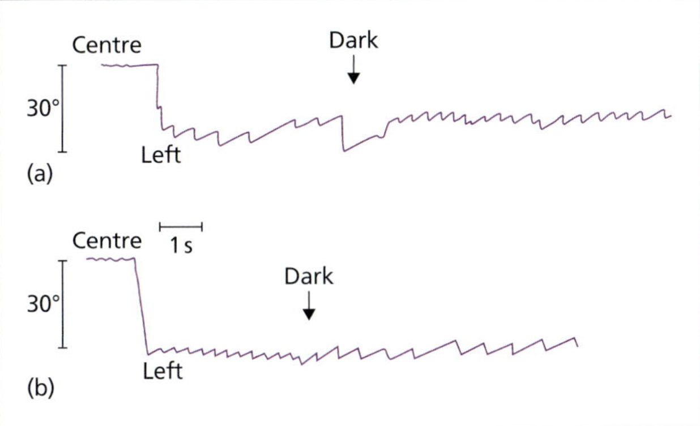

Figure 15.13 Electro-nystagmogram (ENG): effect of removing optical fixation. (a) The effects of gaze testing in a patient with a peripheral vestibular deficit: the spontaneous nystagmus enhances in the absence of optic fixation; (b) a central, gaze-evoked nystagmus: the nystagmus decreases in frequency and slow component velocity in the absence of optic fixation. Source: Luxon 1988. Reproduced with permission of Taylor & Francis.

Rotary chair testing

Rotary chair testing allows measurement and recording of eye movement responses to precise vestibular stimuli. This can be of immense clinical value. The VOR provides a simple example of a reflex arc comprising the vestibular sense organ, the primary, secondary and tertiary vestibular neurones and the effector organs, the oculomotor muscles. Angular acceleration in the plane of the semicircular canal leads to endolymph displacement in a direction opposite to that of rotation. As a consequence, the cupula of that canal deviates in the same direction as the endolymph, resulting in a change of vestibular tonus, an excitatory stimulus being matched by an inhibitory stimulus from the opposite side. As a result there is an impact on the pair of muscles producing the compensatory eye movement (i.e. excitation of the antagonist muscle and disinhibition of the agonist muscle). An acceleration to the right in the plane of the horizontal canal will produce deviation of the eyes to the left.

Types of rotary chair stimuli

Impulsive (step velocity) stimuli Constant velocities such as 40, 60, 80 or 120°/s are attained with an abrupt acceleration of the chair, brought to constant velocity within 1 s. This constant velocity is maintained for up to 2 min while the nystagmic response dies away. The chair is suddenly brought to rest with the same deceleration and the normal limits of nystagmus intensity are established with normal subjects. This provides a rapid assessment of gain (peak slow component velocity ÷ change in chair velocity) and the time constant (time for the slow component velocity to fall to 37% of its initial value) of the canal reflex.

Sinusoidal stimuli To and fro swinging movements of the chair around its vertical axis are programmed with variable stimulus parameters (e.g. frequency and amplitude). The threshold for recordable nystagmus, defined as the angular acceleration maintained for 20 s that will produce nystagmus is $0.15°/s^2$ in the absence of optic fixation. With optic fixation the nystagmus threshold is raised and is normally about $1°/s^2$. Rotational testing is normally performed in darkness but sinusoidal rotation can also be performed with the eyes focused on a target that revolves with the patient, around the vertical axis. This has the purpose of allowing VOR suppression to be assessed. This is an important test of central vestibular function, as visual suppression of the VOR is mediated by central vestibular pathways.

Clinical relevance of rotary chair testing

Rotational stimuli can be used to demonstrate a directional preponderance as determined by the ratio of the duration of nystagmus following the onset of acceleration to that following deceleration. A disadvantage is that both labyrinths are tested simultaneously; unilateral dysfunction may be difficult to identify if the lesion is old and the patient is well-compensated. Rotary chair testing is of particular value in the following situations:

- A negative caloric test, where high frequency oscillation/high intensity acceleration may give evidence of some residual vestibular function.
- Investigation of visuo-vestibular interactions – when failure to suppress the vestibulo-ocular reflex with fixation is evidence of central vestibular dysfunction.

With computerised analysis of responses to rotary chair testing, results can be depicted in a quadrantic fashion following the sequence of start–stop stimuli in a clockwise then anticlockwise direction.

These displays include a mathematical computation of directional preponderance using slow phase velocity and/or durational criteria. Multivariate analysis of sinusoidal harmonic accelerations, asymptotic gain and the time constant have demonstrated a minimal misclassification rate when comparing normal people with patients with total canal paresis.

Video-oculography

Video-oculography is a technique for observing and recording eye movements. An infra-red camera is mounted within goggles and connected to a video monitor. Observation and recordings of the eye movements in the absence of optic fixation can be made in response to a variety of stimuli. This technique is now a standard investigative tool in many departments. A test protocol can be performed which allows video recording of the following:

- Spontaneous nystagmus
- Head-shaking nystagmus
- Passive head tilt
- Head rotation through 180°.

VOG is valuable for identifying and classifying peripheral vestibular lesions and is commonly used in audio-vestibular investigation suites nationally.

Caloric testing

This is the most widely available of all vestibular tests and for many otologists is the cornerstone of vestibular diagnosis. Its great value is that it allows each labyrinth to be tested separately and is a method of demonstrating a peripheral vestibular deficit. The stimulus is easy to apply and involves inexpensive methodology.

Principles of caloric testing

After irrigation of the ear with water 7°C below (30°), and then 7°C above (44°) body temperature, a gradient is set up between the external auditory meatus (EAM) and the two limbs of the horizontal canal. This is by virtue of the position of the patient, whose head is at 30° to the horizontal on the couch. This means that the horizontal semicircular canal becomes vertical and the temperature gradient crosses from one limb of the canal to the other. It is commonly believed that the endolymph circulates because of the difference in the specific gravity on the two sides of the canal. With warm water, there is ampullo-petal flow, with cupular deflection towards the utricle, resulting in activation of the VOR, a sensation of vertigo and horizontal nystagmus directed towards the stimulated ear. However, there remains some doubt about this convection theory, because caloric nystagmus under micro-gravity conditions still occurs (e.g. in space).

The Hallpike–Fitzgerald bithermal caloric test has been available to clinicians for more than 60 years. Each ear is irrigated in turn for 40 s first with water at 30°C and then at 44°C. Inspection of the tympanic membrane after warm irrigation confirms an adequate stimulus if a red flush is seen on the membrane. Direct observation of the eyes allows the endpoint of the nystagmic reaction to be measured. During the procedure, the patient is asked to direct gaze on a fixation point on the ceiling, making the endpoint easier to determine. At this point the lights are switched off and the eyes observed with Frenzel's glasses or infra-red gun. Under normal situations the vestibular nystagmus would be expected to reappear. The endpoints of each test are graphically recorded. More commonly used now is the VNG caloric where an infra-red camera is mounted within goggles and connected to a video monitor to record and analyse responses to thermal irrigations (Figure 15.14).

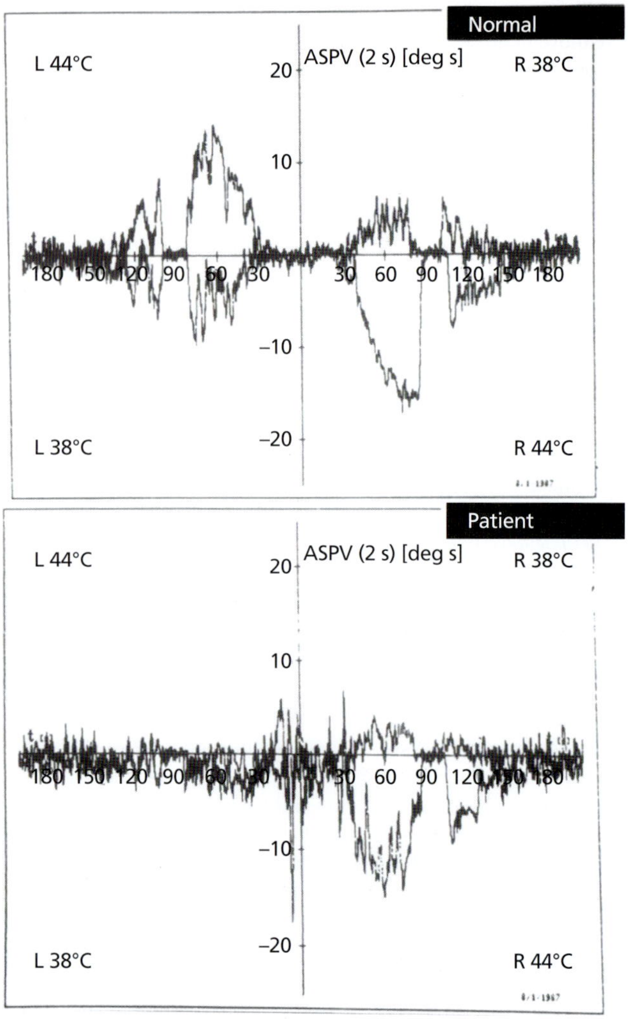

Figure 15.14 Four-quadrant display of caloric irrigations: (a) the four-quadrant display of a set of normal responses to caloric irrigations in a normal subject; (b) the four-quadrant display of responses in a patient demonstrating a left canal paresis. Source: Davies 2004. Reproduced with permission of BMJ.

Quantitative analysis

Normally, nystagmus ceases 90–140 s after onset of irrigation and returns for up to a further 60 s after removal of optic fixation. Two abnormal patterns may appear, either separately or in combination, and are of diagnostic importance.

1. *Total canal paresis:* this is the complete loss of labyrinthine function in one ear, seen when there is a total absence of nystagmus following both 30° and 44° irrigations, even in the absence of optic fixation. Ideally, the test should be repeated using cold water at 20° for 60 seconds to confirm the result. It may reflect an ipsilateral lesion of the labyrinth, VIIIth nerve or brainstem vestibular nuclei, and confirms unilateral vestibular hypofunction.
2. *Directional preponderance:* this occurs when the responses to thermal irrigations produce an excess of nystagmus in one direction (i.e. towards either the right or the left). This indicates

imbalance of vestibular tone arriving at the oculomotor nuclei, a result of either a peripheral vestibular lesion (labyrinth, VIIIth nerve or nuclei) or from a central vestibular lesion, within the cerebellum or brainstem. With more pronounced degrees of vestibular tone imbalance, spontaneous nystagmus makes its appearance.

Figures for duration of nystagmic responses in seconds can be entered into the Jongkees formula, which calculates a percentage figure expressing either the degree of canal paresis or directional preponderance.

Another measurement, the optic fixation index (OFI) is calculated by dividing the summed durations in the light by the summed durations in the dark. If there is no enhancement in the absence of optic fixation (i.e. the OFI is 1.0), the cause may be central – within the cerebellum or vestibulo-cerebellar tracts. Bilateral decreased caloric responses indicate either bilateral vestibular impairment, or vestibular habituation. The latter is seen in acrobats, ice skaters and ballet dancers (OFI <0.5).

There are some disadvantages of VNG calorics when compared with the Fitzgerald–Hallpike technique: it is difficult to detect the endpoint of nystagmus as accurately as with direct vision, but hard copy data are recorded. Other nystagmic components in the vertical direction (e.g. torsional nystagmus) can be seen with VOG calorics. A direct comparison has been made between the maximum slow component velocity and the durations of the four caloric responses in normal subjects. The durations were relatively stable as a parameter, whereas the slow component velocities showed considerable variations in some subjects. Further analysis showed that the test–retest unreliability of the slow component velocity was unacceptably high. Direct visual observation has the advantage that the endpoint of the nystagmus can be estimated more reliably both with and without optic fixation, but does rely on an experienced observer.

Closed-circuit and air caloric testing

Some commercial caloric testing kits use closed irrigation systems to warm and cool the EAM or use air instead of water. The problem with the former is that the tube in which the water flows does not fully occupy the EAM, thus reducing the effectiveness of the stimulus. With the latter, the specific heat of air is much lower than that of water; this means a greater temperature differential is required to effect the same temperature gradient across the labyrinth (i.e. a hot air stimulus of 50°C which needs to be delivered for 60 s will give an equivalent to the 44°C water stimulus). This may be unpleasant and tolerated poorly. Air calorics are generally regarded as less reliable than traditional hot and cold water calorics.

Clinical value of caloric testing

Caloric testing is an essential part of the evaluation of the vestibular system. It tests each labyrinth individually and does not require any sophisticated instruments if water irrigation is used. The quantification and normal values of the measured parameters of the caloric induced nystagmus have been well established. The Jongkees formula is a validated measure, to calculate both canal paresis and directional preponderance. However, caloric test results do not correlate with the degree of dizziness or vertigo and are thus not a measure of discomfort or distress caused by these physiological abnormalities. Also, if a patient has a degree of directional preponderance or canal paresis, this may reflect a vestibular insult at some time even in the distant past, and one from which clinical recovery would be usual. This can have particular relevance in legal claims.

Posturography

It is well known that alterations in vestibular function can profoundly affect posture. Postural control is a vital physiological function if we are to continue any daily activity and is determined by a complex sensorimotor feedback system dependent on a variety of coordinated reflexes. Only in the last three decades have objective measures of vestibulo-spinal postural reflexes been possible. Clinically, the Romberg test has been used to assess postural stability. During normal standing, the body is in continuous motion (i.e. physiological sway), even when attempting to remain still. This is an active process, whereby any loss of balance is compensated by movement of the body's centre of gravity (CoG). These movements result in visually detectable sway movements that maintain the CoG vertically over the base of support.

Static force-plate posturography was an early method of measuring body sway. A typical force-plate consists of a flat rigid surface supported on three or more points by independent force-measuring devices. As the patient stands on the plate, the vertical forces recorded by the measuring devices are used to calculate the position of the centre of the vertical forces exerted on the force-plate over time. With the height and weight of the patient, a computer model of body dynamics can be used to derive the CoG sway angle over time.

Moving platform posturography has been designed to overcome the limitations of the static force platform by controlling the relative contributions of visual, somato sensory and vestibular input. Commercially available platforms calculate body sway based on changes in horizontally (sheer) and vertically oriented (torque) strain gauges mounted under the support surface. The Equitest platform (Figure 15.15) utilises the concept of sway-referencing (i.e. both the support surface and the visual surround can be modulated in phase with the patient's own body sway).

This coupling of either the platform or visual surround to the sway of the subject allows the angle between the foot and the lower leg to be maintained at a constant value, thus minimising somatosensory input with visual input remaining constant despite the subject's sway, respectively.

Six conditions are used in the sensory organisation testing and analysis of the sway scores allowing each of the three principal balance sensors to be isolated and comparisons made to assess sensory preference. The sensory organisation test battery identifies abnormal patterns of postural control, not adequately assessed by studies of the vestibulo-ocular reflex alone and examines the utilisation and integration of visual and somatosensory input with vestibular information, especially under conditions of sensory conflict.

The moving platform has been shown to be of great benefit with individual serial measurement in rehabilitation but of limited value as a diagnostic test.

Vestibular evoked myogenic potentials

Cervical vestibular evoked myogenic potentials (cVEMP) is a neural-event related potential. The cVEMP is an ipsilateral vestibulo-collic reflex with a short latency (<10 ms) which has a regulatory role (i.e. fine tuning of the voluntary motor commands directed to the neck muscles). Its origin is a loud acoustic stimulus which provokes a saccular response via the inferior vestibular nerve, lateral vestibular nucleus, lateral/medial vestibulo-spinal tract and motor neurones of the sternocleidomastoid (SCM) muscle. The clinical relevance is still being fully evaluated but an absent cVEMP is pathologic, if the patient is below the age of 60 years and the appropriate stimulus has been used. It tests the integrity of the

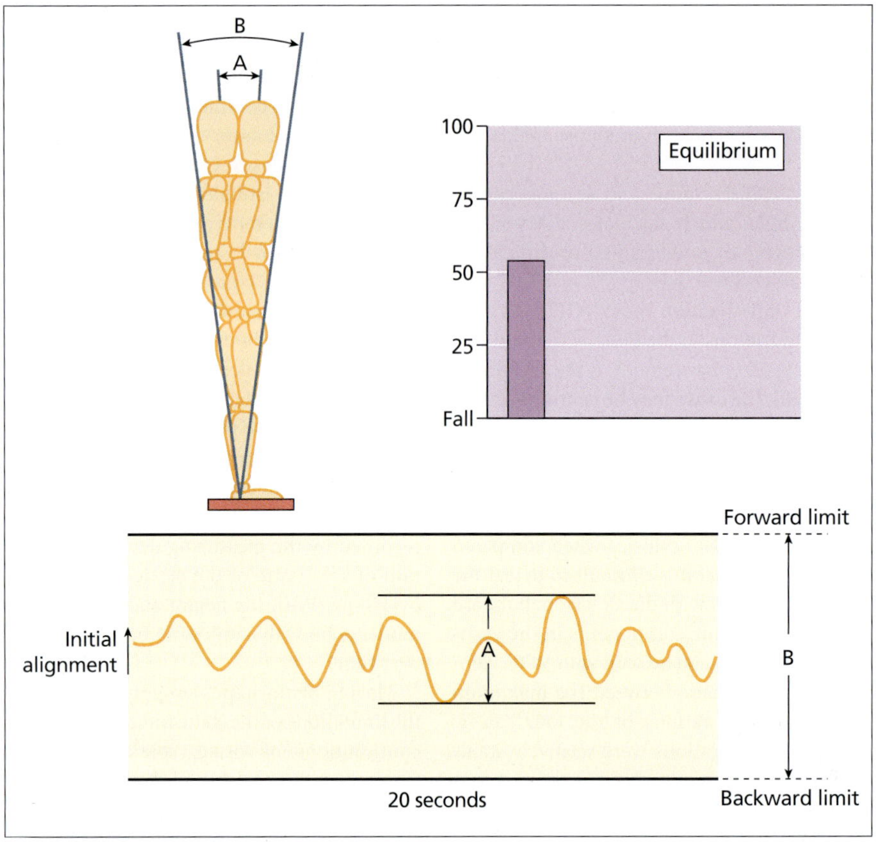

Figure 15.15 The Equitest balance platform – derivation of equilibrium score. The equilibrium score compares patient sway (a) with the theoretical limits of stability for normal subjects (b). Patient sway is calculated from the maximum peak-to-peak anterior to posterior sway occurring over the 20-second trial period.

vestibulo-collic reflex (i.e. saccule, inferior vestibular nerve) and can be abnormal in cases of acoustic neuroma, vestibular neuritis, Tullio and dehiscence of the superior semicircular canal (characterised by an abnormally lowered cVEMP threshold) and Ménière's disease.

Ocular VEMP (oVEMP) has emerged as a useful test in the clinical arena and is a manifestation of the utricular–ocular reflex which stabilises the eyes in response to linear head movements. The potential is recorded from surface electrodes beneath the eyes (placed on the belly of the superior oblique muscle) in response to bone conducted vibration and has a short latency negative (excitatory) component with a latency of 10 ms to peak, identified as n10. Again, this is a relatively new tool and its test sensitivity and specificity in different vestibular disorders is still to be fully evaluated.

Limitations of vestibular tests A major disadvantage of all types of vestibular test is that normative data have to be established for each laboratory before they can be used, as they depend on equipment and exact methodology. The equipment for the rotary chair and posturography is expensive and requires space and in the former case complete blackout of the room. There is no gold standard for vestibular testing and the results of all the tests in the battery must be collated alongside the clinical picture. A further limitation is that while vestibular testing may show an abnormality, not infrequently the site of the lesion cannot be indicated with certainty.

Clinical disorders

The major peripheral vestibular syndromes are described here.

Vestibular neuritis

Vestibular neuritis is one of the three most common causes of acute vertigo. It can be thought of as an acute unilateral vestibular paresis and has variously been known as vestibular neuronitis, vestibular neuro-labyrinthitis or acute vestibulopathy. The syndrome is also often referred to as labyrinthitis, considered a misnomer as there is neither hearing loss nor tinnitus. Vestibular neuritis is a well-recognised syndrome rather than a clearly defined clinico-pathological entity, and is characterised by:

- Acute rotary vertigo (sense of movement away from the side of the lesion)
- Blurred vision/oscillopsia (fast phase of nystagmus directed contralaterally)
- Postural imbalance (positive Romberg and falling towards the side of lesion), and
- Nausea and vomiting.

The onset of vestibular neuritis is typically sudden, without prelude and the degree of real distress out of proportion to the seriousness of the condition. Resolution is usual within a matter of weeks. The clinical picture may be sufficiently clear for further investigation to be unnecessary. For confirmation of diagnosis, unilateral peripheral vestibular hypofunction needs to be identified either at the bedside (Halmagyi head impulse test) or in the balance clinic (using a caloric test). The caloric test shows ipsilateral hypo-responsiveness or non-responsiveness, a sign of horizontal semicircular canal dysfunction.

Aetiology

The possible aetiologies of vestibular neuritis include viral and vascular insults, although in practice a cause is rarely established. Pointers toward a viral aetiology or viral re-activation are:

- Frequency of preceding upper respiratory tract infection
- Postmortem studies – cell degeneration of one or more vestibular nerve trunks, and
- Demonstration of latent herpes simplex virus type I in human vestibular ganglia.

Vestibular neuritis is thought to have a predilection for the superior division of the vestibular nerve, but the dysfunction may equally involve the sensory hair cells of the vestibular end organ and hence the term 'neuritis' is used. Similar presentations can be caused by:

- Multiple sclerosis when a plaque is within the VIIIth nerve root entry zone, and
- Cerebellar vascular disease.

Clinical assessment

Nystagmus is caused by an imbalance between afferent vestibular tone from the two labyrinths. Decrease in afferent activity from the affected ear is integrated with unaltered activity from the normal ear to produce the vestibular, or slow, phase of the nystagmus which is directed towards the affected ear. The fast or saccadic phase, which re-fixes the target on the fovea is towards the unaffected labyrinth. The acute nystagmus is predominantly horizontal-torsional. The reason for this is considered to be the net effect of the three unopposed semicircular canals (i.e. horizontal, posterior and anterior canals). Activity of the two vertical canals cancels out the vertical effect – the posterior canal tending to drive the eyes upwards and the anterior canal tending to drive the eyes downward. The patient senses movement across the retina only during the slow phase of nystagmus and because of the inverting effect of the lens, the sense of movement appears to be in the same direction as the fast phase of the nystagmus.

The postural reactions initiated by the vestibulo-spinal reflexes are usually opposite to the direction of vertigo. This results in Romberg's and Unterberger's tests being directed towards the side of the lesion. The patient's subjective sense of straight ahead and perceived visual vertical represents perceptual consequences of vestibular tone imbalance in yaw and roll planes.

Neuro-otological investigations

If investigation is necessary, VNG confirms a spontaneous vestibular nystagmus directed towards the unaffected ear that increases with removal of optic fixation. With gaze towards the unaffected side (i.e. in the direction of the fast phase), the nystagmus increases in frequency and amplitude. On gaze towards the affected ear, the nystagmus decreases in amplitude and frequency. This effect on the nystagmus by direction of gaze (Alexander's law; see Gaze evoked nystagmus) may be first degree, second degree or third degree.

Course

Throughout the acute phase (1–3 days), patients feel intensely unwell and tend to stay in bed. All head movements exacerbate vertigo, nausea and imbalance. After some 3 days, the spontaneous nystagmus is usually suppressed by optic fixation in the primary position but can still be detected with gaze towards the unaffected ear, and in the absence of optic fixation (e.g. with Frenzel's glasses). After 1–6 weeks, most patients become asymptomatic, experiencing dizziness only with rapid head movements. Some 50–70% show complete recovery as assessed by caloric testing.

Differential diagnosis of vestibular neuritis

When a patient presents acutely with symptoms of severe persistent isolated vertigo with imbalance, the distinct likelihood is that vestibular neuritis is the cause. However, the possibility of cerebellar infarction must also be considered. Symptoms typical of vestibular neuritis can be the sole manifestation of the cerebellar infarction but a three-step bedside oculomotor examination with the acronym 'HINTS' (head impulse–nystagmus–test of skew) appears to be sensitive for detecting stroke. The term pseudovestibular neuritis (PVN) for isolated vertigo of cerebellar origin has also been coined (Table 15.4). The territory most commonly involved is supplied by the medial branch of the posterior inferior cerebellar artery (mPICA). MRI of the brain may be necessary to distinguish between the two conditions and with the tendency towards defensive practice, imaging is becoming hard to avoid.

Benign paroxysmal positional vertigo

Barany first described benign positional vertigo in 1921, recognising it as a lesion of the vestibular end organ involving the otolith, but not until 1952 was it redefined and renamed as benign paroxysmal positional vertigo (BPPV). BPPV, when it affects the posterior semicircular canal (p-BPPV) is characterised by brief attacks of rotary vertigo and concomitant, positioning (aka positional), rotary-vertical/geotropic nystagmus, elicited by changes in head position in the plane of the posterior semicircular canal.

Incidence of BPPV

BPPV is probably the most common cause of vertigo, particularly in the elderly. One survey reported that by the age of 70 years, 30% of the population had experienced BPPV at least once. However,

Table 15.4 Features of cerebellar infarction presenting as apparent vestibular neuritis.

Findings in 24 patients with mPICA cerebellar infarction and PVN	
Halmagyi headthrust test	Normal
[1]Spontaneous nystagmus*	15
[1]Gaze-evoked nystagmus	24
Unidirectional†	7
Bidirectional:	
direction changing‡	13
direction unchanging	4
[1]Asymmetric smooth pursuit	6
[1]Asymmetric OKN	4
[1]Canal paresis	None

mPICA, medial branch of the posterior inferior cerebellar artery; OKN, optokinetic nystagmus; PVN, pseudovestibular neuritis.
[1] Performed using electro-nystagmography (ENG) 1 week after onset of vertigo.
* Beating towards lesion side.
† Only on gaze towards lesion side.
‡ Maximal to lesion side.
Source: Adapted from McKeith 2005. Reproduced with permission of AAN/LWW.

patients of any age can be affected, the overall mean age of onset being in the fifth decade, with a peak incidence around the mid-sixties, women outnumbering men by nearly 2 : 1. There is a slight female predominance in a presumed post-viral group, a higher female : male ratio in an idiopathic group and no sex predominance in a post-traumatic group. The peak age of onset is the fourth decade for the presumed post-viral group, the sixth decade for the idiopathic and an even distribution through the second to sixth decades in the post-traumatic group.

Posterior semicircular canal BPPV

The diagnosis of p-BPPV is made by a typical history of severe vertigo lasting less than 1 minute, triggered by specific head movements (e.g. lying back or rolling over in bed, extending the neck to change a light bulb or pick a book from a high shelf, or bending forwards to wash the hair). It is thought to be caused by an accumulation of otolith debris which has become displaced from the otolith membrane of the utricle and has settled as a bolus of crystals in the most gravity-dependent part of the inner ear, the posterior semicircular canal. The bolus is heavier than the surrounding endolymph and gravitates to the most dependent part of the canal during changes in head position (canalolithiasis; Figure 15.16).

Acting like a plunger, the bolus exerts an ampullo-fugal pull on the cupula, triggering the BPPV attack. The diagnosis is confirmed by characteristic nystagmus on Dix–Hallpike manoeuvre (i.e. ampullo-fugal stimulation of the cupula of the posterior semicircular canal causes excitation of the ipsilateral superior oblique and the contralateral inferior rectus muscle, causing both eyes to move downward). The refixating fast phase of the nystagmus is upbeat and is combined with a torsional component because of the different angles of insertion of the oblique and rectus muscles.

The diagnostic criteria for nystagmus typical of p-BPPV are:

- *Latency*: vertigo and nystagmus commence between several and 20 s after the head-hanging position is reached
- *Duration*: nystagmus gradually reduces after 10–40 s, before it disappears
- *Rotary-vertical (upbeat) nystagmus* is present with the fast phase beating toward the undermost ear (geotropic)
- *Reversal*: on returning to the upright position the vertigo and nystagmus may reoccur less violently in the opposite direction
- *Fatiguability*: on repeating the manoeuvre, the vertigo and nystagmus lessen.

The initial Dix–Hallpike test should be directed toward the ear assumed to be affected, as the nystagmus will become less evident on subsequent manoeuvres, demonstrating fatiguability.

Horizontal canal BPPV – geometric type

Between 5% and 20% of patients with BPPV are thought to suffer from horizontal canalolithiasis (h-BPPV). It may be combined with p-BPPV of the same ear or represent a transition from p-BPPV to h-BPPV as a result of a therapeutic manoeuvre. These two varieties of BPPV are thought to have similar aetiological bases. Symptomatically patients experience episodic vertigo when turning the head from side to side or on lying back in bed. When the Dix–Hallpike manoeuvre provokes a purely horizontal nystagmus, h-BPPV should be suspected. However, the Dix–Hallpike test is positive for horizontal nystagmus in only 80% of h-BPPV cases. The supine roll test is diagnostic of h-BPPV. When h-BPPV occurs as the result of loose otolith crystals in the canal itself (i.e. canalolithiasis), the nystagmus is geotropic – it beats towards the undermost ear.

Apogeotropic horizontal canal BPPV

Atypical h-BPPV is caused by cupulolithiasis (i.e. otolith crystals are adherent to the cupula rather than remaining free-floating in the horizontal canal endolymph). This causes apogeotropic positional nystagmus – nystagmus in the direction opposite to rotation.

The diagnostic manoeuvres are the same for h-BPPV cupulolithiasis and h-BPPV canalolithiasis. The difference is that in cupulolithiasis the nystagmus is apogeotropic: with right h-BPPV caused by cupulolithiasis, when the head is rolled to the right this will elicit left-beating nystagmus. In both types, the nystagmus is direction changing (i.e. when the direction of the head roll is reversed, so is the direction of the nystagmus). The nystagmus of horizontal canalolithiasis is often quite prolonged, distressing and may take some 2 minutes to settle. The nystagmus depends on the assumed head position and not on the net angle of rotation.

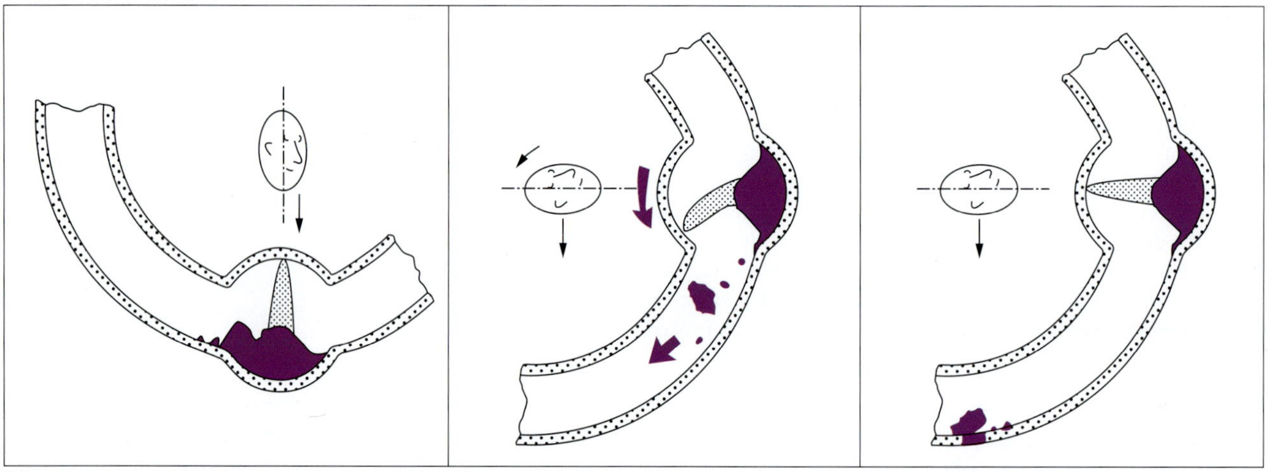

(a) (b) (c)

Figure 15.16 Canalolithiasis. Schematic representation of a free-floating 'heavy clot' of otoconial debris acting like a plunger on the endolymph and cupula of the posterior semicircular canal with a head movement in the plane of the canal. Source: Brandt and Steddin 1993.

Anterior canal BPPV

BPPV of the anterior canal (a-BPPV) is a rare variant, and poorly characterised. It sometimes occurs as an unwanted effect of a particle repositioning manoeuvre (see Head Impulse Test further on) for p-BPPV (i.e. when the otolith debris is inadvertently redirected into the anterior canal from the common crus at the final stage of an Epley manoeuvre). One proposed model is that positional downbeating nystagmus can be caused by anterior semicircular canalithiasis, assuming central causes are excluded. This is because of the ampullo-fugal effects of anterior canal stimulation. Extrapolating to nystagmus induced by the Dix–Hallpike manoeuvre, any downbeating nystagmus could be explained by anterior canalithiasis in the uppermost ear. However, the differential diagnosis of positional downbeating nystagmus must always include central involvement and hence brain imaging.

The frequency of the different varieties of BPPV is shown in Table 15.5.

Migraine-related dizziness

Migraine and vertigo are both common disorders and the possibility of a causal link between the two has been postulated for well over a century, but patho-mechanisms have been difficult to elucidate. The lifetime prevalence of vertigo, both vestibular and non-vestibular, is around 25%. Prevalence studies show that migraine affects at least 16% of the adult population at some time in their lives, with women having a higher prevalence than men. In a dizziness clinic, the prevalence of migraine is over 30%. Of note is that the co-incidence of migraine and vertigo is three times higher than would be expected by a merely statistical interaction of common disorders.

Several studies have characterised the clinical features and temporal association of dizziness and headache in patients with both. One study found that in more than 150 dizzy patients, over 35% had a verifiable diagnosis of migraine; 88% of these had dizziness both with and between migraine attacks; dizziness and/or vertigo could occur at any time during a migraine attack (i.e. as part of an aura or with the headache); often it was head movement or visual motion related. The initial dizziness coincided with the first migraine in 23%; and vestibular testing showed a directional preponderance in 50% and a canal paresis in 25%.

Definitions

Dizziness is a symptom in the following migraine syndromes basilar migraine; benign paroxysmal vertigo of childhood; benign recurrent vertigo. More recently, a plethora of names has been introduced to better characterise the link and hence migraine-associated dizziness, migraine-related vestibulopathy, vestibular migraine and migrainous vertigo have all been used. Questionnaires exist to simplify classification of migraine-related dizziness, but the cornerstones are to make an accurate diagnosis of migraine using established criteria (International Headache Society; Chapter 12) and, in the absence of an alternative explanation, to diagnose migraine linked temporally with dizziness as vestibular migraine using the Neuhauser *et al.* (2001) (and subsequently Lempart *et al.* 2009) criterion.

This link between migraine and dizziness has now formally incorporated into International Headache Society (IHS) terminology, and there is acceptance that dizziness can be related to migraine in other ways than exclusively as one of the aura symptoms of basilar migraine. Less than 10% of the patients with dizziness and migraine meet basilar type migraine criteria.

Basilar migraine

It is common experience that many patients with migrainous headaches describe dizziness, and occasionally vertigo, prior to the onset of headache. If two or more aura symptoms as defined in Table 15.6 are present prior to a typical migraine headache, basilar migraine may be diagnosed.

Vestibular migraine

Vestibular migraine is described as recurrent episodes of vestibular symptoms which are associated with migraine or migrainous features when other vestibular and headache disorders have been ruled out (Table 15.7). The diagnosis of 'possible vestibular migraine' is as for definite, but requires that only one of the criteria B or C for vestibular migraine is fulfilled.

Benign recurrent vertigo

Benign recurrent vertigo was first described in patients who had attacks of sudden intense vertigo, postural imbalance with or without nausea, spontaneous or positional nystagmus lasting several hours, but without headache. Because it is agreed that migraine is not exclusively a headache syndrome, such stereotyped attacks of vertigo with a timescale equivalent to migraine could be regarded as a migraine equivalent.

Ménière's disease

Ménière's disease, also known as endolymphatic hydrops, is an inner ear disorder characterised by prolonged attacks of vertigo, fluctuating hearing loss, tinnitus and aural fullness. To make a definite diagnosis American Academy of Otolaryngology

Table 15.5 Distribution of types of benign paroxysmal positional vertigo (BPPV) in patients with positional vertigo/nystagmus.

Source	n (%)	Posterior (%)	Horizontal		Anterior (%)	Others
			Geotropic (%)	Apogeotropic (%)		
Herdman et al. (1994)	77	63	1		12	24% undetermined
Honrubia et al. (1999)	292	93	6	9	4	0
Korres et al. (2004)	168	90	14		3	0
Nakayama and Epley (2005)	833	66	10		2	21%
Bertholon et al. (2006)	100	61	11	7	1	1% (posterior and horizontal BPPV) 3% (peripheral nystagmus) 12% (central nystagmus) 4% (peripheral and central)

Source: Adapted from Bertholon 2006. Reproduced with permission of Sage.

Table 15.6 Diagnostic criteria for basilar migraine as defined by the International Headache Society (IHS).

Diagnostic criteria for basilar migraine:

A At least two attacks fulfilling criteria B–D

B Aura consisting of at least two of the following fully reversible symptoms, but no motor weakness:
- Dysarthria
- Vertigo
- Tinnitus
- Hypacusia
- Diplopia
- Visual symptoms simultaneously in both temporal and nasal fields of both eyes
- Ataxia
- Decreased level of consciousness
- Simultaneously bilateral paraesthesias

C At least one of the following:
1 At least one aura symptom develops gradually over ≥5 minutes and/or different aura symptoms occur in succession over ≥5 minutes
2 Each aura symptom lasts ≥5 and ≤60 minutes

D Headache fulfilling criteria B–D for IHS diagnostic criteria of migraine without aura (Chapter 12) begins during the aura or follows aura within 60 minutes

Table 15.7 Diagnostic criteria for definite vestibular migraine (International Headache Society and Bárány Society 2012).

A At least five episodes of vestibular symptoms, of moderate or severe intensity, lasting 5 min to 72 hours, e.g.
- Rotational vertigo
- Illusory self or object motion
- Positional vertigo
- Head motion intolerance

B Current or previous history of migraine with or without aura according to the International Classification of Headache Disorders (ICHD)

C One or more migraine features with at least 50% of the vestibular episodes:
- Headache with at least two of the following characteristics: one-sided location, pulsating quality, moderate or severe pain intensity, aggravation by routine physical activity
- Photophobia and phonophobia
- Visual aura

D Not better accounted for by another vestibular or ICHD diagnosis

1995 criteria are commonly used. Nonetheless, monosymptomatic cochlear or vestibular variants are possible depending on whether the endolymphatic hydrops affects predominantly the auditory or vestibular part of the labyrinth, and with time these patients may develop the full disorder. This is a reminder to keep a watching brief on those patients whose initial symptoms do not match the full criteria.

The mechanism underlying the disorder is thought to be a failure of resorption of endolymph by the endolymphatic sac. This view is supported by electromyographic studies, by the finding of peri-saccular fibrosis of the endolymphatic duct and by high resolution MRI. With Ménière's cases, the endolymphatic duct can be visualised on MRI less often than in control subjects. This over-accumulation of endolymph leads to distortion of the membranous labyrinth (i.e. endolymphatic hydrops).

Ménière's disease can rarely be congenital, for example associated with Mondini dysplasia. It is usually acquired (e.g. after an evident inflammatory or traumatic insult to the labyrinth, when it is sometimes known as delayed endolymphatic hydrops), or idiopathic, when it occurs in about 21/100 000 of the population, presenting at 40–60 years of age. The endolymphatic hydrops starts in the helicotrema leading to ruptures of Reissner's membrane separating perilymph from the endolymph and accounting for the symptoms of fullness of the ear during an attack. With these periodic ruptures of Reissner's membrane there is endolymph discharge with a flux of potassium ions across the breached membrane (from 150 mmol/L in endolymph to 8 mmol/L in perilymph). This causes a temporary palsy of the vestibulo-cochlear nerve fibres located in the perilymph space. There is an initial excitation of the nerves leading to severe vertigo and an irritative nystagmus (i.e. beating towards the affected ear). Later, there is blockade of action potentials leading to inactivation of the axonal sodium channels and nystagmus (known as destructive nystgamus) beating toward the unaffected ear. Initially, the ruptures heal, but with disease progression, there are permanent alterations in the morphological features of the membranous labyrinth with loss of cochlear and vestibular neurones. Eventually there is atrophy of the organ of Corti and the vestibular end organ.

Typically, the major loss of hearing occurs in the first few years. In the early stages the hearing loss tends to be reversible, affecting the low frequencies only, but with advancing cochlear involvement, a peaked audiogram can be seen (best threshold at 2000 Hz) and eventually a flat loss is found in a majority of patients. The hearing loss is typically recruiting as identified by stapedius reflex thresholds within 60 dBHL of the pure tone audiometric thresholds at the same frequencies. In general, the longer the patients are followed, the greater the percentage of those who develop bilateral disease. A total of 15% have bilateral disease by 2 years, and by 20 years 30–60% are bilateral. At autopsy, 30% of the temporal bones in patients with Ménière's disease have bilateral involvement.

The early attacks of vertigo are severe, often associated with vomiting. These prostrate the patient for between 2 and 24 hours. About 6% of patients develop drop attacks (Tumarkin's crises) and occasionally there is a loss of consciousness from secondary syncope. The differential diagnosis of the attacks of vertigo can be difficult and includes vestibular migraine, benign recurrent vertigo and other causes of acute vertigo. With disease progression a canal paresis of the affected ear can be seen on caloric testing.

Bilateral vestibular failure

Bilateral vestibular failure (BVF) in adults is a rare clinical entity characterised by unsteadiness, particularly in the dark, and oscillopsia. BVF is defined by the absence of a nystagmic response to both caloric and rotary stimuli.

There are many causes. Some cases have associated neurological disease, such as a progressive cerebellar syndrome, or other cranial neuropathies. Gentamicin ototoxicity, vasculitis and malignant meningitis are also causes. Some cases follow bacterial meningitis.

Clinical presentation depends on whether BVF is very longstanding or recently acquired, and if acquired whether this has been a sequential process or had a sudden onset simultaneously affecting both ears. When the loss is sequential, there are episodes of vertigo lasting from minutes to days. These preceding symptoms may be entirely absent in patients with sudden bilateral BVF. Oscillopsia is a common feature, particularly when walking or travelling in a car. It is a result of the loss of the vestibulo-ocular reflex, particularly at high frequencies (i.e. 1 Hz) associated with physiological head movements. Unsteadiness in the dark or on rough ground is also typical and patients feel most stable when walking in good lighting conditions and on firm ground. When BVF has been present from infancy (e.g. following neonatal meningitis), the absence of peripheral vestibular function is surprisingly well tolerated. There may be some delay in developmental milestones; eventually, young children may learn to ride a bike. Caution is advised for patients with BVF in certain situations (e.g. swimming underwater).

The diagnosis is suspected when the Halmagyi headthrust test is positive to both right and left. In patients with BVF, gaze shifts with the head (doll's eye movement) and only after the head movement is there a corrective saccade to bring the object of interest back on to the fovea. The diagnosis is confirmed with caloric and rotary chair testing: no nystagmic response is elicited with ice cold water and chair accelerations of $120°/s^2$, respectively.

Vestibular paroxysmia

The very existence of this clinical entity has been questioned but it is supported strongly by the prompt response to treatment with carbamazepine. There is paroxysmal hyperactivity to vestibular stimulation combined with a functional defect between attacks. The neuro-pathophysiology is attributed to neurovascular compression, much in the same way as trigeminal neuralgia; ephaptic transmission has also been proposed as a mechanism. The following features define the syndrome:

- Short intense attacks of rotational or to-and-fro vertigo lasting seconds to minutes
- Attacks frequently provoked by particular head positions
- Impaired hearing permanently or during an attack
- Audio-vestibular deficits on testing, and
- Exclusion of a central cause.

Motion sickness

This common problem is caused by repetitive stimulation of the vestibular system. Motion sickness occurs frequently at sea and in cars (especially in children), but also with less usual forms of travel such as on a camel or an elephant. Motion sickness is now rare during commercial flights, but it is a problem during space travel, and one reason why the airship industry did not flourish.

Nausea, sweating, dizziness, vertigo and profuse vomiting develop over several hours or less, accompanied by an irresistible desire either to stop moving or return to land. Prostration and intense incapacitating malaise frequently follow, seen typically in seasickness. The distress, incapacity and dehydration caused by severe seasickness should not be underestimated.

Early symptoms at sea are sometimes helped by maintaining visual contact with the horizon, eating and avoiding the stuffy atmosphere of a cabin. Alcohol tends to make matters worse. However, the motion of a vessel is less dramatic close to its centre of gravity, and hence many sufferers, once symptoms have become established, are averse to remaining on deck, and prefer to 'go below'.

Prophylactic antihistamines, vestibular sedatives (hyoscine, cyclizine or cinnarizine) and stem ginger are of some value. Recovery and habituation with no further attacks usually take place between several hours and several days. However, some individuals remain especially prone to recurent bouts of seasickness, and prefer to remain on dry land.

The precise pathogenesis and neuronal circuitry of motion sickness remains relatively little studied – but there is no doubt that its origin is within the semicircular canals, when they are subjected to particular combinations of pitch, roll and yaw.

Management of vestibular disorders

Management of vestibular pathology requires a clear understanding of normal physiology, the mechanisms of dysfunction and compensation, together with the autonomic and psychological sequelae of vestibular pathology. This leads to accurate diagnosis in the majority, therapy for systemic disorders with vestibular features, prompt intervention for emergencies and rehabilitation for chronic vestibular symptoms, both peripheral and central.

The treatment of vestibular pathology involves:

- Specific therapy for systemic disorders with vestibular manifestations
- Specific pharmacological therapies for labyrinthine disorders
- Vestibular rehabilitation physiotherapy, including canalith repositioning procedures (CRPs)
- Psychological support, and
- Surgical interventions.

A plan should be established for each patient, to include an explanation of the symptoms. These are often bizarre and not easily understood in the context of ear disease (e.g. visual vertigo in a supermarket). The importance of the patient understanding the rationale of the management programme cannot be overemphasised; this ensures compliance.

Concurrent drug regimens should be evaluated during the general medical assessment. This will allow appropriate management of conditions exacerbating or preventing recovery of vestibular symptoms (e.g. hypertension, diabetes, hyperlipidaemia, arthritis or ophthalmological conditions and drug effects). Treatment for specific vestibular disorders (e.g. Ménière's disease and BPPV) should be undertaken. Persistent vertiginous symptoms are managed by intensive vestibular rehabilitation physiotherapy. A regular exercise programme compatible with the patient's age and physical abilities should be commenced. Psychological factors will be addressed by psychotherapy or drugs.

Monitoring of recovery following treatment can prove difficult, as there is a marked discrepancy between vestibular symptoms and signs and vestibular test results. Therefore, outcome measures of recovery have been developed including validated questionnaires documenting vestibular symptomatology, disability and handicap (e.g. the Dizziness Handicap Inventory and the Vertigo Symptom Scale). In addition, validated psychological questionnaires such as the Beck Anxiety and Depression Scales and quality of life evaluations such as the Short Form 36, are commonly used. Functional measurements such as the Dynamic Gait Index, the Functional Gait Index and the Timed Get-Up-and-Go Test may also provide valuable evidence of improvement. In addition, objective resolution of positional nystagmus in BPPV may be of value. Posturographic results can demonstrate improving CoG measurements and more appropriate balance strategies as symptomatic recovery occurs in both peripheral and central vestibular pathology. The ultimate aim is to discharge the patient with full integration into occupational and personal activities.

Drug treatment

Recent developments in neurochemistry have begun to clarify the role of neurotransmitters within the vestibular system, but despite these developments, few of the recent advances have led to the development of new antivertiginous drugs. The treatment of vestibular disorders remains primarily empirical, because of the paucity of high quality clinical drug trials and an evidence-based approach. There are four arms to the pharmacological treatment of vertigo:

1 Vestibular suppressant drugs for acute vertigo
2 Specific treatment of vestibular disorders (e.g. Ménière's disease, migrainous vertigo and central vestibular disorders)
3 Drugs used to treat systemic diseases that cause vertigo
4 Experimental drugs (e.g. drugs that may accelerate compensation).

Symptomatic treatment of acute vestibular symptoms

Acute unilateral loss of vestibular function gives rise to symptoms of vertigo, nausea, vomiting, sweating, pallor and diarrhoea. Patients find such symptoms alarming and commonly fear a serious neurological condition such as a brain tumour or a stroke. Simple reassurance is highly effective, but should be followed by an explanation of the underlying pathology giving rise to such symptoms, and appropriate treatment with antiemetics such as hyoscine, prochlorperazine, promethazine, cyclizine or metoclopramide. Buccal administration of prochlorperazine is effective, but intramuscular therapy can be administered if oral preparations cannot be tolerated because of vomiting. Hyoscine may be administered transdermally. In general, antiemetic drugs act by blocking the afferent pathways from the chemoreceptor zone in the area postrema, the gastrointestinal tract and the labyrinth to the medullary vomiting centre.

Secondly, vestibular sedative drugs should be administered acutely. However, there is good evidence that such medication should be prescribed for the minimum period as the drugs interfere with vestibular compensation. Such drugs include anticholinergics (hyoscine, scopolamine), antihistamines (promethazine, prochlorperazine, cyclizine and metoclopramide) and the calcium-channel antagonists (cinnarizine, flunarizine). These latter two drugs, together with prochlorperazine, may give rise to extrapyramidal side effects, and their dosage should be carefully titrated against symptomatic response, especially in the elderly. In addition, flunarizine has been associated with depression.

Diazepam has been widely used, particularly in North America, in the management of acute unilateral vestibular deafferentation and has been reported to be effective as a consequence of the reduction of neural activity, and inhibition throughout the CNS, including the vestibular nerve and nuclei. Benzodiazepines may be of value in the treatment of vertigo, to counter the anxiety commonly associated with acute vestibular crises. Recent work would suggest the value of steroids in promoting recovery of labyrinthine function in the initial phases of an acute vestibular episode.

Specific treatment of vestibular disorders

Ménière's disease is a commonly misdiagnosed vestibular syndrome, and appropriate treatment requires accurate diagnosis. There are few double-blind randomised studies assessing treatment efficacy in this condition, and it is important to recall the 80% placebo response rate. Medical treatment is either symptomatic, or aimed at influencing the presumed underlying pathological process of endolymphatic hydrops, or sometimes at the hypothesised immunological pathogenesis; surgical treatment aims first to decompress the hydrops (e.g. saccus decompression). Other, destructive procedures in intractable cases include intratympanic gentamicin (so-called medical labyrinthectomy), surgical labyrinthectomy or vestibular neurectomy.

No evidence-based standard treatment protocols exist, and general measures may include lifestyle adaptations such as stress reduction, food elimination and even allergy immunotherapy. Medical therapy commonly includes a low-salt diet and diuretics, although to date there is no clinical trial of sufficient quality to confirm the efficacy of diuretic treatment. Bendroflumethiazide is the thiazide diuretic of choice, although chlorthalidone has been reported to be beneficial in early uncontrolled studies; both diazide and acetazolamide have also been advocated.

Betahistine is a histamine analogue that has been reported to bring about a reduction of the asymmetric functioning of the vestibular end-organs, improve microvascular circulation in the stria vascularis of the cochlea and inhibit the activity of the vestibular nuclei. A systematic review identified major flaws in the clinical trials of betahistine and Ménière's disease. With these limitations, the review noted that betahistine may bring about a reduction in vertigo and tinnitus, but no specific therapeutic effect could be confirmed.

Steroids have been used in the treatment of Ménière's disease on the assumption that they may ameliorate an autoimmune diathesis, but there are no double-blind controlled trials to prove their efficacy. Treatment may be taken orally, or topical application via tympanostomy tubes into the middle ear, which may achieve better drug penetration with less side effects than systemic administration. The outcome of steroid treatment and methotrexate remains controversial.

In patients with intractable vertigo, but preserved auditory function, the instillation of intratympanic gentamicin was popularised in the 1990s and has become a common treatment particularly in North America. Gentamicin is predominantly vestibulo-toxic, but no standard treatment protocol or dose has been defined. High rates of therapeutic success in the control of vertigo have been reported, but sensorineural hearing loss has been reported in up to 30% of cases. Moreover, recurrence of vertiginous symptoms may develop in up to one-third of treated cases within 24 months. Careful consideration of this form of management is required, in view of the significant percentage of patients who develop bilateral involvement with Ménière's disease.

Hyperbaric oxygen therapy with continuous variations in pressure has been reported to be of benefit, as has treatment with the Meniett device, which delivers intermittent micropressure pulse waves to the inner ear through a tympanostomy tube. In a prospective randomised placebo-controlled multicentre clinical trial, the Meniett device was reported to show significant improvement in terms of frequency and intensity of vertigo, dizziness, aural pressure and tinnitus, but further scientific evaluation is required.

Surgical management of Ménière's disease includes prophylactic measures such as endolymphatic sac decompression, for which there is no firm evidence of efficacy and destructive surgical procedures. These latter techniques are primarily reserved for patients with intractable vertigo and profound hearing loss, with clear evidence of the side of lesion giving rise to symptoms. Surgical options include vestibular nerve section and labyrinthectomy. However, such procedures should be undertaken with extreme caution, not only because of the possibility of bilateral pathology in Ménière's disease, but also because of the possible failure of compensation for a total unilateral vestibular loss.

Migraine

The treatment of migrainous vertigo parallels that of migrainous headache (Chapter 12). Dietary measures, lifestyle adaptation and stress reduction techniques are important first measures, together with psychological management and intensive vestibular rehabilitation physiotherapy, for the 25–30% of patients with migrainous vertigo who demonstrate peripheral vestibular dysfunction.

The pharmacological treatment of migraine includes both prophylactic and acute symptomatic management. Prophylactic treatment should be considered in recurrent acute episodes of vertigo in which symptomatic treatment is inadequate. Beta-blockers such as propranolol, calcium-channel blockers such as cinnarazine, serotonin antagonists such as pizotifen, in addition to tricyclic antidepressants such as amitriptyline, have all been shown to be effective in some cases. Symptomatic treatment may include antivertiginous and antiemetic drugs as well as specific treatment for headache. Triptans have been shown to be highly effective in ameliorating both dizziness and headache and may also relieve nausea, vomiting and phonophobia. Sublingual, subcutaneous or rectal zolmitriptan have been recommended as the duration of migrainous vertigo may be too short to warrant treatment with oral triptans. Ergot drugs and acetazolamide have also been reported to be effective in controlling migrainous vertigo.

Episodic ataxia

Episodic ataxia type 2 (Chapter 17) can present with acute vertigo and ataxia, with or without interval symptoms. Both acetazolamide and 4-amino-pyridine have been reported to help.

Central vestibular dysfunction

Central vestibular dysfunction associated with neurological disease is exceedingly difficult to help. It commonly presents with ataxia and disordered oculomotor function, including bi-directional, dysconjugate, rotatory, vertical, periodic, alternating, see-saw or pendular nystagmus. No single treatment is of benefit to all patients, but an understanding of ocular physiology and the neurochemistry of the vestibular system have enabled a rational approach to specific treatments.

Both clonazepam and 3,4-diaminopyridine have been reported to help downbeat nystagmus, while acquired pendular nystagmus may respond to gabapentin. Baclofen has some effect in periodic alternating nystagmus. No specific treatment regimes have been defined; frequently, drugs are used empirically and doses titrated against response and side effects.

For patients with chronic instability and ataxia of central vestibular origin there is some evidence that intensive vestibular rehabilitation physiotherapy and gait retraining strategies may help both stability and confidence.

Treatment of chronic peripheral vertigo

Vestibular rehabilitation physiotherapy

The majority of patients with persistent chronic vestibular symptoms demonstrate uncompensated unilateral peripheral vestibular dysfunction. Less commonly, patients may present with chronic symptoms caused by bilateral vestibular hypofunction, and for both unilateral and bilateral dysfunction, intensive vestibular rehabilitation physiotherapy is the mainstay of treatment. Every effort should be made to ensure optimal sensory input for balance: correction of visual/ophthalmological disorders such as cataracts, aggressive management of joint/orthopaedic problems (e.g. arthritis) and medical management of fluctuating vestibular conditions such as Ménière's disease or BPPV.

Compensation cannot be effective in the face of inadequate sensory input or fluctuating vestibular activity. Importantly, antiemetics and/or vestibular sedative drugs should not be used for chronic symptoms – there is evidence that they impair vestibular compensation. Notwithstanding this fact, there is widespread and inappropriate prescription of these drugs for chronic vestibular symptoms both in primary and tertiary care.

CNS plasticity underpins vestibular rehabilitation and symptomatic vestibular compensation. The Cawthorne–Cooksey exercises are systematic exercises aimed at stimulating visual, vestibular and proprioceptive input on a repetitive basis to enhance compensation. They were initially introduced empirically in the 1940s. In the 1970s and 1980s, animal experimentation provided a scientific basis for their value, providing evidence to support the rationale for specific physiotherapy for chronic vestibular symptoms. Subsequently, a range of vestibular rehabilitation programmes has been devised, containing a number of key elements:

- A detailed explanation of the rationale of exercises, and the aim of therapy to ensure patient motivation and compliance
- A graded approach, with increasing sensory input and speed of task, to expedite compensation
- Emphasis upon exercises that are functionally relevant and that actually provoke dizziness in individual patients, and
- Repeated short but frequent repetitions of individual exercises to promote habituation.

Many studies have shown the efficacy of these regimes. Recent research has highlighted that customised exercises with a programme devised specifically for each patient, based on individual vestibular limitations, is most effective. Mechanical exercise programmes including optokinetic stimulation, visual flow stimuli and rotational stimuli have been shown to be especially helpful and to optimise vestibular compensation. Other strategies shown to enhance compensation include virtual reality t'ai chi and support surface translations.

Traditionally, vestibular rehabilitation physiotherapy has been used in the treatment of unilateral peripheral vestibular disorders that have failed to compensate. Many factors are associated with failure of compensation (Figure 15.17) and most can be targeted with physiotherapy, by specific evaluations including standardised health report questionnaires, scored balance assessment tests and dynamic posturography. These measures also document recovery, support patient motivation and cooperation and direct ongoing physiotherapy.

It cannot be overemphasised that a detailed explanation of the underlying pathological processes, with a basic understanding of vestibular compensation, is crucial if the patient is to accept that

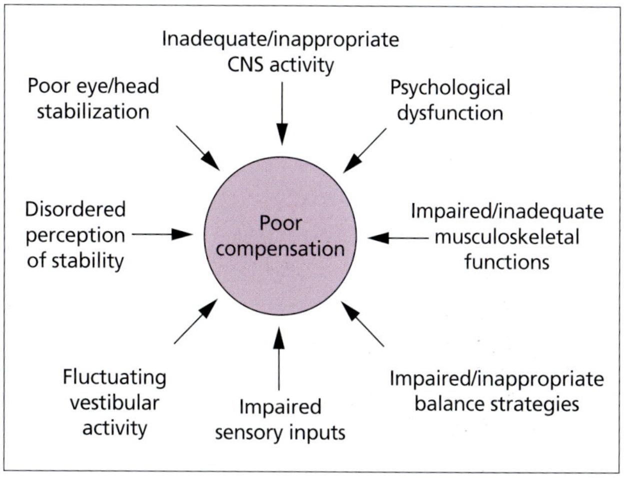

Figure 15.17 Factors predisposing to decompensation.

physiotherapy rather than some alternative, technically sophisticated option is more appropriate. Early intervention may be beneficial, but neither long-standing symptoms nor old age are negative prognostic factors – enthusiastic treatment is always worth trying.

Recent work has also confirmed the value of vestibular rehabilitation physiotherapy in the management of migraine, bilateral vestibular failure and central vestibular pathologies including brainstem and cerebellar disease. An important group of patients, whose symptoms are frequently found to be intractable to standard rehabilitation techniques, are those with visual dependence and visual vertigo. In this group, optokinetic training and mechanical rehabilitative interventions have been shown to be of value. Virtual reality stimulation may be of specific value in this group. A further subset of patients with persistent dizziness are those with vestibular pathology associated with psychological symptoms. This group undoubtedly benefit from vestibular rehabilitation physiotherapy, although a range of psychological support measures should be provided in parallel.

Particle repositioning procedures

BPPV is the most common vestibular syndrome and requires specific particle repositioning procedures aimed at addressing the underlying mechanism of cupulo- or canalithiasis. Accurate diagnosis is crucial for three reasons:

1 Central positional nystagmus, although rare, may indicate serious life-threatening neurological pathology.
2 Management of cupulolithiasis and/or canalithiasis of each of the three semicircular canals requires specific different interventions.
3 The correct specific particle-repositioning procedure is highly successful for these debilitating conditions.

The symptoms associated with BPPV commonly abate over several weeks, but in some 30% symptoms persist, with significant disability and distress. Many different procedures for BPPV have been described, but the two established techniques are the Semont liberatory manoeuvre and the Epley particle-repositioning procedure.

The Brandt–Daroff exercises were devised for the treatment of cupulolithiasis, and consist of rapid movements of the body and head from one lateral position to the other. However, the movement is not tightly aligned to the plane of posterior canal and is repetitive, displacing repositioned crystals and is less used than formerly to manage p-BPPV.

The Semont manoeuvre, developed to liberate otolithic deposits from the cupula of the posterior semicircular canal, is conducted by lying the patient on the affected side with the face turned 45° towards the ceiling. The patient is then rapidly swung in an arc through the sitting position, to lie on the opposite side with the face turned downwards by 45°. This latter position should be maintained for 5 minutes prior to the patient being brought slowly up to the sitting position (Figure 15.18).

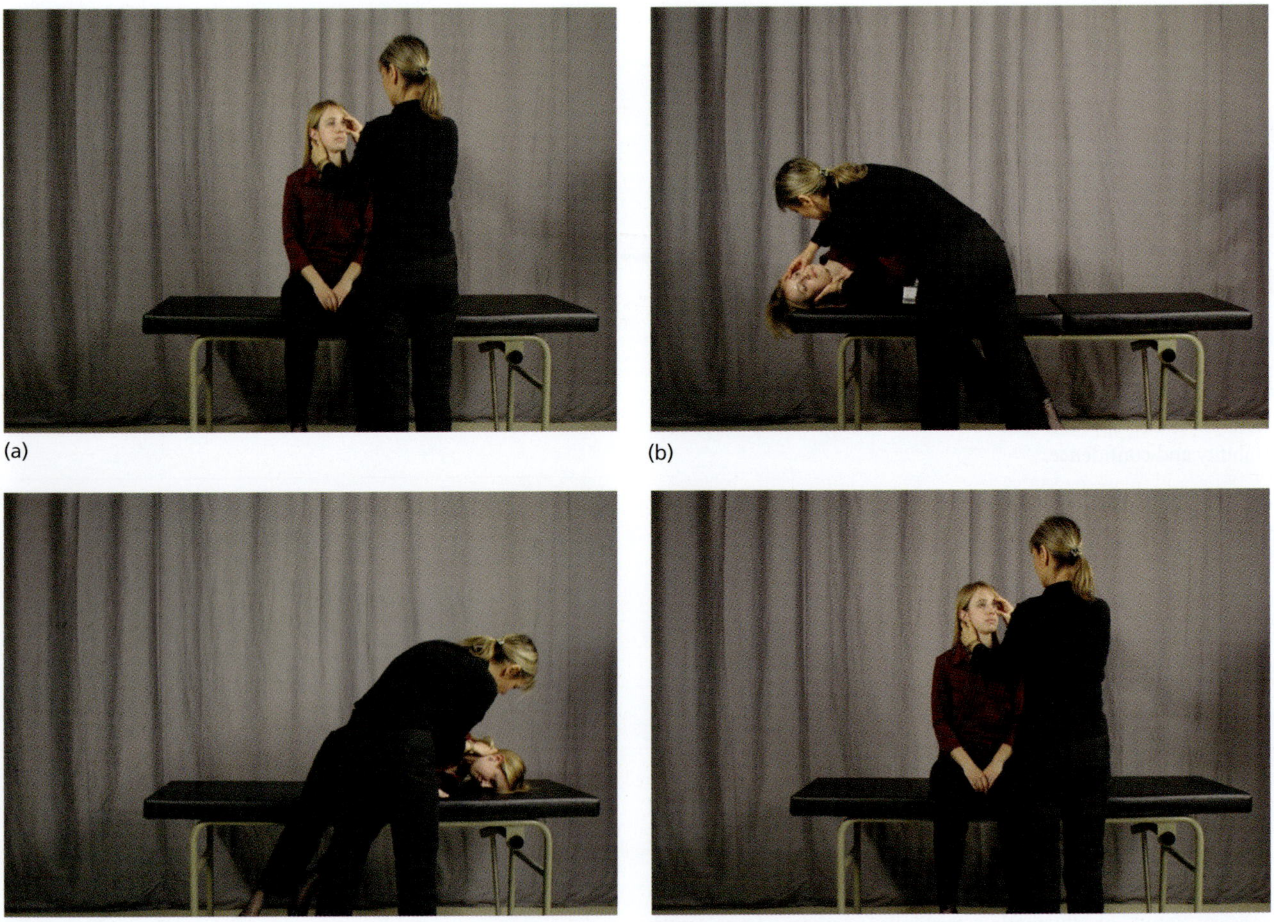

(a) (b) (c) (d)

Figure 15.18 Semont manoeuvre (see text).

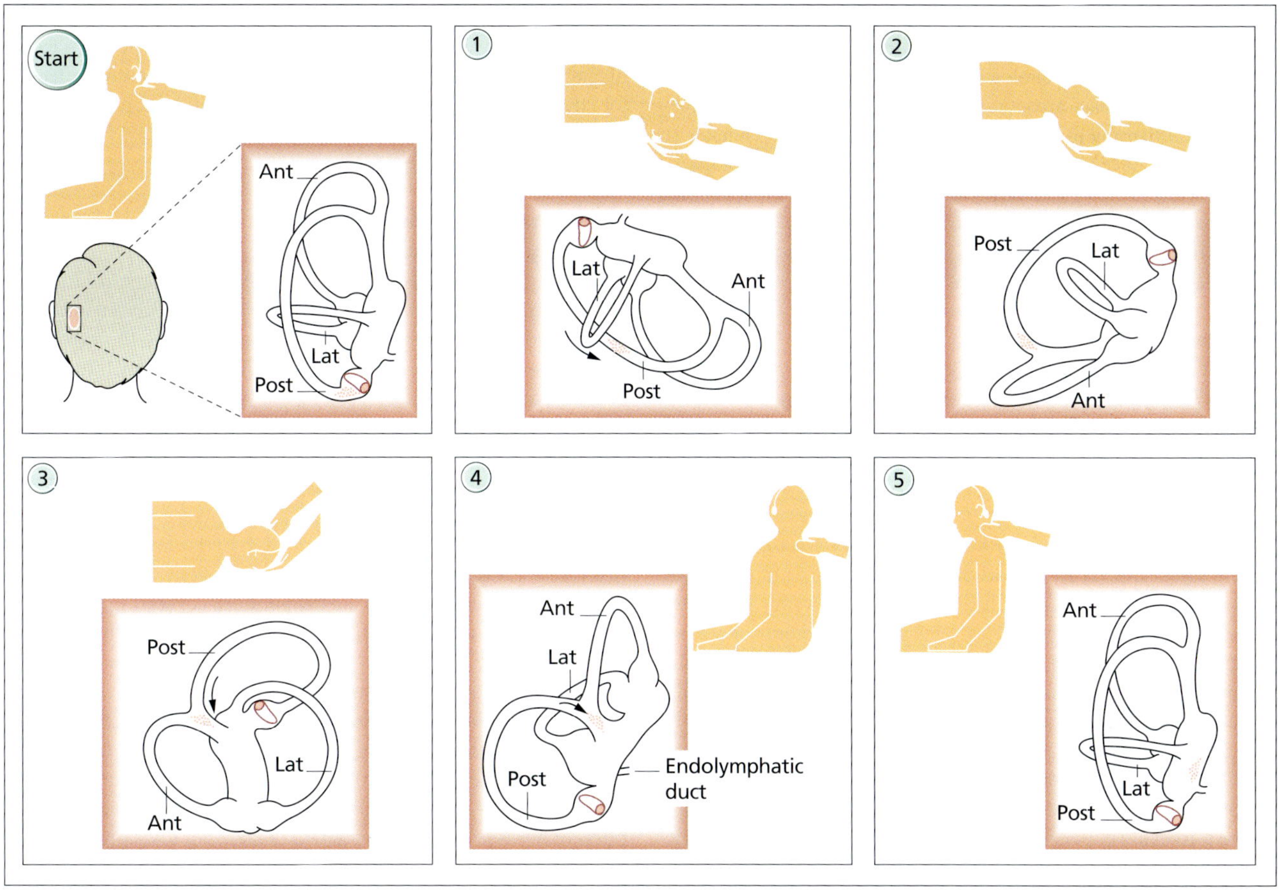

Figure 15.19 Epley manoeuvre (see text).

The Epley particle repositioning procedure (1992) was introduced as a successful technique for treating p-BPPV (Figure 15.19). Subsequently, the technique has been adapted for the treatment of a-BPPV. The manoeuvre is comprised of five separate positions, the first being the Dix–Hallpike manoeuvre for the identification of p-BPPV. The various positions that are then assumed result in the otoconial debris moving to the most dependent part of the posterior canal, and from there to the common crus and then out of the canal into the vestibule where, upon assuming the critical head position, debris does not fall on to the cupula of the posterior canal.

Both the Epley and Semont manoeuvres have been widely evaluated, for both subjective outcome and objective absence of positional nystagmus. They are highly effective, with around 90% of patients becoming symptom-free after repeated manoeuvres. Some evidence suggests the best recovery rate is in cases where vertigo has been caused by vestibular neuritis, while those cases caused by trauma have a poorer outcome, with a recurrence rate of some 50% at 5 years. Importantly, it is well recognised that p-BPPV can convert to a-BPPV or hBPPV after a particle repositioning procedure; careful observation of nystagmus is required to ensure that an appropriate second procedure is conducted where the first appears to have failed.

Specific treatments for h-BPPV and a-BPPV have been described. Horizontal dysfunction resulring from canalolithiasis may be treated with a 12-hour prolonged positioning on the healthy side (Vannuchi manoeuvre) while the barbeque roll (Lempert roll manoeuvre) with 270° rotation in the direction opposite to the affected ear, around the longitudinal axis, have both been reported to be effective. a-BPPV can be treated with a reverse Epley particle repositioning procedure (i.e. a right a-BPPV can be treated with a left posterior canal repositioning procedure). Physical treatments for BPPV are highly effective, and <1% require surgical intervention. Historically, vestibular nerve section has been carried out, but the surgical treatment of choice in intractable cases is now considered to be occlusion of the posterior semicircular canal.

Psychological treatment

Psychological symptoms in association with vestibular pathology are well recognised and frequently result in intense and protracted symptoms when there has been failure to compensate from a vestibular deficit. Many studies have highlighted the association of agoraphobia, anxiety states, panic attacks, depression and avoidance behaviour, together with phobias such as space and motion phobia in patients with vestibular symptoms. Recent work has outlined a possible underlying neurological basis for the relationship between anxiety and vestibular symptoms. Psychological support is a key factor in rehabilitation of many patients with vestibular symptoms and should always be considered when there is no satisfactory explanation either for failure to recover, or decompensation following earlier improvement.

Importantly, the clinician should understand the interaction of psychological and vestibular factors, in order to provide a satisfactory and understandable explanation of the way in which the patient's symptoms are compounded by the interaction of these two aspects of the illness. The specific mode of treatment will depend on the primary underlying psychological disorder: avoidance behaviour, panic attacks, phobias, anxiety states and/or depression. Cognitive–behavioural therapy in parallel with physiotherapy is invaluable in patients who have developed avoidance behaviour and/or panic attacks, while formal psychiatric intervention is required in patients with anxiety states and depression. The index of suspicion of an underlying psychological problem should be high in patients with vestibular dysfunction.

Surgical management of vertigo

Surgical intervention for the treatment of isolated vertigo is rarely needed. The conditions most usually requiring surgical intervention are the life-threatening complications of otitis media, cerebellopontine angle tumours and perilymph fistulae. Surgical procedures may be divided into those aimed at alleviating underlying pathophysiology (e.g. canal-plugging procedures in BPPV and endolymphatic sac decompression for Ménière's disease), although there is little evidence to support the value of the latter intervention. Intractable vertigo with good hearing in Ménière's may be treated by destructive procedures such as vestibular neurectomy or chemical labyrinthectomy (gentamicin), while intractable vertigo with profound hearing loss may be treated with surgical labyrinthectomy. It should be reiterated that destructive procedures should be undertaken with great caution, for two reasons:

1 The possibility of the development of bilateral vestibular dysfunction (e.g. in the case of Ménière's disease or head trauma), and
2 The possibility of persistent vertigo from poor vestibular compensation: there is scant evidence to suggest that total vestibular loss will compensate more effectively than partial vestibular failure.

In conclusion, simple treatment strategies are highly effective for the majority with these distressing and incapacitating symptoms. This is particularly important for the neurologist, who is frequently referred a patient whose symptoms have defied diagnosis and management by an otological colleague. A rational approach to the diagnosis and management of vestibular symptoms is cost-effective for the health care system and has significant personal and occupational benefits for the patient.

Hearing disorders

Anatomy and physiology

Anatomically, the ear is divided into the external, the middle and the internal ears (Chapter 2). Physiologically, the external and middle ears collect, enhance and amplify sound, while the inner hair cells of the organ of Corti transduce mechanical energy into electrical activity. The outer hair cells of the organ of Corti act as both modulators and amplifiers, capable of fine tuning the receptor function of the cochlea. Auditory signals from the organ of Corti are transmitted along the afferent auditory pathway (Figure 15.20): auditory nerve to the ipsilateral cochlear nucleus, from where the majority of afferent auditory fibres project to the contralateral superior olivary complex, lateral lemniscus, inferior colliculus, medial geniculate body and onwards to the auditory cortex.

The auditory efferent pathway (Figure 15.21) arises in the auditory cortex and descends in parallel to the afferent pathway. The anatomy of the higher efferent auditory system remains ill-defined, but within the brainstem the olivo-cochlear bundle projects from the superior olivary complex to the cochlea via the medial and lateral olivo-cochlear system to the contralateral outer hair cells and the ipsilateral inner hair cells of the organ of Corti, respectively. Efferent fibres leave the brainstem in the inferior division of the vestibular nerve. The precise functions of the efferent auditory system remain poorly understood, but amongst the suggested hypotheses are shifts of the dynamic range of hearing to enhance signal detection and frequency selectivity, protection from excessive noise and facilitation of selective attention.

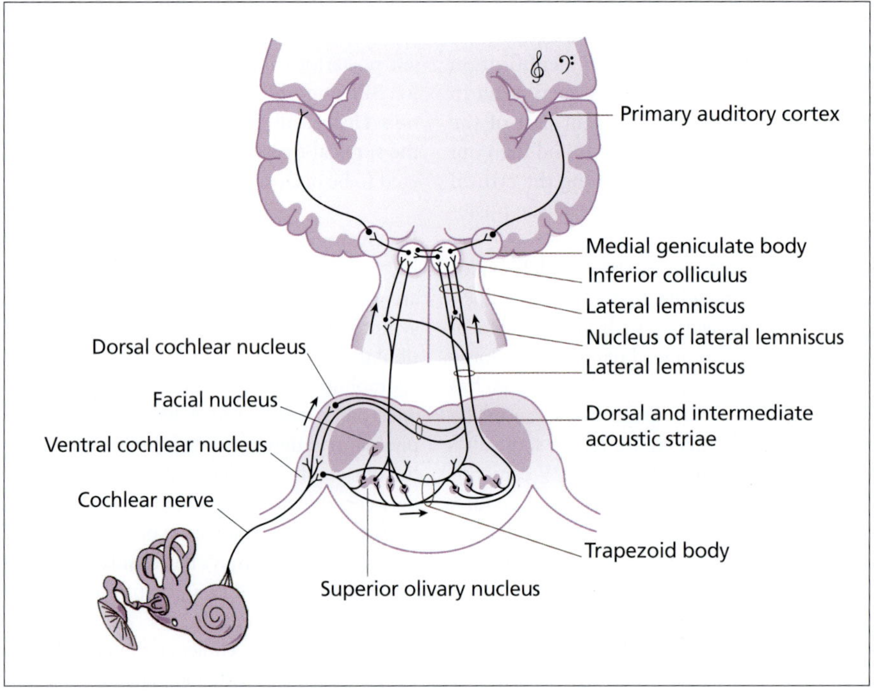

Figure 15.20 Afferent auditory pathway. Source: Noback 1981. Reproduced with permission of Springer Science + Business Media.

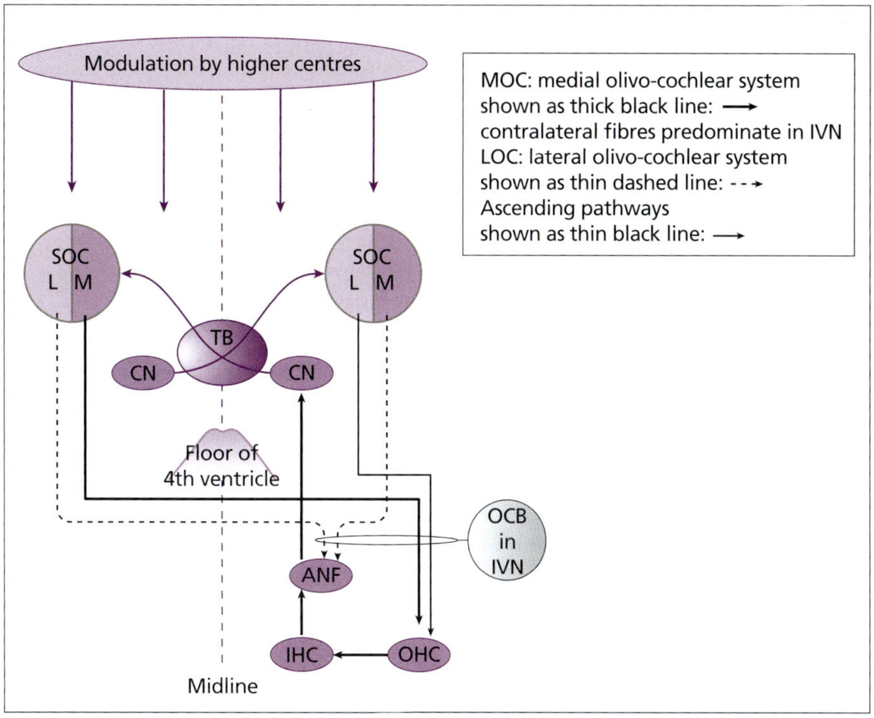

Figure 15.21 Efferent auditory system. Ascending pathways shown as double lines; ANF, auditory nerve fibre; CN, cochlear nucleus; IHC, inner hair cell; IVN, inferior vestibular nerve; LOC, lateral olivo-cochlear system shown as thin dashed line, ipsilateral fibres predominate in IVN; MOC, medial olivo-cochlear system shown as thick black line, contralateral fibres predominate in IVN; OCB, olivo-cochlear bundle; OHC, outer hair cell; SOC, superior olivary complex; TB, trapezoid body. Adapted from Murdin 2008. Reproduced with permission of Informa Healthcare and R. Davies. Also adapted from Ceranic 1998. Reproduced with permission of the BMJ.

Definitions and introduction

Disorders of the ear represent 24% of all disabilities in the adult UK population.

Hearing loss is the most common sensory disability worldwide and in the UK population over 50 years, 35% have at least mild loss of hearing. This may be the result of pathology in the external, middle or internal ear or eighth nerve or central auditory pathways. In the United Kingdom, 1.1/1000 babies are born with permanent bilateral hearing impairment; but this figure doubles by the age of 16. Hearing impairment and deafness have profound socio-economic and psychological consequences. Without appropriate care, children may fail to develop normal speech, language and cognitive skills which limit educational and occupational choices, while adults are less likely to be in skilled employment and suffer social stigmatisation, isolation and a high incidence of psychiatric illness.

Tinnitus is a perception of a sound that originates from within the body rather than the external world. It affects about 10% of most populations studied; about half find tinnitus sufficiently intrusive to seek help. If perceived solely by the patient tinnitus is called subjective and is commonly related to hearing impairment. Objective tinnitus refers to sound audible externally – it has a physical source, such as palatal myoclonus, an arteriovenous fistula or turbulent flow through a stenotic artery. Occasional tinnitus is an almost universal perception, but the prevalence of persistent tinnitus is positively correlated with age and female gender and its intrusiveness is correlated with psychological factors.

Hyperacusis, reduced tolerance to noise or an increased sensitivity to sounds at levels that would not cause discomfort in a normal individual, is the most common dysacusis, occurring in some 6–7% of the population. It is generally associated with normal hearing, but it is reported in 40–80% of people with tinnitus. Hyperacusis differs from loudness recruitment, which refers to oversensitivity to loud sounds.

Impaired structure and/or function of the eighth nerve and auditory brain may have little or no effect on hearing thresholds, but may cause deficits in other aspects of hearing such as distortion of hearing and auditory localisation deficits.

Basic concepts

Hearing loss and tinnitus most commonly indicate middle ear or cochlear dysfunction, but may reflect VIIIth nerve or central auditory pathology as part of a neurological disorder. These latter pathologies characteristically present with difficulties with sound localisation or hearing in conditions of poor signal to noise ratio (e.g. in the presence of background noise).

Conductive hearing loss

Pathology affecting the external and middle ear causes abnormalities of mechanical transmission of sound waves from the environment to the cochlea, known as conductive hearing loss. Typically, there is middle ear enhancement of the auditory signal, but pure conductive hearing losses do not exceed 60 dBHL across the speech frequencies on audiometry.

Sensorineural hearing loss

Cochlear and VIIIth nerve pathology results in sensorineural hearing loss with an inability to transduce the mechanical energy of sound waves into electrical activity within the cochlea or transmit the signals along the VIIIth nerve (Figure 15.20). The precise site may be distinguished on the basis of two pathophysiological phenomena:

1 *Loudness recruitment*: an abnormally rapid increase in loudness with an increase of intensity of stimulus, characteristic of cochlear dysfunction.
2 *Abnormal auditory adaptation*: a decline in discharge frequency with time, observed following an initial burst of neural activity in response to an adequate continuing auditory stimulus, characteristic of VIIIth nerve or brainstem dysfunction.

Auditory neuropathy

Auditory neuropathy or dyssynchrony describes patients in whom hearing impairment is characterised by disordered processing of sound, commonly the result of retro-cochlear pathology from the inner hair cells of the cochlea distally, through to the auditory brainstem pathways centrally. Characteristically, pure tone audiometric thresholds are relatively well preserved, but speech perception is markedly impaired, and acoustic brainstem evoked responses (ABR) are found to be delayed or absent. Cases are not uncommon – some 5–12% of those previously considered to have severe hearing disorder in paediatric populations. The importance of recognising these patients is well established as they have specific management requirements.

Brainstem auditory dysfunction

The auditory nuclei in the brainstem extract signals from background noise and allow binaural integration of auditory information. Electrophysiological and behavioural tests of auditory separation and binaural interaction are of particular value in assessment and include: masked speech, the synthetic sentence identification with ipsilateral computing message test, the masking level difference test and the binaural fusion test.

Auditory processing disorder

Auditory processing disorder (APD) is recognised as a distinct entity, but diagnosis remains a challenge, not only because of the complexity of the auditory brain, but also because of the lack of accepted diagnostic criteria, and a systematic diagnostic test battery. The British Society of Audiology has proposed that APD 'results from impaired neural function and is characterised by poor recognition, discrimination, separation, grouping, localisation, or ordering of non-speech sounds. APD does not result solely from a deficit in general attention, language or other cognitive processes.' Similarly, the American Speech-Language-Hearing Association (ASHA, 1996) proposed that the term 'central' should precede the term APD, because 'most definitions of the disorder focus on the central auditory nervous system' and thus defined (C)APD as 'a deficit in neural processing of auditory stimuli that is not due to higher order language, cognitive, or related factors'.

Patients with APD may demonstrate normal audiograms but show deficits in sound localisation, auditory pattern recognition and sound discrimination, temporal processing, processing of degraded auditory signals or processing of the auditory signal when embedded in competing acoustic signals.

Clinical examination of the ear and hearing

Otoscopy

Pathology of the auricle, the external auditory meatus and the tympanic membrane (TM) may be identified by direct examination with an otoscope or using a head-worn light source, leaving the hands free. Importantly, cholesteatoma should be excluded. A Siegel speculum can be fitted to vary intra-meatal pressure and provide evidence of a labyrinthine fistula (Table 15.8). A stiff TM secondary to a middle ear effusion results or a flaccid TM, secondary to a healed perforation.

Table 15.8 Fistula sign.

This comprises the following:
- Raised pressure causes a conjugate deviation of the eyes towards the opposite ear
- With maintenance of pressure, a corrective fast eye movement (nystagmus) will be introduced towards the affected ear

Depending on where the fistula has developed, the nystagmus will be:
- Horizontal (horizontal semicircular canal)
- Torsional (anterior canal)
- Vertical (posterior canal)

External auditory meatus pressure can be raised by pressure on the tragus, but more accurately by tympanometry. Hennebert's sign is a positive fistula sign in the presence of an intact tympanic membrane

Auricle (pinna)

Congenital abnormalities of the auricle may be associated with findings of middle and inner ear abnormalities.

External auditory meatus

Wax can be removed using a head-light by probe or syringing, after softening if necessary with ceruminolytics (e.g.olive oil).

Congenital conditions include a stenosed or atretic EAM. Acquired abnormalities include foreign body obstruction; otitis externa – caused by *Staphylococcus*, *Pseudomonas* and diphtheroids, fungal infections such *Aspergillus* and *Candida*, and viral infections such as zoster (Ramsay-Hunt syndrome). Exostoses are small rounded bony outgrowths, common in those who swim or dive frequently.

Tympanic membrane and middle ear

The normal eardrum has the appearance of mother-of-pearl with a light reflex, seen antero-inferiorly, but this may be lost if the membrane is thickened. White patches of tympanosclerosis are a result of hyaline secondary to old middle ear disease. Blood may be seen behind the TM, and manifestations of infection may be visible. Retraction of the membrane occurs when there is chronic lowering of pressure within the middle ear (i.e. with chronic obstruction of the Eustachian tube). A fluid level may be visible if secretory otitis media has resulted from reduction of pressure. A bulging drum may occur with raised middle ear pressure (normal colour) or with acute suppurative otitis media (cherry red). Perforations may be marginal (unsafe) or central (safe) perforations in the pars tensa, and attic perforations, which may indicate the presence of cholesteatoma.

Tuning fork tests

Tuning fork tests using 256 and 512 Hz forks (Tables 15.9 and 15.10; Chapter 4) were traditionally used to distinguish conductive from sensorineural hearing loss, and also to identify functional hearing loss. The principles of tuning fork tests are:

- The inner ear is more sensitive to sound conducted by air than bone;
- In pure conductive hearing loss, the affected ear is subject to less environmental noise and is more sensitive to bone-conducted sound.

Table 15.9 Rinne tuning fork test.

Heinrich Rinne described his tuning fork test in 1855:

1 The fork is struck and held with the tines perpendicular to the long axis of the external auditory meatus with the closest tine 1 cm from the entrance to the meatus
2 The patient is asked to report if they can hear the sound (AC)
3 The fork is immediately transferred behind the ear with the base firmly pressed to the bone overlying the mastoid (BC)
4 The patient is asked which sound is louder: that in front of the ear, or that behind the ear?

The Rinne test is positive if AC > BC (i.e. the sound in front of the ear is reported as the louder). This indicates:

- Normal hearing, or
- An ear with a sensorineural hearing loss

The Rinne test is negative if BC > AC (i.e. the sound in front of the ear is reported as the quieter). This identifies:

- A significant conductive component of hearing loss of >15 db
- But, a false negative Rinne test can occur if there is severe sensorineural hearing loss in the tested ear; the BC stimulus is heard in the non-tested ear because of transcranial transmission, and thus will be louder than AC sound. This can be overcome by masking the non-affected ear with a Barany noise box

The Rinne test has a high specificity for conductive hearing loss, but a low sensitivity, this not reaching 90% until the air–bone gap >30 db

Table 15.10 Weber tuning fork test.

The aim of Ernst Weber's test (1934) is to identify the better hearing cochlea. It is used in conjunction with the Rinne test and is of most use in patients with unilateral hearing loss:

1 The 512-Hz tuning fork is struck and placed to the head in the midline, either at the vertex or on the forehead
2 The patient is asked to say whether the sound is heard better in one ear, or equally in both ears

A central Weber is described if the tone is heard centrally:

- This identifies a patient with normal hearing

A lateralising Weber is when the tone is heard to one side:

- This identifies the side of the better hearing cochlea
- But, if there is a conductive component to the hearing loss, the tone may be heard in the poorer-hearing ear (Table 15.9)

Results need interpretation with care and only in conjunction with further hearing tests

Audiological investigations

Auditory tests aim to define pathology within the auditory system, and to site the level of the lesion. A battery of audiological tests is required to:

- Quantify the audiometric threshold at each frequency
- Differentiate conductive from sensorineural hearing loss
- Differentiate cochlear from retro-cochlear abnormality
- Identify central auditory dysfunction in the brainstem, mid-brain or auditory cortex, and
- Identify any non-organic hearing impairment.

Baseline audiometric tests

Pure-tone audiometry

The cornerstone of audiological testing is the pure-tone audiogram (PTA) which measures subjective hearing thresholds and demonstrates the severity, configuration and type of hearing loss, provided there is good patient cooperation. If the patient is unable or unwilling to cooperate, additional audiological investigation, such as oto-acoustic emissions and auditory evoked responses are essential to provide objective measures of hearing.

Pure tone audiometry is performed in a sound-proofed room with a standardised protocol across auditory frequencies of 125–8000 Hz in each ear. Electrically generated pure tones are delivered through headphones or a bone conductor applied to the mastoid process, and the subject is required to respond to the quietest tone, this being recorded as the air or bone conducted hearing threshold for that frequency. For bone conduction, because the intra-aural attenuation for bone conducted sound is negligible, the ear not being tested is masked with narrow-band noise centred on the test frequency. For clinical purposes, air conduction threshold values better than 20 dBHL are considered to be normal. Bone conduction thresholds significantly better than air conduction thresholds indicate a disorder affecting transmission of sound through the middle ear into the inner ear (i.e. conductive hearing loss), whereas bone conduction and air conduction thresholds that are similar imply sensorineural hearing loss.

Acoustic impedance measurements

Tympanometric measurements provide information about pressure within the middle ear and TM compliance. Passive measurements are made of the change in acoustic impedance or immittance of the TM as a function of the pressure in the sealed external acoustic meatus. High impedance abnormalities include middle ear effusion, retracted TM or ossicular fixation. Low impedance abnormalities include thin atrophic TMs and ossicular disruption following head trauma.

Stapedius reflex measurements provide information about the inner ear, in addition to the VIIIth nerve and brainstem function. Dynamic changes are measured, resulting from contraction of stapedius, and stapedial reflex thresholds, in response to stimuli of 500, 1000, 2000 and 4000 Hz, at intensities of 70–100 dB sound pressure level. These provide evidence of recruitment and abnormal auditory adaptation.

Speech audiometry

Speech audiometry assesses auditory discrimination as opposed to auditory acuity, requiring the subject to repeat standard word lists delivered through headphones at varying intensities. The responses are scored to provide an assessment of auditory discrimination which, together with other tests, is valuable in distinguishing conductive and sensorineural hearing impairment. This is of particular value in assessing efficacy of hearing aids. Speech recognition tests are also an essential item of the test battery for identification of auditory neuropathy, as speech intelligibility scores are poorer than can be explained by pure tone thresholds.

Electro-acoustic and electrophysiological tests

Event-related potentials provide the most objective technique of assessing auditory function and the functional integrity of their generators, and help to site pathology within the auditory system and include:

- Oto-acoustic emissions (OAE)
- Electro-cochleography (ECochG)
- Acoustic brainstem evoked responses (ABR)
- Middle latency responses, and
- Cortical evoked responses.

Oto-acoustic emissions

OAEs, first characterised in 1978, are low-intensity sounds generated by the contractile elements of the outer hair cells in the cochlea in response to acoustic stimuli (Figure 15.22). Typically, 260 transients (clicks) at 80–86 dBSPL are presented to evoke a response captured over a time frame of 20 ms after stimulus application and known as transient evoked OAE (TEOAE).

A defining feature of patients with auditory neuropathy is the clearly recognisable waveforms of the TEOAE in the absence of ABR, indicating normal cochlear outer hair cell function. Various studies have reported the lack of contralateral suppression of TEOAE in patients with auditory neuropathy, consistent with VIIIth nerve pathology occurring in the contralateral afferent pathway.

Cochlear microphonics and electro-cochleography

Cochlear microphonics are the early components of the ABR generated in the cochlea. They occur in the 0.7–1 ms window post-stimulus and show similar waveform characteristics to the stimulus itself. Typically, this response is cancelled out when performing ABR by using alternate polarity clicks, thereby generating a 'microphonic-free' ABR. Trans-tympanic ECochG indicate that the phase reversal to the click stimulus occurs at the level of the cochlea itself, and therefore the presence of cochlear microphonics is indicative of a preneural response to sound. ECochG is used to measure the summating and action potentials and is most commonly used in the diagnosis of Ménière's disease, when the summating potential to action potential ratio is greater than 30% (in the normal population it is significantly smaller).

Acoustic brainstem evoked responses

ABR are detected by surface electrodes, and represent electrical activity transmitted by the VIIIth nerve and brainstem auditory relay centres in the 10 s immediately after an acoustic stimulus. Waves I and II are thought to arise from the VIIIth nerve, while waves III, IV and V from generator sites within the brainstem auditory pathways (Figure 15.23). Prolongation of the I–III interval can be seen in auditory nerve and cochlear nucleus pathology. Prolongation of the III–V is usually indicated when pathology is sited above the level of the cochlear nucleus, while absent IV and/or V waves are found in cases with involvement of the mid-upper pons. Inter-aural latency comparisons of wave V are of value in diagnosis of acoustic neurinoma, but may not be useful in detecting brainstem involvement. An absent ABR of the patient with auditory neuropathy may be explained by the altered temporal synchrony of the auditory brainstem pathway.

Middle latency response

The middle latency response generator sites are presumed to be within thalamo-cortical pathways to the auditory cortex. Sensitivity and specificity of middle latency responses for central auditory pathology is reasonably good, and the test is therefore valid and objective in assessment of central auditory dysfunction, but sleep and sedation may affect responses.

Cortical-evoked auditory responses

Cortical- or late-evoked auditory responses are the most effective method of defining auditory thresholds at each frequency in a patient who is unable or unwilling to cooperate; they are essential in legal cases, in which non-organic loss should always be considered.

Aetiology of hearing loss

Conductive hearing loss

Disorders of the tympanic membrane and middle ear

Acquired disorders include acute otitis media, chronic otitis media, serous otitis media, cholesteatoma and ossicular abnormalities.

Acute otitis media is most prevalent in children. Chronic active otitis media unassociated with cholesteatoma is characterised by recurrent infections rather than persistent infections and by odourless, rather than offensive discharge. A central TM perforation and a break in the ossicular chain or malleus fixation are regarded as safe, and unlikely to be associated with cholesteatoma. Serous otitis media is recognised by an air–fluid level in the middle ear, or a bluish discoloration of the drum. Other effusions into the middle ear include blood (e.g. haemo-tympanum after head trauma) or cerebrospinal fluid (CSF) within the middle ear space.

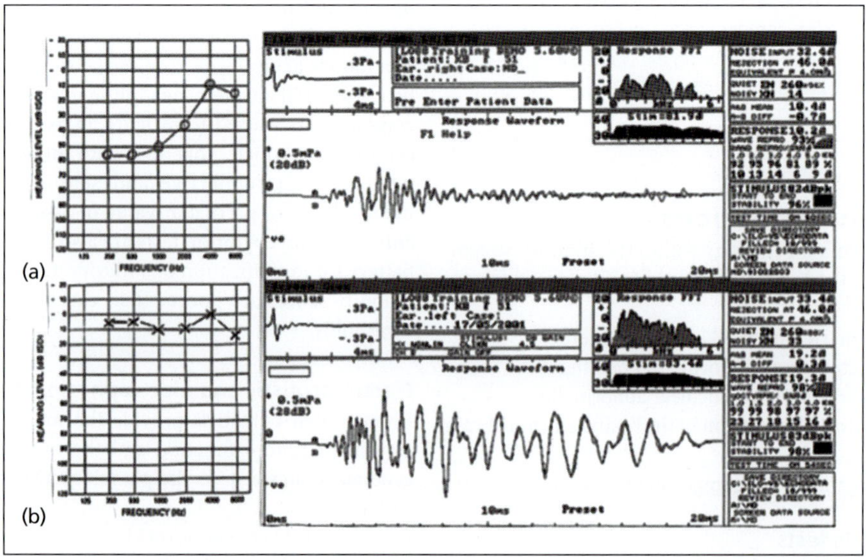

Figure 15.22 Oto-acoustic emissions in a patient with Ménière's disease. (a) Right ear of patient: pure-tone audiogram (PTA) showing typical low frequency hearing loss; transient evoked oto-acoustic emissions (TEOAE) showing reduced response. (b) Left ear of patient: PTA showing normal hearing; TEOAE showing normal response.

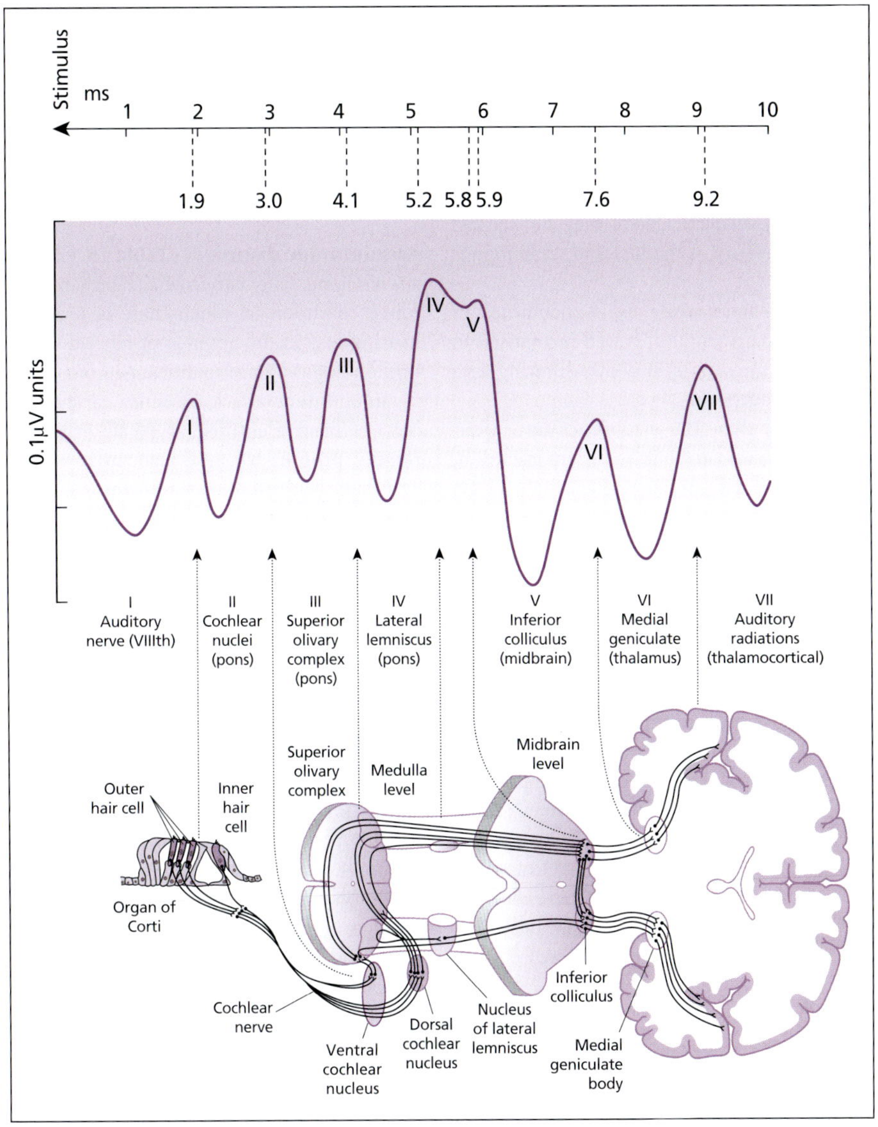

Figure 15.23 Acoustic brainstem evoked responses. Showing the series of neurogenic potentials in the 10-second post click stimulus and the putative generator sites in the VIIIth nerve, brainstem and thalamus. Source: Duane 1977.

Cholesteatoma commonly arises in ears undergoing long periods of negative middle ear pressure and persisting middle ear infection (i.e. following chronic suppurative otitis media). They are potentially serious and requires surgical removal, as they slowly increase in size and may erode the surrounding bone producing intracranial complications. Diagnosis is made from a history of perforation, chronic foul-smelling discharge and keratin debris in the pars flaccida area on otoscopic examination.

Otosclerosis is an inherited autosomal dominant hearing disorder, developing in later childhood or adulthood, associated with the *TGBF1* gene. Deposition of bone leads to fixation of the stapes footplate and a conductive hearing loss. The otosclerotic process can extend to involve the otic capsule, to cause additional sensorineural hearing loss and vertigo.

Glomus tumours are jugulo-tympanic paraganglionomas that tend to expand within the petrous temporal bone and may also extend into the labyrinth, or present as cranial nerve abnormalities. A glomus tumour can present with pulsatile tinnitus and a vascular mass lying behind the TM can sometimes be seen (Chapter 12).

Sensorineural hearing loss

Interest in sensorineural hearing loss has flourished in recent years, because of both the earlier detection of infants with profound hearing loss through newborn hearing screening programmes and because of effective prosthetic, pharmacological and genetic developments.

Genetic hearing loss

There have been significant strides in the understanding of genetic and environmental causes of both cochlear and retrocochlear hearing loss. A plethora of genes with autosomal dominant, recessive and mitochondrial inheritance have been reported, in addition to genetic aberrations giving rise to X-linked hearing loss (Hereditary Hearing Loss Homepage http://hereditaryhearingloss.org). Many of these forms of genetic hearing impairment present either in a non-syndromal or syndromal pattern.

Age-related hearing loss, characterised by progressive deterioration of auditory sensitivity with age, is the leading cause of adult auditory impairment. Until recently it had been attributed to a variety of factors including genetic, nutritional, socio-economic and environmental variables but recent research has suggested that specific genes predispose individuals to environmental triggers affecting various molecular mechanisms underlying changes in auditory function. Specifically, a mitochondrial mutation associated with aminoglycoside-induced hearing loss has been reported.

Autosomal recessive hearing loss accounts for approximately 40% of all cases of childhood hearing loss and manifests as stable, profound, congenital/prelingual impairment. There may be marked intra-familial variation in the severity of the loss and audiology is generally normal.

Autosomal dominant sensorineural hearing loss is uncommon in prelingual profound hearing impairment, but is well recognised in families with hearing loss of various configurations, differing ages of onset and differing rates of progression.

Syndromic hearing loss: more than 100 syndromes have been reported with associated hearing impairment; the more common, with their predominant features, are summarised in Table 15.11. Many of these present in childhood, but hearing loss associated with certain syndromes can progress or indeed become apparent in adult life.

Metabolic disease

Diabetes mellitus: there is no clear evidence indicating whether or not patients with diabetes mellitus have auditory and/or vestibular abnormalities as a consequence of neuropathy, angiopathy or both pathologies. Genetic studies have defined the relationship of diabetes and hearing loss in mitochondrial mutations and in mutations of the *WFS1* gene in the Wolfram syndrome of hearing impairment, diabetes mellitus and optic atrophy.

Renal failure is commonly associated with hearing loss. Ototoxicity from disease, drugs and axonal uraemic neuropathy have all been implicated as possible aetiologies, while both dialysis and renal transplantation have been reported to be associated with recovery of hearing impairment.

Drugs

Many drugs produce ototoxicity, including chloroquine, loop diuretics, aminoglycosides and salicylates. Platinum-based chemotherapeutic agents, in addition to the aminoglycosides, have been shown to damage the hair cells of the inner ear, while vincristine sulfate has been shown to produce bilateral cochlear nerve damage. Thalidomide has been demonstrated to produce aplasia of the VIIIth nerve in association with a Michel aplasia of the inner ear. In neurological practice, intrathecal streptomycin used for the treatment of meningitis, is a cause of deafness. Regular blood level estimations are helpful in preventing ototoxicity.

Acoustic trauma

Noise-induced permanent threshold shift is a common and preventable cause of sensorineural hearing loss, associated with hazardous occupational and/or recreational exposure to noise or acoustic trauma (e.g. gunfire and explosions). Characteristically, the maximal loss is at 4000 Hz, with a notched configuration to the audiogram. With time, the adjacent frequencies gradually deteriorate, but it is rare for a hearing loss greater than 70 dB to be the result of occupational noise exposure.

Acute barotrauma associated with diving, depressurisation in aircraft and explosions may give rise to tympanic membrane haemorrhage into the middle ear, with conductive hearing loss or perilymph fistula which is commonly associated with auditory and vestibular symptoms.

Physical trauma (head injury) may lead to middle ear, inner ear, VIIIth nerve and/or central auditory loss. In mild and moderate head injuries auditory abnormalities, commonly high frequency sensorineural loss, is found in 50% of cases. Labyrinthine concussion and both longitudinal and transverse fractures of the petrous temporal bone may result in sensorineural and/or conductive hearing loss.

Autoimmune disorders (Table 15.12)

Autoimmune inner ear disease (AIED) refers to a presumed autoimmune condition in which there is sudden or rapidly progressive hearing loss in the absence of any other neurological or systemic immunological abnormalities. Although AIED seems to be caused by autoimmune attack on inner ear proteins, no specific antigen has yet been identified. Typically, the hearing loss is bilateral, rapidly progressive and associated with vestibular symptoms. Treatment with steroids (both intra-tympanic and orally administered), methotrexate, plasmapheresis, cyclophosphamide or azathioprine may be effective.

Cogan's syndrome is a rare, presumed autoimmune disorder, affecting the eye and the ear that develops usually in children and young adults in the aftermath of an upper respiratory tract infection. No infectious agent has been conclusively identified as a cause. Inflammatory ocular symptoms, together with vestibular symptoms and hearing loss with rapid progression to total bilateral deafness, are common. Systemic manifestations include lymphadenopathy, night sweats and cardiorespiratory involvement including aortitis, aortic valve insufficiency, pericardial effusion and coronary arteritis, pleuritis and myocardial infarction.

Vogt–Koyanagi–Harada syndrome (VKH) syndrome is a rare condition characterised by bilateral uveitis with cutaneous lesions (vitiligo, alopecia and poliosis), neurological features (CSF pleocytosis) and auditory abnormalities. It is essentially a disorder of melanocyte-containing organs, and occurs more frequently in individuals with darker skins. It is more common in females and usually presents in children or young adults.

Behçet's syndrome commonly presents with oro-genital ulceration, arthritis and headache (Chapter 26) but about one-third of cases have predominantly high-frequency cochlear hearing loss and vestibular involvement.

Susac's syndrome is a rare micro-angiopathy resulting in encephalopathy, retinopathy and hearing loss, and is assumed to have an autoimmune basis (Chapters 5 and 26). It occurs mainly in young adult women and has an acute or subacute presentation. Low frequency, unilateral or bilateral sensorineural hearing loss is often the presenting feature, associated usually with tinnitus and vestibular disturbance. The encephalopathy causes prominent headache, personality change, paranoia, confusion and cognitive impairment.

Other autoimmune conditions associated with deafness include systemic lupus erythematosus (SLE), ulcerative colitis, scleroderma, polyarteritis nodosa, Sjögren's syndrome, giant cell arteritis and Wegener's granulomatosis. Treatment is of the underlying condition.

Retro-cochlear hearing disorders

Retro-cochlear hearing loss is either genetic, acquired congenitally or postnatally (Tables 15.13 and 15.14). In addition to genetic cochlear dysfunction, a small number of children have isolated autosomal recessive auditory neuropathy related to mutations of the otoferlin gene. Mutations in *12SrRna* gene are also associated with auditory neuropathy.

Table 15.11 Inheritance, predominant features, auditory and vestibular abnormalities and CNS findings in syndromes associated with hearing loss.

Syndrome	Mode of inheritance	Predominant features	Auditory and vestibular features	CNS status
Treacher–Collins	AD	Mandibulofacial dysostasis	Severe dysplasia middle and internal ear (A + V)	N
Branchio-otorenal	AD	Branchial cysts/fistulae Structural ± functional renal abnormalities	Anomalies of external ear CHL 20%, SNHL 30%, mixed 50%	N
CHARGE	Occasional AD Rare AR Most sporadic	**C**oloboma, **h**eart defect, **a**tresia of choanae, **r**etarded growth and development, **g**enital hypoplasia, **e**ar anomalies	Structural labyrinth (A + V) dysplasia VIII nerve involvement Absent semicircular canals SNHL ± CHL	Impaired IQ and development
Usher's	AR	Retinitis pigmentosa	Type I: A + V failure Type II: A failure Type III: Variable	N
Alstrom's	AR	Pigmentary retinopathy Diabetes mellitus Obesity	SNHL	N
Apert's	Mainly sporadic. Some AD	Craniosynostosis + oral manifestations Brachydactyly	CHL ME anomalies	Frequent low IQ CNS manifestations
Crouzon's	AD	Craniosynostosis Shallow orbits Ocular proptosis	CHL ME anomalies	Generally N
Osteogenesis imperfecta	AD	Blue sclera Opalescent teeth Deformities of long bone and spine, Hyperextensibility	Type 1 Mild CHL >10 years of age Progressive mixed hearing loss	Generally N
Stickler's	AD	Flat midface and cleft palate High myopia and retinal detachment and cataracts Arthopathy Spondylo-epiphyseal dysplasia	Progressive SNHL	N
Wildervanck's	Sporadic	Fused cervical vertebrae Abducens palsy and retracted globe	SNHL, CHL or mixed in ~30%. Vestibular failure common	Usually N

(continued)

Table 15.11 (continued)

Syndrome	Mode of inheritance	Predominant features	Auditory and vestibular features	CNS status
Alport's	Usually X-linked dominant, rarely AR	Progressive glomerulonephritis Bilateral anterior lenticonus and macular flecks or peripheral coalescing flecks	Progressive SNHL in >10 years in approximately 50% of cases	Usually N
Jervell–Lange–Nielsen	AR	Prolonged Q-T interval Fainting spells/sudden death	Profound SNHL Scheibe anomaly	N
Pendred's	AR	Goitre	Mondini defect Dilated vestibular aqueduct Severe-profound SNHL Vestibular failure 30%	N
Mucopolysaccharidoses: Hurler's Hunter's	AR except Hunter's syndrome which is X-linked	Growth failure. Death <10 years Craniofacial dysmorphism Lysomal storage Excess excretion of dermatomes and heparin sulphates Severe form <ARR>→ death at 4–14 years Mild form <ARR>→ less severe than Hurler's syndrome	Progressive CHL Central auditory dysfunction Mixed HL in ~50%	Impaired IQ and development
Refsum's	AR	Retinitis pigmentosa HMSN (Cardiac enlargement/dysrhthymias Ichthyosis)	Progressive SNHL Vestibular function: normal	Anosmia Progressive weakness + sensory neuropathy, cerebellar signs
Down's	Trisomy 21	Short stature Dysmorphic facial features Hypotonia Single palmar crease Cardiac anomalies Delayed mental development	Abnormal external ear morphology CHL and/or SNHL in majority	Impaired IQ and development

A, auditory; AD, autosomal dominant; AR, autosomal recessive; CHL, conductive hearing loss; HL, hearing loss; ME, middle ear; SNHL, sensorineural hearing loss; V, vestibular.
Source: Luxon 2007. Reproduced with permission of Oxford University Press.

Table 15.12 Autoimmune syndromes associated with hearing loss.

Condition/ syndrome	Neuro-otologic syndrome	Associated findings	Epidemiology	Laboratory markers/diagnostic tests
Cogan's syndrome	'Ménière-like': attacks of vertigo, nausea, tinnitus, and hearing loss	Eye inflammation (keratitis, scleritis, conjunctivitis, uveitis, retinal vasculitis); systemic vasculitis in 10%	Young adults and older children (median 25 years)	Neutrophilia, raised ESR/CRP, MRI enhancement of vestibulocochlear structures
Wegener's granulomatosis	Usually conductive hearing loss; often have otitis media; SNHL reported, but usually as part of mixed picture	Rhinorrhoea and sinusitis; pulmonary, renal, joint manifestations; peripheral nervous system involvement	40–50 years; males and females equally affected	Raised ESR/CRP, raised ANCA (proteinase 3), granulomatous infiltration on MRI, biopsy
Polyarteritis nodosa	Rapid SNHL	Systemic vasculitis (kidney, gut); constitutional symptoms; mononeuritis multiplex	Male > female; older age of onset	Leukocytosis, raised ESR, visceral angiography, organ/nerve/muscle biopsy
Systemic lupus erythematosus	Subacute SNHL; often subclinical (NSAIDs and antimalarials may complicate picture – both may cause SNHL)	Skin, joint, renal, neuropsychiatric; constitutional symptoms	Female > male (5 : 1); age 15–40 years	Raised ESR, ANA, dsDNA antibodies, antiphospholipid antibodies, complement consumption
Sjögren's syndrome	Often subclinical	Dry eyes, dry mouth; Raynaud's and joint symptoms; neuropathies (axonal, sensory-ataxic, trigeminal)	Female > male	ANA, Ro, La, Schirmer's test, lip biopsy

ANA, antinuclear antibody; ANCA, antineutrophil cytoplasmic antibody; CRP, C-reactive protein; ESR, erythrocyte sedimentation rate; MRI, magnetic resonance imaging; NSAIDs, non-steroidal anti-inflammatory drugs; SNHL, sensorineural hearing loss.

Source: Overell 2004. Reproduced with permission of the BMJ.

Table 15.13 Genetic/congenitally acquired retro-cochlear hearing disorders.

Genetic	Non-syndromal	Non-syndromal recessive auditory neuropathy due to mutations in the otoferlin gene	
		Delayed maturation of auditory pathways in neonates	
Genetic	Syndromal	With peripheral neuropathy	Hereditary sensorimotor neuropathy, e.g. Roma (gypsy) families Friedreich's ataxia Neurofibromatosis type 2 Refsum's disease
Genetic	Syndromal	Without peripheral neuropathy	Arnold–Chiari Usher's syndrome Mitochondrial myopathies: MELAS Chronic progressive external ophthalmoplegia Mohr–Tranebjaerg's syndrome (deafness/ dystonia peptide) Skeletal syndromes: Branchio-otorenal Wildervanck's Bone dysplasias: Osteopetroses Hyperostosis cranialis Cammurati–Engelmann's disease Gaucher's
Congenital/toxic/metabolic			Perinatal risk factors: Asphyxia Respiratory distress syndrome Low birth weight Cerebral palsy Hyperbilirubinaemia Thalidomide

MELAS, mitochondrial encephalomyopathy, lactic acidosis and stroke-like episodes.

Charcot–Marie–Tooth disease

Domed-shaped sensorineural hearing loss occurs in Charcot–Marie–Tooth disease (Chapter 10) type 1a and hereditary neuropathy with liability to pressure palsies (HNPP). In the latter, half are thought to have the common PMP22 deletion, and half a PMP22 frameshift mutation. In HNPP cases, data suggest excessive presbyacusis.

Neurofibromatosis type 2

This autosomal dominant genetic disorder, associated with acoustic neuromas, commonly causes retro-cochlear hearing loss, as the presenting symptom. Neurofibromatosis type 2 (NF2) is 10 times less common than NF1 and occurs in 1/30 000–40 000 people. Mutations are found in the NF2 gene (neurofibromin 2; merlin), a tumour suppressor gene located on chromosome 22. Over 50% of NF2 cases are a result of new mutations. The clinical manifestations include peripheral neurocutaneous manifestations (café-au-lait spots and peripheral nerve neurofibromas), ocular abnormalities (juvenile posterior subcapsular lens opacity, retinal hamartomas and optic nerve sheath meningiomas) and both CNS and spinal tumours. CNS tumours include meningiomas (often multiple), vestibular schwannomas (acoustic neuromas), schwannomas in other locations, optic nerve gliomas, ependymomas and neurofibromas. Ninety per cent of NF2 patients have vestibular schwannomas, often bilateral; 50% develop meningiomas or other cranial nerve tumours, 40% develop spinal ependymomas or astrocytomas and 90% ocular manifestations, when examined in detail.

The type of genetic defect influences prognosis: nonsense or frameshift mutations generally cause severe disease, and missense mutations, in-frame deletions or large deletions cause milder disease. Severity varies in those with splice site mutations. The growth rate of VIIIth nerve tumours in NF2 is variable; for very slow growing tumours there is a case for non-operative management. However, the majority of patients with NF2 will develop severe deafness, and some will also become blind. Mean survival after diagnosis is some 15 years and the mean age of death in NF2 around 40 years.

Friedreich's ataxia

Friedreich's is the most common inherited ataxia (Chapter 17), and is frequently caused by a large expansion of an intronic GAA repeat, resulting in decreased expression of the gene product frataxin. The condition is usually inherited in an autosomal recessive pattern, and as frataxin is a mitochondrial protein, it suggests that dysfunction in Friedreich's ataxia is caused by a mitochondrial abnormality. Hearing impairment is an associated but unusual feature.

Refsum's disease

Refsum's disease (Chapter 19) is characterised by defective peroxisomal alpha oxidation of phytanic acid, with clinical features of retinitis pigmentosa, polyneuropathy, anosmia and hearing loss. Adult Refsum's disease is a recessive disorder of the phytanoyl CoA hydroxylase, *PAHX* gene on chromosome 10p30. Although hearing loss in Refsum's disease is common, only a few detailed assessments

Table 15.14 Acquired retro-cochlear hearing disorders.

Acquired infection	Viral	Herpes zoster/herpes simplex: Ramsay-Hunt syndrome Bell's palsy CMV, varicella, mumps
		HIV/AIDS
	Bacterial Fungal/protozoan Spirochaetal	Basal meningitis Pneumococcal Meningococcal Haemophilus Tuberculosis Cryptococcosis Coccidiomycosis
		Toxoplasmosis
		Syphilis, borrelia
Immune-mediated	Post-infective	Guillain–Barré
	Vasculitic/granulomatous	SLE, rheumatoid, sarcoid, Behçet's syndrome
Demyelination	Multiple sclerosis VIIIth nerve Brainstem	
Neoplasia/neoplasia related	Vestibular schwannoma Meningioma Cerebellopontine angle lesions Carcinomatosis Malignant meningitis Radiotherapy	
Metabolic/toxic	Uraemia Paget's disease Organic mercury Cisplatin Superficial siderosis	
Vascular	?Migraine Posterior inferior cerebellar artery syndrome Posterior fossa aneurysms AVM Vascular loops	

AVM, arteriovenous malformations; CMV, cytomegalovirus; SLE, systemic lupus erythematosus.

exist. One report demonstrates that seven of nine adults with Refsum's had a mild to moderate sensorineural hearing loss, predominantly of high-frequency type, and subtle auditory nerve involvement was identified in seven on the basis of ABR.

Mitochondrial disorders

Mitochondrial conditions have a propensity to cause sensorineural hearing loss (Table 15.15). Kearns–Sayre syndrome and MELAS (mitochondrial encephalomyopathy, lactic acidosis and stroke-like episodes) cases tend to have progressive hearing loss of both cochlear and retro-cochlear origin. No correlation between the type and severity of hearing loss and number or severity of other clinical neurological findings is found. In one study of adult patients with 3243A < G mutation, 13 of 16 had a sensorineural hearing loss that was progressive, and both this feature and the severity were correlated with the mutation heteroplasmy in muscle at entry and at end of follow-up. Sensorineural deafness is also a feature of MERRF (myoclonic epilepsy with ragged red fibres) as well as the other less common syndromes (Chapter 10).

Inherited muscle disorders

Inherited muscle disorders can be associated with hearing loss, including facioscapulohumeral dystrophy and myotonic dystrophy. In this latter condition, the hearing loss is reported to resemble 'precocious presbyacusis', or an excessive high-frequency hearing loss characteristic of presbyacusis, and genetic anticipation.

Acquired retro-cochlear hearing disorders (Table 15.14)

Infections Bacterial, viral and mycotic infections may give rise to hearing impairment by direct invasion, blood-borne transmission or via CSF.

Viral infections Sudden sensorineural hearing loss in adults is often presumed to be viral in origin. The Ramsay-Hunt syndrome is characterised by facial palsy, hearing loss, and characteristic herpetic vesicles around the pinna and in the external auditory meatus. Sensorineural hearing loss occurs in half to two-thirds of cases and is the result of cochlear or retro-cochlear involvement.

Table 15.15 Clinical features of mitochondrial syndromes associated with deafness.

Condition/ syndrome	Neuro-otological syndrome	Main clinical features	Additional features	Epidemiology	Laboratory markers
MELAS	Cochlear origin; symmetric gradual onset SNHL	Encephalopathy (seizures ± dementia); stroke-like episodes; mitochondrial myopathy	Short stature; normal early psychomotor development; recurrent headache and vomiting	Usually first decade; sometimes 10–40 years	Ragged red fibres on muscle biopsy; increased lactate
MERRF	Symmetric gradual onset SNHL	Myoclonus; epilepsy; cerebellar syndrome; myopathy	Short stature; dementia; optic atrophy; cardiomyopathy; Wolff–Parkinson–White syndrome; peripheral neuropathy	Usually childhood onset, but may be adults	Ragged red fibres on muscle biopsy; increased lactate
KSS	Symmetric gradual onset SNHL	Retinitis pigmentosa; ophthalmoplegia	Cardiac conduction block; cerebellar syndrome; short stature; impaired intellect	Onset <20 years; majority are sporadic	Ragged red fibres on muscle biopsy; increased lactate, raised CSF protein

CSF, cerebrospinal fluid; KSS, Kearns–Sayre syndrome; MELAS, mitochondrial encephalomyopathy, lactic acidosis and stroke-like episodes; MERRF, myoclonic epilepsy with ragged red fibres; SNHL, sensorineural hearing loss.
Source: Overell 2004. Reproduced with permission of the BMJ.

HIV/AIDS and syphilis A variety of auditory abnormalities have been reported in HIV infection, ranging from conductive to sensorineural hearing loss, with mild audiometric changes, abnormalities in ABR and central auditory dysfunction. A study of HIV revealed a prevalence of hearing impairment of 23%, which may may have been associated with opportunistic infections such as otosyphilis, cytomegalovirus or streptococcal meningitis, or treatment.

In otosyphilis, various presentations are seen, including sudden sensorineural hearing loss and a pattern suggestive of Ménière's disease. Importantly, this is one form of treatable hearing loss and this diagnosis should be sought in any unexplained case of sensorineural hearing loss, particularly in HIV-positive patients. Treatment of otosyphilis with penicillin and corticosteroids may improve tinnitus and vertigo in some cases.

Bacterial meningitis Sensorineural hearing loss in children during or following bacterial meningitis, including TB, is well known, with prevalence of 5–30%. There is little evidence that any single bacterial infection causes greater loss of hearing, either in frequency or degree. Treatment with antibiotics and adjuvant corticosteroids reduces fatalities and also lowers rates of severe hearing loss and other long-term neurological sequelae.

Lyme disease Lyme disease (*Borrelia burgdorferi* infection) causes a spreading erythematous rash on the trunk followed by meningoradiculitis and hearing loss. Elevated antibodies to *Borrelia* antigen have been found in 17% of 98 subjects with a unilateral sudden or fluctuating sensorineural hearing loss. Treatment with intravenous penicillin results in improvement of high-frequency hearing loss in some cases.

Extrinsic and intrinsic tumours of the cerebellopontine angle

Cerebellopontine angle (CPA) tumours (cerebellar medulloblastoma, vestibular schwannoma, meningioma, cholesteatoma, ependymoma, glomus jugulare tumour and metastasis) present commonly with retro-cochlear hearing loss and are diagnosed by MRI. Malignant meningitis and paraneoplastic syndromes can also present with hearing loss (Chapter 21).

Vestibular schwannoma The prevalence of vestibular schwannoma is about 1/100 000 persons, with a peak incidence in the fifth and sixth decades. Vestibular schwannomas account for 10% of intracranial tumours, and more than 75% of CPA lesions. Ninety per cent of cases appear to develop spontaneously and tend to be unilateral, arising from the vestibular portion of the VIIIth cranial nerve just within the internal auditory canal. The earliest features are sensorineural hearing loss (50%), tinnitus (21%), dizziness (9%) and rotary vertigo (5%). Later symptoms resulting from compression of adjacent structures include ipsilateral facial weakness, ipsilateral facial sensory loss, ataxia, headache, vomiting and signs of raised intracranial pressure (Chapters 13 and 21).

Although most of these tumours arise on the superior division of the vestibular nerve, the most common presenting features are deafness and tinnitus. In all patients with unilateral sensorineural hearing impairment, asymmetric bilateral sensorineural loss or unilateral tinnitus, it is essential to exclude a small vestibular schwannoma by detailed MRI.

Multiple sclerosis

About 5–10% of patients with MS experience significant hearing loss, but subtle hearing loss is more common. MS plaques have been identified in the VIIIth nerve root entry zone, cochlear nucleus and in the pons. Sudden hearing loss in MS is rare but typically improves. An ABR abnormality provides clinical evidence of a brainstem lesion in over 75% of cases of MS, but in over half of those there is an absence of clinical brainstem signs.

Sarcoidosis

Bilateral deafness is a feature of neurosarcoidosis (Chapter 26), which can present with cranial nerve dysfunction, typically bilateral facial nerve lesions, including the auditory nerve in about 5% of cases. The deafness is usually of VIIIth nerve origin, although cases are described of granulomatous processes causing necrosis of the incus and encasing the chorda tympani. Treatment of the deafness is with conventional immunosuppressive agents; there is one case report of effectiveness of infliximab.

Vascular disease

Stroke, both haemorrhagic and ischaemic, can cause hearing disorders at many levels within the brain, although these are rare. Cavernomas in the brainstem can sometimes cause deafness, either by small haemorrhages or increase in size. Aneurysms of the anterior inferior cerebellar artery (AICA) constitute less than 1% of all intracranial aneurysms with those of the distal portion (d-AICA) accounting for less than 0.1%. Because of the proximity of the d-AICA to the CPA and the VII–VIIIth nerve complex, aneurysms can mimic vestibular schwannoma, with auditory symptoms – tinnitus and hearing loss. Neuro-otological features related to AICA aneurysms depend on the arterial segment involved, and the relation to the CPA and IAM. Mechanisms include brainstem compression, rupture and post-embolisation infarction.

Posterior circulation ischaemia Sudden deafness occurs following inferior collicular infarction, vertebral artery dissection, infarction of the anterior–inferior cerebellar artery and, rarely, migraine. In one study, 8% of 364 cases of vertebro-basilar insufficiency demonstrated sensorineural hearing loss, the majority being unilateral. Vertigo was associated with hearing loss in most cases. Approximately 50% showed a cochlear type of hearing loss, with approximately half improving over 1 year.

Pontine vascular lesions typically have the greatest effect on hearing. Two overlapping syndromes are recognised: inferior pontine and lateral pontine. Both comprise ipsilateral facial palsy, hearing loss, loss of taste in the anterior two-thirds of the tongue with loss of lateral conjugate gaze. In the lateral pontine syndrome there is also facial sensory loss.

Vascular loops There is no definitive evidence to conclude that vascular loops compress the VIIIth nerve, to produce vestibular or auditory symptoms.

Superficial siderosis

Superficial siderosis is an insidious, progressive, rare disorder (Chapter 17). Symptoms include sensorineural deafness (95%), cerebellar ataxia (88%) and pyramidal signs (76%), dementia (24%), bladder disturbance (24%), anosmia (in >17%), aniscoria (>10%) and sensory signs (13%). Clinical features appear to be caused by chronic subarachnoid haemorrhage from a dural arteriovenous malformation or fistula, dural cyst, other dural pathology, vascular tumour or unknown source. If untreated, the condition results in severe disability and premature death. Diagnosis is confirmed by CSF examination, which shows various breakdown products of haemoglobin, and by MRI, which shows a prominent black rim around posterior fossa structures and sulci on T2 imaging. Treatment is identification and ablation of the source of bleeding, if this is possible.

Auditory processing disorders

Auditory processing disorders (APD) can manifest in both children and adults with difficulties with word recognition, environmental sounds or music and with uncertainty about what an individual hears, despite the presence of normal hearing thresholds. Patients may experience difficulties listening in a background of noise or with people conversing, difficulties in understanding degraded or rapid speech, following oral instructions, localising sounds or with the perception of music. They may also have language and other disorders, professional and academic problems and behavioural, emotional, social and other difficulties.

A detailed history of the auditory complaints is vital. First, this is so because patients may deny the presence of hearing complaints, unless questioned in detail – they do not always attribute difficulties to hearing problems. Secondly, features of auditory complaints may help define the diagnosis (e.g. in cases of cortical deafness), in which the patient has abnormal hearing thresholds because of bilateral auditory cortex lesions, and in auditory agnosias, of speech, music and environmental sounds, which may isolated or in combination. Thirdly, identification of specific auditory complaints (e.g. specific pitch difficulties or music-related problems) guides the choice of tests and provides some clues to the site of the lesion.

Aetiology of APD

There are no robust epidemiological data. However, APD is believed to affect 7% of children and prevalence may be even higher in adults. Disordered auditory processing may occur in the presence of the following:

- Genetic causes. These include syndromes that affect brain structure or make the brain more susceptible to damage. The genetic basis of these auditory processing deficits observed with other developmental disorders remains unclear.
- Neurological conditions such as tumours, stroke and MS.
- Auditory deprivation (e.g. following otitis media with effusion or other type of peripheral hearing loss).
- In the presence of other higher order disorders such as attention deficit disorder, dyslexia, specific language impairment – although in these cases no causal link has been established.
- Age-related changes of the central auditory system, distinct from age-related cochlear hearing loss or cognitive decline.
- Some forms of tinnitus and musical hallucinations, attributed to abnormal activity of the auditory brain may be examples of 'positive' disorders of auditory processing.

The following examples illustrate well-recognised presentations of these pathologies. Recent work with insular stroke cases has demonstrated more subtle defects of central processing.

Cortical hearing impairment

Cortical hearing loss is rare, but is most commonly associated with vascular disease or trauma affecting both temporal lobes. Additional and more dramatic neurological sequelae, including hemiparesis and dysphasia, are the rule. The primary auditory cortex lies in the anterior–posterior transverse temporal gyrus of Heschl. Each ear has bilateral representation in the auditory cortex, and thus it is possible to remove the non-dominant hemisphere in humans without significant effect on either the pure-tone audiogram or the discrimination of distorted speech.

In some cases, the primary auditory deficit predominates, and these cases are described as true cortical deafness. In this situation, a patient may present with no subjective experience of hearing, and demonstrate profound hearing loss on pure-tone audiometry. This may be misdiagnosed as peripheral if electroacoustic and electrophysiological testing are not conducted. For example, oto-acoustic emissions and ABR will demonstrate normal peripheral auditory function. However, abnormal central auditory function will be identified by the later auditory evoked potentials, specifically the middle latency response N1 and P2 waves.

Auditory agnosia

Auditory agnosia was defined originally as a selective disorder of sound recognition: 'I can hear you talking, but I cannot translate it.' This group can be further subdivided into several different clinical presentations: those who are unable to recognise a particular type of sound (e.g. speech, music or particular environmental noises, such as a dog barking), and those who are unable to discriminate at all between verbal and non-verbal sounds. Most cases correspond to the wider definition with impairment of all modalities of auditory function. Nonetheless, there are also cases of verbal auditory agnosia ('word deafness') in which speech perception is severely impaired, while recognition of non-verbal material such as musical tunes embedded within environmental noise remains intact.

Interhemispheric lesions

Patients with surgical section of the posterior corpus callosum demonstrate a typical pattern of auditory processing test results termed the Auditory Disconnection Profile. Characteristically, they have normal performance on monaural low-redundancy speech tests, left ear deficits on dichotic speech tests and bilateral deficits on temporal pattern testing.

Management of auditory disorders

Management of hearing impairment includes:

- Prevention to ensure protection from noise hazards, and avoidance of ototoxic drugs
- Medical management of systemic medical conditions that may be causing or exacerbating auditory dysfunction
- Auditory rehabilitation – a problem-solving exercise centred on each individual patient
- Hearing aids.

Many cases of cochlear hearing impairment are helped by hearing aids, but additional impairments such as arthritis or cerebellar dysfunction confound the fitting process. Importantly, provision of a hearing aid is only effective when the patient wishes to pursue this line of management, rather than it being the suggestion of well-meaning family members or others. The value of environmental aids and instruction in communication skills also helps long-term rehabilitation.

Hearing aids

Hearing aids have a pivotal role in audiological rehabilitation; precise details of their prescription is outside the scope of this chapter. Conventional aids may be body-worn, head-worn by mounting in spectacles, or mounted in or around the ear. The major advantage of body-worn aids is the very high gain and maximum output achieved, whereas the disadvantage is the obvious and unsightly nature of the device, and the poor microphone placement. Post-aural, in-the-ear or in-the-canal hearing aids are often highly effective, but some patients will require additional environmental aids (e.g. amplification systems attached to TVs or telephones, alerting warning devices, such as flashing lights connected to a door bell or an alarm clock).

The need for counselling of hearing-impaired people and their relatives or carers cannot be overemphasised. Simple tactics such as ensuring that light is always on the speaker's face, with the better ear tilted towards the speaker, and minimising background noise can really help communication. Psychological support should always be considered, and social and occupational support offered.

Conductive hearing loss

Any obstruction to the transmission of sound through the external ear by a foreign body, wax, polyp, tumour or infection must be corrected. Acute otitis externa requires suction clearance under microscopy, culture and sensitivity of the organism, and appropriate medication, with or without steroids. Acute otitis media requires pain relief, re-establishment of Eustachian tube function using nasal drops, inhalations or decongestants, mucolytics and systemic antibiotics: amoxicillin is the usual drug of choice. Vaccines have been introduced against *Streptococcus pneumoniae, Neisseria catarrhalis*, respiratory syncytial virus, adenovirus, influenza A and parainfluenza viruses. Chronic suppurative otitis media requires antibiotics to eliminate infection, followed by surgical repair of a perforated ear drum or damage to the ossicles; this helps prevent reinfection and improve sound transmission.

Conductive hearing loss caused by otosclerosis or hereditary osseous dysplasias may be managed conservatively using hearing aids, or surgically by stapedectomy. The procedure carries a small risk of complication of late sudden sensorineural hearing loss, and for this reason stapedectomy is not generally undertaken on both ears. Congenital malformations of the auditory canal and the middle ear may be treated conservatively with bone conduction or bone-anchored hearing aids or may be surgically remediable.

Sensorineural hearing loss

The management of sudden sensorineural hearing loss is a medical emergency requiring hospital admission, bed rest and investigation of possible causes. In the case of bilateral hearing loss, psychological and aggressive auditory rehabilitation are required. There is no universally evidence-based treatment, and a spontaneous recovery rate of approximately 65% is usual. Proposed therapies include inhalation of carbogen (CO_2–oxygen mixtures), hyperbaric oxygen, antiviral treatment, immunosuppression, calcium-channel blockers, steroids, blood volume expanders and various combinations of these different treatment strategies. Randomised controlled studies have demonstrated the efficacy of systemic steroids, but follow-up has questioned their benefit. Steroid therapy is often contraindicated in the presence of bacterial infection, recent surgery, peptic ulceration, a history of TB, poorly controlled hypertension or diabetes.

The management of progressive hearing impairment depends on the underlying aetiology. Syphilitic labyrinthitis is treated with steroids and penicillin, while rapidly expanding CPA tumours are surgically removed or treated with laser therapy. In the majority of cases of small tumours, however, a 'watch, wait and monitor' policy is effective. Immune-mediated sensorineural hearing loss requires urgent management with steroids and/or immunosuppressives following diagnosis. The treatment of Ménière's disease remains empirical. Therapies can be divided into medical regimes, including dietary modifications, drugs (diuretics, vestibular sedatives, drugs aimed at improving the circulation of the inner ear and immunosuppressives), psychological support, physiotherapy and auditory rehabilitation. A recent low-pressure pulse generator (Meniett device) has been advocated as a non-invasive effective treatment for Ménière's disease, but there is no definite evidence of efficacy. Conventional surgical treatment is considered when medical management has failed to control vertigo. Chemical labyrinthectomy using intra-tympanic gentamicin has superceded surgical interventions as a method of controlling severe vestibular symptoms, although no clear treatment protocol has been established and cochleo-toxicity is a significant risk. Chronic symptoms of dizziness resulting from vestibular dysfunction and hearing impairment may be treated with auditory and vestibular rehabilitation.

Chronic sensorineural hearing impairment is managed by appropriate treatment of any relevant medical condition and audiological rehabilitation of residual hearing. The selection and fitting of hearing aids is the key element of rehabilitation for the majority of patients with hearing impairment, but in the last two decades implantable devices have revolutionised auditory rehabilitation. Middle ear implants (vibrators on one of the ossicles or on the tympanic membrane) may be used with all types of hearing loss, although their value is not yet clearly defined. Cochlear implants, in one or both ears, are widely used in profound hearing impairment (e.g. congenital loss or secondary to meningitis, superficial siderosis, mitochondrial disease and head trauma). As with all hearing aid provision, the patient requires long-term auditory training within a specialised multi-disciplinary team following implantation.

VIIIth nerve disorders

Patients whose test results fulfil the criteria for auditory neuropathy represent a heterogeneous group in whom degraded speech perception inconsistent with pure tone sensitivity remains the common feature. Management strategies will be determined by the age of the patient.

Amplification and rehabilitation strategies

Early language intervention For children with auditory neural dyssynchrony (AN), the onsets of plosive consonants and transitions – which make speech intelligible – are lost, preventing these children from categorising or sequencing sounds. A phoneme-based language therapy known as cued speech is used. This is a method whereby cues to vowel and consonant sounds that are difficult to perceive from lip-reading, can be given by synchronous handshapes presented alongside either the mouth or pharynx of the speaker. These cues will give syntax and phonological structure to language and are more easily learned by parents.

Hearing aids Various studies have examined the benefits of hearing aids, and shown variable results. The main concern regarding the use of hearing aids in patients with AN is that they can cause significant noise exposure and permanent threshold shift (up to as much as 20 dBHL). The use of an algorithmic approach to hearing aid fitting and real ear measures to verify parameters of the hearing aid needs to be calculated in much the same way as for the risk–benefit analysis for children with sensorineural hearing loss.

Gap detection and modulation transfer function are abnormal in patients with AN, and a speech-processing type of hearing aid with a high-frequency emphasis to enhance high-frequency transient speech sounds (i.e. consonants) has been recommended. Also, the use of directional microphones and personal FM systems to improve the signal : noise ratio in those patients with pronounced difficulties with speech in background noise has been proposed.

Use of cochlear implants Studies are now being published as to the benefit of cochlear implantation. Studies report small numbers only in children, all of whom had undergone a trial period of powerful behind-the-ear aid use. Neural response telemetry (NRT) is used to assess neural synchrony and temporal coding post-cochlear implant. The presence of the electrically evoked compound action potential (ECAP) is interpreted as indicating that electrical stimulation has restored some degree of synchrony and temporal encoding at the level of the cochlear nerve. Generally, authors conclude that cochlear implantation should be performed only after a trial of conventional amplification and that each decision to implant must be based on the individual circumstances. Auditory brainstem implants have been used in profoundly deaf patients in whom there is complete dysfunction of the VIIIth nerve (e.g. in NF2).

Auditory processing disorders

Intervention for APD is multidisciplinary. Test results help to determine appropriate strategies for each patient. Intervention strategies include environmental modifications, signal enhancement, speaker adaptations, auditory training and compensatory strategies. While there is some evidence to suggest that these manoeuvres help, there are no robust trials to support them. Management is currently based on clinical judgement, and there is much individual variation between units. APD is an expanding field, and there is need for systematic, validated tests, and for studies to assess efficacy of interventions.

Environmental modifications

Noise and sound reflections from surfaces within a room distort and degrade acoustic signals. A noise survey of the acoustic environment (e.g. the classroom) may help determine first whether it adheres to UK building regulations that define the upper limit of noise and, secondly, identify potential corrective measures, such as carpets, curtains, acoustic panelling and sealing of doors and windows.

Signal enhancement strategies

Personal or soundfield FM systems are devices that receive and amplify speech, via a microphone/transmitter, both worn by the speaker. The amplified signal is then transmitted via FM wireless waves to loudspeakers (soundfield) or a special receiver (personal system) that the listener wears in or over the ears. These systems help counteract background noise, sound reflections and loss of acoustic energy over distance.

Relatives and carers: speaker-based adaptations

Speakers (i.e. those in contact with the patient) should be taught how to deliver speech at a slightly slower pace than normal, segment speech and stress different speech segments in order to enhance a message. In addition, rephrasing rather than repetition, and use of visual or other cues may be of help.

Auditory training programmes and compensatory strategies

Auditory training can help in both auditory and non-auditory performance, such as language and reading, and may actually modify cortical neural representation. Informal auditory training does not require technical resources; activities are chosen from the patient's complaints and test results. Patients can perform these programmes unaided or with help of a therapist. Auditory training tasks can be in computer game format, with adaptive procedures (i.e. tasks become more difficult as the listener improves). Examples of computer-based auditory programmes include:

- Earobics (www.earobics.com)
- FastForWord (www.scilearn.com)
- Phonomena (www.mindweavers.co.uk)
- Brain Fitness for older adults (www.positscience.com).

The Brain Fitness programme consists of six adaptive exercises that aim to enhance fidelity in auditory sensory input and language representations during hour-long sessions, 5 days/week over 8 weeks. One study of patients >60 years showed that those who completed the programme improved significantly in trained tasks and in auditory memory and that improvement was maintained for 3 months. Compensatory strategies include active listening, auditory vigilance training, auditory memory enhancement, metacognitive, linguistic, metalinguistic and other strategies.

References

American Speech-Language-Hearing Association. Central auditory processing: current status and implications for clinical practice. *Am J Audiol* 1996; **5:** 41–54.

Bertholon P, Tringali S, Faye MB, Antoine JC, Martin C. Prospective study of positional nystagmus in 100 consecutive patients. *Ann Otol Rhinol Laryngol* 2006; **115:** 587–594.

Halmagyi GM, Curthoys IS. A clinical sign of canal paresis. *Arch Neurol* 1988; **45**: 737–739.
Herdman S, Tusa R, Zee DS, *et al.* Single treatment approaches of benign paroxysmal positional vertigo. *Arch Otolaryngol Head Neck Surg* 1994; **104**: 450–454.
Honrubia V, *et al.* Benign positional vertigo syndrome. *N Engl J Med* 1999; **18**: 1590–1596.
Korres S, Balatsouras DG, Kaberos A, Economou C, Kandiloros D, Ferekidis E. Occurrence of semicircular canal involvement in benign paroxysmal positional vertigo. *Otol Neurotol* 2002; **23**: 926–932.
Lempert T, Neuhauser H, Daroff RB. Vertigo as a symptom of migraine. *Ann N Y Acad Sci* 2009; **1164**: 242–251.
Nakayama M, Epley JL. BPPV and variants: improved treatment results with automated, nystagmus-based repositioning. *Otolaryngol Head Neck Surg* 2005; **133**: 107–112.
Neuhauser H, Leopold M, von Brevern M, Arnold G, Lempert T. The interrelations of migraine, vertigo, and migrainous vertigo. *Neurology* 2001; **56**: 436–441.

Further reading

Agrup C, Luxon LM. Immune-mediated inner-ear disorders in neuro-otology. *Curr Opin Neurol* 2006; **19**: 26–32.
American Academy of Otolaryngology and Head and Neck Surgery Committee of Hearing and Equilibrium. Guidelines for the diagnosis and evaluation of therapy in Ménière's disease. *Otolaryngol Head Neck Surg* 1995; **113**: 181–185.
Baloh RW, Halmagyi GM, eds. *Disorders of the Vestibular System*. New York: Oxford University Press, 1996.
Baloh RW, Honrubia V, eds. *Clinical Neurophysiology of the Vestibular System*, 3rd edn. Philadelphia: Davis, 2001.
Bamiou D, Luxon LM. Vertigo: clinical management and rehabilitation. In: Gleeson M, Jones NS, Clarke R, Luxon L, Hibbert J, Watkinson J, eds. *Scott-Brown's Otolaryngology*, 7th edn. London: Hodder, 2008.
Bamiou DE, Musiek FE, Luxon LM. Aetiology and clinical presentations of auditory processing disorders: a review. *Arch Dis Child* 2001; **85**: 361–365.
Bertholon P, Bronstein AM, Davies RA, Rudge P, Thilo KV. Positional down beating nystagmus in 50 patients: cerebellar disorders and possible anterior semicircular canalithiasis. *J Neurol Neurosurg Psychiatry* 2002; **72**: 366–372.
Bottrill I, Wills A, Mitchell AL. Intratympanic gentamicin for unilateral Ménière's disease: results of therapy. *Clin Otolaryngol Allied Sci* 2003; **28**: 133–141.
Bovo R, Aimoni C, Martini A. Immune-mediated inner ear disease. *Acta Otolaryngol* 2006; **126**: 1012–1021.
Brandt T. *Vertigo: Its Multi-sensory Syndromes*, 2nd edn. London: Springer Verlag, 1999.
Brandt T, Steddin S. Current view of the mechanism of benign paroxysmal positioning vertigo: cupulolithiasis or canalothiasis? *J Vestib Res* 1993; **3**: 373–382.
Brandt T, Steddin S, Daroff RB. Therapy for benign paroxysmal positioning vertigo (BPPV). *J Vestib Res* 1993; **3**: 373–382.
Bronstein A, Lempert T. *Dizziness: A Practical Approach to Diagnosis and Management*. Cambridge: Cambridge University Press, 2007.
Ceranic BJ, Prasher DK, Raglan E, Luxon LM. Tinnitus after head injury: evidence from otoacoustic emissions. *J Neurol Neurosurg Psychiatry* 1998; **65**: 523–529.
Davies R. Bedside neuro-otological examination and interpretation of commonly used investigations. *J Neurol Neurosurg Psychiatry* 2004; 75:iv32–iv44. doi:10.1136/jnnp.2004.054478.
Davies RA. Clinical and audiometric assessment of hearing. In: Luxon LM, ed. *Textbook of Audiological Medicine*. London: Martin Dunitz, 2003.
Davies RA. The essentials of bedside neuro-otological examination and interpretation of commonly used investigations. Neurology in Practice Review. *J Neurol Neurosurg Psych* 2004; **75** (Suppl IV): 32–44.
Davies RA. Retrocochlear hearing disorders. In: Gleeson M, Jones NS, Clarke R, Luxon L, Hibbert J, Watkinson J, eds. *Scott-Brown's Otolaryngology*, 7th edn. London: Hodder, 2008.
Duane D. A neurologic perspective of central auditory dysfunction. In: Keith RW, ed. *Central Auditory Dysfunction*. New York: Grune and Stratton, 1977.
Epley JM. The canalith repositioning procedure: for treatment of benign paroxysmal positional vertigo. *Otolaryngol Head Neck Surg* 1992; **107**: 399–404.
Froehling DA, Bowen JM, Mohr DN, *et al.* The canalith repositioning procedure for the treatment of benign paroxysmal positional vertigo: a randomized controlled trial. *Mayo Clin Proc* 2000; **75**: 695–700.
Furman JM, Balaban CD, Jacob RG, *et al.* Migraine-anxiety related dizziness (MARD): a new disorder? *J Neurol Neurosurg Psychiatry* 2005; **76**: 1–8.
Furman JM, Cass SP. *Vestibular Disorders: A Case-study Approach*, 2nd edn. New York: Oxford University Press, 2003.
Halmagyi GM. Diagnosis and management of vertigo. *Clin Med* 2005; **5**: 159–165.
Hood JD. Tests of vestibular dysfunction. In: Dix MR, Hood JD, eds. *Vertigo*. Chichester: John Wiley and Sons, 1984
Jacob RG, Furman JM, Cass SP. Psychiatric consequences of vestibular dysfunction. In: Luxon LM, Furman J, Martini A, Stephens SDG, eds. *A Textbook of Audiological Medicine: Clinical Aspects of Hearing and Balance*. London: Martin Dunitz, 2003.
James AL, Burton MJ. Betahistine for Ménière's disease or syndrome. *Cochrane Database Syst Rev* 2001; **1**: CD001873.
Kerber KA. The genetics of vertigo. *Semin Neurol* 2006; **26**: 484–491.
Lee H, Sohn S-I, Cho Y-W, Lee S-R, Ahn B-H, Park B-R, *et al.* Cerebellar infarction presenting as isolated vertigo: frequency and vascular topographical patterns. *Neurology* 2006; **67**: 1178–1183.
Leigh RJ, Zee DS. *The Neurology of Eye Movements*, 4th edn. New York: Oxford University Press, 2006.
Luxon LM. Disorders of hearing. In: Donaghy M, ed. *Brain's Diseases of the Nervous System*, 12th edn. Oxford: Oxford University Press, 2008.
Luxon LM. Methods of examination: audiological and vestibular. In: Ludman H, Mawson S, eds. *Edward Arnold's Diseases of the Ear*, 5th edn. Oxford: Oxford University Press, 1988.
Luxon LM. *Textbook of Audiological Medicine*. London: Martin Dunitz, 2003.
Luxon, LM. Vestibular compensation. In: Luxon LM, Davies RA, eds. *Handbook of Vestibular Rehabilitation*. London: Whurr, 1997.
Luxon LM, Bamiou DE. Vestibular system disorders. In: Schapira A, Byrne E, Silberstein S, Frackowiak R, Wszolek Z, DiMauro B, eds. *Neurology: Basic and Clinical Neurosciences*. Philadelphia: Elsevier, 2006.
Murdin L, Davies RA. Otoacoustic emission suppression testing: a clinician's window onto the auditory efferent pathway. *Audiological Med* 2008; **6**: 238–248.
Nance WE. The genetics of deafness. *Ment Retard Dev Disabil Res Rev* 2003; **9**: 109–119.
Neuhauser H, Radtke A, Von Brevern M, Lempert T. Zolmitriptan for treatment of migrainous vertigo: a pilot randomized placebo-controlled trial. *Neurology* 2003; **60**: 882–883.
Noback CR, Demarest RJ. *The Human Nervous System*, 3rd edn. New York: McGraw Hill, 1981.
Overell J, Lindhall AA. Neuro-otological syndromes for the neurologist. *J Neurol Neurosurg Psychiatry* 2004; **75** (Suppl. 4): 53–59.
Pavlou M, Lingeswaran A, Davies RA, *et al.* Simulator based rehabilitation in refractory dizziness. *J Neurol* 2004; **251**: 983–995.
Pavlou M, Bronstein A, Davies RA. Randomized trial of supervised versus unsupervised optokinetic exercise in persons with peripheral vestibular disorders. *Neurorehabil Neural Repair* 2012; **27**: 208–218.
Rudge P. *Clinical Neuro-otology*. Edinburgh: Churchill Livingstone, 1983.
Savundra P, Luxon LM. The physiology of equilibrium and its application to the dizzy patient. In: Scott-Brown WG. *Scott-Brown's Otolaryngology*, vols I–VI, 6th edn. Oxford: Butterworths, 1997.
Schubert MC, Tusa RJ, Grine LE, Herdman SJ. Optimizing the sensitivity of the head thrust test for identifying vestibular hypofunction. *Phys Ther* 2004; **84**: 151–158.
Shumway-Cook A, Horak FB. Rehabilitation strategies for patients with vestibular deficits. *Neurol Clin North Am* 1998; **8**: 441–457.
Starr A, Picton TW, Sininger Y, Hood LJ, Berlin CI. Auditory neuropathy. *Brain* 1996; **119**: 741–753.
Straube A. Pharmacology of vertigo/nystagmus/oscillopsia. *Curr Opin Neurol* 2005; **18**: 11–14.
Strupp M, Brandt T. Pharmacological advances in the treatment of neuro-otological and eye movement disorders. *Curr Opin Neurol* 2006; **19**: 33–40.
Thirlwall AS, Kundu S. Diuretics for Ménière's disease or syndrome. *Cochrane Database Syst Rev* 2006; **3**: CD003599.
Willems PJ. Genetic causes of hearing loss. *N Engl J Med* 2000; **342**: 1101–1109.
Zee D. The management of patients with vestibular disorders. In: Barber HO, Sharpe JA, eds. *Vestibular Disorders*. Chicago, IL: Year Book Medical, 1988: 254–274.

CHAPTER 16

Spinal Column and Spinal Cord Disorders

Simon Farmer and David Choi
National Hospital for Neurology & Neurosurgery

Clinicians involved in the diagnosis and management of spinal disease face formidable challenges. While advances in neuroimaging have provided great insight into the disordered anatomy that underlies many conditions especially those of interest to spinal surgeons there is still much to be learnt about the basic mechanisms of disordered development, the physiology and pathophysiology of spinal cord function along with the mechanisms of spinal repair and the most effective management strategies. In this chapter there is much of common interest with the sub-specialities of neuro-rehabilitation, neuro-inflammation, neuro-infection, neuro-genetics and neuro-muscular disorders.

Spinal surgery from the neurosurgical and orthopaedic perspectives is a rapidly developing field. Spinal disease is a multi-disciplinary subject with important contributions from neurologists, neurosurgeons, orthopaedic surgeons, rheumatologists, neuroradiologists, neurophysiologists, pain specialists, rehabilitationists and the multi-disciplinary team.

This chapter is broadly divided into four sections: (i) spinal embryology anatomy and physiology; (ii) diagnosis of spinal column and cord disorders; and (iii) specific diseases of the spinal column and spinal cord and (iv) their clinical management including medical and surgical approaches.

Spinal embryology, anatomy and physiology

Embryology of the spine

The adult spine is divided anatomically into the cranio-cervical junction, and the cervical, thoracic, lumbar and sacro-coccygeal spine. Developmental abnormalities may arise at each level. Interpretation of congenital and acquired anomalies of the vertebral column is aided by an understanding of normal development. In early fetal life the ectodermal germ layer gives rise to the primitive neural tube which, in turn, gives rise to the entire nervous system during primary neurulation. This normally closes by the end of the fourth intrauterine week; failure of this primary neurulation results in fusion defects such as anencephaly or spina bifida. By this time the primary brain vesicles are present, representing forebrain, midbrain and hindbrain. Mesoderm lies around the neural tube and by the end of the fifth intrauterine week will have completed segmentation into recognisable somite pairs (occipital to coccygeal). Once established, the epithelioid cells of these somites rapidly transform and migrate towards the notochord where they differentiate into three distinct cell lines: sclerotomes (from which connective tissue, cartilage and bone are derived), myotomes (providing segmental muscle) and dermatomes (providing segmental skin). Chondrification of the sclerotomes leads to the development of ossification centres, with an anterior and posterior centre for each vertebral body and a pair for each arch. The process is largely complete by the end of the third month of fetal development.

Disruption during these early stages accounts for many of the vertebral and cranio-cervical anomalies. After the third month of gestation the vertebral column and dura lengthen more rapidly than the spinal cord resulting in regression of the cord tip, leaving the filum terminale below. By term, the cord tip typically lies at the L2–3 interspace. Failure of distension of the brain vesicle results in abnormal brain cavities (including the ventricles) and may result from a failure of the central canal of the spinal cord to obliterate. Secondary neurulation arises in the distal sacral and coccygeal segments but does not produce functioning neural elements. Problems with secondary neurulation may give rise to lipomas of the filum terminale and tethering which prevents the normal ascent of the spinal cord during vertebral growth. Therefore, the conus medullaris continues to lie below its normal position at the L1–2 border.

The fetal spine can be reliably identified on ultrasound at 12 weeks and an accurate assessment of its integrity can be determined by 20 weeks.

Genetic control of spinal development

The notochord provides the template for spinal development although only remnants of it persist in the nucleus pulposus of the cartilaginous discs. The notochord orchestrates the production of numerous signalling molecules between it and the neural tube and somites, initiated by the production of the protein product of a notochord gene called 'Sonic Hedgehog'. Sonic Hedgehog induces differentiation in the ventral and lateral neural tube as well as sclerotome differentiation in the somites. Mesoderm around the neural tube segments into 44 somite pairs (4 occipital, 8 cervical, 12 thoracic, 5 lumbar, 5 sacral and 10 coccygeal) by the end of the fifth week. The segmentation process itself is complex. In the chick, mouse and human embryos segments are formed sequentially. The driver for presomitic mesoderm segmentation may involve an intrinsic

Neurology: A Queen Square Textbook, Second Edition. Edited by Charles Clarke, Robin Howard, Martin Rossor and Simon Shorvon.

molecular oscillator: 'the segmentation clock'. There is rhythmic production of mRNA from several genes related to the NOTCH gene-signalling pathway. In chick embryos, the periodicity is approximately 90 minutes with new somites being formed sequentially. The NOTCH-related genes include '*Lunatic Fringe (LFNG)*', *Delta-like (DLL)*, *Presenilin and Mesoderm Posterior 2 (MESP2;* Figure 16.1). Failure of oscillatory signalling may lead to failure of segmentation in a rostral–caudal direction where the first most caudal somites (whose ultimate fate is to be at vertebral level) are formed normally but then there is progressive loss of segmentation because of degradation of the molecular rhythmicity leading to anomalies of the most rostral vertebra. So far, mutations causing skeletal and spinal abnormality have been identified in the human homologues of three genes associated to the mouse segmentation clock: MESP2 and LFNG – associated with AR spondylocostal dysostosis II and DLL3 AR spondylocostal dysostosis 1 – also known as Jarcho–Levin syndrome.

While the NOTCH genes specify longitudinal segmentation of the developing spinal cord, another group of genes, the *Hox* (homeobox) family, specifies axial development including vertebral shape. In humans there are four families of *Hox* genes (*Hox A-D*) which are also expressed caudally to rostrally, but with differing rostral extents. A rostro-caudal signal is therefore created in the developing embryo, which specifies positional values to each spinal level. Abnormal expression can be demonstrated in transgenic mice, for example mutation of *Hox-b4* results in duplication of the atlas, such that a second atlas replaces the axis vertebra. *Hox* genes have been associated with human congenital anomaly (e.g. the hand-foot-genital syndrome). Often, large *Hox* mutations produce a severely disrupted body habitus incompatible with intrauterine life.

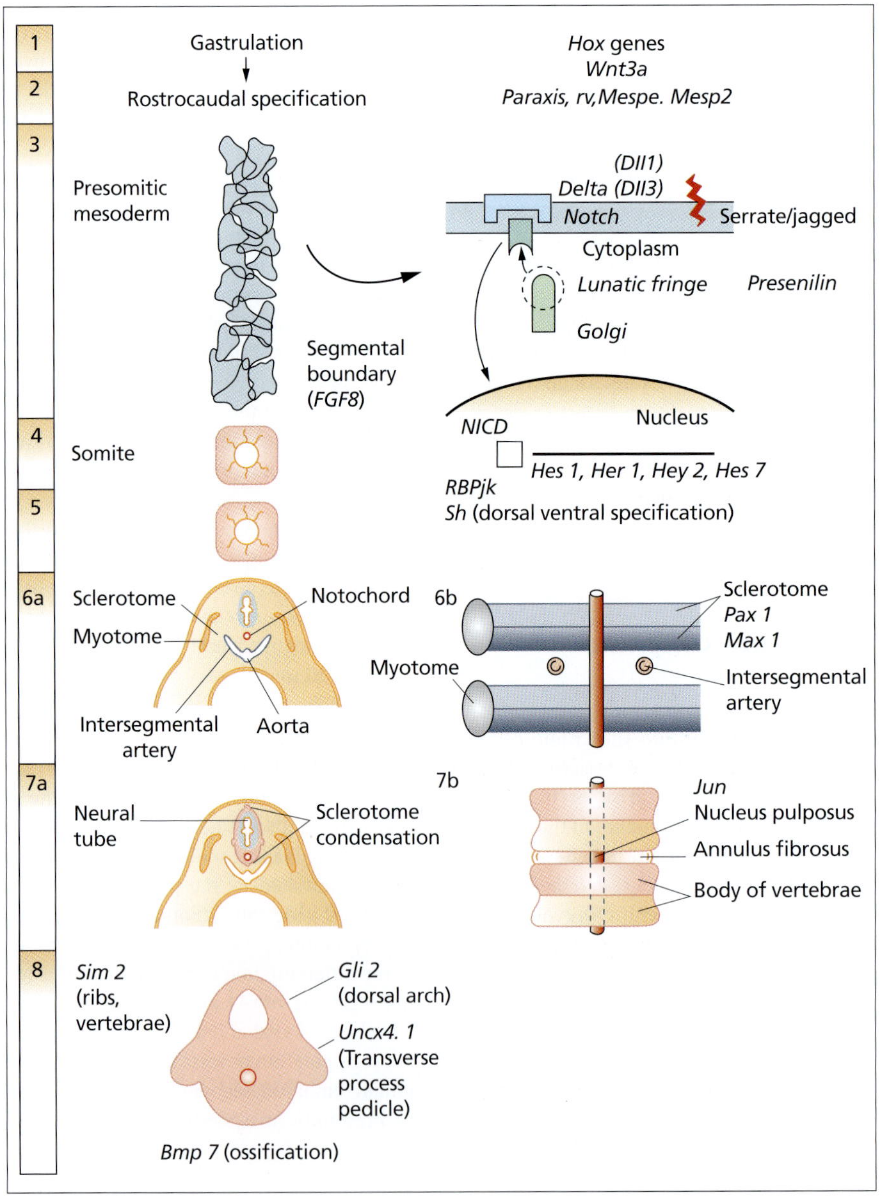

Figure 16.1 Possible steps in mouse spinal development with relevant genes (in text).

Identifying genetic mutations involved in spinal anomaly

Much of the research effort into understanding the genetics of spinal developmental anomaly involves the study of conservation of genes during evolution. Possibly only 200 chromosomal rearrangements have occurred in total because the mouse and human lineages diverged. This means that detailed study of the mouse genome may yield important homologues of human genetically determined spinal maldevelopment. Syntegy conservation may be used to identify fruitful areas of the mouse and human genome in which mutations may produce phenotypes recognisable in human developmental disorders. This allows the search for causative genetic mutations in human malformations to be narrowed. From analysis of mouse developmental abnormalities and comparison with homologous human malformations which include spinal malformation, the following genes have been identified: *Hox, Notch, Pax1, Mox1, Gli, Unex4.1, BMP-7* and *Jun*. Mutations in the *Pax1* gene have been associated with vertebral anomalies in humans.

A new technique of Cre-recombinase-mediated transgenesis mapping has been used to map the destinations of embyronic neural crest and mesodermal stem cells. This mapping has been resolved at the single cell level and it reveals that the boundaries traverse homogeneous skeleton of neck and shoulders. From this mapping it has been discovered that in vertebrates the neural crest anchors the head to the anterior shoulder girdle. Mesoderm, which is controlled by expression of a *Hox* gene, links trunk muscles to the posterior neck and shoulder skeleton. It has been suggested that muscle attachments may be a new way of defining homologous pieces of skeleton. The skeleton identified using the Cre-recombinase technique is abnormal in Klippel–Feil and Chiari malformations. This genetic mapping technique may greatly increase our understanding of head, neck and shoulder morphology; furthermore, it situates human, head, neck and shoulder anomalies in a context that reflects the known complexity of neck and shoulder evolution in vertebrate lineages (Figure 16.1). The genetics of complex skeletal and spinal deformity is beyond the scope of this chapter but is broad terms the syndromes are divided into those that affect bone and those that affect cartilage.

Anatomy and physiology of spinal maldevelopment

Disorders of axonal guidance

In this section of the chapter we discuss conditions that have yielded insight into spinal cord maldevelopment. Consideration of the details of Klippel–Feil syndrome, X-linked Kallmann syndrome and congenital hemiplegia pathophysiology has led to a wider appreciation of corticospinal tract development. While there are many tracts within the spinal cord, the normal development of which is crucial to function, much is known about the development and maldevelopment of the pyramidal tract and thus work in this area has led to an understanding of developmental anomalies.

The pyramidal tract develops late in humans: in the embryo the fibres have reached the pyramidal decussation by the eighth week post-fertilisation; however, the subsequent development is slow, with tract myelination continuing into the child's third year of life. Our understanding of human pyramidal tract development is highly dependent on data from rodents and subhuman primates. In rat, the corticospinal growth cone must navigate through the internal capsule, cerebral peduncle, pons and medulla to reach the spinal grey matter. At a number of points in the journey there are 'choice points' at which chemo-attractants and repellents can influence the journey. Mutations in genes coding for these molecules lead to gross developmental anomalies. The corticospinal tract reaches the cervical cord shortly after birth and then gradually extends to the lumbosacral regions. Initially, there are exuberant collaterals such that most parts of the cortex, including the occipital cortex, innervate the spinal cord. There is then a rapid withdrawal of collaterals and loss of fibres from the corticospinal tract. Whether this process is activity dependant is not fully known. Failure of pyramidal decussation occurs in a number of conditions including Klippel–Feil and X-linked Kallmann syndromes. In animal models, mutations in oligodendrite membrane-bound neurite growth inhibitors appear to lead to a loss of the normal channelling of myelinated fibres leading to abnormalities of growth; furthermore, a midline anchored repellent (ephrin-B3) prevents the cortico-spinal tract from recrossing into the ipsilateral spine.

In humans, malformations of the corticospinal tract may be caused by:

1 Induction failure, disruption during early spinal development (see Klippel–Feil syndrome)
2 Abnormal cell proliferation
3 Abnormal neural migration
4 Abnormal guidance mechanisms
5 Acquired injury.

In all of these cases there are abnormalities of the pyramidal tract, the pyramids and the pyramidal decussation with abnormal ipsilateral corticospinal pathways. Mirror movements are a common feature of a number of these conditions and have been described in all the categories of pyramidal tract malformation set out later. The characteristic neurophysiology described in detail for Klippel–Feil syndrome has been discovered also for X-linked Kallmann's syndrome, disorders of neural migration and prenatally acquired hemiplegia. In addition, ipsilateral transcranial magnetic brain stimulation (TMS) responses indicating an abnormal ipsilateral cortico-spinal tract have been described in patients with familial horizontal gaze palsy with progressive scoliosis (HGPPS). In these subjects, deletions in the *ROBO3* gene cause failure of pyramidal decussation. *L1CAM* disorders, which are associated with a variety of phenotypes including X-linked hydrocephalus, have also been studied using TMS and, surprisingly, given that in animal models a misdirected pyramidal tract in usually the result of *L1CAM* mutations, no TMS evidence of an abnormal ipsilateral pathway was detected in humans. However, in the only neurophysiological study to have been performed, subjects with *L1CAM* mutations were not studied in the ways set out above, instead the focus of the investigation was on proximal rather than distal upper limb muscles. Recently, congenital mirror movements have been found to be caused by mutations in the *DCC* gene.

Congenital mirror movements

These are intense involuntary movements, primarily of distal upper limb muscles, that mirror the voluntary unilateral movement. They cannot be suppressed and typically do not occur during passive movement. Mirror movements occur normally during a child's motor development; however, they are rarely intense and disappear by the age of 6years. Pathological mirror movements are rarely disabling and patients learn adaptive proximal movements so as to avoid inappropriate finger movements (e.g. wrong key strikes while typing). Neurophysiological study of mirror movements has provided striking insights into central motor control and aberrant neural pathways.

In the first study of its kind, a single subject with Klippel–Feil syndrome and mirror movements was found to have abnormal simultaneous bilateral short-latency responses to focal electrical stimulation of unilateral focal electrical stimulation or right primary motor cortex indicating that in the presence of an aberrant fast conducting ipsilateral corticospinal tract. In this subject the spinal (short) latency cutaneomuscular (CMR) and stretch reflexes are confined, as in normal subjects, to the stimulated side but the long-latency components of the CMR and stretch reflexes were found at equal latency in both the stimulated and non-stimulated limbs. Cross-correlation analysis of electromyographic (EMG) activity recorded simultaneously from homologous muscles of left and right hands reveals, in contrast to healthy subjects, the presence of a short duration peak at time zero indicating that during normal muscle contraction both hands receive abnormal common presynaptic drive. This abnormal drive can be shown to be highly muscle specific, indicating that abnormal bilateral corticospinal axons innervate the equivalent motor neurone. This result suggested that the abnormality is at the level of the pyramidal decussation with normal neuronal guidance mechanisms to the spinal motor neurone pools thereafter. Recent studies using EMG–EMG coherence analysis and EEG–EMG coherence analysis in subjects with X-linked Kallmann's syndrome with mirror movements have shown that aberrant corticospinal pathways provide abnormal oscillatory drive from cortex to muscle. Taken together, these findings indicate that voluntary and long-loop reflex activity in abnormal central motor pathways produces the mirror movements seen in Klippel–Feil syndrome and other neurodevelopmental conditions. Similar finding have been reported a number of other patient groups in which intense mirror movements are a feature (e.g. congenital hemiplegic cerebral palsy, X-linked Kallmann's syndrome, RBO3-HGPPS).

The findings in hemiplegic cerebral palsy are of particular interest for they indicate that the corticospinal axons reach both sides of the spinal cord from the undamaged motor cortex. The presence of mirror movements with characteristic neurophysiological findings is associated with MRI scans in which there is no gliosis in response to the cerebral injury, suggesting that antenatal insults before gestational age of 28 weeks causing hemiplegia are associated with very significant pyramidal tract reorganisation and mirror movements. This remarkable central nervous reorganisation may help to sustain function of the child's hemiplegic hand, albeit at the expense of mirror movements. Studies in the cat have shown that lesioning or even functional inactivation of one corticospinal tract at a time in development when there are naturally bilateral innervations of both sides of the spinal cord from both hemispheres induces abnormal persistence of ipsilateral corticospinal pathways suggesting that activity dependence is important for corticospinal function. These neurophysiologcal findings draw attention to early life syndromes of disordered axonal guidance and abnormal lesion induced corticospinal persistence.

Human vertebral segmentation defects

Numerous congenital defects of the spinal column have been identified that result from segmental disruption, for example Klippel–Feil syndrome, Alagille's syndrome, spondylocostal dysostosis (Jarcho–Levin syndrome), congenital scoliosis and kyphosis, Goldenhar's syndrome and the VATER (vertebro-anal-tracheo-esophageal-renal) and VACTERL (vertebral-anal-cardiac-tracheo-esophageal-renal-limb) syndromes. In many of these syndromes there are severe abnormalities affecting a number of body parts. The vertebral segmentation abnormalities may be generalised, regionalised or localised. The vertebral abnormalities (including wedge, hemi or butterfly vertebrae) that give rise to congenital scoliosis and kyphosis are likely to involve problems of somitogenesis. Two mutations in the Notch signalling pathway have been identified these are *Delta-like 3* in spondylocostal dysostosis and *Jag1* in Alagille's syndrome. Spondylocostal dysostosis is dominantly and recessively inherited with multiple segmentation abnormalities of vertebra, axial skeleton and ribs leading to a non-progressive kyphoscoliosis. Alagille's syndrome is a severe multi-organ disorder affecting the liver, heart, eyes, facial bones associated with vertebral segmentation defects. It is likely that Klippel–Feil syndrome results from a disorder either in *Notch* gene signalling or the *PAX* gene but as yet the genetic aetiology is unknown. Furthermore, the syndrome may also be caused by non-genetic errors of development (e.g. resulting from teratogens) and the long narrow shape of the unsegmented vertebral bodies might suggest a problem around the time of chondrification.

Split-cord malformations may occur during development, either anteriorly resulting from a split notochord, or posteriorly because of incomplete closure of the neural tube. A split notochord is likely to induce the development of split vertebral bodies, separated by invaginating gut endoderm or an accessory neuroenteric canal.

Abnormalities of the atlas and axis vertebrae probably also occur because of intrauterine trauma rather than abnormalities of genetic expression. Anterior and posterior spina bifida of the atlas occur in mucopolysaccharidoses and Down's syndrome where excessive movement at the stage of chondrification of the atlas probably results in an incomplete bony ring.

Diagnosis of spinal column and spinal cord disorders

Clinical assessment of spinal disorders

In this section the primary focus is on those symptoms and physical signs that are of particular value in helping the experienced clinician achieve an accurate and timely diagnosis and an assessment that allows a coherent plan of management to be formulated.

Craniocervical junction

Symptoms and signs may be insidious or rapid in onset. Clinical presentation is diverse depending on the level affected.

The lower brainstem, cranial nerves, cervical roots and upper cervical cord may be compromised by pressure from bone or soft tissue, there also may be indirect compromise of the blood supply. Congenital anomalies of the craniocervical junction are often associated with dysmorphic features and obvious skeletal anomalies. Patients most commonly complain of headache and neck pain worsened by movement and coughing. Pain characteristically originates in the suboccipital region and radiates to the vertex in a C2 distribution. Head tilt and 'torticollis' are more common in children, but may sometimes occur in adults. In children with cranio-cervical junction anomalies, hearing loss is the most common cranial nerve symptom. In adults, trigeminal distribution pain and neuralgia can result from direct compression of the Vth nerve or compression of the Vth nerve nuclei in the upper cervical cord. Lesions of other cranial nerves, particularly IX, X, XI and XII, are also seen. Spinal cord compression produces a myelopathic picture with upper motor neurone features, which may progress to involve bladder and bowel control. Occasionally, the myelopathy is confined to the upper limbs. There can be a predilection for the dorsal columns, producing marked joint position sense loss. Brainstem involvement produces dysphagia, dysarthria, internuclear ophthalmoplegia and nystagmus (most commonly horizontal but more classically down-beating). Central apnoea, vivid nightmares associated with sleep apnoea, drop attacks and syncope are important additional features. The intimate relationship of the vertebral arteries to the upper cervical spine and foramen magnum can increase the risk of vertebrobasilar ischaemia. Sequential 'clock-face' involvement of limbs may occur with neural compression at the foramen magnum: spastic weakness of the extremities with progression of motor symptoms, which may begin in the ipsilateral upper limb, followed by weakness of the ipsilateral lower limb, contralateral lower limb and progressing to the contralateral upper limb, caused by compression of the pyramidal decussations. Cruciate paralysis (bilateral upper limb weakness with relative sparing of the lower limbs) and dissociated sensory loss are often associated with pressure on the upper portion of the pyramidal tracts and an intramedullary process, respectively.

Syringobulbia and syringomyelia

Cavitation of the spinal cord sometimes extending into the brainstem is an association of cranio-cervical junction anomalies. The symptoms and physical signs reflect a pathology that starts centrally and expands outwards. The patient complains of painless injuries, muscle wasting and weakness and, more rarely, limb weakness. More unusual presentations, for instance central apnoea, also occur. The classic onion skin sensory loss of syringobulbia is caused by involvement of the spinal nucleus or the tract of the trigeminal nerve and may be associated with tongue wasting, trigeminal pain, palatal and laryngeal weakness and symptoms of medullary involvement. The cavity in syringomyelia affects crossing spinothalamic fibres producing a half-cape or cape loss of pain and temperature sensation; posterior column function is relatively preserved but abnormalities can occasionally be found. There is amyotrophy at the level of the cavity with tendon reflex loss. In advanced stages, neuropathic Charcot joints develop. Below the cavity there can be upper motor neurone symptoms and signs with disturbances of sphincter function, which contrast with the lower motor neurone symptoms and signs at the level of the syrinx.

Cervical spine

The presenting symptoms of cervical spine disease reflect the aetiology. As degenerative disease is the most common condition affecting the cervical spine, pain is the most frequent presenting symptom. The nature and distribution of the pain is a useful pointer to the site and nature of the pathology. In spondylotic disease, typically there is a dull ache in the neck worsened by movement. Spurling's sign is a reliable test of mechanical root compression (the examiner turns and flexes the patient's head to the affected side while applying downward pressure to the top of the patient's head). The sign is considered positive when the pain arising in the neck radiates in the direction of the corresponding dermatome ipsilaterally. The radicular component of the pain is often a dull ache with sharper exacerbations. Cough impulse pain may frequently accompany disc protrusion or prolapse. The symptoms and signs of weakness and numbness may localise a particular radicular level, but the spinal level of traditional dermatomes and myotomes may vary by a level up or down. Below the pathological level there may be upper motor neurone symptoms, signs and a spinal sensory level reflecting cord compression. The patient's complaints can often suggest cervical instability: 'My head feels loose' or 'I have to hold my head' and should not be discounted as an anxiety disorder. Lhermitte's symptoms resulting from posterior column compressions may also occur as a result of cervical instability. Hand weakness in high cervical cord compression may be caused by a combination of pyramidal tract compression and de-afferentation from dorsal column involvement. It can be difficult to describe by a patient. When asked to explain their symptoms, the patient with chronic cervical myelopathy looks at their hands while trying to articulate what is wrong: 'They just don't work'.

Thoracic spine

Degenerative thoracic spine disease typically presents with local or radicular pain but few other symptoms or signs until spinal cord compromise develops, at which point there is usually a combination of upper motor neurone weakness, a spinal sensory level and sphincter disturbance. Thoracic arteriovenous malformations (AVMs) and fistulas may initially present with chronic subtle or intermittent symptoms which progress with time.

Lumbar and sacrococcygeal spine

Degenerative disease is the most common pathology at this site, therefore pain, which may be localised and radicular, is the most common presenting complaint. This pain is usually a dull ache with exacerbations which are often movement sensitive. The anatomical distribution of the radicular component of the pain and the physical signs demonstrate the site of the pathology. In nerve root lesions, lower motor neurone signs reflect the myotomes innervated by the root. For example, wasting of extensor digitorum brevis over the dorsum of the foot indicates an L5 innervated muscle. Tendon reflex loss is a further important indicator of the nerve roots involvement. Sensory loss reflects the dermatomal distribution of the affected root.

Degenerative lumbar canal stenosis presents with low back pain, leg pain, heaviness or weakness often worsened by exercise and standing straight. Patients with spinal claudication prefer to adopt a slightly flexed posture and may find it easier to walk leaning on a shopping trolley, or frequently squat down as if to tie a shoelace. They may be able to ride a bicycle for a longer period of time than they can walk, again because of the flexed riding position. Leg weakness and tendon reflex loss may be exercise-dependent and therefore patients should be examined after they have walked. These findings are important in distinguishing spinal claudication from vascular claudication, which is worse with increased muscular activity, affecting more often the calf muscles, does not vary with posture and is associated with trophic skin changes. Cauda equina syndromes are an acute neurological emergence presenting with low back pain, sciatic-type pain, saddle sensory loss, leg weakness, sphincter and sexual dysfunction. The most important physical signs are those of lower motor neurone weakness in the affected myotomes, sensory loss (especially S3-S5), pain on straight leg raising, tendon reflex loss (ankle jerks) and poor anal tone/voluntary sphincter contraction. Cauda equina symptoms also present insidiously and the clinician needs to be alert for gradual onset sphincteric involvement, disturbances of sexual function and saddle sensory loss, either resulting from degenerative lumbar stenosis or sometimes intrinsic spinal cord pathology affecting the conus.

Other clinical features of spinal disease

It is important to examine for spinal deformity especially scoliosis and kyphosis. If a spinal deformity is evident then the examination should, as well as seeking evidence for local spinal disease, also consider generalised neuromuscular conditions and neurocutaneous conditions. Neurofibromatosis type 1 (Chapters 14 and 26) in particular can be readily diagnosed by the presence of café-au-lait spots, Lisch nodules of the iris, axillary freckling and cutaneous neurofibromas. Papilloedema is an uncommon but recognised sign of spinal pathology and is associated with high cerebrospinal fluid (CSF) protein. Autonomic symptoms and signs are of limited localising value but are seen in severe spinal lesions in which there is loss of temperature control and disturbances of sweating.

Diagnosis of spinal tumours

Clinical presentation is typically with pain and neurological dysfunction. Night pain or pain at rest is characteristic. Nocturnal pain is related to disturbances in CSF venous outflow causing engorgement and swelling of the spinal cord. Axial spinal pain not located in the lumbosacral region should be regarded as a red flag and warrants further investigation, particularly if it is associated with weight loss, decreased appetite or previous medical history of malignancy.

Investigations include blood tests, urine analysis for Bence-Jones protein, and other tumour markers. Radiologically plain X-rays, computed tomography (CT), magnetic resonance imaging (MRI), isotope bone scan, positron emission tomography (PET) scan are all potential imaging technologies. For primary bone tumours it is desirable to have maximal information prior to treatment. A biopsy (hollow needle core biopsy or fine needle aspiration under CT scan guidance) can be very helpful in treatment decisions. For example, the prognosis from Ewing's tumour is better if chemotherapy is given pre-operatively. Similar treatment protocols should be for treatment of osteosarcoma. Other tumours are best dealt with by an en bloc dissection. Identification of tumour type at an early stage is of vital importance in planning definitive treatment.

Pre-operative MRI in many cases allows a diagnosis to be made. It is now an essential part of tumour localisation and characterisation necessary for pre-operative planning. MRI features helpful for diagnosis are shown in Table 16.1.

Table 16.1 Magnetic resonance imaging (MRI) characteristics of intradural spinal tumours.

Ependymoma
T1-weighted images – isointense signal with spinal cord
T2-weighted images – hyperintense signal
Strong homogeneous enhancement with contrast
Astrocytoma
T1-weighted images – isointense or hypointense signal with spinal cord
T2-weighted images – hyperintense signal
Cyst formation
Heterogeneous enhancement with contrast
Haemangioblastoma
T1-weighted images – isointense signal to spinal cord
T2-weighted images – hyperintense signal
Cystic with tumour nodule (50–70%)
Enhances strongly with contrast
Extramedullary extension in 15%

Clinical features of vascular disorders of the spine

Spinal cord infarction usually presents acutely, often with pain followed by paralysis and sensory loss. The most common arterial territory involved is the anterior spinal artery. In anterior spinal artery occlusion the anterior two-thirds of the spinal cord is affected. The spinal level is determined by where in its course the supply from the anterior spinal artery is interrupted. The patient presents with an acute flaccid paraparesis with loss of sphincter control and anaesthesia to temperature and pain but classically with preservation of posterior column functions of joint position and vibration sense. The most typical level is the upper thoracic cord but involvement of the cervical spine and even the caudal brainstem can occur. Anterior spinal artery infarction can be partial. The syndromes of posterior spinal artery infarction, watershed infarction, venous infection, transverse infarction, central cord infarction and lacunar infarction are far more rare. Watershed infarcts and spinal artery hypoperfusion causing spinal transient ischaemic attack (TIA) and 'claudication' may occur because of atheromatous disease of the aorta and its branches. The most common site of hypoperfusion syndromes is the mid thoracic area T4–9 where perfusion is relatively poor. Common causes of spinal cord infarction are listed in Table 16.2.

Haemorrhage in the spine is classified according to the spinal level and anatomical site. Haemorrhages may be intramedullary, subarachnoid, epidural and subdural. The presentation is usually acute with severe spinal pain and myelopathy with a motor and

Table 16.2 Causes of spinal cord infarction.

Artherosclerosis	Diabetes, hypertension, hyperlipidaemia
Inflammatory	Sarcoidosis, arachnoiditis
Infective	Syphillis, TB, herpes zoster, HIV, bacterial meningitis
Vasculitis	SLE, giant cell polyarteritis
Aortic disease	Dissecting abdominal aortic aneurysm, aortic occlusion, trauma, Takayasu syndrome
Arteriopathy	Connective tissue disease, Marfan's syndrome, fibromuscular dysplasia
Embolic disease	Cardiac embolism, decompression sickness
Hypoperfusion states	Cardiac arrest, hypovolemia, cardiopulmonary bypass
Vertebral artery disease	Dissection, trauma
Hypercoagulable states	Clotting factor disorders, antiphospholipid antibodies, blood transfusion
Drug abuse	Cocaine, heroin, ecstasy
Miscellaneous medical	Anaemia, sickle cell, Moyamoya, CADASIL, Paget's disease
Iatrogenic	Vascular surgery, cardiac surgery, spinal surgery, diagnostic catheter radiology, interventional radiology, spinal/epidural anaesthesia; intrathecal drugs

CADASIL, cerebral autosomal dominant arteriopathy with subcortical infarcts and leukoencephalopathy; SLE, systemic lupus erythematosus; TB, tuberculosis.

sensory level and sphincter loss. Spinal subarachnoid haemorrhage presents with severe back pain, radicular pain followed by the classic signs and symptoms of subarachnoid bleeding (i.e. obtundation, neck stiffness and photophobia). Myelopathy may be present but, unlike other causes of spinal haemorrhage, is not necessarily severe.

Diagnosis of spinal vascular disease

The differential diagnosis of spinal cord vascular diseases is influenced primarily by the rapidity of symptom presentation. Severe infectious, para-infectious and inflammatory myelitis including Devic's disease may present acutely. However, hyperacute presentations are more suggestive of vascular disease. Subacute and chronic presentations, either without haemorrhage as in dural AVMs or with small venous haemorrhage as with cavernomas, need to be differentiated from the causes of progressive myelopathy, particularly structural causes and spinal demyelination.

MRI is the primary diagnostic investigation. Spinal MRI will detect over 90% of acute spinal cord ischaemic lesions. Diffusion-weighted and contrast-enhanced MRI may increase the yield further. MRI usually excludes compressive lesions and often will find evidence of demyelination especially if cranial MRI is also performed. Imaging of the aorta with abdominal CT, CT and MR angiography is very important. Subdural and epidural haematomas are detectable but need to be distinguished from abscesses and other causes of fluid collection. AVMs and dural fistulae are usually detectable with expert neuroradiological interpretation of T1.5 MRI. The vessels of the malformation are seen a serpiginous flow voids. In addition, there is usually T2-weighted signal change within the spinal cord substance. However, AVMs and dural fistulae can be missed on MRI. Spinal myelography has detected the vessels of AVMs and dural fistulae that are not visible on MRI. Finally, spinal angiography may be required both for definitive diagnosis and to plan treatment with interventional radiological occlusion either through embolisation or gluing techniques.

In suspected spinal subarachnoid haemorrhage cranial CT often detects subarachnoid blood and a lumbar puncture will provide definitive evidence of subarachnoid haemorrhage. Other investigations are directed towards detection of the cause or contributing factors of the infarct or haemorrhage (e.g. looking for infections such as syphilis, hypercoagulant and hypocoagulant states and vasculitis).

Radiological assessment of spinal disorders

The mainstay of radiological investigation involves X-rays, CT and MRI. Plain and dynamic X-rays are useful for assessing spinal stability, range of movements, and reducibility if deformity is present. CT scans are very useful to assess bone integrity, degenerative changes, bone fracture, and provide a good assessment of mechanical stability. MRI is better at visualising the spinal cord and nerve roots, soft tissues (including discs and interspinous muscles and ligaments), facet joint effusions, spinal tumours and vascular abnormalities.

Specific diseases of the spinal column and spinal cord and their management

Skeletal disorders affecting the spine

Idiopathic scoliosis

Scoliosis refers to a lateral deviation of the spine in the coronal plane and is always abnormal. Idiopathic scoliosis is a disorder unique to humans and is therefore felt to relate to fully erect bipedelism. Only secondary forms of scoliosis are seen in even our nearest primate cousins. It may be classified on the basis of clinical examination into structural and non-structural forms. In a structural scoliosis there is a rotational component to the curve, which is best seen on forward flexion when prominence of rib or loin musculature becomes apparent. This is not the case in non-structural scoliosis, where there is no rotational element. Non-structural scoliosis may be a marker of other pathology such as leg length discrepancy or muscle spasm but is rarely of clinical significance in itself. However, if associated with underlying neurological disease it may progress to a structural deformity.

Once a structural scoliosis is diagnosed, the severity and potential for progression must be assessed. Erect posterior–anterior and lateral X-rays should be taken in a standardised manner so that serial films can be compared. The severity of the curve is given by the Cobb angle, which describes the angle created by the intersection of lines drawn across the end-plates of the upper and lowermost vertebrae delineating the curve (i.e. those with the greatest opposing tilt as illustrated in Figure 16.2). Angles >20° in skeletally immature children demand particular vigilance for it is during periods of rapid growth that scoliosis may progress significantly. Scoliosis presenting in younger children thus has a greater risk of progression. Progression of scoliosis in adults is less common, although underlying neuromuscular disease, pregnancy and osteoporosis pose increased risks. In general, 25% of scolioses do not progress, 25% progress slowly and 25% progress rapidly.

The major causes of structural scoliosis are given in Table 16.3. The most common type is idiopathic scoliosis, accounting for around 70% of all cases. The child is otherwise healthy and no underlying pathology is found. The prevalence of adolescent scoliosis, the most common form, is approximately 4% of the population if mild cases are included. The majority of idiopathic scoliosis are right-sided, thoracic and painless.

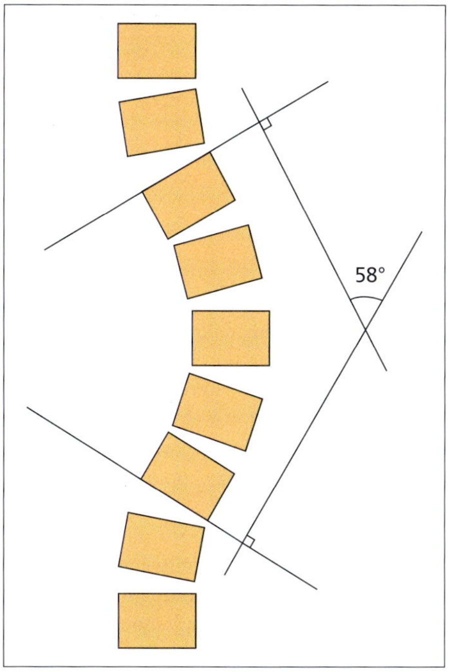

Figure 16.2 Cobb angle. Diagram illustrating method of calculating the Cobb angle to guide treatment of scoliosis.

Table 16.3 Causes of structural scoliosis.

Idiopathic scoliosis
Infantile <3 years
Juvenile 3–10 years
Adolescent >10 years
Congenital scoliosis
Failure of vertebral segmentation and/or formation
Neuromuscular scoliosis
Neuropathic
Upper motor neurone
Cerebral palsy
Lower motor neurone
Spinal muscular atrophy, poliomyelitis, hereditary neuropathies and dysautonomias
Mixed
Myelomeningocoele, spinal dysraphism, tethered cord, syrinx
Myopathic
Congential myopathies
Muscular dystrophies (e.g. Duchenne's)
Miscellaneous causes
Skeletal dysplasias
Marfan's syndrome
Neurofibromatosis
Spinocerebellar degenerations including Friedreich's ataxia
Arthrogryposis
Rett's syndrome
Metabolic bone disease
Dystonia
Parkinson's disease and parkinsonian syndromes
Cranio-cervical junction anomalies especially if associated with syringomyelia
Spinal tumours/trauma/irradiation

The cause of idiopathic scoliosis is multi-factorial and the development and progression of the scoliosis may have different mechanisms. There is often a positive family history of scoliosis, with girls eight times more likely than boys to require treatment. The pattern of inheritance is consistent with a dominant major gene diallele model (the gene is as yet unidentified) with incomplete penetrance. Progression of the curve is more common in thoracic or large curves (>35°) with skeletal maturity another important consideration. The consequences of severe idiopathic scoliosis are cosmetic deformity, cardiopulmonary compromise and back pain.

In adolescents with suspected idiopathic scoliosis, standing lateral and posterior–anterior X-rays should be performed and those patients with curves greater than 20° should be followed by repeat X-rays every 4–6 months. Curves progressing more than 5° in 4–6 months, or exceeding 30°, should be treated with a brace which may delay or arrest scoliosis progression in the skeletally immature child. A thoracolumbar spinal orthosis is generally used, with an added cervical extension (as in the Milwaukee brace) if the apex of the curve is above T8. Bracing is rarely effective once the curve exceeds 45° and it is in these patients that surgery is recommended. Surgery may also be advised if there is a significant thoracic lordosis or rotational deformity that impairs pulmonary function.

Congenital scoliosis

In congenital scoliosis the vertebrae are anomalous either because of a failure of natural segmentation, leading to asymmetric fusion, or to failure of formation, in which only part of the vertebra is formed (see Human vertebral segmentation defects). Often there is a combination of both pathologies. Failure of segmentation may lead to a unilateral fused bar with scoliosis away from the fused side, or a block vertebra. Abnormalities in mesenchymal formation may lead to mild wedging or absence of half a vertebra producing a hemivertebra with a single pedicle and lamina with subsequent scoliosis. In congenital scoliosis there is a high incidence of associated anomalies: neuraxis anomalies in up to 40% of patients, renal and gastrointestinal tract abnormalities in 20% and congenital heart defects in approximately 10%. Sometimes the scoliosis is part of a syndromic diagnosis such as in the Klippel–Feil and Noonan syndromes. Clinically, the scoliosis may vary from a mild non-progressive deformity to a severe and rapidly progressive curve that compromises the spinal cord.

Neuropathic scoliosis is often associated with rapidly progressing curves in juveniles (3- to 10-year-olds) with pain and neurological findings that reflect the underlying disease, such as a tethered cord, diastematomyelia or lipoma. It is important to look for signs of a skin dimple, sinus, haemangioma or hairy patch in all children with a scoliosis, and to perform an MRI scan. Early treatment of the underlying disorder can arrest the progression of the scoliosis, but if treatment is delayed then the curve may reach the point where altered biomechanical forces take effect and the curve continues to progress despite treatment.

If a neurogenic cause for scoliosis is overlooked and the curve is incorrectly believed to be idiopathic, then neurological damage may occur during surgical correction. For example, a tethered cord can be stretched further during instrumentation and straightening of the spine.

Neuromuscular scoliosis

Spinal deformity is common in many of the neuromuscular disorders. In the developed world cerebral palsy, spina bifida and Duchenne muscular dystrophy are the most common causes of neuromuscular scoliosis, although poliomyelitis is still an important cause in developing countries. Because of the underlying condition, the spinal curvature, in contrast to idiopathic scoliosis, generally presents earlier, is more extensive and is more likely to deteriorate through childhood and into adult life, particularly during the 'growth spurt'. Other systems are often already compromised, for example there may be muscle imbalance, cardiopulmonary insufficiency, poor nutrition, insensate skin and osteoporosis. The physical and functional effects of the scoliosis often exacerbate these problems. In addition, the scoliosis may adversely affect walking and seating and cause pain as the ribs abut the iliac crest. This is often compounded by coexisting pelvic obliquity, particularly in the non-ambulant patient.

In congenital or neuromuscular scoliosis there may be a role for bracing but, given the relentless progression of the scoliosis in many of these conditions, early surgery is often indicated. In non-ambulant patients the spinal fusion should involve the pelvis. Surgical risk, particularly of haemostasis and postoperative chest infection, is high in this patient group.

Kyphosis and lordosis

The spine naturally shows some curvature in the anteroposterior plane, seen as a kyphosis in the thoracic region and lordosis at the lumbar spine. A normal lumbar lordosis shows full correction on forward flexion. A kyphosis greater than 40° is abnormal. It may be congenital, caused by a lack of fusion of the vertebral bodies anteriorly or a lack of formation of one or more anterior bodies. Although less common than congenital scoliosis it carries a more severe prognosis, as a higher proportion of patients will develop progressive deformity and myelopathy, particularly during the adolescent growth spurt. Patients with anterior failure of vertebral body formation who present with a sharp angle kyphosis are at particular risk of rapid progression and spinal cord compression. Early arthrodesis is indicated in these cases. Other causes of abnormal kyphosis include Scheuermann's kyphosis, post-trauma, osteomalacia, osteoporosis and tumour infiltration. Scheuermann's kyphosis is the most common form of acquired kyphosis. Presenting in adolescents, it is generally benign and may be corrected with a brace if applied during the adolescent growth spurt. Kyphosis only occasionally progresses once skeletal maturity is reached.

In kyphosis, bracing is advocated for skeletally immature patients with progressive curves less than 60° (normal range 25–40°). Surgery is often required if the curve exceeds 60°. Correction of a kyphosis should be performed at the lowest level possible to minimise risk, and the presence of any fixed flexion deformity at the hips should be noted and corrected first, because this will affect the overall sagittal balance of the spine.

Miscellaneous causes of spinal deformity

A number of primary diseases of bone and connective tissue produce pathology of the spine and cranio-cervical junction. Those that present neurological problems are classified into four broad categories.

Osteopenic disorders In osteopenic disorders bone mineralisation is reduced. These include endocrine diseases such as hypoparathyroidism, Cushing's disease, osteomalacia, primary osteoporosis and osteogensis imperfecta.

Osteogenesis imperfecta (OI) is a heritable disorder of collagen that results in osteopenia and increased bone fragility. In 95% of patients mutations are found in the genes (*COLIA1* and *COLIA2*) encoding the α1 and α2 collagen chains. This results in reduced amounts of collagen which is often structurally abnormal. To date, over 200 mutations have been found; however, there is no close correlation between the molecular abnormalities and the clinical manifestations which are highly variable.

Prenatal diagnosis is available for some forms of the disease. The Sillence classification delineates four major phenotypes on the basis of bone fragility, growth and the presence or absence of additional features such as blue sclerae, dentinogenesis imperfecta and presenile hearing loss. Progressive skeletal deformity is a particular feature of OI type 111 and often requires orthopaedic intervention. Basilar invagination is a rare but important complication of OI in which the skull base develops abnormally and appears to 'fold in' like the undersurface of a closed-cup mushroom, and the C2 odontoid peg translocates upwards. This may be associated with ventral brainstem compression, hydromyelia and hydrocephalus. It generally presents in early adult life with progressive neurological symptoms and signs, the most common being headache and lower cranial nerve dysfunction, particularly atypical trigeminal neuralgia. A range of other features occur from nystagmus to ataxia and quadriparesis. Trigeminal pain, if intractable, may require stereotactic surgery. The treatment of myelopathy involves ventral decompression and occipito-cervical fusion, with or without decompression of the foramen magnum.

Currently, there is much interest in the role of bisphosphonates in the management of OI. They reduce bone pain, improve both bone density and vertebral height, and may improve mobility through reducing spinal deformity. They are recommended in children but very long-term benefits on disease progression, function and quality of life have yet to be fully demonstrated and there are concerns about long-term adverse consequences of the treatment. Bisphosphonate treatment of mild OI is not indicated because of the potential long-term risks of therapy.

Osteoporosis is a progressive decrease in bone mass and density that can predispose to vertebral body fracture. The most common spinal manifestation is a compression or wedge fracture presenting with back pain or radicular pain, and very occasionally cauda equina or spinal cord compression. Multiple wedge fractures can lead to chronic pain and kyphotic deformity. Management includes conservative options (pain control, bracing, steroid injections), minimally invasive techniques (vertebroplasty) or surgery (pedicle screw fixation).

Skeletal dysplasias The two largest categories of these disease are the osteochondrodysplasias and the dysostoses. Osteochondrodysplasias are defined as abnormalities of cartilage or bone growth and development. They generally present as short-limbed dwarfism, with autosomal dominant achondroplasia resulting from mutations in fibrobast growth factor pathways with two mutations in the *FGFR3* gene causing around 99% of cases. Approximately 50% of children with achondroplasia have a thoracolumbar kyphosis in infancy and there is a risk of spinal cord stenosis. Patients characteristically have macrocephaly but a small mid face and small foramen magnum. These abnormalities place them at risk of symptomatic stenosis and hydrocephalus. Sleep apnoea is seen in the majority of patients, which may have a central or respiratory cause. Cervicomedullary decompression with resection of the foramen magnum may be necessary. Atlanto-axial instability has been increasingly recognised in the skeletal dysplasias.

The dysostoses are defined as malformations of individual bones singly or in combination. These include the craniosynostoses (Crouzon and Apert syndromes) in which vertebral anomalies are commonly recognised and Klippel–Feil syndrome (see Klippel–Feil syndrome).

Metabolic storage disorders Metabolic storage diseases include the mucopolysaccharidoses, the glycoprotein storage disorders, the gangliosidoses and the mucolipodoses. These neurodegenerative diseases vary in their severity but show characteristic skeletal dysplasias, such as 'hooked' vertebrae, broad ribs and flared pelvis. Thoracolumbar kyphosis is common, with a risk of spinal cord compression. Other neurological complications include cognitive deterioration, carpal tunnel syndrome and deafness. In Morquio's syndrome (mucopolysaccharidosis IV) the os odonteum is dysplastic or absent. These patients also have striking ligamentous laxity which gives a particularly high risk of atlanto-axial instablity and spinal cord compression.

Mesenchymal and connective tissue disorders Around 30% of patients with neurofibromatosis will develop scoliosis, of which 40% will have associated cervical spine abnormalities. The scoliosis often manifests as an acute-angled short segment kyphoscoliosis, which will inevitably progress unless fusion is performed. Approximately 50% of patients with Marfan's syndrome develop significant scoliosis.

Management of spinal deformity

Patient management varies from case to case and will be influenced by the underlying diagnosis, current levels of function, especially ambulatory abilities, life expectancy and concomitant medical problems. In broad terms, surgery may be performed for progressive deformity, neurological symptoms or pain, but is associated with risks, including infection (2–5%) and neurological damage (1–2%). The primary goal of corrective surgery is to produce a balanced spine in the coronal and sagittal planes when non-operative measures have been unsuccessful. However, it should be remembered that a deformity in one part of the spine will often be coupled with a compensatory scoliosis or kyphosis in another, and correction of the primary deformity should be performed in the context of the overall balance of the spine. A lumbar scoliosis, for example, should not be corrected in isolation if it would lead to overall coronal imbalance as a result of persisting 'compensatory' scoliosis elsewhere.

Degenerative scoliosis In adults, scoliosis may occur in later years because of asymmetric degeneration in discs, facet joints or osteoporotic wedging of vertebral bodies. Surgical fixation might be considered in the presence of pain or progressive deformity.

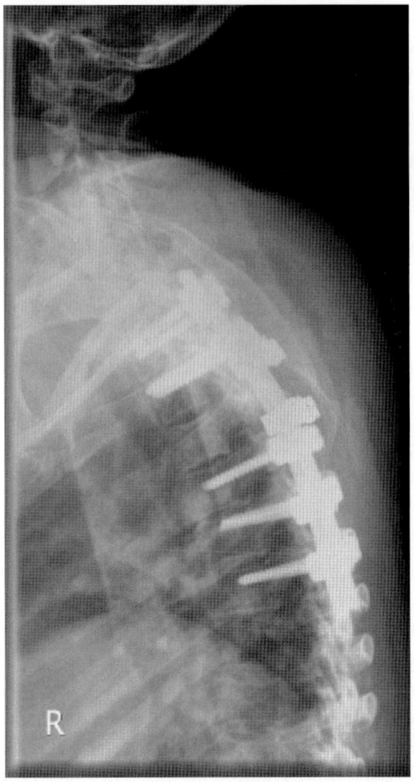

Figure 16.3 Lateral spine X-ray showing pedicle screw fixation for correction of spinal deformity resulting from tumour.

Surgical correction of spinal deformity

Good results are dependent on meticulous patient selection at all stages, with multi-disciplinary pre-operative assessment, experienced specialised spinal surgeons, intraoperative neurophysiological spinal cord monitoring and intensive care support postoperatively. Complications in the immediate peri-operative period include haemorrhage, respiratory and cardiovascular problems. Infection occurs in 2–5% of patients. Paraplegia occurs in 1% of patients and nerve root damage in 1–2%. Up to 5% of patients experience failure of fusion.

In the past, Harrington rods were used to correct deformity by a posterior approach to the spine: these are steel rods with laminar hooks used to open out the concave side of the scoliosis. This technique of unilateral distraction was useful in correcting coronal balance, but not kyphotic deformity. Now the most common surgical technique for correction of deformity is the insertion of pedicle screws, which can be manipulated to good alignment and secured to titanium rods, supplemented with sublaminar and transverse process hooks if required (Figure 16.3). These newer systems of instrumentation allow simultaneous correction of imbalances in the sagittal, coronal and axial planes. Iliac crest bone graft is placed over the construct and between transverse processes to produce a solid fusion.

Standing posterior–anterior and lateral X-rays are required for surgical planning, and primary curves may be identified. Specific categories of primary deformities and compensatory curves have been described. The endpoints for the fusion and the positions of the pedicle screw and hook anchor points can be planned depending on the curve type and degree of flexibility.

Thoracolumbar kyphosis may be corrected by a similar posterior approach, but requires a wedge excision of vertebral body or a subtraction osteotomy of pedicles, to allow sufficient movement for reduction of the deformity. An anterior release operation (e.g. via a thoracotomy) may need to be performed to allow sufficient movement to reduce the kyphosis.

Other approaches include thoracotomy and thoracoscopy for antero-lateral correction of a thoracic deformity, and the retroperitoneal approach to the antero-lateral lumbar spine. Indications for these approaches include congenital malformation of vertebrae, rigid deformities requiring release, pseudoarthrosis after posterior fixation and in children less than 10 years old. Posterior fixation in the skeletally immature patient causes growth arrest of the posterior elements, but growth may continue at the vertebral endplates resulting in progression of the primary curve. For antero-lateral approaches, the convex side of the spine is exposed and screws placed into the vertebral bodies. The screw-heads are attached to a rod, and compression of the screws then reduces the deformity.

Cranio-cervical junction anomalies

The pathophysiology of the cranio-cervical junction anomalies is complex. An important classification has been proposed by Menezes (1999), reproduced in Table 16.4. This subdivides the anomalies into congenital, developmental and acquired causes.

Clinical features of cranio-cervical junction anomaly There are three principal mechanisms by which the cranio-cervical junction anomalies lead to neurological signs. Frequently, more than one mechanism coexists.

Direct compression This may result from developmental abnormalities of the odontoid process. Of particular importance is the condition os odontoideum where the odontoid and the body of the axis are not fused. Atlas assimilation, where there is failure of segmentation

Table 16.4 Causes of craniocervical anomalies.

Congenital anomalies and malformations
Occipital sclerotome malformations – atlas assimilation, pro-atlas remnants
Atlas malformations – bifid atlas, assimilation, fusion, absent arches
Axis malformations – segmentation defects, odontoid dysplasias
Developmental and acquired anomalies
Foramen magnum abnormalities
Foramen stenosis, e.g. achondroplasia (AD *FGFR3* gene)
Secondary invagination (e.g. ostoeogenesis impefecta, Paget's disease)
Atlantoaxial instability
Down's syndrome
Metabolic disorders (e.g. Morquio's, Hurler's syndromes)
Infections (e.g. Grisel's syndrome, tuberculosis)
Trauma
Inflammation (e.g. rheumatoid arthritis, Reiter's syndrome)
Tumour (e.g. osteoblastoma, neurofibromatosis, chordoma, meningioma)
Miscellaneous (e.g. syringomyelia)

AD, autosomal dominant.

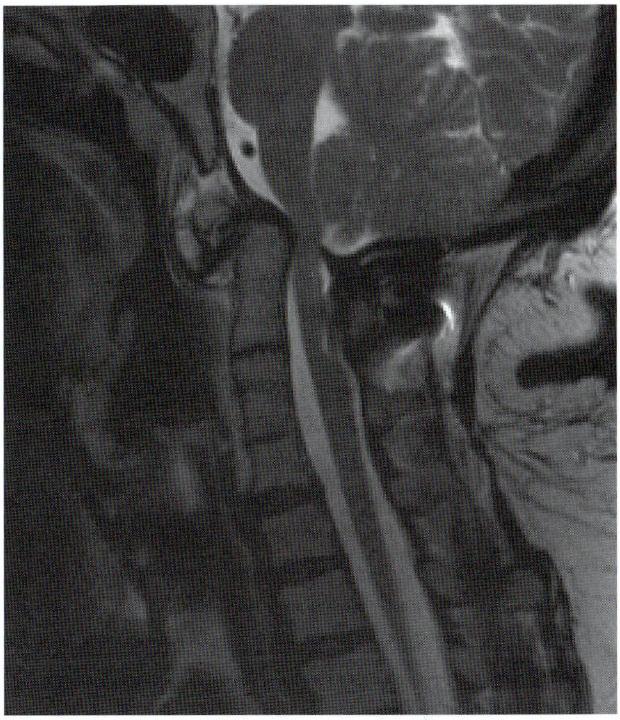

Figure 16.4 Congenital basal impression. T2-weighted sagittal MRI showing odontoid peg compression of cranio-cervical junction.

between the fourth occipital and first spinal sclerotomes, is relatively common and is particularly associated with the Chiari malformations. Direct compression may also result from abnormal articulation around cervical vertebral blocks as is seen in the Klippel–Feil syndrome.

Structural Basilar invagination describes deformity of the osseous structures of the skull base that leads to upward displacement of the edge of the foramen magnum. In its primary congenital form it is often associated with platybasia where the clivus and anterior skull base are abnormally flattened. It can be associated with more subtle developmental bony anomalies and associated neurodysgeneses such as hindbrain herniation (particularly Chiari malformations) and syringohydromyelia. The foramen magnum itself may be narrow, usually as a feature of underlying skeletal dysplasia, as in achondroplasia. Acquired forms of basilar invagination are more common and result from any bone softening condition. The most important causes are osteogenesis imperfecta and Paget's disease. Diagnosis of basilar invagination on cervical spine X-ray historically involved measuring the position of the odontoid tip with respect to either the foramen magnum itself (McRae line) or from lines drawn between the roof of the hard palate and either the posterior lip of the foramen magnum (Chamberlin line) or the caudal part of the occipital bone (McGregor line), although now the diagnosis is more commonly made by CT or MRI scan (Figure 16.4).

Atlanto-axial instability Atlanto-axial dislocation results from incompetence of the transverse ligaments or abnormalities of the dens itself. Instability is defined by an atlanto-dens interval >4 mm, and is demonstrated by flexion/extension X-rays of cervical spine or sagittal CT reconstruction. Three-dimensional CT allows assessment of any rotational component. Instability may occur spontaneously or develop secondarily to inflammation or trauma. It is a recognised feature of the complex developmental cranio-facial and cranio-vertebral anomalies, particularly if there is atlas assimilation and segmentation failure as in the Klippel–Feil syndrome. Syndromes that are also associated with ligamentous laxity carry a particular risk of dislocation (e.g. the mucopolysaccharidoses and Down's syndrome).

Down's syndrome

Trisomy 21 occurs in around 1/650 live births and is the single most common cause of severe learning difficulties. Patients initially present with characteristic dysmorphic features and hypotonia, often with associated cardiac and gastrointestinal anomalies. It is estimated that up to 25% of patients with Down's syndrome have asymptomatic atlanto-axial instability. Only around 1% are symptomatic. Recognised presentations include mild pyramidal tract signs with gait disturbance or the precipitous onset of cord compression. In the absence of signs or symptoms, screening of the atlanto-dens interval is no longer routine.

Chiari malformations

There are four types of hindbrain malformation.

The Chiari I malformation is demonstrated on neuroimaging by the dorsal extension of the cerebellar tonsils below the level of the foramen magnum. The prevalence of Chiari I in asymptomatic individuals is probably less than 1%, but higher if tonsillar descent on sagittal MRI is associated with appropriate symptoms or other hindbrain anomalies and in around 50% of cases of true cerebellar ectopia there is elongation of the medulla. Approximately 50% of Chiari I malformations are associated with cranio-cervical anomalies and syringomyelia. The development of Chiari I is likely to be multifactorial. It has been postulated on the basis of familial aggregation that Chiari I is a disorder of para-axial mesoderm. Chiari I is present in renal–coloboma syndrome in which mutations in the *PAX-2* gene have been identified. However, unlike Chiari II–IV there are clear examples of acquired Chiari I in which serial MRI has demonstrated postnatal development of the anomaly. Furthermore, lowering of CSF pressure following lumbar puncture or lumbar peritoneal shunting may be a risk factor for cerebellar tonsil descent. Chiari I has occurred during baclofen-pump insertion. There are well-documented examples of 'Chiari' or 'pseudo-Chiari' malformations improving following treatment of abnormally low CSF pressure caused by CSF leakage (Figure 16.5 and Figure 16.6).

The symptoms and signs resulting from Chiari I overlap with those associated with other cranio-cervical anomalies. These include headache, especially cough headache, nystagmus and quadriplegia. Additional symptoms and signs may result from associated hydrocephalus or syringomyelia. The condition is rarely symptomatic in childhood. Unusual presentations of Chiari I have been described: sudden death, syncope, ventricular fibrillation resulting from head movement, lingual myoclonus, pulsatile tinnitus, Ménière-type symptoms, acquired esotropia, central apnoea and paroxysmal rage.

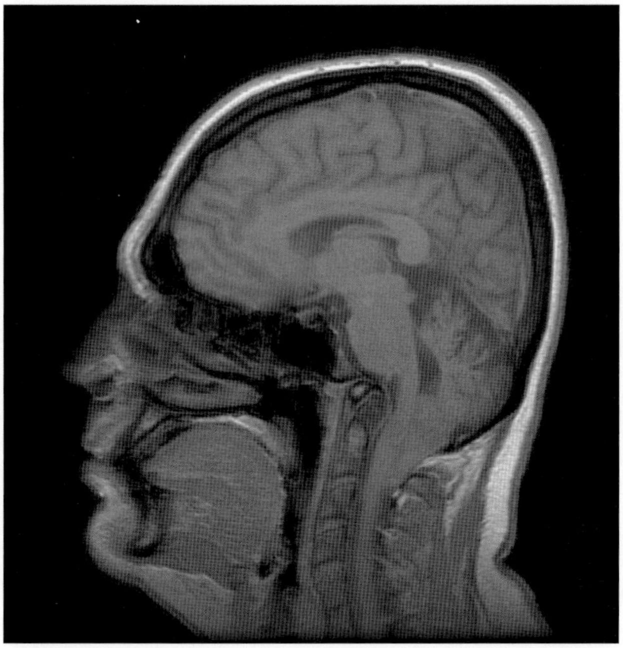

Figure 16.5 Chiari I malformation. MRI showing pre-operative appearances.

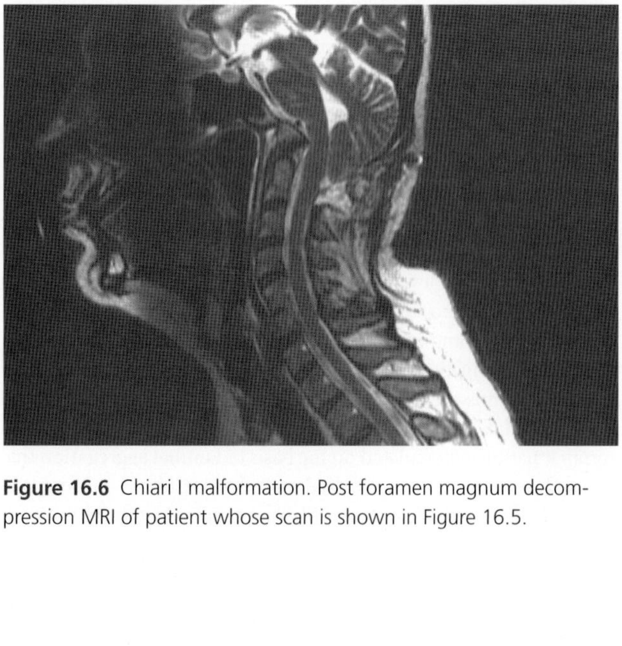

Figure 16.6 Chiari I malformation. Post foramen magnum decompression MRI of patient whose scan is shown in Figure 16.5.

Chiari II malformation is a congenital anomaly that is associated with myelomeningocoele and hydrocephalus in >90% of cases and generally manifests in the neonatal period. It consists of caudal displacement of the medulla and cerebellum (particularly vermis) into the cervical canal overriding the spinal cord often accompanied by partial herniation of the fourth ventricle and distortion of midbrain tectum. Associated abnormalities of supratentorial and midbrain structures are common.

Chiari III is analogous to type II but describes downward displacement of the cerebellum into a posterior encephalocoele, again with elongation and herniation of the fourth ventricle. Clinical features are severe and often life-threatening, particularly where there is cranial nerve dysfunction.

The Chiari IV malformation describes cerebellar hypoplasia and on current understanding is not part of the Chiari spectrum.

Asymptomatic Chiari I malformations can be treated conservatively. There have been case reports of sudden death in some patients with untreated malformations, but majority of these were not truly asymptomatic. Pregnancy in patients with significant Chiari I needs to be monitored and managed with care. Pushing during the second stage of labour causing further tonsillar descent and inadvertent dural puncture during epidural anaesthesia producing coning are two risks that need to be carefully considered. Some neurologists and neurosurgeons recommend that the baby be delivered by caesarean section and under general anaesthetic. Planned pregnancy is not an indication for prophylactic foramen magnum decompression.

Surgical treatment involves decompression of the foramen magnum and should be offered on the basis of significant and relevant symptoms (e.g. severe cough headache), or the presence of physical signs indicating neurological compromise. Posterior suboccipital decompression is the standard surgical management for symptomatic malformations, although there is much debate over how much bone to remove, whether the dura should be opened, scored or left intact, whether to use a dural patch graft or leave the dura widely open, and whether to resect the cerebellar tonsils to encourage good CSF flow. Surgery aims to prevent progression of symptoms, and improvement is seen in more than 80% of patients. Coexistent hydrocephalus usually improves after decompression of the foramen magnum, but if persistent, ventriculo-peritoneal shunting can be performed. Persistent syringomyelia may be treated by syringostomy, or by syringo-subarachnoid, syringopleural or syringo-peritoneal shunting. After foramen magnum decompression it can take several weeks for a patient to become accustomed to their altered CSF dynamics, and the patient may feel unsteady or experience low-pressure headaches. Aseptic meningitis occurs in a minority, and usually responds to a tapered course of steroids over a few weeks.

Congenital basilar invagination

Congenital basilar invagination results from a defect in the development of the cartilaginous skull base, producing elevation of the foramen magnum in relation to the occipital bone, with invagination of the lip of the foramen, along with flattening of the angle between the clivus and anterior fossa floor. This may be associated with other anomalies including occipitalisation of the atlas, Klippel–Feil segmentation defects, Chiari malformation and syringomyelia. Basilar invagination should be distinguished from basilar impression, which is an acquired vertical translocation of the odontoid process into the foramen magnum occurring in conditions such as rheumatoid disease. Basilar impression is not usually associated with moulding of the skull base.

Os odontoideum

Congenital atlanto-axial instability is sometimes caused by aplasia or hypoplasia of the odontoid process, but is more commonly the result of an os odontoideum. This is an independent ossicle located above the centrum of the axis vertebra in the position of the odontoid process, which may be associated with a hypoplastic or completely absent dens. The abnormality is more common in Down's syndrome, spondylo-epiphyseal dysplasias and Morquio's syndrome. The cause is thought to be *in utero*, neonatal or childhood fracture of the odontoid process with subsequent non-union and remodelling. If there is significant instability in a physically active patient, surgical fusion of C1 and C2 is recommended to minimise the risk of damage to the spinal cord in the future. Radiological instability is seen in 15–30% of people with Down's syndrome, but the instability is symptomatic in only 1–2% of patients, often because of learning difficulties. The current recommendation for patients with Down's syndrome and atlanto-axial instability is to restrict sporting activities if asymptomatic and to fuse patients who develop symptoms.

Management of craniocervical junction anomalies

The surgical treatment of cranio-cervical junction anomaly is complex and complete description is beyond the scope of this chapter. If neurological symptoms and signs of brainstem compression occur, or abnormal movement at C1–2 generates significant pain, then surgery is usually indicated. The aim of surgery is twofold: first to decompress and secondly to stabilise the cranio-cervical junction when necessary. Anterior decompressive surgery is commonly performed by the transoral approach, for example for tumours, rheumatoid pannus, os odontoideum and non-united odontoid fractures (Figure 16.7). Posterior decompression may be performed for Chiari malformations.

Horizontal atlantoaxial instability is commonly treated by posterior C1–2 fixation and bone graft, whereas vertical instability or 'cranial settling', analogous to a toffee apple on a stick, requires posterior occipito-cervical fusion.

Syringomyelia

A syrinx is a cystic cavity in the spinal cord (syringomyelia) or brainstem (syringobulbia) that is lined by spinal cord parenchyma, as distinct from a cystic cavity which is in continuity with the central canal and lined by ependymal cells (hydromyelia). It is caused by abnormal transmission of raised CSF pressure through the spinal cord parenchyma during coughing and raised intra-abdominal or thoracic pressure, as a result of pathologically altered CSF dynamics. Syringomyelia can be caused by several conditions:

1 Trauma, with or without spinal cord injury, often with spinal deformity. Around 2–8% of patients with spinal cord injury develop a syrinx over time, usually several years after the injury.
2 Congenital conditions such as Chiari malformations, basilar invagination and Dandy–Walker syndrome.

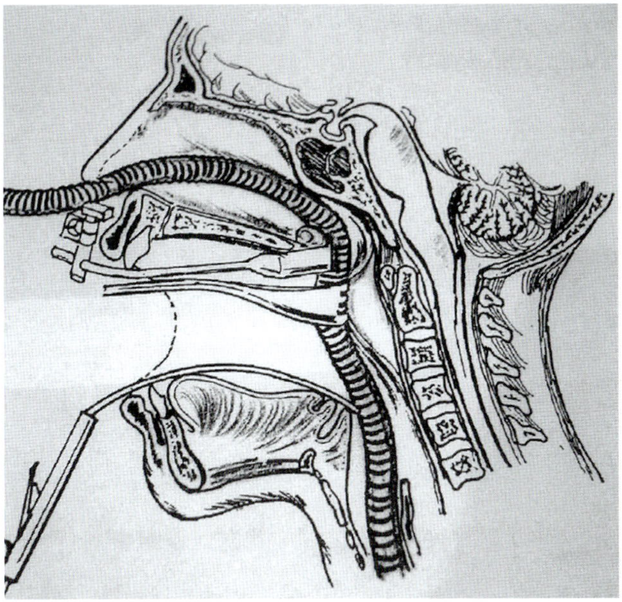

Figure 16.7 The transoral approach to the anterior craniocervical junction.

3 Tumours, especially intramedullary tumours such as astrocytomas and ependymomas. Investigation of syringomyelia should always include a gadolinium-enhanced MRI scan to exclude a tumour as the cause.
4 Arachnoiditis, particularly when affecting thoracic and cervical spine.
5 Spinal infections such as pyogenic meningitis and tuberculosis.

The symptoms and signs of syringomyelia typically progress gradually over time, and are discussed in the section above. Diagnosis is usually made from the clinical features and typical appearance on MRI of the spine (Figure 16.8). A cause for the syrinx (e.g. Chiari malformation, spinal tumour or arachnoiditis) should be actively sought.

Treatment of syringomyelia Non-progressive post-traumatic syringomyelia or hydromyelia causing mild clinical features is best managed conservatively. Progressive symptoms of syringomyelia need to be treated. As far as possible, the cause of the syrinx should be treated first (e.g. posterior fossa decompression for Chiari malformation). If the syrinx progresses and is symptomatic, treatment includes percutaneous drainage or open syringotomy. However, these techniques are associated with a high rate of syrinx recurrence, and a more permanent measure is to inset a shunt between the syrinx and the subarachnoid space, pleural or peritoneal cavities (Figure 16.9). Seventy-five per cent of patients were stabilised or improved in one surgical series by shunting, but because of the rarity of the condition and the variability in the surgical techniques available it is difficult to compare the outcomes of specific surgical options.

Spinal dysraphsim

Spinal dysraphic states are caused by localised failure of neural tube closure during fetal development. Myelomeningocoele is the most common form, with an incidence of 0.8/1000 live births. Neural tube defects are caused by a variety of mechanisms: chromosomal abnormalities, single gene defects and teratogens (including valproate and carbamazepine). There are marked regional

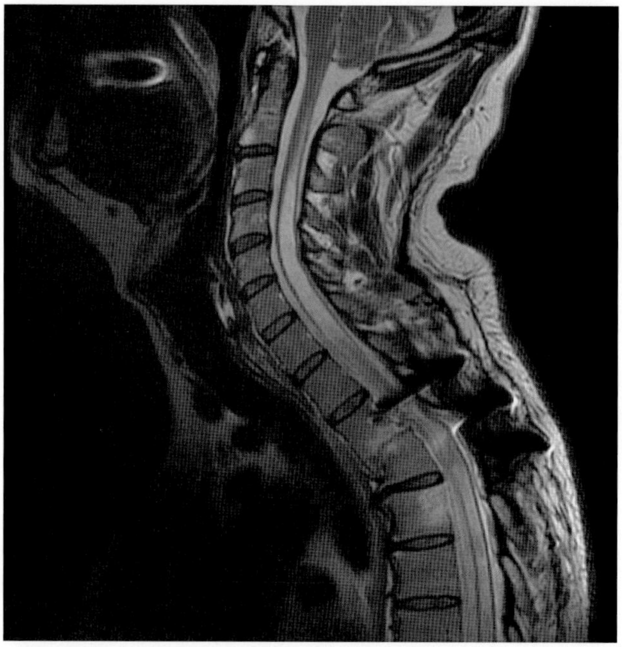

Figure 16.8 Syringomyelia. MRI showing post-traumatic cervico-thoracic syrinx (note T2–3 trauma and artefact resulting from pedicle screws).

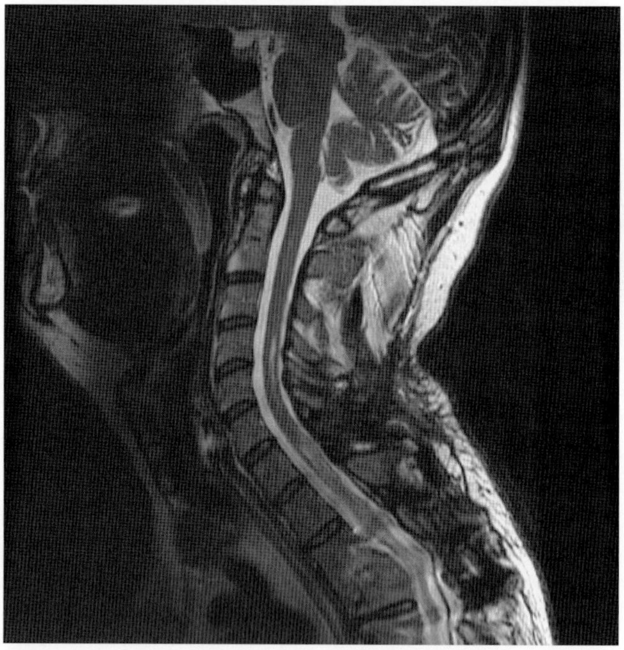

Figure 16.9 Syringomyelia. MRI of patient whose scan is shown in Figure 16.8 following insertion of syringopleural shunt resulting is successful syrinx decompression.

variations in its incidence and the condition is heterogeneous. There are strong genetic components and recurrence risks rise from 1–2% after one affected child to 10% with two affected children. Certain polymorphisms in genes involved in gene repair and folic acid metabolic pathways are associated with an increased risk of neural tube defect. The process of neuralation may be disrupted by teratogenic agents and in particular by maternal and/or fetal folate deficiency. Early folic acid supplementation reduces the incidence of neural tube defects, so that all women are recommended to take supplemental folate prior to conception and during the first trimester. It is estimated that approximately 70% of neural tube defects are preventable through maternal folic acid supplementation (400 μg/day). This advice is especially important for women with a previously affected pregnancy or those taking anticonvulsants in whom the incidence of neural tube defects is around 1% of pregnancies; larger amounts of folic acid are recommended for these women (5 mg/day). Folic acid supplementation should be started pre-conception. Routine antenatal screening provides a prenatal diagnosis in many cases; raised maternal serum alphafetoprotein is associated with open neural tube defects and fetal ultrasonography allows cranial and vertebral structures to be visualised directly. Prenatal counselling and pregnancy termination can then be offered.

Myelomeningocoele and myeloscisis account for 95% of cases of spinal dysraphism, with exposed neural tissue a common feature. In a meningocoele and in spina bifida occulta neural elements are covered by skin. The clinical features are determined by the extent of the myelocoele and the presence of associated abnormalities, which may include both neural and extraneural anomalies. Progressive hydrocephalus requiring surgical treatment is present in 90% of cases and around 70% have a Chiari II malformation. Learning difficulties are common, one-third have an IQ <80. Syringomyelia is present in up to 75% of cases and is often associated with severe scoliosis. Approximately one-third of patients have diastematomyelia.

Approximately 80% of open spina bifida defects are located in the lumbosacral area. The sensory level indicates the upper level of the lesion. Lesions above L3 result in complete paraplegia, but motor deficits may otherwise be patchy with a mixed pattern of upper and lower motor neurone signs. Sphincter and detrusor function is always compromised and careful urological assessment is required. Surgical closure is undertaken within 48–72 hours of delivery to reduce the risk of ascending infection and protect viable neural tissue within the placode. Following closure delayed hydrocephalus is likely. Patients generally require ongoing medical care by a multidisciplinary team.

Spina bifida occulta is a term used for occult dysraphism, where neural structures have not herniated through the mesenchymal defect. It includes diastematomyelia, terminal myelocystocoele and tight filum terminale. Lipomyelomeningocoele and dermal sinuses are often included in this category as they also result from abnormal secondary neurulation. Spina bifida occulta is usually neurologically asymptomatic. The majority of patients have associated cutaneous abnormalities such as a tuft of hair or a dimple over the region, and plain X-rays show underlying vertebral anomalies. MRI scan then confirms the diagnosis. Two neurological presentations are recognised. First, a congenital asymmetric weakness and atrophy of the lower limbs and second the 'tethered cord syndrome' with progressive and sometimes precipitous onset of weakness and spasticity. The latter often presents in childhood or during the adolescent growth spurt and is an important cause of toe walking in childhood. Both presentations may be associated with sphincter disturbance. Treatment is primarily neurosurgical, with release of the spinal cord from the tethering lesion, with full preoperative neurological and urological assessment. Orthopaedic, othortic and physiotherapy management of lower limb deformity is also important.

Klippel–Feil syndrome

Described in 1912, the disorder is characterised by a short neck, impaired neck mobility and a low hairline. The incidence is approximately 1/42 000 births. Three types of Klippel–Feil syndrome are described. The skeletal abnormalities include fusion of two or more cervical or cervico-thoracic vertebrae (Figure 16.10). The syndrome is heterogeneous; differing numbers and positions of fused vertebrae are described and the associated anomalies are highly variable. The condition may be familial: dominant, recessive and X-linked inheritance patterns have been proposed and mutations in the *PAX1* gene may be associated with the condition. Despite the sometimes dramatic spinal abnormalities, a follow-up study over a 10-year period has indicated that only 20% of patients experienced significant cervical spine symptoms and only 6% required surgical intervention.

Extravertebral anomalies associated with Klippel–Feil syndrome affect multiple systems. Skeletal and systemic abnormalities include scoliosis, scapula elevation, rib anomalies, cranio-facial dysmorphology, pulmonary, cardiac, gastrointestinal and urogenital anomalies. Neurological problems include syringomyelia, cranial nerve abnormalities, Duane retraction syndrome, deafness, acquired myelopathy resulting from the spinal abnormality, thin corpus callosum, split cervical spinal cord (Figure 16.11) and failure of pyramidal tract decussation. The latter anomaly is particularly interesting as it may underlie the intense congenital mirror movements that affect a number of these patients. Table 16.5 gives examples of pyramidal tract malformation and misdirection.

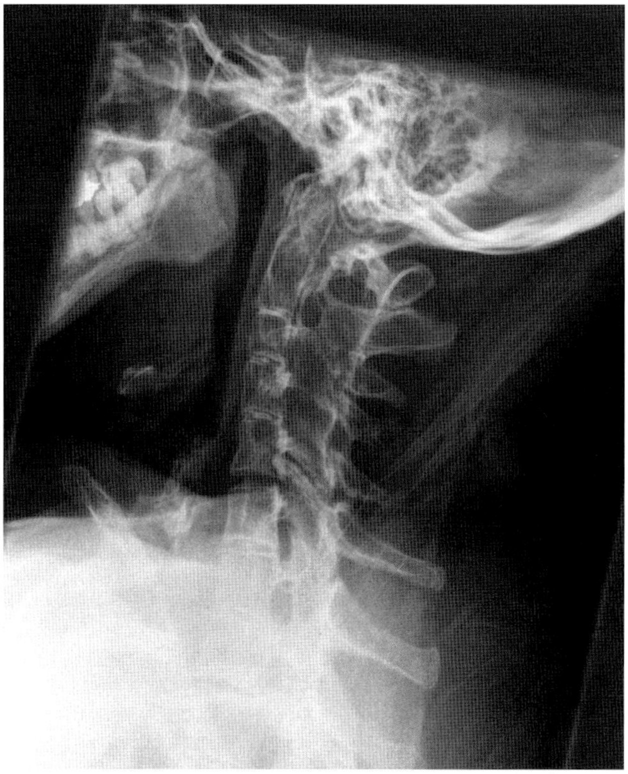

Figure 16.10 Lateral X-ray of patient with Klippel–Feil syndrome showing vertebral segmentation anomaly.

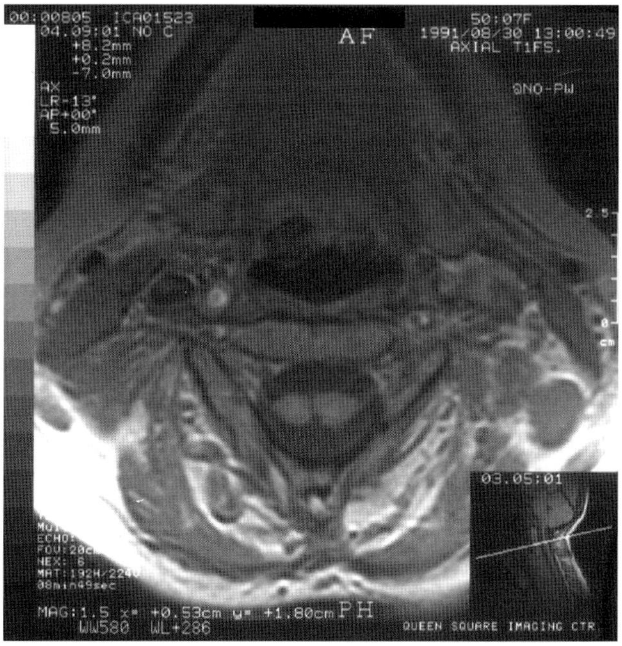

Figure 16.11 Axial MRI showing split cervical spinal cord in patient with Klippel–Feil syndrome.

Table 16.5 Pyramidal tract malformations. (After ten Donkelaar *et al.* 2004.)

Induction defect	Cell proliferation	Neural migration	Guidance	Acquired
Anencephaly	?X-linked Kallmann's syndrome	Lissencephaly	X-linked	Hypoxic–ischaemic damage
Encephaloceles	Hemimegalencephaly	Walker–Warburg	hydrocephalus and	(e.g. hemihydranencephaly)
Meckel–Gruber		Polymicrogyria	other phenotypes	Peri-venticular leukomalacia
Apert		Schizencephaly	associated with	Congenital infections
?Klippel–Feil		Zellweger's syndrome	*L1CAM* mutations	
			HGPPS	
			(*ROBO3* mutations)	

HGPPS, horizontal gaze palsy with progressive scoliosis.

Rheumatological disorders affecting the spine and spinal cord

Paget's disease The disorder is rare before the age of 40 but becomes increasingly common with time, affecting 10% of 90-year-olds. The clinical features are those of bone pain, local deformity, bone enlargement, pathological fracture and a predisposition to sarcomatous change. The disorder often affects the skull and spine and as a result neurological involvement is common. Typical radiological appearances and the finding of an elevated serum alkaline phosphatase confirm a diagnosis of Paget's disease. The disease is one of excessive bone desorption with excessive osteoblastic and osteolytic activity. A genetic predisposition is described and some familial cases have been linked to chromosome 18q. A syndrome of Paget's disease with inclusion body myositis and dementia has been described. Pagetic osteoclasts contain nuclear inclusions and osteoclastic infection is one proposed mechanism although firm evidence for a causative paramyxovirus infection is lacking.

There are numerous potential neurological sequelae of Paget's disease. Direct compression by pagetic bone may lead to headache, dementia, brainstem and cerebellar dysfunction, cranial neuropathies, myelopathy, cauda equina syndrome and radiculopathies. The most common cranial neuropathy is sensori-neural deafness. Optic atrophy, trigeminal neuralgia and hemifacial spasm may occur also. Pagetic softening of the skull may lead to basilar invagination resulting in brainstem and high cervical compression syndromes and occasionally hydrocephalus. The brain and spinal cord can become acutely compressed from epidural haematoma. The vascularity of pagetic bone may lead to cerebral ischaemia as part of a steal syndrome (compared with normal bone, blood flow in pagetic bone is increased threefold). Neurological syndromes may also develop because of compression of blood vessels.

Paget's disease generally responds to treatment with bisphosphonates although a relative resistance to these drugs is described. First line treatment is with potent oral bisphosphonates. Second line treatment regimes include calcitonin, etidronate and intravenous bisphosphonates. Bone pain in particular can resolve within 1–2 weeks of commencement of treatment. Treatment efficacy may be monitored by serum alkaline phosphatase levels and a therapeutic response is expected in approximately 80% of patients treated. Neurological syndromes often improve with medical treatment. Rapidly progressive neurological syndromes require high-dose intravenous bisphosphonate therapy and/or treatment with calcitonin. However, hydrocephalus generally requires shunting. Surgical decompression for basilar invagination, cranial nerve lesions, spinal cord and root compression is indicated if neurological symptoms and signs progress rapidly or despite best medical treatment. Medical treatment prior to surgical intervention may reduce bone vascularity and thus the risk of peri-operative haemorrhage.

Rheumatoid arthritis Rheumatoid arthritis is a chronic inflammatory immune-mediated symmetrical polyarthritis with a predilection for the distal joints. Females are affected twice as commonly as males and the prevalance ranges between 0.2% and 2% of the population in Europe and North America. The inflamed synovium is termed the pannus; it is characterised by T- and B-cell activation, cytokine release, immune complex deposition, angiogenesis and cellular proliferation. This inflammatory process leads to damage and destruction of bone, cartilage and ligaments. Aggressive immunosuppressive therapy with disease-modifying drugs (in particular sulfasalazine and methotrexate) improves the prognosis of rheumatoid arthritis. The newer immune-modifying drugs, such as antitumour necrosis factor and anti-interleukin 1 agents, have further improved prognosis, and compared with past decades, fewer rheumatoid patients are now presenting for surgery to the cervical spine and large joints.

Neurological manifestations of rheumatoid arthritis include entrapment neuropathy, vasculitic neuropathy, myopathy and ischaemic syndromes caused by vasculitis; these are discussed further in Chapter 26. The spinal cord manifestations result from ligamentous disruption, bone destruction and secondary osteoporosis. A rare syndrome of diffuse dural infiltration with inflammatory cells producing a pachymeningitis has been described.

Patients with rheumatoid arthritis of the cervical spine frequently experience headache and neck pain; however, the most feared neurological complication of rheumatoid arthritis is upper cervical cord and brainstem compression. Neurological symptoms usually result from one of three processes: atlanto-axial subluxation, basilar impression (vertical translocation) or subaxial subluxation.

Involvement of the atlanto-axial ligament often combined with local pannus formation and bone destruction produces subluxation. Atlanto-axial subluxation affects 25% of rheumatoid patients of whom 25% have neurological signs. Atlanto-axial subluxation may occur in lateral, rotational, anterior, posterior and vertical directions; the latter three directions being the most neurologically significant. Rheumatoid arthritis may affect the spinal cord caudal to the C1–2 level independently or in association with a high cord lesion. Postmortem studies of myelopathy show necrosis, gliosis and Wallerian degeneration within ascending and descending white matter. Cervical myelopathy is caused by repetitive minor trauma to the spinal cord because of excessive movement of the unstable level. The degree of atlanto-axial subluxation is well characterised by plain flexion–extension radiography; however, because a large part of the compression is caused by inflammatory soft tissue proper assessment requires MRI (Figure 16.12).

Natural history In a series of 235 rheumatoid patients referred for neurosurgical assessment of cranio-cervical junction instability, 60% had myelopathy, the majority of these either had motor or mixed motor and sensory long-tract signs; in approximately 10% the predominant deficits were loss of joint position and Rombergism, indicating a mainly posterior compression. Cranial nerve signs and nystagmus were rare and in this series were associated with other pathologies, especially Chiari malformation.

Rheumatoid arthritis initially involves the hands and feet, and large joints usually require surgery before the neck. Casey *et al.* (1996) discovered that cervical disease requiring surgical treatment tended to occur in patients who had had between two and four previous large joint arthroplasties. This implies that the greater degrees of mobility in rheumatoid joints leads to accelerated degeneration and instability. Hence, the cervical spine is affected commonly, particularly the atlanto-axial joint and the cranio-cervical junction, and the lower spine is usually spared. The percentage of rheumatoid patients who develop atlanto-axial subluxation varies between series, and reported frequencies are biased by the source of data collection. There are few large population-based cohort studies in the literature. Non-surgical studies over the past few decades report that 14–73% of patients with rheumatoid develop atlanto-axial subluxation, with a mean incidence of 35% (21% horizontal and 14% vertical subluxation). More than 30% will have symptomatic atlanto-axial subluxation 5–7 years after the onset of the disease. Five per cent then become myelopathic a decade later, 14–17 years after onset. Once myelopathy has developed the outlook is poor, with up to 50% mortality within a year.

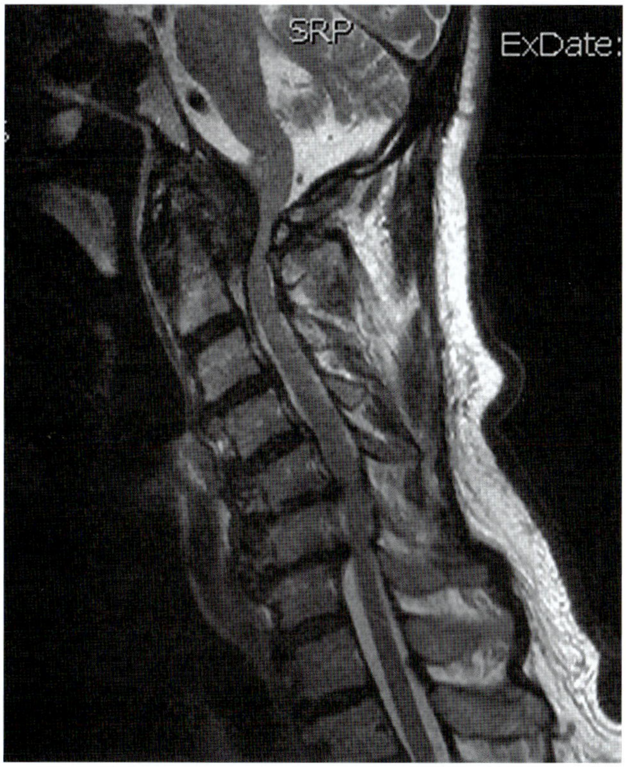

Figure 16.12 Sagittal T2-weighted MRI scan of cervical spine in rheumatoid disease, showing odontoid pseudo-tumour causing cord compression, and kyphotic subluxation of the sub-axial spine.

Indications for surgical management of the rheumatoid spine

A study of surgical outcome comparing the 1970s with the 1990s found an improvement in surgical mortality from 9% to 0%, a decrease in complication rate from 50% to 22%, and improvement of symptoms in 89% of patients who had surgery. Improved outcomes have been a result of better instrumentation and the trend towards earlier surgery; it is now accepted that operations for non-ambulant myelopathic patients are associated with an unacceptably high complication rate, and poor functional improvement. Atlanto-axial fusion is now more commonly performed for instability causing pain, early neurological symptoms and signs, occipital neuralgia or progressive radiological appearances (Figure 16.13).

Selection of appropriate patients for surgical intervention is difficult. The policy of waiting until rheumatoid patients with atlanto-axial subluxation develop signs of serious myelopathy has been strongly challenged on the basis that once spinal cord damage has been sustained it is rarely reversible. In a prospective trial it has been shown that following surgical stabilisation, with or without transoral anterior decompression, approximately 60% of ambulant patients will show stabilisation or improvement of their functional status; in contrast only 20% of non-ambulant patients will show any recovery. Furthermore, surgical morbidity and mortality was found to be significantly higher in the non-ambulant (12.7%) than the ambulant group (8.9%). In the past, major surgery was often performed for patients with end-stage myelopathy, often with poor results. Now surgical stabilisation is generally performed at an

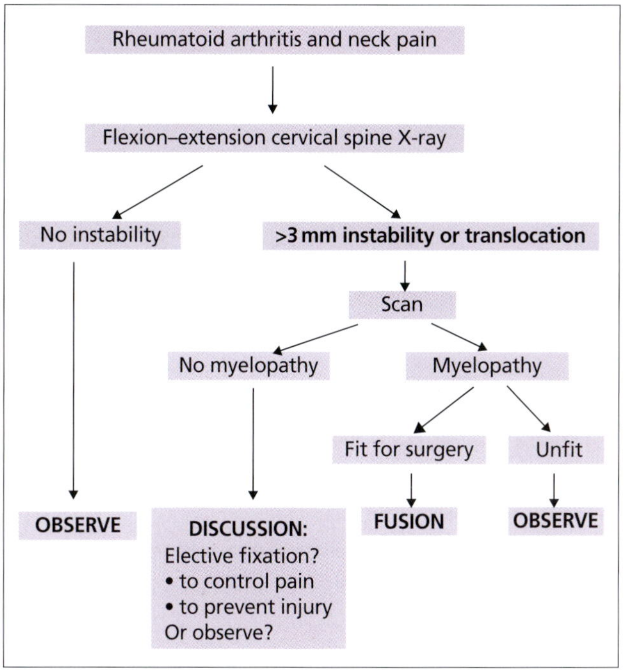

Figure 16.13 Algorithm for assessment and treatment of rheumatoid atlanto-axial disease (in text).

earlier stage once instability has been demonstrated. Early surgery is associated with a better outcome, lower risk and prevents further deterioration in the diseased joint.

It should be noted that the combination of mild neurological impairment and rheumatological/orthopaedic problems puts rheumatoid patients at increased risk of falls and even minor cervical injury can produce catastrophic neurological deterioration. Atlanto-axial subluxation increases the anaesthetic risk because of neck extension during artificial ventilation (Table 16.6).

Spondyloarthropathies

The inflammatory spondyloarthropathies include ankylosing spondylitis, psoriatic arthritis; arthritis associated with inflammatory bowel disease and reactive arthritis (for instance in Reiter disease). Low back pain is common to all conditions. The primary neurological manifestations are best described by a consideration of ankylosing spondylitis, and similar features occur in the other spondyloarthritides.

Ankylosing spondylitis is the most common of the seronegative spondyloarthritides, affecting up to 2% of the population in the West. It usually presents with gradual onset low back pain and stiffness of the large joints. The condition can affect other organ systems. Men are affected more than women. Disease onset is typically before age 40. HLA B27 is strongly associated with >90% of patients expressing the antigen. Unlike rheumatoid disease, it commonly affects the spine and sacroiliac joints, rather than the peripheral joints, and the disease progresses in a caudal–rostral direction, resulting in flexion deformities in posture. The pathological hallmark is the development of enthesopathy, that is inflammation around sites of tendonous insertion. Syndesmophytes form in the spinal column points where spinal ligaments attach to the vertebral bodies.

Table 16.6 Indications for different types of surgical stabilization in rheumatoid disease.

C1–2 fixation should be considered for
Instability and intractable pain
Clinical myelopathy
Occipital neuralgia
Progressive radiological subluxation
Anteroposterior spinal cord diameter less than 6 mm on flexion MRI
PADI less than 10 mm on CT
Patients with instability who are unable to wear a hard collar or brace
Fixation of the occiput to cervical spine should be considered for
Vertical translocation
Excessive degeneration or instability of the occipito-atlantal joints
When C1 or C2 bone quality does not allow adequate screw purchase or fixation of a short segment
Disruption of the ring of C1 by fracture or after transoral odontoidectomy
When there is a significant 'staircase' deformity or instability in the subaxial spine, requiring a longer construct to simultaneously fuse lower levels
Transoral decompression and posterior fixation should be considered
When there is irreducible atlanto-axial subluxation causing ventral compression of the neuraxis
When there is marked vertical translocation (>5 mm) causing brainstem compression
When an anterior soft tissue mass causes compression around the cranio-cervical junction

MRI, magnetic resonance imaging; PADI, posterior atlantodental interval.

The neurological manifestations of ankylosing spondylitis are usually a late stage complication. Loss of spinal movement is associated with vertebral body squaring and extensive loss of ligamentous laxity because of syndesmophyte formation. This process produces a rigid spine with kyphosis. Spinal involvement may produce atlanto-axial subluxation, pathological vertebral fracture, disco-vertebral destruction, spinal canal especially lumbar canal stenosis and a cauda equina syndrome (Figure 16.14). Atlanto-axial subluxation occurs more rarely than in rheumatoid arthritis; however, the management issues are similar. Spinal rigidity and disco-vertebral problems predispose to cord compression. Acute spinal cord compression resulting from epidural haematoma is a recognised problem. Spinal fractures are more common because of the rigidity of the spine, and the use of a rigid collar in the emergency department is often prevented by the degree of kyphotic deformity. Forcing the neck into a collar can itself result in a cervical fracture. Despite the tendency to ankylosis in these patients, conservative management often results in a pseudoarthrosis, and anterior or posterior fusion with surgical fixation is required.

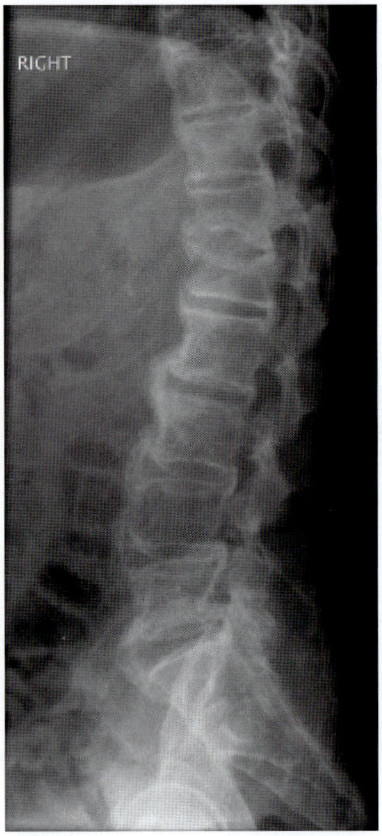

Figure 16.14 Lateral X-ray of thoro-columbar spine in a patient with ankylosing spondylitis.

The cauda equina syndrome is a rare late stage complication of ankylosing spondylitis. It presents gradually with leg pain, leg weakness, sensory disturbance and sphincteric dysfunction. On imaging studies posterior lumbar-sacral diverticulae are present. An arachnoiditis may also contribute to the development of the cauda equina syndrome; however, the presence of the diverticulae indicates that ankylosing spondylitis is the likely cause rather than some other form of arachnoiditis (Figure 16.15). It is important to remember that spinal irradiation was used to treat ankylosing spondylitis and late radiation neurological damage and bone sarcoma may result.

Spinal trauma

The most common cause for spinal injury is vehicle accidents, followed by violent assault, falls and sports injury, especially high board diving. Severity of injury may be classified using the American Spinal Injury Association (ASIA) Score for quantitative assessment of motor and sensory function, or the ASIA/Frankel grading system, A–E for clinical grading:

A The most severe with no motor or sensory function below the level of the lesion, and with no preservation of sensation in sacral dermatomes S4–S5.

B 'Incomplete' in which there is no motor function below the lesion but there is preservation of sensory function (in this group sacral preservation of pinprick sensation indicates a better prognosis for functional recovery).

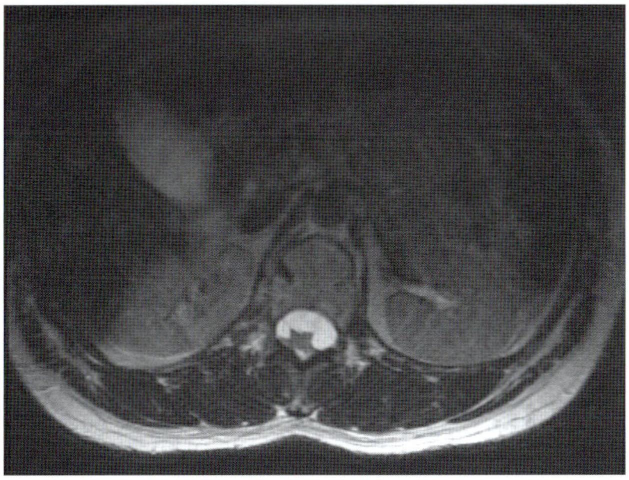

Figure 16.15 Axial MRI of thoracic spine showing deformation of thoracic cord caused by arachnoiditis.

C 'Incomplete' motor function is preserved below level of lesion (MRC <3).
D 'Incomplete' motor function is preserved below level of the lesion with 50% muscles MRC grade 3 or above.
E Normal motor and sensory function.

The majority of grade A patients will show some recovery of motor function (increase in one level) especially in the first 6 months, although later improvement does occur. Between 20% and 30% of grade B patients recover to grade D or E, 50–70% of grade C patients recover to grade D or E. Ambulation is normally achieved in patients who recover to grade D. In severe spinal cord lesions the level of the lesion critically determines the functional outcome with preservation of arm function (lesion below C6) being important for maintenance of transfers and activities of daily living. Assisted ventilation is required for patients with severe spinal cord lesions above C3. Independence of bowel and bladder function, albeit with intermittent self-catheterisation, may be expected if upper limb function is preserved.

Acute management of spinal injury

Resuscitation of the patient and treatment of life-threatening injuries are the initial priorities. Immobilisation of the spine at the scene of the trauma, especially the neck, should be performed until the neurological and mechanical integrity of the spine can be established. A cervical injury should be assumed until proven otherwise in all patients with a significant force of injury or those who are unconscious.

The investigators of the National Acute Spinal Cord Injury Studies (NASCIS) advocated the use of methylprednisolone within 8 hours of the injury, a bolus of 30 mg/kg followed by 23 hours of IV methylprednisolone 5.4 mg/kg/hour. Its effects are not completely understood but as well as reducing oedema steroids may prevent lipid peroxidation, which disrupts myelin. Other drugs that prevent lipid peroxidation are also under trial. However, there is a body of evidence that the side effects of steroids outweigh the benefits in head injuries. The CRASH trial (Corticosteroid Randomisation After Significant Head Injury) looked at the 6-month outcomes of over 10 000 randomised patients and found that mortality in those given high-dose steroids was greater than in those receiving placebo. The majority of data for the use of steroids in spinal cord injury do not show a beneficial effect, and questions have been raised about the handling of data in the NASCIS 2 subgroup analysis. A systematic review of 157 studies of methylprednisolone infusion in spinal cord injuries concluded that there is insufficient evidence to support the use of steroids as a treatment standard. Opinions differ but most surgeons and physicians feel that there is no clinical evidence to support use of high-dose intravenous methylprednisolone during the acute phase of traumatic spinal cord injury.

Surgery should be performed for incomplete lesions with cord compression and progressive neurological signs, mechanical instability preventing mobilisation, and if internal reduction of dislocation is required. Wound débridement may be necessary for dirty penetrating injuries. However, surgery will not improve a fixed neurological deficit that has been present from the time of injury.

The optimal surgical management of spinal fractures and cord injury remains controversial. Traditionally, patients were treated with 6–12 weeks of bed rest, traction and then mobilisation with external orthotic stabilisation. Proponents of conservative management argue that bed rest improves perfusion of the spinal cord at this very vulnerable stage following injury. Neurological outcome was studied in 63 consecutive patients with incomplete cervical cord injuries and was found to be dependent on the initial presenting neurological level of function. The neurological deficit at presentation and also the extent of recovery were not associated with the degree of spinal canal compromise. However, prolonged bed rest is associated with deep venous thrombosis, pulmonary embolism, chest infections, pressure sores and muscle atrophy. The development of titanium constructs and instrumentation over the past few decades have allowed surgeons to produce robust fixation and fusion at an early stage, facilitating early mobilisation, vigorous physiotherapy and avoidance of these complications. A review of the evidence for surgical management of spinal injuries concluded that many animal studies and class II and III human studies supported early intervention in improving neurological outcome. However, there is no class I evidence to support conservative or surgical management of acute spinal injuries, and most clinicians seem to base their judgement on belief, logic and individual experience.

There is a significant trend towards early surgical intervention to minimise the risks of immobilisation and maximise spinal stability for the future, as well as for reasons of health economics. Surgery should be performed in the controlled environment of the next available daytime list. The risks of surgery itself have decreased with the widespread use of modern technology and operating microscopes and, broadly speaking, there is a 1% chance of irreversible cord damage and a 5% chance of other problems including infection, failure of fusion and anaesthetic risks.

Central cord contusion of the cervical spine without instability may occur, especially if there is a background of spondylotic spinal canal stenosis. Some surgeons recommend non-operative management of these patients because of the theoretical risk of worsening their function if surgery is performed within 4–6 weeks of the injury. The evidence for this traditional approach is weak, and originates from a small series of eight patients, two of whom deteriorated after surgery to decompress the cord and section the dentate ligaments. The authors recommend early surgery in this group of patients if there is no spontaneous improvement and the spinal cord is compressed, or if a patient improves but then deteriorates. If there is no active cord compression or instability, then early decompression is not warranted. Of patients with a central cord contusion and tetraplegia or severe paresis, 50% eventually walk again and sphincter control usually recovers but manual dexterity tends recover less satisfactorily.

Experimental therapy for spinal cord injuries In the last three decades there has been much research interest, searching for a cure for paralysis after spinal cord injury. Animal models have demonstrated positive effects of many strategies, but clinical studies have so far failed to produce a significant benefit. Several strategies are presently being studied:

1 Neuroprotection and anti-inflammatory agents (e.g. riluzole, minocycline)
2 Neuroregeneration and the use of nerve growth factors (e.g. Cethrin)
3 Inactivating inhibitory cues in the glial scar, myelin or extracellular matrix (e.g. anti-Nogo-A antibodies, chondroitin sulfate proteoglycan inhibition)
4 Stem cell or regenerative cell techniques (various stem cells, olfactory ensheathing cells, cultured Schwann cells, peripheral nerve grafts)
5 Enhancing local plasticity (monoamine agonists, cellular therapies)
6 Rehabilitation and training, functional electrical stimulation (rehabilitation techniques, method, amount, timing, and epidural spinal cord stimulation)
7 Surgical stabilisation and decompression (method of surgery, timing of decompression).

The olfactory system as a model for nerve repair Until the 1970s it had been thought that no new nerve cells are formed in the adult brain, but with the new labelling technique it was found that in one part of the nervous system – the olfactory system – new nerve cells are being continually generated by division of an adult stem cell located in the nasal mucosa. Throughout normal life, and also at a much accelerated rate after injury to the olfactory nerves, the adult olfactory nerve cells die and are completely replaced by the progeny of adult stem cells lying in the olfactory mucosa. The nerve fibres belonging to the new nerve cells grow through the cribriform plate of the base of the skull and enter the brain. Olfactory ensheathing cells (OECs) are responsible for promoting this regeneration, and have been shown to improve the outcome when transplanted into experimental spinal cord and nerve root injuries in rodent and canine models.

Clinical application of olfactory ensheathing cell transplantation The encouraging reparative results in animal experiments have led to a clinical safety trial in Brisbane, Australia, which has shown no adverse side effects following transplantation of OECs cultured from biopsy samples from the patient's own olfactory mucosa and injected as a suspension at multiple sites in spinal cord injuries. But even with autografts of OECs cultured from biopsy samples of the patient's own nasal mucosa, there remains a need to characterise the human cells and establish a standard culture technology. Although typically located posteriorly on the superior turbinate and adjacent lining of the spheno-ethmoidal recess and nasal septum, considerable variability has been reported in the distribution of the human olfactory area and its histology, probably as a result of the inevitable accumulation throughout life of the effects of periodic infectious and allergenic insults, as well as continuous exposure to damaging agents in the air we breathe. At Queen Square, a project is underway to characterise the OECs that are cultured from human olfactory mucosa, grow the cells under standardised conditions and perform autologous cell transplantation for patients with acute brachial plexus avulsion.

Surgical management of spinal fractures The authors advocate early internal stabilisation once the patient is well enough, with reduction or decompression if required. Specific management is tailored to the patient, neurological and radiological findings.

Cervical fractures Fractures of C1 may be caused by a vertical blow to the vertex of the head, resulting in at least two fractures of the ring of the C1 vertebra (Jefferson fracture). The fragments tend to displace outwards, and usually there is no neurological deficit. Jefferson fractures are usually managed by immobilisation in a halo brace or rigid collar, depending on the degree of instability. Fusion is usually achieved by immobilisation alone, and surgical fixation is rarely required.

Occasionally, rotation of a C1 facet may occur beyond the articular surface of the C2 facet below, resulting in rotatory subluxation and locking of the facet. This may occur because of trauma, in rheumatoid disease or may occur spontaneously, especially in children. Patients present with a characteristic 'cock robin' posture: rotation away from the dislocated side, slight flexion and lateral tilt towards the dislocated side, with contralateral spasm of the sternocleidomastoid muscle.

Reduction may be achieved by gentle traction and manipulation under anaesthetic, or if it is more long-standing, open reduction may be required, using the far lateral approach to the cranio-cervical junction.

Atlanto-occipital dislocation may occur with extreme longitudinal distraction, with or without horizontal dislocation of the cranio-cervical junction. This often results in cardiopulmonary arrest and death. Traction will worsen the situation. Treatment involves internal fixation

Fractures of C2 include the 'hangman's fracture' through the pars interarticularis of the C2 pedicles. The resulting spondylolisthesis is more commonly caused by hyperextension and axial loading during a road traffic accident. These fractures rarely cause a neurological deficit provided there is no significant dislocation, because the diameter of the spinal canal at C2 is effectively increased by the fracture. Instability is indicated by excessive subluxation or angulation of C2 on C3, which is exaggerated on flexion and extension X-rays. Reduction may be achieved by skull traction. Most of these fractures heal with immobilisation using a halo brace or rigid orthosis. Surgery is indicated if the fracture will not reduce adequately, if there is cord compression, or if fusion is not achieved by non-operative measures. The most common operation involves an anterior approach, C2–3 discectomy, fusion and insertion of an anterior plate.

Road traffic accidents and falls from a height are a common cause of odontoid fractures in young people. However, they may occur in older people by seemingly minor falls, hitting the forehead on the ground. Acute symptoms are usually pain and occipital neuralgia, but cervical myelopathy may occur with long-standing fractures and instability. They may be classified into three types:

1 Type I fractures are through the tip of the peg, are rare, and usually stable.
2 Type II fractures are through the base of the peg, and are unstable. These are the most common peg fractures, and the least likely to fuse with immobilisation alone.
3 Type III fractures involve the body of C2, are usually stable and heal with immobilisation alone.

Surgery is usually indicated in type II fractures with excessive displacement of the peg (>4–6 mm in any direction), in older age groups when spontaneous fusion is less likely, or with chronic non-union of the fracture. Within 6 weeks of the accident, a type II peg fracture may be fixed with anterior odontoid peg screws (Figure 16.16), but after longer intervals soft tissue becomes interposed between the bone fragments and posterior C1–2 fixation and bone grafting is required (Figure 16.17). This latter operation will limit cervical rotation by 30%.

Injuries associated with hyperflexion and rotation of the neck can result in a unilateral facet joint dislocation in the subaxial cervical spine. This does not usually cause neurological deficits, nor is instability seen on flexion–extension X-rays. However, extreme hyperflexion injuries may result in bilateral dislocation of the facet joints, usually associated with more extensive disruption of joint capsules, discs and posterior ligaments. CT scanning should be performed to inspect the integrity of the facets, and traction is used to reduce bilateral dislocations. If traction is unsuccessful, then open reduction is required, either by an anterior or posterior approach, followed by fixation and bone graft fusion.

Thoracolumbar fractures The stability of thoracolumbar fractures is well described by the Denis three-column model. The spine is considered as three columns of stability: the anterior, middle and posterior columns. The anterior column consists of the anterior half of the vertebral bodies, discs and the anterior longitudinal ligament. The middle column includes the posterior half of the vertebral bodies, discs and the posterior longitudinal ligament. The posterior column is made up of the facet joints, joint capsules, laminae, spinous processes and adjoining ligaments. Disruption of two of the three columns is considered to be mechanically unstable and probably requires operative fixation, whereas disruption of a single column is likely to be stable and can be treated with bed rest. If surgery is required, posterior instrumentation with pedicle screws is the most common fixation technique, although thoracotomy or retroperitoneal approaches are sometimes required for stabilisation of the thoracic and lumbar spines, respectively.

Non-surgical management of spinal trauma

Whiplash injury Whiplash is a traumatic injury to the cervical soft tissues (including joint capsules, ligaments and muscles) resulting from hyperflexion or hyperextension, in the absence of fractures or instability. Symptoms of pain usually start several hours after the injury, and may be associated with tension headache and poor concentration. Diagnosis is by exclusion of instability, disc herniation or spinal cord injury. The extent to which the symptoms have an organic basis is controversial and medico-legal practice is swamped with claims of disabling symptoms caused by whiplash many of which probably have no justification. It is interesting to note the findings of a Lithuanian study, where few drivers have insurance and disability compensation is unlikely. In this survey there was no significant difference in the incidence of chronic neck pain in people who were involved in a road traffic accident and the general population.

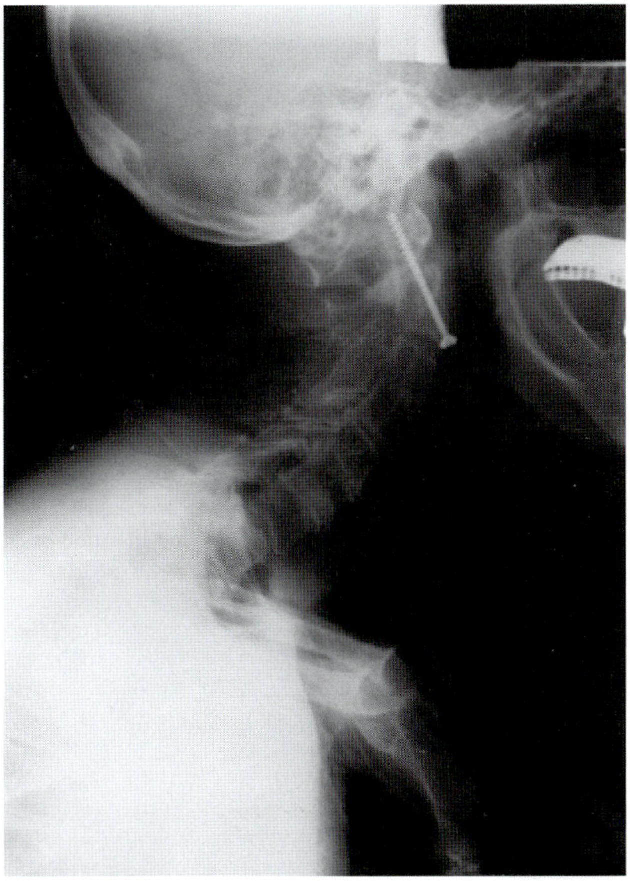

Figure 16.16 Lateral cervical X-ray showing a screw inserted to stabilise an acutely fractured odontoid peg.

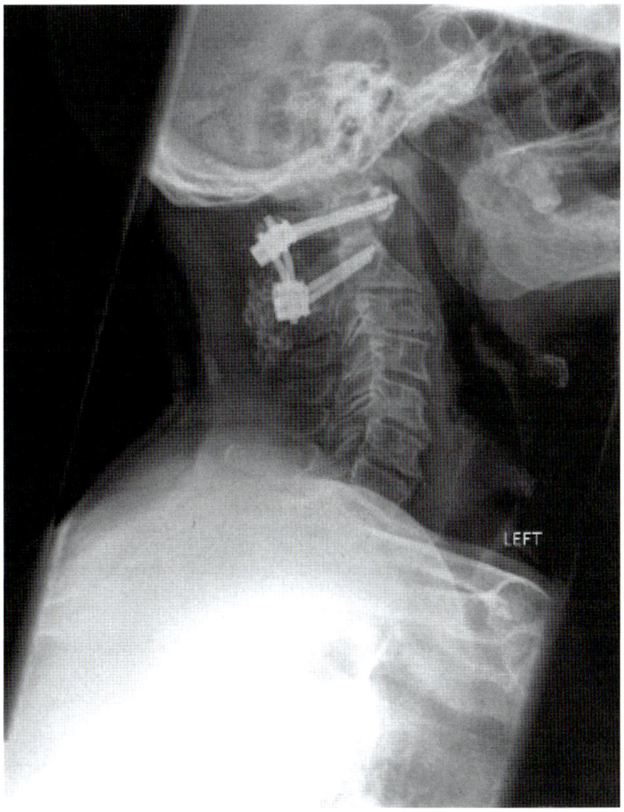

Figure 16.17 Lateral cervical X-ray showing C1–2 fixation for chronic odontoid peg fracture.

Rehabilitation Rehabilitation is covered in detail in Chapter 18. The primary goal of rehabilitation should be to increase functional capability, especially in walking and standing. Weight-supported treadmill training has shown promise in partial spinal cord lesions. In contrast to studies in the cat, at present there is little evidence in humans for a spinal central pattern generator that in the absence of descending control will drive limb movements and posture capable of supporting functional gait. Spinal pattern generators are favourably influenced by afferent feedback from the limbs and centrally by neurotransmitters, especially adrenergic transmitters. This raises the possibility that functional gains in spinal cord injured humans can be achieved through use of treadmill training supplemented by afferent stimulation and adrenergic drugs.

Long-term care of spinal cord injured patients This is considered in more detail in Chapter 18. Complications of long-term management include pressure sores, autonomic dysreflexia, spasticity, syringomyelia, deep vein thrombosis and respiratory problems. Regular turning and good standards of nursing care, physiotherapy, compression stockings, subcutaneous low molecular weight heparin and antispasmodic medications minimise these risks. Autonomic dysreflexia is an exaggerated response to normally innocuous stimuli, occurring in patients with spinal cord injury above T6, and resulting in tachycardia, hypertensive surges, sweating, anxiety and headache. The most common causes are bladder distension, faecal impaction, urinary tract and other infections, tight clothing and mild pain (pressure sores or ulcers). Treatment involves identifying and eliminating the stimulus, and pharmacological control of blood pressure and anxiety if required.

Spinal tumours

Spinal tumours may be benign or malignant, primary or secondary (Chapter 21). Consideration should always be given to the tissue of origin. Most spinal tumours are metastatic malignant tumours. Breast, bronchus, kidney, prostate, thyroid, multiple myeloma and malignant melanoma are the most primary sites.

Tumours can also be categorised by their anatomical location (i.e. extradural or intradural). Intradural tumours may be extramedullary or intramedullary (Tables 16.7 and 16.8). Intramedullary spinal cord tumours account for approximately 2% of adult and 10% of paediatric CNS neoplasms. In adults, 85–90% of intramedullary tumours are astrocytomas or ependymomas. Ependymomas account for approximately 60–70% of all spinal cord tumours found in adults, while in children 55–65% of intramedullary spinal cord tumours are astrocytomas. Haemangioblastomas account for 5% of tumours, whereas paragangliomas, oligodendrogliomas and gangliogliomas account for the remainder. Astrocytomas and ependymomas are more common in patients with neurofibromatosis type 2, which is caused by mutations in the *NF2* (neurofibromin 2 or Merlin) gene (over 200 different mutations have been described). Spinal haemangioblastomas occur in 30% of patients with von Hippel–Lindau syndrome, an autosomal dominant condition caused by mutations in the *VHL* (von Hippel–Lindau tumor suppressor) gene on 3p25.3.

Intradural tumours are now dealt with by microsurgical excision. This is aided in certain cases by the use of an ultrasonic aspirator where an en bloc excision is not feasible. Spinal cord monitoring using somato-sensory evoked potentials and motor evoked potentials improves the operative safety margin.

Ependymomas are usually resectable. Primary astrocytomas can occasionally be completely resected. Surgical excision is easier in children than adults. Complications for intramedullary tumours are common with most patients experiencing short-term neurological deterioration. The role of radiotherapy for intramedullary tumours is controversial. Repeat surgery should probably be considered first for tumour progression. Many of these tumours are slow growing so treatment effects are difficult to judge. In Brotchi's series of 239 patients with low-grade spinal tumours, 5% worsened, 50% stabilised and 40% improved. A patient's neurological function after surgical intervention depends on his or her pre-operative neurological condition. The goal of surgery is to prevent further neurologic dysfunction and to cure the neoplastic condition with complete resection.

Neurofibromas (schwannomas) are relatively easy to remove, with very low morbidity. This is because schwannomas usually arise from the sensory nerve root and the resulting spinal compression is slowly progressive.

Meningiomas arise from the meninges (Figure 16.18), are more common in women and most often affect the thoracic region. Surgical results are generally very good. Operative morbidity most commonly arises from dural defects producing leakage of CSF. Radical excision of the dural origin of the tumour will give the best chance of cure, minimising the risk of tumour recurrence.

Metastatic spinal tumours Secondary bone tumours are becoming more common, partly as a result of an increasingly ageing population, and partly because of better treatments and longer survival for the primary tumour types. The goal of treatment for metastatic spinal tumours is to improve quality of life and functional independence,

Table 16.7 Classification of intradural intramedullary spinal tumours.

Tumour type	Incidence in adults
Ependymoma	65%
Astrocytoma (fibrillary or pilocytic) WHO 2	30–35%
Glioblastoma WHO 4	1.5%
Haemangioblastoma	1–3%
(25% of patients have von Hipplel–Lindau)	
Other glial tumours	Very rare
(Oligodendroglioma, ganglioglioma)	
Metastases	Rare
Cavernomas	Rare

Table 16.8 Classsification of intradural extramedullary tumours.

Meningioma
Neurofibroma/schwannoma including dumb-bell tumours
Paraganglioma
Metastatic including lepromeningeal disease
Arachnoid cyst
Perineural cysts including Tarlov cysts
Epidermoid

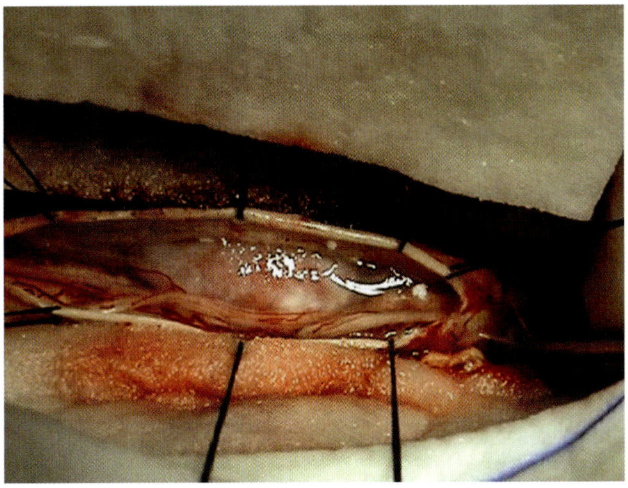

Figure 16.18 Operative photograph of intradural microscopic exploration of spinal meningioma with overlying arachnoid intact. Stay sutures hold dura open, tumour arises from anterolateral dura mater.

rather than a definitive removal of the spinal tumour. Life expectancy is not generally increased by treating metastatic spinal tumours, but quality of life can be improved by treating spinal pain, instability or neurological compression. It is important to balance the potential gain in quality of life provided by surgery, chemotherapy and/or radiotherapy, with the known side effects of these treatments which are not insignificant, taking into account the prognosis and opinion of the individual patient.

Historically, surgery involved laminectomy for resection of posterior elements and extradural tumours. While this approach decompressed the spinal cord it further destabilised the spinal column. Most tumours metastasise to the vertebral body and therefore resection of the posterior elements removes the only sound bone in the vertebral complex therefore leading to instability, and deformity with ensuing neurological deterioration and pain. Findlay (1984) found that surgery (laminectomy) provided no better results than radiotherapy alone, and was associated with more complications. However, in a multi-centre randomised controlled series, Patchell *et al.* have recently demonstrated that surgery and radiotherapy are superior to radiotherapy alone. This study was stopped after planned interim analysis showed superiority of the surgical treatment arm. Outcome measures included pain, ambulation, neurological recovery and bladder control. All outcomes were better with surgical treatment. Other studies have shown surgery should precede radiotherapy. Radiotherapy followed by surgery is associated with a doubling of wound complications breakdown or infection.

Spinal manifestations of neurofibromatosis type 1 Neurofibromatosis is dealt with elsewhere in this book (Chapter 26) but its spinal manifestations are especially important and so are outlined here. These include various tumour types but also varied and complex spinal deformities (kyphoscoliosis) and dural ectasia.

Neurofibromas The typical spinal nerve sheath tumours seen in neurofibratosis type 1 (NF1) patients are benign neurofibromas. They consist of fibroblasts, nerve sheaths and nerve cells. The nerve cells are incorporated into the tumour mass, which complicates surgical removal of the tumour. The spinal nerve root neurofibromas in NF1 are often asymptomatic. A rapid increase in size may be a sign of malignant change, albeit a rare complication; less than 5% of patients with NF1 develop neurofibrosarcomas. In most instances, malignant progression of the fibroblast component appears to be responsible for the development of malignancy, and molecular genetic studies suggest that inactivation of the p53 tumour suppressor gene is a important factor in the sarcomatous progression of neurofibromas.

Fusiform neurofibromas of spinal nerves are usually bilateral, extend to the branch fibres of the nerve and exceed 30 cm in length. They are seen on CT scans as tumours of low attenuation with areas of higher density, which enhance with intravenous contrast medium. MRI shows nerve sheath tumours to be iso-intense or slightly hyperintense with respect to muscle on T1, enhanced T1 and T2 sequences. In approximately 50% of cases, a target pattern with a peripheral hyperintense rim and central low intensity may be seen. This pattern corresponds histologically to peripheral myxomatous tissue and central fibrocollagenous tissue. This pattern is absent in lesions with cystic, haemorrhagic or necrotic changes.

Benign nerve sheath tumours usually have intradural extramedullary location. They extend extradurally and have a dumb-bell configuration through the intervertebral foramen in as many as half of cases. Solitary tumours may involve individual nerves, or multiple nerves may be involved in a plexiform fashion. The tumours are usually multiple, appear at different levels and show different stages of growth. Plexiform neurofibromas involve long segments of the spinal nerves and extend into the spinal cord. They appear more frequently in the second and third decades of life, and the cervical and thoracic segments are primarily affected.

In 1999, Thakkar *et al.* reported 54 patients with NF1 aged 5–56 years and found spinal tumours in 65%. A tumour was discovered in almost all symptomatic patients and in 40% of asymptomatic patients. The site of the tumour was intramedullary in 6%, intraspinal extramedullary in 33% and intraforaminal in 57%.

Lesions of the bony spine in NF1 Spinal and skeletal changes are observed in up to 71% of NF1 patients. They can be classified as:

1 Bony erosions caused by a tumour
2 Pressure damage from intradural, extradural and paravertebral nerve sheath tumours affecting mainly the intervertebral foramen and the spinal canal
3 Osteomalacia from a genetic tubular defect
4 Congenital abnormalities, such as macrocranium, and
5 Mesodermal dysplasias, such as pseudoarthrosis of the extremities, local gigantism and scoliosis.

Abnormal spinal curvature is detected in up to 40% of patients with NF1. The majority of cases develop problems between 11 and 16 years of age. A short segment of angular scoliosis with five or fewer vertebrae primarily involved, usually located in the lower thoracic region, is diagnostic of NF1.

Kyphosis of varying degrees is usually associated with NF1 scoliosis. Kyphosis has been considered a poor prognostic sign because of its tendency to rapid progression and resistance to all types of treatment. Localised or multi-level dural ectasia with enlargement of the spinal canal is also a relatively common finding in neurofibromatosis and is strongly associated with kyphoscoliosis. On X-ray, dural ectasia is associated with vertebral scalloping or concavity of vertebral bodies. The cause of dural ectasia may be a congenital weakness of the dura, in which case the constant pulsation of CSF causes progressive enlargement of the dural sac with resultant scalloping of the posterior portions of the vertebral bodies and erosion of the pedicles. Scalloping of bone may also result from

NF1-related primary bone dysplasia. The damaged vertebra result in disorders of spinal alignment and are interestingly not necessarily directly related to an underlying neurofibroma.

Primary bone tumours These are comparatively rare. They may be benign (e.g. aneurysmal bone cyst, osteoid osteoma, osteoblastoma) or malignant. Some tumours occur much more commonly in younger age groups (e.g. aneurysmal bone cyst or Ewing's tumour). Osteosarcoma has a bimodal age distribution affecting young children and older patients, the latter being associated with malignant changes in Paget's disease. The most common tumours are those arising from the bone marrow, particularly multiple myeloma. A more detailed description of these tumours is outside the remit of this chapter. A working classification is based on tissue origin with tumour types differentiated into bone forming, cartilage forming, giant cell tumours, bone marrow tumours, vascular tumours, other connective tissue tumours, other tumours and tumour-like lesions. The simplified list in Table 16.9 contains examples of each tumour type and is based on the World Health Organization (WHO) classification.

Table 16.9 Modified World Health Organization (WHO) classification of primary skeletal tumours.

Tissue type	Examples of lesion type
Bone	Osteoma (B)
	Osteoid osteoma (B)
	Osteosarcoma – central and peripheral (M)
Cartilage	Chondroma (B)
	Osteochondroma (B)
	Chondrosarcoma (different types) (M)
Giant cell	Osteoblastoma (B)
Bone marrow	Ewing's sarcoma (M)
	Lymphoma (M)
	Myeloma (M)
Vascular	Haemangioma (B)
	Lymphangioma (B)
	Glomus tumour (B)
	Angiosarcoma (M)
Other connective	Fibroma (B)
	Lipoma (B)
	Fibrosarcoma (M)
	Liposarcoma (M)
	Leiomyosarcoma (M)
Other tumours	Neurofibroma (B)
	Neurilemmoma (B)
	Adamantinoma (M)
	Chordoma (M)
Tumour-like	Simple + aneurysmal cysts
	Fibrous dysplasia
	Eosinophilic granuloma

B, benign; M, malignant.

With the exception of Ewing's tumour, primary spine tumours are usually treated by excisional surgery. En bloc resection is useful for chordoma but is often not technically possible. Chordomas arise from the notochord remnants. The majority arise from the most rostral and caudal notochord remnants (craniocervical/clivus and sacral; Figure 16.19).

With the development of more reliable spinal fixation and reconstruction techniques, removal of the whole vertebra is now technically feasible either piecemeal or en bloc. However, in the cervical spine the vertebral artery prevents such an aggressive approach. In the thoracic and lumbar spine posterior en bloc resection is a favoured approach. Titanium mesh expandable cages or stackable carbon fibres cages allow reconstruction of the vertebral body. Spinal stability is also assisted by pedicle screw fixation (Figure 16.20)

Degenerative disease of the spine

Cervical spine Age-related degenerative disease in the cervical spine most commonly affects the mid cervical levels, reflecting the distribution of stress in the neck with upright posture and loading. In younger people, more movement occurs at C5–6 and C6–7 and these levels are the most commonly affected, whereas in older age groups C4–5 and C3–4 become affected in addition. Occasionally, involvement of the atlanto-axial joints and ligaments can produce instability and a soft tissue mass, or 'pseudotumour', in the position of the degenerate odontoid process. Cervical disc degeneration is associated with the formation of osteophytes around the annular attachments to the end-plates, with reciprocal degeneration and hypertrophy of the facet joints. Dehydration of the discs may result in reversal of the normal lordosis to produce a straight neck or even kyphotic deformity. Vertebral subluxations may occur.

Atlanto-axial instability may occur because of degenerative changes in the joints and ligaments at the cranio-cervical junction producing a pseudotumour around the degenerate odontoid process (Figure 16.21). When this occurs, treatment involves fusion of

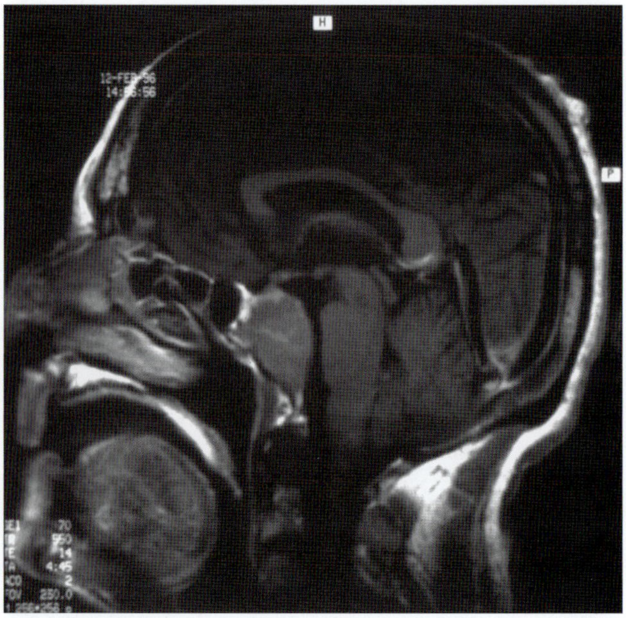

Figure 16.19 MRI showing clival chordoma.

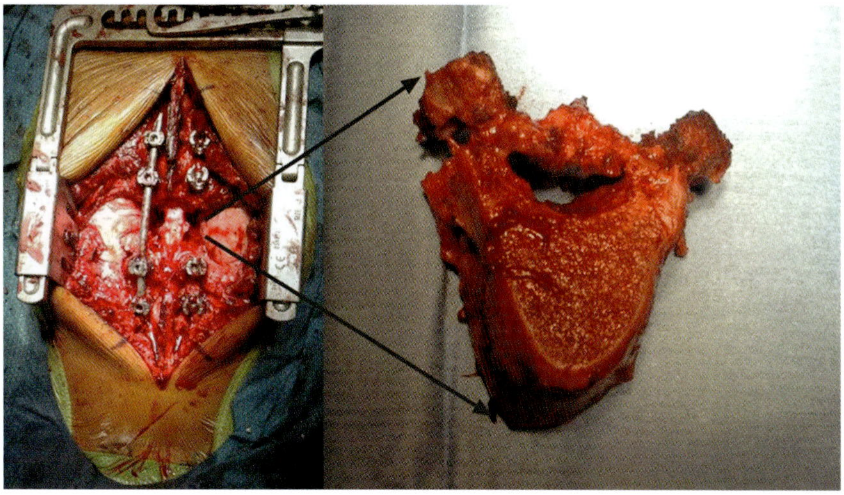

Figure 16.20 Showing spinal fixation and specimen.

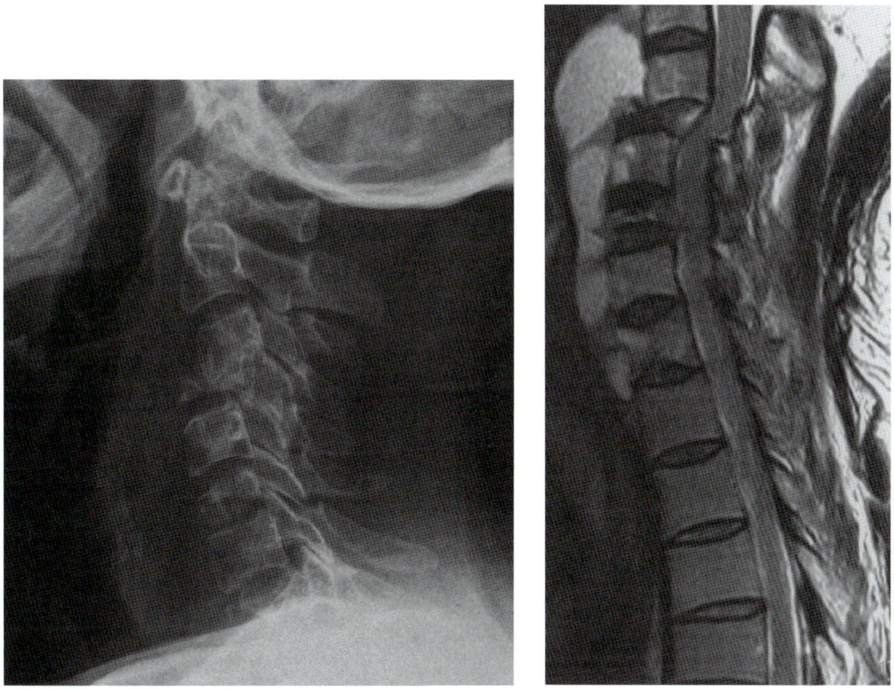

(a) (b)

Figure 16.21 (a) Lateral cervical; spine with pathological collapse C34 disc space and C6 vertebra with retropharyngeal swelling. (b) T2- weighted sagittal MRI showing pre-vertebral swelling, kyphosis.

C1 and C2, with surveillance MRI to ensure the size of the odontoid mass does not increase. If the diagnosis is in doubt then a transoral biopsy should be taken. In the subaxial spine, osteophytosis can cause radiculopathy if stenosis of nerve root canals develops, or myelopathy if the spinal canal is sufficiently compromised.

Radicular pain usually follows a waxing and waning course, with intermittent exacerbations but, like lumbar radiculopathy, most symptoms of brachalgia settle down with time and surgery is often not required. Cervical myelopathy may occur because of disc herniation and osteophytic compression of the cervical cord. Furthermore, the anterior horn cells of the cervical expansion are affected by direct compression, arterial insufficiency, venous congestion, repetitive minor trauma or a combination of these events. In general, 25% of patients with spondylotic cervical cord compression remain static, but 75% progressively deteriorate.

Non-surgical management of cervical degenerative disease
Treatment of musculoskeletal axial spinal pain initially involves removing exacerbating factors such as heavy lifting, and improving posture and muscles of core stability with physiotherapy and allied techniques. The patient should be encouraged to stay active with gentle exercise, such as walking, as far as possible. Simple back pain is usually self-limiting, and the majority of patients improve within a few weeks with conservative measures. Paracetamol and non-steroidal

anti-inflammatory medication are helpful, and occasionally stronger analgesics or benzodiazepine muscle relaxants may be required for short durations. Acupuncture, transcutaneous electrical nerve stimulation (TENS), ultrasound, heat or cold treatments, massage, hydrotherapy, chiropractic treatment or osteopathy may also be useful. If back pain persists for more than 6 weeks, the patient should be reviewed by a clinician to exclude other causes of pain including neoplasia, arthritides, osteoporotic fractures, infection or nerve root compression. Persistent mechanical pain may be treated with steroid injection to the facet joints, nerve roots, or epidural space depending on the presenting features and MRI findings.

Spinal cord or nerve root compression may require surgical management. Spinal cord compression (e.g. because of cervical disc prolapse) is likely to require decompression because patients tend to deteriorate with time. However, nerve root compression is common with increasing age and is not always associated with pain. Decompression should be performed for persistent or severe radicular pain that does not respond to conservative measures. The evidence for the benefit of nerve root decompression for the treatment of motor radiculopathy (in the absence of pain) is unclear.

Surgical management of cervical degenerative disease For cervical degenerative disease, surgery may be considered if symptoms fail to improve after 2–3 months, or if neurological signs progress. Surgery to decompress cervical roots may be by anterior or posterior approaches. Anterior cervical discectomy with decompression of the nerve roots is performed if there is any coexistent cord compression, or if the majority of root compression is caused by disc prolapse. Posterior foraminotomy is a simpler operation that may be used if there is no cord compression. This approach avoids the small risk of recurrent laryngeal nerve palsy that may occur with anterior operations, and does not require fusion of a motion segment, but is associated with more postoperative neck pain in the short term. There is an overall risk of spinal cord or nerve root injury during surgery, in approximately 1% of patients to varying extents, and this together with other possible complications need to be taken into consideration when deciding to proceed with surgical treatment.

In cervical myelopathy it is common to observe an initial deterioration followed by a period of stabilisation, but most patients will later progress further if untreated. The main aim of surgery is to prevent deterioration; however, improvement can occur. Surgical treatment may be performed anteriorly, by cervical discectomy and sometimes corpectomy, or posteriorly by laminectomy or laminoplasty. The method of decompression depends on the degree of lordosis or kyphosis of the spine, the main cause of the cord compression and surgeons' preference. If the cord compression is mainly caused by a disc prolapse in a kyphotic neck, then anterior decompression is preferable. Compression from hypertrophy of the ligamentum flavum in a lordotic neck is best treated by posterior decompression. After laminectomy there is a risk of progressive kyphosis because of removal of the posterior tension-band elements of the cervical spine, leading many surgeons to adopt the technique of spinal canal augmentation by laminoplasty which was originally developed in Japan for treatment of patients with ossification of the posterior longitudinal ligament

The overall results of anterior and posterior decompressive surgery for myelopathy are similar, although it should be remembered that the indications for each approach are different and therefore not directly comparable. After laminectomy in one series, 56% of patients improved, 25% were unchanged and 19% slightly worse, and with anterior decompression 75% of patients improved.

Fusion after cervical discectomy has been the standard treatment for a number of years, but there is an increased incidence of accelerated degenerative disease in adjacent discs, because of the added mechanical stresses placed on adjacent discs after fusion of a previously mobile segment. Within 10 years of fusion, around 29% of adjacent discs will degenerate and require surgery. To avoid this complication, a number of different artificial disc implants have been developed that do not restrict movement after anterior decompression, and thereby minimise the development of adjacent segment disease (Figure 16.22). The short-term results of artificial disc implants have been favourable, but in the longer term it is unclear as to whether they will require replacement within a lifetime.

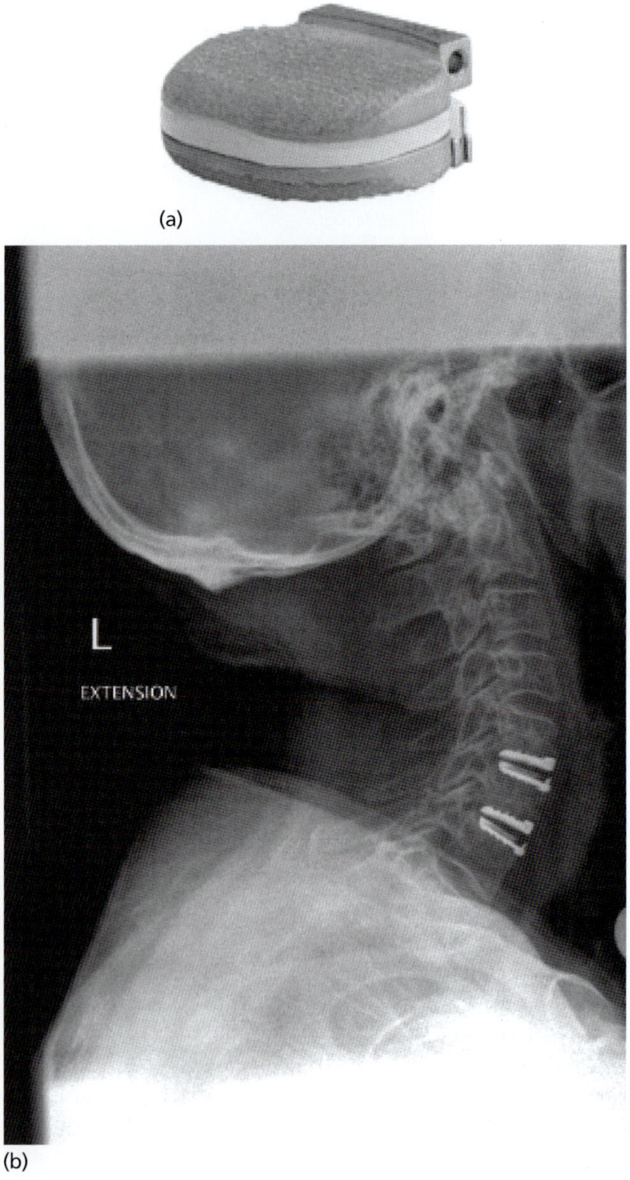

Figure 16.22 (a) Photograph of artificial cervical disc implant. (b) Lateral cervical spine X-ray showing artificial disc implants at two levels.

Thoracic spine Degenerative disease in the thoracic spine is less common than in the cervical and lumbar spine because of the decreased movement that occurs at thoracic levels. Thoracic disc prolapses account for only 0.5% of all disc prolapses and usually occur in younger age groups (third to fifth decades) at T8–12 levels. Patients often present with a history of chronic pain with only subtle sensory or motor changes.

Surgical treatment of thoracic disc disease In symptomatic patients, discectomy is performed by an anterolateral approach, most commonly by thoracotomy. Direct posterior approaches are associated with a high risk of mechanical cord damage and should be avoided, although in some cases a posterolateral approach (transpedicular or costotransversectomy) may be appropriate. The spinal fusion is achieved in a similar way to cervical spine surgery if required.

Lumbar spine Lumbar canal stenosis may occur because of acquired degenerative changes such as hypertrophy of facet joints, ligamentum flavum, disc prolapse or spondylolisthesis, or congenital causes such as achondroplasia. If the spinal canal cross-sectional area diminishes below a critical value then radicular symptoms or neurogenic claudication may occur, either because of direct compression or ischaemia of nerve roots. Neurological examination may be normal, including straight-leg raising. The natural history if untreated is a slowly progressive course with most symptoms remaining the same, or gradually worsening over the next few years after diagnosis. Treatment is by laminectomy with or without discectomy; 60–80% of claudication improves after surgery.

Lumbar disc prolapse is a common cause of radicular leg pain, and is present in 1–3% of people with lower back pain. Approximately 80–90% of patients with radicular leg pain improve over the following few months without surgery. Long periods of immobilisation should be discouraged and gentle mobilisation and exercise can aid recovery. 'Red flags' of urinary incontinence, urinary retention, faecal incontinence, peri-anal numbness and leg weakness should prompt urgent referral for an MRI scan to exclude a central disc prolapse and cauda equina compression. Otherwise, unless the pain is refractory to medical treatment, 2–3 months of pain management is recommended before consideration of surgery.

The L4–5 and L5–S1 vertebral discs are the most common levels of disc prolapse. They produce L5 and S1 radiculopathies, respectively. A disc prolapse more commonly involves the nerve root of the level below. For example, at L4–5, although the L4 nerve root exits at that level, it has already exited lateral to the common position of a disc bulge and will not be caught by it unless the bulge is more laterally placed. Instead, the L4–5 disc bulge will usually catch the L5 nerve root *en passant*.

Surgical treatment of lumbar disc disease Lumbar microdiscectomy is the standard surgical technique for removing disc prolapses, although percutaneous techniques (using laser, thermocoagulation, chymopapain or mechanical disruption with a nucleotome) and minimally invasive techniques are now sometimes used with limited efficacy. In a randomised controlled trial of microdiscectomy versus non-surgical therapies, surgically treated patients had better outcomes at 1 year, but the difference was not significant by 4 and 10 years.

Low back pain and degenerative disc disease

Low back pain affects 70–85% of population at some point in their lives, with an incidence of 15% and point prevalence of 30%. The primary risk factor is age-related degenerative changes in the lumbar spine. The intervertebral discs in particular show degeneration which can be appreciated as loss of hydration on MRI. By the age of 50 years 90% of the population show loss of hydration of the nucleus pulposus.

The disc comprises the nucleus pulposus, a gelatinous structure surrounded by the annulus fibrosus. With ageing there are changes in the collagen matrix, loss of hydration, apoptosis and loss of the blood supply. The hydrostatic mechanisms for dissipation of force are lost. This, coupled with weakening of the annulus, leads to an increased risk of rupture of the nucleus pulposus through the annulus fibrosus. This is most likely to occur during loading of the spine in flexion and torsion. Importantly, the nucleus pulposus is likely to be an immune privileged site. The evidence for this is that it expresses the FAS ligand like other immune privileged tissues, which induces apoptosis of FAS-positive invading T cells. The annulus fibrosus and notochord elements do not express FAS ligand. Extrusion of the disc into the epidural space sets up an intense inflammatory process with autoimmune reaction and inflammatory cell infiltration. There is a resulting increase in inflammatory cytokines especially interleukin 1, tumour necrosis factor α (TNF-α), interleukin 6 along with increased levels of prostaglandin E2. In degenerate discs there is an increase in matrix metalloproteinases (MMPs). MMPs are zinc-dependent enzymes that are involved in modelling of connective tissue. Experimental data implicates MMPs 1 and 2 in the pathogenesis of disc herniation. Ultimately, spontaneous resorption of herniated disc material may occur as the result of action of MMPs and cytokines.

The pain in degenerative spinal disease results from a variety of interacting mechanisms. A major contributor to the pain is the inflammatory response evoked by the disc herniation. There are important nociceptive contributions from the facet joints, vertebrae, muscles, ligaments and facia. Nociceptive pathways involve the sinovertebral nerve, which arises from the ventral root and grey rami near the dorsal root ganglion to innervate a number of structures, particularly the posterior longitudinal ligament. There is also a noiceptive contribution from the dorsal root ganglion.

Management of lower back pain Pain may be managed by conservative and surgical methods. If radicular pain is very severe, then bed rest may be advised to minimise loading of the lumbar spine and nerve root foramina, with analgesia (including paracetamol and non-steroid anti-inflammatory drugs), and sometimes benzodiazepine muscle relaxants. However, prolonged bed rest beyond 3–4 days should be discouraged because it is usually associated with a worse outcome than a gradual return to normal activities and work. Heavy lifting, prolonged sitting and abnormal postures should be discouraged, and a program of gentle exercise and education established, often supplemented with physiotherapy. Correct posture, sleeping position and lifting techniques are important.

Chiropractics and osteopathy, acupuncture, epidural steroid and facet joint injections may help in the short term, but there is little evidence of long-term benefits. Spinal manipulation should not be performed in the presence of severe or progressive neurological deficit.

Surgical lumbar fusion is accepted practice in the presence of instability resulting from tumour, trauma, infection or degenerative disease, but its use for mechanical back pain alone is controversial. A randomised controlled trial comparing surgical fusion with an intensive rehabilitation programme revealed improvements in both groups after treatment, but no significant difference between surgery and rehabilitation. Whereas surgical fixation was associated with an improved outcome, there is limited evidence to support the use of surgery in the absence of instability. In fact, surgical fusion of a mobile segment is associated with exaggerated adjacent disc disease in 20% of patients over the next 10 years after surgery. This has stimulated interest in artificial disc replacements, such as the 'ProDisc' and 'Charite' prosthetic lumbar discs, which have been associated with good outcomes in back pain and patient satisfaction after 2 years from operation. However, recent reports suggest that some of these disc replacements actually result in a fusion anyway, without changing the patient outcome.

Spinal infections

All components of the spine are vulnerable to attack by bacterial, fungal, viral and parasitical infections. The structures involved include the vertebral column, most commonly the intervertebral disc (discitis) and the vertebra (osteomyelitis). Infection can spread to the extradural space with abscess formation and the intradural contents can also be affected. Intramedullary infection is very rare. Further detailed discussion of infectious disease of the nervous system and spine can be found in Chapter 9.

Bacterial infections of the spine In adults, lumbar bacterial infections often originate from urinary tract infections which drain via the Batson venous plexus. The respiratory system is a common source of blood-borne infection with spinal infection usually following the initial infection by some 1–8 weeks. Purulent material may break out of cortex of the bone anteriorly to form a paravertebral abscess or posteriorly to form an epidural abscess. Infection-related weakening of the bone may cause vertebral body collapse. Haematogenous osteomyelitis is seen more often in children than in adults. This is believed to be because the epiphyseal plate present in the growing skeleton of a child and absent in adults is more vulnerable than mature bone to blood-borne infection. Risk factors for bacterial spinal infection include an immunocompromised state, including diabetes, TB, HIV, malnutrition and intravenous drug use.

The risk factors for bacterial discitis are the same as those for osteomyelitis. Iatrogenic cases occur after disc surgery, therapeutic injections, lumbar puncture and epidural anaesthesia. The most common organism is *Staphylococcus aureus*, particularly *Staphylococcus epidermidis*. Methicillin-resistant *Staphylococcus aureus* (MRSA) can occur. *Streptococcus viridans* is the next most common infecting organism.

Treatment of pyogenic discitis and spinal osteomyelitis Blood cultures often identify the infecting organism and guide appropriate antibiotics use. Because of difficulty in obtaining a culture from blood, CT-guided biopsy of the infected area should always be considered prior to antibiotics. Epidural abscesses are usually considered to be a surgical problem but in a debilitated patient with a small thin abscess and a bacteriological diagnosis-appropriate antibiotic, chemotherapy alone is a reasonable approach.

Antibiotics are given for variable lengths of time and 2–3 months of parenteral therapy may be required. Before parenteral antibiotics are discontinued, the erythrocyte sedimentation rate (ESR) should have fallen to at least two-thirds of the pre-treatment level. In addition, the patient should be afebrile, without pain on mobilisation, and ideally improving from disease-related neurological complications. A persistently high ESR or C-reactive protein implies continuing infection, and additional intravenous antibiotics are indicated. In such an instance, additional biopsies for microbial culture may need to be taken.

Bracing or other forms of orthosis is strongly recommended to provide stability for the spine while the infection is being treated and the tissues are healing. The goal of spinal immobilisation is to provide opportunity for the affected spinal level(s) to fuse in an anatomically aligned position. Bracing is usually continued for 6–12 weeks, until either a bony fusion is seen on radiography or until the patient's pain subsides. A rigid brace is optimal and only need be worn when the patient is upright or mobile. Surgical fixation may be required if mechanical instability develops, or if the infection is refractory to conservative measures.

Spinal tuberculosis Mycobacterium tuberculosis (TB) of the spine is an uncommon form of tuberculosis occurring in less than 1% of patients with tuberculosis. TB typically first affects the intervertebral discs. The primary risk factors for TB infection in the United Kingdom are ethnicity and/or immunocompromise.

TB infection typically presents with local pain, fever, night sweats and general ill health including weight loss. If the disease spreads from the disc into the vertebral body osteomyelitis will occur with epidural abscess formation and/or vertebral body collapse. Pathological fractures will cause pain, deformity (kyphosis) and in some cases spinal cord compression.

The diagnosis is difficult in patients with no evidence of extraspinal TB. The clinical presentation together with the radiological appearances (plain X-ray, CT and MRI scan) of spinal TB and a positive tuberculin test usually suggest a diagnosis of spinal tuberculosis.

In Pott's disease, the spinal cord may become involved either because of compression by disrupted bone and/or disc and ligaments, expansion of a TB abscess or by direct invasion of cord and leptomeninges by granulation tissue. Primary tuberculoma of the spinal cord is rare. Neurological deficits when present usually develop gradually. A positive diagnosis is made from detection and culture of acid-fast bacilli from the bone or body fluids. Polymerase chain reaction (PCR) detection of mycobacterium DNA may speed the diagnosis but initiation of effective treatment should not be delayed if the clinical index of suspicion is high.

With the advent of effective combination chemotherapy in the early 1950s, the mortality rate among patients with spinal TB decreased from nearly 100% to 3%. It is important to note that while triple and quadruple therapy drug regimens remain highly effective for most cases of spinal TB, in immuno-compromised patients, especially those with HIV/AIDs, drug-resistant TB is an increasing problem.

Role of surgery in spinal tuberculosis The initial procedure introduced for the surgical treatment of spinal infections was laminectomy. However, this procedure did not allow access to anterior abscesses and contributed to spinal instability, which often resulted in progressive deformity. In 1960, Hodgson and Stock extensively reported on this procedure in the treatment of TB of the spine. Late spinal deformity was prevented with spinal fusion and instrumentation. The need for an anterior approach (by thoracotomy) was stimulated by the failures of posterior fusion in some of their patients, many of whom had TB involving four to eight vertebrae and such pronounced kyphosis as to make posterior fusion mechanically unsound. The current surgical management of spinal TB requires of radical débridement and anterior fusion. The anterior approach gives a wide access to the disease. The removal of all avascular bone is essential to ensure rapid sound bone fusion. Anterior fusion by bone transplantation after a thorough excision of the disease focus is successful in a very high proportion of cases.

The Medical Research Council (MRC) examined the role of surgery for spinal TB with antibiotic chemotherapy versus antibiotic chemotherapy alone. The first MRC trial, published in 1974, of the treatment of spinal TB revealed equivalent results at 5 years when chemotherapy alone was compared with radical surgical treatment combined with chemotherapy. The primary advantage of anterior spinal arthrodesis was a decreased tendency for progression of deformity. The role of surgery for spinal TB has been re-examined in a recent Cochrane review which concluded that the data were insufficient to be clear whether surgery with chemotherapy is better than chemotherapy alone. However, it is very important to note that very few patients in the MRC trial were neurologically affected. Furthermore, it is important to appreciate that the surgical approach analysed by the original MRC trials is not comparable to modern spinal surgery performed by specialist spinal surgeons with high-quality spinal instrumentation, modern anaesthesia, intraoperative neurophysiological monitoring with decisions informed by neurologists and infectious diseases specialists and by modern radiology (MRI and CT scanning). Surgery may be indicated in certain subgroups of patients, particularly those presenting with a significant neurological deficit, with progressive neurological deficits, those who develop neurological deficits on appropriate antibiotic therapy and those with an initial kyphosis angle greater than 30°, especially in a child with further skeletal growth potential.

Fungal infections Fungal infections of the spine are rare. Fungi such as *Cryptococcus*, *Candida* and *Aspergillus* are found worldwide, whereas *Coccidioides immitis* and *Blastomyces dermatitidis* are limited to specific geographical areas. *Aspergillus* and many *Candida* species are normal commensals of the body and produce disease in susceptible individuals when they gain access to the vascular system through intravenous lines, during implantation of prosthetic devices or during surgery. Other fungi produce spinal involvement usually as a result of haematogenous or direct spread of organisms from an initial pulmonary source of infection. Involvement of the vertebral bodies can lead to vertebral compression fractures and gross deformity of the spine. Spread of infection along the anterior longitudinal ligament can lead to psoas or paravertebral abscesses, similar to tuberculosis. Recognition of the disease requires a high index of suspicion, proper travel history and a detailed physical examination. Treatment relies on the early and effective pharmacotherapy and constant monitoring of clinical progress and is discussed in Chapter 9. Resistance to medical therapy, spinal instability and neurologic deficits are indications for spinal débridement and stabilisation with spinal fusion. Prognosis depends on the premorbid state of the patient, the type of fungal organism and the timing of treatment. Immuno-compromised patients fare badly.

Acute viral infections These are covered in greater details in Chapter 9. Acute myelitis may result from direct infection with a number of virus including the herpes group (herpes simplex virus 1 and 2, herpes zoster virus, cytomegalovirus and Epstein–Barr virus), enteroviruses and, especially in the United States, the flavivirus family.

Subacute infections These subdivide into bacterial viral and other. Typically, pyogenic bacterial infections are acute or subacute. Tuberculosis, syphilis, fungal infections, Lyme disease and *Mycoplasma* are subacute or chronic.

Specific viral infections causing myelopathy are human T-cell lymphotropic virus 1 and 2 (HTLV-1 and 2) and HIV. Para-infectious and post-vaccine myelopathies have been described following exposure to herpes zoster virus, *Mycoplasma*, mumps, hepatitis B and rabies.

Chronic viral infections of the spinal cord Tropical spastic paraparesis (TSP) is a viral infection of the spinal cord that causes weakness in the legs due to HTLV-1 and 2 retrovirus. Symptoms may begin years after infection. In response to the infection, the body's immune response may injure nerve tissue, causing symptoms that include neurogenic bladder problems, leg pain and loss of feeling in the feet, tingling sensations and unpleasant sensations when the skin is touched. Patients with TSP may also exhibit uveitis, arthritis, pulmonary lymphocytic alveolitis, polymyositis, keratoconjunctivitis sicca and infectious dermatitis. Some factors that might have a role in transmitting the disorder include being a recipient of transfusion blood products (especially before 1989), breast milk feeding from a seropositive mother, intravenous drug use or being the sexual partner of a seropositive individual for several years. Not every HTLV-1 seropositive carrier will develop TSP; fewer than 5% will exhibit neurological dysfunction or, eventually, haematological malignancy such as adult T-cell leukaemia/lymphoma.

Treatment of tropical spastic paraparesis Initial trials of treatment using antiretroviral drugs have not produced neurological improvement nor have they convincingly shown a slowing of disease progression. Essentially there are two approaches. The first is to try to inhibit viral replication. This has been attempted with antiviral drugs: the reverse transcriptase inhibitor zidovudine (AZT) and the cytosine analogue lamivudine alone and in combination. However, in contrast to HIV, the virus replicates without the need for reverse transcription and although these drugs can produce a reduction in HTLV-1 pro-viral load, little clinical response was seen in a randomised double-blind placebo controlled trial of Combivir (zidovudine + lamivudine). The second approach has been to suppress the immune response both with steroids, steroid-sparing drugs and interferon-1α. Although short-term improvements have been noted, no sustained clinical improvement or measurable reduction in disease progression is yet reported in rigorous analysis of the effects of these approaches. Future trials are in progress and are planned to assess the affects of ciclosporin, anti-TNFα and alemtuzumab (Campath 1H).

There are numerous acute viral causes of transverse myelitis which are discussed in the following section and in Chapter 9.

Spinal cord inflammation

Devic disease (neuromyelitis optica) There is strong evidence that this disease is a separate entity from multiple sclerosis. It is characterised by episodes of myelopathy and optic neuropathy which are often severe. It is more common amongst the Japanese. The involvement of optic nerve and spinal cord is selective. The condition is discussed in Chapter 11. In the spinal cord the critical radiological differential diagnosis is from multiple sclerosis. It is strongly suspected if there is a contiguous segment of central spinal cord inflammation extending over three or more vertebral segments.

A Devic-like syndrome is also described in association with other autoimmune diseases including systemic lupus erythematosus (SLE). Neurological sarcoidosis may also present with a Devic-like picture of spinal and optic nerve inflammation (Figure 16.23). In these conditions there is a myelitis sometimes associated with optic neuropathy. Often, extensive investigation is required to look for evidence of SLE, CNS sarcoid, Behçet's disease, vasculitis,

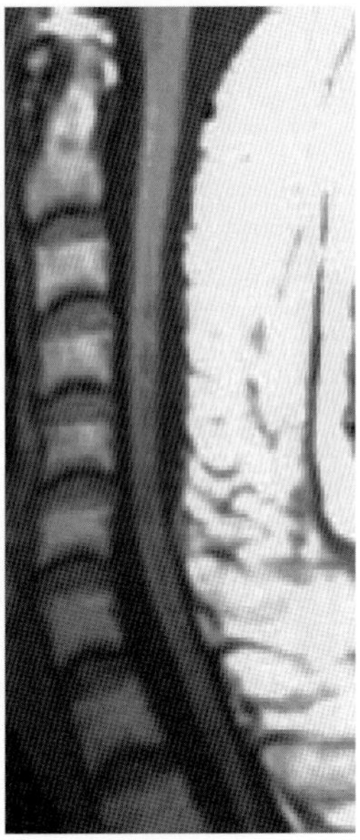

Figure 16.23 Sagittal MRI of cervical cord (T1-weighted) showing extensive intrinsic cord lesion with cavitation in case of Devic's disease.

infectious and para-infectious myelitis including acute disseminated encephalomyelitis (ADEM) and post-vaccine myelitis and para-neoplastic conditions. The differential diagnosis of transverse myelitis is very extensive (Table 16.10).

NMO antibodies are present in 50–70% of patients with NMO or NMO spectrum disorder (in constrast to multiple sclerosis, which is not an antibody-mediated condition). These antibodies target the protein aquaporin 4 which is found astrocyte membranes, and which as a channel for water transfer across the cell membrane. Originally felt to be highly specific, it has now been detected in patients with SLE, Sjögren's syndrome, Hashimoto's thyroiditis and paraneoplastic myelopathy. Nevertheless, in the appropriate clinical context NMO antibody determination is a very useful test.

Vascular disorders of the spine

Vascular diseases including those of the spinal cord are discussed further in Chapters 5 and 26. Like vascular disease of the brain, the syndromes can be thought of in terms of infarction, haemorrhage, transient loss of vascular supply and vascular malformations.

Vascular malformations Spinal vascular malformations usually present subacutely unless there is acute haemorrhage (this does not happen with dural AVMs or fistulae). Dural fistulae present as a myelopathy with progressive motor sensory and sphincteric loss. There may be radicular involvement and lower motor neurone signs because of impairment of dorsal and ventral root blood supply as well as anterior horn cell loss. Intradural fistulae more typically present acutely with the effects of intramedullary or subarachnoid bleeding. Adhesive arachnoiditis of the spine may be a late complication of spinal haemorrhage but rarely is a presenting feature leading to the diagnosis of a vascular malformation that has bled previously. Cavernous malformations may present acutely with large intramedullary haemorrhage or with a subacute myelopathy resulting from venous bleeding and consequent spinal damage. The presentation of cavernomas is often with stepwise neurological deterioration.

Neoplastic vascular lesions Cavernous angiomas (also known as cavernomas, cavernous haemangiomas or malformations) consist of a mass of endothelial cells which form sinusoidal spaces filled with blood, without intervening parenchyma, surrounded by haemosiderin-stained spinal parenchyma. They may present with focal haemorrhage or with mass effect and spinal cord syndromes. Symptomatic cavernous angiomas should be treated by surgical excision to prevent further haemorrhage and progression of deficits, whereas asymptomatic lesions should be observed because the natural history of these lesions is unclear. Definitive treatment should take into account the accessibility of the lesion, age of the patient and degree of neurological deficit.

Haemangioblastomas are neoplastic masses consisting of endothelial cells, pericytes and stromal cells. They may occur sporadically, or as part of von Hippel–Lindau syndrome. They usually are intramedullary, but have contact with the pial surface, and may have an associated cystic component or syrinx. Prior to surgery it is important to localise the large feeding vessels supplying the tumour by angiography, to minimise bleeding during resection. Treatment is by surgical resection, staying on the tumour capsule and dividing feeding vessels as they are exposed, similar to the technique of AVM resection.

Arteriovenous malformations AVMs account for about 4% of primary intraspinal masses, and may be classified into the following four types (Table 16.11).

Type I Dural arteriovenous fistulas (AVFs) are the most common type of AVM. AVFs do not have a nidus of abnormal vessels like classic AVMs. Instead, there is a direct connection between an artery and vein, with either single or multiple feeders. The dural fistula is in the root sleeve at an intervertebral foramen, feeding directly into spinal draining veins which may be intradural or extradural (Figures 16.24 and 16.25). They usually present with progressive myelopathy in middle-aged adults, resulting from venous congestion and hypoperfusion of the spinal cord, and are more common in the thoracic spine. Treatment of AVFs involves occlusion of the fistula by surgery or embolisation by interventional radiology.

Type II Glomus AVMs consist of a nidus of compacted abnormal arteries and veins within the spinal cord which may be fed by multiple normal vessels, such as the anterior and posterior spinal arteries (Figure 16.26). The abnormal vessels are intramedullary, and are similar to the vessels seen in intracranial AVMs, either in a compact mass or diffusely arranged. The vessels in the nidus are usually high flow, resulting in myelopathy from the mass effect or steal phenomena. Treatment is by surgical excision of the nidus, embolisation, or both.

Type III Juvenile or metameric AVMs are large AVMs that are intradural and extradural, fed by multiple vessels, often involving neighbouring bone and soft tissues (Figure 16.27). They are very difficult to treat and require a multi-modal approach.

Type IV These are AVFs on the surface of the cord that are intradural but extramedullary.

Most AVMs present with a progressive neurological deficit over months to years as a result of venous congestion or arterial steal, but may also present with sudden parenchymal haemorrhage, subarachnoid haemorrhage, mass effect or cord infarction. A spinal AVM is an important differential diagnosis for patients with subarachnoid haemorrhage and normal intracranial angiography, especially when neck stiffness and pain is more of a feature than

Table 16.10 Causes of transverse myelitis (Chapters 9 and 11).

Infections	Bacterial	Especially staphylococcus including epidural abscess *Mycoplasma* TB *Borrelia* *Rickettsia* Syphilis Tetanus
	Viral	Enterovirus – coxsackie, poliovius, enterovirus 71 Flavivirus – West Nile HZV, HSV 1, 2 HIV, HTLV-1 CMV, EBV Influenza
	Parasites	Schistosomiasis Toxoplasma Malaria Cysticercosis
	Fungal	
Post-infectious		Acute disseminated encephalomyelitis
Post-vaccination		Especially rabies vaccine, (numerous other case reports)
Primary demyelination		Multiple sclerosis Devic's disease
Inflammatory disorders		Systemic lupus erythematosus Mixed connective tissue disease Sjögen's disease Scleroderma Rheumatoid disease Antiphospholipid syndrome Sarcoid Vasculitides Ulcerative colitis Behçet's disease Serum sickness Post-haemopaeotic stem cell infusion GVH Immune dysregulation and immune reconstitution in AIDS
Primary neoplasia		Gliomas Ependymomas
Secondary neoplasia		Especially lymphomas, metastases
Paraneoplastic		Especially associated with small cell carcinoma of lung and lymphoma (anti CRMP-5 and anti-amphiphysin)
Drugs		Heroin
Toxins		Subacute combined degeneration (B_{12} deficiency) Snake and spider bite Arsenic Diethylene glycol Nitrous oxide Cynanide Intrathecal chemotherapy
Radiation		Dose-dependent. Acute and delayed
Miscellaneous		Decompression sickness Electrical injury

CMV, cytomegalovirus; EBV, Epstein–Barr virus; GVH, graft-versus-host disease; HSV, herpes simplex virus; HTLV, human T-cell lymphotropic virus; HZV, herpes zoster virus; TB, tuberculosis.

Table 16.11 Vascular malformations affecting the spinal cord.

Type	Anatomy	Demographics	Clinical presentation	Treatment
Dural fistula (Type 1 SDAVF)	Dural supply	Age 40–70 Male predominance	Progressive myelopathy from venous hypertension	Embolisation Surgery
Arteriovenous malformation (Type 2, 3 SCAVM)	Intramedullary Compact nidus or Diffuse nidus or 'Juvenile-type 3'	Age 5–40 Complex lesions associated with genetic risk factors and developmental anomalies	Acute neurological deficit from haemorrhage. Spinal aneurysms can cause subarachnoid haemorrhage	Embolisation Surgery Conservative management
Perimedullary fistula (Type 4 SCAVM or PMAVF)	Perimedullary Type I compact lesion on pial surface Medullaris with aneurysms Type III giant complex lesions	Type I: age 30–70 Type II: age 20–40 Type III: age 2–30 Congenital and genetic disorders	Progressive myelopathy from venous hypertension. Acute neurological symptoms from aneurysmal rupture (Type II, III)	Surgery for smaller lesions Embolisation or surgery for larger lesions
Epidural fistula (EAVF)	Epidural venous plexus involvement	Any age Complex lesions		Embolisation Surgery Conservative or partial treatment for complex lesions
Cavernous malformation (CM)	Intramedullary	Any age Multiple cavernomas associated with genetic disorder	Acute neurologic deficit from intralesional microbleed	Surgery or observation Radiosurgery?

EAVF, epidural arteriovenous fistula; PMAVF, perimedullary arteriovenous fistula; SCAVM, spinal cord arteriovenous malformation; SDAVF, spinal dural arteriovenous malformation.

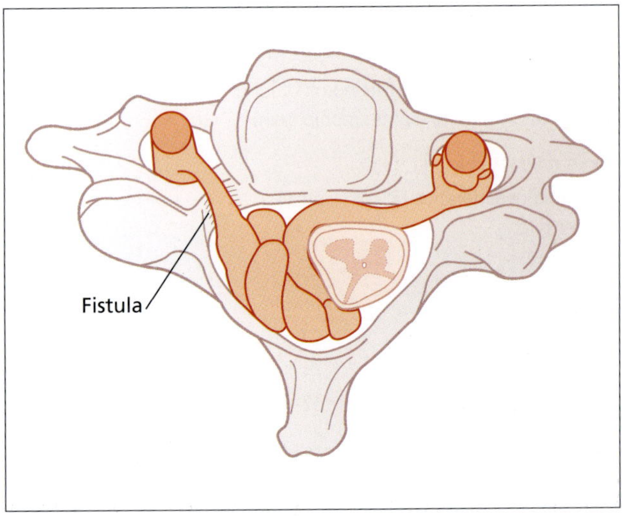

Figure 16.24 Diagram of extradural spinal arteriovenous (AV) fistula.

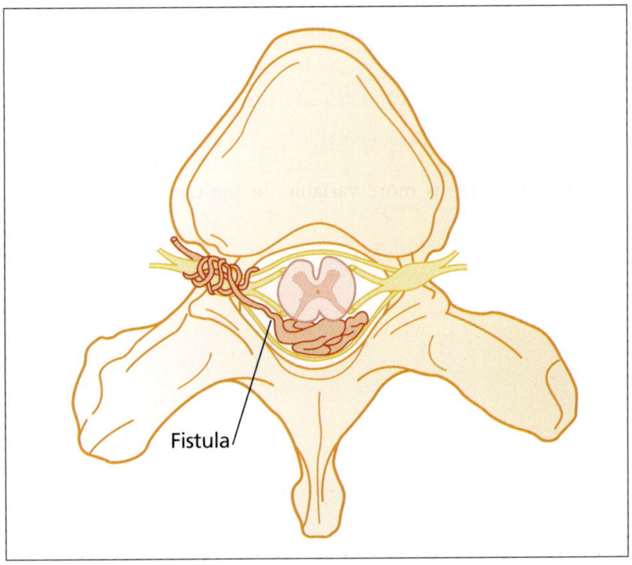

Figure 16.25 Diagram of intradural spinal AV fistula.

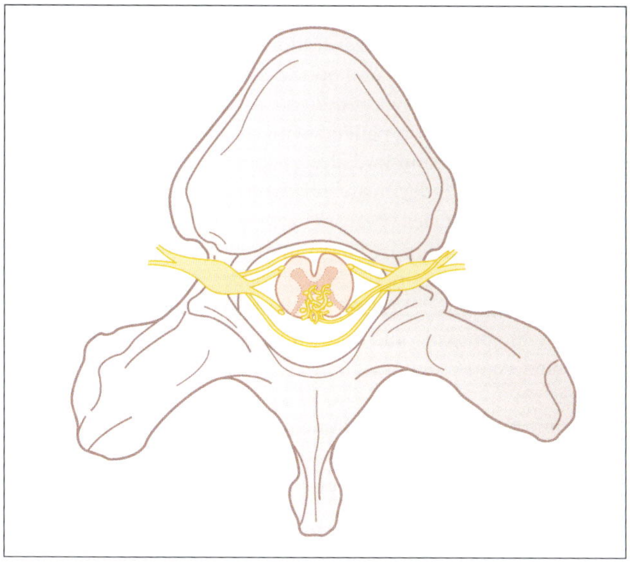

Figure 16.26 Diagram of glomus or nidus spinal arteriovenous malformation (AVM).

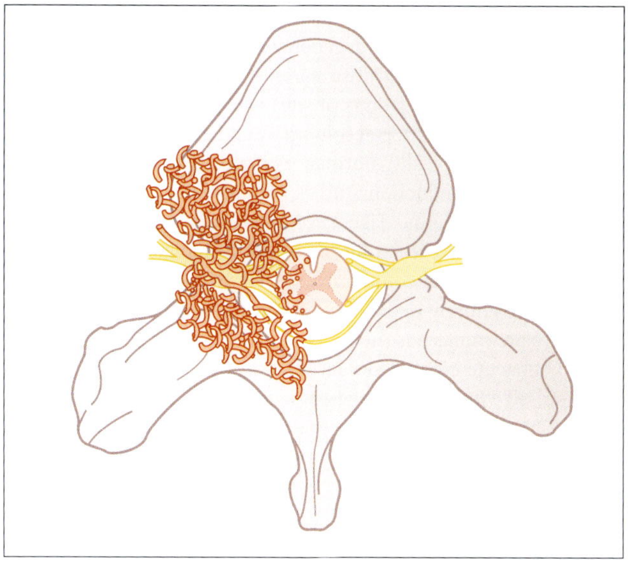

Figure 16.27 Diagram of juvenile type AVM.

headache. MRI and spinal angiography are the investigations of choice for diagnosis and treatment planning.

Management of spinal vascular disease

There is no active treatment for acute spinal cord infarction. During high-risk vascular procedures pre-treatment with steroids and opiate antagonists has been advocated and neuroprotective agents have been examined experimentally. However, there is no clinical evidence for effectiveness of any of these approaches. Some vascular surgeons advocate spinal fluid drainage during surgery believing that through the lowering of CSF pressure spinal perfusion may be maintained during critical moments such as placing of the aortic cross-clamp during aortic aneurysm repair. The best safeguard against iatrogenic spinal cord infarction, however, is highly skilled surgical and anaesthetic practice.

Spinal epidural and subdural haematomas should be decompressed acutely by a spinal surgeon or neurosurgeon. Spinal AVMs and cavernomas can be excised. However, the majority are not amenable to this approach. Interventional radiology is the treatment of choice for dural fistulae and intradural AVMs.

The prognosis for functional recovery in established spinal infarction is poor with significant functional recovery leading to ambulation in well under 50% of those affected. The prognosis for spinal haemorrhage is more variable. In the case of compressive epidural and subdural haematomas it is dependent on the rapidity of decompression. In intradural bleeding it depends greatly on the site and source of bleeding. Haematomas caused by high-flow intradural AVMs are often catastrophic. The effects of bleeding from cavernomas may be milder and disability often progresses over many years. The natural history of cavernomas is still poorly understood and therefore the decision when and whether or not to intervene remains problematic.

Metabolic diseases of the spinal cord (Table 16.12; Chapter 19)

Subacute combined degeneration of the cord resulting from vitamin B_{12} (hydroxylcobalamin) deficiency presents as a myelopathy with prominent dorsal column symptoms and signs. The characteristic clinical picture is of a patient complaining of paraesthesiae

Table 16.12 Metabolic spinal syndromes.

Metabolic myelopathies due to a nutrient deficiency
B deficiency
Nitrous oxide toxicity
AIDS-associated myelopathy (AIDS associated with impaired B_{12} metabolism)
Folate deficiency
Copper deficiency
Vitamin E deficiency
Metabolic myelopathies due to a possible toxin (geographical predilection)
Cassava toxicity
Lathyrism
Fluorosis
Subacute myelo-optico neuropathy (clioquinol toxicity)
Tropical myeloneuropathies
Metabolic myelopathies due to possible toxins (without a geographical predilection)
Chemotherapy-related myelopathy
Hepatic myelopathy
Heroin myelopathy
Organophosphate toxicity

and unsteadiness with mild upper motor neurone leg weakness, depressed knee and ankle jerks with extensor plantar responses and, most importantly, impaired joint position sense with Rombergism will lead many neurologists to recommend immediate vitamin B_{12} administration before the serum vitamin B_{12} levels are known. The treatment should be minimum of $5 \times 1000\,\mu g$ in the first 2 weeks followed by maintenance injections of $1000\,\mu g$/month for 3 months and then 1000 μg every 3 months for life. There are case reports of severe subacute combined degeneration of the cord being helped by administration of high-dose steroids.

Neurological investigations of subacute combined degeneration of the cord may reveal dorsal column T2 signal change on MRI. The spinal fluid is typically normal. Somatosensory potentials are delayed. Nerve conduction studies may reveal an axonal sensorimotor polyneuropathy. Haematological and gastroenterological investigations can reveal a megaloblastic anaemia and vitamin B_{12} malabsorption most commonly caused by pernicious anaemia. Humans are entirely dependent on dietary sources of vitamin B_{12} and there are numerous dietary and malaborption states that may lead to subacute combined degeneration of the cord. Risk factors for acquired vitamin B_{12} deficiency include malabsorption states, pregnancy, drug use including anti-peptic ulcer treatments, HIV-AIDS and haematological conditions leading to increased haemopoesis.

The spinal cord pathology of subacute combined degeneration of the cord reveals degeneration of myelin and axons. Gliosis is not prominent unless the case is very long-standing. These changes may be reversed with vitamin B_{12} administration. The exact mechanism of spinal cord damage in vitamin B_{12} deficiency is not known. However, vitamin B_{12} is the cofactor for conversion of homocysteine to methionine and it is essential for conversion of methylmalonyl-CoA to succinyl-CoA. Unlike folate, vitamin B_{12} is not known to participate directly in purine metabolism and thus DNA synthesis. While secondary effects are possible, administering high levels of folate can circumvent DNA synthesis impairment because of vitamin B_{12} deficiency. Therefore, because neurological manifestations can develop independently of megaloblastic anaemia, it seems unlikely that problems with purine synthesis are responsible for the neuropathology. It is possible that abnormal myelination results from abnormal incorporation of methymalonate and methylpropionate (these are precursors of cobalamin-dependent synthesis of succinyl-CoA) into branched-chain fatty acids. Furthermore, methionine deficiency secondary to failed conversion from homocysteine may lead to impaired synthesis of myelin phospholipids. However, these ideas remain speculative.

An important consideration is that of subacute combined degeneration with normal serum vitamin B_{12} levels. Cases of 'functional' B_{12} deficiency in which serum levels are normal but there is neurological damage because of B_{12} lack are well described. In these syndromes there is elevation of the serum homocystine and methylmalonic acid levels. Furthermore, cases in which nitrous oxide anaesthesia or during recreational use have provoked neurological vitamin B_{12} deficiency are described. Exposure to nitrous oxide irreversibly inactivates cobalamin. Detailed metabolic investigation of the B_{12} pathway is indicated in cases of 'functional' vitamin B_{12} deficiency. The most important lesson is that the correlation between serum vitamin B_{12} levels and the neurological syndrome is weak for complex reasons and the clinician should not be discouraged by normal initial serum B_{12} levels from giving vitamin B_{12} in a neurologically impaired patient with physical signs characteristic of subacute combined degeneration of the cord.

Folic acid deficiency could in theory produce a similar syndrome to that caused by vitamin B_{12} deficiency. However, in practice, there is little evidence that isolated folate deficiency in absence of other risk factors (e.g. alcohol excess) actually causes neurological impairment. Folic acid supplementation, providing this does not induce vitamin B_{12} deficiency, is straightforward.

Acquired copper deficiency causes a syndrome not dissimilar from subacute combined degeneration of the cord, with dorsal column and pyramidal signs and optic neuropathy. It can also cause a lower motor neurone syndrome and peripheral neuropathy. It is most commonly seen in patients with malabsorption states, those on enteral nutrition and in dialysis patients. Zinc ingestion lowers copper levels and indeed is a treatment of patients with Wilson's disease. Copper deficiency causes haematological as well neurological features and is diagnosed by estimation of serum copper, serum caeruloplasmin and 24-hour urinary copper. Zinc levels and excretion should also be checked. Treatment involves stopping zinc ingestion if present and providing copper supplementation. Congenital copper deficiency (Menkes syndrome is discussed in Chapter 19).

Vitamin E deficiency may be acquired as part of malabsorption state and typically presents as a spino-cerebellar degeneration. Genetic causes of a vitamin E deficiency are covered in Chapter 19.

Rare additional metabolic and toxic causes of myelopathy include hepatic failure, chemotherapy especially intrathecal drugs, heroin toxicity, organophosphate poisoning, nitrous oxide poisoning, flourosis (via skeletal deformity), lathyrism (probably caused by beta-*N*-oxalyl-L-alpha, beta-diaminopropionic acid (ODAP) poisoning from a chickpea staple diet) and cassava poisoning (probable cyanotoxin ingestion).

Hereditary spastic paraplegia

Hereditary spastic paraplegia (HSP) is a term covering a genetically and clinically heterogeneous group of inherited disorders characterised by progressive spasticity and weakness predominantly affecting the lower limbs. The transmission of the conditions may be X-linked, autosomal dominant or recessive and they may be divided into pure (uncomplicated) and complicated forms (Table 16.13). In the former there is only spinal involvement but the latter are associated with other neurological abnormalities. To date, linkage to 56 loci and mutations in at least 41 genes have been described resulting in this syndrome.

In pure HSP, patients present with steadily progressive gait disturbance or, in childhood, with delayed motor milestones. There is usually progressive spasticity of the lower limbs with hyperreflexia and extensor plantar responses. However, there may be little or no pyramidal limb weakness and the examination continues to be characterised by dissociation between the severity of the spasticity and relatively mild weakness. Rarely, there may be wasting of the intrinsic muscles of the feet, urinary disturbance with urgency, frequency and hesitancy, anal sphincter disturbance, sexual dysfunction, pes cavus or mild proprioceptive sensory impairment, particularly in long-standing disease. Spasticity predominantly affects the lower limbs with brisk reflexes and ankle clonus but there may be mild signs in the upper limbs and pes cavus may be present.

In complicated HSP, spastic paraparesis is associated with a variety of other neurological manifestations in a variable phenotype: optic atrophy and retinopathy; extrapyramidal involvement (choreoathetosis, dystonia and rigidity); cerebellar signs (ataxia, dysarthria and nystagmus); cognitive impairment (dementia, mental retardation and neuropsychiatric manifestations); sensori-neural deafness and epilepsy (myoclonic, simple or complex partial, absence, atonic or grand mal). Peripheral neuropathy and amyotrophy, icthyosis and cardiac deficits may also be associated.

Table 16.13 Hereditary spastic paraplegia (HSP).

Gene	Inheritance	Locus	Protein	Notes
SPG1/L1CAM	X-linked	Xq28	L1 cell adhesion molecule	MASA syndrome, hydrocephalus, MR, hypoplasia of corpus callosum
SPG2/PLP1	X-linked	Xq22	Proteolipoprotein 1	Nystagmus, dysarthria, sensory disturbance, MR, optic atrophy; allelic to Pelizaeus–Merzbacher
SPG3A/ATL1	AD	14q11-q21	Atlastin 1	Early onset, pure HSP; 10% AD HSP
SPG4/SPAST	AD	2p22-p21	Spastin	Pure HSP; 40% pure AD HSP
SPG5A/CYP7B1	AR	8q21.3	Cytochrome P450–7B1	Pure HSP
SPG6/NIPA1	AD	15q11	Non-imprinted in Prader–Willi/ Angelman's syndrome 1	Pure HSP
SPG7	AR	16q24.3	Paraplegin	Optic atrophy, nystagmus, cerebellar signs
SPG8/KIAA0196	AD	8q24.13	Strumpellin	Adult-onset pure HSP
SPG9	AD	10q23.3-q24.1		Cataracts, motor neuropathy, short stature, MR, skeletal abnormalities
SPG10/KIF5A	AD	12q13	Kinesin-5A	Pure HSP
SPG11	AR	15q21.1	Spatacsin	MR, thin corpus callosum, dysarthria
SPG12	AD	19q13		Pure HSP, rapidly progressive
SPG13/HSPD1	AD	2q33.1	Heat shock protein 60	Pure HSP
SPG14	AR	3q27-q28		Motor neuropathy, MR
SPG15/ZYFVE26	AR	14q24.1	Spastizin	Retinal degeneration, MR, amyotrophy
SPG16	X-linked	Xq11.2		Quadriplegia, aphasia, visual impairment, MR
SPG17/BSCL2	AD	11q13	Seipin	Silver syndrome, amyotrophy of distal upper limbs
SPG18	AR	8p12-p11.21		MR, hypoplasia of corpus callosum, epilepsy
SPG19	AD	9q		Pure HSP, slow progression
SPG20	AR	13q12.3	Spartin	Troyer's syndrome; distal amyotrophy, dysarthria, MR
SPG21	AR	15q21-q22	Maspardin/ACP33	Mast syndrome; adult onset, cognitive decline, extrapyramidal features
SPG23	AR	1q24-q32		Lison syndrome; abnormal skin pigmentation, neuropathy
SPG24	AR	13q14		Pure HSP
SPG25	AR	6q23-q24.1		Adult onset, intervertebral disk herniation
SPG26	AR	12p11.1-q14		Distal amyotrophy, mild MR
SPG27	AR	10q22.1-q24.1		Adult onset pure HSP
SPG28	AR	14q21.3-q22.3		Pure HSP
SPG29	AD	1–31.1-p21.1		Sensorineural deafness, neonatal hyperbilirubinaemia, hiatal hernia
SPG30	AR	2q37.3		Peripheral neuropathy, cerebellar atrophy
SPG31/REEP1	AD	2p11.2	Receptor expression-enhancing protein 1	Pure HSP
SPG32	AR	14q12-q21		Mild MR, thin corpus callosum, cerebellar atrophy
SPG33/ZFYVE27*	AD	10q24.2	Protrudin	Controversial – described mutation may be noncausative polymorphism
SPG34	X-linked	Xq24-q25		Pure HSP
SPG35/FA2H	AR	16q21-q23.1	Fatty acid 2-hydroxylase	MR, epilepsy, white matter abnormalities on MRI
SPG36	AD	12q23-q24		Pure HSP

(continued)

Table 16.13 (continued)

Gene	Inheritance	Locus	Protein	Notes
SPG37	AD	8p21.1-q13.3		Pure HSP
SPG38	AD	4p16-p15		Silver syndrome; distal amyotrophy
SPG39/PNPLA6	AR	19p13.3	Neuropathy target esterase	Motor neuropathy with distal wasting
SPG41	AD	11p14.1-p11.2		Pure HSP
SPG42/SLC33A1	AD	3q25.31	Acetyl-CoA Transporter	Pure HSP
SPG43	AR	19p13.11-q12		Distal amyotrophy
SPG44/GJC2	AR	1q41-q42	Gap junction protein gamma 2	Allelic with Pelizaeus–Merzbacher like disease, hypomyelination
SPG45	AR	10q24.3-q25.1		MR, nystagmus, optic atrophy
SPG46	AR	9p21.2-q21.12		MR, thin corpus callosum
SPG48/KIAA0415	AR	7p21	Putative DNA helicase	Pure HSP, putative-based on 2 individuals

AD, autosomal dominant; AR, autosomal recessive; HSP, hereditary spastic paraplegia; MASA, mental retardation, aphasia, shuffling gait and adducted thumbs; MR, mental retardation.

Cranial and spinal MRI scans are usually normal but there may be spinal atrophy in some forms (e.g. SPG6 and 8). In complicated forms, imaging may show cerebral and cerebellar atrophy or hypoplasia of the corpus callosum.

The age of onset of the conditions varies from infancy to the eighth decade but is usually between the second and fourth decade. The prognosis is variable between families and to a lesser extent within families. Early onset HSP (>35 years) tends to be slower in its progression and most patients remain ambulant throughout their lives. However, the later onset forms of the condition (>35 years) tend to be associated with more rapid disease progression, with many patients becoming wheelchair bound in their sixties and seventies. However, there is no effect on prognosis according to the mode of transmission.

The management is entirely symptomatic with spasticity being treated with appropriate antispastic medication including baclofen, dantrolene and tizanidine. Severe spasticity may be helped by local injection of botulinum toxin. Early and regular physiotherapy is required to maintain the range of movements, strength and flexibility and to avoid the development of contractures. In complicated forms, cardiomyopathy can occur and requires specific treatment.

Table 16.14 Causes of superficial siderosis.

Neurosurgery	Including late effects of CNS tumour removal in childhood
SAH	Caused by aneurysm, AVM or angiogram negative; SAH due to transthyretin (Asp18Gly TTR mutation) leptomeningeal amyloidosis; intracerebral and spinal cavernomas
Tumours	Pituitary, cerebellar, spinal astrocytomas, spinal teratoma, ependymoma, filum terminale preganglionomas, spinal meningeal melanocytoma
Nerve root trauma	Avulsion, pseudomeningocoele
Miscellaneous causes	Neurofibromatosis type 1, CNS vasculitis, anticoagulation

AVM, arteriovenous malformation; CNS, central nervous system; SAH, subarachnoid haemorrhage.

Miscellaneous conditions affecting the spine and spinal cord

Superficial siderosis This is a condition in which there is abnormal subarchnoid haemosiderin deposition (Chapter 26). The condition affects many neurological systems and when taken together the symptoms and signs form a coherent and recognisable clinical picture. A literature review of 87 cases revealed the following clinical features: sensorineural deafness (95%), cerebellar ataxia (88%), pyramidal signs (76%), dementia (24%), bladder disturbance (24%), anosmia (at least 17%), aniscoria (at least 10%) and sensory signs (13%). Less frequent features included extraocular motor palsies, movement disorders and lower motor neurone signs secondary to anterior horn cell damage (5–10% each). Neck pain, low back pain and sciatic type pain are recognised clinical features. T2-weighted MRI studies are diagnostic, and reveal a dark rim, representing the paramagnetic affects of iron deposition, particularly around posterior fossa structures, the spinal cord and occasionally the cerebral hemispheres.

Previous spinal surgery is a recognised cause of superficial siderosis with chronic subarachnoid bleeding resulting from small blood vessel anomaly. Local spinal pathology affecting the dura such as a root lesion/avulsion or vascular anomaly are also recognised causes of the condition. The remainder of cases in which a cause may be identified usually result from subarachnoid haemorrhage or the late consequences of a major neurosurgical procedure such as hemispherectomy. However, as shown in Table 16.14, there are a number of other conditions implicated in the development of superficial siderosis. The serious long-term prognosis of the disorder means an exhaustive search for a bleeding source and CSF leak should be undertaken. A lumbar puncture can indicate recent bleeding but given that the problem can be intermittent, a clear CSF does not guarantee that there is no ongoing tendency to accumulate more blood products and therefore iron. Thorough investigation requires MRI of brain and whole spine and often a CT myelogram looking for a dural tear. Exploratory surgery of a region from which chronic bleeding could occur may be indicated (e.g. the site of previous surgery or a root avulsion). Successful surgical ablation of a bleeding source can arrest further iron deposition but will not affect the neurotoxicity of the iron already deposited. A blood patch is

Table 16.15 Causes of arachnoiditis.

Iatrogenic: spinal surgery, multiple lumbar punctures and spinal anaesthesia
Trauma
SAH including spinal SAH
Spinal infection, especially tuberculosis and suppurative pyogenic meningitis
Myodil (Pantopaque) radiological contrast agent (this has not been used in the United Kingdom since 1984)

SAH, subarachnoid haemorrhage.

also considered if there is evidence of a non-surgical CSF leak. The role of medical treatment with chelation therapy has not yet been established by randomised controlled trials. Trientine is almost certainly not helpful. There are recent data suggesting that the iron chelator deferiprone (Ferriprox), which crosses the blood–brain barrier, can reduce iron load on MRI. It is to be hoped that this MRI finding will translate into clinical benefit in an otherwise untreatable condition.

Cochlear transplants have been successfully performed for the hearing loss associated with siderosis and should be undertaken before VIIIth nerve function is lost.

Arachnoiditis Fibrosis and adhesions of the intradural space can occur after trauma, infection, surgery or subarachnoid bleeding, and usually involve the pia and theca as well as the arachnoid layers around the cord (Table 16.15). Pain and radicular symptoms arise because of involvement of the lumbar nerve roots, or myelopathy if the cord becomes tethered by these adhesions at any point or if the cord vasculature is compromised.

The diagnosis involves the exclusion of other causes of radicular pain or myelopathy, and the demonstration of arachnoiditis on MRI. The differential diagnosis includes intrinsic tumours and carcinomatous meningitis. Radiological arachnoiditis is seen in many asymptomatic patients who have had spinal surgery or myelography, and there is no clear evidence to associate radiological findings directly with symptoms. In postoperative patients therefore, arachnoiditis should not necessarily be assumed to be the cause of new symptoms.

In the lumbar region, nerve roots adhere to form bundles, or lie centrifugally in contact with the thecal sac, producing the appearance of an empty sac. In the thoracic spine, arachnoiditis produces intramedullary cystic changes with syrinx and cavity formation. The MRI appearances can be confusing (Figure 16.15). When arachnoiditis occurs in the thoracic regions, the cord may be tethered to the theca (e.g. at the point of surgical durotomy) or may produce arachnoid cysts as a result of poor communication of the CSF spaces.

Surgical detethering may treat a tethered cord in a patient with progressive neurological symptoms. Arachnoid cysts producing cord compression may be marsupialised or shunted but the problem is often recurrent. Lumbar arachnoiditis producing radicular pain is usually best treated by symptomatic control, including epidural injections of local anaesthetic and steroid, pain management techniques and analgesics. Despite attempts to inhibit fibrosis as yet no successful medical therapies capable of reversing arachnoiditis have been developed and the condition can relentlessly progress causing severe pain and disability.

Further reading

Physiology

Carr LJ, Harrison LM, Evans AL, Stephens JA. Patterns of central nervous reorganization in hemiplegic cerebral palsy. *Brain* 1993; **116**: 1223–1247.

Dobson CB, Villagra F, Clowry GJ, Smith M, Kenwrick S, Donnai D, *et al.* Abnormal corticospinal function but normal axonal guidance in human *L1CAM* mutations. *Brain* 2001; **124**: 2393–2406.

Farmer SF, Ingram DA, Stephens JA. Mirror movements studied in a patient with Klippel–Feil syndrome. *J Physiol* 1990; **428**: 467–484.

Spinal cord development and repair

Agarwal AK, Peppelman WC, Kraus DR, Pollock BH, Stolzer BL, Eisenbeis CH Jr, *et al.* Recurrence of cervical spine instability in rheumatoid arthritis following previous fusion: can disease progression be prevented by early surgery? *J Rheumatol* 1992; **19**: 1364–1370.

David KM, Copp AJ, Stevens JM, Hayward RD, Crockard HA. Split cervical spinal cord with Klippel–Feil syndrome: seven cases. *Brain* 1996; **119**: 1859–1872.

David KM, McLachlan JC, Aiton JF, Whiten SC, Smart SD, Thorogood PV, *et al.* Cartilaginous development of the human craniovertebral junction as visualised by a new three-dimensional computer reconstruction technique. *J Anat* 1998; **192**: 269–277.

David KM, Thorogood P, Stevens JM, Einstein S, Ransford AO, Crockard HA. The onse bone spine: a failure of notochord/sclerotome signalling. *Clin Dysmorphol* 1997; **64**: 303–314.

Feron F, Perry C, Cochrane J, Licina P, Nowitzke A, Urquhart S, *et al.* Autologous olfactory ensheathing cell transplantation in human spinal cord injury. *Brain* 2005; **128**: 2951–2960.

Fili L, Schwab ME. The rocky road to translation in spinal cord repair. *Ann Neurol* 2012; **72**: 491–501.

Huang PP, Constantine S. 'Acquired' *Chiari I malformations. J Neurosurg* 1994; **80**: 1099–1102.

Louvi A, Artavanis-Tsakonas S. Notch signalling in vertebrate neural development. *Nat Rev Neurosci* 2006; **7**: 93–102.

McGaughran JM, Oates A, Donnai D, Read AP, Tassabehji M. Mutations in PAX1 may be associated with Klippel–Feil syndrome. *Eur J Hum Genet* 2003; **11**: 468–474.

Matsuoka T, Ahlberg PE, Kessaris N, Iannarelli P, Dennehy U, Richardson WD, *et al.* Neural crest origins of the neck and shoulder. *Nature* 2005; **436**: 347–355.

Menezes AH. Craniocervical anomalies and syringomyelia. In Choux M, DiRocco C, Hockley A, Walker M, eds. *Pediatric Neurosurgery*. New York: Churchill Livingstone, 1999: 151–184.

Pourquie O, Kusumi K. When body segmentation goes wrong. *Clin Genet* 2001; **60**: 409–416.

Pueschal SM, Scola F. Atlantoaxial instability in individuals with Down's syndrome: epidemiologic, radiographic and clinical studies. *Pediatrics* 1987; **80**: 555.

Ramón-Cueto A, Nieto-Sampedro M. Regeneration into the spinal cord of transected dorsal root axons is promoted by ensheathing glia transplants. *Exp Neurol* 1994; **127**: 232–244.

Samii C, Mobius E, Weber E, Heinbrok HW, Berlit P. Pseudo Chiari type I malformation secondary to cerebrospinal fluid leakage. *J Neurol* 1999; **246**: 162–164.

ten Donkelaar HJ, Lammens M, Wesseling P, Hori A, Keyser A, Rotteveel J. Development and malformations of the human pyramidal tract. *J Neurol* 2004; **251**: 1429–1442.

Theiss SM, Smith MD, Winter RB. The long-term follow up of patients with Klippel–Feil syndrome and congenital scoliosis. *Spine* 1997; **22**: 1219–1222.

Spinal cord trauma

Bracken MB, Shepard MJ, Collins WF, *et al.* A randomized, controlled trial of methylprednisolone or naloxone in the treatment of acute spinal-cord injury. *N Engl J Med* 1990; **322**: 1405–1411.

Denis F. The three column spine and its significance in the classification of acute thoracolumbar spinal injuries. *Spine* 1983; **8**: 817–831.

Edwards P, Arango M, Balica L, *et al.* Final results of MRC CRASH, a randomised placebo-controlled trial of intravenous corticosteroid in adults with head injury-outcomes at 6 months. *Lancet* 2005; **365**: 1957–1959.

Hugenholtz H, Cass DE, Dvorak MF, Fewer DH, Fox RJ, Izukawa DM, *et al.* High-dose methylprednisolone for acute closed spinal cord injury: only a treatment option. *Can J Neurosci* 2002; **29**: 227–235.

Katoh S, el Masry WS, Jaffray D, McCall IW, Eisenstein SM, Pringle RG, *et al.* Neurologic outcome in conservatively treated patients with incomplete closed traumatic cervical spinal cord injuries. *Spine* 1996; **21**: 2345–2351.

Tator CH. Review of treatment trials in human spinal cord injury: issues, difficulties and recommendations. *Neurosurgery* 2006; **59**: 957–982.

Spinal tumours

Brotchi J, Bruneau M, Lefranc F, Baleriaux D. Surgery of intraspinal cord tumors. *Clin Neurosurg* 2006; **53**: 209–216.

Findlay GF. Adverse effects of the management of malignant spinal cord compression. *J Neurol Neurosurg Psychiatry* 1984; **47**: 761–768.

Patchell RA, Tibbs PA, Regine WF, Payne R, Saris S, Kryscio RJ. Direct decompressive surgical resection in the treatment of spinal cord compression caused by metastatic cancer: a randomised trial. *Lancet* 2005; **366**: 643–648.

Thakkar SD, Feigen U, Mautner VF. Spinal tumours in neurofibromatosis type 1: an MRI study of frequency, multiplicity and variety. *Neuroradiology* 1999; **41**: 625–629.

Varma DG, Moulopoulos A, Sara AS, Leeds N, Kumar R, Kim EE. MR imaging of extracranial nerve sheath tumors. *J Comput Assist Tomogr* 1992; **16**: 448–453.

Rheumatoid diseases

Casey AT, Crockard HA, Bland JM, Stevens J, Moskovich R, Ransford AO. Surgery on the rheumatoid cervical spine for the non-ambulant myelopathic patient: too much, too late? *Lancet* 1996; **347**: 1004–1007.

Choi D, Casey ATHC, Crockard HA. Neck problems in rheumatoid arthritis: changing disease patterns, surgical treatments and patients' expectations. *Rheumatology* 2006; **45**: 1183–1184.

Cody JD, Singer FR, Roodman GD, Otterund B, Lewis TB, Leppert M, *et al.* Genetic linkage of Paget's disease of bone to chromosome 18q. *Am J Hum Genet* 1997; **61**: 1117–1122.

Fujiwara K, Fujimoto M, Yonenobu K, Ochi, A. A clinico-pathological study of cervical myelopathy in rheumatoid arthritis: post-mortem analysis of two cases. *Eur Spine J* 1999; **8**: 46–53.

Gibson JN, Waddell G. Surgery for degenerative lumbar spondylosis. *Cochrane Database Syst Rev* 2005; **4**: CD001352.

Henderson FC, Geddes JF, Crockard HA. Neuropathology of the brainstem and spinal cord in end stage rheumatoid arthritis: implications for treatment. *Ann Rheum Dis* 1993; **52**: 629–637.

Hamilton JD, Gordon MM, McInnes IB, Johnston RA, Madhok R, Capell HA. Improved medical and surgical management of cervical spine disease in patients with rheumatoid arthritis over 10 years. *Ann Rheum Dis* 2000; **59**: 434–438.

Poncelet A. The neurological complications of Paget's disease. *J Bone Min Res* 1999; **14** (Suppl. 2): 88-91

Wolfe F, Michaud K, Olaf G, Choi HK. Predicting mortality in patients with rheumatoid arthritis. *Arthritis Rheum* 2003; **48**: 1530–1542.

Infections

Ho E. Infectious etiologies of myelopathy. *Semin Neurol* 2012; **32:** 154–160.

Hodgson AR, Stock FE. Anterior spine fusion for the treatment of tuberculosis of the spine: the operative findings and results of treatment in the first one hundred cases. *J Bone Joint Surg Am* 1960; **42**: 295–310.

Jutte PC, Van Loenhout-Tooyackers JH. Routine surgery in addition to chemotherapy for treating spinal tuberculosis. *Cochrane Database Syst Rev* 2006; **1**: CD004532.

Medical Research Council Working Party on Tuberculosis of the Spine. A controlled trial of anterior spinal fusion and debridement in the surgical management of tuberculosis of the spine in patients on standard chemotherapy: a study in Hong Kong. *Br J Surg* 1974; **61**: 853–866.

Other medical conditions affecting the spinal cord

Fearnley JM, Stevens JM, Rudge P. Superficial siderosis of the central nervous system. *Brain* 1995; **118**: 1051–1066.

Glorieux FH, Bishop NJ, Plotkin H, Chabot G, Lanque G, Travers R. Cyclic administration of pamidronate in children with severe osteogensis imperfecta. *N Engl J Med* 1998; **339**: 947–952.

Gutteridge DH, Ward LC, Stewart GO, Retallack RW, Will RK, Prince RL, *et al.* Paget's disease: acquired resistance to one aminobisphosphonate with retained response to another. *J Bone Miner Res* 1999; **14** (Suppl. 2): 79–84.

Kumar N. Metabolic and toxic myelopathies. *Semin Neurol* 2012; **32:** 123–136.

Lennon VA, Wingerchuk DM, Kryzer TJ, Pittock SJ, Lucchinetti CF, Fujihara K, *et al.* A serum autoantibody marker of neuromyelitis optica: distinction from multiple sclerosis. *Lancet* 2004; **364**: 2106–2112.

Lucchinetti CF, Mandler RN, McGavern D, Bruck W, Gleich G, Ransohoff RM, *et al.* A role for humoral mechanisms in the pathogenesis of Devic's neuromyelitis optica. *Brain* 2002; **125**: 1450–1461.

Mass J. Inherited myelopathies. *Semin Neurol* 2012; **32:** 114–122.

Moftaka P, Hetts S, Ko, N. Vascular myelopathies. *Semin Neurol* 2012; **32:** 146–153.

O'Riordan JI. Central nervous system white matter diseases other than multiple sclerosis. *Curr Opin Neurol* 1997; **10**: 211–214.

Rauch F, Glorieux FH. Treatment of children with osteogenesis imperfecta. *Curr Osteoporos Rep* 2006; **4**: 159–164.

Sawin PD, Menezes AH. Basilar invagination in osteogenesis imperfecta and related osteochondrodysplastias: medical and surgical management. *J Neurosurg* 1997; **86**: 950–960.

Scoliosis

Giampietro PF, Blank RD, Raggio CL, Merchant S, Jacobsen FS, Faciszewski T, *et al.* Congenital and idiopathic scoliosis: clinical and genetic aspects. *Clin Med Res* 2003; **1**: 125–136.

Lenke LG, Edwards CC, Bridwell KH. The Lenke classification of adolescent idiopathic scoliosis: how it organizes curve patterns as a template to perform selective fusions of the spine. *Spine* 2003; **28**: S199–207.

McMaster MJ, Singh H. Natural history of congenital kyphosis and kyphoscoliosis. *J Bone Joint Surg* 1999; **81A**: 1367–1383.

Other surgical

Dickens DRV. The spine. In Broughton NS, ed. *A Textbook of Paediatric Orthopaedics.* London: WB Saunders, 1997: 267–281.

Fagan LH, Ferguson S, Yassari R, Frim DM. The Chiari pseudotumour cerebri syndrome: symptom recurrence after decompressive surgery for Chiari malformation type I. *Pediatr Neurosurg* 2006; **42**: 14–19.

Fairbank J, Frost H, Wilson-MacDonald J, Yu LM, Barker K, Collins R, Spine Stabilisation Trial Group. Randomised controlled trial to compare surgical stabilisation of the lumbar spine with an intensive rehabilitation programme for patients with chronic low back pain: the MRC spine stabilisation trial. *Br Med J* 2005; **330**: 1485.

Degenerative spine disease

Hillibrand AS, Carlson GD, Palumbo MA, Jones PK, Bohlman HH. Radiculopathy and myelopathy at segments adjacent to the sites of a previous anterior cervical arthrodesis. *J Bone Joint Surg Am* 1999; **81**: 519–528.

Levy M, Llinas, R. Pilot safety trial of deferiprone in 10 subjects with superficial siderosis. *Stroke* 2012; **43:** 120–124.

Logue V, Edwards MR. Syringomyelia and its surgical treatment-an analysis of 75 patients. *J Neurol Neurosurg Psychiatry* 1981; **44**: 273–284.

Lunsford LD, Bissonette DJ, Zorub DS. Anterior surgery for cervical disc disease. Part 2: Treatment of cervical spondylotic myelopathy in 32 cases. *J Neurosurg* 1980; **53**: 12–19.

Lynch JJ, Crockard HH. Primary bone disease of the skull base. In Robertson J, Coakham H, eds. *Cranial Base Surgery: Management, Complications and Outcome.* New York: Churchill Livingstone, 1999: 659–673.

Schrader H, Obelieniene D, Bovim G. Natural evolution of late whiplash syndrome outside the medicolegal context. *Lancet* 1996; **347**: 1207–1211.

CHAPTER 17

Cerebellar Ataxias and Related Conditions

Nicholas W. Wood
UCL Institute of Neurology

Ataxia derives from the Greek, meaning quite simply, disorder. In neurology the word is used to describe incoordination of muscular activity associated with dysfunction of the cerebellum and its connections. The causes of cerebellar dysfunction are numerous and impossible to cover in great depth here. This chapter thus adopts a structured approach to assessment and management of the ataxic patient, with descriptions of the main disorders affecting the cerebellum. There have been numerous classifications applied to the ataxias; none is without significant drawbacks. The approach used here is clinical, describing how one can sort through the differential diagnosis of an ataxic syndrome in a way that is systematic, robust and efficient.

Approach to the patient with ataxia

Symptoms

The assessment of patients with possible ataxia begins as they are seen to walk, when one can observe the gait and the ability, or otherwise, to sit down smoothly into the chair. As the symptoms are elucidated there is time to catch the explosive cerebellar dysarthria. However, many patients with ataxia have abnormalities in other neurological pathways in addition to those in the cerebellar system, so one may hear a spastic or dysphonic quality to the speech that can complicate the picture. The specific symptoms of cerebellar disease are problems with balance and general coordination of limbs. This can be described as a feeling of disequilibrium, sometimes called dizziness by the patient. Patients often have noticed a speech disturbance themselves or quite frequently this has been pointed out by family or friends. Limb ataxia may first be hinted at by the patient's deteriorating handwriting or that there is difficulty carrying a glass of fluid, or a tremor. Vertigo is generally more suggestive of neoplastic, inflammatory and vascular disease rather than the more slowly progressive degenerative processes.

It is useful to determine the age at onset and the course, including the mode of onset (e.g. a sudden rather than insidious course). An acute history may suggest a cerebellar haemorrhage. A haematoma is often associated with acute raised intracranial pressure symptoms and appropriate signs. If these features develop more slowly in the ataxic patient, then space-occupying lesions including a tumour or even an abscess should be considered and excluded by imaging.

The age at onset helps focus the differential diagnosis. Table 17.1 gives an outline of the broad range of diseases to consider in each category. In the field of ataxia, any symptom occurring in a patient over the age of 25 years is classed as late onset. The pattern of onset and subsequent course also helps in sifting the diagnostic possibilities. The length of the history should be established and it is worth asking about early motor milestones and athletic ability at school, which can indicate a much earlier onset than previously appreciated.

Having determined the mode and age at onset, concentrate on quantifying the current problems, how and when they emerged, with a particular emphasis on any extracerebellar features. This should include assessment of cognitive, sensory and any neuromuscular features.

Genetics has a significant role in the aetiology of ataxia: a detailed family history is required, even in the case of apparently sporadic ataxia. The family history needs to be elicited in detail as many of the inherited ataxias are complicated and it is possible that an affected relative may have presented with a clinical picture very different from the proband.

Vomiting, headache or vertigo frequently suggest a posterior fossa mass lesion. Direct questioning should also cover the urinary system, skeletal deformities and cardiac disease. A detailed enquiry of drug ingestion, for both medical and recreational purposes, including alcohol, and occupational exposure is also required.

Physical signs

The examination has two main aims: to establish and delineate the cerebellar features and to determine the involvement of other systems both in the central nervous system (CNS) and other organs.

The range of potential diagnoses is usually evident from the clinical history and examination. More formal gait assessment should include any additional features, such as signs of parkinsonism or dystonia, Rombergism and any suggestion of pyramidal or neuropathic signs.

At the bedside the assessment of the extraocular movements is vital. It is extremely rare to see a patient with a cerebellar cause for their symptoms who does not have some abnormality in their extraocular movements. However, it may be necessary to search hard for such signs. In the primary position the presence of square wave jerks should be assessed. The assessment of ocular pursuit usually

Neurology: A Queen Square Textbook, Second Edition. Edited by Charles Clarke, Robin Howard, Martin Rossor and Simon Shorvon.

Table 17.1 Differential diagnosis of ataxia based on age and pattern of onset.

Course	Chronic/insidious onset ataxia	Subacute cerebellar syndrome	Acute cerebellar syndrome
Early	Congenital ARCA	Infective e.g. abscess Raised ICP Post-infectious Some drugs/toxins	Some infections and vascular causes
Adult	Alcohol ILOCA ADCA MSA-C Gluten ataxia FXTAS	Paraneoplasia SOL	Vascular causes

ADCA, autosomal dominant cerebellar ataxia; ARCA, autosomal recessive cerebellar ataxia; FXTAS, fragile X tremor ataxia syndrome; ICP, intracranial pressure; ILOCA, idiopathic late onset ataxia; MSA-C, multiple system atrophy type C; SOL, space-occupying lesion.

reveals a broken jerky quality, because of insertion of saccades into attempted pursuit. At its most extreme, normal pursuit is entirely absent and the eyes move entirely by use of the saccadic system. One can choose to stress this system more by assessment of the ability to inhibit the vestibular ocular reflex. Nystagmus may be found, and although this is the best known of the cerebellar eye signs, it is far from invariably present. The saccadic system should also be assessed both by eliciting voluntary saccades – with the instructions 'look left, look right' – and reflex saccades where one presents a target. Using these two methods one can assess the speed of initiation, the accuracy and the velocity of the saccades. Typically, in the patient with cerebellar dysfunction there are dysmetric saccades, either hyper- or hypo-, which are demonstrated by overshoot or undershoot, with a small corrective saccade to reach the target. A discrepancy between voluntary and reflex saccades may indicate a supranuclear gaze palsy or oculomotor apraxia. Some of these assessments at the bedside can be difficult and a true quantification can only be obtained by electrophysiological testing, but this is only rarely necessary. In some of the rarer complicated ataxias one may observe ophthalmoparesis – this is most common in mitochondrial disease and autosomal dominant cerebellar ataxias (ADCAs). The presence of opsoclonus may suggest paraneoplastic disease in an appropriate clinical setting. Downbeat nystagmus with symptoms of vertical oscillopsia suggests a structural lesion at the foramen magnum.

Ophthalmoscopy is necessary to assess the optic nerve, retina and macula, looking for signs of atrophy or pigmentary changes.

The classic limb signs of cerebellar disease in the upper limbs include intention tremor, dysdiadochokinesis, rebound and finger–nose incoordination, where one may observe dysmetria and past pointing. In the legs an assessment of heel–shin coordination usually suffices. It is quite usual to find that the legs are more severely affected than the arms (Chapter 4).

Additional signs

Assessment of other systems should include signs of dysmorphism, skeletal abnormalities especially pes cavus and scoliosis, skin rashes and organomegaly. Neurologically, a full analysis of the other systems should include assessment of the pyramidal tracts, sensory impairment, neuropathy, extrapyramidal and autonomic features. The latter can be quickly assessed at the bedside by measuring supine and standing blood pressure (BP). It is best to measure BP at 1-minute intervals, for 3 minutes. If there is further concern more formal autonomic testing can be performed.

Investigations

In certain ataxic disorders specialised ancillary tests are required; these are discussed later in the chapter. Here the broad approaches to investigating the ataxic patient are mentioned.

Imaging

High-quality magnetic resonance imaging (MRI) has revolutionised practice in this area. MRI is useful in determining the presence and often nature of any space-occupying lesion, it can readily identify haemorrhage and is the investigation of choice if inflammatory causes are being considered. However, once these more common aetiologies are excluded, imaging plays a relatively small part in the assessment of the ataxic patient. In the long differential of the degenerative forms of ataxia, MRI will often show non-specific cerebellar atrophy, with or without brainstem or more generalised atrophy, all too often not providing specific diagnostic refinement. Research imaging methods are being developed to address some of these deficiencies, but they are not yet in clinical service.

Electrophysiological tests

While imaging helps to define structural anatomy, a range of electrophysiological tools can be used to clarify the functional integrity of the nervous system, and can help delineate the involvement of other neurological systems. In assessing a complicated ataxia of uncertain origin, appropriate neurophysiological tests can be helpful. Neurophysiology is also helpful in considering:

- Is there a subclinical neuropathy?
- Visual system function, with evoked responses or electroretinography?
- Motor/sensory function, with somatosensory evoked responses and central motor conduction times.

The finding of an associated neuropathy may indicate a degenerative cause. For example, early onset ataxia with a significant sensory neuropathy may suggest either Friedreich's ataxia (FRDA), ataxia telangiectasia or abetalipoproteinaemia. In later onset cases, and some rare genetic forms of ataxia, an inflammatory cause such as Sjögren's disease needs to be excluded. It is helpful to differentiate axonal from demyelinating neuropathies. The vast majority of associated neuropathies in the degenerative ataxias are axonal. Occasionally, an early onset ataxia is associated with a demyelinating neuropathy and this might indicate the diagnosis of autosomal recessive ataxia of Charlevoix-Sagueney (ARSACS). This disorder is also associated with retinal layer hypertrophy which is best identified using optical coherence tomography.

Table 17.2 Blood tests and the ataxic patient.

Blood test	Purpose	Notes
Routine blood tests (including thyroid function)	General investigation, and may show evidence of multi-system disease	Hypothyroidism is a very rare but treatable cause of ataxia
Autoantibodies and anticardiolipin	SLE, Sjögren's and antiphospholipid syndromes	Often subacute and complicated phenotype
Antigliadin and endomysial antibodies	Coeliac disease and gluten ataxia	Common in general population, so care not to overinterpret
Vitamins, especially B and E	Thiamine, B_{12} and vitamin E deficiencies	All associated with ataxia
Antineuronal antibodies	Various cancers associated with subacute and/or aggressive cerebellar syndromes	(see Table 17.7 and Chapter 21)
Leukocyte enzymes	In particular, hexosaminidase A	Often concomitant LMN syndrome
Very long chain fatty acids	A variant of adrenomyeloneuropathy	Gene test is also available
Ammonia and lactic acid	Metabolic ataxias	Consider in early onset often subacute and variable phenotypes
Gene tests	See text for specific details	Becoming increasingly important for sporadic ataxia cases; SCA 6 and FRDA should be considered

FRDA, Friedreich's ataxia; LMN, lower motor neurone; SLE, systemic lupus erythematosus.

Blood tests

There is a long list of potential tests that can be considered in a case of undiagnosed ataxia (Table 17.2), much as one would for complicated neurological disease of other causes, but some deserve special mention here. Despite their rarity, it is always worthwhile considering the treatable, so an assessment of B vitamins and vitamin E should not be forgotten. Hypothyroidism is frequently mentioned as a cause of ataxia; this is extremely rare. A range of antibody tests are now frequently employed, including an autoantibody screen, antiphospholipid syndrome, antineuronal antibodies and assessment for sensitivity to gluten. An assessment of lysosomal and other enzymes may also point to a specific neurometabolic disorder; hexosaminidase A is of particular relevance to the ataxic patient. There are now numerous gene tests widely available; these are discussed in more detail later.

Ancillary tests

If an inflammatory disorder of the nervous system is being considered an assessment of intrathecal oligoclonal immunoglobulins may help (Chapter 11). These are found not only in cases of multiple sclerosis, but also in paraneoplastic disorders (Chapter 21) and other rarer inflammatory conditions such as neurosarcoidosis (Chapter 26). Autonomic features, such as postural dizziness and urinary urgency, may require a detailed assessment of the autonomic system, to both aid the diagnosis and guide treatment. Occasionally, electrophysiological assessment of anal sphincter denervation is helpful and may point towards a diagnosis of multiple system atrophy. In patients with early onset ataxia of a complicated nature, including severe epilepsy, myoclonus and/or cognitive decline, it may be necessary to perform biopsies of axillary skin and muscle.

The ataxic disorders

There are several different ways of structuring discussion of the causes of ataxia. Here, whether or not a condition is inherited or acquired is used as the main dividing line, but even this is not always straightforward. As new genes are discovered, some patients previously thought to have sporadic acquired disorders move into the inherited group. Similarly there are intrauterine events or processes that can produce a syndrome reminiscent of ataxias of other patients with ataxias of genetic origin.

Inherited ataxia syndromes

Congenital ataxias

This group of disorders, as the name implies, encompasses ataxic disorders of early onset; generally these are non-progressive. The clear identification of such early life onset in a developing infant is not always easy, and similarly the definition of non-progression in the growing child also presents difficulties. Moreover, as improvements in our understanding of the genetic bases of these disorders have developed it has become clear that the majority of these disorders have a genetic cause.

There are a number of well-recognised syndromes (Table 17.3) with a range of additional features including involvement of other organs and dysmorphism. The clinical clues that one might be dealing with a congenital problem include developmental motor delay; this can sometimes become apparent by a longer time than normal that a toddler spends crawling before taking independent steps. The demonstration of non-progression is difficult because as a child develops they acquire motor skills. Frequently, the history is that of a child, who although able to acquire new skills is always behind

Table 17.3 Congenital inherited ataxic disorders. This is an incomplete list; numerous reports of often singular families. There is also some overlap with the autosomal recessive ataxias, some of which have congenital features (e.g. deafness), but have a progressive ataxia. The conditions listed here have, as far as it is possible to determine, non-progressive ataxia.

Syndrome	Additional features	Mode of inheritance	Gene defect
Joubert's syndrome	Episodic hyperpnoea, abnormal eye movements and mental retardation	Autosomal recessive Genetically heterogeneous	*AHI1* gene *NPHP1* gene *CEP290* Plus others with established and distinct loci
Gillespie's syndrome	Mental retardation and partial aniridia	Autosomal recessive	Pax 6
Congenital nystagmus	Hypoplasia of the macula in some cases	Autosomal recessive and X-linked	*NYS1–6p* *NYS2*, X-linked and others
Congential hypoplasia and quadripedal gait	Mental retardation and seizures	Autosomal recessive	17p
Paine's syndrome	Spasticity, mental retardation and microcephaly	X-linked recessive ataxia	No gene identified

their peers and described as clumsy. As motor skills are acquired the child may actually report fewer problems with unsteadiness. Imaging can sometime help in some syndromes and there may be significant reduction in cerebellar volume, including signs such as 'molar tooth' an abnormally deep interpeduncular fossa with elongated, thick and maloriented superior cerebellar peduncles as seen with Joubert's syndrome. The combination of a very small cerebellum and associated structures on imaging in a child who is not profoundly ataxic points strongly towards a congenital explanation.

Other possibilities to be considered in these early onset cases are those caused by developmental abnormalities. Most of these are readily diagnosed with modern imaging techniques and include Arnold–Chiari malformation and Dandy–Walker cysts. These are discussed in more detail in Chapter 16.

Autosomal recessive cerebellar ataxias

There is a long list of mutations inherited in an autosomal recessive manner and, as a general rule, onset of the autosomal recessive ataxias is before the age of 20 years (Table 17.4). FRDA is by far and away the most common cause, accounting for approximately 40% of autosomal recessive cerebellar ataxia (ARCA) cases. The remainder are all individually rare. Improvements in gene sequencing technologies are revolutionising the gene testing environment and its is likely that many previously untestable genes will become available soon.

Friedreich's ataxia

This has an estimated prevalence of approximately 2/100 000. The condition is characterised by a progressive gait and limb ataxia and a number of additional features including an axonal sensorimotor neuropathy, pyramidal tract involvement, hypertrophic cardiomyopathy, skeletal abnormalities, optic atrophy, deafness and diabetes. Typically, it begins between the ages of 8 and 15 years. There are reported instances of later onset, even as late as the seventh decade; these are the exception. The chief invariable additional feature is the neuropathy, predominantly sensory and progressive.

Following the identification of the gene frataxin in 1996, it was shown that the predominant mutation is a trinucleotide repeat (GAA) in intron 1. Expansion of both alleles is found in over 96% of patients. The remaining patients have point mutations on one allele in association with an expansion on the other. This has permitted the introduction of a specific and sensitive diagnostic test, as it is a relatively simple matter to measure the repeat size. The normal GAA repeat length varies from 7 to 22 units, whereas the disease range is around 100–2000 repeats; the shorter the length of the repeat the later the onset and generally the milder the disease phenotype.

The frataxin protein has been shown to be involved in iron metabolism within the mitochondria and a number of therapeutic strategies based around improving mitochondrial function are being developed. No treatment to date has been shown to influence disease progression.

Ataxic disorders associated with defective DNA repair

There are several rare disorders characterised at a molecular level by a reduced capacity to repair DNA. The most well known and most studied is ataxia telangiectasia (AT). This produces a mixed movement disorder with the presence of dystonia and chorea in addition to the progressive ataxia. Growth and sexual development can be delayed and mild learning difficulties are common but not invariable. The typical skin and eye lesions (Figure 17.1) usually develop between the ages of 3 and 6 years and are best seen on the conjunctival surface and the ear. AT is associated with abnormalities of both humoral and cell-mediated immunity and is caused by mutations in the *ATM* gene. There are variants of this clinical phenotype with absence of telangiectasia and later onset, also caused by mutations in *ATM*.

A rarer clinically similar disease caused by mutations in *hMRE11* has been identified and is termed AT-like disorder. Clinically related conditions xeroderma pigmentosum and Cockayne's syndrome (Table 17.4) are also caused by defects in DNA repair; they are much rarer and associated with additional features, most frequently skin abnormalities.

Table 17.4 Autosomal recessive cerebellar ataxias (ARCAs).

Syndrome	Gene defect	Clinical pointers	Notes
Friedreich's ataxia (FRDA)	GAA repeat (and some point mutations in *FRDA* gene)	Neuropathy, pyramidal signs, skeletal abnormalities, diabetes and cardiomyopathy	Most common ARCA
Ataxia telangiectasia (AT) AT-like disorder	*ATM* *hMRE11*	Oculomotor apraxia, mixed movement disorder, humoral immune deficiencies, increased cancer risk	Telangiectasia not always present or easily identified
Cockayne's syndrome	CS type A – *ERCC8* gene CS type B – *ERCC6* gene	'Cachectic dwarfism' Mental retardation Pigmentary retinopathy	
Xeroderma pigmentosum (XP)		Increased skin cancer in XP but not Cockayne's	
AOA1	Aprataxin	Oculomotor apraxia	
AOA2	Senataxin	Oculomotor apraxia	Probably second most common ARCA
ARSACS	Sacsin	Demyelinating neuropathy, hypertrophy of the retinal layer (detected using OCT)	Along with senataxin second in frequency to FRDA
Hypogonadism	RNF216	Hypogonadotrophic hypogonadism	a.k.a. Gordon Holmes' syndrome
Marinesco–Sjögren's syndrome	*SIL1* on chr 5q31	Cataracts and mental retardation	
Progressive myoclonic ataxia (Ramsay-Hunt syndrome)	Genetically complex	Epilepsy is frequently associated	Overlaps with differential of progressive myoclonic epilepsy
Behr's and related syndromes, e.g. 3-methylglutaconic aciduria type III (Costeff's syndrome)	No gene for Behr's yet identified *OPA3* gene	Optic atrophy (OA), spasticity and mental retardation	There are other cases with OA but not Behr's syndrome
Congenital or childhood onset deafness	Genetically complex	Several different families/ syndromes reported	May cause overlap with Usher's syndrome
Autosomal recessive late onset ataxia	Heterogeneous	Clinically variable with a range of additional features	Relatively rare

Ataxias associated with oculomotor apraxia

There are two genetically distinct but clinically similar disorders associated with the distinctive feature of oculomotor apraxia: ataxia associated with oculomotor apraxia (AOA) types 1 and 2. AOA is used to describe intermittent failure of the voluntary saccadic system, and should be suspected where the patient uses head thrusts or synkinetic blinking to help initiate a voluntary saccade. AOA1 has been shown to be caused by mutations in the aprataxin gene on chromosome 9p13. This is characterised by the association of ataxia with chorea early in the disease course, oculomotor apraxia, peripheral neuropathy and variable but mild learning difficulties. MRI reveals cerebellar atrophy; serum analysis may show hypercholesterolaemia and hypoalbuminaemia.

AOA2 is very similar clinically and also overlaps with the AT phenotype. Mutations in senataxin have been shown to cause this syndrome. Alpha-fetoprotein (AFP) is elevated in virtually all cases and is therefore a useful screen for this disorder. AOA2 appears to be more common than either AT or AOA1, accounting for approximately 8% of autosomal recessive ataxia.

Ataxia caused by vitamin E deficiency

A relationship between spino-cerebellar dysfunction and vitamin E deficiency has been recognised for many years. Many cases have a demonstrable cause for their vitamin E deficiency such as abetalipoproteinaemia, chronic liver disease and malabsorptive states secondary to cystic fibrosis or bowel resection. In 1985, Harding *et al.* described

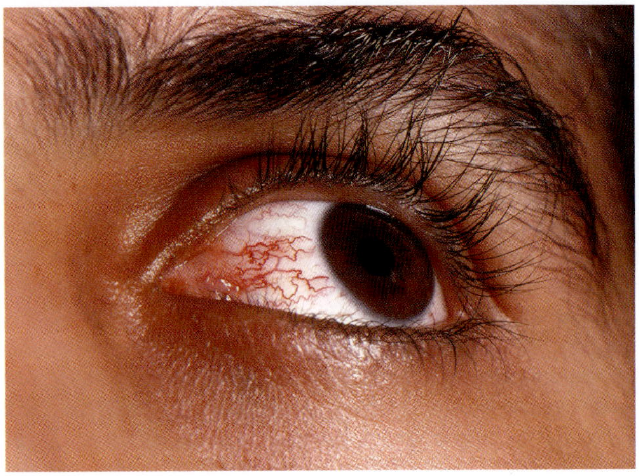

Figure 17.1 Conjunctival telangiectasia in a patient with ataxia telangiectasia. (Courtesy of The Audio Visual Services Unit, National Hospital for Neurology and Neurosurgery.)

a patient with a progressive spino-cerebellar disorder who had isolated vitamin E deficiency with no evidence of malabsorption. The clinical features of this syndrome include progressive gait ataxia, incoordination of the limbs, areflexia and large fibre sensory loss. Homozygosity mapping led to the identification of a gene α-tocopherol transfer protein (αTTP) on chromosome 8q. These patients have an impaired ability to incorporate vitamin E (α-tocopherol) into very low density lipoproteins in the liver. This function is necessary to maintain the adequate circulation of α-tocopherol. A number of mutations have been described, but the mainstay of diagnosis is the measurement of serum vitamin E rather than genetic analysis. Despite its rarity, it is imperative not to miss such a diagnosis because replacement therapy helps to stabilise the situation and in some cases produces improvements. Generally, vitamin E deficiency caused by malabsortion requires substantially higher doses of replacement therapy than those caused by αTTP mutations.

The most severe vitamin E deficiency state occurring in humans is abetalipoproteinaemia. The typical presentation is in the second decade, with progressive ataxia, areflexia, posterior column signs; a pigmentary retinopathy may also be seen. It is caused by mutations in the gene encoding a subunit of the microsomal triglyceride transfer protein and is associated with low levels of apoprotein B, which normally carries lipid from the intestinal cell to the plasma. This results in very low levels of circulating lipids, particularly cholesterol, and severe malabsorption of the fat-soluble vitamins A, D, E and K. Serum vitamin E concentrations are either low or undetectable from birth; acanthocytes are usually present in the peripheral blood.

Hypobetalipoproteinaemia is a molecularly related but genetically distinct disorder inherited in an autosomal dominant manner and characterised by moderately reduced serum concentrations of cholesterol, triglyceride and low-density lipoproteins. Most patients are asymptomatic but neurologically they may present with ataxia, absent reflexes and proprioceptive deficits.

Autosomal recessive spastic ataxia of Charlevoix-Saguenay

This condition was thought to be extremely rare and probably confined to a region of Quebec. However, following identification of the gene it is now recognised to be the second most common ARCA (with a similar frequency to mutations of senataxin) after FRDA. Clinically, it is distinguished by the presence of a demyelinating neuropathy and hypertrophy of the retinal layer.

Other metabolic causes of ataxia

These are nearly all autosomal recessive disorders unless otherwise stated.

Intermittent metabolic ataxias

These may be caused by abnormalities in the urea cycle, aminoacidurias and disorders of pyruvate metabolism. Most commonly, a high ammonia as a marker of urea cycle dysfunction is the explanation. All these conditions have a similar phenotype with ataxia, dysarthria, vomiting, confusion and involuntary movements. Seizures and a variable degree of learning difficulties may also be seen. Precipitants are not always identified but a history of prodromal illness or a large protein load should be sought. Treatment consists of protein restriction and intravenous fluid administration during acute episodes.

Ornithine transcarbamylase (OTC) deficiency is X-linked and is the most common urea cycle enzyme defect. Affected males die in the neonatal period, but severity varies considerably in females, from the presence of severe neurological deficit to no symptoms apart from mild protein intolerance. It can present in adult or even late adult life. A heavy protein meal, infection or the prescription of valproic acid therapy can precipitate an encephalopathy in an asymptomatic case.

Amino acidurias including Hartnup's disease also need to be considered in the intermittent ataxias. There is often a super-added involuntary movement disorder, psychiatric disturbance and a variable degree of cognitive decline. A pellagra-like rash may also be seen in this condition. Hartnup's disease is caused by mutations in *SLC6A19* which encodes a neutral amino acid transporter. Some amino-acidurias, including intermittent branched-chain ketoaciduria and isovaleric acidaemia, present in a similar clinical pattern to the hyperammonaemias. In contrast to the urea cycle disorders, a high-protein diet and oral nicotinamide therapy may help.

Pyruvate dehydrogenase deficiency (PDH) is rare and genetically heterogeneous, although the majority of cases are caused by mutations in the gene for X-linked E1 α subunit of the enzyme. However, there is a high frequency of manifesting female heterozygotes with a wide spectrum of disease severity because of variable X chromosome inactivation. Generally, it is a disease with an infantile onset although in manifesting females later onset and slightly more benign course can be seen. In addition to the complicated clinical picture of spasticity, seizures and severe learning difficulties, dysplastic features on brain MRI may be seen. The diagnosis is made most readily by assay of PDH activity in cultured fibroblasts.

Very rarely, intermittent ataxia has been reported as a result of multiple biotin-dependent carboxylase deficiencies. The picture is complicated, with generalised seizures, myoclonus, nystagmus and hypotonia. There are associated defects of humoral and cell-mediated immunity. It is important to diagnose by checking serum biotinidase activity as biotin therapy may result in clinical improvement.

Progressive metabolic ataxias

There is a long list of storage and other metabolic disease that can produce ataxia as a component of the presenting features, usually minor. Also, as awareness and diagnostic accuracy is improving most of these patients are identified in early life, in paediatric clinics. The list includes the sphingomyelin lipidoses, metachromatic leukodystrophy, galactosylceramide lipidosis (Krabbe's disease) and the hexosaminidase deficiencies. Also within this group is adrenoleuko-myeloneuropathy, discussed later in this chapter.

A late onset form of hexosaminidase A deficiency may result in a progressive ataxia with predominantly proximal neurogenic weakness. On imaging there is striking and selective atrophy of the cerebellum. Ataxia may also be seen in Niemann–Pick disease type C, combined with a supranuclear gaze palsy. Sphingomyelinase activity is usually within the normal range, but foamy storage cells are found in the bone marrow. Unlike Niemann–Pick types A and B, type C is not caused by abnormalities in the sphingomyelin gene but in the *NPC* gene on chromosome 18. The exact molecular events leading to the mishandling of lipid and cholesterol are unclear.

Cholestanolosis (also called cerebrotendinous xanthomatosis, CTX) is a rare autosomal recessive disorder caused by defective bile salt metabolism, resulting from a deficiency of mitochondrial sterol 27 hydroxylase encoded by *CYP27A1* gene. It usually begins after puberty and gives rise to ataxia, dementia, spasticity and peripheral neuropathy. Systemically, it leads to premature atherosclerosis, cataracts and tendon xanthomas. Treatment with chenodeoxycholic acid and a statin appears to improve serological parameters and stabilisation of the disease.

Autosomal dominant cerebellar ataxias

This is clinically and genetically a heterogeneous group of disorders. There are currently some 30 identified loci for the dominant ataxias. These are numbered in the sequence of each locus as it is found. Spinocerebellar ataxia type 1 (SCA 1) was one of the first neurological diseases to have its gene mapped, reported in 1977. Not all the genes have been identified (Table 17.5). Some common themes at both a clinical and molecular level emerge. The molecular consequences of the most common type of mutation is an expanded CAG repeat and the salient points are made in Table 17.6.

The dominant ataxias have two broad classification systems, one clinical and the other based on the underlying SCA mutation. Despite the progress in the genetic field, the clinical classification system proposed by Harding in 1984 remains useful for structuring diagnostic thoughts and the approach to genetic investigation. This clinical classification is divided into three parts, with a roman numeral for each.

ADCA I is characterised by a progressive ataxic syndrome complicated, variably, by cognitive impairment, pyramidal signs, supranuclear gaze abnormalities, neuropathy and extrapyramidal signs. It is extremely rare to see all these features in one patient; the burden of involvement within each system varies both within and between families. One needs to bear this in mind when taking a family history. The disease usually starts after the age of 25, although occasional childhood onset has been reported – a feature that is a consequence of anticipation, the result of the unstable and expanding nature of the underlying repeating mutations (Table 17.6).

ADCA II is also complicated; some of the features of ADCA I may also be seen but it is the macular dystrophy that singles out this disease. This is the rarest of the clinical subtypes; virtually all cases are caused by mutations in the *SCA7* gene.

ADCA III is generally of later onset than the other two subtypes and is a so-called 'pure' ataxia. A note of caution, however: the signs in ADCA I and II emerge with disease progression, so it is sometimes difficult to be sure that a patient and/or their family are truly 'pure' without the benefit of a long history and/or examining other affected relatives. As a rule of thumb, a progressive ataxia without additional features after 10 years' duration is strong clinical evidence of ADCA III. The tests most widely used and available are detailed in Table 17.7.

As a rough rule of thumb, testing for SCA 1, 2, 3, 6 and 7 identifies the causative mutation in 50% of those with a clinical diagnosis of probable ADCA. The remaining 50% is comprised of the rarer SCAs including SCA 12, 14 and 17 and of course those yet to be identified.

Dentato-rubro-pallido-luysian atrophy

Dentato-rubro-pallido-luysian atrophy (DRPLA), an autosomal dominant disorder found mainly in Japan but reported worldwide, has a variable clinical presentation comprising various combinations of ataxia, dystonia, myoclonus, seizures, dementia and parkinsonism. This disorder is another expanded CAG repeat (Table 17.6).

Investigations

The main investigation involves the identification of the underlying mutation. A fairly widely available and relatively simple panel of gene tests is now available and should be the first investigation undertaken in suspected cases. However, the clinician should explain to the patient, and family if appropriate, the implications of a positive test. This should include the facts that it is inherited in an autosomal dominant fashion, so siblings and offspring are at 50% risk and that the penetrance is high – close to 100%.

Research imaging studies have highlighted some regional differences in patterns of brain atrophy, but none of these is currently useful in the clinical setting. Neurophysiological techniques may be helpful in identifying peripheral nerve. A detailed neuro-ophthalmological assessment can be helpful.

Treatment

All these diseases are progressive, currently incurable and with no proven disease-modifying therapies available. The predominant mutations accounting for at least 50% of cases are caused by an expanded CAG repeat in the coding segment of the gene. This triplet encodes glutamine and these diseases are known as the polyglutamine disorders. As discussed in Chapters 8 and 10, this mutation is also found in other neurological disorders, Huntington's disease and Kennedy's syndrome. This indicates that there is something common in the pathway of neurodegeneration between these clinically distinct disorders; this raises hope that discoveries in one of these diseases will have an impact upon the others.

Genetic forms of episodic ataxia

This heterogeneous group of disorders is characterised by a marked periodicity in attacks of ataxia. There are many of these patients who describe paroxysmal worsening of their disorder. Some will have clearly defined metabolic syndromes, as described earlier. Some have a familial disorder with an autosomal dominant pattern: these are described here. Many more have an ill-defined syndrome without a clear reason for these episodes. The unusual history of such episodes, if their nature is not recognised, often leads to the mistaken view that these are psychological in origin. At a molecular and genetic level, it is perhaps unsurprising that ion channel mutations have been implicated in many of these disorders.

Episodic ataxia type 1

This is a rare disorder characterised by attacks of brief duration, lasting seconds or a few minutes. The attacks may be frequent; some patients may experience many attacks each day. Attacks may be precipitated by sudden movement or shocks. The condition classically presents in childhood and attack frequency lessens with age, so it is important to seek early life history in older relatives. They are most often associated with peripheral myokymia which can be seen clinically in some, but may require electromyography (EMG) to diagnose.

Mutations in a potassium channel *KCNA1* gene have been shown to cause this syndrome. This channel is closely related to the peripheral neuromuscular potassium channel, attacked by autoantibodies in neuromyotonia (Chapters 10 and 21), which also causes myokymia. Treatment success is variable; acetazolamide may help.

Table 17.5 The autosomal dominant cerebellar ataxias.

SCA no.	Genetic locus	Gene	Clinical pointers	Notes
1	6p22.3	Ataxin 1 CAG repeat	Complicated, including: neuropathy, cognitive decline, pyramidal and extrapyramidal features	
2	12q24.13	Ataxin 2 CAG repeat	As above, plus slow saccades and neuropathy	
3	14q32.12	Ataxin 3 CAG repeat	As above but a stronger extrapyramidal phenotype	Probably most common worldwide
4	16q24-qter	N/K	Associated with a neuropathy	
5	11q13.2	SPTBN2 beta-III spectrin D		Very rare
6	19p13.13	CACNAIA CAG repeat	Later onset (>45 years) and relatively pure	Point mutations in this gene produce either familial hemiplegic migraine or EA2
7	3p14.1	Ataxin 7 CAG repeat	Complicated, with slow saccades and prominent macular dystrophy	Shows the most marked anti-cipation in the known SCAs
8	13q21	Kelch-like 1 CTG repeat		Uncertain pathogenicity
9	SCA9	Reserved		
10	22q13.31	Ataxin 10 ATTCT repeat		
11	15q14–q21.3	Tau-tubulin kinase 2 point mutation		Pure ataxia
12	5q32	PPP2R2B CAG repeat	Prominent tremor	
13	19q13.33	KCNC3 point mutations		
14	19q13.42	PRKCG point mutations	Prominent dystonia	
15	3p24.2-pter	ITPR 1		
16	8q23–q24.1	Not known (NK)		
17	6q27 TBP	TBP CAG repeat	HD-like features	Rare
18	7q31–q32	N/K		Additional sensor-motor neuropathy
19	1p21–q21	KCND3		Allelic to SCA 22
20	11q12	Heterozygous duplication		A contiguous gene duplication syndrome
21	7p21.3-p15.1	TMEM230	Cognitive Impairment	
22	1p21–q23	KCND3		Allelic to SCA 19
23	20p13-p12.2	PDYN		
24	1p36	N/K		1 Family
25	2p21-p15	N/K		1 Family
26	19p13.3	EEF2		1 Family
27	13q33.1	FGF14 point mutations		
28	18p11.22–q11.2	AFG3L2		Can also cause AR spastic ataxia 5
Unspecified	16q22.1	Puratrophin 1 point mutations		Overlaps SCA 4 region, but not definitively SCA 4 gene

Table 17.6 Core principles of the polyglutamine tract disorders.

- Several neurodegenerative disease are caused by the same type of mutation; namely, an expanded encoded CAG repeat – Huntington's disease, SCAs 1–3, 6, 7, 17, dentato-rubro-pallido-luysian atrophy (DRPLA) and Kennedy's disease
- The CAG repeat is polymorphic in both normal and disease-associated chromosomes. However, once above a critical threshold the repeat becomes more unstable and may expand from one generation to the next
- There is a tight inverse correlation of length of repeat and age at onset
- Anticipation is seen: this is the phenomena of earlier onset and often more severe disease in succeeding generations
- The greatest instability is seen in the paternal line and most cases of anticipation and *de novo* mutation occur on transmission of an allele from father to offspring
- The CAG codon encodes glutamine and this expanded glutamine tract is in some way 'toxic' to adult neurones

The prevalence of the individual disease varies worldwide and is in part determined by the proportion of high normal repeats in the general population. It is believed that this high normal repeat is an occasional feeder of the *de novo* mutations.

Table 17.7 Clinical impact of the autosomal dominant cerebellar ataxias (ADCAs).

ADCA type	Genetic tests (widely available)	Relative contribution to each subclass (%)
ADCA I	SCA 1–3	50
ADCA II	SCA 7	99
ADCA III	SCA 6	50

Episodic ataxia type 2

This is more common than EA1; clinically these attacks resemble a form of vertebro-basilar migraine attack. The attacks generally last hours, build up over several minutes and are associated with nausea, vertigo and often vomiting. The patients look pale and unwell. There may be an associated mild headache. The attacks may vary from daily to several months between. Again, attacks become less frequent as the patient enters adulthood. However, unlike EA1 a slowly progressive ataxia usually develops over the years. The typical picture is to see children or adolescents with episodes, with a parent with a more progressive permanent ataxia.

This disorder is caused by point mutations, usually of nonsense type, in the calcium channel gene *CACN1A*. This is the same gene that may cause familial hemiplegic migraine (Chapter 12) and SCA 6 (see Autosomal dominant cerebellar ataxias). This phenomenon, where different clinical disorders are caused by different mutations in the same gene, is called allelic heterogeneity.

Treatment by acetazolamide may be useful, but some have had more success with dichlorphenamide. There is no evidence currently that preventing attacks impacts on the progressive component of the illness, but as EA2 is a rare disorder this is hard evidence to obtain.

Other episodic ataxias

There are families reported with episodic ataxia but no evidence of mutations in either of the above genes. EA3 describes a family with vertigo and tinnitus; there is evidence that the disease causing mutation lies on 1q42. EA4 has been used to describe a family with periodic vestibulo-cerebellar ataxia (PATX). There are several other novel genes for EA recently described.

X-linked ataxia syndromes

The ataxic syndromes associated with mutations on the X chromosome are generally rare and usually complicated. Moreover, the clinical picture points to the underlying diagnosis. A variant of adrenoleukodystrophy may produce ataxic features; the presence of a pyramidal leukodystrophic phenotype with a demyelinating neuropathy usually points to the correct diagnosis. A measurement of serum very long chain fatty acids is a useful screening tool and mutations in the underlying gene can be sought. Pelizaeus–Merzbacher disease can produce an early life onset complicated ataxia; mutations or rearrangements of the *PLP* gene can be detected. Neuro-acanthocytosis is described in more detail in Chapter 6; usually ataxia is overshadowed by the involuntary movements of chorea and dystonia. Autosomal dominant, autosomal recessive and X-linked forms have all been described. A wet blood film looking for 'thorny' red cells (acanthocytes) should be requested. The X-linked form, also called McLeod's syndrome, is associated with abnormalities of the Kell antigen.

Fragile X tremor ataxia syndrome (FXTAS) is a recent addition to the differential diagnosis of mid to late life onset progressive ataxia. Fragile X syndrome is the most common cause of mental retardation in males and is caused by an expanded (non-coding) repeat in the *FMR1* gene. In the 'normal' range of repeats there is a high normal or premutation repeat length (55–200 CGG repeats). Hitherto, this has been considered purely as a substrate for occasional expansion into the disease-associated range and the production of fragile X syndrome in male descendents. Jacquemont *et al.* (2004) reported an excess of pre-mutation carriers in patients with a late onset ataxia syndrome with prominent tremor and associated cognitive decline. Others have confirmed these findings and pathological examination has revealed the presences of novel proteinaceous nuclear inclusions in both neurones and astrocytes. They are ubiquitin positive but dissimilar to the inclusions of Parkinson's disease, Alzheimer's disease and other tauopathies, nor do they resemble the nuclear inclusions seen in CAG repeat disease. Imaging reveals generalised volume loss of cerebrum and cerebellum and signal changes in the middle cerebellar peduncles. Diagnosis of FXTAS in appropriately selected clinical cases is by genetic analysis of the *FMR1* repeat.

Mitochondrial ataxia syndromes

The range of disorders that can be caused by mitochondrial DNA (mtDNA) mutations is described in Chapter 10. In brief, mtDNA is entirely maternal in origin so inheritance of any traits caused by mutations in the 16.5 kb circular DNA molecule is through the maternal line. Mitochondria are vital for oxidative phosphorylation and any defects in this system can have wide-ranging multi-systemic features. Ataxia is quite common in a number of well-characterised mtDNA syndromes. Kearns–Sayre syndrome is an early life (<20 years) disorder of ataxia, progressive external ophthalmoplegia, pigmentary retinopathy and raised cerebrospinal fluid (CSF) protein. Most commonly it is caused by a deletion of approximately 5 kb of the mtDNA molecule. This usually arises spontaneously and is non-transmissible and therefore is generally non-familial. Missense mutations may also cause complicated ataxia phenotypes including neurogenic ataxia and retinitis pigmentosa (NARP), caused by a mutation at 8993 and the point mutations at 3243 (MELAS) and 8344 (MERRF) syndromes. As a general rule, a complicated multi-systemic disturbance particularly those involving dementia, deafness and visual problems with or without lactic acidosis suggests a mitochondrial disease. A muscle biopsy may be required (Chapter 10).

There is also overlap with the so-called Ramsay-Hunt syndrome of ataxia and myoclonus. The differential diagnosis includes MERRF, DRPLA, ceroid lipofuscinosis, sialidosis, and Unverricht–Lundborg disease. Usually, seizures are common in these latter disorders.

Many of these disorders are now amenable to direct gene testing for the underlying mutation and it is worth checking with the local genetic laboratory for available tests.

Next generation gene sequencing

The revolution in technologies that has allowed a huge increase in speed and accuracy of genetic testing coupled with a consequent massive reduction in cost has not only had a major impact on gene identification, but is also starting to influence the range of gene tests available. It is by the nature of this innovation that any statements in textbooks will be out of a date by the time of publication and it is often necessary to use the variety of genetic information available on the internet for the most up-to-date information. It is likely that over the next few years the remaining genetic disorders, including the ataxias, will be identified and there is also great optimism that genome sequencing will be made more available for diagnostic use.

Acquired ataxia syndromes

Of the many acquired cerebellar disorders, chronic alcohol abuse is probably the most common, followed by various nutritional deficiencies. The more common acquired disorders are mentioned here.

Infective disease

In this section, only those infections that give rise to prominent cerebellar dysfunction are discussed. For a more detailed account of CNS infections, see Chapter 9.

Acute or subacute onset

Acute cerebellar ataxia of childhood is the most common acute ataxia and although attributed to a viral infection, serological evidence is usually lacking. The usual viral causes include echoviruses, coxsackie groups A and B, poliovirus, Epstein–Barr and herpes simplex virus. Very occasionally some bacteria produce a similar syndrome.

The condition usually presents between the ages of 1 and 8 years and a mild prodromal illness is sometimes reported. The illness worsens over hours or occasionally days; the child presents with severe ataxia particularly of the midline, with the limbs relatively spared. Additional features include myoclonus, opsoclonus or ocular flutter. Despite this dramatic presentation the outlook is good although it may take several months for full recovery.

Post-infective processes may also affect the cerebellum and its connections. Ataxia is particularly well recognised as part of the syndrome of post-infectious disseminated encephalomyelitis after varicella infection. It has also been reported following measles, rubella and mumps. There are a number of brainstem syndromes including Bickerstaff's encephalitis and the Fisher variant of acute inflammatory polyradiculoneuropathy, which may present with ataxia, but the clinical picture is complicated by brainstem signs such as ophthalmoplegia.

Progressive ataxia with a chronic or subacute course

Infections causing progressive ataxia are all rare. In childhood, one needs to consider the post-measles complication of subacute sclerosing panencephalitis. This rare but serious condition has a number of other features including myoclonus and cognitive decline. Congenital rubella may produce a pancerebellar syndrome in association with dementia, optic atrophy and occasionally multifocal myoclonus with onset between the ages of 8 and 19 years. HIV infection has become the great mimic and may produce an encephalopathy with ataxic features.

In adulthood there are very few infective agents that produce a progressive cerebellar presentation. Of most importance are the various presentations of prion disease. These are discussed in more detail in Chapter 8. Ataxic features are most commonly found in the familial Gerstmann–Sträussler–Scheinker syndrome and in variant Creutzfeldt–Jakob disease. The iatrogenic form of spongiform encephalopathy also produces a predominant ataxic phenotype. This disease resulted from erroneous contamination and inoculation by a variety of means, including growth hormone replacement therapy, corneal and dural grafts. It has become rare, following its identification and the important public health measures that ensued.

Cerebellar involvement has also been described following infection by *Mycoplasma pneumoniae*, *Legionella pneumoniae* and *Toxoplasma gondii*, as well as in typhoid fever and tick paralysis. Lyme disease can produce an ataxic picture complicated by bilateral facial palsy and CSF lymphocytic pleocytosis. A number of tropical infections also need consideration in the appropriate clinical setting. A transient cerebellar syndrome lasting several weeks and resembling acute cerebellar ataxia of childhood has been reported following *Plasmodium falciparum* infection. Cerebellar signs, particularly gait ataxia, are common in the racemose form of neuro-cysticercosis (Chapter 9).

'Vanishing white matter disease' is one of the more prevalent inherited childhood leukoencephalopathies and is characterised by progressive neurological decline, and in particular cerebellar ataxia (Chapter 11). However, there is wide phenotypic variability and it may present in adulthood. It is an unusual disease in which there is a genetic defect (in one of five subunits of a translation initiation factor eIF2B) and yet its sensitivity to febrile infections is striking. MRI is usually extremely helpful in establishing the diagnosis.

Space-occupying lesions of the posterior fossa associated with fever require urgent imaging to identify the possibility of a cerebellar abscess. These usually present relatively subacutely with headache and symptoms and signs of raised intracranial pressure. TB may produce a more indolent condition.

Inflammatory disease

An isolated cerebellar syndrome is a rare presentation of multiple sclerosis. MRI shows white matter lesions, which is usually the reason multiple sclerosis is considered. The differential diagnosis of possible demyelinating disease or other inflammatory conditions are discussed in Chapter 11. They include sarcoidosis, systemic lupus erythematosus (SLE) and similar syndromes, antiphospholipid and Sjögren's disease. Investigation needs to be tailored to the clinical impression and but involves appropriate antibody tests, CSF examination, and ancillary tests such as lip biopsy in the case of sicca syndrome.

Vascular disease

Degenerative cerebrovascular disease can present with an abrupt onset cerebellar and/or brainstem syndrome. The presence of severe headache, raised intracranial pressure and impairment of consciousness suggest the possibility of a posterior fossa haematoma. This is a neurological emergency and requires urgent imaging to determine the necessity for neurosurgical intervention. Outcome is worse if diagnosis is delayed.

Thrombotic and embolic events cause an isolated cerebellar syndrome relatively rarely; commonly there are associated brainstem signs, such as diplopia and vertigo. These conditions are discussed in Chapter 5.

Vascular anomalies

Cerebellar haemangioblastomas are vascular and cystic tumours that can present as mass lesions with a consequent cerebellar syndrome. The lesion usually takes the form of an expanding cyst, which causes the subacute deterioration. Appropriate imaging reveals the anatomy and extent of the cyst, and neurosurgical management is usually effective in resolving the symptoms. These tumours rarely bleed spontaneously, but once this has happened, they do need to be monitored. Generally growth results in progressive symptoms and signs and thus regular imaging is not always required.

These tumours can occur throughout life, but the development of a haemangioblastoma before the age of 40 raises the possibility of von Hippel–Lindau disease (VHL). The presence of two haemagioblastomas or a family history are almost diagnostic of this condition. This is important to establish, as the patient and at risk family members will need to be considered for genetic screening. Because VHL is a multisystem disorder, further investigation is required which should include neuro-ophthalmological examination for the retinal angiomas, abdominal imaging for multiple organ cysts, renal cell carcinomas and phaeochromocytomas. Twenty-four hour urinary catecholamines should be measured in all cases. VHL is inherited in an autosomal dominant manner although there is a significant new mutation rate, so the absence of a family history does not exclude the diagnosis nor the need for relative screening once the diagnosis is confirmed.

Other vascular anomalies such as dural fistulae and arteriovenous malformations are discussed in Chapter 5; they are relatively rare causes of an ataxic syndrome.

Chronic bleeding, often from an unknown cause can result in superficial siderosis. This is a rare disorder, more common in males than females (3 : 1) that causes slowly progressive cerebellar ataxia, mainly of gait, and sensorineural deafness, often combined with pyramidal signs. It may also be complicated by dementia, bladder disturbance, anosmia, anisocoria and sensory signs. The MRI features are diagnostic, showing a dark rim around the posterior fossa structures and spinal cord on T2 images. These signal changes represent encrustation of the brain surfaces with haemosiderin. Treatment when possible relies on identifying the source of bleeding (Figure 17.2).

Acquired metabolic disorders

These disorders includes Wernicke's encephalopathy, hepatic encephalopathy, pontine and extrapontine myelinolysis related to hyponatraemia, and hypothyroidism. The latter is only very rarely a cause of a cerebellar syndrome, but as it is potentially treatable it should always be considered. Generally, the other clinical features of these conditions point towards the appropriate investigation and although rare they are all potentially treatable, modifiable or avoidable.

Toxins and physical agents

A large variety of toxins, drugs and other physical agents have been implicated in the pathogenesis of cerebellar disorders. They predominantly cause an insidious onset, slowly progressive clinical syndrome with variable degrees of atrophy on imaging. Direct evidence for causation is not always found and one is often left to take a pragmatic approach to toxin exclusion, where this is possible.

Ethyl alcohol (ethanol)

Ethanol is by far the most common toxin producing a cerebellar ataxia (Chapter 19). Acute toxicity produces the well-known effects of staggering gait and slurred speech. Chronic abuse may produce an insidious, slowly progressive gait and limb ataxia with associated dysarthria. This is generally a pure ataxia without pyramidal signs. However, an alcohol-induced neuropathy is frequently also present and this may only be detected with neurophysiology. Imaging usually shows cerebellar atrophy. Lifelong abstinence is strongly advised but even then the disease may continue to progress. However, there is usually some stabilisation and very occasionally mild improvement. Thiamine supplementation is advisable.

Drugs

Antiepileptic medication, especially phenytoin, carbamazepine and the barbiturates, can all cause an acute or subacute cerebellar syndrome when the dose is too high. This susceptibility varies from patient to patient and cannot be judged by serum level alone but should be based on symptoms and signs. The latter include nystagmus, dysarthria and gait ataxia. The symptoms may be transient and reflect peak dose levels. There is some evidence that chronic exposure may result in a permanent and progressive cerebellar syndrome in a small minority of cases. This syndrome is usually irreversible although cessation may stop or slow progression.

Lithium toxicity, or as a sequelae to an acute encephalopathy, may produce an irreversible and persistent deficit. There may be a history of an acute precipitant such as starvation or fever.

There is a rare reversible ataxia associated with a variety of drugs, including piperazine (for threadworm), high dose 5-fluorouracil and cytosine arabinoside.

Solvents and solvent abuse

Acute exposure to solvents (Chapter 19) can produce a reversible syndrome but prolonged exposure has been reported to produce a persistent deficit. Additional features such as behavioural problems, confusion, cognitive deficits and even psychosis may be seen.

Heavy metals

In the developed world this is an increasingly rare explanation of the usual progressive and complicated ataxias produced by heavy metals including thallium, lead and methyl mercury (Chapter 19). Features and complications vary. These include distal parasthesiae and cortical blindness (Hg), neuropathic features (Pb and Th) and hair loss (Th). Although often coming on abruptly, features may develop some weeks after exposure.

Physical agents

Hypoxia, heat stroke and hypothermia (Chapter 19) may all produce cerebellar features and at autopsy quite profound Purkinje cell loss may be seen. However, these significant insults often produce generalised cerebral dysfunction that usually dominates the clinical picture.

Paraneoplastic cerebellar degeneration

This syndrome is quite distinctive (Chapter 21), with generally a subacute onset, over weeks and months, of midline cerebellar ataxia, usually profound. Typically, patients lose independent mobility within 12–18 months. They may also have chaotic eye movements and oscillopsia. The diagnosis should be suspected in such aggressive cases with onset in later life. Imaging is helpful in that it is typically virtually normal: there are few conditions that produce such unimpressive imaging findings in the face of a major clinical syndrome. Another disease area to consider in this situation is prion-related ataxia.

General health questioning may reveal symptoms such as weight loss, general debility or symptoms suggestive of a primary tumour. There has been substantial progress in our understanding of these disorders and at the time of writing nine specific antibodies have been identified in patients with paraneoplastic cerebellar degeneration

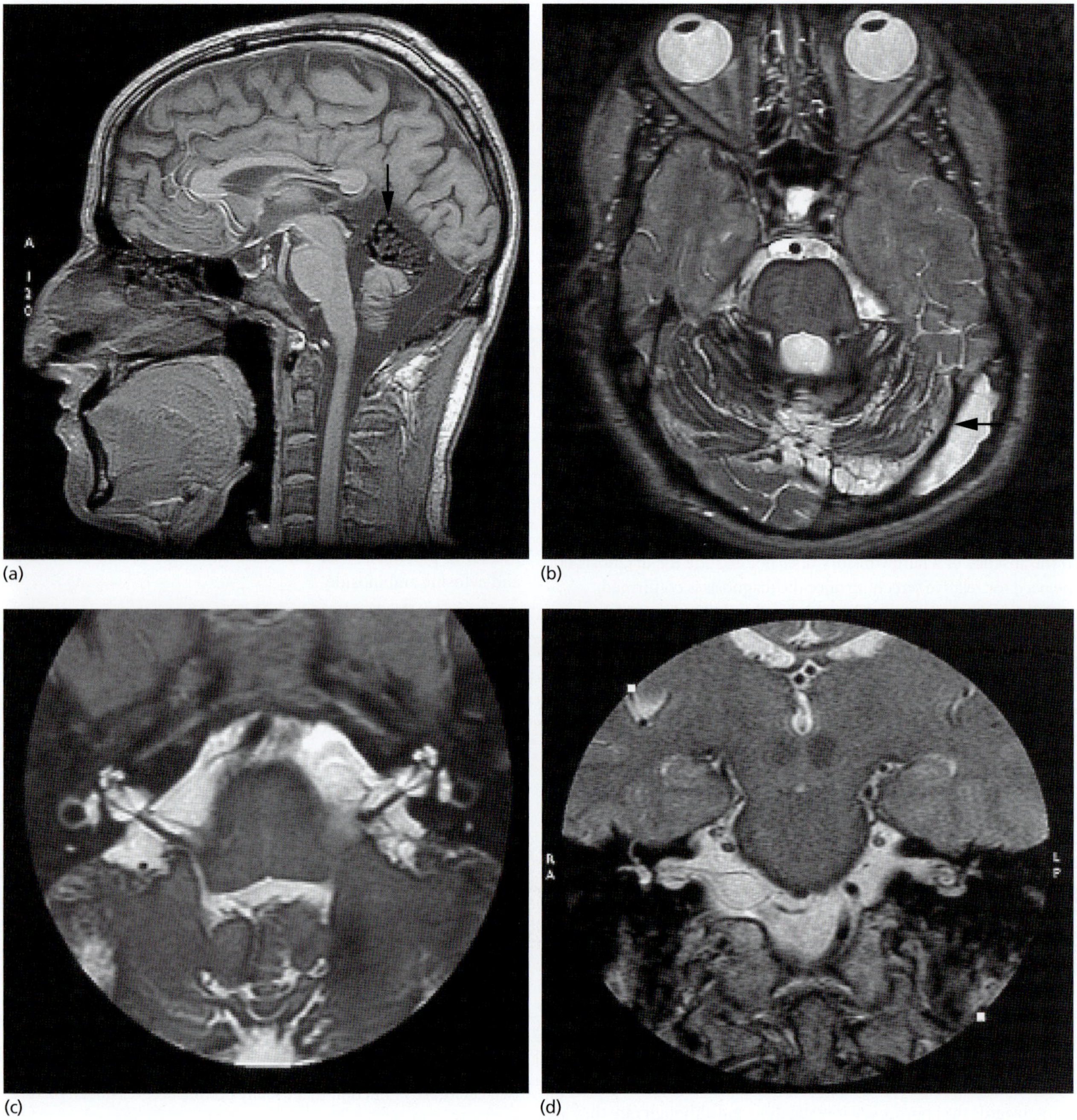

Figure 17.2 Magnetic resonance imaging (MRI) of siderosis in a 38-year-old man with progressive tinnitus, deafness and ataxia (courtesy of Queen Square Imaging Centre). (a) Sagittal MR showing hypointensity in cerebellum, with cerebellar atrophy. (b) T2-weighted axial MRI showing superficial hypointensity surrounding cerebellum. (c, d) T2-weighted MRIshowing superficial hypointensity surrounding VIII and V.

(PCD). These are shown in Table 17.8. The major tumours associated with PCD are gynaecological, breast, lung and testicular cancers and Hodgkin's lymphoma. Frequently, the tumours are small and difficult to identify. The role of antibodies (if any) in causation is not clear. It would appear that there is an autoimmune response to the cancer, which may keep the tumour in check, and that this response produces antibodies that cross-react with cerebellar antigens. Management is based on identification and treatment of the underlying malignancy. Immunomodulation, mostly with intravenous immunoglobulin or plasma exchange, has been tried but with variable success.

There are some patients who present with a sub-acute ataxic syndrome in whom no neoplastic lesion can be found. A minority of these patients have evidence of an immunological process (e.g. CSF oligoclonal bands ± antibodies). The pathogenic role of the immunlogicla dysfunction is frequently unclear. In some instances there are reports of an antibody association with cerebellar ataxia (e.g. anti GAD) the pathogenic role in such cases remains unclear.

Late onset cerebellar degenerations

These conditions are probably the largest and least understood group of ataxias that present in adulthood to the neurologist. The aetiology is almost certainly heterogeneous and the syndromes that are recognised vary in some of their features.

Table 17.8 Antineuronal antibodies (after Shams'ili *et al.* 2003).

Antibody	Clinical syndrome	Associated cancer	Immunohistochemistry
Anti-Yo	Cerebellar ataxia	Ovarian, breast	Cytoplasm of Purkinje cells and large brainstem neurones
Anti-Hu	Cerebellar ataxia, PEM/SN	SCLC	Nuclei of all neurones, nucleolar sparing
Anti-Ri	Cerebellar ataxia, OM	Breast, gynaecological, SCLC	Nuclei of all central neurones, with nucleolar sparing
Anti-Tr	Cerebellar ataxia	Hodgkin's lymphoma	Cytoplasm and dendrites of Purkinje cells
Anti-VGCC	Cerebellar ataxia, LEMS	SCLC (60%)	–
Anti-Ma	Cerebellar ataxia, brainstem dysfunction	Numerous	Nuclei and cytoplasm of neurones
Anti-Ta/Ma2	Limbic encephalopathy, cerebellar ataxia	Testicular	Nuclei and cytoplasm of neurones
Anti-CRMP5/CV2	PEM/SN, cerebellar ataxia	SCLC, thymoma, gynaecological	Cytoplasm of oligodendrocytes
Anti-mGluR1	Cerebellar ataxia	Hodgkin's lymphoma	Cytoplasm of Purkinje cells and brush cells, climbing fibres

LEMS, Lambert–Eaton myasthenic syndrome; OM, opsoclonus/myoclonus; PEM, paraneoplastic encephalomyelitis; SCLC, small cell lung cancer; SN, sensory neuronopathy; VGCC, voltage gated calcium channels.

Multiple system atrophy

This is the most common clearly defined syndrome, accounting for up to 50% of the late onset cases. Multi-system atrophy (MSA) usually starts in the sixth to seventh decades and unfortunately is relentlessly progressive, with severe disability within 5–7 years. It may present with a parkinsonian syndrome (Chapter 6), with autonomic dysfunction (Chapter 24) or as a cerebellar syndrome. Whatever the initial presentation other features tend to develop with time, although usually one set of clinical features predominates. Associated extra features include urinary symptoms, postural dizziness and REM sleep disturbance. Additional clinical signs include signs of extrapyramidal disease; these may be mild and need careful clinical assessment to determine, lying and standing BP, antecollis and mini-myoclonus in the fingers.

There is no absolute diagnostic formulation for MSA; the internationally agreed criteria require typical pathological features for a definite diagnosis. MRI may reveal signs of brainstem and cerebellar atrophy and also the 'hot cross bun sign'. This is not entirely specific, but in the right clinical setting does strongly support the diagnosis. Sphincter EMG may also show evidence of denervation, and autonomic function assessment may help both diagnostically and to allow appropriate symptom management.

The management of MSA involves a coordination of expertise with input from a multi-disciplinary team. There is no satisfactory drug treatment for the cerebellar features but physiotherapy and other support services can be of benefit.

Ataxia and sensitivity to gluten

This is the relatively newly described syndrome in which patients with mid and later life onset of progressive ataxia have been reported either to have clinical signs or intestinal biopsy features of gluten enteropathy (e.g. coeliac disease), or have a range of antibodies (principally antigliadin) suggesting sensitivity to gluten. This manifests itself as a neurological disease, termed gluten ataxia. However, antigliadin antibodies are non-specific and relatively common in the general population; their actual role in the ataxia remains uncertain. Anecdotally, it is said that gluten exclusion does not appear to impact on the progression, but well-designed studies are needed to confirm this.

Idiopathic late onset ataxia

This is an heterogeneous syndrome encompassing the significant proportion of cases of presumed degenerative ataxia in which no cause is found. Typically, the symptoms start in the sixth decade and beyond; patients present with a slowly progressive relatively pure ataxia. There are exceptions, and in particular mild pyramidal signs can be found, but the cerebellar features predominate. The prognosis in this group is generally somewhat better than those with the cerebellar presentation of MSA.

Conclusions

The differential diagnosis of the ataxias is long, and often complex. However, there are some basic rules that are a valuable guide: the age at onset, pattern of onset and course provide a quick and fairly reliable initial screen. After these specific questions, the family history, alcohol exposure and additional neurological symptoms often lead to a clear diagnostic shortlist, even before examination. Examination is focused on delineating the cerebellar features and seeking evidence of involvement in other systems. Investigation is then tailored to the emergent differential list.

Unfortunately, the drug treatment of ataxia for either symptoms or disease modification is still very poor. However, there are a small number of treatable or modifiable diseases; these should be rigorously excluded whenever they are suspected. Established balance problems are very resistant to any pharmacological intervention. Supportive therapies such as speech therapy and physical interventions are frequently required. It is hoped that as we further our understanding of the molecular and cellular processes involved that more targeted and rational therapies will emerge.

References

Harding AE, Matthews S, Jones S, Ellis CJ, Booth IW, Muller DP. Spinocerebellar degeneration associated with a selective defect of vitamin E absorption. *N Engl J Med* 1985; **313**: 32–35.

Jacquemont S, Hagerman RJ, Leehey MA, Hall DA, Levine RA, Brunberg JA, *et al.* Penetrance of the fragile X-associated tremor/ataxia syndrome in a premutation carrier population. *JAMA* 2004; **291**: 460–469.

Shams'ili S, Grefkens J, de Leeuw B, van den Bent M, Hooijkaas H, van der Holt B, *et al.* Paraneoplastic cerebellar degeneration associated with antineuronal antibodies: analysis of 50 patients. *Brain* 2003; **126**: 1409–1418.

Further reading

Araki W, Hirose S, Mimori Y, Nakamura S, Kimura J, Ohno K, *et al.* Familial hypobetalipoproteinaemia complicated by cerebellar ataxia and steatocystoma multiplex. *J Intern Med* 1991; **229**: 197–199.

Bomont P, Watanabe M, Gershoni-Barush R, Shizuka M, Tananka M, Sugano J, *et al.* Homozygosity mapping of spinocerebellar ataxia with cerebellar atrophy and peripheral neuropathy to 9q33–34, and with hearing impairment and optic atrophy to 6p21–23. *Eur J Hum Genet* 2000; **8**: 986–990.

Bootsma D, Kraemer KH, Cleaver J, Hoeijmakers JHJ. Nucleotide excision repair syndromes: xeroderma pigmentosum, Cockayne syndrome and trichothiodystrophy. In *The Metabolic Basis of Inherited Disease*, 8th edn. Scriver CR, Beaudet AL, Sly WS, Valle D, eds. New York: McGraw Hill, 1998: 245–274.

Brain R, Wilkinson M. Subacute cerebellar degeneration associated with neoplasms. *Brain* 1965; **88**: 465–477.

Brown GK. Pyruvate dehydrogenase E1 alpha deficiency. *J Inherited Metab Dis* 1992; **15**: 625–633.

Browne DL, Gancher ST, Nutt JG, Brunt ER, Smith EA, Kramer P, *et al.* Episodic ataxia/myokymia syndrome is associated with point mutations in the human potassium channel gene, *KCNA1*. *Nat Genet* 1994; **8**: 136–140.

Cader MZ, Steckley JL, Dyment DA, McLachlan RS, Ebers GC. A genome-wide screen and linkage mapping for a large pedigree with episodic ataxia. *Neurology* 2005; **65**: 156–158.

Campuzano V, Montermini L, Molto MD, *et al.* Friedreich's ataxia: autosomal recessive disease caused by an intronic GAA triplet repeat expansion. *Science* 1996; **271**: 1423–1427.

Chance PF, Cavalier L, Satran D, Pellegrino JE, Koenig M, Dobyns WB. Clinical nosologic and genetic aspects of Joubert and related syndromes. *J Child Neurol* 1999; **14**: 660–666; discussion 669–672.

Danek A, Jung HH, Melone MA, Rampoldi L, Broccoli V, Walker RH. Neuroacanthocytosis: new developments in a neglected group of dementing disorders. *J Neurol Sci* 2005; **15**: 171–186, 229–230.

Date H, Onodera O, Tanaka H, Iwabuchi K, Uekawa K, Igarashi S, *et al.* Early-onset ataxia with ocular motor apraxia and hypoalbuminemia is caused by mutations in a new HIT superfamily gene. *Nat Genet* 2001; **29**: 184–188.

Di Prospero NA, Fischbeck KH. Therapeutics development for triplet repeat expansion diseases. *Nat Rev Genet* 2005; **6**: 756–765.

Durr A, Cossee M, Agid Y, *et al.* Clinical and genetic abnormalities in patients with Friedreich's ataxia. *N Engl J Med* 1996; **335**: 1169–1175.

Enevoldson PG, Sanders MD, Harding AE. Autosomal dominant cerebellar ataxia with pigmentary macular dystrophy: a clinical and genetic study of eight families. *Brain* 1994; **117**: 445–460.

Everett CM, Wood NW. Trinucleotide repeats and neurodegenerative disease. *Brain* 2004; **127**: 2385–2405.

Fearnley JM, Stevens JM, Rudge P. Superficial siderosis of the central nervous system. *Brain* 1995; **118**: 1051–1066.

Gallus GN, Dotti MT, Federico A. Clinical and molecular diagnosis of cerebrotendinous xanthomatosis with a review of the mutations in the *CYP27A1* gene. *Neurol Sci* 2006; **27**: 143–149.

Gotoda T, Arita M, Arai H, Inoue K, Yokota T, Fukuo Y, *et al.* Adult-onset spinocerebellar dysfunction caused by a mutation in the gene for the α-tocopherol transfer protein. *N Engl J Med* 1995; **333**: 1313–1318.

Hadjivassiliou M, Grunewald R, Sharrack B, Sanders D, Lobo A, Williamson C, *et al.* Gluten ataxia in perspective: epidemiology, genetic susceptibility and clinical characteristics. *Brain* 2003; **126**: 685–691.

Hanna MG, Wood NW, Kullmann D. The neurological channelopathies. *J Neurol Neurosurg Psychiatry* 1998; **65**: 427–431.

Harding AE. Friedreich's ataxia: a clinical and genetic study of 90 families with an analysis of early diagnostic criteria and intrafamilial clustering of clinical features. *Brain* 1981; **104**: 589–620.

Harding AE. *The Hereditary Ataxias and Related Disorders*. Edinburgh: Churchill Livingstone, 1984.

Jackson JF, Currier RD, Terasaki PI, Morton NE. Spinocerebellar ataxia and HLA linkage: risk prediction by HLA typing. *N Engl J Med* 1977; **296**: 1138–1141.

Kleta R, Romeo E, Ristic Z, Ohura T, Stuart C, Arcos-Burgos M, *et al.* Mutations in SLC6A19, encoding B0AT1, cause Hartnup disorder. *Nat Genet* 2004; **36**: 999–1002.

Klockgether T, Ludtke R, Kramer B, Abele M, Burk K, Schols L, *et al.* The natural history of degenerative ataxia: a retrospective study in 466 patients. *Brain* 1998; **121**: 589–600.

Lock RJ, Pengiran Tengah DS, Unsworth DJ, Ward JJ, Wills AJ. Ataxia, peripheral neuropathy, and anti-gliadin antibody. Guilt by association? *J Neurol Neurosurg Psychiatry* 2005; **76**: 1601–1603.

Le Ber I, Bouslam N, Rivaud-Pechoux S, Guimaraes J, Benomar A, Chamayou C, *et al.* Frequency and phenotypic spectrum of ataxia with oculomotor apraxia 2: a clinical and genetic study in 18 patients. *Brain* 2004; **127**: 759–767.

Marsden CD, Harding AE, Obeso JA, Lu C-S. Progressive myoclonic ataxia (the Ramsay-Hunt syndrome). *Arch Neurol* 1990; **47**: 1121–1125.

Matilla-Duenas A, Goold R, Giunti P. Molecular pathogenesis of spinocerebellar ataxias. *Brain* 2006; **129**: 1357–1370.

Moreira MC, Klur S, Watanabe M, Nemeth AH, Le Ber I, Moniz JC, *et al.* Senataxin, the ortholog of a yeast RNA helicase, is mutant in ataxia-ocular apraxia 2. *Nat Genet* 2004; **36**: 225–227.

Muller DP, Lloyd JK, Wolff OH. Vitamin E and neurological function. *Lancet* 1983; **i**: 225–228.

Ophoff RA, Terwindt GM, Vergouwe MN, van Eijk R, Oefner PJ, Hoffman SM, *et al.* Familial hemiplegic migraine and episodic ataxia type-2 are caused by mutations in the Ca^{2+} channel gene *CACNL1A4*. *Cell* 1996; **87**: 543–552.

Parker CC, Evans OB. Metabolic disorders causing childhood ataxia. *Semin Pediatr Neurol* 2003; **10**: 193–199.

Quinn NP, Marsden CD. The motor disorder of multiple system atrophy. *J Neurol Neurosurg Psychiatry* 1993; **56**: 1239–1242.

Rees J. Paraneoplastic syndromes. *Curr Opin Neurol* 1998; **11**: 633–637.

Ryan MM, Engle EC. Acute ataxia in childhood. *J Child Neurol* 2003; **18**: 309–316.

Savitsky K, Bar-Shira A, Gilad S, Rotman G, Ziv Y, Vanagaite L, *et al.* A single ataxia telangiectasia gene with a product similar to PI-3 kinase. *Science* 1995; **268**: 1749–1753.

Sawaishi Y, Takada G. Acute cerebellitis. *Cerebellum* 2002; **1**: 223–228.

Seow HF, Broer S, Broer A, Bailey CG, Potter SJ, Cavanaugh JA, *et al.* Hartnup disorder is caused by mutations in the gene encoding the neutral amino acid transporter SLC6A19. *Nat Genet* 2004; **36**: 1003–1007.

Sistermans EA, de Coo RF, De Wijs IJ, Van Oost BA. Duplication of the proteolipid protein gene is the major cause of Pelizaeus–Merzbacher disease. *Neurology* 1998; **50**: 1749–1754.

Shoulders CC, Brett DJ, Bayliss JD, *et al.* Abetalipoproteinaemia is caused by defects of the gene encoding the 97 kDa subunit of a microsomal triglyceride transfer protein. *Hum Mol Genet* 1993; **2**: 2109–2116.

Steckley JL, Ebers GC, Cader MZ, McLachlan RS. An autosomal dominant disorder with episodic ataxia, vertigo, and tinnitus. *Neurology* 2001; **57**: 1499–1502.

Steinlin M. Non-progressive congenital ataxias. *Brain Dev* 1998; **20**: 199–208.

Stewart GS, Maser RS, Stankovic T, Bressan DA, Kaplan MI, Jaspers NG, *et al.* The DNA double-strand break repair gene *hMRE11* is mutated in individuals with an ataxia-telangiectasia-like disorder. *Cell* 1999; **99**: 577–587.

Tranchant C, Fleury M, Moreira MC, Koenig M, Warter JM. Phenotypic variability of aprataxin gene mutations. *Neurology* 2003; **60**: 868–870.

van der Knaap MS, Pronk JC, Scheper GC. Vanishing white matter disease. *Lancet Neurol* 2006: **413–423**.

Vedanarayanan VV. Mitochondrial disorders and ataxia. *Semin Pediatr Neurol* 2003; **10**: 200–209.

Wadsworth JD, Hill AF, Beck JA, Collinge J. Molecular and clinical classification of human prion disease. *Br Med Bull* 2003; **66**: 241–254.

Watanabe H, Saito Y, Terao S, Ando T, Kachi T, Mukai E, *et al.* Progression and prognosis in multiple system atrophy: an analysis of 230 Japanese patients. *Brain* 2002; **125**: 1070–1083.

Yamamoto T, Ninomiya H, Matsumoto M, Ohta Y, Nanba E, Tsutsumi Y, *et al.* Genotype–phenotype relationship of Niemann-Pick disease type C: a possible correlation between clinical onset and levels of NPC1 protein in isolated skin fibroblasts. *J Med Genet* 2000; **37**: 707–711.

CHAPTER 18

Restorative Neurology, Rehabilitation and Brain Injury

Richard Greenwood[1], Diana Caine[1], Ulrike Hammerbeck[2], Alexander Leff[2], Diane Playford[2], Valerie Stevenson[1] and Nick Ward[2]

[1] National Hospital for Neurology & Neurosurgery

[2] UCL Institute of Neurology

There are many opportunities for the prevention or reversal of disease, but health care systems worldwide are dominated by people with chronic diseases and conditions that in general have not been prevented and cannot be reversed. In the United States, patients with chronic conditions account for nearly 80% of health care costs. In the United Kingdom, neurological damage accounts for 40% of people who are severely disabled and require daily help, and for most of those with complex disabilities resulting from a combination of physical, cognitive and behavioural problems. Any health care system is thus confronted on a daily basis with a demand to meet this need from finite resources. This chapter addresses the nature of disability, how it can best be ameliorated, which training techniques and medical treatments are most effective, particularly after single incident brain injury, and the organisational structures required for their optimal delivery.

The nature of disability and its optimal management

When reversal of pathology is incomplete, profound life changes may result from the consequences of a disease or condition, classified in a framework by the WHO International Classification of Functioning (ICF) in 2001 as:

1 Loss of physiological and psychological function or anatomical structure, collectively known as impairments,
2 Limitations in functional activities, and
3 Restrictions of participation in social roles (Figure 18.1).

In these circumstances, the majority of disabled people benefit from the goal-focused learning and problem-solving process termed rehabilitation, delivered by skilled multi-disciplinary rehabilitation teams. Although often not made explicit, aspects of this process are integral to the optimal management of many chronic disorders. In the context of neurological disease, rehabilitation goals are achieved via:

1 The prevention of avoidable secondary systemic, neurological and psychological complications of a disease
2 Functional compensation via behavioural adaptation and substitution, and modification of personal, environmental and social contextual factors, and
3 Neural restoration and substitution (Table 18.1), delivered by organised complex polymodal inpatient, residential or community-based intervention programmes.

As a result, functional independence is increased, or at least maintained, and avoidable deterioration prevented. In addition, the difficult process of adjustment to loss and change is made possible, so that life quality and personhood is subjectively improved, to make life really 'worth living'. These crucially important outcomes are easily forgotten during investigation and assessment at the level of impairment, for example during a functional imaging study, the injection of botulinum toxin or a physiotherapy session in the gym.

Key aspects of multi-dimensional rehabilitation

A holistic biopsychosocial individualised multi-dimensional rehabilitation programme includes:

- Reiterative multi-disciplinary assessment,
- Problem definition and measurement,
- Goal-setting and treatment planning,
- Treatment delivery,
- Evaluation of effectiveness, and
- Reassessment with a view to further treatment.

Medical and surgical pathological diagnoses and treatments are combined with interventions, acutely and longer term, in parallel rather than in series (Figure 18.2), involving training and skill learning, in order to achieve attitudinal and behavioural change, reduce impairment and functional dependence, and facilitate social roles and life quality. Skill retraining is largely delivered via physical, occupational, speech and language and cognitive therapies, and may include facilitation of adaptation to loss by both the patient and family, the prescription of appliances and environmental modifications, and the development and application of new technologies and service delivery systems. In the context of disorders that affect brain function, and therefore learning, particularly well-defined and structured treatments are required to achieve skill learning.

Rehabilitation is a thus a complex intervention, and is delivered via a menu of multi-disciplinary inpatient and community-based service delivery systems which differ by plant, personnel and process (Figure 18.3). A classification of these different service options, as a rehabilitation typology, remains to be agreed nationally and internationally, let alone cross-culturally but would facilitate the development of service delivery systems or networks via comparison

Neurology: A Queen Square Textbook, Second Edition. Edited by Charles Clarke, Robin Howard, Martin Rossor and Simon Shorvon.

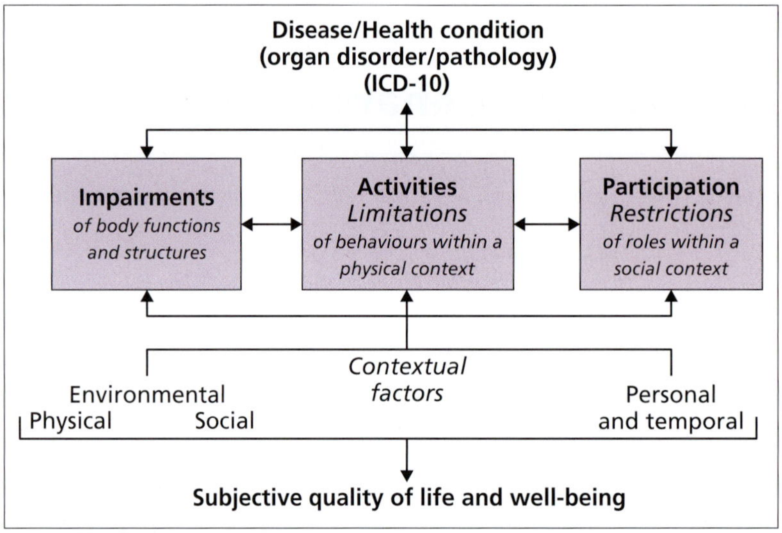

Figure 18.1 A holistic biopsychosocial model of illness and health via an interactive classification of disease (ICD-10), function (ICF 2001) and subjective quality of life (sQoL).

Table 18.1 Mechanisms of recovery after neurological damage.

Prevention of neural and systemic complications and Functional compensation via • Behavioural adaptation and substitution and • Modification of personal, environmental and social contextual factors allow
Allow neural restoration and substitution via • Resolution of oedema, mass effects and toxic–metabolic dysfunction, and diaschisis (i.e. functional changes in brain areas remote from an area of damage) • Neural replacement, regrowth and • Reorganisation of use-dependent neuronal networks

studies and audit of agreed guidelines. The use of each component of such a network is driven by a number of factors:

- Patient need
- Pre-injury characteristics
- Co-morbidities
- Time since injury
- Level of dependency
- Characteristics of the residual impairments
- Age
- Social back-up, and
- Resources available.

Natural histories of neurological damage

The ways in which the inpatient and community-based components of rehabilitation service systems are configured, used and linked are driven largely by three differing natural histories of neurological disease and injury:

1 Single incident brain and spinal cord damage, and acute peripheral paralyses;
2 Deteriorating conditions including late stage multiple sclerosis, degenerative dementias, and motor neurone and Parkinson's disease;

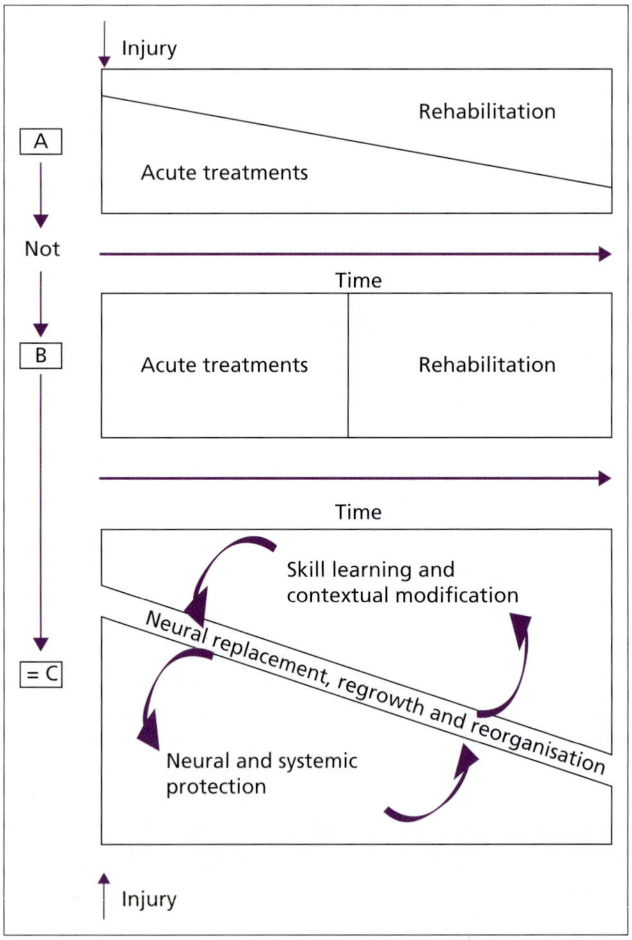

Figure 18.2 Acute treatments focus on neural and systemic protection, while rehabilitative strategies involve skill learning and contextual modification. Their use in parallel (a) rather than in series (b), combined with care and over time, is most likely to prevent complications and entrain the neurobiological processes contributing to neural restoration so that outcomes are optimised (c).

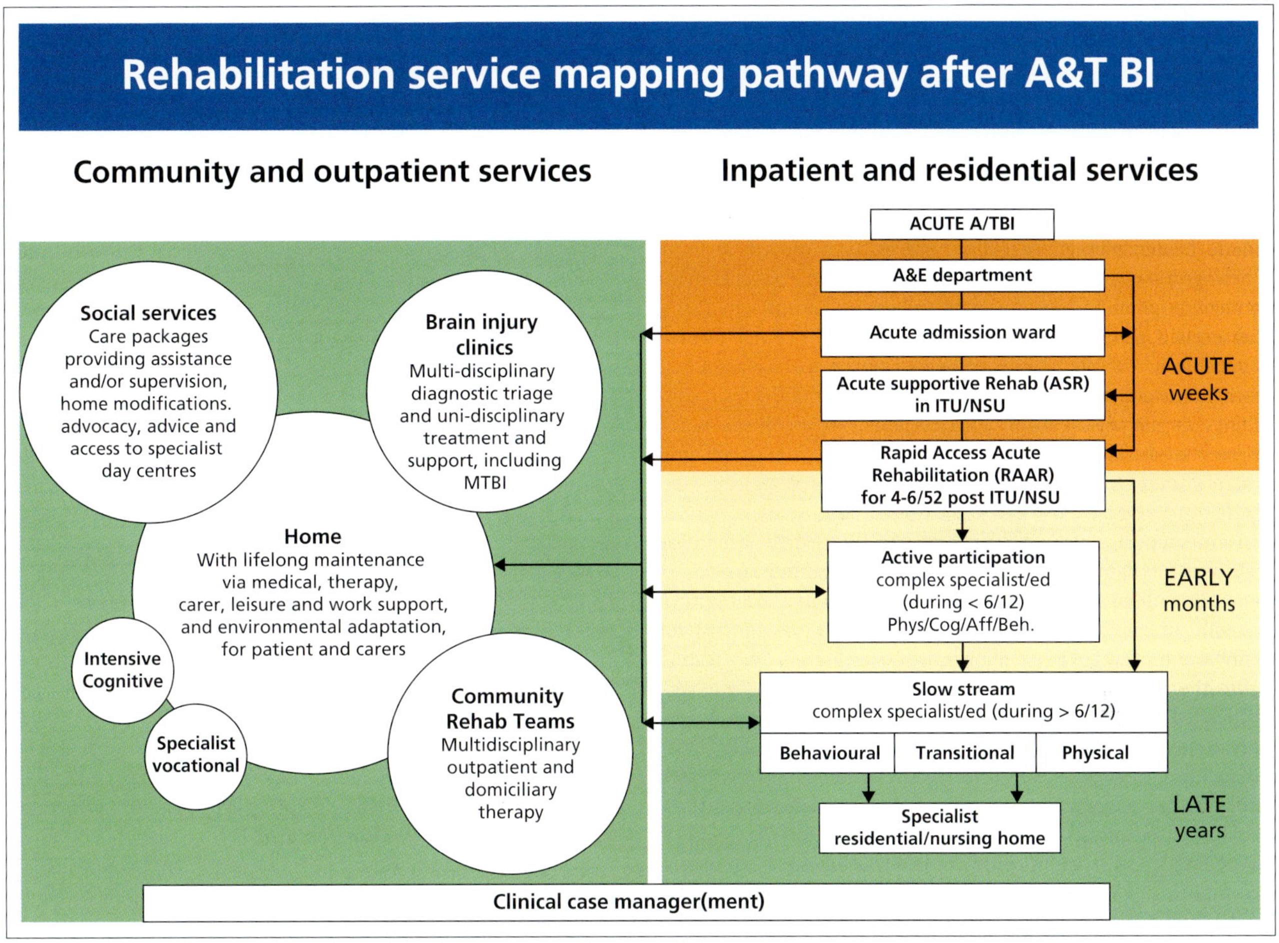

Figure 18.3 Classification of rehabilitation services after single incident acquired and traumatic (A&T) brain injury (BI) by time, severity and need. Acute medical and surgical management varies by pathology and is described elsewhere. The rehabilitation options illustrated can be defined and coded to clarify gaps in service provision and clinical pathways. MTBI, mild traumatic brain injury.

3 Initially static conditions such as cerebral palsy, post-polio syndrome and the late effects of other single incident events sometimes acquired in childhood.

Inpatient and community-based components in each of these three clinical pathways should provide both regional (high-cost, low-volume) and local service options for patients with more or less severe and complex disability. Provision of a coordinated menu of services across health and social care boundaries is very difficult but essential because most of the work associated with managing any long-term condition is done in the individual's home and community, with only a small fraction occurring in a hospital or other residential environment. Both the affected individual and their family, if involved, require informed encouragement, support and advice to maintain a balanced access to different management strategies. This may fail at certain points during the disease trajectory and require specialist input.

The key to effective longitudinal management is to ensure that interventions are appropriate and timely. This requires effective and interactive verbal and written communication across health and social care sectors, and ongoing involvement with the individual and family. There are many benchmarks and models to guide best practice for the longitudinal provision of inpatient and community-based rehabilitation, work (re)entry, personal care and support, equipment and accommodation, palliative care, and support for family and carers in the context of long-term neurological conditions.

Resources, integrated care pathways, effectiveness and evidence base

In the United Kingdom, these were summarised in 2005 by the Department of Health's National Service Framework (NSF) for long-term neurological conditions, which sets out 11 evidence-based quality requirements 'to improve health and social care services for people with long-term neurological conditions and their carers', with the aim to promote quality of life and independence by ensuring patients received timely coordinated care and support planned around their needs and choices. Whether problems with the implementation of these recommendations, discussed by the UK National Audit Office in 2011, can be at least partially resolved by specialist nurses or clinical or organisational case managers, remains to be investigated.

The composition of the multi-disciplinary teams that deliver these complex interventions differs depending on clinical need. Cohesive engagement of such a team requires a framework that makes explicit 'who does what, when, where and how' to achieve a commonly agreed aim, via a series of long and short-term goals, agreed, if possible, with the patient. Linguistic harmonisation between disciplines, particularly between doctors, nursing and the therapies in an inpatient setting, and health and social services in the community, is crucial to success. In a clinical setting, this framework is provided by both generic and individualisable documentation that reflects, and thus measures, a classification of the consequences of a disease.

Integrated Care Pathways provide a multi-disciplinary team with generic evidence-based checklists, process and disease focused, which describe core clinical activities that underpin a patient's management longitudinally, and prompt and educate health care teams at all levels. A generic checklist of this type should be complemented by a regularly reiterated individualised formulation of a plan of care in which the patient, if possible, and each member of the team contributes in discussion to an Interdisciplinary Care Plan, which defines and documents at regular intervals the patient's problems, their needs and the action plans necessary to achieve agreed short and long-term goals en-route to an overall aim. Audit of clinical decision support systems of this type can be used to incentivise improvements in quality of care, reduce clinical risk and variation in standards, and minimise resource utilisation, and have been shown to significantly improve clinical practice in a variety of contexts, for example at the level of prescribing practices and serious medication errors, the delivery of preventive treatments and adherence to recommended care standards. This has been exemplified in the United Kingdom, since 1998, by a series of national audits which aim to improve the quality of stroke care by auditing the provision of care against evidence based standards (http://www.rcplondon.ac.uk/projects/sentinel-stroke-national-audit-programme).

The effectiveness, compared with historical controls, of organised multi-disciplinary care and rehabilitation, was demonstrated initially following spinal injuries sustained in the Second World War (1939–1945). Since then the opportunity to trial the effectiveness of the rehabilitation process has been provided by the high incidence and prevalence of stroke. Trials of different models of inpatient and community based care and rehabilitation after stroke have shown convincingly that organised care produces better outcomes than disorganised care, a result that has far-reaching implications for health care systems in general (Figure 18.4). Rigorous evidence to support complex interventions in the context of other single incident neurological conditions, or as a result of deteriorating or static neurological disorders, is sparse by comparison. The top-down systems approach, often using prospective randomised and blinded group methodologies, has been complemented by bottom-up and largely proof-of-principle investigation of neural reorganisation after neurological damage. After initially demonstrating the ubiquity of use-dependent plasticity in healthy controls, these studies have shown that the same process underpins later neurological recovery in the context of disease, and are beginning to explore how drivers of neural reorganisation can contribute to improved outcomes.

Interest in investigating the process of rehabilitation has arisen from two directions. One has resulted from the need to demonstrate how rehabilitation can maintain or improve quality of care without increasing resource use, often by using project and systems management techniques originally derived from industry, and more recently the implementation sciences, which emphasise cognitive and behavioural techniques to generate organisational and individual behavioural changes in professionals that achieve best practice. By contrast, advances in the basic and clinical neurosciences (Table 18.2) have provided explanations about how traditional rehabilitative treatments might work. They have been instrumental over the last 20 years in changing clinicians' perceptions from a view that therapies from physiotherapy to psychotherapy offered little more than homeopathy, to an acceptance of the need to explore and develop rehabilitation interventions at the level of impairment. We explore in this chapter the delivery and effectiveness of these two components of the rehabilitation process in neurological disease.

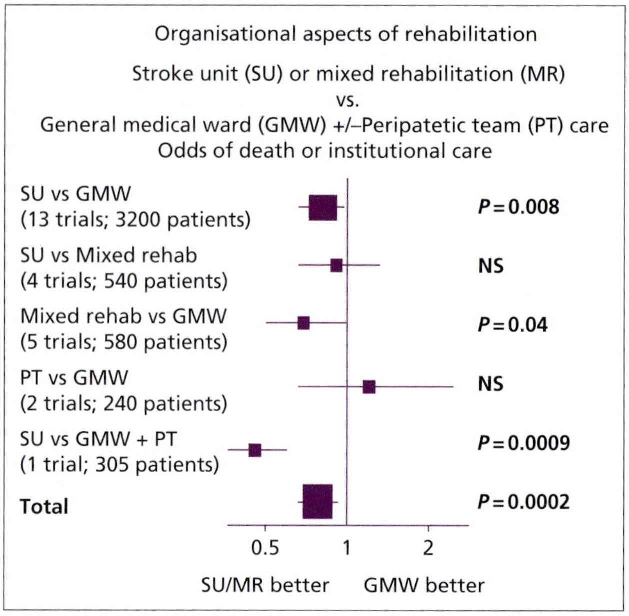

Figure 18.4 Care in stroke (SU) or mixed rehabilitation units can be organised and is thus more effective than in general medical wards (GMW) with or without input from a peripatetic team (PT), where it remains disorganised. Source: Stroke Unit Trialists' Collaboration 2001. Reproduced with permission of Elsevier.

Table 18.2 Evidence from the basic sciences over the last century initially denied and subsequently confirmed the suggestion that neural repair and reorganisation occurred in the central nervous system (CNS) after damage. This repair process is facilitated by the prevention of complications and driven by goal-focused task-related training during rehabilitation.

- Donaldson (1895): 'In the central nervous system the cell elements are plastic in the sense that their connections are not rigidly fixed, and they remember. By virtue of these powers, the cells can adjust themselves to new surroundings'
- Cajal (1928): 'In adult centres, the nerve paths are something fixed, ended, immutable; everything may die, nothing may be regenerated. It is for the science of the future to change, if possible, this harsh decree'
- Raisman (1969): 'The finding of heterotypic re-innervation in the septum implies that the nervous system can no longer be considered incapable of reconstruction in the face of damage'
- Finger and Stein (1982): 'Until very recently, prevailing concepts of brain function precluded the possibility of structural and neurochemical reorganisation of function; theoretically, once damage occurred, the possibility for rehabilitation was to train the patient to use alternative, but less effective, behavioral strategies'
- Neural reorganisation in lesioned animals (e.g. Jenkins and Merzenich 1987; Nudo et al. 1996) confirmed longitudinally by brain mapping techniques in humans after stroke.

Neural reorganisation and restoration

At present, clinical experience still emphasises that the most obvious functional gains following neurological damage result from the prevention of complications, whether physical, cognitive, behavioural or emotional, and from adaptive interventions that include environmental modification and personal adjustment, rather than from neural restoration. However, if complications are prevented, so that use can be allowed or even forced, then neural reorganisation in remaining neural structures and networks can follow, though for the foreseeable future still result in 'alternative, but (inevitably) less effective, behavioural strategies', and functional gain may still be largely the result of a learned increase in compensatory rather than normal behaviours.

After neural damage, successful restorative therapies depend on approaches that (i) encourage neural protection to minimise secondary neural damage and enhance neuronal survival, and (ii) facilitate three restorative treatment strategies:

1 Neural replacement
2 Neural regrowth and regeneration, and
3 Reorganisation of functionally useful activity-dependent neuronal maps and networks.

Damaged neurones in the adult mammalian spinal cord can regenerate with treatments that provide an environment that promotes growth via:

1 Cell-based therapies, which may operate largely via neurotrophic and anti-inflammatory mechanisms, and
2 Neurotrophic factors and inhibitors of axonal growth inhibitors, to facilitate neuronal survival and axonal sprouting.

Similar approaches are under consideration in the treatment of brain damage and/or degeneration, whether progressive as in Parkinson's disease or multiple sclerosis, or single incident following stroke or head injury. The successful application of techniques designed to promote neural replacement and/or repair is likely also to require an understanding of the drivers of use-dependent cellular and network remodelling that that are needed to incorporate new tissue into functionally useful networks.

What encourages scientists and clinicians to believe that neural reorganisation is an important tool in the restorative therapies? There is now a wealth of evidence suggesting that central nervous system (CNS) reorganisation at least accompanies and often underpins much of the improvement in impairment that is frequently seen after injury, and during skill learning in healthy individuals. Experiments in both animals and humans show that many regions in the normal adult CNS, particularly the cortex but also in the spinal cord, have a capacity, which is learning dependent, to change structure and function in response to environmental change and memorise this change. This process, often referred to as plasticity, is the basis for skill learning and is now firmly grounded in evidence.

Work on focal brain damage in animal models has clearly demonstrated that for some months after injury, peri-lesional and distant brain regions have an increased capacity for plastic change. Developmental proteins not normally expressed in the adult brain re-emerge in the hours and days following focal brain injury. These proteins are involved in neuronal growth, apoptosis, angiogenesis and cellular differentiation. Structural changes, which include increased dendritic branching and synaptogenesis, occur. There is also evidence of peri-lesional and distant cortical hyperexcitability following focal cortical damage, which results from down-regulation of the α1-GABA receptor subunit and a decrease in GABAergic inhibition. Taken together, these changes suggest, particularly shortly after injury, that damaged brain is more amenable to activity-driven changes in structure and function, and that the potential for plastic change is greater than in the normal adult brain.

In the human brain, similar injury-induced changes appear to occur. Research in humans is performed largely at the systems level, rather than the molecular or cellular level, using techniques such as functional magnetic resonance imaging (fMRI) and transcranial magnetic stimulation (TMS), often using stroke as a model. One of the most common and most devastating consequences of stroke is the loss of both power and dexterity in the limbs contralateral to the injury. This occurs as a result of damage to the cortico-spinal pathway (Chapter 2). The majority of corticospinal fibres originate in the primary motor cortex (M1), but there are smaller contributions from other cortical regions. In primates, M1, the dorsolateral premotor area (PMd) and the supplementary motor area (SMA) are each part of parallel independent motor networks with separate projections to spinal cord motor neurones as well as connections to one another at the level of the cortex, and to subcortical reticulospinal and rubrospinal pathways originating at brainstem level.

These observations have led to the suggestion that a number of motor networks acting in parallel generate an output to the spinal cord necessary for movement. It is possible that damage in one of these networks could be compensated for by altered activity in another. Functional imaging experiments have demonstrated that stroke patients rely on secondary motor regions in the brain including PMd, SMA, and subcortical pathways to a greater degree when there is damage to the main motor output from M1. However, the projections from these brain regions to spinal cord motor neurones are less numerous and less efficient than those from M1 and thus, although these patients improve as a result of recruitment of these secondary motor regions, they are unlikely to regain premorbid performance levels.

Thus, the extent of recovery of motor function is at least partially dependent on how much of the normal network is left intact. In the brain of a patient after stroke there is a new configuration of motor networks, less effective than that in the intact brain but able nevertheless to generate some form of motor signal to spinal cord motor neurones in the most efficient way possible. Longitudinal fMRI studies of stroke patients reveal an initial overactivation of many primary and non-primary cortical motor regions during the performance of a motor task. Thereafter, functional recovery is associated with a focusing of task-related brain activation patterns, as is seen during motor skill learning in healthy subjects. The brain activation patterns do not return to normal in all cases but, at least in the motor system, the focusing of activation will tend towards the most efficient system available. One of the roles of restorative treatments is to help this focusing process.

The functional organisation of skill systems post-injury will depend most obviously on the extent of the anatomical damage, but within these anatomical constraints there is room for more or less efficient reconfiguration of these networks. Alterations in this efficiency by reorganisation, rather than regeneration of tissue, are most likely to underlie therapy-driven reductions in impairment. There are a number of other factors that contribute to this process: how much and what type of treatment is delivered, the biological age of the subject, the premorbid state of their brain, current drug treatments, and probably their genetic status. All of these factors will influence the potential for skill-dependent and learning-dependent changes within intact brain networks – the proposed mechanism by which functionally relevant brain reorganisation occurs.

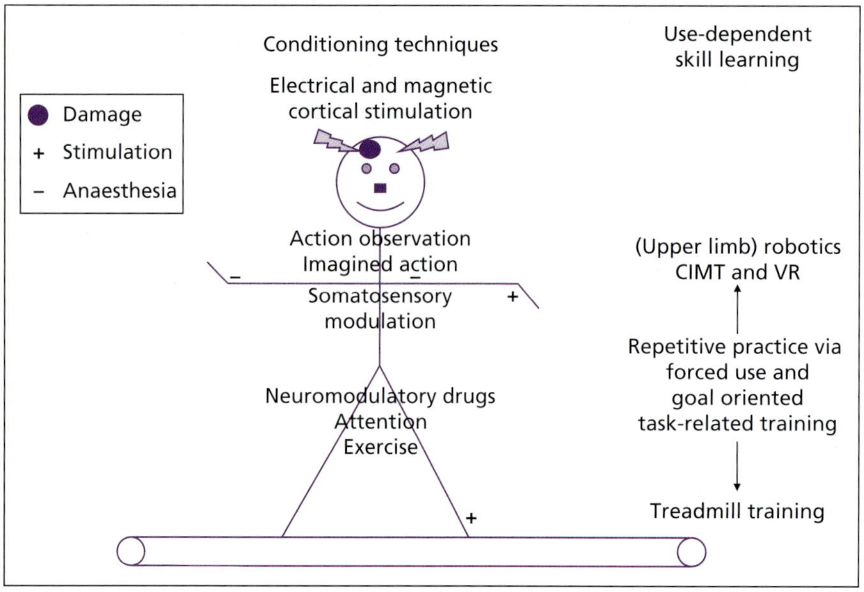

Figure 18.5 Use-dependent and conditioning drivers of neural reorganisation that have the potential to enhance functional recovery after neural injury. CIMT, constraint induced movement therapy; VR, virtual reality.

Therapies, and other conditioning techniques (Figure 18.5), can be considered as inputs that interact with a system, in this case the damaged brain. The aim of this input is generally to optimise the functional reorganisation of the damaged system. It will succeed in driving functionally useful change only to the extent that the brain regions and networks with which it interacts are intact and able to influence output pathways. Adjuvant treatments are designed to condition the brain to make activity-driven change in response to afferent input more likely and more effective, and enhance the effect of therapy if delivered shortly before or during a treatment session:

- Non-invasive Brain Stimulation (NIBS) including repetitive Transcranial Magnetic Stimulation (rTMS) and trancranial Direct Current Stimulation (tDCS), and
- Drugs, for example monoaminergic noradrenergic, dopaminergic and serotoninergic drugs such as amphetamine, levodopa or fluoxetine.

The success of these adjuvant treatments, which can be used either singly or together, will depend on a number of factors including whether the networks with which the therapy interacts are intact. Thus, non-invasive excitatory stimulation of the affected M1 is unlikely to have any success in patients with large middle cerebral artery territory infarcts, while inhibitory stimulation of a normal contralesional homologue may restore inter-hemispheric balance and improve motor or language function. As yet, the mechanisms of action of these interventions are not well understood, but the notion of residual functional anatomy may provide a model with which to improve prediction of outcome, and facilitate realistic expectations and goal setting, as well as the exploration of whether and how interventions of different types work in different patients (Figure 18.6).

In summary therefore, successful restorative therapies for patients with impairments secondary to either brain or spinal cord damage are likely to consist of multiple approaches that:

- Minimise secondary damage,
- Enhance neuronal survival,
- Facilitate axonal regeneration, and
- Organise activity into functionally useful neuronal networks by behavioural training.

These therapeutic approaches need to be targeted, either singly or in combination, at those impairments that underlie a particular functional limitation. For example, mobility may be affected by leg weakness resulting from either a lack of descending neural drive, spasticity, sensory loss, ataxia and imbalance, or secondary muscle atrophy, or to biomechanical changes and compensatory strategies that have developed over time since the initial destructive lesion. Treatment strategies to help patients compensate for and adapt to their functional limitations have been used for many years, whereas those aimed at minimising impairments have received less attention. In order to effectively implement current and new treatments for impairment, it is imperative to ask whether and how coexisting impairments contribute to a given functional limitation, a task to which the clinical neurosciences can make a unique contribution.

Treatment of neurological impairments and functional limitations

Restorative and compensatory approaches, skill learning and task-related training

Non-invasive therapy interventions and task-related training in the context of neural damage are an integral part of the rehabilitation process after a neurological event, and aim to optimise a person's functional ability. They may be broadly divided into those that are restorative and those that are compensatory. Restorative approaches aim to improve function via measurable improvement in an underlying impairment of an aspect of body function and structure, for example muscle weakness or dysphasia, and can be contrasted with strategies that aim to improve function by compensating for an underlying impairment, which may not change despite measurable improvements in functional activities and social participation (Figure 18.1). Both strategies may be associated with recordable adaptive changes within neural systems. Compensatory strategies

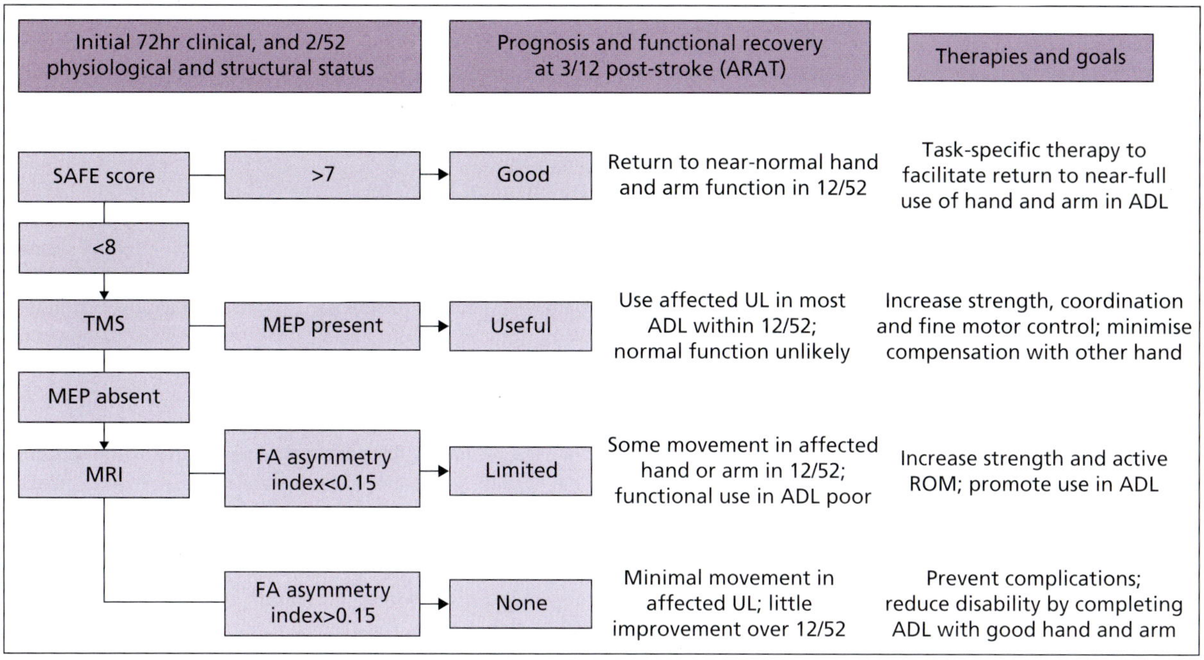

Figure 18.6 An algorithm predicting recovery potential (PREP) to enable reliable subacute prediction of functional recovery of the upper limb at 3 months post-stroke. First, the shoulder abduction and finger extension (SAFE) MRC score (range 0–10) is rated at 72 hours. Then, if the SAFE score is <8, at 2 weeks post-stroke the integrity of the cortico-spinal tract is assessed, initially physiologically using the TMS MEP from extensor carpi radialis in the affected limb, followed if necessary by a measure of the structural integrity of the affected posterior limb of the internal capsule using the fractional anisotropy asymmetry index.
ARAT, action research arm test; TMS, transcranial magnetic stimulation; MEP, motor evoked potential; MRI, magnetic resonance imaging; FA, fractional anisotropy; ROM, range of movement.

may be external, for example an ankle-foot orthosis (AFO) for a foot drop or a communication aid for dysarthria. These improve function while being used but have no effect on behaviour once removed. Alternatively, they may be internal and improve function by changing behaviour (strategy-based therapy), so that gains transfer to function outside the periods of therapy, for example hip circumduction during walking or alternative dressing strategies to achieve independence in personal activities of daily living (ADL). Compensation for the underlying deficit is by no means always detrimental, and may be the most efficient means of moving or communicating, and particularly important to people with long-term progressive conditions.

Early trials investigating specific therapy approaches failed to find clear evidence of effectiveness. This has resulted over the last 20 years in the investigation of the efficacy of individual components and principles of training, and of the underlying type, structure, timing and intensity of therapy interventions. Functional imaging studies in both animals and humans have shown that adaptive changes within the CNS result not only from repetition, but also task-orientation, attention and reward.

Both task-related practice and impairment based intervention may promote functional gain, sometimes via the use of compensatory strategies. The severity of the neurological deficit may influence the effectiveness of these approaches. In a study comparing task-related reaching to strengthening, patients with poor motor recovery only improved their paretic limb coordination with task-related practice. By contrast, in patients with better recovery whose kinematics were fairly normal, only progressive resistance training resulted in a decrease in the compensatory trunk movements that often accompany reaching with the paretic limb.

Studies on healthy subjects suggest that skill learning may also be optimised by varying practice structure, and the instructions and support given by the therapist. Skills are mostly performed in an unpredictable environment, so-called open skills. Many factors can vary even during the performance of a simple task such as speaking a sentence or picking up a cup: the location of the cup, its orientation, weight and frictional qualities, as well the presence of adjacent objects, the availability of sensory cues and the subsequent action such as drinking or placing the cup in a cupboard, all affect the planning and execution of the task. Coordination between reaching and grasping phases, and grip and load forces while manipulating the object all need to be adapted. Acquisition of these open skills requires variable practice in which task parameters are randomly changed to reflect the normal variation in the environment. By contrast, skills performed in a predictable environment, closed skills, benefit from constant practice conditions. The type of skill to be achieved can also determine practice structure. The interdependence of successive stages of a skill determine whether breaking a skill into simpler constituent parts, which are then practiced individually, termed part practice, will result in an overall improvement in the parent task. This may be effective for certain serial skills that are composed of a string of discrete stages, while it may not be as effective for continuous skills, such as walking, where each stage is interdependent.

During the initial stages of learning, feedback involving verbal instruction, manual guidance and demonstration of skill may be required as the learner determines what to do, what the goals are and how to achieve saturation of gains achieved in-session in order to optimise between-session consolidation. However, the use of continuous therapist-derived or augmented feedback about task performance in the later stages of learning may result in the learner becoming reliant on this type of feedback to the detriment of using their own internal feedback via visual, vestibular and somatosensory information. Fading the amount of therapist feedback across trials, or providing feedback only if the task falls outside preset criteria can avoid this. In addition, the type of therapist-derived feedback required for optimal learning in the context of deficits in motor programming or sensory feedback may be determined by lesion location: for example following a sensorimotor cortex or basal ganglia stroke, explicit instruction may disrupt implicit motor learning, a problem that does not occur in healthy controls or following cerebellar stroke.

Evidence for the optimal timing of intervention in humans is scant but thought to be within the first 3 months after insult, based on evidence from animal studies that show a brief window of heightened plasticity between roughly 5 days to 3–4 weeks post brain infarct. The point at which therapy should be terminated is equally unclear. After stroke it is often recommended that therapy should finish when patients reach a plateau and fail to respond to rehabilitation. However, this may be partly the result of adaptation to a therapy programme and, as in healthy subjects, the performance of an exercise regime over time. Further improvements may be observed after a modification in intensity and/or specific intervention. It is now recognised that the potential for reorganisation and improvement in function exists in health as well as in the chronic stage post injury.

Animal and, more recently, human studies suggest that high intensity of therapy is beneficial, but at present clear-cut guidelines for intensity of intervention in humans are seldom available. Overall, an increased intensity of a motivating and appropriate therapy seems beneficial. Possible cost-effective means of doing this include the use of group training rather than individual therapy, constraint of the non-affected limb during waking hours, or a conversation partner. Greater intensity might also be provided by emerging interventions such as the use of automated robotics, virtual environment practice, mental imagery and the use of telerehabilitation described later.

Physical therapeutic interventions for motor disorders

Bobath approach and Motor Relearning Programme

In the past 60 years, various physiotherapy treatment approaches have been adopted which use different underlying theoretical assumptions about the control of movement and the mechanisms underlying recovery. Early approaches proposed by Rood, Brunstromm, Knott, Voss and Bobath were underpinned by neurophysiological theory, in particular the role of afferent information in facilitating movement. In the last 20 years, theoretical assumptions and knowledge gleaned from biomechanics and motor learning have resulted in the modification of existing approaches and the development of other approaches such as the Motor Relearning Progamme (MRP). In the United Kingdom, the long-favoured Bobath approach now tends to be integrated with new evidence into a more eclectic approach, while the motor re-learning approach is more commonly used in Australia, its country of origin. Techniques used in the Bobath and motor re-learning approaches have many similarities. Both emphasise the need for task-specific practice and maintenance of muscle length and joint alignment. The motor re-learning approach emphasises time spent practicing task-specific activities and strength training, with verbal instructions to direct and correct movement performance. By contrast, the Bobath approach emphasises the need to manually facilitate components of normal movement that are absent, and to normalise tone. Despite these differences, studies comparing the effectiveness of these and other approaches have revealed no difference in their efficacy. This may be because of similarities in the techniques, or the fact that therapy only forms a small part of a patient's day.

Impairment based treatment techniques

Muscle weakness after a CNS lesion is common and is often the result of a primary deficit in central control. A lack of descending control results in alterations in motor unit recruitment, firing patterns and inappropriate agonist–antagonist co-activation. With time, changes in muscle fibre type, and alterations in muscle length and the length–tension relationship occur; disuse atrophy may also develop as sensorimotor deficits limit a person's normal level of activity. Muscle weakness in turn predicts poor function; for example lower limb weakness is associated with reduced walking speeds and stair climbing ability post-stroke. Progressive resisted strength training post-stroke can result in an increase in upper and lower limb muscle strength without any increase in spasticity. Such strength gains can in turn lead to functional improvements. Optimal strength training is thought to be achieved by 2 × 8 repetitions at 80% of 1 repetition maximum (1RM), but whether this is best performed as concentric or eccentric movements during open or closed kinetic chain exercises has not been fully established.

Muscle strength can also be maintained and improved by electrical stimulation in upper and lower limbs, but effects on ADL may be minimal. Most studies have assessed the effects of stimulating distal musculature such as the wrist extensors and tibialis anterior. Neuromuscular stimulation may also be initiated by electromyography (EMG) signals recorded from the target muscle. This technique may result in larger gains in motor control because active participation optimises motor relearning, but in clinical trials transfer of these improvements to functional abilities has been minimal.

Sensory facilitation techniques use the application of stimuli such as muscle stretch, tactile input and weight-bearing through the affected limb to achieve muscle activation. Many of these inputs modulate spinal cord circuitry, as the effects are seen in paretic muscle of people with complete spinal cord lesions, and supraspinal modulation may also occur. These passive sensory stimuli facilitate muscle responses less than voluntary activation, and therefore active participation should be encouraged wherever possible.

In the management of upper motor neurone induced hypertonia, the contribution of neural and non-neural components needs to be established as their treatments differ and should be addressed separately. Although this is possible experimentally, it is not an easy task in the clinical setting, and there are no good outcome measures available. Neural contributions to hypertonia, caused by an increase in stretch reflex evoked muscle activity, as spasticity, are amenable to pharmacological interventions, which should be given in conjunction with therapeutic goals and follow-up. Although the severity of spasticity correlates with functional limitations it is still not clear to what extent this is causal.

Physical interventions focus on the non-neural aspect of hypertonia, namely increased stiffness of the intramuscular and periarticular connective tissue. Maintenance and restoration of muscle length and muscle compliance may be achieved using a variety of techniques including active and passive stretches, standing regimes, splinting, orthoses and optimising sitting posture in a wheelchair.

However, the evidence to support this is limited, and the best type and duration of stretches remains unclear. These interventions are likely to influence the enhancement in stretch evoked activity, possibly via inhibitory sensory input resulting from the patient's active movement and positioning, in much the same way as transcutaneous electrical stimulation (TENS) and specific cutaneous nerve stimulation have been shown to inhibit stretch reflexes in people with spasticity, possibly via modulation of presynaptic inhibitory interneurones.

Constraint induced movement therapy

Constraint induced movement therapy (CIMT) following stroke or traumatic brain injury (TBI) involves constraining the non-paretic upper limb for up to 90% of waking hours while performing intensive (forced use) task-oriented therapy on the paretic limb. The training involves general task practice and shaping, part practice when the behavioural goal is approached in small steps, and feedback about task performance is given at each step. Only 20–25% of stroke survivors have sufficient sensori-motor function for inclusion in CIMT studies. Large-scale studies investigating this approach have shown significant improvements in functional ability and motor impairment in both chronic and acute stroke patients. The EXCITE trial recruited 222 stroke patients 3–9 months post-stroke to CIMT versus usual care and found significant gains in affected upper limb function which persisted at 1 year. Subsequently, TMS and fMRI studies have demonstrated that alterations in cortico-spinal conduction, motor maps and movement-related activation patterns accompany the behavioural changes. The time spent training during CIMT is longer than reported for other approaches, up to 6 hours of practice for 10 out of 14 days, and may explain the large effect size. One study has reported no difference in the degree of motor recovery when this technique was compared with conventional therapy of a similar intensity level.

Modified CIMT (mCIMT), in which the training hours and the constraint time are reduced to 1 or 2 hours and 3–4 hours a day respectively, but over a longer period of 10 weeks, in a distributed rather than massed practice schedule, has been reported in a number of studies to produce similar benefits when given to patients at various time points after stroke, to patients with various stroke severities, after TBI, and in combination with other interventions, including botulinum toxin injections. Further studies are ongoing to determine the optimal protocol and time-frame of intervention.

Balance and posture

Balance, posture and mobility require the integration of multisensory information (visual, vestibular and somato-sensory) at multiple levels of the CNS, and as a result of this distributed control are often affected by neural damage. Postural stability is a vital prerequisite for all functional movements, and without postural stability the upper limbs are often used to aid balance. Positioning and specialised seating may be required to substitute for impaired mechanisms of postural control, and can improve limb function, and prevent progression of deformity such as scoliosis and windswept limbs, as well as spread pressure distribution and thus prevent pressure sores and associated complications. The provision of an appropriate manual or electric wheelchair can also greatly improve mobility. Compensatory approaches to gait rehabilitation and mobility include the use of walking aids and orthoses. Such interventions may not increase gait asymmetry, as previously thought, and can reduce energy expenditure.

Treadmill training, functional electrical stimulation, cueing, fitness and mental imagery

Treadmill training with body weight support via a harness system and robotic assisted step trainers allow safe, repetitive practice of the entire act of walking. The task can be progressed by varying the treadmill speed and incline, and decreasing the assistance given by the therapist and the amount of body weight support. This increases balance requirements and the need for antigravity muscle activity. Unexpectedly, to date these techniques have produced equivalent rather than greater benefit in trials, for example the Spinal Cord Injury Locomotor Trial (SCILT) and the Locomotor Experience Applied Post Stroke (LEAPS) trials, when compared with similar amounts of conventional over-ground therapist-led gait training in patients with stroke, spinal cord injury, multiple sclerosis, cerebral palsy and Parkinson's disease, and the place of these technologies needs further exploration.

Functional electrical stimulation (FES) of a peripheral motor nerve and the muscles supplied may be used to compensate for muscle weakness. A variety of foot-drop stimulators are available which compensate for the presence of foot drop. Onset of swing phase is detected either by a heel switch or a goniometer that detects knee position and triggers common peroneal nerve stimulation via surface, cuff or subcutaneous electrodes. The contraction of the tibialis anterior muscle results in dorsiflexion during the swing phase and can result in increased walking speed following stroke and multiple sclerosis. With prolonged use, an increase in walking speeds without the stimulator may also be observed, possibly by increasing muscle strength.

Multi-channel FES has also been used to retrain standing, weight transference and gait. Stimulation may be via surface or subcutaneous electrodes, and more recently direct stimulation of the nerves via cuff electrodes. In people with paraplegia a minimum of four channels are required for ambulation when used in combination with a walking aid. Stepping can be induced via common peroneal stimulation resulting in ankle dorsiflexion and a flexor withdrawal reflex, while stimulation of the quadriceps provides knee control during the stance phase. Hand or foot switches are used to trigger alternate leg movements and the person requires sufficient arm strength to provide balance via a walking aid. Multi-channel FES systems have been used in combination with orthoses, providing hybrid assistive systems with greater external symmetry. Reports of people with paraplegia achieving independent stance and gait have been described. However, many use such systems for exercise and the physiological and psychological benefits of standing rather than for functional tasks. Muscle fatigue, high energy expenditure with the use of this system, abnormal muscle activation patterns due to hypertonia, and the time to don and doff these systems still fail to make them a realistic clinical tool, and, as a result of unrealistic expectations, many people discontinue the systems within a year.

In Parkinson's disease gait cadence, stride length and velocity have been shown to be improved by cueing. Cues can be provided either internally, by paying attention to step length, or externally as auditory or visual cues. These have been used as well as treadmill training to overcome freezing, festination and falls of patients with Parkinson's disease. Six to eight weeks of physiotherapy and exercise training, with or without auditory cueing, improve mobility and independence, but permanent cueing systems and follow-up training are needed to sustain these improvements in the longer term.

Cardio-respiratory training and exercise classes may reverse the detraining effects of immobility and reduced activity seen in many chronic conditions. One month after stroke, aerobic capacity, measured by peak oxygen consumption on maximal exercise testing, is reduced to about 60% of normal, making the performance of ADL effortful and fatiguing. Although ADL exert a training effect so that exercise capacity improves, aerobic capacity remains reduced at 6 months and probably in the long term. Activity intolerance is thus common among stroke survivors who may work close to their individual maximal exercise capacity, compared with age- and weight-matched controls, while engaged in only domestic chores. Aerobic training, muscle strengthening or both usually improve targeted outcomes including balance and walking speed and distance, although not consistently ADL. Various recommendations have been made by the British Association of Sports and Exercise Sciences. All adults should perform at least 150 minutes of moderate or 75 minutes of vigorous activity per week. In people with mild to moderate static MS, mild to moderate endurance exercise as well as moderate resistance exercises are well tolerated and have a beneficial effect. Even 3 minutes of very strenuous exercise three times a week appears to be very helpful for some people, and is a realistic target for all.

Mental imagery and sensory stimulation techniques can be used to facilitate motor retraining. Mental imagery of an action activates areas of the brain that overlap with those involved in motor control. Imagined motor tasks have been trialled as an adjunct to help the rehabilitation of functional movements. After stroke, improvements in upper limb use and of ADL have been reported after mental imagery of the paretic limb, but further evidence is needed to establish which patients benefit and what protocol is most effective. Evidence to support sensory retraining post-stroke is still limited. Training regimes vary but tend to include a progression from localising to discriminating different tactile and proprioceptive stimuli, and practice in tasks requiring stereognosis. Functional gains in upper limb tasks have not been demonstrated.

Robotics and virtual reality

Two emerging technologies, robotics and virtual reality, are likely to provide new opportunities for skill retraining after neural injury, and may be used to increase and/or prolong the amount of therapy, but they have not yet been shown to produce better results than conventional therapies delivered at the same intensity. Robotic devices may be used to provide appropriate assistance or resistance to a movement depending on the person's level of impairment. They have the advantage of being able to control and record movement-associated forces and kinematics, and so the intensity of therapy can be accurately determined instead of simply stating the total duration of therapy. Studies using robotic devices to retrain proximal upper limb movements in stroke have demonstrated significant improvements in motor impairment, which have not always translated into improved functional ability. Similarly, robotic gait machines are now being used to aid walking rehabilitation in people with stroke and incomplete spinal cord injury. Such devices are as effective as treadmill training but significantly reduce the need for the therapist to facilitate paretic leg swing and weight transference on to the paretic stance limb.

Virtual reality technology provides a virtual two- or three-dimensional visual environment. The display may be head mounted or movement of the head can be used to produce movements of the visual scene as in the real world, and it is also possible to give haptic (touch) force feedback from a virtual object via a manipulandum. It is thus possible to create a complex variable environment for intensive retraining of sensori-motor function, factors lacking in many conventional therapy approaches. Upper limb training in a virtual environment after stroke has resulted in improvements in motor function that transfer to the natural situation. The ability to manipulate the visual scene is also an advantage for the rehabilitation of balance, particularly in those subjects who have over-relied on visual information to balance while not using remaining vestibular and somato-sensory information, for example after central and peripheral vestibular lesions.

Language disorders: speech and language therapy and communication aids

Normal language function is usually dependent on an intact left hemisphere. However, current neuroscientific evidence points to a network of nodes and connections, both within and between hemispheres, that support individual language operations. For instance, naming is subserved by an extensive network that is vulnerable to damage at many of its nodes, which is why most aphasic patients suffer from anomia. It is beyond the scope of this chapter to review the evidence for and utility of the behavioural classification of aphasia subtypes, but we believe that documentation of impairments in the main language areas (speaking, writing, listening and reading) is more useful for guiding therapies than clinical classification. Descriptions of the various classical speech disorders are given in Chapter 4, and neuroanatomy is outlined in Chapter 2.

Acquired language impairment (dysarthria or aphasia) is the second most common major symptom caused by stroke and is common in all major forms of dementia, with a prevalence of more than 90% once patients have reached the moderately affected phase. The treatment evidence base is derived almost solely from post-stroke aphasia studies although trials in dementia are ongoing, particularly in patients with progressive non-fluent aphasia.

Despite occasional high profile papers that appear to show that speech and language therapy (SALT) is no better than non-specialist interventions, the evidence for the overall effectiveness of SALT in post-stroke aphasia is pretty clear. A Cochrane review indicates: 'We identified 39 trials involving 2518 randomised participants that were suitable for inclusion in this review. Overall, the review shows evidence from randomised trials to suggest there may be a benefit from speech and language therapy but there was insufficient evidence to indicate the best approach to delivering speech and language therapy.'

Bhogal *et al.* took a different approach, segregating positive from negative SALT studies and asking what the systematic differences between them were. The answer was compelling: positive studies had on average 100 hours of therapy (delivered at a rate of 9 hours each week) while patients in negative studies clocked-up only 45 hours in total (at a rate of 2 hours/week). Intensity was clearly conflated with total dose, but the weight of evidence from other studies, including those into expert human performance, suggests that dose is the more important of the two. The issues over exactly what type of therapy to give (phonological or semantic cues) or how to provide feedback to patients (error-full, errorless or error-reducing learning) remain unanswered, but the key principles are clear. These are:

- Outcome-based therapy, be it at the level of impairment or activities and participation,
- Mass practice,
- Adaptive, that is, appropriate to the patients current abilities, not too easy or difficult, and
- Feedback to promote learning, especially as some patients with aphasia have difficulty recognising their own errors.

One solution to the dose issue is to utilise computer-based therapy programmes. Many exist and at least one has proved effective in a small-scale clinical trial. A list of current electronic therapy packages of varying quality can be found here (www.aphasiasoftwarefinder.org).

A large range of drugs have been trialled in aphasia. A thorough review is beyond the scope of this chapter, but well-designed studies (placebo-controlled, double-blind) have been carried out that show significant improvements when levodopa, memantine or donepezil are used. In studies where the drug was paired with behavioural therapy, the SALT effect sizes average at a fairly consistent 0.3 while the drug effects can be substantially higher than this but are patchy by comparison.

Another promising adjuvant is NIBS as tDCS, when a small current is passed through the brain using a battery and scalp electrodes. Because the current is continuous, there is no sensory stimulation to the scalp which makes this an easy technique to double blind. It is not clear which regime to use (strength of current, exact placement of leads, activation of left, right or both hemispheres) but if tDCS effects on language follow in the footsteps of motor systems research, then modest gains of about a third can be expected, compared with the effect of practice alone.

The therapies discussed thus far are all aimed at improving standard language communication, and can be considered under the rubric of restorative techniques. Some patients with a severe speech output aphasia (often a mixture of anomia and apraxia of speech) may not be able to mount much of a vocabulary even with mass practice. Such patients tend to have intact semantics and non-verbal communication skills and so can benefit from using a different mode of communication, such as gesture therapy. The evidence is weaker than for conventional speech therapy, but in a sub-set of the more severely impaired patients this may represent the best approach. In neuroscience terms this is a strategy-based compensatory therapy but one that changes both behaviour and brain connectivity.

There are many types of communication aids available. These change patients' interactions with other people but, when the aid is removed, performance falls back to previous levels, as no neuroplastic changes are induced. Some aids require an intact language system (e.g. Lightwriter SL40) and are for patients with isolated articulatory failure, such as motor neurone disease. Others use pictures for patients to point at. Modern mobile devices are moving the field forward quickly and software tools such as text-to-speech, e-readers and a variety of other apps are taking over from the older, more bulky aids (http://www.stroke.org.uk/sites/default/files/Communication%20aids%20&%20computer%20therapy.pdf).

Visual loss and restorative therapies

We cover this large and complex field by anatomical site of visual impairment, and results from damage to the retina, the visual tract causing hemianopia, and the association visual cortices to cause neglect and visual-perceptual disorders.

There are myriad causes of primary visual failure which can be congenital (rare) or acquired. In older age the leading cause of visual loss is macular degeneration which is age-related and affects people in their fifth decade and beyond. The dry form is most common and progression can be slowed with antioxidants plus zinc. The wet form (associated with the formation of neovascular membranes) can be treated with the monoclonal antibody ranibizumab, which is recommended by the National Institute for Health and Care Excellence (NICE) for a sub-set of patients. There is good evidence that low vision services improve outcomes in such patients. These interventions include counselling and prescription, provision of low-vision devices with some sessions provided by a low-vision therapist to teach use of assistive devices and adaptive strategies to perform daily living tasks independently. An interesting strategy-based therapy for patients with severe visual loss is echo location. Patients make ingressive tongue clicks and, with training, learn to interpret the resulting echoes which allows them to construct a 3D image from the reflected echoes of objects; a sensation referred to as 'flash sonar' by the developers. Functional neuroimaging studies have shown that skilled users recruit occipital cortex when performing echo-location tasks; this effect is larger in congenitally or early blind individuals.

Hemianopia is a loss of vision to one side of fixation and is usually caused by damage to the visual tracts after they have partially crossed (decussated) at the optic chiasm. The most common causes are stroke, traumatic brain injury and tumors. From stroke alone the incidence in the United Kingdom is ~10 000–15 000 people per year. The best estimate for its prevalence comes from an Australian study that found 0.8% of adults 49 years or older had a hemianopia, which equates to at least 80 000 in the United Kingdom. The visual field defect rarely improves 6 months after the onset and affects a whole host of activities of daily living.

There are three main approaches to treatment: visual restoration, eye movement strategies and prisms. There are two main types of visual restoration and each comes with its own patented hardware. One aims to improve high acuity, conscious vision at the borders of the field defect, NovaVision VRT (visual restoration therapy), while the other, Neuro-Eye therapy, improves vision deep into the impaired field. Both rely on mass practice of detecting stimuli at the border of the blind field (NovaVision) or deep within the blind field (Neuro-Eye therapy). There has been much controversy over whether NovaVision VRT really is effective, and, if so, by what mechanism; this will be dealt with later. Neuro-Eye therapy is less controversial, as the stimuli (Gabor patches) are presented deep in the blind field and probably rely on sparse, non-V1 pathways by which visual stimuli can be processed but do not always reach conscious perception (the definition of blindsight). The practice effects are retinotopic; that is, performance gains are only seen in those parts of the visual field where stimuli were shown although this requires thousands or tens-of-thousands of trials. The problem for visual rehabilitation is this: how functionally useful *is* blindsight? It is certainly better than nothing and may help reduce collision rates, but to date there have been no studies addressing the carryover or impact that these training regimes may have on patients' ADL.

Visual restitution therapy appears much more promising in terms of potential carryover as the claim is that, with sufficient practice, patients can restore high acuity, conscious vision. The main problem has been that any visual field gains have only been seen on using the visual field test that is bundled with the therapy package. This is an issue, as the visual field test relies on the same stimuli that are used in the training or therapy part of the programme. Obviously, if vision is really being restored, it should not matter what method is being used to test any visual field gains. The prevailing view is that the training results in more efficient eye movements into the damaged field and not genuine field expansion. Patients care much less about the mechanism of action than duelling scientists, and there is good evidence that the therapy does improve visual function.

The most convincing and consistent evidence for improving visual function in patients with hemianopia comes from studies that retrain eye movements. This involves mass practice using stimuli that provoke a specific type of eye movement. Unlike the visual restitution therapies, these have a clear carryover effect on to untrained stimuli. There are over 10 published studies in this area and a recent Cochrane review of the more rigorous ones concluded: 'There is limited evidence which supports the use of compensatory scanning training for patients with visual field defects.' A further study published since then very nicely demonstrated the specificity of these techniques. In a randomised, cross-over design, reading therapy and 'visual exploration training' were provided to 36 patients with homonymous visual field defects. The results were very clear and showed that the training-related improvements in reading and visual exploration were specific and task dependent; the combined effect size was 0.47 for visual search and 0.28 for reading speed. Interestingly, the cross-over therapy had no effect (positive or negative) on the other task; that is, when undergoing the second therapy block, gains made from the first block remained stable, suggesting that therapy gains persist in the short to medium term. While the specificity was no great surprise (although this was the first study to explicitly test this), it is good news that there was no interference. There are now two, free-to-use, web-based therapies for patients with hemianopia causing hemianopic alexia (www.readright.ucl.ac.uk or problems with visual search: www.eyesearch.ucl.ac.uk). Both contain testing and therapy materials and are designed for home use by patients.

The evidence for therapeutic interventions in more complex perceptual disorders (pure alexia, prosopagnosia, simultanagnosia) is sporadic and weak and it is difficult to make any specific recommendations. Spatial neglect or inattention is more common and has a stronger evidence base although the presumed efficacy for the main therapy (prism adaptation) has been questioned in a recent well-conducted review. Drug therapies have also been tried, with a recent study showing a small but significant (10%) improvement in table-top tests of selective attention when transdermal rotigotine, a dopamine agonist, was compared with placebo.

Cognitive impairments

The cognitive sequelae of neurological disorders are evaluated by means of detailed neuropsychological assessment which identifies both strengths and weaknesses in the patient's profile. This section focuses on intervention relating to attention, memory and executive deficits. Neuropsychological interventions invariably involve a preliminary phase of psycho-education as part of 'brain-injury education': an explanation in terms of brain–behaviour relations, to patients and/or their carers of the nature of and reason for the deficits the patient is experiencing. This is important, not least in providing them with a vocabulary with which to speak about symptomatology that is unfamiliar and often bewildering. Following this didactic phase, intervention may comprise any or all of the three approaches described elsewhere in this chapter: environmental manipulation (adaptive interventions); training in the use of compensatory strategies; and retraining with the aim of restoring specific impairments.

Environmental manipulation and compensatory strategies

Environmental manipulation involves modifications that improve well-being by changing living, training or working conditions. These may include such things as provision of a quiet, relatively distraction free space; the overt breaking down of tasks into their components with smaller sub-goals; and external monitoring of performance and feedback to aid adjustment of behaviour to goals. Such modifications are reliant on others for their implementation, but while quite simple in themselves can significantly improve the patient's ability to perform a task.

Compensatory strategies focus on trying to make good the functional deficit rather than resolving or reversing the problem impairment. This may include non-technological aids including use of a diary or calendar for daily routines, appointments, special occasions, or future events; and a daily checklist in a prominent place as a reminder to complete certain tasks, such as 'lock the door', 'turn off the iron', and so on. Assistive technologies for patients with severe cognitive deficits include prospective memory aids such as the NeuroPage system, which uses automated radio-paging or SMS (text message) technology to send reminders of things to do, such as taking medication, or non-specific alerting messages ('STOP') to reduce goal neglect. Small voice recorders can be loaded with reminder messages including appointments, telephone numbers, grocery lists or prescription refills, while mobile phones with touch screen capability allow easy input and access to notes, telephone numbers, dates, daily reminders and to-do lists. There is good evidence that prospective prompting devices of this sort are useful for people with memory impairment, and similar evidence is being acquired to support the use of devices (e.g. the SenseCam), which support retrospective autobiographical memory.

Restorative approaches

Restorative approaches aim at recovery of lost function through re-training and practice of specific cognitive skills. Attention training is based on the premise that attentional abilities can be improved by activating particular aspects of attention through a stimulus drill approach. The repeated stimulation of attentional systems via graded attention exercises is hypothesised to facilitate changes in attentional functioning. Memory re-training is based on the demonstrated link between encoding and retrieval processes in normal subjects. Training focuses on visual imagery or elaborative encoding including acronyms or rhymes to aid recall of new information. Sometimes, retraining strategies combine some of these elements.

Executive function, retraining and behavioural modification

The term executive function describes a set of cognitive abilities, for which the pre-frontal cortex is key, that are necessary for behavioural regulation in the context of goal-directed behaviour: the ability to initiate and stop actions, to monitor and change behaviour as needed, and to plan, and execute, future behaviours when faced with novel tasks and situations. These skills are closely allied to those involved in social cognition, which involves the ability to empathise, and recognise emotions and mental states in other people, and if damaged result in 'personality' changes and inappropriate social behaviours, including disinhibition or emotional indifference. Both skill sets are crucial to independent living, community re-entry and the resumption of social roles.

Because of the extensive connectivity of the prefrontal cortex, executive and social cognition deficits frequently result from abnormal functional connectivity after brain injury, irrespective of the precise location of pathology. At the same time, the complexity of this aspect of cognition – still an area of considerable theoretical discussion – makes targeted re-training difficult. Some strategies focus on goal maintenance. Goal Management Training (GMT), for example, is a method of remediating executive dysfunction that is based on theories of sustained attention, and addresses higher order executive deficits. When sustained attention is compromised following a brain injury, a person may become distracted from achieving their goals by either habits or environmental influences. The primary focus of GMT is to teach the patient to periodically stop ongoing behaviour, in order to monitor and adjust goals in order to stay on task. Other interventions are based on problem-solving: patients are trained to reduce the complexity of a multi-stage problem by breaking it down to sub-goals.

Although the training tasks in each cognitive domain may bear little resemblance to tasks encountered in everyday life, it is argued that re-training the cognitive processes underlying functional activities will result in generalisable gains. In general, there has been some evidence of improvement on tasks practiced, and some other neuropsychological measures tapping similar functions, especially in patients with focal rather than diffuse pathology, but to date there has been no consistent evidence that such training has a significant impact upon the everyday functioning of the brain-injured person.

The cognitive rehabilitation of patients with brain injury must address not only the specific focal neuropsychological deficits that result from localised brain lesions, but also more generalised complaints that are common to most kinds of cerebral pathology, irrespective of aetiology, lesion location or distribution of pathology. These include cognitive fatigue and reduced speed of information processing, both of which also impact upon one another to the detriment of cognitive efficacy and stamina.

Finally, it is impossible to think about the cognitive rehabilitation of a brain-injured patient without also thinking about the person's psychological status more generally. Even mild residual problems following a head injury can constitute a significant trauma to the person's sense of self. In addition to whatever other kind of rehabilitation strategy is used, psychological support is then also required to assist the person with brain injury or illness and their close others in coming to terms with lasting personality and lifestyle changes, and forming a new post-injury identity.

Telerehabilitation

We know that behavioural therapies are effective, but patients' responses are critically dependent on the amount of time spent practicing with them. Given this, rehabilitation at a distance, or telerehabilitation, and using social media seem promising strategies to ensure that patients receive the correct dose of the right sort of therapy. This is a rapidly growing topic and so we can only touch on the main issues here, but telerehabilitation can be applied to all the main areas of neurological rehabilitation. We cover: information sharing and peer-to-peer support; assessment at-a-distance; and teletherapy, either with or without a therapist's direct involvement.

Peer-to-peer support via the provision of information is an important part of rehabilitation as it helps patients and their carers adjust to and self-manage their condition. There are a large number of websites offering information didactically, but the more interactive ones allow patients to share information with each other, either via chat rooms or in a more innovative manner such as utilised by the forum PatientsLikeMe (www.patientslikeme.com). This site allows patients to share experiences of their symptoms and also their evaluations of interventions. While claiming to cover all disorders, the site was historically built up by patients with motor neurone disease and this currently remains the best-covered disorder. The number of patients adding their own data is impressive; the totality of their experiences is very likely to speak to any incoming patient's situation. For example, one can type in a symptom such as spasticity and see how many patients using the site have reported this symptom, what their underlying condition is, what they are using to treat it and, crucially, how effective they perceive the given therapy to be. This symptom alone has 20 000 ratings (Figure 18.7).

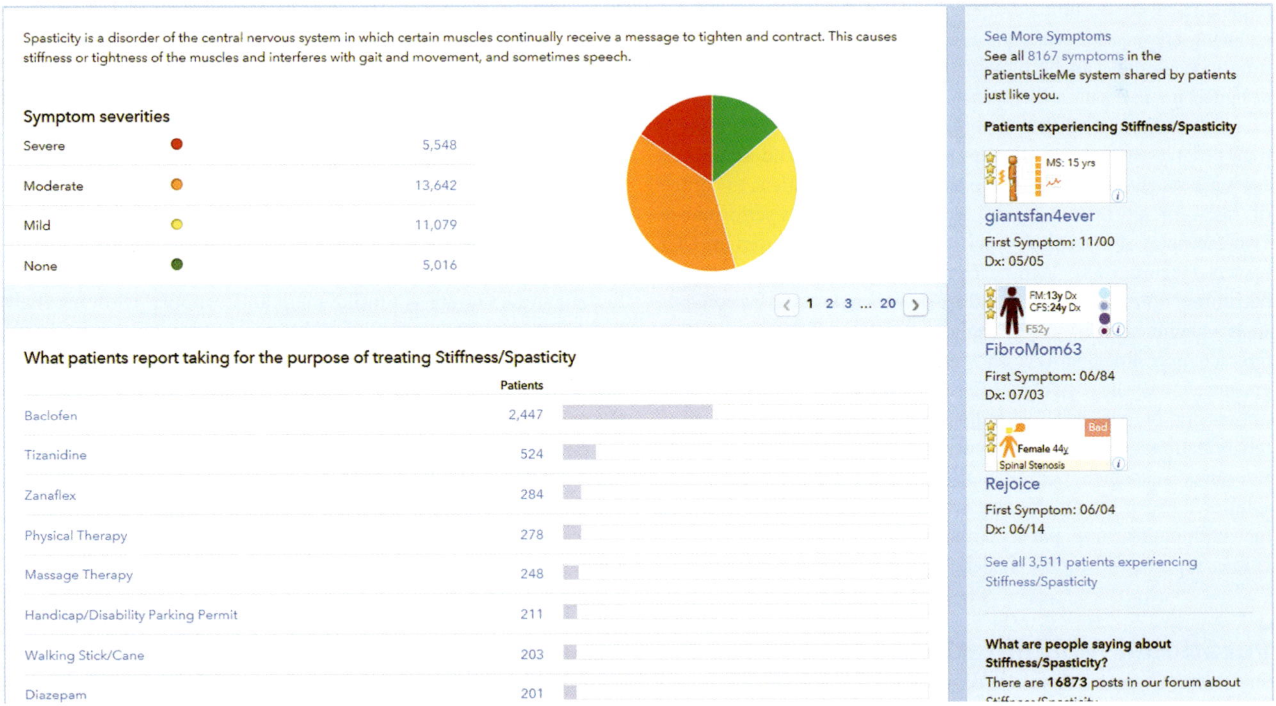

Figure 18.7 Snapshot from the spasticity page of PatientsLikeMe taken on 11 April 2016: http://www.patientslikeme.com/symptoms/show/5. Source: PatientsLikeMe, Inc. 2015. Reproduced with permission.

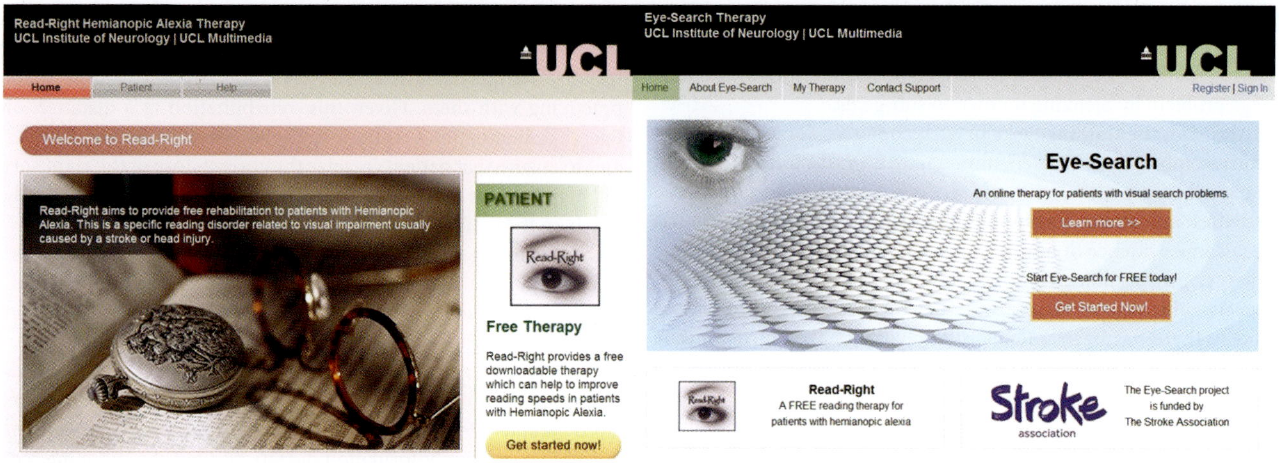

Figure 18.8 Homepages of Read-Right and Eye-Search: adaptive, web-based therapy for patients with acquired visual field defects. Source: Reproduced with permission of UCL.

Most tele-assessment provides a specialist clinical opinion without the clinician having to be in the same place as the patient. There often needs to be a therapist/clinician alongside the patient and two-way visual and auditory links are important. An example of how this works can be seen on www.bbc.co.uk/news/health-11644278. There are now many other examples, such as speech and language therapy and real-time, internet-based, remote, telefluoroscopic evaluation of oro-pharyngeal swallowing. There are ongoing trials assessing the effectiveness of this new practice. Therapy as well as assessment can be delivered in this way; however, these examples all require therapists and clinicians to interact directly with the patient, in real-time. While this solves the problem of having to transport patients to specialists, it does not solve the problem of how to deliver a greater dose of therapy to patients given the limited number of therapists.

There are a wide variety of digital or electronic teletherapy programmes that can be bought for home use. The majority are designed for use with a therapist; that is, patients get on with their exercises at home and then meet up with a therapist who reviews their progress and sets new therapy goals. However, stand-alone therapies are also available and these either allow the patient to control the task difficulty or automatically adapt to the patient's performance. Two examples of this sort of web-based therapy are housed on UCL servers (Figure 18.8). Web-based and other digital therapies are becoming more sophisticated and are increasingly using 'peripherals' such as hand-held devices or motion detectors to allow patients to interact more imaginatively and realistically with the therapy programme. Given the costs of one-to-one therapy, and given the amount of time and practice required to make improvements in neurological rehabilitation, 'smart' digital packages that can sense patients' responses and help them to adapt their behaviour look like promising solutions. Providing an effective form of feedback, which is critical for volitional learning, particularly for patients with cognitive difficulties, is perhaps the most challenging yet exciting issue.

Vocational rehabilitation

Sir Ludwig Guttman, a pioneer of spinal injury rehabilitation in the United Kingdom in the 1940s, stated that the successful outcome of rehabilitation was the return of the patient to tax-paying status. This approach may be welcomed by the Exchequer, but it reflects assumptions that may be erroneous, both about the relative value that an individual places on return to work, and about the fact that resumption of employment can only be achieved at the expense of a reduction in other valued aspects of life, such as social, sexual and leisure activities. A broader definition recognises that adults need meaningful occupation, and covers voluntary activity as well as education, home-making and leisure activities. Although a popular view is that work is onerous and stressful, there is clear evidence that work leads to better quality of life, improved mood and greater life expectancy. Nevertheless, until recently, proactive vocational rehabilitation has been neglected.

The following paragraphs reflect the situation in the United Kingdom, but the principles are widely applicable. At diagnosis, 98% of people with progressive neurological conditions such as MS are in work. Within 10 years most are unemployed. With stroke 30% are under 65 years of age. Most do not return to work. The rate of work return for people with spinal cord injury and paraplegia is 15% in the United Kingdom and 60% in Canada. In the United Kingdom, most people receiving state financial benefit have relatively minor disability and expect at some time to return to work. Only 0.7% of recipients of incapacity benefit have had a stroke, 0.2% have tetraplegia and 0.9% have MS.

The chances of returning to work after 1 year on UK incapacity benefit (now known as Employment and Support Allowance) are less than 20%. The reasons for this are complex but include the demands imposed by the job itself, the limitations imposed by illness or disability and the barriers and expectations created by the society we live in. Vocational rehabilitation aims to overcome the barriers faced by an individual with an injury, illness or disability when retraining, returning to or starting work. It includes the support needed by both the individual and by the employer. Typically, this involves:

1. Retraining (e.g. for a bricklayer who has become paraplegic).
2. Capacity building (e.g. increasing exercise tolerance in an individual who has become physically unfit).
3. Return to work management by employers (e.g. a graded return to work over a period of weeks or months following meningitis).
4. Disability awareness – being aware of how society and individuals perceive people with disability, how this is reflected in the media, literature and the arts and how this influences behaviours.

5 Symptom management (e.g. being aware of the roles of other professionals such as occupational therapists and physiotherapists in vocational rehabilitation).
6 Adjustment counselling.
7 Reasonable adjustments at work.

Such adjustments include:

- Changing recruitment and selection procedures.
- Modifying work premises (e.g. making ramps, modifying toilets).
- Changing job design, work schedules or other work practices (e.g. swapping duties among staff, permitting people to work from home or regular breaks for those with fatigue).
- Modifying equipment (e.g. the provision of voice-activated software for those with upper limb problems or an amplifier-adapted telephone for the hearing impaired).
- Providing training or other assistance (e.g. induction programmes for staff with a disability and co-workers who ensure staff with a disability can gain access to training).

Most adults who acquire disability through neurological disease use the hospital consultant or the general practitioner as their first point of contact. Early and mild disability such as fatigue, or more effortful walking, can impact on work before impacting on other areas of life. No matter how good individuals' clinical treatment may be, if they lose their job unnecessarily then treatment has, in part, failed them. Early intervention has two main advantages. The individual can identify the best way to disclose their illness and disability within the workplace which is very different from disclosure to family and friends. Secondly, means of ameliorating the impact of disability can be identified, so work performance can be maintained and loss of goodwill within the workplace avoided. The individual's ability to access timely advice and support therefore depends upon clinicians, who should consider the following steps:

- Ask about work, the impact of work on the disease and the disease upon work.
- Discuss disclosure, and support them in explaining their needs to an employer when they decide to disclose.
- Identify if the individual has access to an occupational health department.
- Remind and inform the patient of the terms of the Equality Act.

One of the major roles of the occupational health physician is assessment of disability and fitness to work. In the United Kingdom, as few as 30% of employees have access to a specialist occupational health service. The UK Equality Act enshrined in law that disabled people should not be treated less favourably than others for a reason related to their disability. Employers have to make reasonable adjustments for disabled people. Such adjustments include making adjustments to premises, such as removing physical barriers or providing distraction free environments; altering hours of working or training; assigning people to a different place of work or training; allowing absence during working or training hours for rehabilitation, assessment or treatment; acquiring or modifying equipment such as voice-activated software; modifying instructions or reference manuals; modifying procedures for testing or assessment; providing a reader or interpreter; providing supervision or other support. Schools, colleges, universities and providers of adult education and youth services also have to ensure that they do not discriminate against disabled people.

Other practical measures include:

- Referral to vocational rehabilitation or occupational therapy services. As few as 10% of people with long long-term neurological conditions access any form of vocational rehabilitation. Such services should perform a comprehensive assessment, and deliver job retention interventions, which include clarification of the responsibilities of all parties under the Equality Act, and work site visits to meet employers and other interested parties to discuss needs and adjustments, design vocational rehabilitation interventions including practice of specific tasks, and adjustment counselling.
- Making individuals aware of the role of Disability Employment Advisors (DEAs) and the Access to Work scheme. DEAs provide specialist support for those wishing to move into employment or retain an existing job in the event of disability and are based in JobCentrePlus. The Access to Work scheme provides funding for costs that an employer may incur because of an employee's disability, and most commonly is used to provide support with transport costs to work for individuals who cannot use public transport or drive. Other support can be provided such as a powered wheelchair for use at work, adapted desks, specialist software or adaptations to premises.
- Supporting people who decide to decrease their hours, or retire, by signposting access to benefits and financial advice, and providing support with identifying other forms of occupation.

Medical treatments for specific problems

Symptoms related to neurological impairments caused by either single incident or chronic progressive conditions can cause distress and impact on function. Each person's needs differ and their optimal function and well-being will only be attained if individualised treatment goals, functionally relevant to the patient, are defined. This approach facilitates learning and self-management techniques, skills that do not result from generic prescription for a given impairment. Optimal management often involve several different disciplines working across health and social care sectors to enable the individual to incorporate treatment strategies into their daily life, and to ensure that interventions take place in an effective and timely fashion.

Spasticity

The impact of spasticity on an individual is extremely varied. On one level it may be useful, perhaps to allow standing or walking when weakness would otherwise preclude it, but it can also cause discomfort, pain and sleeplessness, or result in devastating loss of function with development of long-term problems such as pressure sores and contractures. The impact on function is variable; walking may be slower, falls more frequent, the ability to self-propel a wheelchair or transfer reduced, and many ADL such as washing, dressing, toileting and sexual activity compromised. Poorly managed spasticity can also have serious long-term physical consequences. Muscle shortening and tendon or soft tissue contractures can lead to restriction of passive movement and physical deformity, and can have major functional implications, causing difficulties with personal hygiene or dressing, problems in positioning and seating, and thus restricted community mobility and social isolation. The development of pressure sores may in turn increase spasticity and spasms, to cause a vicious circle of further contractures and dependency. Early identification of these factors enables timely intervention to minimise development of secondary complications.

The mainstay of management of spasticity is education of the individual and, if applicable, their family or carers in strategies to self-manage; these include the implementation of an effective regime of physical therapy including stretching and, if possible, standing with or without assistance. Knowledge of the triggers and aggravating factors detailed in Table 18.3 is particularly important to prevent exacerbation of spasticity and its associated features, and ensure drugs are used at appropriate times and dosages.

There is no agreed evidence-based model available for the systematic pharmacological management of spasticity and much of what is done is based on a logical and pragmatic approach. The identification of appropriate treatment goals will help optimise choice of agent, and also timing and dose. For example, painful nocturnal spasms may best be managed with a long-acting agent that has sedative side-effects taken at night-time. Alternatively, stiffness and spasms that interfere with an individual's morning transfers and personal care may benefit from medication taken on waking, prior to transferring out of bed. Dosages for those who are walking, and who may rely on their spasticity to do so, are often lower than in those who use a wheelchair for mobility. The general rule to 'start low and go slow' will limit any deleterious effects on function or unwanted side effects. The most common side effects reported are drowsiness, and weakness caused by unmasking underlying weakness by removing tone and reducing spasticity which was functionally useful.

The oral agents most commonly used are baclofen, tizanidine, benzodiazepines, dantrolene, gabapentin, pregabalin and canabinoids; all can be used alone as monotherapy or in combination (Table 18.4). Most of the clinical trials of baclofen, tizanidine, dantrolene and benzodiazepines in the management of spasticity took place over 20 years ago. Most involved patients with either multiple sclerosis (MS) or spinal cord injury. Although most studies have shown a positive effect in reducing hypertonia and spasms, little attention has been paid to functional benefit. Four small double-blind placebo-controlled randomised studies of gabapentin have been performed to date. Two of these were in patients with MS, one was in spinal cord injury alone and another included patients with any cause of upper motor neurone syndrome. All showed a beneficial effect for gabapentin on measures of spasticity without excessive side effects. There are no placebo controlled trials of pregabalin in those with spasticity, but case series and anecdotal reports have suggested a positive effect. Nabiximols (Sativex®) is an oromucosal spray that delivers 2.7 mg delta-9-tetrahydrocannabinol (THC) and 2.5 mg cannabidiol (CBD) in each 100 μLspray. Sativex has been licensed on the basis of an enriched study which

Table 18.3 Common cutaneous and visceral stimuli that may aggravate spasticity.

Cutaneous stimuli	Visceral stimuli
Altered skin integrity: Red or inflamed skin Broken skin Infected skin Pressure sores Ingrown toenails	Any systemic or localised infection Bowel dysfunction (e.g. constipation, overflow or diarrhoea) Bladder dysfunction (e.g. infections or incomplete emptying) Deep vein thrombosis
Tight fitting clothes or urinary leg bag appliances	
Uncomfortable orthotics or seating	

Table 18.4 Oral antispasticity agents.

Drug	Starting dose	Maximum dose	Side sffects
Baclofen	5–10 mg/day	120 mg/day, usually in 3 divided doses	Drowsiness, weakness, parasthesiae, nausea, vomiting
Tizanidine	2 mg/day	36 mg/day, usually in 3 or 4 divided doses	Drowsiness, weakness, dry mouth, postural hypotension * Monitor liver function
Dantrolene	25 mg/day	400 mg/day, usually in 4 divided doses	Anorexia, nausea, vomiting, drowsiness, weakness, dizziness, parasthesiae * Monitor liver function
Diazepam	2 mg/day	40–60 mg/day, usually in 3 or 4 divided doses	Drowsiness, reduced attention, memory impairment * Dependency and withdrawal syndromes
Clonazepam	0.25–0.5 mg, usually at night-time	3 mg, usually in 3 divided doses	Same as diazepam
Gabapentin	300 mg/day (can start at 100 mg/day)	3600 mg/day, usually in 3 divided doses	Drowsiness, somnolence, dizziness, weight gain
Pregabalin	5–75 mg/day	600 mg/day in 2 doses	Drowsiness, somnolence, dizziness, weight gain
Cannabis and cannabinoids, e.g. nabiximols (Sativex)	1 oromucosal mouth spray nocte	12 sprays/day	Dizziness, drowsiness, disorientation

Table 18.5 Goal-based outcome measures.

Outcome measure	Author	Date	Description
Self Identified Goals Assessment (SIGA)	Melville and Nelson	2001	Developed from research in older people, this is designed for occupational therapists to use with clients in subacute rehabilitation and nursing homes. It is the only goal-based outcome measure that provides a protocol to elicit patient identified goals, based on an exploratory interview. Each goal is assigned a rating 0 (unable to do) – 10 (can do) on a visual analogue scale. Post-therapy intervention the patient rates their performance and change scores are compared
Goal Attainment Scaling (GAS)	Kirusek *et al.*	1994	A five-point scale. The expected outcome (goal) is assigned the position of zero on the scale. Better than expected and much better than expected levels of outcome are +1 and +2, respectively. Worse and much worse than expected are −1 and −2. A high level of skill needed on part of the therapist to quantify various levels of goal achievement. This has been used in a variety of settings, demonstrating acceptable inter-rater reliability and concurrent validity (Emmerson and Neely 1988)
Canadian Occupational Performance Measure (COPM)	Baptiste *et al.*	1993	Designed for occupational therapists to use with clients to set goals. Standardised instrument with semi-structured interview format that elicits patient identified goals and quantitative patient ratings of these goals. Change scores between assessment and reassessment are the most meaningful scores derived from this assessment
Self Assessment of Occupational Functioning (SAOF)	Baron and Curtin	1990	Based on the Model of Human Occupation (Kielhofner 1995) which promotes collaborative treatment planning between patient and occupational therapist. This instrument elicits written responses to predetermined items
Satisfaction with Performance Questionnaire	Yerxa and Baum	1986	Quantitative scale of satisfaction with performance in daily occupations and community living. The scores highlight areas of decreased satisfaction with performance. Goals are negotiated between the therapist and patient on that basis

demonstrated a 50% responder rate defined as a 20% improvement in a numerical rating scale, and is usually trialled over 4 weeks to assess responder status. While not a therapy for spasticity, two Phase III studies have demonstrated that prolonged release fampridine improves walking speed by 20% in about one-third of people with MS resulting in a European Medicines license being issued in 2011. Two recent studies have failed to show a specific effect on spasticity in spinal cord injury but further studies are underway to explore the role of prolonged-release fampridine in other conditions such as cerebral palsy and stroke.

Botulinum toxin (BTX) type A is the most widely used focal treatment for spasticity. The toxin irreversibly inhibits release of acetylcholine at the neuromuscular junction, but its clinical effect is reversed by nerve sprouting and re-innervation which leads to functional recovery of the muscle over a few months. The toxin is injected directly into the targeted muscle and takes 10–14 days to have a visible effect. Several studies have shown BTX is effective at reducing tone and improving passive function; benefits in active function have been more difficult to demonstrate. It is essential that BTX injections are followed by goal-focused physiotherapy to obtain the maximum benefit (Table 18.5). Common goals include hand and perineal hygiene, dressing, pain, hand movement and limb position. Local injection of ethyl alcohol or, more commonly, phenol is an alternative option to BTX for focal management of spasticity. Chemical neurolysis is irreversible and results in destruction of neural tissue by protein coagulation. Injections may be targeted at peripheral nerves or motor points, areas of muscle most sensitive to electrical stimulation. Partial nerve regeneration and sprouting may subsequently occur so that the clinical effect may wane after several weeks or months. If necessary the injections can be repeated. Those most commonly applied are medial popliteal blocks to aid spastic foot drop, or obturator nerve blocks either in ambulatory patients with scissoring gait or with the aim of improving ease of perineal hygiene and seating posture in more dependent patients.

Intrathecal therapies should be considered if oral medication in combination with appropriate physical measures is not tolerated or fails to control lower limb spasticity, for example to enable safe seating or hoist transfers. The concentration of GABA receptors in the lumbar spinal cord allows very small dosages of intrathecal baclofen (ITB) to be effective without causing any systemic side effects. A programmable pump is implanted into the abdomen and a catheter conveys the baclofen into the intrathecal space. ITB has been shown to be an effective treatment option in the management of severe spasticity of either cerebral or spinal origin; more recently it has been shown to be effective in improving gait. Intrathecal phenol is a cheap and less invasive treatment than ITB and can be extremely effective. As phenol is a destructive agent that indiscriminately damages motor and sensory nerves, it is reserved for those individuals who have no functional movement in their legs, who have lost bladder and bowel function and who have impaired sensation to their legs. The effect of a single injection is usually permanent though if wearing off is seen it can be repeated if necessary. Selective dorsal root rhizotomies involve sectioning some of the rootlets of each targeted dorsal root to reduce the afferent input while preserving sensory and sphincter function. This is generally reserved for children with cerebral palsy.

Ataxia

Cerebellar ataxia is unfortunately an extremely challenging symptom to manage. The effects on the individual are variable and may cause only minor problems with finger dexterity in some patients but in others catastrophic loss of upper limb function, mobility and even loss of sitting balance. Severe tremor and head titubation may occur and can be very distressing. Physio- and occupational therapy are the mainstay of management. By optimising the individual's sitting position, posture and the provision of distal supportive aids, the ease and quality of functional tasks such as feeding, self-care and keyboard use can be improved. Drug therapy is of limited value because of poor efficacy and adverse effects; drugs that are often tried with variable success include isoniazid (with pyridoxine), clonazepam, carbamazepine, gabapentin, mirtazepine and propranolol.

For severe cases it may be appropriate to consider deep brain stimulation, historically of the ventral intermediate (VIM) nucleus of the thalamus and more recently the ventralis oralis posterior (Vop) a basal ganglia outflow nucleus, and zona incerta (ZI); nearly 90% of patients report at least some sustained improvement in tremor control. Effects on function have been less consistently reported, and preoperative patient education about what functional changes are realistically likely to occur is extremely important. Although a potentially useful technique, side effects can include hemiplegia and dysphagia; complete cessation of tremor is rarely achieved, and frequent reprogramming is often necessary.

Pain

Pain is common in neurological conditions and can be very debilitating for the individual, interfering with mobility and sleep and contributing to depression. It may be neurogenic in origin or secondary to mechanical factors. Back pain is particularly common in wheelchair users, in whom spasticity, immobility, abnormal postures, and often an extremely effortful and abnormal gait affect the paravertebral musculature and lumbar spine. Early physiotherapy is essential to aid in spasticity management, to correct posture and/or gait and to limit further damage. Pain relief should include local measures such as heat pads and transcutaneous electrical nerve stimulation (TENS), though medication may be necessary and includes short-term use of non-steroidal anti-inflammatory drugs and simple analgesia. During the first 6 months after stroke, shoulder pain occurs in over 60% of patients and may increase in incidence after discharge. It causes considerable morbidity and once established is difficult to treat. Its occurrence correlates with pre-stroke shoulder pain, severe upper limb weakness, neglect, sensory loss, visual field defects and gleno-humeral subluxation, but their role in its pathogenesis remains uncertain and shoulder subluxation is not clearly a cause. Autonomic changes in the limb, shoulder–hand syndrome and reflex sympathetic dystrophy may also be seen but should not be confused with the painful shoulder. Other disorders of the shoulder including fractures should be excluded. Prevention, particularly in patients at high risk, should include support of the flaccid arm when in bed or a wheelchair, and appropriate handling techniques to avoid traction injury; patients may benefit from neuromuscular electrical stimulation (NMES). Local steroid injection should be avoided unless there is clear evidence of an inflammatory component to the pain, and supra-scapular nerve block has been shown to be an effective treatment.

Neurogenic pain results from injury to peripheral or central afferent pathways. Its characteristics and management are summarised elsewhere (Chapter 23). It is seen in 60–70% of patients with spinal cord damage, usually of traumatic origin, when it is treated in the same way as central pain following stroke or other brain injury. If refractory, patients may be considered for spinal or deep brain stimulation. Pain is reported in 28–86% of patients with MS. Most have chronic pain but an estimated 10% have acute paroxysmal pains, the most common of which is trigeminal neuralgia which occurs more commonly in MS patients than in the general population. It usually responds well particularly to carbamazepine, but also to gabapentin. Other paroxysmal pains also occur in MS and include dysaesthetic burning pains precipitated by touch, movement or hyperventilation, sometimes with painful tonic spasms, which may be helped by carbamazepine, gabapentin or lamotrigine.

Central post-stroke pain (CPSP) is reported to develop in about 8% of stroke patients, and is moderate to severe in 5% of patients. Usually, individuals present with CPSP within 1–2 months after a stroke, but occasionally it may be as long as 1–6 years after injury. Symptoms may be vague and hard to characterise, making an early diagnosis difficult. Failure to make the diagnosis can cause prolonged suffering and reduce the potential for successful rehabilitation. The pathophysiology is thought to involve altered somato-sensory processing at thalamic and cortical levels. The clinical features are extremely varied and include muscular sensations, dysaesthesias, hyperpathia, allodynia, shooting pains or visceral pain such as bloating or fullness of the bladder. Treatment is similarly varied and may include opioids, tricyclic antidepressants, anticonvulsants and even intravenous lidocaine.

Bladder, bowel and sexual dysfunction

Bladder and bowel dysfunction is extremely common in neurological conditions, particularly when there is autonomic involvement or spinal cord damage (Chapters 16 and 25) . Urinary incontinence after stroke or head injury is usually the result of disruption of the suprapontine inhibition of bladder contractility, causing detrusor hyper-reflexia; detrusor hypo-reflexia and retention may occur after damage to the micturition centre in the dorso-lateral pons. Occasionally, frontal lobe damage causes inability to suppress the urge to void (a frontal function in health) leading to uninhibited sphincter relaxation. To these difficulties may be added functional incontinence caused by cognitive and communication difficulties and mobility problems. Evidence for the effectiveness of methods promoting continence after brain damage is currently derived largely from trials in other patient groups and after exclusion of outflow obstruction, as a result of prostatic hypertrophy or occasionally of stricture caused by previous catheter traction in acutely agitated patients. Management often includes a combination of specialist assessment, anticholinergic drug therapy and behavioural management, most commonly used in residential settings for elderly or demented people, by prompted and/or timed voiding.

In MS, estimates of bladder dysfunction are of the order of 75% and bowel dysfunction approximately 50%. Common bladder symptoms are those of frequency, urgency and nocturia. As bladder dysfunction increases, incontinence, retention and urinary tract infections occur. Most of these are a result of a combination of detrusor hyper-reflexia causing urgency and incontinence, and sphincter dyssynergia causing failure to empty and thus increased residual volumes. As urinary symptoms are often of mixed aetiology it is essential to assess bladder emptying by measuring the post-micturition residual volume, by either catheterisation or preferably trans-abdominal ultrasound, before initiating any therapy. If there is no residual volume, then detrusor hyper-reflexia can be treated with anticholinergic agents such as oxybutynin or tolterodine. If nocturia fails to be controlled with anticholinergics, the use of desmopressin (DDAVP) delivered by a nasal spray can be considered, although caution must be taken to avoid overdose and potentially dangerous hyponatraemia. When urgency or incontinence cannot be managed medically, patients should be offered intravesical botulinum toxin type A, but it is important to note that this may cause incomplete emptying or retention requiring catheterisation. Detrusor sphincter dyssynergia can be treated using clean intermittent self-catheterisation (CISC). Often, patients require a combination of CISC and an anticholinergic but bladder control is usually greatly improved. Occasionally, control remains poor and modulation of somatic afferents by either percutaneous posterior tibial nerve stimulation (PTNS) or sacral nerve stimulation, or an indwelling catheter need to be considered. In the event of long-term catheterisation, a suprapubic catheter is usually preferred.

Bowel dysfunction is less frequent than urinary dysfunction in the context of MS or stroke but can be extremely distressing and may occasionally result in bowel perforation or lead to pseudo-obstruction. Usually, individuals complain of constipation and urgency; incontinence is less frequent. Management of constipation is easier than incontinence and may be helped by avoiding the use of constipating anticholinergic drugs, improving toilet access and education. The establishment of a routine is probably important. Often, treatment with oral agents including lactulose, senna or stool softeners (macrogol) used regularly is enough, but glycerine suppositories and micro-enemas can be extremely useful, and trans-anal rectal irrigation may be needed paricularly after spinal injury. Incontinence often linked to urgency can be helped with loperamide, and more recently PTNS has been shown to be an effective treatment.

Sexual dysfunction is a problem often overlooked by health professionals but is common in people with neurological disorders (Chapter 25) and is often accompanied by bladder dysfunction. Hyposexual behaviours are most commonly reported after stroke and TBI, and in the context of Parkinson's disease and MS, in which the incidence of erectile dysfunction is in the order of 70%. Psychological factors in either patient or partner may play a part. Psychosexual counselling should be considered in all cases alone or in combination with other therapies. The advent of the phosphodiesterase-5 inhibitors such as sildenafil, tadalafil and vardenafil, which are fast-acting oral drugs, have reduced the need for more invasive techniques such as intracavernosal injection of alprostadil (prostaglandin E1). Women complain most frequently of vaginal dryness and difficulty reaching orgasm. The use of lubricating gels may be helpful and there is some evidence that sildenafil may help some women although the response is less clear than in men.

Fatigue

Fatigue is particularly problematic for people with MS, TBI and stroke. Patient-derived stroke-specific health-related quality of life (HRQoL) measures identify lack of energy as one of the four most impacting problem areas following stroke. If severe, fatigue may limit education, employment and social opportunities. Its occurrence following stroke is predicted by pre-stroke fatigue and the degree of dependence and depression post-stroke, but it occurs independently in some patients as primary post-stroke fatigue, and often results from stroke-disordered attention in association either with physical impairment, sleep-disordered breathing and obstructive sleep apnoea, or incidental systemic co-morbidities. Initial therapy for all causes of fatigue should be aimed at optimising sleep pattern, by treating nocturnal spasms, nocturia or depression and instigating a personalised fatigue management programme. Occupational therapists can be of help in devising such programmes, which include looking at the individual's daily routine to incorporate fatigue-limiting strategies and introducing regular rest periods. In MS, amantadine has been shown in small studies to be of some benefit as has aerobic exercise. CNS stimulants such as pemoline are best avoided because of side effects and dependency. Other agents such as modafanil and 3, 4-diaminopyridine have been investigated but efficacy is not clear and side effects limit routine clinical use.

Dysphagia

The importance of effective dysphagia management, to prevent its attendant and sometimes life-threatening risks of dehydration, malnutrition, aspiration and chest infections in the context of single incident or deteriorating neurological conditions, is difficult to overemphasise. It occurs clinically in about 50% of all stroke patients admitted to hospital, with video-fluoroscopic and instrumental evidence of a swallowing abnormality in some 80% of patients. Aspiration, particularly silently, predicts chest infection. Video-fluoroscopic and flexible endoscopic evaluation of swallowing increase the reliability with which aspiration can be identified when selecting which patients need tube feeding. After stroke, the FOOD trials in 859 stroke patients, randomised to nasogastric feeding within 1 week versus more than 1 week post-stroke, found that absolute mortality was reduced by 5.8% in the early group. Percutaneous endoscopic gastrostomy (PEG) feeding was associated with an absolute increase in risk of death of 1.0% and an increased risk of death or poor outcome of 7.8% in 321 patients randomised to PEG versus nasogastric tube a median of 1 week post-stroke. Thus, nasogastric feeding should be used for dysphagic patients early post-stroke, although it may not prevent chest infections, while PEG feeding is reserved for patients in whom nasogastric feeding is not tolerated or is required in the longer term. Non-invasive swallowing therapies in adults with neurogenic dysphagia, using modification of posture or the consistency of food and fluid, oral motor exercises, pharyngeal stimulation, or a combination of techniques may reduce aspiration on clinical testing. However, there is still no robust evidence to show that these therapies reduce the incidence of chest infections or improve nutritional status in the context of either single incident or progressive neurological conditions.

Neuropsychiatric problems

Psychiatric disorders are covered in detail in Chapter 22. There is a high cumulative incidence of psychiatric disorders in any physical illness, predicted by physical and social inactivity and a premorbid history of depression and mental disorder. It is important that they are recognised, as they may impact on participation, stall progress in rehabilitation, and determine outcome and placement. After brain injury, additional factors relating to lesion location may also be relevant, for example left anterior damage affecting frontal–subcortical circuits resulting from stroke, head injury and MS predisposing to depression (Table 18.6). Disordered mood may be complicated by organic cognitive and behavioural problems, and can be difficult to diagnose in the presence of a language disturbance, anosognosia, abulia or confused agitation.

Depression after stroke is probably under-recognised and undertreated. In one recent meta-analysis, the frequency in 51 studies was 29–36% with a mean of 33%. In the majority of patients, depression resolved spontaneously within a few months. The main predictors for its development are premorbid vulnerability, and stroke severity measured by physical disability and cognitive impairment. Its presence predicts increased mortality and resource

Table 18.6 Avoidable generic and specific complications after brain injury and their management.

Complication	Management
Co-morbidities	
Hyper-/hypo-tension	Antihypertensives/treat cause
Cardiac events	Specific medical treatments
Fever	Antipyretics
Gastrointestinal bleeding	? Prophylaxis; avoid NSAIDs
Drug side-effects	Drug withdrawal
Musculoskeletal pain	Physical therapies
Polytrauma	Refer to other specialties
Physical dependency ± neural injury	
Pressure sores and skin breaks	Pressure care, and 24-hour handling
Contractures and shoulder pain	Handling, positioning, NMES, steroid or botulinum toxin injection, suprascapular nerve block
PEs and DVTs	Thromboprophylaxis
Falls	Risk assessment
Constipation and faecal impaction	Bowel regime and toiletting programme
Aspiration and chest infections	Tracheostomy and dysphagia management
Urinary tract infections	Toiletting programme, ± drugs
Malnutrition and dehydration	Dysphagia management and dietetics
Detraining	Aerobic exercise programmes
Brain injury	
Hydrocephalus, mass effects and re-bleeds	Neurosurgical management
Confusion and agitation	Environmental management ± drugs
Autonomic storms	Time and drugs
Epilepsy	AEDs if no other trigger
Sleep-disordered breathing	CPAP ventilation
Spasticity	Spasticity management
Vegetative and minimally aware states	Avoid misdiagnosis
Emotionalism	Time and antidepressants
Heterotopic ossification	Etidronate ± NSAIDs
Syndrome of the trephined	Timely cranioplasty
Late maladaptive behaviours	Behaviour modification programmes
Involuntary movements	Drugs and DBS
Central pain	Pain management techniques
Fatigue	Exclusion of treatable causes; fatigue management
Hypothalamic–pituitary axis dysfunction	Endocrine testing and replacement
Catastrophic illness	
Critical illness neuromyopathy	Multi-disciplinary retraining
PTSD, depression and anxiety	CBT ± drugs
Family breakdown	Information + training

AEDs, antiepileptic drugs; CBT, cognitive–behaviour therapy; CPAP, continuous positive airway pressure; DBS, deep brain stimulation; DVT, deep vein thrombosis; NSAID, non-steroidal anti-inflammatory drug; PE, pulmonary embolism; PTSD, post traumatic stress disorder.

utilisation, and early treatment has been reported to benefit functional outcomes. The functional gains reported in the recent FLAME study to result from the early prescription for 3 months of fluoxetine after stroke are not obviously the result of an antidepressant effect.

There is an increased risk, often initially evident at 6–12 months but also in the very long term, of a number of psychiatric disorders after mild, moderate and severe TBI. Major depression occurs in about 15% of patients after mild head injury and about one-third of patients after moderate and severe TBI, when it is predicted by pre-injury educational or employment difficulties, psychiatric illness, and alcohol and substance abuse. The risk of anxiety disorders, including obsessive-compulsive, but also panic and post-traumatic stress disorders, is also increased. Psychosis and suicide are more common in people who have had a TBI than in the general population but usually occur in individuals who were vulnerable to these problems pre-injury, and thus at risk of injury including TBI. Drug treatment with a selective serotonin re-uptake inhibitor (SSRI), sometimes combined with a mood regulator such as carbamazepine for accompanying anxiety disorders, may be useful but should take into account the increased susceptibility to drug side effects of patients with TBI. Although cognitive and psychotherapeutic interventions are advocated after severe TBI, rigorous evidence for their efficacy is lacking to date; cognitive–behavioural therapy reduced anxiety and depression up to 5 years after mild and moderate injury in a small randomised waiting-listed controlled study. Endocrine replacement, as a result of hypothalamic–pituitary axis dysfunction, is necessary in about 5% of patient after moderate and severe TBI, but appears to be more common after blast injury.

Psychiatric symptoms may also develop in patients with MS but are usually mild and commonly include low mood, irritability, poor concentration and anxiety. Rates of depression in community samples have ranged between 25% and 40% and tend to be higher in nursing home settings. Psychological support or cognitive–behavioural therapy is often helpful. If medication is indicated it should be used as it is in the healthy population but with greater attention to possible adverse effects, particularly exacerbation of bladder or sexual dysfunction.

Single incident brain injury

Stroke and traumatic brain injury (TBI), the most common causes of focal and diffuse acquired brain injury (ABI), respectively, are also two of the most prevalent neurological conditions affecting the CNS. They involve very different populations, with contrasting clinical needs and expectations, and highlight important questions relating to neural protection and restoration, delivery of rehabilitation, and routes to improving participation and life quality. In white populations, about 90% of stroke patients are over 65 years of age compared with some 20% of patients following TBI. Both conditions result in an annual incidence of hospital admission of 1–3/1000 adults. Following TBI, only 10–20% of patients remain in hospital for more than 3 days, because 80–90% of injuries are mild, while after stroke such brief admission is now the exception. Because younger age groups are over-represented in the TBI population, and usually have a near-normal life expectancy of 30–40 years even after severe injury, the prevalence of stroke and TBI related disability is similar at about 1%.

Not only are the personal costs of single incident brain injury enormous, but also the economic consequences. In the United Kingdom the annual costs of direct and informal care and lost productivity after stroke was estimated by the National Audit Office in 2005 at £7.0 billion; these costs will increase as the population ages. Similar data describing the overall economic burden of head injury in the United Kingdom are not available but must be of at least similar magnitude assuming the prevalence outlined above; costs estimated at about $60 billion annually in the United States are very similar to those after stroke.

Guidelines for hyperacute thrombolysis and neurosurgical management, and intensive and high dependency care after stroke and head injury are established and continue to evolve (Chapter 5). High dependency care, following that required for thrombolysis, is now being investigated acutely after stroke, to assess the benefits of providing continuous rather than manual monitoring for hypoxia, hyperglycaemia, hypotension, cardiac arrhythmias and elevated body temperature during the first 48–72 hours after admission. Whether these new technologies will improve outcome at discharge in previously more dependent patients, and reduce mortality in patients with severe injury without increasing the prevalence of dependency, is not at present obvious.

During the first few weeks after a significant single incident brain injury of any cause, acute inpatient rehabilitation should focus on the prevention of systemic and neurological complications, while resolution of cerebral oedema, toxic metabolic dysfunction and intracranial mass effects take place, and provide a basis for ongoing neuro-protection in parallel rather than in series with the initiation of preventative and restorative strategies (Figure 18.2).

During the subsequent several months, early rehabilitation programmes focus on skill learning to reduce dependency in personal care and domestic and community-based ADL, while late programmes particularly address social and work related roles, and issues of life quality. The time post-injury when the components of these programmes (Figure 18.3) should begin and end varies with a number of factors, particularly injury severity. Many of these issues are addressed in evidence and expert opinion based guidelines produced in relation to stroke, and accessible via www.strokecenter.org/prof/guidelines.htm, and, in the United Kingdom, http://publications.nice.org.uk/stroke-rehabilitation-cg162, and head injury and other acquired single incident brain injuries in the Department of Health's National Service Framework (NSF) for Long-term Conditions (2005). Evidence, summarised later, for the effectiveness of components of these systems is largely derived from trials after stroke. Its application to rehabilitation after head injury is tempting but largely unproven.

Stroke

In the United Kingdom, stroke is the most common single cause of severe physical disablement in people living at home, and is likely to become more prevalent as the population ages. Motor impairment is the most common impairment post-stroke, and 6–12 months post-stroke only 60% of patients presenting with hemiplegic stroke have achieved independence in personal care. Of survivors, 30–40% are depressed, 10–15% severely so. Over half need help with housework, meal preparation or shopping. A similar number lack a meaningful social, recreational or occupational activity during the day.

These disabilities, or limitations in activities and restrictions in participation (Figure 18.1), are the result not only of motor impairments, but also impairments in sensory, perceptual, cognitive, communication and affective function, which can be measured by standardised stroke-specific or generic rating scales, perhaps drawn from the ICF, or, for example, a stroke-specific battery of impairments, the National Institute of Health Stroke Scale (NIHSS), combined with a generic neuro-cognitive score, which can be combined with physiological and anatomical, and possibly biochemical, measures of damage, and used to monitor progress and the effect and choice of interventions, and to predict outcome.

Organised acute and early inpatient, and increasingly community-based, rehabilitation, via a reiterative multi-disciplinary goal-setting process, has been investigated in depth after stroke. A Cochrane meta-analysis of 21 trials (n = 3994) comparing care and rehabilitation in a stroke unit (SU) with an alternative services, usually in a general medical or geriatric ward with or without a visiting stroke team, showed that patients who receive unit-based inpatient care, particularly in a discrete ward, do not stay longer in hospital and are more likely to be alive, independent and living at home 1 year after the stroke, regardless of gender, age and stroke severity (Figure 18.4). Subsequent secondary analysis has shown that similar benefits occur after either ischaemic or haemorrhagic stroke. Compliance with post-acute SU guidelines (Table 18.7) has been shown to correlate with outcome. The reduction in SU deaths probably results from fewer complications of immobility rather than neurological or cardiovascular complications. The increased number of patients discharged home, rather than to institutional care from SUs, is largely attributable to an increase in the number of patients returning home physically independent (Rankin score 0–2), rather than dependent (Rankin score 3–5).

Aspects of care common to acute and rehabilitation SUs include:

- Comprehensive medical, nursing and therapy assessments,
- Integration of nursing care within the multi-disciplinary team,
- Early mobilisation and treatment of hypoxia, hyperglycaemia, and suspected infection and avoidance of urinary catheterisation, and
- Formalised goal-orientated multi-disciplinary team care, with early discharge planning and education and involvement of carers.

Table 18.7 Compliance with these dimensions of process during post-acute rehabilitation correlates with functional outcome after stroke.

1	Multi-disciplinary team coordination
2	Baseline assessment
3	Goal setting
4	Treatment plan
5	Monitoring of progress
6	Management of impairments/disabilities
7	Prevention of complications
8	Prevention of recurrent stroke
9	Family involvement
10	Patient and family education
11	Discharge planning

Many of these aspects of care are not delivered by a peripatetic specialist stroke team (PSST). In one study, complications including stroke progression, chest infections and dehydration were less frequent in the SU. More patients were dead or institutionalised (30% vs. 14%; $P < 0.001$) and fewer were alive without severe disability (66% vs. 85%; $P < 0.001$) in the group allocated to the PSST.

Remarkably, the differences between SU and alternative care persist for many years. Even 10 years after randomisation to an acute and rehabilitation SU or a general ward, fewer SU patients had died (75.5% vs. 87.3%; $P = 0.008$), and more were at home (19.1% vs. 8.2%; $P = 0.018$). More were at least partly independent with a Barthel Index (BI) score of ≥60 (20.0% vs. 8.2%; $P = 0.012$), if not independent with a BI score of ≥95 (12.7% vs. 5.4%; $P = 0.061$). Increased survival times have been observed 5 years after randomisation to a SU versus a general medical or geriatric ward.

Early discharge of medically stable patients with support by a multi-disciplinary outreach team after mild and moderate stroke, with an admission BI of >9/20, adds to initial SU gains. A meta-analysis of individual patient data from 14 trials of early supported discharge (ESD) versus conventional care in patients moderately disabled at discharge (median discharge BI 15/20) showed:

- A reduced risk of death or dependency ($P = 0.02$) in the ESD group,
- Hospital stay shortened by 7 days ($P < 0.0001$), and
- Significant improvement in extended ADL ($P = 0.05$), although not in subjective health status or mood in either patients or carers.

Two other studies found that these gains can include better life quality, assessed by the Nottingham Health Profile, at 1 year, and that gains in domestic and extended ADL are still evident after 5 years.

Once in the community, patients are known to be at risk of deteriorating after stroke as a result of multiple health problems including falls, depression, physical and social inactivity, and isolation, in addition to age-related co-morbidities. HRQoL declines in the 6 months after discharge. The place for, and optimal process in, residential service systems other than SUs for patients later after stroke remains to be examined. A meta-analysis of trials of therapy-based outpatient or domiciliary rehabilitation, delivered by either a multi-disciplinary team or by a physiotherapist or occupational therapist, with the goal of improving task-orientated behaviours, has shown that deterioration is prevented ($P = 0.009$) and dependency in personal care reduced ($P = 0.02$). The effective components and best location for this type of service need further exploration, but benefit has been consistent in trials of community-based occupational therapy. A meta-analysis of eight trials showed that intervention was associated with improved personal, extended and leisure-based ADL depending on the intervention target. These findings are confirmed in more wide-ranging systematic reviews of occupational therapy for stroke patients. Most studies of physiotherapy in patients in the community after stroke investigate the effect of a particular physiotherapy treatment on improving upper or lower limb function at the level of impairment and mobility, which may improve, rather than limitations in activity and independence, which if examined may not. Domiciliary physiotherapy within 6 months post-stroke has been shown to reduce risk of re-admission after an average of only 2.9 (range 1–8) visits and reduces dependency at less cost compared with day hospital attendance. In patients more than 1 year post-stroke as few as 4–5 physiotherapy sessions produced a clinically small but significant improvement in mobility.

Informal carers should be recognised as an important resource. They enable patients to remain in the community and their support is likely to facilitate patient outcomes. The levels of depression in the patient are greater in those who feel poorly supported. Formal support for carers, rather than assistance for patients, is often more difficult to obtain. Trials of psychosocial interventions to support stroke carers using information packages, specialist nurses, a mental health worker or family support workers have failed to show functional or psychological benefit in patients and only modest psychosocial benefit for carers. By contrast, there is evidence to suggest that carer adjustment is increased by education and counselling or by training in social problem-solving skills. Training informal carers in basic nursing skills and facilitation of personal care techniques reduces costs and caregiver burden; this improves psychosocial outcomes for both carer and patient, although there is no change in patient mortality, institutionalisation and disability.

Traumatic brain injury

It seems likely, although unproven, that many of the lessons learned from trials of programs providing acute, early and later rehabilitation after stroke are applicable to those required after diffuse, rather than focal, ABI (Figure 18.3). This is most frequently traumatic in origin, though there is now an increasing number of disabled patients surviving after hypoxic-ischaemic brain injury. However the evidence base derived from group studies of TBI is meagre by comparison with that after stroke. This reflects both the relatively small numbers of patients requiring inpatient care for more than a few days after head injury, and the difficulties involved in community follow-up of the larger number of patients with less severe injuries, many of whom are disadvantaged and peripatetic pre-injury and additionally cognitively impaired post-injury.

By contrast with stroke, long-term disability after diffuse ABI results largely from cognitive, affective and behavioural, rather than physical, impairments in a younger population with a longer life expectancy. A number of studies over the last 20 years have shown how over time post-injury, mobility and independence in personal care are least affected while the ability to fulfil social and work-related roles remains problematic. There is thus a high incidence of TBI in the prison and homeless populations, and, in the community, after TBI people often require supervision rather than hands-on care; their needs thus impact on less easily identifiable impairments and budgets than stroke, over a longer period. Whether the increased long-term mortality seen after even mild TBI is caused by an ongoing inflammatory or degenerative process initiated by injury, or the difficulties there are in delivering effective rehabilitation and 'an enriched environment' in these circumstances, or other factors, for example the long-term effects of hypothalamic–pituitary axis dysfunction or the metabolic syndrome, is not known.

As long-term functional outcomes depend largely on residual cognitive and behavioural problems, which in turn are usually dependent on the initial severity of injury, unsurprisingly measures of the severity of cognitive and behavioural impairment early post injury, using the initial Glasgow Coma Scale score, and the duration of unconsciousness or unawareness (absence of command following), and of post-traumatic amnesia (PTA), estimated either prospectively or retrospectively, are still the most reliable predictors of long-term outcome after TBI, while imaging characteristics, and neurophysiological and biochemical markers of injury remain unhelpful except possibly in hyper-acute settings. When pre-injury factors, particularly related to disadvantaged or elite performance, and ongoing co-morbidities, particularly those caused by pain and psychiatric problems, are also taken into account, these data enable the realistic prediction, and thus discussion with family members and carers, and some patients, of probable ceilings to achievable functional recovery long-term. This in turn assists engagement in realistic short and long-term goal setting and rehabilitation planning.

For those patients initially in low awareness states, longitudinal studies of outcome show that some who achieve partial independence in the longer term may not have begun to improve until 4–5 months post-injury, and of patients in a low awareness state at 1 month post injury, about 20% will achieve independence in the community by 5 years. In the long term, in general a PTA of:

- 10 days is almost invariably associated with residual cognitive problems, but does not preclude a return to a person's old job, possibly with some restrictions,
- 4 weeks precludes a return to a previous, but not to an altered, work role, and
- 3 months precludes a return to regular paid work, but not to voluntary work or community independence.

After coma emergence there is initially a period of agitated and combative behaviour during PTA, similar to that seen during hyperactive delirium, followed by confusion and anxiety without aggression, before the ability to form continuous memories is restored despite longer term background cognitive deficits, which often particularly involve executive and attentional skills rather than memory. These behaviours put patients, and sometimes their carers, at risk of injury as a result of falls and absconsion, and prevent participation in training. Hitherto patients have been policed largely pharmacologically, but drug side effects and their prolongation of PTA, particularly as a result of the protracted use of sedative doses of neuroleptics, especially haloperidol, which down-regulate dopaminergic brain function, has meant that management now focuses on environmental adjustments and behavioural techniques, rather than the administration of drugs, to reduce stimulation and unpredictability via a framework of timetabled activities and interventions including rest periods, while restraint is minimised, and measures to prevent falls and their consequences are put in place. Early institution of these measures possibly shortens the duration of PTA and time for which high dependency and hospital care is required. Extreme acute agitation can leave little choice about the use of an intramuscular or intravenous sedative, usually using either a shorter acting benzodiazepine or a neuroleptic, often as lorazepam or haloperidol, respectively. In less extreme circumstances, if initial environmental modification fails to reduce hypervigilance and over-arousal, once pain, infection and other co-morbidities have been treated, and the sleep–wake cycle optimised, most authors recommend minimal doses of an atypical neuroleptic rather than a benzodiazepine (e.g. quetiapine) to optimise compliance in training and procedural learning. Whether other drugs that contain agitated behaviours and reduce anxiety late after severe head injury (e.g. beta-blockers, mood-stabilising anticonvulsants or antidepressants) also have a part to play during PTA remains virtually unexplored.

For those patients requiring protracted inpatient rehabilitation after severe TBI, historical evidence emphasises the importance of preventing the physical complications of immobility, just as it does after spinal injury. Studies in the late 1960s from the United States documented frequent pressure sores, joint contractures and frozen shoulders in patients late after severe head injury, problems that should now not be seen. Since then, a few small studies, mostly retrospective and comparison, rather than prospective and randomised, have investigated whether organised acute rehabilitation (AR), on discharge from ITU, with or without subsequent facilitation of the rehabilitation care pathway, improves long-term outcome, at less cost, than delayed or less organised care. They include a recent prospective but non-randomised Norwegian study which compared outcomes in two groups of patients, all of whom received acute rehabilitation, before being transferred either seamlessly to sub-acute rehabilitation or, as a result of bed availability, via a local hospital or nursing home, and found shorter hospital stays (88 vs. 124 days; $P = 0.07$) and, at 12 months post-injury, better functional outcomes (Extended Glasgow Outcome Scale [GOSE] 6–8 71% vs. 37%; $P = 0.007$) and more frequent home discharge (Home/NH 81/13 vs. 53/23; $P = 0.06$) in the 'seamless' group.

Other group studies of inpatient rehabilitation after head injury address the benefits of early (sub-acute) inpatient rehabilitation, which in the United Kingdom still starts 1–4 months or more after injury, rather than acute rehabilitation in parallel with and immediately after neurosurgical treatment. Most, from North America or the United Kingdom, are non-randomised retrospective or prospective comparisons of two groups. They still emphasise the economies in resource use resulting from reduced lengths of hospital stay in rehabilitation rather than acute care, with at least equivalent (if not improved) functional outcomes that are said to result from early transfer to rehabilitation. One two-centre study investigated outcome after moderate and severe injury in 24 patients who were randomised prospectively to receive supplemented inpatient rehabilitation versus 27 patients who received the usual programme. The supplemented group made greater gains in functional independence by the time of discharge during a similar length of stay.

Prospective randomisation of the far greater number of less severely injured patients early after injury presents fewer methodological problems because there are more patients and cheaper treatment options. These patients have usually mobilised and moved into the community but experience many cognitive, affective, behavioural and somatic post-concussional symptoms. However, compliance with follow-up and treatments is difficult to ascertain unless trial entry is limited to patients who are not premorbidly disadvantaged (e.g. athletes or military personnel). A US trial prospectively randomised military personnel, who had recovered independent mobility and returned home with supervision within 3 months of moderate and severe head injury, to either 8 weeks of an inpatient cognitive–behavioural community and vocational re-entry programme costing \$51 840 ($n = 67$) or a low cost (\$504) cognitive and exercise-based home programme with weekly telephone support from a psychiatric nurse ($n = 53$). Both treatments were followed by a 6-month graded return to limited military duties. About 40% of patients recruited to the study had a PTA of 7 days or more and 35% had been unconscious for 24 hours or more. At 1 year post-treatment, overall there was no difference in the two groups in return to work or quality of life measures, but of patients unconscious for more than 1 hour initially (n = 75), 80% were fit for duty in the hospital group versus 58% in the home-based group (P = 0.05). There was a trend (P = 0.13) in favour of the home-based group in patients (n = 44) unconscious for an hour or less.

Other prospective randomised group studies early after injury have recruited less severely injured patients and investigated the effect on post-concussional symptoms of psychological interventions including reassurance, information giving and advice. These have found that intervention is associated with significant reduction in the intensity and number of symptoms and quicker return to work. One study investigated outcome at 6 months in all patients admitted to hospital after head injury. Cases were randomised to usual care or a programme of face-to-face interviews with written advice about likely prognosis and recovery times, and the management of post-concussional symptoms. These included reduced speed of information processing, memory problems, the interaction of cognitive and emotional stress, post-concussion symptoms, post-traumatic stress and a graduated return to normal levels of activity. This found that in patients with a PTA between 1 hour and 7 days, intervention was associated with significant reduction of concentration difficulties, headaches, fatigue, sleep disturbance and irritability with improvement in the patient's relationship with a partner, ability to cope with family demands, participate in social activities and enjoyment of leisure activities. Only 12% had more than one face-to-face contact. The economic benefits of this relatively low cost intervention in these patients, 70% of whom still had post-concussional symptoms and/or psychosocial problems at 6 months post-injury, has not been investigated. Other studies after mild TBI have also found early single educational interventions effective in reducing later anxiety and complaints. The cornerstones of treatment after mild traumatic brain injury (concussion) sustained in sport are physical and cognitive rest until symptoms resolve, followed by a graded program of exercise prior to return to play, preceded and accompanied by an explanation of the mechanism of symptom generation, with specific treatment, if needed, for example of the symptoms of post-traumatic migraine or a traumatic peripheral vestibulopathy.

Late after moderate and severe injury, gains in community and vocational function and life quality are usually limited by residual cognitive, affective and behavioural problems, rather than physical difficulties. However, adaptive change may continue for years, especially in younger patients, and with the judicious prescription of goal-focused interventions and ongoing support, which may need to be life-long. A United Kingdom study prospectively randomised 110 patients a median of 1.37 years after largely severe injury to either a multi-disciplinary outreach programme twice a week for a mean of 27 weeks or to written advice. Two years after recruitment there were still significant gains in outreach treated patients in measures of community independence and self-organisation but not in socialising, productive employment or mood. After severe injury, the high rate of unemployment in this young population of 50–70% compared with rates of 10–20% pre-injury is now well documented. Work retraining and supported employment models have been described over the last 20 years. Their efficacy, sometimes achieving employment rates of above 50% late after severe injury, has so far been gauged against a pre-intervention baseline rather than a prospectively randomised control and tends to assume rather than demonstrate improved life quality with employment. Nevertheless, specialist programmes of this sort are important aspects of the rehabilitation menu in clinical practice.

Residual cognitive problems most commonly involve speed, attention, executive function and memory, and are often accompanied by irritability, impulsivity and verbal aggression, triggered by anxiety resulting from difficulties problem solving in the context of increases in environmental demand. They may be containable by informed family and non-specialist support in the community, but may become complicated by late secondary depression as insight increases. Less frequently, neurobehavioural disability is caused by more obvious disorders of behaviour and social cognition, which result in reports of the subject's personality being 'changed', as described in Phineas Gage, and also occurs after other types of damage that particularly involves ventro-medial prefrontal cortices. These affective and behavioural problems may deteriorate with time, particularly in the absence of rehabilitation provision. Problem behaviours are more difficult for carers to tolerate and manage than long-term physical and cognitive deficits, and are well-recognised causes of marital breakdown, social isolation and recurrent unemployment. Management is advocated with programmes of various intensities on an outpatient, day-patient or residential basis to deliver cognitive rehabilitation, cognitive–behavioural therapy and psychotherapeutic strategies, sometimes with adjunctive drug treatment such as carbamazepine or an antidepressant. These programmes are intended to promote insight and a self-managed framework within which it is possible to plan and set realistic goals, and thus reduce anxiety, indifference and other maladaptive and isolating antisocial behaviours. The clinical usefulness of other drug treatments, for example amantadine or methylphenidate to improve attentional skills and speed of processing, and reduce irritability, or modafinil to reduce excessive day time sleepiness, remains unpredictable. Aggressive or sexual behaviours sufficiently aberrant to require residential behaviour modification are uncommon although resource demanding, particularly when accompanied by psychiatric disorders, which may be pre-existing. They require the application of behavioural frameworks that can modify and reduce aggressive behaviour even years post-injury. Improvement in life quality resulting from these complex cognitive and behavioural interventions has so far proved difficult to demonstrate.

The long-term change in independence and social roles that occurs as a result of severe brain injury may require support life-long if optimal function is to be maintained and deterioration prevented. Complications such as falls and further injuries, depression and social isolation, fits or substance abuse are largely avoidable, given adequate support. Provision for those patients who are mobile in the community should include low cost specialist day centres, as Headway Houses in the United Kingdom, and if possible access to a professional with experience of the consequences of acquired brain injury to provide case management and support, particularly at times of change, and to facilitate change over extended periods of time.

Over the last 10–15 years, the use of advanced imaging techniques to investigate the capacity for category specific mental imagery has shown how the responsiveness of some patients apparently in low awareness states, particularly after traumatic rather than hypoxic-ischaemic brain injury, is limited by failure of motor outflow rather than a failure of understanding or the ability to reason, even years after injury. These findings have encouraged a reappraisal of the neurological basis of consciousness, ethical decisions about the withdrawal of nutrition and hydration, and real-time communication with these patients using brain–computer interfaces. Recent reports of patients in low awareness states, either vegetative or minimally conscious, regaining the ability to demonstrate reliable awareness after very long periods, with or without neural stimulation or drugs, confirms that late and slow, albeit functionally relatively minor, improvement in less disabled patients may also occur over many years, and begs the question as to whether the changes seen are the result of structural plasticity, how much these changes depend on the quality and level of training and care provided, and, if so, whether and how this input can be afforded.

Service delivery

Organisational behaviours and interdisciplinary assessment

Delivery of any organised complex multi-disciplinary service, especially involving disciplines with different professional training backgrounds and languages, as is the case in rehabilitation, demands definition not only of structure, as plant and personnel, but also process, which has the following key elements:

- Inter-disciplinary assessment and problem definition
- Treatment planning and delivery
- Evaluation of effectiveness and reassessment.

Assessment

An interdisciplinary assessment is very different from that offered by a physician working independently. Patients with complex disability, when multiple factors affecting functional performance present as a single problem, benefit from comprehensive assessment by a rehabilitation team. These teams can work in different ways depending on the setting, and on the needs of the individual. Multi-disciplinary working involves a group of different professionals working alongside one another towards a common overall long-term aim, with different disciplines delivering interventions to achieve goals in parallel rather than in close collaboration. A more integrated approach is offered by an interdisciplinary team that works together to achieve a series of agreed goals toward a long-term aim. Team members have a fuller understanding of each other's roles and skills and work together in a holistic way, ensuring that different interventions complement each other. This approach is encouraged by settings in which staff are in geographical contact on a regular basis, either in inpatient rehabilitation units or in the community.

The advantages of an interdisciplinary assessment are that different disciplines identify different contributing problems, and can develop an appropriately ordered plan to deal with these contributing causes. For example, a patient with MS may present with a small sacral pressure sore. The contributing factors include immobility, incontinence, under-nutrition, lack of insight and motivation, low mood and spasms. The spasms may be aggravated by constipation and incomplete bladder emptying, as well as pain caused by the pressure sore; the tone problems can be ameliorated by seating the patient correctly; the provision of a pressure-relieving cushion may counter the impact of immobility; and cognitive–behavioural therapy or an antidepressant may help depression. This analysis of the problems demands nursing, psychology, medical, occupational therapy and physiotherapy diagnoses. Interdisciplinary teams provide a more accurate assessment, and decrease the need for hospital admission.

When a team of different disciplines work together they need a framework for assessment and description of an individual's abilities and difficulties. The ICF (Figure 18.1) provides such a framework. It classifies health at the level of body functions or structure, the whole person, and the whole person in a social context. Disabilities, formerly termed disablements, result from:

- Impairments (losses or abnormalities of body functions and structures)
- Activity limitations (previously disabilities), and
- Participation restrictions (formerly termed handicaps).

A person's disabilities and their level of functioning are outcomes of multiple interactions between health conditions and contextual factors. Two sorts of contextual factors are identified:

- Social and physical environmental factors (e.g. social attitudes, access to buildings, legal protection), and
- Personal factors which include gender, age, other health conditions, social background, education, overall behaviour pattern and other factors that influence how disability is experienced by the individual.

These interactions help explain why apparently similar patients have different outcomes. An individual patient may complain of difficulty walking, and not only the causes but also the consequences of the problem, including their subjective perception of life quality, are likely to differ in different individuals.

Goal-setting

Having completed an interdisciplinary assessment and identified the individual's capabilities, disabilities and priorities, the next step is to devise a treatment plan. This treatment plan is usually articulated as a treatment goal. Goal setting may therefore be regarded as a key skill for rehabilitation professionals, and indeed any professional involved in complex interventions. There is a growing clinical literature on the subject of goal-setting, but the evidence base for goal-setting was originally derived from the organisational psychology literature of the 1970s.

In 2002, Locke and Latham synthesised studies of over 40 000 participants and 100 different tasks in eight countries and in field, laboratory and simulated settings into a theory of goal-setting. They define a goal core, mechanisms, moderators and other factors. The goal core defines the task, the level of difficulty and specifics of how, and in what timeframe, the goal should be completed. In other words, goals need to be formulated to be SMART: specific, measurable, achievable, relevant, and time-limited. Goals affect performance via a number of mechanisms, including directing attention and effort toward goal-related activities and increasing effort and persistence. Challenging goals have been demonstrated to lead to greater effort than low-level goals. The benefits of goal-setting can be moderated by factors such as the individual's commitment to the goal, the importance of the goal to them, their belief that the goal can be attained (self-efficacy), the extent of feedback about goal progress and performance, and the complexity of the task. Thus, the final outcome of goal-setting will depend on the balance between these mechanisms and moderators of the goal-setting process, and their satisfaction with the process. Thus, when considering the specifics of goal-setting it is important to recognise a number of other factors, including the importance of the individual's relationships and their previous experience of health service professionals, the impact of the disease itself, particularly in relation to prognosis and disease course, and the views of their family.

A number of studies of goal-setting in the rehabilitation environment have been reported. Earlier studies suggested that people with disabilities and particularly those with TBI should be allocated goals and treatment interventions. In a randomised control trial of 16 adults with TBI, the experimental group were actively involved to a high level in the goal-setting process, by prioritising wooden blocks that had activities of daily living written on them. In contrast, the controls were involved at a low level. Although both groups initially improved in goal attainment (as measured by Goal Attainment Scaling), at the assessment 2 months following discharge, those experiencing the higher level of involvement had maintained their therapeutic gains in contrast to the low involvement group, who had returned to pre-test level.

The part played by goal difficulty and goal origin (self-set goals versus assigned goals) on the performance of adults with brain injury has been assessed by a simple arithmetical task. Eighty-seven patients with a diagnosis of stroke or TBI were randomly assigned to one of three groups: a specific high goal was assigned; a 'do your best' goal was given; or a personal goal had to be stated. Results showed that assigned difficult goals led to better performance than assigned easy goals, and that self-setting a goal did not increase performance to the same level as the assignment of a difficult goal. These findings suggest that goal origin (assigned or self-set), and

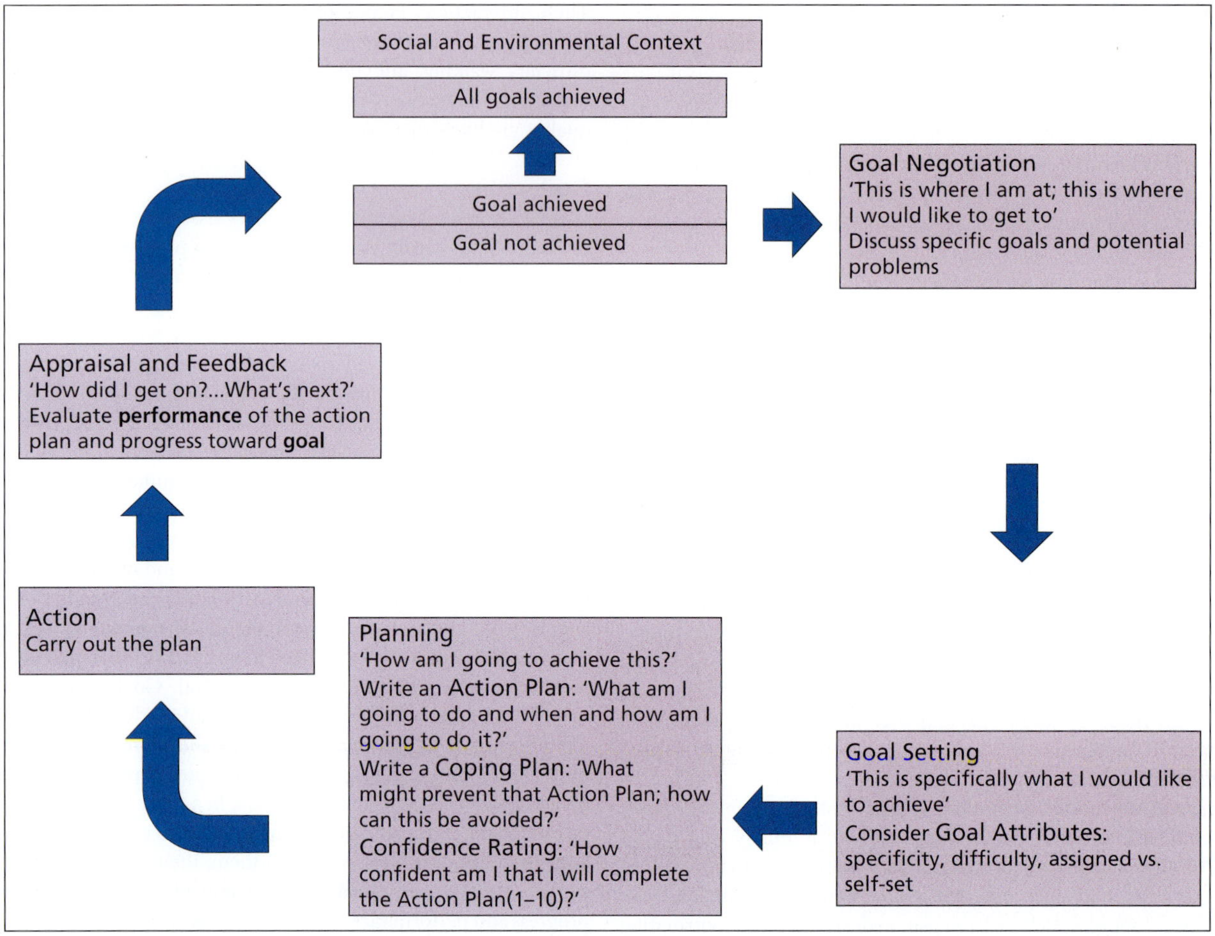

Figure 18.9 Goal setting and action planning practice framework. Source: Scobbie 2011. Reproduced with permission of Sage.

goal difficulty are important moderators in the goal-setting process and influence performance.

In addition, the association between participation in goal-specific outpatient occupational therapy and improvement in self-identified goals in adults with brain injury has been investigated. Using a repeated measures design, standard therapy designed to achieve specific goals was followed by a period of no treatment. Thirty-one participants with brain injury were recruited at three sites located in different regions of the United States. Participants completed the Canadian Occupational Performance Measure (COPM) and the Community Integration Questionnaire (CIQ) at admission, discharge and 1 and 18 weeks after discharge. In addition, Goal Attainment Scales were developed at admission and scored on discharge. Of the 149 goals identified by participants, 81% were achieved. Goal Attainment Scores improved significantly (z = 7.52; P <0.001), with a large effect size (r = 0.94). The COPM scales showed significantly greater gains during the treatment (average 15.3 weeks) compared with the no treatment period (average 9.9 weeks). It was concluded that participation in goal-specific outpatient occupational therapy that focuses on teaching compensatory strategies was strongly associated with achievement of self-identified goals and reduction of disability in adults with mild to moderate brain injury. However, these results may not be generalisable to the broader brain-injured population.

More recently, recognising the difficulties of establishing patient centred goal-setting in practice, qualitative studies have focused on barriers to goal setting and perceived benefits. These studies suggest that patients perceive that monitoring progress towards meaningful goals helps achieve practical goals, such as independence and returning to work, reduce emotional impact and support coping. Patient-related barriers to goal setting may result from poor understanding of and lack of information about the process, so that patients avoid exposing their incompetence at setting goals that results from not knowing or understanding prognosis, cognitive impairment and distress about the impact of a sudden onset disabling condition such as stroke. System-related barriers include issues such as limited time set aside for goal setting, and the prioritisation of 'hands on' treatment. As a result, most studies suggest that goal setting is not patient centred.

These qualitative studies have highlighted the need for a good underpinning theory of goal-setting in rehabilitation, which is reflected in clinical practice by developing structures and processes that support staff to deliver patient-centred goal-setting and patients to participate. Recently, Scobbie *et al.* have identified the theoretical constructs that are thought to influence patient behaviour in relationship to goal-setting as self-efficacy, outcome expectancies, goal attributes (specificity, difficulty), action planning and coping planning, and appraisal and feedback (Figure 18.9). In practical terms, this converts to a framework with four key intervention points:

1 Developing goal intentions by appraising their current situation, when staff work with the patient to increase patient self-efficacy and motivation.
2 Setting a specific goal.
3 Activating goal-related behaviour by defining an action plan specifying who will do what when, and a coping plan that details potential barriers and how these will be managed.
4 Appraisal and feedback.

The variables hypothesised to effect change in patient outcomes were self-efficacy and the action plan. Work of this sort, combined with goal setting timetabled into the working week, as recommended by the 2013 NICE stroke rehabilitation guidelines (Clinical guideline 162), should lead to greater understanding and implementation of patient-centred goal-setting.

Outcome measurement

Outcome evaluation of the success of any rehabilitation can examine process or functional outcomes. At the simplest level, achieving a specified goal is a measure of outcome. The difficulty of using goals as outcome measures is that because when they are unique to an individual patient, they cannot be used to describe groups or compare outcomes between groups. Where suitable outcome measures exist, and are appropriate to both the disorder and the intervention, it may be preferable to examine outcomes other than goal achievement.

Traditionally, physicians have used measures to tell them something about the presence, natural history and severity of a disease. Direct measurement of the extent of the pathology is often impossible, but often there are markers of the disease activity, for example MRI changes in MS or [^{18}F]dopa positron emission tomography (PET) in Parkinson's disease. There is now increasing interest in patient-based outcomes that focus on aspects of health considered important by the patient. These measures typically focus on HRQoL. Rating scales measure either generic aspects of health or focus on one particular aspect. Generic measures, such as the Medical Outcomes Study Short Form 36 (MOS SF-36) health status scale, allow different patient populations to be compared and allow the inclusion of a control population in a study. Typically, the usefulness of such scales may be limited by their inability to capture a range of outcomes relevant to the particular patient populations studied, and so they may be unresponsive to change in a clinical condition. Alternatives include disease-specific measures such as the Parkinson's Disease Questionnaire-39 (PDQ-39) or the Multiple Sclerosis Impact Scale (MSIS); site-specific scales such as the Disabilities of the Arm, Shoulder and Hand (DASH) outcome questionnaire; or dimension-specific measures that measure one aspect of quality of life such as well-being (e.g. the General Health Questionnaire [GHQ]).

Clinically useful instruments should be easy to administer, clinically appropriate, brief, cheap and easy to analyse, and measure the outcome that is relevant to the intervention and to that disease group. They should also be acceptable to patients, being neither intrusive nor upsetting. Since about 1990 there has been a marked increase in the numbers of papers that address outcome. Typically, these papers report a new or previously described scale in terms of its psychometric properties. Traditional psychometric approaches inform users about the scientific properties of the scales. Scientifically sound instruments are valid, reliable and responsive. A valid instrument measures what it is intended to measure. Validity cannot be proven but evidence in support of validity can be gathered. Content validity is the extent to which the measure represents the full range of the conceptual domain it addresses. Criterion-related validity compares the measure against a gold standard. Construct validity compares the measure in different situations. Does it correlate with other measures of related entities (convergent validity)? Does it fail to correlate with measures that purport to measure a different concept (discriminant validity)? Does it detect differences in groups known to be different in the concept measured?

A reliable instrument performs in an accurate, consistent and reproducible manner that is stable over time. The purpose of reliability testing is to determine the extent to which random error is present in the measurement. To be reliable, scales need clear descriptions of the meaning of individual points on the scale. There is evidence that idiosyncrasies of performance represent a major source of variability in rating scales. Stability of the scale over time is assessed using test–retest reliability. Inter-rater reliability is the agreement between two or more raters, intra-rater reliability is the agreement between two ratings made at different times by a single observer on the same patients. Responsiveness describes the ability of the scale to measure clinically relevant change, such as the impact of rehabilitation, or the effect of a new drug.

Indices of outcome

There is now a range of measures used commonly in rehabilitation. The Barthel Index (BI) is the most commonly used assessment of limitations in personal ADL. It consists of 10 items measured on either a two, three or four point scale, with a maximum score of 20. The BI has been well studied in a number of settings and its general validity has been established. It correlates well with clinical impression, with motor loss after stroke and with scores on other ADL scales. It is reliable and simple to use but its content is only relevant to people with moderate and severe disability – it has a floor and ceiling, which need to be populated by other measures. However, despite being widely used and having been evaluated using traditional psychometric approaches, it is clear that there remain a number of problems. First, the Barthel is an ordinal scale and is typically reported using a summed score out of the maximum total summed score of 20. However, the raw scores are simply ordered points. The intervals between them are not equal, thus a total score of 16 may represent many different patterns of disability. In addition, because the scale is not linear, it is not possible to compare scores from two different scales (e.g. the BI and Functional Independence Measure [FIM]), which measure the same construct, because the relationship between the scales will vary according to the level of disability being measured.

More recently, scales have been assessed using two new psychometric methods: Rasch analysis and Item Response Theory, which overcome some of these difficulties. Both approaches model the probability of an individual's response to an item, in that a person with high levels of function will have an increased probability, relative to an individual with low levels of function, of scoring more than zero on any item, whether rating, for example, dressing or toileting. These psychometric methods use statistical techniques that can be used to transform ordinal scales into interval scales. Thus, the relationship between one point and another can be given a specific value. This has a number of potentially exciting consequences. First, it will allow different scales to be anchored to a common point thus allowing large item banks to be created from scales that address the same underlying construct (e.g. upper limb function). Secondly, when a calibrated item bank is developed, testing programs can be made more flexible and appropriate, which allows more accurate measurement of both individuals and groups, and makes it easier to assess the impact of treatment. The ability to measure change more accurately means that the numbers needed to detect significant differences between groups may be smaller. Thirdly, it will be possible to compare groups measured using different scales, with enormous impact on our ability to interpret systematic reviews and perform meta-analyses.

Service quality

One of the difficulties in evaluating a rehabilitation service is that many markers of a quality service may not directly affect outcome. Given the difficulty in running efficient coordinated services, systems that allow the evaluation of the rehabilitation process are invaluable. Evaluating process is facilitated by the development of an Integrated Care Pathway (ICP). An ICP is a document that maps the interventions that should occur during a specific episode of patient care. Typically, the ICP allows evidence-based practice to be operationalised for a specific setting. The benefits of ICPs lie in specifying the best possible method of delivering care and in describing the patterns of variances. A variance sheet may be used to record either departures from the pathway as a procedural variance or the reasons for non-achievement of goals. Individual variances are neither good nor bad; they are simply a method of recording what happened to a specific patient and the reasons for it, thus allowing for individualised patient care. The patterns of variances across a group of patients will identify strengths and weaknesses in the processes around particular episodes of care, and permit incorporation of new ideas and remediation of problems. When combined with measurement tools it is possible to identify which aspects of care impact positively or adversely on outcome.

Conclusions

Adequate widespread longitudinal provision of strategies that prevent complications and secondary deterioration, and drive neural reorganisation have not yet been achieved even by health services in industrialised economies. To do so requires major structural reorganisation, so that goal-focused care and retraining programmes using individualised current best practice can be routinely provided, life-long if needed. A regime change of this sort would probably result in further significant reduction in morbidity and mortality long term after neural injury. It is likely to be facilitated by an increase in the translation of examples of effective delivery of complex treatments in other clinical areas, and of ideas from the science of organisational behaviour, into the implementation of clinical networks, multi-disciplinary team working and individualised treatment programmes.

This clinical process will benefit from, and can initiate, continued investigation of new technologies and restorative treatments, studied in cohorts triaged by robust subject and disease-related variables. Treatments that simultaneously prevent complications and drive the induction of structural plasticity in useful directions are likely to produce most functional gain. Such a conjunction fortuitously occurs in CIMT, which uses both constraint to induce, or force, use of an underused motor system, and movement therapy, as massed practice, to drive motor output and shape use. This was shown to be functionally effective in the ground-breaking Phase III EXCITE trial in the United States, at a cost of $7.5 million over 5 years. Its clinical implementation is inevitably limited by its functional entry criteria and intensive treatment schedule, which requires constraint of the less affected hand for most of 14 consecutive days, and one-to-one training of the affected hand for 6 hours a day for 10 of those days; as a result, even patient recruitment to the trial occurred at a rate of only one patient per month per site. Thus, the perception, at least in the United Kingdom, that CIMT has failed to translate into routine clinical practice may be more apparent than real, although if modified CIMT, for shorter sessions over longer periods, proves equally effective, clinical use might increase.

Similar delivery issues, relating to questions of therapy intensity and duration, real-world effectiveness and when post-injury treatments should be given, apply to many other efficacious training therapies and techniques, as well as robotic training, drugs that modulate neural replacement, regrowth and reorganisation, and non-invasive magnetic and electrical stimulation techniques of the central and peripheral nervous system, all of which might increase the effectiveness of training therapies and their longer term effects.

Chosen therapies and conditioning techniques need first to be standardised and then investigated in proof-of-concept and mechanistic Phase II studies before Phase III trials can be achieved, after which clinical implementation requires further investigation. This framework potentially underpins an industrial number of studies, at national and international levels, using both impairment based and functional entry and outcome measures, to define which treatment or treatment combinations work, how and when to use them following neural injury, and for what type and level of impairment. Just as functional imaging's major, if inadvertent, contribution to clinical practice has been to change attitudes to the prescription as well as the practice of rehabilitation, so the demonstration in small studies in the laboratory that restorative treatments can result in useful functional change is likely to encourage the addition of an exploratory element to many patients' coping strategies, and increase recruitment to Phase II and III trials intended to translate these treatments into the clinical domain.

Further reading

General texts

Cramer SC, Nudo RJ, eds. *Brain Repair After Stroke*. Cambridge: Cambridge University Press, 2010.

Dobkin BH. Neurobiology of rehabilitation. *Ann N Y Acad Sci* 2005; **1038**: 148–170.

Greenwood RJ, Barnes MP, McMillan TM, Ward CD, eds. *Handbook of Neurological Rehabilitation*. Hove and New York: Psychology Press, 2003.

Zasler ND, Katz DI, Zafonte RD, eds. *Brain Injury Medicine: Principles and Practice*, 2nd edn. New York: Demos Medical Publishing, 2013.

Epidemiology

Corrigan JD, Selassie AW. Orman JA. The epidemiology of traumatic brain injury. *J Head Trauma Rehabil* 2010; **25**: 72–80.

Hoffman C, Rice D, Sung HY. Persons with chronic conditions: their prevalence and costs. *JAMA* 1996; **276**: 1473–1479.

Thornhill S, Teasdale GM, Murray G, *et al.* Disability in young adults one year after head injury: a prospective cohort study. *Br Med J* 2000; **320**: 1631–1635.

Guidelines

Department of Health. *National Service Framework for Long-term Conditions*. London: The Stationary Office, 2005.

Intercollegiate Stroke Working Party. *National Clinical Guidelines for Stroke*, 4th edn. London: Royal College of Physicians, 2012.

Medical Research Council. Developing and evaluating complex interventions: new guidance. 2008. http://www.mrc.ac.uk/complexinterventionsguidance (accessed 15 January 2016).

Stroke Guidelines and Consensus Statements. www.strokecenter.org/prof/guidelines.htm (accessed 15 January 2016).

Restorative neurology

Aboody K, Capella A, Niazi N, *et al.* Translating stem cell studies to the clinic for CNS repair: current state of the art and the need for a Rosetta stone. *Neuron* 2011; **70**: 597–613.

Dancause N, Nudo RJ. Shaping plasticity to enhance recovery after injury. *Prog Brain Res* 2011; **192**: 273–295.

Donaldson HH. *The Growth of the Brain: A Study of the Nervous System in Relation to Education*. London: Walter Scott, 1895.

Finger S, Stein DG. *Brain Damage and Recovery of Function: Research and Clinical Implications*. New York: Academic Press, 1982.

Grefkes C, Fink GR. Disruption of motor network connectivity post-stroke and its noninvasive neuromodulation. *Curr Opin Neurol* 2012; **25**: 670–675.

Grefkes C, Ward NS. Cortical reorganization after stroke: how much and how fuctional? *Neuroscientist* 2014; **20**: 56–70. doi:10.1177/1073858413491147.

Ham TE, Sharp DJ. How can investigation of network function inform rehabilitation after traumatic brain injury. *Curr Opin Neurol* 2012; **25**: 662–669.

Hermann D, Chopp M. Promoting brain remodelling and plasticity for stroke recovery: therapeutic promise and potential pitfalls of clinical translation. *Lancet Neurol* 2012; **11**: 369–380.

Jenkins WM, Merzenich MM. Reorganization of neocortical representations after brain injury: a neurophysiological model of the bases of recovery from stroke. *Prog Brain Res* 1987; **71**: 249–266.

Krakauer JW, Carmichael ST, Corbett D, *et al.* Getting neurorehabilitation right: what can be learned from animal models? *Neurorehabil Neural Repair* 2012; **26**: 923–931.

Levin MF, Kleim JA, Wolf SL. What do motor 'recovery' and 'compensation' mean in patients following stroke? *Neurorehabil Neural Repair* 2009; **23**: 313–319.

Nudo RJ, Wise BM, SiFuentes F, Milliken GW. Neural substrates for the effects of rehabilitative training on motor recovery after ischemic infarct. *Science* 1996; **272**: 1791–1794.

Pekna M, Pekny M, Nilsson M. Modulation of neural plasticity as a basis for stroke rehabilitation. *Stroke* 2012; **43**: 2819–2828. doi:10.1161/STROKEAHA.112.654228.

Raisman G. Neuronal plasticity in the septal nuclei of the adult brain. *Brain Res* 1969; **14**: 25–48.

Ramon y Cajal S. *Degeneration and regeneration of the nervous system*, Vol. **2**. New York: Haffner, 1928: 750.

Reis J, Fritsch B. Modulation of motor performance and motor learning by transcranial direct current stimulation. *Curr Opin Neurol* 2011; **24**: 590–596.

Stinear CM, Barber PA, Petoe M, *et al.* The PREP algorhithm predicts the potential for upper limb recovery after stroke. *Brain* 2012; **135**: 2027–2035.

Skill learning and task-related training

Boyd LA, Winstein CJ. Providing explicit information disrupts implicit motor learning after basal ganglia stroke. *Learn Mem* 2004; **11**: 388–396.

Dayan E, Cohen LG. Neuroplasticity subserving motor skill learning. *Neuron* 2011; **72**: 443–454.

Kitago T, Krakauer J.W. Motor learning principles for neurorehabilitation. *Handb Clin Neurol* 2013; **110**: 93–103.

Physical therapeutic interventions for motor disorders

Burridge JH, Hughes AM. Potential for new technologies in clinical practice. *Curr Opin Neurol* 2010; **23**: 671–677.

Dobkin BH, Duncan PW. Should body weight-supported treadmill training and robotic-assistive steppers for locomotor training trot back to the starting gate? *Neurorehabil Neural Repair* 2012; **26**: 308–317.

Lang KC, Thompson PA, Wolf SL. The EXCITE Trial: reacquiring upper-extremity task performance with early versus late delivery of constraint therapy. *Neurorehabil Neural Repair* 2013; **27**: 654–663.

O'Donovan G, Blazevich AJ, Boreham C, *et al.* The ABC of Physical Activity for Health: A consensus statement from the British Association of Sport and Exercise Sciences. *J Sports Sciences* 2010: **28**: 573–591.

Page SJ, Boe S, Levine P. What are the 'ingredients' of modified constraint-induced therapy? An evidence-based review, recipe, and recommendations. *Restorative Neurol Neurosci* 2013; **31**: 299–309.

Wolf SL, Winstein CJ, Miller JP, *et al.* Effect of constraint-induced movement therapy on upper extremity function 3 to 9 months after stroke: the EXCITE randomized clinical trial. *JAMA* 2006; **296**: 2095–2104.

Language disorders

Berthier ML, Pulvermuller F. Neuroscience insights improve neurorehabilitation of poststroke aphasia. *Nat Rev Neurol* 2011; **7**: 86–97.

Bhogal SK, Teasell R, Speechley M. Intensity of aphasia therapy, impact on recovery. *Stroke* 2003; **34**: 987–993.

Brady MC, Kelly H, Godwin J, *et al.* Speech and language therapy for aphasia following stroke. *Cochrane Database Syst Rev* 2012; **5**: CD000425.

Caute A, Pring T, Cocks N, *et al.* Enhancing communication through gesture and naming therapy. *J Speech Lang Hear Res* 2013; **56**: 337–351.

Howard D. The treatment of acquired aphasia. *Philos Trans R Soc Lond B Biol Sci* 1994; **346**: 113–120.

Price CJ. The anatomy of language: a review of 100 fMRI studies published in 2009. *Ann N Y Acad Sci* 2010; **1191**: 62–88.

Seniow J, Litwin M, Litwin T, Lesniak M, *et al.* New approach to the rehabilitation of post-stroke focal cognitive syndrome: effect of levodopa combined with speech and language therapy on functional recovery from aphasia. *J Neurol Sci* 2009; **283**: 214–218.

Visual loss

Barrett AM, Goedert KM, Basso JC. Prism adaptation for spatial neglect after stroke: translational practice gaps. *Nature Rev Neurol* 2012; **8**: 567–577.

Mueller I, Mast H, Sabel BA. Recovery of visual field defects: a large clinical observational study using vision restoration therapy. *Restor Neurol Neurosci* 2007; **25**: 563–572.

Pollock A, Hazelton C, Henderson CA, *et al.* Interventions for visual field defects in patients with stroke. *Cochrane Database Syst Rev* 2011; **10**: CD008388.

Schuett S, Heywood CA, Kentridge RW, *et al.* Rehabilitation of reading and visual exploration in visual field disorders: transfer or specificity? *Brain* 2012; **135**: 912–921.

Stelmack JA, Tang XC, Reda DJ, *et al.* Outcomes of the veterans affairs low vision intervention trial (LOVIT). *Arch Ophthalmol* 2008; **126**: 608–617.

Teng S, Puri A, Whitney D. Ultrafine spatial acuity of blind expert human echolocators. *Exp Brain Res* 2012; **216**: 483–488.

Warren M. Pilot study on activities of daily living limitations in adults with hemianopsia. *Am J Occup Ther* 2009; **63**: 626–633.

Cognitive impairments

Boelen DH, Spikman JM, Fasotti L. Rehabilitation of executive disorders after brain injury: are interventions effective? *J Neuropsychol* 2011; **5**: 73–113.

Bowen C, Yeates G, Palmer S. *A Relational Approach to Rehabilitation: Thinking About Relationships After Brain Injury*. London: Karnac, 2010.

Chen AJ, Novakovic-Agopian, Nycum TJ, *et al.* Training of goal-directed attention regulation enhances control over neural processing for individuals with brain injury. *Brain* 2011; **134**: 1541–1554.

Chung CS, Pollock A, Campbell T, *et al.* Cognitive rehabilitation for executive dysfunction in adults with stroke or other adult non-progressive acquired brain damage. *Cochrane Database Syst Rev* 2013; **4**: CD008391.

Driscoll DM, Dal Monte O, Grafman J. A need for improved training interventions for the remediation of social functioning following brain injury. *J Neurotrauma* 2011; **28**: 319–326.

Jamieson M, Cullen B, McGee-Lennon M, *et al.* The efficacy of cognitive prosthetic technology for people with memory impairments: a systematic review and meta-analysis. *Neuropsych Rehabil* 2014; **24**: 419–444. doi: 10.1080/09602011.2013.825632.

Johansson B, Berglund P, Rönnbäck L. Mental fatigue and impaired information processing after mild and moderate traumatic brain injury. *Brain Inj* 2009; **23**: 1027–1040.

Krasny-Pacini A, Chevignard M, Evans J. Goal management training for rehabilitation of executive functions: a systematic review of effectiveness in patients with acquired brain injury. *Disabil Rehabil* 2014; **36**: 105–116. doi: 10.1080/09602011.2013.825632.

Manly T, Murphy FC. Rehabilitation of executive function and social cognition impairments after brain injury. *Curr Opin Neurol* 2012; **25**: 656–661.

Piras F, Borella E, Incoccia C, Carlesimo GA. Evidence-based practice recommendations for memory rehabilitation. *Eur J Phys Rehabil Med* 2011; **47**: 149–175.

Sohlberg M, Avery J, Kennedy MRT, *et al.* Practice guidelines for direct attention training. *J Med Speech-Lang Pathol* 2003; **11**: xix–xxxix.

Spikman JM, Boelen DHE, Lamberts LF, *et al.* Effects of a multifaceted treatment programme for executive dysfunction after acquired brain injury on indications of executive functioning in daily life. *J Int Neuropsychol Soc* 2010; **16**: 118–129.

Spikman JM, Boelen DHE, Pijnenborg GH, *et al.* Who benefits from treatment for executive dysfunction after brain injury? Negative effects of emotion recognition deficits. *Neuropsychol Rehab* 2013; **23**: 824–845. doi: 10.1080/09602011.2013.826138.

Telerehabilitation

Chang YJ, Chen SF, Huang JD. A Kinect-based system for physical rehabilitation: a pilot study for young adults with motor disabilities. *Res Dev Disabil* 2011; **32**: 2566–2570.

Ericsson KA, Lehamnn AC. Expert and exceptional performance; evidence of maximal adaptation to task constraints. *Ann Rev Psychol* 1996; **47**: 273–305.

Malandraki GA, McCullough G, He XM, *et al.* Teledynamic evaluation of oropharyngeal swallowing. *J Speech Lang Hearing Res* 2011; **54**: 1497–1505.

Saywell N, Vandal AC, Brown P, *et al.* Telerehabilitation to improve outcome for people with stroke: protocol for randomised controlled trial. *Trials* 2012; **13**: 233.

Theodoros DG. Telerehabilitation for service delivery in speech–language pathology. *J Telemed Telecare* 2008; **14**: 221–224.

Medical treatments

Adey-Wakeling Z, Crotty M, Shanahan EM. Suprascapular nerve block for shoulder pain in the first year after stroke: a randomized controlled trial. *Stroke* 2013; **44**: 3136–3141.

Alderfer BS, Arciniegas DB, Silver J. Treatment of depression following traumatic brain injury. *J Head Trauma Rehabil* 2005; **20**: 544–562.

Choi-Kwon S, Han SW, Kwon SU, *et al.* Poststroke fatigue: characteristics and related factors. *Cerebrovasc Dis* 2005; **19**: 84–90.

DasGupta R, Fowler CJ. Bladder, bowel and sexual dysfunction in multiple sclerosis: management strategies. *Drugs* 2003; **63**: 153–166.

Erwin A, Gudesblatt M, Bethoux F, *et al.* Intrathecal baclofen in multiple sclerosis: too little, too late? *Mult Scler* 2011; **17**: 623–629.

Goodman AD, Brown TR, Edwards KR, *et al.* A phase 3 trial of extended release oral dalfampridine in multiple sclerosis. *Ann Neurol* 2010; **68**: 494–502.

Induruwa I, Constantinescu CS, Gran B. Fatigue in multiple sclerosis: a brief review. *J Neurol Sci* 2012; **323**: 9–15.

Irving GA. Contemporary assessment and management of neuropathic pain. *Neurology* 2005; **64** (Suppl 3): S21–S27.

Oddy M. Sexual relationships following brain injury. *Sex Relat Ther* 2001; **16**: 247–259.

Panicker JN, de Sèze M, Fowler CJ. Rehabilitation in practice: neurogenic lower urinary tract dysfunction and its management. *Clin Rehabil* 2010; **24**: 579–589.

Rickards H. Depression in neurological disorders: Parkinson's disease, multiple sclerosis, and stroke. *J Neurol Neurosurg Psychiatry* 2005; **76**: 148–152.

Stevenson VL. Rehabilitation in practice: spasticity management. *Clin Rehabil* 2010; **24**: 293–304.

Single incident brain injury

Stroke

Chollet F, Tardy J, Albucher JF, *et al.* Fluoxetine for motor recovery after acute ischaemic stroke (FLAME): a randomised placebo-controlled trial. *Lancet Neurol* 2011; **10**: 123–130.

Cumming TB, Marshall RS, Lazar RM. Stroke, cognitive deficits, and rehabilitation: still an incomplete picture. *Int J Stroke* 2013; **8**: 38–45.

Dennis MS, Lewis SC, Warlow C. Effect of timing and method of enteral tube feeding for dysphagic stroke patients (FOOD): a multicentre randomised controlled trial. *Lancet* 2005; **365**: 764–772.

Dong YH, Slavin MJ, Chan BP-L, *et al.* Cognitive screening improves the predictive value of stroke severity scores for functional outcome 3–6 months after mild stroke and transient ischaemic attack: an observational study. *BMJ Open* 2013; **3**: e003105. doi:10.1136/bmjopen-2013-003105.

Fearon P, Langhorne P. Early Supported Discharge Trialists. Services for reducing hospital care for acute stroke patients. *Cochrane Database Syst Rev* 2012; **9**: CD000443. doi:10.1002/14651858.CD000443.pub3.

Indredavik B, Bakke F, Slordahl SA, *et al.* Stroke unit treatment: 10-year follow-up. *Stroke* 1999; **30**: 1524–1527.

Kalra L, Evans A, Perez I, *et al.* Training carers of stroke patients: randomised controlled trial. *Br Med J* 2004; **328**: 1099–1101.

Kwakkel G, Kollen BJ. Predicting activities after stroke: what is clinically relevant? *Int J Stroke* 2013; **8**: 25–32.

Langhorne P, Fearon P, Ronning OM, *et al;* on behalf of the Stroke Unit Trialists' Collaboration. Stroke unit care benefits patients with intracebral haemorrhage. Systematic review and meta-analysis. *Stroke* 2013; **44**: 3044–3049.

National Audit Office. Progress in improving stroke care. *Department of Health*, 2010. www.nao.org.uk/stroke2010 (accessed 15 January 2016).

Nijland RH, van Wegen EE, Harmeling-van der Wael BC, *et al.* Presence of finger extension and shoulder abduction 72 hours after stroke predicts functional recovery. Early prediction of functional outcome after stroke: the EPOS cohort study. *Stroke* 2010; **41**: 745–750.

Saposnik G, Kapral MK, Coutts SB, *et al.* Do all age groups benefit from organised inpatient stroke care. *Stroke* 2009; **40**: 3321–3327.

Stroke Unit Trialists' Collaboration. Organised inpatient (stroke unit) care for stroke. *Cochrane Database Syst Rev* 2013; **9**: CD000197. doi: 10.1002/14651858. CD000197.pub3.

Thorsén AM, Holmqvist LW, de-Pedro CJ, *et al.* A randomized controlled trial of early supported discharge and continued rehabilitation at home after stroke: five-year follow-up of patient outcome. *Stroke* 2005; **36**: 297–303.

Traumatic brain injury

Andelic N, Bautz-Holter E, Ronning P, *et al.* Does an early onset and continuous chain of rehabilitation improve the long-term functional outcome of patients with severe traumatic brain injury. *J Neurotrauma* 2012; **29**: 66–74.

Brown AW, Malec JF, Mandrekar J et al. Predictive utility of weekly post-traumatic amnesia assessments after brain injury: a multicentre analysis. *Brain Inj* 2010; **24**: 472–478.

Fridman EA, Schiff ND. Neuromodulation of the conscious state following severe brain injuries. *Curr Opin Neurobiol.* 2014;**29**:172-7.

Giacino JT, Whyte J, Bagiella E, *et al.* Placebo controlled trial of amantadine for severe traumatic brain injury. *N Engl J Med* 2012; **366**: 819–826.

Giles GM, Wager J, Fong L, *et al.* Twenty-month effectiveness of a non-aversive, long-term, low-cost programme for persons with persisting neurobehavioural disability. *Brain Injury* 2005; **19**: 753–764.

Hammond FM, Sherer M, Malec JF, et al. Amantadine irritability multisite study group. Amantadine effect on perceptions of irritability after traumatic brain injury: results from the amantadine irritability multisite study. *J Neurotrauma* 2015;**32**:1230-1238.

Laureys S, Schiff ND. Coma and consciousness: paradigms (re)framed by neuroimaging. *Neuroimage* 2012; **61**: 478–491.

Marshman LAG , Jakabek D, Hennessy M, *et al.* Post-traumatic amnesia. *J Clin Neurosci* 2013; **20**: 1475–1481.

McMillan TM, Teasdale GM, Stewart E. Disability in young people and adults after head injury: 12–14 year follow-up of a prospective cohort. *J Neurol Neurosurg Psychiatry* 2012; **83**: 1086–1091.

McMillan TM, Teasdale GM, Weir CJ et al. Death after head injury: the 13 year outcome of a case control study. *J Neurol Neurosurg Psychiatry* 2011; **82**: 931–935.

McMillan TM. Outcome of rehabilitation for neurobehavioural disorders. *NeuroRehabilitation* 2013; **32**: 791–801.

Monti MM, Vanhaudenhuyse A, Coleman MR, *et al.* Willful modulation of brain activity in disorders of consciousness. *N Engl J Med* 2010; **362**: 579–589.

Moreau OK, Mollin E, Merlen E, *et al.* Lasting pituitary hormone deficiency after traumatic brain injury. *J Neurotrauma* 2012; **29**: 81–89.

Mysiw WJ, Bogner J, Corrigan J, *et al.* The impact of acute care medications on rehabilitation outcome after traumatic brain injury. *Brain Inj.* 2006;**20**:905–11.

Nakase-Richardson R, Whyte J, Giacino JT, *et al.* Longitudinal outcome of patients with disordered consciousness in the NIDRR model systems programmes. *J Neurotrauma* 2012; **29**: 59–65.

Ponsford J. Rehabilitation interventions after mild head injury. *Curr Opin Neurol* 2005; **18**: 692–697.

Ponsford J, Janzen S, McIntyre A, *et al.* INCOG recommendations for management of cognition following traumatic brain injury, part I: Post Traumatic Amnesia/ Delirium. *J Head Trauma Rehabil* 2014;**29**:307-20.

Powell J, Heslin J, Greenwood R. Community based rehabilitation after severe traumatic brain injury: a randomised controlled trial. *J Neurol Neurosurg Psychiatry* 2002; **72**: 193–202.

Salazar AM, Warden DL, Schwab K, *et al.* Cognitive rehabilitation for traumatic brain injury: a randomized trial. Defense and Veterans Head Injury Program (DVHIP) Study Group. *JAMA* 2000; **283**: 3075–3308.

Shiel A, Burn JP, Henry D, *et al.* The effects of increased rehabilitation therapy after brain injury: results of a prospective controlled trial. *Clin Rehabil* 2001; **15**: 501–514.

Spikman JM, Timmerman ME, Milders MV, *et al.* Social cognition impairments in relation to general cognitive deficits, injury severity and prefrontal lesions in traumatic brain injury patients. *J Neurotrauama* 2012; **29**: 101–111.

Stuss DT, Binns MA, Carruth FG, *et al.* The acute period of recovery from traumatic brain injury: posttraumatic amnesia or posttraumatic confusional state? *J Neurosurg* 1999; **90**: 635–643.

Wade DT, King NS, Wenden FJ, *et al.* Routine follow up after head injury: a second randomised controlled trial. *J Neurol Neurosurg Psychiatry* 1998; **65**: 177–183.

Wehman P, Targett P, West M, *et al.* Productive work and employment for persons with traumatic brain injury: what have we learned after 20 years? *J Head Trauma Rehabil* 2005; **20**: 115–127.

Wheaton P, Mathias JL, Vink R. Impact of pharmacological treatments on cognitive and behavioural outcomes in the postacute stages of adult traumatic brain injury: a meta-analysis. *J Clin Psychopharmacol* 2011; **31**: 745–757.

Organisational behaviours

Catchpole KR, De Leval MR, McEwan A, *et al.* Patient handover from surgery to intensive care: using Formula 1 pit-stop and aviation models to improve safety and quality. *Pediatr Anesth* 2007; **17**: 470–478.

Emmerson GJ, Neely MA. Two adaptable, valid, and reliable data-collection measures: goal attainment scaling and the semantic differential. *Counselling Psychologist* 1988; **16**: 261–271.

Grol R, Grimshaw J. From best evidence to best practice: effective implementation of change in patients' care. *Lancet* 2003; **362**: 1225–1223.

Kielhofner G. *A Model of Human Occupation: Theory and Application.* Williams & Wilkins, 1995.

Leplege A, Hunt S. The problem of quality of life in medicine. *JAMA* 1997; **278**: 47–50.

Locke EA, Latham GP. Building a practically useful theory of goal setting and task motivation: a 35-year odyssey. *Am Psychol* 2002; **57**: 705–717.

Pearson SD, Goulart-Fisher D, Lee TH. Critical pathways as a strategy for improving care: problems and potential. *Ann Intern Med* 1995; **123**: 941–948.

Scobbie L, Dixon D, Wyke S. Goal setting and action planning in the rehabilitation setting: development of a theoretically informed practice framework. *Clin Rehabil* 2011; **25**: 468–482.

World Health Organization. *International Classification of Functioning, Disability and Health.* Geneva, WHO, 2001. http://www3.who.int/icf/icftemplate.cfm (accessed 16 January 2016).

CHAPTER 19

Toxic, Metabolic and Physical Insults to the Nervous System and Inherited Disorders of Metabolism

Robin Howard[1], Jeremy Chataway[1], Mark Edwards[2], Simon Heales[1], Robin Lachmann[1], Alexander Leff[2] and Elaine Murphy[1]

[1] National Hospital for Neurology & Neurosurgery

[2] UCL Institute of Neurology

Toxic, nutritional and metabolic derangements can cause damage to the nervous system by a variety of mechanisms and lead to a wide spectrum of characteristic neurological disorders. Exposure to toxic substances, which can be accidental or deliberate in the context of substance abuse, can cause encephalopathy, stroke, seizures or neuropathy. Nutritional deficiencies are probably the most common worldwide cause of neurological disease and are manifest as a number of well-characterised, usually reversible but potentially serious neurological disorders. Metabolic encephalopathy is brought about by the consequences of organ failure or exposure to endogenous or exogenous toxins or drugs that can affect the central nervous system (CNS). The cause of these conditions can be unclear at presentation and often requires detailed clinical and laboratory analyses before the correct diagnosis is made and appropriate therapy instituted. Similarly, neuromuscular abnormalities can occur as a consequence of toxic exposure or nutritional deficiency.

Neurological disorders associated with exposure to toxic substances

Environmental factors and toxins are important causes of neurological disease. They are often under-recognised and are difficult to diagnose as the onset of symptoms can be slow and the clinical pattern can mimic other common conditions. This chapter includes a review of the effects of accidental and deliberate exposure to industrial and environmental toxins and drugs of addiction including alcohol. Some of the more important toxins that affect the nervous system are shown in Table 19.1 and the patterns of neurological involvement in Table 19.2.

Heavy metals

Exposure to heavy metals or industrial toxins is usually cumulative, developing over a prolonged period of months or years as a consequence of environmental or occupational exposure. However, these agents can be acutely toxic with accidental or deliberate ingestion of excessive amounts. The adverse effects of acute or chronic exposure develop earlier and more rapidly in the young and the consequences differ from those in adults. Heavy metals impair the function of the nuclei or cytoplasmic structures, particularly mitochondria. Acute exposure often leads to encephalopathy with confusion, attention deficit and seizures, while chronic involvement is of a more insidious onset with mood disturbance, memory and cognitive impairment. Systemic features usually accompany neurological manifestations.

Lead

Lead is the most common source of heavy metal intoxication because of its extensive commercial use and presence in Ayurvedic medication. Occupational exposure occurs in workers in smelting and metal foundries, battery manufacture and industrial plants. Accidental ingestion occurs in children with pica (eating dirt and the coating of pipes); however, exposure has diminished with the phasing out of leaded petrol and diminished use of lead-based paints. Inorganic lead is absorbed from the gastrointestinal tract and children are particularly vulnerable.

Lead binds to erythrocytes and is distributed throughout the body. It is incorporated into the brain and other soft tissues where it may persist for prolonged periods. It is toxic to the nervous system and leads to altered migration of neurones during development. It also interferes with cell membranes, myelin, neurotransmitter function and calcium metabolism.

Lead toxicity has a number of effects in the nervous system leading to acute encephalopathy (particularly in children) and polyneuropathy in adults. Lead encephalopathy may follow gastrointestinal symptoms and patients present with headache and fatigue leading to confusion, altered level of consciousness, behavioural change and focal or generalised seizures. Other signs include ataxia, impaired motor function and coma. In children, lead is a significant neurodevelopmental toxin, which produces mild learning difficulties. In adults, chronic exposure leads to a similar but slower onset encephalopathy characterised by headache, myalgia, paraesthesia, irritability, sleep disturbance and loss of libido evolving into progressive confusion and stupor. Pure motor neuropathy can occur affecting the upper more than the lower limbs. The onset is usually symmetrical and often associated with prominent gastrointestinal disturbance. There can be bilateral wrist or foot drop with marked atrophy and occasional fasciculation, which can mimic motor neurone disease. Although the sensory component is usually minor, the neuropathy may be particularly painful. Lead toxicity can cause a blue line at the gingival margin (Figure 19.1).

Investigations will show elevated concentrations of lead in the blood, there is a hypochromic microcytic anaemia with basophilic

Neurology: A Queen Square Textbook, Second Edition. Edited by Charles Clarke, Robin Howard, Martin Rossor and Simon Shorvon.

Table 19.1 Toxins that can affect the nervous system.

Metals
Lead
Mercury
Arsenic
Manganese
Aluminium
Thallium
Tin
Bismuth
Solvents and small molecule toxins
Ethanol
Methanol
Toluene
Trichloroethylene (TCE)
Tetrachlorethylene (perchlorethylene, PCE)
Ethylene oxide
Hexacarbon solvents include n-hexane and methyl n-butyl ketone (MnBK)
Xylene and styrene
Carbon disulfide
Cyanide
Acrylamide
Allyl chloride
Methyl bromide
Methyl chloride
Nitrous oxide
Organophosphates
Carbon monoxide
Natural toxins
Plant toxins
Fungal toxins
Marine toxins
Insect and animal toxins
Snake venom
Spider toxins
Scorpion toxin
Botulinum toxin

stippling of the red cells (Figure 19.1), hyperuricaemia, reduced blood γ-amino-laevulinic acid and raised zinc and lead protoporphyrins. Nerve conduction studies show a marked axonal neuropathy with denervation although there can be mild motor conduction slowing. Nerve biopsy confirms axonal degeneration although paranodal demyelination can be present.

The mortality of acute severe lead encephalopathy can be >25%. Treatment is initially supportive and involves eliminating the source of lead exposure. Chelation therapy is used, if lead concentrations are markedly elevated, to remove lead before it can be incorporated into the CNS or soft tissues. This involves treatment with EDTA, dimercaprol (2,3-dimercaptopropanol) or BAL (British anti-Lewisite). Early treatment usually leads to improvement in the neuropathy but the prognosis of the encephalopathy is less certain.

Mercury

Mercury exists in an elemental inorganic or organic form. The inorganic form is absorbed rapidly following inhalation during industrial exposure in the production of thermometers, barometers or batteries and historically was also accidentally ingested during hat-making. The organic form, methylmercury, is far more toxic and occasionally poisons water supplies, as was the case in the Minamata outbreak in Japan in the 1950s and 1960s.

Chronic industrial exposure to elemental or inorganic mercury causes systemic manifestations with renal, skin, pulmonary and gastrointestinal involvement including gingivitis, cutaneous erythema (Pink's disease), anaemia and proteinuria. Patients develop progressive rest and intention tremor ('hatter's shakes'), ataxia and myopathy; there is memory and cognitive impairment, social withdrawal, personality change with anxiety, excitability, emotional lability and insomnia. Eventually, drowsiness, confusion and stupor supervene. Methylmercury is bio-amplified by aquatic species and following ingestion causes paraesthesiae, tremor, ataxia, spasticity, progressive visual field and hearing loss with encephalopathy, progressing to stupor, coma and death.

The diagnosis is confirmed by demonstrating elevated blood and urine mercury. Treatment is by facilitating the elimination of mercury with prompt chelation using penicillamine and providing supportive care. The role of chelation therapy with dimercaprol is controversial.

Arsenic

Inorganic arsenic has been extensively employed in herbicides and pesticides and as a timber preservative in the past, although current use is mainly restricted to the production of glass, electronics and computer microchips. It also occurs in a non-toxic organic form in seafood. Exposure occurs by drinking contaminated well water, especially in the Indian subcontinent, or as a consequence of mining lead or copper smelting; arsenic is sometimes found in herbal medications. It has been used as a poison because it is odourless, tasteless and highly toxic.

Arsenic disrupts protein structure and enzyme activity leading to inhibition of mitochondrial function and oxidative metabolism. Acute or subacute exposure is associated with nausea, vomiting, abdominal pain and bloody diarrhoea, followed by progressive encephalopathy. Autonomic features including hypotension, tachycardia and vasomotor collapse develop culminating in arrhythmia, myoglobinuria, acute renal failure, obtundation, acute confusional state, coma and death. Low dose chronic exposure causes weight loss, severe alopecia and white horizontal striations on the nails (Mees' lines) (Figure 19.2). There is usually severe gastrointestinal disturbance and skin changes include melanosis, keratosis and malignancy. There can be personality disturbances with confusion, irritability, delusions and visual hallucinations; optic nerve and spinal cord involvement can also occur. Arsenic neuropathy is a sensori-motor neuropathy which is predominantly axonal although demyelinating features occur soon after exposure. It usually develops within several weeks of the acute exposure and is characterised by distal pain and progressive weakness initially in the lower limbs,

Table 19.2 Patterns of neurological involvement caused by toxins.

Syndrome	Clinical features	Causes
Acute encephalopathy	Non-specific – headache, nausea and vomiting, fatigue, irritability Confusion, disorientation Amnesia Cerebellar – ataxia, slurred speech Seizures, clouding of consciousness, coma	Organic solvents inc. toluene (acute exposure) Lead, arsenic, thallium, manganese, mercury
Chronic behavioural and cognitive impairment	Non-specific – headache, nausea and vomiting, fatigue, irritability Mood disturbance, anxiety, psychosis	Lead, cholorinated hydrocarbons
Delayed post-exposure encephalopathy	Delayed development of confusion and unresponsiveness	Carbon monoxide
Extrapyramidal	Tremor Rigidity Parkinsonism – bradykinesis Postural instability	Manganese
Myelopathy / myeloneuropathy	Gait ataxia Pyramidal signs – slow movement, weakness, hyperreflexia, extensor plantar responses Distal weakness and sensory loss	Cobalamine deficiency, nitrous oxide, copper deficiency
Polyneuropathy	Distal weakness and sensory loss	Lead, Arsenic, Thallium, Toluene

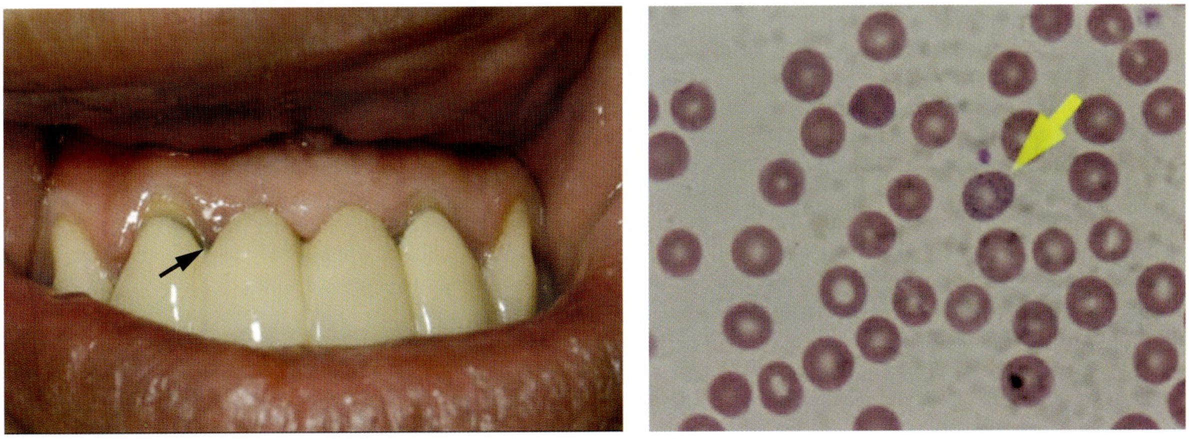

(a) (b)

Figure 19.1 (a) Lead lines (blue pigmentation seen along gum lines, arrow). (b) Basophilic stippling seen within the red blood cell. Source: Tsutsui 2013. Reproduced with permission of the New Zealand Medical Journal.

subsequently spreading to the upper limbs with areflexia and distal sensory loss. The neuropathy is associated with respiratory muscle weakness.

There can be anaemia, pancytopenia, basophilic stippling, myoglobinuria, elevated liver enzymes and raised cerebrospinal fluid (CSF) protein. Arsenic binds to keratin and therefore can be detected in hair, nail, bone, teeth or urine. It is cleared rapidly from the circulation so urine levels are a better guide to toxity than are serum levels. Nerve conduction studies show motor and sensory axonal neuropathy with occasional demyelinating features. Nerve biopsy confirms axonal degeneration.

The treatment involves removal of exposure, decontamination of the gastrointestinal tract and aggressive support. Chelation therapy can be undertaken with derivatives of dimercaprol such as DMSA (2,3-dimercaptosuccinic acid), DMPS (2,3-dimercapto-1-propanesulfonic acid) (Unithiol), BAL or D-penicillamine but there is little evidence to suggest this helps in the later stages of arsenic neuropathy. Exchange transfusion and forced alkaline diuresis can be necessary.

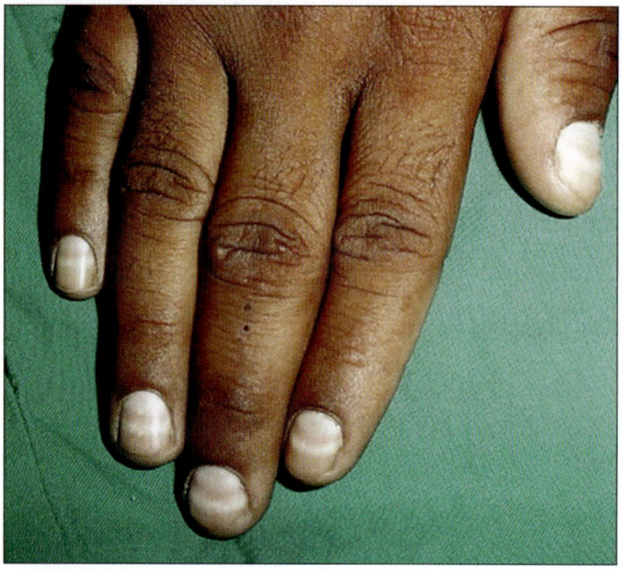

Figure 19.2 Mee's lines. Source: Chauhan 2008. Reproduced with permission of Elsevier.

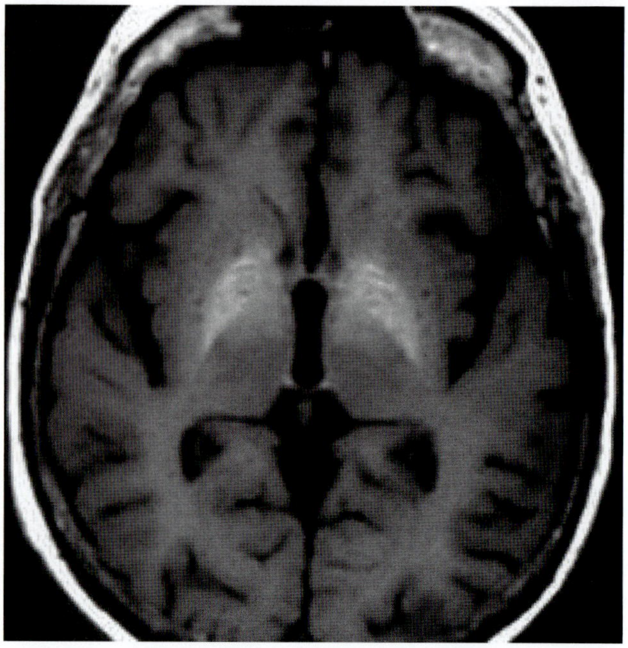

Figure 19.3 Manganese toxicity: bilateral and symmetric high signal intensity in globus pallidus on T1-weighted images.

Manganese

Manganese is present in all living organisms and functions as an enzyme cofactor. It is widely used as a fuel additive and also in fertilisers and fireworks. Toxicity occurs as a consequence of its industrial use in iron and steel manufacturing and in welding but exposure can also be iatrogenic as a consequence of poorly balanced total parenteral nutrition.

Acute exposure can lead to a progressive encephalopathy ('manganese madness') characterised by fatigue, apathy, insomnia, auditory and visual hallucinations, personality change, compulsive behaviour, irritability and aggression culminating in progressive memory disturbance. More chronic exposure leads to a characteristic pattern of extrapyramidal abnormalities with selective degeneration of the pallidum but relative sparing of the substantia nigra, characterised by parkinsonian facies, hypersalivation, micrographia, bradykinesis, rigidity and severe dystonia with occasional myoclonic jerking. The tremor is characteristically of low amplitude, bilateral and symmetrical, present on action and posture. There is often early development of speech and gait abnormalities, dystonia and action myoclonus with a poor response to levodopa. There can be an associated encephalopathic component including emotional lability and progressive cognitive impairment.

The diagnosis is confirmed by the presence of elevated serum manganese, and urine concentrations can also be helpful. Magnetic resonance imaging (MRI) scan can show abnormal signal intensities in the globus pallidus and subthalamic nucleus (Figure 19.3).

Management necessitates removal of the toxic sources and chelation with EDTA is occasionally helpful. The response to levodopa is variable. Dialysis may be necessary and liver transplantation has been reported to result in the reversal of parkinsonism.

Aluminium

Aluminium is abundant and is extensively used in packaging, food containers and cooking utensils and in water treatment. Industrial exposure can occasionally occur after smelting or inhalation of aluminium dust but this is rare.

Acute intoxication leads to progressive agitation, confusion and myoclonic jerking, sometimes with generalised tonic–clonic seizures progressing to coma and death. More chronic exposure causes a progressive tremor, incoordination and ataxia with the development of focal epilepsy. Dialysis dementia (Chapter 20) is at least partly brought about by the toxic effects of aluminium in the dialysis fluid and in phosphate binders. Aluminium retention occurs in the uraemic state and progressive cognitive impairment, dysarthria and encephalopathy can develop after several years of dialysis.

The treatment includes de-ionisation of the dialysate and avoidance of aluminium-containing phosphate binders. However, aluminium intoxication can occur as a consequence of chelation therapy that actually displaces sequested aluminium from bone and this should therefore be avoided.

Thallium

Exposure to thallium is now relatively rare as its use has been banned in pesticides. There is still an occasional incidence of deliberate exposure by attempted murder or suicide.

Acute exposure can lead to an encephalopathy characterised by hallucinations, paranoia and cognitive impairment. Systemic involvement is similar to arsenic in causing abdominal cramps, vomiting and diarrhoea. Alopecia develops after several weeks and is a key diagnostic clue, and Mees' lines are seen in the nails. There can be a progressive encephalopathy with ataxia, chorea and confusion culminating in cardiac and respiratory failure and coma. Chronic exposure leads to a progressive predominantly sensory axonal neuropathy which is painful and associated with distal sensory loss, weakness and areflexia. Neurophysiology confirms progressive axonal loss. High thallium levels can be detected in blood, urine and hair samples.

The treatment is with gastric lavage, laxatives and haemodialysis. Absorption from the gastrointestinal tract can also be reduced by Prussian blue or activated charcoal, both of which bind thallium.

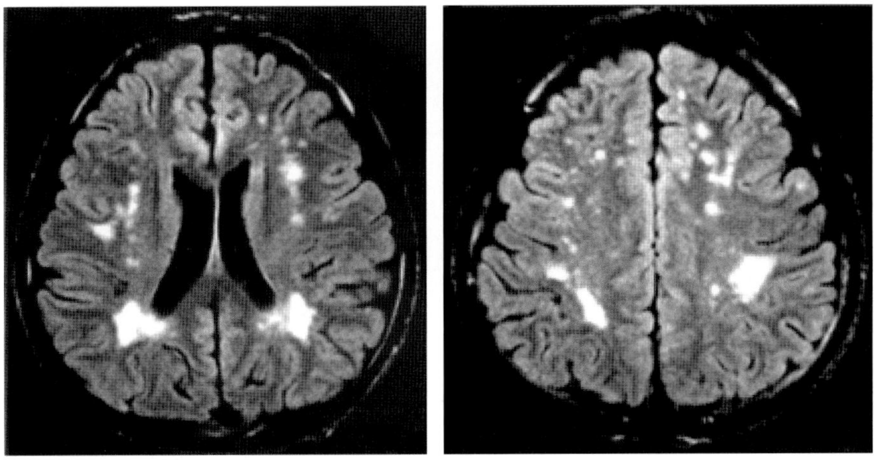

Figure 19.4 Toluene exposure: MRI Tl-weighted scan showing extensive white matter change.

Tin

Tin is extensively used in the manufacture of electronics and in soldering. The inorganic form is not associated with any abnormal neurological features but the organic forms (in particular triethyl tin), which can be inhaled, lead to progressive neurological dysfunction characterised by raised intracranial pressure with headache, apathy, cognitive impairment and hallucinosis culminating in seizures and coma. There may also be behavioural disturbances including emotional lability and cognitive impairment with confusion and disorientation. Abnormal eye movements, papilloedema and a cerebellar syndrome also occur.

Blood levels are a poor guide; urine levels may be more reliable. Treatment is by use of chelating agents, plasma exchange and D-penicillamine.

Bismuth

Bismuth is contained in some surgical dressings and is sometimes used in the treatement of peptic ulcers and to bulk stools after colostomy. Excessive intake can lead to a progressive behavioural disturbance including depression, apathy and irritability, culminating in a florid encephalopathy with hallucinosis, tremor, myoclonus, ataxia and dysarthria leading to convulsions and coma. The myoclonus is characteristically stimulus-sensitive and can be multi-focal or generalised. Chelation treatment with dimercaprol is often effective.

Solvents and toxins

CNS dysfunction can occur as a consequence of an accidental exposure to a high dose of industrial solvents or to more prolonged chronic exposure to moderate levels in the workplace or as a drug of abuse. The long-term symptoms of prolonged exposure to solvent vapour include progressive cognitive deficits affecting attention, memory and executive function and causing visuo-spatial disturbance with subsequent cerebellar or motor involvement.

Toluene

Toluene (methyl benzene) is a volatile hydrocarbon solvent used in the manufacture of paints, glues and petrol. Exposure occurs relatively commonly during manufacture or industrial processes and the condition can be unrecognised. However, much of toluene poisoning is attributable to deliberate inhalation, such as in glue sniffing.

Toluene is highly lipid-soluble and so crosses the blood–brain barrier readily. It causes CNS demyelination, with secondary neuronal damage. It also causes a mixed axonal–demyelinating neuropathy. Acute exposure leads to progressive headache, nausea, vomiting and dizziness. There can be cardiorespiratory symptoms secondary to pulmonary hypertension before the development of cognitive impairment including euphoria, disorientation, memory loss and focal neurological signs such as dysarthria, ataxia and intention tremor with progression to stupor and coma. Long-term exposure is associated with toxic encephalopathy, progressive intention tremor and stimulus-sensitive myoclonus, dementia and there can be a progressive optic neuropathy with opsoclonus.

MRI scan may show cerebral atrophy or diffuse symmetrical abnormalities in the basal ganglia, thalamus or cingulate gyrus or extensive white matter high signal change (Figure 19.4). There are elevated urinary hippuric acid levels and blood toluene can also be a valuable guide.

Treatment is by removal of the source of the exposure and supportive care.

Trichloroethylene and tetrachlorethylene

The chlorinated hydrocarbons, trichloroethylene (TCE) and tetrachlorethylene (perchlorethylene; PCE) are industrial solvents particularly used as degreasers and in dry-cleaning fluids. Exposure occurs by inhalation, contamination of drinking water or in recreational abuse because of their euphoric effects. Acute toxicity causes encephalopathy characterised by progressive nausea, dizziness and headache leading to disorientation, stupor and coma. Chronic exposure is associated with trigeminal neuropathy causing progressive sensory impairment spreading from the nose in a trigeminal distribution leading to facial and buccal numbness. Weakness of the muscles of mastication and facial expression may then develop with progressive ptosis, ophthalmoplegia, retrobulbar neuritis, optic atrophy and vocal cord involvement. Further exposure leads to a chronic sensorimotor neuropathy with mixed axonal and demyelinating features and progressive impairment of attention, memory and orientation.

The level of TCE metabolite tricholorethanol can be measured to monitor exposure.

Treatment is by removal from exposure. Patients who have been acutely exposed should have oxygen administered and be treated with gastric lavage and haemodialysis. Improvement in trigeminal and other cranial nerve involvement is usually incomplete.

Ethylene oxide

Ethylene oxide is used to sterilise heat-sensitive medical equipment and as an alkylating agent in industrial synthesis. It is highly toxic, causing a severe progressive reversible encephalopathy. Long-term exposure leads to a sensorimotor axonal neuropathy and mild cognitive change. Improvement generally follows discontinuation of exposure.

Hexacarbon solvents

Hexacarbon solvents, and in particular n-hexane and methyl n-butyl ketone (MnBK), are commonly used in industrial solvents and household glues. They are neurotoxic and are liberated during petrol production and refining. They are also present in most glues and solvents and are widely abused for recreational reasons.

A reversible acute encephalopathy is common in those who take solvents for recreational reasons, leading to euphoria, dizziness, ataxia and progressive cognitive impairments, encephalopathy and coma. However, chronic exposure causes a progressive distal sensorimotor axonal peripheral neuropathy associated with autonomic involvement and parkinsonism. N-hexane exposure also causes facial numbness, maculopathy or optic neuropathy. The management is cessation of exposure.

Xylene and styrene

Xylene and styrene are structurally similar to toluene and found in solvents, paints and varnishes. Acute exposure occurs by inhalation or absorption from the skin and can lead to acute encephalopathy with disturbances of cognition, attention and behaviour. Chronic exposure to lower levels can cause mild but progressive disturbance of behaviour, psychomotor performance and visual function.

Carbon disulfide

Carbon disulfide is used as a solvent in varnishes and insecticides, in the manufacture of plastics including rayon and cellophane as well as the vulcanisation of rubber. It is a potent neurotoxin with exposure caused by inhalation and oral ingestion rather than by transdermal exposure. Acute exposure to high levels leads to encephalopathy with progressive drowsiness and disruption of behaviour with mood swings, hallucinations, psychotic disturbances and memory loss. A similar encephalopathy occurs with chronic exposure but a distal demyelinating sensori-motor peripheral neuropathy may occur and there may also be parkinsonism, retinopathy, optic neuropathy, cerebellar involvement and a small vessel vasculopathy.

Blood and urine carbon disulfide levels give a guide to exposure. The treatment is removal from the source but no agent is available to neutralise the effects of carbon disulfide which can be present for many years.

Cyanide

Cyanide blocks trivalent iron in cellular respiration enzymes and inactivates cytochrome oxidase. This leads to an immediate cessation of cell respiration with hypoxia and respiratory arrest. Exposure usually occurs as a consequence of deliberate poisoning. However, cyanide poisoning can also occur during accidental smoke inhalation or from ingestion of incorrectly prepared cassava flour (see Konzo). Acute exposure affects structures with high oxygen requirements leading to haemorrhage necrosis. Presentation is with dizziness, headache, vertigo and agitation, culminating in seizures, respiratory arrest and death. Chronic ingestion can cause progressive cognitive impairment, parkinsonism and delayed dystonia. MRI shows bilateral areas of hyperintensity in the lentiform and caudate nuclei also the striatum and globus pallidus.

Treatment involves immediate administration of 100% oxygen followed by hydroxycobalamin and sodium thiosulfate.

Acrylamide and acylonitrile

Acrylamide is used as an adhesive and grouting agent. Inhalation or cutaneous exposure can occur during manufacture or in the polymerisation process. Acute high-dose exposure can cause an encephalopathy characterised by confusion, hallucinations, drowsiness and ataxia. More commonly, however, chronic exposure leads to a characteristic progressive distal sensorimotor axonal neuropathy which initially develops in the lower limbs before affecting the upper limbs. Autonomic involvement is common with hyperhidrosis and dermatitis. There can be a progressive cerebellar ataxia and occasionally pyramidal signs occur. It is associated with dermatitis, palmar erythema, fatigue and weight loss.

Nerve conduction studies confirm the presence of an axonal sensorimotor polyneuropathy initially affecting large myelinated fibres and biopsy shows distal axonal degeneration. Acrylonitrile is used to make plastics for pipes and building components. It is absorbed by inhalation and through the skin and converted to cyanide which is responsible for the associated acute toxicity. Chronic toxicity is associated with fatigue, headache, nausea and nasal irritation.

Allyl chloride

Allyl chloride is used in the preparation of epoxy resins and insecticides. It can cause a mixed motor and sensory distal axonal neuropathy which only recovers after prolonged discontinuation.

Methyl bromide

Methyl bromide is widely used as a refrigerant, in fire extinguishers and as a soil fumigant. Acute exposure causes a progressive encephalopathy with convulsions and delirium leading to hyperpyrexia, coma and death. Chronic exposure to lower levels causes systemic features including nausea, vomiting, headache and mucosal irritation before CNS deficits develop which can include progressive speech disturbance and cerebellar ataxia, incoordination, seizures and myoclonus. Long-term exposure leads to a distal sensorimotor polyneuropathy, occasionally upper motor neurone signs, and visual disturbance including optic atrophy.

Management is supportive but dialysis can be necessary to remove bromide.

Methyl chloride

Methyl chloride is a methylating agent used in the production of lead, rubber or polystyrene foam. Toxicity is associated with inhalation or absorption through the skin. There is CNS depression which can cause headache, dizziness, confusion, speech abnormalities and diplopia with incoordination. Severe prolonged exposure can lead to seizures or stimulus-sensitive myoclonus.

Methyl alcohol (Methanol)

Methyl alcohol is used as an industrial solvent and as an adulterant to denature ethanol and prevent its abuse. Toxicity results from the formation of formaldehyde and formate. Acute toxicity causes

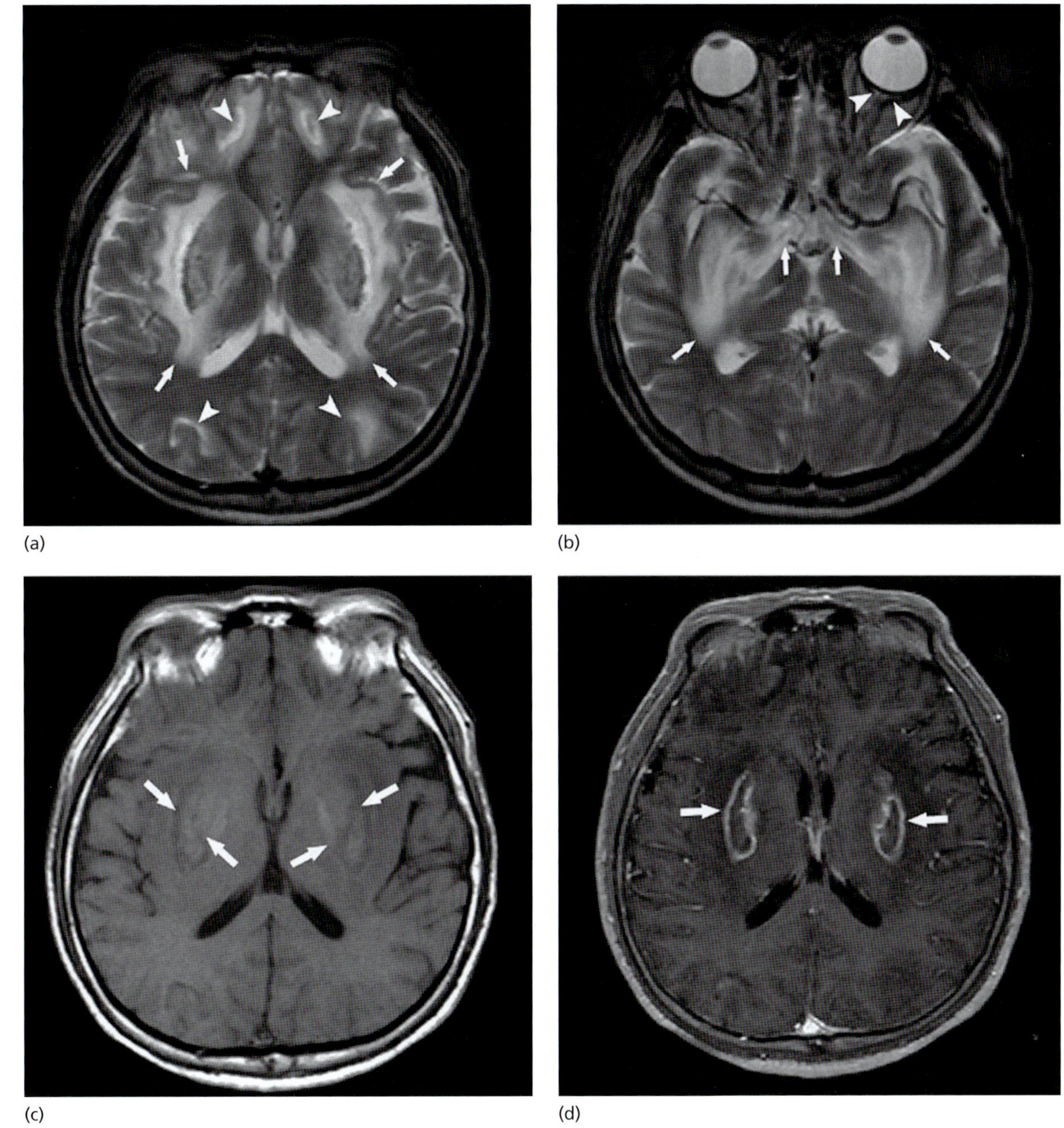

Figure 19.5 MRI on day 15 after methanol intoxication. (a) T2-weighted image showed high signal abnormalities in bilateral basal ganglia (arrows), frontal, and occipital subcortical white matter (arrowheads), consistent with oedematous change. (b) T2-weighted image showed oedematous change involving bilateral optic tracts and optic radiations (arrows). High signal oedematous change was also noted in the optic disc of left eye (arrowheads). (c) T1-weighted image showed slightly high signal component in bilateral basal ganglia, indicating the haemorrhage (arrows). (d) T1-weighted image with gadolinium administration showed marginal enhancement in bilateral putamen, indicating breakdown of the blood–brain barrier. Source: Yang 2005. Reproduced with permission of Macmillan.

encephalopathy with prominent visual symptoms due to toxic optic neuropathy, and seizures. It is associated with headache, abdominal pain, nausea and vomiting (see Alcohol abuse). MRI shows characteristic infarction or haemorrhage in the putamen (Figure 19.5).

Treatment is with haemodialysis and inhibition of the conversion to formaldehyde by fornepizole or ethanol and correction of the accompanying metabolic acidosis with sodium bicarbonate.

Nitrous oxide

Exposure to nitrous oxide (N_2O; 'laughing gas') occurs in patients receiving prolonged general anaesthesia or by intentional inhalational abuse. Nitrous oxide oxidises cobalamin and therefore disrupts B_{12}-dependent pathways rendering methycobalamine inactive; this inhibits methylation reactions, which are in turn important for production of myelin. The clinical pattern of toxicity is therefore identical to subacute combined degeneration with extensive spinal cord, brain and peripheral nerve demyelination. There is a progressive distal sensory neuropathy beginning in the hands with proprioceptive loss secondary to involvement of large sensory nerves and dorsal columns. Progressive spasticity and hyper-reflexia due to a myelopathy then develops.

Nerve conduction confirms slowing of motor and sensory conduction velocities with secondary axonal loss. Vitamin B_{12} replacement may help in the management but this does not always reverse the neuropathy. MRI findings include hyperintense T2 signal in the dorsal and lateral columns.

Organophosphates

Forty per cent of pesticides contain organophosphates; they are also found in herbicides, lubricants, flame retardants and as a petroleum additive. Exposure usually occurs in agricultural settings although ingestion may occur in children or in suicide attempts. Organophosphates inhibit cholinesterases leading to cholinergic toxicity and in acute exposure this is typically manifest within 4 days and resolves over 3–4 weeks. Presentation is with salivation, lacrimation, diarrhoea, urinary frequency, mydriasis, bradycardia, bronchoconstriction and diffuse muscle weakness involving respiratory, bulbar and proximal limb musculature leading to respiratory failure. Acute central effects are also seen causing confusion, dizziness, ataxia, blurred vision and impaired memory culminating in seizures and coma. Chronic exposure ('sheep dipper flu') is characterised by transient symptoms including headache, rhinitis, pharyngitis and myalgia. However, a longer term mild impairment of cognitive and memory functions occasionally occurs. Prolonged exposures can also lead to a late onset sensorimotor axonal peripheral neuropathy and occasionally ataxia and upper motor neurone involvement with spasticity.

Organophosphates are easily absorbed through the skin and therefore it is important that those with potential exposures use protective masks, gloves and appropriate clothing. The skin should be carefully washed following exposures and it is essential to maintain the airway because of the risk of aspiration. Prolonged treatment with atropine, pralidoxime or obidoxime and benzodiazepines can be necessary.

Carbon monoxide

Carbon monoxide (CO) is clear, colourless and odourless. It is commonly used in attempted suicide but exposure also occurs from leaking car exhausts or incorrectly installed domestic gas-powered boilers. Occasional exposure occurs in miners and gas workers. Carbon monoxide has a greater affinity for haemoglobin than does oxygen itself and therefore binds preferentially to oxygen-binding sites to form carboxyhaemoglobin. This limits dissociation of oxygen in the tissues resulting in relative tissue hypoxia. Carboxyhaemoglobin also inhibits oxygen binding and oxidative phosphorylation in the mitochondria, further exacerbating functional hypoxia in tissues with a high metabolic demand. Acute exposure causes headache, dizziness, confusion, disturbance of consciousness and behavioural change. Visual disturbance and progressive shortness of breath develop rapidly with subsequent loss of consciousness, seizures, coma and cardiac arrest. Exposed individuals can have pink –red skin, or may be cyanosed. Prolonged acute intoxication is fatal in 25% of exposed individuals. A high proportion of survivors have residual neurological features including extrapyramidal signs. Patients with initial transient choreiform movements can develop progressive tremor, parkinsonism, dystonia and urinary incontinence. A delayed onset encephalopathy may develop after a period of apparent partial or complete recovery with cognitive and personality impairment with memory dysfunction, apathy, mutism, pyramidal signs and the progressive development of vegetative features. There may be elevated levels of carboxyhaemoglobin and MRI shows diffuse symmetrical high intensity white matter change also involving the caudate with bilateral pallidal necrosis (Figure 19.6).

Treatment of acute exposure is by removal from the source and the provision of 100% oxygen. Hyperbaric oxygen can enhance recovery from acute symptoms. However, the prognosis for neurological recovery after carbon monoxide exposure is poor. Insidious chronic low-grade exposure to carbon monoxide can be associated with industrial exposure or badly ventilated and faulty household heating appliances. The syndrome of chronic occult carbon monoxide poisoning is manifest as headache, fatigue, dizziness, paraesthesiae, visual disturbance with chest pain and palpitation associated with ventricular arrhythmias. The diagnosis of low-grade exposure depends on recognition of the syndrome and demonstration of elevated levels of carboxyhaemoglobin. Management depends on identifying the source of carbon monoxide and prompt removal. Oxygen therapy, as discussed earlier, may be necessary.

Marine toxins

Marine toxins are difficult to detect as they are often without colour, taste or odour. Furthermore, most are unaffected by cooking, freezing or salting. They can be divided into:

- *Ingested:* elaborated by marine micro-organisms and ingested in seafood (i.e. ciguatera, puffer fish [tetrodotoxin] and shellfish).
- *Contact* (jellyfish, sea anemone, venomous fish and stingrays)
- *Envenomation toxins* (sea snakes and cone snails): neuropeptides secreted directly by marine creatures which then sting or bite to kill prey or envenomate humans.

Ingested toxins

Ciguatera Ciguatera is the most common form of poisoning associated with seafood. The toxin (ciguatoxin) occurs in reef fish (e.g. snapper or barracuda) who consume an apophytic dinoflagellate which then elaborates the toxin. There are at least four neurotoxins which cause voltage-gated sodium channels to open.

Poisoning leads to the rapid development of acute abdominal cramp, nausea, vomiting and diarrhoea. Peri-oral, limb and trunk paraesthesiae develop 12–48 hours after ingestion of contaminated fish. In the most severe cases there is a characteristic cold allodynia ('temperature reversal'). Cranial nerve palsies, polymyositis or a rapidly progressive sensorimotor and autonomic polyneuropathy affecting bulbar and respiratory muscles can occur. This rarely progresses to limb weakness, flaccid quadriplegia, areflexia and respiratory muscle impairment. Although the condition generally resolves spontaneously within a few days, fatalities are caused by respiratory insufficiency and cardiac dysfunction may occur. Bioassay of the toxin is possible.

Treatment is supportive although parenteral mannitol may prevent the obligate influx of intracellular water as intracellular sodium increases.

Tetrodotoxin Tetrodotoxin (TTX) occurs in the liver and ovaries of puffer fish, toad fish and some types of crabs. The toxin is elaborated by marine bacteria and blocks the action potential of voltage-gated sodium channels in skeletal and cardiac muscle and sensory and motor nerves. TTX blocks voltage-gated sodium

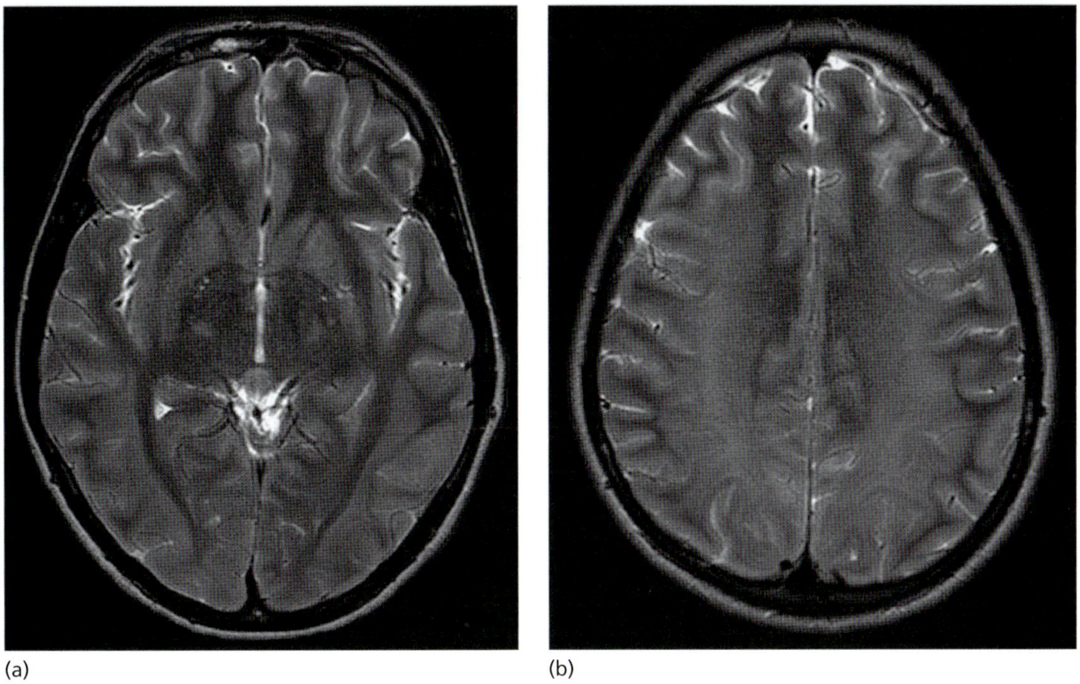

Figure 19.6 Carbon monoxide poisoning following domestic radiator leak. MRI showing (a) symmetrical high intensity basal ganglia and (b) white matter change (axial T2-weighted image).

channels at nanomolar concentrations. Onset is with numbness of the lips and tongue followed by worsening paraesthesiae in the face and limbs with a sense of euphoria and systemic features including gastrointestinal and cardiac disturbance. With ingestion of large amounts of TTX there is worsening neuromuscular paralysis involving the limbs, trunk, cranial nerves bulbar and respiratory muscles leading to death if artificial ventilation is not instituted.

The early fatality rate is high (50–80%). Supportive treatment is successful in most cases because the condition is fully reversible, although it is important to note that patients can be fully conscious in spite of total paralysis. Atropine treatment can be necessary to treat bradycardia.

Scombroid Scombroid poisoning is common as it is caused by poor storage of tuna and similar fish. Toxicity differs from the other marine toxins as it has a histamine-like effect. The onset is rapid and resembles an acute anaphylactic response with pruritus, throbbing headache, erythema, urticaria, paraesthesiae and palpitation; poisoning tends to be self-limiting.

Treatment is with intravenous histamine receptor blockers and supportive care.

Shellfish

- Saxitoxin is a heat-stable water-soluble toxin that is concentrated in shellfish and acts by blocking voltage-gated sodium channels. There is a rapid onset of paraesthesiae, particularly peri-orbital, and limb weakness. There may be severe respiratory involvement including the diaphragm with significant mortality.
- Shellfish toxicity may be caused by secondary infectious agents such as *Vibrio cholerae* and hepatitis A and occurs with bivalve molluscs including clams, mussels, scallops and oysters.
- Neurotoxic shellfish poisoning is caused by brevetoxins which act by opening slow sodium channels. There is simultaneous onset of gastrointestinal and neurological symptoms including tremor, dysphagia, pupillary paralysis and hyporeflexia. The features are similar to ciguatera but milder.
- Amnestic shellfish poisoning, due to associated algal blooms, is caused by the toxin domoic acid which stimulates kainate-type glutamate receptors and has a toxic action on the limbic system leading to severe anterograde and retrograde amnesia, myoclonus, seizures and status epilepticus and coma. Systemic symptoms include labile blood pressure, cardiac dysrhythmia and myoglobinuria. The syndrome can improve gradually over 3 months but permanent residual profound amnestic deficits occur.

Contact toxins contain multiple substances including small polypeptides, large proteins, phospoholipids, glycoproteins, amines and carbohydrates. These venoms are generally thermally instable and act by blocking sodium channels.

Other biological toxins

Snake venom

Snake venom from many members of the Elapidae family, which includes the banded krait and sea snakes, contains toxins that cause neuromuscular junction blockade resulting in a myasthenia-like syndrome, particularly affecting the muscles of neck flexion and the ocular, bulbar and proximal limb muscles, occasionally leading to respiratory paralysis. Onset is often with local pain, swelling and erythema in the region of the bite with local lymph node involvement. The onset of systemic symptoms depends upon the site of the bite and the species, but over 1–12 hours muscle fasciculation, weakness and hypotension can develop with eventual shock.

Presynaptic neuromuscular junction dysfunction occurs with β-bungarotoxin envenomation by banded kraits while α-bungarotoxin causes an additional post-synaptic neuromuscular junction blockade. Snake bites generally cause death not because of the paralysis but because of the systemic effects of proteolytic toxins acting on blood constituents and tissues, often causing extensive haemorrhagic or thrombotic change. Nevertheless, the neurological features can aid diagnosis and choice of appropriate anti-venom.

Spider toxins

The female black widow spider produces a neurotoxin (α-latrotoxin) which acts presynaptically to trigger massive spontaneous neurotransmitter release, from the neuromuscular junction as well as other synapses. There may be intense pain in the region of the bite with a characteristic erythematous target lesion. This is followed by the development of involuntary spasms in the abdominal muscles which spreads to involve the limbs. The funnel-web spider, indigenous to parts of Australia, produces a toxin that affects sodium channels and causes a severe dysautonomia, piloerection, sweating and diaphragm involvement culminating in respiratory arrest.

Treatment is by supportive care in intensive care with anti-venom if available. Muscle spasm is treated with benzodiazepines.

Scorpion toxin

Scorpions elaborate a toxin that has both presynaptic and postsynaptic effects. These may lead to local symptoms followed by the development of progressive severe autonomic impairment with muscle fasciculation and progressive bulbar, respiratory and cardiac involvement. Occasionally, encephalopathy may occur secondary to CNS involvement.

Ticks

Tick toxin has not been isolated or characterised. It causes a rapidly developing, progressive flaccid motor weakness affecting ocular, bulbar, respiratory and limb musculature because of presynaptic inhibition of acetylcholine. It is essential for the tick to be removed immediately.

Fungal poisons

Fungal poisons are highly diverse, and neurotoxic compounds occur in several of the most toxic species. Some members of the Amanitae family such as the fly agaric (*Amanita muscaria*) contain molecules that act at GABA, glutamate and acetylcholine receptors (muscimol, ibotenic acid and muscarine). However, the high fatality associated with death cap (*Amanita phalloides*) ingestion is mainly associated with amatoxin, which inhibits mRNA synthesis and leads to hepatic and nephrotic toxicity. Some members of the Psycilocybe family are used recreationally because of their psychoactive effects. Psilocybins are structural analogues of serotonin and produce LSD-like effects with euphoria, hallucination, tachycardia and eventually seizures.

Lathyrism

Lathyrism occurs in countries where the chickling pea (grass pea) *Lathyrus sativus* is grown, and generally only under conditions of food deprivation. It is endemic in parts of Bangladesh, India and Ethiopia. It is caused by the neurotoxic amino acid β-*N*-oxalylamino-L-alanine (BOAA), which acts as an agonist at the AMPA subclass of glutamate receptors. There is prominent degeneration in Betz cells of the motor cortex and pyramidal tracts. The condition develops with an insidious onset of gait unsteadiness characterised as a lurching and scissoring gait and development of a spastic paraparesis with normal sensory examination. There is no involvement of cognition or cerebellar function. A peripheral sensory neuropathy, which is predominantly demyelinating, can occur in a minority of patients. A related toxin, β-methylamino-L-alanine (BMAA) is present in the fruit of the cycad palm, and has been implicated in the amyotrophic lateral sclerosis–parkinsonism–dementia complex amongst the Chamorro population. However, it remains unclear whether the epidemiological evidence can be explained by consumption of this toxin. Neurolathyrism can be prevented by mixing grass peas with cereal or detoxification by aqueous leaching.

Konzo

Konzo occurs in epidemics in East and Central Africa. It affects children above the age of 3 years and women of childbearing age, causing sudden-onset symmetrical non-progressive permanent spastic paralysis, predominantly affecting the lower limbs but spreading to involve the upper limbs and the optic nerves. The pathology resembles lathyrism with involvement of cortical Betz cells directed towards the lower extremities and their corresponding corticospinal tracts. It is believed to be associated with high dietary levels of cyanide caused by the intake of poorly prepared bitter cassava, particularly if there is protein malnutrition, but the aetiology of Konzo continues to be debated.

Subacute myelo-optico neuropathy

Subacute myelo-optico neuropathy (SMON) is a myeloneuropathy with optic nerve involvement which occurred in Japan between 1955 and 1970. Epidemiological studies suggest that SMON was caused by the antiparasitic drug clioquinol which is a copper chelator and may have led to copper deficiency.

Tropical myelo-neuropathy

This term has been used to describe a number of syndromes caused by various nutritional and toxic causes including malnutrition, cyanide intoxication from cassava consumption and lathyrism. A particular epidemic in Cuba was associated with optic neuropathy, sensori-neural deafness, dorsolateral myelopathy, dysautonomia, bulbar weakness and axonal neuropathy. The condition was associated with an irregular diet, heavy smoking, alcohol and excessive sugar consumption. Treatment with B-group vitamins and folic acid led to marked improvement.

Radiation-induced neurological disease

Exposure to radiation occurs naturally but this is low intensity and carries few risks. Increased levels are associated with exposure to occupational or therapeutic radiation and, rarely, to nuclear weapons. Radiation can be divided to non-ionising and ionising. Non-ionising radiation (e.g. ultraviolet, infra-red, microwaves, radio waves, laser radiation and visible light) has low energy and is therefore unable to break chemical bonds and cause ionisation; thus, injury is caused by local heat production and is generally mild, although damage to retinal and optic nerve fibres can occur. However, ionising radiation is considerably more serious. This radiation is caused by high energy particles or electromagnetic waves (X-rays and gamma rays) which can break chemical bonds and therefore produce ionisation within tissues leading to DNA damage and mutation. Ionising particulate radiation is caused by α particles, electrons, neutrons or protons. Alpha particles (composed of two protons and two neutrons) are produced by uranium, radium and polonium. They lead to high levels of ionising radiation but are usually blocked by paper or clothing and are therefore only toxic if ingested or inhaled (see Neurobiological weapons). Beta particles are high energy electrons emitted from decaying isotopes of strontium 90 which are commonly used to generate X-rays and radiotherapy. Toxicity also occurs with ingestion. High energy neutrons are only produced with nuclear fission but are a serious radiation risk following detonation of a nuclear reaction or if a reactor becomes critical. Proton exposure also occurs naturally from cosmic radiation.

The early effects of radiation, seen after exposure to large doses delivered over a short period of time (>1 Gy), affect rapidly dividing tissues including skin, bone marrow and gut epithelium. The onset is with prodromal gastrointestinal symptoms before the condition manifests with bone marrow suppression, loss of intestinal mucosal cells leading to bowel disturbance and sepsis, and finally cerebrovascular involvement. Management involves meticulous decontamination at the site of exposure and supportive care with transfusion and treatment of sepsis.

Late toxicity following accidental or therapeutic exposure to radiation is usually seen in organs with slowly dividing cells such as the CNS, kidney and liver, causing radiation necrosis. The characteristic delayed complication is malignancy, particularly of the thyroid gland, breast or leukaemia.

Therapeutic radiation

Therapeutic radiotherapy creates ionised oxygen which reacts with cellular DNA. Healthy cells have a greater ability than tumour cells for DNA repair and therefore the cumulative effects of unrepaired DNA result in cell death (apoptosis of tumour cells while healthy cells are more able to repair themselves). Acute complications of therapeutic radiotherapy include encephalopathy which can occur during or up to 1 month after radiotherapy has commenced. It is associated with headaches, nausea, changes in mental state and symptoms suggestive of increased intracranial pressure because of breakdown of the blood–brain barrier and secondary cerebral oedema. The acute effects of therapeutic radiotherapy also include hypersomnolence, encephalopathy, memory disturbance and there can also be gastrointestinal symptoms. MRI shows increased oedema with contrast enhancement which resolves over several months. The condition is caused by damage of the blood–brain barrier and is steroid responsive (Chapter 21).

Early-delayed radiation encephalopathy

Early-delayed radiation encephalopathy develops 1–4 months after radiotherapy and is caused by injury to oligodendroglia producing demyelination and vasogenic oedema. This can present with somnolence, decline in long-term memory and encephalopathy. There can also be brainstem involvement with diplopia, nystagmus, dysarthria and ataxia. This form of radiation encephalopathy resolves over several weeks but occasionally may progress to profound encephalopathy, coma and death. Subacute encephalopathy can also be associated with a myelopathy and a transient brachial plexopathy.

Late-delayed radiation encephalopathy

Late-delayed radiation encephalopathy develops several months or years after cranial irradiation and is associated with diffuse cerebral atrophy, focal radiation necrosis or secondary vascular change. The pathological findings are of demyelination. There can also be signs of raised intracranial pressure. The patient presents with cognitive decline, personality change and gait disturbance developing 6–18 months or more after total brain irradiation. There can be a more indolent intellectual impairment leading to dementia. Delayed effects of radiotherapy also include endocrine dysfunction because of hypothalamic impairment, optic neuropathy, progressive cranial neuropathy, myopathy or chronic progressive myelopathy. The incidence of delayed radiotherapy effects is related to total radiation dosage and the size of fractionated doses. A total dose of >5500 Gy carries a 5% chance of developing radiation necrosis. Risk is increased with a higher daily dosage, if there has been concurrent chemotherapy or if there are underlying vascular risk factors. It can be extremely difficult to distinguish brain radiation injury from the effects of brain tumours by conventional imaging. The hypometabolic state of radiation necrosis may be reflected in metabolic imaging such as fluorodeoxyglucose positron emission tomography (FDG-PET). Brain biopsy will show extensive necrotic tissue without predominance of malignant cells. There is involvement of the white matter with loss of oligodendrocytes and demyelination. There may also be thickened vessels with endothelial proliferation, fibrosis and moderate infiltration of lymphocytes and macrophages (Chapter 21).

Transient radiotherapy myelopathy

Transient radiotherapy myelopathy usually occurs within the first 6 months of treatment, particularly to the cervical spinal cord, although it can continue to develop for 2 years after treatment. It is most commonly seen in patients treated for lymphoma or neck and thoracic neoplasms. Presentation is with mild sensory impairment and Lhermitte's phenomenon. The condition itself is self-limiting and relates to demyelination in the posterior columns. Chronic, usually progressive, myelopathy is a delayed syndrome which develops more than one year after radiotherapy for tumours in the head and neck, cervical or mediastinal region. Focal neurological deficits related to spinal cord involvement include progressive sensory impairment in the lower limbs followed by progressive myelopathy. There may be a transverse myelitis or Brown-Séquard syndrome with sphincter disturbance.

Treatment is with corticosteroids but this only leads to a temporary improvement and there is generally secondary necrosis and atrophy of the cord because of vasculopathy.

Radiation plexopathy

Plexopathy can affect the brachial or lumbar plexus and follows radiotherapy in these regions. It is important to distinguish the development of progressive radiation plexopathy from direct neoplastic involvement of the plexus. The onset is characterised by paraesthesiae and dysaesthesiae with pain and progressive atrophy and weakness developing over several months. It develops 1–3 years or longer after radiotherapy and is particularly associated with high doses of radiotherapy (>6000 Gy), large daily fractionations, lymphoedema, induration of the supraclavicular fossa and myokymia on electromyography (EMG). The condition seems to be caused by small vessel damage and fibrosis; it responds poorly to steroids. Positron emission tomography (PET) imaging of the brachial plexus can distinguish malignant infiltration from radiotherapy-induced plexopathy.

Radiation administered to the neck can also accelerate the development of carotid artery atherosclerosis. This can develop as early as 1 year after treatment but is often delayed by 10 years or more. It is associated with a high treating dose and daily fractionated dose. Cerebral ischaemia can be caused by atherosclerotic embolisation to the brain or haemodynamically significant arterial stenosis. Histologically arterial damage cannot be distinguished from typical atherosclerosis but it occurs in the radiotherapy field.

Lightning and electrical damage to the nervous system

Fifty people are struck by lightning in the United Kingdom each year, with three fatalities. In the United States there are around 100 fatalities per year. For injuries related to technical electricity (at work and at home), the UK annual estimate is approximately 3000 incidents with 30 fatalities. There are some 1500 deaths from electrocution annually in the United States.

Mechanisms of lightning and other electrical damage

Lightning: initiation and pattern of contact

Intra-cloud lightning is the most common form of lightning, but it is cloud-to-ground lightning that causes human injury. Usually, a highly branched discharge, known as the stepped leader, appears below the cloud base and heads toward the ground at a speed of 10^6 m/s. When the tip of the leader approaches within 30 m of the ground, the induced electric field produces an upward connecting discharge, usually from the nearest tallest object(s). When the two discharges meet, the first return stroke begins; this is an intense wave of ionisation that propagates up the leader into the cloud at close to the speed of light. This is followed by a series of further ionising strokes between the cloud and the ground each lasting some 500 ms with 40–80 ms gaps. These gaps are long enough to allow for retinal resolution of the individual strokes – which is why lightning is seen to flicker. The repeated earthbound strokes do not always follow the path of the initial leader, which is why lightning can appear forked. The large current of the return stroke causes the air in the surrounding channel to heat up to about 30 000°K in a microsecond, the channel pressure rises to 20 atmospheres or more; the decay of this pressure wave is heard as thunder.

Although the electrical forces associated with lightning strike are enormous (10^6 V, 30 000 amps), the damage caused to a person struck is limited by the very short duration of the passage of current. In contrast, in accidental electrical injury, the power sources are much less, but contact can last for seconds or even minutes leading to severe thermal injury of tissues in and around the current path.

The prelude to a strike, familiar to many mountaineers, is the build-up of atmospheric charge with buzzing of metallic equipment, skin tingling and hair standing on end. This is a signal for immediate evacuation from prominent features such as a summit or crest of a ridge, if this is feasible. It is unusual for lightning strikes to occur in aircraft, cars or ships at sea because these vehicles act as 'faradic cages'; that is, containers made from a conductor that shields its contents from external electric fields. Because the conductor is an equipotential there is no potential difference within the container.

A major factor that determines injury in lightning strikes is whether the heart or CNS is involved in the current path (either can result in cardiorespiratory arrest), this in turn depends on the way the strike reaches the subject.

1. Direct strikes are the most damaging as the head is usually involved.
2. Side flash occurs when lightning strikes a nearby object such as a tree, and the current arcs to flow through the subject.
3. Ground current injuries are caused by lightning striking the ground near the subject; as the current dissipates, it reaches the subject and passes through them, usually via the legs if they are standing.
4. Most indoor injuries are minor and occur when the subject is shocked by current dissipating along telephone or other wiring.

Many people can be injured at the same time as all of the above mechanisms of current transfer can occur in a single strike; at Ascot racecourse, United Kingdom, in 1956, 46 people were injured, two of them fatally.

Electrical injuries: high and low-voltage

Electrical injuries are usually categorised on the basis of the voltage exposure: high (>1000 V) or low. Low-voltage injuries usually result from exposure in the home, are relatively common but rarely severe (although death can occur from contact with as little as 25 V). High-voltage injuries usually affect those whose occupations bring them into contact with high-tension power lines or electrified rails. Members of the public can be involved in accidents that bring them into contact with these sources – children, anglers carrying their rods, those erecting or using aerials, parachutists and those attempting deliberate self-harm. High-voltage exposure is the cause of some 70% of electrical injuries and death. The voltages and currents associated with electrical exposure are much less than with lightning; however, the period of exposure is longer which magnifies the heating effects of current passage through the body leading to deep tissue necrosis, a complication rarely encountered in lightning strikes. Alternating current can increase this effect if tetanic contraction is induced in flexor muscles of the grasping hand, with periods of exposure approaching a minute or beyond in some cases.

Nervous system complications of lightning and electrical injury

Neurological sequelae can be split into four categories:

1. Immediate and transient (IT)
2. Immediate and prolonged/permanent (IP)
3. Delayed and progressive (DP)
4. Secondary trauma caused by lightning or electrical exposure (e.g. head or spinal injury caused by falls, usually secondary to a loss of consciousness). Complications are generally shared by both types of exposure.

Transient loss of consciousness is the most common symptom associated with both types of electrical exposure, occurring in 70–80% of patients. Confusion, amnesia, paraesthesiae and limb weakness are also common IT symptoms. A specific IT syndrome said to be pathognomic of lightning strike is known as keraunoparalysis (*kerauno*, Greek for thunderbolt; literally, 'smasher'). This is sometimes known as Charcot paralysis; he provided the first description – of short-lived complete lower limb paralysis with spared sphincter function and marked vasoconstriction with limb coolness, lividity and peripheral cyanosis. The symptoms abate over hours or, rarely, days. The pathophysiology is poorly understood. This syndrome should be differentiated from the much rarer true spinal cord syndromes that complicate lightning or electrical injury, which are usually of the IP or DP type.

The neuropathological mechanisms that result in IP or DP symptoms are not fully understood, but probably comprise a mixture of thermal and non-thermal effects of current passage through affected tissues culminating in cell membrane breakdown. Thermally driven cell membrane damage occurs at temperatures as low as 43 °C, although exposure needs to be for 4 hours or more to cause thermal disruption of the bilipid layer. Non-thermal mechanisms include electroporation, a process driven by supraphysiological rises in transmembrane electric potential that causes permanent holes in the cell membrane leading to fatal loss of the ionic gradient. Micropathological CNS lesions vary and include haemorrhage (both gross and petechial), neuronal cell death, myelin breakdown and glial proliferation. Cerebral oedema is seen in cases complicated by hypoxic brain injury secondary to cardiopulmonary arrest. The three most reported DP syndromes affect motor neurones, basal ganglia and the spinal cord. Stroke-like syndromes (particularly venous sinus thrombosis), seizures, extrapyramidal syndromes, isolated cerebellar dysfunction (rare) and spinal cord syndromes at any level (also rare) are all described.

Delayed syndromes are the least common. There is often doubt over any causative link, especially as the time since exposure can be many years. This is well illustrated by a study of psychological morbidity in a series of 165 patients with chronic sequelae of lightning and electrical injury. The mean symptom lag from time of exposure was 4.5 years; the majority of the symptoms reported were suggestive of depression.

There is even less evidence for IP or DP syndromes affecting the peripheral nervous system causing a mononeuropathy or polyneuropathy, with the exception of direct thermal damage causing full-thickness burns through individual nerves. Complex regional pain syndromes are also described and are hard to evaluate.

Non-nervous system complications of lightning and electrical injury

Cardiac

Cardiopulmonary arrest is the most common cause of death in lightning and electrical injuries. Although this can be neurogenic, it is usually caused by the direct effect of current passing through the heart leading to asystole or ventricular fibrillation. Cardiopulmonary resuscitation in these circumstances is often much more successful than out-of-hospital arrests from other causes.

Skin and muscle damage

Fern-shaped superficial cutaneous burns are sometimes seen following lightning strikes; these heal, but discoloration can persist for some years, or even permanently. Lightning rarely causes major skin or deep tissue burns; however, electrical injury, especially of high-voltage type, can be devastating to deep tissues. It is not possible to predict the amount of deep tissue injury from the overlying skin involvement. Striated muscle is particularly sensitive to AC current and high-voltage exposure is often complicated by rhabdomyolysis, subsequent renal failure, compartment syndromes and surgical amputation following overwhelming limb damage. Cataracts complicate lightning and electrical injuries that involve the head and neck in the current path, including lightning strikes that dissipate along telephone wires.

Management

Initial management includes basic resuscitation and CPR. All patients suffering lightning strike or high-voltage electric injury require transfer to hospital for appropriate therapy and, in some cases, ECG monitoring. Asymptomatic patients with low-voltage injuries in the absence of nervous system, cardiac or skin involvement need not be admitted. The neurologist, like members of other specialist teams, is most likely to be called upon to help with patients with moderate to severe injuries following lightning or electrical injury. There is no good evidence base for particular treatment of neurological symptoms caused by electrical current exposure; symptoms should be treated on their own merits.

Heat stroke

Heat stroke is present if the core body temperature exceeds 40 °C (104 °F). It can occur either as a result of vigorous and prolonged exertion or during excessively hot weather, when it affects those who have difficulty with heat regulation including children, the elderly or those with chronic medical problems causing impairment of the mechanisms of heat loss (e.g. dermatological disease or following ingestion of anticholinergic drugs).

In non-exertional heat stroke, presentation is usually with progressive impairment of consciousness manifest as irritability, confusion, delusions and hallucinations culminating in coma. There is usually anhidrosis and patients can also develop cranial nerve abnormalities, early cerebellar dysfunction (ataxia, tremor and dysarthria), seizures and opisthotonus, and the development of cerebral oedema with decerebrate posturing and status epilepticus. Systemic involvement leads to a hyperdynamic circulation with tachycardia and postural hypotension (caused by vasodilatation of cutaneous vessels and venous pooling), dehydration, congestive cardiac failure, systemic inflammatory response syndrome, multi-organ failure, myocardial damage and rhabdomyolysis.

Following exertional heat stroke, non-specific symptoms of heat exhaustion are often unrecognised before impairment of consciousness develops: fatigue, weakness, nausea, vomiting, abdominal pain, muscular cramp, headache and syncope. Predisposing factors include exercise in inappropriate clothing (e.g. wet-suits), viral illness, obesity, dehydration, poor physical fitness, excessive alcohol and illicit drugs (e.g. cocaine and amphetamines). When heat stroke becomes established the clinical features are identical to those patients with non-exertional causes.

Treatment is with rest, removal from the hot environment and correction of dehydration and electrolyte disturbances. Gentle cooling and oral rehydration is adequate in mild cases but in more severe cases ventilatory support, intravenous fluids and intensive monitoring of fluid, electrolyte balance and cardiac and neurological function is necessary. Cold gastric or peritoneal lavage or the use of cooling devices or controlled hypothermia can be of value. Iced water immersion is an efficient form of reducing the core temperature rapidly but is usually impracticable in patients with impaired consciousness and highly uncomfortable for those patients who are awake. Evaporation techniques are safer and as effective as immersion.

A poor prognosis is suggested by the development of lactic acidosis, acute renal failure, hypercalcaemia, coagulopathy or prolonged coma (>4 hours). Muscle necrosis may lead to a grossly elevated creatine kinase level. Death occurs as a consequence of cerebral oedema and herniation. It is essential to recognise persons at risk of heat stroke and to ensure they are not exposed to excessive heat and maintain adequate fluid replacement.

Hypothermia and non-freezing cold injury

Accidental hypothermia is the unintentional decline in core temperature below 35 °C (95 °F). Primary hypothermia is caused by exposure to cold; secondary hypothermia occurs when a disease causes failure of thermoregulation (e.g. CNS tumour leading to hypothalamic impairment, exposure to toxins or neurodegenerative disorders). Hypothermia causes bradycardia because of decreased depolarisation of cardiac pacemaker cells which is not mediated by the vagus and is resistant to therapies such as atropine. Hypothermia progressively depresses the CNS. With mild hypothermia there is confusion, lethargy, loss of fine motor coordination with ataxia, dysarthria and slowed reflexes. Severe hypothermia (<28 °C) is characterised by rigidity, areflexia, reduced consciousness and eventually coma. At core temperatures <25 °C, brain electrical activity becomes abnormal and below 20 °C the EEG can be flat and consistent with brain death.

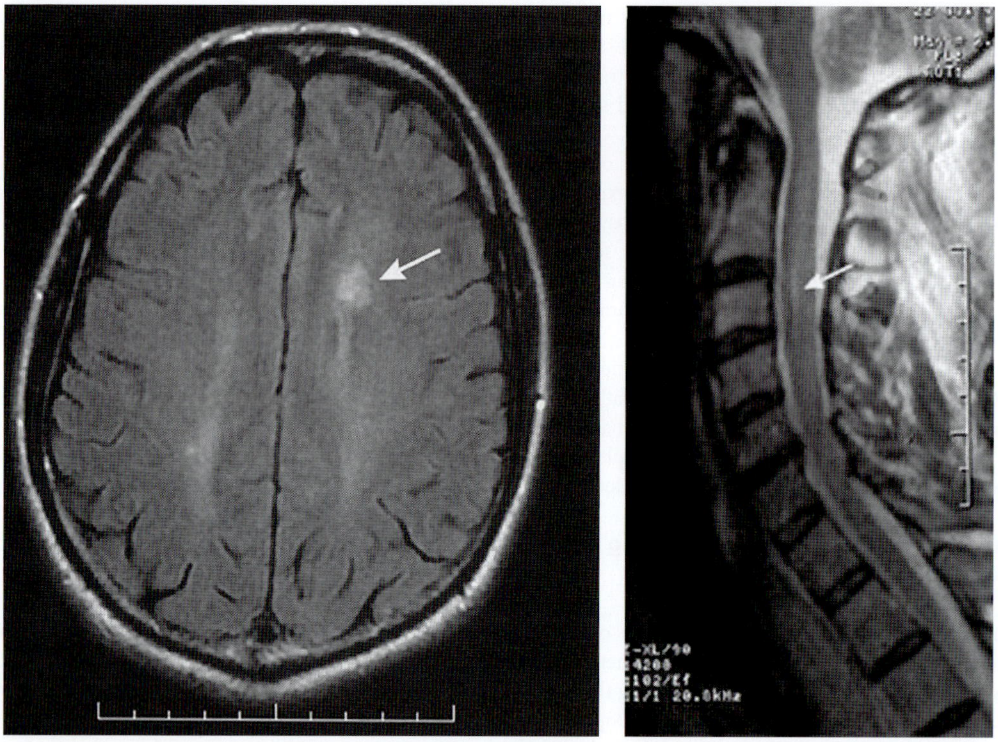

(a) (b)

Figure 19.7 Decompression sickness: (a) MRI T2 high signal lesion (arrow); (b) high signal at C3–C4 (sagittal (arrow) T2WI). Source: Jallul 2007. Reproduced with permission of Macmillan.

Management is aimed at preventing arrhythmias, particularly ventricular fibrillation, ensuring adequate oxygenation and initiating external and core rewarming using warm intravenous fluid, abdominal lavage and, if necessary, cardiopulmonary bypass. Intensive intervention is indicated, even in those who appear dead. Hypothermia is neuroprotective; some patients recover completely.

Non-freezing cold injury describes persistent painful and autonomic symptoms, usually in the feet, following exposure to temperatures approaching 0 °C. Symptoms can persist for many years and are occasionally permanent.

Diving

The effects of diving relate to the high pressure environment and the consequences of decompression. Barotrauma occurs when divers descend beyond a depth of 100 m breathing gas mixtures of helium and oxygen. Damage occurs because the volume of a gas decreases under a high pressure (Boyle's law). At depth, the body space fails to equate with the external environmental pressure. Barotrauma can also affect the middle or inner ear, sinuses, teeth or gastrointestinal tract causing headache, facial pain, vertigo, hearing loss and abdominal pain. Direct high pressure injury to the CNS leads to a progressive rest or intention tremor, myoclonus, hyper-reflexia and transient cognitive and memory disturbance.

Decompression sickness

Decompression sickness (DCS) occurs because the solubility of a gas increases under high pressure (Henry's law). Therefore, nitrogen dissolved in the tissues at depth will be released as gas as the diver ascends to a higher atmospheric pressure. DCS ('the bends') occurs when surfacing to a lower pressure causes the release of air bubbles (usually composed of nitrogen) into the bloodstream and tissues. DCS usually develops within 2 hours of surfacing but can be delayed by up to 36 hours. DCS type I is characterised by limb and joint pain, while DCS type II causes cardiorespiratory impairment and involvement of the CNS because of direct mechanical effects of the air bubbles or because of arterial gas emboli. Cerebral DCS usually involves the arterial circulation leading to alteration in the level of consciousness, weakness, headache, gait disturbance, fatigue, diplopia or visual loss. There can be acute hemispheric dysfunction causing hemiparesis, aphasia and hemianopia and/or progressive encephalopathy, coma and death. Pathologically, the condition is characterised by oedema, haemorrhagic infarction and axonal degeneration with demyelination. Occasionally, brainstem involvement may lead to vestibular disturbance. Spinal cord DCS presents with partial myelopathy that localises to the thoracic cord although the level can vary from C4 to L1. The onset is often acute (<3 minutes of surfacing) with the development of weakness, paraesthesiae and numbness of the legs with early bladder involvement. The severity can vary from mild sensory involvement to dense limb weakness. MRI may show high signal lesions on T2-weighted imaging (Figure 19.7).

The treatment of established DCS requires the urgent provision of hyperbaric oxygen. While most cases resolve, the prognosis is uncertain and residual deficits occur in some patients.

Arterial and venous gas emboli

Arterial gas emboli formed in the tissues can also enter the venous circulation. There is a particular risk, even following a shallow dive, if there is a patent foramen ovale with a right to left cardiac shunt that air will enter the systemic arterial circulation resulting in cerebral air embolism.

Altitude medicine

Acute mountain sickness and cerebral oedema

Acute mountain sickness (AMS) is a relatively common condition occurring in unacclimatised subjects ascending rapidly to 2500 m or above. It is usually self-limiting with appropriate management. A small proportion of patients develop the far more serious complications of cerebral and pulmonary oedema (usually >4000 m). AMS is manifest as headache, fatigue, weakness, dizziness, difficulty sleeping and gastrointestinal symptoms such as anorexia, vomiting and nausea. A chronic form can occur as a consequence of persisting hypobaric hypoxia causing persistent malaise and headache. AMS may be prevented by slow ascent (height should be gained slowly above 2500 m at the rate of 300–500 m/day) carrying little and with frequent rests. Symptomatic treatment includes analgesics and antiemetics. Acetazolamide, a carbonic anhydrase inhibitor, is also widely used for prevention but is associated with significant toxicity and it is recommended that a therapeutic trial should be undertaken at sea level before use. Dexamethasone may also help.

With continued ascent, pulmonary and cerebral oedema can occur. On a 6000-m peak there is only 50% of sea level oxygen and the arterial pO_2 is approximately 50 mmHg. Brain perfusion (cerebral blood flow) increases at even modest altitude to 3500 m in response to hypobaric hypoxia and can lead to the development of cerebral oedema. Presentation can be gradual or acute. Onset is usually with severe headache and progressive ataxia. There can be neuropsychological effects including impairment of short-term memory, defects in verbal fluency and cognitive function with the development of hallucinations. Papilloedema (Figure 19.8) and focal signs including cranial nerve palsies, hemiplegia and seizures can develop and impaired consciousness evolving from drowsiness to coma may develop over 12–72 hours. Sudden devastating altitude-related cerebral oedema may develop unpredictably at extreme altitude (usually >7000 m) in climbers who have been well acclimatised.

Investigations are not usually possible but where MRI has been undertaken in high altitude cerebral oedema there are features of brain oedema (Figure 19.9) and posterior reversible leukoencephalopathy with changes in the splenium of the corpus callosum. In fatal cases there are ring micro-haemorrhages in the brain, arterial and venous thrombosis (Figure 19.10).

It is essential to have a high index of suspicion for these conditions. Exercise should be avoided and the patient should descend as soon

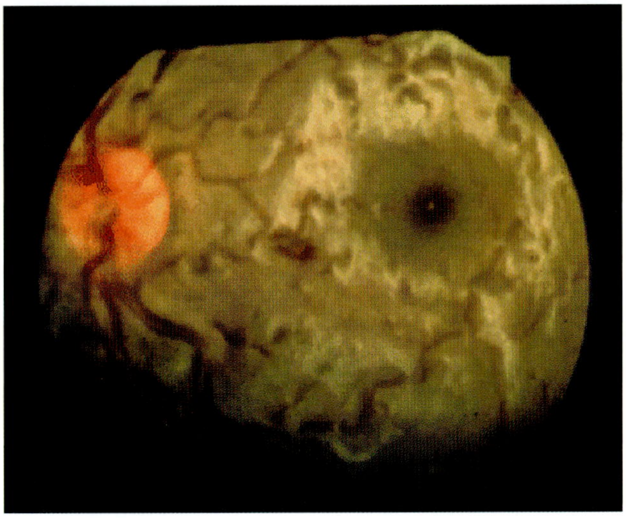

Figure 19.8 Abrupt retinal oedema at extreme altitude: papilloedema, retinal oedema and venous congestion.

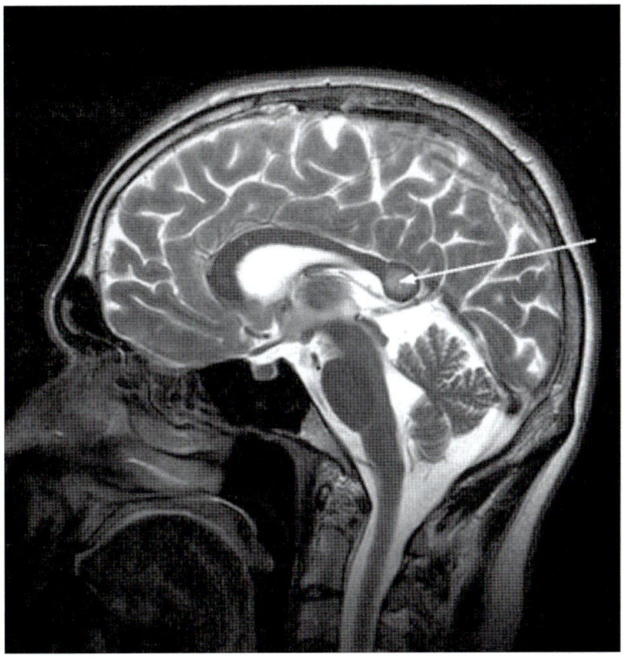

Figure 19.9 High altitude cerebral oedema: T2-weighted MR scan showing oedema of splenium of corpus callosum (arrow). Courtesy of Dr S. Wong.

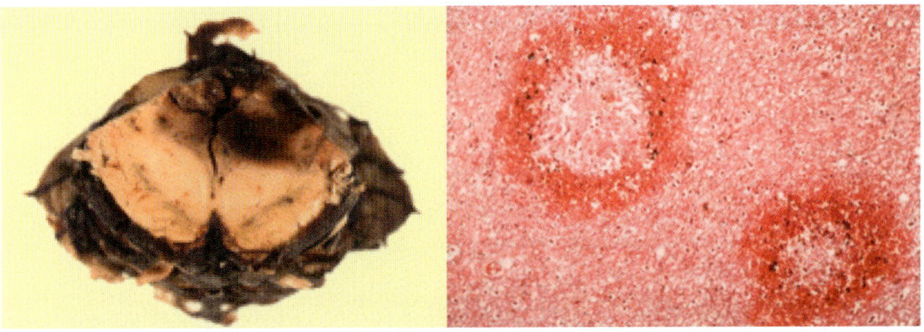

(a) (b)

Figure 19.10 Acute mountain sickness developing gradually into fatal cerebral oedema: (a) brainstem showing haemorrhagic infarction; (b) ring haemorrhages in cerebral white matter. Courtesy of Professor D. Heath.

Table 19.3 Treatments for severe forms of altitude illness.

Manouevre/drug	Regimen	Comment
Descent	250 m as a minimum	Essential, if possible
Dexamethasone	8 mg + 4 mg every 6 h (IV, IM, oral)	Often helpful in minutes, used primarily for brain oedema
Nifedipine	10 mg + 20 mg sustained release every 12 h	Mainly for pulmonary oedema
Oxygen	2–4 L/min by mask or cannula	Always helpful, calming
Portable chamber	2–4 psi for 2–3 h	Never truly portable/claustrophobia

IM, intramuscular; IV, intravenous.

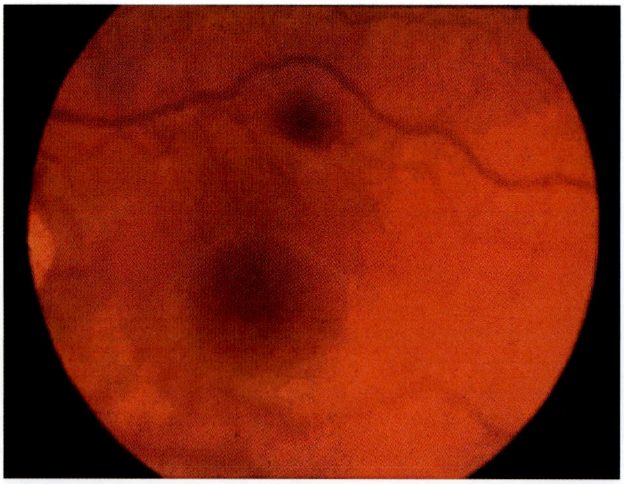

Figure 19.11 Symptomless retinal haemorrhages at 5500 m.

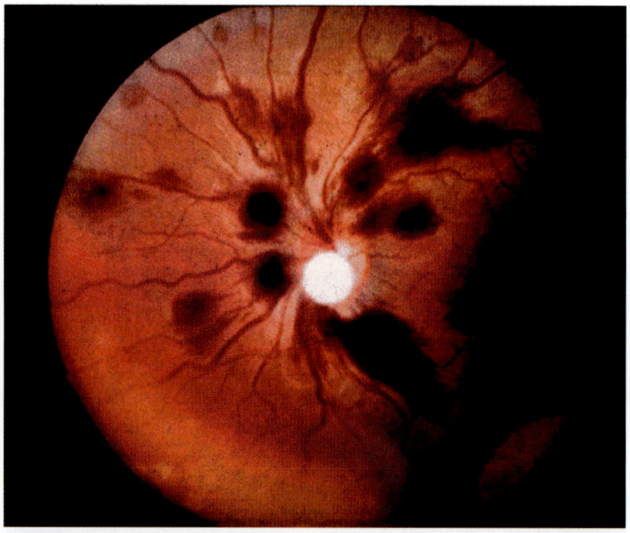

Figure 19.12 High altitude retinopathy with permanent visual loss. Retina showing extensive haemorrhagic change.

and as fast as feasible – most deaths occur because the subject remains at a high altitude. Treatment is with 8 mg dexamethasone by mouth or injection and then 4 mg dexamethasone 4-hourly for several days before gradually weaning the dose over a week. Oxygen inhalation (6 L/minute initially) or hyperbaric oxygen administered by a portable pressure chamber should be used if available (Table 19.3).

Retinal haemorrhages are common at >5000 m but rarely cause visual loss and usually resolve spontaneously (Figure 19.11). They are not a manifestation of high altitude cerebral oedema. Cerebral infarction manifest as stroke or transient ischaemic attack (TIA) occurs more commonly than expected and is probably related to dehydration and polycythaemia secondary to hypoxia. Retinopathy with permanent visual loss can occur (Figure 19.12).

High altitude pulmonary oedema

High altitude pulmonary oedema is also caused by hypoxia but is often less obvious than cerebral oedema. It is manifest as breathlessness at rest, dry cough, dyspnoea, crackles in the lung bases and the production of copious pink frothy sputum. Once again the patient must be evacuated immediately to a lower altitude and rapidly provided with oxygen inhalation at a minimum of 2 L/min. Acetazolamide 250 mg 6-hourly may also be valuable and nifedipine and prophylactic salmeterol have also been used (Figure 19.13).

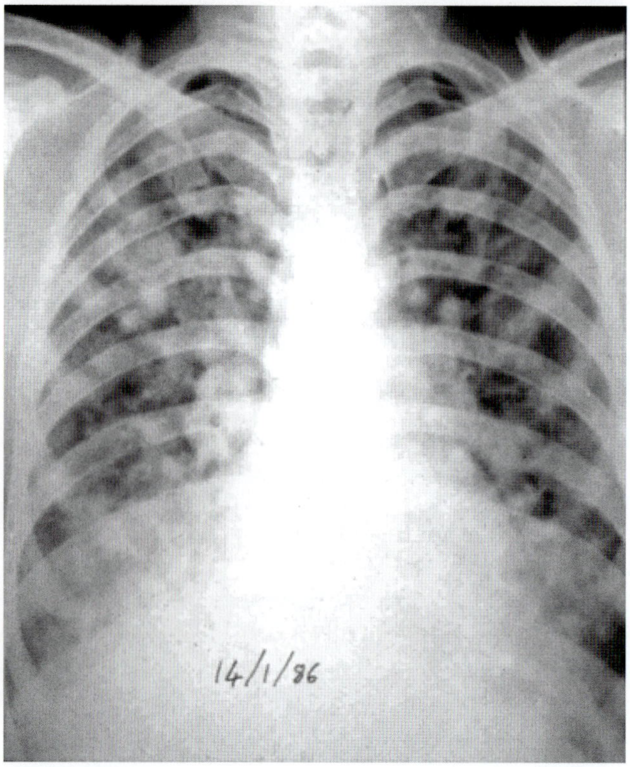

Figure 19.13 Chest X-ray showing high altitude pulmonary oedema.

Neurobiological weapons

Biological weapons, although simple to produce, can be highly potent and difficult to detect. Indeed, recognition that a chemical or biological attack has occurred can be extremely difficult because of the delay before clinical manifestations become apparent. Diagnosis may depend on recognising a pattern of clustering or atypical illness in animals or humans, possibly occurring at an unusual age. Potential biological agents of terrorism are listed in Table 19.4.

Modes of release

Aerosol release of infectious particles is the most efficient form of dissemination and can be accomplished relatively easily and particles remain suspended in the air for many hours increasing the infective capabilities. In contrast, contamination of food and water is more difficult to undertake as large amounts of infective agents are required. Dissemination using bombs or missiles would be of limited value because much of the infective agent is lost at impact or explosion. Contamination of mail items or direct injection can only be undertaken on a small scale and is unreliable. Finally, dissemination of infectious diseases could theoretically be undertaken by infiltrating a contagious person.

Nerve agents

Organophosphates

Organophosphates (see Neurological disorders associated with exposure to toxic substances) act as cholinesterase inhibitors to precipitate the rapid onset of cholinergic crises by hyperstimulation of muscarinic and nicotinic receptors. Unless a specific reactivator (an oxime) is administered, recovery will not occur for several months until acetylcholinesterases can be resynthesised. Organophosphates have been used in attacks in Japan, Iraq and Syria.

Sarin, Sabin, Tabun, Soman, Cyclosarin, VX These nerve agents are all liquids at room temperature and are tasteless and odourless. However, most are spontaneously volatile and evaporate rapidly and spontaneously apart from VX, which is an oily liquid that evaporates more slowly. All are toxic via inhalation or skin absorption. The agent that has been the most likely to be used is sarin, which is usually absorbed by inhalation and has been deployed against civilian populations in recent conflicts.

The onset of symptoms is with headache, pupillary constriction leading to blurred vision and cholinergic symptoms of rhinorrhoea, sialorrhoea and bronchorrhoea with secondary bronchoconstriction and respiratory distress. There may be nausea, vomiting, abdominal cramps and diarrhoea, bradyarrythmias, tachyarrhythmias and hypertensive crisis. Progressive cholinergic muscle involvement leads to fasciculation, weakness and respiratory muscle impairment causing apnoea and respiratory arrest. VX is a viscous liquid that degrades rapidly on exposure to the atmosphere but is easily absorbed through the skin and is extremely toxic, causing rapid involvement of the neuromuscular junction leading to irreversible muscle contraction and a complete paralysis of all musculature. VR, a structural isomer of VX, also leads to cholinergic crisis with profound irreversible cholinergic weakness, seizures and cardiorespiratory arrest.

The management of nerve agents involves decontamination, supportive care and the administration of specific antidotes. Seizures require urgent benzodiazepine therapy with im or buccal midazolam. Decontamination is undertaken by immediate removal of all clothing to prevent continuing exposure and careful scrubbing with water and antiseptic. Supportive care can require intubation and ventilatory support. Atropine is recommended as a first line treatment, this competes with acetylcholine at the post-synaptic muscarinic receptors and may prevent cholinergic crisis, thus drying secretions and resolving bronchoconstriction. It may be necessary to administer repeated doses of atropine every 5–10 minutes and extremely high doses may be required. Oximes (pralidoxime, obidoxime) cleave the nerve agent into harmless and rapidly metabolised fragments, thus restoring normal catalytic activity. They also react directly with acetylcholinesterases and therefore work equally at mixed cholinergic sites. Pralidoxime chloride is the drug of choice but its use is limited because binding leads to a chemical change in the nerve agent that blocks the ability of the oxime to reactivate the complexes. Prior to exposure

Table 19.4 Potential biological agents of terrorism.

Bacteria
Bacillus anthracis
Brucella suis
Francisella tularensis
Rickettsia
Salmonella typhi
Shigella
Vibrio cholerae
Yersinia pestis
Viruses
Encephalomyelitis
Engineered virus
Smallpox
Viral haemorrhagic fever
Chemical agents
Hydrogen cyanide
Zyklon B
Chlorine
Mustard gas
Phosgene
Nerve agents: • Tabun • Sarin • Sabin • Soman • Cyclosarin • VX • VR
Toxin
Aflatoxin
Botulinum
Antitoxin A
Mycotoxins
Ricin
Marine toxins • Tetrodotoxin • Saxitoxin
Radioactive toxins

pyridostigmine can be of value as it reversibly binds a proportion of acetylcholinesterase allowing it to become gradually available to counteract the effects of the permanent blockade caused by the nerve agent. This can be of use for rescue workers. The long-term effects of nerve agents remain unclear.

Other toxins and poisons

Antitoxin A Antitoxin A is elaborated by a freshwater bacterium and is an acetylcholine agonist that causes cholinergic crisis with fixed permanent muscle contraction as it is not released from the receptor. Furthermore, the toxin inhibits acetylcholinesterase leading to a further cholinergic stimulation. A severe flaccid paralysis with respiratory muscle involvement leads to apnoea. Management is with supportive care as there is no specific antidote although oximes may have some value.

Mycotoxin Mycotoxins are produced by fungi and can be used as biological agents as they are resistant to destruction and rapidly absorbed through the skin. The mechanism of action involves the blocking of protein synthesis leading to inhibition of mitochondrial metabolism. There may be rapid cutaneous, respiratory and CNS toxicity. Management requires decontamination and supportive care.

Ricin Ricin is extracted from the bean of the castor plant. It inhibits DNA replication leading to cellular necrosis when internalised in cells. Historically, it has been used to assassinate individuals rather than as a weapon of mass destruction. It can be administered as an aerosol, droplet or by injection and leads to rapid tissue necrosis in the gastrointestinal tract, kidney and heart. Convulsions may occur. Management is supportive.

Marine toxins (see neurological disorders associated with exposure to toxic substances) Marine toxins are discussed above.

Dioxin and Agent Orange These were particularly used during the Vietnam War as defoliants and herbicides. The long-term consequences are now recognised and there may be cognitive and neuropsychiatric impairment as well as a distal sensory peripheral neuropathy particularly affecting the lower limbs.

Radioactive toxins Polonium 210 is an α emitter that is highly toxic and causes damage to organic tissue if ingested, inhaled or absorbed, but does not penetrate epidermis and therefore is not hazardous if the source remains outside the body.

Botulinus toxin Botulism has been discussed in Chapter 9. The toxin is highly potent and can be readily aerosolised and absorbed by inhalation or ingestion into the gastointestinal tract, persisting in this state for many weeks. The toxin is relatively easily degraded by exposure to heat, acidity or sunlight for >12 hours. Recovery follows only after there is regeneration of new axons which can take many months. Presynaptic inhibition of cholinergic autonomic (muscarinic) and motor (nicotinic) receptors leads to an extensive flaccid paralysis.

Anthrax Spores of the Gram-positive organism *Bacillus anthracis* can be inhaled, ingested or absorbed through the skin and cause a severe haemorrhagic bacterial meningitis in addition to primarily pulmonary, cutaneous and gastrointestinal toxicity. The diagnosis is made difficult by the prolonged interval from exposure to presentation. Involvement of the CNS greatly increases the risk of mortality. Ciprofloxacin is the treatment of choice but doxycycline, clindamycin or rifampicin are also effective. Pre-exposure vaccination may have some protective effect. *B. anthracis* is easy to produce, the spores are hardy, highly infectious and remain in the environment for many years. They can be stored almost indefinitely and can only be removed by filtration with small pores or by formaldehyde. Aerosol deployment of dry spores risks secondary infection and spores could be effective in water or food supplies.

Tularemia This is caused by *Francisella tularensis*, a non-motile aerobic Gram-positive coccobacillus that is highly infective and can cause a meningitis or encephalitis although an atypical pneumonia is more frequent. First line treatment is an aminoglycoside antibiotic (streptomycin or gentamycin); alternatives include doxycycline, chloramphenicol and ciprofloxacin.

Smallpox Smallpox is a potentially devastating infection caused by variola, which is a DNA virus and infectious in droplet form. The last known case was in 1977 but intact virus remains in a number of laboratories, and is a potential neurobiological weapon. The Variola virus invades mucosal cells of the respiratory system before viraemic dissemination to bone marrow, spleen and lymph nodes. Immediate vaccination following exposure is essential and the subject should be isolated as soon as possible.

Other viruses Arboviruses, causing viral haemorrhagic fever, might be used as biological weapons because of high infectivity, low infectious dose and the absence of any specific treatment. However, most forms of arbovirus encephalitis are self-limiting. With supportive care patients recover well from these forms of infection although fatal encephalitis can occur. Vaccines are of limited benefit and treatment is with supportive care.

Vitamin deficiencies and toxicity

The vitamin deficiency syndromes are summarised in Table 19.5.

Vitamin A

Vitamin A deficiency occurs in fat malabsorption syndromes and leads to a variety of ophthalmic disorders. Retinol is required for the synthesis of rhodopsin, a visual pigment necessary for normal rod function in the retina; its deficiency leads to night blindness. There can also be corneal ulceration and carotenisation of the conjunctiva. 'Bitot spots' are white foam-like lesions, which appear on the side of the cornea and are characteristic of vitamin A deficiency.

Vitamin A toxicity is associated with ingestion of carotene-rich liver and proprietary treatments and may cause idiopathic intracranial hypertension. The skin is often dry and pruritic and generalised joint and bone pains occur. Serum retinol levels may be helpful to establish the diagnosis.

Vitamin B_1 (thiamine)

Thiamine is found in most food and cereals but reduced intestinal absorption occurs in alcoholism and malabsorption syndromes. Deficiency is also associated with malnutrition, inadequate parenteral nutrition, haemodialysis, uraemia or repeated vomiting.

Table 19.5 Vitamin deficiency syndromes.

Vitamin	Solubility	Name	Principal deficiency syndromes
A	F	Retinol	Night blindness
B_1	W	Thiamine	Congestive cardiac failure (wet beri beri) Sensory axonal neuropathy (dry beri beri) Wernicke–Korsakoff syndrome
B_3	W	Niacin (nicotinic acid)	Pellagra (dermatitis, diarrhoea, dementia)
B_5	W	Pantothenic acid	Paraesthesiae and dysasthaesiae (burning feet syndrome)
B_6	W	Pyridoxine	Peripheral neuropathy (ataxic, axonal, sensorimotor)
B_{12}	W	Cobalamine	Subacute combined degeneration (axonal sensorimotor neuropathy and myelopathy) Optic atrophy Progressive cognitive impairment
Biotin	W		Non-specific – myalgia, dysasthaesiae, anorexia, nausea, dermatitis
Folate	W		Mild cognitive impairment, depression, elevated homocysteine levels (risk factor for vascular disease)
C	W	Ascorbic acid	Scurvy – impaired collagen synthesis with disordered connective tissue – ecchymosis, bleeding gums, petechiae, coiled hair, impaired wound healing, weakness
D	F	Cholecalciferol, ergocalciferol	Proximal myopathy, osteomalacia, rickets
E	F	Tocopherol	Spinocerebellar degeneration with limb ataxia, sensory axonal neuropathy
K	F	Phylloquinone	Haemorrhagic disease

F, fat; W, water.

Thiamine depeletion can develop acutely and is a medical emergency because of the development of congestive cardiac failure and peripheral oedema (wet beri-beri), an axonal sensory neuropathy (dry beri-beri) or Wernicke–Korsakoff syndrome (cerebral beri-beri). The effects of thiamine deficiency are discussed later.

Vitamin B_3 (niacin, nicotinic acid)

Niacin deficiency leads to the syndrome of pellagra. The condition occurs in populations that are dependent on corn but has decreased in frequency as white bread is now enriched with niacin. Clinically, pellagra is characterised by the development of dermatitis, diarrhoea and dementia (the three D's). The onset is usually with gastrointestinal symptoms including anorexia, diarrhoea and stomatitis. Skin changes are also frequently seen and erythema particularly affects the face, chest and dorsal surfaces of the hands and the feet. There can be mood changes, fatigue, malaise, lethargy and confusion with progression to neuropsychiatric disturbances including apathy, inattentiveness and memory loss or the development of spastic paraparesis with startle myoclonus. The cognitive impairment, which occurs in chronic alcoholics even with adequate thiamine replacement, is probably caused by niacin deficiency and is characterised by a defect in recent memory, visuospatial ability, abstract reasoning and speed of information processing. Treatment is with oral niacin replacement, often provided in food supplements.

Vitamin B_6 (pyridoxine)

This is important in the metabolism of many amino acids. Deficiency often occurs in infancy because of feeds containing inadequate levels of B_6. In children there can be hyperirritability, exaggerated auditory startle and recurrent convulsions leading to status epilepticus. Neonatal pyridoxine deficiency can cause seizures and all neonatal seizures should be treated with pyridoxine if the cause is not immediately obvious (Chapter 7). In adults, pyridoxine deficiency is usually secondary to medication including isoniazid, hydralazine and penicillamine. There can be peripheral neuropathy with distal weakness and painful sensory loss, absent tendon reflexes and Romberg's sign. High dose pyridoxine also causes a distal sensory axonal neuropathy with sensory ataxia.

Vitamin B_{12} deficiency (see Chapter 16)

Vitamin B_{12} is abundant in meat, fish and animal by-products. Approximately 90% of total body B_{12} is stored in the liver. Because of the large body stores, even with severe impairment of B_{12} absorption, the symptoms and signs of B_{12} deficiency can take many years to evolve. Daily requirements are small and only rarely can B_{12} deficiency arise because of dietary insufficiency. It is associated with pernicious anaemia caused by defective intrinsic factor production by the gastric parietal cells but can also follow gastrectomy or small intestine disorder including surgical resection of the terminal ileum

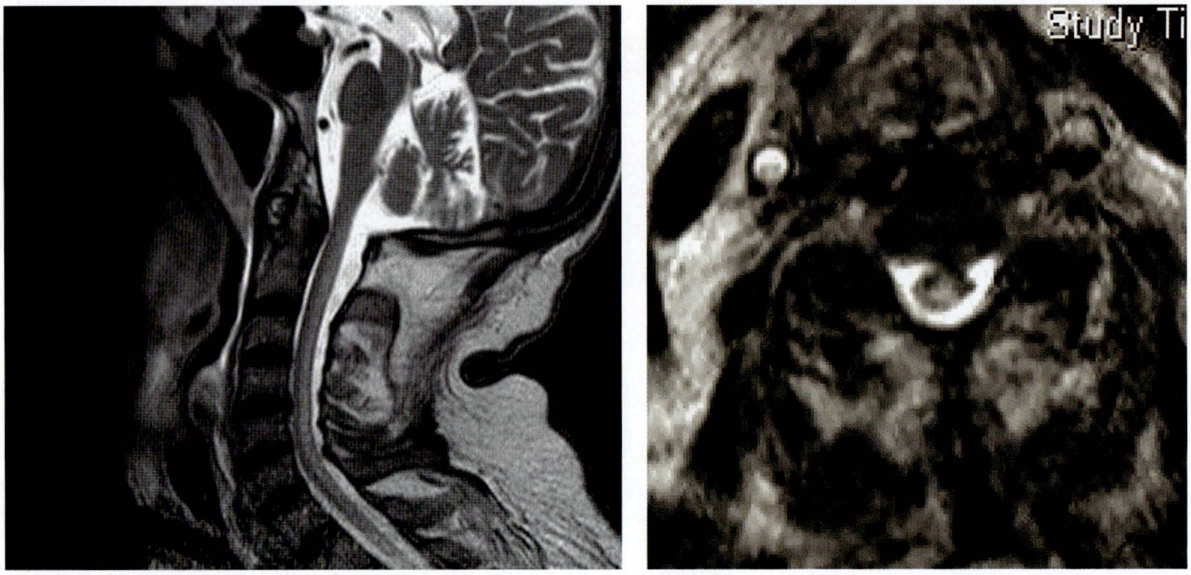

(a) (b)

Figure 19.14 T2-weighted sagittal (a) and axial MRI (b) of the cervical and upper thoracic spinal cord of a patient with subacute combined degeneration of the spinal cord.

and blind loop syndrome. The elderly, vegetarians and patients taking H2 blockers for ulcers are at particularly high risk.

Systemic manifestations of vitamin B_{12} deficiency include gastrointestinal involvement, characterised by the development of glossitis and a pan-enteropathy with diarrhoea and malabsorption of nutrients. Neurological features occur in up to 40% of patients with B_{12} deficiency but these evolve over several months or longer. Symptoms develop insidiously with progressive paraesthesiae in the hands and feet with weakness and unsteadiness of gait culminating in peripheral neuropathy and myelopathy. Central manifestations include confusion, depression, progressive hallucination and mental slowing. Patients occasionally present with isolated cognitive or psychiatric disturbances but any direct relationship between B_{12} and dementia remains unclear. There can also be optic neuropathy.

Subacute combined degeneration of the cord

This effect of B_{12} deficiency is characterised by a sensorimotor axonal neuropathy and myelopathy. Neuropathic manifestations include distal paraesthesiae, numbness, gait ataxia and diminished proprioception in the lower limbs, while the myelopathic component leads to variable motor impairment because of pyramidal tract dysfunction with extensor plantar responses; the reflexes are variable depending on the extent of cord and peripheral nerve involvement. Incontinence of bowel and bladder with impotence and postural hypotension occur as part of the myelopathy. Visual impairment is also associated with B_{12} deficiency with the development of optic atrophy, impaired acuity and centro-caecal scotoma. Brainstem and cerebellar signs are occasionally present.

Progressive cognitive impairment is characterised by memory loss, behavioural affective changes and occasionally stupor and coma. The blood film shows the development of a macrocytic anaemia with hypersegmented neutrophil nuclei and megaloblastic change in the bone marrow. Serum cobalamin levels can be used as a screening test and the Schilling test is valuable in demonstrating impaired absorption of vitamin B_{12} even if serum levels are normal. Elevated levels of methylmalonic acid (MMA) and plasma total homocysteine (HCy) are useful but limited ancilliary tests. MRI may show extensive white matter change which can become confluent with disease progression culminating in leukoencephalopathy. The spinal cord shows abnormalities in the lateral and posterior columns with enhancement and residual changes may persist after treatment (Figure 19.14). Visual and somatosensory evoked potentials are delayed. Nerve conduction studies reveal small or absent sensory action potentials reflecting an axonal neuropathy in approximately 80% of patients.

The clinical features of nitrous oxide intoxication, copper deficiency and the vacuolar myelopathy of AIDS are identical to those of subacute combined degeneration because they are associated with cobalamine inactivity or deficiency.

The pathological changes of subacute combined degeneration of the spinal cord include spongy change with focal loss of myelin and axonal destruction in the white matter of the spinal cord particularly affecting posterior and lateral columns of the cervical and upper thoracic spinal cord. The peripheral nerves show axonal degeneration without significant demyelination. There may also be involvement of the optic nerves and cerebral white matter.

With adequate treatment, some of the deficits of B_{12} deficiency can be reversible with most improvement occurring within the first 6 months of treatment. The myelopathy is least likely to make a complete recovery. B_{12} replacement should be given a minimum of twice weekly for 2 weeks, followed by monthly injections. If there is malabsorption of B_{12} then injections should be continued every three months for life. With full treatment at least partial improvement occurs in most patients but daily oral supplementation with large amounts of cobalamine may be necessary.

Folate deficiency

Absorption of folate takes place in the jejunum and ileum with levels being reduced in chronic alcoholism and following small bowel resection or disease. A number of drugs interfere with folate metabolism including sulfasalazine, methotrexate and azathioprine. Overt neurological deficit is unusual in folate deficiency but there can be mild cognitive impairment, depression and an increased risk of stroke or neural tube deficit in pregnancy. A syndrome resembling subacute combined degeneration of B_{12} deficiency can occur and folate deficiency leads to elevated homocysteine levels, a risk factor for the development of cerebrovascular, cardiovascular and peripheral vascular disease. Folate is administered orally but can be given parenterally in acutely ill patients and in pregnancy.

Vitamin D

Vitamin D deficiency is associated with hypoparathyroidism, hypophosphataemia, chronic renal failure, malabsorption, dietary deficiency or inadequate exposure to sunlight. Neurological presentation is as a proximal myopathy which can be associated with osteomalacia. There is proximal weakness with a characteristic waddling gait but no involvement of bulbar or ocular musculature. Creatine kinase is elevated, EMG shows myopathic change and biopsy will confirm evidence of type II muscle fibre atrophy. Treatment is vitamin D replacement which leads to a slow recovery of the weakness.

Vitamin E

Vitamin E is fat-soluble and acts as a free radical scavenger and antioxidant. It is normally stored in large amounts so that clinical symptoms only become apparent after many years of deficiency, usually secondary to malabsorption in cystic fibrosis, adult coeliac disease or because of abnormalities of specific vitamin E receptors (e.g. aβlipoproteinaemia). There is progressive spinocerebellar degeneration with limb ataxia, because of involvement of the posterior columns, and an axonal, predominantly sensory, peripheral neuropathy with prominent involvement of proprioception. Rarely, pyramidal features can develop with extensor plantar responses and ocular signs including ptosis, nystagmus, external opthalmoplegia and optic neuritis. Investigation shows evidence of spiky red blood cells (acanthocytes) as well as retinal pigment change. Low serum vitamin E can be shown on assay but CSF is normal. Nerve conduction studies confirm a mild axonal neuropathy and occasionally the MRI scan shows high signal in the posterior columns. Treatment is with the recommended daily requirement of vitamin E of 10 mg/day. If the vitamin is deficient then the therapy should be given with water-soluble tocopherol 200–600 mg/day.

Alcohol abuse

Alcohol abuse is extremely common and is associated with important cultural, economic and environmental influences and consequences. It affects all socio-economic strata of society. Primary alcoholism is defined as addiction to alcohol in the absence of an underlying cause. Physical dependence can become such a strong compulsion that psychopathology develops with neglect of self and family. This culminates in severe disruption of general health, behaviour and cognitive function leading to loss of personal relationships and occupation. Secondary alcoholism occurs when excessive drinking is the consequence of other major psychiatric illness (e.g. drug addiction, schizo-affective disorder or manic depression).

Metabolism of alcohol

Alcohol is rapidly absorbed from the gastrointestinal tract and is metabolised in the liver where it is oxidised to acetaldehyde by the action of alcohol dehydrogenase and other enzymes. The role of acetaldehyde in alcohol toxicity is uncertain but it is highly cytotoxic and is also readily metabolised to acetate by the mitochondrial enzyme acetaldehyde dehydrogenase. Tolerance to alcohol is the acquired resistance to its effects. Intoxication occurs because alcohol crosses the blood–brain barrier.

The clinical manifestations of alcohol can be divided into:

1 Effects of acute intoxication
2 Effects of alcohol substitutes
3 Withdrawal syndrome occurring after sudden abstinence, and
4 Chronic disorders associated with prolonged alcohol abuse.

Effects of acute intoxication

The consequences of acute alcohol intoxication are widely tolerated by many societies, particularly amongst young people. The initial behavioural effects of euphoria, social disinhibition, loss of restraint and reduced psychomotor capacity are well-recognised but progression to behaviour disturbance, irritability, slurred speech, ataxic gait, aggression and loss of control can have serious consequences with high levels of intoxication. Depressant effects including drowsiness, stupor and coma can supervene with the risk of vomiting, aspiration and respiratory impairment. Acute intoxication is associated with psychotic disturbances including an acute paranoid state with auditory hallucinations, anxiety, agitation, outbursts of aggression and inappropriate violent or even destructive social behaviour of which the individual can have no recollection. These periods of amnesia, in which there is no ability to retain short-term memories, increase in duration and persist into periods when sober and fully conscious. Symptoms occur with serum levels as low as 50–150 mg/dL (10–31 mmol/L) but in those with previous alcohol intake and induction of the hepatic enzymes, symptoms develop at a higher concentrations of blood alcohol. Extreme intoxication (>300 mg/dL or 65 mmol/L) results in cerebellar impairment (ataxic dysarthria and nystagmus) and coma associated with hypotension, respiratory depression and hypothermia, with death occurring from brainstem depression if the blood alcohol level exceeds 400 mg/100 mL. Because alcohol is rapidly absorbed acute intoxication may require sedation and treatment of agitation with haloperidol or chlorpromazine. Eventually, ventilatory support and haemodialysis may be necessary, especially if there is a suggestion of methanol intake in addition.

Effects of alcohol substitutes

Methyl alcohol (methanol)

This is commonly used as a solvent and in antifreeze. It may be abused as a substitute for ethyl alcohol in 'meths'. It is directly toxic to the CNS as a depressant and is oxidised to formaldehyde and formic acid, which inhibit cytochrome oxidase and have a direct toxic effect on the putamen and optic nerves (see solvents & toxins). Acute intoxication can be delayed for many hours. Delirium can develop at the onset but a rapid progression occurs to cause visual field loss, blindness secondary to retinal oedema, pseudobulbar palsy and cognitive impairment. Severe toxicity culminates in metabolic acidosis and cerebral oedema leading to respiratory failure, coma and death. In patients who recover from acute intoxication there can be residual blindness and parkinsonian features. Treatment involves reversing the acidosis with large doses of sodium bicarbonate, retarding the mechanism of methanol with ethyl alcohol or fomepizole and, where necessary, haemodialysis.

Ethylene glycol

This is also commonly used as a solvent, in antifreeze, air conditioners and fire extinguishers. It can contaminate proprietary alcoholic drinks or be ingested in suicide attempts. Intoxication is associated with lethargy and progressive hypersomnolence, hyperventilation with seizures and hypotension. There is a metabolic acidosis with an anion gap. Anuric renal failure develops which is also associated with seizures. With high levels there can be the delayed onset of a cranial neuropathy, which resolves slowly. Treatment is by haemodialysis with intravenous sodium bicarbonate and, if necessary, ethanol. Fomepizole (4-methylpyrazole) is also used as a competitive inhibitor of alcohol dehydrogenase.

Withdrawal syndromes

The severity of withdrawal symptoms is proportional to the level of previous alcohol intake and the abruptness of cessation. Withdrawal of alcohol in the chronic abuser sometimes leads to the development of delirium tremens (the 'DTs') with CNS hyperexcitability, initially characterised by tremulousness with anxiety, insomnia, confusion, hyperactivity, hallucinations and seizures. The symptoms progressively worsen over several hours before settling, up to 72 hours after the last intake of alcohol. The tremor is generalised, present at rest and on action and can involve the face and tongue. It is associated with irritability and is usually present in the morning, but progressively worsens and increases in duration with prolonged withdrawal. There is usually an associated gastrointestinal disturbance with nausea, vomiting and autonomic hyperactivity with tachycardia, hypertension and sweating. Disturbing vivid auditory and visual hallucinations develop and these can persist for several days after the physical symptoms have settled. The patient frequently awakes lucid with no recollection of the acute delirious phase. Recurrence is common and, in severe cases, death supervenes. It is essential to consider the possibility of alcohol withdrawal in patients who develop confusion, tremor or seizures after being admitted to hospital for more than 12 hours. Severe withdrawal delirium tremens occurs in about 5% of patients and is associated with hyperpyrexia, ketoacidosis and circulatory collapse. Isolated hallucinations may occur in up to one-quarter of patients following withdrawal. They are often visual but occasionally auditory. Patients often lack insight into their hallucinations and their development indicates a poor prognosis with significant mortality.

Withdrawal seizures ('rum fits')

These typically occur within the first 24–48 hours of withdrawal. They are generalised, tonic–clonic convulsive seizures, which usually occur singly or in brief clusters although status may develop. The EEG shows mild changes, sometimes with photosensitivity, and generally reverts to normality within a few days. Even if status develops, the condition is usually self-limiting and patients often do not require antiepileptic medication although acute treatment with lorazepam or diazepam may be necessary.

Management of alcohol withdrawal

Minor symptoms can be managed with simple reassurance and nursing in a calm quiet well-lit environment although benzodiazepines can be helpful. Moderate symptoms, including autonomic hyperactivity and irritability, necessitate an incremental dose of benzodiazepines. Thiamine and glucose should be given to prevent the development of metabolic encephalopathy. Severe symptoms associated with confusion, poor cooperation, restlessness and aggressive behaviour can require intravenous diazepam (Diazemuls) given by slow injection and, if further treatment is necessary, haloperidol 5–10 mg intramuscularly or 5 mg twice daily up to 20 mg/day is the treatment of choice. Chlordiazepoxide, clomethiazole or clonidine are also effective.

Chronic disorders associated with prolonged alcohol abuse

Wernicke's encephalopathy

This is a complex of symptoms and signs resulting from an acquired nutritional deficiency of thiamine (vitamin B_1) rather than any direct toxic effect of alcohol. It is characterised by encephalopathy, oculomotor disturbances and ataxia. Thiamine and other B vitamins act as co-enzymes in glucose and lipid metabolism, amino acid production and neurotransmitter synthesis. Because thiamine stores are relatively small and there is a large daily turnover, deficiency can occur within 2–3 weeks of low intake. The brain is particularly sensitive to disturbance of complex B vitamin-dependent metabolism of glucose.

Wernicke's encephalopathy can present as an acute or slowly evolving disorder, often precipitated by an intercurrent medical event or metabolic stress such as trauma or infection. In addition to alcohol, it is caused by other conditions in which a depletion of thiamine can occur:

- Hyperemesis of pregnancy
- Systemic malignancy
- Haemo- or peritoneal dialysis
- Gastrointestinal surgery
- Prolonged intravenous feeding
- Anorexia,
- AIDS.

The acute syndrome is characterised by apathy, confusion, impairment of ocular motility and cerebellar ataxia lapsing into an encephalopathy with progressive disturbance of behaviour, personality, orientation and cognitive function developing over days or weeks leading to stupor, coma and ultimately death. There can be hallucinations, perceptual disorder and agitation. Ocular signs are characteristic and include ophthalmoplegia, nystagmus and conjugate gaze palsy. The ophthalmoplegia is initially caused by paresis of the lateral recti with subsequent involvement of other ocular muscles leading to total ophthalmoplegia. Nystagmus can be both horizontal and vertical and there is also sluggish pupillary response to light with light-near dissociation. Fundal examination shows small retinal haemorrhages and occasionally optic neuropathy develops. Progressive truncal and gait ataxia is common but the limbs are rarely involved.

MRI shows high T2 signal in the peri-aqueductal and the paraventricular region of the medial thalamus and hypothalamus while the mamillary bodies appear shrunken (Figure 19.15). CSF is characterised by elevated protein, while serum thiamine and erythrocyte transketolase activity are reduced. The pathology in Wernicke's syndrome shows symmetrical haemorrhagic and necrotic change predominantly affecting the mamillary bodies, dorsal medial nucleus of the thalamus and peri-aqueductal region as well as the tegmentum of the pons. Treatment is by thiamine given immediately commencing at 50–100 mg parenterally in the acute stages. Untreated Wernicke's encephalopathy is associated with a significant mortality but with adequate treatment the signs resolve rapidly.

Korsakoff's syndrome

This is a progressive and severe amnestic syndrome that is incompletely reversible. Memory is preferentially involved in comparison to other cognitive function with a profound impairment of both retrograde and antegrade memory with relative preservation of distant past memory, language and calculation abilities. There may also be perceptual difficulties and loss of insight although this is often less marked. Patients show striking loss of memory with

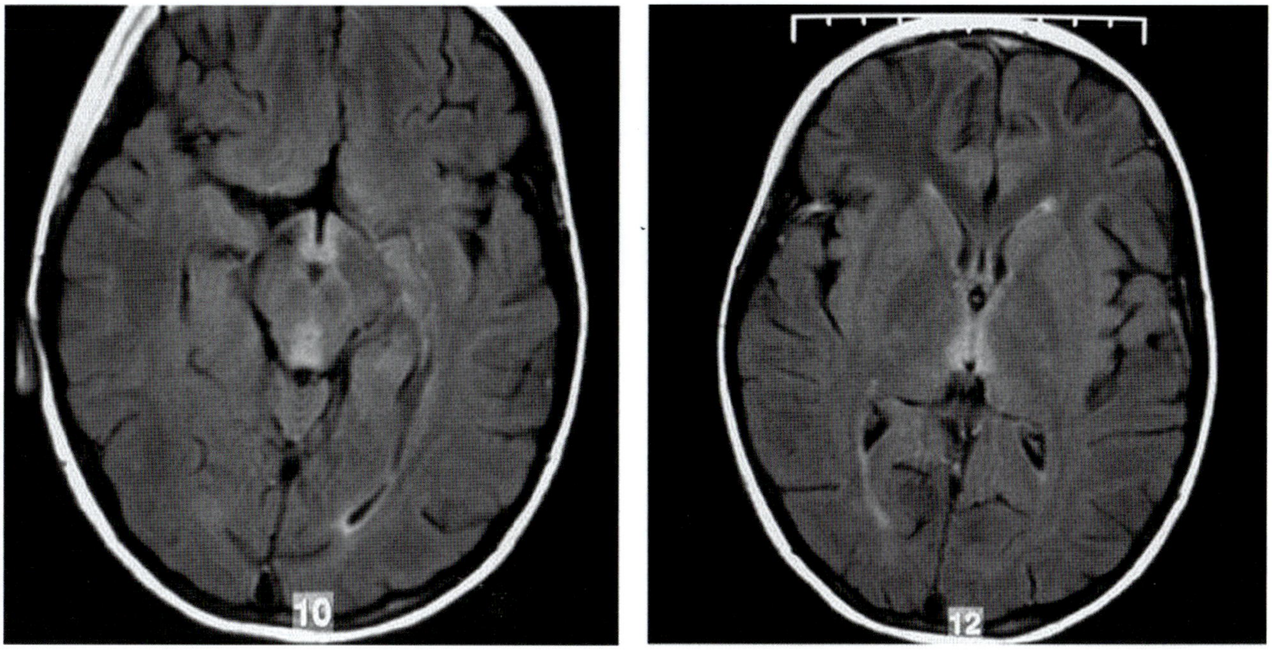

(a) (b)

Figure 19.15 Wernicke syndrome. Axial fluid-attenuated inversion recovery (FLAIR) images showing increased signal in the (a) mamillary bodies and dorsal midbrain and (b) thalami. Source: Cooke 2006. Reproduced with permission of Macmillan.

disorientation in time and place but retain alertness, attention, calculation and, at onset, normal social behaviour. The condition is characterised by confabulation, with intrusion of false memories.

Pathologically, the memory impairment of Korsakoff syndrome is associated with selective necrosis of the basal septal nuclei of the frontal lobes, the temporal lobes and diencephalon (Figures 19.16 and 19.17). In alcoholism, Korsakoff syndrome is caused by thiamine deficiency but can also occur following:

- Infarction
- Anoxia
- Trauma
- Tumours involving the frontotemporal regions
- Herpes simplex encephalitis
- Temporal lobe epilepsy.

Treatment requires urgent and high doses of thiamine replacement and should be continued until a noticeable improvement has occurred and for as long as clinical improvement continues. Improvement in memory function is slow and usually incomplete. Up to one-quarter of patients show no recovery while only slight improvement occurs in the remaining patients. Complete recovery is rare.

Wernicke–Korsakoff syndrome can be difficult to detect and a high index of suspicion is necessary in all patients who abuse alcohol and those with poor diet or gastrointestinal disturbance including diarrhoea and vomiting.

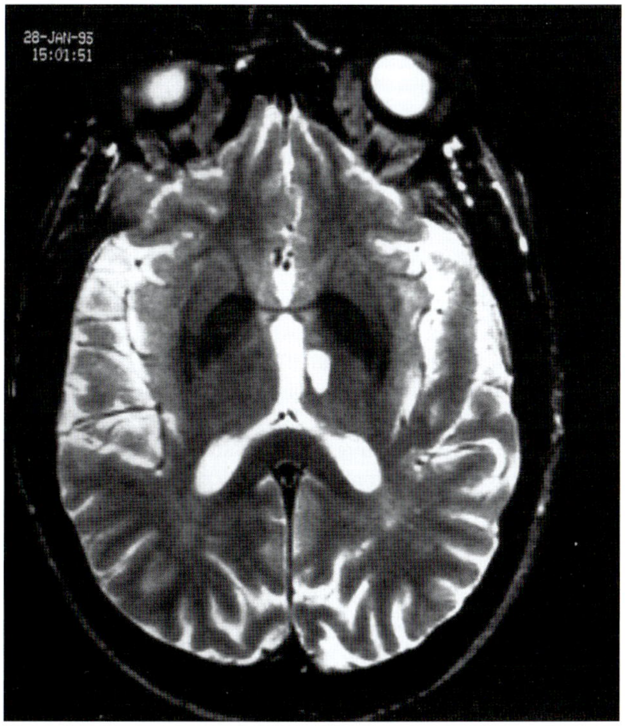

Figure 19.16 Korsakoff's syndrome. T2-weighted axial MRI showing thalamic infarct. Courtesy of Professor M. Kopelman, St. Thomas' Hospital.

Cerebellar ataxia

Chronic alcohol abuse is the most common cause of acquired cerebellar atrophy and is often associated with alcohol polyneuropathy. The ataxia usually affects men and can be so severe that the patient is unable to stand without support. Patients walk with a broad-based gait with slow short steps but limb ataxia and speech disturbance are minimal although cerebellar abnormalities of ocular movement are often present. Progressive unsteadiness evolves over several months with truncal ataxia and mild gait disturbance. Abstinence from alcohol leads to a slow and incomplete improvement. Pathological examination shows selective atrophy

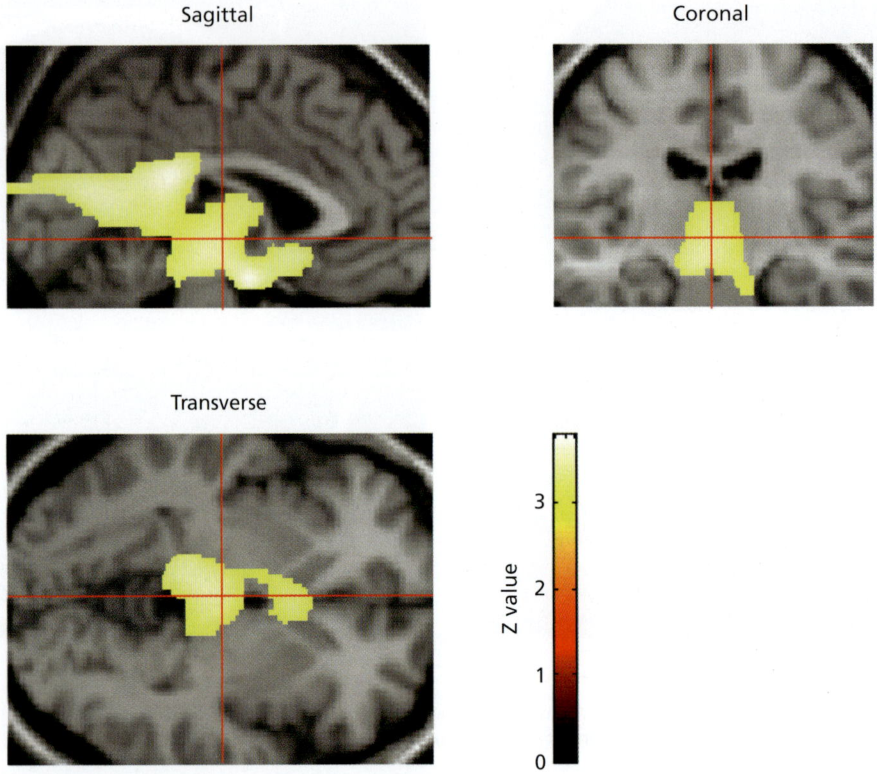

Figure 19.17 FDG PET scan showing hypometabolism in patients with Korsakoff's syndrome with significant reduction of signal in thalamus, ventro-medial cortex and retrosplenium. Source: Reed *et al.* 2003. Reproduced with permission of Elsevier.

of the anterior and superior part of the cerebellar vermis with cell loss particularly involving the Purkinje cells. Cerebellar ataxia can be associated with Wernicke's encephalopathy or occur in isolation.

Confusional state and dementia

Cortical atrophy and ventricular dilatation occur with prolonged alcohol intake. This is associated with a global confusional state characterised by progressive indifference to surroundings and abulia. Patients are easily aroused but are disorientated with cognitive deficits which can worsen and become fixed, interfering with activities of daily living, before evolving into frank dementia which may persist even after discontinuation of alcohol.

Alcoholic peripheral neuropathy

Sensorimotor axonal peripheral neuropathy is a characteristic feature of alcohol abuse, occurring as a consequence of thiamine deficiency in Wernicke's encephalopathy or because of direct alcohol toxicity. The neuropathy is usually insidious in onset, often mild and predominantly sensory. However, rapid progression may occur with motor impairment severe enough to affect gait. Painful symmetrical sensory loss occurs to all modalities, particularly affecting the lower limbs; it is characterised by distal tingling, burning and lancinating pain. Autonomic involvement is manifest as impotence, sweating, pupillary abnormalities and postural hypotension. Investigation shows a macrocytosis and elevation of hepatic enzymes. There may be an elevated CSF protein and nerve conduction studies show an axonal polyneuropathy predominantly affecting sensory and motor action potential with slowing of conduction velocity. Management is discontinuation of alcohol consumption and ensuring adequate nutritional intake with thiamine and vitamin B supplements. However, recovery is generally incomplete and there is often considerable residual weakness and paraesthesiae.

Alcoholic myopathy

Acute myopathy can occur with chronic alcohol abuse but may also follow binge intake. It is secondary to the direct toxic effects of alcohol although other factors including muscle crush, seizures and electrolyte disturbances can contribute. The onset is with acute and severe muscle pain, cramp, swelling and a rise in the creatine kinase level, evolving rapidly into focal or generalised myopathic weakness often with selective involvement of the calves. A cardiomyopathy can coexist. Although recovery usually occurs within days or weeks, rhabdomyolysis and myoglobunuria may occur, leading to hyperkalaemia and renal failure. A more chronic myopathy is associated with prolonged consistent alcohol abuse, characterised by slowly developing, painful proximal myopathy particularly affecting the shoulder and hip girdle muscles. This myopathy can be asymptomatic and noted because of an isolated elevation in creatine kinase levels. EMG shows myopathic features and there can also be a coexisting neuropathy. Biopsy of chronic alcohol myopathy shows no significant muscle fibre necrosis but atrophy affecting type II (especially type IIB) fibres. In the acute form there is scattered muscle fibre necrosis with regeneration. The myopathy can be reversible with many months of abstinence and good nutrition. Recovery is often incomplete.

Other neurological complications of alcohol abuse

Marchiafava–Bignami syndrome

This is a condition associated with drinking strong red wine, usually Chianti, that affects severe and chronic alcoholics in middle or late life. The aetiology is unknown and presentation is variable with a slowly progressive disturbance of cognitive function, personality and behaviour. There is progressive motor slowing with incontinence, frontal release signs and a broad-based gait. There can be cognitive impairment, dysarthria, hemiparesis, apraxia, aphasia and seizures and occasionally a patient can present in stupor or coma. There is selective demyelination of the central portion of the corpus callosum with sparing of the anterior and posterior portions, other white matter tracts are also affected. Treatment is with nutritional support and rehabilitation but recovery is variable. Imaging shows high signal lesions on T2 MRI in the corpus callosum and anterior commissure.

Fetal alcohol syndrome

Prenatal exposure to ethanol impairs fetal growth and neurodevelopment. There may be dysmorphic facial features and microcephaly, mental retardation and learning difficulties including speech delay and hyperactivity.

Psychiatric sequelae

In chronic alcohol abuse depressive illness is common, particularly on withdrawal, and up to one-quarter of patients fulfil the criteria for a major depressive disorder; however, it often remits after several months and rarely requires antidepressant medication. Some patients also have an anxiety disorder which may develop into frank psychotic symptoms during withdrawal.

Traumatic injury

Traumatic injuries to the head may occur during intoxication causing parenchymal contusions, subdural or extradural haematoma, subarachnoid haemorrhage and lead to post-traumatic epilepsy.

Compressive neuropathies (see Chapter 10)

The most common neuropathies occurring in alcohol abuse include compression of the radial nerve at the spiral groove causing 'Saturday night palsy'. Compression of the peroneal nerve at the fibula head can lead to foot drop as can compression of the sciatic nerve in the gluteal region.

Amblyopia (see Chapter 14)

Amblyopia occurs as a consequence of chronic alcoholism and is associated with poor dietary and heavy tobacco use and weight loss. Progressive optic nerve involvement leads to painless visual loss affecting both eyes with diminished visual acuity, a centrocaecal scotoma and mild disc pallor. The treatment is to maintain adequate diet and B vitamins which generally leads to visual recovery.

Alcoholic cirrhosis

It must be emphasised that neurological effects of alcohol abuse run in parallel with systemic factors. Alcohol-related cirrhosis is the most common and serious manifestation. Patients may develop porto-systemic encephalopathy, tremor, myoclonus and asterixis.

Strachan's syndrome

This is a severe painful ataxic sensorimotor neuropathy associated with visual loss resulting from amblyopia, tinnitus, gastritis and stomatitis. The condition is related to nutritional deficits. There have been outbreaks of the condition in Cuba associated with retrobulbar optic neuropathy, peripheral neuropathy, sensori-neural hearing loss and myelopathy with spastic paraparesis and dysphonia. The aetiology remains unclear but a relationship to poor nutrition, heavy alcohol and tobacco exposure has been noted.

Other deficiency states associated with neurological manifestations

Copper deficiency

Copper deficiency is rare because of the low daily requirement and its ubiquitous distribution. This occurs following gastrointestinal disturbance, in particular after gastrectomy but excessive zinc (e.g. dental cream and during chronic haemodialysis) can also cause copper deficiency by chelating free copper. It also occurs in enteropathy and as a complication of total parentral nuitrition. Copper is essential to the nervous system and bone marrow and functions as a prosthetic group in key enzymes involved in catecholamine synthesis, the respiratory chain, folate metabolism and antioxidant function. The most common neurological manifestation of acquired copper deficiency is a myeloneuropathy with sensory ataxia. The MRI shows increased T2 signal in the dorsal columns, particularly in the cervical region. The condition appears clinically and radiologically identical to subacute combined degeneration of the cord associated with B_{12} deficiency or nitrous oxide intoxication.

Magnesium deficiency

This can also occur after gastrointestinal surgery or with chronic use of diuretics. It is an essential co-enzyme involved in the metabolism of thiamine and its deficiency can lead to an impaired response to thiamine in Wernicke's encephalopathy resulting from alcohol or hyperemesis gravidum.

Drugs of abuse

Epidemiology

The clinical assessment of drug abuse is difficult because addicts may use several drugs at one time, or abuse alcohol concurrently. Furthermore, the drug can be contaminated either at source or at the time of administration and the metabolism of drugs of abuse is unpredictable depending on dosage, mode of administration and the ability of the body to metabolise the drug.

Drug dependence is both psychological when drug use is compulsive because of pleasurable or dysphoric effects and physical if discontinuation of the drug will lead to serious and painful symptoms. Drug users develop tolerance and require larger doses to maintain the effects of the drug and to prevent the development of withdrawal symptoms.

There are five major groups of drugs of abuse (Table 19.6):

1 Stimulants
2 Sedatives
3 Hallucinogens
4 Organic solvents, and
5 Drugs used to enhance athletic performance.

Stimulants

Stimulants share the ability to enhance transmission at the catecholaminergic synapse and therefore have common pharmacological and toxic effects and also develop cross-tolerance. Stimulants are abused because they cause elation, increased alertness and enhance stamina and motor activity. Prolonged excessive use is associated with motor manifestations including tics, tremor, myoclonus and an acute dystonic reaction.

Table 19.6 Drugs of abuse that affect the nervous system.

Stimulants
Sympathomimetics
Amphetamines, methamphetamine, dexamphetamine
Crack/cocaine
Methylphenidate (Ritalin)
Ephedrine
Serotoninergics
MDMA and derivatives (Ecstasy, MDMA, MDEA, PMA)
Others
Modafinil, caffeine, nicotine, methcathinone
Sedatives and tranquilisers
Opiates and opioids
Morphine
Heroin
Opium
Codeine
Hydromorphine
Fentanyl
Pethidine
Tramadol
Naloxone
Barbiturates
Benzodiazepines
Others
Methaqualone, GHB, ethanol
Hallucinogens
Psychedelics
Phenylethylamine – MDMA, mescaline
Tryptamins – LSD, psilocybin
Dissociatives
Dextromethorphan
Ketamine
Methoxetamine
Phencyclidine
Deliriants
Atropine
Scopolamine
Cannaboids
Marijuana
(GHB and solvents are also hallucinogens)
Organic solvents
Solvents
Propane
Butane
Toluene
Fuels
Gasoline
Kerosine
Propellant gases
Freon
Nitrous oxide
Drugs used to enhance athletic performance
Steroids
Erythropoietin (EPO)
Diuretics
β-blockers

Amphetamines

Dexamphetamine, the dextro-isomer of amphetamine, is used in clinical practice. Metamphetamine ('crystal meth' or 'ice') is widely abused. Acute intoxication is characterised by increased alertness, a sense of self-confidence and well-being, euphoria and extrovert behaviour, loss of appetite and the desire to sleep, tremor, dilated pupils, tachycardia and hypertension. In extreme cases this results in paranoid delusions, hallucinations and violence. Intoxication can lead to convulsions, hyperthermia, rhabdomyolysis and intracerebral haemorrhage. Stroke resulting from stimulant abuse is discussed later (see Conditions caused by stimulant abuse).

Designer drugs

Designer drugs are synthetic derivatives, usually amphetamine analogues. Ecstasy (MDMA) is a synthetic compound that is a derivative of a stimulant (methamphetamine) and a hallucinogen (mescaline). It is widely abused by the young because of its capacity to induce euphoria, wakefulness, intimacy, sexual arousal and disinhibition. It is erroneously believed to provide a 'safe' high but its unique adverse effects are caused by both the release and uptake block of endogeneous catacholamines and serotoninergic toxicity. In high doses it has an amphetamine-like stimulant effect and unpredictable toxicity, exacerbated by dehydration. It may cause an acute toxic reaction with headache, hypertension, hyperpyrexia, seizures, rhabdomyolysis and the development of hyponatraemia leading to confusion, seizures, cerebral oedema, coma, cerebral herniation and death. A hypertonic state may develop causing hepatotoxicity, coagulopathy, cerebral infarction or haemorrhage. MDMA causes a massive central serotoninergic discharge which accounts for its psychic effects which can be clinically indistinguishable from schizophrenia. There can be permanent impairment of memory. Many substances have been combined with Ecstasy as adulterants: toxic MDMA and piperazine analogues, dextrometamphetamine, ketamine, paracetamol and other non-psychoactive adulterants. Several other amphetamine-derived drugs are widely used, and all have similar effects following acute and prolonged intoxication. Other sympathomimetic drugs of abuse such as cocaine, amphetamine and methamphetamine present with a clinical syndrome that is indistinguishable from that of MDMA.

Methylphenidate (Ritalin)

This can rarely cause an amphetamine-like syndrome with behavioural disturbances, seizures and intracerebral haemorrhage.

Methcathinone analogues – khat

Khat is a flowering plant native to East Africa and the Arabian Peninsula. The leaves contain the alkaloid cathinone, an amphetamine-like stimulant. For many years the leaves have been chewed as a recreational drug within the region where it naturally grows because only fresh leaves are strongly psychoactive. Its stimulatory effects include a feeling of euphoria, excitement, increased alertness and sexual arousal. Toxic effects include anorexia, tremor, tachycardia, arrhythmia, hypotension and respiratory arrest. Increased air transport has led to extensive smuggling of the drug, with a global distribution. Cathinone breaks down to cathine and norephedrine. This occurs after khat has been ingested or if the leaves are left to dry for more than 48 hours.

Methcathinone ('cat' or 'jeff') is a derivative of cathinone. It is inexpensively and easily manufactured as a designer drug from its precursor, ephedrine. It has a similar amphetamine-like stimulant and euphoric effect when snorted, ingested or injected.

Mephedrone is a synthetic stimulant drug of the cathinone and amphetamine class which has received considerable publicity as a 'legal high'. The neurotoxicity remains uncertain but a number of deaths have been reported

MPTP

Methylphenyltetrahydropyridine (MPTP) was developed in the United States as a designer drug with close clinical similarities to amphetamine. The effects of abuse were similar but some abusers developed a moderate to severe parkinsonian syndrome with bradykinesis, freezing, rigidity, instability, dysarthria and a symmetrical parkinsonian tremor. There was a variable response to levodopa with the development of typical motor fluctuations and dyskinesiae. Pathological features include moderate to severe neuronal loss and gliosis in the substantia nigra without Lewy bodies.

Cocaine

Cocaine is the most commonly abused psychomotor stimulant and is administered intranasally, parenterally or smoked as crack. Moderate doses are associated with mood elevation, increased alertness, reduced fatigue and enhanced performance but psychiatric effects develop rapidly including paranoia, delusions, hallucinations, seizures, choreo-athetoid movements and agitation. Chronic abuse can lead to progressive neuropsychiatric features including restlessness, irritability and psychotic, aggressive, paranoid states. These are associated with visual and auditory hallucinations with amphetamine abuse and violent behaviour with the cocaine alkaloid, crack. Long-term abuse of stimulants can lead to toxic encephalopathy or a fixed cognitive dysfunction with cerebral atrophy.

Conditions caused by stimulant abuse

Ischaemic stroke Ischaemic stroke occurs as a consequence of stimulant abuse for several reasons. It is associated with acute hypertension, vasoconstriction, dissection and haemorrhagic vasculitis occurring with amphetamine or cocaine. Furthermore, cardiac thrombus can embolise to the brain in patients with infective endocarditis or cardiomyopathy caused by arrhythmias or because foreign body material may be injected with the drug. Stroke can also be a consequence of infective endocarditis causing mycotic aneurysms or haemorrhagic transformation in cerebral infarction. Crack cocaine is the most important cause of drug-related stroke accounting for about 50% of all cases and being much more common than amphetamine-related stroke. With crack-cocaine, infarction often affects the cortical or deep penetrating arteries, but anterior spinal artery occlusion also occurs. The onset of stroke following use of amphetamine or crack cocaine is rapid because of blood pressure surges. Approximately 50% occur in the middle cerebral artery territory. Imaging shows asymptomatic subcortical white matter lesions in crack and cocaine users.

Haemorrhagic stroke This is particularly associated with cocaine and amphetamine. It seems to occur with intranasal or intravenous usage or smoking crack. Intracerebral haemorrhage is usually in basal ganglia but is occasionally lobar, intraventricular or subarachnoid. Haemorrhage may be associated with hypertension, vasculitis or a pre-existing aneurysm or arteriovenous malformation may rupture.

Vasculitis This is seen more commonly with methamphetamine than cocaine. It usually evolves rapidly with headache, progressive encephalopathy and raised erythrocycte sedimentation rate. Diffuse vasospasm is associated with bleeding or focal narrowing; there can also be a necrotising vasculitis resembling polyarteritis nodosa, involving small calibre vessels and necrosis. Treatment is with high dose steroids.

Other effects of stimulant abuse In addition to stroke and epilepsy, systemic complications of stimulants include the development of hyperthermia, dehydration and rhabdomyolysis with an increased risk of myocardial infarction and cardiac arrhythmia. Cocaine and amphetamine also give rise to movement disorders including vocal and motor tics, chorea, and acute dystonic reaction particularly affecting the head and neck and an oromandibular dyskinesia. Treatment is supportive with attempts to cool the patient, reduce blood pressure and maintain oxygenation. Neuroleptics, anxiolytics and sedatives may be necessary and seizures should be treated appropriately. Withdrawal of cocaine can be difficult as the tolerance develops to the euphoric and anorexic effects of the drug and the psychiatric manifestations may worsen.

Sedatives

Opiates

Heroin and morphine are highly addictive drugs which are usually administered intravenously but can be sniffed, smoked or injected subcutaneously (skin popping). Intravenous administration is often non-sterile and can lead to infective complications (Table 19.7). Fentanyl is an opiate with 100 times the potency of morphine.

The effects of heroin are the same as morphine but more powerful. There is an initial analgesic effect and then a sense of 'rush' with euphoria or dysphoria before drowsiness and hallucinations. Systemic features include pruritus, dry mouth, nausea, vomiting, constipation and urinary retention. There can be severe pupillary constriction before the development of respiratory depression, hypoxic–ischaemic brain injury and post-anoxic encephalopathy. The immediate effects can be reversed with naloxone, a safe and effective antidote which should be given to anyone with a suspected opiate overdose. If the patient has not been discovered for a prolonged period of time there can be extensive

Table 19.7 Infective complications of non-sterile intravenous drug administration.

Local abscess
Cellulitis
Infective endocarditis
Botulism
Tetanus
Embolic infarction
Meningitis
Pyogenic arthritis
Infectious hepatitis
Cerebral abscess
Septic arthritis
Mycotic aneurysms
Osteomyelitis
Discitis
HIV

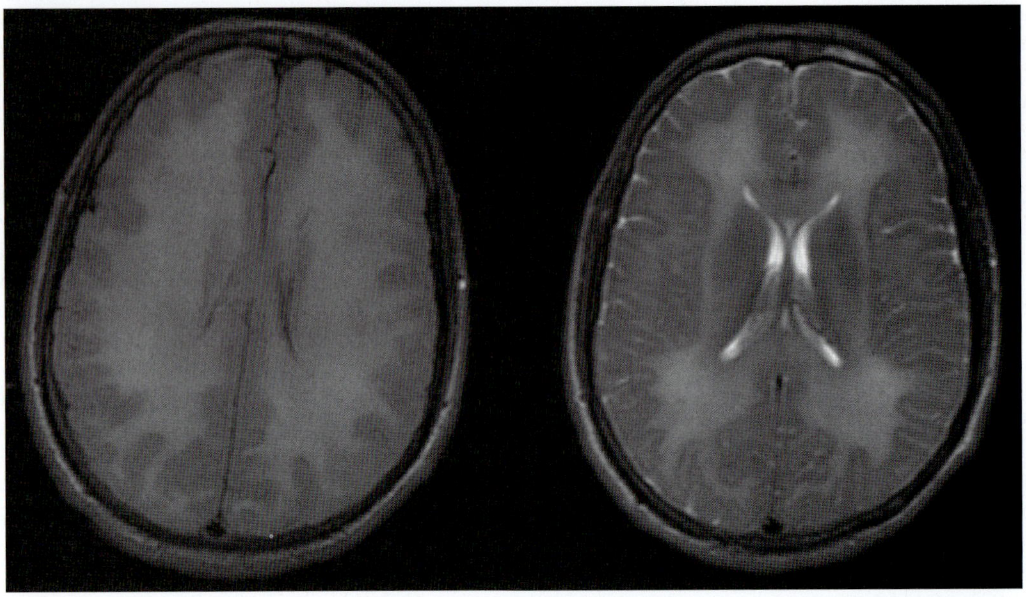

Figure 19.18 Toxic encephalopathy caused by presumed inhalation of heroin pyrolate. T2-weighted MRI scan showing extensive white matter change.

compression and stretching of peripheral nerves and damage to the brachial plexus, common peroneal, ulnar or sciatic nerves with secondary ischaemia. Rhabdomyolysis is caused by a compartment syndrome as a consequence of trauma, hypotension, fever and seizures or brought about by direct opiate toxicity. It occurs after prolonged periods of unconsciousness and leads to myoglobinuria and sometimes renal failure. Repeated intramuscular injections can also lead to focal fibrosis and weakness in injected muscles with contractures. Stroke is secondary to an infective vasculitis or to the development of mycotic aneurysms but infarction can also be a consequence of paradoxical embolism or contaminants. An acute myelopathy can occur with excessive heroin abuse with paraparesis, segmental sensory level, and urinary retention. A distal sensory or sensorimotor neuropathy also occur. Inhalation of heroin pyrolate, particularly if contaminated by heating the drug on aluminium foil, can cause toxic encephalopathy with extensive white matter change on MRI (Figure 19.18).

The symptoms and signs of withdrawal from opioids appear within hours and include the characteristic syndrome of drug craving, restlessness and irritability, followed by the development of autonomic flu-like symptoms, sweating, lacrimation and rhinorrhoea. There may be piloerection, abdominal cramps, diarrhoea and coughing. The symptoms may develop rapidly following administration of naloxone but controlled withdrawal ought not to be dangerous and treatment of symptoms with oral methadone, a long-acting opiate, may ameliorate the symptoms. Clonidine and α_2-adrenergic agonists suppress the autonomic disturbances of opioid withdrawal.

Barbiturates

Barbiturates are abused because of their euphoric and sedative actions which are similar to alcohol. Acute intoxication leads to slurred speech, gait ataxia, coma, hypotension, hypothermia and eventually respiratory depression with apnoea. Treatment is supportive and involves the use of gastric lavage. When barbiturates are withdrawn acutely there may be irritability, tremor, tachycardia and a reduced seizure threshold. It can be necessary to reinstitute the barbiturate before reducing with gradual tapering dosage.

Table 19.8 Hallucinogens commonly used as drugs of abuse.

Phencyclidine
Lysergic acid diethylamide (LSD)
Ketamine
Marijuana
GABA hydroxybutyrate (GHB)
Solvents

Benzodiazepines

Benzodiazepines, when used acutely, induce a comfortable sensation of lassitude, but in excessive doses there is progressive drowsiness, confusion, euphoria and impairment of psychomotor function leading to stupor and coma. The effects of acute overdoses can be reversed by flumazenil which is a specific antagonist, but this is short-lived. Chronic use of benzodiazepines leads to tolerance and physical dependence. Withdrawal symptoms develop within 24 hours of cessation of the use of short-acting benzodiazepines leading to irritability, increased sensitivity to light and sound and autonomic disturbance including tremor and tachycardia which can develop into delirium, hallucinosis and seizures.

Hallucinogens

Hallucinogens are abused because of the heightened and distorted sensory perception with eventual hallucinogenic effects (Table 19.8). The subject experiences perceptual change, decreased pain sensation and autonomic effects which include flushing, sweating, hypertension and tachycardia. Abuse is associated with an acute confusional state, ataxia, dysarthria and nystagmus. Numbness and perceptual change develop with features of self-mutilation, convulsions, dystonia and coma. LSD and Ecstasy can cause the serotonin syndrome.

Lysergic acid diethylamide

Lysergic acid diethylamide (LSD) is a hallucinogen that alters perception, mood and thought. Acute effects are associated with dizziness, blurred vision, nausea and weakness. There is often euphoria, depersonalisation, distortion of time and bizarre behavioural effects, including arousal and depression, which can lead to accidents or suicide. Chronic abuse has been associated with cerebral infarction and cognitive deficits.

Marijuana

Marijuana can be smoked, eaten or taken intravenously. It is widely abused because of its effects on memory, mood, judgement and sense of time. It induces a sense of relaxation with a subjective slowing of time, euphoria and depersonalisation. In high doses there can be a toxic psychosis with hallucination, paranoia and a variable degree of anxiety, aggressiveness or sedation and sleepiness. The long-term consequences of abuse remain uncertain but paranoia and panic reaction do occur. Tolerance leads to a degree of irritability, restlessness and insomnia. Synthetic cannabinoids are analogues of marijuana and have been termed 'legal highs' but many of these are extremely toxic.

Ketamine

Ketamine is primarily used as an anaesthetic but has hallucinogenic properties. It is a drug of abuse and in large doses can lead to coma in humans while moderate doses can cause euphoria, relaxation and paranoia. Prolonged use leads to a long-term syndrome of psychosis, agitation, bizarre behaviour and catatonia.

Phencyclidine (angel dust)

This is taken orally, nasally or by inhalation and has a mixture of effects including a euphoric or dysphoric state, which can lead to catatonia and psychosis especially in chronic abuse.

GABA hydroxybutyrate

GABA hydroxybutyrate (GHB) induces euphoria, disinhibition and loss of short-term memory but its use is associated with sedation, disorientation and vomiting. In higher doses, seizures can develop.

Anticholinergics

These can also be used as recreational drugs because they can cause hallucinations and delirium. Excessive anticholinergic stimulation is associated with mydriasis, dry flushed skin, tachycardia, urinary retention and fever. In severe overdoses there can be myoclonus, seizures, coma and death.

Solvents

Lighter fluids, varnishes and paint thinners are frequently abused as inhalants because they are based on organic solvents including toluene, hexane and benzene. Their use is associated with a characteristic rash with inflammation around the mouth and the nose. Inhalation of low doses leads to a feeling of exhilaration, lightheadedness and giddiness with auditory and visual hallucinations. With more prolonged or severe usage vomiting, tinnitus, headache occur and eventually the development of seizures. Long-term exposure causes toxic encephalopathy with progressive impairment of coordination and cognition, and the development of diplopia and ataxia with increasing disorientation, confusion, respiratory depression and coma. Toluene (see Neurological Disorders associated with exposure to toxic substances) particularly can give rise to ataxia, oculomotor and brainstem dysfunction, pyramidal features and dementia. Long-term complications include cardiac arrhythmias, suffocation from the use of plastic bags during inhalation, vomiting, aspiration and peripheral neuropathy. Sudden death can occur. MRI may show widespread white matter abnormalities.

Athletic performance-enhancing drugs

The neurotoxicity of some of these drugs is uncertain. Anabolic steroids including corticosteroids, insulin and growth hormone have direct physiological effect in building muscle. Stimulants, including amphetamine and cocaine, are also used to heighten alertness, reduce fatigue and prolong endurance. Erythropoietin (EPO) increases haemoglobin and oxygen delivery in endurance sports and β_2-agonists have a fat burning effect. Abuse of these substances is widespread and their effects may be unpredictable.

Investigation of suspected substance abuse

The first line of investigation is a urine toxicology screen, which can become positive within hours of ingestion and remains positive for variable periods depending on the drug used and the presence of coincidental alcohol use. Positivity for amphetamine, cocaine, barbiturates and morphine is relatively short but benzodiazepines and heroin remain detectable for up to 8 weeks.

Adverse reactions to drugs

Adverse reactions to drugs are a common cause of neurological morbidity and mortality. Drug reactions commonly lead to a variety of manifestations that can mimic naturally occurring neurological disease. There are many individual anecdotal case reports suggesting drugs are relevant to the aetiology of individual conditions but a clear causal relationship is much more difficult to establish. Throughout this section only the most important or most common forms of neurological drug toxicity are discussed.

Seizures

Many drugs can cause seizures in healthy individuals or, more commonly, provoke seizures in patients with pre-existing epilepsy or a low seizure threshold (Table 19.9). Iatrogenic seizures can also occur as a consequence of withdrawal of antiepileptic medication or be provoked by other medical procedures such as

Table 19.9 Drugs that may provoke seizures.

Respiratory agents – theophylline, aminophylline, terbutaline
Psychotropic medication – phenothiazines, clozapine, butyrophenones, lithium
Antimicrobial agents – antibiotics (isoniazide, nalidixic acid), antifungal, antituberculous, antihelminthics
CNS stimulants – caffeine, cocaine, amphetamines, methylphenidate
Antineoplastic agents
Opiates and narcotic agents – pethidine, morphine
Vaccines
Radiological contrast agents

Table 19.10 Drugs that may cause headache.

Non-steroidal anti-inflammatory drugs	Ibuprofen, diclofenac, celecoxib
Antimicrobial medication	Sulphonamide, cephalosporin, ciprofloxacin, isoniazid, penicillin
Antiviral agents	valaciclovir
Cytotoxic medication	Cytosine arabinoside
Corticosteroids	
Intravenous immunoglobulin (IVIg)	
Intrathecal medication	Contrast material and cytotoxic medication (e.g. methotrexate)
Others	Antimicrobials, steroids, baclofen, spinal anaesthesia

surgery, electroconvulsive therapy, labour and delivery or intrathecal chemotherapy. Other factors predisposing to drug-induced seizures include metabolic abnormalities, organ failure, water intoxication or electrolyte abnormalities, particularly hyponatraemia.

Headache

Headache can occur either as a direct consequence of medication or because the medication has acted as a trigger in a predisposed individual (Table 19.10). Acute exposure can cause a primary headache often brought about by vasodilatation. The most common drugs causing headaches are non-steroidal anti-inflammatory drugs (indomethacin, diclofenac), nifedipine, cimetidine, ranitidine, β-blockers (atenolol, metoprolol, propranolol) and vasodilatator drugs (including glyceryltrinitrate). A number of drugs also cause or exacerbate a tendency to migraine including cimetidine, the oral contraceptive pill, atenolol, indomethacin and nifedipine. Chronic headache is associated with the overuse of medication or by drug withdrawal. Headaches resulting from transient hypertension occur with monoamine oxidase inhibitors (MAOIs), as a reaction to treatment or when sympathomimetic agents are given concurrently. Intravenous immunoglobulin (IVIg) commonly gives rise to headache particularly in known migraine sufferers, this can be caused by aseptic meningitis. Idiopathic intracranial hypertension occurs predominantly in young women who are overweight and is particularly associated with use of the oral contraceptive drug, vitamin A intoxication or a variety of other medications including antibiotics (tetracycline, ampicillin, nitrofurantoin), non-steroidal anti-inflammatory drugs (naproxen, ibuprofen), retinoids, danazole, amiodarone, perhexiline and thyroxine. Headache can also occur as a consequence of drug-induced aseptic meningitis (e.g. NSAIDs, IVIg).

Confusional states

Drugs are a common cause of a confusional state, manifest as a fluctuating level of consciousness, diminished awareness, impairment of intention and memory, disorientation, hallucination and paranoid delusions. The primary drugs that can be responsible are summarised in Table 19.11.

Table 19.11 Drugs associated with confusional state.

Tranquilisers and hypnotics – barbiturates
Benzodiazepines
Antiparkinsonian medication
Antidepressants including SSRIs
Abrupt withdrawal of drugs

Table 19.12 Drugs associated with encephalopathy.

Lithium	Diffuse disturbance of cerebral function associated with tremor, myoclonus, seizures, ataxia and confusion. The cerebellar dysfunction may persist
Psychotropic medication	Impairment of consciousness and memory with psychomotor activity are common, particularly with neuroleptics (haloperidol and antidepressants), tricyclic drugs, fluoxetine, venlafaxine
Anticholinergic medication	Antiparkinsonian, antipsychotics, antihistamines, antiemetics, benzodiazepines
Drugs of abuse	Cocaine, opiates
Histamine (H2) receptor antagonists	Cimetidine
Non-steroidal anti-inflammatory drugs	
Opioid analgesics	Morphine and heroin
Others	Penicillins, cephalosporins, vigabatrin, valproic acid

Encephalopathy

Clouding of consciousness or delirium is commonly caused by multiple general medical factors but is particularly related to the effects of medication. It can be manifest as a disturbance of consciousness but there can also be changes in cognition or perception. The disturbances develop over a relatively short period of time and fluctuate during the course of the day. A large number of drugs can cause delirium but most reports are anecdotal. The most important medications can have multiple effects (Table 19.12).

Memory disturbance

Memory impairment is commonly associated with the use of medication. This can cause temporary impairment of antegrade and retrograde memory, a transient global amnesia, fugue-like state or, much less commonly, a fixed and irreversible amnesia (Table 19.13).

Neuropsychiatric effects

The behavioural effects of medication can be difficult to assess and be non-specific. The development of listlessness, insomnia, drowsiness, restlessness, anxiety, euphoria or depression can be a

Table 19.13 Drugs that may be associated with memory disturbance.

Chemotherapy (particularly intrathecal methotrexate)
Anticholinergic medication
Antidepressants
Antiepileptic drugs
Analgesic drugs of abuse

manifestation of underlying disease or other metabolic or infective complications but a variety of medications do contribute: tricyclic antidepressants, amphetamines, phenothiazines, barbiturates, hypnotic, anticholinergics, antiepileptic medication and antihistamines. Similar features may be precipitated by acute withdrawal of medication. Affective disorders are less common but may be severe. A depressive reaction can occur during drug treatment. In the past, reserpine and methyldopa were recognised to cause depression. More commonly now, depression occurs with other antihypertensive medication (clonidine, propranolol and calcium channel blocking drugs) but is also seen with corticosteroids, hypnotic agents, NSAIDs, antituberculous medication, H2 antagonists, digoxin, baclofen, anabolic steroids, barbiturates and benzodiazepines. Acute manic or hypomanic psychosis is unusual but can be associated with corticosteroids, thyroid replacement or, rarely, captopril, chloroquine and dopaminergic drugs.

Coma

This usually results from an inadvertent or deliberate overdose with hypnotic sedatives, antidepressants, analgesics or drug combinations. An overdose of insulin will also produce an acute hypoglycaemic coma and other drugs that can be implicated include phenothiazines, salicylates and valproic acid.

Sleep disorders

Sleep disorders resulting from medication may be manifest by excessive sleepiness, insomnia, sleep-related breathing disorders or parasomnias. Excessive drowsiness is associated with sedative, hypnotic or antidepressive medication and may also occur with antiepileptic drugs. Paradoxically, the same medication may also be associated with insomnia as can respiratory drugs including bronchodilators, cardiovascular drugs (antihypertensive medication, calcium channel blockers, beta-blockers and CNS stimulants). Vivid dreams and nightmares are often associated with drugs affecting noradrenaline, serotonin and dopamine neurotransmitters; these include the CNS stimulants, antipsychotic drugs and antiparkinsonian medication. Parasomnias can be related to the introduction of antipsychotic medication, sedatives, hypnotics or antidepressants.

Toxic leukoencephalopthy

This is a disorder associated with a structural alteration of white matter caused by a variety of toxic insults usually related to therapeutic agents, illicit drug use and occupational exposure to toxins. The condition involves white matter tracts serving higher cerebral function and therefore presents with neurobehavioural disturbances including inattention, forgetfulness and changes in personality leading to somnolence, apathy, cognitive impairment and ultimately dementia, coma and death. MRI initially shows hyperintensity in the peri-ventricular white matter but this progresses

Table 19.14 Drugs that may be associated with toxic leukoencephaolopathy.

Antineoplastic treatments	Cranial irradiation, methotrexate, cisplastin, cytarabine, levamisole, interleukin 2, interferon
Immunosuppressants	Tacrolimus, ciclosporin
Antimicrobial	Amphotericin B
Drugs of abuse	Toluene, ethanol, cocaine, amphetamine, ecstasy, heroin (IV or inhaled), psilocybin
Environmental toxins	Carbon monoxide, arsenic, carbon tetrachloride

to a severe hyperintensity involving widespread white matter with necrotic areas. These changes are reflected in the pathology of patchy oedema within myelin which becomes widespread, leading to the destruction of oligodendrocytes, axonal loss and necrosis. The condition is associated with a variety of toxins listed in Table 19.14.

Cerebrovascular disease

Cerebrovascular disease can be associated with the use of drugs by a large number of potential mechanisms. There is a clear risk of haemorrhage as a complication of anticoagulant and thrombolytic therapies. Cerebral blood flow may be reduced particularly in elderly patients in the presence of cerebrovascular disease by any antihypertensive medication that reduces blood pressure below perfusion pressure. This may predispose to cerebral infarction in watershed territories. Cerebrovascular disease may be caused by direct neurotoxicity or indirect mechanisms such as involvement of other systems including cardiovascular, haematological, respiratory, renal, hepatic and metabolic or the presence of predisposing or coexisting general medical risk factors. A variety of medications can cause transiently elevated blood pressure including sildenafil, amphetamines, ephedrine, heroin and other drugs of abuse. Vasospasm may occur with sympathomimetics, triptans and cerebral vasculitis is particularly associated with amphetamines, Ecstasy, penicillin, tacrolimus and, occasionally, allopurinol. There is a small increased risk of thrombo-embolism, ischaemic arterial or cerebral venous occlusion in women taking the oral contraceptive pill; chemotherapeutic agents including cisplatinum can also cause cerebral venous or arterial thrombosis or haemorrhage.

Impairment of taste and small

Disturbances of taste (dysgeusia) and smell (dysosmia) are extremely common manifestations of drug toxicity. They are particularly associated with antidiabetic therapy (oral hypoglycaemics), phosphodiesterase inhibitors, theophylline, caffeine, ethambutol, other antibiotics including penicillin, antirheumatic medication (gold, D-penicillamine), angiotensin converting enzyme inhibitors and many cytotoxic agents.

Drug-induced movement disorders (Chapter 6)

Several movement disorders are caused by commonly prescribed medication (Table 19.15). Acute dystonic and dyskinetic reactions often develop immediately following treatment and can be manifest as oromandibular dystonia, oculogyric crisis and opisthotonus.

Table 19.15 Drug-induced movement disorders.

Acute dystonia	Neuroleptic medication (phenothiazide and butyrophenones) Tricyclic antidepressants Metoclopramide Antiepileptic drugs (phenytoin, carbamazepine) Others (propranolol, ondansetron and fluoxetine)
Akathesia	Phenothiazines Butyrophenones Benzodiazepines Antidepressants, SSRIs (particularly fluoxetine)
Choreoathetosis	Antiepileptic medication Oral contraceptives Drugs of abuse (e.g. crack cocaine) Lithium
Parkinsonism	Dopamine receptor blocking drugs (particularly phenothiazines, butyrophenones and haloperidol) SSRIs may also induce or exacerbate parkinsonian syndromes
Tremor – essential and action	Sympothomometics Tricyclic antidepressants Lithium and levodopa Aminophylline, theophylline Caffeine Hypoglycaemics Antiepileptic drugs (valproate, phenytoin, carbamazepine, primidone) Sedatives Barbiturates Benzodiazepines
Tardive dyskinesia	Dopamine antagonists (especially antipsychotics) Metoclopramide Promethazine Prochlorperazine Antihistamines Tricyclic antidepressants Levodopa Monoamine oxidase inhibitors

Dystonia can be more generalised with slow writhing movements of the limbs or prolonged contractions of the axial and limb musculature. The acute dystonias are usually self-limiting once the drug is discontinued. Akathisia is a state of motor restlessness characterised by an inability to keep the legs still and an urge to constantly move, pace or run. Akathisia usually remits within days or weeks following withdrawal of the neuroleptic drug but can occasionally persist or be permanent. Choreoathetosis is manifest as irregular multifocal non-stereotyped semi-purposeful jerky movements often associated with slower dystonic movements. Drug-induced tics are associated with amphetamine-like drugs, methylphenidate, haloperidol and other antipsychotic medication. Drug-induced parkinsonism is the most common form of iatrogenic movement disorder and can be extremely difficult to distinguish from idiopathic Parkinson's disease. The onset tends to be slow, with bradykinesis being the most prominent feature characterised by variable rigidity, tremor and gait disturbance. The condition is usually reversible after drug withdrawal or dosage reduction over the course of several weeks but drugs may unmask latent idiopathic Parkinson's disease. A number of drugs may aggravate an essential or physiological tremor. Tardive dyskinesia usually develops after more than 12 months of continuous therapy but may evolve over a much shorter period, occasionally developing after cessation of therapy. It is characterised by orofaciobuccal dyskinesia with lip-smacking and pursing, jaw opening, closing and protrusion of the face with writhing movements of the tongue and facial grimacing. The movements tend to be stereotyped and may interfere with speech or swallowing. There can be associated choreoathetotic movements of the limbs and trunk with repetitive foot tapping. Tardive forms of tic, myoclonus and tremor are also described. A variety of dopamine receptor blocking drugs can cause tardive dyskinesiae; the newer atypical dopamine receptor blocking drugs, including clozapine, appear to carry less risk.

All the major classes of conventional neuroleptic drugs (phenothiazines, butyrophenones, thioxanthenes) and the atypical antipsychotic drugs including clozapine, olanzapine, quetiapine and risperidone have been reported to cause extrapyramidal syndromes. All these side effects are idiosyncratic and patients vary greatly in their susceptibility and in the dose necessary to precipitate the side effects; patients with dementia with Lewy bodies are particularly vulnerable.

Ototoxicity

Drug-induced damage to the cochlear and vestibular function is common. The former is manifest as tinnitus and hearing loss and the latter as vertigo, oscillopsia and imbalance. Both are characteristically associated with aminoglycoside antibiotics, gentamicin and streptomicin. Balance is usually preferentially affected. Loop diuretics, salicylates, antimalarials (quinine, chloroquine) and cytotoxic agents including cisplatin and vincristine can be associated with hearing loss (Chapter 15).

Cerebellar disorders

Cerebellar disorders are usually dose-related and reversible but can become fixed deficits after antiepileptic drugs, phenothiazides, lithium or ciclosporin.

Visual disorders

Drug-induced visual disorders can be brought about by a variety of different mechanisms and visual disorders.

- *Pupillary*: miosis is produced by parasympathetic drugs which include cholinergic agents (neostigmine, pyridostigmine) and opiates (morphine) but mydriasis, which may occur with anticholinergic agents (atropine, hyoscine), tricyclic antidepressants and phenothiazines (MAIOs, tricyclics), is a more serious drug effect because of the risk of precipitating closed angle glaucoma.
- *Distortion of the lens* can cause refractory changes because of fluid shifts with diuretics and antidiabetic therapy (insulin, oral hypoglycaemics) and corticosteroids.
- *Drug-induced retinopathy* can be caused by the development of pigmentary change (as occurs with chloroquine-like drugs and cardiac glycosides).

- *Macular oedema* (oral contraceptive) or visual field loss (e.g. ethambutol, indomethacin, vigabatrin) may occur and optic neuropathy has been associated with some antibiotics (e.g. chloramphenicol, isoniazide, ethambutol, cytotoxic medication, opiates and NSAIDs).
- *Nystagmus* is the most common drug-related eye movement disorder and is caused by antiepileptic drugs, tricyclic antidepressants, ototoxic medication, salicylates and MAOIs.

Autonomic effects

Disturbances of autonomic function are commonly caused by drug toxicity. Drug-induced syncope may occur as a consequence of vasovagal disturbances, postural hypotension or cardiac disease. Postural hypotension occurs with a variety of antihypertensive medication (particularly β-blockers, vasodilatators and diuretics), antidepressants and levodopa. In the elderly, syncope is particulary associated with fluoxetine, haloperidol and levodopa. Bladder disturbance occurs with anticholinergic medication (atropine, hyoscine), particularly with pre-existing prostatic outflow tract obstruction. Medication can cause sexual dysfunction at any level of function. Antihypertensive medication (β-blockers) is particularly associated with impotence or impairment of ejaculation, while antidepressant medication can affect libido or cause orgasmic dysfunction. Spinal toxicity can follow intrathecal injection of steroids, cytotoxic medication or contrast material leading to an infective or aseptic meningitis, adhesive arachnoiditis or direct toxic effects on the spinal cord or nerve roots. Epidural injection is not associated with these problems unless there is penetration of the dura.

Neuromuscular drug effects

There are many drugs that can cause non-specific fatigability but peripheral neuropathy is an extremely common manifestation of drug toxicity (Chapter 10).

Peripheral neuropathy

Most drug-related neuropathies are predominantly axonal although demyelination and conduction block can occur. Both motor and sensory patterns are seen. The major categories of drug-induced peripheral neuropathy are summarised in Table 19.16.

Drugs interfering with neuromuscular transmission

These can cause a myasthenic-like syndrome, uncover latent myasthenia or exacerbate the existing disease. These are discussed in Chapter 10; only the most important drugs are listed in Table 19.17.

A large variety of muscle diseases can be caused by drugs (Table 19.18).

Myalgia, stiffness and cramp

Many drugs cause myalgia, stiffness and cramp, often in association with a transiently elevated creatinine kinase level. Drug-induced myopathy may be associated with myotonia, pain or myokymia and may be focal or generalised. The most important drugs causing the different forms of myopathy are listed in Table 19.18.

Malignant hyperthermia

This condition occurs in susceptible individuals following anaesthesia using a halogenated inhaled anaesthetics (including halothane, enflurane and isoflurane) and/or a depolarising muscle relaxant such as succinylcholine. The condition is characterised by the sudden onset of fever and rigidity associated with a high

Table 19.16 Drugs causing peripheral neuropathy.

Antibiotics		Neuropathy
Metronidazole	A/D	Sensory
Nitrofurantoin	A	Sensorimotor or motor
Isoniazide	A	Sensorimotor or sensory
Ethambutol	A	Sensorimotor or motor
Dapsone	A	Motor
Antiviral nucleoside analogues	A	Sensory
Chemotherapeutic agents		
Cisplatin	A	Sensory
Vinca alkaloids	A	Sensorimotor ± autonomic
Cytarabin (high dose)	D	Sensory
Thalidomide	A	Sensory
Cardiovascular drugs		
Statins	A	Sensory > sensory motor
Amiodarone	D/A	Sensorimotor > motor
Enalapril	A	Sensorimotor > sensory
Hydralazine	A	Sensorimotor > sensory
Streptokinase	A	GBS-like syndrome
Antirheumatic drugs		
Gold	A/D	Motor > GBS-like
Chloroquine	D/A	Sensorimotor
Colchichine	A	Sensorimotor
Allopurinol	A/D	Sensorimotor
Others		
Tacrolimus	D	GBS-like
Ciclosporin	A	Sensory
Disulfiram	A	Sensorimotor
Lithium overdose	A/D	GBS-like (sensorimotor)
Phenytoin	A/D	Sensory and motor

A, axonal; D, demyelinating.

Table 19.17 Drugs that may cause disorders of the neuromuscular junction.

Antibitoics – aminoglycosides, tetracycline, ciprofloxacin
Antiarrhythmics – quinidine, procainamide
Antimalarials – chloroquine
Antirheumatics – pencillamine D
Beta-blockers – propranolol, atenolol, metopralol, sotalol
Antiepileptics – phenytoin
Neuroleptics – chlorpromazine, clozapine, flupenthixol, lithium, MAOIs
Neuromuscular junction blocking agents

MAOI, monoaminase oxidase inhibitor.

Table 19.18 Drugs that may cause muscle disease.

Subacute necrotising myopathy

Symmetrical proximal weakness with myalgia and elevated CK
- Amiodarone
- Chloroquine
- Lipid-lowering medication – simvastatin, pravastatin, atorvastatin
- Colchicine
- Corticosteroids
- Zidovudine
- Heroin

Myositis

Inflammatory myopathy indistinguishable from polymyositis with elevated CK
- Chloroquine
- Corticosteroids
- D-penicillamine
- Lipid-lowering drugs – simvastatin, pravastin
- Others – phenytoin, levodopa, cimetidine

Myotonia

Drug either causing the myotonia or unmasking latent myotonic disorders
- Proprofol
- Depolarising muscle relaxants – suxamethonium
- Diuretics – frusemide, acetazolomide
- Vincristine
- Lipid-lowering drugs – simvastatin, pravastatin
- Beta-blockers – propranolol, pindolol

Focal fibrous myopathy following intramuscular drug injection

Caused by needle trauma and local effects of agent injected leading to severe muscle fibrosis and contractures
- Antibiotics
- Chloroquine
- Drug abuse

Myopathy resulting from hypokalaemia
- Diuretics
- Purgative abuse
- Licorice
- Amphoterocin B

Mitochondrial myopathy

Characterised by myalgia, proximal weakness and elevated CK
- Zidovudine

Rhabdomyolysis

Acute and severe necrotising myopathy characterised by severe muscle pain, swelling and weakness leading to myoglobinuria and renal failure
- Anaesthetics
- Lipid lowering drugs – simvastatin, pravastatin
- Diuretics
- Barbiturates
- Opiates – morphine, heroin
- Alcohol
- Other drugs of abuse – amphetamines, LSD

CK, creatine kinase; LSD, lysergic acid diethylamide.

creatine kinase level with metabolic acidosis and myoglobinuria. Liability to malignant hyperthermia is transmitted in an autosomal dominant fashion and occurs in genetically predisposed individuals who have an intrinsic abnormality of the excitation–contraction coupling mechanism in skeletal muscle. This leads to an excessive release of Ca^{2+} from the sarcoplasmic reticulum resulting in myofibrillar contraction. The condition seems to be caused by a defect in the calcium release channel (RYR1) and the genetic basis is a mutation in the *RYR1* gene on chromosome 19q or in other calcium channel genes.

The onset of the condition is variable. In the most florid forms acidosis, rigidity and hyperpyrexia may develop within 30 minutes of anaesthesia but in some patients the onset is slower with the condition developing over several hours with only mild signs. The initial features are tachycardia, raised end tidal carbon dioxide, metabolic acidosis and progressive muscular rigidity. The hyperthermia develops later but can be severe. In its most severe form the condition progresses to rhabdomyolysis and myoglobinuria, disseminated intravascular coagulation (DIC), cardiovascular collapse or hyperpyrexia leading to multi-system failure. There seems to be similar sensitivity to anaesthetic agents in patients with other neuromuscular diseases, in particular Duchenne muscular dystrophy, myotonia congenita, myotonic dystrophy, central core disease, congenital myopathy and osteogenesis imperfecta.

Vulnerability to this syndrome is suggested by a positive family history or previous difficulties during anaesthesia. It can be tested *in vitro* using biopsied muscle and observing a hypercontractile response to caffeine or halothane. Management involves the immediate discontinuation of the triggering anaesthesia and hyperventilation with 100% oxygen at high flow. Dantrolene is recommended as specific therapy in a dose of 2.5 mg/kg IV repeated as necessary. Supportive care of heart rate, temperature and oxygenation are essential. Core temperature can be reduced by ice lavage. Hyperkalaemia is managed by the use of bicarbonate, glucose, insulin and calcium but it is essential to be aware of rebound hypokalaemia which may precipitate further episodes. Myoglobinuria is treated with diuretics, fluid support and bicarbonate as necessary. With rapid and appropriate management the prognosis in an acute episode is good and the syndrome resolves rapidly. It is clearly essential to be aware of any susceptibility to this condition in planning anaesthesia. Complete recovery occurs in general but weakness may last for months after an acute episode.

Neuroleptic malignant syndrome

This is a serious and potentially fatal complication of treatment with antipsychotic agents. The condition is characterised by onset within 2 weeks of initiating or increasing neuroleptic therapy although, rarely, it can develop after months or years of stable treatment. The signs evolve over up to 72 hours although the onset can be more acute and it usually resolves within 2 weeks. The presentation is usually with progressive and severe pyrexia (>40 °C in 40% of patients) although a more insidious prodrome with a modest pyrexia can occur. There is progressive encephalopathy and impairment of conscious state ranging from lethargy to delirium, confusion, agitation and coma. Severe 'lead pipe' rigidity with other extrapyramidal features including bradykinesis, rest tremor and dystonia develop. There is autonomic instability including tachycardia, tachypnoea, diaphoresis, labile blood pressure, skin pallor or flushing, sialorrhoea and urinary disturbance including incontinence. The condition is characterised by grossly elevated creatine kinase level and there is also usually a leukocytosis, metabolic acidosis and elevated CSF protein but muscle biopsy is non-specific.

The most common drugs causing this condition are haloperidol, fluphenazine and chlorpromazine but other phenathiazines, lithium, metoclopramide, tricyclic antidepressants or atypical antidepressants (clozapine,risperidone, olanzapine) can also be responsible. Other risk factors seem to include the use of depot injections, rapid dose increase and the presence of dehydration or agitation. There can also be a genetic predisposition to the condition. Despite treatment, neuroleptic malignant syndrome can progress to the development of rhabdomyolysis leading to myoglobinuria and renal failure, coagulation defects from DIC, respiratory failure, shock, seizures and coma. In some series mortality has been up to 20%, with persisting neurological sequelae in 10% of survivors.

The management is both supportive and specific. The neuroleptic must be immediately discontinued and the core temperature normalised. There must be close attention to hydration, blood pressure, cardiac, respiratory and renal function with adequate anticoagulation. Specific management remains controversial. Dantrolene is a muscle relaxant that inhibits excitation contraction mechanisms and may influence central dopaminergic mechanisms in the active phase of neuroleptic malignant syndrome. It has been reported to be effective but there is a risk of hepatic toxicity. Bromocriptine is a dopamine agonist that works by acting centrally to counter the neuroleptic effects. It has been given in divided doses for up to 10 days after resolution of symptoms but its use is limited by side effects of nausea, hypertension and worsening mental state. Electroconvulsive therapy has been advocated because of its efficacy in treating malignant catatonia but there is little evidence to support its use.

Neuroleptic malignant syndrome probably results from a sudden decrease in central dopaminergic function resulting from profound dopamine receptor blockade at multiple sites including the corpus striatum and thermoregulatory and vasomotor centres in the hypothalamus. However, while the condition usually occurs with dopamine receptor blocking drugs it may also be seen with dopamine depleting drugs or even without exposure to neuroleptics.

Serotonin syndrome

Serotonin syndrome is a variable but potentially life-threatening drug reaction caused by excessive serotonin stimulation of the central and peripheral nervous systems. It results from therapeutic use, intentional self-poisoning or inadvertent interaction between drugs. Clinical manifestations are variable. There is a characteristic triad of mental state change, neuromuscular abnormalities and autonomic hyper-reactivity. The condition is probably more common than was previously thought particularly with increasing use of selective serotonin re-uptake inhibitors (SSRIs).

Presentation can be with mild tachycardia and minor autonomic features including shivering, diaphoresis and mydriasis. These can be considered to be simple drug reactions and the medication is often discontinued. However, in more severe forms the condition may progress to an intermittent tremor or myoclonus with hyper-reflexia. There can be severe hyperthermia, tachycardia and hypertension. Progressive encephalopathy with clouding of consciousness, confusion and hypomania may develop. Autonomic features that may evolve include mydriasis, hyperactive bowel sounds, diaphoresis and neurological involvement including the development of lead pipe rigidity, myoclonus, tremor, incoordination, clonus and hyper-reflexia. The condition usually develops within 24 hours of the initiation of causative medication but the onset can be within minutes or come on after several weeks at stable dosage.

Laboratory investigation may show metabolic acidosis, rhabdomyolysis, abnormalities of liver function and there may be features of DIC or renal failure but most cases are relatively minor and resolve over 12–24 hours. The condition occurs with monotherapy using SSRIs or when there is an interaction between two drugs from this class. These include SSRIs (citalopram, escitalopram, fluoxetine, fluvoxamine, paroxetine and sertraline) or other antidepressant drugs that inhibit the re-uptake of serotonin by other mechanisms including duloxetine, olanzapine, mirtazapine and venlafaxine.

Serotonin syndrome can also be associated with other drugs that inhibit the re-uptake of serotonin and these are listed here. The condition has been reported to follow administration of a serotoninergic agent up to 5 weeks after discontinuation of fluoxetine.

Drugs that can cause serotonin syndrome either in isolation or when combined include:

- SSRIs
- Atypical antidepressants
- MAOIs – phenelzine and selegiline
- Tricyclic antidepressants
- Dopaminergic agents
- Antiepileptic drugs – sodium valproate, carbamazepine
- Lithium
- Anaesthetics
- Opiate analgesics – tramadol, meperidine, pentazocine
- Risperidone
- Over-the-counter cold remedies containing ephedrine and dextromethorphan
- Antiemetics – ondansetron, metoclopramide
- Antimigraine – sumatriptan and other triptans
- Drugs of abuse – Ecstasy, opioids, LSD
- Herbal products – St John's wort
- Withdrawal of medication.

The condition can be transient and not require treatment other than the discontinuation of the relevant medication. However, if the symptoms are severe, management is both supportive and specific. Following discontinuation of the serotoninergic medication it is necessary to control agitation, monitor the level of consciousness, respiratory and cardiac function and to control hyperthermia and autonomic instability. Sedation, neuromuscular paralysis and orotrachial intubation with ventilation can be necessary.

There remains controversy about specific treatment using 5-HT antagonists. A variety of treatments have been used but none is proven. The present recommendations are for the administration of cyproheptadine as it binds to 5-HT receptors. Chlorpromazine has also been used but there is no benefit from other 5-HT antagonists including lorazepam, methysergide and propranolol.

It is important to distinguish this condition from neuroleptic malignant syndrome, malignant hyperthermia, anticholinergic syndrome and the tyramine cheese reaction and this differential diagnosis is summarised in Table 19.19.

Tyramine cheese reaction

The tyramine cheese reaction usually occurs in patients taking non-selective MAOIs. Ingestion of tyramine-containing substances (usually cheese or red wine) or sympathomimetic agents can lead to an acute hypertensive crisis, headache, nausea and vomiting culminating in hyperthermia and rarely DIC, renal

Table 19.19 Comparison of clinical features of serotonin syndrome, neuroleptic malignant syndrome (NMS), malignant hyperpyrexia, tyramine and anticholinergic syndrome.

		Serotonin syndrome	NMS	Malignant hyperpyrexia	Tyramine	Anticholinergic
Medication		Sereotoninergic drugs	Dopamine agonists	Inhalation anaesthetic or succinylcholine	MAOI	Anticholinergic
Onset		<12 hours	1–3 days	30 min – 24 hours	<12 hours	<12 hours
Vital signs	T°	++	+	++	0	+
	BP	+	+	+	++	±
	Pulse (tachycardia)	+	+	+	+	+
Systemic	Diaphoresis/skin	++	++	++	0	Dry
	Bowel sounds	Hyperactive	Normal	Normal/decreased	Normal	Absent
	Headache	+	0	0	+	++
	Flushing	+	+	+	+	++
Neurology	Mental state	++	++	+	0	++
	Mydriasis	+	0	0	0	++
	Rigidity	+	++	++	0	0
	Reflexes	++	+	0	0	Normal
	Myoclonus/tremor	++	+	0	0	0

MAOI, monoamine oxidase inhibitor.

failure and cardiopulmonary arrest. The condition is caused by excessive tyramine that has not been deaminated, leading to the release of catecholamines in nerve endings and the adrenal medulla. There may be progressive confusion and delirium which may evolve into coma. The patient appears flushed and may be pyrexial but there are no extrapyramidal features. Management is by withdrawal of the precipitating medication and supportive care.

Anticholinergic syndrome caused by medication toxicity

In this condition, mental state changes are common, usually beginning as a mild encephalopathy with disorientation but progression to profound clouding of consciousness and coma may occur. Anticholinergic features include mydriasis, dry oral mucosa and hot erythematous skin. In contrast to the serotonin syndrome there are reduced or absent bowel sounds and no extrapyramidal features. There is a tachycardia, increased respiratory rate and occasionally urinary retention. Management is with discontinuation of the causative drugs.

Inherited disorders of metabolism

This section deals with neurological disease seen in adult patients with inherited disorders of metabolism. The clinical presentation, differential diagnosis, investigation and management of adult onset leukodystrophy is also discussed. The conditions described do not make up a fully comprehensive or exhaustive list of all the inherited metabolic defects that can lead to neurological abnormalities in adults, but rather represent the conditions that are more frequently encountered in a large adult metabolic clinic.

Porphyria

The porphyrias are a group of rare conditions caused by abnormal biosynthesis of haem, which is a precursor of haemoglobin and cytochrome P450 enzymes. Most, apart from X-linked protoporphyria, are inherited in an autosomal dominant manner.

Classification is based on the tissue where metabolic intermediates accumulate (hepatic or erythrocytic) or on the clinical

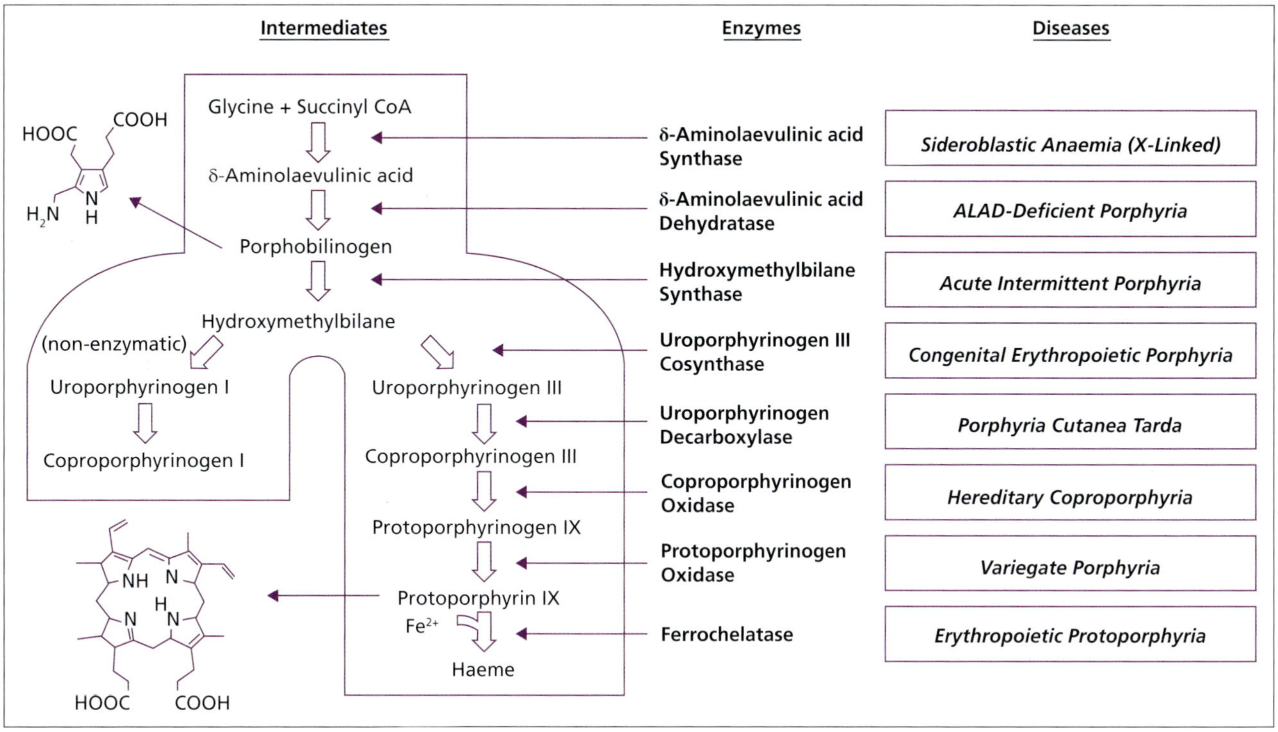

Figure 19.19 Metabolic pathway for the formation of haem.

presentation (neurovisceral or cutaneous). The most common of the acute porphyrias (acute intermittent porphyria; AIP) is caused by deficiency of the enzyme hydroxymethylbilane synthase leading to the overproduction and accumulation of the porphyrin precursors ALA (δ-aminolevulinic acid) and PBG (porphobilinogen) which are neurotoxic. Other forms of porphyria are caused by enzyme defects at other points in the synthetic pathway (Figure 19.19).

Acute intermittent porphyria

Most heterozygotes with this autosomal dominant condition remain asymptomatic throughout life. However, certain precipitants including drugs, a calorie deficient diet, intercurrent infection, surgery or the luteal phase of the menstrual cycle, can trigger an attack.

AIP is characterised by recurrent attacks of acute abdominal pain and neuropsychiatric manifestations, generally from the teenage years onwards. There can be an acute or subacute, predominantly motor, polyneuropathy but no skin photosensitivity. It is characterised by symptom-free periods interrupted by acute neurovisceral attacks occurring with varying frequency. Neurovisceral attacks are characterised by the acute onset of severe abdominal pain which is usually poorly localised and associated with nausea, vomiting, diarrhoea or constipation and features of an ileus. There is a secondary dysautonomia with hypertension, tachycardia, tremor, hyperhidrosis and urinary retention. Neuropsychiatric manifestations include anxiety, confusion, restlessness, agitation, insomnia and psychosis. There can be generalised seizures, sometimes in association with hyponatraemia. The polyneuropathy often follows neurovisceral attacks, but also occurs independently, and can be associated with back pain, prominent wasting and involvement of the proximal and cranial musculature. There can be occasional mild sensory features, but profound muscle weakness sometimes progresses to involve respiratory muscles, particularly the diaphragm.

Diagnosis

The finding of elevated urine porphobilinogen during an attack is a sensitive and specific indicator of an acute porphyria. This usually remains elevated between attacks of acute intermittent porphyria, unless there have been no symptoms for a prolonged period.

For confirmation of the diagnosis, determination of the specific enzyme deficiency, and finding of asymptomatic carriers then total urinary porphyrins, plasma porphyrins, faecal porphyrins, measurement of erythrocyte hydroxymethylbilane synthase activity and/or mutation analysis are useful. To determine the most appropriate samples for investigation discuss with a local specialist porphyria service (contact details available on www.porphyria-europe.org).

Management

The greatest period of risk to patients is prior to the diagnosis being made when they and their physicians are unaware of the potential problems. Management includes the prevention of attacks by avoiding precipitating factors. Treatment during an attack is both symptomatic and specific: symptomatic care involves the use of narcotic analgesics for abdominal pain; treatment of nausea, vomiting and agitation; correction of electrolyte disturbances; maintenance of high carbohydrate intake (IV 10% glucose); and treatment of underlying precipitating factors including infection. Specific

Table 19.20 Examples of disorders with a neurological phenotype that might be encountered in an adult neurology clinic.

Disorders of amino acid metabolism

Phenylketonuria

Maple syrup urine disease

Tyrosinaemia (types I, II, III)

Homocystinuria

Organic acid disorders

Methylmalonic acidemia

Propionic acidemia

Isovaleric acidemia

Glutaric aciduria type I

Urea cycle disorders / disorders associated with hyperammonaemia

N-acetylglutamate synthase deficiency

Carbamoylphosphate synthase deficiency

Ornithine transcarbamylase deficiency

Argininosuccinate synthase deficiency (Citrullinemia type I)

Argininosuccinate lyase deficiency

Arginase deficiency

HHH (hyperammonaemia, hyperornithinaemia, homocitrullinaemia)

Citrin deficiency (Citrullinemia type II)

Fatty acid oxidation disorders

Very long chain acyl-CoA dehydrogenase (VLCAD) deficiency

Short (SCAD), medium (MCAD) and long chain acyl-CoA dehydrogenase (LCHAD) deficiencies

Carnitine translocase deficiency

Carnitine palmitoyltransferase I and II deficiencies

Multipe acyl-CoAdehydrogenase deficiency (Glutaric aciduria type II)

Disorders of carnitine mediated transport and uptake

Carnitine transporter deficiency / primary carnitine deficiency

Disorders of carbohydrate metabolism / transport (with a muscle +/or neurological phenotype)

Galactosemia

Glut-1 deficiency

Glycogen storage disease II (acid maltase deficiency, Pompe disease)

Glycogen storage disease III

Glycogen storage disease V (McArdle disease)

Danon disease

Polyglucosan body disorders

Epilepsy, progressive myoclonic (Lafora)

RBCK1-related polyglucosan body myopathy - E3 ubiquitin ligase

Glycogen storage disease IV / Polyglucosan body disease, adult form

Glycogen storage disease XV

Glycogen storage disease VII (phosphofructokinase deficiency)

Disorders of neurotransmission

Dopa-responsive dystonia (Segawa syndrome)

Lysosomal storage disorders

See Table 19.22

Others

Mitochondrial disease (see Chapter 10)

Porphyria

Congenital disorders of glycosylation

Disorders of homocysteine, B12 and folate metabolism (see Table 19.21)

Wilson disease (see Chapter 6)

Disorders of creatine biosynthesis

Leukodystrophies (see Table 19.24)

treatment involves the use of intravenous haem arginate which acts by inhibiting aminolaevulinic acid (ALA) synthase, the rate-limiting enzyme, allowing further metabolism along the pathway and leading to rapid resolution of symptoms (though weakness and neuropathy may resolve slowly and incompletely, particularly after a prolonged severe attack).

Medications should be checked before administration to ensure that they are not known to be porphyrinogenic (including hormonal contraception, anaesthetic agents and antiepileptic drugs, particularly carbamazepine, phenytoin, phenobarbital, primidone and topiramate). Liver transplant for severe frequent attacks is effective.

Disorders of amino acid metabolism

There are many disorders of amino acid metabolism associated with neurological abnormalities, including enzymatic deficiencies within the degradative pathways of specific amino acids (e.g. phenylketonuria, the organic acidemias, classic homocystinuria), as well as within pathways using common products of catabolism, such as the urea cycle disorders (Table 19.20).

Phenylketonuria

Phenylketonuria (PKU) is one of the most common inherited metabolic disorders, with an incidence of about 1/10 000 live births. For more than 40 years, all newborn babies in the United Kingdom (and other countries) have been screened for PKU, and patients with PKU make up the largest cohort of any adult metabolic clinic. PKU results from a deficiency of phenylalanine hydroxylase, which converts phenylalanine into tyrosine. Hyperphenylalaninaemia can also, rarely, be caused by deficiency of tetrahydrobiopterin (a cofactor of phenylalanine hydroxylase).

The infant brain is sensitive to high phenylalanine levels and, if left untreated, PKU gives rise to severe mental retardation. Microcephaly is common and about 25% of patients with untreated PKU have epilepsy. In older patients, behavioural problems are common and some have psychotic illnesses. A few patients develop movement disorders with pyramidal and extrapyramidal signs. Although most of the pathology is related to brain damage, eczema is also common. Because of a deficiency in melanin formation (secondary to tyrosine deficiency), Caucasian patients tend to be fair-skinned with blond hair and blue eyes.

There is evidence to suggest that phenylalanine itself is toxic to the developing brain. In rare patients who have normal IQ despite very high plasma phenylalanine concentrations, magnetic resonance spectroscopy (MRS) has shown that phenylalanine concentrations in the brain are normal. Like other large neutral amino acids, phenylalanine is actively transported into the brain by the L-type amino acid carrier. It has been suggested that genetic variance in this transport system might account for the phenotypic variability seen between PKU patients with similar plasma concentrations of phenylalanine but, to date, no evidence for this has been found.

There are also secondary deleterious effects of hyperphenylalaninaemia. Because phenyalanine competes with other large neutral amino acids for transport into the brain, high levels of phenylalanine in the CNS are accompanied by low levels of other amino acids such as tyrosine and tryptophan. It has been suggested that this can lead to deficiencies in neurotransmitters, particularly dopamine, which is derived from tyrosine. A relative deficiency of large neutral amino acids can also affect protein synthesis.

MRI studies show signal abnormalities in the periventricular white matter, but these appear to relate directly to the brain concentration of phenylalanine, improving if phenylalanine levels are lowered, and it is questionable whether they have any functional consequences.

Management Blood and brain phenylalanine levels can be lowered by restricting dietary protein intake. Provided this dietary therapy is instituted soon after birth, PKU can be effectively treated, with intellectual outcomes similar to those of unaffected siblings. The low protein diet is highly restrictive: patients must avoid high protein foods such as meat, fish and eggs, and are allowed only limited amounts of many other staple foods such as potatoes and cereals. For normal growth and health it is therefore necessary to prescribe synthetic supplements to provide protein requirements, as a phenylalanine-free amino acid mixture, and all the vitamins, minerals and other micronutrients that are usually obtained from meat and dairy products (e.g. vitamin B_{12}, calcium and iron). The amount of natural dietary protein allowed is titrated against blood phenylalanine concentrations which vary according to residual PAH enzyme activity which in turn is a function of the genotype. In infancy and early childhood, metabolic control needs to be strict in order to protect the developing brain and, in the United Kingdom, practice is to keep the phenylalanine level 360–480 µmol/L (normal range 33–81 µmol/L).

There is evidence that after 10 years of age the IQ of children with PKU is fixed, whether or not they remain on a strict low protein diet, implying that the brain becomes resistant to the toxic effects of phenylalanine as it matures. However, other studies have shown more subtle, reversible cognitive deficits in adult patients not on a protein-restricted diet when compared with those who have followed a diet throughout life. Current recommendations in the United Kingdom are to encourage patients to follow a protein-restricted diet with a more relaxed target phenylalanine level of 700 µmol/L in adults.

In practice, however, many adult patients choose to resume a normal diet, and their phenylalanine levels rise accordingly. There is currently no evidence that this poses any risk of irreversible neurological damage, although higher levels can affect executive function and reaction time. The current uncertainty about the effects of high phenylalanine on the adult brain is reflected in the lack of international consensus on what phenylalanine targets should be in adult patients following a protein restricted diet. Some US authors suggest that patients should maintain levels of less than 360 µmol/L throughout life while French guidelines are for adults to maintain levels under 1300 µmol/L. The authors' current practice is to educate and support patients to achieve the phenylalanine levels where they feel they function best.

There have been some reports of spastic paraparesis developing in untreated patients, but these seem to have been secondary to vitamin B_{12} deficiency. These patients are particularly susceptible to nutritional deficiencies as, even when dietary restrictions have been lifted, many still avoid high protein foods and follow a diet of poor nutritional quality. In these cases, it is important to monitor nutritional status carefully and continue with appropriate vitamin supplementation.

Maternal PKU syndrome Phenylalanine is teratogenic and high maternal levels of phenylalanine will cross the placenta and cause the maternal PKU syndrome in the fetus (intrauterine growth retardation, developmental delay, microcephaly, congenital cardiac disease and dysmorphic features). This syndrome can be prevented by meticulous maternal control of phenylalanine levels in the pre-conception period and throughout pregnancy.

Organic acidemias

These are a group of disorders resulting from impaired activity of specific enzymes involved in the catabolism of the branched-chain amino acids – leucine, isoleucine and valine (Figure 19.20). The most common of these conditions that are seen in the adult metabolic and neurology clinic are maple syrup urine disease (MSUD), isovaleric acidemia (IVA), methylmalonic acidemia (MMA) and propionic acidemia (PA). The disorders can have common clinical presentations:

1. A severe neonatal metabolic decompensation with neurological impairment
2. An acute intermittent form with recurrent episodes of metabolic decompensation
3. A chronic progressive form with developmental delay, failure to thrive and neurological involvement.

Diagnosis is based on plasma amino acid analysis (e.g. MSUD), a urine organic acid profile, and confirmed by measurement of specific enzyme activities in cultured fibroblasts and/or genetic testing. Newborn screening, where available, is carried out by blood spot leucine/isoleucine (e.g. MSUD) or acylcarnitine (e.g. IVA, PA, MMA) measurement.

Maple syrup urine disease

MSUD is caused by a defect in the catabolism of the branched-chain amino acids leucine, isoleucine and valine caused by deficiency of branched-chain α-ketoacid dehydrogenase (BCKD) (Figure 19.20). MSUD derives its name from the aroma of the accumulated ketoacids excreted in urine. Classic untreated MSUD, with complete deficiency of BCKD, usually presents in the first week of life with non-specific symptoms which rapidly progress to encephalopathy and death. Partial enzyme activity results in an intermediate phenotype with intermittent acute encephalopathic episodes, developmental delay and a spastic paraparesis.

Neurotoxicity is directly related to the degree and duration of elevation of the plasma leucine level. Acute leucine intoxication is characterised by confusion, hyperactivity, hallucinations, dystonia, ataxia and eventually coma. There is some evidence to suggest that leucine competitively inhibits transport of other large neutral amino acids (LNAAs), such as tyrosine, across the blood–brain barrier. Low cerebral tyrosine has been implicated in some of the acute symptoms of leucine toxicity. A chronic cerebral protein deficiency, secondary to the effects of leucine on other LNAA levels and on general protein restriction as part of treatment, may result in

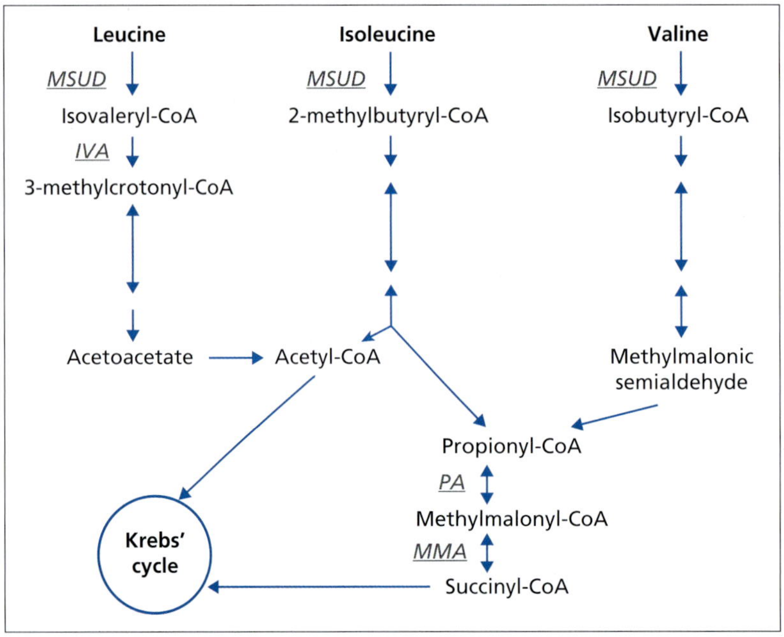

Figure 19.20 Catabolism of the branched chain amino acids (the organic acidurias). The branched chain amino acids, leucine, isoleucine and valine, are initially catabolised by a common pathway. Subsequently, leucine is catabolised to acetoacetate and acetyl-CoA which enters the Krebs' cycle (tricarboxylic acid, TCA). Acetyl CoA and propionyl-CoA are derived from isoleucine. PropionylCoA also enters the Krebs' cycle via conversion to succinyl-CoA. Valine is also metabolised to propionyl-CoA. Maple syrup urine disease (MSUD) is caused by deficiency of the branched-chain 2-ketoacid dehydrogenase complex; isovaleric acidemia (IVA) by isovaleryl-CoA dehydrogenase deficiency; propionic acidemia (PA) by propionyl-CoA carboxylase deficiency; and methylmalonic acidemia (MMA) by methylmalonyl-CoA mutase deficiency or deficiency of its cofactor adenosylcobalamin (see Figure 19.23).

paucity of dendritic branching and suboptimal myelination and contribute to the developmental delay seen in many patients.

Management With timely treatment, death and neurodisability can be avoided even in the severe classic forms of MSUD. In the acute phase, high leucine levels can rapidly be reduced by haemofiltration. Long-term management is dietary. The principles of treatment are to restrict dietary protein to reduce levels of the toxic metabolite, to provide a synthetic amino acid supplement, lacking the toxic metabolite and containing trace elements and vitamins, to replace protein requirements and allow normal growth and development and to prevent protein catabolism at times of fasting or physiological stress using a high carbohydrate emergency regimen. Patients collect regular blood spots at home (using the same Guthrie cards as in newborn screening) so that leucine levels can be monitored and their dietary protein intake adjusted accordingly.

With timely diagnosis and rapid reduction of leucine levels in the newborn period the prognosis can be good. Normal intellectual ability is possible, but is dependent on meticulous long-term dietary treatment with expectant management of intercurrent illnesses. Several countries, including the United Kingdom, now perform newborn screening for MSUD.

Isovaleric acidemia

Isovaleric acidemia (IVA) is caused by deficiency of isovaleryl-CoA dehydrogenase, a mitochondrial flavoenzyme (Figure 19.20). The severity of its clinical phenotype is variable and asymptomatic patients are known. Management is with a restricted protein diet and supplemental glycine and carnitine. Metabolic crisis in adulthood is unlikely.

Propionic acidemia and methylmalonic acidemia

Propionic and methylmalonic acid are biochemical intermediaries of BCAA degradation, and both have fundamental roles in energy production, in the degradation of other amino acids, fatty acid metabolism, the Krebs' cycle, gluconeogenesis and the detoxification of ammonia (Figure 19.20). Complete deficiency of either propionyl CoA carboxylase or methylmalonyl CoA mutase (MUT 0) results in severe neonatal encephalopathy, often fatal. Partial deficiency or defects in the synthesis of a cofactor such as adenosylcobalamin can present either in a similar manner or subacutely, but are more amenable to treatment.

Classic MMA and PA present in the neonatal period with nonspecific signs that rapidly progress to lethargy, seizures and coma. Patients typically demonstrate a severe metabolic acidosis with increased anion gap, ketonuria, a variable pancytopenia and hyperammonaemia. Intermediate phenotypes including cofactor defects can present later in life with acute encephalopathy, developmental delay, a movement disorder or behavioural disturbances. Specific insults to the basal ganglia result in choreoathetosis with compatible radiological findings.

Management Some patients with MMA respond to intramuscular vitamin B_{12} and all patients should be offered a trial of this. Subsequent treatment includes a protein restricted diet, prevention of catabolism, supplementation of vitamins and trace elements, and use of an emergency regimen during periods of acute decompensation.

Long-term complications Both PA and MMA require surveillance for long-term problems: acute pancreatitis, cardiomyopathy, osteopenia, an acute and/or chronic extrapyramidal disorder, premature

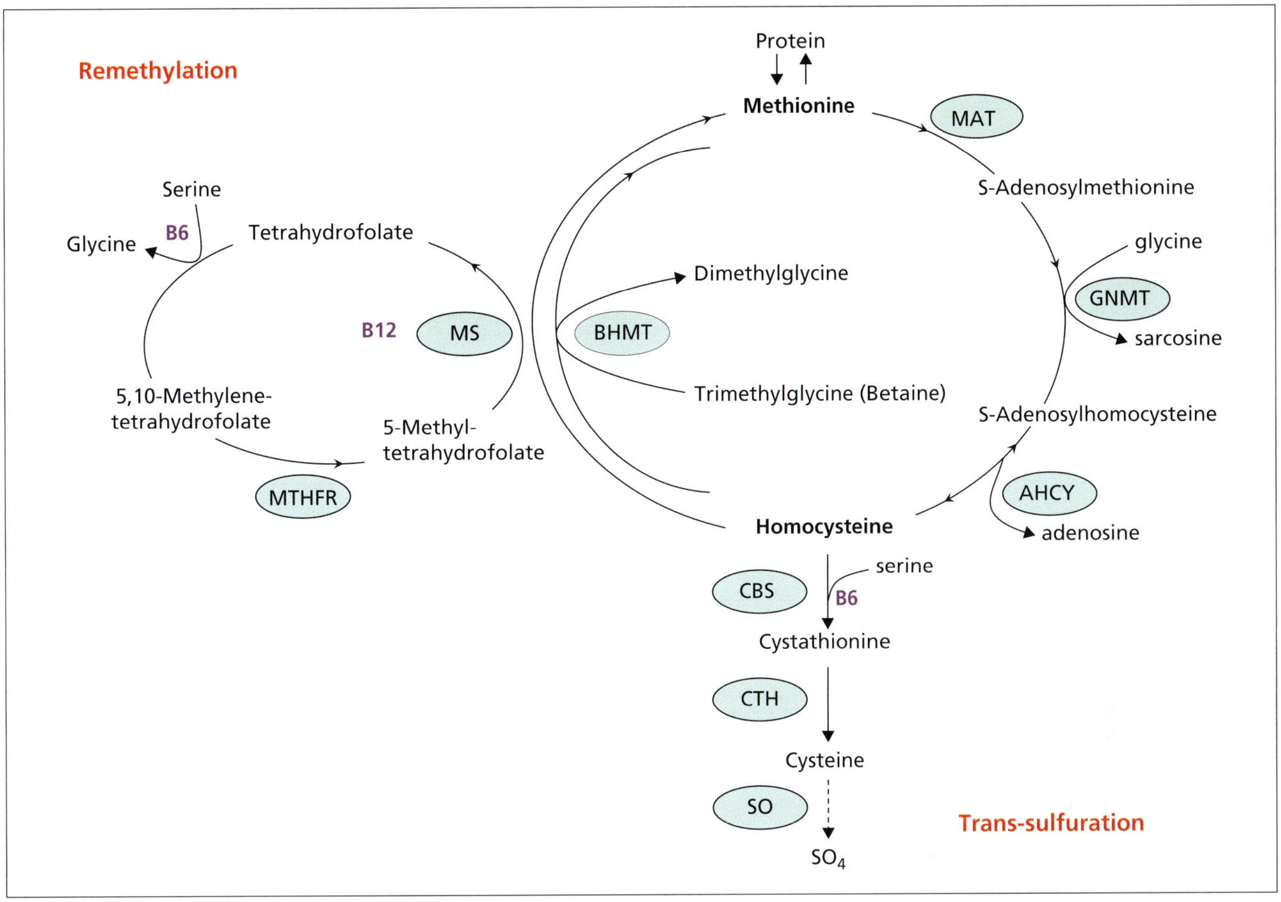

Figure 19.21 Methionine is converted to S-adenosylmethionine by the enzyme methionine S-adenosyltransferase (MAT). S-adenosylmethionine is a methyl-group donor for a number of transmethylation reactions. One of these reactions produces S-adenosylhomocysteine, which is cleaved to adenosine and homocysteine by S-adenosylhomocysteine hydrolase (AHCY). Homocysteine is then either recycled back into methionine or condensed with serine to form cystathionine. The condensation reaction is catalysed by cystathionine beta-synthase (CBS). Remethylation is catalysed by cobalamin-requiring methionine synthase (MS), or by betaine-homocysteine methyltransferase (BHMT). The methyl group is transferred to cobalamin from 5,10-methylenetetrahydrofolate which is regenerated in the folate cycle (requires 5,10-Methylenetetrahydrofolate reductase (MTHFR)). Cystathionine is cleaved to cysteine and alpha-ketobutyrate by cystathionine gamma-lyase (CTH). The final step of trans-sulfuration is catalysed by sulfite oxidase (SO) and converts sulfite to sulfate. GNMT Glycine N-methyltransferase.

ovarian insufficiency, optic atrophy and sensorineural hearing loss. Complications can occur even in the presence of apparently good metabolic control. Progressive renal glomerular and tubular disease are specific features of MMA and in some cases can be very aggressive leading to end-stage renal failure.

Disorders of homocysteine metabolism

The methionine–homocysteine cycle, also known as the single carbon transfer pathway, is found in all tissues and can broadly be divided into transulfuration and remethylation components (Figure 19.21). The cycle aims to conserve methionine and provide sufficient *S*-adenosylmethionine for vital transmethylation reactions. Vitamin B_{12} (cobalamin, Cbl) is important in the effective metabolism of homocysteine and thus defects of cobalamin absorption, transport and intracellular metabolism have biochemical and clinical consequences, similar to HCU.

Transsulfuration defects

Homocystinuria (Table 19.21) Homocystinuria (HCU) is an autosomal recessive defect caused by deficiency of the enzyme cystathione β-synthase (CBS), and characterised biochemically by elevated plasma homocysteine and methionine and decreased cysteine. Classic clinical manifestations involve the eye, skeleton, central nervous and vascular systems, but the age of onset and severity vary widely among affected individuals. Reported neurological involvement includes developmental delay, mental retardation, dystonia, seizures and psychiatric disturbances. As there are effective treatments, neonatal screening is available in some countries.

HCU is a cause of stroke in childhood and adulthood (Chapter 5). Cerebral infarction is caused by arterial or venous sinus thrombosis (Figure 19.22). Occlusive vascular disease results in cognitive decline and is associated with significant morbidity and mortality. Without treatment, just over one-third of patients with HCU will have a thromboembolic event, with cerebrovascular accidents accounting for one-third of these. Pregnancy, the combined oral contraceptive pill and other typical risk factors for thrombosis are well-recognised precipitants in patients with HCU. It is important to remember that thrombosis can be the first and *only* manifestation of Homocystinuria. However, there is an 85% risk reduction in vascular events among adequately treated patients.

Approximately 20% of untreated patients will develop seizures. Again, these are largely preventable by early effective treatment.

Table 19.21 Disorders of homocysteine metabolism.

	Disorder	Enzyme/protein deficiency	Gene	EC number/ gene map locus	Cognitive impairment	Other neurological features	Met	tHcy	MMA	B12	Folate	Treatment options
Defects in the methionine–homocysteine trans-sulfuration pathway	Methionine S-adenosyltransferase deficiency	Methionine S-adenosyltransferase	MAT1A	EC 2.5.1.6	Y	Y	↑	N/↑	N	N	N	None. S-adenosylmethionine
	Glycine N-methyltransferase deficiency	Glycine N-methyltransferase	GNMT	EC 2.1.1.20	N	N	↑	N/↑	NR	N	N	
	S-adenosylhomocysteine hydrolase deficiency	S-adenosylhomocysteine hydrolase	AHCY	EC 3.3.1.1	Y	Y	↑	↑	NR	N	N	Methionine restricted diet, phosphatidylcholine, creatine
	Homocystinuria	Cystathionine β-synthase	CBS	EC 4.2.1.22	Y	Y	↑	↑	N	N	N	Methionine restricted diet, cysteine supplementation, B12, folic acid, betaine, pyridoxine, vitamin C, antithrombotic agents
	γ-Cystathionase deficiency	Cystathionine gamma-lyase	CTH	EC 4.4.1.1	N	N	N	N	N	N	N	None. Pyridoxine
	Isolated sulfite oxidase deficiency	Sulfite oxidase	SUOX	EC 1.8.3.1	Y	Y	N	N	N	N	N	Methionine/cysteine restricted diet
Defects in the methionine remethylation pathway	Methylenetetrahydrofolate reductase deficiency	Methylenetetrahydrofolate reductase	MTHFR	EC 1.5.1.20	Y	Y	↓	↑	N	N	↓/N	Betaine, folic acid, methionine, pyridoxine, B12
	No disorder described	Betaine-homocysteine methyltransferase	BHMT	EC 2.1.1.5								No disorder identified

Defects in cobalamin (B12) absorption and transport	Haptocorrin (R binder) deficiency	Transcobalamin I	TCN1	11q11-q12	N	Y	N	N	N	↓	N	B12
	Hereditary intrinsic factor deficiency	Gastric intrinsic factor, transcobalamin III	GIF	11q13	Y	Y	N	↑/N	↑/N	↓	N	B12
	Megaloblastic anaemia I	Cubilin or amnionless	CUBN/ AMN	10p12.1	Y	Y	N	↑/N	↑/N	↓	N	B12
	Transcobalamin deficiency	Transcobalamin II	TCN2	22q11.2-qter	Y	Y	N	↑/N	↑/N	N/↓	N	B12, folic acid
Defects in intracellular utilization of cobalamin (B12)	Cobalamin deficiency, CblF type	Lysosomal membrane cobalamin exporter	LMBRD1	6q12-q13	Y	Y	↓/N	↑	↑	↓	N	B12
	Cobalamin deficiency, CblC type	Role in cobalamin metabolism/reduction	MMACHC	1p34.1	Y	Y	↓/N	↑	↑	N	N	B12, betaine
	Cobalamin deficiency, CblD type	Role in cobalamin metabolism/reduction	MMADHC	2q23.2	Y	Y	↓	↑/N	↑/N	↓/N	N	B12, betaine, folic acid
	Cobalamin deficiency, CblE type	Methionine synthase reductase	MTRR	5p15.3-p15.2	Y	Y	↓/N	↑	N	N	N	B12, betaine
	Cobalamin deficiency, CblG type	Methionine synthase	MTR	EC 2.1.1.13	Y	Y	↓	↑	N	N	N	B12, betaine, methionine
	Cobalamin deficiency, CblA type	Role in cobalamin metabolism/reduction	MMAA	4q31.1-q31.2	Y	Y	N	N	↑	N	N	B12, protein restriction
	Cobalamin deficiency, CblB type	Role in cobalamin metabolism	MMAB	12q24	Y	Y	N	N	↑	N	N	B12, protein restriction

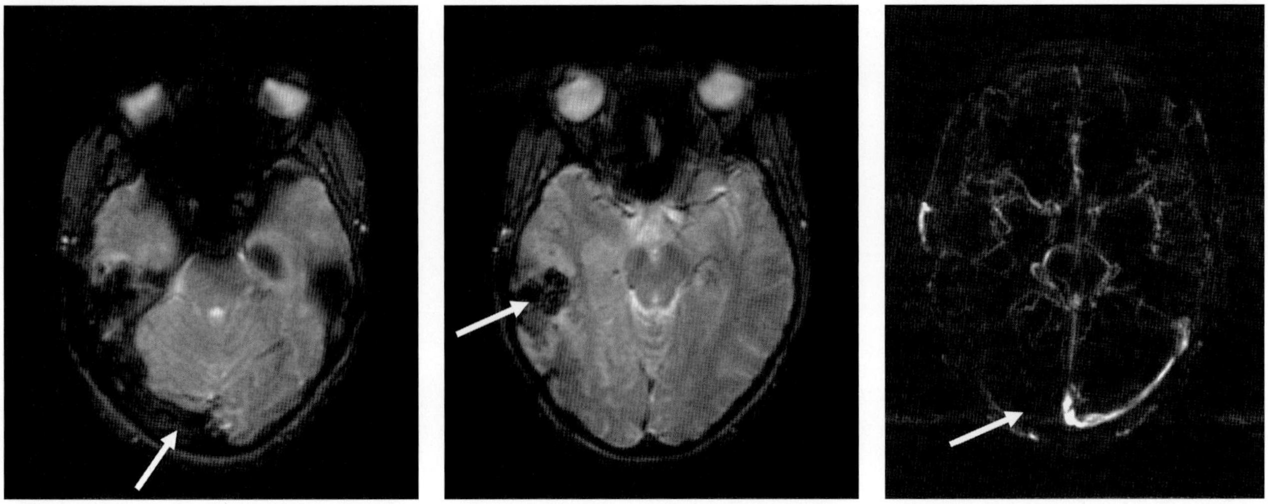

(a) (b) (c)

Figure 19.22 Transverse venous sinus thrombosis presenting in a pregnant women subsequently diagnosed with homocystinuria (HCU). (a) A 33-year-old woman presented at 11 weeks' gestation with a severe headache secondary to a right transverse venous sinus thrombosis. (b) She also had acute haemorrhage in the right posterior temporal lobe (b). (c) On MR venogram she had a filling defect in the right transverse venous sinus. She was found to have severe hyperhomocystinaemia, tHcy 214 μmol/L (reference range 0–15 μmol/L), and was subsequently diagnosed with HCU. She had previously had one miscarriage and one normal pregnancy. She was treated with subcutaneous heparin 7500 units twice daily, folic acid 5 mg/day, oral vitamin B_{12} 50 μg/day and pyridoxine 300 mg/day. By the third trimester her total homocysteine level had fallen to 6 μmol/L. The remainder of pregnancy was uneventful and she delivered a normal, healthy child. Heparin was continued for 2 months post-partum. In addition post-partum warfarin 3.5 mg/day was continued for 2 years until the venous sinus became patent again 2 years later. Source: Murphy 2010. Reproduced with permission of Oxford University Press, USA.

Psychiatric features are frequently reported in patients with HCU, although the precise prevalence is uncertain. Clinically significant diagnoses have included depression, chronic behavioural abnormalities, obsessive–compulsive disorder and personality disorders.

Management The aim of treatment is to reduce total homocysteine levels to at least less than 100 μmol/L and preferably to as close to normal as possible, lifelong. In those patients diagnosed by neonatal screening, the aim is to prevent intellectual impairment, neurological, vascular, ocular and skeletal complications. In later diagnosed patients, the aim is to prevent vascular events and worsening of existing complications.

Adequate B_{12} and folate status should be ensured for all patients with HCU. Vitamin B_6 (pyridoxine) is a cofactor for the enzyme CBS. Hence, some patients with homocystinuria are vitamin B_6 (pyridoxine) responsive. A large international natural history survey identified 629 patients, of whom 36% were classed as B_6-responsive, 36% B_6 non-responsive and the remainder either unclassified or intermediate in response. It is important to ensure adequate folate status before testing for B_6-responsiveness to prevent masking of potential responsiveness by less than optimal N5-methytetrahydrofolate-dependent homocysteine remethylation. To test for pyridoxine responsiveness it is recommended to give 500mg/day, checking homocysteine at baseline and again after 6 weeks. Ideally, once responsiveness has been determined, the dosage should be reduced incrementally until the lowest effective dose for maintenance therapy is reached.

For B_6 non-responsive patients, in those countries where patients are identified by newborn screening, then a natural protein-restricted diet supplemented by a synthetic methionine-free, cystine-supplemented amino acid mixture is introduced. However, starting a low-protein diet is often unpalatable to older children and adults, so that many of these are treated with medications alone. Betaine is a methyl donor that has been shown to reduce homocysteine and raise methionine concentrations by increasing homocysteine methylation via betaine-homocysteine methyltransferase. Doses of betaine up to 9 g/day in divided doses have been given in adults. Plasma methionine increases on betaine therapy, and the dosage is usually adjusted to maintain plasma methionine levels <1000 μmol/L to reduce the risk of cerebral oedema.

Defects in intracellular cobalamin metabolism

Eight distinct defects of the intracellular cobalamin pathway have been identified by fibroblast studies and complementation analysis (Figure 19.23). Dependent on their location in the pathway, these defects can lead to combined hyperhomocysteinaemia and methylmalonic acidemia (cblF, cblC, cblD-hyperhomocysteinaemia and methylmalonic acadaemia), isolated hyperhomocysteinaemia (cblD-hyperhomocysteinaemia, cblE, cblG) or isolated methylmalonic aciduria (cblA, cblB, cblD-methylmalonic acidemia, MUT).

Cobalamin C (CblC) defects Defects in CblC with combined hyperhomocysteinaemia and methylmalonic acidemia are the most common of the disorders of the intracellular cobalamin pathway. Neonatal presentation is associated with progressive neurological deterioration, and ophthalmologic, haematologic and dermatologic abnormalities. Later onset cases have been described with learning difficulties, dementia and gait abnormalities.

Management All Cbl defects can be treated with parenteral B_{12}, although this does not always reverse or prevent clinical complications. Intravenous therapy may be given for the first days following an acute presentation and then switched to frequent intramuscular hydroxocobalamin (the dose required will vary but may be up to 1 mg/daily, lifelong). Betaine and folic acid can also be useful.

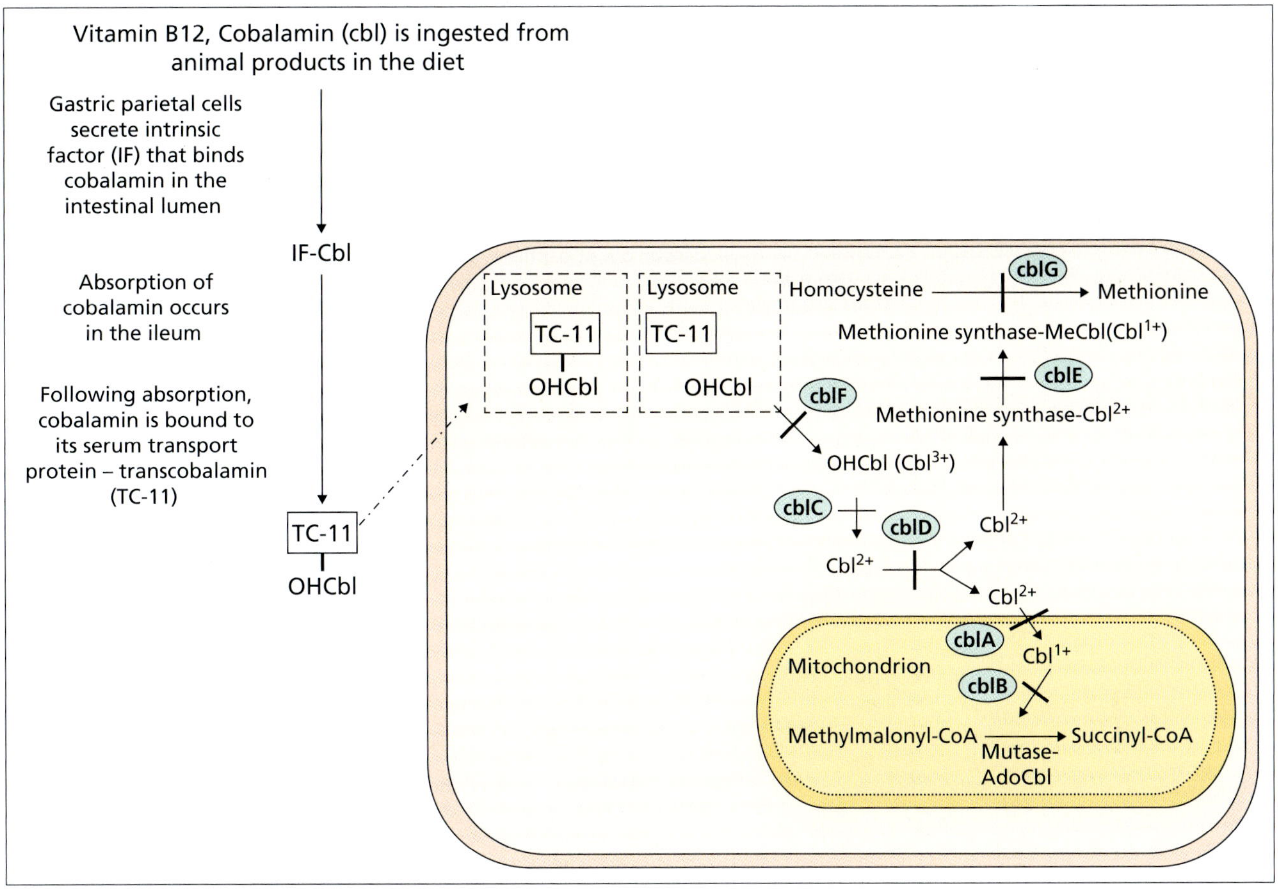

Figure 19.23 Cobalamin (cbl) absorption, transport and intracellular metabolism. Dietary B_{12} (cobalamin) is ingested from foods of animal sources. Cbl is released from its binding proteins in the stomach and forms a complex with intrinsic factor (IF). IF-cbl interacts with a receptor protein, cubulin, in the ileum. Cbl is then transported across the enterocyte into the portal blood system and travels to cells for further metabolism bound to transcobalamin II. Transcobalamin II facilitates uptake of cbl by cells and into lysosomes. Cbl is released into the cytoplasm, the central cobalt atom is reduced and cytosolic methylation forms MeCbl (which is required by the enzyme methionine synthase) or mitochondrial adenosylation forms AdoCbl (which is required by the enzyme methylmalonyl CoA mutase). Source: Murphy 2010. Reproduced with permission of Oxford University Press, USA.

Remethylation defects The remethylation defects all have defective methionine synthesis in common. Broadly speaking, clinical presentation varies with age. In the neonatal and early infancy period, patients present with a rapidly progressive neurological condition with multisystem or haematological involvement. In childhood, the presentation is with developmental delay, gait abnormalities and possibly haematologic abnormalities. In adolescence and adulthood patients the condition can be variable, ranging from asymptomatic to progressive neurological and psychiatric features.

Methylenetetrahydrofolate reductase (MTHFR) deficiency MTHFR is the enzyme that catalyses the reduction of methylenetetrahydrofolate to methyltetrahydrofolate. Methyltetrahydrofolate is a methyl donor for the methylation of homosyteine catalysed by methionine synthase. MTHFR deficiency is characterised by plasma hyperhomocysteinemia and low to normal methionine. Folate levels tend to be low to normal, whereas B_{12} levels are generally normal. A common polymorphism in the MTHFR gene (*C677T*) is associated with increased thermolability of the enzyme *in vitro* and hyperhomocysteinaemia, particularly in individuals with low folate status, and has been the subject of several large epidemiological studies as a risk factor for cardio- and cerebrovascular disease in adults.

Clinical features are variable but include developmental delay, microcephaly, recurrent strokes, arterial and venous thromboses, gait abnormalities, seizures and psychiatric manifestations.

Management Treatment possibilities include folate, B_{12}, betaine and riboflavin (as a source of flavin required by MTHFR).

Urea cycle disorders

The urea cycle disorders (UCDs) are a group of inherited metabolic diseases that affect the liver's ability to incorporate nitrogen into urea (Figure 19.24). This leads to hyperammonaemia. Severe cases present with hyperammonaemic encephalopathy in the neonatal period and this is often fatal and usually results in significant cerebral oedema with damage to the brain and long-term neurological consequences. More attenuated forms, however, only produce hyperammonaemia when the patient is placed under unusual metabolic stress, and these can present in adulthood (see Table 19.20 for a list of the urea cycle disorders).

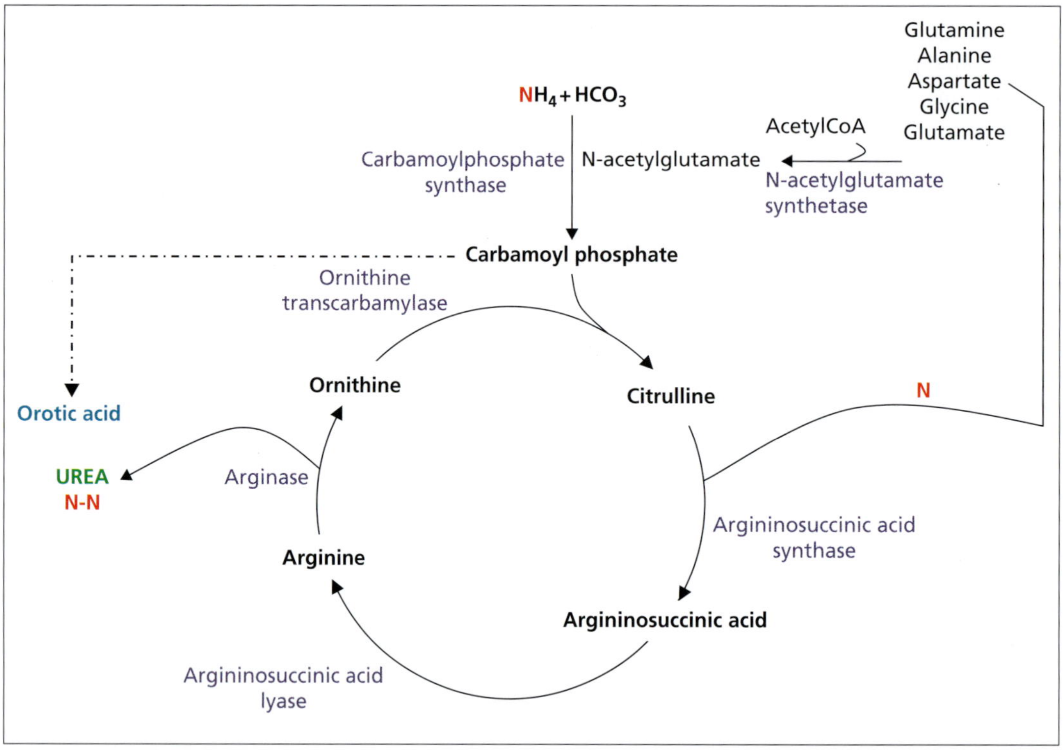

Figure 19.24 The urea cycle. Ammonia, from amino acid catabolism, is detoxified to urea in the liver. Urea is then excreted in the urine. One turn of the urea cycle results in the disposal of two nitrogen atoms, one from NH_3 and one from aspartate. The cycle consists of six enzymatic reactions: three in the mitochondrial matrix (carbamoylphosphate synthetase 1 [CPS1], ornithine transcarbamylase [OTC] and N-acetylglutamate synthetase [NAGS]) and three in the cytosol (argininosuccinate synthetase [ASS], argininosuccinate lyase [ASL] and arginase [ARG]). Defects of all six enzymes have been described. X-linked OTC deficiency is the most common. The other disorders are autosomal recessive in inheritance.

Encephalopathy in the context of an adult patient with an inherited metabolic disease, can be intermittent, fluctuating or rapid and fulminant progressing to coma. Patients can present with reduced cognition and concentration, a change in personality (often agitated and/or aggressive), lethargy, vomiting or decreased consciousness and coma. Neurological findings include seizures, abnormal posturing, abnormal gait and poor coordination. Symptoms are often reversible with early treatment and consideration of a metabolic component should be given to any adult who presents with encephalopathy. Late-onset 'milder' inherited metabolic conditions in adults are often unmasked by intercurrent infection, alcohol or drug (mis)use, and so physicians should be wary of attributing all encephalopathic symptoms to these, particularly if patients are not responding as expected to standard treatments. Information about previous unusual behaviours (e.g. protein aversion, unexplained episodes of confusion or agitation) should be sought from family and friends.

All adults who present with acute or acute-on-chronic encephalopathy in whom there is no obvious cause (e.g. recent trauma or hypoxia) should have a plasma ammonia level measured promptly.

By far the most common cause of hyperammonaemia in adults is hepatic failure, often associated with portosystemic shunting. Once this has been excluded as a cause then consideration should be given to other secondary causes, and defects of the urea cycle are important amongst these. Hyperammonaemia can occur secondary to a fatty acid oxidation disorder or an organic acidemia – but is much more frequently a result of these conditions in infancy or childhood than in adulthood. An important secondary cause of elevated ammonia is valproate therapy, which can precipitate hyperammonaemia, including in individuals with a previously unknown urea cycle defect.

While the precise underlying cause of hyperammonaemia can take some time to elucidate, treatment can be started immediately to avoid death or long-term neurological damage. The aims of treatment are to reduce nitrogenous waste production and lower plasma ammonia before cerebral oedema develops.

Diagnosis

Definite diagnosis should not delay immediate treatment but appropriate samples (including plasma amino acids, an acylcarnitine profile, urine organic acids) should be taken, preferably during the acute presentation, in order that chronic management can be tailored and genetic counselling can be given to both the index patient and other potentially affected family members.

Management

In severe hyperammonaemia with marked encephalopathy, seizures or coma, haemodialysis is the most efficient way to reduce plasma ammonia (peritoneal dialysis is not as efficient and should be avoided). Vascular access should be secured and haemodialysis started as soon as possible in the HDU or ITU setting.

Protein intake should be stopped for 24–48 hours, and a hypercaloric solution (intravenous 10% dextrose; intralipid may also be given) started, with insulin if needed to enhance anabolism. Intravenous arginine and alternative pathway therapies (sodium benzoate and sodium phenylbutyrate) will promote the excretion of nitrogen-containing metabolites in the urine, as an alternative to urea formation.

Long-term management will require input from a specialist centre to ensure appropriate dietary advice (including supplementation of vitamins and minerals in those on a restricted diet) and titration of oral medications to ensure optimal metabolic control. Protocols for the management of hyperammonaemic encephalopathy can be found on the British Inherited Metabolic Disease Group website (www.bimdg.org.uk).

Arginase deficiency

Arginase deficiency is an atypical UCD in that hyperammonaemia is not generally the presenting feature. Instead, there is failure to thrive and children have developmental delay and a progressive spastic diplegia. Epilpesy can also be a feature. In patients diagnosed by newborn screening, if arginine levels are controlled with the use of a low protein diet and essential amino acid supplements, neurological disease can be slowed. In late diagnosed patients, controlling arginine levels can improve symptoms and slow progression.

Disorders of carbohydrate metabolism

Glycogen storage diseases (the GSDs)

Glycogen is a macromolecule composed of up to 60 000 linked glucose molecules. It is the primary energy source between meals, with a series of metabolic reactions releasing stored glucose as needed. Glycogen is found in many tissues, being particularly abundant in liver and muscle. Many disorders of glycogen synthesis or breakdown are described. Clinically, these are broadly divided into those that predominantly affect the liver (e.g. types 0, I, III, VI and IX), those mainly affecting skeletal and/or cardiac muscle (e.g. types II, V, VII, and XV) and those that are associated with neurodegeneration (e.g. Lafora disease and some of the polyglucosan body storage disorders; Table19.20).

Hepatic involvement in glycogen storage diseases

The hepatic forms do not generally have specific neurological manifestations apart from the potential consequences of severe prolonged hypoglycaemia which can cause encephalopathy, seizures and even death.

Skeletal/cardiac muscle involvement in glycogen storage diseases

Pompe disease/acid maltase deficiency (GSD II) GSD II is caused by lysosomal acid maltase deficiency and can either cause infantile Pompe disease with a significant cardiomyopathy and generalised myopathy, or late onset disease with a limb girdle dystrophy presenting in later childhood or adulthood. Without specific therapy, infantile Pompe disease is invariably fatal. Late onset acid maltase deficiency causes progressive weakness with diaphragmatic involvement and leads to death following respiratory failure. Since 2006, enzyme replacement therapy, which is modifying the natural history of the disorder, has been available.

GSD III GSD type III is caused by glycogen debrancher deficiency. An echocardiographic appearance of hypertrophic cardiomyopathy has been documented in many individuals. Its clinical significance is uncertain, however, as most affected individuals are asymptomatic, though severe cardiac dysfunction, congestive heart failure and sudden death have occasionally been reported. There have also been a few case reports of a diet high in protein and limited in carbohydrate reducing severe cardiac hypertrophy.

Skeletal myopathy often becomes prominent in the third to fourth decade of life. Proximal muscles are primarily affected but involvement of the diaphragm and distal muscles including the calves, peroneal muscles and hands is also described. Exercise intolerance is reported.

McArdle disease (GSD V) (Chapter 10) GSD V is characterised by muscle pain that typically comes on within a few minutes of starting exercise. Exercise tolerance (reduction in heart rate) may improve after 7–10 minutes if aerobic exercise (e.g. jogging, cycling) is continued but at a slower, gentler pace – this is called the second-wind phenomenon. Static or isometric exercise (e.g. bench press, shoulder raises, carrying heavy shopping) is poorly tolerated, as is sprinting. Some older patients may have evidence of a fixed proximal myopathy with wasting.

Diagnosis Laboratory tests will show elevated creatine kinase, urate and myoglobinuria and, in severe cases, renal impairment. In up to 85% of patients from northern Europe, a common mutation R50X can be detected, and so, in patients with a typical clinical history, genetic mutation analysis can be used as a first line diagnostic test. GSD V can also be confirmed by muscle biopsy which shows an excess of glycogen and absence of muscle phosphorylase. The ischaemic forearm exercise test, with measurement of lactate and ammonia, the traditional screening test for muscle disorders of carbohydrate metabolism, is less often performed now as it is painful for the patient, not specifically diagnostic for GSD V and has been largely superceded by genetic testing.

Management Acute severe rhabdomyolysis should be treated with prompt fluid (normal saline) replacement and renal support as required. Intravenous dextrose during acute crises and oral sucrose prior to exercise may also be helpful. Patients should be given advice on safe forms of exercise and how to achieve the second-wind phenomenon.

Central nervous system involvement in glycogen storage diseases

Lafora disease Lafora disease is characterised by seizures, often with visual hallucinations that typically start during adolescence, followed by progressive myoclonus, severe dementia with dysarthria and ataxia. Most affected individuals die within 10 years of onset, usually from status epilepticus or from complications related to nervous system degeneration. It is caused by mutations in one of two genes: *EPM2A* (laforin) or *NHLRC1* (malin). Diagnosis is confirmed by mutation analysis. A skin biopsy will show abnormal inclusions – the Lafora bodies.

Adult polyglucosan body disease (GSD IV) GSD type IV, caused by glycogen branching enzyme deficiency, can present in various forms including cirrhosis and liver failure, or, in its adult form, with progressive gait disturbance, urinary incontinence, upper and lower motor neurone dysfunction, distal sensory loss and cerebellar dysfunction. Histopathological findings include large polyglucosan bodies which contain abnormally long and poorly branched glucosyl chains.

Galactosaemia

Classic galactosaemia is an autosomal recessive inborn error of metabolism caused by mutations of the *GALT* gene, resulting in markedly reduced function of the enzyme galactose-1-phosphate

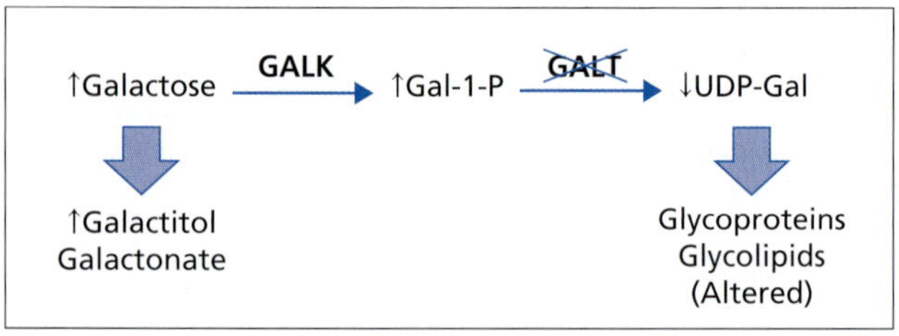

Figure 19.25 Simplified scheme of disturbance of galactose metabolism in classic galactosaemia.
Deficiency of galactose-1-phosphate uridyltransferase (GALT, crossed) leads to altered metabolites with increases in galactose, galactitol, galactonate, and Gal-1-P (galactose-1-phosphate), and reduction in UDP-Gal (uridine diphosphate-galactose), a sugar required for normal galactosylation of glycoproteins and glycolipids. GALK (Galactokinase). Source: Rubio-Agusti 2013. Reproduced with permission of John Wiley & Sons.

uridyltransferase (GALT) and subsequent accumulation of galactose-1-phosphate (Gal-1-P), galactose and derived metabolites, through alternative pathways (Figure 19.25). It has an estimated prevalence of 1/30 000 newborn babies. Diagnosis can be established by demonstrating increased levels of erythrocyte Gal-1-P and decreased activity of erythrocyte GALT (<5%).

Galactosaemia presents almost invariably in the neonatal period with acute multiple organ dysfunction, often involving the liver, after newborn infants are exposed to dietary galactose. Although it can be fatal if untreated, acute symptoms resolve rapidly with galactose restriction. Despite adequate treatment, however, surviving patients can develop long-term complications, such as premature ovarian failure and CNS dysfunction, including cognitive difficulties, psychiatric symptoms, speech and motor problems.

Motor complications have been reported in 18-45% of patients, with the most common features being tremor and cerebellar ataxia. There is a wide spectrum of severity, with some patients showing mild abnormalities on examination and others with disabling symptoms. Following a systematic clinical examination of all patients attending our clinic with galactosaemia, we found a higher proportion of motor dysfunction, reaching 66%, although only 28% of our patients reported symptoms. Mild motor dysfunction might therefore be missed in some patients unless carefully they are carefully examined. Patients with evidence of motor dysfunction also had a higher frequency of other non-motor neurological features, including cognitive impairment, psychiatric problems and speech difficulties, suggesting a common pathogenic mechanism, leading to widespread CNS damage.

Management Current recommendations are that dietary restriction of galactose is continued lifelong. However, there are a few reports of adults on unrestricted or more relaxed diets in whom the outcome is similar to that of patients who have continued on dietary galactose restriction. This remains therefore an active area of research.

Fatty acid oxidation defects

Mitochondrial oxidation of fat is an important energy source for many tissues, especially during fasting or sustained aerobic exercise. At these times, long-chain fatty acids are released from triglyceride stores in adipose tissue and transported to other tissues in the blood. Short- and medium-chain fatty acids can diffuse across the mitochondrial membrane, but long-chain fatty acids require a specific transport mechanism (Figure 19.26). Long-chain acyl-CoA compounds are conjugated with carnitine to form acylcarnitines, which are then transported into the mitochondrial matrix by carnitine palmitoyltransferases (CPTs). Once inside the mitochondria, the carnitine is recycled to the cytoplasm and the acyl-CoA esters enter the β-oxidation pathway. Each β-oxidation cycle shortens the acyl chain by two carbon atoms and results in the production of one molecule of acetyl-CoA which can then enter the tricarboxylic acid (TCA) cycle or, in the liver, be used to generate ketone bodies.

About 15 inherited fatty acid oxidation (FAO) disorders have been described (Table 19.20). Many of these are life-threatening diseases of childhood and present with hypoketotic hypoglycaemia, encephalopathy and hepatic dysfunction. Milder phenotypes can present in adulthood, causing exercise intolerance, episodic rhabdomyolysis and neuropathy.

Although resting skeletal muscle relies on low level FAO for energy, during exercise there is a switch to utilising muscle stores of glycogen. Once these have been depleted (after about 5–10 minutes), the main fuels become the muscles' stores of triglycerides and glucose from the circulation. As exercise continues, the supply of free fatty acids becomes more important and, after about an hour, mitochondrial FAO is once again the major source of energy for muscle. In the milder FAO defects, residual FAO is adequate to supply the resting energy requirements of muscle, but is insufficient during extended exercise, resulting in muscle cell death and rhabdomyolysis.

FAO disorders such as carnitine palmitoyltransferase 2 (CPT2) or very long chain acyl-CoA dehydrogenase (VLCAD) deficiencies can present for the first time in adolescence or adulthood. The presentation is typically with symptoms of myalgia, muscle stiffness and/or rhabdomyolysis after more prolonged exercise (e.g. playing football or marathon running). Prolonged fasting, cold exposure, intercurrent infection or even emotional stress are other well-recognised precipitants. Symptoms may last for a number of weeks following an acute attack, but patients may be completely asymptomatic, with normal muscle strength on examination, between attacks.

Medium-chain acyl-CoA dehydrogenase deficiency (MCADD) is the most common FAO defect with an incidence of 1/10 000 live births. Patients usually present with hypoglycaemic hypoketotic encephalopathy towards the end of the first and into the second year of life. Because a significant number of affected infants either die or have significant cerebral damage in this first episode, neonatal screening is now widely available. Rare patients will present for the first time in adulthood with rhabdomyolysis or cardiomyopathy.

Multiple acyl-CoA dehydrogenase deficiency (MADD), also known as glutaric aciduria type II (GA-II), is caused by mutations in a number of different proteins that are involved in the mitochondrial transport of electrons from acyl-CoA to uniquinone. This results in a functional defect in a number of acyl-CoA dehydrogenases involved both in β-oxidation and in the degradation of branched-chain amino acids. The more severe forms lead to early death with non-ketotic hypoglycaemia and acidosis, but adult onset disease has also been described. This can involve metabolic decompensation, hypotonia, cardiomyopathy and, rarely, leukodystrophy with spastic quadriplegia. In milder cases, there is only a lipid storage myopathy and rhabdomyolysis. Biochemically, organic acids are detectable in the urine and there is a secondary carnitine deficiency.

The final stages of β-oxidation of long-chain fatty acids is catalysed by an enzyme complex termed the mitochondrial trifunctional protein (TFP). Isolated long-chain 3-hydroxyacyl-CoA

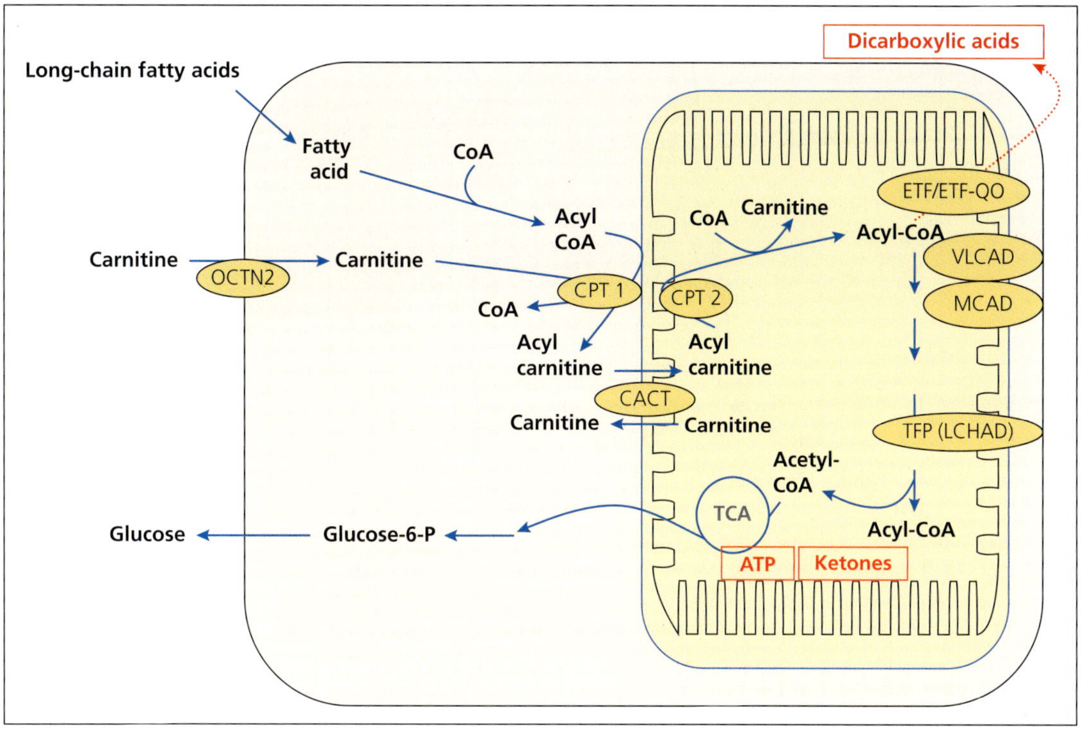

Figure 19.26 Fatty acid oxidation. Fatty acids enter the mitochondria. Medium- and short-chain fatty acids enter independently of carnitine, but long-chain fatty acids need to be activated to coenzyme A and transferred to carnitine (CPT1, carnitine palmitoyltransferase I) in order to cross the inner mitochondrial membrane (CACT, carnitine acylcarnitine translocase). They are then transferred back to CoA esters in the mitochondrial matrix (CPT2, carnitine palmitoyltransferase II). Beta-oxidation is catalyzed by enzymes of different fatty acid chain length specificity (VLCAD, MCAD, TFP(LCHAD)). Electrons are passed to the respiratory chain either directly or via transfer proteins (ETF, ETF-QO). Acetyl-CoA can be oxidized in the tricarboxylic acid (TCA, Krebs) cycle or, in the liver, used to synthesize ketone bodies. ETF: electron transfer flavoprotein; ETF-QO: electron transfer flavoprotein ubiquinone oxidoreductase; MCAD: medium-chain acyl-CoA dehydrogenase; OCTN2: high affinity sodium-dependent carnitine transporter; VLCAD: very-long-chain acyl-CoA dehydrogenase; TFP (LCHAD): mitochondrial trifunctional protein (long chain acyl CoA dehydrogenase).

dehydrogenase deficiency is the most common form of MTP deficiency. Patients present either acutely with hypoglycaemia, liver failure and cardiomyopathy, or more chronically with feeding problems and hypotonia. Long-term complications include retinopathy and peripheral neuropathy. Exercise intolerance and episodic rhabdomyolysis may also occur.

Diagnosis

If there is a strong suspicion of a fatty acid oxidation disorder, then a muscle biopsy should be avoided. Instead a typical acylcarnitine profile (plasma or blood spot) will suggest the condition which can then be confirmed by measurements of fatty acid oxidation and/or CPT2 enzyme activity in skin fibroblasts (grown from a punch skin biopsy). Genetic testing allows screening of other potentially affected family members.

Management

Acute severe rhabdomyolysis (Chapter 10) should be treated with prompt fluid (saline) replacement, intravenous dextrose and renal support as required. Other measures that may be helpful in preventing recurrent symptoms include restriction of dietary long-chain fat, with substitution by medium-chain triglyceride (MCT), carbohydrate or triheptanoin. The lipid lowering agent, bezafibrate (200 mg three times daily) has been shown to increase CPT II enzyme activity in muscle and reduce the number of attacks of rhabdomyolysis. In some patients with fatty acid oxidation disorders cannot achieve the second-wind phenomenon.

Neurotransmitter disorders

The term neurotransmitter disorder usually refers to those disorders that can be identified by analysis of CSF. These include the inherited disorders of dopamine and serotonin metabolism along with disorders affecting the availability of the vitamins, pyridoxal phosphate (PLP) and 5-methyltetrahydrofolate (5-MTHF) (Figure 19.27).

Dopamine and serotonin both require the presence of the cofactor tetrahydrobiopterin (BH4) to catalyse the first committed step of their biosynthesis. The initial enzymes in the pathway, tyrosine and tryptophan hydroxylase, work in concert with BH4 and the substrates tyrosine and tryptophan to generate L-dihydroxyphenylalanine and 5-hydroxytryptophan (5-HTP). A single PLP-dependent enzyme, aromatic amino acid decarboxylase (AADC), then catalyses the conversion of L-dihydroxyphenylalanine and 5-HTP to form dopamine and serotonin. These neurotransmitters can be packaged into synaptic vesicles and liberated in response to an action potential. Upon release, the neurotransmitter can be taken back into the presynaptic neurone and repackaged into vesicles or metabolised further. With regards to dopamine, the action of catechol methyl transferase, monoamine oxidase and aldehyde dehydrogenase results in the formation of homovanillic acid (HVA). For serotonin, the action of monoamine oxidase leads to generation of

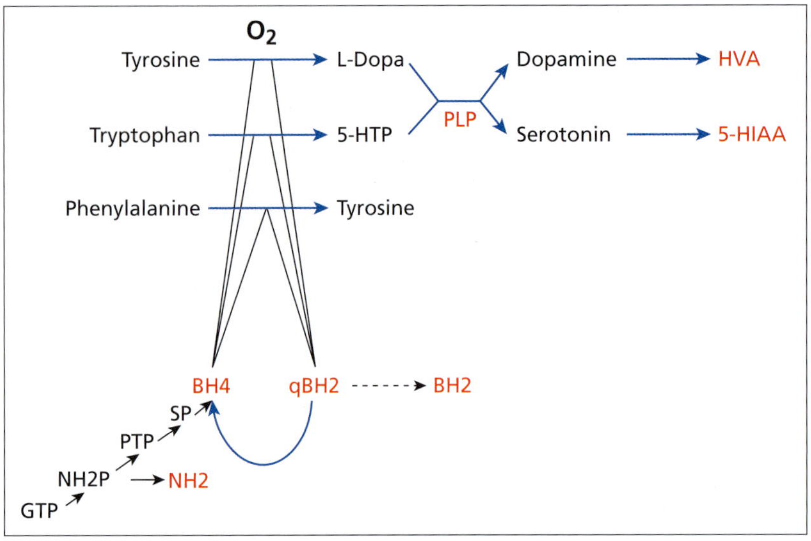

Figure 19.27 Dopamine and serotonin metabolism. Dopamine and serotonin are synthesised via tyrosine hydroxylase and tryptophan hydroxylase and aromatic amino acid decarboxylase activity. Molecular oxygen and BH4 are the obligatory cofactors for these two hydroxylases. BH4 is synthesised, de novo, from guanosine triphosphate (GTP) via a number of enzymatic steps. GTP cyclohydrolase catalyses the conversion of GTP to dihydroneopterin triphosphate (NH2P). 6-pyruvoyaltetrahydropterin (PTP) is formed from NH2P via the action of PTP synthase. Aldose reductase generates sepapterin (SP) from PTP. SP is then transformed to the active BH4 cofactor as a consequence of sepiapterin reductase activity. When acting as a cofactor, BH4 is oxidised to quinonoid dihydrobiopterin (qBH2). A recycling system, comprising of dihydropteridine reductase plus pterin-4a-carbinolamine dehydratase, regenerates BH4 from qBH2. The concentration of the metabolites in red can be quantified in CSF to provide insight into the integrity of dopamine, serotonin, BH4 and PLP metabolism. NH2 is the dephosphorylated from of NH2P and BH2 is the stable rearrangement product of qBH2. Note BH4 is also required for the hepatic metabolism of phenylalanine to tryrosine via phenylalanine hydroxylase.

5-hydroxyindoleacetic acid (5-HIAA). Assessment of HVA and 5-HIAA is used to provide an indication of the integrity of central dopamine and serotonin metabolism, respectively.

Clinical presentations

Dopa-responsive dystonia (DRD, Segawa syndrome) is classically caused by a dominantly inherited mutation in the GTP cyclohydrolase 1 gene. Patients typically present in childhood with lower limb dystonia, parkinsonism and sometimes a degree of spasticity. Symptoms often show diurnal fluctuation so that they get worse as the day goes on. Not all patients represent with this classic phenotype. Some present in infancy with a more severe phenotype, while others present in late teens or early adult life with asymmetric tremor and bradykinesia mimicking early onset Parkinson's disease. Response to small doses of levodopa is typically very dramatic and this response is sustained in the long-term. For this reason all those with young-onset dystonia in whom there is no known cause should be investigated for DRD or at least have a trial of levodopa (Chapter 6).

Patients with other defects in the pterin pathway (e.g. sepiaterin reductase deficiency, tyrosine hydroxolase deficiency, rare patients with homozygous GTP cyclohydrolase 1 mutations) present with an earlier onset and more severe phenotype characterised by oculogyric crises, severe dystonia, spasticity, parkinsonism, myoclonus and cognitive impairment. A similar phenotype is seen in those with AADC deficiency or central folate disorders. Parkinsonism, dystonia, chorea, oculogyric crises, ptosis, hypersalivation, myoclonic epilepsy, epileptic encephalopathy, cognitive decline, microcephaly, swallowing difficulties, pyramidal tract features, temperature instability and sweating can form part of the clinical picture. Additionally, decreased PLP availability is associated with a neonatal epileptic encephalopathy that can be refractive to antiepileptic drugs. White matter changes may also be apparent because of the critical involvement of 5-MTHF and one carbon metabolism in myelin formation.

Laboratory diagnosis

Inherited disorders of dopamine and serotonin metabolism can exhibit a highly informative pattern in CSF. Patients with tyrosine hydroxylase deficiency will have an isolated low CSF HVA concentration while in individuals with AADC deficiency the concentrations of HVA and 5-HIAA will be below the appropriate age-related reference interval. Additionally, for AADC deficiency, elevated levels of 5-hydroxytryptophan and 3-methyl dopa (metabolite of L-dihydroxyphenylalanine) can be demonstrated (i.e. due to substrate accumulation). Patients with disorders of BH4 metabolism can also have decreased concentrations of HVA and 5-HIAA and a characteristic pterin profile that can reflect the nature of the metabolic block (e.g. failure of the BH4 recycling system leads to an increase in the CSF concentration of BH2 while GTP cyclohydrolase 1 deficiency patients have decreased NH2 and BH4 concentrations). Hyperphenylalaninaemia is associated with the majority of BH4 disorders. However, sepiapterin reductase and the autosomal dominant form of GTP cyclohydrolase are not associated with an elevated blood concentration of phenylalanine. These patients will therefore not be identified by a newborn screening programme but can be identified by phenylalanine loading.

Deficiency of PLP, arising from enzyme deficiencies that affect availability of this cofactor (e.g. pyridox(am)ine-5'-oxidase [PNPO] deficiency) can have a low CSF concentration of PLP. As a consequence of this PLP deficiency, dopamine and serotonin metabolism may be compromised, giving a profile comparable to that of AADC deficiency.

5-MTHF is the major transport form of folates and is the species that is quantified in CSF to provide an insight into folate availability and integrity of one carbon metabolism. In addition to the disorders of folate metabolism that directly lead to alterations in

5-MTHF status (e.g. 5,10,-methylene tetrahydrofolate reductase deficiency), other inborn errors of metabolism appear to negatively impact upon 5-MTHF availability: dihydropteridine reductase deficiency and disorders of the mitochondrial electron transport chain. In the latter, the mechanisms responsible for the failure of mitochondrial function leading to a CSF 5-MTHF deficiency have not been fully elucidated but might include a failure of active transport across the blood–brain barrier and an increase of reactive oxygen species generation leading to accelerated 5-MTHF catabolism. A CSF deficiency of 5-MTHF can occur in conjunction with a peripheral folate deficiency (e.g. caused by folate malabsorption and dietary insufficiency) or in isolation. This latter situation is known as cerebral folate deficiency (CFD). An important cause of CFD is mutations affecting the function of folate transporter alpha (FOLR1) which is involved in the transport of 5-MTHF into the CSF compartment. Drugs such as levodopa can also result in a decreased 5-MTHF within CSF. This situation arises as a consequence of excess levodopa being methylated to 3-methyldopa. Consequently, there is a drain on one carbon metabolism resulting in loss, with time, of 5-MTHF.

In addition to the enzyme deficiencies described, perturbation of dopamine metabolism can arise as a result of failure of the dopamine reuptake transporter (SLC6A3). For such patients, a distinctive CSF profile results (i.e. there is a markedly elevated concentration of HVA as a result of the extra-neuronal metabolism of dopamine).

Management

Once identified, patients with 'neurotransmitter' disorders can, in general terms, respond well to appropriate treatment intervention. Knowledge of the biochemical pathways involved coupled with expertise gained in other areas of neurology (e.g. treatment of patients with Parkinson's disease) can lead to effective and targeted options. With regards to tyrosine hydroxylase deficiency, levodopa (in the presence of a peripheral decarboxylase inhibitor) can correct the central dopamine deficiency and is often associated with marked clinical improvement. Disorders of BH4 metabolism are treated with levodopa plus 5-hydroxytryptophan in order to correct both the dopamine and serotonin deficiency. BH4 can also be included in order to correct peripheral phenylalanine metabolism. Alternatively, a phenylalanine restricted diet can be implemented. Treatment of AADC deficiency can be more challenging because of the nature of the metabolic block. PLP administration can be tried in an attempt to stimulate, by its role as a cofactor, any residual AADC activity. Folinic acid is also given to correct any secondary 5-MTHF deficiency arising from the increased methylation of accumulating levodopa to 3-methyldopa. Dopamine agonists and monoamine oxidase inhibitors are also frequently used.

Patients with a PLP deficiency, arising from impaired PNPO activity, need to be treated with PLP, and not pyridoxine, and can respond well to initiation of such treatment. 5-MTHF deficiency should be addressed by administration of folinic acid. Folic acid should not be given as this can exacerbate a CSF 5-MTHF deficiency state.

Currently, there does not appear to be an effective treatment for patients with mutations affecting the functioning of the dopamine transporter. However, some reports suggest a response from the use of dopamine agonists.

Lysosomal storage disorders

Lysosomal storage disorders (LSDs) (Table 19.22) are inherited diseases that affect the ability in a cell to recycle macromolecules (complex lipids, glycoproteins and mucopolysaccharides). Deficiency of lysosomal hydrolases or associated proteins leads to the accumulation of substances proximal to the metabolic block within the lysosomal compartment. This storage leads to ultrastructural changes in the cell and pathological alterations to cell biology. Lysosomal storage disorders are classified according to the type of storage material (e.g. sphingolipidoses, mucopolysaccharidoses, glycoproteinoses). LSDs are a clinically heterogeneous group of conditions, with the phenotype depending on which tissues have the highest turnover of the relevant storage material. For instance, the GM2 gangliosidoses cause storage in neurones and neurodegeneration, while metachromatic leukodystrophy leads to storage in oligodendrocytes and demyelination.

Table 19.22 The lysosomal storage disorders that may be associated with neurological problems.

Mucopolysaccharidosis
Type I (Hurler/Scheie)
Type II (Hunter)
Type III (Sanfilippo types A–D)
Type IV (Morquio types A and B)
Type VI (Maroteaux–Lamy)
Glycosphingolipidoses
GM1 Gangliosidosis (neonatal, juvenile and adult forms)
GM2 Gangliosidosis (Tay–Sachs and Sandhoff's diseases)
Gaucher disease (type I, II and III)
Niemann–Pick disease types A and B
Niemann–Pick disease type C
Fabry disease
Farber disease
Krabbe disease (globoid cell leukodystrophy)
Metachromatic leukodystrophy
Saposin-related disorders (types A, B, C, combined)
Oligosaccharidoses
Fucosidosis
Mannosidosis
(Galacto)sialidosis
Mucolipidoses
ML II (I-cell disease)
ML III
Neuronal ceroidlipofuscinoses
Adult neuronal ceroid lipofuscinosis (NCL) (Kufs disease)

Within each disease there is also marked variability of clinical phenotype. This is thought to relate in large part to the precise nature of the genetic mutation and the degree of residual activity of the affected enzyme. As a rule, the most severe mutations lead to early onset, rapidly progressive disease, while those with residual activity of even a few per cent may have a relatively attenuated, late onset presentation. In mucopolysaccharidosis types I and II (Hurler and Hunter diseases), skeletal involvement with dysostosis multiplex is seen in all patients, but only the most severely affected develop neuronal storage and neurodegeneration.

Many of the lysosomal storage disorders can lead to neurological involvement as summarised in Table 19.23. Some of the more common diseases are discussed in more detail here:

Table 19.23 Neurological involvement in lysosomal storage disorders, clinical features and current treatment options.

Disease	Inheritance	Gene product	Storage material	Incidence	Clinical features	Options for treatment
MPS I (Hurler Scheie's disease)	AR	Alpha-L-iduronidase	Dermatan sulfate	1/75 000–85 000	Dysostosis multiplex resulting in compression neuropathies and myelopathy	Bone marrow transplantation. ERT for systemic features but does not affect CNS disease
			Heparan sulfate		Corneal clouding Hepatosplenomegaly Cardiomyopathy Pneumonia Cognitive impairment	
MPS II (Hunter disease)	X-linked	Iduronate-2-sulfatase	Dermatan sulfate	1/92 000–149 000 (males). Symptomatic females also reported	Dysostosis multiplex resulting in compression neuropathies and myelopathy	Bone marrow transplantation. ERT for systemic features but does not affect CNS disease
			Heparan sulfate		Hepatosplenomegaly Valvular heart disease Obstructive sleep apnoea Cognitive impairment	
MPS III (Sanfilippo disease)	AR	Heparan-N-sulfatase/ Alpha-N-acetylglucosaminidase/ Acetyl-CoA:glucosamine-N-acetyltransferase/ N-acetylglucosamine-6-sulfatase	Heparan sulfate	1/86 000–114 000	Cognitive impairment Behaviour problems	Intrathecal ERT (in clinical trial). Chaperone therapy
Gaucher disease	AR	Beta-glucocerebrosidase	Glucosyl ceramide	1/57 000–86 000	Hypersplenism Hepatomegaly Bone involvement Horizontal supranuclear gaze palsy Dementia Ataxia Spasticity Epilepsy Parkisonism	ERT for systemic features but does not affect CNS disease. Substrate reduction therapy

Fabry disease	X-linked	Alpha-galactosidase A	Ceramide trihexoside	1/80 000–117 000	Peripheral neuropathy Ischaemic stroke Dolichoectasia (elongation/ fusiform dilatation of intracranial vessels)	ERT. Chaperone therapy (in clinical trial)
GM1-gangliosidosis	AR	Beta-galactosidase	GM1	1/161 000–384 000	Dystonia Pyramidal signs Skeletal disease	Currently supportive
GM2-gangliosidosis (Tay–Sachs, Sandhoff diseases)	AR	Beta-hexosaminidase	GM2	1/32 000–384 000	Ataxia Dysarthria Spasticity Dementia	Chaperone therapy
Niemann–Pick C disease	AR	NP-C1/NP-C2	Cholesterol, GSLs	1/45 000–286 000	Ataxia Dystonia Dysarthria Dementia Psychiatric Vertical supranuclear ophthalmoplegia	Cyclodextrin (in clinical trial)
Krabbe disease	AR	Beta-galactocerebrosidase	Galactosylceramide Psychosine	1/74 000–201 000	Paraplegia or hemiplegia Ataxia Visual loss Peripheral neuropathy Dementia	HSCT if performed early
Metachromatic leukodystrophy	AR	Arylsulfatase A	Metachromatic lipid deposits	Overall 1/40 000. 20% adult onset	Personality change Spasticity Seizures Peripheral neuropathy	Intrathecal ERT (in clinical trial)

ERT, enzyme replacement therapy; HSCT, haematopoietic stem cell transplantation.

Glycosphingolipidoses

Glycosphingolipids (GSL) are derived from ceramide by sequential addition of sugar molecules. The glycosphingolipidoses are a group of lysosomal storage disorders that result from an inability to degrade these complex lipids. As a group, they are the most common of the lysosomal storage disorders and all can involve the nervous system.

Gaucher disease Gaucher disease is caused by deficiency of glucocerebrosidase leading to the accumulation of glucosylceramide within lysosomes. As with other LSDs, a broad spectrum of severity is seen in Gaucher disease. Severe mutations that inactivate the glucocerebrosidase enzyme completely are not compatible with life and result in hydrops fetalis. Where there is minimal residual enzyme activity, glucosylceramide accumulates in a wide range of cell types, including neurones, and affected infants suffer a rapidly progressive neurological deterioration, so-called type 2 Gaucher disease. In most patients, there is sufficient residual enzyme activity to fully degrade all glucosylceramide in most cell types, including neurones. Significant storage is only observed in macrophages, which are exposed to a much greater load of GSL than other cells because of their role in phagocytosing senescent erythrocytes. These patients therefore have visceral disease resulting from infiltration of the liver, spleen and bone marrow with lipid-laden macrophages, but they do not have neurological involvement. These patients have type 1 Gaucher disease.

Between these two extremes are a group of patients with often severe visceral disease that is accompanied by more slowly progressive neuropathic disease, traditionally termed type 3 Gaucher disease. These patients often present in childhood with a horizontal supranuclear gaze palsy. In more mildly affected patients this may be the only neurological manifestation, but a wide variety of other syndromes have been reported including myoclonic epilepsy, ataxia and dementia.

More recently, it has been shown that there is a strong association between parkinsonism and heterozygosity for mutations in the glucocerebrosidase gene. The nature of this association is not clear but it seems unlikely to relate to storage of glucosylceramide as the association seems to be stronger for heterozygotes than for homozygote patients who have Gaucher disease.

Gaucher disease was the first lysosomal storage disorder for which enzyme replacement therapy (ERT) became available. Enzyme replacement therapy involves the intravenous infusion of recombinant glucocerebrosidase. This is efficiently taken up by Gaucher macrophages and is a highly effective treatment for non-neuropathic Gaucher disease. However, because the recombinant molecule cannot cross the blood–brain barrier, enzyme replacement therapy has not been effective in treating neuropathic disease.

Fabry disease This is an X-linked disorder caused by a deficiency of the lysosomal enzyme α-galactosidase A, the gene for which is localised at Xp22. This results in the accumulation of ceramide trihexoside (CTH) in many cell types. It is a multi-system disease affecting the heart, kidney and blood vessels. Stroke can be the first clinical manifestation. As in other X-linked diseases, men are generally, but not always, more severely affected than women.

Clinical symptoms usually develop in early adolescence with the initial manifestation often being the development of acroparaesthesiae with severe pain in the hands and feet, commonly triggered by hot weather or pyrexia. Angiokeratoma, hypohidrosis, irritable bowel syndrome, and corneal and lenticular abnormalities are other common features. Progressive renal, cardiac and cerebral involvement then develops. CNS involvement manifests as an increased risk of ischaemic stroke because of the involvement of the cerebral vessels or secondary to cardiac disease. There is a predilection for the vertebro-basilar system with posterior circulation stroke manifesting as hemiparesis, vertigo, diplopia, nystagmus, dysarthria or ataxia.

Diagnosis in men depends on the demonstration of reduced α-galactosidase A enzyme activity in plasma leukocytes or dried blood spots. This test is not useful in women, where genotyping is the investigation of choice. In some cases being investigated for renal impairment, kidney biopsy may show intralysosomal lipid deposition.

Classic Fabry disease has a poor prognosis, with most untreated males dying by the age of 40 years, generally from renal failure although cardiac and cerebrovascular disease can also cause fatal complications. With increased disease awareness, many patients with attenuated phenotypes are now being diagnosed who may not have severe end organ involvement. Life expectancy is reduced only slightly in heterozygous female patients.

Management Carbamazepine, gabapentin, pregabalin or even low doses of opiates are useful for the symptomatic treatment of the painful acroparaesthesiae. Progressive renal failure may require dialysis or transplantation. Angiokeratomata are generally asymptomatic but can be treated by laser coagulation of small and medium sized vessels. Conventional stroke protection with antiplatelet drugs or anticoagulation may have a role. Enzyme replacement therapy has been developed to treat the condition. Some symptoms may respond, but it is not as effective as enzyme replacement therapy for Gaucher in patients with established disease. It is hoped that if enzyme replacement therapy is started early enough, it may be able to prevent the long-term complications.

GM_2 gangliosidosis GM_2 gangliosidosis is caused by mutations in the genes encoding the subunits of β-hexosaminidase (an αβ-heterodimer). Mutations of the *HEXA* gene lead to Tay–Sachs disease and of the *HEXB* gene to Sandhoff disease. β-hexosaminidase cleaves the terminal galactose residue from GM_2 ganglioside. As GM_2 ganglioside is predominantly expressed in neurones, the GM_2 gangliosidoses are predominantly neurodegenerative disorders.

As with the other lysosomal storage disorders, there is a spectrum of disease severity. The classic infantile forms present within the first 6 months of life with seizures, blindness and developmental delay and are rapidly fatal. Although rare in the general population, certain ethnic groups have much higher incidences. In Ashkenazi Jewish populations, where the carrier frequency for Tay–Sachs disease is 1/30 (compared with 1/300 for the general population), carrier screening programmes have dramatically reduced the numbers of babies affected.

The late onset forms of GM_2 gangliosidosis can present in childhood or adulthood with gait problems, dystonia, cognitive decline and pronounced bulbar involvement. The disease is slowly progressive and patients eventually succumb to complications such as respiratory infections secondary to dysphagia.

The diagnosis is made by assaying the activity of β-hexosaminidase in peripheral blood leukocytes. Brain imaging shows striking cerebellar degeneration which is secondary to loss of Purkinje cells. Histologically there is neuraxonal dystrophy, characterised by the formation of axonal spheroids and meganeurites with ectopic dendritogenesis, which is also seen in other lysosomal storage disorders in which there is ganglioside storage within neurones.

Management Currently, therapy is supportive. Substrate reduction therapy with miglustat has been shown to prolong life in a knockout mouse model of Sandhoff disease but a clinical trial in patients with late onset Tay–Sachs disease showed no benefit.

Adult onset inherited leukodystrophies

This complex set of inherited conditions have as their hallmark the progressive destruction or loss of myelin. The adult forms of disease can be an attenuated or frankly different phenotype from that reported in childhood. Reported prevalence varies from 40/million (X-linked adrenoleukodystrophy) to case reports (e.g. Nasu–Hakola disease), with perhaps a total of about 300/million. This is a rapidly evolving field, with easier access to MRI imaging and genetic testing likely to increase the reported incidence and prevalence over the coming years.

As an approach to investigation, we include here a summary of a recent review describing the most commonly presenting leukodystrophies in adults (age >16 years) with their major clinical and MRI features, a logical diagnostic approach and possible treatment options.

Table19.24 lists the most frequent of the adult onset leukodystrophies, with non-classic leukodystrophies, mitochondrial disorders and CADASIL (cerebral autosomal dominant arteriopathy with subcortical infarcts and leukoencephalopathy) also included, as they commonly enter the differential diagnosis of these conditions.

Importantly, before embarking on investigating inherited causes of widespread MRI white matter involvement, there are a number of *acquired* conditions that need to be excluded: inflammatory, vascular, toxic, metabolic, autoimmune, infectious and neoplastic causes. The approaches are standard and similar to the differential diagnosis for example of multiple sclerosis (Chapter 11), and include lymphomatosis, functional B_{12} deficiency, HIV infection and carbon monoxide poisoning. A very rapid onset and progression over months is much more likely to be acquired than genetic, though cerebral adrenoleukodystrophy (ALD) can present abruptly.

After eliminating acquired causes, a suggested structured approach would be to consider the following in turn:

- *Family history.* If a true dominant pattern can be established this is useful as it will reduce the current diagnostic possibilities significantly.
- *Ethnicity.* Some diagnoses are more common, though not exclusive, to certain populations: Ashkenazi Jewish (mucolipidosis, adult onset gangliosidosis and adult polyglucosan body disease); Asia-Indian or Turkish (megalencephalic leukodystrophy with cysts) and adult sialidosis (Finnish).
- *Clinical presentation.* Table 19.25 lists phenotypic features that can guide towards a particular leukodystrophy.
- *MRI pattern* (Table 19.26). This is illustrated schematically in Figure 19.28. There is overlap amongst the conditions and widespread atrophy can be seen in the late stage of many (Figures 19.29 and 19.30).

Initial specialist biochemical investigations include (fasting) very long chain fatty acid (VLCFA) levels, relevant white cell enzyme activities, cholestanol profile, urine bile alcohols and plasma amino acids. As ALD has a relatively high prevalence and potential options for treatment, it should be tested for early. Close liaison with the laboratory is important to optimise the handling of appropriate samples.

If no abnormalities are found on biochemical testing it can be appropriate to proceed to genetic testing, including whole exome sequencing. This is likely to be an area of rapid diagnostic advancement, with the development of DNA chip, exome and genome-based investigative technologies.

Brain biopsy can be considered if the patient is deteriorating and a potentially treatable condition is possible or when the result can have important implications for the management of the family. The yield for brain biopsy can be increased to near 80% by targeting a radiologically identified lesion (with contrast enhancement). The risk of complications including infection, seizures and haemorrhage, is approximately 10–20%, but no long-term neurological sequelae are reported.

There follows a brief description of the clinical and MRI features of some of the leading adult onset leukodystrophies (to be read in conjunction with Table 19.26 and Figures 19.29 and 19.30). The non-classical leukodystrophies, CADASIL and mitochondrial disorders, are described separately in Chapters 6 and 10.

X-linked adrenoleukodystrophy

Clinical presentation The phenotypic expression is wide and varies between and within families. Recognised phenotypes include adrenal insufficiency alone, adult onset cerebral ALD, adult onset adrenomyeloneuropathy (AMN) without cerebral involvement, and AMN with cerebral involvement and/or adrenal insufficiency. Adult onset cerebral ALD usually presents with psychiatric features followed by ataxia, seizures, dementia and death. Adrenal insufficiency should be specifically tested for. The AMN phenotype consists of a slowly progressive spastic paraparesis, with sphincter dysfunction, erectile dysfunction and sensory involvement. At least 20% of heterozygous females also develop symptoms, commonly in their thirties, of an AMN-like phenotype.

MRI features Occipital regions are usually first to be involved, with the corpus callosum, splenium and internal capsule posterior limbs, which then progress anteriorly. In cerebral ALD, peripheral contrast enhancement is seen, and in AMN, cord atrophy. As transplant is now considered an option for very early adult cerebral ALD, annual MRI with contrast and neuropsychometric assessment is suggested.

Krabbe disease

Clinical presentation The adult form (approximately 1 in 10 of all cases) classically presents with a paraparesis with cortical features of visual involvement, dementia and seizures. There can be slowing of peripheral nerve electrophysiology.

MRI features The signal change is posterior, with a pattern of radiating stripes of normal signal intensity. T2 high signal is seen in the posterior internal capsule, brainstem and corticospinal tracts. On CT, thalamic and basal ganglia hyperintensities are seen, which may represent calcification.

Cerebrotendinous xanthomatosis

Clinical presentation Multisystem involvement is common, including cataracts, tendon xanthomata (Achilles tendon typically), osteoporosis, and liver, endocrine and chest involvement. Neurological features are spastic paraparesis, ataxia and a peripheral neuropathy followed by dementia.

MRI features Periventricular white matter change and atrophy, with sparing of the corpus callosum are seen. The T2-weighted signal intensity can be high in the cerebellar white matter and low in the dentate nucleus.

Table 19.24 The most frequently described adult onset inherited leukodystrophies.

Disorder	Age of onset	Incidence	Ethnic predilection	Inheritance	Useful investigation(s)	Gene(s)
X linked adrenoleukodystrophy adrenomyeloneuropathy (ALD/AMN)	Juvenile to adulthood	Overall 1 in 27 000–40 0000. >20% of affected men may have significant brain involvement		X-linked. Heterozygote women can develop spastic paraparesis	Very long chain fatty acid levels	*ABCD1*
Metachromatic leukodystrophy (MLD)	Up to 70 years	Overall 1 in 40 000. 20% adult onset		AR	Arylsulfatase A (ARSA) enzyme activity (leukocytes/fibroblasts)*	*ARSA*
Cerebrotendinous xanthomatosis (CTX)		Overall 1 in 50 000		AR	Sterol profile. Urine bile alcohols	*CYP27A1*
Globoid cell leukodystrophy (Krabbe disease)	Up to 60 years	Overall 1 in 100 000. 10% adult onset.		AR	Galactocerebrosidase (GALC) enzyme activity (leukocytes/fibroblasts)	*GALC; PSAP*
Cerebral autosomal dominant arteriopathy with subcortical infarcts and leukoencephalopathy (CADASIL)	Migraine: mean 30 years (range: 6–48 years). Ischaemic events: mean 50 years (range: 20–70 years)	2–4/100 000 Finland. 1.98/100 000 west Scotland. 1.32/10 000 west England		AD and sporadic	Electron microscopy of skin biopsy	*NOTCH3*
Mitochondrial disorders (see also Chapter 10)				Maternal, AD, AR	Lactate (blood/CSF). Mitochondrial respiratory chain enzyme activity	Various
Hexosaminidase A deficiency (GM2 gangliosidosis, adult-onset Tay–Sachs disease)	20–40 years	64 cases	64% Jewish origin	AR	Beta-hexosaminidase A (HEX A) enzymatic activity (leukocytes)	*HEXA*
Diffuse leukoencephalopathy with neuroaxonal spheroids (HDLS)	Mean 40 years (range 15–78 years)	52 cases		AD and sporadic	Characteristic brain biopsy findings (now superceded by molecular genetic testing)	*CSFR1*
Adult polyglucosan body disease	40–60 years	47 cases	Ashkenazi Jewish	AR	Sural nerve biospy. Glycogen brancher enzyme (GBE) activity (fibroblasts)	*GBE1*
Alexander disease	12–62 years	36 cases		AD and sporadic	Characteristic brain biopsy findings (now superceded by molecular genetic testing)	*GFAP*

Adult onset autosomal dominant leukodystrophy (ADLD)	30–50 years	Unknown: at least 27 cases reported in literature		AD		*LMNB1*
Vanishing white matter disease (VWM)	Mean 30 years (range 16–62 years)	177 cases in total, 25 with onset >16 years		AR		*eIF2B 1-5*
Megalencephalic leukoencephalopathy with subcortical cysts (MLC)	6 months–50 years	11 cases >20 years	Asian-Indian, Turkish	AR		*MLC1; HEPACAM*
MTHFR deficiency	Any age	Limited case reports		AR	Plasma amino acid profile	*MTHFR*
α-mannosidosis	Adolescence, but severe ataxia 30–40 years	Limited case reports		AR	Urine oligosaccharides. Vacuolated lymphocytes. α-mannosidase enzyme activity (leukocytes)	*MAN2B1*
Mucolipidosis type IV	Usually infant childhood, 1 case onset 16 years (14)	Late onset reported because of attenuated phenotype	Ashkenazi Jewish	AR		*MCOLN1*
Adult sialidosis	Usually childhood, but can be 20–30 years	Limited case reports	Finnish	AR	Urine oligosaccharides. Vacuolated lymphocytes. α-neuroaminidase enzyme activity (fibroblasts)	*SLC17A5*
Organic acidurias	Adolescence to adulthood	Limited case reports		AR	Urine organic acid profile (UOA)	
1. Canavan disease					↑ N-acetylaspartic acid (UOA). Aspartoacylase enzyme activity (fibroblasts)	*ASPA*
2. Glutaric acidemia type 1 (16)					↑ Glutaric acid, 3-OH-glutaric acid (UOA). Acylcarnitine profile	*GCDH*
3. L-2-hydroxyglutaric aciduria					↑ 2-hydroxyglutaric acid (UOA). ↑ Lysine (CSF)	*L2HGDH*
4. 3-methylglutaconic aciduria type 1					↑ 3-methylglutaconate, 3-hydroxyisovaleric acid (UOA)	*AUH*

(continued)

Table 19.24 (continued)

Disorder	Age of onset	Incidence	Ethnic predilection	Inheritance	Useful investigation(s)	Gene(s)
Pelizaeus–Merzbacher disease (PMD)	Usually infant-childhood onset, case reports of adult onset up to age 45 years	Limited case reports		X-linked. Heterozygote women can develop spastic paraparesis		*PLP1*
Recessive hypomyelinating leukoencephalopathy (Pelizaeus–Merzbacher-like disease)	Case report of onset age 15 years	Case report		AR		*GJC2; HSPD1; AIMP1*
Leukoencephalopathy with brainstem and spinal cord involvement and lactate elevation (LBSL)	Usually childhood	Case report		AR	MRS: elevated lactate	*DARS2*
Polycystic lipomembranous osteodysplasia with sclerosing leukoencephalopathy (PLOSL; Nasu–Hokola disease)	Mean 30 years (range 10–45 years)	33 cases in Japan	Most reported cases in Finland and Japan, but occurs worldwide	AR	Imaging of the hand	*TYROBP; TREM2*
Cockayne syndrome	Usually infant/childhood	Overall 1.8–2.7 per million births. 4 cases reported with adult onset	Canada (aboriginal residents of Manitoba, Newfoundland), Japan, Middle Eastern and Western Asian countries (35)	AR		*ERCC6; ERCC8*

*ARSA enzyme activity in leukocytes that is 5–20% of normal controls may be caused by pseudodeficiency. Pseudodeficiency may be difficult to distinguish from true ARSA enzyme deficiency by biochemical testing alone. Therefore, the diagnosis of MLD is usually confirmed by molecular genetic testing of *ARSA*. Pseudodeficiency alleles are common polymorphisms that result in lower than average ARSA enzyme activity; however, these alleles are reported to still produce sufficient functional enzyme to avoid sulfatide accumulation and thus do not cause MLD in either the homozygous state or the compound heterozygous state with an MLD allele. For further information on mitochondrial disorders see Chapter 10.

Source: Ahmed et al 2014. Reproduced with permission of the BMJ.

Table 19.25 Clinical features associated with specific adult-onset leukodystrophies.

Suggestive presenting features	Leukodystrophy
Visual involvement	
Optic atrophy	Metachromatic leukodystrophy, Krabbe disease, mitochondrial disorders, Pelizaeus–Merzbacher disease
Cortical blindness	Krabbe disease
Retinal degeneration	Krabbe disease, mitochondrial disorders, Cockayne syndrome
Cataracts	Cerebrotendinous xanthomatosis, mitochondrial respiratory chain disorders
Abnormal eye movements/ nystagmus	Pelizaeus–Merzbacher disease
Neurological features	
Peripheral neuropathy	Metachromatic leukodystrophy Cerebrotendinous xanthomatosis Krabbe disease Adult polyglucosan body disease (GSD IV)
Cerebellar ataxia	Cerebrotendinous xanthomatosis Alexander disease Adult polyglucosan body disease (GSD IV) Vanishing white matter disease
Psychiatric symptoms	Metachromatic leukodystrophy Vanishing white matter disease Cerebral adrenoleukodystrophy Hereditary diffuse leukoencephalopathy with axonal spheroids
Pyramidal weakness/spasticity	Adrenomyeloneuropathy/adrenoleukodystrophy Krabbe disease Cerebrotendinous xanthomatosis Vanishing white matter disease Adult polyglucosan body disease Hereditary diffuse leukoencephalopathy with axonal spheroids
Bulbar dysfunction and palatal myoclonus	Adult onset Alexander disease
Dystonic dyskinetic movement disorder	Glutaric acidemia type 1
Autonomic features	Adult onset autosomal dominant leukodystrophy
Migraine and stroke	CADASIL
Other features	
Primary/secondary amenorrhoea	Vanishing white matter disease
Fractures following minor trauma	Polycystic lipomembranous osteodysplasia with sclerosing leukoencephalopathy (PLOSL; Nasu–Hokola disease)
Macrocephaly	Alexander disease, organic acidurias (Canavan disease, glutaric acidemia type 1, L-2-hydroxyglutaric aciduria), megalencephalic leukoencephalopathy with subcortical cysts
Tendon xanthomas	Cerebrotendinous xanthomatosis

Source: Ahmed et al 2014. Reproduced with permission of the BMJ.

Table 19.26 Specific MRI findings in leukodystrophies.

MRI findings	Leukodystrophy
Pattern of white matter involvement	
Predominantly frontal peri-ventricular	MLD, HDLS
Predominantly parietal	ADLD
Predominantly peri-ventricular	APBD
Predominantly posterior	Krabbe disease
Predominantly occipital	X-ALD
Posterior white matter changes progressing anteriorly	X-ALD
Anterior temporal lobe changes	CADASIL
Contrast enhancement of periphery of lesions	X-ALD, Alexander disease
Sparing of U fibres	MLD, CTX, APBD, CADASIL
Involvement of U fibres	L-2-hydroxyglutaric aciduria
Corpus callosum	
Thinning	ADLD, VWM, HDLS
Hyperintensities	HDLS, VWM
Involvement	MLD, X-ALD, Krabbe disease
Sparing	CTX, APBD
Other findings	
Enhancement of corticospinal tracts	Krabbe disease
Cerebellar/brainstem white matter change	AMN, CTX, Alexander disease
T2 hypointensity of dentate nucleus	CTX, L-2-hydroxyglutaric aciduria
Atrophy medulla oblongata and upper cervical cord	Alexander disease
Spinal cord atrophy	APBD, AMN
Cystic changes	VWM, mitochondrial disease

ADLD, Adult onset autosomal dominant leukodystrophy, ; AMN, adrenomyeloneuropathy; APBD, adult polyglucosan body disease; CADASIL, cerebral autosomal dominant arteriopathy with subcortical infarcts and leukoencephalopathy; CTX, cerebrotendinous xanthomatosis; HDLS, hereditary diffuse leukoencephalopathy with neuroaxonal spheroids; MLD, metachromatic leukodystrophy; VWM, vanishing white matter disease; X-ALD, X-linked adrenoleukodystrophy.
Source: Source: Ahmed et al 2014. Reproduced with permission of the BMJ.

Metachromatic leukodystrophy

Clinical presentation The adult form accounts for approximately 20% of metachromatic leukodystrophy (MLD) presentations. The initial symptoms are often psychiatric, followed by motor involvement (spastic paraparesis), cerebellar ataxia and cognitive decline. Other neurological signs include dystonia, optic atrophy, a demyelinating peripheral neuropathy (though more often seen in children) and seizures.

MRI features These include widespread symmetrical confluent white matter change with a peri-ventricular frontal predominance, a tigroid pattern of radiating stripes in the affected white matter. The subcortical U fibres are typically spared and the corpus callosum is often involved early.

Hereditary diffuse leukoencephalopathy with neuroaxonal spheroids

Clinical presentation Cognitive and personality change, particularly of executive function occur, usually progressing to death within 6 years. CSF1R (colony stimulating factor 1 receptor) is an important mediator of microglial function. Pathologically, loss of myelin, axonal destruction and spheroids and lipid-laden macrophages are seen.

MRI features The T2 signal change is bifrontal, extending to the subcortical regions, posterior limb of the internal capsule and pyramidal tracts of the brainstem. MRI changes can be asymmetrical at outset before becoming symmetrical.

Alexander's disease

Clinical presentation In adults, bulbar and pyramidal tract involvement are well described, as well as sleep disturbance and cerebellar ataxia. This can be combined with autonomic and urinary dysfunction and palatal myoclonus. Cytoplasmic astrocyte inclusion bodies containing the intermediate glial filament acidic protein (GFAP) called Rosenthal fibres are seen.

MRI features Usually contrast enhancement can be seen if the patient is less than 40 years old. Atrophy of the medulla and upper spinal cord, as well as peri-ventricular white matter change is seen. The adult MRI appearances tend to be distinct from those seen in childhood which can include frontal change, peri-ventricular rim and thalamic and/or basal ganglia involvement.

Vanishing white matter disease

Clinical presentation Adult onset disease has been described in at least 25 cases in the literature, with cerebellar, spasticity, dementia, seizures and psychiatric symptoms (one-third) dominating. Ovarian failure is characterisitic.

MRI features The signal change is diffuse hyper/hypo intensity on T2 weighting accompanied by cystic change and atrophy. Corpus callosal and cerebellar atrophy can be present. As the name suggests, ultimately, the hemispheric white matter can disappear.

Pelizaeus–Merzbacher disease and Pelizaeus–Merzbacher-like disease

Clinical features Confined to limited case reports for the adult onset form with ataxia, dementia and tremor; though heterozygote females can present with a progressive cord syndrome. Pelizaeus–Merzbacher disease (PMD) is caused by mutations in the myelin

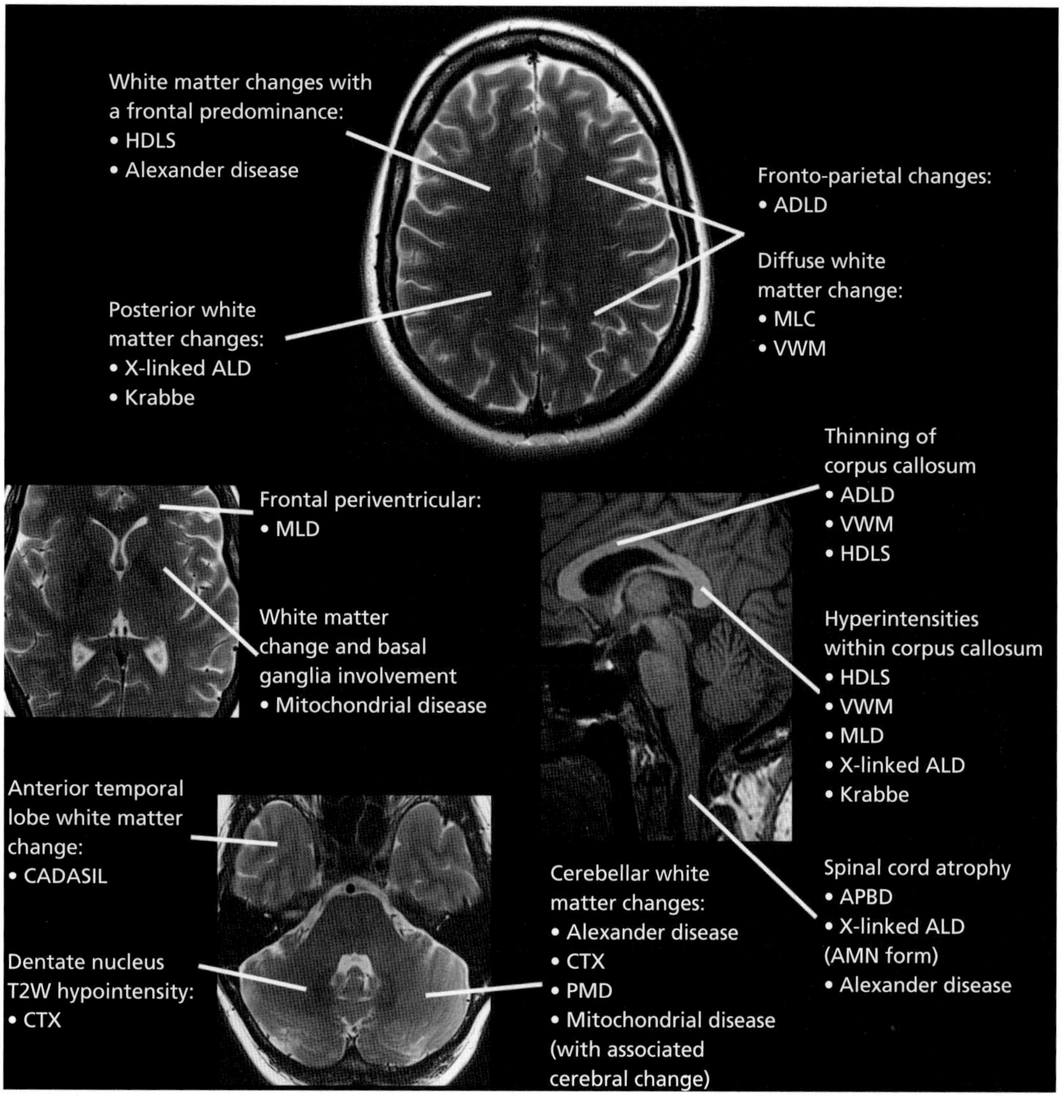

Figure 19.28 Schematic illustration of brain MRI findings in specific leukodystrophies. ADLD, adult onset autosomal dominant leukodystrohy; ALD, adrenoleukodystrophy; AMN, adrenomyeloneuropathy; APBD, adult polyglucosan body disease; CADASIL, cerebral autosomal dominant arteriopathy with subcortical infarcts and leukoencephalopathy; CTX, cerebrotendinous xanthomatosis; HDLS, hereditary diffuse leukoencephalopathy with neuroaxonal spheroids; MLC, megalencephalic leukoencephalopathy with subcortical cysts; MLD, metachromatic leukodystrophy; PMD, Pelizaeus–Merzbacher disease; VWM, vanishing white matter disease. Source: Ahmed *et al.* 2014. Reproduced with permission of BMJ.

proteolipid protein (*PLP*) gene on the long arm of the X chromosome, and is allelic to hereditary spastic paraplegia (HSP) type 2 (Chapter 16). Pelizaeus–Merzbacher-like disease (PMLD) is clinically indistinct from PMD, but *PLP* mutation negative.

MRI features The MRI patterns tend to show diffuse white matter change (hyperintensity) cortically, sparing the U fibres.

Management Current treatment of adult onset leukodystrophies is largely supportive, though chenodeoxycholic acid has been used as therapy for cerebrotendinous xanthomatosis since 1975 (however, its effect in symptomatic adults may be limited). A number of clinical trials are currently underway using interventions such as haematopoietic stem cell transplant, intrathecal enzyme replacement therapy and autologous haematopoietic stem cell transplant transduced with ABCD1 lentiviral vector (for ALD). Further details can be found on www.clinicaltrials.gov.

Peroxisomal disorders

Peroxisomes are cellular organelles found in all human cells except erythrocytes. They have several functions including the synthesis of phospholipids, oxidation of VLCFA, oxidation of phytanic acid, catabolism of lysine and formation of bile acids.

Phenotypes vary considerably but the typical clinical presentation of a peroxisomal disorder is with dysmorphic features, neurological abnormalities, ocular signs, hepatic or gastrointestinal dysfunction.

Diagnosis is suggested by abnormal metabolites in plasma and/or erythrocytes and confirmed by specific fibroblast studies showing abnormalities of peroxisomal biogenesis or reduction in specific

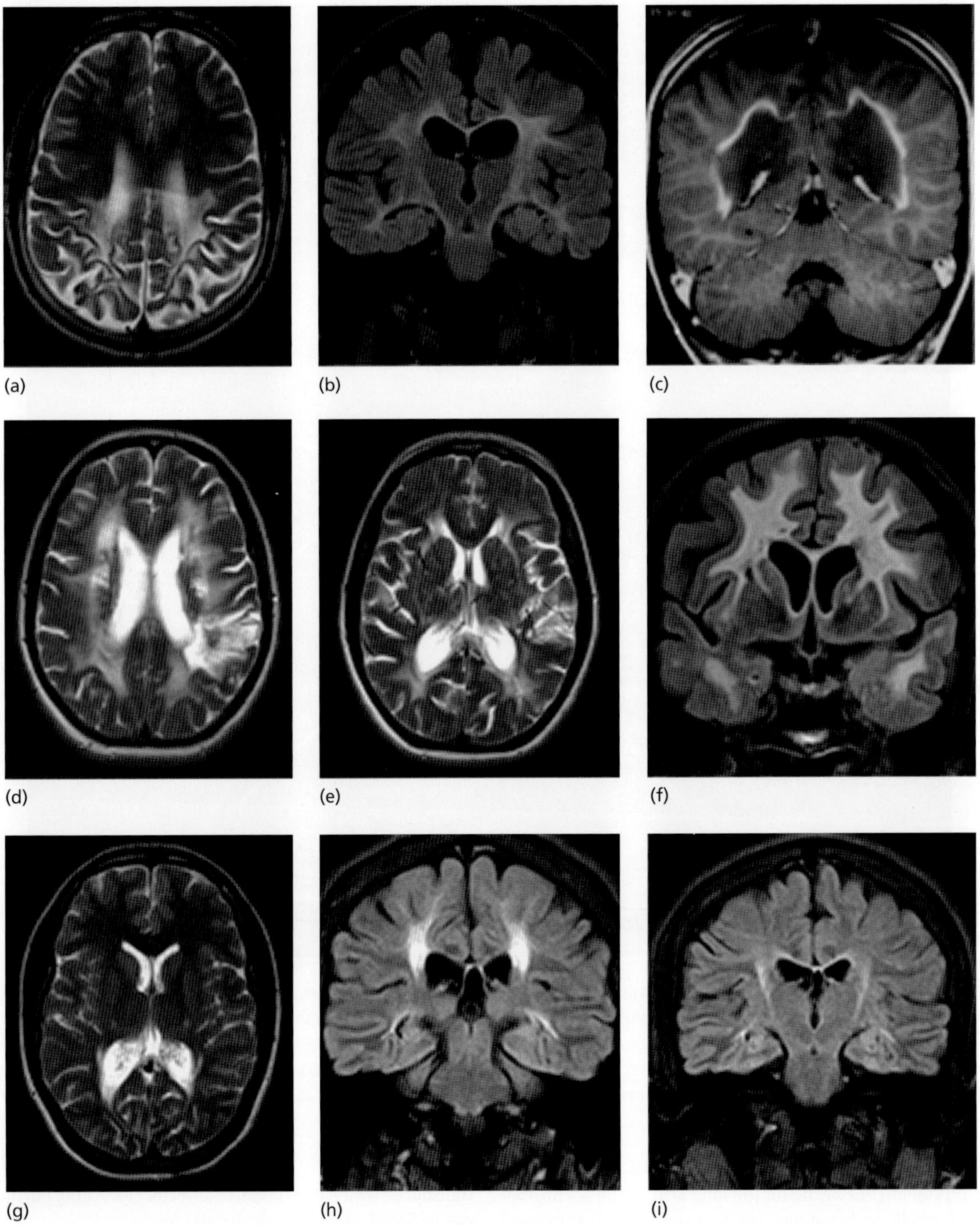

Figure 19.29 MRI brain acquisitions of: X-linked adrenoleukodystrophy on (a) axial T2-weighted, (b) coronal FLAIR and (c) coronal postgadolinium contrast sequences showing diffuse white matter signal T2-weighted hyperintensity and volume loss of the posterior frontal, posterior callosal and parieto-occipital regions, extending along the corticospinal tracts through the internal capsules and temporal peri-ventricular white matter. Peripheral enhancement of the parieto-occiptal confluent symmetrical signal abnormality is demonstrated. Cerebral autosomal dominant arteriopathy with subcortical infarcts and leukoencephalopathy on (d,e) axial T2-weighted and (f) coronal FLAIR sequences showing diffuse symmetrical white matter hyperintensity extending through the external capsules and temporal poles with multiple mature subcortical and a left superior parietal cortical infarcts. Krabbe disease (globoid cell leukodystrophy) on (g) axial T2-weighted and (h,i) coronal FLAIR sequences showing posterior peri-ventricular and deep white matter hyperintensity and volume loss involving the corticospinal tracts and splenium of the corpus callosum. Source: Ahmed *et al.* 2014. Reproduced with permission of BMJ.

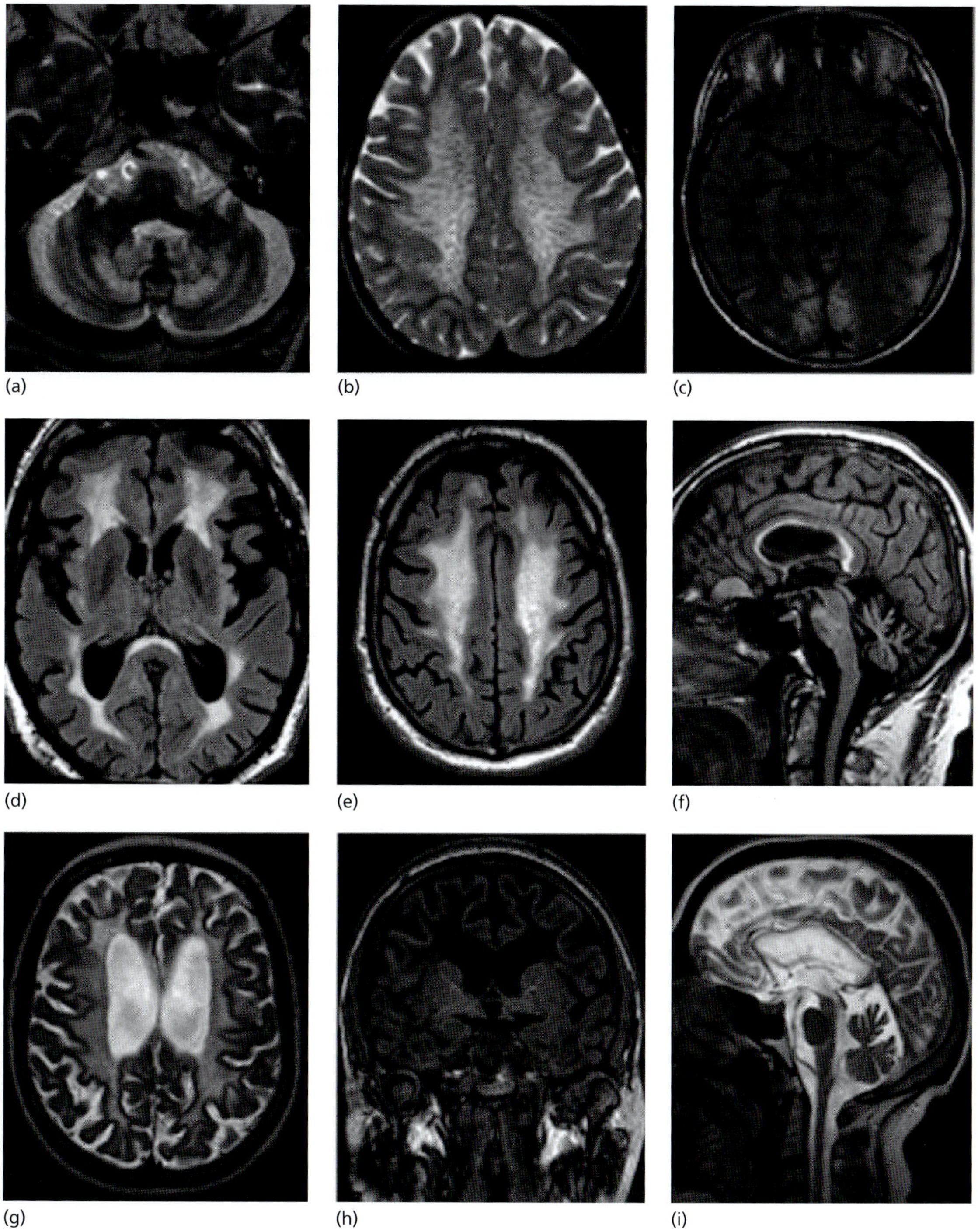

Figure 19.30 MRI brain acquisitions of: cerebrotendinous xanthomatosis on an axial T2-weighted sequence through the posterior fossa (a) demonstrating white matter signal hypointensity involving the dentate nuclei and surrounding hyperintensity. Note the diffuse volume loss of the cerebellum disproportionate to the visible temporal poles. Metachromatic leukodystrophy on an axial T2-weighted sequence through the centra semiovale (b) demonstrating widespread symmetrical white matter signal hyperintensity sparing the subcortical U fibres and radiating transmedullary bands. Mitochondrial encephalopathy lactic acidosis and stroke-like episodes on an axial FLAIR sequence (c) demonstrating swelling and patchy hyperintensity of the cortical and subcortical matter of the occipital, right mesencephalic and left lateral temporal regions during an acute stroke-like episode. Adult polyglucosan body disease on an axial (d,e) and sagittal (f) FLAIR sequences demonstrating diffuse peri-ventricular and inferior callosal white matter hyperintensity and volume loss. There is similarly cerebellar and spinal cord volume loss. An incidental planum sphenoidal meningioma is present. Vanishing white matter disease on axial and sagittal T2-weighted (g,i) as well as coronal T1-weighted (h) sequences demonstrating diffuse white matter T2-weighted hyperintensity and volume loss. Atrophy of the corpus callosum and spinal cord is also present. Source: Ahmed et al 2014. Reproduced with permission of BMJ.

enzyme activities and/or genetic testing. The two most commonly encountered disorders of peroxisomal metabolism in adult practice are X-linked adrenoleukodystrophy/adrenomyeloneuropathy and Refsum disease.

Refsum disease

Refsum disease is a rare inherited autosomal recessive condition caused by a deficiency in phytanoyl CoA-hydroxylase, resulting in the accumulation of phytanic acid. It is characterised by retinopathy, peripheral neuropathy and cerebellar ataxia. The onset of symptoms ranges from late childhood to the sixth decade and can be precipitated or exacerbated by intercurrent infections and pregnancy. Progressive visual failure, often presenting as night blindness, results from a 'salt and pepper' retinopathy and cataract formation. A demyelinating sensorimotor polyneuropathy is prominent, with symmetrical distal sensory impairment, and progressive mild to moderate distal weakness. Other characteristic features include icthyosis, cataracts, anosmia, sensorineural deafness and cardiomyopathy.

The diagnosis is established by finding elevated phytanic acid in the plasma (measured as part of a VLCFA profile) and reduced fibroblast phytanoyl CoA-hydroxylase activity.

Management Refsum disease is treated by restricting the dietary intake of phytanic acid. Although phytanic acid is present in fruit and vegetables, it is tightly bound to chlorophyll and humans do not absorb it efficiently so these foods are not restricted. Ruminants, however, do absorb phytanic acid and it is concentrated in their meat. Therefore beef, lamb, dairy products and fish need to be avoided. With a suitable diet, plasma phytanate levels can be brought into the normal range. If diet is not successful in doing this, plasma exchange can be considered. Unfortunately, even with normal phytanate levels, the disease remains slowly progressive and most patients will lose their sight and develop significant peripheral neuropathy.

Table 19.27 Summary of potential inherited metabolic diseases potentially presenting as an neurological/psychiatric/encephalopathic emergency in adulthood.

Disorder	Emergency presentation	Laboratory tests	Treatment options
Glycogen storage disorders	Rhabdomyolysis Cardiomyopathy	Creatine kinase	Modified diet Exercise advice
Fatty acid oxidation disorders	Rhabdomyolysis Cardiomyopathy	Creatine kinase Acylcarnitine profile Urine organic acids Fibroblast FAO studies	Intervenous dextrose Modified diet Exercise advice Bezafibrate L-carnitine
Urea cycle defects	Encephalopathy Stroke-like episodes Psychiatric features	Ammonia Plasma amino acids Urine orotic acid	Intervenous dextrose Haemofiltration Arginine Sodium benzoate Sodium phenylbutyrate
Organic acidemias	Encephalopathy Cardiac disease Renal impairment	Blood gas Ammonia Acylcarnitine profile Urine organic acids	Intervenous dextrose Haemofiltration L-carnitine
Homocystinuria	Thrombosis Lens dislocation Psychiatric features	Plasma amino acids	Pyridoxine Folate B12 Betaine
Lysosomal storage disorders	Cardiomyopathy Psychiatric features	White cell enzyme activities Filipin staining of fibroblasts	Enzyme replacement therapy Substrate reduction therapy
Adrenoleukodystrophy	Adrenal insufficiency Spastic paraparesis	Very long chain fatty acid levels Synacthen test	Adrenal replacement Consider bone marrow transplant
Mitochondrial disease	Cardiomyopathy Stroke-like episodes	Mitochondrial respiratory chain enzyme activities	Largely supportive
Acute porphyrias	Abdominal pain Psychiatric features Neuropathy	Urine porphobilinogen	Haem arginate infusion

FAO, fatty acid oxidation.

Table 19.28 Systemic features of some inborn errors of metabolism.

Variable	Abnormality	Disorder (with neurological + other features)
Hair	Thinning hair or alopecia	Adrenomyeloneuropathy/adrenoleukodystrophy Argininosuccinic aciduria Biotinidase deficiency
Skin	Eczema	Phenylketonuria
	Photodermatitis	Hartnup disease
	Livedo reticularis	Homocystinuria
	Ichthyosis	Refsum disease
	Angiokeratomas	Fabry disease Oligosaccharidoses
Eye		
Lens	Cataract	Galactosaemia Lowe (oculocerebrorenal) syndrome Mitochondrial disorders Homocystinuria Cerebrotendinous xanthomatosis
	Dislocation	Sulfite oxidase or molybdenum cofactor deficiencies Homocystinuria
Cornea	Clouding	Mucopolysaccharidoses Oligosaccharidoses Mucolipidoses
Retina	Cherry-red spot	Sialidoses Sphingolipidoses
	Pigmentary retinopathy	Refsum disease Zellweger spectrum disorders Pantothenate kinase-associated neurodegeneration Cockayne syndrome Neuronal ceroid lipofuscinoses Mitochondrial disorders *LCHAD* deficiency
Optic nerve	Atrophy	Krabbe's disease Metachromatic leukodystrophy Pelizaeus–Merzbacher disease
Organomegaly	Hepatosplenomegaly	Oligosaccharidoses Mucopolysaccharidoses Gaucher's disease Glycogen storage diseases Cholesterol ester storage disease Niemann–Pick disease
Skeleton	Clinical and radiological dysostoses	Mucopolysaccharidoses Oligosaccharidoses Sphingolipidoses Mucolipidoses
Multi-system involvement		Mitochondrial disorders Lysosomal disorders Peroxisomal disorders Congenital disorders of glycosylation

(continued)

Table 19.28 (continued)

Variable	Abnormality	Disorder (with neurological + other features)
Skeletal muscle	Myopathy	GSD II (Pompe disease, acid maltase deficiency) GSD III (debrancher deficiency)
Kidney	Renal impairment	Fabry disease
Vascular system	Thrombotic events	Homocystinuria Defects of cobalamin metabolism *MTHFR* deficiency
	Stroke/stroke-like events	Fabry disease Mitochondrial disorders Homocystinuria Congenital disorders of glycosylation
Heart	Valve disease	Mucopolysaccharidoses Mucolipidoses
	Cardiomyopathy	Fabry disease Some glycogen storage disorders Some fatty acid oxidation disorders Mucopolysaccharidoses Organic acidemias (methylmalonic and propionic)
	Dysrhythmia	Fabry disease Congenital disorders of glycosylation
Other features	Very early onset severe epilepsy	Pyridoxine, folinic acid, and pyridoxal-5′-phosphate dependent epilepsies Glycine encephalopathy
	Intermittent encephalopathy	Urea cycle disorders Organic acidemias
	Tendon xanthomas	Cerebrotendinous xanthomatosis
	Primary/early ovarian insufficiency	Galactosaemia

Disorders of phospholipid and glycosphingolipid biosynthesis

Phospholipids are important components of cell membranes. Glycosphingolipids are also found in cell membranes, particularly in neurones. Recent advances in laboratory instrumentation and technology, and increased use of whole exome analysis, have allowed identification of an increasing number of disorders in this group. For the majority no specific treatment is available.

Disorders of phospholipid synthesis

Phosphatidate phosphatase 1 deficiency is caused by mutations in the *LIPN1* gene and characterised by episodes of recurrent myoglobinuria (precipitated by fever, anaesthesia or fasting) and muscle weakness.

Barth syndrome (cardiolipin remodelling enzyme deficiency) is an X-linked condition caused by mutations in the *TAZ* gene. Clinical presentation includes cardiomyopathy, skeletal muscle weakness, cyclical neutropenia and growth retardation.

Neurodegeneration with brain iron accumulation (NBIA) is characterised by static encephalopathy in childhood and neurodegeneration in adolescence or adulthood. It is caused by phospholipase A2 deficiency secondary to mutations in the *PLA2G6* gene. Other disorders such fatty acid 2-hydroxylase deficiency (*FA2H* mutations, a cause of SPG35) and pantothenate kinase-associated neurodegeneration (*PANK2* mutations) show overlapping clinical features.

Disorders of glycosphingolipid synthesis

Autosomal dominant serine palmitoyltransferase deficiency (*SPTLC1* or *SPTLC2* mutations) causes hereditary sensory autonomic neuropathy type 1. Mutilating ulcerative complications are a prominent sign.

Acute neurological emergencies caused by inherited metabolic disease

The majority of adults with a rare inherited disorder of metabolism who present to emergency services will have a known diagnosis, usually made in childhood. They may bring with them specific information and guidelines for emergency management of their condition. In the United Kingdom, nationally agreed guidelines are accessible via the internet (www.BIMDG.org.uk).

Other patients present for the first time in adulthood, and while, quite correctly, the emphasis in adulthood tends to be on acquired conditions such as infection or poisoning, the possibility of an late-presenting inherited disorder of metabolism should always be considered for adults with encephalopathy, atypical stroke, psychiatric features, rhabdomyolysis, and/or disturbances of acid–base balance – particularly if these episodes are recurrent and there is no other obvious underlying cause. Hypoglycaemia is an unusual initial presentation of inherited metabolic disease in adulthood. Because of compensatory mechanisms, adults can maintain their blood glucose levels despite significant metabolic disturbance so an adulthood presentation with hypoglycaemia often represents a late event secondary to severe decompensation (e.g. in fatty acid oxidation disorders or organic acidemias). Typically, acute episodes occur following metabolic 'stress' (e.g. fasting, intercurrent infection, major surgery, gastrointestinal illness, excessive alcohol or exercise), but a precise underlying precipitant is not always identified.

Table 19.27 summarises some of the more frequent acute presentations of adults with metabolic disease to emergency services, initial tests and potential treatments. A neurologist's advice is likely to be sought for many of these presentations and so it is important for all physicians to be aware of these disorders as effective treatments are available for many, and, as the disorders are genetic, making the diagnosis has implications both for the affected patient and their relatives. Not all diagnostic tests are readily available in the emergency setting, or even outside specialist laboratories, so thought should be given to the storage of appropriate samples, including DNA, in the acute setting, particularly for patients in a critical condition. Table 19.28 summarises the prominant clinical features of some inborn errors of metabolism.

References

Ahmed RM, Murphy E, Davagnanam I, Parton M, Schott JM, Mummery CJ, *et al.* A practical approach to diagnosing adult onset leukodystrophies. *J Neurol Neurosurg Psychiatry* 2014; **85:** 770–781. doi: 10.1136/jnnp-2013-305888.

Chauhan S, D'Cruz S, Singh R, Sachdev A. Mees' lines. *Lancet* 2008; **372:** 1410.

Cooke CA. An atypical presentation of Wernicke's encephalopathy in an 11-year-old child. *Eye* 2006; **20:** 1418–1420.

Jallul S, Osman A, El-Masry W. Cerebro-spinal decompression sickness: report of two cases. *Spinal Cord* 2007; **45:** 116–120.

Reed LJ, Lasserson D, Marsden P, Stanhope N, Stevens T, Bello F, *et al.* FDG-PET findings in the Wernicke–Korsakoff syndrome. *Cortex* 2003; **39:** 1027–1045.

Tsutsui RS. Lead poisoning from Ayurvedic medicines. *New Zealand Med J* 2013; **126:** 80–83.

Yang CS, Tsai WJ, Lirng JF. Ocular manifestations and MRI findings in a case of methanol poisoning. *Eye* 2005; **19:** 806–809.

Further reading

Toxins

Bradberry S, Vale A. Managegement of poisoning: antidotes. *Medicine* 2007; **35:** 562–565.

Charness ME, Simon RP, Greenberg DA. Ethanol and the nervous system. *N Engl J Med* 1989; **321**: 442–454.

Evison D, Hinsey D, Rice P. Chemical weapons. *Br Med J* 2002; **324**: 332–335.

Gradjean P, Landrigan PJ. Developmental neurotoxicity of industrial chemicals. *Lancet* 2006; **368**: 2167–2178.

Isbister GK, Kiernan MC. Neurotoxic marine poisoning. *Lancet Neurol* 2004; **4**: 219–228.

Kumar N. Industrial and environmental toxins. Continuum Lifelong learning. *Neurology* 2008; **14:** 102–137.

Mayo-Smith MF. Pharmacological management of alcohol withdrawal: a meta-analysis and evidence-based guideline. American Society of Addiction working group on pharmacological management of alcohol withdrawal. *JAMA* 1997; **278**: 144–151.

Roberts DM, Aaron CK. Managing acute organophosphorus pesticide poisoning. *Br Med J* 2007; **334**: 629–634.

Starr JM, Pattie A, Whiteman MC, Deary IJ, Whalley LJ. Vitamin B-12, serum folate, and cognitive change between 11 and 79 years. *J Neurol Neurosurg Psychiatry* 2005; **76**: 291–292.

Victor M, Adams RD, Collins GH. *The Wernicke–Korsakoff Syndrome and Related Neurologic Disorders due to Alcoholism and Malnutrition.* Philadelphia: F.A. Davis, 1989.

Victor M, Ropper A. *Principles of Neurology*. New York: McGraw-Hill, 2001.

Ward PC. Modern approaches to the investigation of vitamin B_{12} deficiency. *Clin Lab Med* 2002; **51**: 435–445.

Warrell DA. Treatment of bites by adders and exotic venomous snakes. *Br Med J* 2005; **331**: 1244–1247.

Warrell DA. Venomous animals. *Medicine* 2012; **40:** 159–163.

Metabolic disorders

Chatterjee A, Yapundich R, Palmer CA, Marson DC, Mitchell GW. Leukoencephalopathy associated with cobalamin deficiency. *Neurology* 1996; **46**: 832–834.

Dhar M, Bellevue R, Carmel R. Pernicious anemia with neuropsychiatric dysfunction in a patient with sickle cell anemia treated with folate supplementation. *N Engl J Med* 2003; **348**: 2204–2207.

Green R, Kinsella LJ. Current concepts in the diagnosis of cobalamin deficiency. *Neurology* 1995; **45**: 1435–1440.

Hemmer B, Glocker FX, Schumacher M, Deuschl G, Lücking CH. Subacute combined degeneration: clinical, electrophysiological and magnetic resonance imaging findings. *J Neurol Neurosurg Psychiatry* 1998; **65**: 822–827.

Lindenbaum J, Healton EB, Savage DG, *et al.* Neuropsychiatric disorders caused by cobalamin deficiency in the absence of anemia or macrocytosis. *N Engl J Med* 1988; **318**: 1720–1728.

Martin RJ. Central pontine and extra-pontine myelinolysis: the osmotic demyelination syndromes. *J Neurol Neurosurg Psychiatry* 2004; **75** (Suppl III): 22–28.

Menger H, Jorg J. Outcome of central pontine and extrapontine myeliolysis. *J Neurol* 1999; **246**: 700–705.

Pruthi RK, Tefferi A. Pernicious anemia revisited. *Mayo Clin Proc* 1994; **69**: 144–150.

Physical insults

Clarke, C. Acute mountain sickness: medical problems associated with acute and subacute exposure to hypobaric hypoxia. *Postgrad Med J* 2006; **82**: 748–753.

Drugs of abuse

Enevoldson TP. Recreational drugs and their neurological consequences. *J Neurol Neurosurg Psychiatry* 2004; **75** (Suppl III): 9–15.

Levine SR, Brust JCM, Futrell N, *et al.* Cerebrovascular complications of the use of the 'crack' form of alkaloidal cocaine. *N Engl J Med* 1990; **323**: 699–704.

Vale A. Substance abuse: routes, hazards and body packing. *Medicine* 2007; **35:** 570–572.

Inborn errors of metabolism

Ahmed RM, Murphy E, Davagnanam I, Parton M, Schott JM, Mummery CJ, *et al.* A practical approach to diagnosing adult onset leukodystrophies. *J Neurol Neurosurg Psychiatry* 2014; **85:** 770–781. doi: 10.1136/jnnp-2013-305888.

Aylett SB, Neergheen V, Hargreaves IP, Eaton S, Land JM, Rahman S, *et al.* Levels of 5-methyltetrahydrofolate and ascorbic acid in cerebrospinal fluid arecorrelated: Implications for the accelerated degradation of folate by reactive oxygen species. *Neurochem Int* 2013; **63:** 750–755.

Bosch AM. Classical galactosaemia revisited. *J Inherit Metab Dis* 2006; **29:** 516–525.

Brady RO. Enzyme replacement for lysosomal diseases. *Annu Rev Med* 2006; **57:** 283–296.

Carecchio M, Schneider SA, Chan H, Lachmann R, Lee PJ, Murphy E, *et al.* Movement disorders in adult surviving patients with maple syrup urine disease. *Mov Disord* 2011; **26:** 1324–1328.

Channon S, Goodman G, Zlotowitz S, *et al.* Effects of dietary management of phenylketonuria on long-term cognitive outcome. *Arch Dis Child* 2007; **92:** 213–218.

Chavany C, Jendoubi M. Biology and potential strategies for the treatment of GM2 gangliosidoses. *Mol Med Today* 1998; **4:** 158–165.

Costello DJ, Eichler AF, Eichler FS. Leukodystrophies: classification, diagnosis and treatment. *Neurologist* 2009; **15:** 319–328.

Cox TM. Gaucher disease: understanding the molecular pathogenesis of sphingolipidoses. *J Inherit Metab Dis* 2001; **24** (Suppl 2): 106–121; discussion 87–88.

Dawson C, Murphy E, Maritz C, Chan H, Ellerton C, Carpenter RH, *et al.* Dietary treatment of phenylketonuria: the effect of phenylalanine on reaction time. *J Inherit Metab Dis* 2011; **34:** 449–454.

Desnick RJ, Ioannou YA, Eng CM. Alpha-galactosidase A deficiency: Fabry disease. In: *The Metabolic and Molecular Bases of Inherited Disease*, 8th edn., vol. **3**. Scriver CR, Beaudet AL, Sly WS, *et al.* eds. McGraw-Hill, 2001: 3733–3774.

Escolar ML, Poe MD, Provenzale JM, *et al.* Transplantation of umbilical-cord blood in babies with infantile Krabbe's disease. *N Engl J Med* 2005; **352**: 2069–2081.

Fellgiebel A, Muller MJ, Ginsberg L. CNS manifestations of Fabry's disease. *Lancet Neurol* 2006; **5**: 791–795.

Gilkes CE, Love S, Hardie RJ, *et al.* Brain biopsy in benign neurological disease. *J Neurol* 2012; **259:** 995–1000.

Hendriksz CJ, Corry PC, Wraith JE, *et al.* Juvenile Sandhoff disease: nine new cases and a review of the literature. *J Inherit Metab Dis* 2004; **27**: 241–249.

Imrie J, Dasgupta S, Besley GT, *et al.* The natural history of Niemann–Pick disease type C in the UK. *J Inherit Metab Dis* 2007; **30**: 51–59.

Kaplan F. Tay-Sachs disease carrier screening: a model for prevention of genetic disease. *Genet Test* 1998; **2**: 271–292.

Kaufman FR, McBride-Chang C, Manis FR, *et al.* Cognitive functioning, neurologic status and brain imaging in classical galactosemia. *Eur J Pediatr* 1995; **154** (Suppl 2): S2–S5.

Kurian MA, Gissen P, Smith M, Heales S J, Clayton PT. The monoamine neurotransmitter disorders: an expanding range of neurological syndromes. *Lancet Neurol* 2011; **10**: 721–733.

Lamari F, Mochel F, Sedel F, Saudubray JM. Disorders of phospholipids, sphingolipids and fatty acids biosynthesis: toward a new category of inherited metabolic diseases. *J Inherit Metab Dis* 2013; **36:** 411–425. doi: 10.1007/s10545-012-9509-7. Review.

Leuzzi V, Tosetti M, Montanaro D, *et al.* The pathogenesis of the white matter abnormalities in phenylketonuria: a multimodal 3.0 tesla MRI and magnetic resonance spectroscopy (1H MRS) study. *J Inherit Metab Dis* 2007, **30**. 209–216.

Lyon G, Kolodny EH, Pastores GM. *Neurology of Heriditary Metabolic Diseases of Children*, 3rd edn. McGraw-Hill, 2006.

Maegawa GH, Stockley T, Tropak M, *et al.* The natural history of juvenile or subacute GM2 gangliosidosis: 21 new cases and literature review of 134 previously reported. *Pediatrics* 2006; **118**: e1550–1562.

Maria BL, Deidrick KM, Moser H, *et al.* Leukodystrophies: pathogenesis, diagnosis, strategies, therapies, and future research directions. *J Clin Neurol* 2003; **15:** 319–328.

Moser HW, Mahmood A, Raymond GVC. X linked adrenoleukodystrophy. *Nat Clin Pract Neurol* 2007; **3:** 140–151.

Moser HW. Adrenoleukodystrophy: phenotype, genetics, pathogenesis and therapy. *Brain* 1997; **120:** 1485–1508.

Oldfors A, DiMauro S. New insights in the field of muscle glycogenoses. *Curr Opin Neurol* 2013; **26:** 544–553. doi: 10.1097/WCO.0b013e328364dbdc.

Renaud DL. Clinical approach to leukoencephalopathies. *Semin Neurol* 2012; **32:** 29–33.

Rubio-Agusti I, Carecchio M, Bhatia KP, Kojovic M, Parees I, Chandrashekar HS, *et al.* Movement disorders in adult patients with classical galactosemia. *Mov Disord* 2013; **28:** 804–810.

Schiffmann R, van der Knapp MS. An MRI based approach to the diagnosis of white matter disorders. *Neurology* 2009; **72:** 750–759.

Schott JM, Reineiger L, Thom M, *et al.* Brain biopsy in dementia: clinical indications and diagnostic approach. *Acta Neuropathol* 2010; **120:** 327–341.

Scriver CR, Kaufman S. Hyperphenylalaninaemia: phenylalanine hydroxylase deficiency. In: Scriver CR, Beaudet AL, Sly WS, *et al.* eds. *The Metabolic and Molecular Bases of Inherited Disease*, 8th edn., vol. **2**. McGraw-Hill, 2001: 1667–1724.

Sedel F, Saudubray JM, Roze E, Agid Y, Vidailhet M. Movement disorders and inborn errors of metabolism in adults: a diagnostic approach. *J Inherit Metab Dis* 2008; **31:** 308–318. doi: 10.1007/s10545-008-0854-5. Review.

Sevin C, Aubourg P, Cartier N. Enzyme, cell and gene-based therapies for metachromatic leukodystrophy. *J Inherit Metab Dis* 2007; **30**: 175–183.

Sevin M, Lesca G, Baumann N, *et al.* The adult form of Niemann–Pick disease type C. *Brain* 2007; **130**: 120–133.

Sidransky E. Gaucher disease: complexity in a 'simple' disorder. *Mol Genet Metab* 2004; **83**: 6–15.

Van der Knapp MS, Valk J, eds. *Magnetic Resonance of Myelination and Myelin Disorders*, 3rd edition. Berlin: Springer; 2005.

Verrips A, Hoefsloot LH, Steenbergen GC, *et al.* Clinical and molecular genetic characteristics of patients with cerebrotendinous xanthomatosis. *Brain* 2000; **123:** 908–919.

Wyatt K, Henley W, Anderson L, Anderson R, Nikolaou V, Stein K, *et al.* The effectiveness and cost-effectiveness of enzyme and substrate replacement therapies: a longitudinal cohort study of people with lysosomal storage disorders. *Health Technol Assess* 2012; **16:** 1–543. doi: 10.3310/hta16390.

Yahalom G, Tsabari R, Molshatzki N, *et al.* Neurological outcome in cerebrotendinous xanthomatosis treated with chenodeoxycholic acid: early versus late diagnosis. *Clin Neuropharmacol* 2013; **36:** 78–83.

CHAPTER 20

Disorders of Consciousness, Intensive Care Neurology and Sleep

Robin Howard[1], Sofia Eriksson[1], Nicholas Hirsch[1], Neil Kitchen[1], Dimitri Kullmann[2], Christopher Taylor[1] and Matthew Walker[2]

[1] National Hospital for Neurology & Neurosurgery

[2] UCL Institute of Neurology

Consciousness

Consciousness is a state of awareness of self and environment that gives significance to stimuli from the internal and external environment. It depends on two critical components: arousal or alertness; and cognitive content of mental functions which allow expression of sensation, emotion and thought.

Arousal reflects the integrity of the ascending reticular activating system and the brainstem, predominantly bilateral tegmental regions of the upper pons and, to a lesser extent, the midbrain while cognitive function is subserved by the cerebral hemispheres. Coma can be caused either by bilateral hemispheric damage, or by a structural or metabolic lesion affecting the brainstem reticular activating system or its projections to the thalamus and cortex. Impairment of arousal leads to a reduced level of consciousness with secondary impairment of cognitive content, which may be temporary or permanent depending on the aetiology. Unilateral dysfunction or disease of the cerebral hemispheres does not, by itself, cause stupor or coma.

States of impaired consciousness

The different patterns of arousal and awareness are complex and variable, but characteristic features do allow the description of a spectrum of states of conscious level. These range from full consciousness to coma. A number of terms have been applied to these intermediate states but overlap inevitably occurs (Table 20.1).

In the 'locked-in syndrome' consciousness and cognition are preserved. The condition is discussed here because it commonly presents diagnostic difficulties as the patient has lost motor function making movement and speech impossible. Horizontal eye movements are lost and the subject is usually only able to communicate by opening and voluntarily moving their eyes in the vertical plane.

Causes of coma

Coma is caused by a large number of neurological and general medical disorders. In clinical practice a useful scheme depends on identifying the following findings in the initial assessment of the patient (Table 20.2):

1. Lateralising signs
2. Meningism
3. Pattern of brainstem reflexes.

Initial assessment and management of coma

Acute initial management is summarised in Table 20.3. The clinical assessment of coma is summarised in Table 20.4.

Medical assessment

It is essential to obtain as detailed and accurate a history as possible from all witnesses and to establish any history of a predisposing event (e.g. previous trauma), pyrexia, prodromal symptoms (e.g. headache, neck stiffness), ataxia, epilepsy or previous episodes as well as medication list and psychiatric history.

Examination

An urgent and detailed general medical examination must be undertaken immediately after resuscitation. The breath may smell of alcohol, ketones, hepatic or renal fetor. Examination of the mucous membranes may show evidence of cyanosis, anaemia, jaundice or carbon monoxide intoxication. Bruising in the mastoid or orbital regions or blood in the external auditory meatus may suggest temporal, orbital or basal skull fractures. Endocarditis is suggested by splinter haemorrhages, and opiate intoxication by hypodermic needle marks. Other relevant skin lesions include a purpuric petechial rash suggesting meningococcal septicaemia or a coagulation disorder, maculopapular lesions indicating viral meningo-encephalitis, endocarditis or fungal infection, or bullous lesions suggesting barbiturate intoxication.

Pyrexia is usually caused by systemic sepsis but its absence does not exclude infection, particularly in elderly or immunocompromised patients. Hyperpyrexia occurs in thyrotoxic crisis, heat stroke, drug toxicity (e.g. Ecstacy) and malignant hyperthermia. Primary neurogenic hyperpyrexia is unusual but can be associated with hypothalamic lesions or subarachnoid haemorrhage (SAH). Rarely, severe hypothermia may be the primary cause of coma, but more commonly hypothermia occurs as a result of coma from environmental (accidental hypothermia) or metabolic causes, endocrine disorders (hypothyroidism, hypopituitarism or hypoadrenalism) or drugs (e.g. alcohol, barbiturates). Profuse sweating suggests cholinergic poisoning, neuroleptic malignant syndrome or serotonin syndrome.

Hypertensive crisis leads to disturbed consciousness, but hypertension is more commonly secondary to cerebral causes such as

Neurology: A Queen Square Textbook, Second Edition. Edited by Charles Clarke, Robin Howard, Martin Rossor and Simon Shorvon.

Table 20.1 Definitions and descriptions of states of altered consciousness.

Clouding of consciousness	Reduced alertness characterised by impaired attention and memory. Patients may be distractible, hyperexcitable and irritable, with slow thought processes
Acute confusional state	Impaired alertness state in which stimuli are intermittently misinterpreted. Patients are drowsy, bewildered and disorientated in time sometimes with day–night reversal. They have poor short-term memory and comprehension and difficulty undertaking complex tasks
Delirium	Rapid onset of a floridly abnormal mental state, with disturbed consciousness, disorientation, severe motor restlessness, fear, irritability, consistent misperception of sensory stimuli and visual hallucinations. There may be lucid periods with hyperactivity during which the patient is agitated, talkative and irritable. There may be hypoactive periods with hypersomnolence and sleep–wake inversion
Obtundation	Mental blunting with apathy and inactivity. The patient is drowsy with reduced alertness and a lessened interest in the environment
Stupor	Similar to deep sleep, from which the patient can be aroused only by vigorous and repeated stimuli. Even when aroused communication is by monosyllabic sounds and simple behaviours, and as soon as the stimulus ceases the stuporose subject lapses back into an unresponsive state
Akinetic mutism	Slowed or virtually absent bodily movements in the absence of paralysis or weakness. The patient is flaccid, does not respond to pain and lies immobile, mute and unresponsive to commands, questions and greetings. Wakefulness, alertness, sleep–wake cycles and self-awareness are preserved
Coma	A state of unrousable unresponsiveness in which the subject lies with eyes closed. There is no understandable response to external stimuli or inner need and the patient does not utter understandable responses nor accurately localises noxious stimuli. Thus, there is a total absence of awareness of self and environment even when the subject is externally stimulated. There is no spontaneous eye opening, response to voice, localisation to painful stimuli or verbal output

Table 20.2 (a) Causes of coma with intact brainstem function, without meningism and without lateralising signs.

Alcohol	
Drugs	All sedatives, anaesthetics and many drugs (e.g. barbiturates, tranquillisers, opioids, psychotropics, salicylates, amphetamines)
Seizures, epilepsy	Convulsive status epilepticus, non-convulsive status epilepticus, post-ictal, non-epileptic status
Hypoxic–ischaemic encephalopathy	
Respiratory	Hypoxaemia, hypercarbia
Electrolyte disturbances	Hyponatraemia, hypernatraemia; hypocalcaemia, hypercalcaemia, hypermagnesaemia
Diabetes mellitus	Hypoglycaemia, ketoacidosis, lactic acidosis, hyperosmolar non-ketotic diabetic coma
Uraemia/dialysis	
Hepatic encephalopathy	
Endocrine	Panhypopituitarism, hypothyroidism, hyperthyroidism, hypoadrenalism, Hashimoto's encephalopathy
Core temperature change	Hypothermia, hyperpyrexia
Nutritional	Wernicke's encephalopathy
Inborn errors of metabolism	Hyperammoniacal states, aminoacidurias, organic acidurias
Toxins	Carbon monoxide, methanol, lead, cyanide, thallium, others
Extrapyramidal	Acute movement disorders (status dystonicus), neuroleptic malignant syndrome, serotonin syndrome
Autoimmune	Steroid responsive encephalopathy, autoimmune encephalitis
Others	e.g. porphyria, Reye's syndrome (hepatic), idiopathic recurrent stupor, mitochondrial disease, hypothalamic lesions, septic encephalopathy, malaria
States that mimic coma	Catatonia, conversion reaction, malingering, psychogenic unresponsiveness

SAH and raised intracranial pressure (ICP). Hypotension resulting in coma may be caused by hypovolaemia, myocardial infarction, septicaemia, diabetes mellitus or deliberate overdose with hypotensive medication.

The presence of meningism suggests infective or carcinomatous meningitis, SAH or herniation (either central, tentorial or cerebellar tonsillar). Meningism is rarely found in patients in deep coma and can be difficult to assess in those who have had tracheal intubation. The pattern of respiration is of some localising value (see Bulbar function), but is also affected by cerebral herniation syndromes, metabolic and toxic conditions including drug overdose, acidosis, diabetes and liver disease.

Fundal examination can show retinopathy due to diabetes or hypertension. Papilloedema suggests raised ICP, hypertensive retinopathy or carbon dioxide retention and subhyaloid haemorrhage indicates aneurysmal SAH (Figure 20.1). Otoscopic examination may reveal otorrhoea or haemotympanum from a basal skull fracture. Cerebrospinal fluid (CSF) rhinorrhoea can be confirmed by the presence of glucose in a watery nasal discharge but testing for 'beta-trace protein' is more specific.

Table 20.2 (b) Typical causes of coma with meningism, with or without brainstem signs and with or without lateralising signs.

Infection	Meningitis, encephalitis, malaria, HIV-related
Vascular	Subarachnoid haemorrhage (spontaneous or traumatic)
Tumour	Malignant meningitis

Table 20.2 (c) Typical causes of coma with intact brainstem function and asymmetrical lateralising signs with or without meningism.

Cerebrovascular
Infarction
Ischaemia
Embolic – cardiac, large vessel, fat
Hypoperfusion/hypotension
Haemorrhage
Extradural
Subdural
Subarachnoid
Intracerebral (primary or secondary)
Congophilic amyloid angiopathy
Intravascular lymphoma
Vasculitis
Venous thrombosis
Mitochondrial disease
Hypertensive encephalopathy
Eclampsia
Endocarditis
Bacterial, Libman–Sacks, marantic
Traumatic brain injury
Cerebral oedema
Infection
Brain abscess and tuberculoma, single or multiple
Subdural empyema
Creutzfeldt–Jakob disease
Malaria, HIV-related
Encephalitis
Inflammatory
Posterior reversible leukoencephalopathy
Brain neoplasms
White matter diseases
Multiple sclerosis
Leukoencephalopathy associated with chemotherapy and/or radiotherapy
Acute disseminated encephalomyelitis
Acute haemorrhagic leukoencephalitis
Posterior reversible leukoencephalopathy
Toxic leukoencephalopathy
Progressive multifocal leukoencephalopathy

Table 20.2 (d) Causes of coma with intact brainstem function and symmetrical lateralising signs with or without meningism (and see Table 20.2c).

Diffuse axonal (traumatic) brain injury
Hypoxic–ischaemic brain injury
Bilateral subdural haematoma/empyema
Cerebrovascular
Subarachnoid haemorrhage
Multiple infarcts due to:
Fat emboli
Cholesterol emboli
Disseminated intravascular coagulation
Thrombotic thrombocytopenic purpura
Vasculitis
Tumour
Multiple metastases
Gliomatosis
Lymphoma
Demyelination
Acute disseminated encephalomyelitis
Acute haemorrhagic leukoencephalitis
Infection
Encephalitis

Table 20.2 (e) Causes of coma with signs of focal brainstem dysfunction (with or without meningism, with or without lateralising signs).

Herniation syndromes
Intrinsic brainstem disease
Advanced metabolic/toxic encephalopathy
Others
Central pontine myelinolysis
Multiple sclerosis
Brainstem encephalitis
Vascular
Vertebrobasilar occlusion, dissection, haemorrhage, AVMs
Basilar artery and brainstem infarction
Mass lesions affecting brainstem or cerebellum
Posterior fossa tumours
Abscesses, tuberculomas
Traumatic brain injury
Cerebellar
Cerebellar infarct, haematoma, abscess, glioma

AVM, arteriovenous malformation.

Level of consciousness

The level of consciousness should be assessed by the ability of the patient to respond to stimuli of varying intensity by speech, eye opening and motor movements. Because of the importance of correctly identifying locked-in patients, the eyelids should be held open and the patient asked to move their eyes in a horizontal and

Table 20.3 The acute management of coma.

Cardiopulmonary resuscitation
Oxygenation (face mask 40% oxygen. Aim for O_2 saturation >95%)
Tracheal intubation to ensure adequate oxygenation and secure airway
Mechanical ventilation where indicated by desaturation, irregular breathing pattern, pooling of secretions or facial injury
Adequate intravenous access
Maintain blood pressure
Fluids (crystalloids – rapid infusion of 500–1000 mL normal saline followed by 150 mL/hr)
Vasopressor agents
Extreme hypertension (systolic BP >250 mmHg, MAP >130 mmHg)
Labetolol 10 mg IV
Hydralazine 10 mg IV
Maintain core temperature
Hypothermia – warming blanket
Hyperpyrexia – cooling blanket, ice pack, ice water levage
Glucose
If hypoglycaemic give glucose 50%, 50 ml IV
Thiamine
100 mg IV
Naloxone
0.4–2 mg every 3 min IV
Flumazenil
Slow infusion of 0.2 mg/min (<5 mg) to reverse benzodiazepine toxicity
Correct electrolyte and acid – base disturbance
Hyponatraemia – 3% hypertonic saline and furosemide after placement of CVP monitor
Hypercalcaemia – saline rehydration
Elimination of toxins
Haemodialysis and/or haemofiltration
Acute treatment of seizures
Raised intracranial pressure
Hydrocephalus – ventriculostomy
Evacuation of mass
Decompressive craniectomy
Osmotic agents – mannitol 1–2 g/kg IV, 2 repeated doses 30–40 mins apart
Infection
Broad-spectrum antibiotic if suspicion of meningitis
Aciclovir or dexamethasone (see text)
Further acute management of the unconscious patient
Includes adequate treatment of seizures
Correction of electrolyte and acid–base disturbances
Supportive treatment including adequate nutrition, nursing and physiotherapy

CVP, central venous pressure; MAP, mean arterial blood pressure.

Table 20.4 The comatose patient: immediate actions and assessment.

1	Resuscitation and emergency treatment
2	Medical assessment
3	Establish level of consciousness (e.g. Glasgow Coma Scale)
	Eye opening
	Motor responses
	Verbal output
4	Identify brainstem activity/brainstem reflexes
	Pupils
	Eye movements
	• Spontaneous
	• Oculocephalic
	• Oculovestibular
	Corneal reflexes and facial movements
	Bulbar
	• Cough
	• Gag
	Respiratory pattern
5	Motor function
	Involuntary movements
	Seizures
	Muscle tone
	Motor responses
	Tendon reflexes
	Plantar responses

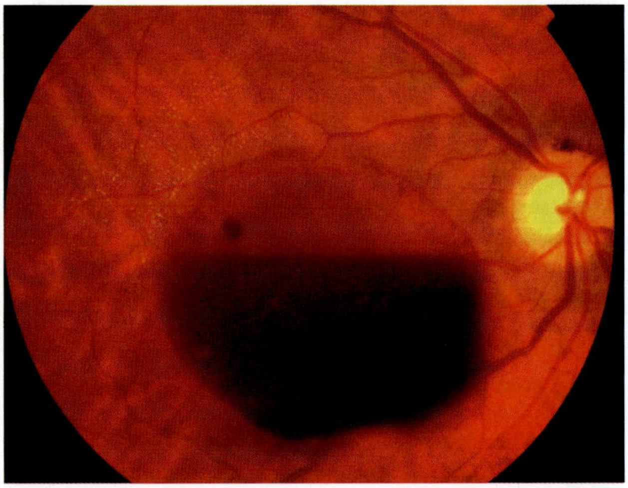

Figure 20.1 Subhyaloid hyaemorrhage in a patient with subarachnoid haemorrhage.

vertical plane. Visual, auditory and painful stimuli of increasing intensity can then be systematically presented bilaterally in cranial nerve and limb territories.

Glasgow Coma Scale

The Glasgow Coma Score (GCS) is the most widely used and reproducible scale to assess the level of consciousness. It is a standard scoring system used for the assessment of the unconscious patient based on their eye opening, motor and verbal responses to external stimuli (Table 20.5). It was designed as an easily used, objective, reproducible scale for patients with head trauma, to assess varying levels of consciousness facilitating the early recognition of deterioration resulting from raised ICP, usually from herniation. It has proved an extremely

Table 20.5 Glasgow Coma Score (GCS).

Eye opening	Motor response	Verbal
4 Spontaneous	6 Obeys command	5 Orientated
3 To speech	5 Localises pain	4 Confused speech
2 To pain	4 Withdrawal	3 Inappropriate words
1 None	3 Flexion posturing	2 Incomprehensible sounds
	2 Extensor posturing	1 None
	1 None	

valuable and durable scale which can be used by medical, nursing and paramedical staff. It requires regular and serial observations.

However, there are several limitations to its use. The scale excludes assessment of many important neurological functions, requires regular and consecutive observations to be effective, and is limited to the best response in a single limb. It therefore cannot represent asymmetry and has poor diagnostic value. Its inter-rater reliability in non-experienced observers is limited because it is difficult to standardise the intensity of maximal auditory, visual and painful stimuli; full assessment cannot be undertaken in intubated patients or when soft tissue swelling prevents eye opening. Furthermore, the scale represents the addition of ordinal values that are not equal and are not independent of each other and it is relatively insensitive to changes in the level of consciousness at higher levels. Although the GCS score is helpful when assessing any change in the level of consciousness, particularly in the context of traumatic brain injury (TBI), it cannot replace detailed and careful neurological examination of the pattern of responsiveness.

Several new scores have been developed. The best is the Full Outline of UnResponsiveness (FOUR) introduced in 2005 to overcome many of the difficulties inherent in the GCS (Table 20.6). Instead of the verbal component, the FOUR score includes pupil reactions and respiratory pattern to reflect brainstem function, thus making it more applicable in the intubated patient. The score provides greater neurological detail than the GCS and it has good inter-observer reliability.

Assessment of neurological function

Eyelids In coma the eyelids are usually closed. Opening by an examiner is followed by slow spontaneous re-closure while, in psychogenic coma, there is usually forceful resistance to eyelid opening and active closure. Rarely, the eyelids may be open in coma ('eyes open coma') because of a failure of inhibition of levator palpebrae associated with lesions in the ponto-mesencephalic region. In this situation, it is difficult to distinguish coma from the vegetative state.

Pupillary responses It is essential to ensure an adequate light source and, if necessary, to examine the pupils with a magnifying glass. Pre-existing ocular or neurological injury, or topical or systemic medication, may cause pupillary asymmetry or even a fixed dilated pupil (Chapter 14).

The pupillary response indicates the functional state of the afferent (II) and efferent (III) pathways and the midbrain tegmentum. The presence of equal, light-reactive pupils indicates that the reflex pathway is intact. A normal pupillary reaction to light in a comatose patient suggests a metabolic rather than structural cause of coma. Unilateral or bilaterally small pupils with normal reactions to light may be caused by Horner's syndrome associated with lesions involving the descending sympathetic pathways in the hypothalamus, midbrain, pontine tegmentum, medulla (e.g. lateral medullary infarction), ventrolateral cervical spine or in the carotid sheath (e.g. carotid artery damage). The extent of constriction makes it difficult to observe responses to light and magnification may be required.

Mid position pupils, which do not respond to light but in which the accommodation reflex is spared, are associated with dorsal tectal, pretectal or tegmental lesions (Argyll Robertson pupils). The pupils may spontaneously and rhythmically fluctuate in size (hippus) and dilate to the ciliospinal reflex. This is a normal phenomenon.

In progressive compressive IIIrd nerve lesions, the initial sign is a sluggish pupillary response followed by the development of fixed dilatation (caused by involvement of the parasympathetic fibres with sparing of the sympathetic pathways). A unilateral IIIrd nerve lesion may also cause an efferent pupillary defect in which a light stimulus elicits a consensual but not a direct constriction response. This can be a sign of impending tentorial coning and is a medical emergency. Widely dilated pupils caused by anticholinergic agents do not reverse with pilocarpine. Irregular oval, unequal pupils follow brainstem transtentorial herniation which leads to midbrain infarction. Fixed and moderately dilated pupils are seen in brain death because of the loss of both sympathetic and parasympathetic influences.

Oculomotor disorders The preservation of normal eye movements means the brainstem is intact – from the oculomotor nucleus rostrally to the vestibular nuclei caudally, and their cerebellar connections (Chapter 14). In the primary ocular position, the eyes may be either dysconjugate, conjugate in the midline or deviated in a conjugate manner. Dysconjugate deviation of the eyes is common in patients with impaired consciousness and often reflects loss of descending voluntary control but may simply be caused by decompensation of a pre-existing strabismus or a cranial nerve palsy.

A complete IIIrd nerve palsy is manifest as pupillary dilatation, ptosis and deviation of the eye downward and laterally. Oculomotor nerve palsies may occur as a consequence of midbrain lesions from direct trauma or as a manifestation of transtentorial herniation but have many other causes (Chapter 14). Internuclear ophthalmoplegia (INO), caused by a lesion of the medial longitudinal fasciculus, causes isolated failure of ocular adduction with nystagmus of the abducting eye but normal vertical eye movements and pupils. Dysconjugate vertical gaze may be caused by IVth nerve palsy (which occurs commonly following trauma, metabolic encephalopathy or drug intoxication) or is caused by a skew deviation associated with otolithic, cerebellar or brainstem lesions. Inward deviation and failure of abduction indicates a VIth nerve palsy which is common and may be caused by trauma or raised ICP but is a poor guide to localisation.

Tonic horizontal conjugate ocular deviation is common in coma. The eyes usually deviate towards the side of a destructive hemispheric lesion (e.g. infarction, haemorrhage or tumour) and away from the hemiparesis. However, the eyes may deviate away from an irritative epileptic focus or from a thalamic lesion. Below the ponto-mesencephalic junction the eyes deviate away from the lesion side, and look towards the hemiparesis (pontine gaze palsy). In hemispheric lesions it is usually possible to drive the eyes across the midline with a vestibular stimulus but this is not true for brainstem gaze palsies. Seizure activity may cause intermittent aversive horizontal deviation although the eyes may deviate to the side of the focus in post-ictal gaze palsy. Tonic downward deviation of the eyes is

Table 20.6 FOUR score (Full Outline of UnResponsiveness).

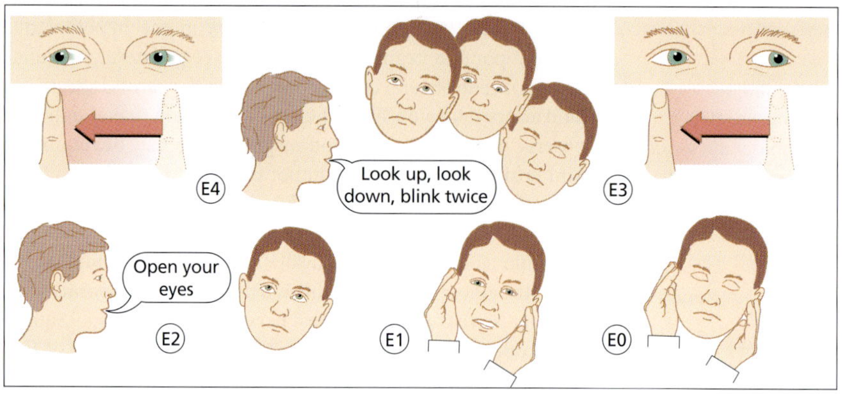

Eye response

4. Eyelids open or opened, tracking or blinking to command
3. Eyelids open but not tracking
2. Eyelids closed but open to a loud voice
1. Eyelids closed but open to pain
0. Eyelids remain closed with pain

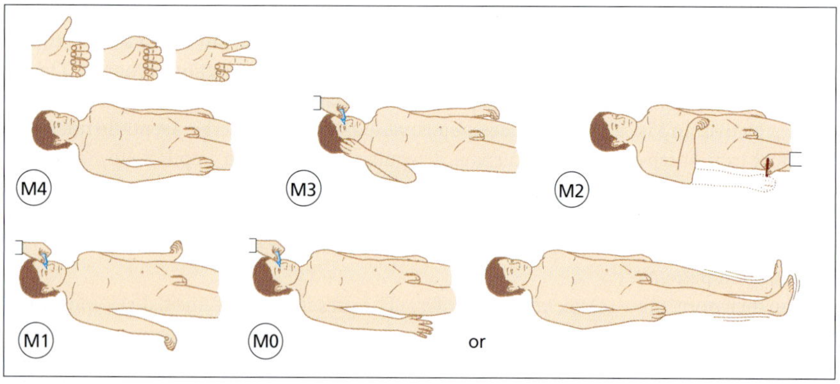

Motor response

4. Thumbs up, fist or peace sign to command
3. Localising to pain
2. Flexion response to pain
1. Extensor posturing
0. No response to pain or generalised myoclonic status epilepticus

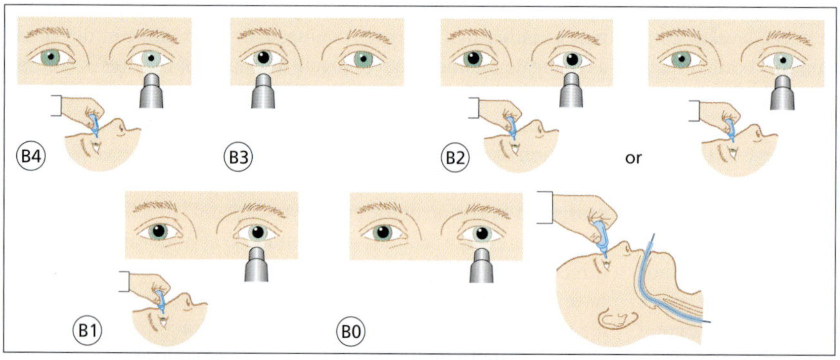

Brain stem reflexes

4. Pupil and corneal reflexes present
3. One pupil wide and fixed
2. Pupil *or* corneal reflexes absent
1. Pupil *and* reflexes absent
0. Absent pupil, corneal and cough reflex

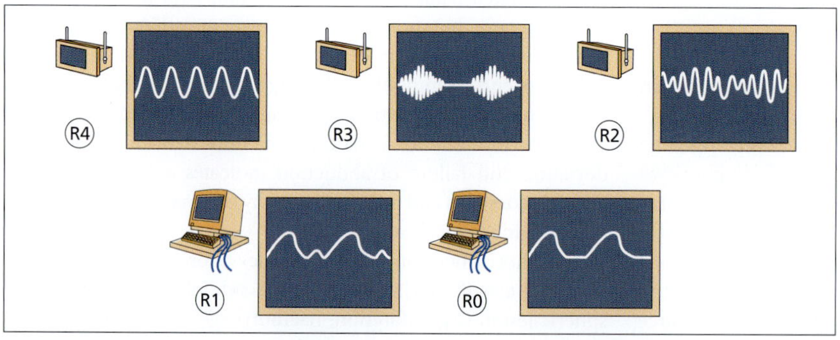

Respiration

4. Not intubated, regular breathing pattern
3. Not intubated, Cheyne–Stokes breathing pattern
2. Not intubated, irregular breathing pattern
1. Breaths above ventilator rate
0. Breaths at ventilator rate or apnoea

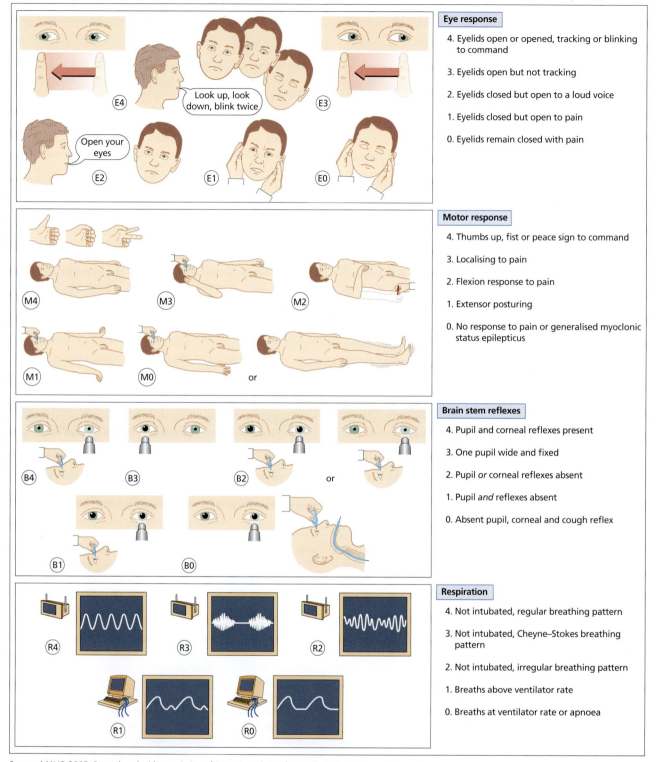

Source: MAYO 2005. Reproduced with permission of Mayo Foundation for Medical Education and Research.

associated with tectal compression caused by thalamic or dorsal midbrain lesions (usually haemorrhagic) but can be seen in metabolic coma or rarely in pseudocoma. Prolonged tonic upward deviation occurs as a consequence of extensive hypoxic–ischaemic damage but may occur transiently in seizures or in oculogyric crises caused by encephalitis lethargica or neuroleptic medication.

Horizontal nystagmus occurring in comatose patients suggests an irritative or a supratentorial aversive epileptic focus, usually associated with other motor manifestations of seizures including movements of the eyelids, face, jaw or tongue. Intermittent unilateral nystagmoid jerks in a horizontal or rotatory fashion indicate mid or lower pontine damage. Parinaud's syndrome (dorsal midbrain syndrome) is characterised by loss of upgaze, light-near dissociation of pupillary responses, convergence-retraction nystagmus and eyelid retraction (Collier's sign). There may also be accommodation or convergence spasm, associated oculomotor palsy (III, IV), skew deviation or internuclear ophthalmoplegia. It is associated with direct compressive lesions in the dorsal midbrain including pineal tumours, obstructive hydrocephalus, mesencephalic haemorrhage, arteriovenous malformation, trauma or multiple sclerosis (MS).

Spontaneous eye movements Spontaneous roving eye movements are intermittent slow random purposeless lateral movements, either conjugate or dysconjugate. Roving eye movements imply intact oculomotor brainstem pathways and indicates light coma, typically resulting from metabolic or toxic causes. Periodic alternating gaze disturbance is characterised by a slow cycle of horizontal gaze deviation in which the eyes are deviated for several minutes before moving to the opposite lateral gaze. This occurs in metabolic coma, particularly hepatic encephalopathy, but can also occur with bilateral hemispheric infarction or diffuse brain injury. Conjugate vertical eye movements are separated into different types according to the relative velocities of the downward and upward phases (Table 20.7). Vertical nystagmus differs from ocular bobbing and dipping because there is no latency between the corrective saccade and the next slow deviation. In the primary position there is a slow downward drift followed by a rapid correcting saccade.

Vestibulo-ocular reflexes Vestibulo-ocular reflexes are the involuntary ocular movements that occur after stimulation of the vestibular apparatus, and can be tested either by mechanical rotation of the head (oculo-cephalic) or caloric irrigation (oculo-vestibular). The oculo-cephalic reflex is tested by sudden passive rotation of the head in either lateral direction, or flexion and extension of the neck, while observing the motion of the eyes (Table 20.8). The manoeuvre should not be performed on any patient in whom cervical instability is suspected. If supranuclear influences are absent the eyes will normally remain fixed in space (i.e. continue to look forward).

Incomplete abduction suggests a VIth nerve palsy while impaired adduction suggests a IIIrd nerve palsy or an INO. Reduced or absent oculo-vestibular reflexes indicate severe intrinsic brainstem impairment. They are tested by irrigation of the tympanic membrane with cold or warm water (30°C or 44°C, respectively). In the awake subject, cold water causes a slow conjugate deviation of the eyes towards

Table 20.7 Involuntary vertical eye movements in coma.

Ocular bobbing	Initial vertical movement is downward Repetitive rapid downbeating saccades followed by a slow return to the mid position Paralysis of both reflex and spontaneous horizontal eye movements	Intrinsic pontine or cerebellar lesion Metabolic and toxic coma Extra-axial posterior fossa masses
Ocular dipping	Initial vertical movement is downward Slow initial downward phase is followed by a relatively rapid return to mid position	Hypoxic-ischaemic brain injury Following status epilepticus
Downbeat nystagmus	Rapid downward saccade followed by slow upward drift It may have a rotatory or circular component and moves with the same frequency as palatal myoclonus It is distinguished from ocular bobbing as there is no latency between the upward phase and the following downward jerk	Impairment of the lower brainstem in the region of the inferior olive and is particularly seen with the Arnold–Chiari malformation.
Reverse ocular bobbing	Initial vertical movement is upward Rapid conjugate upward jerk followed by slow downward drift that carries the eyes past the midposition. Then eyes slowly return to mid position	Non-localising Metabolic Viral encephalitis Pontine haemorrhage
Reverse ocular dipping	Initial vertical movement is upward Slow initial upward phase followed by rapid downward saccade returning the eyes to the mid position	Viral encephalitis Metabolic encephalopathy Pontine infarction
Upbeat Nystagmus	Slow downward drift followed by a rapid upward correcting saccade	Associated with disorders at the ponto-mesencephalic or ponto-medullary junction Cerebrovascular disease Multiple sclerosis Brainstem infarct Wernicke's encephalopathy
Opsoclonus	Intermittent bursts of large amplitude high-velocity multi-directional saccadic eye movements If the movements are entirely horizontal they are called ocular flutter	Paraneoplastic Viral encephalitis Metabolic encephalopathy Drug toxicity

Table 20.8 Oculocephalic responses.

Passive head movement (by examiner)	Response	Cause
Horizontal movement	Eyes remain conjugate and maintain fixation (move in opposite direction to head)	Normal with reduced level of consciousness
	No movement in either eye	Low brainstem lesion Peripheral vestibular lesion Drugs, anaesthesia
	Eyes move appropriately in one direction but do not cross the midline in the other	Gaze palsy (unilateral lesion in pontine gaze centre) Pontine lesion
	One eye abducts but the other fails to adduct	IIIrd nerve palsy Internuclear ophthalmoplegia (lesion of the median longitudinal fasciculus)
	One eye adducts but the other fails to abduct	VIth nerve palsy
Vertical movement	Eyes remain conjugate and maintain fixation (move in direction opposite head movement)	Normal with reduced level of consciousness
	No movement in either eye	Low brainstem lesion Peripheral vestibular lesion Drugs, anaesthesia
	Only one eye moves	IIIrd nerve palsy
	Loss of upward gaze	Pretectal or midbrain tegmental compression

the stimulated ear followed by a corrective saccade towards the midline. Warm water irrigation causes conjugate eye deviation with a slow phase away from the stimulated ear followed by a corrective saccadic phase towards the ear. Simultaneous bilateral warm water application causes a slow upward deviation while simultaneous bilateral cold water application results in slow downward deviation. As with the oculo-cephalic manoeuvre, impaired abduction suggests a VIth nerve palsy while impaired adduction is compatible with a IIIrd nerve lesion or INO. Limited oculo-vestibular movements may be caused by metabolic and/or toxic coma or drug intoxication. Vertical movements are impaired by disorders of the midbrain particularly affecting regions responsible for maintaining consciousness, while pontine lesions lead to loss of horizontal saccadic movements.

Other cranial nerves The eyes are usually closed in coma. However, if the patient is in light coma and if both afferent and efferent limbs of the corneal reflex are intact and the eye is held open, a bilateral blink reflex can be elicited in response to corneal or eyelash stimulation. The blink reflex may be lost with a lesion at the level of the pons, interrupting the afferent pathway along the Vth cranial nerve. However, unilateral absence of blinking indicates a lesion of the VIIth nerve affecting the efferent pathway. In this situation the stimulus may induce deviation of the jaw to the opposite side (corneopterygoid reflex). The corneal reflex has a higher threshold in comatose patients and may be lost with deep sedation. The jaw jerk may be brisk in coma and the presence of clonus suggests involvement of the corticobulbar tract or metabolic encephalopathy but it is also seen during weaning from sedation or in the vegetative state. In coma the facial grimace to painful stimuli reflects VIIth nerve function. Lesions at a pontine level may damage facial nerve nuclei and produce ipsilateral complete facial paralysis. Upper motor neurone lesions produce contralateral facial weakness, but tend to spare the forehead and orbicularis oculi muscles because of the bilateral cortical representation.

Bulbar function The clinical assessment of bulbar function in patients with an altered level of consciousness is difficult and unreliable. Airway protection may be impaired despite the presence of palatal movement and a pharyngeal and cough reflex. In an intubated patient the cough reflex may be tested indirectly by manipulating the tracheal tube or by administering tracheal suction. An impaired cough reflex is manifest as a poor or absent cough response, absence of distress and lack of lacrimation, and implies a central medullary lesion although the response may also be depressed by metabolic encephalopathy or by lesions of the afferent vagal pathway or efferent limb to the respiratory muscles. The pharyngeal (gag) reflex is also difficult to assess in comatose patients as it is suppressed by sedative drugs. However, impairment of palatal and uvula elevation upon pharyngeal and palatal stimulation implies low brainstem impairment.

Several characteristic patterns of respiratory irregularity have been described by Plum and Posner (Figure 20.2) but it is difficult to attribute precise respiratory function to discrete anatomical substrates because lesions are rarely localised and coexisting pulmonary, cardiovascular or autonomic influences may complicate the clinical picture. Furthermore, earlier recognition of respiratory insufficiency has led to rapid therapeutic intervention with controlled ventilation.

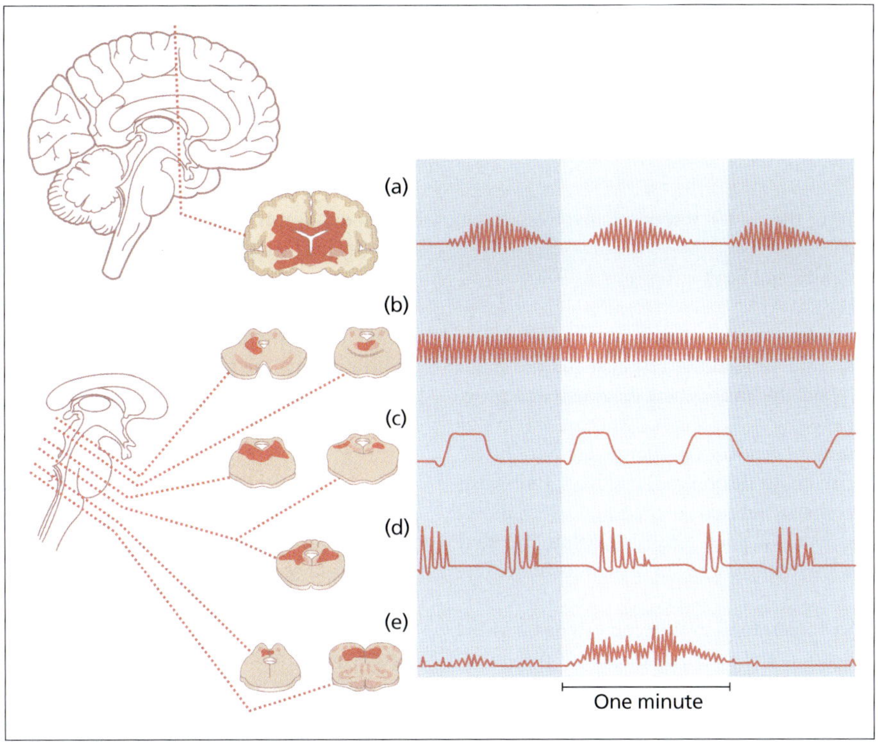

Figure 20.2 Abnormal reapiratory pattern associated with pathological lesions (shaded area) at various levels of the brain. tracings by chest-abdominal pneumograph, inspiration reads up. (a) Cheyne-Stokes respiration. (b) Central neurogenic hyperventilation. (c) Apneusis. (d) Cluster breathin. (e) Ataxic breathing. Source: Plum and Posner 1983. Reproduced with permission of Oxford University Press.

Primary central neurogenic hyperventilation is a rare condition characterised by rapid regular hyperventilation that persists in the face of alkalosis, elevated PaO_2, low $PaCO_2$ and in the absence of any pulmonary or airway disorder. However, in the critically ill patient, an increased respiratory rate in coma is more commonly secondary to intrinsic lung involvement, especially aspiration pneumonia.

Apneustic breathing consists of sustained inspiratory cramps with prolonged pauses at full inspiration or alternating brief end-inspiratory and expiratory pauses. The pattern is associated with bilateral tegmental infarcts or demyelination in the pons (Figure 20.3).

In ataxic respiration there is a completely irregular respiratory cycle of variable frequency and tidal volume alternating with periods of apnoea; it is particularly associated with medullary impairment, either caused by brainstem stroke or compression and it is important to recognise as it may herald impending respiratory arrest.

Hiccups consist of brief bursts of intense inspiratory activity involving the diaphragm and inspiratory intercostal muscles. Intractable hiccups can be the result of structural or functional disturbances of the medulla or its afferent or efferent connections with the respiratory muscles. The presence of hiccups in this context can also presage the development of respiratory arrhythmia culminating in respiratory arrest.

Voluntary control of breathing can be impaired by bilateral lesions affecting the descending corticospinal or corticobulbar tracts, and is particularly seen in association with destructive vascular lesions of the basal pons or of the medullary pyramids which may result in the 'locked-in' syndrome. Selective interruption of the voluntary pathways leads to a strikingly regular and unvarying respiratory pattern, with loss of the ability to take a deep breath, hold the breath, cough voluntarily or initiate any kind of volitional respiratory movement although the respiratory pattern may vary with emotional stimuli. These patients can often be weaned from artificial ventilation.

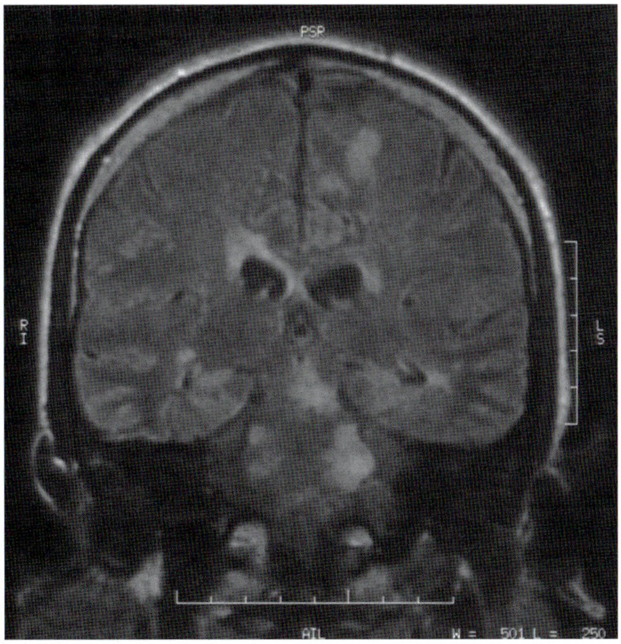

Figure 20.3 Extensive plaques of demyelination in the brainstem of a patient with ataxic breathing and progressive central apnoea requiring ventilatory support (MRI, coronal, FLAIR).

Cheyne–Stokes respiration (CSR) is characterised by a smooth waxing and waning of breath volume and frequency separated by periods of central apnoea. The respiratory oscillations are associated with phasic changes in cerebral blood flow (CBF), CSF pressure,

PaO_2 and alveolar oxygen and carbon dioxide, level of alertness and pupillary size; periodic heart block and ventricular arrhythmias are also common. Neurogenic CSR is associated with diffuse metabolic encephalopathy, cerebrovascular disease and raised ICP and may occur with supratentorial or, less commonly, infratentorial structural lesions.

Motor responses Examining the motor responses involves assessment of the:

- Resting posture of the limbs and head
- Involuntary movements
- Spontaneous movements (purposeful or non-purposeful)
- Response to external stimuli – the motor response to deep painful stimuli is extremely valuable in assessing diagnosis and prognosis of coma.

Two characteristic patterns of generalised reponses are recognised:

1 Decorticate posturing refers to flexion at the elbows and wrists with shoulder adduction and internal rotation and extension of the lower extremities. It has a poor localising value and may result from lesions of the hemispheres or thalamus above the diencephalon.
2 Decerebrate posture is characterised by bilateral extension of the lower extremities, adduction and internal rotation of the shoulders and extension at the elbows. It is usually caused by brainstem lesions, particularly of the bilateral midbrain or pons, and carries a poor prognosis. Occasionally, decerebrate posturing occurs as a result of severe metabolic encephalopathy (e.g. caused by hypoglycaemia or liver failure) or bilateral supratentorial lesions involving the motor pathways.

In clinical practice the pattern of motor response to stimuli is often mixed within the same patient with localising, flexion or extension movements occurring in different limbs and varying with recovery.

Tone The pattern and asymmetry of muscle tone may be helpful in localising focal structural lesions, and may help in differentiating metabolic from structural coma. The presence of spasticity implies established lesions while acute structural damage affecting the spinal cord or metabolic encephalopathy usually leads to hypotonia and flaccidity. The presence of a unilateral grasp reflex indicates an ipsilateral frontal lobe disturbance. Plucking or clutching movements of the limbs indicate light coma and intact corticospinal pathways.

Involuntary movements Tonic–clonic or other stereotyped movements suggest generalised or focal seizures or epilepsia partialis continuans (EPC). Myoclonic jerking (non-rhythmic jerking movements in single or multiple muscle groups) is seen with hypoxic–ischaemic encephalopathy or metabolic coma (e.g. hepatic encephalopathy). Rhythmic myoclonus must be distinguished from epilepsia partialis continua.

Distinction of metabolic and toxic coma from structural coma

It is often possible to distinguish metabolic encephalopathy from structural causes on the basis of clinical examination although non-convulsive status epilepticus can resemble both causes. The preceding medical history may suggest a metabolic abnormality and the onset is more likely to be acute in the presence of a toxic or structural lesion. Metabolic or toxic lesions usually result in coma without lateralising or brainstem signs while structural lesions may be suggested by asymmetrical motor signs. Metabolic encephalopathy is favoured by the presence of involuntary limb movements (tremor, myoclonus and asterixis), abnormalities of the respiratory pattern (hypoventilation or hyperventilation) and the presence of acid–base disturbances. The level of consciousness tends to fluctuate and be lighter in patients with metabolic disorders. However, these clinical features are merely indicators.

Psychogenic unresponsiveness

This may be distinguished by history, examination and, if necessary, investigations. There are often atypical factors in the history and occasionally obvious psychiatric precipitating factors. Examination reveals inconsistent volitional responses, particularly on eyelid opening. When the patient's hand is held in front of their face and then loosened it may drop and slide next to the face rather than fall directly. Tickling the hair cells with a vibrating fork may cause the eyes to open. There may be forced upward or downward gaze which suddenly changes direction. Spontaneous saccadic eye movements are often present, and pupillary constriction will occur on eye opening. Oculo-vestibular stimulation with cold stimulus will show preservation of the fast phase away from the stimulated side and the electroencephalography (EEG) will show responsive alpha rhythms.

Outcome from coma

Most patients who survive the initial insult emerge from coma within 2–4 weeks, although the pattern and extent of recovery is highly variable, ranging from vegetative state to full recovery. It is not possible to assess the prognosis of a patient in coma with accuracy but a number of clinical factors help in predicting the likely outcome. Most data are based on the assessment of patients with hypoxic–ischaemic brain injury (HIBI).

Aetiology

Coma associated with drug and alcohol ingestion or metabolic disturbance generally carries a good prognosis for recovery providing there is no severe underlying disorder. The prognosis for a patient in traumatic coma is better than that for a patient at a similar level of coma from non-traumatic causes. Patients in coma caused by structural cerebral disease (e.g. cerebrovascular disease or SAH) and HIBI is poor.

Depth of coma

The depth of coma, as determined by GCS and by the presence or absence of reflexes in the cranial nerve territory, is a sensitive guide to outcome.

Duration of coma

Survival following cardiorespiratory arrest is closely correlated with the duration of coma. Only 12% of patients comatose more than 6 hours after cardiac arrest survive with a good outcome or moderate deficits and, if there is no eye opening, vocal response or motor function after 6 hours the patient has only a 6% chance of making a moderate or good recovery.

Presence of seizures

The presence of focal or generalized seizures and convulsive and non-convulsive status epilepticus are all associated with a poorer outcome.

Co-morbidity

Following cardiac arrest there is a clear correlation between outcome and age at cardiac arrest. The presence of coexisting general medical disorders are also associated with a poor outcome: ischaemic heart disease, structural cardiac disease, hypertension, diabetes mellitus, impaired renal function and the presence of pneumonia or sepsis.

Investigations

A poor prognosis is indicated by:

- Imaging showing either anteroseptal shift, extensive subcortical change (Figure 20.4), temporal lobe infarction and hydrocephalus implies a worse outlook.
- Raised ICP.
- An iso-electric EEG, burst-suppression or 'alpha coma' (8–12 Hz rhythm, which is not localised to the occipital lobe, and which does not suppress upon eye opening).
- Absent cortical somatosensory evoked potentials performed >12–24 hours after cardiorespiratory arrest.

Following TBI, the most important predictive features for survival of patients in coma >6 hours are:

- Depth of coma on GCS
- Age
- The extent of injury, presence of skull fracture, hemispheric damage or extracranial injury.

Following a cardiorespiratory arrest, the most accurate guides to a poor prognosis at 3 days are:

- Absence of pupillary light reflexes, corneal reflexes and motor responses (except extensor plantar responses)
- Absence of other brainstem reflexes
- Loss of cortical N20 response on short latency somatosensory evoked potential (SSEPs) at 1–3 days
- Elevated serum neurone-specific enolase
- EEG showing alpha coma, burst suppression or an isoelectric trace

These features provide some prognostic information to allow discussion with relatives about the patient's wishes and likely outcome. However, these indicators are by no means specific or reliable. A poor outcome may also occur even if the initial signs suggest recovery. It must be emphasised too that many of these statements relate to studies that were undertaken several years ago. With better techniques of intensive care, physiological measurement and cerebral protection these data should only be used as a general guide.

Locked-in syndrome

The locked-in syndrome is characterised by preservation of consciousness with dissociation between automatic and volitional control of lower cranial nerve and limb function. Volitional respiratory, facial, bulbar and limb control is lost but there may be involuntary movements including ocular bobbing, facial grimacing, oral automatisms and trismus, palatal myoclonus and emotional responses including laughing and crying. There is preserved awareness of the environment and self, and patients can usually communicate through vertical eye movements, with synergistic elevation of the upper eyelids when looking upwards. These vertical eye movements are often slow and incomplete, but are the only way in which the patient can communicate because there is a horizontal gaze palsy, anarthria and tetraplegia. These patients are not in coma so it is essential to establish a consistent form of communication, however laborious for the patient and their carers.

The most frequent cause of locked-in syndrome is vertebro-basilar occlusion, usually in the rostral or middle segments (Figure 20.5). Pontine haemorrhage or embolism may also cause the condition. Other causes of the syndrome have been described in which the lesion was situated in the ventral pontine tegmentum, basis pontis or in the mesencephalic region at the level of the cerebral peduncles.

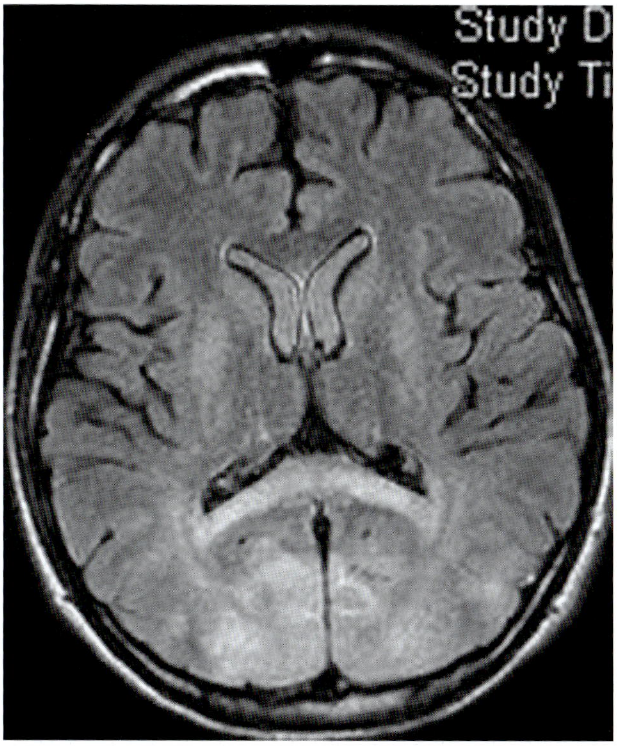

Figure 20.4 Global ischaemic–hypoxic brain lesions (MRI, axial, FLAIR).

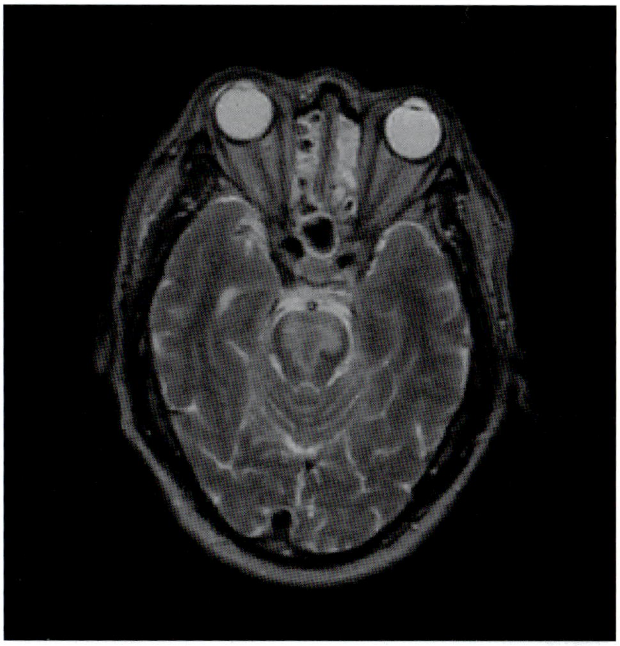

Figure 20.5 Extensive pontine infarction caused by vertebrobasilar occlusion in a patient with locked-in syndrome (MRI, T2-weighted).

The aetiology of non-vascular cases include central pontine myelinolysis, trauma, encephalitis, tumour, pontine abscess, MS and heroin abuse. Peripheral lesions (i.e. severe neuropathy such as Guillain–Barré syndrome) may cause an apparent locked-in syndrome with severe limb, facial and bulbar paresis, although respiration is frequently affected because of respiratory muscle involvement. In addition, vertical eye movements are not selectively spared in the same way as with the classic syndrome.

Functional recovery is possible in both vascular and non-vascular groups of locked-in patients and therefore an aggressive rehabilitation programme should be instituted as early as possible to allow the patient to achieve the highest possible level of recovery as rapidly as possible. However, the prognosis for most patients in locked-in syndromes is poor, with severe residual disability. The mortality rate is high with most deaths occurring in the first 4 months, either from extension of the lesion or from respiratory complications (pneumonia, respiratory arrest or pulmonary embolus).

Vegetative state

Patients in a vegetative state appear to be awake with their eyes open but show no evidence of awareness of self or environment, are unable to interact with others and have no evidence of sustained reproducible purposeful or voluntary behavioural responses to visual, auditory, tactile or noxious stimuli. There is no evidence of language comprehension or expression. Patients are able to breathe spontaneously and the papillary, ocular, gag, cough, sucking and swallowing reflexes are usually present. Sleep–wake cycles are preserved as are hypothalamic and brainstem autonomic responses. There is bladder and bowel incontinence. Inconsistent non-purposive movements, facial grimacing, smiling and frowning, chewing, swallowing, bruxism, vocalisation, grasping and inconsistent auditory and oculomotor orientating reflexes to peripheral sounds or movement may occur. The diagnosis of vegetative state is not tenable if there is any degree of voluntary movement, sustained visual pursuit, consistent and reproducible visual fixation or response to threatening gestures.

The vegetative state usually develops after a variable period of coma; it may be partially or totally reversible or may become established. Persistent vegetative state is defined as a vegetative state that has continued for at least 1 month. This definition does not imply permanency or irreversibility. It has been recommended that the term "permanent vegetative state (PVS)" be used to describe patients who remain in a vegetative state for more than 3 months after a hypoxic brain injury or 12 months after cranial trauma as improvement after this time is highly unlikely. However, the term is best avoided because there is a high rate of misdiagnosis.

It has recently been shown by functional imaging techniques that exposure to personally meaningful information or verbal instructions activates the cerebral cortex in some patients in a vegetative state and in some exceptional instances patients in a vegetative state can retain a degree of awareness or even communication shown by reproducible changes on functional imaging in response to stimuli. These patients have generally sustained TBI and some emerge into a minimally conscious state. This finding emphasises the difficulty in establishing a diagnosis of permanent vegetative state. Functional imaging techniques may be used to supplement clinical observation of the unconscious patients but it is important to recognise that activation does not necessarily reveal conscious experience, memory or self-awareness. The clinical implication of these studies is that patients in a vegetative state cannot any more be considered to be totally lacking in awareness. This has led to the naming of the condition unresponsive wakefulness syndrome (UWS) rather than vegetative state.

Minimally conscious state

Patients in a minimally conscious state (MCS) are no longer in coma nor in a vegetative state because they demonstrate low level behavioural responses consistent with severe neurological impairment and disability. MCS is much more common than vegetative state 6 months after brain injury. This condition includes a wide variety of responses. Patients who are minimally responsive may be able to show consistent evidence of awareness of themselves or their environments by making eye contact, or turning their heads to sound, following simple commands, gestural or verbal yes/no responses, intelligible speech or purposeful behaviour. They are not able to communicate consistently. These patients may remain in minimally responsive states or eventually recover some ability to communicate reliably or use objects functionally. Positron emission tomography (PET) and functional magnetic resonance imaging (fMRI) studies show that patients in MCS can have more extended cerebral processing in response to external stimuli or various modalities such as noxious or self-related auditory stimuli. The extent of activation in individual brain damage patients in response to complex stimuli sometimes correlates with clinical outcome and functional imaging may be helpful as a prognostic indicator.

Determining brain death

Cardiac and respiratory function can be maintained artificially for prolonged periods after the brain has ceased to function. The diagnosis of brain death is necessary when withdrawal of artificial life support is considered and if the possibility of organ donation exists. These are both delicate issues.

Brain death is diagnosed in three stages.

1. It must be established that the patient has suffered an event of known aetiology resulting in irreversible brain damage with apnoeic coma (i.e. the patient is deeply unconscious, mechanically ventilated with no spontaneous respiratory movement)
2. Reversible causes of coma must be excluded, and
3. A set of bedside clinical tests of brainstem function are undertaken to confirm the diagnosis of brainstem death and to exclude any relevant metabolic derangement.

The procedure is as follows:

1. The cause of coma must be known to be irremediable brain damage of known aetiology. This may be obvious within hours of a primary intracranial event such as a severe head injury or spontaneous intracranial haemorrhage, but diagnosis may be more difficult following hypoxic brain injury or encephalitis.
2. There should be no evidence that coma could be caused by depressant drugs or neuromuscular blocking agents. Narcotics, hypnotics and tranquillisers may have prolonged action, particularly when hypothermia coexists or in the context of renal or hepatic failure. Determination of sedative drug levels and tests of neuromuscular function may be necessary.
3. Primary hypothermia (<35°C) as the cause of unconsciousness must have been excluded. It is important to recognise that the previously widespread adoption of therapeutic hypothermia can further complicate the determination of brain death.
4. Potentially reversible circulatory, metabolic and endocrine disturbances must have been excluded as the cause of the continuation of unconsciousness.
5. The patient is being maintained on the ventilator because spontaneous respiration has ceased.

6 All brainstem reflexes are absent:
- The pupils are fixed, dilated and do not respond to sharp changes in the intensity of light.
- There is no corneal reflex (care should be taken to avoid damage to the cornea because this may be used for organ donation).
- The vestibulo-ocular reflexes are absent. No eye movements are seen during or following the slow injection of at least 50 mL ice cold water over 1 minute into each external auditory meatus in turn. Wait several minutes before testing the other side. Clear access to the tympanic membrane must be established by direct inspection and the head should be flexed at 30°.
- There is no gag reflex or reflex response to bronchial stimulation when a suction catheter is passed into the trachea.
- No motor responses can be elicited following painful stimulation applied to an area within the cranial nerve distribution.
- No respiratory movements occur when the patient is disconnected from the mechanical ventilator. During this test the $PaCO_2$ should reach 6.65 kPa. This should be ensured by arterial blood gas measurement. Hypoxaemia following disconnection from the ventilator should be prevented by pre-oxygenating the patient with 100% oxygen for 10 minutes while on the ventilator and then delivering oxygen at 6 L/minute through a catheter situated in the tracheal tube when mechanical ventilation is temporarily removed. This test examines the function of the respiratory centre.

Repetition of testing

In the United Kingdom, the diagnosis of death by brainstem testing should be made by at least two medical practitioners who have been registered for more than 5 years, have been trained in this field and are not members of the transplant team. The complete set of tests should always be performed on two separate occasions by the two practitioners working alone or together. The interval between tests has not been defined in adults, and usually the tests are repeated within a short period to avoid further distress to the patient's relatives. In legal terms, the time of death is taken as the time of the first failed brainstem test. Confirmatory ancillary tests (EEG, transcranial Doppler, CBF scanning or cerebral angiography) are not required in the United Kingdom, United States or most European countries.

It is essential that relatives, partners and carers be kept fully informed of the clinical condition of the patient and that explanation be given to them regarding the condition and prognosis. They should be given explanation of the investigations being undertaken and of their interpretation throughout the process of the determination of death of the brainstem in a sympathetic, timely and appropriate fashion by those concerned.

Neurological intensive care

Dedicated neurological intensive care units (NICUs) are predominantly involved with the management of patients with primary encephalopathies, the control of raised ICP, the management of ventilatory, autonomic and bulbar insufficiency, and the consequences of profound neuromuscular weakness. The increasing availability of NICUs in Europe and the United States has allowed a focus on all critical needs of the neurological patient as well as the management of peri-operative instability of patients with neurosurgical or interventional neuroradiology. In general, critical illness resulting from primary neurological diseases such as myasthenia gravis, Guillain–Barré syndrome, CNS infections, status epilepticus and stroke have a better outcome than those patients with neurological disease secondary to general medical disorders seen on general ICUs. However, such patients can remain dependent on ICU support for very much longer periods of time. This results in significant psychological demands on the patients, their carers, nurses, physicians and other health care professionals. There is sound evidence that patients with critical neurological disease have better outcomes when cared for in dedicated NICUs.

Indications for intensive care management of neurological patients

The major indications for considering admission to NICU include the management of coma, bulbar or generalised weakness, autonomic failure, raised ICP and/or status epilepticus.

The aim of neurological intensive care is monitoring, early detection and management of impending neurological or systemic deterioration, as well as the minimisation of such risk that will potentially lead to deterioration or poor outcome. There are general principles of intensive care management including meticulous nursing and medical care, monitoring of a range of physiological variables and early and aggressive physiotherapy, including frequent alterations of limb positioning, passive limb movements and appropriate splinting which helps to maintain joint mobility and prevents limb contractures and pain while awaiting neurological improvement. Other aspects of general ICU care include the management of agitation and pain, maintenance of an adequate airway and ventilation, cardiovascular stability, nutrition and prophylaxis against thromboembolism.

Many patients with impaired consciousness or severe neuromuscular weakness are not able to communicate adequately. It is essential that satisfactory means of communication are established as soon as possible. Furthermore, when communication is difficult, the family often represents the patient's interests and they must therefore have comprehensive access to medical and nursing staff throughout so that they understand the immediate clinical situation, management and outlook.

Ventilatory failure associated with neurological disease

The central and peripheral causes of ventilatory insufficiency or failure that may require admission to the NICU are listed in Tables 20.9 and 20.10. It is essential to anticipate the development of respiratory failure before the emergence of hypoxia and/or hypercapnia. Thus, the threshold for tracheal intubation is lower in the context of rapidly progressive neuromuscular weakness. Patients with acute neurological disorders require tracheal intubation and ventilation because of the development of acute respiratory insufficiency or because they are unable to protect their upper airway from obstruction as a consequence of impaired consciousness or bulbar weakness. The latter predisposes to pulmonary aspiration of saliva and food that cannot be cleared by the patient because of an inadequate cough secondary to poor diaphragmatic and anterior abdominal wall musculature. Bronchopneumonia often results.

The most useful and reproducible bedside test of ventilatory function is the measurement of the forced vital capacity (FVC). The normal value is approximately 10–15 mL/kg. Serial measurements often indicate whether respiratory muscle function is stable or deteriorating and are especially important in fluctuating diseases such as myasthenia gravis. By the time arterial blood gas

Table 20.9 Central causes of ventilatory insufficiency or failure that may require admission to a neurological intensive care unit (NICU).

Cortical	**Foramen magnum and upper cervical cord**
Epilepsy	Arnold–Chiari malformation – cerebellar ectopia
Vascular	Achondroplasia, osteogenesis imperfecta
Tumour	Rheumatoid arthritis – odontoid peg compression
Metabolic	Trauma
Infection	Vascular
Brainstem	**Cervical and upper thoracic spinal cord**
Congenital (Ondine's curse) – primary alveolar hypoventilation	Acute epidural compression: neoplasm or infection
Tumour	Acute transverse myelitis
Vascular	Cord infarction
Multiple sclerosis and acute disseminated encephalomyelitis	Other myelopathies (including traumatic)
Motor neurone disease	Tetanus
Infection:	**Autonomic**
Borrelia	Multi-system atrophy
Listeria	**Extrapyramidal**
Post varicella encephalomyelitis	Status dystonicus
Poliomyelitis	
Rabies	
Encephalitis lethargica	
Western equine encephalitis	
Paraneoplastic	
Leigh's disease	
Reye's syndrome	
Hypoxaemia	

Source: Howard 2003. Reproduced with permission of BMJ.

tensions have become abnormal respiratory muscle function is often severely compromised.

Neurological indications for tracheal intubation and mechanical ventilation

The nature of neurological respiratory failure can dictate a prolonged period of mechanical ventilation. When this is the case, the orotracheal tube should be replaced by a tracheostomy as soon as possible. Tracheostomy allows greater patient comfort, easier nursing management (including suction) and the possibility of oral nutrition and speech, as well as aiding weaning from mechanical ventilation by reducing respiratory dead space. Indications for tracheal intubation are shown in Table 20.11.

Mechanical ventilation

Mechanical ventilation of the lungs may be provided by intermittent negative pressure ventilation or intermittent positive pressure ventilation. The former is delivered using devices such as tank ventilators (iron lungs) and cuirass ventilators; apart from in a few specialised units, these devices are rarely used nowadays. Modes of ventilation are summarised in Table 20.12.

Weaning

Weaning of patients from mechanical ventilation may start as soon as respiratory muscle function returns; the patient needs to be able to maintain adequate oxygenation, a normal respiratory rate and appropriate spontaneous tidal volumes with minimal mechanical support. In addition, the patient needs to maintain a patent airway, to initiate cough and gag reflexes and to clear secretions independently. Sophisticated ventilatory modes (Table 20.12) aid weaning, but many units prefer to wean by allowing patients to breathe spontaneously off the ventilator for increasing periods solely with continuous positive airway pressure (CPAP).

Conditions requiring neurointensive care support

Raised intracranial pressure

ICP is the pressure exerted by the CSF in the frontal horns of the lateral ventricles of the brain. It is normally 7–17 mmHg (1–2 kPa) when supine. Because the skull, in an adult, is a rigid box and its contents are incompressible, the ICP depends on the volume of intracranial contents, normally approximately 100 mL blood (5–7%), 50–120 mL CSF (5–12%) and 1.4 L brain tissue (80–85%). The Monro–Kellie doctrine states that because the total intracranial volume remains constant, an increase in the volume of one of the components of the intracranial cavity (e.g. brain) requires a compensatory reduction in another (e.g. CSF) to maintain a constant pressure. Because brain tissue is essentially incompressible, any additional volume results in movement of CSF into the spinal subarachnoid space, reduction of CSF volume by increased absorption in the arachnoid villi and removal of blood from the cerebrovascular bed. As mass effect worsens, compensatory mechanisms are pushed to exhaustion and a relatively small increase in volume will precipitate a large rise in ICP.

ICP has a key role in determining cerebral perfusion pressure (CPP) and CBF. As the ICP rises, CPP and CBF decrease, particularly when cerebral autoregulation is impaired. This may lead to obstruction of venous blood vessels, brain swelling, regional ischaemia, structural distortion and the development of brainstem compression. Recent studies show that ICP elevation itself (in the presence of well-controlled CPP <60) was independently associated with neurological deterioration; so even if CPP is maintained, an elevated ICP state can still aggravate neurological injury.

Raised ICP can be caused by:

- Mass effect (e.g. tumour, infarction with oedema, contusion, intracerebral haemorrhage, haematoma – extradural or subdural).
- Generalised cerebral oedema (e.g hypertensive encephalopathy, following hypoxic ischaemic brain injury and status epilepticus, liver failure or hypercapnia).
- Increase in venous pressure (e.g. venous sinus thrombosis, superior vena cava obstruction).
- Obstruction to CSF flow and/or absorption (e.g. obstructive hydrocephalus, extensive meningeal infiltration, SAH).
- Increased CSF production (e.g. choroid plexus tumour, meningitis, SAH).

Raised ICP in the conscious patient is characterised by headache, which may be exacerbated by coughing, sneezing or straining. It is often worse on wakening and associated with nausea and vomiting. The diurnal variation in headache is caused by raised ICP when recumbent and associated raised $PaCO_2$ and reduced CSF absorption during sleep.

Table 20.10 Peripheral causes of ventilatory insufficiency or failure that may require admission to a neurological intensive care unit (NICU).

Anterior horn cell	**Neuromuscular transmission defects**
Motor neurone disease	Myasthenia gravis
Poliomyelitis or post polio syndromes	Lambert–Eaton myasthenic syndrome
Multiple radiculopathies	Neuromuscular blocking agents
Carcinomatous meningitis	Other:
AIDS polyradiculitis	Botulism
Polyneuropathy	Toxins
Acute inflammatory demyelinating polyneuropathy (AIDP)	Hypermagnesaemia
Acute motor and sensory axonal neuropathy (AMSAN)	Organophosphate poisoning
Acute motor axonal neuropathy (AMAN)	**Muscle**
Critical illness polyneuropathy	Dystrophy
Other polyneuropathies:	Duchenne, Becker, limb girdle, Emery–Dreyfuss
Hereditary sensorimotor	Inflammatory
Acute porphyria	Myotonic dystrophy
Organophosphate poisoning	Metabolic
Herpes zoster/varicella	Acid maltase deficiency
Neuralgic amyotrophy	Mitochondrial myopathies
	Myopathies associated with neuromuscular blocking agents and steroids
	Acute quadriplegic myopathy
	Myopathy and sepsis
	Cachectic myopathy
	HIV-related myopathy
	Sarcoid myopathy
	Hypokalaemic myopathy
	Rhabdomyolysis
	Periodic paralysis

Source: Howard 2003. Reproduced with permission of BMJ.

Table 20.11 Indications for tracheal intubation.

A decreasing forced vital capacity in the presence of bulbar dysfunction
Impending neuromuscular respiratory failure (forced vital capacity <15 mL/kg, tachypnoea, poor cough, dyspnoea at rest, use of accessory muscles, staccato speech)
Respiratory failure (PaO_2 <8 kPa (60 mmHg) breathing room air) with or without hypercarbia
Inability to protect airway
Failure of central regulation of respiration (apnoea, ataxic or cluster breathing)
Brain swelling with depressed level of consciousness (Glasgow Coma Score <9)
To provide control of $PaCO_2$ in patients with raised intracranial pressure
Bulbar failure (in order to protect the airway from pulmonary aspiration)
Encephalopathy/coma
Cardiovascular instability (e.g. hypotension)

Reduced level of consciousness is an almost universal finding in patients who have significant acute herniation syndromes; with or without ICP elevation. In severely raised ICP this is accompanied by Cushing's triad (bradycardia, hypertension and respiratory irregularity). It is important to note that raised ICP is not always observed in herniation.

Raised ICP may be unvarying, particularly following head injury when the level reflects the severity of the insult (severe >20 mmHg). However, the presence of fluctuations and, in particular, A and B waves, indicates rapid deterioration because of vasogenic change and suggests that intracranial hypertension leading to herniation will develop unless urgent intervention is undertaken (Figure 20.6).

Measurement of intracranial pressure

A variety of different techniques are available for the measurement of ICP. Intraventricular fluid filled catheter transducer systems require an external pressure transducer connected to a catheter placed in the lateral ventricle to allow direct pressure management. The system is the most accurate technique for ICP measurement as it can be recalibrated as required and allows drainage of CSF. It is not limited by intercompartment pressure gradients provided all

Table 20.12 Modes of ventilatory support.

Controlled mechanical ventilation (CMV)	Preset tidal volume at a preset respiratory rate, independent of the patient's respiratory effort Patient is completely dependent on the ventilator Used for patients who are unable to breathe or who have received neuromuscular blocking agents
Intermittent mandatory ventilation (IMV)	A mandatory minute volume is preset and delivered by the ventilator, but the patient is allowed to breathe spontaneously from a gas source between ventilator breaths
Synchronised intermittent mandatory ventilation (SIMV)	As for IMV but with coordination of the positive pressure ventilation by the ventilator so that it coincides with a spontaneous breath
Inspiratory pressure support	The patient's spontaneous breath is augmented with supplementary gas flow
Inspiratory volume support	Ventilator automatically monitors the lung properties and modifies the inspiratory pressure support in order to deliver a predetermined tidal volume
Positive end expiratory pressure (PEEP)	An adjunct to intermittent positive pressure ventilation (IPPV) and maintains a positive pressure during expiration. Helps minimise alveolar collapse and improves lung compliance
Continuous positive airway pressure (CPAP)	The application of positive airway pressure throughout all phases of spontaneous ventilation. Helps prevent airway and alveolar collapse

the ventricles are in communication. However, these catheters are associated with a risk of infection, blockage, haematoma formation and seizures and are difficult to place in small ventricles which are a common problem if raised ICP is caused by brain swelling.

More commonly, a catheter tip transducer system is used to record from the ventricle, subdural or subarachnoid space or parenchyma. This is usually undertaken with a catheter tip transducer inserted via an airtight support bolt (e.g. Codman© or Camino©). These systems are slightly less reliable, require pre-insertion calibration and may fail after several days, but the ease of placement has led to their widespread use in patients with cerebral trauma.

Indications for intracranial pressure monitoring

ICP monitoring is undertaken as a guide to treatment or, less commonly, as a diagnostic investigation. Clinical and radiological evidence is not always a reliable guide to raised ICP and monitoring is necessary if there is an unstable haemodynamic state or a mass lesion indicating the possibility of incipient herniation.

Evidence supports the routine use of ICP monitoring in patients with severe head injury (GCS 3–8) and an abnormal CT scan, significant focal motor signs or hypotension. ICP monitoring may be helpful following SAH, intracerebral haemorrhage, venous sinus thrombosis or following hypoxic brain injury, encephalitis or hepatic encephalopathy. It may also be of diagnostic value in patients with normal pressure hydrocephalus, idiopathic intracranial hypertension or decompensated hydrocephalus.

Management

The management of raised ICP following TBI is summarised in (Figure 20.7). Urgent treatment of raised ICP may be necessary to avoid development and progression of herniation and subsequent brain ischaemia, infarction and death. If ICP exceeds 20 mmHg treatment is mandatory.

The first line of management of raised ICP is to ensure a secure airway and maintain oxygenation and systemic mean arterial blood

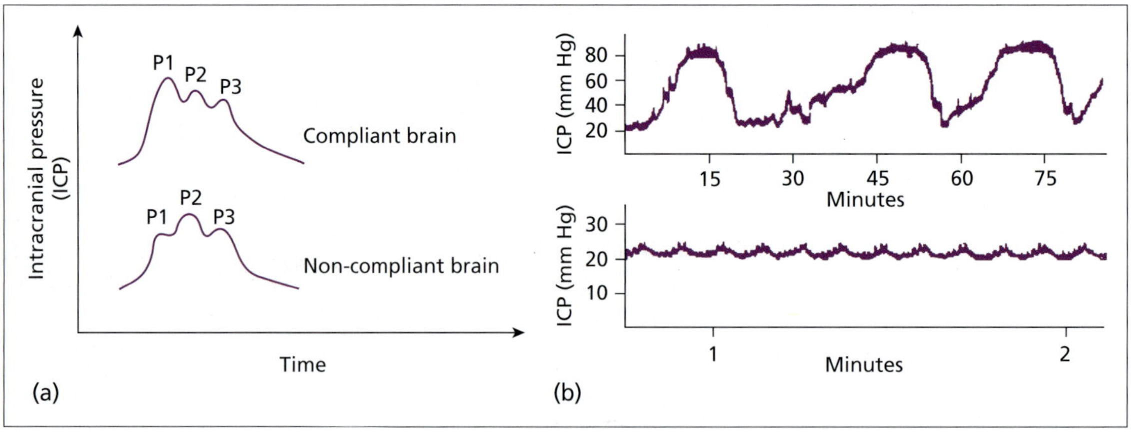

Figure 20.6 (a) The ICP waveform is essentially a modified arterial pressure trace and has characteristic elements. In the normal brain, the first peak (P1, the percussive wave) is a result of arterial pressure transmitted from the choroid plexus. P2 is the 'tidal' wave and reflects brain compliance. P3 is caused by closure of the aortic valve (i.e. the dicrotic notch). In the non-compliant brain, the amplitude of P2 typically exceeds P1.
(b) More useful information is gained by recording ICP waveforms over time and certain patterns may be seen. Lundberg A (plateau) waves consist of rapid rises in ICP lasting 5–10 minutes (upper trace). They are always pathological and represent severe intracranial hypertension. Lundberg B waves are oscillations in ICP of 0.5–2 waves/min and represent unstable ICP, possibly related to cerebral vasospasm. Intracranial pressure (ICP) trace for a patient with a plateau of high ICP (lower trace).

ICP directed therapy in Traumatic Brain Injury (TBI)

Basic Measures

- Sedation and analgesia – **propofol** and **fentanyl** infusions
- Artificial ventilation – **PaO_2 > 13 kPa, $PaCO_2$ 4.5–5.0 kPa, PEEP 5 cm H_2O**
- **MAP ≥ 90 mmHg** or SBP ≥120mmHg
- Blood glucose **5.5–9 mmol/l**
- Temperature **35.5–37°C**
- **Head up 30°** – *provided not hypotensive and thoracic/lumbar spine cleared*
- Commence **spine clearance** algorithm – *straight bed tilt until thoracic/lumbar spine cleared*

***Hyperventilation** reserved for acute rises in ICP*

*Use of **PEEP** and effect on ICP should be individualised to achieve PaO_2 target*

Therapeutic goals once ICP monitoring commenced

ICP < 20–25 mmHg

CPP = 60 mmHg

To attain CPP ensure adequate fluid resuscitation before starting vasopressors
Insert oesophageal Doppler if indicated to guide fluid management
Doppler mandatory when vasopressors > 0.2 mcg/kg/min or when requirements increasing

ICP < 20 mmHg

Continue current therapy

Neurosurgeon may consider 'waking' patient to assess
Consider C-spine clearance and need for further imaging prior to 'wake up'

ICP 20–25 mmHg

Check

√ Pupils – equal and reacting
√ ET tapes
not tight/impeding venous drainage
√ Head & neck in neutral alignment
return to supine position
√ ICP waveform
√ $PaCO_2$ within parameters/adequate PaO_2
√ Sedation infusions intact

Ensure

Adequate sedation – *give bolus and observe effect*

Consider

√ Increasing rate of sedation
√ Bolus of muscle relaxant – *if effective start infusion*

ICP > 25 mmHg

Repeat checks and consider

√ Reducing $PaCO_2$ to 4.0–4.5 kPa
√ Active cooling to 35°C
√ Thiopentone *(see Protocol)*
√ Insertion of $SjvO_2$ to allow further manipulation of PCO_2

☎ Neurosurgeon
to obtain further management plan
(e.g. CSF drainage or decompressive craniectomy)

Neuromuscular blocking agents

NMBAs have no direct effect on ICP but prevent rises produced by coughing on ET tube

Atracurium

- Give bolus and observe effect on ICP
- If effective commence infusion
- If history of asthma use **vecuronium**
- Propofol and NMBAs **not** compatible *(infuse as per UCLH guidelines)*
- Seizures difficult to detect if paralysed *(may be signalled by bilateral pupillary dilatation, small ↑ ABP + ↑ ICP)*

Propofol infusion syndrome (PRIS)

- Rare but lethal complication of propofol infusion *(particularly in association with use of vasopressors)*
- Common clinical features include: hyperkalemia, hepatomegaly, lipemia, metabolic acidosis, myocardial failure, rhabdomyolysis, renal failure
- Always consider the diagnosis in patients receiving propofol, but particularly when using doses >75 mcg/kg/min or when usage at any dose exceeds 48h
- ***Daily screen** for ↑ CK, unexplained acidosis, ECG changes*

Dosing for analgesics and sedatives

Propofol	0.5 mg/kg test bolus 20–75 mcg/kg/min infusion
Fentanyl	2 mcg/kg test dose 2–5 mcg/kg/h infusion
Midazolam	2mg test dose 2–4 mg/h infusion

Neurocritical Care NHNN 2010

University College London Hospitals NHS
NHS Foundation Trust

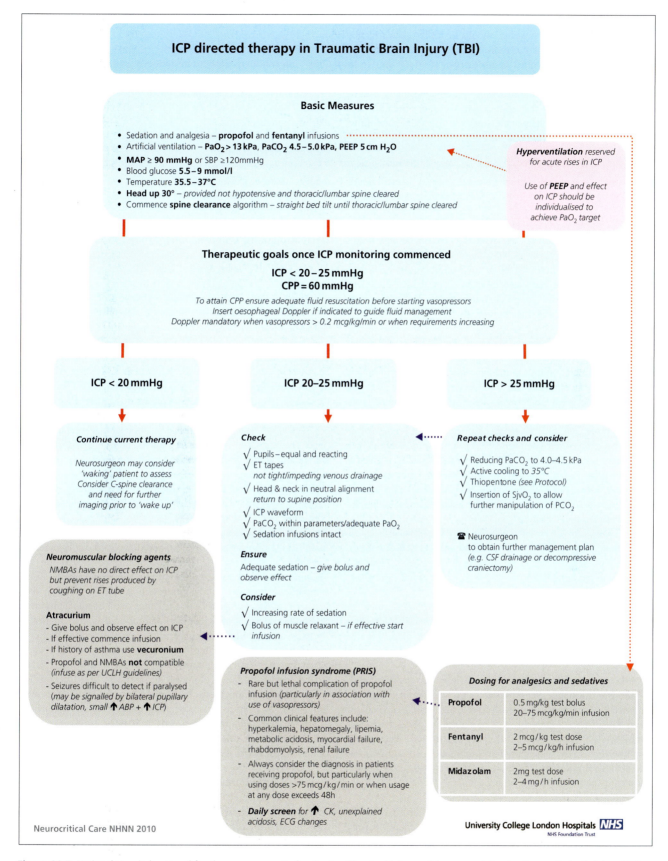

Figure 20.7 National Hospital protocol for the management of patients with raised intracranial pressure following traumatic brain injury (TBI).

pressure (MAP >80 mmHg should be targeted). Treatment of the underlying cause, where possible, should be undertaken urgently and aggressive control of metabolic derangements, seizures and pyrexia is essential. CPP must be maintained at 50–70 mmHg by ensuring optimal arterial blood pressure with avoidance of hypotension; this requires careful intravenous fluid management and the use of inotropic agents. Neuromuscular blockade, sedation and analgesia are needed to help avoid surges in ICP from suctioning, coughing or other interventions such as physiotherapy.

Head positioning The head should be elevated to 30° to facilitate venous drainage. Any constriction around the neck (e.g. tracheal tube ties) must be avoided as this may obstruct cerebral venous drainage.

Controlled hyperventilation Hyperventilation lowers $PaCO_2$ and induces cerebral vasoconstriction reducing cerebral blood volume. This is a rapid, effective way of reducing elevated ICP but is limited by a contingent reduction in CBF to any area of critical perfusion. Patients are therefore ventilated to a $PaCO_2$ of 4 kPa. Beneficial effects of hyperventilation are often transient and it should only be used for 10–20 hours and then weaned slowly.

Osmotic agents Mannitol is a hyperosmolar diuretic that lowers ICP and increases CBF by drawing free water out of the brain tissue and into the circulation thus reducing interstitial water content and dehydrating brain parenchyma. This effect is achieved by establishing an osmotic gradient between blood and brain parenchyma. However, with prolonged therapy, mannitol may diffuse into damaged brain cells and exacerbate tissue oedema. It is also associated with a hyperosmotic state and leads to a profound diuresis with consequent fluid management difficulties. Mannitol 20% is given as a bolus 1 g/kg. Repeat doses are given at 0.25–0.5 g/kg as needed every 6–8 hours. Furosemide and thiazide diuretics may also be used to increase osmolarity in the vascular compartment and maintain the intravascular volume.

Inotropic support Augmentation of MAP may help delivery of oxygen and glucose to the brain averting the progression to cytotoxic oedema and reducing ICP.

CSF drainage via an intraventricular catheter This may be undertaken intermittently in response to elevations in ICP. However, ventriculostomy is associated with a risk of peri-operative haemorrhage and secondary infection thereafter.

Hypothermia Hypothermia can lower ICP by decreasing cerebral metabolism. Moderate hypothermia (35°C) decreases raised ICP but lower body temperatures cause cardiac arrhythmias and coagulation disturbances. Raised body temperature is deleterious as it increases ICP and must therefore be treated aggressively. Hypothermia is now widely used in combination with other therapies for lowering raised ICP; however, there remains considerable uncertainty about the long-term benefits.

Fever control Temperature elevation causes more harm, by vasodilatation, an increase in intracranial mass and thus more neuronal injury. Adequate control of pyrexia is essential.

Decompressive surgery This has been increasingly used following extensive TBI and middle cerebral artery occlusion, intracranial haemorrhage, SAH or severe encephalitis. Some reports suggest good recovery but there is a high incidence of severe residual morbidity.

Other interventions Barbiturate-induced coma reduces cerebral metabolic activity and causes cerebral vasoconstriction which leads to a reduction in CBF, cerebral blood volume and consequently ICP but may be accompanied by a high incidence of side effects, particularly hypotension.

Cerebral herniation

Cerebral herniation is an important mechanism of coma and permanent neurological impairment. It occurs when raised ICP leads to torsion and compression of the brainstem against the tentorium, falx and bony structures.

Herniation of the temporal lobe through the tentorium (uncal herniation)

This is caused by asymmetrical mass effect causing the temporal lobe, uncus and hippocampus to shift towards the midline leading to compression of the midbrain against the tentorial edge (Figure 20.8). The initial manifestation of incipient uncal herniation is involvement of the IIIrd nerve ipsilateral to the mass lesion, causing a sluggish reaction to light which is followed by fixed pupillary dilatation. This occurs because the parasympathetic fibres lie outermost and are therefore involved at an early stage. Alteration of consciousness occurs because of involvement of the anterior reticular activating system (RAS). Following this there may be compression of the ipsilateral posterior cerebral artery against the tentorial edge which may lead to occlusion and haemorrhagic infarction of the occipital lobe. The herniated uncus causes the midbrain to be shifted and compressed against the rigid dura on the contralateral side causing damage to the cerebral peduncles, particularly affecting fibres that project to the leg leading to a hemiparesis ipsilateral to the lesion and a worsening IIIrd nerve palsy. The rigid tentorium carves out a notch on the lateral aspect of the midbrain (Kernohan's notch). Tearing of the paramedian perforating vessels is caused by torsion, anteroposterior elongation and downward displacement of the midbrain and leads to consequent brainstem infarction and haemorrhage. The dilated pupil may become a little smaller as the sympathetic pathway in the brainstem is damaged, while with further brainstem compression the other pupil becomes midsized and unresponsive. Established oculomotor paresis appears, first in the eye originally involved and shortly afterwards in the other eye.

Survivors of tentorial herniation may be left in a locked-in or vegetative state or may demonstrate other signs of residual brainstem damage including oculomotor nerve dysfunction, INO, vertical gaze paresis, homonymous hemianopia or blindness, pyramidal limb weakness, parkinsonism or other extrapyramidal syndromes. Tentorial herniation may occasionally be arrested and reversed without residual deficit. Imaging may show the presence of small intrinsic brainstem haemorrhages (Duret haemorrhages) (Figure 20.8).

Central herniation of the brainstem

This occurs as a result of diffuse symmetrical raised ICP often because of cerebral oedema or obstructive hydrocephalus. Downward displacement of the hemispheres leads to compression of the diencephalon and midbrain and descent through the tentorial notch. Characteristic patterns of brainstem descent were described by Plum and Posner, but these are now rarely observed in practice because of early therapeutic intervention. They outlined that initially compression of the midbrain leads to impairment of

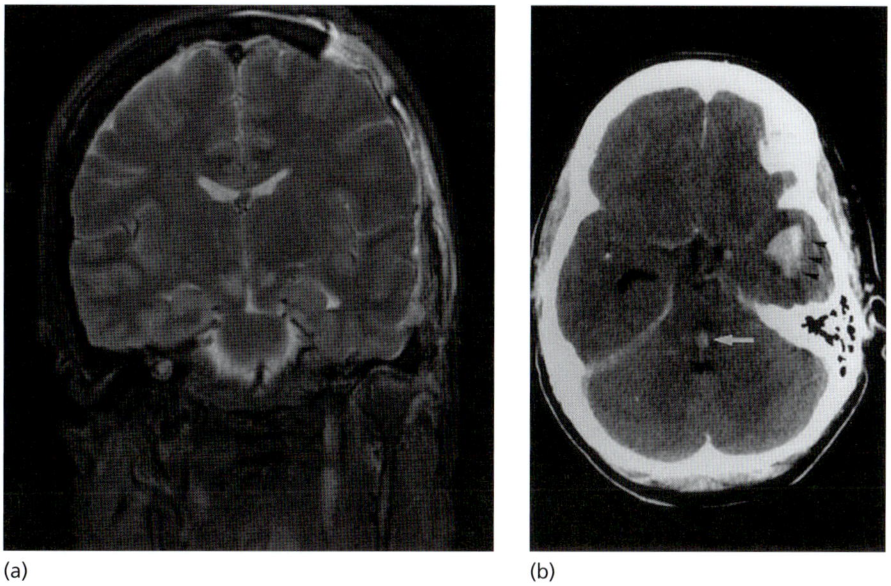

Figure 20.8 (a) Uncal herniation (MRI, T2-weighted coronal); (b) Duret haemorrhage (arrow) (CT scan). Source: Parizel 2002. Reproduced with permission of Springer Science + Business Media.

concentration and alertness leading to progressive somnolence and reduced levels of consciousness. The pupils remain reactive but constricted, because of involvement of sympathetic pathways, and roving eye movements are gradually lost with progressive compression. With increasing supratentorial pressure there is a further downward shift leading to compression and torsion of the pons with rupture of the paramedian perforating arteries. With progressive descent of the brainstem the patient becomes deeply unconscious with abnormal patterns of respiration and temperature control. The pupils are unequal, unreactive, midsized and irregular. Vestibulo-ocular reflexes may elicit restricted vertical gaze, but then a progressive total ophthalmoplegia develops. Eventually there may be decerebrate posturing to painful stimuli prior to the development of hypotension, apnoea, cardiac arrhythmia and death.

Subfalcine herniation

This occurs when the cingulate gyrus is displaced across the midline and under the falx. It is usually caused by a structural lesion in the frontal lobe but may follow a traumatic injury. There may be compression of the ipsilateral anterior cerebral artery with secondary frontal infarction and oedema.

Upward transtentorial herniation

Upward transtentorial hernation of the brainstem may rarely occur as a result of lesions that compress the upper brainstem including tumour or haemorrhage in the pons, cerebellum or region of the 4th ventricle, particularly if any resulting hydrocephalus is drained. The tectum of the midbrain and the anterior cerebellar lobules are forced upwards through the tentorium leading to signs of brainstem dysfunction: small, asymmetrical and fixed pupils, vertical ophthalmoplegia and abnormal respiratory patterns leading to decerebrate posturing and coma.

Tonsillar herniation

Tonsillar herniation occurs if there is downward displacement of inferior medial cerebellar tonsils into the foramen magnum. This may be caused by an Arnold–Chiari malformation or a posterior fossa mass lesion. There may be progressive medullary compression and ischaemia characterised by a sudden respiratory arrest with quadriplegia or the development of a stiff neck, vomiting, skew deviation of the eyes, respiratory irregularity, coma and death.

Traumatic brain injury

Head injury causes acceleration and deceleration of the skull which results in rotational forces on the supratentorial brain exerting shearing forces on the grey and white matter tracts and vessels, and traction on the midbrain and hypothalamic reticular neurones. Damage to the brain following trauma includes the immediate, or primary, injury caused at the moment of impact, and the secondary injury that develops in the first few hours or days after the impact which may result from extracranial or intracranial causes.

The consequences of severe TBI are summarised below:

1 *Primary brain injury*
- Disruption of brain vessels
- Haemorrhagic contusion
- Diffuse axonal injury

2 *Secondary brain injury*

Intracranial causes:
- Lobar contusion
- Intracranial haemorrhage (extradural, subdural or intracerebral) causing raised ICP or herniation
- Raised ICP caused by to brain swelling around a contusion or diffusely within the brain.

Extracranial causes:
- Systemic hypotension (systolic BP <90 mmHg)
- Hypoxaemia (PaO_2 <60 mmHg)
- Hypercarbia (high blood CO_2)
- Disturbances of blood coagulation.

Early management should follow Advanced Trauma Life Support guidelines:
- Stabilisation of the airway, breathing and circulation
- Attention to cervical spine trauma
- Neurological assessment.

At present, no neuroprotective agent has been shown to reduce primary brain injury. However, secondary insults, which further exacerbate neuronal injury and lead to a worse outcome, are often preventable with prompt intervention. Over one-third of all patients with severe TBI develop hypoxia and/or hypotension during the acute post-injury period. These secondary insults are correlated with a large increase in morbidity and mortality.

Skull fractures

Skull fractures occur three times more commonly in the vault than the base of the skull and are associated with a high incidence of intracranial haematomas. If the fracture is open (involves the basal air sinuses) or depressed, then surgical intervention is required. Clinical indicators of a base of skull fracture include periorbital bruising (panda or racoon eyes), retro-auricular bruising over the mastoid process (Battle sign), blood in the tympanic membrane (haemotympanum) and an associated CSF leak from the nose (rhinorrhoea) or the ears (otorrhoea). Eighty per cent of CSF leaks close spontaneously but bacterial meningitis may complicate some cases. There is no evidence to support the use of routine antibiotic prophylaxis for skull fractures.

Extradural haematoma

An extradural haematoma (Figure 20.9) is an accumulation of blood in the extradural space between the inner side of the skull and the dura mater. Most (>90%) are associated with skull fracture and are caused by injury of the middle meningeal artery, therefore affecting the parietal and tempero-parietal areas. Rarely, a fracture may be associated with tearing of large veins at the vertex of the skull or of the venous sinuses. Associated brain contusion is less common than with subdural haematoma (SDH). There is typically a lucid interval after the injury in which the patient temporarily regains consciousness. The outcome depends on the level of consciousness at the time of surgery, with mortality approaching 20% if the patient is unconscious prior to surgery.

Subdural haematoma

A subdural haematoma (SDH) is an accumulation of blood between the inner side of the dura and the arachnoid layer (Figure 20.10). It is either due to tearing of cortical veins when the haemotoma is usually frontal, or small arteries, when it is more often temporo-parietal. Most patients with acute SDH have an accompanying brain injury and their prognosis is worse than those with extradural haematoma. The patient is usually unconscious or there is impaired alertness, cognition with focal signs – continued deterioration is usual. Acute SDH can present with seizures. A poor outcome is more likely if the trauma is severe with underlying brain contusion, the SDHs are bilateral, accumulated rapidly, or if there was >4 hours delay in surgical management. CT imaging allows assessment of skull fracture, contusion and haemorrhage

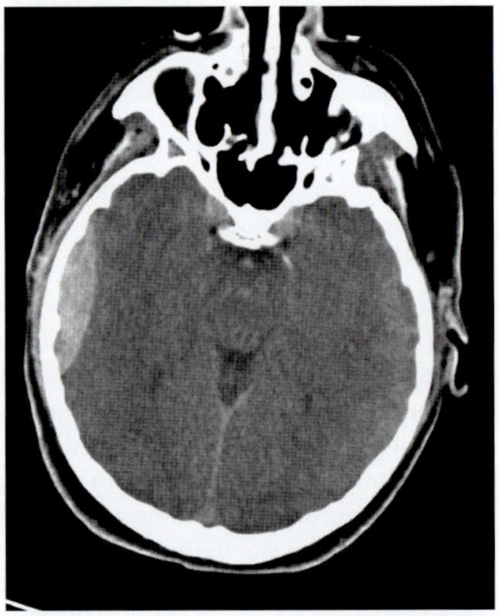

Figure 20.9 CT scan showing acute extradural haematoma.

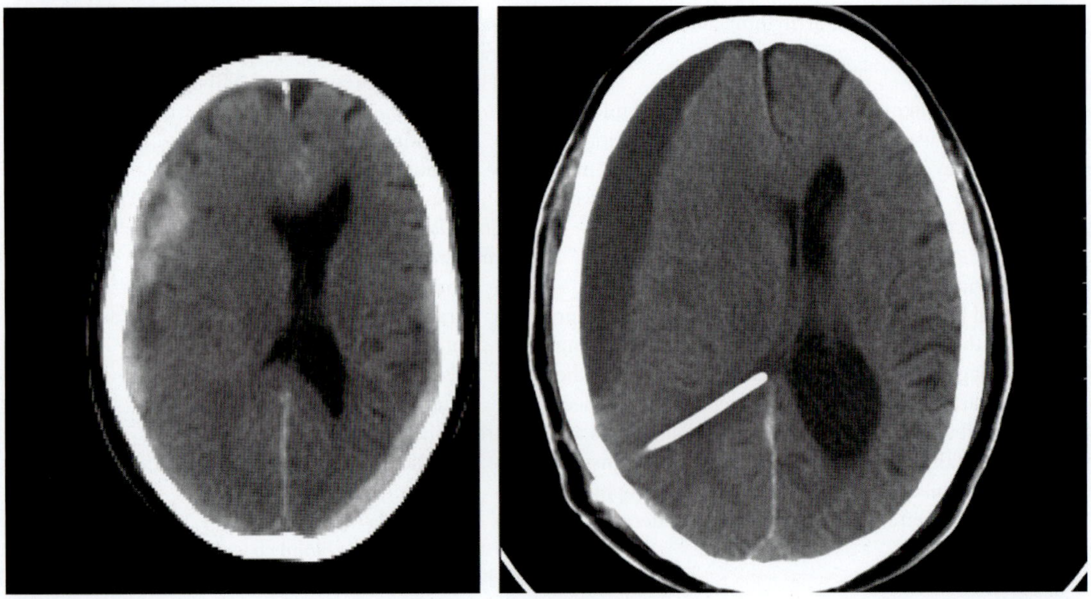

(a) (b)

Figure 20.10 CT scan showing: (a) extensive fresh bilateral acute subdural haematoma with midline shift; and (b) large chronic subdural haematoma following insertion of intraventricular shunt.

but SDH can become isodense 1–3 weeks after onset or in the presence of anaemia; therefore, in the subacute or chronic state MRI is preferable to CT.

Chronic SDH can develop many weeks or even months after head injury. The injury may be minor and the patient may not remember a particular event. Predisposing factors include increasing age, alcoholism, coagulopathy, epilepsy and the presence of ventricular drains. The most common symptom is headache, which worsens progressively and is associated with a fluctuating level of consciousness, focal signs, seizures and raised ICP. The treatment of choice is evacuation of the subdural collection and irrigation with isotonic saline at body temperature. Many small SDHs are treated conservatively.

Traumatic subarachnoid haemorrhage

Traumatic SAH is seen in 30–40% of patients following severe TBI but must be quantified on early CT scan because later scans underestimate its incidence and severity. Its presence indicates a poor outcome following TBI (Figure 20.11). It is important to ensure that the SAH was not the primary event leading to a fall and secondary head trauma by excluding the presence of an aneurysm.

Haemorrhagic contusions and lacerations

Haemorrhagic contusions and lacerations are superficial areas of haemorrhage usually affecting the frontal and temporal lobes although they may involve deeper structures (Figure 20.12). They are usually caused by venous injury sustained as the brain hits the bony protruberances of the skull at the site of impact and then the opposite side during deceleration (contrecoup injury). The term contusion is used when the pia mater has not been breached, and laceration when the pia mater is torn. Local areas of contusion with no or minimal blood flow are common after severe TBI and the centre of the contusion is often irreversibly damaged. However, areas around the contusion (known as penumbra) are associated with localised cerebral oedema and have survival potential if the oxygen supply to this region is maintained. Focal contusions can be associated with cerebral oedema and raised ICP leading to delayed neurological deterioration and surgical evacuation may be necessary.

Intracerebral haematoma

Intracerebral haematoma usually occurs as a result of direct trauma to intracranial vessels and affects the frontal and temporal lobes or basal ganglia. It is a cause of delayed neurological deterioration in <20% of patients with severe TBI particularly if there is a coagulopathy.

Diffuse axonal injury

Diffuse axonal injury (DAI) occurs in 50–60% of patients with severe head injury and is the most common cause of coma, vegetative state and subsequent disability (Figure 20.13). Severe DAI has three neuropathological components:

1. A focal lesion in the corpus callosum, often associated with traumatic intraventricular haemorrhage
2. Focal lesions in the brainstem, and
3. Widespread microscopic damage to axons, often associated with scattered small haemorrhages, mainly located along or near the grey–white matter interface.

Cerebral ischaemia

Cerebral ischaemia, whether brought about by hypoxia, hypotension or intracranial hypertension, dominates severe TBI and is the single most important factor in determining outcome, with ischaemic lesions being found in 90% of patients at postmortem. Areas of

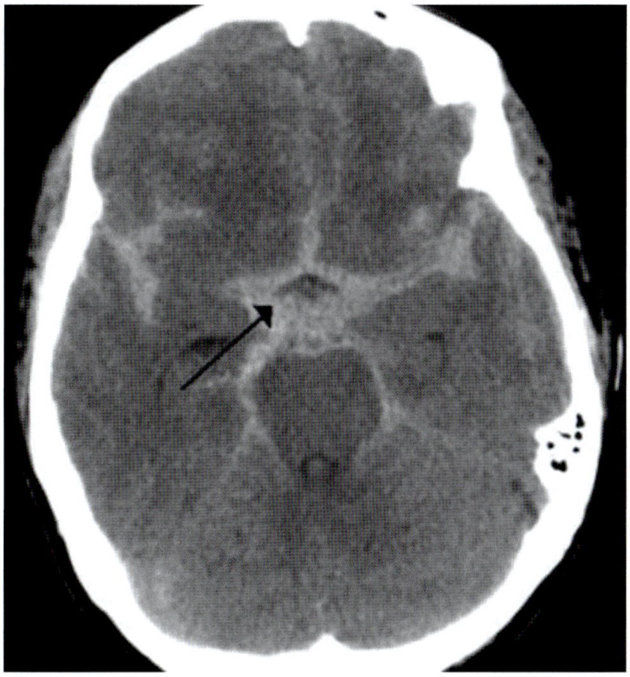

Figure 20.11 CT scan showing traumatic subarachnoid haemorrhage (arrow).

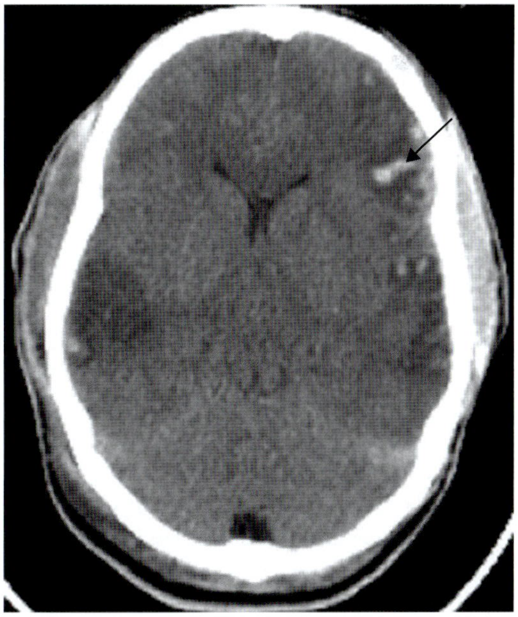

Figure 20.12 CT scan of patient with traumatic brain injury (TBI) showing extensive left temporal contusion (arrow) and laceration with contrecoup injury in right temporal region.

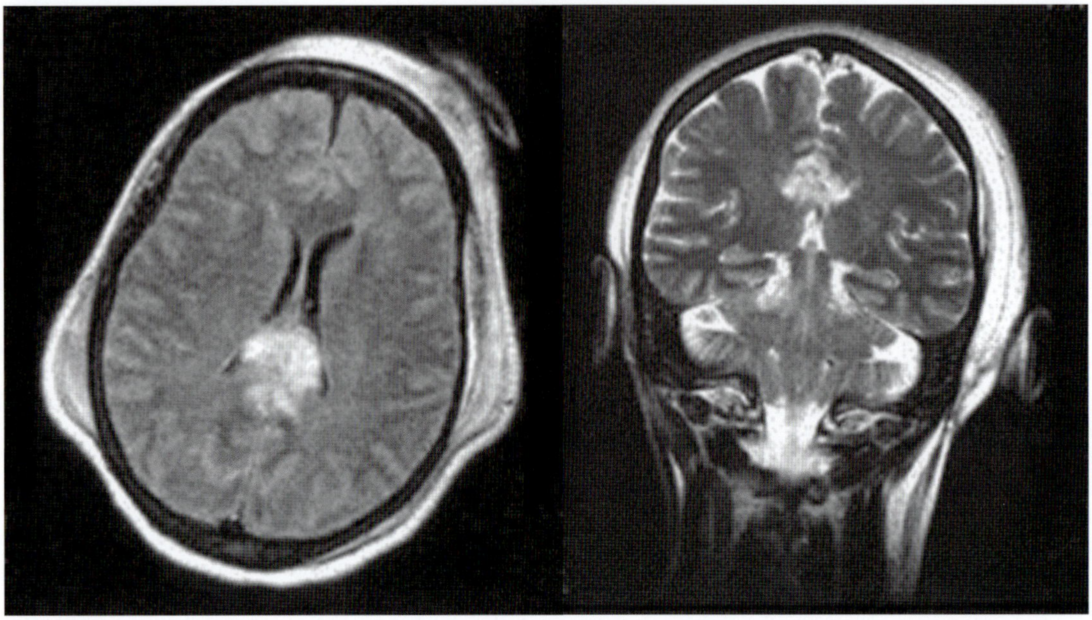

Figure 20.13 Diffuse axonal injury showing extensive haemorrhagic change in the region of the splenium (MRI T1-weighted axial and T2-weighted coronal).

focal ischaemia occur in <50% of patients with SDH or DAI but are rare in patients with extradural haematoma or normal imaging. Blood flow in and around areas of brain tissue damaged by trauma may be abnormal because of vasomotor paralysis with loss of autoregulation leading to impaired blood pressure control and reduced reactivity to carbon dioxide. CBF becomes pressure-dependent, rendering this area of brain more susceptible to ischaemia at lower blood pressures and more likely to sustain injury at higher pressures.

Intensive care management of TBI

The aim of intensive care management of the head-injured patient is to prevent and treat secondary physiological insults.

Monitoring Monitoring of ECG, direct arterial blood pressure, central venous pressure and pulse oximetry is mandatory in all patients. An oesophageal Doppler monitor or pulmonary artery catheter may assist in directing therapy in those patients with haemodynamic instability. Regular arterial blood gas analysis, measurement of blood glucose and sodium and core temperature monitoring are also required to optimise treatment strategies. Cerebral monitoring allows measurement of CPP, estimation of CBF and assessment of the adequacy of oxygen delivery to the brain. This allows therapy to be targeted to specific changes in brain function and to ensure a balance between cerebral metabolic supply and demand. Monitoring may include measurement of ICP, transcranial Doppler ultrasonography (TCD) of blood flow velocity in the middle cerebral artery and jugular venous bulb oximetry to assess the balance between cerebral oxygen supply and demand after head injury.

Paroxysmal sympathetic hyperactivity Episodes of paroxysmal sympathetic hyperactivity (autonomic storms) occur in patients with severe TBI particularly with diffuse axonal injury, following HIBI, SAH, intracerebral haemorrhage and hydrocephalus. Manifestations typically include fluctuation in temperature, blood pressure, heart rate, respiratory rate, sweating and muscle tone. Pupillary dilatation, intense flushing and severe dystonia may also be present. The episodes recur regularly and last for between 1 and 10 hours. They tend to reduce in frequency with time. It is suggested that the episodes are caused by activity of the diencephalic or brainstem sympathoexcitatory regions as a result of direct activation or inhibition secondary to loss of cortical and subcortical control. The episodes may be induced by stimulation or may occur spontaneously. They may be confused with seizures or other paroxysmal syndromes including malignant hyperthermia, neurologic malignant syndrome, sepsis or the response to raised ICP. The management includes ensuring adequate hydration, exclusion of mimicking conditions (infection, pulmonary embolism, hydrocephalus, epilepsy), effective analgesia and avoidance of triggers. The most useful pharmacological agents are non-selective beta-blockers (e.g. propranolol), opiates and clonidine.

ICP after TBI ICP monitoring is indicated for all patients with head injury with any abnormality on CT scan who do not obey commands. Conventional approaches to the management of patients with head injury have concentrated on a reduction in ICP to prevent secondary ischaemic insults. ICP >20 mmHg and CPP <60 mmHg are powerful predictors of outcome together with age, admission GCS and pupillary signs. Aggressive management, based on ICP monitoring, significantly reduces the overall mortality rate without causing a disproportionate number of severely disabled or vegetative patients.

Decompressive craniectomy Decompressive craniectomy is based on the concept of reducing the pressure buildup within the intracranial bony compartment resulting from brain swelling (compartment syndrome) by removal of skull bone (at least 12 cm flap) and opening the dural membranes. This allows improved compliance, reduced ICP and improved blood supply to the brain. Craniectomy decreases the mean ICP and the duration of both

Table 20.13 Indications for decompressive surgery.

Intracranial mass lesions with midline shift or basal cistern compression on CT scan
A surgically significant EDH or acute SDH needs evacuation within 2–4 hours of injury to achieve optimal chance of recovery
For small haemorrhagic contusions or other small intracerebral lesions a conservative approach is generally adopted but operation should be considered urgent for a large ICH (>20–30 mL) based on position, clinical condition and ICP
Skull fractures that are depressed > skull thickness and compound fractures with torn dura require surgery

CT, computed tomography; EDH, extradural haematoma; ICH, intracerebral haematoma; ICP, intracranial pressure; SDH, subdural haematoma.

ventilatory support and ICU stay but is associated with a significantly worse outcome at 6 months so the role of decompressive surgery remains uncertain. The indications for decompressive surgery are summarised in Table 20.13.

Hydrocephalus and shunts

Hydrocephalus may be defined as excessive CSF. It can be caused by excess production, altered flow through the ventricular system and/or impaired reabsorption into the venous system circulation via the arachnoid granulations. Such is the importance of CSF that Harvey Cushing, one of the founders of neurosurgery, called it the 'fourth circulation'.

Clinically, hydrocephalus can be divided into communicating and non-communicating. Communicating (non-obstructive) hydrocephalus denotes an enlarged ventricular system but normal communication and flow between the ventricles and the extracerebral CSF. The aetiology is impaired absorption while non -communicating (obstructive) hydrocephalus results from obstruction to the normal CSF pathways.

Sometimes both categories of hydrocephalus are distinct (e.g. communicating hydrocephalus secondary to SAH and non-communicating hydrocephalus secondary to a colloid cyst of the 3rd ventricle). However, they may coexist (e.g. an intraventricular or skull base tumour causing some obstruction but also producing a highly proteinaceous CSF or chronic meningitis leading to impaired reabsorption of CSF). It is also important to differentiate between acute hydrocephalus (which has more rapid and devastating consequences including herniation and death) and chronic hydrocephalus.

Arrested hydrocephalus applies to those adult patients who have some developmental hydrocephalus and abnormality of the brain development resulting in large ventricles and often large heads but who are well. Occasionally, these patients decompensate later in life and can present with headaches and/or ataxia or more acutely following what would otherwise be a minor head injury. Hydrocephalus *ex vacuo* describes apparent enlargement secondary to cerebral volume loss for any reason. Normal pressure hydrocephalus (NPH) describes a mild degree of hydrocephalus where the CSF pressure is intermittently raised. Clearly, this condition of NPH and hydrocephalus *ex vacuo* would need to be distinguished in the elderly population where the rare triad of cognitive failure, urinary incontinence and gait apraxia associated with NPH may be incomplete.

The presenting features of hydrocephalus depend on its aetiology and rate of development and the presence of raised ICP. For example, a sudden collapse into coma and even sudden death can occur in rare instances of colloid cysts obstructing the 3rd ventricle outflow, whereas the gradual development of non-communicating hydrocephalus will result in headache and papilloedema progressing to a gait disturbance before more obvious symptoms and signs of raised ICP develop.

Investigations

Imaging (CT or MRI) will define ventricular size and therefore show enlargement. Imaging also gives an indirect indication of raised ICP (e.g. periventricular lucency, ventricular to sulcal effacement and differential size of the different parts of the ventricular system). It is important to reflect on both the ventricular volume and the presumptive pressure before deciding on a management plan. Investigation of patients with suspected NPH is controversial. Walking tests following lumbar puncture, lumbar infusion and concomitant ICP measurements as well as isotope cisternography have been used to determine the pressure–volume relationship.

Management

Frequently, conservative management is appropriate, particularly in those cases of arrested hydrocephalus. The mainstay of active treatment involves either a shunt or third ventriculostomy. With a shunt procedure CSF is channelled via a hollow silicon tube between the ventricular system and the peritoneum. Other sites can be used such as the right atrium and occasionally the pleura. Shunts have the advantage of being simple and relatively reliable. However, they do have a failure rate that accumulates over time secondary to blockage and they can also become infected despite the numerous proprietary attempts to either impregnate them with antibiotics and/or the use of non-touch techniques by surgeons and peri-operative antibiotics. The shunts themselves range from the very simple to those with anti-siphon devices and programmable options where the flow may be altered to suit the response of the patient. These may be particularly appropriate in those patients with relatively low raised pressure, typically NPH, where over-drainage would be a serious complication.

Endoscopic third ventriculostomy is an increasingly used technique in which a hole is fashioned in the thinned floor of the 3rd ventricle such that the ventricular CSF communicates directly with the basal cisterns. This is particularly useful in cases of aqueduct stenosis or tumours in the posterior fossa and midbrain and thus this technique is far more commonly used in paediatric than in adult patients. In the acute clinical situation, such as hydrocephalus secondary to meningitis or SAH, particularly where the protein level is very high and/or when intrathecal antibiotics are to be administered, then a temporary shunt or external ventricular drain is inserted, which may be converted to a shunt at a later date. Finally, lumboperitoneal shunts are used on occasion, particularly when there is a technical issue in cannulating the ventricular system, usually when the ventricles are small and the pressures are high and very typically in idiopathic intracranial hypertension.

Stroke (Chapter 5)

The principles of assessment and resuscitation from acute stroke are similar regardless of the underlying cause and include the following:

- Airway management – tracheal intubation is indicated when there is:
  - impaired level of consciousness (GCS <9)
  - progressive respiratory impairment or respiratory failure

  - impaired cough and airway clearance
  - pulmonary oedema/aspiration
  - seizure activity
  - a need for diagnostic or therapeutic procedures such as MRI or thrombolysis
- Maintenance of adequate arterial blood pressure–cerebral perfusion pressure
- Intravenous fluid management
- Temperature control
- Control of seizures
- Institution of enteral nutrition
- ICP management
- Medical treatment of complications (e.g. sepsis)
- Other management related to the underlying cause (e.g. anticoagulation, thrombolysis, evacuation of haematoma, clipping and coiling of intracerebral aneurysms)
- Decompressive hemicraniectomy (Figure 20.14).

Late deterioration following stroke occurs for a number of reasons.

Middle cerebral artery occlusion

Late clinical deterioration following middle cerebral artery (MCA) occlusion is common and depends on the severity, localisation and pathology. It is associated with cerebral oedema, which usually develops after 2–7 days and causes a mass effect leading to horizontal and vertical distortion and shift of the brainstem. This change in dynamics may not be reflected by ICP monitors. Other causes of deterioration include haemorrhagic conversion of the infarct, which may produce diencephalic brain herniation, the development of seizures and systemic factors including congestive cardiac failure, pulmonary oedema, cardiac arrhythmias or pulmonary emboli.

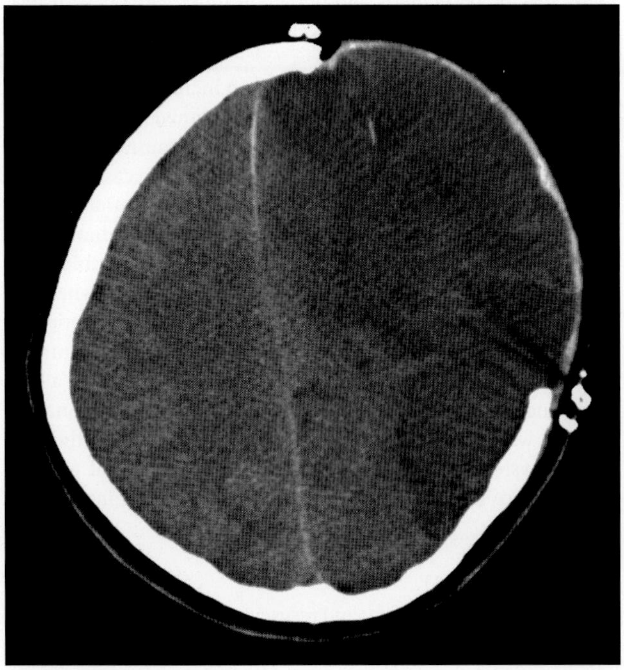

Figure 20.14 Maligant middle cerebral artery (MCA) syndrome. Axial CT demonstrating a large left MCA infarct with a decompressive frontal craniectomy and herniation of swollen brain through the defect.

Acute basilar occlusion

Following acute basilar occlusion, late deterioration occurs in up to one-third of patients because of extension of the thrombus causing successive occlusion of the perforating arteries or because of emboli arising from the occluded vessel.

Artery of Percheron

This is a rare vascular variant in which a single dominant thalamoperforating artery arises from one posterior cerebral artery and supplies both paramedian thalami. Occlusion of this vessel results in bilateral paramedian thalamic infarction with or without mesencephalic infarction. This is an uncommon but important cause of altered consciousness or coma.

Cerebellar infarcts

These are associated with progression of infarction leading to brainstem involvement and herniation, late brainstem compression arising from cerebral oedema around the infarct, the development of hydrocephalus from obstruction of 3rd and 4th ventricles, aqueduct or outflow and systemic complications. Occasionally, decompressive surgery is necessary.

Subarachnoid haemorrhage

The acute management of SAH is summarised in Table 20.14. Sudden death may occur following SAH in up to 10% because of early rebleeding, intraventricular extension of the haemorrhage or complications including pulmonary aspiration, cardiac arrhythmias and neurogenic pulmonary oedema. Clinical deterioration may also develop because of delayed cerebral ischaemia from progressive vasospasm, enlargement of intracerebral haematoma or the development of hydrocephalus.

Supratentorial intracerebral haemorrhage (basal ganglia or lobar)

This is associated with enlargement of the haematoma, development of surrounding oedema, obstructive hydrocephalus or systemic complications including aspiration pneumonia, sepsis or cardiac arrhythmias.

Infratentorial intracranial haemorrhage (cerebellar or brainstem)

Following infratentorial intracranial haemorrhage (cerebellar or brainstem), clinical deterioration is commonly caused by direct brainstem compression accompanied by cerebellar herniation rather than obstructive hydrocephalus. Rebleeding is a neurosurgical emergency and the high mortality often justifies surgical evacuation. The management of intracerebral haemorrhage is summarised in Table 20.15.

Cerebral venous thrombosis

Late complications of cerebral venous thrombosis include extension of the thrombosis, development of haemorrhagic infarction, raised ICP secondary to cerebral oedema, seizures, the development of systemic complications including aspiration pneumonia, pulmonary emboli and sepsis and complications of a hypercoagulable state (Figure 20.15). Deep cerebral venous thrombosis due to involvement of the deep cerebral veins causes venous infarction and oedema of the thalamus which can be markedly asymmetric and can also involve the basal ganglia. There may be severe impairment of consciousness or coma, particularly if there is bilateral thalamic swelling causing 3rd ventricular compression and hydrocephalus.

Table 20.14 Acute management of subarachnoid haemorrhage (SAH) (SBP Systolic blood pressure; MAP, Mean arterial blood pressure; SIADH, Syndrome of Inappropriate ADH secretion; CSF, cerebrospinal fluid).

Airway management
Investigation and monitoring
Treatment of systemic complications
Hypoxaemia
Metabolic Acidosis
Hypovolaemia
Hyper / Hypoglycaemia
Cardiac – arrhythmia, stunned myocardium
Pulmonary – neurogenic pulmonary oedema
Hyponatraemia due to haemodilution, SIADH, cerebral salt wasting
Pyrexia, anaemia, pain, constipation
DVT prophylaxis
Reverse anticoagulation
Treatment of ruptured aneurysm
Endovascular coiling
Surgical clipping
Prevention of rebleeding
Definitive endovascular or surgical aneurysm repair
Treatment of acute hypertension and predisposing factors (pain, anxiety, agitation)
Role of antifibrinolytic agents (controversial)
Cardiovascular
Maintain BP in high normal range (SBP <160; MAP<110mmHg)
Hypotension - IV crystalloids and vasopressors (metaraminol / noradrenaline)
If systolic BP> 160mmHg treat with antihypertensives (labetolol / hydaralazine/nicardipine)
Treatment of seizures (prophylaxis not indicated)
Treatment of hydrocephalus
Temporary external ventricular drainage
CSF diversion via ventricular shunts
Prevention of delayed cerebral ischaemia / vasospasm
Nimdipine (60mg 4hrly for 21 days)
(Triple 'H' therapy) if aneurysm secured
Prevention of hypovolaemia – IV crystalloid and colloids (>300ml/24hr)
Hypertension - supranormal bp is maintained using IV crystalloids, vasopressors
Haemodilution – (controversial)
Others – statins, removal of subarachnoid blood

Seizures (Chapter 7)

Seizures on the ICU are usually focal or generalised motor convulsions, although all seizure types occur. Common precipitants are hypoxia–ischaemia, drug toxicity, narcotic withdrawal and metabolic abnormalities (Table 20.16). It is essential to diagnose the seizure type and cause to ensure early appropriate treatment and

Table 20.15 ICU management of intracerebral haemorrhage (ICH).

Airway management
Investigation and monitoring
BP control – controversial
Systolic BP (SBP)>180mmHg or mean arterial pressure (MAP) > 130mmHg - continuous infusion of antihypertensive (labetolol or nicardipine)
Do not reduce MAP > 25% in first 24 hours or below baseline BP
Haemostatic therapy
Reversal of anticoagulation (iv vitamin K., fresh frozen plasma or coagulation factors)
Recombinant factor VII (rFVII) is unproven
Raised intracranial pressure (ICP)/ cerebral oedema
Positioning (head up >30°)
Anaesthesia and sedation
ICP monitor (if coma, mass effect, intraventricular extension, hydrocephalus)
Pressor agents to optimise cerebral perfusion pressure (CPP)
Osmotherapy (20% mannitol 1.0-1.5g/kg IVI)
Hyperventilation (PaO_2 3.5-4.0KPa)
Hypothermia (unproven)
Surgical intervention (ventricular drainage or definitive intervention)
Control of:
Seizures (prophylactic antiepileptic drugs not indicated)
Temperature (>38°)
Hypoglycaemia (Aim for glucose 8-10mm/L)
Swallowing & aspiration (nil by mouth, nasogastric tube)
DVT prophylaxis (stockings, pneumatic compression, low MW heparin introduced 1-4 days after ICH)
BP management – aim for SBP 160, MAP 110 mmHg (controversial)
SBP>200 or MAP>150 – aggressive bp reduction (labetalol)
SBP>180 or MAP>130 and raised ICP –maintain CPP between 61–80mmHg
SBP>180 or MAP>130 – modest reduction in bp
Surgical intervention (controversial)
Extraventricular drainage for hydrocephalus
Craniotomy and clot evacuation (e.g. cerebellar haematoma)
Endoscopic guidance techniques
Hemicraniectomy

CPP, cerebral perfusion pressure; ICP, intracranial pressure; MAP, mean arterial blood pressure.

differentiation from metabolic myoclonus and extrapyramidal movement disorders. Non-convulsive status epilepticus (NCSE) is common and a poorly recognised cause of coma. Classic ictal signs may be absent and diagnosis may depend on the observation of subtle movements of fingers, eyes or lips. NCSE should be considered where there is abrupt deterioration in conscious level without explanation, often following a recognised seizure or after anoxic ischaemic insult with preserved brainstem reflexes. Convulsive status is less common. EEG monitoring can be helpful.

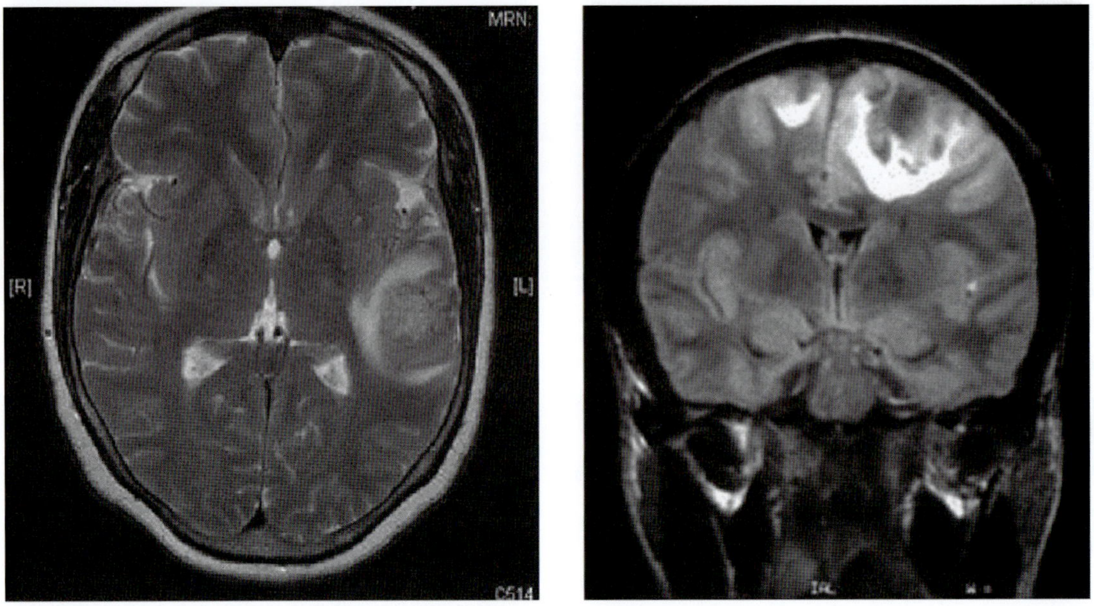

(a) (b)

Figure 20.15 Extensive haemorrhagic venous infarction. (a) T2 axial MRI; (b) FLAIR coronal MRI.

Table 20.16 Causes of partial or generalised status epilepticus in an ITU setting.

Acute	Chronic
Head injury	Pre-existing epilepsy
CNS infection (encephalitis, meningitis)	Poor antiepilepsy drug compliance
Cerebrovascular accident	Dosage alteration
Renal failure	Chronic alcoholism/alcohol withdrawal
Sepsis syndrome	Cerebral space-occupying lesion
Drug toxicity	
Electrolyte imbalance	
Hypoglycaemia	
Hypoxic – ischaemic brain injury	
Pseudostatus	
Benzodiazepine or other suppressant withdrawal	

Myoclonic status and Lance-Adams syndrome are discussed later.

Status epilepticus (SE)

Following adequate resuscitation, the treatment of status epilepticus (Chapter 7) in the NICU has four simultaneous aims:

- termination of seizures;
- prevention of seizure recurrence once status is controlled;
- management of the precipitating causes;
- management of the complications.

Monitoring respiratory and cardiac function and continuous EEG (cEEG) recording is necessary in prolonged and refractory status. The appropriate titration of anaesthetic agents during status epilepticus may be based on the appearance of burst or, preferably, total suppression on the EEG. cEEG recording will give an indication of worsening or recurrent status epilepticus regardless of the presence or absence of sedating drugs or paralysing agents.

The underlying cause of SE can require urgent treatment. Causes include acute bacterial meningitis or viral encephalitis, cerebral vascular disease due to emboli, arterial occlusion or venous sinus thrombosis, withdrawal of anti-epilepsy drugs or alcohol. Autoimmune limbic or brainstem encephalitides (e.g. *N*-methyl-D-aspartate [NMDA] and VGKCAb) can cause SE and can require immunomodulatory treatment.

The complications of status epilepticus relate either to the cerebral and metabolic consequences of prolonged seizures or to the effects of medical treatment. Cardiopulmonary problems include the development of aspiration pneumonia, adult respiratory distress syndrome, deep vein thrombosis, pulmonary emboli, myocardial ischaemia and cardiac arrhythmia. Hyperthermia is common and rhabdomyolysis may develop. Prolonged hypoxia may cause cerebral damage whilst electrolyte disturbance, and metabolic acidosis may contribute to the development of multi-organ failure. Many drug treatments used in status epilepticus cause sedation, respiratory depression and hypotension. Artificial ventilation is required if general anaesthesia is indicated or if the seizures remain difficult to control. It is also necessary to maintain systemic blood pressure at normal or supranormal levels to ensure adequate cerebral perfusion. Fluid resuscitation and/or inotropic support should be guided by appropriate cardiovascular monitoring.

Acute bacterial meningitis

The mortality and morbidity of acute meningitis in adults remain substantial, particularly if there is a delay in initiating treatment and monitoring complications (Chapter 9). Patients with meningitis are usually admitted to an ICU when in coma, with complications such as seizures, cerebral oedema and tentorial herniation, or because they have developed systemic problems including septicaemia, pulmonary aspiration or cardiopulmonary compromise. Late deterioration

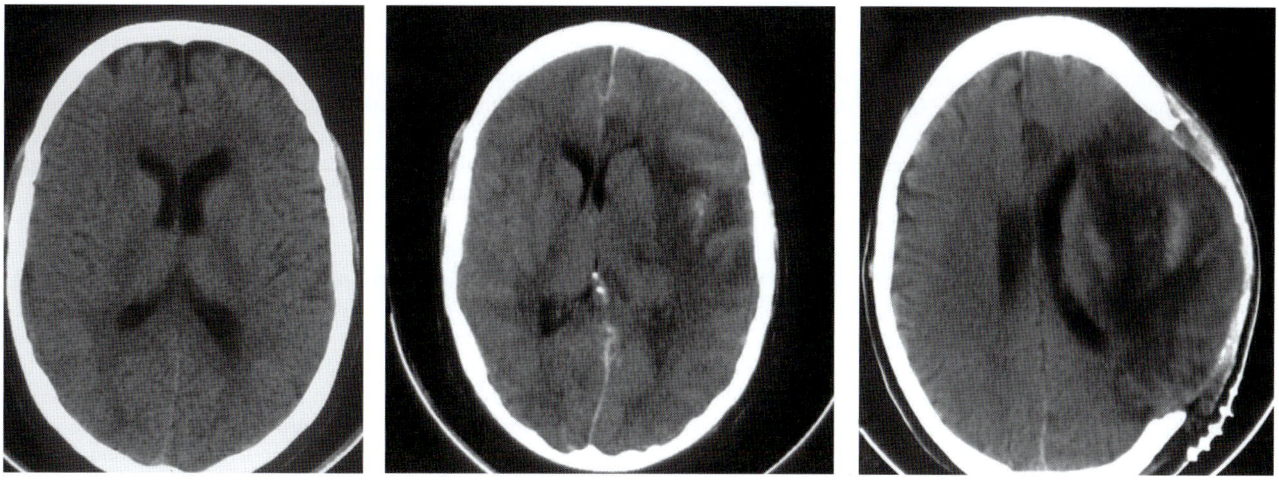

Figure 20.16 Sequence of CT scans in a patient with herpes simplex encephalitis showing progressive hemispheric swelling and decompression.

following acute bacterial meningitis may be caused by antibiotic resistance or by the development of cerebral oedema, subdural effusion or empyema, superior sagittal sinus thrombosis, hydrocephalus, vasculitis, or systemic complications including pericardial effusion and polyarteritis.

Herpes simplex encephalitis

Clinical deterioration in this condition is usually the result of severe cerebral oedema with diencephalic herniation or systemic complications, including generalised sepsis and aspiration (Chapter 9). Furthermore, progressive worsening of focal seizures may lead to status epilepticus. Aggressive treatment including tracheal intubation and mechanical ventilation with appropriate sedation should be instituted and seizures treated. Prolonged sedation or general anaesthesia may be necessary. Decompressive craniotomy may be successful in cases where there is rapid swelling of a non-dominant temporal lobe (Figure 20.16).

Autoimmune encephalopathy

Antibodies directed against cell-surface neuronal antigens are associated with central nervous system disorders which present with encephalopathy or seizures requiring intensive care. They often respond to immunotherapies.

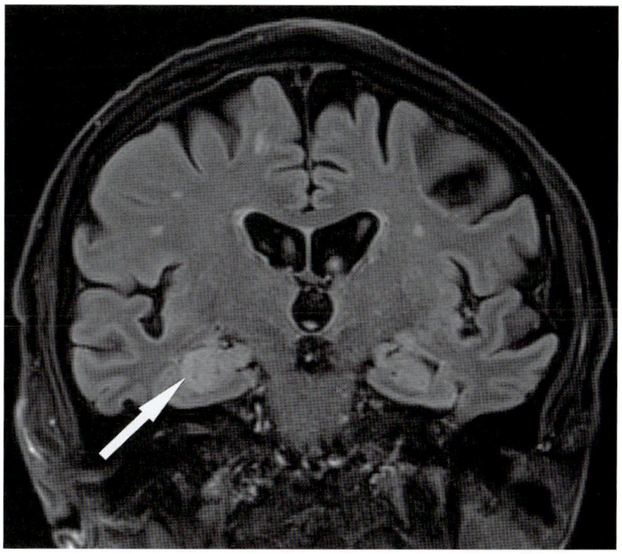

Figure 20.17 Limbic encephalitis. FLAIR coronal image showing swelling and abnormally high signal within the right hippocampal formation (arrow).

Limbic encephalitis associated with neuronal surface antigens

Limbic encephalitis (LE) typically present with acute to subacute onset of memory loss, confusion and seizures. There may be psychiatric/behavioural disturbances. Patients with VGKC-complex-antibodies (generally LGI1Ab) may present to intensive care because of worsening encephalopathy with hyponatraemia due to inappropriate antidiuretic hormone (ADH) secretion or because of seizures. MRI typically shows evidence of hippocampal swelling, inflammation and high signal in the medial temporal lobes (Figure 20.17). The EEG is abnormal with diffuse slowing and occasional temporal epileptogenic foci and CSF may be normal or show a mild lymphocytosis with unmatched oligoclonal bands. Encephalopathy due to VGKC-complex antibodies may be amenable to immunotherapy and some patients respond well to high-dose oral corticosteroids, pulsed methyl prednisolone, plasma exchange and/or immunoglobulin. The seizures often cease and hyponatraemia resolves but patients may be left with prolonged encephalopathy and late-onset hippocampal sclerosis. LE may also be associated with AMPA receptor and $GABA_B$ antibodies, there is often a tendency for these forms to relapse and require longer term immunosuppression.

Morvan's syndrome

Morvan's syndrome is characterised by muscle fasciculation and cramp. However, the presence of autonomic disturbance and CNS involvement manifests as sleep disturbance, particularly insomnia, and hallucinations may require admission to intensive care. Patients with antibodies to the VGKC-complex-protein CASPR2 commonly have neuromyotonia and there is a significant incidence of underlying tumour (often thymoma).

Encephalitis due to NMDA receptor antibodies

This condition is distinct from LE with much more extensive involvement of brain function. The onset is generally with psychiatric or behavioural disturbances. Seizures develop and worsen over 2 to 3 weeks before evolving into severe and, occasionally life-threatening, dyskinesia (orofacial grimacing, dystonic posturing and choreoathetoid movements). There is often autonomic instability and reduced consciousness which may require prolonged ventilatory support. The CSF may show pleocytosis, intrathecal synthesis of oligoclonal bands and positive antibodies. MRI is generally normal but may show mild abnormalities in the cerebral cortex, meninges or basal ganglia. The condition is often associated with ovarian tumour (usually teratoma) in women, or other tumours in men and women (e.g. lymphoma) but this is not invariable and there is a separate autoimmune form of the condition. The syndrome often responds to removal of the tumour and immunotherapy but recovery may be prolonged and in some cases the outcome is very poor with a significant mortality amongst patients who require prolonged intensive care. Treatment is with immunomodulation with steroids, plasma exchange or IVIg but long-term immunosuppression with cyclophosphamide or rituximab is often necessary and relapses can occur in up to 25% of non-paraneoplastic patients.

Steroid responsive encephalopathy

This condition is often associated with raised thyroid antibodies and was previously called Hashimoto's encephalopathy. There is a slow impairment of consciousness with episodic confusion often associated with agitation, hallucinations, tremor, recurrent stroke-like episodes and cognitive impairment. There may be raised microsomal, peroxidase or anti-thyroglobulin thyroid antibodies at variable titres. The condition may be prolonged but responds well to steroids and is likely to be autoimmune mediated although the thyroid antibodies are unlikely to be pathogenic.

Other antibody-mediated encephalomyelopathies

Stiff person syndrome and PERM (progressive encephalomyelopathy with rigidity and myoclonus) are discussed in Movement disorder emergencies.

Metabolic encephalopathy

Acute metabolic encephalopathy can be considered as an acute condition of global cerebral dysfunction in the absence of primary structural brain disease. The diagnosis includes delirium and acute confusional states. The pathophysiology of metabolic encephalopathy varies according to the cause but all forms interfere with the function of the ascending reticular activating system and its cortical projections leading to impairment of arousal and awareness. All causes of metabolic encephalopathy are characterised by impaired and fluctuating attention and cognition from mild memory loss to severe delirium or coma. Marked variation in the mental status over times is characteristic. While metabolic encephalopathy is often treatable, the clinical course can be protracted, with neurological recovery often lagging behind recovery of the underlying condition.

If prolonged sedation has been excluded, the most common cause of depressed consciousness is a metabolic encephalopathy which may be a result of one or more causes. The diagnosis can be difficult in an unconscious patient and careful assessment of medication, sepsis, metabolic status and fluid balance is essential.

Metabolic encephalopathy presents as an acute confusional state, decreased level of arousal, delirium (characterised by a fluctuating level of attentiveness) or coma. It is associated with a variety of conditions including hepatic and renal failure, sepsis, electrolyte imbalance, endocrine dysfunction or HIBI. There may be a lack of fixed focal deficit, tremor, asterixis, multifocal myoclonus and relative sparing of the cranial nerves.

Septic encephalopathy

Septic encephalopathy is the most common form of encephalopathy encountered in intensive care medicine and is present in 50–70% of septic patients. It is characterised by disorientation, delirium, impaired consciousness or coma. There may be rigidity, tremors and seizures. Usually, an extracranial site of infection can be identified and appropriate treatment commenced, but in less than <50% of cases is an organism isolated from blood cultures. EEG is a sensitive diagnostic investigation for septic encephalopathy; the findings lack specificity but correlate well with the severity of encephalopathy and mortality.

Uraemic encephalopathy

Uraemic encephalopathy, dialysis disequilibrium and dialysis dementia are distinct conditions. Uraemic encephalopathy can occur as a consequence of renal failure particularly if the onset is acute or if there is coexisting hepatic failure. Clinical features of uraemic encephalopathy are non-specific with fatigue, insomnia, pruritus and progressive cognitive impairment culminating in asterixis, tetany, myoclonus, confusion, seizures, stupor and coma. Progression mirrors the severity of uraemia although coexisting metabolic and endocrine factors may also be present (e.g. hypocalcaemia, hyperphosphotaemia, hypokalaemia and metabolic acidosis). Uraemic encephalopathy is easily reversible with dialysis or transplantation.

Dialysis disequilibrium syndrome generally follows the initiation of treatment with haemodialysis and is probably caused by the development of cerebral oedema resulting from a urea gradient in which brain urea concentration exceeds that in the blood. It may be associated with milder manifestations including disorientation, tremor or more severe features such as seizures and coma. Dialysis dementia is now extremely rare. It was thought to be related to aluminium toxicity incurred through dialysis. This led to progressive and permanent memory loss, dysarthria, facial grimacing, myoclonus and psychiatric sequelae.

Hepatic encephalopathy

Hepatic encephalopathy presents with lethargy, somnolence and disorientation leading to coma associated with slurred speech, a flapping tremor (asterixis) and foetor culminating in coma. Cerebral oedema is caused by ammonia-induced vasodilation and leads to impaired autoregulation. Features of raised ICP and seizures may occur before the development of deep coma. There are no specific diagnostic liver function test abnormalities although elevated blood ammonia levels and an abnormal EEG (bilateral synchronous delta waves and triphasic waves) indicate hepatic encephalopathy and portal–systemic shunting. The management of chronic hepatic encephalopathy requires avoidance of precipitating factors, and the use of lactulose and antibiotics, particularly neomycin.

Severe acute hepatic encephalopathy caused by fulminant hepatic failure is an ICU emergency involving the management of cerebral oedema, acute elevated ICP and seizures. It requires monitoring, ventilation and osmotherapy with mannitol. Hypothermia and hyperbaric oxygen have also been used. The only proven therapy to improve outcome is orthotopic liver transplantation.

Hyperpyrexia and hyperthermia

Hyperpyrexia is most commonly caused by sepsis but may be brought about by inflammation, drug reaction (e.g. Ecstacy), malignant hyperpyrexia, heatstroke or injury (e.g. stroke), SAH and TBI. It leads to tachycardia, elevated cardiac output, hypotension, an increase in tissue oxygen demand associated with an increase in metabolic rate. Neurological involvement includes altered consciousness and seizures associated with the development of multiorgan dysfunction (rhabdomyolysis, disorders of clotting, renal and liver failure).

Management involves:

- Minimise heat gain – controlled temperature, avoid ambient environmental warming
- Reduce shivering – magnesium, meperidine, benzodiazepines or propofol
- Treat underlying cause – antibiotics, drain sepsis
- Drug treatment of pyrexia – antipyretics, muscle relaxation
- Cooling – external, extracorporeal, intravascular.

Hypernatraemia

Hypernatraemia may be caused by unreplaced water loss (e.g. insensible sweat loss), gastrointestinal loss, cranial or nephrogenic diabetes insipidus, osmotic diuresis (e.g. glucose in uncontrolled diabetes mellitus or mannitol). It may also be caused by sodium overload (intake of hypertonic sodium solution). Slowly developing hypernatraemia is not a concern because brain cells maintain volume but patients with serum osmolality >350 MOsm/kg or with serum sodium >160 mEq/L may develop lethargy, confusion, decreased mental status and occasionally seizures. Severe hypernatraemia causes of water movement out of the brain resulting in a decrease in brain volume which may cause new focal intracerebral, and SAH and venous sinus thrombosis. The rate of correction should be slow.

Hyponatraemia

Hyponatraemia is a common problem on NICU and is defined as serum sodium level <135 mmol/L. The causes of hyponatraemia are classified according to the extracellular fluid osmolality, intravascular volume and pressure status. Normal serum osmolality ($2[Na^+]$ + urea + glucose [mmol/L]) is in the range of 285–295 mOsm/kg. Encephalopathy resulting from hyponatraemia depends on the rate of development and the absolute sodium levels. Rapidly evolving hyponatraemia results in confusion, seizures (generalised tonic–clonic seizures), muscle cramps, generalised weakness and coma. Hypertonic hyponatraemia is caused by the presence of osmotically active solutes other than sodium (e.g. glucose and mannitol), which lead to shifts of free water from the intracellular to the extracellular component. Normotonic hyponatraemia is usually caused by retention of large volumes of isotonic solutes that dilute sodium (e.g. hyperlipidaemia). Hypotonic hyponatraemia (serum osmolality <260 mOsm/kg) is by far the most common abnormality seen in neurological patients. It occurs when there is excessive water retention in relation to sodium ions and may be classified according to the intravascular volume state of the patient. Hypervolaemic hypotonic hyponatraemia is associated with excessive body fluid load as may be seen with cirrhosis, ascites, congestive cardiac failure, nephrotic syndrome and severe hypoproteinaemia. Hypovolaemic hypotonic hyponatraemia is caused by excessive extrarenal loss (e.g. diarrhoea, vomiting, sweating, pancreatitis, burns) or renal loss (e.g. use of diuretics or as occurs in renal failure) or centrally mediated cerebral salt wasting.

In normovolaemic hypotonic hyponatraemia (inappropriate secretion of ADH SIADH) there is excessive water retention by the kidneys leading to dilutional hyponatraemia with mild expansion of the extracellular fluid. This occurs because appropriate secretion of ADH is not appropriately suppressed by low plasma osmolality. This leads to further reabsorption of free water in the distal renal tubules; however, in SIADH sodium handling remains unaffected so that there is a paradoxical increase in sodium excretion attempting to return the intravascular volume to normal levels. Therefore, increased urinary sodium excretion continues despite the increase in free water.

The features of SIADH are summarised in Table 20.17. Inappropriate ADH secretion is associated with a variety of neurological and systemic causes summarised in Table 20.18.

Table 20.17 Criteria for the diagnosis of syndrome of inappropriate antidiuretic hormone (ADH) secretion.

Hyponatraemia (serum sodium <135 mOsm/L)
Plasma hypotonicity (plasma osmolality <280 mmol/kg)
Inappropriately concentrated urine (osmolality >100 mL/kg)
Continued sodium excretion (urinary sodium >20 mOsm/L)
The patient is clinically normovolaemic
Exclusion of cardiac, renal or endocrine disease

Inappropriate ADH secretion is associated with a variety of neurological and systemic causes summarised in Table 20.18.

Table 20.18 Causes of syndrome of inappropriate ADH secretion.

Neurological disorders
Head injury, trauma
Cerebrovascular – infarction, ICH, SAH
Tumours
Abscess, meningitis, encephalitis
Guillain–Barré syndrome, acute intermittent porphyria
Pulmonary disorders – pneumonia, TB, COPD, asthma
Malignancy – bronchus, lymphoma, prostate, pancreas
Endocrine – hypothyroidism, Addison's disease
Drugs
Analgesics – NSAIDs, opiates
Antiepileptics – carbamazepine
Antidepressants – SSRIs, tricyclics, monoamine oxidase inhibitors
Chemotherapy agents – vincristine, vinblastine, cyclophosphamide
Antipsychotics – haloperidol, thioridazine
Hypoglycaemic agents – chlorpropamide, tolbutamide
Postoperative

COPD, chronic obstructive pulmonary disease; ICH, intracerebral haematoma; NSAID, non-steroidal anti-inflammatory drug; SAH, subarachnoid haemorrhage; SSRI, selective serotonin re-uptake inhibitor; TB, tuberculosis.

Cerebral salt wasting

Hypovolaemic hyponatraemia may also occur in association with the condition of cerebral salt wasting (CSW). In this condition a centrally mediated process leads to increased sodium and water excretion and hypovolaemia, in contrast to SIADH which is characterised by excessive sodium loss with water retention by the kidneys. In clinical practice the only reliable way of distinguishing SIADH from CSW is assessment of the volume status. Hypovolaemia, as seen in CSW, is associated with orthostatic hypotension, tachycardia, dry mucous membranes, poor skin turgor and reduced central venous pressure but none of these signs is entirely reliable.

The distinction between SIADH and CSW is essential because the management of SIADH involves reduction in the intake of electrolyte-free water to reduce the expansion of intracellular volume. The administration of saline would simply increase the extracellular fluid as sodium continues to be lost as a consequence of ongoing ADH secretion and the shift of sodium from the extracellular fluid to the intracellular fluid would cause progressive cerebral oedema. Conversely, in CSW, where there is a hypovolaemic state, treatment is the administration of both salt and water with isotonic or hypertonic saline to counteract the primary abnormality of renal salt wasting. In this situation, fluid restriction actually worsens the hypovolaemia and hyponatraemia as the salt wasting continues and would cause cerebral infarction.The situation is particularly complex in SAH where there appear to be features of both SIADH and CSW. However, the hypovolaemic state exacerbates vascular spasm and therefore it is now widely accepted that hypervolaemic therapy is appropriate to prevent further vascular spasm.

In general clinical practice, acute symptomatic hyponatraemia is often brought about by hypervolaemic states such that occur in congestive cardiac failure or nephrotic syndrome and treatment is therefore with loop diuretics to promote renal loss of water in excess of sodium. Treatment of asymptomatic hyponatraemia should be cautious with mild free water restriction if the patient is isovolaemic or hypovolaemic.

Central pontine myelinolysis

Central pontine myelinolysis is a demyelinating syndrome, initially described in alcohol or malnourished patients. The condition is associated with rapid correction of hyponatraemia which leads to shift of fluid from the intracellular to the extracellular compartments causing dehydration of the brain resulting in non-inflammatory damage to the myelin sheath and the oligodendrocytes with relative sparing of neurones and axons.

The condition may present with a severe and unexplained encephalopathy or seizures occurring secondary to hyponatraemia but it may progress to flaccid quadriparesis, pseudobulbar palsy manifest as dysarthria, dysphagia with pupillary and oculomotor abnormalities and occasionally patients may present with a locked-in syndrome. The presence of extrapontine myelinolysis leads to a more diffuse neurological pattern with movement disorders including parkinsonism, choreoathetosis, dystonia and spasmodic dysphonia.

Demyelination is most frequently seen in the central pons, but may extend into the midbrain; however, extrapontine myelinolysis is often symmetrical and may occur in the cerebral cortex, external capsule, limbic system or basal ganglia. MRI confirms the presence of hyperintense, 'bat-wing' lesions on T2-weighted images, which do not enhance and are seen primarily in the central pons (Figure 20.18). Diffusion-weighted imaging is a more sensitive technique to show these abnormalities.

The outcome is variable and the prognosis depends on the severity and extent of demyelination in the pons. Some patients may recover from the condition despite extensive radiological or clinical involvement.

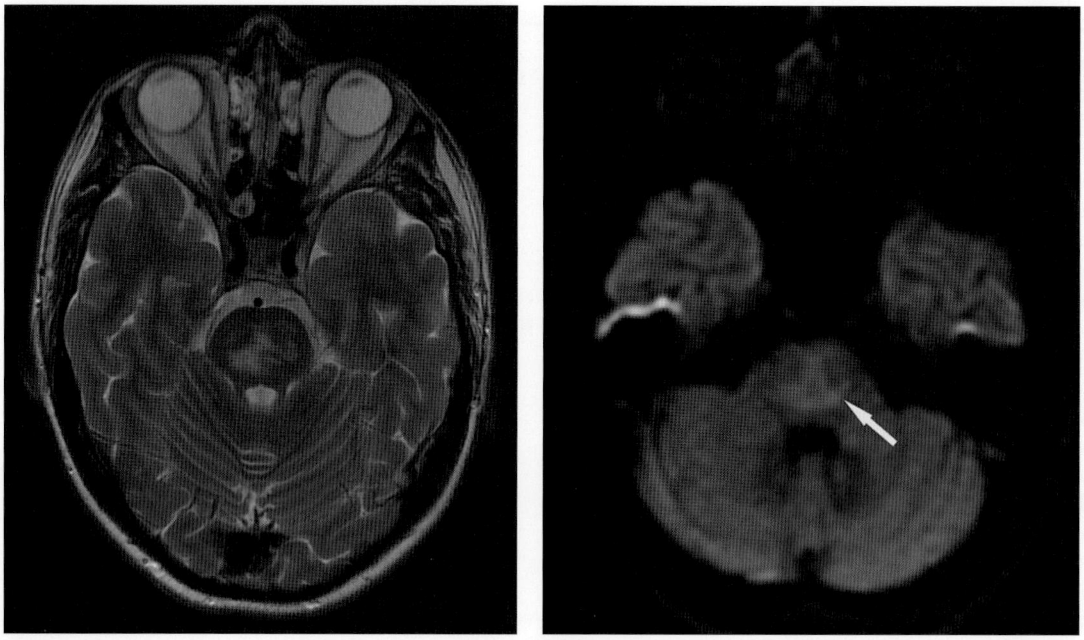
(a) (b)

Figure 20.18 Central Pontine myelinolysis. T2-weighted (a) and diffusion weighted (b) axial images demonstrating abnormally high signal and restricted diffusion (white arrow) within the central pons in a typical trident pattern.

Posterior reversible encephalopathy syndrome

Posterior reversible encephalopathy syndrome (PRES) occurs as a result of acute hypertensive encephalopathy, eclampsia or immunosuppression. The onset is with headache, vomiting and a progressive encephalopathy characterised by confusion and disorientation. There may be seizures and visual disturbance, in particular cortical blindness. The condition is associated with immunosuppressive therapy particularly after transplantation using ciclosporin, cisplatinum, 5-fluouracil, amphotericin B, methotrexate, tacrolimus or interferon-α. Reversible posterior leukoencephalopathy seems to arise from a mechanical disruption of the blood–brain barrier, either by overwhelming hydrostatic factors (e.g. hypertension) or dysfunction of the endothelial cells of the barrier because of toxins. The MRI shows characteristic high intensity white matter abnormalities on T2-weighted sequences in the parieto-occipital white matter. Fluid attenuated inversion recovery (FLAIR) sequences show a similar predominantly white matter pattern of hyperintensity consistent with vasogenic oedema (Figure 20.19). In general, changes are confined to the posterior circulation territory. It is suggested this is because the vascular blood in this area has lower pressure and less sympathetic innervation compared with the anterior circulation and is therefore more easily affected by systemic hypertension. However, there are increasing reports of anterior territory or asymmetrical changes occurring. Management is with antihypertensive agents, withdrawal of immunosuppression and supportive care. This condition is reversible with treatment and the MRI scan may normalise but there may be residual focal cerebral haemorrhage or permanent injury.

Hypoxic–ischaemic brain injury

HIBI usually follows cardiac arrest and carries a very poor prognosis. The history of the event and the presence of pre-arrest morbidity are important prognostic factors but detailed examination of the patient remains the mainstay of assessment. The assessment of HIBI remains primarily clinical and is made more difficult by the use of ever more sophisticated techniques of sedation, ventilation, hypothermia, neuromuscular blockade and haemodynamic management (Figure 20.20).

Hypoxia and ischaemia should be considered as pathologically and clinically distinct patterns of brain injury although they usually coexist. Ischaemia describes a reduction in blood supply leading to decreased oxygen delivery and limited or no removal of damaging cellular metabolites which therefore accumulate (e.g. lactate, H^+, glutamate) leading to severe brain injury. Hypoxia refers to a reduction of either oxygen supply or utilisation. It can develop as a direct consequence of reduced oxygen supply, reduced ambient oxygen pO_2, low haemoglobin or impaired tissue utilisation following poisoning of the mitochondrial cytochrome enzymes (e.g. due to cyanide). The pathophysiology of carbon monoxide poisoning is complex with components of both anaemic and histotoxic hypoxia and occasionally global ischaemia caused by cardiac failure. Following isolated hypoxia there is an increase in CBF which allows continuing delivery of glucose to the brain and clearance of toxic metabolites from the brain. Therefore, hypoxia that occurs in isolation, even if prolonged, rarely causes severe brain injury, provided the systemic circulation is preserved.

Prognostic factors following cardiac arrest

The long-term outcome is critically dependent on the cause of arrest and the peri-arrest management. The outcome is best for patients with ventricular tachycardia or fibrillation in whom resuscitation is commenced rapidly. The likelihood of successful resuscitation in asystole or pulseless electrical activity is much lower. In primary hypoxic arrest immediate restoration of oxygenation is of overwhelming importance to outcome.

The most important prognostic factors following out-of-hospital cardiac arrests are:

- Age
- Co-morbidity
- Circumstances of arrest
- Witness/immediate bystander resuscitation

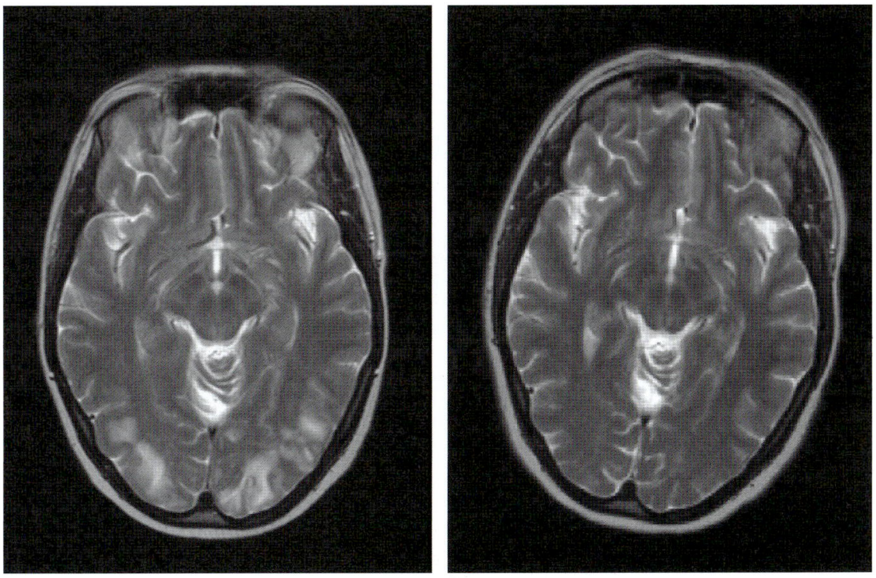

(a) (b)

Figure 20.19 Posterior reversible leukoencephalopathy in a patient who was hypertensive following the administration of intrathecal methotrexate. MRI T2-weighted: (a) following intrathecal methotrexate; and (b) 3 months later showing complete resolution. Courtesy of Dr Paul Holmes, St Thomas' Hospital.

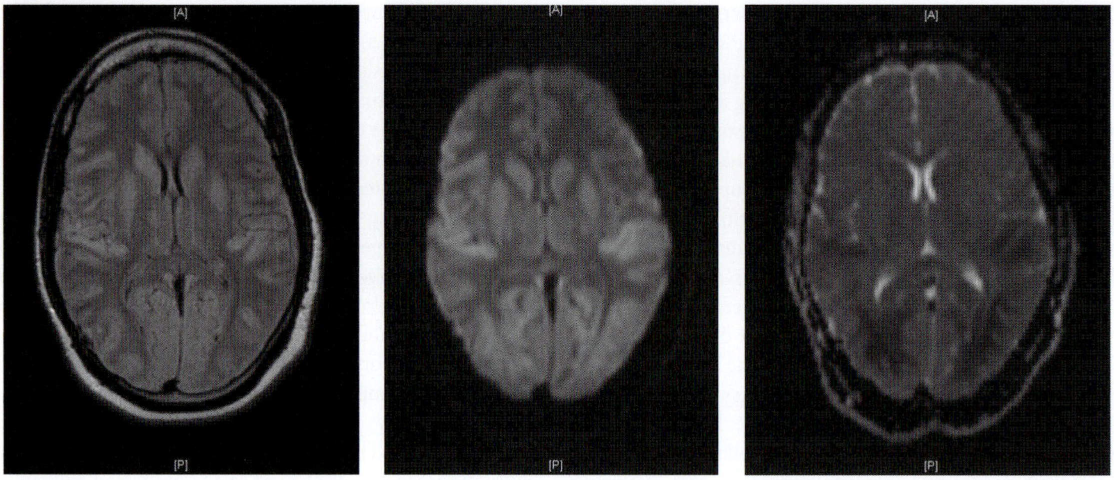

Figure 20.20 After hypoxic-ischaemic brain injury, MRI changes include high signal in the caudate and putamen, less so in the thalami (a) T1 (b) DWI sagittal with restricted diffusion on ADC (c) in the occipital regions and peri-rolandic cortex.

- Effective CPR
- Early attendance of paramedics
- Cardiac rhythm
- Resuscitation
- Fever within first 48 hours
- Duration of cardiac arrest
- Advanced directive.

It is well recognised that a good outcome may result after prolonged cardiac arrest occurring in hypothermic conditions. This led to the use of induced controlled hypothermia following cardiac arrest associated with ventricular fibrillation. However, induced controlled hypothermia can be difficult to apply and uncomfortable, patients require sedation and a neuromuscular blocking agent (vecuronium or pancuronium) to prevent shivering. Recent studies have suggested that induced controlled hypothermia has no effect on outcome and the treatment is now being abandoned in both TBI and following HIBI.

The outcome of HIBI worsens if:

- The patient has been in coma (i.e. unresponsive) for >6 hours.
- Lack of spontaneous limb movements or failure to localise painful stimuli in the initial stages.
- Prolonged loss of pupillary responses (if atropine has not been administered).
- Sustained conjugate eye deviation (upgaze or downgaze).
- Specific forms of abnormal eye movements (including upbeat and downbeat nystagmus, ping pong gaze or period alternating nystagmus).
- Myoclonic seizures.
- Involvement of lower cranial nerve function.

However, these signs are variable and dependent on medication used during resuscitation.

Seizures

Focal or generalised convulsive tonic–clonic seizures are relatively unusual in the initial stages following HIBI but may evolve during the recovery period. Status epilepticus occurring after HIBI responds poorly to conventional antiepileptic drugs including phenytoin.

Post-hypoxic myoclonic status may develop immediately after resuscitation when it typically causes bilateral synchronous local or generalised multifocal jerking of the face, limbs, trunk or diaphragm. The EEG shows limited background activity with a burst suppression pattern and intermittent generalised periodic complexes with no cortical focus. It responds poorly to medication and carries a uniformly bad prognosis.

Another form of myoclonus (Lance–Adams syndrome) comes on after a latent period of 24–48 hours after resuscitation. It often follows a primary respiratory arrest or anaesthetic event and usually occurs in a younger age group. Consciousness is usually less deeply impaired, and focal myoclonus is often action or startle sensitive. The prognosis of the Lance–Adams form of post-hypoxic myoclonus is generally favourable and these patients continue to improve over time although cerebellar signs including ataxia, dysarthria and intention tremor may persist. The EEG shows a focal cortical origin with responsive cortical rhythms which progressively regain normal patterns. The condition responds reasonably well to antiepileptic drugs including valproate, piracetam, levetiracetam and clonazepam.

The EEG has been widely used over many years to assess the level of consciousness and to guide prognosis after HIBI. A number of patterns suggest a poor prognosis:

- Generalised electrical suppression
- Generalised burst suppression
- Unresponsive alpha, theta or delta rhythms
- Periodic patterns
  - periodic lateralised epileptiform discharges (PLEDS)
  - bilateral independent or synchronous PLEDS (BiPLEDS).

SSEPs are valuable in assessing the prognosis following HIBI. Bilateral absence of the cortical N20 response represents widespread cortical injury after cardiac arrest with a high specificity for poor outcome.

In the first 2 days after HIBI, CT scans may show diffuse swelling with effacement of the basal cisterns, ventricles and sulci, attenuation of the grey–white matter interface and hypodensity of the cortical grey matter and basal ganglia (caudate, lenticular nucleus, thalamus and putamen) resulting from cytotoxic oedema. Focal areas of infarction may develop in the basal ganglia or cortical watershed territories.

MRI is undertaken less commonly following HIBI because patients often require sedation, ventilation and airway protection. In

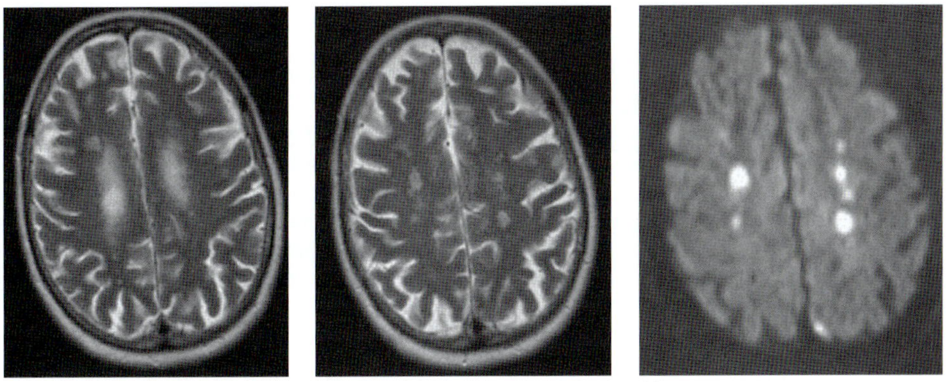

Figure 20.21 After severe circulatory compromise, for example following problematic cardiac surgery, a pattern of border-zone ischaemia may occur. MRI shows high signal on T2 (a) and FLAIR (b) in the deep border-zone regions, as well as high signal on diffusion weighted imaging (c).

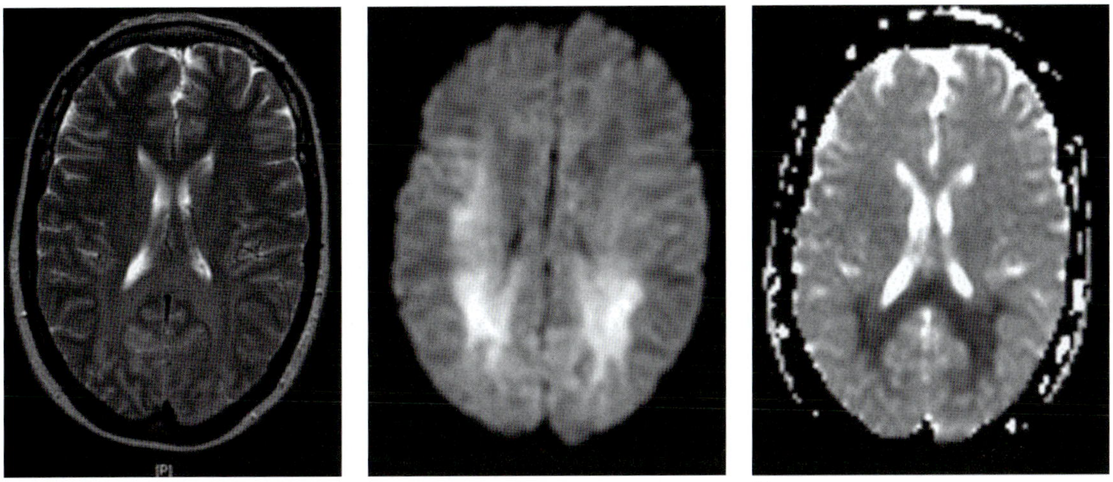

Figure 20.22 Diffuse white matter high signal following hypoxic–ischaemic brain injury (HIBI). T2 (a), DWI (b), ADC map (c).

the acute stages (first few days) after severe HIBI, diffusion-weighted and FLAIR images show widespread hyperintensity initially involving the basal ganglia, caudate, striatum and thalamus followed by the cortex and subcortical white matter, cerebellum and hippocampus. Conventional T1 and T2 weighted scans are normal. Diffusely abnormal findings on diffusion-weighted images and fluid attenuated inversion recovery correlate with a poor outcome (Figures 20.21 and 20.22).

Longer-term complications of HIBI

Following resuscitation after a severe HIBI the patient generally remains in coma for several days although, rarely, this may persist for longer. The level of consciousness may improve but many patients remain in a vegetative or minimally aware state for prolonged periods. Recovery is often associated with a variable level of residual cognitive impairment.

Movement disorders A variety of movement disorders may develop after HIBI because the basal ganglia are particularly vulnerable to injury. In younger patients with predominantly hypoxic brain injury later onset dystonia develops after several weeks, while in older patients with predominantly ischaemic insults an akinetic rigid syndrome may occur.

Border-zone infarction Border-zone infarction is associated with HIBI resulting from cardiac arrest, it is also seen after prolonged cardiac bypass associated with hypotension but can also be caused by multiple emboli particularly following aortic procedures with prolonged bypass time. The vulnerable border-zone regions lie between the territories of brain supplied by the three major cerebral arteries (Figure 20.21). Unilateral border-zone infarction may develop with severe stenosis or occlusion of an internal carotid artery. The syndromes of border-zone infarction are summarised in Table 20.19.

Delayed post-hypoxic encephalopathy Delayed post-hypoxic encephalopathy is a rare condition that follows primarily hypoxic injury such as carbon monoxide poisoning, drowning, hanging, strangulation, drug overdose and respiratory depression. Patients seem to have made a complete recovery from hypoxic coma with normal cognitive function for 1–4 weeks before a relapse occurs with cognitive deterioration, frontal lobe (urinary incontinence and gait disturbance) and

Table 20.19 Syndromes of border-zone infarction.

Border zone	Clinical syndrome
Anterior and middle cerebral arteries	Bi-brachial weakness and sensory loss. Initially, this involves the whole limb but later becomes confined to the hands and forearms ('man in a barrel') Mild spasticity and brisk reflexes, particularly the finger jerks Superficial sensation is retained but there is cortical sensory loss in the fingers Disturbance of volitional eye movement caused by lesions in both frontal eye fields Rarely, fluctuating cortical ischaemic over the frontal parasaggital border-zone may lead to non-epileptic myoclonic limb jerking, during which the EEG shows diffuse slow waves with no focal or ictal features
Middle and posterior cerebral arteries	Initial period of cortical blindness that rapidly improves although visual acuity may be reduced for some weeks Dyslexia, dysgraphia and dyscalculia and often a memory deficit for both verbal and non-verbal material
Common border zone of the three vessels	Lower altitudinal field defect Difficulty in visual judgement of size, distance and movement and a disorder of smooth occulomotor pursuit Restriction of visual attention and an absence of blink reaction to visual threat Difficulty with movements performed under visual guidance (optic ataxia)
Cerebellum	Unusual because the extensive anastomosis on the cerebellar cortex Border-zone between the territories of supply of the superior cerebellar and posterior inferior cerebellar arteries May present as dizziness, vertigo and ataxia
Spinal cord	Longitudinal and horizontal border-zone Anterior spinal artery has a highly variable segmental supply and discontinuity between cervical, thoracic and lumbar levels Infarction in the thoracic cord may occur at the border-zone territories between the cervical and thoracic supply (T3/T4) or between the mid thoracic and lumbar enlargement at approximately T9. However, the entire mid thoracic region (T4–T9) is vulnerable Anterior spinal artery syndrome or border zone infarction restricted to deep grey matter causing amyotrophy

extrapyramidal signs from basal ganglia involvement (short stooping gait, parkinsonian faces and rigidity). MRI shows extensive white matter change and involvement of the basal ganglia (globus pallidus and occasionally putamen, caudate nucleus, thalamus and hippocampus). The outcome is variable. Up to 50% are said to make a good recovery but residual cognitive and extrapyramidal deficits are also common and delayed post-hypoxic encephalopathy may culminate in an unresponsive vegetative state.

Movement disorder emergencies

Movement disorder emergencies are characterised by inadequate voluntary movements (hypokinetic) or the presence of abnormal involuntary movements (hyperkinetic). Occasionally, movement disorders may become severe and prolonged enough to threaten respiratory function or risk aspiration, and severe exhaustion with metabolic derangements (status dystonicus).

Acute parkinsonism is most commonly caused by dopamine blocking drugs. Toxic causes are usually associated with severe encephalopathy often leading to akinesis which is poorly responsive to levodopa. Acute illnesses worsen parkinsonism and require correction of the underlying medical condition, while maintaining Parkinson's disease medication. Abrupt discontinuation of treatment may also result in disastrous and even fatal consequences and can be prevented by the administration of Parkinson's disease medication entrally or parentrally. The use of transdermal delivery of dopamine agonists allows more flexibility for the delivery of Parkinson's disease medication on the ICU. The parkinsonism–hyperpyrexia syndrome is usually indistinguishable from neuroleptic malignant syndrome and is probably caused by a central dopamine deficiency.

Hyperkinetic movement disorders are typically categorised by the predominant type of abnormal involuntary movement:

- Tremor
- Dystonia
- Myoclonus
- Chorea
- Athetosis
- Ballism
- Tardive dyskinesia

Hyperkinetic emergencies, because of fulminant muscle activity, carry a risk of hyperthermia and rhabdomyolysis. Close monitoring of serum creatine kinase (CK), electrolyte and renal function is essential for the early detection of rhabdomyolysis and intravenous hydration is critical in preventing acute renal failure. Severe pain may be a feature and adequate analgesia is necessary.

Symptomatic treatment is often necessary:

- Sedation – benzodiazepines.
- Anaesthesia – propofol is an ideal choice because of the short half-life.
- Neuromuscular blockade – required if sedation fails to control hypokinetic movement adequately. Non-depolarising paralytic agents (e.g. atracurium) are preferable to depolarising agents (succinylcholine) because the latter may induce or worsen rhabdomyolysis.

Lethal catatonia is a rare condition with features of neuroleptic malignant syndrome but no exposure to dopamine blocking drugs. Clinically there is agitation, stereotypes, psychosis and autonomic disturbance leading to the development of catatonia in which patient adopt fixed abnormal postures in association with major behavioural disturbances. Rigidity and mutism occur with periods of intense agitation and bizarre repetitive movements. The condition is usually associated with major psychiatric disturbances, especially schizophrenia, but may occur following stroke, meningitis, head trauma and metabolic disturbance. Treatment is with electroconvulsive therapy (ECT) which is tolerated even by severely debilitated patients.

Stiff person syndromes and progressive encephalopathy with rigidity and myoclonus

Stiff person syndrome is associated with severe pain and spasms in the lumbar paraspinal muscles and lower limbs with an exaggerated lumbar lordosis. Muscle spasms can occur spontaneously or be provoked by noise or movement but may be so forceful as to produce femoral fractures or joint subluxation and are associated with life-threatening autonomic dysfunction. It is particularly associated with anti-GAD antibodies, and is amenable to immunomodulatory treatment with plasma exchange or immunoglobulin (IVIg). A more aggressive variant is PERM (progressive encephalopathy with rigidity and myoclonus) which is associated with muscle rigidity, stimulus sensitive spasms and brainstem dysfunction. There may also be hyperekplexia and cerebellar ataxia with autonomic dysfunction. Breathing and swallowing difficulties may contribute to the development of respiratory failure.The condition is associated with antiglycine receptor antibodies. Treatment is with immunomodulation using corticosteroids, IVIg, plasma exchange or cyclophosphamide. Intrathecal baclofen has also been used.

Acute dystonia

Acute dystonia is usually precipitated by neuroleptics or other dopamine blocking drugs such as antiemetics. It may be life-threatening if the airway or breathing are compromised. It includes conditions such as oculogyric crisis, laryngeal dystonia, blepharospasm, torticollis, trismus, dysarthria and dystonia. Dystonia is usually short-lived and easily reversed by procyclidine but it may recur. Acute dystonia may evolve into status dystonicus in which there is a life-threatening disorder of unremitting severe generalised dystonic spasms (dystonic storms). Drug treatment is very difficult but involves the use of dopamine blockers and dopamine depletors including benzhexol, tetrabenezine and pimozide. Treatment also often involves introducing sedation, paralysis and ventilation. Intrathecal baclofen has been used. Functional surgery is often recommended (e.g. bilateral ventral lateral thalamotomy, unilateral pallidotomy, bilateral pallidal stimulation).

Stridor

The development of stridor in MSA can be the presenting feature. It results from failure of the vocal cords to abduct normally. The incidence of sudden death is high because of respiratory obstruction possibly associated with autonomic failure and central apnoea. Treatment has included nasal CPAP and botulinum toxin injection into the laryngeal adductors but tracheostomy is treatment of choice. Acute laryngeal dystonia can also present with nocturnal; stridor that interferes with the normal breathing pattern.

Cervical cord disorders (Chapter 16)

Traumatic, demyelinating or vascular lesions of the spinal cord, particularly at high cervical levels, may cause acute flaccid tetraplegia, selectively affecting respiratory control. Patients with previously unsuspected Arnold–Chiari malformation with cerebellar ectopia may present with acute ventilatory failure and tetraparesis following a cervical spine hyperextesion injury. Cervical myelitis or structural lesions of the cord may selectively affect respiratory control, in particular the automatic generation of the respiratory rhythm leading to central apnoea. Examples of conditions that may lead to impaired respiratory control as a consequence of lesions of the cervical cord are shown in Figures 20.23, 20.24 and 20.25.

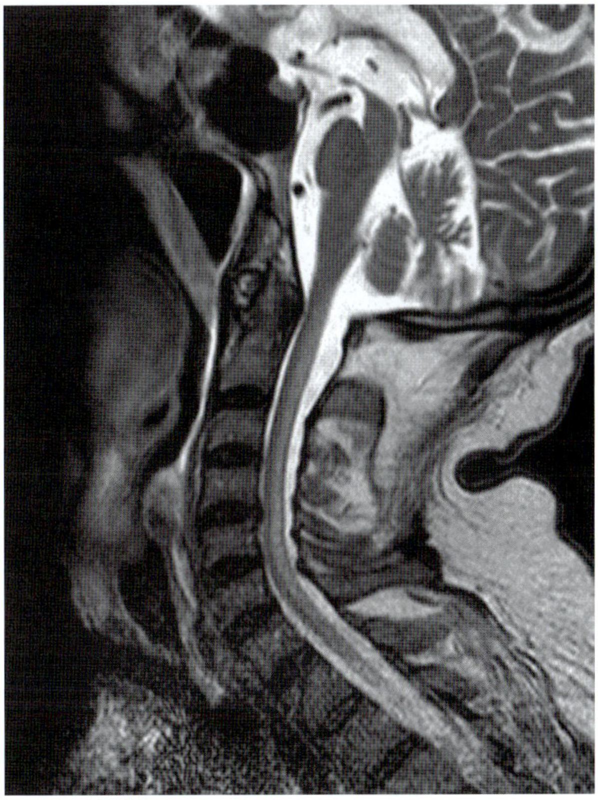

Figure 20.23 Subacute combined degeneration (MRI, T2-weighted sagittal).

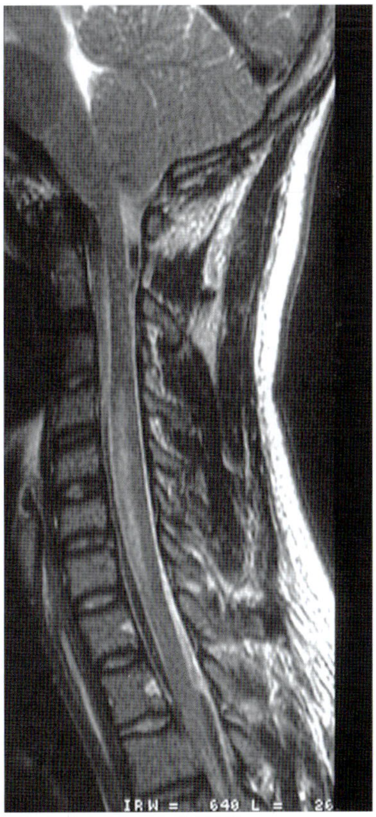

Figure 20.24 Spinal cord infarction (MRI, T2-weighted sagittal).

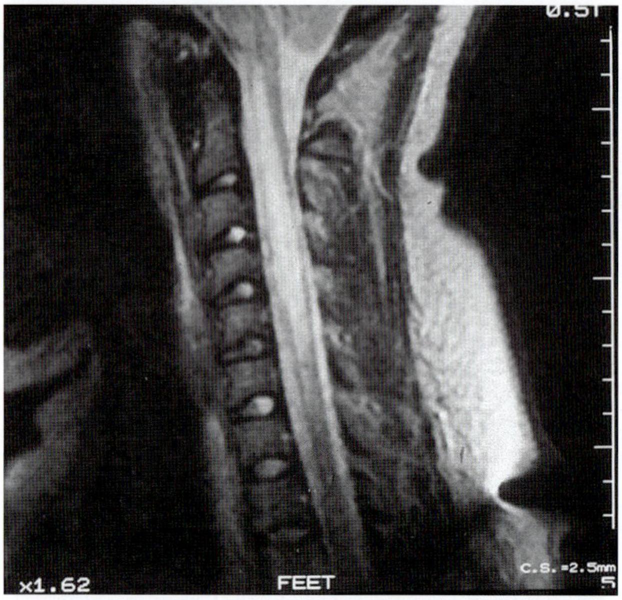

Figure 20.25 Neuromyelitis optica (MRI, T2-weighted sagittal).

Anterior horn cell disease

Patients with motor neurone disease can present with acute respiratory weakness, or develop this early in the course of their disease – often associated with infection. These patients may be intubated and ventilated before the diagnosis has been made. The progressive nature of the condition means that weaning to non-invasive ventilatory support may be impossible. Patients with late post-polio functional deterioration may also present with progressive nocturnal hypoventilation or acute respiratory failure and acute flaccid paralysis may be caused by poliomyelitis and West Nile virus, or occur as a paraneoplastic syndrome.

Neuromuscular disease

Patients with neuromuscular disease (Chapter 10) require NICU care when they develop acute or acute on chronic respiratory failure or acute bulbar or limb weakness. They may develop severe and unexpected deterioration of respiratory, bulbar and limb function as a consequence of intercurrent events including systemic infection, disease exacerbation and increased pulmonary load (e.g. pregnancy or obesity).

Neuropathies (Chapter 10)

Patients can be admitted because of a severe, primary neuropathy which recovers slowly (e.g. acute inflammatory demyelinating neuropathy), or develop neuropathy related to therapeutic agents (e.g. acute intermittent porphyria) or nutritional deficiencies. The intensive care patient is at particular risk of developing critical illness polyneuropathy.

Acute inflammatory demyelinating polyneuropathy About one-third of patients with Guillain–Barré syndrome require admission to ICU because of respiratory insufficiency requiring mechanical ventilation, severe bulbar weakness threatening pulmonary aspiration or autonomic instability, causing cardiac arrhythmias or fluctuations in blood pressure (Chapter 10); often there is a combination of factors. Ventilatory failure is primarily caused by inspiratory muscle weakness, although weakness of the abdominal and accessory muscles of respiration, retained airway secretions leading to pulmonary aspiration and atelectasis are all contributory factors. The associated bulbar weakness and autonomic instability reinforce the need for control of the airway and ventilation. Patients with acute motor and sensory axonal neuropathy (the axonal form of Guillain–Barré syndrome) usually present with a rapidly developing paralysis developing over hours leading to respiratory failure requiring tracheal intubation and ventilation. There may be total paralysis of all voluntary muscles of the body, including the cranial musculature, the ocular muscles and the pupils. Prolonged paralysis and incomplete recovery are more likely and prolonged ventilatory support may be necessary.

The diagnosis of neuropathy may be difficult to recognise because of the presence of multi-organ impairment or other general medical factors. Occasionally, some patients may actually develop acute demyelinating polyneuropathy during the course of a critical illness; not surprisingly, when this occurs the rapid development of inexplicable weakness and its cause may not be recognised.

Miller Fisher syndrome Ataxia, areflexia and ophthalmoplegia are the classic features. Diplopia is the most common initial complaint (in about one-third), while ataxia is evident in about one-fifth of patients at onset. Facial weakness, bulbar impairments with dysphagia and dysarthria, along with facial or limb paraesthesias, may also occur and mild proximal limb weakness is found in approximately one-third of patients.

Bickerstaff's brainstem encephalitis Bickerstaff's brainstem encephalitis is a closely related condition in which progressive ophthalmoplegia and ataxia, maximal at less than 4 weeks, are associated with drowsiness and coma, and upper motor neurone signs. MRI shows high intensity abnormalities in the posterior fossa, white matter or thalami in 30% of patients. The course is monophasic with complete recovery at 6 months in 66%.

Acute intermittent porphyria (Chapter 19) Acute intermittent porphyria is an uncommon autosomal dominant disease, characterised by recurrent episodes of abdominal pain, psychiatric disturbances, seizures and acute, predominantly motor axonal, neuropathy with autonomic features, which may mimic the Guillain–Barré syndrome causing bulbar and ventilatory failure with patchy sensory involvement. Attacks can be precipitated by heavy alcohol consumption and by numerous medications, many of which are commonly administered in the ICU, such as diazepam, theophylline and barbiturates.

Phrenic nerve neuropathies Phrenic nerve neuropathies may lead to ventilatory failure and admission to ICU (Table 20.20).

Critical illness polyneuropathy Critical illness polyneuropathy (CIP) is an acute sensorimotor axonal neuropathy that develops in the setting of systemic inflammatory response syndrome (SIRS) and/or multi-organ failure, particularly in the presence of hypoalbuminaemia, hyperglycaemia and insulin deficiency with or without corticosteroids and neuromuscular blocking agents. Up to 70% of patients with sepsis and multi-organ failure develop abnormalities on nerve conduction studies. CIP is characterised by delayed weaning, severe flaccid wasting and weakness; areflexia and sensory impairment may be seen in patients who are able to cooperate with the examination. However, the signs are variable and difficult to elicit because of sedation or coexistent septic encephalopathy. CIP is self-limiting but the overall prognosis is influenced by the severity of the underlying condition and this accounts for most of the mortality. The outcome is also related to the severity of the sepsis and other factors including the extent and severity of the neuropathy, the time on ICU and the presence of hyperglycaemia, hyperosmolality or hypoalbuminaemia. When the neuropathy is mild or moderate, recovery is relatively rapid and complete. In those with more severe polyneuropathy, recovery is limited; persisting weakness and sensory deficits are common in long-term survivors of protracted critical illness, even up to 4 years after discharge.

The differential diagnosis of CIP includes other neuropathies, neuromuscular transmission defects and myopathies, of which the most important one is critical illness myopathy. The diagnosis of neuromuscular blockade can be established by repetitive nerve stimulation studies. Differentiating CIP from critical illness myopathy is more difficult and sometimes these two diseases can occur simultaneously.

Table 20.20 Causes of phrenic nerve neuropathy.

Brachial neuritis
Brachial plexopathy
Following thoracotomy, cardiac surgery
Trauma
Heavy metal intoxication – lead, thallium, arsenic
Metabolic – hypophosphataemia, renal failure
Infections – Borrelia, HIV
Neuropathies:
Chronic inflammatory demyelinating neuropathy
Multi-focal motor neuropathy
Hereditary neuropathy with liability to pressure palsy
Hereditary sensorimotor neuropathy
Diabetes

Neuromuscular junction disease

Disruption of neuromuscular transmission is an important cause for weakness and failure to wean in critically ill patients.

Prolonged neuromuscular blockade Prolonged neuromuscular blockade after either short- or long-term blockade with non-depolarising neuromuscular blocking agents (NMBAs; Table 20.21) may occur in association with metabolic acidosis, hepatic or renal insufficiency and elevated levels of magnesium. Weakness should not persist beyond 2 weeks after stopping the blocking agent and typically lasts for only a few days. Prolonged blockade should be considered in any patient who remains weak after discontinuation of NMBAs. The condition occurs in the context of cumulative doses of NMBAs often given with corticosteroids, aminoglycosides or other anaesthetic agents. Repetitive nerve stimulation is abnormal with a decremental response in the compound muscle potential amplitude but the CK levels are normal. Recovery usually occurs within several days of discontinuation of the NMBA.

Neuromuscular disorders resulting from the disruption of neuromuscular transmission should be considered as a cause for neuromuscular weakness and failure to wean in critically ill patients. Patients with myasthenia gravis or the Lambert–Eaton myasthenic syndrome have an extremely high sensitivity to even low doses of NMBAs and other agents such as aminoglycoside antibiotics and antiarrhythmic agents (Table 20.21).

Myasthenia gravis In myasthenia gravis admission to the NICU is indicated by the development of incipient ventilatory failure, progressive bulbar weakness leading to failure of airway protection or severe limb and truncal weakness causing extensive paralysis (Chapter 10). Admission should be determined by the rate of progression, the presence of bulbar weakness and the clinical state of the patient rather than an absolute level of FVC alone. Respiratory failure often results from a myasthenic crisis (usually precipitated by infection, surgery or inadequate treatment), but may also more rarely be precipitated by a cholinergic crisis. The associated bulbar weakness predisposes to pulmonary aspiration and acute respiratory failure necessitating urgent tracheal intubation and ventilation. Patients with recent onset generalised myasthenia gravis started on

Table 20.21 Drugs that may affect the neuromuscular junction.

Neuromuscular blocking agents (non-depolarising)	Aminosteroidal (pancuronium, vecuronium, pipecuronium, rocuronium) Benzylisoquinolinium (D-tubocurarine, atracurium, cisatracurium, doxacurium, mivacurium)
Antibiotics	Aminoglycosides, clindamycin, tetracycline, quinolones, polymyxin, erythromycin
Local anaesthetics	Lidocaine
Antiarrhythmics	Quinidine, procainamide
Beta-blocking agents	Propranolol, atenolol, acebutolol, bisoprolol, labetalol, metoprolol, oxprenolol, pindolol, sotalol, timolol
Calcium channel blockers	Verapamil, diltiazem
Immunosuppressive agents	Cyclophosphamide, ciclosporin
Diuretics	
Corticosteroids	
Statins	
Antiretrovirals	Zidovudine, lamivudine
Others	D-penicillamine, phenytoin, dantrolene, lithium carbonate, interferon α

a high-dose daily corticosteroid regimen are particularly at risk for acute paradoxical deterioration during the first 48–96 hours of treatment. Thymectomy should be coordinated by an NICU with experience of the procedure and the postoperative care of patients with myasthenia.

Botulism This is caused by toxins produced by *Clostridium botulinum,* an anaerobic Gram-positive organism. These act at the presynaptic region of the neuromuscular junction causing failure of release of acetylcholine from the terminal. The classic form occurs after ingestion of food that contains toxin, but increasing numbers of patients are being seen who have developed botulism as a consequence of using contaminated opiates or unclean needles to inject drugs of abuse into infected skin lesions (skin popping).

Patients develop cranial nerve deficits, including blurred vision, diplopia, ptosis, dysarthria and dysphagia. The weakness often affects the arms before progressesing to the legs. Autonomic symptoms, including dry mouth, unreactive pupils and ileus, are frequent. The condition may be suspected by prominent and early ocular signs (dilated sluggishly reactive pupils and ophthalmoplegia) and dysphagia. Management is described in Chapter 9.

Other neuromuscular transmission disorders that may cause confusion in ICU include organophosphate poisoning, tick paralysis, black widow spider and certain types of snake envenomation.

Muscle disease

Myopathies occur much more frequently during critical illness than previously recognised. Three main types have been identified:

1. Diffuse non-necrotising cachectic myopathy
2. Myopathy with selective loss of thick (myosin) filaments ('critical illness myopathy')
3. Acute necrotising myopathy of intensive care.

Diffuse non-necrotising cachectic myopathy This is common and presents as muscle wasting with associated weakness. However, the CK levels and electromyograms (EMG) are normal or show only mild changes. It is associated with prolonged ICU admission, sedation or paralysis causing muscle disuse, and poor nutrition with protein catabolism during critical illness. There is proximal or general weakness. Biopsy shows type 2 fibre atrophy and neurogenic atrophy. The outcome depends on the underlying critical illness.

Critical illness myopathy (myopathy with selective loss of thick [myosin] filaments) This is a distinct form of myopathy that occurs in patients with critical illness on ICU. It is under-recognised and is one of the most common forms of generalised weakness on the ICU, being considerably more frequent than critical illness polyneuropathy. It is sometimes associated with prolonged exposure to high doses of corticosteroids and non-depolarising muscle blocking agents (e.g. pancuronium, vecuronium or atracurium) used to treat acute pulmonary disorders, such as asthma. However, it can occur in other situations including SIRS, major organ transplantation – particularly liver – and it does not seem to correlate with the duration of intensive care. Other factors that may contribute include nutritional deficiencies, concurrent drug administration with aminoglycosides or ciclosporin, hyperglycaemia, renal and hepatic dysfunction, fever, severe metabolic and electrolyte disorders.

The problem tends to be recognised as the acute illness resolves, when it becomes apparent that the patient cannot wean from ventilatory support because of limb and respiratory muscle weakness. The limb weakness may be mild or severe and is predominantly proximal although it may be generalised. There may be facial and neck weakness but the extraocular movements are often spared, reflexes are reduced and sensation is not affected.

Blood CK levels are elevated in <50%. Needle EMG may show myopathic features but is often unhelpful in distinguishing between myopathy and polyneuropathy because insufficient motor units are obtained. Muscle biopsy is necessary to establish the diagnosis. Histological changes include abnormal variation of muscle fibre size, fibre atrophy, angulated fibres, internalised nuclei, rimmed vacuoles, fatty degeneration of muscle fibres, fibrosis and single fibre necrosis. Inflammatory changes are absent (Figure 20.26). There is selective loss of thick (myosin) myofilaments and preservation of thin (actin) myofilaments and Z discs (Figure 20.27).

The outcome from critical illness myopathy is generally better than after critical illness polyneuropathy and most patients make a full recovery unless there has been severe and prolonged paralysis.

Acute necrotising myopathy of intensive care This is a rare condition which may be a form of rhabdomyolysis. It develops after exposure to neuromuscular blocking agents with or without steroid therapy but may be associated with other infective or metabolic insults. The serum CK is markedly elevated, there is usually associated myoglobinuria. EMG confirms a severe myopathy and biopsy shows patchy or widespread necrosis with occasionally vasculitis or infarction within the muscle. The prognosis for recovery of weakness is poor.

Other myopathies Almost any form of myopathy may be responsible for prolonged respiratory failure in critical care units. Patients with weakness and asthma and others who have been exposed to corticosteroids alone may have acute steroid myopathy. This is a slowly evolving mild to moderate proximal weakness with mild elevation of CK and type 2 fibre atrophy. Occasionally, direct sepsis may affect the muscle causing pyomyositis resulting from septic micrometastases.

Inflammatory myopathies may cause respiratory muscle weakness. Patients with dermatomyositis may have a characteristic skin rash. The EMG may be misleading, showing numerous fibrillation potentials and positive sharp waves that are more characteristic of denervation from neuropathy. The CK is elevated and muscle biopsy of an involved muscle is necessary to make the diagnosis. Other inflammatory myopathies include viral myositis, acute alcoholic rhabdomyolysis and myopathy secondary to hypophosphataemia. Trichinosis caused by the ingestion of raw contaminated pork may cause an acute and severe myopathy with diaphragm and intercostal muscle involvement.

Patients with muscular dystrophy may present with ventilatory failure or develop respiratory insufficiency either as an early manifestation or as an inevitable feature of disease progression. Myotonic dystrophy is occasionally identified for the first time in the ICU. In adults, acid maltase deficiency may present with proximal weakness, scoliosis and diaphragmatic paralysis. The apparently abrupt respiratory insufficiency probably occurs on the background of long-standing unrecognised disease. Progressive respiratory impairment occurs in all patients with Duchenne muscular dystrophy, and acute deterioration may occur because of intercurrent events such as aspiration pneumonia.

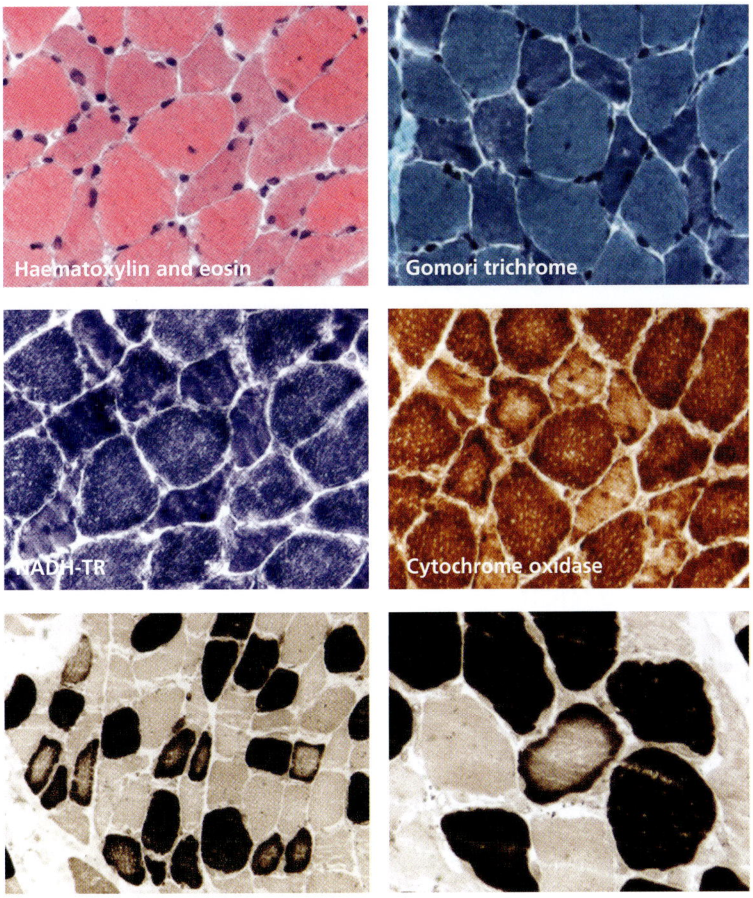

Figure 20.26 Muscle biopsy in critical illness myopathy showing abnormal variation in fibre size with dark atrophic fibres. Courtesy of Prof Janice Holton, Professor of Neuropathology, Institute of Neurology, Queen Square.

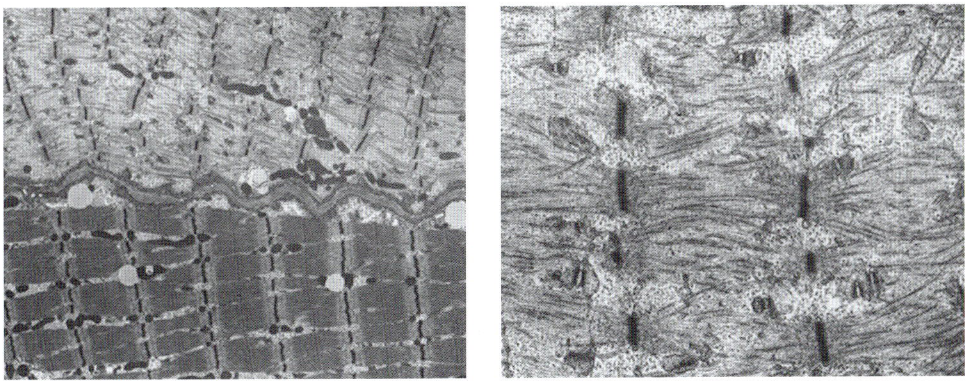

Figure 20.27 Electron microscope of muscle biopsy: (a) in normal; (b) in critical illness myopathy showing loss of myosin thick filaments. Courtesy of Prof Janice Holton, Professor of Neuropathology, Institute of Neurology, Queen Square.

Rhabdomyolysis may be precipitated by trauma, compartment syndrome, ischaemic arterial occlusion or drugs and is associated with high serum CK levels, myoglobinuria and general weakness. There are reports of respiratory decompensation associated with mitochondrial myopathies, limb girdle muscular dystrophy, HIV-related myopathy and sarcoid myopathy involving the diaphagm.

Tetanus (Chapter 9)

Most patients with established tetanus will be admitted to an NICU because of increased muscle tone and spasms that typically begin in the masseter muscles, resulting in the classic finding of trismus. Respiratory compromise is caused by spasm of respiratory muscles or laryngospasm. Autonomic dysfunction occurs in severe cases and results in heart rate and blood pressure lability, arrhythmias, fever, profuse sweating, peripheral vasoconstriction and ileus. Muscle rupture and rhabdomyolysis can complicate extreme cases.

Supportive care consists of treatment in a quiet ICU setting to allow cardiorespiratory monitoring with minimal stimulation. Intubation may be required owing to hypoventilation caused by muscular rigidity or laryngospasm and should be performed in a controlled elective manner if possible. Therapeutic paralysis with neuromuscular blocking agents may be necessary in severe cases. Treatment in the ICU has resulted in a pronounced improvement in prognosis for patients with tetanus. Modern mortality is approximately 10%.

Rabies (Chapter 9)

Paralytic rabies, produces neuromuscular weakness that can be difficult to differentiate from other causes of weakness such as Guillain–Barré syndrome. Rabies may begin with local wound pain and paraesthesias followed by fasciculations near the site of inoculation.

General medical care on the NICU

The role of an ICU is to maintain normal physiological homeostasis while actively treating the underlying cause of any physiological derangement. The following general medical complications may arise during the care of patients on an NICU (Table 20.22).

Nosocomial infection and infection surveillance

Sepsis (and the systemic inflammatory response to sepsis) remains the major cause of organ failure and death in the ICU, being either directly or indirectly responsible for 75% of all deaths. Common sites of infection include the urinary tract, respiratory tract (especially ventilator-associated pneumonia) and catheter-related sepsis. Placement of intravenous catheters requires meticulous aseptic technique and regular changing of lines. It is important to ensure that the tips of catheters that have been removed are sent for culture. Catheter-related infections are usually caused by coagulase-negative staphylococci (*Staphylococcus epidermidis* or *S. aureus*) and treatment should be directed by sensitivities determined by culture. The importance of infection control in the NICU cannot be overstated. This involves the isolation of the infected patient whenever possible, meticulous staff hygiene (e.g. hand-washing before and after each patient contact, aseptic techniques for invasive procedures), early identification and treatment of infection by routine blood, urine, sputum culture, use of disposable equipment and, most importantly, joint ward rounds between microbiologists and the ICU team (Table 20.23).

Anticoagulation

Prophylaxis against venous thrombosis is essential and all patients should wear graduated compression stockings and have regular active or passive leg exercises. Unless contraindicated, low molecular weight heparin should be routinely administered.

Delirium

Delirium is characterised by alteration in the level of consciousness ranging from paradoxical agitation to sedation and stupor. Impairment of attention may be manifest as distractibility or difficulty shifting the focus of attention (perseveration), distorted thinking and memory impairment. Symptoms fluctuate and are worse at night with sleep wake reversal, often associated with the development of hallucinations, visual illusions, disorientation and perceptual distortion. Delirium is common in ICU patients and is associated with increased mortality and poor cognitive outcome. Risk factors for the development of delirium are summarised in Table 20.24.

Primary prevention of delirium may need to be balanced against the requirements for sedation, analgesia and general ITU management. Prevention is multi-factorial and the principles are summarised in Table 20.25.

Patient comfort

Agitation is common in the NICU and is distinct from delirium. It has a variety of causes (Table 20.26). It may manifest as discomfort, pulling at intravenous and bladder catheters, tracheal and nasogastric tubes, shouting, aggressive behaviour, extreme restlessness and confusion. Pain is particularly common and often unrecognised because of confusion and the difficulties with communication in the aphonic or paralysed patient.

Many patients require sedation but there is a natural reluctance to sedate patients with an evolving CNS disorder. The first line of management is to reassure and calm the patient in a quiet environment and to ensure a normal diurnal cycle. There should be careful nursing and treatment of the underlying causes, including positioning, splinting, bed cages, catheterisation and physical treatments. Nonetheless, sedative and analgesic drugs are often necessary to reduce distress, anxiety and pain and to aid toleration of tracheal tubes, intermittent positive pressure ventilation (IPPV), tracheal suction and physiotherapy.

Pain

Pain is a prominent feature of many neurological conditions seen in the NICU and needs to be recognised and treated effectively, particularly in patients with a reduced level of consciousness or who are mechanically ventilated and unable to communicate. Combinations of opioid and non-opioid drug treatment, including agents directed towards neuropathic pain (e.g. amitriptyline, gabapentin), may be required. These provide effective analgesia, induce euphoria and aid toleration of IPPV. Side effects of opiates include hypotension, respiratory depression, nausea and vomiting, and decreased gut motility; the fear of addiction is vastly exaggerated. Intravenous administration is more easily controlled and predictable. Commonly used drugs include morphine and fentanyl but short-acting drugs such as remifentanil may be valuable.

Communication

Speech is often possible even in patients who are mechanically ventilated via a tracheostomy. It requires speaking valves and, more importantly, the expertise of an experienced speech and language therapist. Where speech is impossible, other communication aids should be used.

Sleep

Sleep deprivation almost invariably occurs in patients nursed in an ICU setting. Factors include disruption of day–night cycles, environmental factors such as noise and patient fear. The disruption is associated with agitation, confusion and the development of ICU psychosis. Furthermore, sleep deprivation has a direct effect on respiratory muscle function, catabolism and the immune response. It is essential to re-establish a normal pattern of sleep by the use of hypnotic drugs (e.g. benzodiazepines, sedative tricyclic antidepressants, zopiclone). The use of melatonin has proved useful in resistant insomnia.

Table 20.22 General medical complications of the neurological intensive care unit (NICU).

Pulmonary complications	Acute hypoxaemic respiratory failure caused by ventilation–perfusion mismatch from infection (often secondary to aspiration), atelectasis, pulmonary oedema or pulmonary embolus
	Nosocomial or aspiration pneumonia
	Ventilator-associated pneumonia caused by gastro-oesophageal reflux and cross-colonisation from other patients, hospital personnel or equipment
	Acute lung injury and acute respiratory distress syndrome are associated with sepsis, trauma, aspiration pneumonitis and fat embolism
	Neurogenic pulmonary oedema
	Pulmonary emboli
Cardiovascular system	The principal function of monitoring the cardiovascular system in NICU is the maintenance of arterial blood pressure and blood volume to ensure adequate organ perfusion
	Hypotension may be the result of an inadequate circulating blood volume, poor myocardial contractility, a decreased SVR or a combination of these factors
	Hypovolaemia
	Decreased myocardial contractility may be the result of many factors including ischaemic heart disease, sepsis, hypoxaemia, hypercarbia, acidosis, cardiac disease, electrolyte disturbance and drugs
	Hypertension is a common consequence of acute neurological events
	Cardiac arrhythmias are associated with aneurysmal SAH, head injury, acute ischaemic or haemorrhagic stroke, status epilepticus, Guillain–Barré syndrome and impending or established brain death
	Sinus bradycardia is due to sympathetic blockade and/or increased vagal tone and occurs in Guillain–Barré syndrome
	Sinus tachycardia is extremely common in acute neurological illness and may be associated with hypoxaemia, hypercapnia and neuromuscular blockade or as a compensatory mechanism in anaemia, hypovolaemia and pulmonary emboli
	Atrial fibrillation with a rapid ventricular response is common, as either a cause or a consequence, in acute stroke
	Atrial flutter may compromise ventricular filling and increase the risk of ischaemia
	Heart block
	Ventricular tachycardia is common in SAH and may predispose to the development of torsade de pointes, ventricular flutter and ventricular fibrillation

Table 20.22 (continued)

Alimentary system	Protein catabolism is almost invariable in patients nursed on the ICU and is often caused by an inadequate supply of calories and an increased energy and oxygen consumption associated with the stress response to injury and sepsis
	Enteral feeding via a nasogastric tube should be started as soon as possible as this decreases catabolism, provides protection against peptic ulceration and maintains intestinal integrity, thus decreasing the occurrence of bacterial translocation (see nosocomial infection) • Adynamic ileus • Gastrointestinal bleeding • Constipation occurs as a result of opioid drug administration, immobility and a lack of fibre in some enteral feeds • Diarrhoea has many causes but infection (including that by *Clostridium difficile*), malabsorption and diarrhoea associated with enteral feeds are the most important

SAH, subarachnoid haemorrhage; SVR, systemic vascular resistance.

Table 20.23 Risk factors for nosocomial infections.

Age over 70 years
Widespread use of broad-spectrum antibacterial drugs
Mechanical ventilation and endotracheal tube
Presence of foreign bodies (e.g. intravascular cannulae, bladder catheter, pacemaker)
Immunodeficiency states and immunosuppressant medication
Colonisation of the oropharynx
Use of H_2 receptor antagonists
Underlying chronic lung disease and reintubation

Table 20.24 Delirium.

The development of delirium is related to: • The degree of sedative exposure (especially benzodiazepines) • Pain caused by suboptimal analgesia • Sleep disruption • Age • Pre-existing cognitive dysfunction • Sensory impairment • Poor nutrition – multiple surgical procedures, malnutrition, dehydration, alcohol • Systemic infection • Surgery

Communication with the family

Communication with family and friends on the ICU presents great challenges for medical and nursing staff. It is essential that staff should be consistent in their assessment and honest in the appraisal of the uncertainties in management and prognosis. It is preferable if only one or two clinicians act as the primary source of information.

It is important to recognise that the family may experience acute stress reactions which may be manifest as anger, frustration, bitterness and guilt. There must be adequate and patient discussion, often on a daily basis.

End of life issues on intensive care

In the final stages of severe illness when treatment fails, or no longer provides a net benefit to patients, the primary goal of medicine – to restore a person's health – cannot be achieved. This is a common situation on ICU where many patients are unable to communicate their wishes to family or doctors.

There must always be a heavy presumption in favour of administering life-prolonging treatments when they are considered of potential benefit (e.g. cardiopulmonary resuscitation, mechanical ventilation, renal support, artificial nutrition and hydration, drug infusions, blood products and antibiotics). However, the decision to withdraw such treatment is difficult and depends on the assessment of best interest given the possibility of meaningful recovery, the sanctity of life and the right of each individual to be treated with dignity, compassion and respect. Withdrawal of life prolonging treatment is entirely distinct from euthanasia and physician assisted suicide; rather it switches attention to palliation and allows the already dying patient to achieve a peaceful, natural and dignified death.

When patients are competent to make decisions themselves the overriding principle of autonomy to determine their wishes must be respected. If the patient is not competent to make a decision on his or her own behalf then that decision rests with the medical carers made in the best interest of the patient. The responsible doctors must not transpose their own beliefs, values or priorities on to the patient and must make a concerted effort to ascertain the wishes of the patient from the family or caregivers.

The ethical issues of withholding and withdrawing life-prolonging medical treatment are complex and demanding. When treatment is futile and modern technology is simply prolonging the dying process, it is often in the best interest of the patient to withdraw life-prolonging medical treatment and to allow the illness to run its natural course. However, such decisions require meticulous and sensitive communication and a deep understanding of the emotional turmoil experienced by the family or caregivers. Ultimately, the clinician's primary duty is always to the patient and his or her best interests. These issues continue to be extensively debated. While patients are insentient as a consequence of the disease or its treatment, the family are their advocate. Frequently, families are involved in end-of-life decisions for patients in coma or vegetative state in whom there is no hope of recovery. It is essential to establish, if possible, the patient's own preference for management through living wills, advanced directives or simply by having voiced a clear preference to family or the surrogate decision-makers. The autonomy of the patient must be maintained by respecting these preferences, although a consensus agreement of family members must always be sought by careful explanation and education.

Table 20.25 Management of delirium.

Non-pharmacological
Treat hypoxia, infection and pain
Provide support and orientation (natural daylight, news, TV)
Allow clear day–night cycles
Maintain afferent sensory input (glasses, hearing aids)
Pharmacological
Avoid medication particularly antimuscarinic agents, phenothiazides, amitriptyline, hyoscine, prednisolone, ranitidine, dopaminergic (levodopa), GABAminergic (benzodiazepines) and drugs that suppress REM sleep (e.g. opioids, benzodiazepines, tricyclic antidepressants)
Hyperactive/mixed delirium
Haloperidol – but risk of extrapyramidal side effects and QT_c prolongation
Atypical antipsychotics (preferred) – olanzapine, risperidone, quetiapine
α-2 agonists – particularly clonidine in hyperactive delirium
Propofol
Benzodiazepines – should be avoided because they may exacerbated the delirium but short acting midazalam is useful in the management of alcohol withdrawal

Table 20.26 Causes of agitation and restlessness on the neurological intensive care unit (NICU).

Pain
Anxiety
Confusion
Sleep deprivation
Sepsis
Drugs and withdrawal
Metabolic – hypoglycaemia, hyperglycaemia, hyponatraemia, uraemia, hepatic
Respiratory – infection, hypoxaemia, hypercarbia
Cardiac – low output state, hypotension

Neurology of general critical care

The majority of neurologists work in district general or teaching hospitals with large general ICUs. In this setting, ICUs require an increasing input from neurologists, especially with regard to the assessment of hypoxic brain damage and the neurological complications of organ failure, critical illness and sepsis.

Neurological complications on the ICU are usually caused by metabolic encephalopathy, seizures, hypoxic–ischaemic encephalopathy, stroke or neuromuscular disorders but multiple complications are common.

Failure to awaken/depressed conscious state

Sudden or gradual deterioration in consciousness may occur during an ICU stay or reflect failure to awaken after general anaesthesia for several reasons (Table 20.27). Sedation and analgesia are

Table 20.27 Causes of failure to awaken on ICU after sedation or anaesthetic.

Drugs – sedation, analgesia, neuromuscular paralysis
Hypoxic – ischaemic injury
Sepsis
Metabolic encephalopathy – renal, hepatic, electrolyte, endocrine
Stroke
Primary CNS inflammation
Multi-factorial – most common

Table 20.28 Causes of persistent weakness on the ICU.

Disorders of the cortex and brainstem
Epilepsy – status epilepticus (convulsive & non-convulsive)
Vascular – brainstem infarction or haemorrhage, subarachnoid haemorrhage, intracerebral haemorrhage
Infection – brainstem encephalitis, herpes simplex encephalitis, poliomyelitis
Inflammatory – Multiple sclerosis (MS), acute disseminated encephalomyelitis (ADEM), acute haemorrhagic leukoencephalopathy (AHL)
Metabolic – central pontine myelinolysis
Hypoxic–ischaemic encephalopathy
White matter disease – posterior reversible leukoencephalopathy, toxic leukoencephalopathy
Autoimmune encephalitis – paraneoplastic, Morvan's, Hashimoto's
Disorders of the spinal cord
Arnold–Chiari malformation, cerebellar ectopic
Trauma • Acute epidural compression due to neoplasm, infection, haematoma • Acute transverse myelitis (demyelination, infective) • Cord infarction
Anterior horn cell
Motor neurone disease
Poliomyelitis and post polio syndrome
Spinal muscular atrophy
Multiple radiculopathies
Carcinomatous meningitis
AIDS polyradiculitis
Acute polyneuropathy
Acute inflammatory demyelinating polyneuropathy (AIDP)
Acute motor and sensory axonal neuropathy (AMSAN)
Acute motor axonal neuropathy (AMAN)
Phrenic neuropathies
Critical illness polyneuropathy (CIP)
Others – toxic neuropathies, vasculitis, diphtheria, porphyria
Chronic polyneuropathies
Chronic inflammatory demyelinating polyneuropathy (CIDP)
Diabetic polyneuropathy
Neuromuscular transmission defects
Myasthenia gravis
Lambert–Eaton myasthenic syndrome
Congenital myasthenic syndromes
Neuromuscular blocking agents
Other: botulism, snake bites, fish toxins, organophosphates, hypermagnesaemia, poisoning

Table 20.28 (continued)

Myopathy
Congenital
Myotonic dystrophy
Acid maltase deficiency
Mitochondrial
Periodic paralysis
Acquired
Inflammatory myopathies – polymyositis, dermatomyositis
Critical illness myopathy • Associated with neuromuscular blocking agents and steroids • Associated with sepsis
Non-necrotic cachectic myopathy
Rhabdomyolysis
Others: HIV-related, sarcoid, hypokalaemia, hypophosphataemia

confounding factors in those with depressed consciousness. These drugs are used to reduce agitation and pain, with the goals of diminishing discomfort, oxygen demand, ventilator asynchrony and self-removal of catheters and other devices. They also induce amnesia and reduce the risk of a post-traumatic stress disorder. Withdrawal of sedation before review is essential for reliable neurological assessment and it is important to realise that the effects of sedative drugs may take several days to clear; any of them may accumulate if there is multi-organ failure, and even with apparently normal metabolic function their half-life may be abnormally long in patients who have been critically ill. Deep sedation leads to prolonged recovery time, difficulty weaning, ileus and a confusional state. Other drugs used for sedation or analgesia may also contribute to apparent neuromuscular weakness; opioids (particularly morphine, fentanyl, alfentanyl), benzodiazepines and other anxiolytic and hypnotic agents.

Weakness and failure to wean from mechanical ventilation

Weakness on the ICU often presents as difficulty in weaning from ventilation but there may also be reduced movements in an obtunded patient, or generalised or focal weakness in an alert patient. This must be distinguished from the non-specific weakness of fatigue secondary to systemic illness (Table 20.28).

Weakness may be central or peripheral. In the comatose patient, a central cause should be suspected if there are upper motor neurone signs, if the distribution of the weakness is pyramidal or if there is a hemiparesis. Paraparesis is often caused by nerve or muscle disorders, and less often spinal disorders (infarction secondary to a hypotensive or embolic episode). Monoparesis may occasionally be a manifestation of a stroke but more often a consequence of pressure or positioning palsy (femoral or common peroneal nerve palsies).

Neuromuscular disease may occur in the ICU patient as:

- A complication of a non-neurological illness (e.g. critical illness polyneuropathy associated with SIRS)
- A primary neurological disorder (e.g. Guillain–Barré syndrome)
- An acute exacerbation of an underlying neuromuscular condition (e.g. myasthenia gravis)

- Progression of a previously diagnosed neuromuscular disease (e.g. Duchenne muscular dystrophy, motor neurone disease, acid maltase deficiency), or
- A complication of treatment (e.g. acute quadriplegic myopathy).

Sleep and its disorders

Structure of normal sleep

Sleep is a highly organised and regular process which is divided into stages defined by changes in EEG, electro-oculogram (EOG) and muscle tone (EMG). Four principal states of consciousness – wakefulness, light sleep, slow wave sleep (SWS) and rapid eye movement (REM) sleep – can be distinguished (Figure 20.28).

The onset of sleep is characterised by a brief transitional phase (stage 1) in which the alert and wakeful alpha rhythm (8–13 Hz) begins to slow, and slow theta (4–7 Hz) waves appear. EOG usually demonstrates rolling eye movements. EMG activity may be reduced from that during wakefulness but is still present. Stage 2 sleep is characterised by the appearance on the EEG of episodic bursts of central, 14–16 Hz rhythms (sleep spindles) and 0.5–1 second high-amplitude central sharp waves (K complexes). EMG activity is similar to that in stage 1. In stages 3 and 4 sleep (SWS) the EEG is dominated by high-amplitude delta activity (>4 Hz). SWS is associated with slowing of cardiac and respiratory rate, lowered blood pressure, marked muscular relaxation and a reduction in metabolic rate by approximately 70% of normal levels. Normal values for sleep parameters in an adult are summarised in Table 20.29.

Table 20.29 Approximate normal values for sleep parameters in an adult.

Sleep efficiency	>90%
Stage 1	10%
Stage 2	50%
Stage 3/4	20%
REM sleep	20%
Sleep onset	>10 minutes
REM sleep onset	90 minutes

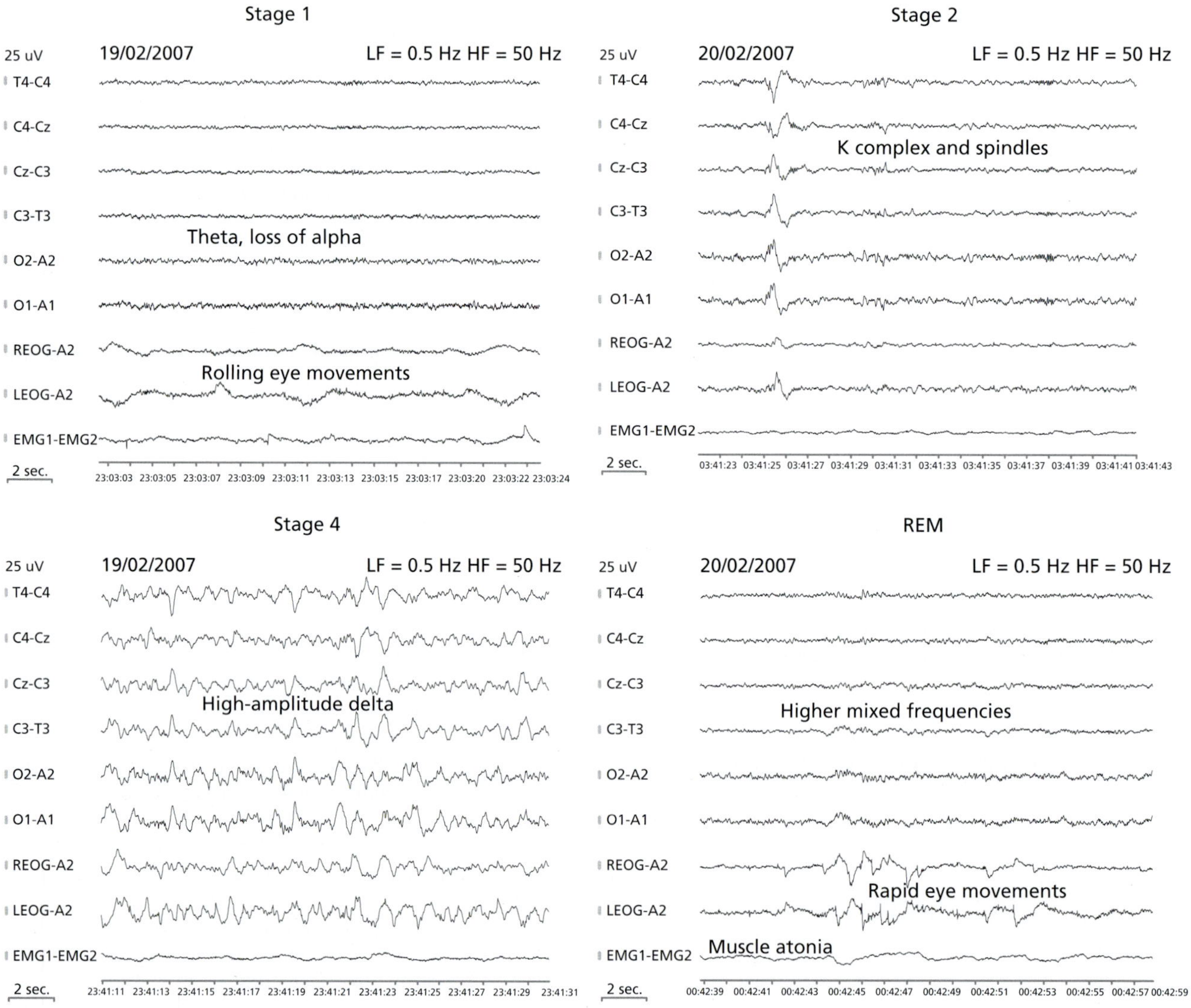

Figure 20.28 EEG recordings showing sleep stages.

REM sleep

REM sleep is characterised by desynchronisation of the EEG with the appearances of faster frequency rhythms. There are bursts of saccadic eye movements and profound relaxation of muscle tone in most major muscle groups of the limbs, neck and trunk including the diaphragm. Functional imaging during REM sleep shows that limbic regions, associated with emotional behavioural and experience, are activated during REM sleep, while regions of the frontal cortex are less active. Descending neuromuscular inhibition leads to profound muscular relaxation (atonia) of REM sleep. This may be important in preventing dream enactment.

Patterns of sleep

As a subject falls asleep there is descent through four stages of deepening non-REM sleep during the first hour which is accompanied by a gradual slowing of the EEG rhythms. This is followed by ascent through the same stages culminating in REM sleep. The process is then repeated several times during the night. The first episode of REM sleep generally occurs as the sleep stages ascend through light sleep after about 60–90 minutes following sleep onset and it is often relatively short. As rhythmic cycling continues, the length of time spent in REM sleep tends to increase throughout the night while the time spent in SWS progressively decreases.

Regulation of wakefulness and sleep

The regulation of wakefulness and sleep depends on complex neuronal and biochemical interactions involving the cortex (basal forebrain), diencephalon (thalamus and hypothalamus) and brainstem. A number of neurochemicals are involved in the regulation of sleep including those that are wake promoting (e.g. noradrenaline, acetylcholine, histamine, and dopamine); sleep promoting (e.g. melatonin and GABA); and both sleep and wake promoting (e.g. serotonin). More recently, the hypocretin (orexin) system has been shown to have a critical role in sleep regulation. The occurrence of REM sleep depends on the interaction between REM-inhibiting nuclei (raphe nucleus secreting serotonin, locus coeruleus secreting noradrenaline) and REM-promoting nuclei (laterodorsal and pedunculo-pontine tegmental nuclei secreting acetylcholine).

Regulation of the timing of the sleep cycles involves two mechanisms:

1 Central rhythm generation which is determined by a circadian oscillator located in the suprachiasmatic nucleus of the hypothalamus. This is influenced by light detected in the retina and melatonin. The oscillations are mediated by the cyclical transcription and translation of specific genes, so-called clock genes. The circadian rhythm affects not only sleep, but also other functions via the diurnal secretion of hormones from the pituitary and pineal gland.
2 Independent homeostatic mechanisms which are controlled by the time spent awake. It is suggested that the 'sleep debt' which builds up during long periods of wakefulness depends on the accumulation of 'somnogens', possibly adenosine, in the brain.

Functions of sleep

The functions of sleep remain unclear. The traditional role of sleep has been thought to be restorative but there is evidence to suggest a more complex mechanism in information processing such as memory consolidation. Even minor degrees of sleep deprivation have significant effects on cognition, memory and behaviour.

Sleep and breathing

SWS sleep leads to an increase in parasympathetic tone and decrease in sympathetic tone leading to a reduction in heart rate, blood pressure and respiratory rate. REM sleep is associated with autonomic instability causing fluctuations in heart rate and blood pressure. The muscles of the upper airway relax during all stages of sleep (especially in REM sleep) causing snoring and predisposing to the significant airway obstruction that underlies sleep apnoea or hypopnoea syndrome. Respiratory failure resulting from neuromuscular weakness is also exacerbated during REM sleep because of the muscular relaxation involving upper airway, intercostal muscles and the diaphragm.

Classification of sleep disorders

Sleep medicine is an evolving field with wide variability in knowledge of each individual sleep disorder. Table 20.30 lists the most recent classification that is based on common complaints (e.g. insomnia or hypersomnias) as well as presumed aetiological basis (e.g. circadian rhythm disorders) or organ system from which problems arise (e.g. sleep-related breathing disorders). The classification system is currently under review.

Insomnia

Insomnia is the complaint of 'poor sleep'; the duration or subjective quality of sleep is inadequate and non-restorative. Insomnia is extremely common and is said to merit treatment in 8–14% of the normal population. It is often associated with daytime fatigue but rarely daytime sleepiness. Although insomnia can be idiopathic, in many instances there is an underlying cause.

Several factors may contribute to insomnia: psychological difficulties, a variety of prescribed medications (particularly beta-blockers) and non-prescribed drugs including caffeine, alcohol and substances of abuse, particularly cocaine and amphetamine. Sleep is also disrupted by depression, anxiety, stress, pain, cognitive impairment, pregnancy, nocturia and other medical disorders (especially respiratory and cardiac disorders). Insomnia may occur as a consequence of other sleep disorders (e.g. restless legs syndrome) causing interrupted sleep architecture. Neurological conditions that cause insomnia include those in which sleep is disrupted because of pain or discomfort (e.g. MS); those in which there is interference with sleep onset or maintenance; and those in which a structural lesion may interfere with sleep generation. In addition to the economic and social effects, chronic unremitting insomnia predisposes to

Table 20.30 Classification of sleep disorders.

1	Insomnias
2	Sleep-related breathing disorders
3	Hypersomnias of central origin not due to a circadian rhythm sleep disorder, sleep-related breathing disorder or other cause of disturbed nocturnal sleep
4	Circadian rhythm sleep disorders
5	Parasomnias
6	Sleep-related movement disorders
7	Isolated symptoms, apparent normal variants and unresolved issues
8	Other sleep disorders

Source: American Academy of Sleep Medicine 2005. Reproduced with permission of AASM.

psychiatric disorders including depression, anxiety and substance abuse.

Insomnia can, exceptionally, result from prion disease. Fatal familial insomnia is a very rare hereditary prion disease caused by a mutation in codon 178 of the prion protein gene. It is characterised by insomnia, loss of slow wave sleep, oneiric episodes (daytime dream episodes and enactment) and progressive neurological decline.

Management

A critical aspect of management is to treat the underlying cause (e.g. anxiety, depression). In addition, the first line is to teach, establish and maintain good sleep hygiene with a regular bedtime, the avoidance of nocturnal stimulants, stressful activity or exercise close to bedtime and daytime napping and establishing comfortable and regular sleep arrangements. Regular exercise not close to bedtime can increase and consolidate deep sleep. Cognitive–behavioural therapy (CBT) has been shown to be the most effective treatment for chronic insomnia and can be administered either individually or in group sessions. Access to appropriate CBT for insomnia may be limited and a number of internet based applications are currently being developed.

Most drugs used in insomnia act as agonists at the benzodiazepine site of the $GABA_A$ receptor; these drugs have effects other than their sedating action, including muscle relaxation, antiepileptic effects, anxiolytic effects, memory impairment, behavioural disturbance (especially in children) and ataxia. Some drugs have a more specific action (e.g. zolpidem, zaleplon and zopiclone) by targeting only specific $GABA_A$ receptor subtypes. Drugs with longer duration of action may affect psychomotor performance, memory and concentration, and also have prolonged anxiolytic and muscle relaxing effects. Alternatively, benzodiazepines with too short a half-life may result in rebound insomnia and daytime hyperexcitability. Hypnotic drugs such as zolpidem and specific benzodiazepines are indicated for the management of acute insomnia or in the short-term management of chronic insomnia. There is a growing use of sedative antidepressants (e.g. mirtazapine, trazodone and amitriptyline) for longer term treatment of insomnia, and in some melatonin may be helpful.

Sleep-related breathing disorders

Obstructive sleep apnoea/hypopnoea syndrome

Obstructive sleep apnoea/hypopnoea syndrome (OSAHS) is the most common medical cause of daytime hypersomnolence and is associated with significant morbidity including an increased incidence of hypertension, cerebrovascular disease and road traffic accidents. It is associated with nocturnal sleep disturbance, unrefreshing sleep, difficulty in concentration and nocturnal choking. Sleep apnoea refers to a cessation in airflow during sleep >10 seconds while hypopnoea is defined as >50% reduction in airflow associated with oxygen desaturation >4% or arousal on EEG. More than five apnoeas/hypopnoeas per hour (apnoea/hypopnoea index, AHI) is considered significant with AHI 5–15/hour representing mild, AHI 15–30/hour moderate and AHI >30/hour severe OSAHS.

Obstruction of the upper airway usually occurs between the caudal soft palate and epiglottis. It is worsened during sleep when reduced upper airway muscle tone leads to collapse of the upper airway and obstruction. This is exacerbated by obesity (body mass index >28 kg/m^2), a narrow palate, crowding of the oropharynx and jaw or facial structural anomalies. Patients have difficulty with falling asleep, loud snoring, stridor, coughing spells during sleep and restless sleep with frequent wakenings. There may be snoring and irregular breathing patterns and prolonged apnoea. Severe obstructive sleep apnoea is associated with morning headache, impaired memory, nocturia, anxiety and the development of Pickwickian features with cor pulmonale.

Management The first line management is weight loss, establishing regular sleep patterns and avoidance of alcohol, nicotine, caffeine and sedatives in the evening. Investigation and appropriate treatment of co-morbidity, particularly hypothyroidism, is mandatory. CPAP by nasal or face mask is effective in OSAHS, improving sleep architecture, nocturnal oxygenation and the symptoms of sleepiness, impaired cognition, mood and driving ability and cardiovascular function. However, its use requires considerable educational support and technical back-up. Compliance may be variable in the less severe forms of the condition because of poor mask fitting, dryness of the mouth and airways, claustrophobia, aerophagia and social difficulties. Oral appliances such as mandibular advancement splints may be valuable in improving excessive daytime somnolence (EDS) and the cardiovascular complications of mild OSAHS. They work by holding the mandible forward, thus increasing the upper airway space by advancing the tongue and possibly changing genioglossus activity. Surgical treatment (uvulo-palato-pharyngoplasty) does not have a role. Tracheostomy may be necessary in patients with incipient cor pulmonale.

Hypersomnias of central origin

Primary (idiopathic) hypersomnia

Primary (idiopathic) hypersomnia is a rare disorder characterised by EDS but without cataplexy or nocturnal sleep disruption which usually starts in adolescence. The aetiology is unknown but there is a rare familial incidence. This can be associated with prolonged nocturnal sleep times in which the person often sleeps through an alarm clock. Sleep drunkenness is a common feature in the morning when the person may be disorientated, confused, slow, unsteady and sleepy. EDS is unaffected by prolonged sleep or frequent naps. Polysomnography shows shortened sleep latency, increased total sleep time and an absence of sleep onset REM periods. Primary hypersomnia is associated with low or normal levels of CSF orexin/hypocretin. However, it must be distinguished from narcolepsy without cataplexy or other causes of EDS.

Recurrent hypersomnia

Recurrent hypersomnia may occur in the Kleine–Levin syndrome. This condition usually occurs in adolescence and in males. The episodes of hypersomnolence are associated with hyper(mega)phagia, cognitive change, aggression and hypersexuality; prognosis is guarded as it does not respond well to treatment with stimulants, carbamazepine, lamotrigine or lithium, but it usually resolves within a decade of onset.

Idiopathic recurring stupor

Idiopathic recurring stupor is a rare syndrome occurring in males over 30 years and characterised by episodes of stupor and coma lasting hours to days with no obvious precipitating factors. The EEG demonstrates beta rhythms and the condition responds to the benzodiazepine antagonist flumazenil, raising the possibility that this condition results from endogenous benzodiazepine agonists.

Excessive daytime somnolence in neurological disease

EDS can also occur as a consequence of structural brain lesions, following head injury or encephalitis (particularly encephalitis lethargica) and is a complication of neurodegenerative conditions (e.g. Alzheimer's disease and idiopathic Parkinson's disease) and also MS and myotonic dystrophy.

Narcolepsy

Narcolepsy is the most cause of central hypersomnia. A primary disorder of alertness with an estimated prevalence of 3–5/10 000, it may develop at any age but the peak onset is between 15 and 30 years with a secondary peak in the fourth decade. Narcolepsy is rarely familial. However, the lifetime risk for developing narcolepsy is increased in first degree relatives of narcoleptic patients to 1%. The presenting symptoms are usually EDS, with irresistible sleep attacks during the day often occurring at inappropriate times. Other symptoms of this syndrome are cataplexy, sleep paralysis, hypnogogic hallucinations or vivid dream-like images, which characteristically occur at sleep onset, disrupted sleep (including occurrence of REM sleep behavioural disorder) and short periods of automatic behaviour during daytime (micro-sleeps).

There may be a range of secondary symptoms related to sleepiness including visual blurring, diplopia and difficulties with memory and concentration. In combination, the symptoms of narcolepsy often have a major impact on relationships, education, employment, driving, mood and quality of life.

Cataplexy

Cataplexy is the occurrence of brief episodes of muscle weakness or paralysis precipitated by strong emotion, such as laughter, anger or surprise. There is a partial or complete loss of bilateral muscle tone. In its less severe form, cataplexy leads to transient bilateral ptosis, head droop, slurred speech or dropping things from the hands. Cataplexy may be severe enough to lead to complete collapse. The episodes are brief, lasting for seconds or minutes, but they may be followed by a sleep episode or occur recurrently (especially following sudden medication withdrawal) leading to status cataplecticus. Cataplexy is present in over 70% of people who have narcolepsy and can predate or follow the onset of other symptoms.

Hypnogogic/hypnopompic hallucinations

These are brief vivid dream-like episodes that occur at sleep onset or immediately before waking, and are often frightening or disturbing in nature. They are characterised by brief visual, tactile or auditory events, which continue for several minutes. They can occur during daytime naps.

Sleep paralysis and automatic behaviours

Sleep paralysis is the inability to move on waking from sleep. The episode can last from a few seconds to minutes but diaphragm and respiratory muscle activity continues. It is caused by the persistence of REM-related atonia on waking. Sleep paralysis is often associated with a hypnic hallucination often of someone pressing down on the chest or choking the person.

Short periods of automatic behaviour occur on wakening, characterised by absent-minded behaviour, nonsense speech or writing nonsense, reflecting the intrusion of sleep into the awake state. Nocturnal sleep disruption is also common, resulting paradoxically in insomnia.

Pathophysiology of narcolepsy

Narcolepsy is associated with abnormalities of the hypocretin–orexin neurotransmitter system. Low or undetectable levels of CSF orexin/hypocretin are found in most patients although some may have normal or raised levels (low hypocretin levels best correlate with the presence of cataplexy). This has led to one hypothesis that in most patients there is a deficiency of hypocretin resulting from hypocretin neuronal loss in the hypothalamus. In most, it is likely this is an autoimmune condition – narcolepsy is strongly associated with HLA type and recently it has been found to be associated with anti-tribble homolg 2 (a protein found in hypocretin secreting neurons) autoantibodies (TRIB2). In addition, there has been an association beytween narcolepsy and the H1N1 influenza vaccination. There may also be a form with 'hypocretin resistance' caused by abnormal hypocretin receptor–post-receptor dynamics leading to overproduction of hypocretin. Narcolepsy can also rarely occur secondary to tumours, encephalitis, head injury and MS. Narcolepsy-type symptoms can develop with inherited conditions such as Niemann–Pick type C disease, Norrie disease, Möbius syndrome and Prader–Willi syndrome.

Investigations

Polysomnography (PSG) is important in excluding other causes of EDS including obstructive sleep apnoea, periodic limb movement disorder and REM-related behavioural disorder; however, all are more common in people with narcolepsy. Polysomnography may also demonstrate early onset sleep (<10 minutes) and early onset REM sleep (<20 minutes). The Multiple Sleep Latency Test (MSLT) is used to confirm the diagnosis. In this test the patient is allowed to fall asleep 4–5 times at 2-hourly intervals throughout the day and the latency to onset of sleep and REM sleep is measured. In narcolepsy, about 70% of patients will have a mean sleep latency of <5 minutes and a latency to REM sleep of <15 minutes on at least two occasions. These criteria have a specificity of 97% and a positive predictive value of approximately 70%. Most accepted diagnostic criteria require, as a minimum, a mean sleep latency on MSLT of ≤8 min and two or more sleep onset REM periods following a satisfactory nocturnal sleep (minimum 6 hours) during the night prior to the test. The presence of EDS, cataplexy and a typical MSLT allows a definite diagnosis of narcolepsy. The presence of two of these features renders the diagnosis probable, and other factors (such as the presence of other symptoms) need to be taken into account. Narcolepsy without cataplexy remains a diagnostic challenge and diagnosis is critically dependent on the MSLT and/or polysomnography. MSLT needs to be interpreted with care and the clinical context always needs to be considered. It can be affected by concomitant medication and psychiatric disease (e.g. depression); indeed, studies in the general population have brought into question its specificity.

There is a strong correlation between narcolepsy (with cataplexy) and the HLA-DQB1*06:02 variant but this subtype is common in the general population and therefore the positive predictive value is low. Measurement of CSF hypocretin levels can be used to make a diagnosis of narcolepsy, but normal levels does not exclude a diagnosis of narcolepsy without cataplexy.

Management of narcolepsy

General management Narcolepsy is a life-long condition with potentially wide-ranging implications. It is essential that patients and their relatives should have access to relevant and accurate information. Narcolepsy is entirely compatible with success both at school and in the workplace, but appropriate supportive provision may be necessary and career choices should take account of the possible hazards caused by EDS and cataplexy. Regular nocturnal sleep habits and attention to sleep hygiene help to minimise EDS, and planned naps can be used to optimise daytime performance.

People with narcolepsy are required to declare the diagnosis to the Driver and Vehicle Licensing Authority and are advised not to drive until satisfactory control of symptoms is achieved.

Sleepiness EDS is reduced by amphetamine-like stimulants (usually dexamfetamine, which is licensed for this use, or methylphenidate), and modafinil. The use of modafinil is supported by randomised controlled trials. Advantages of amphetamine-like drugs include long experience, low cost, a possible action against cataplexy and higher efficacy; modafinil has the advantage that tolerance does not develop (which can occur with amphetamines) and possibly a lower rate of side effects. Common side effects of amphetamine-like drugs include irritability and insomnia while modafinil may cause headache, nausea and rhinitis, and may interact with the oral contraceptive pill; a pill with higher dose ethinylestradiol (at least 50 μg) is required.

Cataplexy Cataplexy can often resolve with an improvement in nocturnal sleep and daytime somnolence. In addition, cataplectic symptoms often improve with age. Specific treatments include the tricyclic antidepressants (clomipramine) and the serotonin uptake inhibitors (fluoxetine). Other antidepressants, such as venlafaxine, can also be useful. These drugs also treat other narcolepsy symptoms. More recently, sodium oxybate (the sodium salt of gamma-hydroxybutyrate) has shown to be effective in cataplexy and also improves daytime somnolence.

Circadian rhythm disorders

Intrinsic circadian rhythms maintain a sleep–wake cycle of approximately 24 hours. They are set by environmental day length and are influenced by social activity, which can adjust timings. A mismatch between the internal circadian cycle and the external environment leads to insomnia, EDS and disruptive sleep function and activities of daily living. These may occur because of alterations in the internal circadian cycle (i.e. delayed or advanced sleep phase syndrome) or to changes in the environment (e.g. jet lag). Circadian rhythm disorders have also been associated with neurological and psychiatric disease such as encephalitis lethargica (in which there is circadian rhythm reversal) and schizophrenia (in which there can be a severely disrupted circadian rhythm).

Delayed or advanced sleep phase syndrome

These conditions are characterised by an inability to fall asleep or remain asleep at a conventional time. The persistence of the pattern distinguishes the condition from alterations in sleep rhythms, change in work timetables or travel across time zones. Advanced sleep syndrome (early to bed and early to wake) has been associated with mutations in clock genes. These conditions may be difficult to manage as attempts to regularise rhythms can lead to prolonged sleep latency and chronic insomnia, resulting in the excessive use of stimulants, hypnotics or alcohol. These conditions can be helped by CBT, and a regimen of planned advancement of bedtime. Bright light therapy and melatonin may also be of some benefit.

Shift work and jet lag

These conditions occur when the physical environment is altered and there is a mismatch with the internal circadian cycle. Many social factors influence the ability to acclimatise to a change in routine or travel including age, community, work responsibility and stress. They may lead to EDS or insomnia and a deterioration in the performance at work and a dependence on medication. Melatonin (2 mg 1 hour before bedtime) has been shown to have a benefit in these conditions.

Parasomnias

Parasomnias are undesirable physical events that occur during the sleep period and may be considered disorders of sleep state transition, partial arousal or arousal. The parasomnias are usually classified according to sleep state of origin (Table 20.31).

Non-REM parasomnias

The arousal disorders are abnormal non-REM sleep phenomena and include confusional arousal, sleep walking and sleep terrors. They represent incomplete awakenings from sleep, most commonly deep slow wave sleep (stage 3 and 4), which is preponderant in the first third of the night. These disorders share common underlying pathophysiological and phenotypic features. The onset is usually in childhood and symptoms often resolve spontaneously during adolescence. However, a significant proportion continues to have episodes in adulthood (up to 4%). There is often a family history, autosomal dominant inheritance with reduced penetrance has been suggested, and the first genetic locus was recently identified on chromosome 20.

Sleep walking is common in children, but also occurs in adults. It arises from a deep sleep, typically in the first third of the night, and may be either calm or agitated, with varying degrees of complexity and duration. Repetitive behaviours may occur and occasionally eating may be a feature. The episodes usually last 1–2 minutes but prolonged complex behaviours including driving have been reported. It is often very difficult to awaken the patient who is then confused with variable amnesia for the event. The most important

Table 20.31 A classification of parasomnias according to ICSD 2.

Disorders of arousal (from non-REM sleep)
Confusional arousals
Sleepwalking (somnambulism)
Sleep terrors (night terrors)
Parasomnias usually associated with REM sleep
REM sleep behaviour disorder
Recurrent isolated sleep paralysis
Nightmare disorder
Other parasomnias
Sleep-related dissociative disorders
Sleep enuresis (bedwetting)
Sleep-related groaning (catathrenia)
Exploding head syndrome
Sleep-related hallucinations
Sleep-related eating disorders
Parasomnia, unspecified
Parasomnia due to drug or substance
Parasomnia due to medical condition

American Academy of Sleep Medicine 2005. Reproduced with permission of AASM.

consideration is protection from injury. Treatment is often unnecessary but precipitating factors such as sleep deprivation and alcohol should be avoided; drug treatment with benzodiazepines or antidepressant medication may be valuable.

Sleep terrors are the most disturbing disorder of arousal for the patient and family. They are often characterised by a loud scream associated with extreme panic and prominent, occasionally violent, motor activity, resulting in bodily injury or property damage. The patient is inconsolable during the terror and amnesic for the event, which may be complete. Often, people report dream-like episodes in which they are being attacked or chased. The patient appears to be in a state of acute terror with tachycardia, tachypnoea, mydriasis and increased muscle tone. They last between 30 seconds and 3 minutes and can occur from early childhood. Treatment is rarely necessary but clonazepam and antidepressant medication are helpful. Sleep terrors characteristically begin during the deep sleep of the first third of the night; however, when episodes are very frequent they may be diffusely distributed across the sleep period and occur in any non-REM stage. Sleep terrors are sometimes familial and are associated with increased incidence of sleep walking and confusional arousals.

Confusional arousals are characterised by partial awakening movements in bed, occasional thrashing about or inconsolable crying and associated with confusion and impaired mentation, disorientation in time and place, and perceptual impairment. Behaviour is often inappropriate and can be aggressive. Confusional episodes are usually brief but may last up to 30 minutes. Confusional arousals can be associated with disorders causing deep or disturbed sleep, including metabolic, toxic and other encephalopathies; idiopathic hypersomnia; symptomatic hypersomnia and sleep apnoea syndrome.

In adults, more complex action may be carried out during non-REM parasomnias including sexual acts (sexsomnia), sleep eating, driving and violent acts. These are of forensic importance, because if a criminal act is committed during sleep then the defence of the act being an 'automatism' can be used.

Disorders of arousal may be triggered by pyrexia, prior sleep deprivation, emotional stress or a variety of medications including sedatives and hypnotics, neuroleptics, minor tranquillisers, stimulants and antihistamines. For some people, alcohol may also be a trigger to episodes or may make the episodes more elaborate. For the majority of people with non-REM parasomnias, identification and avoidance of triggers as well as reassurance are usually sufficient. However, antidepressants and benzodiazepines may be effective if the behaviours are dangerous to persons or property or are disruptive to the family. Safety aspects are important, such as making sure doors and windows are properly locked and that objects people can hurt themselves or others with are not by the bedside.

REM sleep disorders

REM-related parasomnias include nightmares, sleep paralysis and REM sleep behaviour disorder. Nightmares are dreams with frightening content. They usually last only a few minutes and are associated with movements, mumbling and vocalisation before awakening. They often occur in the second half of the night during REM sleep (in contrast to non-REM parasomnia) and may be related to REM rebound during a period of recuperation after REM sleep deprivation from either stress, drugs or surgery. Terrifying hypnagogic hallucinations (sleep onset nightmares) are part of the narcoleptic tetrad but may also occur in isolation. They are nightmares occurring at sleep onset in association with sleep onset REM. Tricyclic antidepressants especially clomipramine may be effective both for episodes in non-REM and in REM sleep onsets. Sleep paralysis may also occur as part of narcolepsy or as an isolated phenomenon sometimes running in families. Episodes may be frightening but are harmless and can be triggered by sleep deprivation.

REM sleep behaviour disorder (RBD) is a condition characterised by loss of normal atonia during REM sleep and motor activity causing abnormal behaviour during REM sleep, 'dream enactment'. Movements include generalised limb or truncal jerking which may progress to prominent, violent or more complex disruptive sleep behaviours, which are often aggressive, confrontational and may be violent with patients enacting intense dreams occasionally leading to self-injury. The duration is seconds to minutes. Episodes occur most nights and there may be several episodes per night with varying severity. As opposed to non-REM parasomnias which are more common in childhood, RBD is more common in older patients and there is a male predominance. The condition may be idiopathic in younger adults. However, in older adults, it is very commonly associated with neurodegenerative disorders (parkinsonism, multisystem atrophy, Lewy body dementia), narcolepsy, cerebrovascular disease, MS or Guillain–Barré syndrome. RBD may develop months or years before the onset of any underlying neurological disorder and with prolonged follow-up the proportion of patients developing some neurodegenerative disorder increases up to 40–60%. RBD may also emerge during withdrawal from alcohol or sedative-hypnotic abuse and with anticholinergic and other drug intoxication states leading to loss of REM atonia. Antidepressant medication can also induce RBD and may need to be discontinued if possible. Clonazepam is an effective treatment in RBD in suppressing both the violent behaviour and the intense subjective dream recall by suppression of phasic EMG activity during REM sleep rather than by restoration of REM atonia. Adjunctive or alternative medication may involve melatonin or, less frequently, dopa agonists. Safety measures are important to avoid injury to patient and bed partner.

Other forms of parasomnia

The exploding head syndrome is also a form of parasomnia and may represent a form of sleep start in which there is a sudden arousal during transition into sleep with a sensation of a loud noise 'bursting' in the head. They can also occur during REM sleep. Hypnic headache is rare, occurring in older patients, regularly at constant times at night. The headache is diffuse, protracted and relatively mild.

Catathrenia (sleep groaning) predominantly occurs during REM sleep and is characterised by apparent breath holding followed by prolonged expiration associated with a groaning sound presumed to be caused by vibration of the vocal cords. The sound can sometimes be high pitched and although the patient is usually unaware of the noise, this often disturbs the bed partner. Desaturations are rare. The cause is unknown and there is no known effective treatment although CPAP and benzodiazepines have been tried, usually with little effect.

Bruxism is intermittent repeated grinding or clenching of teeth during sleep, which is common in children and also in the severely disabled and may appear at any sleep stage. It can be associated with other movement disorders during sleep. Sleep bruxism may be a manifestation of mild REM sleep behaviour disorder. There is no satisfactory treatment although attempts are made at occlusal adjustment and splints particularly if there are signs of dental wear. Bruxism can result in tongue biting, which we have seen confused with tongue biting that can occur during nocturnal seizures.

Facio-mandibular myoclonus is a distinct syndrome and is different from bruxism. It consists of myoclonic jerks involving the masticatory and facial muscles occurring mainly during non-REM sleep. Tooth grinding and temporomandibular pain, which are often associated with bruxism, are usually absent. This syndrome is benign and is only of importance as it can result in lip and tongue biting which can also lead to a misdiagnosis of nocturnal seizures.

Sleep-related movement disorders

Restless legs syndrome

Restless legs syndrome (RLS) affects 2–15% of the population, depending on case ascertainment and is more frequent in the older age group. It is twice as common in females as males and there is often a significant family history. There are four essential criteria for diagnosis:

1. An urge to move the legs, usually accompanied by uncomfortable dysaesthesiae
2. The urge to move or the sensations worsen during periods of rest or inactivity
3. The urge to move or the sensations are partially or totally relieved by movement
4. The urge to move or the sensations are worse in the evening or during the night.

Symptoms may lead to difficulty getting to sleep, frequent awakenings, reduced sleep efficiency and insomnia. Leg jerking may also occur during wakefulness and be independent of the dysaesthesiae. RLS usually follows a chronic and often progressive course with intermittent fluctuations, but there may be prolonged periods of remission. Periodic limb movements of sleep are commonly associated with RLS. The condition may be idiopathic or secondary to iron deficiency, pregnancy, uraemia or other neurological conditions such as neuropathy and spinal cord disease.

RLS may be difficult to relieve completely. Any underlying cause should be sought and treated. In particular, all patients should be screened for iron store status and iron supplementation should be considered if serum ferritin is below 112 pmol/L (50 μg/L). There are several drugs that can cause or exacerbate RLS including antipsychotics and antidepressants and patients may benefit from discontinuation of these drugs if possible. Non-pharmacological treatment measures include avoidance of alcohol, caffeine and smoking. For patients with severe symptoms, medication may be necessary. Dopamine agonists (ropinirole, pramipexole and rotigotine) are the only agents licensed in the United Kingdom. Although effective, these drugs may be associated with problems including augmentation (the onset of symptoms earlier in the day; increased severity of symptoms). Augmentation may be more likely to occur in those with iron deficiency (emphasising the need to treat this). Pregabalin has also been shown to be effective in placebo controlled trials. Other treatment options include gabapentin, benzodiazepines and opioids. Benzodiazepines have a greater effect on maintaining sleep rather than treating movements. Opioids can be be particularly effective when augmentation has occurred and there are reports of the successful use of codeine, morphine, methadone and fentanyl patches.

Periodic limb movements of sleep

Periodic limb movements of sleep (PLM) are common, with more than 30% of individuals over 65 years having a significant number of periodic limb movements. The movements most commonly affect the legs and are characterised by dorsiflexion of toes, ankles and sometimes also hips. However, movements can also affect the head and arms. Movements occur periodically every 5–90 seconds and a series of more than four in a row is needed for diagnosis. People with severe PLM have more than 50 per hour. Although PLM may be asymptomatic, patients may have complaints of difficulty falling asleep, frequent awakenings, daytime sleepiness (PLM disorder, PLMD). Further, bed partners may also complain about the movements. PLM can be associated with other sleep disorders in particular RLS, but also sleep apnoea, narcolepsy or REM sleep behavioural disorders. It is most commonly an isolated phenomenon; most people with RLS have PLM but most people with PLMD do not have RLS. Treatment is only justified if periodic limb movements are symptomatic (e.g. causing excessive daytime somnolence) and follows the same principles as RLS.

Rhythmic movement disorders

Rhythmic movement disorders (*jactatio capitis nocturna*) are a group of behaviours characterised by stereotyped movements (rhythmic oscillation of the head or limbs, head banging or body rocking) which typically occur just before sleep onset and persist into light sleep. They most commonly occur in infants and young children, often associated with autism and mental retardation but have been described in adults with normal IQ. Significant complications include scalp and body wounds, subdural haematoma, retinal petechiae, skull callus formation and significant family and psychosocial problems. There are no EEG signs of arousal during the rocking movements. Behavioural therapy and medication that results in more rapid sleep onset (e.g. benzodiazepines) can be helpful, but often treatment is difficult.

Isolated symptoms, apparently normal variants

Sleep–wake transition disorders occur in the transition between waking and sleeping. Hypnic jerks (sleep starts) and nocturnal leg cramps all commonly occur in otherwise healthy individuals and are regarded as physiological alterations rather than pathological conditions. Hypnic jerks are brief body jerks at sleep onset, which may involve limbs, trunk or head. The jerks may be single or repetitive and may be spontaneous or provoked by stimuli. Visual, auditory or somatosensory sleep starts may also occur. In non-REM sleep, small flickering movements called sleep myoclonus are associated with very brief, highly localised EMG potentials. In some cases, the amplitude and frequency of these movements increase, at which points they are called fragmentary myoclonus.

Other sleep disturbances in extrapyramidal disease

In extrapyramidal disorders, particularly idiopathic Parkinson's disease (PD), Huntington's, Tourette's syndrome and torsion dystonia, involuntary movements may persist during sleep. These usually occur during stage 1, 2 and REM sleep and are less common in stage 3 and 4 sleep. Sleep difficulties are particularly frequent in patients with PD and these include difficulty getting to sleep, inadequate time asleep, disrupted sleep and daytime sleepiness which may occur as a result of nocturia, inability to turn over during the nights or on waking, inability to get out of bed unaided, leg cramps and jerks, dystonic spasms of the limbs or face and back pain during the night. There may be an increased prevalence of PLMD, RLS and RBD in association with PD.

The treatment of PD itself may alleviate abnormal motor activity during sleep but separate treatment may be necessary and clonazepam is particularly valuable. Respiratory disturbances, characterised by involuntary movements of laryngeal or respiratory muscles and impaired volitional control, are common in PD, progressive supranuclear palsy (PSP) and multi-system atrophy. There are also sleep-fragmenting respiratory disorders, such as sleep apnoea or upper airway resistance syndrome, a restrictive type of lung defect caused by an intrinsic defect in breathing control, impaired respiratory muscle function caused by rigidity and faulty autonomic control of the lungs. Patients with PD may also have obstructive respiratory defect, stridor or laryngeal spasm associated with off states or dystonic episodes, diaphragmatic dyskinesiae, drug-induced respiratory arrhythmias and dyspnoea and upper airway dysfunction with tremor-like oscillations. Dystonic movements and tics may persist during sleep at a reduced frequency and amplitude but are maximally active during stage 1 and 2 and REM sleep episodes.

Epilepsy syndromes associated with sleep

It is essential to distinguish the sleep-related paroxysmal events described earlier from nocturnal epilepsy and it may be difficult on history alone to distinguish epilepsy from non-REM parasomnia and RBD, necessitating further investigation with video-EEG telemetry. Epilepsy has a complex association with sleep. Certain seizures are more common during sleep such as frontal lobe seizures that occur from light non-REM sleep. Rarely, nocturnal seizures may be the only manifestation of an epileptic disorder and these can be confused with a parasomnia – this has been especially true for autosomal dominant nocturnal frontal lobe epilepsy (some of which are caused by mutations in the nicotinic acetylcholine receptor), the seizures of which were thought originally to represent a nocturnal paroxysmal dyskinesia. Nocturnal frontal lobe seizures are brief, stereotypical, cluster and occur at any time of night. These features may help to distinguish frontal lobe seizures from parasomnia. In addition, frontal lobe seizures can result in bilateral posturing and head version (rarely seen in parasomnia) and a distinct cessation (in contrast to non-REM parasomnia). Certain features such as fear and confusion are poor distinguishing features. Many cases of episodic nocturnal wanderings are possibly seizures or post-ictal confusion. Rarely, non-convulsive status epilepticus can occur during slow wave sleep (epileptic status epilepticus during sleep, ESES), particularly in children; the clinical manifestation of this is usually intellectual regression and autism and can occur in Landau–Kleffner syndrome (characterised by language regression) and also 'benign' epilepsy with centro-temporal spikes. Lack of sleep can precipitate seizures, especially in the idiopathic generalised epilepsies, and sleep apnoea has been reported to worsen seizure control. Sleep disturbances also commonly occur in people with epilepsy in whom there is a higher incidence of sleep apnoea, fragmented sleep and insomnia as well as daytime somnolence (often drug-related).

Traumatic brain injury and sleep

Sleep–wake disturbances are common after TBI and in prospective studies have been shown to affect between half and three-quarters of patients. Occurrence of sleep–wake disturbances does not appear to be related to the location or severity of the injury. A variety of sleep-wake disturbances occur, but excessive daytime somnolence, either with reduced ability to stay awake during the day or increased sleep need per 24 hours (increased by more than 2 hours compared with before injury), is the most common. Occasionally, this is caused by disrupted nocturnal sleep; for example, by sleep apnoea or periodic limb movements. Slightly reduced levels of hypocretin have also been found in patients following TBI and may contribute to excessive daytime somnolence. Modafinil can be tried but is rarely helpful. Other stimulants have not been studied systematically but may be beneficial. Fatigue (lack of energy or exhaustion) can also be seen after TBI and an association with other symptoms such as pain and depression has been noted. A similar association has been found in patients developing insomnia after TBI; this is most common in patients with mild head injuries, anxiety and depression. Screening for and treating concomitant psychiatric disorders should be performed in all patients with post-traumatic insomnia and CBT is also a useful treatment option. Circadian rhythm disorders have been described following TBI; either delayed sleep phase syndrome or irregular sleep–wake patterns. Melatonin and light-box treatment can be used to normalise sleep patterns.

Acknowledgement

The authors are grateful to BMJ Publications for permission to reproduce sections from Howard R. *et al.* Admission to neurological intensive care: who, when and why? *J Neurol Neurosurg Psychiatry* 2003; **74**: 2–16.

References

Parizel PM, Makkat S, Jorens PG, *et al.* Brainstem haemorrhage in descending tentorial herniation. *Intensive Care Med* 2002; **28:** 85–88.

Plum F, Posner JR. *Diagnosis of Stupor and Coma*, 3rd edn. Philadelphia: FA Davis, 1983.

Further reading

States of impaired consciousness

Andrews K, Murphy L, Munday R, *et al.* Misdiagnosis of the vegetative state: a retrospective study in a rehabilitation unit. *Br Med J* 1996; **313:** 13–16.

Boly M. Measuring the fading consciousness in the human brain. *Curr Opin Neurol* 2011; **24:** 394–400.

Multi-Society Task Force on PVS. Medical aspects of the persistent vegetative state. *N Engl J Med* 1994; **330:** 1499.

Multi-Society Task Force on PVS. Medical aspects of the persistent vegetative state. *N Engl J Med* 1994; **330:** 1572.

Owen AM, Coleman MR. Functional neuroimaging of the vegetative state. *Nat Rev Neurosci* 2008; **9:** 235–243.

Wijdicks EFM, Bamlet WR, Maramattom BV, Manno EM, McClelland RL. Validation of a new coma scale: the FOUR score. *Ann Neurol* 2005; **58**: 585–593.

Brain death

Monti MM, Vanhaudenhuyse A, Coleman MR, *et al.* Willfull modulation of brain activity in disorders of consciousness. *N Engl J Med* 2010; **362:** 579–589.

Webb A, Samuels O. Brain death dilemmas and the use of ancillary testing. *Continuum Lifelong learning. Neurol* 2012; **18:** 659–668.

Wijdicks EF. Brain death worldwide: accepted fact but no global consensus in diagnostic criteria. *Neurology* 2002; **58**: 20–25.

Wijdicks EF. Determining brain death in adults. *Neurology* 1995; **45**: 1003–1011.

Working Party of the Royal College of Physicians, UK. A code of practice for the diagnosis of brainstem death including guidelines for the identification and management of potential organ and tissue donors. Department of Health, UK: 1998. Available online at: http://webarchive.nationalarchives.gov.uk/+/www.dh.gov.uk/en/Publicationsandstatistics/Publications/PublicationsPolicyAndGuidance/DH_4009696 (accessed 10 February 2016).

Neurological intensive care

Al-Shahi Salman R, Labovitz DL, Stapf C. Spontaneous intracerebral haemorrhage. *Br Med J* 2009; **339:** 284–287.

Bacon D, Williams MA, Gordon J. Position statement on laws and regulations concerning life-sustaining treatment, including artificial respiration and hydration, for patients lacking decision-making capacity. *Neurology* 2007; **68**: 1097–1100.

Bleck TP, Smith MC, Pierre-Louis SJ, *et al.* Neurologic complications of critical medical illnesses. *Crit Care Med* 1993; **21**: 98–103.

Diringer MN, Zazulia AR. Hyponatraemia in neurologic patients: consequences and approaches to treatment. *Neurologist* 2006; **12**: 117–126.

Freeman WD, Tan KM, Glass GA, *et al.* ICU management of patients with Parkinson's disease or parkinsonism. *Curr Anaesthesia Crit Care* 2007; **18:** 227–236.

Heany M, Foot C, Freeman WD, Fraser J. Ethical issues in withholding and withdrawing life-prolonging medical treatment in the ICU. *Curr Anaesthesia Crit Care* 2007; **18:** 277–283.

Holzer M. Targeted temperature management for comatose survivors of cardiac arrest. *N Engl J Med* 2010; **363:** 1256–1264.

Kipps CM, Fung VSC, Gratten-Smith P, *et al.* Movement disorder emergencies. *Movement Disord* 2005; **20:** 322–334.

Leach R. Fluid management on hospital medical wards. *Clin Med* 2010; **10:** 611–615.

Mendelow AD, Timothy J, Steere JW, *et al.* Management of patients with head injury. *Lancet* 2008; **372:** 680–687.

Nielsen N, Wetterslev J, Cronberg T, *et al.* Targeted temperature management at 33°C versus36°C after cardiac arrest. *N Engl J Med* 2013; **369:** 2197–2206.

Parizel PM, Makkat S, Jorens PG, *et al.* Brainstem haemorrhage in descending tentorial herniation. *Intensive Care Med* 2002; **28:** 85–88.

Rabinstein AA, Wijdicks, EFM. Hyponatraemia in critically ill neurological patients. *Neurologist* 2003; **9**: 290–300.

Razvi SSM, Bone I. Neurological consultations in the medical intensive care unit. *J Neurol Neurosurg Psychiatry* 2003; **74** (Suppl. 3): 16–23.

Rossetti AO, Lowenstein DH. Management of refractory satus epilepticus in adults. *Lancet Neurol* 2011; **10:** 922–930.

Sequader F. Clinical value of decompressive craniectomy. *N Engl J Med* 2011; **364:** 16–17.

Shorvon S. The management of status epilepticus. *J Neurol Neurosurg Psychiatry* 2001; **70** (Suppl. 2): 22–27.

Towne AR, Waterhouse EJ, Boggs JG, *et al.* Prevalence of nonconvulsive status epilepticus in comatose patients. *Neurology* 2000; **54**: 340–345.

Van den Berghe G, Wouters P, Weekers F, *et al.* Intensive insulin therapy in critically ill patients. *N Engl J Med* 2001; **345**: 1359–1367.

Wijdicks EFM, Rabinstein AA. The family conference: end-of-life guidlines at work for the comatose patient. *Neurology* 2007; **68:** 1092–1094.

Yentis SM, Hirsch NP, Smith GB. *A to Z of Anaesthesia and Intensive Care*, 4th edn. Oxford: Butterworth, Heinemann, 2008.

Encephalopathy

Bolton CF, Young GB, Zochodne DW. The neurological complications of sepsis. *Ann Neurol* 1993; **33**: 94–100.

Bolton CF. Sepsis and the systemic inflammatory response syndrome: neuromuscular manifestations. *Crit Care Med* 1996; **24**: 1408–1416.

Diringer MN, Zazulia AR. Hyponatraemia in neurologic patients: consequences and approaches to treatment. *Neurologist* 2006; **12**: 117–126.

Evans TW. Hemodynamic and metabolic therapy in critically ill patients. *N Engl J Med* 2001; **345**: 1417–1418.

Guidelines for the management of severe traumatic brain injury. *J Neurotrauma* 2007; **24** (Suppl 1): S1–S108.

Holzer M, Bernard SA, Hachimi-Idrissi S, *et al.* Hypothermia for neuroprotection after cardiac arrest: systematic review and individual patient data meta-analysis. *Crit Care Med* 2005; **33:** 414–418.

Howard RS, Kullmann DM, Hirsch NP. Admission to neurological intensive care: who, when and why? *J Neurol Neurosurg Psychiatry* 2003; **74** (Suppl. 3): 2–9.

Howard RS, Radcliffe J, Hirsch NP. General medical care on the neuromedical intensive care unit. *J Neurol Neurosurg Psychiatry* 2003; **74** (Suppl. 3): 10–16.

Kaplan PW. Electrophysiological prognostication and brain injury from cardiac arrest. *Semin Neurol* 2006; **26:** 403–412.

Lee VH, Wijdicks EFM, Manno EM, Rabinstein AA. Clinical spectrum of reversible posterior leukoencephalopathy syndrome. *Arch Neurol* 2008; **65:** 205–210.

Lee YC, Phan TG, Jolley DJ, *et al.* Accuracy of clinical signs, SEP, and EEG in predicting outcome of hypoxic coma: a meta-analysis. *Neurology* 2010; **74:** 572–580.

Morris HR, Howard R, Brown P. Early myoclonic status and outcome following cardiorespiratory arrest. *J Neurol Neurosurg Psychiatry* 1998; **64**: 267–268.

Nolan JP, Laver SR, Welch CA, Harrison DA, Gupta V, Rowan K. Outcome following admission to UK intensive care units after cardiac arrests: a secondary analysis of the ICNARC Case Mix Programme Database. *Anaesthesia* 2008; **62:** 1207–1216.

Wijdicks EF, Young GB. Myoclonus status in comatose patients after cardiac arrest. *Lancet* 1994; **343**: 1642–1643.

Young GB. Neurologic prognosis after cardiac arrest. *N Engl J Med* 2009; **361:** 605–611.

Zandbergen EG, de Haan RJ, Stoutenbeek CP, *et al.* Systematic review of early prediction of poor outcome in anoxic-ischaemic coma. *Lancet* 1998; **352**: 1808–1812.

Neuromuscular

Campellone JV, Lacomis D, Kramer DJ, *et al.* Acute myopathy after liver transplantation. *Neurology* 1998; **50**: 46–53.

Case Records of the Massachusetts General Hospital. Case 11–1997: A 51-year-old man with chronic obstructive pulmonary disease and generalized muscle weakness. *N Engl J Med* 1997; **15**: 1079–1088.

Dhar R. Neuromuscular respiratory failure. *Continuum Lifelong Learning. Neurology* 2009; **15**: 40–67.

Hudson LD, Lee CM. Neuromuscular sequelae of critical illness. *N Engl J Med* 2003; **8**: 745–747.

Hughes RA, Cornblath DR. Guillain–Barré syndromes. *Lancet* 2005; **366**: 1653–1666.

Hund E. Critical illness polyneuropathy. *Curr Opin Neurol* 2001; **14**: 649–653.

Hurford WE. Sedation and paralysis during mechanical ventilation. *Respir Care* 2002; **47**: 334–346.

Jacobi J, Fraser GL, Coursin DB, *et al.* Clinical practice guidelines for the sustained use of sedatives and analgesics in the critically ill adult. *Crit Care Med* 2002; **30**: 119–141.

Lacomis D, Giuliani MJ, Van Cott A, *et al.* Acute myopathy of intensive care: clinical, electromyographic, and pathological aspects. *Ann Neurol* 1996; **40**: 645–654.

Lacomis D, Petrella JT, Giuliani MJ. Causes of neuromuscular weakness in the intensive care unit: a study of ninety-two patients. *Muscle Nerve* 1998; **21**: 610–617.

Lacomis D, Zochodne D, Bird SJ. Critical illness myopathy. *Muscle Nerve* 2000; **23**: 2785–1788.

Leijten FS, Harinck-de Weerd JE, Poortvliet DC, *et al.* The role of polyneuropathy in motor convalescence after prolonged mechanical ventilation. *JAMA* 1995; **274**: 1221–1225.

Lorin S, Nierman DM. Critical illness neuromuscular abnormalities. *Crit Care Clin* 2002; **18**: 553–568.

Wijdicks EEF, Litchy WI, Weisner RH, Krom RAF. Neuromuscular complications associated with liver transplantation. *Muscle Nerve* 1996; **19**: 696–700.

Zochodne DW, Rarnsay DA, Saly V, Shelley S, Moffatt S. Acute necrotizing myopathy of intensive care: electrophysiological studies. *Muscle Nerve* 1994; **17**: 285–292.

Sleep

Bassetti C, Aldrich MS. Idiopathic hypersomnia. A series of 42 patients. *Brain* 1997; **120**: 1423–1435.

Lesage S, Hening WA. The restless legs syndrome and periodic limb movement disorder: a review of management. *Semin Neurol* 2004; **24**: 249–260.

Mahowald MW, Bornemann MC, Schenk CH. Parasomnias. *Semin Neurol* 2004; **24**: 283–292.

Olson EJ, Boeve BF, Silber MH. Rapid eye movement sleep behaviour disorder: demographic, clinical and laboratory findings in 93 cases. *Brain* 2000; **123**: 331–339.

Zaman A, Britton T, Douglas N, *et al.* Narcolepsy and excessive daytime sleepiness. *Br Med J* 2004; **329**: 724–728.

CHAPTER 21

Neuro-Oncology

Jeremy Rees[1], Robert Bradford[1], Sebastian Brandner[2], Naomi Fersht[1], Rolf Jäger[2] and Elena Wilson[1]

[1]National Hospital for Neurology & Neurosurgery

[2]UCL Institute of Neurology

Neuro-oncology covers both the scientific and clinical aspects of central nervous system (CNS) tumours and neurological complications of cancer. In common with many other areas of medicine, a multi-disciplinary approach provides optimal standards of care. The emergence of new therapies throughout neurology has changed the role of neurologists from diagnostic to therapeutic clinicians. This is especially relevant in neuro-oncology. Improvements in radiological and histological diagnosis and surgical technique, advances in molecular neuro-oncology, the application of new biological agents and increasing use of combined radiotherapy and chemotherapy for tumours such as gliomas have led to small but definite improvements in survival.

There is increasing awareness of the large array of CNS tumour types, the spectrum of neurological complications of cancer, particularly paraneoplasia, and the neurotoxicity of chemotherapy and radiotherapy, making it essential to have up-to-date knowledge. This chapter provides a clinically dominated guide to the key issues in neuro-oncology. The initial sections reflect the highly specialised nature of disciplines within neuro-oncology. The multi-disciplinary aspects of care are outlined in the sections on clinical management.

Epidemiology of common primary intracranial tumours

Incidence

Brain tumours include primary tumours arising from intracranial structures and metastases from outside the CNS. Primary CNS tumours account for approximately 2% of all cancers in adults and 20% in childhood. They have a high case fatality ratio; broadly, there is a 25% chance of any adult patient who has a brain tumour dying from it. In adults they are second only to stroke as a cause of neurological death. They place a considerable burden of suffering on patients, their families and carers.

Incidence figures for brain tumours depend much on methods of case ascertainment. Incidence of specific tumour types is believed to be much the same worldwide. The crude UK incidence for primary tumours is 15.3/100 000/year and for secondary tumours 14.3/100 000/year. It is likely that the true incidence is higher. One study from the south-west of England ascertaining data mainly from radiology records found the crude incidence for primary tumours to be 21/100 000/year. There are some suggestions that the incidence of glioma and CNS lymphoma is increasing, particularly in elderly patients. This may simply be because of better case ascertainment and the increasing use of imaging (e.g. for patients presenting with stroke).

Different tumour types present in different age groups. Supratentorial gliomas are uncommon below the age of 30 years but become increasingly prevalent thereafter. They account for over 60% of primary tumours. The most frequent tumours of adolescence are germ cell tumours and astrocytomas, those in middle life astrocytomas, meningiomas and pituitary adenomas and in later life, high-grade gliomas and metastases. Infratentorial tumours are more common in childhood. Seventy per cent of paediatric primary intracranial tumours arise in the cerebellum and brainstem, specifically astrocytomas, ependymomas and medulloblastomas. Meningiomas and schwannomas occur more frequently in women; the reverse is true for astrocytomas.

Survival

Although brain tumours account for only 2% of all cancers, they are responsible for more years of life lost per patient before the age of 70 years than any other cancer. The latest survival trends have shown only modest improvement over the last 10 years The prognosis of a brain tumour is largely related to age, performance status, histological type, grade, molecular signature and tumour location. Intra-axial tumours are associated with poorer survival than extra-axial tumours as are tumours growing in eloquent regions of the brain. Although there has been some improvement over the last 30 years, only about 36% of adults with malignant brain tumours in the United Kingdom survive 1 year and 19% survive 5 years or more. This compares to a 5-year survival rate of 17–20% in Europe and 25% in the United States. These discrepancies may be partly because of inclusion of benign brain tumours, certainly in US registries. As a general rule, young patients fare better than older with the same histological types. The 5-year survival is around 50% for patients under 40 years and 60% for children.

Patients with benign tumours (e.g. meningiomas) may survive many decades or be cured permanently. Children with brain tumours survive for longer than adults: 5-year survival in children is around 60%. Histological grading has particular prognostic implications and is an essential part of the neuropathological assessment. This is especially so because brain tumours rarely spread outside the nervous

Neurology: A Queen Square Textbook, Second Edition. Edited by Charles Clarke, Robin Howard, Martin Rossor and Simon Shorvon.

system. They are therefore not staged according to the familiar TNM (tumour, node, metastasis) system. Prognosis is usually expressed in terms of percentage survival at 5 years. For astrocytomas, 5-year survival is over 90% for World Health Organization (WHO) Grade I tumours, around 50% for WHO Grade II tumours, 30% for WHO Grade III tumours and less than 5% for WHO Grade IV tumours.

Risk factors

The cause of most brain tumours remains unknown. The only definite environmental risk factor is ionising radiation, either following nuclear explosions or therapeutic radiation. Cranial radiotherapy (RT) at low doses has been shown to increase the relative risk of meningiomas by a factor of 10 and of gliomas by a factor of 3. Other RT-induced tumours include sarcomas and schwannomas. They have been described following RT for tinea capitis, craniopharyngioma, pituitary adenomas and prophylactic cranial irradiation for acute lymphoblastic leukaemia. Secondary tumours tend to lie within the radiation field, usually within lower dose regions, and develop from a few years to many decades after RT. The median time to the development of gliomas is 7 years. Sarcomas develop with a longer lag time and meningiomas may be seen 30–40 years later. Radiation induced meningiomas are more likely than spontaneous tumours to have atypical histology.

No other environmental risk factor has been clearly identified. There has been widespread concern about mobile (cellular) phones. Case–control studies have shown a consistent association between long-term use of mobile and cordless phones and glioma and vestibular schwannoma, but not meningioma, providing support for the hypothesis that radiofrequency electromagnetic fields play a part in the initiation and promotion stages of carcinogenesis. Given the almost universal use of mobile phones nowadays, it is important that brain tumour trends continue to be surveyed.

Genetic causes of brain tumours are rare but important. Occasionally, brain tumours occur in successive generations without any other tumour predisposition. Typically, they are associated with neurocutaneous syndromes such as neurofibromatosis (optic nerve glioma, meningioma, vestibular schwannoma), tuberous sclerosis (subependymal giant cell astrocytoma) and von Hippel–Lindau syndrome (haemangioblastoma). There are also rare familial tumour syndromes, for example Li–Fraumeni syndrome (glioma) and Cowden's disease (dysplastic cerebellar gangliocytoma or Lhermitte–Duclos disease).

Clinical features

The clinical presentation of a brain tumour depends on location, rate of growth and pathology. Any tumour has the potential to produce a focal deficit and raised intracranial pressure although this is most commonly seen with high-grade tumours because of rapid growth and brain tissue necrosis and with posterior fossa mass lesions. In contrast, low-grade tumours are infiltrative, less destructive than their high-grade counterparts and present more frequently with a seizure disorder.

There are no clinical features that are unique to brain tumours and the first suspicion of a brain tumour can only come from imaging. Even then, there are a number of tumour mimics on computed tomography (CT) and magnetic resonance imaging (MRI) scans for both low-grade and high-grade tumours. Examples of high-grade mimics include brain abscesses, tumefactive multiple sclerosis (MS), tuberculosis and toxoplasmosis; examples of low-grade mimics include cortical dysplasia, viral encephalitis and neurocysticercosis. Close liaison with neuroradiology is therefore important before subjecting the patient to an invasive procedure such as a biopsy.

Several hospital-based studies have examined the clinical features of brain tumours. A study of over 300 brain mass lesions showed that headache and seizures were the most frequent symptoms followed by neurological deficit and cognitive behavioural changes. Patients with cognitive decline tended to be diagnosed late and had developed focal or multiple symptoms by the time they were seen. Asymptomatic papilloedema and hemianopia was noted in particular, pointing to the need for careful fundoscopy and visual field testing.

Headache

Tumours can produce raised intracranial pressure either by the mass effect of a rapidly growing lesion with associated vasogenic oedema or by blockage of cerebrospinal fluid (CSF) pathways, typically seen with posterior fossa tumours and with intraventricular tumours. Stretching or distortion of the meninges can give rise to headache without raised pressure. Intra-tumoural haemorrhage can produce an acute rise in pressure leading to severe headache with coma or reduced consciousness. This clinical picture is also sometimes seen with large tumours without any evidence for a bleed, particularly in peri-ventricular locations where encystment of a horn of the lateral ventricles can occur.

Severity of headache is not a helpful diagnostic pointer – indeed, the most severe headaches encountered are almost invariably caused by primary headache syndromes such as migraine or cluster headache. A study of over 100 patients with brain tumours revealed that headaches were present in under 50%, equally for both primary and metastatic tumours, and that the headaches were similar to tension-type headaches or migraine in over 80% of those (i.e. not clinically sinister in themselves). The typical tumour headache was bi-frontal, worse on one side but it was the most prominent symptom in under half of the patients. Brain tumour headaches were made worse by bending in around one-third, unlike true tension-type headaches. Nausea or vomiting was present in 40%. Early morning headache was uncommon. Nausea and vomiting, abnormal physical signs or a significant change in prior headache pattern were particular risk factors for a tumour.

What usually distinguishes headaches of a brain tumour from benign headaches is the gradual evolution of associated symptoms (i.e. focal deficit, seizures, ataxia and vomiting), the latter being seen particularly with posterior fossa tumours. It is quite exceptional for a patient with a brain tumour to present with headache alone.

Seizures

Tumour-associated seizures may be partial and/or generalised. There is an inverse relationship between tumour grade and occurrence of seizures and certain low-grade tumours (e.g. oligodendrogliomas and gangliogliomas) are associated with seizures in over 90% of cases. The type of seizure is dependent on tumour location and there are no distinguishing features of focal seizures to distinguish a tumour from a non-neoplastic process. In a recent retrospective study of over 80 adults with supratentorial low-grade gliomas, seizures occurred in all but one and only 30% of patients became seizure-free on anticonvulsants. There was no clear association between severity of the seizure disorder and behaviour of the underlying tumour, in particular the return of seizures after a period of seizure freedom did not invariably indicate tumour recurrence.

Focal deficits

Focal deficits depend on the location of the tumour and are usually gradually progressive. However, stroke-like presentations, and even apparent transient ischaemic attacks (TIAs), are well recognised.

These are sometimes caused by intra-tumoural haemorrhage and sometimes by presumed vascular changes associated with the tumour. Progressive focal deficits occur typically in patients with high-grade tumours (e.g. glioblastoma and brain metastases) rather than with low-grade tumours, presumably because of the ability of the latter to infiltrate normal tissue without interfering with function. Parasagittal tumours (e.g. meningiomas) may present with a spastic paraparesis or monoparesis.

Brainstem symptoms

Vertigo and disequilibrium are common presenting symptoms of posterior fossa tumours. In cerebellopontine angle tumours (e.g. vestibular schwannomas), unilateral hearing loss is usually the first and only symptom; later symptoms arise from trigeminal, facial nerve and brainstem compression. Facial numbness occurs in about 25% of these patients and is more common at the time of presentation than facial weakness. Objective hypoesthesia involving the teeth, buccal mucosa or skin of the face is associated with larger tumours, but a subjective reduction in sensation that cannot be documented on objective examination occurs commonly with medium-sized and small tumours. Depression of the corneal reflex generally occurs earlier and more commonly than objective facial hypoesthesia. Tumours of the pineal and tectal plate may present with Parinaud's syndrome and hydrocephalus caused by obstruction of the aqueduct.

Cognitive and behavioural symptoms

A minority of patients with tumours present with cognitive symptoms and/or a behavioural disorder (e.g. abulia or depression caused by a subfrontal meningioma). Specific focal cognitive deficits (e.g. alexia, acalculia) may be seen in tumours affecting the dominant parietal lobe particularly around the angular gyrus. Neuropsychiatric symptoms such as depression, paranoid delusions and personality changes are all well recognised and stress the need for imaging in patients with atypical affective disorders. By contrast, psychosis is a very rare presenting symptom.

Endocrine symptoms

Patients with pituitary and hypothalamic tumours may present with endocrine disturbances brought about by anterior or posterior pituitary failure or oversecretion (e.g. acromegaly). These may also cause visual failure typically commencing with bitemporal quadrantanopia or hemianopia as the optic chiasm is compressed.

Rare presentations

Patients with orbital plate tumours (Chapter 13) may present with anosmia without any other symptoms caused by compression of olfactory nerves in the anterior cranial fossa. Visual failure is discussed in Chapter 14. In children, hypothalamic and thalamic tumours may present as a diencephalic syndrome, with failure to gain weight and to grow as expected, and emaciation. Affected infants and children may behave in an alert, happy and outgoing manner, in contrast to their outward appearance. Precocious puberty, particularly in boys, may be caused by a number of tumours including gliomas, pineal tumours and germ cell tumours.

Histogenesis of brain cancer

The nomenclature of brain tumours according to the WHO classification is still largely based on the historical resemblance of tumour cell shape, morphology and localisation to those of differentiated cells of the brain or expression of glial or neuronal proteins, identified by immunohistochemical techniques. Thus, gliomas were thought to arise from neoplastic transformation of astrocytes, oligodendrocytes or their precursors. Currently, it is impossible to demonstrate directly which cell of origin gives rise to which specific glioma in humans. This remains a fundamental question in glioma biology. The most likely candidates to give rise to intrinsic brain tumours are cells originating from the stem and progenitor cell compartments of the developing brain (e.g. medulloblastoma) and adult brain (e.g. glioblastoma, oligodendroglioma). A combination of the cell type of origin and the combination of genomic or mutations or epigenetic changes are the most likely determinant of the tumour type.

The increasing interest in the role of stem cells in the origins of brain tumours is the basis of many research programmes. Stem cells are defined as having the ability to perpetuate themselves through self-renewal and to generate mature cells of a particular tissue through differentiation. There are numerous parallels between somatic stem cells and cancer stem cells. Both show self-renewal, differentiation and capacity for histogenesis. Somatic stem cells self-renew in a highly controlled manner and differentiate into mature cells which go on to form normal tissues, whereas cancer cells show poorly controlled self-renewal, often abortive differentiation and go on to form abnormal tissues (i.e. tumours). The observation that only a small minority of tumour cells show an indefinite potential for self-renewal *in vitro* or *in vivo* gave rise to the hypothesis that tumours are composed of both cancer stem cells and more differentiated cells. The existence of a cancer stem cell has been proven for acute myeloid leukaemia, breast cancer ($CD44^+/CD24^-$ cells), glioblastoma and medulloblastoma ($CD133^+$ cells). Implications of the cancer stem cell hypothesis are:

- Cancer cells can be organised hierarchically in that they range from poorly differentiated, highly proliferative cells to more mature, less proliferative forms.
- Cancer cells share cell cycle pathways that are relevant to normal human development and control of growth.

Molecular mechanisms involved in tumour formation

An intrinsic difficulty in the study of signalling pathways involved in oncogenesis is the multitude of genetic and epigenetic changes that accrue during the multi-step process of malignant transformation of normal cells into tumour cells. An additional obstacle is the heterogeneity of mutations within a single tumour which suggests separate subpopulations of cells are capable of promoting growth in the same malignancy.

Genomics describe the changes in the genetic information of a cell, whilst epigenetic modifications are reversible modifications on the DNA that affect gene expression without altering the DNA sequence.

Three types of genes are involved in tumorigenesis:

1. Oncogenes
2. Tumour suppressor genes, and
3. Repair/stability genes.

The two most common epigenetic changes are:

1. DNA methylation, leading to inactivation or attenuation of gene expression, and
2. Histone modification, which regulates gene expression by disruption of the contact between nucleosomes and by recruiting chromatin remodelling ATPases.

The more important genetic and epigenetic mutations associated with brain tumours are summarised in Table 21.1.

Table 21.1 Summary of relevant markers of intrinsic brain tumours.

Tumour	WHO Grade	Mutation	Frequency (%)	Relevance
Pilocytic astrocytoma	I	*KIAA:BRAF* fusion gene	75, in cerebellar location	D
Pleomorphic xanthoastrocytoma	I	*BRAF V600E*	66	D
Pleomorphic xanthoastrocytoma with anaplasia	n/a	*BRAF V600E*	65	D
Gangliogliomas	I		30	D
Diffuse astrocytoma	II	*IDH1,2* *ATRX* loss	100	D, P
Oligoastrocytoma	II	*IDH1,2* 1p/19q codeletion or *ATRX* loss	82 50–70	D, P P
Oligodendroglioma	II	*IDH1,2* 1p/19q codeletion	100 100	D, P P
Anaplastic astrocytoma	III	*IDH1,2* *ATRX* loss	90	D, P P
Anaplastic oligoastrocytoma	III	*IDH1,2* 1p/19q codeletion	66 50	D, P D, P
Anaplastic oligodendroglioma	III	*IDH1,2* 1p/19q codeletion or *ATRX* loss	100 100	D, P D, P
Primary glioblastoma	IV	*MGMT* methylation* 7p gain, 10q loss *EGFR* amplification	40 70 30%	P – –
Secondary glioblastoma (GBM-IDH) (progression from anaplastic astrocytoma)	IV	*IDH1,2* *ATRX* loss	100	D, P
Ependymoma and anaplastic ependymoma, post fossa	II, III	*LAMA2*† *NELL2*† *LAMA2+NELL2*†	32 52 8	P P P
Medulloblastoma	IV	Wnt‡ SHH‡ Group 3‡ Group 4‡		P P P P

D, diagnostic; P, prognostic.

* The degree of methylation varies from low to high.

† These markers are differentially expressed in Group A and B ependymomas, and *not* mutated.

‡ These are prognostically relevant subgroups of medulloblastoma.

Genetic components in oncogenesis

The most common genetic components are oncogenes and tumour suppressor genes, which regulate cell division, control apoptosis or cell cycle arrest. Repair/stability genes become tumorigenic by loss of their DNA repair function. Oncogenes are genes that under normal conditions (i.e. development and cell self-renewal) promote cell birth and growth but when disinhibited (unleashed) become autonomously active. For example, a point mutation in *c-kit*, which codes for a tyrosine kinase, leads to constitutive activation in the kinase domain and is causally implicated in the pathogenesis of gastrointestinal stroma tumours which arise from interstitial cells of Cajal in the gut. In contrast, tumour suppressor genes are gatekeepers of cell cycle function and under physiological conditions exert a negative regulation on processes promoting the cell cycle. They may also control apoptosis and therefore mutations in these genes can lead to a failure of apoptosis. Typical examples are:

- *p53:* the 'guardian of the genome' which causes induction of apoptosis in response to cell damage. Inactivation leads to less apoptosis of cells that should have undergone programmed cell death.
- *Retinoblastoma (Rb):* the prototypic tumour suppressor gene that controls the cell cycle at G1.
- *PTEN* (phosphatase and tensin homologue): germ-line mutations are associated with Cowden's syndrome and other hamartomatous disorders.
- *BRAF* (v-RAF murine sarcoma viral oncogene homologue B1 (BRAF) gene): missense mutations (BRAF V600E) occur in primary nervous system tumours, such as pleomorphic xanthoastrocytomas (PXA) and gangliogliomas, and a fusion between two transcripts (*KIAA:BRAF*) are seen in about 60% of pilocytic astrocytomas.

Repair and/or stability genes normally function by repairing DNA damage–mismatch repair, nucleotide excision repair and base excision repair. Under normal conditions, DNA damage is kept to a minimum, but loss of function results in accumulation of DNA mutations and eventually tumour formation. A commonly observed alteration of a DNA repair gene is the suppression of the DNA repair enzyme MGMT (*O*-6-methylguanine-DNA methyltransferase), which results in a reduction of repair processes of damaged (mutated) tumour DNA. The epigenetic mechanism of DNA methylation of the promoter region of the *MGMT* gene leads to reduction of MGMT expression and DNA repair in response to alkylating chemotherapy agents (e.g. temozolomide).

Mutations in oncogenes, tumour suppressors and repair/stability genes can occur in the germ line, resulting in hereditary tumour syndromes or in somatic cells, causing sporadic tumours. The initial event in the neoplastic process is a single somatic mutation resulting in a growth advantage of a clonally expanding cell population. Additional mutations then accrue and cause further series of clonal expansions, eventually resulting in a tumour.

The cell cycle is controlled by a cascade of genes, which may either promote or suppress it: for example, mutations of cdk4 and cyclin D1 in the Rb pathway are oncogenic (i.e. activating), while mutations of Rb and p16, both tumour suppressor genes, lead to inactivation. Hence, the combinations of these mutations result in activation of the same pathway. However, despite the detailed knowledge of pathway function, it still remains unclear what eventually determines the phenotype of a brain tumour – is it the initial mutation, the sequence of subsequent mutations or the differentiation state of the cell in which the initial genetic event occurs? As a corollary of this complexity and multiplicity of mutations in an advanced tumour, it is impossible to track back to the primary event. Hence, *in vivo* models are needed in which specific pathways in stem cells can be altered to study the genotype–phenotype correlation of brain tumours.

Epigenetic events in oncogenesis

Epigenetic events are important mechanisms underlying cancer development and progression, the most common of which are DNA methylation and histone modification. DNA methylation occurs almost exclusively at CpG dinucleotides. Some CpG dinucleotides are clustered in CpG islands, and are often associated with the promoter region, causing downstream gene activation. Generally, unmethylated, promoter CpG island permits initiation of transcription, whereas a methylated promoter CpG island represses promoter activity. In cancer, global hypomethylation and local hypermethylation can occur. One of these biomarkers, MGMT (see Genetic components in oncogenesis), is now important in clinical decision-making. If MGMT is inactivated, DNA damage is not repaired, cells that do not undergo apoptosis develop a mutator phenotype that drives tumour evolution. However, methylation of the MGMT gene renders tumours susceptible to the DNA damaging effects of alkylating drugs and glioblastoma patients with a methylated MGMT gene show a survival benefit when treated with the alkylating drug temozolomide in addition to radiation.

Histone modifications and other epigenetic mechanisms establish and maintain gene activity, and regulate a wide range of cellular processes, including gene transcription, DNA replication and DNA repair. Alterations in the function of histone-modifying complexes can disrupt the pattern and levels of histone markers and thus deregulate the control of chromatin-based processes, ultimately leading to oncogenic transformation and the development of cancer. A DNA mutation encoding an enzyme of the anaerobic glucose metabolic pathway, isocitrate dehydrogenase 1 and 2 (IDH1 and IDH2) genes result in the loss of normal catalytic activity necessary for the production of α-ketoglutarate (α-KG), and gain of a new activity, the production of an oncometabolite, R-2-hydroxylglutarate (R-2-HG). R-2-HG acts as an antagonist of α-KG and competitively inhibits the activity of multiple α-KG-dependent dioxygenases, including both histones and DNA demethylases involved in epigenetic control of gene expression and cell differentiation. It has been shown that cells with mutant IDH show stemness properties and a delay in differentiation. IDH mutations are present in 70–80% of WHO Grades II and III astrocytomas and oligodendrogliomas. Astrocytomas with mutant IDH show a global hypermethylator phenotype, which includes high rates of MGMT methylation.

WHO classification of CNS tumours

Most brain tumour classifications are based on the work of Bailey and Cushing (1926) who named tumours after the cell type in the developing embryo, fetus or adult that most resembled the tumour histologically. The classification system now most widely accepted is that of the World Health Organization (WHO 2007) which recognises more than 120 different tumour types, and is shown in Table 21.2. Consensus guidelines have been recently developed following a meeting in Haarlem, the Netherlands in 2014, in which histology, WHO grade and molecular information will be incorporated to provide an 'integrated diagnosis' and this will be introduced into the fourth edition of the WHO classification.

Neuroepithelial tumours

Neuroepithelial tumours form the vast majority of intrinsic brain tumours and encompass a broad spectrum of neoplasms that arise from or share morphological properties of neuro-epithelial cells. Accordingly, they are further subgrouped into:

- Glial neoplasms, collectively classified as gliomas, which include astrocytic, oligodendroglial and ependymal tumours
- Tumours with predominant neuronal phenotype, such as ganglioglioma, dysembryoplastic neuro-epithelial tumour and central neurocytoma
- Neuroblastic tumours
- Pineal tumours
- Embryonal tumours such as medulloblastoma
- Choroid plexus tumours.

The grading of gliomas and other tumours in the WHO scheme is based on the presence of certain morphological characteristics within the tumour: cellular and nuclear atypia, mitotic activity, vascular endothelial proliferation and necrosis. These features reflect the malignant potential of the tumour in terms of invasion and growth rate. Tumours without any of these features are WHO

Table 21.2 WHO 2007 classification of nervous system tumours (Grades I, II, III, IV).

TUMOURS OF NEUROEPITHELIAL TISSUE

A. Astrocytic tumours
- i. Pilocytic astrocytoma (I)
  - pilomyxoid astrocytoma (II)
- ii. Subependymal giant cell astrocytoma (I)
- iii. Pleomorphic xanthoastrocytoma (II)
- iv. Diffuse astrocytoma (II)
  - fibrillary astrocytoma, gemistocytic astrocytoma
  - protoplasmic astrocytoma
- v. Anaplastic astrocytoma (III)
- vi. Glioblastoma (IV)
  - giant cell glioblastoma, gliosarcoma
- vii. Gliomatosis cerebri (III)

B. Oligodendroglial tumours
- i. Oligodendroglioma (II)
- ii. Anaplastic oligodendroglioma (III)

C. Mixed gliomas (oligoastrocytic tumours)
- i. Oligoastrocytoma (II)
- ii. Anaplastic oligoastrocytoma (III)

D. Ependymal tumours
- i. Subependymoma (I)
- ii. Myxopapillary ependymoma (I)
- iii. Ependymoma (II)
  - cellular, papillary, clear cell, tanycytic
- iv. Anaplastic ependymoma (III)

E. Choroid plexus tumours
- i. Choroid plexus papilloma (I)
- ii. Atypical choroid plexus papilloma (II)
- iii. Choroid plexus carcinoma (III)

F. Other neuroepithelial tumours
- i. Astroblastoma (IV)
- ii. Chordoid glioma of third ventricle (II)
- iii. Angiocentric glioma (I)

G. Neuronal and mixed neuronal–glial tumours
- i. Dysplastic gangliocytoma of cerebellum (Lhermitte–Duclos disease, Grade I)
- ii. Desmoplastic infantile astrocytoma/ganglioglioma (I)
- iii. Dysembryoplastic neuroepithelial tumour (I)
- iv. Gangliocytoma (I)
- v. Ganglioglioma (I)
- vi. Anaplastic ganglioglioma (III)
- vii. Central neurocytoma (II)
- viii. Extraventricular neurocytoma (II)
- ix. Cerebellar liponeurocytoma (II)
- x. Papillary glioneuronal tumour (I)
- xi. Rosette-forming glioneuronal tumour of the fourth ventricle (I)
- xii. Paraganglioma of the spinal cord (I)

H. Tumours of the pineal region
- i. Pineocytoma (I)
- ii. Pineal parenchymal tumour of intermediate differentiation (II, III)
- iii. Pineoblastoma (IV)
- iv. Papillary tumour of the pineal region (II, III)

I. Embryonal tumours
- i. Medulloblastoma (IV)
  - desmoplastic/nodular medulloblastoma,
  - medulloblastoma with extensive nodularity,
  - anaplastic medulloblastoma,
  - large cell medulloblastoma
- ii. CNS primitive neuroectodermal tumour (IV)
  - CNS neuroblastoma, CNS ganglioneuroblastoma,
  - medulloepithelioma,
  - ependymoblastoma
- iii. Atypical teratoid/rhabdoid tumour (IV)

TUMOURS OF CRANIAL AND PARASPINAL NERVES

Schwannoma (I)
- cellular, plexiform, melanotic

Neurofibroma (I)
- plexiform

Perineurioma (I)
- perineurioma (NOS, I–III),
- malignant perineurioma (II-IV)

Malignant peripheral nerve sheath tumour (MPNST, II–IV)
- epithelioid MPNST, MPNST with mesenchymal differentiation, melanotic MPNST,
- MPNST with glandular differentiation

TUMOURS OF MENINGES

A. Tumours of meningothelial cells
- i. Meningioma
  - meningothelial (I), fibrous (fibroblastic, I), transitional (mixed, I), psammomatous (I),
  - angiomatous (I), microcystic (I),
  - secretory (I),
  - lymphoplasmacyte-rich (I),
  - metaplastic (I),
  - chordoid (II), clear cell (II), atypical (II),
  - papillary (III), rhabdoid (III),
  - anaplastic/malignant (III)

B. Mesenchymal tumours (I–IV)
- i. Lipoma
- ii. Angiolipoma
- iii. Hibernoma
- iv. Liposarcoma
- v. Solitary fibrous tumour
- vi. Fibrosarcoma
- vii. Malignant fibrous histiocytoma
- viii. Leiomyoma
- ix. Leiomyosarcoma
- x. Rhabdomyoma
- xi. Rhabdomyosarcoma
- xii. Chondroma
- xiii. Chondrosarcoma
- xiv. Osteoma
- xv. Osteosarcoma
- xvi. Osteochondroma
- xvii. Haemangioma
- xviii. Epithelioid haemangioendothelioma (II)
- xix. Haemangiopericytoma (II)
- xx. Anaplastic haemangiopericytoma (III)
- xxi. Angiosarcoma
- xxii. Kaposi's sarcoma
- xxiii. Ewing's sarcoma – PNET

C. Primary melanocytic lesions

Diffuse melanocytosis, melanocytoma, malignant melanoma, meningeal melanomatosis

D. Other neoplasms related to the meninges

Haemangioblastoma (I)

LYMPHOMAS AND HAEMATOPOIETIC NEOPLASMS

Malignant lymphomas, plasmacytoma, granulocytic sarcoma

GERM CELL TUMOURS

Germinoma

Embryonal carcinoma

Yolk sac tumour

Choriocarcinoma

Teratoma
- mature, immature, teratoma with malignant transformation

Mixed germ cell tumour

TUMOURS OF THE SELLAR REGION

Craniopharyngioma (I)
- adamantinomatous, papillary

Granular cell tumour of the neurohypophysis (I)

Pituicytoma (I)

Spindle cell oncocytoma of adenohypophysis (I)

METASTATIC TUMOURS (IV)

Grade I; those with atypia alone are WHO Grade II. Those tumours with atypia and mitosis are WHO Grade III and those with vascular proliferation or necrosis or both are WHO Grade IV. Grade I and II tumours are termed low grade and Grade III and IV tumours high grade. In one subset of astrocytomas the usual four-featured grading system is not used, because of their distinctive cell appearance. Tumours in this subset may have endothelial proliferation and marked cellular atypia; nevertheless, they are slow growing, well circumscribed and thus low grade:

- Juvenile pilocytic astrocytoma
- PXA, and
- Subependymal giant-cell astrocytoma.

Figures 21.1 and 21.2 illustrate the histological features of some common tumours showing the microscopic H&E features on the left and the key pathological pointers to the diagnosis on the right.

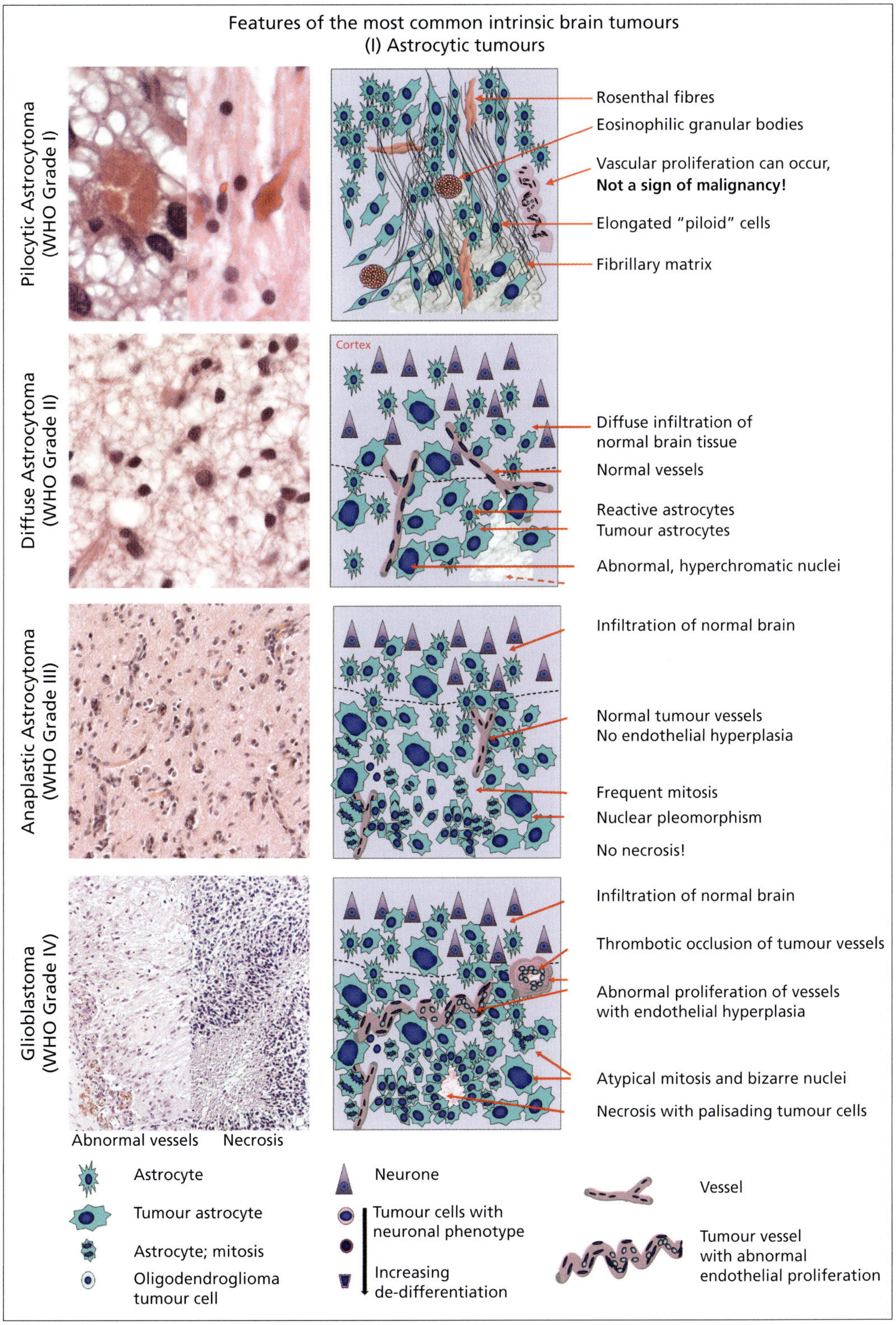

Figure 21.1 Histological features of Grade I–IV astrocytomas.

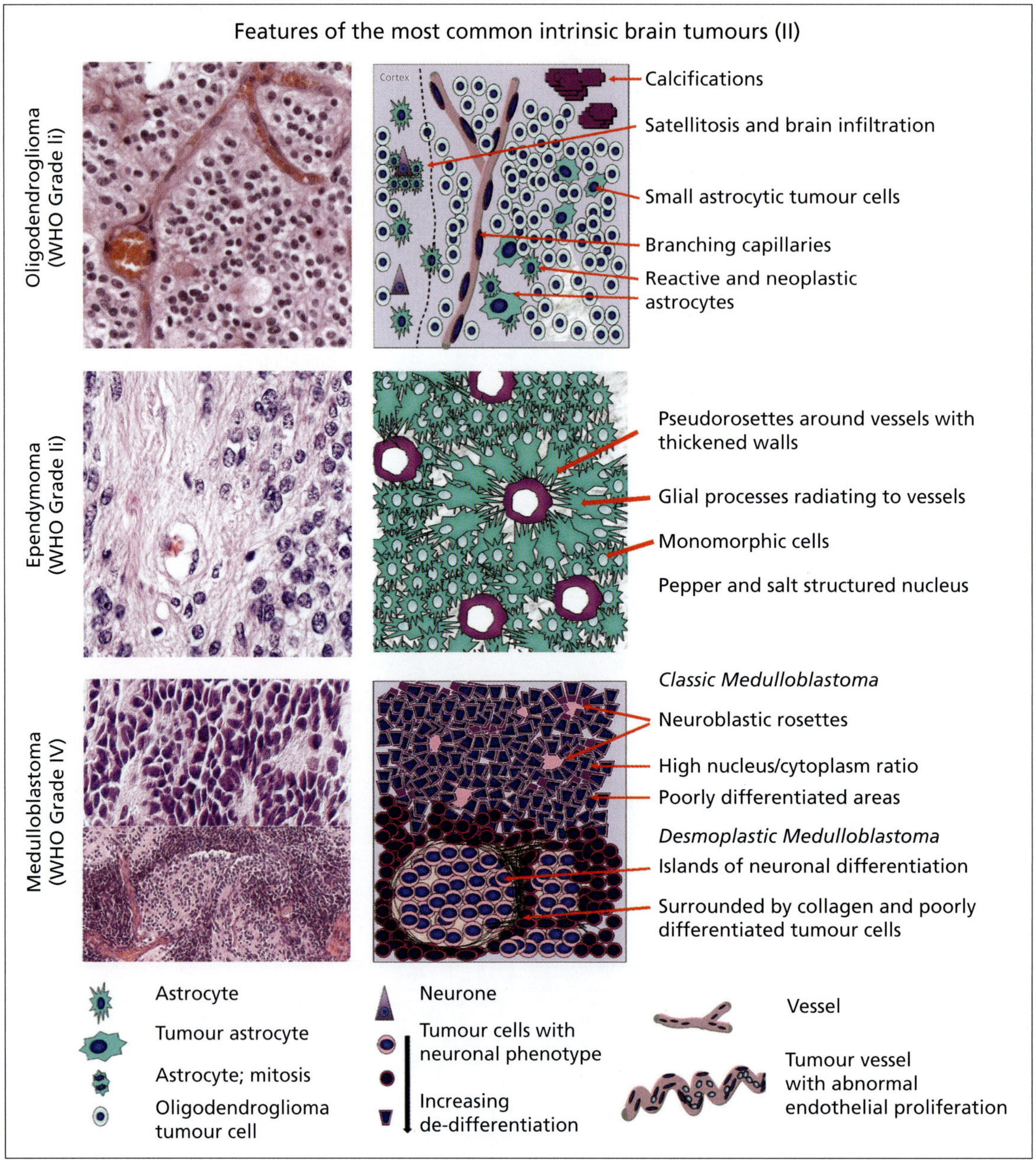

Figure 21.2 Histological features of common intrinsic brain tumours.

Imaging of brain tumours

Structural imaging

MRI is the preferred modality for structural imaging of brain tumours (Chapter 4). MRI provides better soft tissue differentiation and tumour delineation than CT. However, CT demonstrates tumour calcification better than MRI: on MRI, the signal may be difficult to distinguish from intra-tumoural haemorrhage. Structural MRI of brain tumours should include T2-weighted, fluid-attenuated inversion recovery (FLAIR) and T1-weighted images before and after injection of gadolinium. The general imaging and macroscopic appearance of common intracranial tumours are shown in Figures 21.3 and 21.4.

Most tumours appear hypodense on CT, hypointense on T1 and hyperintense on FLAIR and T2 MRI. Highly cellular tumours such as lymphomas, primitive neuro-ectodermal tumours and central neurocytomas have decreased water content and therefore appear hyperdense on CT and relatively hypointense on T2 MRI. Intra-tumoural haemorrhage and tumour calcification appear usually hypointense on T2 images and become more conspicuous on T2* gradient echo images. Hyperintensities on T1 images can be because of haemorrhage, calcification, melanin or fat.

Contrast enhancement on CT or MRI is either seen in highly vascular extra-axial tumours such as meningiomas (Figure 21.5a) or in intra-axial tumours disrupting the blood–brain barrier such as cerebral lymphomas (Figure 21.6). Enhancement is generally a feature of malignant tumours such as high-grade gliomas and metastases but can also be present in certain low-grade tumours, such as pilocytic astrocytomas, ganglioneuromas and WHO Grade II oligodendrogliomas. The visibility of contrast enhancement on MRI can be improved by magnetisation transfer imaging, by doubling or tripling the gadolinium dose or by using high relaxivity gadolinium compounds.

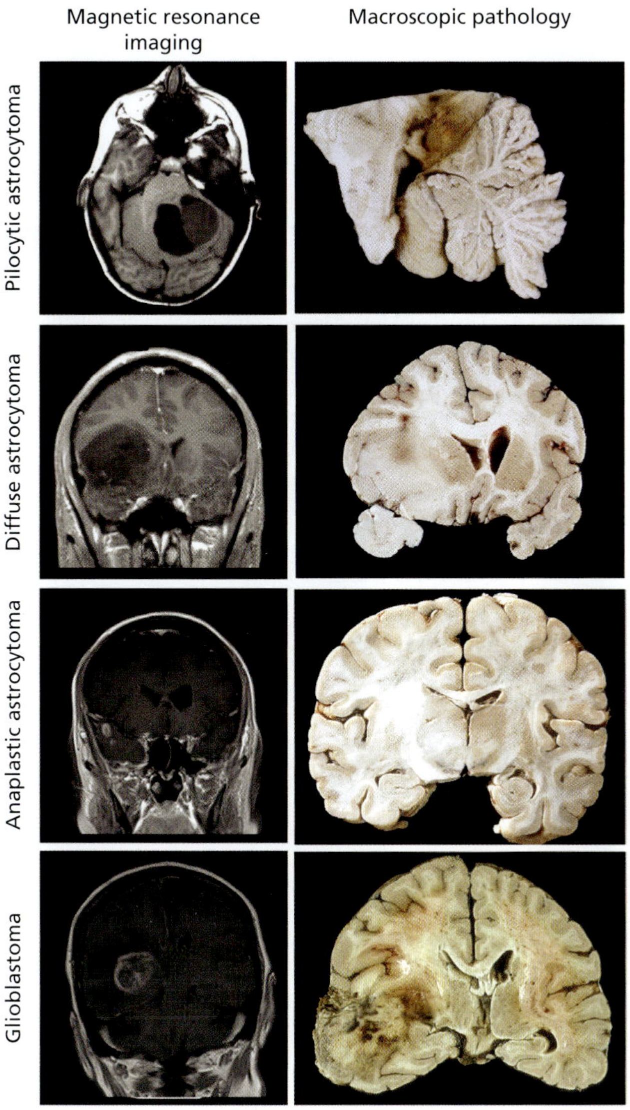

Figure 21.3 Imaging and macroscopic appearance of gliomas.

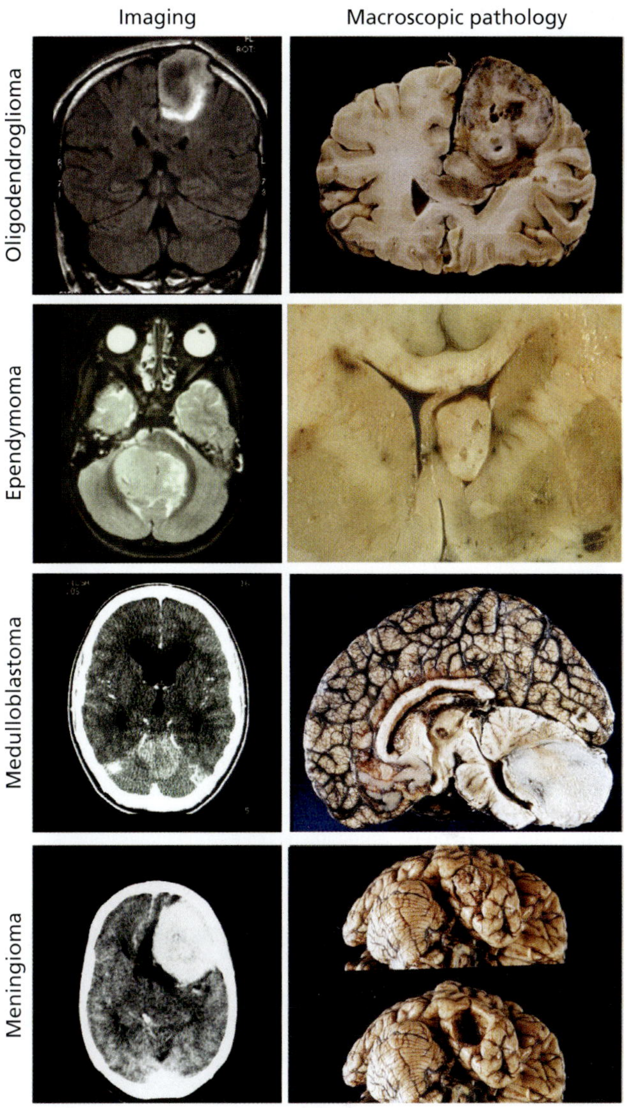

Figure 21.4 Imaging and macroscopic appearance of common brain tumours.

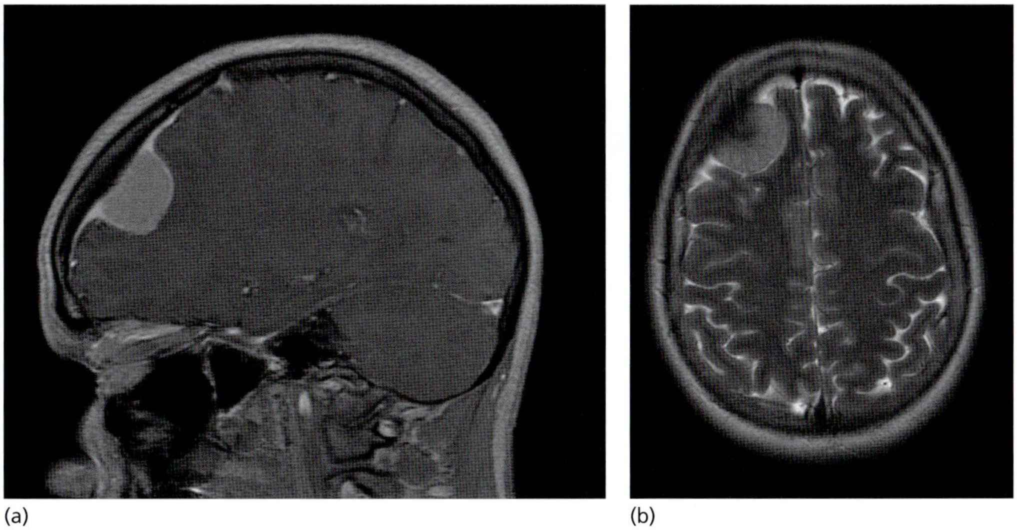

Figure 21.5 (a) Frontal meningioma. Sagittal contrast-enhanced T1 images of a meningioma showing typical appearances of an enhancing durally based mass associated with bony hyperostosis and a dural tail sign. (b) Corresponding axial T2 images demonstrating a grey matter iso-intense mass displacing the frontal lobe with hyperostosis but no associated oedema.

Physiological imaging

Physiological imaging, as its name implies, provides information about physiological and metabolic processes not seen with standard MRI sequences. Much of the recent progress in tumour imaging is based on these methods, which are now being increasingly implemented in practice. The most frequently used physiological sequences include diffusion-weighted imaging (DWI), perfusion-weighted imaging (PWI), MR spectroscopy (MRS) and functional MRI (fMRI). More recently, CT perfusion imaging has emerged as another technique to assess the relative cerebral blood volume (rCBV) and permeability changes in brain tumours. Compared with MR perfusion techniques it brings limited diagnostic focus to the region of interest despite progress in multi-detector technology.

Diffusion-weighted imaging

DWI measures Brownian motion of water molecules within tissue. Images are obtained by measuring the signal loss typically on MR T2 images following the application of diffusion gradients (Figure 21.6). The signal loss depends on several factors including the gradient strength and apparent diffusion coefficient (ADC)

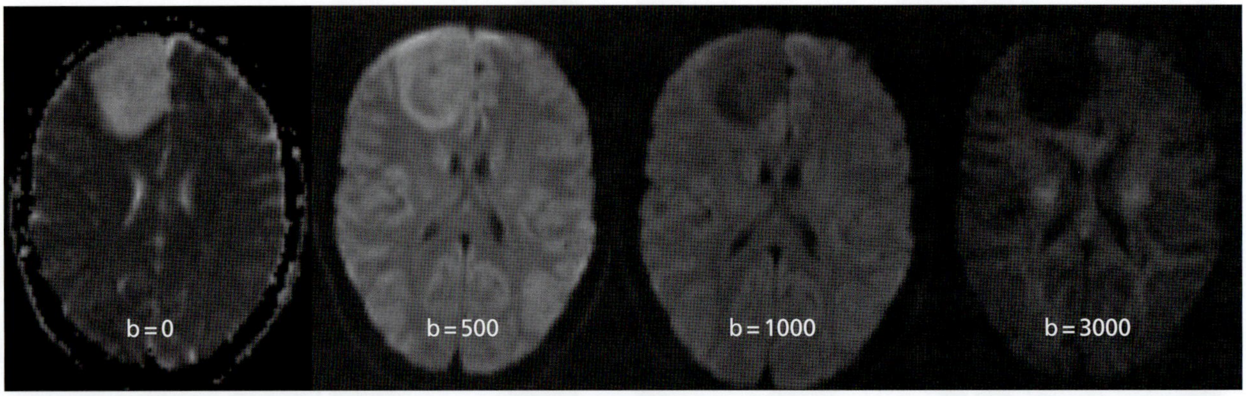

Figure 21.6 Diffusion-weighted images of a frontal low-grade glioma. With increasing diffusion weighting (higher b values) progressive signal loss occurs, first in areas of high water mobility, such as cerebrospinal fluid (CSF) and subsequently also in the tumour.

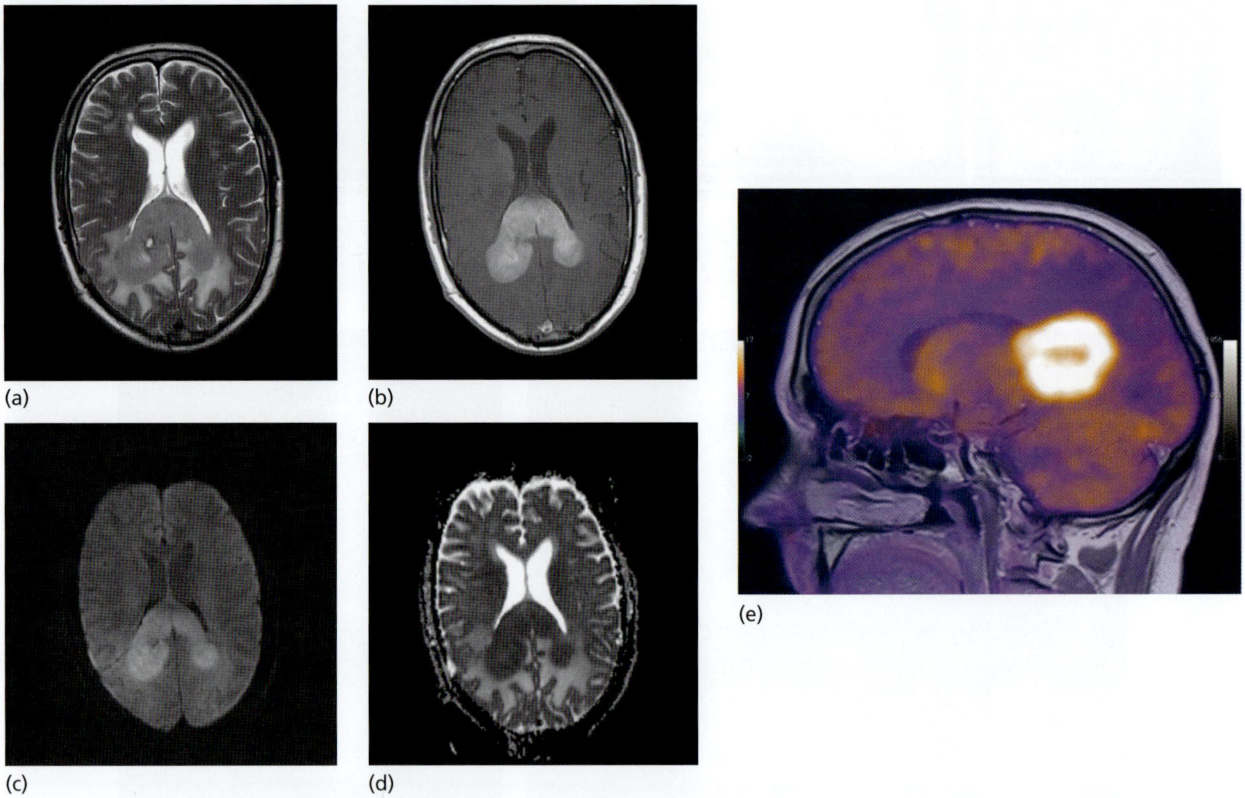

Figure 21.7 Primary central nervous system (CNS) lymphoma. A relatively T2 hypointense (a), uniformly enhancing mass (b) is expanding the splenium of the corpus callosum and extends into the peritrigonal regions of both hemispheres. The solid tumour parts appear bright on diffusion-weighted images (DWI) (c) and dark on the apparent diffusion coefficient (ADC) map (d), in keeping with restricted water diffusion in a highly cellular tumour. The sagittal image of a fluorodeoxyglucose positron emission tomography (FDG PET) MRI (e) shows marked uptake of the tracer in the mass centred on the splenium of the corpus callosum.

which describes water diffusion within tissue. As a general rule, the more mobile the water molecules, the higher the ADC and the lower the signal on DWI. DWI is still influenced by T2 effects, which can lead to artefacts known as T2 shinethrough, whereas ADC maps provide a quantitative representation of water movement. Therefore, highly cellular tumours (e.g. lymphoma), which are associated with limited water mobility, show up as dark on ADC and bright on DWI (Figure 21.7).

Visual inspection of DWI has a limited role in the diagnosis of brain tumours. However, it may be valuable to identify lesions with severely restricted diffusion, such as acute infarcts or abscesses that can occasionally mimic brain tumours on standard MRI but which appear as high-intensity lesions on DWI and low intensity on ADC maps (Figure 21.8).

ADC measurements provide more detailed information about brain tumours and have been shown to correlate with the histological cell count and with the presence of hydrophilic substances in the tumour matrix. Diffusion tensor imaging (DTI) provides additional information about the direction of water diffusion. Anisotropy is the tendency of water to move in some directions more than others, and can be quantified using parameters such as fractional anisotropy (FA). Compact white matter tracts normally show a high degree of anisotropy which can be lost if they are infiltrated by tumour cells destroying ultrastructural boundaries. Tractography is an application of DTI which depicts white matter tracts and their connections on direction-encoded colour images. Tractography is useful in the pre-operative assessment of brain tumours and can differentiate between displacement and infiltration of white matter tracts.

Perfusion-weighted imaging

Dynamic susceptibility-weighted contrast-enhanced (DSC) MRI is the most widely used technique of PWI in brain tumours. It can analyse a series of images acquired during the first pass of an intravenously injected bolus of gadolinium (Figure 21.9). rCBV measurement provides an indirect measure of tumour neovascularity. This correlates closely with angiographic and histological markers of tumour vascularity and the expression of vascular endothelial growth factor (VEGF). High-grade glial tumours tend to have higher rCBV values than low-grade tumours and PWI significantly increases the specificity and sensitivity of conventional MRI in the classification of gliomas. Maps of rCBV can also be a useful adjunct for stereotactic tumour biopsies, directing tissue sampling towards areas of maximal angiogenesis. PWI can also be

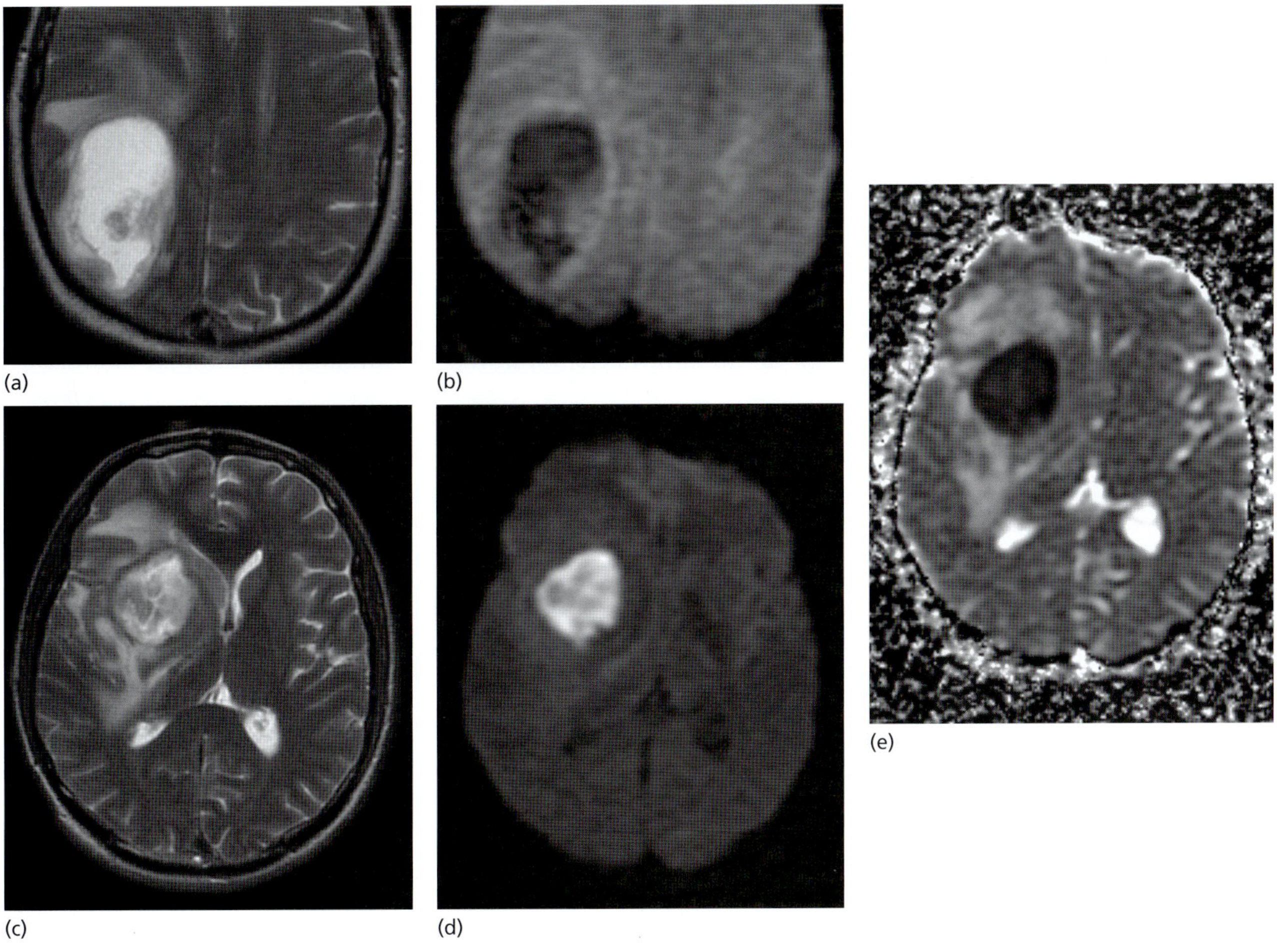

Figure 21.8 (a) T2 image of a cystic high-grade glioma with a hyperintense centre, irregularly thickened rim and vasogenic oedema. (b) The diffusion-weighted image shows loss of signal in the central portion, typical of a necrotic centre in a cystic neoplasm. (c) T2 image of another, undiagnosed cystic frontal lobe mass lesion with a hyperintense centre and surrounding vasogenic oedema. (d) Diffusion-weighted image shows markedly restricted diffusion in this case, typical of an abscess confirmed at biopsy. (e) On the corresponding ADC map the abscess cavity appears dark and vasogenic oedema appears bright.

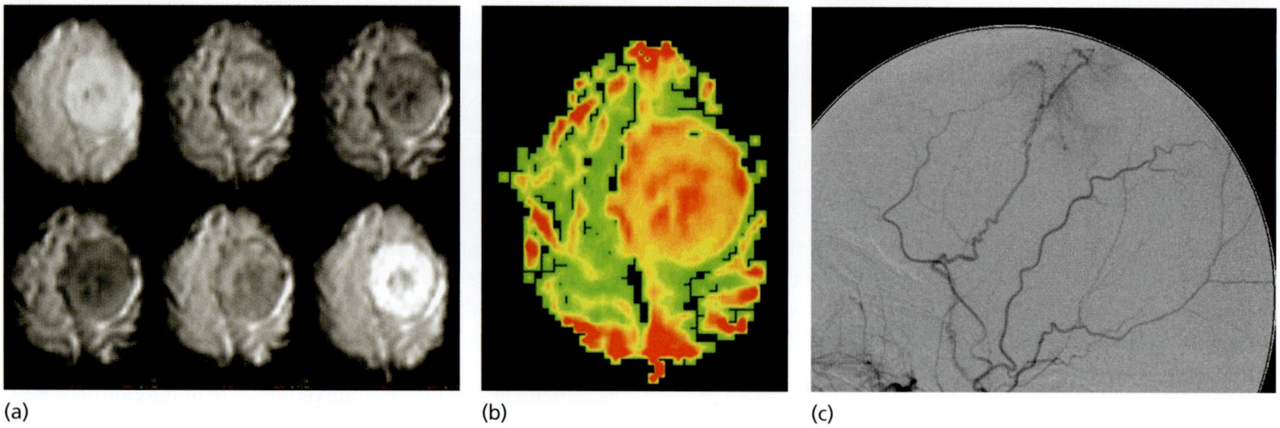

Figure 21.9 Parasagittal meningioma. (a) Dynamic susceptibility contrast perfusion weighted sequences in a patient with a left parasagittal frontal meningioma, showing marked loss of signal intensity within the tumour during the first pass of contrast medium bolus. (b) Corresponding colour overlay map showing increased relative cerebral blood volume (rCBV). Red areas indicate regions of most elevated rCBV within the tumour and over brain surface vessels. (c) Digital subtraction angiogram of the external carotid artery showing a tumour blush confirming increased vascularity of the meningioma.

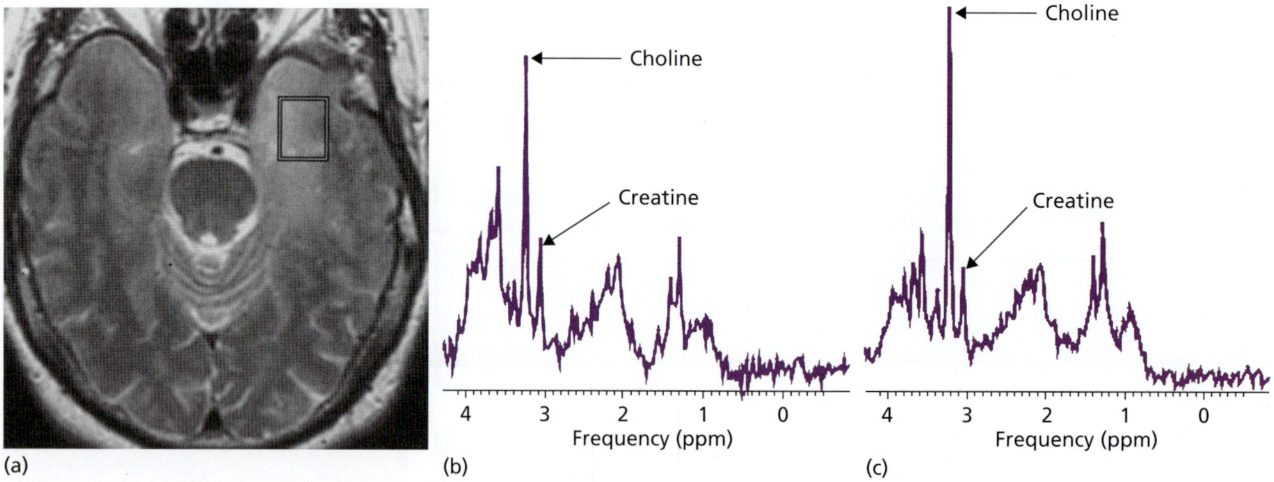

Figure 21.10 (a) Single voxel magnetic resonance (MR) spectroscopy of a left temporal lobe tumour demonstrating region of interest. (b) Initial MR spectrum of a low-grade primary tumour showing a high choline : creatine ratio. (c) MR spectrum 6 months later, following transformation into a high-grade tumour shows a further increase in the choline peak compared to the baseline study (from 1.6 to 3.1 mmol/L).

used to help distinguish between pseudoprogression and true progression in patients with glioblastoma after treatment with chemoradiation.

Permeability imaging (K^{trans})

Microvascular permeability of brain tumours can be quantified by measuring the transfer coefficient K^{trans} which is influenced by endothelial permeability, vascular surface area and flow. This can be measured using a T1 steady state or a first pass T2* gradient echo technique. The former has a higher spatial resolution and is more accurate but requires longer acquisition times and more complicated post-processing; the latter can be combined with DSC perfusion imaging. K^{trans} correlates with tumour grade and is probably more sensitive than rCBV measurements for glioma grading. However, because of the complex post-processing analysis, this technique is rarely used in clinical practice.

MR spectroscopy

Proton MRS analyses aspects of the biochemical make-up of a brain tumour and provides semi-quantitative information about major metabolites. A common pattern in brain tumours is a decrease in *N*-acetyl-aspartate (NAA), a neurone-specific marker, with an increase in choline, lactate and lipids. The concentration of choline is a reflection of the turnover of cell membranes and is more elevated in regions with a high neoplastic activity (Figure 21.10). Lactate is the end product of non-oxidative glycolysis and a marker of hypoxia in tumour tissue, now recognised as a major promoter of tumour angiogenesis and invasion. Lactate probably indicates

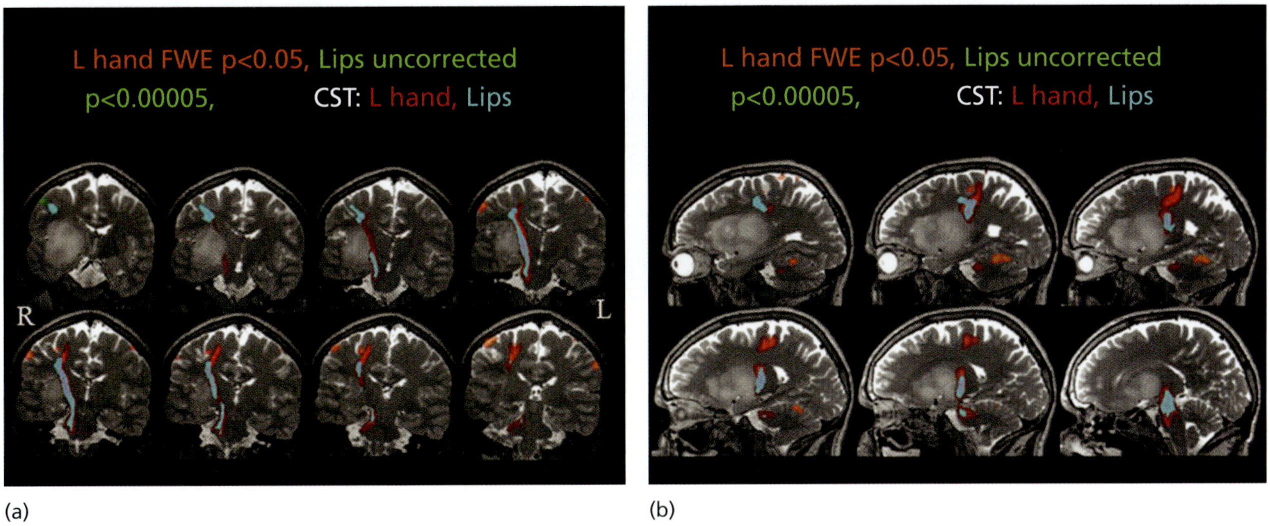

Figure 21.11 (a) Coronal and (b) sagittal fMRI of a motor task involving the left hand in a patient with a right temporal glioma showing activation of motor pathways and relationship with corticospinal tract anatomy showing close approximation of the posterior medial tumour border with motor pathways.

viable but hypoxic tissue, whereas mobile lipids reflect tissue necrosis and breakdown of cell membranes. MRS with a short echo times (20–40 ms) can demonstrate additional metabolites, such as myo-inositol, glutamate and/or glutamine and mobile lipids but is hampered by baseline distortion and artefactual NAA peaks. Chemical shift imaging (CSI) or MRS provides spectral information across a whole tumour region and has been used to inform surgical biopsy targets.

Functional MRI

Blood oxygen level-dependent (BOLD) imaging detects changes in regional cerebral blood flow during various forms of brain activity (Chapter 4). Paradigms using motor tasks, language and speech production and memory are able to show recruitment of activation within relevant cortical areas. The main use of fMRI in tumour imaging is the pre-operative localisation of eloquent cortical regions which may have been displaced, distorted or compressed by the tumour (Figure 21.11). This can both improve the safety of surgery and allow for a more radical resection. Ideally, fMRI should be combined with MR tractography in order to minimise intra-operative injury to white matter tracts connected to eloquent cortical areas.

Applications of physiological imaging

Distinguishing between astrocytomas and oligodendrogliomas

PWI and DWI can help to differentiate between low-grade astrocytic and oligodendroglial tumours. WHO Grade II oligodendrogliomas have significantly higher rCBV than WHO Grade II astrocytomas with median values of 3.68 and 0.92, respectively, which concurs with the histological findings of increased vascular density in oligodendrogliomas (Figure 21.12). In addition, rCBV of oligodendrogliomas appears dependent on their genotype, the loss of 1p/19q being associated with significantly higher rCBV values. Measurement of the ADC, using a whole tumour histogram analysis, appears promising for differentiating between astrocytomas and oligodendrogliomas, but requires complex post-processing analysis. Oligodendrogliomas have significantly lower ADC values than astrocytomas (Figure 21.13), reflecting higher cellular density and differences in tumour matrix composition. However, there is considerable overlap between the oligodendrogliomas and astrocytomas that it cannot be reliably used as a substitute for histology.

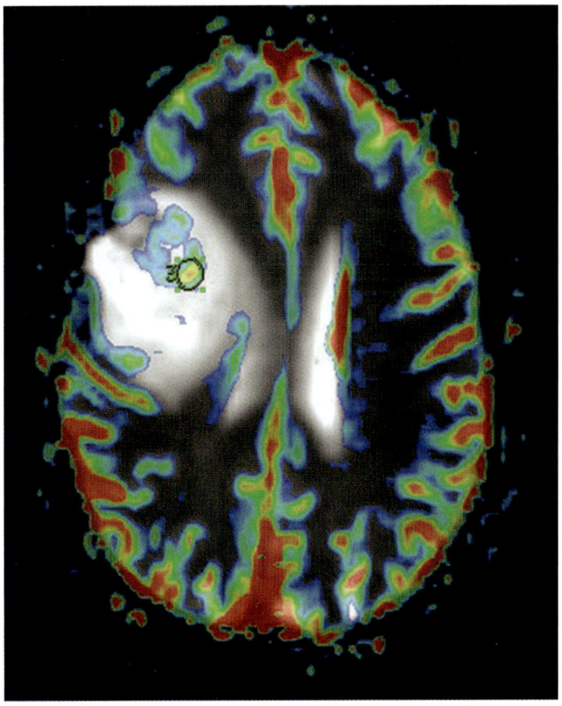

Figure 21.12 rCBV colour overlay of a right frontal oligodendroglioma showing elevated rCBV within the anterior part of the tumour. This is commonly seen in oligodendrogliomas and does not represent malignant transformation.

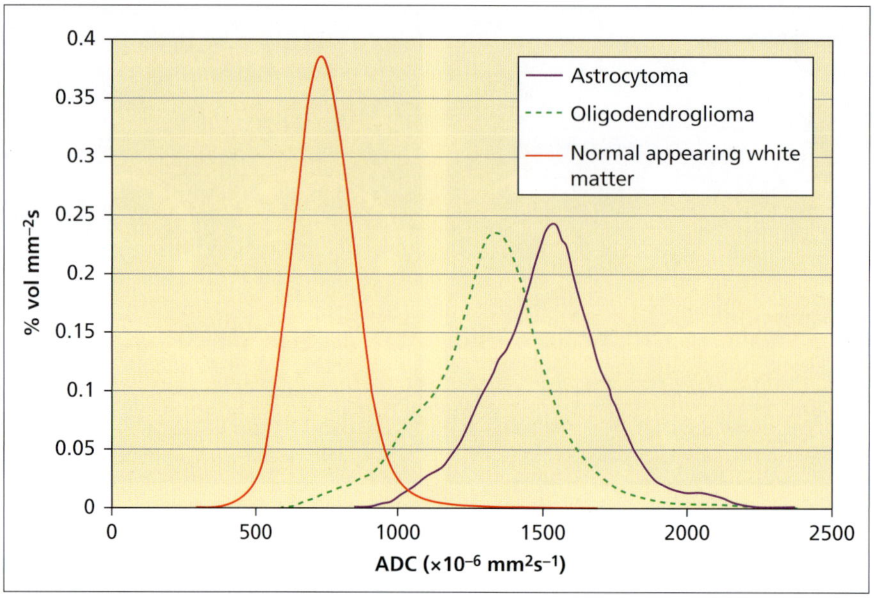

Figure 21.13 Whole tumour ADC histograms of a low-grade astrocytoma and a low-grade oligodendroglioma. Both have higher ADC values than normal white matter. Histogram of the oligodendroglial tumour is shifted to the left compared to histogram of the astrocytic tumour, indicating overall lower ADC values in the former.

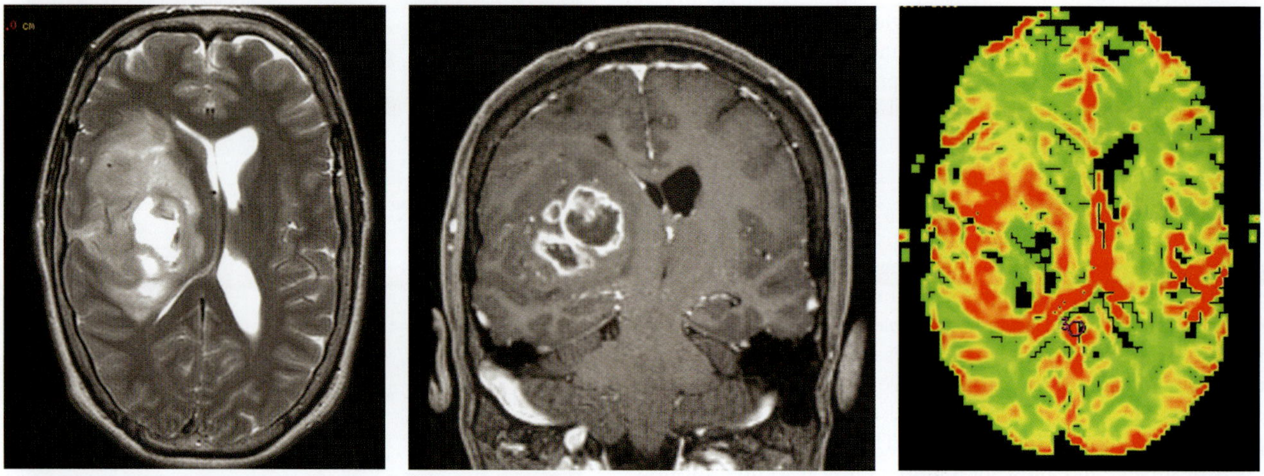

Figure 21.14 Right frontal anaplastic oligodendroglioma. (a) Axial T2-weighted sequence showing a heterogeneous mass with a necrotic centre. (b) Coronal T1W MR slices post contrast demonstrates irregular ring enhancement within the mass, central necrosis, mass effect and vasogenic oedema. (c) rCBV map shows large intra-tumoural areas of increased rCBV (red) reflecting new vessel formation (angiogenesis), suggesting areas of high-grade transformation within a previous low-grade tumour.

Distinguishing between low-grade and high-grade gliomas

Advanced MRI can help distinguish between low-grade and high-grade gliomas. Formation of new blood vessel (angiogenesis) represents an important aspect of glial tumour progression and mean maximum rCBV values correlate closely with histological grades. PWI is also valuable (Figure 21.14). DWI can be disappointing in helping to differentiate high-grade from low-grade gliomas (Figure 21.15).

Imaging of peri-tumoural tissue

Investigation of peri-tumoural regions with physiology-based MR techniques is of similar importance to the radiological assessment of the tumour itself. Differences in the peri-tumoural tissues of low-grade and high-grade gliomas have been demonstrated with DWI, PWI and MRS. The peri-tumoural regions of high-grade gliomas show a more marked decrease in ADC, FA and NAA and increase in rCBV than low-grade tumours. This is a reflection of the more invasive nature of these tumours which infiltrate the adjacent brain tissue leading to an increase in rCBV, destroy ultrastructural boundaries to produce a decrease both in ADC and FA, and replace normal brain tissue with a corresponding fall in NAA. Metastases, on the other hand, are surrounded by pure vasogenic oedema that contains no infiltrating tumour cells. Therefore, peri-tumoural regions in metastases typically show neither increase in rCBV nor decrease in FA.

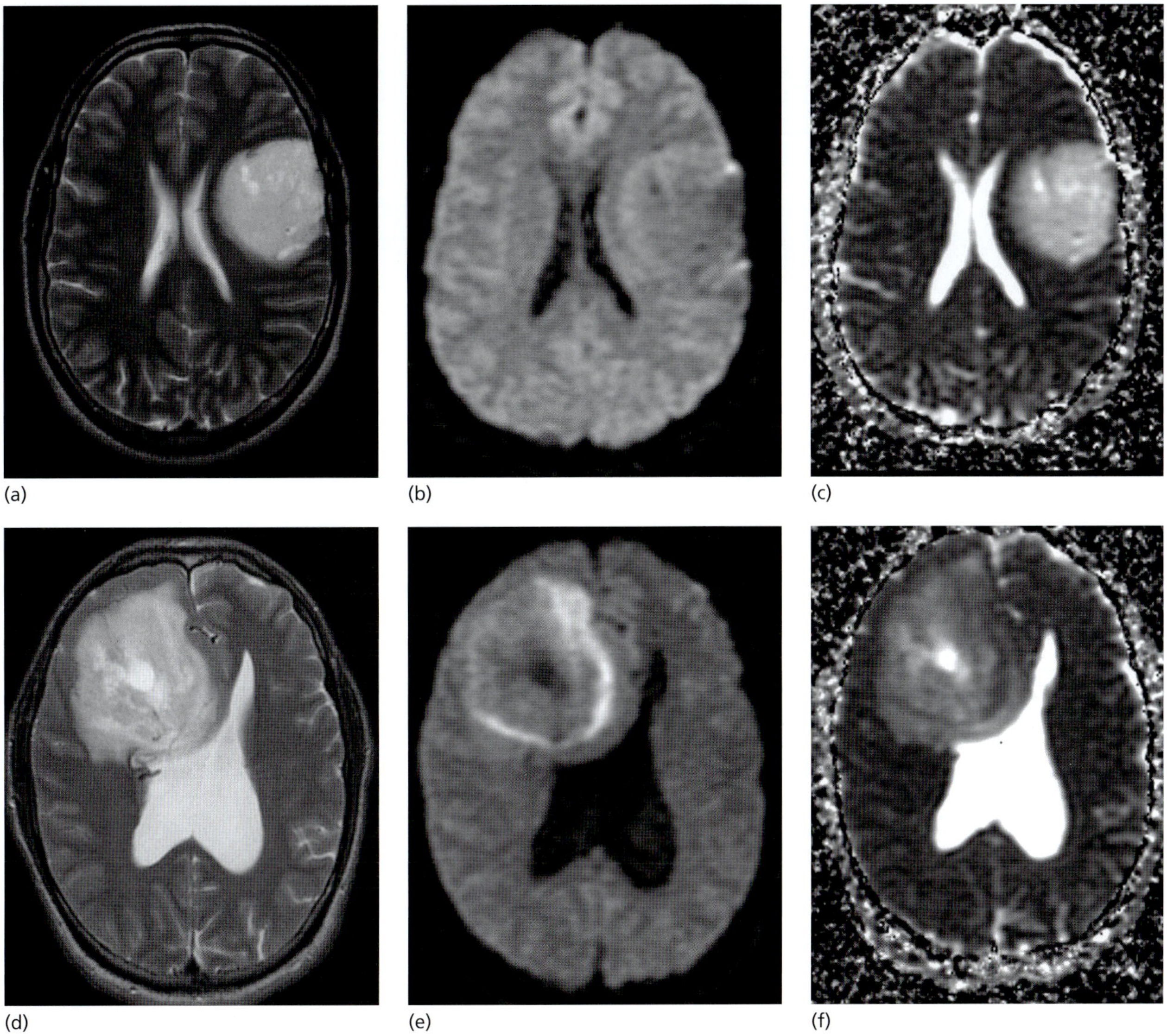

Figure 21.15 (a) T2 image of a homogeneously appearing left frontal low-grade astrocytoma. (b) The tumour is not very conspicuous on diffusion-weighted images as diffusion and T2 effects cancel each other out (T2 masking). (c) Tumour becomes very conspicuous on the ADC map because of its relatively increased water diffusivity. Overall appearance on the ADC map is also homogeneous. (d) T2 image of a high-grade right frontal anaplastic astrocytoma with a heterogeneous appearance. Note enlarged vessels at posterior aspect of mass. (e) Diffusion-weighted image shows a peripheral hyperintense rim, confirmed to be of restricted diffusion on the ADC map with a cystic necrotic centre. (f) ADC map confirms a centre of increased diffusivity (bright) and rim of decreased diffusivity (dark) as well as surrounding oedema (bright).

Monitoring tumour growth and response to treatment

Change in tumour size is still the most important imaging criterion for the evaluation of treatment response. Many treatment protocols for solid tumours recommend unidimensional or bi-dimensional measurements of tumour size. Volumetric (three-dimensional) tumour measurements are better predictors of patient survival than linear or two-dimensional tumour measurements. Volumetric contrast-enhanced T1 images are valuable in any serial imaging protocol that aims to assess tumour progression or treatment response. The assessment of tumour response and progression in glioblastoma (GBM) had traditionally been based on measurements of enhancing tumour portions known as Macdonald criteria. With the advent of combined chemo-radiation as standard therapy and antiangiogentic drugs as second line treatment for GBM, new phenomena such as pseudoprogression and pseudoresponse have to be taken into account and have made an assessment solely based on assessment of enhancing tumour portion unreliable. The Response Assessment in Neuro-Oncology (RANO) Working Group has published recommendations for updated response criteria for high-grade gliomas, which incorporate measurements of non-enhancing signal change seen on T2W and FLAIR sequences, in recognition of the fact that high-grade gliomas are infiltrative in nature, and do not always cause disruption of the blood–brain barrier.

Parameters detectable with physiological MRI have an increasing role in monitoring disease progression and early effects of treatment. This pertains particularly to measurements of rCBV and K^{trans}. The strength of these perfusion techniques lies in their ability

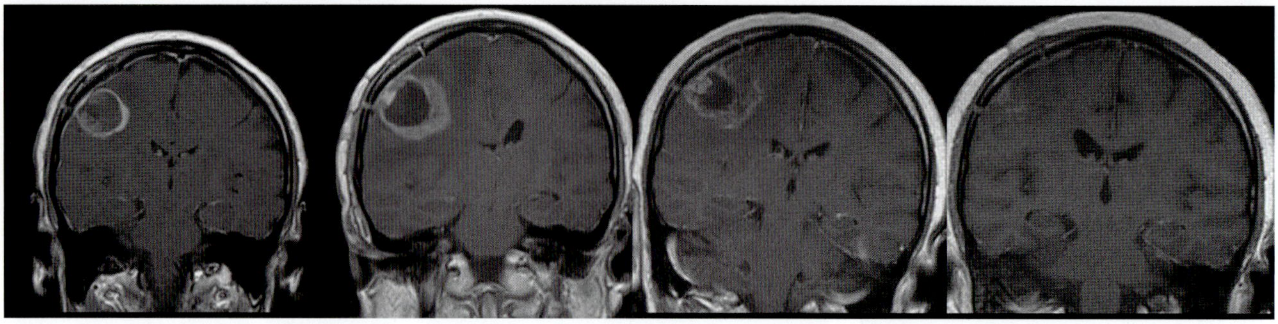

Figure 21.16 Pseudoprogression after treatment of GBM. Contrast-enhanced coronal T1weighted images in a patient with a glioblastoma before and at 6 weeks, 16 weeks and 6 months after treatment with chemoradiation (60 Gy in 30 fractions over 6 weeks with concomitant temozolomide). The baseline image shows an irregular ring-enhancing mass in the right posterior frontal lobe. At 6 weeks after treatment the mass has enlarged and shows increased enhancement with thickening of its rim. The enhancement decreases subsequently at 16 weeks and 6 months without altering the treatment. The time course of these appearances is typical for 'pseudoprogression'.

to detect changes within internal tumour architecture in the absence of or prior to an overall change in tumour size.

Serial PWI of conservatively treated low-grade gliomas show an increase in rCBV 12 months before visible tumour enhancement, the conventional marker of tumour progression. PWI and permeability measurements have also been used to monitor antiangiogenic therapy. A significant fall in rCBV occurs within 48 hours of administration of antiangiogenic drugs (e.g. bevacizumab). Measurements of rCBV also correlate better with clinical status than conventional MRI. PWI has also demonstrated a significant reduction of rCBV in enhancing cerebral mass lesions treated with dexamethasone, an important fact to consider when comparing different treatment regimens.

Pseudoprogression and pseudoresponse

Pseudoprogression is caused by an inflammatory reaction, which results in a temporary increase of contrast enhancement and oedema, usually within 12 weeks of chemoradiation, and subsides subsequently without additional treatment of GBM (Figure 21.16). Pseudoprogression is more frequently observed in patients with methylation of the DNA repair gene *MGMT*, and is associated with a longer overall survival. There are certain histological similarities between the inflammatory response in pseudoprogression and radiation necrosis, the delayed complication of radiotherapy occurring 6–12 months after treatment. Advanced MRI such as DSC and DCE perfusion imaging are helpful in differentiating these two conditions from true tumour progression.

Pseudoresponse is characterised by a decrease of enhancement and oedema following the administration of antiangiogenic drugs without any effect on tumour growth or survival. In pseudoresponse, the tumour continues to progress by an infiltrative pattern without angiogenesis, resulting in an increase of non-enhancing T2/FLAIR hyperintense tumour portions (Figure 21.17). Antiangiogenic treatment can also be associated with non-enhancing areas of markedly decreased ADC, which appear to correspond to atypical gelatinous necrotic tissue rather than tumour, with improved outcome.

Imaging the effects of radiotherapy

The effect of radiation on the brain has a time-dependent course, with a distinction between acute, early-delayed and late-delayed radiation injury (Chapter 19). Severity depends on the total radiation dose, individual fraction size and volume of brain irradiated. Imaging is especially helpful in the diagnosis of late-delayed radiation-induced leukoencephalopathy and radiation necrosis.

Radiation-induced leukoencephalopathy

Radiation-induced leukoencephalopathy is a late-delayed demyelinating process that involves the peri-ventricular region and can extend into the juxtacortical region in more severe cases. On MRI, leukoencephalopathy appears as non-enhancing, confluent, usually symmetrical areas of T2 hyperintensity, typically 6 months or more following radiotherapy (Figure 21.18).

Radiation necrosis

Radiation necrosis is also a late-delayed complication of radiotherapy and radiosurgery, which can appear as an enhancing mass lesion and thus be difficult to distinguish from recurrent tumour on conventional imaging. PWI and DWI may help to distinguish between radiation necrosis and tumour recurrence (Figure 21.19). In radiation necrosis, the enhancing lesion has a low rCBV, whereas this tends to be high in tumour recurrence as a consequence of increased new vessel formation. ADC measurements of the enhancing components in recurrent tumour are significantly lower than in radiation necrosis, mirroring the higher cellular density in recurrent neoplasm.

Optic neuropathy

Optic neuropathy is most commonly seen following radiotherapy of sellar and parasellar lesions and is a late-delayed complication of radiotherapy, with T2 hyperintense signal change typically in the intracranial portion of the optic nerve.

Radiation-induced tumours

Meningiomas are the most commonly encountered radiation-induced tumours, with typical latency periods over 10 years. Gliomas and schwannomas are also seen, developing many years after radiotherapy. Radiation-induced cavernomas are more common than previously assumed; their detection rate is significantly increased with the use of haemorrhage-sensitive gradient echo MR sequences.

Imaging complications of chemotherapy

Many chemotherapeutic agents are neurotoxic. Combining chemotherapy and radiotherapy can result in additive and synergistic effects. The most frequent imaging findings are leukoencephalopathy

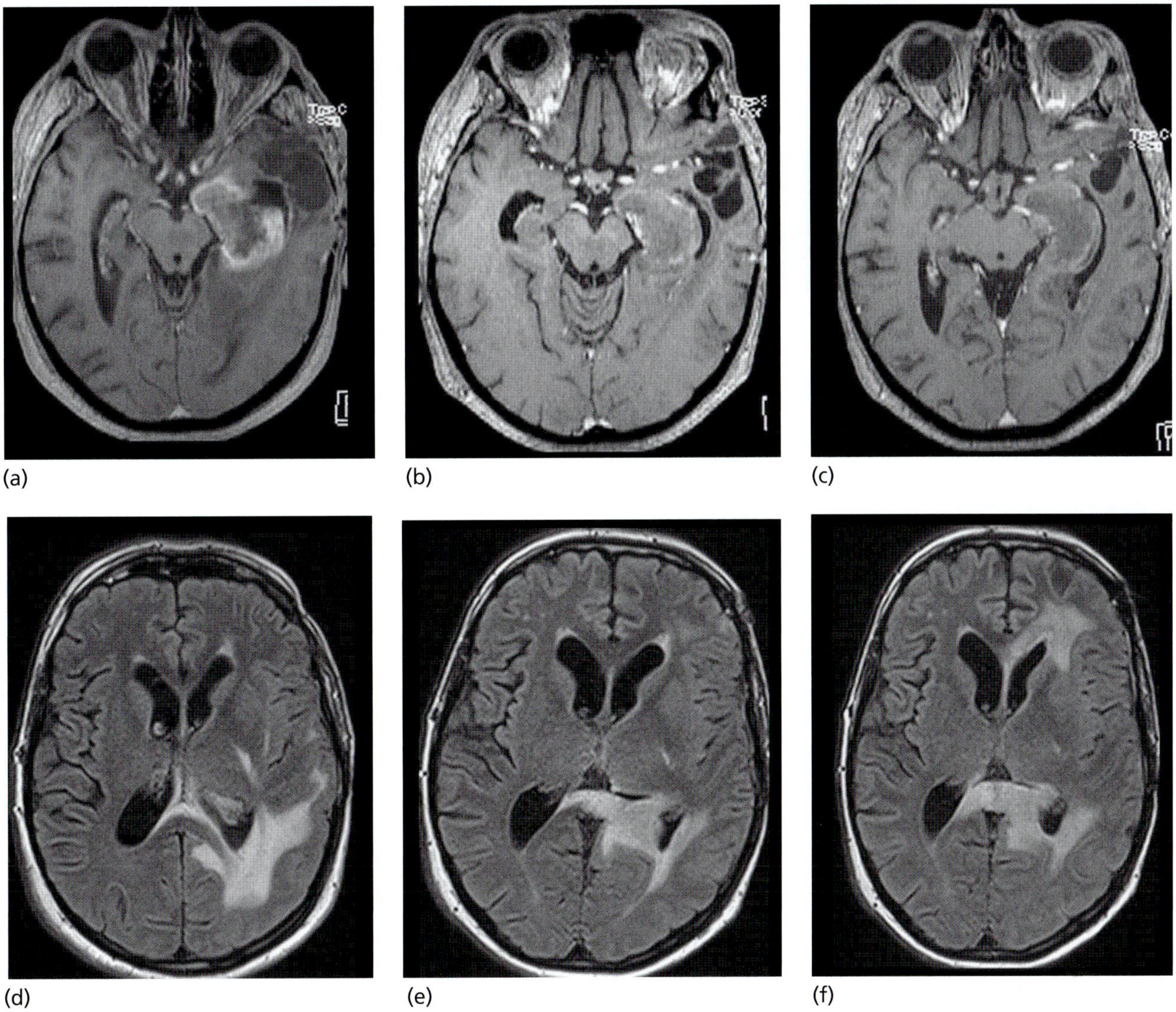

Figure 21.17 Pseudoresponse after treatment with bevacizumab. Contrast-enhanced T1-weighted image (a,b,c) and FLAIR images (d,e,f) in a patient with glioblastoma receiving anti-vascular endothelial growth factor (anti-VEGF) therapy as second-line treatment. The baseline images show an enhancing tumour component in the left temporal lobe and a non-enhancing FLAIR hyperintense component in the left peritrigonal region (d). Six weeks after anti-angiogenesis treatment there is marked decrease of enhancement (b) and some resolution of oedema in the left peritrigonal region (e) but there is now thickening and increased signal intensity of the splenium of the corpus callosum. 16 weeks post treatment the enhancement remains minimal (c) but there has been a further increase in the non-enhancing infiltrative tumour in the splenium of the corpus callosum and also around the frontal horn of the left lateral ventricle. (f) These appearances are typical for 'pseudoresponse' with progression of the non-enhancing tumour components.

(Chapters 19 and 20), with bilateral, typically symmetrical white matter lesions of low density on CT and T2-hyperintense on MRI (Figure 21.18). These are most commonly seen following methotrexate, even when given alone. In acute methotrexate encephalopathy, abnormalities can be undetectable on T2 images and only become apparent on DWI and ADC maps (Figure 21.20).

Multidisciplinary management of brain tumours

The optimal management of CNS tumours requires a multidisciplinary approach incorporating the disciplines of clinical neurology, neuroradiology, neuropathology, neurosurgery, radiotherapy, medical oncology, specialist nursing, general practice and palliative care. Multi-disciplinary working is essential to improve both outcome and experience for these patients, to provide access to specialist services through close collaboration, to recruit patients into clinical trials and to standardise management across regions. The ideal model of service provision promotes a unified care pathway, incorporating medical, psychological, supportive and palliative care for patients and carers. Within the last decade a further dimension has been clearly defined – an approach that unites these disciplines into therapy that is focused on improving not just survival but also the quality of life, with real involvement of both patient and carers in the therapeutic process. There are decisions to be made about treatment for diagnoses of the utmost gravity. One significant advance, sometimes painful to all, is to discuss frankly the prognosis, the limited choice of therapy and the uncertain but often dismal outlook in many a case.

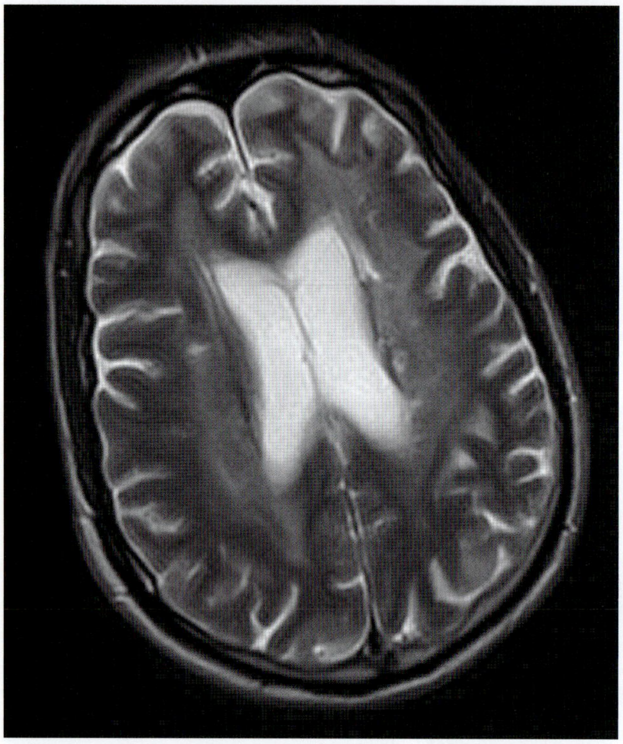

Figure 21.18 Radiation-induced leukoencephalopathy. Axial T2 image of patient treated with radiotherapy for frontal oligodendroglioma who developed progressive cognitive decline 1 year after radiotherapy treatment. MRI shows confluent periventricular high signal change and ventricular dilatation.

Improving outcome and quality of life

The impact of a diagnosis of a brain tumour upon a person's life is profound and multi-faceted. Patients experience both physical and cognitive effects of the tumour and side effects of treatment. They and their carers have to cope with the emotional impact and psychological effects of living with a life-threatening illness. The diagnosis is likely to be the major life event to date and to colour every aspect of the remaining months or years. Cognitive deficits of memory, speech and language, behavioural changes and physical decline combine to produce a formidable burden. When cognitive problems are prominent, recovery from or preservation of cognitive function has been shown to be, in the main, more important to patients than loss of physical function. To plan treatment and gain consent from patients with cognitive impairment is difficult. Progressive cognitive decline presents a continuing challenge for patients, carers and all involved in providing care.

Quality of life can be enhanced by skilled key workers, good communication with patients and carers, access to high-quality information, specialist rehabilitation, supportive and palliative care. Above all, patient and carer need a central point of contact and a plan for action in emergencies and for intercurrent problems. The development of charitable support networks has helped towards providing non-hospital based support for patients, families and carers.

It is often the neuro-oncology clinical nurse specialist who has a primary role in providing information, advice and support to patients and carers at the time of diagnosis, during treatment and disease progression and who facilitates continuity of care across the disciplines involved.

Surgical management

Surgery remains the mainstay of brain tumour management, providing stereotactic biopsy, open craniotomy and tumour resection in some patients. The aims are to obtain the histological diagnosis, relieve mass effect and improve focal deficits, with an ultimate

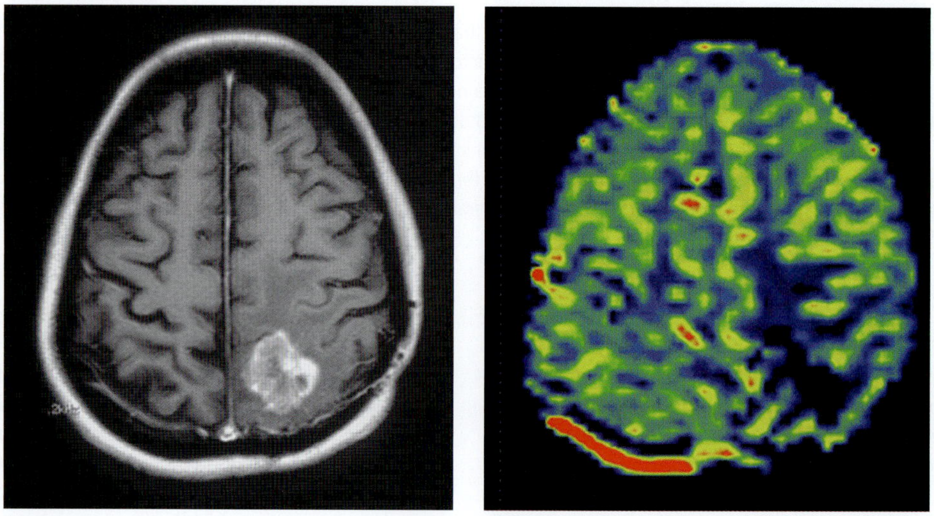

(a) (b)

Figure 21.19 Radiation necrosis following radiotherapy 2 years previously for a high-grade glioma. (a) T1-weighted post gadolinium shows typical appearances of irregular contrast enhancement and central necrosis suggestive of tumour recurrence. (b) rCBV map shows mass has a decreased blood volume compared with normal white matter and appears dark, in keeping with radiation necrosis. A recurrent high-grade glioma is likely to have shown an elevated rCBV.

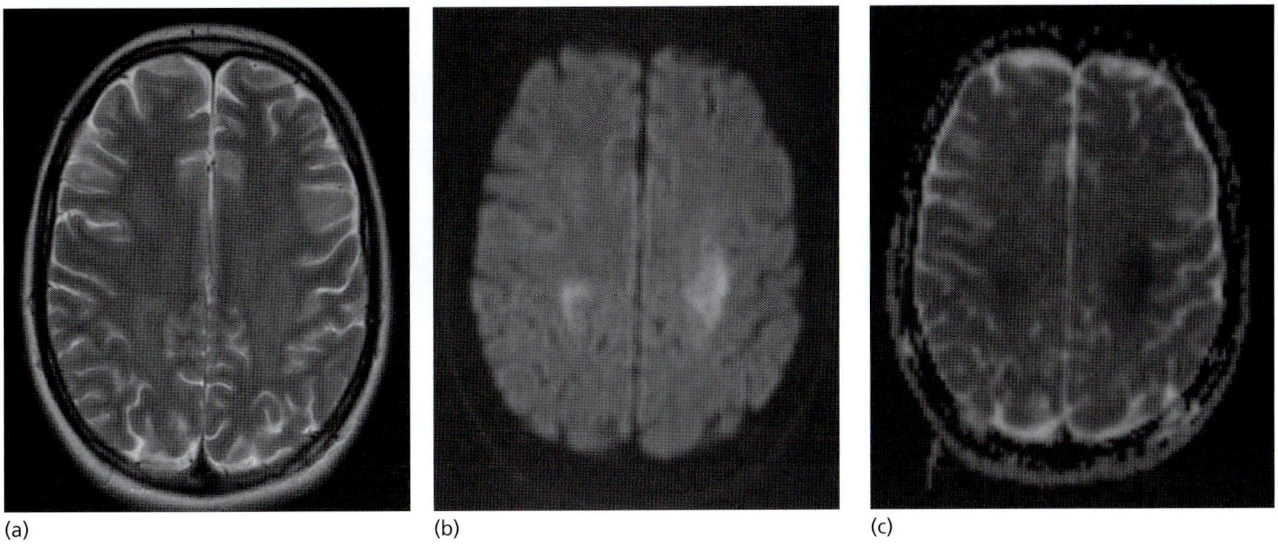

Figure 21.20 Methotrexate encephalopathy. (a) T2 MR in a 6-year-old child following intrathecal methotrexate for acute lymphoblastic leukaemia (ALL) shows very subtle signal increase in parietal white matter. (b) Diffusion-weighted images show much more conspicuous increase of signal intensity in the posterior part of the centrum semiovale. (c) ADC map confirms restricted diffusion in the posterior white matter, a feature of methotrexate toxicity, potentially reversible.

curative goal in selected cases. Technological advances such as neuro-navigation guided biopsy and resection, awake craniotomies with neurophysiological monitoring, cortical mapping, microsurgical techniques, and intra-operative real-time imaging have made some impact on morbidity and mortality. However, more often than not, radical surgery for highly malignant tumours is inappropriate, as the survival benefit over biopsy and adjuvant therapy is modest in elderly patients with poor performance status, who make up the majority of patients with malignant brain tumours.

General principles

The neurosurgical techniques used for brain tumours include image-directed biopsy, either by frame-based, stereotactic methods or by frameless methods using neuro-navigation techniques, with craniotomy for partial or gross total tumour resection. In addition, specific subspecialty tumour surgery include skull base, pituitary and sellar tumours, which have all benefited from use of neuro-endoscopy and allowed for extensive operative techniques to be converted to minimally invasive surgery, with significantly lower morbidity and mortality.

With all tumours, total macroscopic excision is the surgical aim, but this is only realistic in a limited proportion, given the high eloquence of brain structure. Tumours frequently either infiltrate eloquent brain anatomy or are intimately involved with sensitive anatomical structures such as the optic nerve, cavernous sinus or the petro-clival region. Complete resection is commonly possible with extra-axial tumours, in particular meningiomas or sometimes metastatic tumours, but rarely possible with intrinsic tumours. The most difficult of this category are the low-grade gliomas, given the extensive invasive nature often into eloquent cortical structures. Tumours of the middle and posterior skull base require highly specialised surgical avenues such as trans-oral, maxillotomy, retro- or trans-labrynthine routes to make access possible, while avoiding injury to critical neural structures, such as specific cranial nerves and sensitive vascular anatomy.

Surgical instrumentation and methods

Stereotactic frames A large variety of CT and MRI compatible rigid stereotactic frames are available which can be applied to the patient's head for biopsy by pins affixed to the outer table of the skull. Frame-based stereotactic biopsy renders an accuracy of about 1–2 mm, with the most accuracy achieved for deep-seated lesions versus more superficial lesions. Frame-based stereotactic biopsy can be used to obtain a histopathological diagnosis of all regions of the brain, including deep structures such as the thalamus, basal ganglia or brainstem. The complication rate associated with stereotactic biopsy is low; the most major complications are a consequence of bleeding. Overall risks include a 1% risk of death, 5% risk of minor reversible morbidity and 2–3% risk of serious morbidity. The method generally achieves a definite histological diagnosis in 95% of cases. The final diagnosis is significantly different from the initial neuroradiological diagnosis in 5–10%.

Neuro-navigation and frameless stereotaxy In the past decade stereotactic biopsy techniques have gradually been replaced by frameless stereotaxy, a technique that employs neuro-navigation technology. Neuro-navigation involves computer-assisted technologies to guide or navigate the neurosurgical approach. Using mathematical coordinates to identify structures within a defined space (e.g. the skull), neuro-navigation allows highly accurate localisation of structures. This is achieved by real-time fusion of pre-operative imaging of the patient's brain, using either CT or MRI, which includes fiducial markers on the patient's scalp to define a coordinate system of the desired space. The patient can be registered to the neuro-navigation system pre-operatively; this provides the surgeon with the ability to relate the position of a real surgical instrument within the surgeon's hand or microscope's focal point to the location of the imaged pathology, updated in real time. The neurosurgeon is able to create a three-dimensional model that can be manipulated to examine and explore the location of the tumour in relation to normal anatomical structures, in addition to examine alternative surgical approaches prior to the definitive surgery. Virtual images are displayed on a

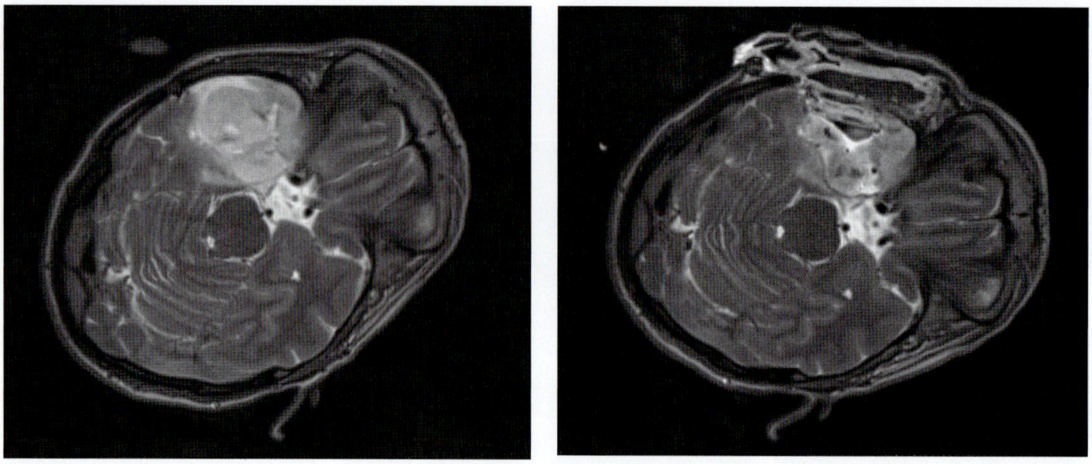

(a) (b)

Figure 21.21 Intraoperative MRI. (a) T2 images of patient with right temporal tumour before and (b) after resection, while the patient is still anaesthetised. There has been an extensive resection with a small triangle of signal change remaining medially.

monitor visible to the surgeon, who can interact with this image with a sterile pointer during the operation. Regions of exposed brain can be touched by the pointer and the position in space correlated with the position of the tumour shown on the peri-operative scan. This method is slightly less spatially accurate than frame-based stereotaxy, within the region of 3 mm variation, particularly as there is inevitably some brain shift when the skull and dura are opened; the overall accuracy is within 10 mm.

Neuro-navigation can be used both for biopsy and gross tumour resection. It has been shown to be efficient for biopsy, except for deep small targets in the brain. For tumour resection, its main advantage is being able to tailor and fashion the craniotomy and surgical approach for individual tumours, providing increased confidence, and giving a rough guide to determine extent of tumour resection intra-operatively. Operative mortality is about 2%, with serious morbidity of about 5–6% and minor morbidity of a further 5–6%. The limitations of neuro-navigation are that it is based on previously acquired imaging datasets; the system does not allow for correction of brain shift, a result of dura being opened, pressure changes occurring within intracranial space, CSF leaking out and brain oedema. In an attempt to eliminate the short-comings of neuro-navigation systems, real-time imaging modalities have evolved, such as intra-operative diagnostic ultrasound and intra-operative MRI.

Intra-operative diagnostic ultrasound Ultrasound has been used in neurosurgery for over two decades. Precise localisation of lesions in the brain is a challenge, and methods to minimise and eliminate exploration and dissection in the brain parenchyma are constantly being sought. Pre-operative CT and MRI images provide ideal road-maps for surgical planning; however, they are limited in their ability to determine the precise location of lesions intra-operatively, in particular deep lesions beneath the cortical surface. Real-time images obtained from intra-operative ultrasound provide dynamic information on localisation, in depth, orientation, mass effect and presence of cystic components; ultrasound can facilitate cyst drainage and alleviate pressure prior to tumour excision. Ultrasound can also be used to confirm extent of tumour resection.

Intra-operative MRI Interventional MRI (iMRI) is a real-time intra-operative adjunct for guiding surgery without ionising radiation, providing exquisitely detailed imaging compared to CT. Surgical navigation can be repeatedly updated by intra-operative and dynamic images of the brain and lesion while surgery is proceeding, and account for the changes that occur as a result of CSF leakage, oedema and hemorrhage. The main advantage of iMRI is that it allows the surgeon to identify the extent of residual tumour that can still be resected (Figure 21.21). The use of physiological iMRI to understand more clearly the pathology of brain tumours is promising. However, iMRI suites are only available in very few neurosurgical centres. Its real value as an operative adjunct has yet to be established.

Neuro-endoscopy Technological advances in neuro-endoscopy, improved optics, video and camera systems have made neuro-endsocopy and minimally invasive neurosurgery a routine technique not only for pituitary but also for skull base tumours. Large and extensive exposures are required for upper cervical spine and clivus lesions, through trans-oral or 'open door' maxillotomy approaches and resection of the odontoid which have in the past been associated with significant morbidity. These areas can now be approached using endoscopic trans-nasal approaches. The endoscopic approach possesses some inherent advantages, including decreased exposure to oral flora and excellent visualisation, while at the same time minimising prolonged retraction. Most surgeons who incorporate neuro-endoscopy and minimally invasive surgery do so in close collaboration with their head and neck, and ENT colleagues.

Radiotherapy

The benefits of surgical treatment for the majority of intrinsic malignant tumours are limited by their aggressive biological behaviour together with considerations surrounding neurological deficits following removal of tumour tissue from infiltrated normal brain or spinal cord. Many CNS tumours, even benign WHO Grade I meningiomas, may recur many years after removal particularly if initial resection is incomplete. For these reasons, radiotherapy and chemotherapy play an important part in the overall management of primary CNS tumours.

Radiotherapy planning

Conformal radiotherapy Radiotherapy planning based on CT and MRI is now the standard approach to primary brain tumour treatment. CT-based planning allows accurate tumour dose localisation and relative sparing of normal brain. The patient is immobilised in a plastic mask. CT slices (0.3 cm) are obtained in the treatment position. MRI data from diagnostic studies are then fused with CT data, to define the precise volumes to be treated to high dose. The patient is usually treated in the supine position. This position is most easily reproducible and the most comfortable. The field arrangement is chosen to encompass the tumour volume with maximal sparing of surrounding brain, usually utilising 2–3 fixed fields. Using modern conformal radiotherapy techniques, scanning and planning software permits reconstruction of three-dimensional anatomy. The tumour and target volumes are visualised from the plane of the incoming radiation beams. Using these data the radiotherapist can then design shielding that conforms closely to the tumour volume, giving a steep dose gradient between tumour and normal brain. Total radiation doses given are usually in the range 45–60 Gy, with typical daily fractions of 1.8–2 Gy.

Stereotactic radiotherapy A refinement of conventional brain radiotherapy is to combine conformal planning with stereotactic techniques for both immobilisation and tumour localisation. This enables a further reduction in the treatment volume because of increased accuracy of tumour localisation; relocation error is often reduced to below 1 mm. Relocatable stereotactic frames permit the dose to be given in a conventionally fractionated regime. These techniques are used more in the treatment of benign brain tumours, such as pituitary adenomas, meningiomas and vestibular schwannomas, with the aim of reducing the amount of normal brain tissue in the high dose treatment volume.

Radiosurgery Radiosurgery harnesses image-directed surgical planning with focused high-dose radiation delivery to the selected target. In this sense it is more akin to surgical ablation than to radiotherapy. The technique is used increasingly for cerebral metastases and for relatively inaccessible skull base tumours such as chordomas, meningiomas and vestibular schwannomas.

Intensity modulated radiotherapy Intensity modulated radiotherapy (IMRT) enables the radiation dose to be modified throughout the treatment volume. This permits treatment of concave volumes, sparing of nearby critical structures (such as the optic pathways), and reduction of dose to areas such as the temporal lobes. This sparing may reduce the late side-effects of radiation when treating benign brain tumours, and allow dose escalation when treating malignant brain tumours.

Spinal radiotherapy For spinal tumour masses, developments in radiotherapy planning have improved accurate delineation using MRI data superimposed on CT scans in the proposed treatment position. In most cases, MRI will be used to define the target lesion and fields designed to encompass this volume with 3–5 cm margins. Attention should be paid to anatomical influences on tumour spread, for example when treating disease in the conus medullaris the anatomical boundary to spread is at S3. Treating below this level will only add toxicity. In most cases, treatment fields do not need to extend further laterally than the lateral processes of the vertebral bodies (to ensure adequate coverage of the exiting nerve roots), that is, some 2 cm lateral to the border of the vertebral body. Patient positioning and immobilisation for treatment are important to prevent dose inaccuracies or inhomogeneity. Radiotherapy doses to the ovaries and uterus in young female patients need to be reduced as far as possible to minimise effects on fertility. Three-dimensional conformal planning with appropriate shielding will help with this. It is generally safe to irradiate limited volumes of spinal cord to doses of 50–55 Gy. Animal data suggest a relatively small effect of volume once treatment lengths of 8 mm are exceeded. Estimates of the total dose to give 5% toxicity rate at 5 years (TD 5/5) using 2 Gy fractions are between 57 and 61 Gy; previously damaged spinal cord probably has a lower radiation tolerance.

Radiation neurotoxicity

Radiotherapy-induced neurotoxicity is seen commonly following treatment of even relatively benign CNS tumours, both in children and adults. Radiation damage to the brain and spinal cord is categorised according to the time at which the clinical features develop. Acute, early-delayed and late-delayed radiation effects must be considered. As a general rule, acute and early-delayed toxicity are reversible and improve spontaneously and/or with steroids while late-delayed toxicity is irreversible.

Diagnosis Damaging effects of radiotherapy, suspected from symptoms and signs should only be ascribed to it if the following conditions are met:

- Anatomy of the clinical signs corresponds to the radiation portals.
- Dosage and fractionation are sufficient to damage that particular area of the nervous system.
- Time elapsed between radiotherapy and development of the neurological syndrome is compatible with known effects of radiotherapy on the nervous system.
- Tumour recurrence has been excluded, particularly in the brain where clinical and radiological features of radiotherapy necrosis can be hard to differentiate.
- Other differential diagnoses (e.g. spinal intramedullary metastasis, paraneoplastic syndromes, CNS infection and malignant meningitis) have been excluded.

Acute toxicity Common acute effects include alopecia, scalp erythema, fatigue, headache, nausea and sometimes vomiting. Neuronal toxicity is thought to underlie the feelings of intense lethargy seen commonly within 2 weeks of starting treatment. The usual daily radiation dose is 1.8–2 Gy.

Early-delayed toxicity Acute toxicity can be followed by a longer period of lethargy and exhaustion ('somnolence syndrome') lasting up to 3 months after treatment, known as early-delayed toxicity. Worsening of pre-existing deficits and seizures can occur. This condition is usually reversible with steroids but improvement is sometimes slow, over many weeks.

Late-delayed toxicity Late-delayed effects include cognitive decline resulting from leukoencephalopathy, vascular damage and radiation necrosis. These late-delayed effects become apparent between 6 months and even up to 20 years following treatment. Other late effects include changes in taste, hearing and vestibular function. Radiation necrosis, usually apparent between 6 and 24 months after radiation, can mimic tumour recurrence both clinically and radiologically. The estimated risk of brain necrosis is 5% following 64 Gy; some data suggest a lower threshold dose of 50–58 Gy. Modern imaging techniques such as PWI and DWI MRI sequences and fluorodeoxyglucose positron emission tomography (FDG PET) scanning can help distinguish between necrosis and tumour recurrence.

ADC and rCBV measurements are also of some value (see Imaging the effects of radiotherapy).

Other complications of cranial radiotherapy

Cataract, chiasm, pituitary and skin The lens is commonly treated to near-tolerance in frontal tumours, with a substantial risk of cataract development. Other late toxicity may become relevant if other normal structures are included in the high radiation dose volume (e.g. the optic chiasm, pituitary and skin). These toxicities can be avoided to some extent by planning and accurate shielding of normal structures. In some instances, moderate dose irradiation will be unavoidable and patients must be warned of possible consequences.

Secondary tumours Radiotherapy also can cause second brain and exceptionally spinal tumours. Meningiomas, gliomas, schwannomas and cavernomas can develop many years after treatment.

Vascular disease Radiotherapy can lead to accelerated large vessel arterial disease, most commonly seen in young adults presenting with internal carotid artery occlusion and moya-moya disease following treatment in childhood for optic nerve or hypothalamic gliomas.

Myelopathy, radiculopathy and plexopathy Myelopathy may ensue in the months following radiotherapy treatment of head and neck cancer. Radiotherapy to the cord rarely causes acute toxicity. Radiation myelopathy is usually late-delayed and presents either as a progressive myelopathy or as a lower motor neurone syndrome. This is most commonly seen in patients with Hodgkin's disease given mantle radiotherapy. Some patients seem especially susceptible to myelotoxic effects of radiotherapy and develop a severe cord syndrome after radiation doses well below usual tolerance. Patients treated with axillary radiotherapy for breast cancer may develop a late-delayed radiation brachial plexopathy, distinguished from tumour recurrence by the absence of pain and sometimes the presence of myokymic discharges on electromyography.

High-grade gliomas

The most common primary brain tumours are the high-grade glioma, which are either WHO Grade III anaplastic gliomas (astrocytoma, oligodendroglioma or oligoastrocytoma) or WHO Grade IV, glioblastoma, GBM or gliosarcoma. Of these, GBM is the most frequent malignant primary CNS tumour, accounting for about 30% of all primary brain tumours and 60% of all gliomas. Despite aggressive multi-modality treatment, median survival times are poor. GBM tends to occur in older people (peak incidence 60–70 years) and arise in the cerebral hemispheres, most commonly temporal, parietal and frontal lobes. Histological diagnosis is mandatory, except in situations where the condition of the patient is so poor that oncological treatment is not warranted and palliative care is all that can be offered. In all other situations where MRI is suggestive of a high-grade glioma, the main differential is a metastasis or a primary CNS lymphoma; histological diagnosis is essential, to provide clear prognostic information and tissue for molecular analysis.

Pathology

Anaplastic astrocytoma

Anaplastic astrocytomas (WHO Grade III) show an infiltrative behaviour with focal or generalised increase in proliferative potential. These tumours may progress from a low-grade astrocytoma but they are also seen at first biopsy without evidence for an underlying low-grade lesion. They have an intrinsic propensity to progress to GBM. They are characterised histologically by increased cellularity, higher mitotic activity and more distinct nuclear atypia than WHO Grade II gliomas, but there is no necrosis or vascular proliferation as seen with GBM.

Glioblastoma

Typical histological features of GBM include poorly differentiated, often highly pleomorphic glial tumour cells with marked nuclear atypia and brisk mitotic activity. Necrosis and/or microvascular proliferation are essential for diagnosis and in most cases both are present. GBM can vary considerably in their histological appearance, ranging from highly cellular and monotonous to very variable and heterogeneous. This may present a challenge when histological diagnosis is based on small needle biopsies.

Molecular genetics Genetic studies suggest that primary GBM (*de novo*) and secondary GBM (evolving from low-grade gliomas by multi-step progression) are different entities. Primary GBMs arise in older patients and are strongly associated with loss of chromosome 10q, gain in chromosome 7, amplification and over-expression of the epidermal growth factor receptor gene (*EGFR*), and show increased murine double minute 2 promoter (*MDM2*) oncogene activity. In contrast, secondary GBMs arise from previous low-grade gliomas, occur in younger individuals and are associated with early p53 loss, *IDH* mutations and over-expression of platelet-derived growth factor gene (*PDGF*).

The identification of *IDH1/2* mutations has been a breakthrough because these mutations are frequent in secondary glioblastomas (80%) but very rare in primary glioblastomas (5%). Primary and secondary glioblastomas with *IDH1* mutations have similar gene expression profiles. These observations suggest that primary glioblastomas with *IDH1/2* mutations have progressed from less malignant precursor lesions (low grade or anaplastic astrocytoma) which escaped clinical diagnosis and were thus misclassified as primary.

MGMT promoter methylation has become the most powerful molecular test in malignant gliomas and is predictive for response to alkylating agent chemotherapy in glioblastoma. As a result, the MGMT status has become a parameter for stratification of patients with glioma within clinical trials.

H3 histone family 3A (*H3F3A*) mutations, initially detected in paediatric malignant brainstem glioma (diffuse intrinsic pontine glioma), also occur in young adult GBM and in locations other than brainstem. The frequency has not yet been established but an estimate ranges around 5% of all adult GBM harbouring this alteration.

Telomerase reverse transcriptase (*TERT*) is essential in maintaining telomere length and its activity is pathologically increased in a number of human cancers, including GBM. *TERT* and *IDH* mutations are mutually exclusive in GBM, but co-occur in oligodendrogliomas. Two large studies show conflicting results with regard to *TERT* mutation status and survival, but it is possible that *TERT* may in the future become a useful prognostic marker. Approximately 50% of primary GBM carry a *TERT* promoter mutation.

Imaging

Anaplastic astrocytoma

Anaplastic astrocytomas (WHO Grade III) usually show contrast enhancement and more extensive infiltration of the peri-tumoral

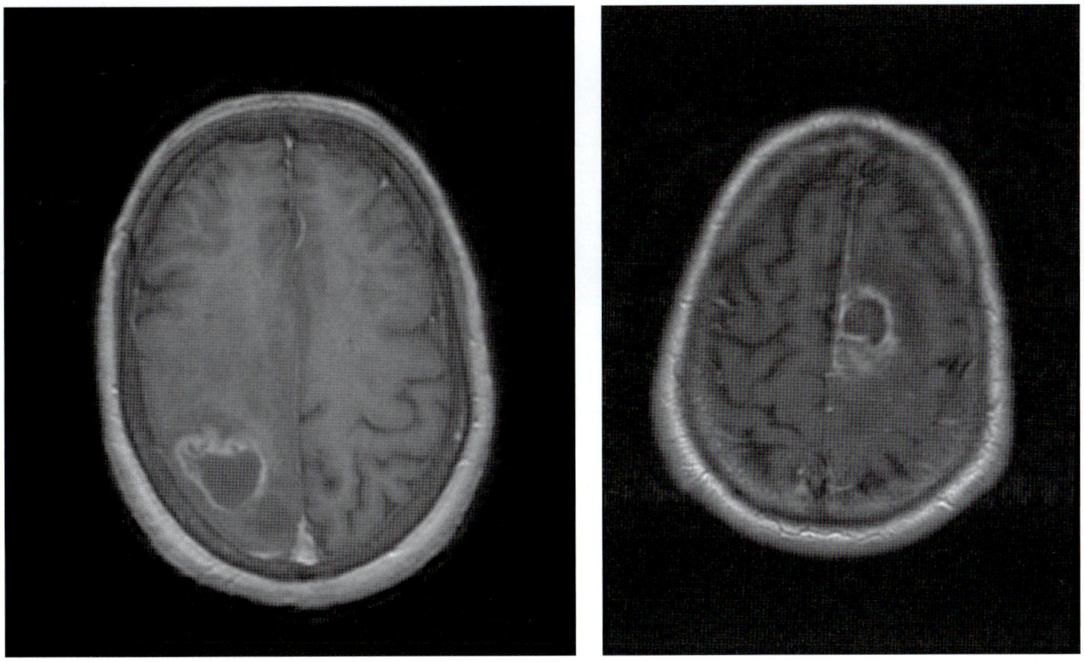

(a) (b)

Figure 21.22 (a) T1-weighted image plus gadolinium MR showing right frontal glioblastoma multiforme with irregular enhancing rim and central area of necrosis, with diffuse hemispheric swelling caused by surrounding vasogenic oedema. (b) Almost identical appearing lesion in left frontal lobe which turned out to be toxoplasma abscess.

tissues than WHO Grade II lesions. They may also be accompanied by vasogenic oedema. In many cases, however, it is not possible to distinguish radiologically between Grade II and Grade III tumours: absence of enhancement does not rule out a high-grade tumour.

Glioblastoma

As noted earlier, GBM is a poorly differentiated, highly pleomorphic tumour with vascular proliferation and necrosis. Vasogenic oedema and contrast enhancement are more extensive than in anaplastic (WHO Grade III) astrocytomas. Tumour necrosis appears as intra-tumoural areas of approximately CSF signal intensity, frequently surrounded by an irregularly enhancing rim corresponding to regions of active mitosis. Intra-tumoural haemorrhage with T1 hyperintense and T2 hypointense areas contributes to the heterogeneous MR appearance of GBMs. The differential diagnosis includes brain metastases (vasogenic oedema is usually more extensive than in GBM), tumefactive MS, pyogenic abscess, and TB, the latter an important consideration in developing countries (Figure 21.22).

Surgery

Malignant gliomas infiltrate surrounding normal brain and surgical cure is therefore not possible, even with very extensive resections. Indications for debulking of a tumour are for symptomatic relief of raised intracranial pressure or focal deficits, caused by tumour mass effect and compression of eloquent cortical structures. Invasion of eloquent brain areas is the limiting factor in achieving a complete gross tumour resection. The principle of 'oncological cytoreduction' enhancing the efficacy of adjuvant therapies is invoked in support of macroscopic complete resections and is therefore offered to patients at the better end of the prognostic spectrum (i.e. younger age and higher performance status). There is mounting evidence for survival benefits in patients who have had gross macroscopic resections. Recently, fluorescence-guided surgery using Gliolan (5-aminolaevulinic acid) has been shown to improve the extent of resection in high-grade gliomas from an estimated 36% to 65% with improvement in progression-free survival at 6 months from 21% to 41%. This is based on the principle that malignant cells take up 5-ALA and are then visible under UV light using a dedicated microscope which circumvents the problems of identifying tumour margins intra-operatively (Figure 21.23). The volume of tumour that could be resected had previously been limited because of the risk of neurological deficits. In general, it is accepted that 80% tumour resection provides oncological advantage by providing cytoreduction and improving response to adjuvant chemo- and radiation therapy. A few centres suggest that resection of 98% is an independent variable associated with longer survival, with an approximate 3-month survival advantage compared to patients with 80% resection. In a small proportion of patients with recurrent disease, a second resection (11%) or a third resection (4%) is performed, again in younger patients with high performance status who have responded well to first line treatment.

Radiotherapy

The addition of radiotherapy to surgery is standard palliative management for patients with high-grade gliomas. The degree of benefit varies between different prognostic groups; it is typically modest and measured in months. Several studies have demonstrated a dose response to radiation, with improved median survival when fractionated doses of around 60 Gy in 30 daily fractions are given compared to lower doses in the 45 Gy range. No convincing further improvement is apparent when doses are increased above 60 Gy, using either external beam or brachytherapy boost doses. This may be because a potential increase in tumour control is obscured by an increase in early radiation toxicity or because high doses given to a

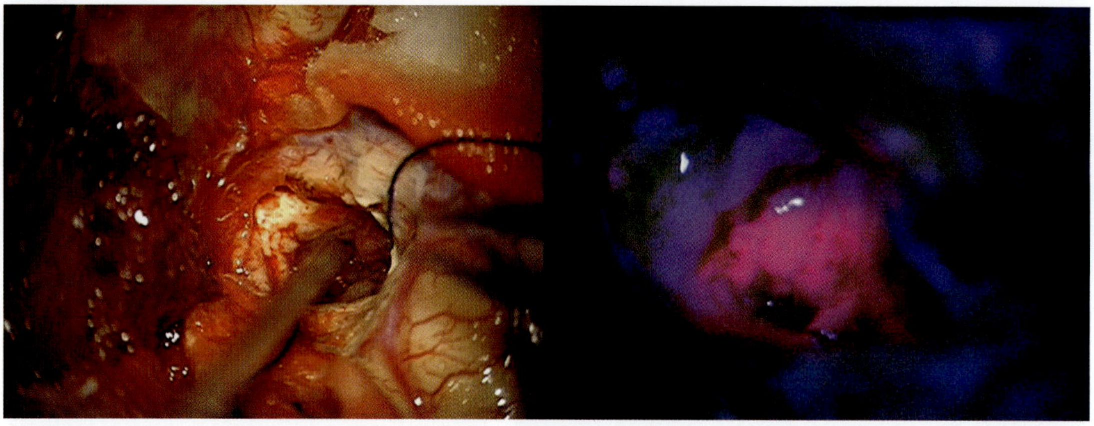

Figure 21.23 Intraoperative appearance of glioblastoma multiforme (GBM) in white light and UV light with patient preloaded with 5-aminolaevulinic acid showing 'burning embers' of pink viable tumour cells, not visible in white light.

very localised field do not encompass the whole area at risk for recurrence. For patients in the best prognostic groups with WHO Grade IV gliomas (i.e. those with little deficit), addition of radiotherapy improves survival by 5–6 months but only to a median figure of 9–12 months. In patients with lower than median expected survival, the impact of radiotherapy is even more modest and may be only a matter of weeks. Overall, functional deficit improves in one-third of patients and stabilises the situation, if briefly, in half. In the poorest prognostic groups an alternative approach using shortened course, high-dose palliative radiotherapy regimes is sometimes advocated on the basis that this impinges less on quality of life in the remaining months. When discussing relative risks and benefits of radiotherapy, it is important to take into consideration the limited symptomatic improvement that can be anticipated, the rarity of a prolonged response and the lethargy, hair loss and risks of neurological deterioration resulting from radiation. Very occasionally, radiosurgery (highly focused radiotherapy) using either linear accelerator or gamma knife machines are used for small nodular recurrences.

Chemoradiation

In GBM, temozolomide chemotherapy given concurrently with radiotherapy and then adjuvantly for a further 6 months has been shown to increase survival when compared with radiotherapy alone. High quality trial data now support the use of daily low-dose temozolomide (75 mg/m^2) throughout a 6-week course of radiotherapy followed by monthly 5-day courses (150–200 mg/m^2) for 6 months. Overall median survival, although modest, increased from 12.1 to 14.6 months; however, 2-year survival increased from 10% to 26% and 5-year survival from 2% to 10%. The addition of chemotherapy produced some increased toxicity, although mild with no measurable impact on quality of life. An important issue was a high incidence of *Pneumocystis carinii* pneumonia during concomitant treatment necessitating prophylaxis with co-trimoxazole or pentamidine. This regime has rapidly become standard treatment for good performance patients with GBM who are considered to be able to tolerate combined treatment. The benefits occur in all clinical prognostic subgroups, including patients aged 60–70 years, with methylation of the MGMT promoter the strongest predictor for outcome and additional survival from the additional temozolomide chemotherapy.

Grade III tumours have a better prognosis than WHO Grade IV and therefore may experience late-delayed toxicity from combined chemo-radiation that offsets any potential survival benefits. A trial (BR14) is currently underway to assess whether chemoradiation with either concomitant temozolomide, adjuvant temozolomide or both are superior to radiation alone in anaplastic gliomas without the 1p19q deletion, typically seen in anaplastic oligodendrogliomas (which carry a much better prognosis irrespective of treatment modality and timing of chemotherapy). An additional question is whether molecular analysis will enable identification of patients with glioma who are more likely to respond to temozolomide. The mechanism of cytotoxicity of temozolomide relies on DNA base damage that can be repaired by a specific enzyme, O^6-methylguanine-DNA methyltransferase (MGMT). MGMT is responsible for removal of O^6-alkylguanine from DNA induced by alkylating mutagens/carcinogens. Levels of MGMT within tumour cells vary between patients with GBM and depend on whether the MGMT promoter sequence is methylated (and therefore inactivated). Data suggest that patients with high levels of MGMT repair enzymes are unlikely to benefit from the addition of temozolomide chemotherapy. Molecular and chromosomal analysis of all high-grade gliomas is likely to become a standard part of management.

Chemotherapy

The place of chemotherapy in first line treatment of high-grade gliomas has been assessed in many studies since the 1960s. These have included regimes in which chemotherapy is administered adjuvantly (following surgery and radiotherapy) or neoadjuvantly (prior to radiotherapy). Few have demonstrated a significant benefit in terms of survival compared with surgery and radiotherapy alone. The MRC Glioma Meta-analysis Group concluded that adjuvant chemotherapy given at or around the time of surgery and radiotherapy had a marginal benefit of 6% absolute improved survival at 1 year. The chemotherapy regimes were most commonly procarbazine, CCNU (lomustine) with vincristine (PCV), the most active combination of traditional chemotherapy in this disease. Common UK practice, prior to temozolamide, was to give chemotherapy at first relapse rather than around the time of initial radiotherapy.

Relapsed high-grade gliomas

Chemotherapy was until recently used almost exclusively in the United Kingdom at the time of relapse of high-grade gliomas. The standard approach in the United Kingdom has been the PCV combination regime in 6-weekly cycles. Response rates, meaning here temporary symptomatic benefit, are 20–30%. A recent trial has shown that PCV is equivalent in efficacy and tolerability to temozolomide. Radiological improvement and clinical response are associated with increased time to further progression. However, there are no data that suggest significant improvement in overall survival for the majority of patients. Toxicities from this regime include bone marrow suppression, liver function test abnormalities, neuropathy, skin rash and gastrointestinal upset. In most patients the regime is well tolerated; if it is not, it is rarely appropriate to continue in view of the poor response rates. Optimal chemotherapy for patients who have previously received adjuvant treatment with temozolomide is also not resolved. This situation is difficult because of the relative paucity of agents with well-documented response rates in this situation. An alternative approach if the recurrence is operable is to debulk and insert carmustine (Gliadel) wafers into the resection cavity. This tends to avoid systemic side effects but may cause cerebral oedema and poor wound healing. Other potentially useful agents include carboplatin and taxol. Novel agents are being assessed, including antiangiogenic agents. The most interesting agent, bevacizumab (Avastin), has now been tested in two randomised controlled trials in newly diagnosed GBM and has shown a modest improvement in progression-free survival but not overall survival. Because of its antiangiogenic properties, it produces dramatic radiological responses with reduction in contrast enhancement and oedema and reduces steroid requirements, but does not prevent tumour cell migration and infiltration (Figure 21.7).

Anaplastic oligodendrogliomas

Anaplastic oligodendrogliomas are known to have a better prognosis than other high-grade gliomas. There is clear evidence for an association between deletion of chromosomes 1p and 19q and response to either chemotherapy or radiotherapy. Because many older studies did not distinguish this subgroup, these treatment-sensitive patients were probably an important source of heterogeneity in randomised trials. Current data suggest that response rates to nitrosurea-based chemotherapy in anaplastic oligodendrogliomas are 60–70%. This is compared to figures of 20–30% for other high-grade gliomas and reflects the fact that about 70% of anaplastic oligodendrogliomas have loss of heterozygosity (LOH) at chromosomes 1p/19q associated with 100% chemosensitivity. The exact relationship between these chromosomal losses and the mechanisms underlying the chemo-sensitivity is unclear. Despite this, large clinical studies were not able initially to demonstrate a survival benefit for either neoadjuvant or adjuvant chemotherapy in this patient group when compared with patients given their first chemotherapy at relapse. A more recent review of long-term follow-up data looking at patients with anaplastic oligodendrogliomas and oligoastrocytomas have now shown a survival benefit after 12 years but only in patients with co-deletion of 1p and 19q chromosomes treated with adjuvant PCV chemotherapy after radiotherapy compared with radiotherapy alone. However, the toxicity of PCV is not to be underestimated and only 30% of patients managed to complete the six cycles of adjuvant chemotherapy as originally prescribed. Current practice for anaplastic oligodendroglioma is therefore to assess chromosome loss as a prognostic rather than a predictive factor. Based on these data, there is now more enthusiasm for adjuvant PCV in 1p19q deleted anaplastic oligodendrogliomas for patients fit enough to tolerate this extra treatment.

Low-grade gliomas

Low-grade gliomas are a heterogeneous group of slow-growing primary brain tumours (WHO Grades I and II) and account for 15– 20–30% of all gliomas. They occur in both children and adults, with a peak incidence in the second and third decades of life. The most common low-grade gliomas are pilocytic astrocytomas (WHO Grade I) and diffuse astrocytomas/oligodendrogliomas and oligoastrocytomas (WHO Grade II). Pilocytic astrocyomas are mostly seen in children and young adults, and are associated with a 90% cure rate with surgery and/or radiotherapy. In contrast, Grade II gliomas are less histologically stable than Grade I tumours, with the majority transforming to higher grades over time. Median survival varies according to histology – the prognosis for WHO Grade I tumours is so good that median survival is never reached while for WHO Grade II tumours, it varies from 5–7 years for astrocytic tumours to 10–15 years for oligodendroglial tumours.

Pathology

Pilocytic astrocytoma

Pilocytic astrocytomas are composed of bipolar cells with long hairlike GFAP-positive processes, leading to the term pilocytic. Some pilocytic astrocytomas may be more fibrillary and dense in composition. Rosenthal fibres, eosinophilic granular bodies and microcysts are often present. Myxoid foci and oligodendroglioma-like cells may also be present, though non-specific. Long-standing lesions may show haemosiderin-laden macrophages and calcifications.

Molecular genetics The *KIAA:BRAF* fusion in pilocytic astrocytomas has been detected across all age groups and in various tumour locations, including cerebellum, cerebral hemispheres, hypothalamus, optic nerve and brainstem. *BRAF* duplication/fusion is more frequently present in cerebellar pilocytic astrocytomas. It is a very rare event in diffusely infiltrating gliomas, which may rarely contain *BRAF* point mutations.

Diffuse astrocytoma

Diffuse astrocytomas (WHO Grade II) tend to develop within the cerebral hemispheres, especially in the frontal and temporal lobes. These account for 10–15% of all gliomas and occur predominantly in adults. This tumour is further subdivided into fibrillary, gemistocytic (i.e. large swollen cytoplasm) and the very rare protoplasmic variant. They are slowly growing tumours that typically affect young adults and have an intrinsic tendency to progress into higher grades (WHO Grades III and IV). This process, known as malignant transformation, distinguishes WHO Grade II tumours from WHO Grade I tumours with more stable histology and a considerably better prognosis.

The characteristic morphology of the cells of WHO Grade II astrocytomas resembles well-differentiated astrocytes, embedded in a fibrillary or microcystic matrix. Mitotic activity is rarely present and there is no microvascular proliferation or necrosis. The gemistocytic astrocytoma is a more aggressive subtype and is particularly prone to progress to high-grade glioma.

Molecular genetics of diffuse and anaplastic astrocytomas Molecular classification of low-grade gliomas is increasing in importance, mainly because the histological diagnosis of diffuse gliomas can be difficult in a substantial number of cases, with marked interobserver variability. Diffuse astrocytomas show mutations at the codon 132 in the isocitrate dehydrogenase 1 (*IDH1*) genes, primarily of the *IDH1R132H* type, and less commonly in the *IDH2* gene.

These mutations occur early, with a high frequency, in WHO Grade II and III astrocytic and oligodendroglial tumours and in secondary GBMs, which develop from astrocytomas. *IDH* mutations in gliomas are early, if not initiating events in their pathogenesis, and are associated with several clinically relevant parameters including patient age, histopathological diagnosis, combined 1p/19q deletion, TP53 mutation, MGMT promoter hypermethylation and patient survival. Another useful biomarker is ATRX (alpha-thalassemia/mental retardation syndrome X-linked), which when lost can aid in the refinement of the diagnosis of IDH mutant astrocytomas, and may be used to delineate these tumours from oligoastrocytomas and oligodendrogliomas. ATRX loss and IDH mutant anaplastic astrocytomas have a favourable prognosis compared to anaplastic astrocytomas with *IDH* mutation only. Overall, the integration of genomic data has delineated three molecular classes of LGG: those with *IDH* mutation and either 1p/19q codeletion (best prognosis); those with IDH mutation and *TP53* mutation (intermediate prognosis); and those with an *IDH* mutation that had the worst prognosis as they were molecularly and clinically similar to glioblastoma.

Oligodendroglioma

Oligodendrogliomas (WHO Grades II and III) are diffusely infiltrating neoplasms found almost exclusively in the cerebral hemispheres, most commonly in the frontal lobes and typically involving subcortical white matter and cortex. Despite their name, their origin from oligodendrocytes or their precursors has not been proven. They comprise a continuous spectrum ranging from well-differentiated tumours to highly malignant neoplasms. The WHO grading system distinguishes two malignancy grades. Grade II oligodendrogliomas are slowly growing, well-defined hemispheric tumours composed of rounded homogeneous nuclei. Paraffin embedding results in a reproducible artefact, the formation of clear cytoplasm around the nuclear giving rise to a perinuclear halo, often referred to as fried egg or honeycomb cells. Further typical features are branching capillaries and calcification. Grade III oligodendrogliomas show increased tumour cell density, mitotic activity, presence of microvascular proliferation and necrosis. These are graded WHO Grade III rather than Grade IV.

Molecular genetics of oligodendroglioma Oligodendrogliomas carry *IDH1* or *IDH2* mutations, and are characterised by the codeletion of chromosomal arms 1p/19q, in the past often also referred to as combined loss of chromosomal arms (LOH). 1p19q codeletions are frequent in oligodendrogliomas (50–70%), less common in oligoastrocytomas (30–50%) and rare in astrocytomas (0–15%). Numerous studies on this genotype–phenotype correlation have subsequently shown that 1p/19q co-deletion is related to survival. This improved prognosis (and response to radiotherapy and chemotherapy) is present whether observed at initial diagnosis or at recurrence. Oligodendrogliomas with 1p/19q co-deletion also tend to progress more slowly at recurrence. *TP53* mutations are the most frequent in astrocytomas (50–90%) and oligoastrocytomas (40–50%) but are uncommon in oligodendrogliomas (5–10%).

Oligoastrocytoma

Some gliomas have intermixtures of astrocytic and oligodendroglial cellular elements and are appropriately called oligoastrocytomas or mixed gliomas. Like astrocytomas and oligodendrogliomas, they have a propensity to transform into high-grade gliomas. However, this entity, based on morpohological assessment, is likely to be phased out, as the combination of the *IDH* mutation with ATRX loss defines astrocytomas, and the combined *IDH* mutation and 1p/19q co-deletion defines oligodendrogliomas (i.e. ATRX loss and 1p/19q co-deletion are almost always mutually exclusive).

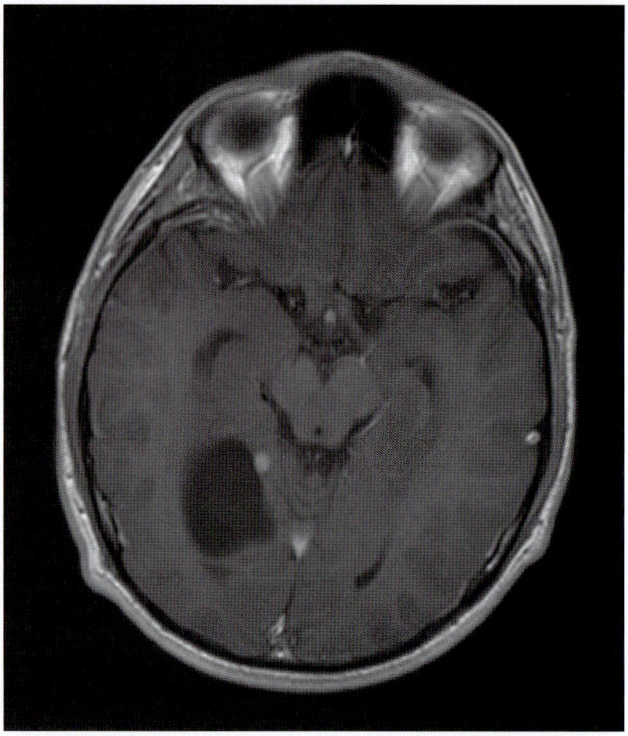

Figure 21.24 Pilocytic astrocytoma. Contrast-enhanced T1 image of an adult patient with a pilocytic astrocytoma showing a cystic lesion with a small enhancing mural nodule anteromedially.

Imaging

Pilocytic astrocytoma

Pilocytic astrocytomas (WHO Grade I) have a predilection for the cerebellum and midline structures such as the hypothalamus, thalamus, optic chiasm and brainstem. Optic pathway gliomas (OPG) are seen commonly in neurofibromatosis type 1 (NF1). In adults they may be also found in the cerebral hemispheres. They usually have a significant cystic component and show mural enhancement which can be nodular or ring-like (Figure 21.24). Infratentorial pilocytic astrocytomas in adults may be mistaken for haemangioblastomas.

Diffuse astrocytoma

Diffuse astrocytomas (WHO Grade II) typically occur in the cerebral hemispheres of young adults, involve cortex and white matter and have less well-defined borders than pilocytic astrocytomas. Mass effect is variable and contrast enhancement usually absent. They appear isodense or hypodense on CT which shows areas of calcification in up to 20%. On MRI, diffuse astrocytomas are hypointense or isointense on T1 images and hyperintense on T2 and FLAIR images, which provide the best contrast between tumour and normal brain tissue. WHO Grade II astrocytomas show a low mitotic activity but have a propensity to progress to a higher histological grade, as suggested by the development of new gadolinium enhancement (Figure 21.25).

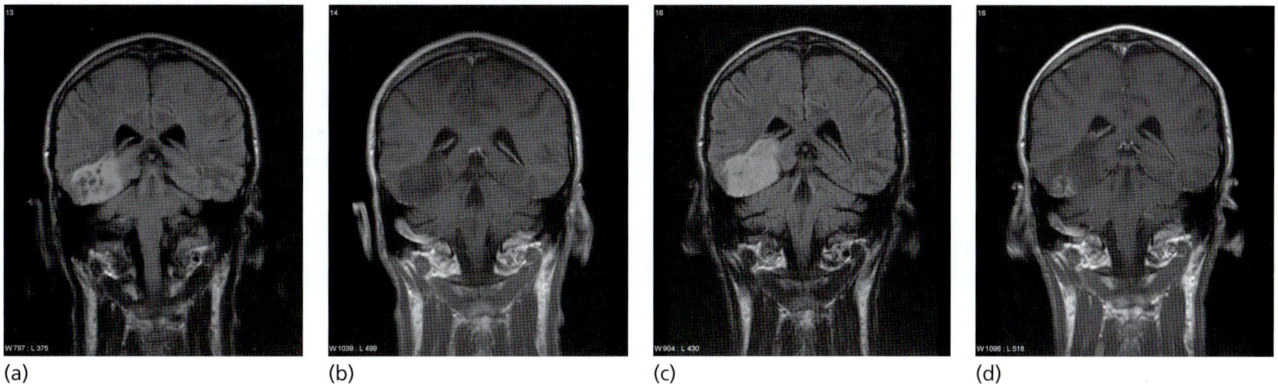

Figure 21.25 (a) Coronal FLAIR image of a WHO Grade II astrocytoma presenting as well-demarcated hyperintense temporal lobe mass containing small cysts. (b) Corresponding contrast-enhanced T1 image does not demonstrate any pathological enhancement. (c) 12 months' follow-up FLAIR image demonstrates tumour enlargement with disappearance of cystic elements. (d) 12 months' follow-up contrast-enhanced T1 image: pathological enhancement at the inferior aspect of tumour. Repeat biopsy confirmed progression to WHO Grade III astrocytoma.

Oligodendroglioma

Up to 90% of oligodendrogliomas contain calcification visible on CT, central, peripheral or ribbon-like. Both low and high-grade oligodendroglial tumours express pro-angiogenic mitogens and may contain regions of increased vascular density with finely branching capillaries which have a chickenwire appearance seen as contrast enhancement on MRI and increased rCBV on PWI. However, contrast enhancement is variable and often heterogeneous. It is a much less reliable indicator of tumour grade than in astrocytic tumours. Oligodendrogliomas with intact 1p/19q tend to have a more homogeneous signal on T1 and T2 images with sharper borders than tumours with 1p/19q co-deletions.

Surgery for low-grade gliomas

Pilocytic astrocytoma

Maximal resective surgery (with minimal morbidity) is the mainstay of treatment and results in a greater than 90% 10-year survival. The choice between focal radiotherapy and chemotherapy depends upon the age of the patient and consequent risk of radiation-induced cognitive deficits. Chemotherapy is now preferred up to the age of 8; previously the cut-off was up to 3 years.

Optic pathway gliomas in NF1 follow a very indolent course. Surveillance is preferred for these cases, with surgery and radiotherapy or chemotherapy reserved for progression with symptomatic visual impairment. These children with NF1 have a higher risk of long-term effects of radiation, especially vasculopathy and second tumours, so radiation is avoided where possible.

Diffuse astrocytoma and oligodendroglioma

In adults, the optimal management of diffuse astrocytomas and oligodendrogliomas is uncertain. The typical patient is a young adult presenting with seizures without neurological deficit or raised intracranial pressure. Management is difficult because of the tremendous variability in natural history of these tumours. Although morphologically and radiologically indistinguishable at diagnosis, some low-grade gliomas transform within a few months while others remain low-grade for several years. Radiologically, a high-grade glioma may present as a low-grade glioma and so early tissue diagnosis should be obtained if there is any suspicion that the tumour may be higher-grade (e.g. tumour growth within 3 months), the presence of contrast enhancement, presentation in an older (>40 years) patient, or with neurological deficits or raised intracranial pressure.

The timing of neurosurgical intervention, either in the form of image-directed biopsy or tumour resection, depends on many factors. However, with technical advances in pre-operative structural and functional imaging, there is a trend towards earlier and more extensive tumour resection, particularly as research has shown that all low-grade gliomas grow steadily and that the vast majority transform into high-grade gliomas at some point in their natural history. A recent study comparing outcomes between two Norwegian university hospitals with different treatment philosophies suggests that early resection is associated with significantly improved survival rates compared with watch-and-wait. Five year survival was 60% in the watch-and-wait group compared with 74% in the surgical group. This difference increased to 24% at 7 years. Importantly, there were no significant differences in surgical complications between the two hospitals or acquired neurological deficits. These data suggest that all patients with low-grade gliomas should be thoroughly evaluated after radiological diagnosis with additional physiological sequences and functional imaging to consider whether the surgical option is feasible. Following this, a thorough discussion with a surgeon who has experience in low-grade glioma surgery, including awake craniotomy, should be the standard of care.

Many tumours can be resected via a standard craniotomy performed under general anaesthesia. Awake craniotomy is advocated for tumours that are located in eloquent cortex or adjacent subcortical white matter. Management of low-grade gliomas is therefore best carried out in centres that support awake craniotomies and cortical mapping. A battery of diagnostic tests can be performed pre-operatively to aid in characterising the relationship of tumour to eloquent cortex. MRI is helpful in defining the anatomical sulcal and gyral patterns correlating tumour location to motor, sensory and speech cortex. In addition, MRA may be helpful in defining critical vascular structures surrounding and often involving tumour boundaries. fMRI provides more accurate localisation of motor and sensory cortex in addition to expressive speech centres, with receptive speech or comprehension being less accurately identified (Figure 21.11). DTI can identify white matter tracts adjacent to or infiltrated by tumour, which can help planning surgery pre-operatively. Neuropsychological testing is used to establish dominance for speech and memory, in addition whether any functional compromise has occurred from mass effect or infiltration by tumour into the mesial temporal structures.

Information gathered from pre-operative diagnostic tests is combined with data obtained during intra-operative neurophysiological testing to identify areas of critical function, the area of pathology and safe corridors of entry into the cortex. Therefore the surgeon is given greater confidence, because great variability exists in the morphology of cortical structures and their landmarks, and recognition of sulcal and gyral patterns intra-operatively is rarely straightforward. During cortical stimulation, the patient is asked to perform tasks testing motor and sensory function. Language testing is more accurately carried out using specific language paradigms and visual cards than counting or naming of objects, days or the alphabet. If the patient is under general anaesthesia, although the extent of cortical mapping will not be to the same accuracy as in awake craniotomy, somatosensory evoked potentials can be used to identify motor and/or sensory cortex. Patient preference, the surgeon's considered view and experience, availability of pre-operative and intra-operative tests along with a skilled neuro-anaesthesia team are key factors for performing awake craniotomies.

In any event, fewer than 30% of adult low-grade gliomas are truly resectable in their entirety either because of location or diffuse infiltration. Partial resections provide tissue for histological diagnosis and prognostication but have not been shown to be of prognostic benefit. Many patients are therefore treated with antiepileptic drugs and remain well for many years. This group is monitored closely with imaging surveillance, usually at 6-month intervals. Treatment at progression may include biopsy and radiotherapy/chemotherapy or partial resection particularly where there is mass effect.

Radiotherapy for low-grade gliomas

The role of radiotherapy early in the course of disease is still not clear. Several trials have examined dose–response and timing of radiotherapy for WHO Grade II gliomas. WHO Grade I tumours are rarely treated with radiotherapy. Contrary to the situation in high-grade gliomas, there is little evidence with WHO Grade II tumours for a dose response beyond 50 Gy. The timing of radiotherapy for these patients has also been contentious. Some centres have advocated early postoperative radiotherapy on the basis that it is likely to be radio-biologically most effective when tumour volume is small and that the incidence of malignant transformation will be reduced. Others have felt that the long natural history of the disease means that such early intervention is unwarranted. This issue has been addressed in a randomised trial. The results suggest that while time to progression is improved from 3.4 to 4.8 years in the treated group, early irradiation to 54 Gy does not improve overall survival. Thus, many oncologists advocate early treatment only for those patients at highest risk of progression, such as those with tumours in eloquent areas or for whom surveillance is inappropriate.

Radiotherapy is also used in patients with intractable seizures in the absence of tumour progression. In about 75% seizures improve. In a trial comparing radiotherapy with no radiotherapy in low-grade gliomas with seizures, 25% of patients who had been irradiated had had seizures at 1 year, compared to nearly 50% who had not been irradiated.

Chemotherapy for low-grade gliomas

The role of chemotherapy in adult low-grade gliomas has also not yet been fully established, and is usually reserved for large tumours requiring extensive radiation fields. However, both low and high-grade oligodendrogliomas are more chemo- and radiosensitive than astrocytomas, attributed to a specific chromosomal loss of both 1p and 19q.

Two small prospective Phase II trials have shown radiological and clinical response to single agent temozolomide chemotherapy. Although the objective response rates were quite different between the two trials (10% in the British compared with 47% in the Italian trial), the tumour regression rates were almost identical (57% and 56%, respectively) when minor responses were also considered. A recently published North American trial has shown a highly significant survival advantage of 5 years with the addition of PCV chemotherapy to radiotherapy in patients with low-grade gliomas, particularly in oligodendrogliomas and tumours with IDH mutations. On this basis, adjuvant chemotherapy should become the standard of care for LGG patients treated with radiotherapy.

An international multi-centre trial comparing chemotherapy with temozolomide against radiotherapy for patients with low-grade gliomas, stratified for chromosomal 1p loss. Preliminary results suggest that radiotherapy is superior to chemotherapy.

Other low-grade tumours in childhood

There are a number of other rarer tumours in childhood that often present with seizures and behave in a benign fashion. They are usually treated with surgery alone. The likelihood of recurrence is highly dependent on the amount of residual tumuor.

Tumours of predominantly neuronal cell origin

Gangioglioma and gangliocytoma

Gangiogliomas and gangliocytomas (WHO Grade I) are slow-growing tumours that grow preferentially within the temporal lobes of children and young adults. CT and MRI show peripherally located mixed solid and/or cystic lesions that commonly calcify. Enhancement is variable and often peripheral.

Central neurocytoma

Central neurocytomas (WHO Grade II) occur predominantly in the second and third decades of life and are the most common masses within the lateral ventricles in this age group. They typically arise from the septum pellucidum and occupy the frontal horns and bodies of the ventricles and sometimes extend through the foramen of Monro. Obstructive hydrocephalus is common. CT frequently demonstrates calcification and small cysts. MRI shows a heterogeneously enhancing mass with septated cysts and isointense grey matter nodules with susceptibility artefact from calcification. These tumours also show restricted water diffusion (Figure 21.26).

Dysembryoplastic neuroepithelial tumour

Dysembryoplastic neuroepithelial tumours (DNET) are WHO Grade I and usually located in the cerebral cortex. On CT, DNET are usually hypodense. On MRI they are T1-hypointense and T2-hyperintense. Small intra-tumoural cysts may cause a bubbly appearance; calcification is seen in about 25% and enhancement is uncommon. Thinning of the overlying bone is present in approximately half of the cases, reflecting the extremely slow growth of these tumours which allows bone remodelling to occur (Figure 21.27).

Molecular genetics of low-grade glioneuronal tumours A range of low-grade glial and glioneuronal tumours, many clinically presenting

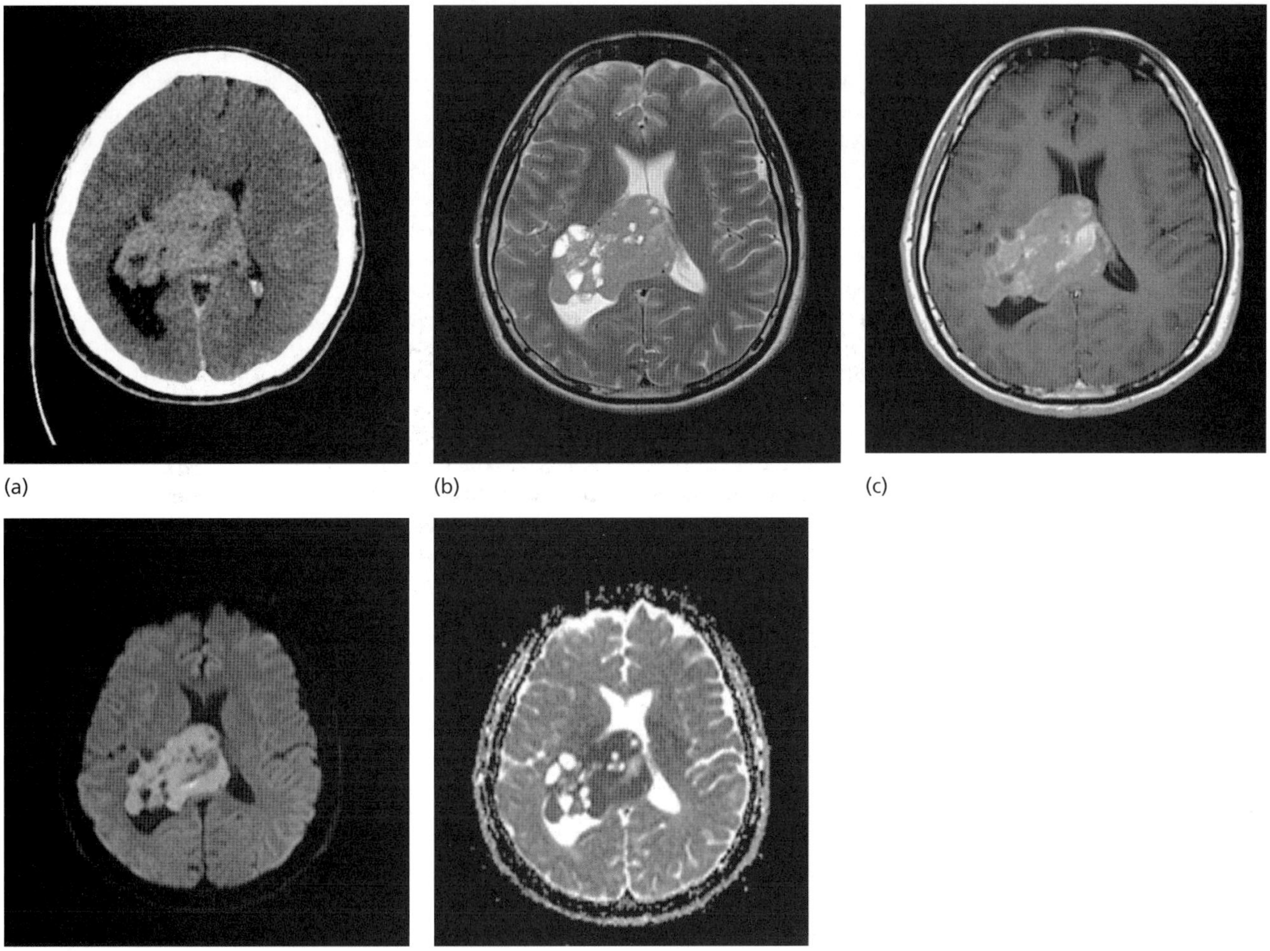

(a) (b) (c) (d) (e)

Figure 21.26 Central neurocytoma. (a) Unenhanced CT shows a hyperdense intraventricular mass containing small cysts. (b) It has a relatively low signal intensity on T2-weighted images and enhances with intravenous gadolinium (c). The solid tumour parts appear bright on DWI images (d) and dark on the ADC map (e), which indicates restricted water diffusion in a highly cellular tumour.

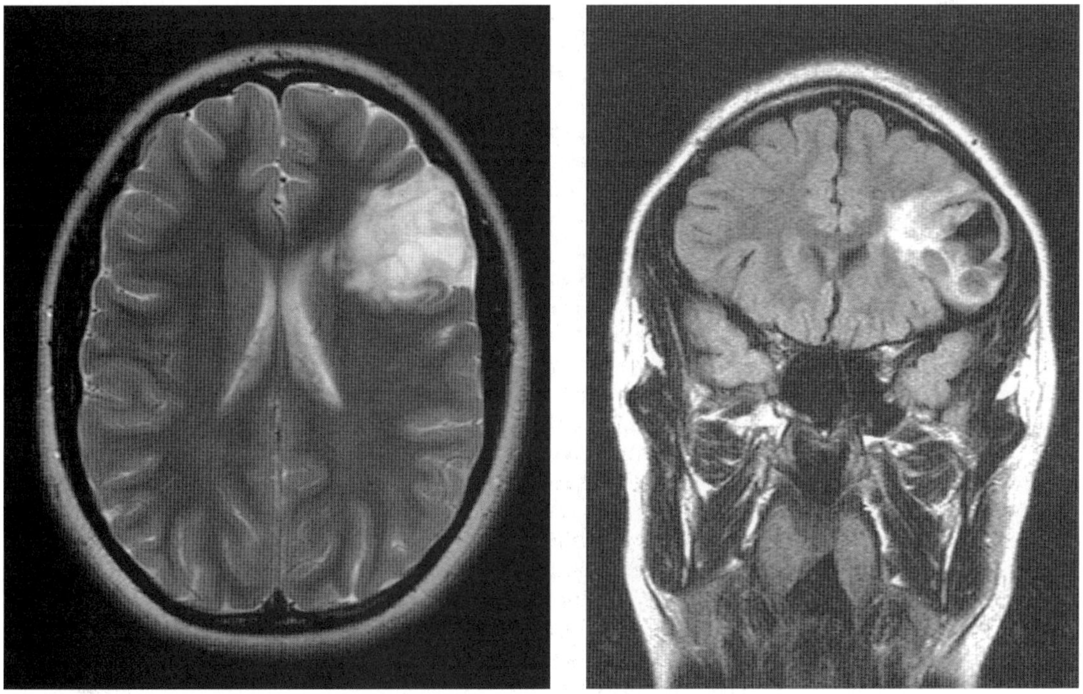

(a) (b)

Figure 21.27 Left frontal dysembryoplastic neuroepithelial tumour (DNET). (a) T2 image of left frontal hyperintense mass that proved to be a DNET. (b) Coronal FLAIR image shows cystic components within DNET giving rise to the classical 'soapbubble appearance'.

with long-standing epilepsy in children and adults have been identified as *BRAF V600E* mutant. The mutation is most commonly seen in PXA and the anaplastic form of PXA (65%), followed by gangliogliomas (25%) and DNETs (30%). It is occasionally seen in desmoplastic infantile ganglioglioma/astrocytoma (16%) and rarely pilocytic astrocytomas (10% or less). The prognostic value of the *BRAF V600E* mutation is less well established than that of *IDH* mutations in astrocytomas and oligodendrogliomas

Choroid plexus tumours

Choroid plexus tumours are either papillomas or carcinomas, papillomas being much more common than carcinomas. The location and incidence of choroid plexus papillomas varies with age. They are more common in childhood, presenting as a cauliflower-like mass in the trigone of the lateral ventricle. In adults, papillomas occur predominantly in the 4th ventricle. CT shows an isodense to hyperdense mass with punctate calcification and homogeneous enhancement. On MRI, the papillomas appear as lobulated, intraventricular masses of heterogeneous, predominantly intermediate signal intensity on T1 and T2 images with intense contrast enhancement.

Meningiomas

Pathology

Meningiomas are common extra-axial intracranial tumours that grow slowly, are well demarcated and usually do not infiltrate the brain. They originate from meningothelial cells which are most abundant in the arachnoid villi and occasionally from the craniospinal arachnoid. They are most common in elderly patients with a peak in the sixth and seventh decade, with a slight predominance for female gender. The most common meningioma types are meningothelial, fibrous/fibroblastic, transitional and psammomatous (abundant whorls with calcifications), and more than 10 additional variants are listed in the WHO classification. Most of them correspond to WHO Grade I and behave similarly. Atypical features in meningioma are increased mitotic activity (greater than 4 mitoses per 10 high-powered field [HPF]), patternless growth and necrosis corresponding to WHO Grade II (atypical) or WHO Grade III (anaplastic meningioma), when there are greater than 20 mitoses per 10 HPF. The higher grade meningiomas have a propensity for recurrence, as one might expect. In rare cases they behave almost as aggressively as malignant gliomas.

Imaging

Meningiomas (WHO Grades I–III) can be spherical and well-circumscribed, craggy and irregular or flat, infiltrating en plaque lesions. They arise within the parasagittal area, convexities, sphenoid wing, tuberculum sellae, olfactory groove, tentorium and foramen magnum. Spinal meningiomas usually arise dorsally in the thoracic spine and almost exclusively in women. On CT, 60% of meningiomas are hyperdense without contrast and some 20% contain calcification. Hyperostosis, best seen on bone window settings indicates the site of the tumour attachment to the meninges. On MRI, meningiomas frequently appear isointense to cerebral cortex on both T1 and T2 images and may occasionally be difficult to detect without IV contrast. They can have capping cysts of CSF signal intensity. Associated vasogenic oedema is not infrequent and often disproportionate to tumour size.

Meningiomas enhance vividly and usually homogeneously on MRI. Linear enhancement can extend along the adjacent dura mater (Figure 21.5). This sign, known as the dural tail, was once thought to be pathognomonic for meningioma but can also be seen with other tumours such as schwannomas or even metastases. MRS may show an alanine peak, characteristic for meningioma though seen in less than 50% of cases. PWI of meningiomas shows typically a markedly elevated rCBV, which can be of help in differentiating these benign tumours from dural metastases which tend to have a lower rCBV. PET CT using a somatostatin analogue can help differentiate meningiomas from other extra-axial masses, because of the high density of somatostatin receptors in meningiomas (Figure 21.28).

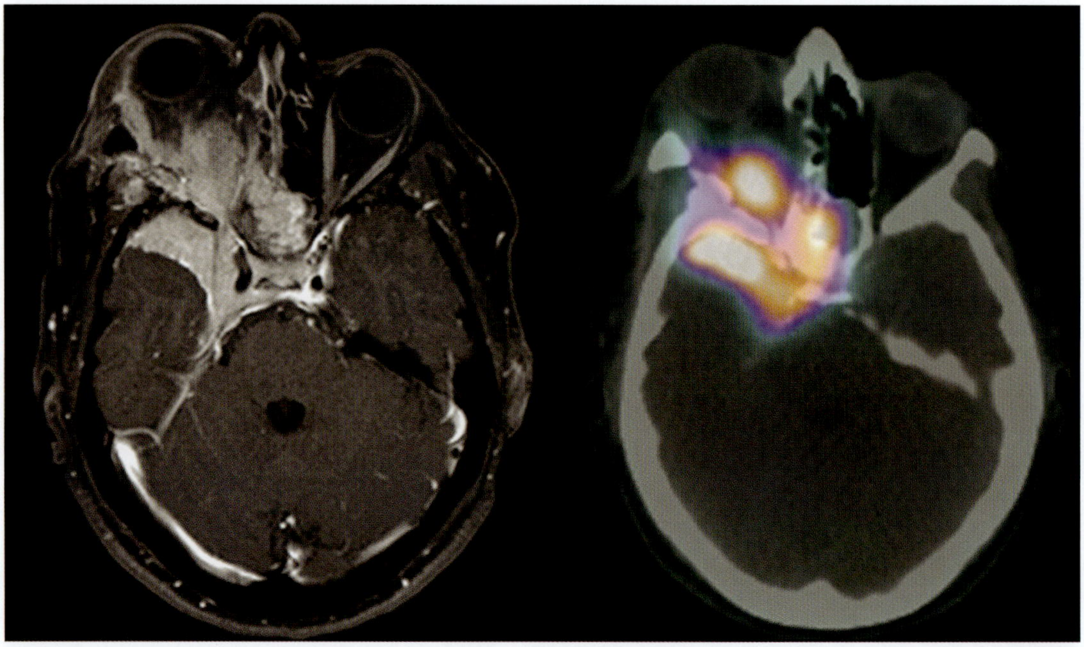

Figure 21.28 Meningioma. Contrast-enhanced fat-saturated T1-weighted axial MRI (a) show a right sphenoid wing meningioma extending into the cavernous sinus and orbit. (b) PET CT using the somatostatin analogue 68Ga-DOTATOC shows high uptake of the tracer in the enhancing extra-axial tumour.

Surgery

The majority of meningiomas are benign, with recurrence rates frequently less than 10% after total excision. Radical surgery remains the mainstay of treatment. Pre-operative embolisation in very vascular meningiomas is sometimes advocated to reduce peri-operative blood loss. A minority of meningiomas present management problems if they cannot be fully excised or if there are aggressive histological features. Various characteristics of meningiomas have been used to predict tumour recurrunce, such as anatomical location, extent of tumour resection and histopathological features, with the single most important prognostic factor being the completeness of surgical resection. Simpson introduced a classification system that predicts recurrence rates based on extent of tumour resection (Table 21.3). Tumour histology is also an important factor in predicting recurrence, if the tumour exhibits anaplastic and malignant features (WHO Grade II–III), the rate of recurrence is significantly higher, with 3% recurrence predicted for benign meningiomas, 40% for atypical and 80% for malignant meningiomas over a 5-year period.

Radiotherapy

Several retrospective series have suggested that radiotherapy improves local control when these tumours are aggressive, but no randomised series are available. In one retrospective series of WHO Grade I meningiomas, local recurrence rates following presumed total resection and subtotal resection were 52% and 77%, respectively at 7 years median follow-up. Subtotal resection with radiotherapy achieved local control rates of 91% compared to 38% with subtotal resection alone. There was no influence on survival with adjuvant radiotherapy treatment. Although these data argue in favour of radiotherapy as adjuvant treatment after subtotal resection, they do not address its long-term side effects, particularly in younger age groups. Long-term risks include induction of a second tumour, pituitary failure and cognitive decline. Radiotherapy is therefore not offered routinely after subtotal resection of meningiomas because of these concerns. A common approach is to reserve radiotherapy for adjuvant treatment at first or subsequent relapse or in subgroups with higher risks of local relapse, including Grade II and Grade III meningiomas.

Newer radiotherapy planning techniques, such as iMRT and radiosurgery can be used to reduce the volumes of normal brain irradiated in these patients, as these tumours can often be treated with a very small margin (5–7 mm) beyond visible tumour on MRI.

Table 21.3 Simpson classification for prediction of recurrence rates for meningiomas.

Recurrence (%)	Grade	Description
10	I	Macroscopically complete removal, excision of dural attachment
20	II	Macroscopically complete removal, coagulation of dural attachment
30	III	Macroscopically complete removal, without resection or coagulation of dural attachment
40	IV	Partial removal
	V	Decompression/biopsy

However, there are no data that show the reduction in late toxicity by this approach.

Chemotherapy

There are no chemotherapy agents that are routinely used in meningiomas, not amenable to either surgery or radiotherapy (e.g. multiple or recurrent tumours). A number of drugs including hydroxyurea and mifepristone have been shown to have modest efficacy and can be tried in individual cases.

Brain metastases

Pathology

Metastases are macroscopically well demarcated. The tumour is often firm because of the growth of fibrous tissue from without; the surrounding oedematous brain is soft. Microscopically they are discrete and well demarcated in the brain; they tend to have an architecture of septa and often lymphocytic infiltrates. Diffuse infiltration can occasionally be seen in small cell carcinomas of the lung, melanoma and with lymphomas. Necrosis is a feature of many metastases. Carcinoma of the lung may be squamous, glandular or undifferentiated. Breast carcinoma metastases can reproduce architectural features of the primary lesion, with ducts, chords and cellular columns. Gastrointestinal metastases can show features of intestinal epithelium. Melanoma metastases are often haemorrhagic; they may contain melanin and can appear with a diffuse growth pattern. Most metastatic carcinomas are reactive for cytokeratins. Antibodies to thyroid transcription factor 1 can be useful in identifying metastatic lung cancer. Melanomas express S-100, HMB-45 and Melan-A.

Imaging

Brain metastases most commonly arise from carcinoma of the lung, breast, kidney and malignant melanoma. Most metastases enhance strongly with contrast media, either uniformly or they are seen as ring-like structures if the metastasis has outgrown its blood supply. Metastases are frequently associated with vasogenic oedema, often disproportionate to the size of the tumour. Haemorrhage occurs in about 10% of metastases, resulting in high signal on T1 images and low signal on T2 images. Similar signal characteristics can also occur in non-haemorrhagic metastases from melanoma, because of the paramagnetic properties of melanin. Increasing the dose or relaxivity of gadolinium compounds can improve the sensitivity for detection of metastases on MRI.

DWI may help to predict the histology of brain metastases. Small cell lung cancer metastases and neuro-endocrine metastases have a lower ADC than adenocarcinoma metastases and appear bright on DWI (Figures 21.29). PWI and MRS of the peri-tumoural rather than intra-tumoural region help to differentiate a single metastasis from a high-grade glioma. DWI is helpful in distinguishing cystic metastases from cerebral abscesses. Abscesses contain more viscous fluid and pus; they show a more marked restriction of water diffusion than necrotic tumours.

Brain metastases have traditionally been considered as terminal event, carrying a very poor prognosis, with only palliative measures appropriate. Even today, the treatment for most brain metastases is purely palliative. However, the last two decades have seen both increased early diagnosis, as improvements in systemic chemotherapy have led to more patients surviving and developing brain metastases, and the emergence of a younger, fitter population suitable for more aggressive approaches. Diagnostic imaging advances are allowing earlier, asymptomatic diagnosis.

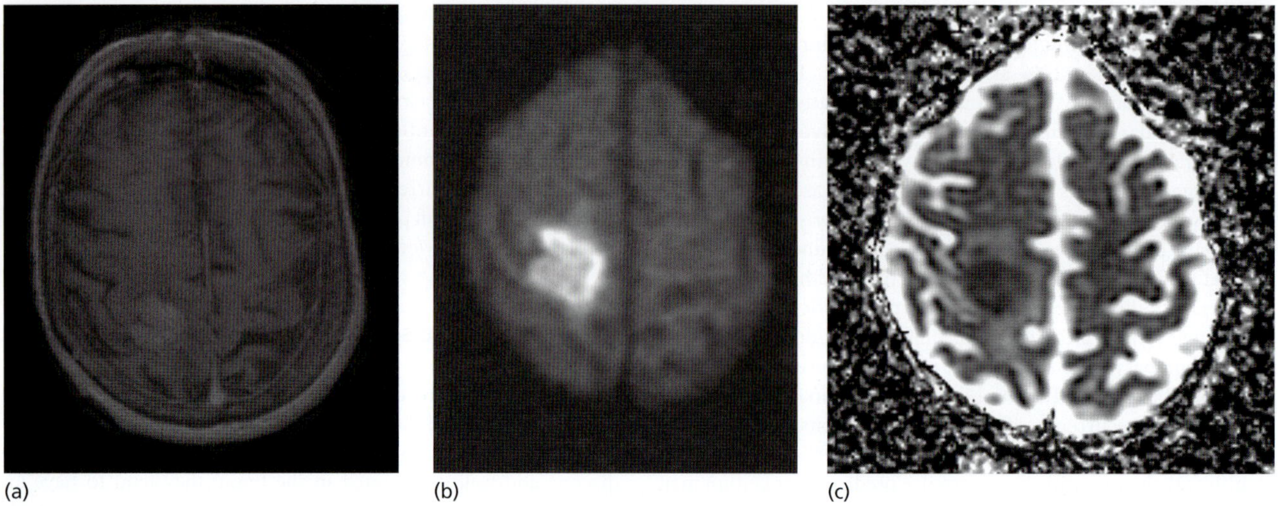

Figure 21.29 SCLC metastasis. (a) Contrast-enhanced T1 image of a right parietal metastasis from a small cell lung carcinoma. (b) Mass appears markedly hyperintense on diffusion-weighted image. (c) ADC map confirms decreased water diffusivity within the tumour (dark), consistent with a highly cellular metastasis.

As a result management options and paradigms for patients with brain metastases are evolving.

Surgery and/or radiotherapy

Brain metastases can be treated focally, by surgical excision and radiosurgery, or with the well-established standard treatment of whole-brain radiotherapy (WBRT). Chemotherapy may have a role in certain chemo-sensitive tumours, such as germ cell neoplasms and trophoblastic disease, which are rare examples in which cure may be achieved with aggressive treatment. Novel treatment paradigms should combine these various treatment modalities in order to provide the most comprehensive and tailored therapeutic option for individual patients. Management of these patients must be carefully considered in the context of their overall disease burden and prognosis. Several oncology groups have attempted to categorise these patients into prognostic groups with the aim of predicting those most likely to benefit from treatment. Clearly, these decisions depend on having accurate and up-to-date information about disease status within and outside the brain and a careful assessment of the patient's performance status.

Surgery has a role in the management of brain metastases in both diagnosis and treatment. In some patients with no previous malignant history or in whom there is diagnostic doubt, biopsy may be necessary to confirm the diagnosis even if no other surgical intervention is planned. The most difficult group in this respect are elderly patients with concurrent medical conditions and no obvious primary site. In these cases even biopsy may not be appropriate. However, caution in diagnosis is essential: about 10% of patients with suspected brain metastases harbour unsuspected histology including abscesses, inflammatory/infective lesions such as neurocysticercosis or gliomas.

Surgical resection may be used for the definitive treatment of oligometastases (one, two or three lesions) or solitary metastases unsuitable for radiosurgery, for example with significant associated oedema and mass effect, greater than 3 cm diameter and in the setting of low volume or controlled extracranial disease. Palliative debulking may be appropriate for symptomatic relief, improved quality of life and to allow tapering of steroids. Some patients may need treatment of hydrocephalus. Surgery is usually contraindicated in cases with several brain lesions, as surgical results are so poor, a reflection that many patients will die in any event from uncontrolled disease outside the brain within a few months of surgery.

Stereotactic radiosurgery with either a cobalt source (gamma knife) or linear accelerator (LINAC based) may be used as an alternative to surgery, particularly for solitary metastases in eloquent regions of the brain or oligometastases. Outcome is considered equivalent, although no head-to-head comparison with surgery has ever been carried out. Most radiotherapists limit the size of lesions to be treated to those less than 3 cm diameter because of the high radiation doses administered.

There is now a move away from routine use of adjuvant WBRT following surgery or radiosurgery as a result of randomised trial data confirming neurocognitive deficits as early as 4 months following WBRT, and no survival benefit. Previously, the standard approach was to add a short course of palliative radiotherapy (e.g. 20 Gy given in five daily fractions of 4 Gy in 1 week). The European EORTC 22952-26001 study addressed whether adjuvant WBRT increased the duration of functional independence after either surgery or radiosurgeryn good performance status patients with up to three brain metastases and with controlled extracranial disease. Although the addition of WBRT reduced both local and distant recurrence in the brain, there was no impact upon duration of functional independence or survival. It was concluded that when using regular MRI-based follow-up, salvage treatment is effective in preventing neurologic progression as a cause of death.

Radiotherapy alone to the whole brain has also been standard treatment for patients with unresectable metastatic brain lesions and/or with uncontrolled systemic disease. However, the palliative value of short course radiotherapy is dubious and it is hard to know whether improvements are a result of the radiation or concomitant use of steroids.

Chemotherapy

In all CNS malignancies the blood–brain barrier is at least a theoretical limitation to drug penetration, but the exact contribution that this makes to the poor response to chemotherapy is unclear.

A distinct minority of tumour types presenting as brain metastases are known to demonstrate clinically useful chemo-sensitivity. These metastases include small cell lung cancer (SCLC), germ cell tumours and breast cancer. Response rates up to 66% at first treatment in SCLC have been documented. Some studies have shown that breast cancer brain metastases can respond to agents used for systemic disease in over 50% of cases. Median survivals after chemotherapy are similar to those after WBRT. Therefore, chemotherapy is probably most appropriate for those who are relatively chemo-naïve, as many patients will have been exposed to multiple chemotherapy agents prior to presenting with brain metastases.

New approaches are clearly needed in the treatment of brain metastases. Combinations of conventional chemotherapy agents with molecularly targeted drugs such as gefitinib (Iressa), a tyrosine kinase inhibitor, have been shown to produce responses at primary tumour sites such as lung tumours and may help metastases. Temozolomide has also been studied alone or in combination with radiotherapy.

The use of dexamethasone to improve symptoms of raised intracranial pressure, brain oedema and focal deficits is part of standard treatment of brain metastases and brain malignancies generally. The optimal dose has not been defined but some data suggest that low-dose dexamethasone (4 mg/day) is as effective as the usual higher dose (16 mg/day) in the majority.

Primary spinal cord tumours

In comparison with brain tumours, primary spinal cord gliomas (Figure 21.30) are relatively rare and are usually astrocytomas or ependymomas, usually low-grade, affecting commonly the cervical cord or, in the case of ependymomas, the conus. Other more common primary spinal tumours are meningiomas arising from the dura, and schwannomas arising from the spinal nerve roots and lipomas, either intramedullary or extramedullary. The symptoms and signs at presentation are a combination of the effects of nerve root involvement at the level of the tumour (e.g. girdle pain), and the effects of long tract involvement at that level (e.g. paraparesis or tetraparesis). MRI is usually diagnostic.

Surgery

Radical surgery is indicated for presumed extramedullary tumours via laminectomy at the appropriate level(s). Occasionally, more extensive approaches are required (e.g. with dumb-bell schwannomas), where thoracotomy or abdominal surgery may be required. With intramedullary astrocytomas, it is sometimes possible to enter the spinal cord posteriorly in the midline, between the posterior columns, or alternatively through the dorsal root zone and removed the tumour without encroaching on functioning pathways. Tumours associated with a cyst can occasionally be dissected free from the normal structures with little morbidity, with an apparently total macroscopic removal.

Chemotherapy for intrinsic cord tumours

Overall, there are few data about the chemo-sensitivity of intrinsic cord malignancies. The literature addressing responses to chemotherapy in intracranial ependymoma suggests a low response rate to combination chemotherapy regimes and no evidence that it improves survival. Low chemo-sensitivity has been attributed to over-expression of *MDR1* (multi-drug resistance gene) in ependymoma tissue. Paediatric literature suggests a modest response to chemotherapy in high-grade spinal astrocytomas. However, these small studies do not allow firm conclusions to be drawn about responses in adult patients.

Spinal ependymomas

The most common primary spinal intramedullary tumour in adults is ependymoma, some 50–60% of such neoplasms which occurs most commonly in mid adult life. It is common for the diagnosis to be made after months or years of slowly progressing symptoms. Surgery is usually the first treatment, to make a histological

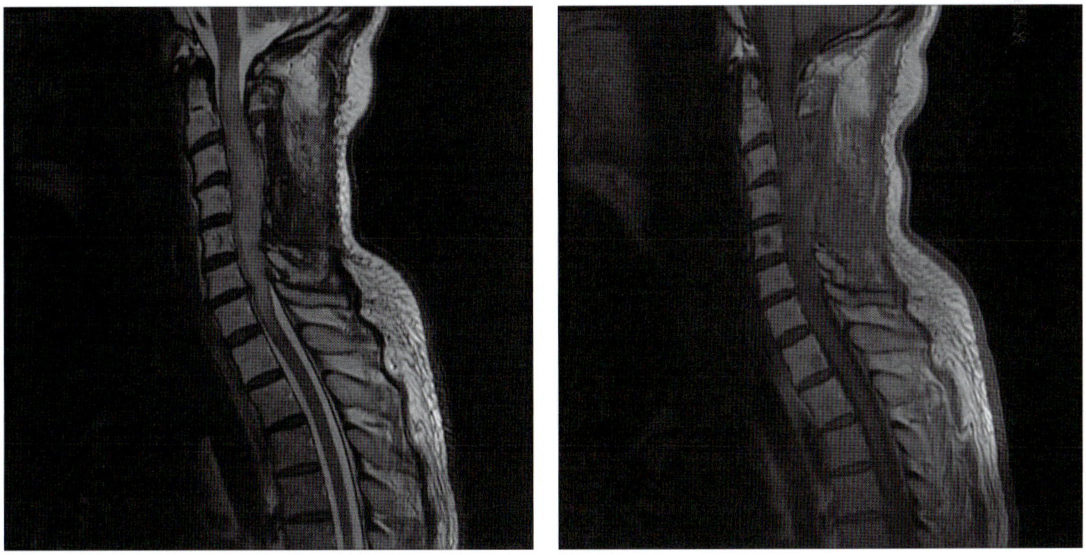

(a) (b)

Figure 21.30 Intramedullary cervical cord glioma. (a) Sagittal T2-weighted image of expansile high signal intrinsic cord lesion extending from cervicomedullary junction down to C7, occupying the whole spinal canal. An extensive laminectomy has been performed to decompress the cord. (b) Sagittal T1-weighted post gadolinium images showing faint central enhancement. A biopsy of the tumour showed an anaplastic astrocytoma.

diagnosis and attempt gross removal. A postoperative MRI at 2–3 months is often recommended to record residual disease and serve as a baseline for follow-up. In low-grade fully resected tumours, recurrence rates are low, in the region of 5–10%. However, this does not fully take in to account the problems of defining grade and extent of resection in these tumours. A recent series suggests that local relapse rates may be higher than generally appreciated at long-term follow-up: there is a significant recurrence rate beyond 5 years, with only 50% of patients progression free at 10 years. Local postoperative radiotherapy is usually recommended in all patients. There are not enough data available to be able to assess whether there is a dose response to radiation in these circumstances. Most studies reporting outcome after radiotherapy are small series that use a narrow range of doses. It is clear though that recurrences distant from the original ependymoma site are very rare, therefore extended field or cranio-spinal treatments are not recommended unless there is evidence of distant spread. The maximum radiation dose that can be administered is limited by the tolerance of the spinal cord. Current practice is to treat low-grade ependymomas to a dose of 50 Gy in 1.8 Gy fractions and higher grade tumours to 54 Gy.

Spinal astrocytomas

Primary spinal cord astrocytomas are most often low-grade fibrillary subtypes. Clinically and radiologically these tumours often present in a very similar way to ependymomas although they may be less well defined than a typical ependymoma. Surgery is often not appropriate in patients with significant neurological deficit or with high-grade lesions for whom extensive resection does not improve survival. Prognosis is less good than in ependymoma. High-grade astrocytomas have a median survival of around 20 months.

No large studies have addressed the role of radiotherapy in spinal glioma patients. Small series suggest that less extensive surgery plus postoperative radiotherapy can produce local control in around 50% of patients with low-grade tumours, with 5-year survival rates of around 60%.

Spinal meningiomas and schwannomas

With spinal meningiomas, excision is usually curative and recurrence is uncommon, even when it has not been feasible to excise the dura widely. Schwannomas affecting spinal nerve roots can usually be cured by total excision. However, in some cases these tumours may have an aggressive course and not be surgically curable.

Metastatic spinal cord compression

The spine is a common site for metastatic disease, commonly with bony involvement, but sometimes with extradural deposits and, rarely, with intramedullary spread. These tumours usually spread haematogenously into the vertebral bodies and cause epidural spinal cord compression. Typically, the clinical history is much shorter than with primary spinal tumours. Thus, patients may present as an emergency, with rapidly progressing paraparesis with urinary incontinence and/or retention. Referral may be delayed when there is no previous history of cancer, unless the true nature of the problem is identified. Oncologists are well aware of syndromes caused by spinal metastases, and in patients with a previous known history of malignancy, the diagnosis tends to be made promptly.

Speed of diagnosis followed by urgent imaging is of the essence in preventing or minimising permanent neurological deficit. Where there has been a short clinical history and the patient has a severe paraparesis with sphincter function lost for more than 12 hours, the results of surgical decompression are poor. A randomised trial of surgery followed by radiotherapy against radiotherapy alone for metastatic spinal cord compression showed that significantly more patients in the surgery group were able to walk after treatment and retained the ability to walk significantly longer than in the radiotherapy group. The benefits of this trial cannot be applied to patients with multiple metastases and in this group urgent radiotherapy is usually offered, particularly where the tumour is likely to be radiosensitive and the patient is deemed sufficiently well to survive for a number of months.

Patients with rapidly advancing neurological deficits and with severe cord compression by tumour, as well as spinal disease, generally need urgent surgery if stabilisation of their deficits is to be achieved. There has been a clear trend towards adjusting the surgical approach to the exact site of the metastatic tumour in order to obtain maximum decompression, coupled with fixation to stabilise the diseased spine. Major anterior or lateral approaches are suitable for anteriorly or laterally placed spinal metastases, but these often require a neurosurgeon to have assistance from a thoracic or abdominal surgeon. Single or multiple level corpectomy of the vertebral body with subsequent repair by bone cement, titanium-based cages or bone graft and concomitant posterior spinal fixation with metal instrumentation are performed more frequently than in the past. Posterior decompression should not be performed for anteriorly placed tumours as the resulting laminectomy can lead to spinal instability and rapid neurological deterioration when the patient is mobilised.

Skull base tumours

Chordoma

These are rare tumours arising from remnants of the embryonic notochord and may therefore develop at any point along the length of the neuraxis, in particular the skull base and clivus, vertebral column and sacrum. They are locally aggressive malignant tumours that invade into bone and soft tissues and occasionally metastasise to distant sites. Patients usually die of locally recurrent disease. Clival chordomas present with headache and diplopia caused by VIth nerve palsy. This may progress to involve the Vth nerve and then the lower cranial nerves with vertigo, tinnitus and bulbar palsy causing dysphagia and hoarseness. Rarely, brainstem compression may occur with pyramidal tract dysfunction, ataxia and emotional lability. Chordoma is the most common neoplasm of the sacrum and it may often be extensive before diagnosis. Slowly progressive low back pain with radicular or sciatic radiation involves the sacral nerve roots leading to peri-anal numbness, sphincter disturbance with urinary retention, incontinence and impotence. Involvement of the true vertebrae is uncommon. There may be bone destruction and infiltration into the paraspinal soft tissues. Dorsal expansion leads to nerve root displacement with severe localised radicular pain and sensory loss. Chordomas arising in the cervical region may cause direct oesophageal compression and rarely myelopathy.

Pathology

There are three histological types of chordoma: classic, chondroid and dedifferentiated. The histological appearance (Figure 21.31) of classic chordoma is of a lobulated tumour composed of groups of cells separated by fibrous septa against a background of myxoid stroma (Figure 21.31d). Typical immunohistochemical profiles include positive labelling of the tumour cells with cytokeratin (Figure 21.31e) S100 protein (Figure 21.31f). The cells have small round nuclei and abundant vacuolated cytoplasm, sometimes

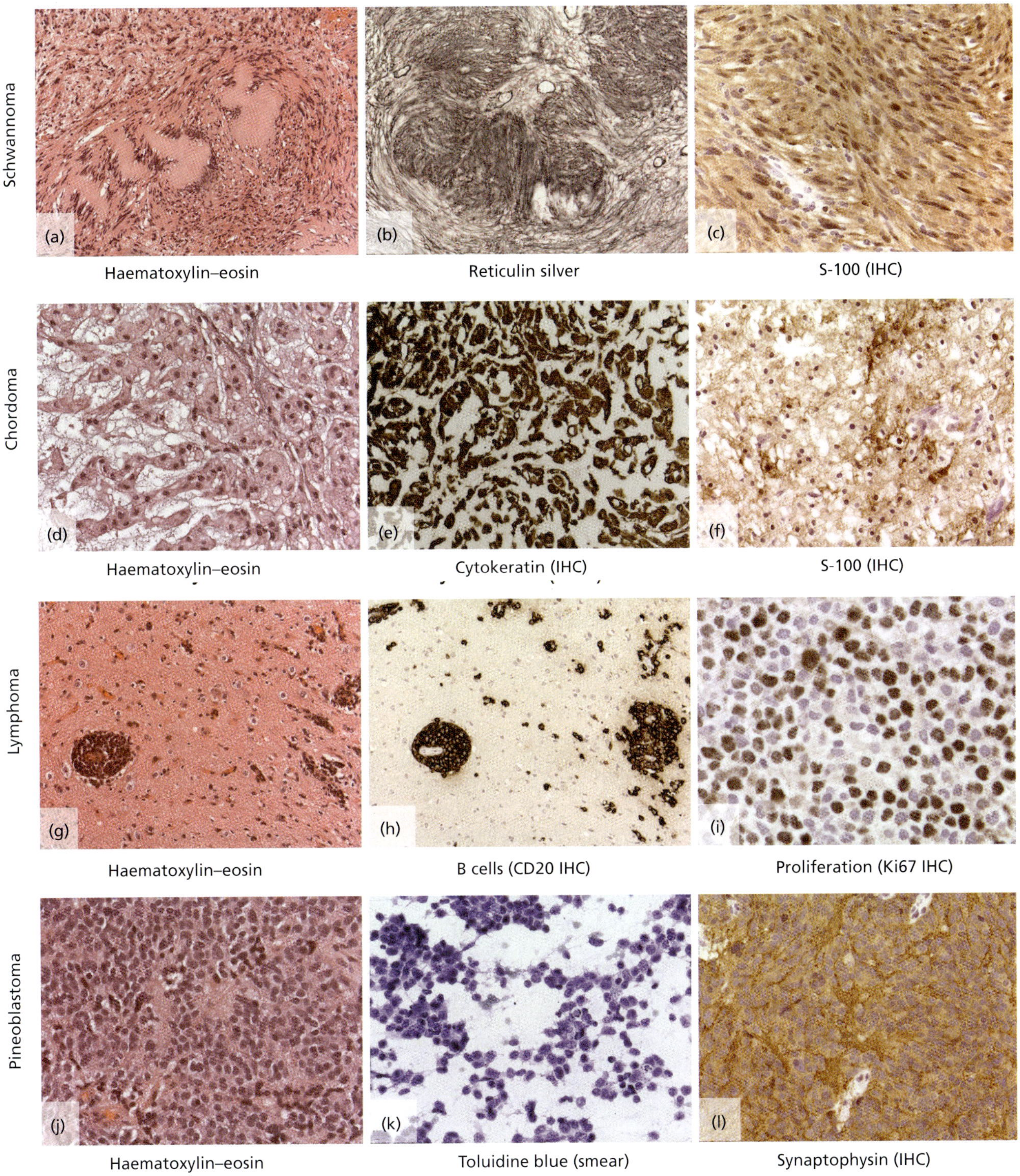

Figure 21.31 Histological features of schwannoma, chordoma, lymphoma and pineoblastoma.

described as physaliferous. Chondroid chordomas histologically show features of both chordoma and chondrosarcoma.

Imaging

Imaging of clival chordomas on CT shows tumour calcification, eroded bone and focal areas of hyperintensity and hypointensity within the tumour. On MRI, the margins are clearly delineated; T2 shows hyperintense areas with extension either anteriorly into the paranasal sinuses and nasopharynx or posteriorly towards the brainstem.

Treatment

Chordomas are difficult to treat because of their infiltrative behaviour and complete resection is rarely feasible. Partial resection is usually combined with radiotherapy to try to eradicate residual disease, but these tumours are highly radio-resistant. Chordomas require doses in excess of 75 Gy for local control rates of around 80% at 5 years. For this reason, there is interest in the use of high-energy proton beam therapy. The specific characteristics of proton beam therapy, with very sharp dose fall off, allow the delivery of such high doses adjacent to critical structures (such as the brainstem and optic pathways). This is not possible with standard conformal radiotherapy from a linear accelerator, but doses of up to 65–70 Gy may be delivered using intensity modulated radiotherapy (IMRT). However, there are no convincing data that suggest protons are superior to standard radiotherapy in terms of overall survival. The overall 5-year survival is approximately 65%; older women with large tumours tend to have the worst prognosis. The prognosis is variable with a better outlook for chordomas in the clivus or sacrum than in the vertebral column. Morbidity and mortality occurs because of the erosive nature of the tumour and the location within eloquent regions of the brain and skull base.

Chondrosarcoma

Chondrosarcomas are rare slowly growing tumours thought to arise from embryonal rest cells, most commonly in the petro-occipital synchondrosis. They resemble chordomas superficially in that they present as a locally aggressive skull-base tumour causing cranial nerve compression with facial weakness or sensory loss, hearing impairment, vertigo or bulbar involvement, but they have a consistently better prognosis. Although they are similar in management, distinction between the two is important because of the different prognoses and outcome. The majority of chondrosarcomas of the skull base are located off the midline, a helpful sign when compared with chordomas which are usually midline. The primary treatment is surgical resection, as with chordomas. These tumours are relatively resistant to radiotherapy, and again preferably treated with proton beam therapy.

Neurofibromatosis and schwannomas

Schwannomas are benign tumours derived from Schwann cells (Chapter 20) and account for about 8% of primary intracranial neoplasms. Their most common location is in the cerebellopontine angle but they can occur on any cranial nerve as well as on spinal nerve roots and peripheral nerves.

Pathology

The schwannoma shown in Figure 21.31 has typical arrangements of palisading nuclei against a fibrillary background, with formations known as Verocay bodies. Around those structures are loosely textured tumour areas: Antoni B areas (Figure 21.31a). Reticulin silver stain visualises the dense pericellular basement membranes (Figure 21.31b). S100 immunohistochemistry typically shows nuclear and cytoplasmic staining in schwannoma (Figure 21.31c).

Molecular genetics

Bilateral vestibular schwannomas are the hallmark of neurofibromatosis type 2 (NF2). NF2 occurs in individuals who have a defective tumour suppressor gene located on chromosome 22q12.2. The defective protein produced by the gene is called merlin or schwannomin. Other manifestations, including peripheral neurofibroma, mengingioma, glioma and juvenile posterior subcapsular lenticular opacities, are often present as well. Many patients with NF2 present in late adolescence or early adulthood but occasionally may present later in the fifth to seventh decade with slowly growing tumors. Peripheral neurofibromata and café-au-lait spots are much less frequently observed than with neurofibromatosis type 1 (NF1).

NF1 is associated with a mutation on chromosome 17, and presents with more peripheral tumours as well as optic pathway gliomas and spinal neurofibromas. These patients also have Lisch nodules in the iris (Chapter 14), café-au-lait patches, subcutaneous schwannomas or neurofibromas and possibly other intracranial or intraspinal tumours, such as gliomas and meningiomas.

Clinical features

Clinical features of vestibular schwannomas include progressive hearing loss, tinnitus and vertigo. Unilateral hearing loss is overwhelmingly the most common symptom present at the time of diagnosis and is generally the symptom that leads to diagnosis. Assume that any unilateral sensorineural hearing loss is caused by a vestibular schwannoma until proven otherwise. An MRI is mandatory in patients of any age presenting with unilateral sensorineural hearing loss. Headaches are present in 50–60% of patients at the time of diagnosis, but fewer than 10% of patients have headache as their presenting symptom. Headache appears to become more common as tumour size increases and is a prominent feature in patients who develop obstructive hydrocephalus associated with a very large tumour. Large tumours (>4 cm) can obstruct the flow of spinal fluid through the ventricular system by distorting and obstructing the 4th ventricle. In the early decades of the twentieth century, most patients are said to have presented with hydrocephalus and papilloedema.

Vestibular schwannomas are managed in three ways:

1. Serial observation (wait, scan, surveillance)
2. Stereotactic radiosurgery
3. Microsurgical excision.

Management depends on multiple factors: patient age, the size and growth rate of the tumour, hearing status, co-morbidities and patient preference. Patients should be seen in a multi-disciplinary team so that all management options can be discussed. In older patients, serial imaging with 12-monthly MRI is appropriate, particularly if hearing has been lost. In younger patients with a tumour that has been shown to be growing, treatment is necessary. The majority of patients will have active treatment and, in this respect, the pendulum has swung heavily away from surgical microdissection to stereotactic radiosurgery or fractionated stereotactic radiotherapy. This can be performed with either the multiple source cobalt unit (gamma knife, often used to deliver single fraction radiosurgery treatments) or a linear accelerator (LINAC) which can deliver single or multiple fraction radiotherapy using either frameless or relocatable frame-based systems. Both are carried out in an outpatient setting without the need for a general anaesthetic. The goal is to deliver a high dose of radiation to the tumour volume with minimal doses to surrounding structures (i.e. cranial nerves, brainstem and vessels). This will slow down or stop the growth but does not cause the tumour to disappear. Single fraction radiosurgery can only be applied to tumours up to 3.5 cm in diameter. Tumour reduction occurs in 70–90% of cases although there is a temporary volume increase in about 25% of patients. Facial nerve damage occurs in about 10–15% but hearing is preserved (in small tumours) in more than 50% of cases. The main disadvantages of radiosurgery include its limitation to small tumours, the possibility of deteriorating cranial nerve function after treatment and potential risk of malignant change within the remaining schwannoma. Risks of developing a secondary malignancy from radiosurgery are small – 1 in 1000 patients followed over 30 years.

In contrast, microsurgical tumour resection remains the treatment of choice for tumour eradication and potential cure. It is the only treatment option for large tumours (>3.5 cm). Three surgical approaches are used: retrosigmoid, translabyrinthine and middle fossa. The retrosigmoid approach can be used for any tumour but is advantageous for large vestibular schwannoma or for small tumours where hearing preservation is attempted. In translabyrinthine surgery, the cerebellum is hardly ever retracted and facial nerve preservation rates may be higher. The middle fossa approach has largely been abandoned in the United Kingdom. The main long-term complication is facial paralysis. Incomplete facial recovery occurs in about 20% of patients and there is a 5% rate of complete facial palsy, which may require facial nerve reconstruction.

Skull base meningiomas

Skull base meningiomas account for approximately 25–30% of all intracranial meningiomas. They occur in the olfactory groove/planum sphenoidale, parasellar region, cavernous sinus, sphenoid wing and petroclivus/petrous apex. The clinical presentation, typically insidious, is caused either by involvement of the cranial nerves or mass effect on the cerebellum and/or brainstem. Raised intracranial pressure can result from the tumour mass or obstructive hydrocephalus. Patients with small asymptomatic meningiomas who are elderly, who have medical co-morbidities or both may be observed and treatment initiated if and when tumour progression is documented.

Surgery is the treatment of choice for patients with apparently resectable meningiomas. The likelihood of accomplishing a complete resection depends upon the site and extent of the tumour. Skull base meningiomas can be particularly challenging because they often cannot be completely resected, and surgery is associated with significant complications. The overall recurrence rate is therefore disproportionately high. Like vestibular schwannomas, skull base meningiomas can be treated with stereotactic radiosurgery. Conformal radiotherapy can also be used and is indicated if the tumour is irregular, too large to be treated with radiosurgery, or both.

Pituitary tumours

The pituitary is a tiny organ, uniquely supplied by two separate circulations: the systemic and portal systems. The sellar and parasellar regions are the sites of many disease processes (Table 21.4) of which pituitary tumours account for the majority. Pituitary tumours represent 10–15% of all intracranial neoplasms. They can be classified by biological behaviour, size or histological and functional criteria (Tables 21.5 and 21.6).

Biological behaviour

Tumours may be either benign, invasive adenomas or carcinomas. Benign forms are most common but up to 50% show evidence of capsule invasion and about one-third invade the dura or the sphenoid sinus. Pituitary carcinomas are exceedingly rare.

Size

Microadenomas are less than 10 mm and macroadenomas greater than 10 mm in diameter. Microadenomas are the more common and typically lie within the sella but can extend into the suprasellar space. Macroadenomas erode the sellar floor as they enlarge and eventually cause its destruction. The anatomy of adenomas is defined most accurately by MRI which clearly displays anterior and posterior lobes of the pituitary and its relation to the paranasal air and venous sinuses.

Table 21.4 Lesions of the sellar region.

1 Tumours
Primary pituitary tumours
Craniopharyngioma
Meningioma
Germ cell tumours
Glioma – hypothalamic, optic nerve
Granular cell tumours
Lymphoma
Ependymoma
Metastases
2 Others
Cysts – Rathke's pouch, epidermoid, dermoid
Empty sella syndrome
Carotid and anterior communicating artery aneurysm
Lymphocytic hypophysitis
3 Granulomatous disease
Sarcoidosis
Wegener's granulomatosis
Histiocytosis X
4 Infections
Pituitary abscess – bacterial or fungal infection
Tuberculosis
Syphilis

Histology

Cells forming a pituitary adenoma are defined by histological, hormonal and immunological characteristics. Acidophilic and chromophobe cells usually produce prolactin, growth hormone (GH) or thyroid-stimulating hormone (TSH). Basophilic cells produce adrenocorticotrophic hormone (ACTH), β-lipotrophin, luteinising hormone (LH) and follicle-stimulating hormone (FSH).

Functional criteria

Radioimmunoassay allows precise measurement of pituitary hormones. The most common type of pituitary adenoma (approximately 30%) are functionally inactive and typically chromophobe adenomas. Of those adenomas that secrete hormones, 60–70% produce prolactin, 10–15% secrete growth hormone and some 5% secrete ACTH. Gonadotrophin and TSH secreting tumours are exceptionally rare.

Clinical presentation

Patients with pituitary adenomas present typically with chronic mass effects, particularly affecting visual structures, chronic headaches, endocrine abnormalities resulting from hormonal hypersecretion and/or hyposecretion, or a combination of these factors. Occasionally, acute pituitary apoplexy occurs. Macroadenomas are the most common cause of chiasmal compression in adults and cause bi-temporal hemianopia. Partial patterns of visual loss develop, depending on the anatomical relationship of the tumour and the chiasm, leading to asymmetrical superior bi-temporal hemianopia or optic nerve

Table 21.5 Classification of pituitary tumours.

Cell of origin	Hormone	Clinical features
Non-functioning	None	Cause symptoms only when they extend beyond the sella Most common type of macro-adenoma (30–35%)
Lactotroph	Prolactin	Typically intrasellar but may enlarge The most common hormone producing pituitary adenoma (40% of cases)
Corticotroph	ACTH	Secretion of ACTH leading to Cushing's syndrome (approx. 10% of cases) Usually confined to sella. May enlarge and become invasive particularly after adrenalectomy (Nelson's syndrome)
Somatotroph	GH	Gigantism in children and adolescents; acromegaly in adults Suprasellar extension relatively common Approximately 15% of cases
Thyrotroph	TSH (also occasionally GH and Prl)	Hyperthyroidism without TSH suppression May be large and invasive Rare, approx. 1–2%
Gonadotrophin	FSH or LH	Usually non-functioning May result in ovarian overstimulation, increases testosterone level, testicular enlargement or pituitary insufficiency due to compression of the stalk or destruction of pituitary tissue by the tumour Uncommon
Plurihormonal	More than one hormone	May have one cell population producing two or more hormones or two or more distinct cell types
Carcinoma		Usually functional (ACTH and Prl producing) Varying degrees of nuclear atypia and cellular polymorphism but often high mitotic rate and cell proliferation Rare (<0.2%)
Metastatic		Breast and lung cancer are most common neoplasms metastasing to pituitary. Also lymphoma, leukaemia, melanoma and prostate

ACTH, adenocorticotrophic hormone; FSH, follicle-stimulating hormone; GH, growth hormone; LH, luteinising hormone; Prl, prolactin; TSH, thyroid-stimulating hormone.

Table 21.6 Endocrine syndromes associated with pituitary tumours.

Prolactinoma (hyperprolactinaemia)	Amenorrhoea, infertility, galactorrhoea, loss of libido, erectile dysfunction
Corticotroph (Cushing's syndrome)	Obesity with centripetal fat distribution, hirsutism, abdominal striae, acne, hypertension, glucose intolerance, muscle wasting and weakness, osteoporosis, neuropsychiatric disturbance, immunosuppression
Nelson's syndrome	Due to growth of residual tumour after bilateral adrenalectomy in Cushing's patients Occurs when high plasma ACTH levels persist despite adequate glucocorticoid replacement Hyperpigmentation, mass effect. Tumours resistant to therapy
Growth hormone (acromegaly or gigantism)	Growth of hands and feet, prognathism, coarsening of facial features, carpal tunnel syndrome, diabetes, osteoarthritis, arthralgia, excessive sweating, obstructive sleep apnoea
TSH (thyrotoxicosis)	Features of thyrotoxicosis, weight loss, anxiety, palpitations, tremor, insomnia, menorrhagia
Gonadotrophin	Rare: testicular enlargement, ovarian stimulation

ACTH, adenocorticotrophic hormone;TSH, thyroid-stimulating hormone.

involvement. Oculomotor palsies develop if the pituitary adenoma extends laterally into the cavernous sinus through which pass cranial nerves III, IV and VI, the first two divisions of V and the sympathetic nerves to the eyes. Extension into a temporal lobe can lead to epilepsy. Rarely, hydrocephalus may occur because of direct compression of the 3rd ventricle leading to raised intracranial pressure or erosion through the sella to cause CSF rhinorrhoea. Compression of the internal carotid artery may lead to cerebral ischaemia. Hypothalamic invasion may affect temperature regulation and cause hypersomnolence, autonomic dysregulation and diabetes insipidus. Hormonal abnormalities caused by pituitary adenomas depend on the cell type and hormone produced (Table 21.6).

Pituitary apoplexy

Pituitary apoplexy results from acute haemorrhagic or ischaemic infarction of the pituitary, often with a previously unrecognised secreting or non-functioning pituitary adenoma, and is believed to occur because a tumour has outgrown its blood supply. Extensive haemorrhagic infarction leads to mass effect in the suprasellar space and cavernous sinus. Apoplexy is rare and presents with sudden headache, meningism, vomiting, visual loss, ophthalmoplegia, visual field defect and occasionally impairment of consciousness. Secondary pituitary dysfunction and hyponatraemia can follow. The CSF shows evidence of haemorrhage with a pleocytosis and elevated protein. Predisposing factors include pregnancy, postpartum haemorrhage, trauma, diabetic ketoacidosis, radiotherapy and angiography. The condition may occur after bromocriptine has been started. Steroids are required urgently to treat pituitary apoplexy. Surgery may be necessary. Pan-hypopituitarism commonly follows and requires lifelong replacement therapy.

Drug therapy and surgery

Management of pituitary tumours is directed at normalising hormonal secretion, reversing endocrine manifestations of excess secretion and preventing progressive neurological deficit, especially visual loss. Treatment options include surgery, medical management and radiotherapy. The choice is determined by the histological typing of the tumour, the nature of its hormonal expression, the size and its extension into surrounding structures. Surgical treatment is preferred for GH, TSH and ACTH producing and endocrinologically inactive tumours. Transphenoidal pituitary surgery is the most widely employed approach, particularly for non-functioning macroadenomas causing chiasmal compression. It allows direct visualisation of the gland and tumour and is well tolerated. It is successful in debulking tumours even if there is a considerable suprasellar extension and regrowth is uncommon. Advances in MRI, using high-field techniques, allow peri-operative assessment of the completeness of surgery and the planning of postoperative management. However, transphenoidal surgery is less effective if there is an hour-glass narrowing between the intrasellar and suprasellar component of the tumour or if there is infection within the sphenoid sinus. In these situations, surgery via a craniotomy using a subfrontal approach may be necessary.

GH secreting tumours may be treated initially with medical treatment using the GH receptor antagonist, pegvisomant, or somatostatin analogues (e.g. octreotide, lanreotide) which normalise GH level and decrease the tumour size in refractory acromegaly. Prolactinomas are usually treated medically with dopamine agonists (e.g. cabergoline or bromocriptine), which are effective in shrinking the size of the adenoma and lowering serum prolactin levels. Prolactin levels are often maintained after the drug has been discontinued but if medical therapy fails then transphenoidal surgery and radiotherapy may be indicated.

Radiotherapy

Radiotherapy is an effective adjunct to the treatment of pituitary tumours and contributes to the high rates of cure. Radiotherapy is indicated where surgery is contraindicated, following incomplete removal, especially around the cavernous sinus, when there is a large tumour mass at diagnosis (the large silent corticotrophs are at high risk of early local recurrence), following recurrent disease or where surgery has failed to cure a hormone producing tumour. Pituitary carcinoma requires radical resection followed by adjuvant radiotherapy and the consideration of temozolomide chemotherapy, dependent on histological subtype.

Hormonal responses to radiotherapy are typically slow over months to years. Radiotherapy may eventually lead to hypopituitarism and the need for full hormonal replacement. This risk needs to balanced against the risk of further recurrence, and take patient preference into account – especially in young patients wanting to maintain fertility and with longer to develop a radiation-induced second tumour. The risk to visual function from conventionally fractionated radiotherapy is very low. Radiotherapy is usually CT-planned and conventionally fractionated. A stereotactic set-up or radiosurgery may be able to exclude the hypothalamus from the high dose volume and reduce the risk of hypopituitarism in small tumours confined to the sella. More rapid falls in hormone levels have been seen with radiosurgery but there are concerns about radiation-induced optic neuropathy.

Craniopharyngioma

These are slow-growing benign extra-axial cystic tumours in the parasellar region. Cysts, sometimes multiple, contain thick proteinaceous material, often shiny because of a high content of cholesterol crystals. A cyst can extend in any direction and project into the hypothalamus, basal cisterns, 3rd ventricle, cerebellopontine angle, posterior fossa or the foramen magnum. Presentation is usually as a slow-growing tumour but there may be a sudden onset with rapid deterioration because of increase in volume or rupture causing a chemical meningitis or ventriculitis. The most common symptoms are headaches, visual disturbance and endocrine dysfunction. The clinical features may be similar to pituitary adenoma with progressive chiasmal compression except that craniopharyngiomas typically compress the superior aspects of the chiasm and cause inferior field defects. There may also be involvement of the optic nerves if the tumour is pre-chiasmal causing progressive optic atrophy with impaired acuity and constriction of the fields. Endocrine dysfunction is brought about by involvement of the pituitary stalk leading to hypothyroidism, adrenal insufficiency, diabetes insipidus, growth failure and reduced sexual drive. Compression of the 3rd ventricle leads to hydrocephalus and raised intracranial pressure with headache and papilloedema. Secondary hypothalamic involvement is common leading to hyperphagia and obesity. Craniopharyngiomas can infiltrate the frontal lobes, mammillary bodies and limbic system, eventually spreading to the Sylvian fissure leading to emotional, psychiatric and behavioural disturbances, apathy and short-term memory deficits.

Radical cure is the exception – the cysts are often multiple, adherent and inaccessible. Surgical resection is rarely possible and in any event surgery carries considerable morbidity, with risks of cyst rupture and hypothalamic damage. Recurrence is common. Incomplete removal must be followed by radiotherapy. The risks of side effects related to radiotherapy are relatively low but intellectual decline, optic neuropathy and hypothalamic damage may occur. There may also be residual endocrine deficits including diabetes insipidus and cognitive impairments. New techniques of intracyst chemotherapy, stereotactic radiotherapy or internal irradiation are also used. Prognosis is highly variable with a significant morbidity and mortality from local extension. A poor outcome may be predicted by a young age of onset, preoperative visual impairment, papilloedema, hydrocephalus and hypothalamic involvement. Subtotal resection, tumour calcification and adhesive tumour wall also predict a poor outcome.

Primary CNS lymphomas

The term lymphoma encompasses a large heterogeneous group of malignant lymphoid neoplasms. When these tumours are confined to the brain, spinal cord or leptomeninges they are known as primary CNS lymphomas (PCNSL). These account for about 3% of primary CNS tumours, occurring predominantly in older people with a slight male preponderance. Immunosuppressed patients, most commonly HIV-positive, are about 1000 times more likely to develop PCNSL than immunocompetent adults. Indeed, PCNSL were rarely seen at all before the AIDS epidemic. However, there is also sound evidence that the incidence of PCNSL has increased in the immunocompetent population over the last two decades, particularly in those over 65 years.

Imaging

PCNSL usually present as a single, lobulated enhancing mass, often abutting an ependymal (Figure 21.7) or meningeal surface. Occasionally, PCNSL are multiple. Enhancement is uniform in immunocompetent patients but tends to be ring-like in immunocompromised patients because of areas of central necrosis. The high cellular density of PCNSL accounts for its hyperdensity on CT and hypointensity on T2 MRI. The ADC of PCNSL is lower than in gliomas or toxoplasmosis which is an important differential diagnosis in immunocompromised patients. PCNSL grows in an angiocentric fashion around existing blood vessels without extensive new vessel formation. PWI therefore shows only a modest increase in rCBV, much less marked than in high-grade gliomas where angiogenesis is a prominent feature. In contrast to PCNSL which presents as an intraparenchymal mass, secondary CNS lymphoma (i.e. arising as relapse in the CNS from a previously treated extracranial lymphoma) involves more frequently the dura, ependymal, leptomeninges and cranial nerves, which show pathological enhancement with gadolinium (Figure 21.32). Both PCNSL and secondary CNS lymphomas show avid tracer uptake on FDG PET imaging.

Pathology

Lymphomas are arranged in dense patternless sheets and infiltrate adjacent brain tissue diffusely and also in characteristic peri-vascular arrangements (Figure 21.31 g). Most primary intracerebral lymphomas are of B-cell type and are positive for the B-cell marker CD20 (Figure 21.31 h). These tumours are highly malignant and exhibit a very high mitotic index; Ki67 proliferation can be as high as 90%. The lymphoma shown in Figure 21.31(i) has a proliferation index of approximately 50%. Anaplastic large cell and T-cell variants are also described. They rarely metastasise outside the CNS but may spread along CSF pathways into the spinal cord. Approximately 20% of cases have intraocular involvement at diagnosis. Even in the majority of patients who have a single supratentorial mass lesion, the disease should be regarded as multifocal from outset. There is therefore no benefit in resection of the tumour except where there is life-threatening intracranial hypertension.

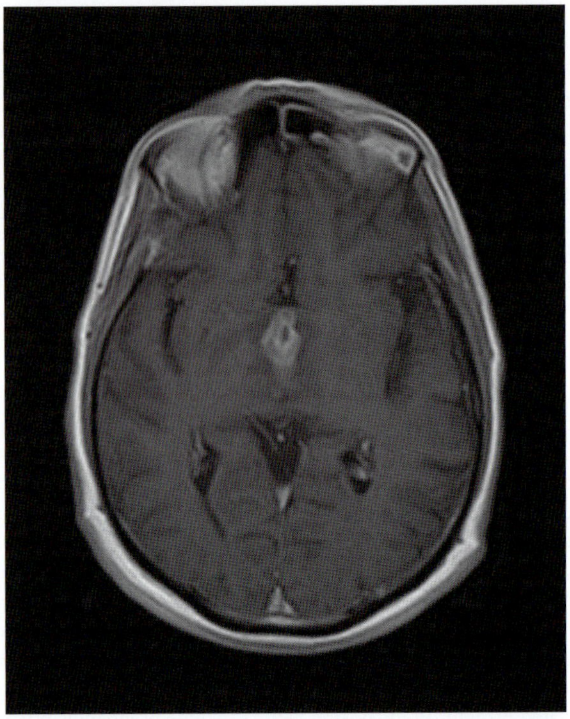

Figure 21.32 Secondary CNS lymphoma. Axial T1-weighted image post gadolinium showing enhancing tumour within the 3rd ventricle lining the ependymal surfaces in a patient who had received treatment for Stage IV non-Hodgkin's lymphoma and who had relapsed in the brain.

Clinical presentation

PCNSL usually present as either solitary or multiple mass lesions with raised intracranial pressure, progressive focal neurological deficit and seizures. Intracranial lesions are usually supratentorial; more than 60% are peri-ventricular, involving the splenium, corpus callosum, basal ganglia and the thalamus. Rarely, the tumour invades and proliferates within the small vessels of the brain, spreading along intravascular spaces. This is known as intravascular lymphoma or malignant angioendotheliomatosis. This presents as either progressive multifocal cerebrovascular events or as a subacute encephalopathy. Very rarely, PCNSL develop in the meninges, leading to a progressive leptomeningeal syndrome with cranial nerve palsies, hydrocephalus and myelopathy. Ocular lymphoma presenting with visual loss can predate the appearance of intracranial lymphoma.

Diagnosis

Diagnosis is usually suspected from initial imaging which typically shows one or several homogeneously enhancing masses, often in a peri-ventricular location. In immunocompetent patients, in about 30% of cases the tumours are multiple, rising to some 50% in patients with AIDS. Once the diagnosis is suspected, steroids should be withheld because of their lympholytic properties until a stereotactic biopsy has been carried out, unless the patient has life-threatening intracranial symptoms. There are many reported cases of these tumours disappearing after even a few days on steroids. This phenomenon is not diagnostic of CNS lymphoma; it is seen also with inflammatory masses (e.g. acute demyelination) and even with gliomas.

The diagnosis may be confirmed from a CSF sample if the brain lesion is sufficiently small to allow safe lumbar puncture. CSF cytology is positive in about 30% of cases and the sensitivity increases with two or three lumbar punctures. Flow cytometric studies and polymerase chain reaction (PCR) looking for clonal rearrangements of immunoglobulin heavy chains can improve sensitivity but are not universally available. In situations where CSF is negative or a lumbar puncture cannot be carried out for fear of coning, a stereotactic biopsy will usually establish the diagnosis. A contrast-enhanced MRI of the spine should also be carried out to look for leptomeningeal tumour deposits. Open craniotomy and resection can lead to seeding of tumour cells into the leptomeningeal space and does not confer any survival benefit. Once the diagnosis is suspected, the patient's HIV status should be determined and the eyes examined by an experienced ophthalmologist for evidence of intraocular disease. Asymptomatic ocular involvement occurs in some 20% of patients and specific additional treatment may be required. Staging body CT and bone marrow aspirate are seldom required as systemic lymphoma is found rarely in PCNSL. Such a finding has no effect on subsequent disease course. Serum lactate dehydrogenase is often greatly raised, sometimes useful as a diagnostic pointer and as a prognostic factor in PCNSL.

Treatment

Current treatment of PCNSL is based around the use of high-dose intravenous methotrexate (HDMTX: $3\,g/m^2$) regimens followed by whole brain with or without spinal or ocular radiotherapy, in contrast to systemic non-Hodgkin's lymphoma where the standard first line regimen is R-CHOP. In an effort to intensify chemotherapy and avoid the use of radiotherapy altogether (to minimise neurotoxicity), some centres have treated good performance patients with HDMTX alone followed by myeloablative chemotherapy and then autologous stem cell rescue. Long-term data have not been published. The additional benefit of intrathecal chemotherapy either via the lumbar route or via an Ommaya–Rickman reservoir directly into the ventricles is also not proven. WBRT in combination with corticosteroids leads to a response in about 70% of patients. This regimen is best reserved for elderly patients with poor performance status who would otherwise not tolerate HDMTX-based therapies.

The major dilemma facing oncologists arises in patients over the age of 60 years in whom the combination of methotrexate and WBRT is associated with an almost 100% risk of cognitive decline, ataxia and incontinence 1–2 years after treatment. This has led to the development of protocols based around chemotherapy alone although there is a risk of renal and bone marrow failure with these intensive regimens. Furthermore, as there are no randomised Phase III studies that prove that this can produce a long-term survival benefit, our own practice has been to irradiate to a dose of 30 Gy after obtaining radiological remission with chemotherapy.

The prognosis depends on age and performance status, as with other CNS tumours, but also on the extent of spread along CSF pathways and whether or not the patient is HIV-positive. Average survival of elderly patients treated with steroids alone is in the region of 6 months, increasing to 1 year with the addition of radiotherapy. This rises to 2 years in those under the age of 60 years. The combination of HDMTX chemotherapy followed by radiotherapy in patients under the age of 60 years is associated with 5-year survival rates of 65%, clearly much higher than any survival for high-grade gliomas.

Primitive neuroepithelial tumours and medulloblastomas

Primitive neuroepithelial tumours (PNET) account for about 20% of childhood brain tumours overall and are the second most frequent childhood primary brain tumour after the relatively benign cystic astrocytomas. They are rare (less than 1% of brain tumours) in adults. They are highly malignant (WHO Grade IV) with a propensity for spread through the CSF. They are called medulloblastoma when found in the posterior fossa, pineoblastoma in the pineal region, and supratentorial PNET when presentin the cerebral hemispheres. Medulloblastomas typically occur in children, declining sharply in incidence after the age of 15 years; they are the most common highly malignant brain tumour of childhood. About 1 in 20 metastasise outside the CNS. Overall 5-year mortality of medulloblastoma cases is 60%. Supratentorial PNETs carry a significantly worse prognosis than medulloblastoma with only about 50% surviving 3 years, thought to be to the result of a combination of biological differences and the difficulty of complete surgical resection.

Pathology

Macroscopically, these tumours vary in growth pattern, ranging from firm and discrete to soft and less well-defined masses. Medulloblastomas mostly arise in the cerebellar vermis, but with increasing age tend to develop within the cerebellar hemispheres. There is increasing experimental evidence that most medulloblastomas originate from the external granular layer (EGL) of the cerebellum. Histologically, they vary in their appearance. The undifferentiated or classic medulloblastoma is the most common form, characterised by densely packed, round or oval cells with a high nucleus to cytoplasm ratio and showing neuroblastic rosettes formed by circular arrangements of tumour cells around a virtual centre (Figure 21.2c). The nodular or desmoplastic variant is characterised by extensive formation of nodules that show neuronal differentiation and are surrounded by thin collagenous septae and undifferentiated cells. A more recently defined entity is the large cell anaplastic variant (approximately 4%) composed of markedly irregularity and atypia, frequent mitoses and apoptosis. This variant is associated with a particularly poor prognosis. Medulloblastoma can show a variable degree of differentiation into neuronal, and rarely glial, ependymal, muscular (medullomyoblastoma) or melanocytic (melanotic medulloblastoma) lineages.

Molecular genetics and histogenesis of medulloblastoma

Four major subgroups have been identified: Wnt, sonic hedgehog (Shh), Group 3 and Group 4.

The best known of the medulloblastoma subgroups is the Wnt subgroup because of its very good long-term prognosis in comparison to other subgroups, with long-term survival exceeding 90%. The Shh group of medulloblastomas are named after the sonic hedgehog signalling pathway, which is thought to drive tumour initiation in many, if not all such cases; it is frequent in both infants (0–3 years) and adults (>16 years), but much less frequent in children (3–16 years). The prognosis of Shh medulloblastoma is similar to Group 4 medulloblastomas, and intermediate between that Wnt medulloblastomas (good prognosis) and Group 3 medulloblastomas (poor prognosis). Group 3 tumours are mostly 'classic' medulloblastomas, but they also encompass the majority of the large cell anaplastic histological type. They have a poor prognosis. The molecular pathogenesis of Group 4 tumours is currently not well understood. The title Group 4 has been chosen for the current consensus nomenclature until further analysis has been done. Group 4 patients have an intermediate prognosis, similar to individuals with Shh tumors.

There are several histological variants including the classic (undifferentiated) medulloblastoma, which is the most common in adults, desmoplastic nodular and large cell (anaplastic), the latter associated with a particularly poor prognosis.

Imaging

Medulloblastomas usually arise in the cerebellar midline in children and the cerebellar hemispheres in adults. In contrast, PNETs are usually supratentorial. The high nuclear : cytoplasmic ratio of both these tumours is responsible for their hyperdense appearance on CT and hyperintense appearance on DWI. A three- to fourfold elevation of choline and lipid on MRS is caused by their intense cellularity and cell turnover. PNETs enhance and have a propensity for dissemination in the subarachnoid space with leptomeningeal deposits. Staging of these tumours requires contrast-enhanced MRI of the entire neuraxis.

Clinical features

Clinical features include gait ataxia, headache, vomiting and visual loss resulting from hydrocephalus. Children tend to have midline tumours that are well-defined and enhance homogeneously, whereas in adults tumours usually arise within the cerebellar hemispheres and are poorly enhancing. All patients require staging with MRI of the spine, ideally prior to surgery, as well as CSF examination either prior to surgery or 10–14 days after. Postoperative imaging to determine the extent of resection should be carried out ideally within 24–48 hours after surgery.

Treatment

The main adverse factors in children are: age less than 3 years; postoperative macroscopic residual disease >1.5 mL; anatomical site; anaplastic and large cell variants; and CSF metastases. These factors are used to determine the standard and high risk groups for prognosis and management. Current therapy for good prognosis, standard risk children comprises cranio-spinal irradiation (CSI) and adjuvant chemotherapy. An 85% 5-year survival is now seen in the standard risk group, but this falls to between 30 and 50% in those with adverse factors. Aggressive chemotherapy schedules and hyperfractionation of CSI (treating twice a day) are being investigated in the high risk population to try and improve the poor survival rates.

Surgery has three aims – histological diagnosis, maximal safe tumour resection and relief of hydrocephalus – thus avoiding the need for a CSF diversion procedure with attendant risks of upward brainstem herniation, CSF dissemination and infection. Mortality should be less than 1%, morbidity 5–10%, with an unusual complication being cerebellar mutism. This is thought to arise from damage to the dentate nuclei but it gradually improves; it should not delay the start of adjuvant radiotherapy.

All patients are then treated with CSI. In adults the dose is usually 36 Gy to the whole neuraxis followed by a boost to the posterior fossa of 18 Gy. The CSI dose has been safely reduced to 24 Gy in the standard risk group in children, in an attempt to avoid the significant cognitive, endocrine and growth deficits, with the addition of Packer chemotherapy (cisplatin, vincristine and CCNU). However, chemotherapy brings its own side effects of hearing loss, infertility, renal failure, peripheral neuropathy and myelosupression. Higher doses (46 Gy) are given to nodular metastases in the spine. The delivery of CSI is complex and the technical quality of radiotherapy shown to be closely related to outcome in PNET. It has been proposed that it should only be delivered in designated paediatric and young adult radiotherapy centres as these have the necessary expertise through treating a significant number of cases.

The majority of reported cases of adult medulloblastoma (MB) come from retrospective studies from single institutions spanning many decades. It is therefore difficult to draw firm conclusions about the best treatment. Being an adult is itself considered an adverse factor and therefore immediately high risk. Certain principles are clear, namely the need for maximal resective surgery followed by CSI. The role of chemotherapy is not yet established for adults with MB, as standard treatment (surgery plus CSI) yields a 60% 5-year progression-free survival. There is a perception that radiotherapy is less harmful to adults than to children in the long term and that survival benefit from chemotherapy in adults is less convincing than in children. However, most neuro-oncologists would treat high-risk adult patients with MB with adjuvant chemotherapy.

Relapse in adult patients with MB occurs in 20–50% by 5 years and is usually in the posterior fossa or in the spine. Treatment at relapse is therefore directed at resection or highly focused radiotherapy (e.g. stereotactic radiosurgery) to the posterior fossa followed by high-dose myeloablative chemotherapy and stem cell rescue. Unfortunately, almost all patients experience eventual recurrence either in the CNS or at distant non-CNS sites and succumb. Overall survival ranges are 25–85% at 5 years and 35–50% at 10 years. Clinical trials are needed for adult patients, but until further results become available we must be guided by paediatric trials.

Pineal region tumours

Introduction

A variety of tumours occur in the pineal region (Table 21.7), including germ cell tumours (germinomas and non-germinamotous germ cell tumours), pineal parenchymal tumours (pineocytoma and pineoblastoma) as well as gliomas and metastases.

Table 21.7 Tumours of the pineal region.

Tumours of pineal origin (20%)
Pineocytoma
Pineoblastoma
Tumours of germ cell origin (>50%)
Germinoma
Non-germinomatous germ cell tumours
Teratoma
Embryonal carcinoma
Choriocarcinoma
Yolk sac tumour
Tumours of supporting or adjacent tissues
Glioma
Ganglioneuroma
Ganglioglioma
Meningioma
Non-neoplastic cysts
Arachnoid cyst
Pineal cyst
Vascular lesions
Aneurysm of vein of Galen
AVM
Cavernous malformation

AVM, arteriovenous malformation.

Pathology

Pineoblastomas belong to the group of PNETs and arise in the pineal region. Histological features include the formation of neuroblastic rosettes as shown in (Figure 21.31j). In intraoperative smear preparations, these tumours typically spread out to monolayers with fine synaptic networks (Figure 21.31k). They almost invariably express the neuronal marker synaptophysin, as shown in (Figure 21.31l).

Clinical features

The clinical syndromes associated with pineal region tumours are determined by the close anatomical relationship of the gland with the quadrigeminal plate and midbrain tectum ventrally, the 3rd ventricle rostrally and the cerebellar vermis caudally. Typical syndromes include:

- *Obstructive hydrocephalus:* headache, nausea, vomiting and obtundation
- *Parinaud's syndrome:* vertical gaze palsy, light-near dissociation mid-point pupils, loss of convergence and convergence–retraction nystagmus (Chapter 14), and
- *Ataxia:* caused by involvement of the superior cerebellar peduncle.

Germ cell tumours can produce diabetes insipidus, amenorrhoea, growth arrest and pseudo-precocious puberty. The diagnostic work-up of a pineal region tumour includes a gadolinium-enhanced MRI scan and tumour markers in serum and CSF alpha-fetoprotein (AFP) and human chorionic gonadotrophin (β-HCG). High levels are pathognomic of malignant germ cell tumours and obviate the need for biopsy.

Treatment

There is a high morbidity and mortality associated with pineal region surgery and thus debate about the pros and cons of biopsy alone versus open resection. The ultimate choice of procedure will depend largely on the individual surgeon but, as a general rule, a stereotactic biopsy is preferred where there is disseminated disease, clearly invasive malignant tumour or the patient has multiple other medical problems. The mortality and morbidity of stereotactic biopsy in modern series is around 1.3% and <1.0%, respectively. In contrast, open resection should be reserved for patients with benign lesions, in whom surgery can be curative or rarely for debulking of malignant tumours, particularly where the biopsy diagnosis has been hampered by small amounts of tissue or has been inconclusive.

The subsequent treatment and prognosis depends much on histology. Germinomas are exquisitely sensitive to radiotherapy and are associated with good long-term survival. Patients with non-germinomatous germ cell tumours have a significantly worse prognosis and are usually treated with a combination of chemotherapy and radiotherapy. Pineoblastomas are managed like medulloblastomas with a pre-operative MRI spine and CSF, which if negative should be followed by maximal tumour resection, followed by CSI and chemotherapy. If either of these is positive, then the risks of surgery probably outweigh the benefits and patients should be treated with upfront CSI and chemotherapy.

Germ cell tumours

Germ cell tumours (GCT) arise from primitive embryonic cells and usually present as ovarian or testicular tumours. The CNS is the second most common extragonadal site for germ cell tumours (after the mediastinum). They generally arise in the midline in the region of the pineal gland and the suprasellar region, accounting for approximately 50% of pineal tumours. Each of the histological germ cell variants are derived from cells of a normal stage of embryonal development and may be classified as follows:

1 Undifferentiated germ cell tumours derived from primordial germ cells:
   - Germinoma
2 Differentiated non-germinomatous germ cell tumours (NGGCT):
   - Teratoma
   - Embryonal carcinoma
   - Endodermal sinus tumour (yolk sac tumour)
   - Choriocarcinoma.

When a GCT is suspected, MRI of the cranio-spinal axis, serum tumour markers, and CSF sampling for tumour markers and cytology are required for diagnosis, management and staging. High levels of AFP and β-HCG in either compartment are pathognomic of secreting NGGCTs. They replace the need for biopsy and can be used to monitor response to chemotherapy and remission status on surveillance. However, these tumour markers are not sensitive as many tumours do not produce them and others are of mixed histology. β-HCG is elevated in choriocarcinoma. Bifocal disease (concurrent primary tumours in the suprasellar/parasellar and pineal regions) is seen in 30% of germinomas and is also considered pathognomic. Less than 10% of GCTs have metastatic disease at presentation.

The diagnosis determines the prognosis. Germinomas (Figure 21.33) are histologically identical to testicular seminomas and are not usually associated with raised CSF tumour markers. They are extremely radio-sensitive with a 90% cure rate with cranio-spinal radiotherapy alone, and this is the mainstay of treatment. NGGCTs have a worse prognosis than germinomas and require multi-modality therapy to attain a 5-year survival around 70%. The standard regimen is for platinum-based chemotherapy, followed by surgery and/or radiotherapy. The radiotherapy is focal in localised disease and cranio-spinal for metastatic disease. Teratomas require surgery only.

NGGCTs have a mixed density on MRI and CT and often present as large cysts or areas of calcification with distinct margins. Occasionally, formed tissue may be identified within the cyst and more aggressive NGGCT show heterogeneous enhancement. Choriocarcinoma may show extensive haemorrhagic change.

Optic pathway glioma

Optic pathway gliomas (OPG) are rare astrocytic neoplasms arising from the optic pathway that occur most commonly in children. They comprise 0.6–1.5% of all intracranial tumours, 1.7–7% of all gliomas, 3.5% of all orbital tumours and 66% of all optic nerve tumours. They usually have an indolent but progressive nature, which may result in blindness and eventually death, despite attempts at timely treatment.

The majority of patients are diagnosed below the age of 10 and the most common histology in this group is pilocytic astrocytoma. There is an association with neurofibromatosis type 1 (NF1) and in this group the prognosis is more favourable. Approximately half of all patients with OPG have NF1. Adult patients with optic nerve gliomas are thought to represent a separate group of glioma with a highly aggressive phenotype that presents with signs and symptoms of acute optic neuropathy, progresses to blindness within a few weeks and death within a few months. There is a relationship between age of diagnosis and tumour grade, with a tendency to high grade tumours in older patients. Many patients are diagnosed on the basis of imaging as the tumours are intrinsic to the axons of the visual pathway and are therefore not easily amenable to biopsy unless there is an extrinsic component. On MRI, optic nerve gliomas appear as diffuse enlargement of the

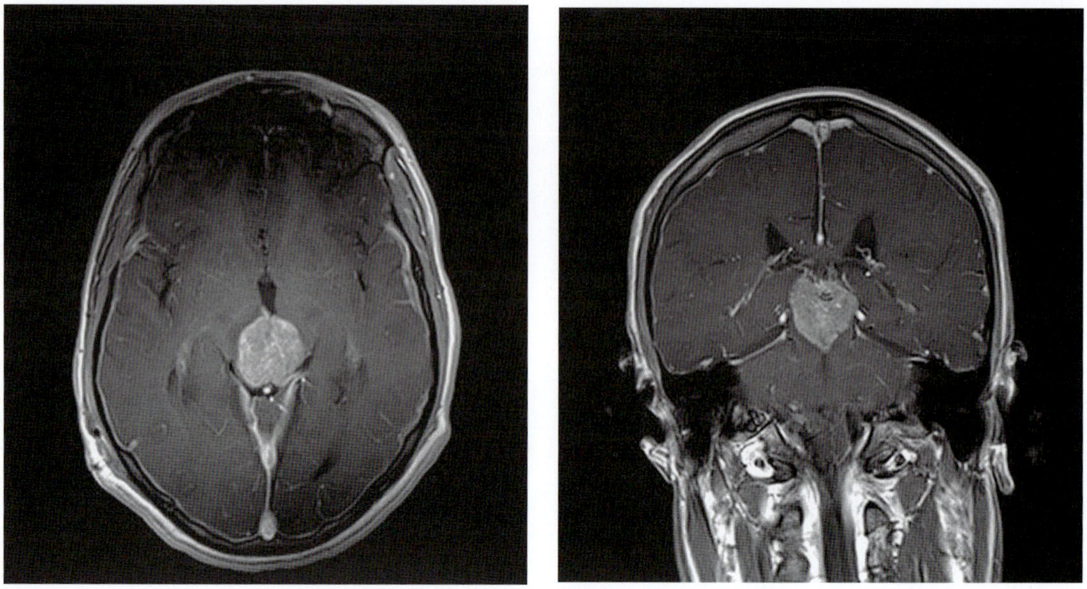

(a) (b)

Figure 21.33 Germinoma. (a) Axial and (b) coronal T1-weighted post gadolinium images of midline germinoma presenting with bi-ventricular hydrocephalus.

optic nerves with spread into the chiasm and the optic radiation. There may be a fusiform appearance and commonly the lesions are isointense on T1-weighted images and iso- to hyper-intense on T2 sequences. Those not related to NF1 usually enhance with gadolinium.

Treatment of optic pathway glioma

For children younger than 8 years of age and those with NF1, primary chemotherapy treatment is recommended, to delay or obviate the need for radiotherapy and the associated morbidity. Response rates are good and endocrine, intellectual and overall neurological function may be preserved. The recommended agents are vincristine and carboplatin given for 18 months. For those children having radiotherapy, protons are advised to avoid morbidity to normal tissues. It is unusual for surgery to be used in children with low grade OPG.

For the majority of adult patients the untreated clinical course is that of progressive blindness and death from local tumour progression. Lesions that are localised to the optic nerve can be cured by surgical excision and postoperative radiotherapy is not given if the lesion has been completely excised unless it recurs. In the care of posterior lesions extending into the chiasm, hypothalamus and contiguous structures, total resection is not possible without substantial morbidity; the role of surgery is to provide histological confirmation and to perform shunting if necessary.

Radiotherapy is an effective treatment in those unsuitable for surgery, after partial resection and in patients who progress after surgery alone. Local failure rates after radiotherapy are greater for posterior than for anterior tumours. Fractionated stereotactic radiotherapy with MRI and CT fusion to assist treatment planning has the advantage of delivering a higher dose more accurately to the tumour and a lower dose to adjacent normal brain tissues and is recommended if available. The advantage of this treatment is that it spares the pituitary gland in optic chiasm lesions. A dose of 50.4–52.2 Gy in 1.8 Gy fractions, aiming to keep within normal tissue tolerance for the eyes and optic apparatus is recommended. Intensity modulated radiotherapy may also be used to good effect to reduce morbidity. Following treatment visual fields and endocrine function should be monitored.

Ependymomas

Ependymomas are slowly growing tumours, derived from the ependymal lining cells, which present at any age but are most common in the first and second decades of life. They account for 4–9% of neuroepithelial tumours. They occur at any site along the ventricular system, most commonly in the 4th ventricle in children and the cervical spine or conus medullaris in adults.

Pathology

They are well-defined but can encase peripheral nerves when they grow laterally from the 4th ventricle. Characteristic histological features are the formation of pseudorosettes, the concentric arrangement of ependymal cells around a vessel. Fibrillary glial processes of ependymal cells radiate to centrally located vessels and form a nuclei-free area, which creates this distinctive histological appearance. There are further variants of ependymoma which are named according to prevailing features such as cellular, papillary, clear cell and tanycytic but these distinctions have little or no clinical importance. A distinct variant is the WHO Grade I myxopapillary ependymoma of the spinal filum terminale.

Grade II ependymomas are well defined, show monomorphic nuclei and rare mitotic activity while Grade III (anaplastic) ependymomas show increased cellularity, increased mitotic rate and often vascular proliferation and necrosis. In adults, ependymomas account for about 2% of all intracranial tumours and are associated with a high survival rate compared with other glial tumours (5 and 10-year survival 85% and 76%, respectively). Overall survival correlates well with histological grade, extent of resection, age and performance status.

Molecular genetics of ependymomas Despite histological similarities, ependymomas arising from the spinal cord and the infratentorial and supratentorial compartments of the CNS show diverse clinical behaviour. Using unsupervised clustering, two distinct molecular subtypes of infratentorial ependymoma were identified. These correlated by differences in progression-free survival and overall survival. Expression of the markers laminin alpha 2 (LAMA2) and neural epidermal growth like factor 2 (NELL2) in the transcriptome subgroups showed the following pattern: LAMA2 is over expressed in Group A ependymomas, occur in younger patients (mainly children) and have a better progression free and overall survival and a longer time to metastasis. Group A ependymomas often have Chr 1q amplifications. NELL2 expression is significantly higher in Group B ependymomas, with poorer progression-free survival, overall survival and shorter time to metastasise.

Imaging

Ependymomas (WHO Grades II and III) in the brain are usually intraventricular, although extraventricular rests of ependymal cells may also give rise to hemisphere tumours. They are well-demarcated lobulated mass lesions with calcification on CT in over 50% and mixed signal intensity on MRI (predominantly hyperintense on T2 and isointense to hypointense on T1 images). Enhancement is mild to moderate and often heterogeneous.

Treatment

All patients should have staging with MRI of the whole cranio-spinal axis and CSF obtained either preoperatively or more commonly 2 weeks post surgery. The goal of surgery for ependymomas is gross total resection, which is achievable in 70–90% of cases, and should be confirmed with an early postoperative scan (<24 hours). The rates of long-term tumour control are high after gross total resection. Radiotherapy is typically indicated for subtotally resected tumours, irrespective of grade and for completely resected anaplastic ependymomas. Cranio-spinal treatment is now only used now for patients with disseminated disease as evidenced by MRI 'drop metastases' or positive CSF, as the risk of relapse down the cranio-spinal axis for local disease is less than 3%. Areas of bulky disease can be boosted to 50 Gy for spinal metastases or to 55–60 Gy for primary tumours and brain metatases. Chemotherapy with cisplatin and/or etoposide may be indicated for relapsed disease but is not usually effective. In rare cases of localised relapse, radiosurgery or re-irradiation may be considered on a case by case basis.

Dermoids and epidermoid cysts

These are cystic lesions arising from inclusion of ectodermal tissue during neural tube development and sequestration cysts which may accompany dysraphism (e.g. spina bifida) with communication to the skin surface through a sinus tract. Dermoid cysts contain hair follicles, sweat glands and sebaceous glands. They arise in the posterior fossa in the region of the midline, vermis or 4th ventricle or in the suprasellar cistern and present with local mass effects or by rupture of their contents into the CSF causing granulomatous meningitis. Management is by total surgical excision. Incompletely resected cysts may recur.

Epidermoid cysts are more common and arise in the cerebello-pontine angle or middle cranial fossa causing mass effect, facial pain and cranial nerve deficits. Surgical removal of epidermoid cysts may be difficult because of their tendency to spread along cranial nerves but is usually curative. Very rarely epidermoid cysts undergo malignant transformation.

Imaging

Intracranial dermoid cysts lie usually near the midline and contain all skin elements, including fat, which appears as very low density on CT and high signal intensity on MR T1 images. Epidermoid cysts, formerly known as pearly tumours, grow slowly over many years by accumulating desquamated epithelium. They conform to the contour of the subarachnoid space they occupy, sometimes invaginating into the brain parenchyma. On CT and standard T1 and T2 MRI, epidermoid cysts are non-enhancing lesions of signal intensity to CSF, a reason why they can be confused with arachnoid cysts. DWI easily distinguishes epidermoid tumours from arachnoid cysts, as water diffusion is markedly restricted in the former but not in the latter (Figure 21.34).

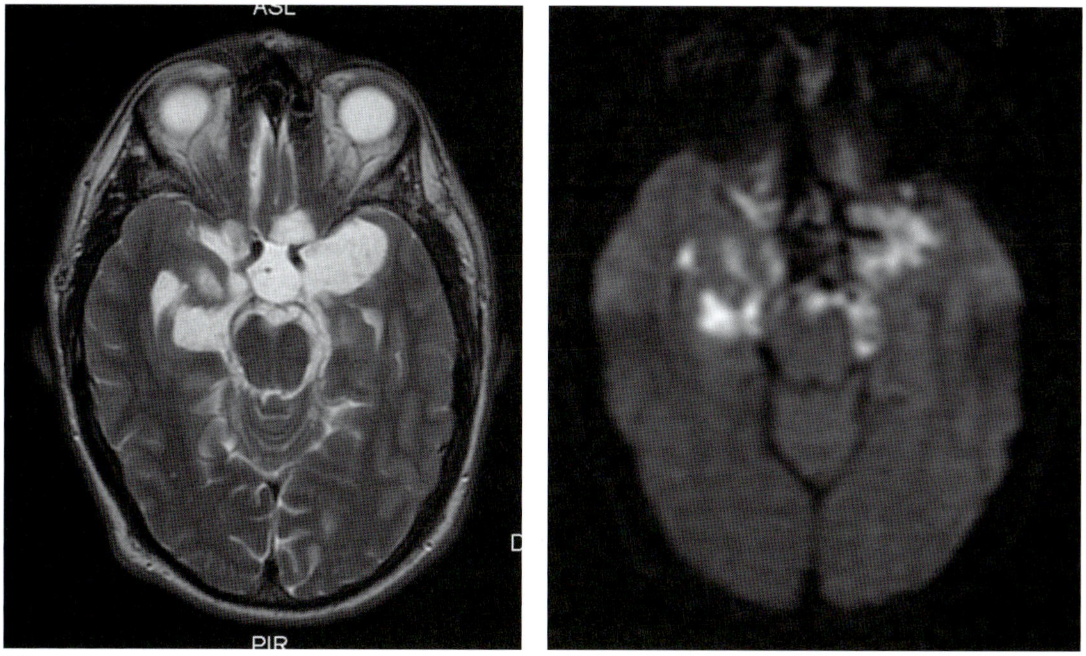

(a) (b)

Figure 21.34 (a) T2 image of an extensive epidermoid tumour spreading through the basal cisterns and invading the temporal lobes. (b) Diffusion-weighted image of the epidermoid tumour: characteristically bright and well delineated from surrounding CSF and brain parenchyma.

Haemangioblastomas

These are benign, cystic, highly vascular tumours. They are formed by vessels that range in size from small capillaries to large vessels and there may be one or more associated cysts. They generally arise in the posterior fossa and cause symptoms either because of raised intracranial pressure or cerebellar dysfunction. Less commonly there may be brainstem involvement leading to motor and sensory deficits. Polycythaemia may occur in 10% of patients from tumour production of erythropoietin. They may also arise within the spinal cord causing radicular pain, posterior column loss and pyramidal involvement with weakness, spasticity and bladder disturbance. There may be an associated cavity within the cord and clinical syringomyelia. Rarely, haemangiomas arise supratentorially.

Haemangioblastomas are most commonly associated with von Hippel–Landau (VHL) syndrome (Chapter 26). This condition is caused by a germ line defect in a tumour suppressor gene on chromosome 3p25. VHL is associated with multiple haemangiomas which may be asymptomatic. There is also retinal angiomatosis, renal cell carcinoma, visceral cysts and phaeochromocytoma.

Haemangioblastomas are relatively sharply demarcated: invasion and remote metastases are rare. Surgical resection is generally possible and total resection curative. Residual or inoperable tumours may be treated with external beam radiotherapy or stereotactic radiosurgery. The overall outcome is good with 5-year survival of 75%, particularly with small tumours and complete surgical removal. Screening for VHL is necessary in all patients with haemangioblastoma.

Colloid cysts, Rathke's pouch tumours and neuro-enteric cysts

These benign cystic lesions represent developmental malformations. The cysts are lined by columnar, mucin-producing epithelial cells which resemble respiratory or enteric lining. Colloid cysts are characteristically located in the roof of the 3rd ventricle and may block the foramen of Monro leading to obstructive hydrocephalus. Characteristically, this may be postural with intermittent headache and drop attacks. Rathke's pouch cysts arise in the sellar region. Neuro-enteric cysts arise in the spinal cord or within the brain. Imaging shows isodense or hypodense lesions on CT and MRI. Symptomatic lesions require surgical excision and a ventriculoperitoneal shunt may be necessary if there is hydrocephalus.

Neurological complications of cancer

Neurological complications of cancer (NCC) are common, serious, potentially disabling and often treatable when correctly diagnosed. The most frequent neurological complaints in patients with cancer overall are pain, confusion, headache and weakness. NCC are common reasons for admission to hospital. Many oncologists have had little formal training in neurological assessment. Many neurologists see relatively few cancer patients and are unlikely to know in detail the recent advances in cancer management and the way in which the nervous system can be affected by them, especially neurotoxicity of modern biological agents. Radiation treatment can lead to delayed neurological problems which may emerge years after the original treatment, possibly when the original cancer has been cured. It is thus essential that neurologists have a broad overview of NCC in order to focus on the differential diagnosis and appropriate tests, that they can gain access to specialist neuro-oncologcial advice, often in liaison with an oncologist. Table 21.8 outlines the main neurological problems in cancer patients.

Table 21.8 Neurological complications of cancer.

Direct effects
Infiltration by primary tumour or draining lymph nodes: e.g.
Nasopharyngeal carcinoma – multiple cranial nerve palsies
Lung cancer, e.g. Pancoast tumour causing T1 radiculopathy with Horner's
Breast cancer – brachial plexus lesions
Metastases
Brain
Skull base and vault
Dura
Spinal cord – extradural, intradural, intramedullary
Leptomeninges (malignant meningitis)
Brachial and lumbar plexus
Perineural
Indirect effects
Metabolic encephalopathies (e.g. hyponatraemia due to SIADH)
Vascular disorders (e.g. hypercoagulable states, haemorrhage and non-bacterial thrombotic endocarditis)
CNS infections
Paraneoplastic neurological disorders
Unwanted effects of treatment
Chemotherapy neurotoxicity
Radiotherapy neurotoxicity
Intrathecal administration
Compression neuropathies (e.g. after surgery)

SIADH, syndrome of inappropriate antidiuretic hormone.

As with any neurological presentation, the history is key. With respect to patients with known cancer the following points should be ascertained: details of the histology and staging (Tumour Node Metastasis) of the primary tumour, site, presence of known metastases, treatment received to date including hormonal treatments and current medication, both for the cancer, for pain and any other symptoms (e.g. vomiting).

Direct effects and infiltration

The majority of NCC are caused by direct invasion of the nervous system or metastatic spread. This is usually easily diagnosed clinically and/or with appropriate imaging. As the sensitivity of imaging increases, it has become evident that the highest resolution imaging is frequently needed to reach a diagnosis. MRI with contrast enhancement or PET may well be necessary if less sophisticated imaging is negative. Although there are common patterns of tumour spread (e.g. bony metastases with breast, bronchus, prostate, kidney and thyroid cancer), almost any malignancy can spread anywhere within the neuraxis.

Invasion or compression of neurological structures occurs when a primary or secondary tumour or draining lymph node is in direct contact with a nerve, nerve root, spinal cord or brain. Tumour invasion of nerve roots is sometimes associated with severe pain: this may be helpful to differentiate malignant infiltration from effects of

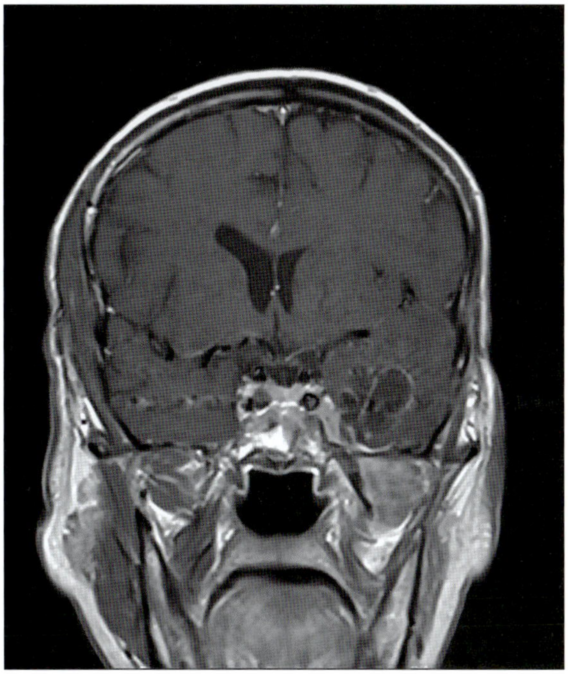

Figure 21.35 Perineural spread. Coronal T1-weighted post gadolinium images of squamous cell carcinoma extending across the base of skull into the left cavernous sinus and intradurally into the left temporal lobe. Note high signal change within left pterygoid resulting from denervation.

previous treatment. In some cases (e.g. Pancoast tumour), neurological symptoms of radiculopathy can be the presenting complaint. Less commonly, microscopic growth of tumour cells, particularly lymphoma along nerve sheaths, occurs after the primary tumour has been treated. Examples of direct perineural invasion include multiple cranial nerve palsies with nasopharyngeal carcinoma or squamous cell head and neck cancer (Figure 21.35), brachial plexopathy from breast cancer in the axillary tail, T1 radiculopathy with Horner's syndrome from apical lung cancer (Pancoast's syndrome) and, in children, paraganglioma and/or neuroblastoma causing spinal cord compression via paravertebral spread through the neural foramina into the epidural space.

Metastases

Metastases are a major cause of neurological problems in patients with cancer. They are commonly fatal when they involve the CNS. They occur by haematogenous spread, the usual mechanism of brain metastases; by lymphatic dissemination, usually to peripheral nerves; or by dissemination through the CSF, producing leptomeningeal metastases. The likelihood of metastasis increases with increasing primary tumour size and the duration of patient survival following treatment to the primary site. The site to which a tumour metastasises depends on the anatomy of the venous and lymphatic drainage of the organ harbouring the tumour, the micro-environment of the receiving organ and the molecular phenotype of the tumour, particularly the propensity to express surface adhesion molecules. As an example, colorectal cancer usually metastases to the posterior fossa and prostate cancer to the epidural space via Batson's venous plexus, a system of paravertebral veins that connect pelvic and thoracic vessels to the intraspinal veins.

Malignant meningitis

Malignant meningitis (MM) is one of the most sinister complications of any cancer, occurring in 3–8% of patients often at the later stages of the disease but occasionally presenting in a patient with no known tumour. The median survival is typically 2–3 months, although patients with breast cancer can survive for up to 2 years, as this is a more chemosensitive tumour. MM is becoming more frequent because of the improved prognosis of patients with systemic cancer and earlier diagnosis with MRI. It is characterised by invasion of the leptomeninges and/or CSF by cancer cells and can affect either brain, the spinal cord and nerve roots. Tumours that commonly cause MM are lung and breast cancer, melanoma and leukaemia/lymphoma, where bloodstream spread is the route into the CNS. However, almost any tumour can cause MM, including colorectal and urogenital cancer. MM occurs, if rarely, as a complication of primary brain tumours. This is seen in paediatric practice with medulloblastomas, ependymomas and oligodendrogliomas and in adult practice in the terminal stages of glioblastoma.

In adult practice, breast is the most common solid tumour associated with MM followed by lung cancer, both small cell and non-small cell. In some 5% of these cases, the patient presents *de novo* with MM. In some cases the primary may never be found. Although haematogenous invasion is the most common route for cancer cells to reach the leptomeninges, direct invasion from metastases in contact with the meninges (i.e dural), subdural and intraparenchymal metastases and perineural invasion occurs. Iatrogenic seeding during surgical resection of posterior fossa metastases has even been implicated in the pathogenesis of MM.

Clinical features

MM can present with cerebral, cranial nerve, spinal and/or radicular symptoms and signs (Table 21.9), either in isolation or as a multifocal process. The initial symptoms are often vague: unexplained nausea, vomiting, drowsiness and intermittent confusion. Patients may then develop combinations of cranial nerve palsies, sensorineural deafness, papilloedema resulting from communicating hydrocephalus, seizures or patchy radiculopathy. Patients should be asked about numb patches in the body and examined for evidence of nerve root involvement.

Diagnosis

Gadolinium-enhanced MRI provides the most sensitive imaging modality. Abnormal enhancement, which may be linear or nodular, is seen in 70% of patients with MM, compared to about 30% with contrast-enhanced CT. Linear enhancement may be seen in cerebral sulci and within the ponto-medullary cisterns. This gives rise to a characteristic pattern of sugar coating of the brainstem, within the cerebellar folia or along the spinal cord appearing as tramlines over the cord or nodular meningeal deposits (Figure 21.36). Communicating hydrocephalus occurs in 10% of patients. A meningitic syndrome is sometimes seen but not commonly. Many MM patients simply feel generally unwell. Imaging should always be carried out prior to lumbar puncture as the procedure itself may lead to artefactual meningeal enhancement. In contrast to its role in diagnosis, MRI is of little use for monitoring the response to therapy.

CSF examination with cytology of a large volume (at least 10 mL) of fluid is the single most useful investigation both for diagnosis and monitoring treatment. CSF biochemistry is nearly always abnormal in MM irrespective of the CSF cytology. Abnormalities include raised CSF protein (usually <2 g/dL except in cases of spinal block),

Table 21.9 Clinical presentations of malignant meningitis.

Location in neuraxis	Symptoms	Signs
Cerebral	Headache, nausea and vomiting	Papilloedema
	Cognitive changes, impaired consciousness	Encephalopathy
	Gait problems	Hemiparesis, ataxia
	Seizures	
	Focal deficits	
Cranial nerves	Diplopia	III, IV, VI lesions
	Visual loss	Optic neuropathy
	Facial weakness/numbness	V, VII lesions
	Deafness/vertigo	Sensorineural hearing loss, nystagmus
	Dysphagia, dysarthria	IX, X, XII nerve lesions
Spinal cord and roots	Back/neck/radicular pain	Nuchal rigidity
	Weakness	LMN weakness, reflex asymmetry
	Patches of numbness	Dermatomal sensory loss
	Sphincter dysfunction	e.g. Urinary incontinence, constipation

LMN, lower motor neurone.

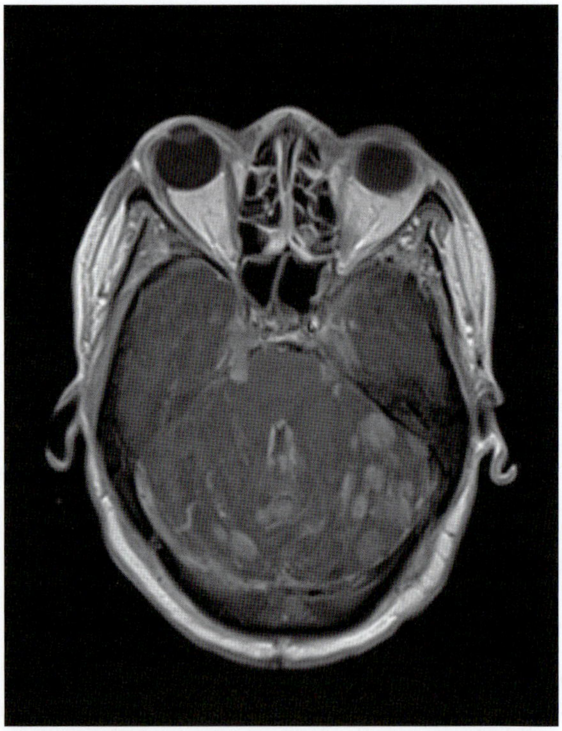

Figure 21.36 Malignant meningitis. Axial T1-weighted image post gadolinium showing extensive nodular leptomeningeal enhancement from metastatic breast cancer.

low CSF : plasma glucose ratio and elevated CSF white count. There is little correlation between CSF white cell count and the likelihood of detecting malignant cells. Sensitivity of CSF cytology rises from 65% after one lumbar puncture to 90% after three punctures. Ideally, fluid should be taken to the cytology laboratory immediately after collection in order to minimise cell autolysis. Certain tumours (e.g. leukaemias) are more likely to shed cells into the CSF than others – in cytology negative cases flow cytometry using specific lymphoma markers may be helpful in suggesting the diagnosis. There is no benefit in measuring tumour markers within the CSF.

Treatment

Treatment of MM is solely palliative. Thus, the decision to treat a patient with MM and metastatic disease depends on the patient's tumour status in the rest of the body and their overall physical condition. In general, MM once diagnosed has a median survival of 2–6 months. Particularly poor prognostic factors include low performance status, presence of encephalopathy and melanoma/lung cancer/brain tumour as the primary. Patients with breast cancer and MM have a median survival of 7.5 months and are therefore more often eligible for aggressive treatment.

Corticosteroids, non-steroidal anti-inflammatory drugs and opiates form the basis of palliative treatment. Anticonvulsants may be needed. Cranio-spinal radiotherapy is rarely indicated because of significant morbidity associated with treatment, particularly myelosuppression and the time taken for planning and carrying out treatment. More commonly, radiotherapy is used for treatment of isolated sites of symptomatic bulky disease, particularly in the posterior fossa and spinal cord.

Drug therapy, when appropriate, consists of systemic and intrathecal chemotherapy and hormonal therapy (e.g. tamoxifen for breast cancer). Systemic chemotherapy is often ineffective because of difficulties in achieving significant levels of cytotoxic drug within the CSF and the intrinsic chemoresistance of the underlying primary tumour. It is limited largely to treatment of chemosensitive tumours such as breast cancer and lymphoma. High dose methotrexate (3–8 g/m^2) or cytarabine (3 g/m^2) produce high enough serum levels to allow for therapeutic levels in the CSF, despite their low permeability.

Intrathecal chemotherapy via an Ommaya reservoir connected to the lateral ventricles or via repeated lumbar punctures is usually reserved for patients with good performance status and no or limited evidence of systemic disease. It is not useful in patients with bulky tumour deposits or where there is partial or complete obstruction to CSF flow. In cases of doubt, CSF flow studies may be helpful in evaluating CSF dynamics. It is debatable whether intrathecal chemotherapy offers any advantages over standard therapy for breast cancer and so is rarely used by medical oncologists.

The most commonly used intrathecal drugs are methotrexate and cytarabine, active against leukaemia and lymphoma, and methotrexate and thiotepa for breast cancer. Cytarabine is now available in a depot liposomal formulation which reduces the need for lumbar punctures from two per week to one every 2 weeks. None of these agents has intrinsic activity against melanoma and lung cancer. Novel agents that have been used intrathecally include topotecan and gemcitabine. The most serious toxicity is acute aseptic meningitis, which can be treated or prevented by corticosteroids.

Indirect effects of cancer

Toxic and metabolic encephalopathy

Toxic and metabolic encephalopathy is a frequent occurrence in cancer patients, particularly in the terminal phases, and presents when fully developed with delirium or an acute confusional state. There are numerous causes (Table 21.10). A thorough evaluation is required: many causes are reversible. The earliest manifestations are subtle deficits of concentration and attention which progress through towards inappropriate behaviour, cognitive disturbance and into a full-blown state of delirium, characterised by either a state of lethargy and apathy (quiet delirium) or by hyperactivity and restlessness, similar to that seen in the delirium tremens of alcohol withdrawal. These symptoms may be initially mistaken for anxiety and depression, particularly as neurological signs are often absent and rarely focal. The neurological examination reveals deficits in orientation, attention, concentration and language, short-term memory problems and visuo-spatial disorientation. Tremor, myoclonus and asterixis are also sometimes seen. Investigation of these patients consists of excluding a primary neurological cause such as brain metastases or MM and identifying any treatable extracerebral or metabolic condition. A careful drug history is mandatory.

Table 21.10 Causes of toxic/metabolic encephalopathy with cancer.

Tumour	Brain or meningeal metastases
Drugs	Opioids, benzodiazepines, corticosteroids, chemotherapy
Infections	Pneumonia, UTI, intra-abdominal abscess, CNS infection
Hypoxia	Pneumonia, pulmonary emboli
Electrolytes	Hypercalcaemia, hyponatraemia, hypophosphataemia
Endocrine	Adrenal insufficiency (e.g. rapid steroid withdrawal)
Hepato-renal	Uraemia, hepatic failure
Nutritional	Thiamine deficiency (Wernicke's encephalopathy)
Unrelated	Alcohol or drug abuse or withdrawal, cardiac/respiratory co-morbidity

UTI, urinary tract infection.

Vascular disorders

Cerebrovascular problems are relatively common in cancer patients. They are brought about either by direct effects of a tumour and/or its treatment on blood vessels, or by a coagulopathy caused indirectly by the neoplasm. Cerebral haemorrhage can be the presenting symptom of a primary intracranial tumour or, more commonly, metastases, particularly from melanoma, extracranial germ cell tumours and rarely colonic carcinoma. The most common primary brain tumours associated with intra-tumoral haemorrhage are oligodendrogliomas, glioblastomas and germ cell tumours. Bleeding is also sometimes seen in meningiomas, medulloblastomas, choroid plexus papillomas and ependymomas. Intracerebral haemorrhage can also follow thrombocytopaenia caused by either tumour or leukaemic invasion of bone marrow, chemotherapy or radiotherapy.

A hypercoagulable state leading to arterial or venous thrombosis is sometimes seen in patients with widespread metastatic disease caused by multiple pro-coagulant effects of cancer on platelet function and coagulation factors. This was first described in 1865 by Trousseau who noted accelerated clotting times and thrombophlebitis in more than 60% of the cancer patients he saw. Haemostatic abnormalities occur in more than 90% of cancer patients, most commonly presenting as deep vein thrombosis or disseminated intravascular coagulation (DIC) with depletion of platelets and clotting factors. In general, venous thrombo-embolism is more frequent in solid tumours while DIC causes both venous and arterial occlusions and is seen in widespread metastatic cancer and haematological malignancies. Occasionally, drug therapy causes abnormal coagulation (e.g. cerebral vein thrombosis associated with L-asparaginase in acute leukaemia). Rarer causes of cerebral infarction include tumour emboli (usually intracardiac tumours such as atrial myxoma), non-bacterial thrombotic endocarditis (NBTE) and cerebral vasculitis. A diffuse brain syndrome with multiple small infarcts can develop. Occlusion of venous sinuses may also result from compression or invasion by metastatic tumour, particularly breast cancer and lymphoma. Other causes of hypercoagulability include hyperfibrinogenaemia, seen in some 50% of cancer patients, and antiphospholipid syndrome.

Non-bacterial thrombotic endocarditis

This form of endocarditis, also known as marantic endocarditis, is a rare but well-recognised cause of ischaemic stroke in the cancer population, particularly patients with mucinous adenocarcinomas from the lung, pancreas, stomach and ovary. This condition is poorly understood. NBTE results from predisposition for platelets and fibrin plugs to deposit on cardiac valves, usually aortic and mitral, giving rise to sterile vegetations, which can cause arterial emboli. One-third of patients with NBTE have a purely neurological presentation either with a diffuse encephalopathy, focal signs, including transient ischaemic attacks or rarely spinal cord infarction. Coagulation testing is usually normal although a few cases have evidence of DIC. In some cases, NBTE may precede the diagnosis of malignancy and can thus be the first presentation of an occult tumour. Treatment is directed to the underlying cause. Anticogulation is rarely helpful and carries substantial risks of haemorrhage.

CNS infections in cancer patients

Infections of the CNS occur more frequently in patients with cancer than in the general population. They are one of the least common neurological complications of cancer and are usually seen in patients with haematological malignancies. Nevertheless, they are important to keep in mind because these patients rarely have the florid symptoms and signs of infection seen in immunocompetent patients. The most common presentation of CNS infection in a cancer patient is simply an altered mental state with headache and fever. Neck stiffness can be mild or absent. There should be a low threshold for imaging and lumbar puncture in such patients presenting with drowsiness and irritability. The causative organisms are different from those in the general population. In some 40% of patients, multiple pathogens infect the CNS simultaneously. *Cryptococcus neoformans* and *Listeria monocytogenes* are the major causes of meningitis in cancer patients while enteric Gram-negative bacilli, *Toxoplasma gondii, Aspergillus fumigatus* and *Nocardia asteroides* are major causes of brain abscesses. Gram-negative organisms such as *Pseudomonas aeruginosa* and *Escherichia coli* are common causes of meningitis in neutropenic patients: the paranasal sinuses should always be considered as possible sources of CNS infection. Accurate microbiological diagnosis is essential in order to institute vigorous and appropriate antibiotic therapy. Despite this, treatment of CNS infections in this patient group is far less successful than in immunocompetent patients. There is a mortality of some 85% in neutropenic patients with CNS infection. Survival depends on bone marrow recovery in addition to correct antibiotic treatment. Even when antibiotic treatment cures the infection, relapse and superinfection are common. The treatment of individual infections is discussed in Chapter 9.

Paraneoplastic neurological disorders

Paraneoplastic neurological disorders (PND) are uncommon neurological complications of cancer. They are important because they frequently present before the malignancy becomes symptomatic, because they cause severe neurological disability and because of the putative immunological mechanism by which some forms of PND have been shown to arise. Tumours can cause neurological symptoms through indirect mechanisms such as hyponatraemia and hypercalcaemia. However, the term paraneoplastic is usually reserved for disorders thought to be caused by autoimmune attack triggered by tumour antigens against nervous system components. Because PND are much less common than direct, metastatic and treatment-related complications of cancer, a neurological condition should only be regarded as paraneoplastic if a particular neoplasm associates with a remote but specific effect on the nervous system more frequently than would be expected by chance. For example, subacute cerebellar ataxia in the setting of ovarian cancer is sufficiently characteristic to be called paraneoplastic cerebellar degeneration (PCD), so long as other causes have been excluded. Conversely, carpal tunnel syndrome in a cancer patient is not paraneoplastic because both conditions, being reasonably common, are likely to coexist. In patients without known cancer, the more common causes of neurological problems such as inflammatory and/or autoimmune conditions and hitherto undiagnosed tumours or metastases should be excluded before concluding that a patient is likely to have a PND.

Incidence and prevalence

The precise incidence and prevalence of PND in the overall cancer population remains largely unknown. Certain common cancers that frequently associate with PND (e.g. SCLC), have been extensively investigated, but the majority of studies tend to concentrate on specific antineuronal antibodies and their neurological and tumour associations rather than provide prospective data on PND frequency.

The incidence of PND depends on the stringency of criteria used. In one early systematic study of PND, the term carcinomatous neuromyopathy was used to describe cancer patients with a combination of neuromuscular abnormalities, usually proximal muscle weakness, ataxia and distal sensory loss. Some 4% of women with breast cancer, 7% of patients with all cancers and 16% of men with lung cancer had evidence of PND compared with 2% of age-matched controls. The most frequent PND is Lambert–Eaton myasthenic syndrome (LEMS): this occurs in 2–3% of patients with SCLC. Overall, PND affect less than 1% of all patients with cancer. Cerebellar degeneration with ovarian cancer is the next most common form of PND occurring in about 1% of cases.

The median age of onset of PND is over 60 years. Less than 10% of cases are in those under 50 years. PND occur relatively rarely in young people – except with the typical tumours of the 20–40 age group – Hodgkin's disease (PCD), testicular cancer (brainstem and limbic encephalitis), breast cancer (many different syndromes) and in children, neuroblastoma (opsoclonus-myoclonus). The sex ratio of patients with PND is variable and probably depends on the underlying syndrome. In most studies there is a female preponderance of around 3 : 1 which cannot be accounted for by association with breast and ovarian gynaecological cancer alone.

Detailed long-term observational data for PND are not available. Response to treatment is frequently disappointing but LEMS may respond well. Spontaneous resolution of PND has occasionally been reported. PND cause serious disability. Most patients who do not succumb to either the neurological syndrome or the underlying tumour usually remain dependent on their carers.

Clinical features

PND are summarised in an anatomical classification in Table 21.11. Some CNS syndromes such as cerebellar degeneration are typically focal at presentation but frequently progress to involve other anatomical structures. Other PND are characterised by patterns of widespread dysfunction early on, for example the combination of limbic encephalitis of the medial temporal lobes and projections with a sensory neuropathy affecting dorsal root ganglia. As more antibodies are recognised, the range of PND phenotypes is ever widening. Atypical forms (e.g. parkinsonism and other movement disorders) are being reported increasingly.

PND usually begin abruptly and present within days to weeks, progressing rapidly. Stroke-like presentations are seen; imaging is usually negative. Most patients become significantly disabled within a few weeks of onset and then plateau. Urgent investigation is indicated, especially in CNS syndromes, so that tumour therapy is started early to prevent progressive neuronal death and irreversible disability. Less frequently, patients may develop a second PND clinically different from the first.

There are no unique clinical features that define a syndrome as paraneoplastic but certain clinical syndromes in association with

Table 21.11 Classification of paraneoplastic neurological disorders by anatomical location within the nervous system.

Site	Syndrome	Typical primary tumours
Brain	Cerebellar degeneration	SCLC, breast, ovarian, Hodgkin's disease
Brain	Limbic encephalitis	SCLC, ovarian teratoma, testicular tumours
Brainstem	Brainstem encephalitis	SCLC
Brain and cord	Encephalomyelitis with rigidity	Breast, SCLC
Brain	Opsoclonus-myoclonus	SCLC, neuroblastoma, breast
Retina	Retinopathy	SCLC
Cord	Necrotising myelopathy	Any
Cord and anterior horn cells	Motor neurone syndromes	Any
Dorsal root ganglia	Sensory neuronopathy	SCLC
Motor neurones	Subacute motor neuronopathy	Non-Hodgkin's lymphoma
Peripheral nerves	Vasculitic neuropathy	B-cell lymphoma
Peripheral nerves and roots	Acute inflammatory demyelinating polyradiculoneuropathy (as Guillain–Barré syndrome)	Hodgkin's disease
Peripheral nerves	Sensory/sensorimotor neuropathy	Any
Peripheral nerves	Mononeuritis multiplex	Any
Autonomic system	Autonomic neuropathy	SCLC
Peripheral nerves	Neuromyotonia	SCLC
Gut	Neurogastrointestinal enteropathy	SCLC
Neuromuscular junction	Lambert–Eaton myasthenic syndrome	SCLC
Neuromuscular junction	Myasthenia gravis	Thymoma
Muscle	Polymyositis and dermatomyositis	Any
Muscle	Acute necrotising myopathy	Any

SCLC, small cell lung cancer.

tumours are so recognisable as to be called classic. A recent study carried out by the PNS Euronetwork consortium of 979 patients found that 78% of patients had such classic syndromes, the most frequent being paraneoplastic cerebellar degeneration, sensory neuronopathy and limbic encephalitis. These well-recognised syndromes are as follow:

1 Encephalomyelitis
2 Limbic encephalitis
3 Subacute cerebellar degeneration
4 Opsoclonus-myoclonus
5 Sensory neuronopathy (dorsal root ganglionopathy)
6 Lambert–Eaton myasthenic syndrome
7 Dermatomyositis
8 Chronic gastrointestinal pseudo-obstruction.

Paraneoplastic cerebellar degeneration

Patients with paraneoplastic cerebellar degeneration (PCD) typically present with the subacute onset of disequilibrium with increasing ataxia of gait, trunk and limbs. Complex eye movement abnormalities are seen with combinations of disordered pursuit movements, multi-directional nystagmus (often down-beating) and gaze palsies. Severe disability develops rapidly with dysphagia and dysarthria. The condition usually stabilises within 6 months although PCD sometimes evolves into a multi-focal neurological degeneration particularly in patients with anti-Hu antibodies. PCD occurs in a variety of tumours, most commonly ovarian and breast cancer, lung cancer and Hodgkin's disease. Tumours, if not previously diagnosed, usually appear within weeks to months of the onset of symptoms, although there may be a lead time bias because of the neurological diagnosis prompting a search for an underlying tumour.

Long intervals between PCD and tumour appearance are rarely seen, for example PCD with characteristic clinical features and high titre anti-Yo antibodies has been diagnosed 13 years before breast cancer became evident. Occasionally, PCD occurs after tumour diagnosis and treatment and in the case of Hodgkin's disease may be a harbinger of relapse.

A diagnosis of PCD is usually suspected when imaging of the posterior fossa is unremarkable in the presence of severe cerebellar ataxia. Unusual imaging abnormalities include diffuse oedema of the cerebellum and very early cerebellar atrophy. In PCD, the cerebellum gradually becomes atrophic, over months. Other investigations (e.g. CSF examination) are rarely helpful but are useful to rule out leptomeningeal metastases which can occasionally cause isolated gait ataxia. CSF oligoclonal bands are usually positive in PCD.

The diagnosis of PCD is usually supported by finding antineuronal antibodies, specifically anti-Yo (38%), anti-Hu (32%), anti-Tr (14%), anti-Ri (12%) and anti-mGluR (4%). In a study of PCD, the functional outcome was better with anti-Ri and anti-Tr and worse with anti-Yo and anti-Hu. Patients receiving antitumour treatment, with or without immunosuppressive therapy, lived significantly longer than those who remained untreated.

Pathologically there is severe and sometimes complete loss of cerebellar Purkinje cells with relatively minor thinning of the molecular layer. The deep cerebellar nuclei are spared except in cases of encephalomyelitis, when extensive inflammatory changes are seen.

Paraneoplastic encephalomyelitis and limbic encephalitis

Paraneoplastic encephalomyelitis (PEM) syndromes are one of the more common PND affecting the CNS and characterised by multi-focal inflammation with predilection for limbic and brainstem structures. This process may occur with or without sensory neuropathy, autonomic neuropathy and LEMS.

Limbic encephalitis is usually seen in association with SCLC and presents with personality changes, irritability, depression, seizures, memory loss and sometimes dementia. The majority of these patients have anti-Hu antibodies. The main finding on examination is severe impairment of episodic memory. This can improve with treatment of the underlying tumour. Investigations are usually non-specific – CSF may be inflammatory with pleocytosis and an elevated protein concentration. MRI may show high signal change within one or both medial temporal lobes. Epileptic discharges may be seen on EEG. Pathological changes affecting limbic and basal ganglia structures include neuronal cell loss, reactive microglial proliferation and peri-vascular lymphocytic infiltration. Other commonly associated tumours are testicular cancer (approximately 20%) and breast cancer (approximately 10%). Neurological symptoms precede cancer diagnosis in around half of cases by several months.

In one series over half of limbic encephalitis patients had antineuronal antibodies: most commonly, anti-Hu, anti-Ma1 and anti-Ma2. Anti-Hu antibodies usually associated with SCLC patients, multifocal neurological symptoms and a poor outcome. Patients with anti-Ma2 antibodies tend to be young men with testicular tumours, hypothalamic involvement and a poor outcome. In patients with neither anti-Hu nor anti-Ta antibodies, lung cancer remains the most common tumour.

Recent studies have identified new antibodies against cell surface antigens that are associated with diffuse and limbic encephalitis. The most frequent example is encephalitis associated with the NR1 subunit of the *N*-methyl-D-aspartate (NMDA) receptor (Chapter 20) which is characterised by dramatic neuropsychiatric presentation, limbic and then diffuse encephalitis, autonomic instability and stereotyped movement disorders particularly orofacial dyskinesias. Unlike the classic paraneoplastic syndromes, this disease most commonly occurs in young women with ovarian teratomas, and responds to immunotherapy. Occasionally, children may be affected and usually present with seizures and abnormal movements.

Brainstem encephalitis

Brainstem encephalitis accounts for some 15% of cases of PEM. The clinical syndrome is characterised by brainstem dysfunction, cranial nerve palsies, long tract signs and cerebellar ataxia. Less common features include movement disorders such as parkinsonism, chorea, jaw-opening dystonia and laryngospasm, the latter sometimes seen in association with anti-Ri antibodies. Occasionally, brainstem encephalitis can cause central alveolar hypoventilation with recurrent respiratory failure or coma. As with limbic encephalitis, imaging and CSF examination are usually non-specific. The diagnosis is usually confirmed by finding antineuronal antibodies. An important differential diagnosis is *Listeria monocytogenes* rhombencephalitis.

Paraneoplastic encephalomyelitis with rigidity

This rare syndrome causes truncal and limb rigidity, stimulus-sensitive myoclonus, painful spasms and brainstem and spinal cord inflammatory involvement. It is usually fatal. By contrast, the typical (non-paraneoplastic) stiff person syndrome with anti-GAD antibodies (Chapter 6), characterised by axial and proximal lower limb stiffness, spasms with continuous motor unit activity on EMG behaves in a more indolent fashion. However, typical stiff person syndrome may rarely be a presenting feature of breast cancer and associated with antiamphiphysin antibodies.

Paraneoplastic opsoclonus-myoclonus

Paraneoplastic opsoclonus-myoclonus (POM), often called dancing eyes syndrome, is a rare syndrome seen typically in young children with neuroblastoma. It also occurs in adults with breast cancer and SCLC. Dramatic, chaotic, saccadic, multi-directional eye movements (opsoclonus) are associated with myoclonus of the trunk, limbs and head including the diaphragm and palate. There is also cerebellar ataxia. This syndrome is associated with cancer in about 20% of adults. As with other PND affecting the CNS, routine investigations are usually normal or non-specifically abnormal. Several autoantibodies have been described in POM, particularly anti-Ri (breast, SCLC) and antineurofilament antibodies in children with neuroblastoma. POM can also follow viral infections, drug overdoese and as part of a post-infective encephalitis.

Paraneoplastic retinal degeneration

PND can cause visual failure. Retinal photoreceptors, rods, cones and optic nerves can all be affected. Paraneoplastic retinal degeneration, otherwise known as cancer-associated retinopathy, is usually seen in SCLC and gynaecological tumours and associated with antibodies against recoverin, a photoreceptor protein. Visual loss is painless, bilateral and presents with loss of colour vision, night blindness and initial photosensitivity. There is loss of visual acuity. Field testing shows peripheral and ring scotomas. There may be arteriolar narrowing and mottling of the fundus caused by changes in the retinal pigment epithelium.

Necrotising myelopathy

The spinal cord can be the main target of paraneoplastic autoimmunity, in most cases as part of an encephalomyelitis. Rarely, patients develop a rapidly progressive isolated necrotising myelopathy, characterised pathologically by extensive necrosis of both white and grey matter, most marked in the thoracic segments. This is usually associated with a CSF pleocytosis and extensive (more than three segments) T2 signal abnormality on MRI, with gadolinium enhancement. The most common antineuronal antibodies are antiamphiphysin and CV2 (CRMP5), associated with breast cancer and SCLC. The prognosis is very poor.

Motor neurone syndromes

There is controversy and generally doubt about whether typical motor neurone disease (MND) can be regarded as a paraneoplastic syndrome. However, three motor neurone syndromes are seen in patients with cancer. The first is a rapidly progressive MND-like condition with anti-Hu antibodies, presenting with subacute motor paralysis resulting from anterior horn cell damage (subacute motor neuronopathy). The second is primary lateral sclerosis with breast cancer, lymphoma and myeloma. The third is apparently typical MND developing some years after a diagnosis of cancer. It seems likely that the first two groups are indeed paraneoplastic: the third is probably not, reflecting the occurrence of two reasonably common diseases in the same patient.

Paraneoplastic sensory neuronopathy

Also known as dorsal root ganglionitis, paraneoplastic sensory neuropathy (PSN) causes subacute, rapidly progessive asymmetric and painful sensory symptoms dominated by severe proprioceptive loss, which affects upper limbs more than lower limbs. All sensory modalities are affected. In contrast, motor function is preserved. Nerve conduction studies show absent sensory action potentials but normal motor velocities. The CSF is typically inflammatory, particularly if the neuropathy is associated with encephalomyelitis. The differential diagnosis includes Sjögren's syndrome and cisplatin toxicity. The pathology centres on dorsal root ganglia where there are lymphocytic infiltrates and loss of ganglion cells.

Paraneoplastic neuropathies

The peripheral nervous system is more commonly involved by PND than the CNS. Distal, predominantly sensory neuropathies are seen frequently in cancer patients and are more commonly caused by metabolic, nutritional and treatment-related axonal degeneration than paraneoplastic disease. However, in any patient presenting with a severe peripheral, predominantly sensory neuropathy in whom standard investigations are negative, about 10% will eventually be diagnosed with cancer, particularly if there is rapid progression to severe disability and absence of regeneration in a sural nerve biopsy (Chapter 10).

Paraneoplastic neuropathies are clinical and immunologically heterogeneous and are associated with antineuronal antibodies in over 50% of cases. Anti-Hu antibodies are the most frequently identified. Patients with sensorimotor neuropathies also tend to have anti-CV2 antibodies in association with SCLC or high-titre antinuclear antibodies in association with breast cancer.

Sensory and sensorimotor neuropathy Paraneoplastic sensory and sensorimotor neuropathy is well recognised in many different cancers. Nerve conduction studies typically show a mixed sensory and motor axonal neuropathy. An occasional case may have typical demyelinating features and respond to intravenous immunoglobulin. Patients with an apparent chronic inflammatory demyelinating polyradiculoneuropathy with atypical features including resistance to first line treatments, an unusually aggressive course or the presence of myopathy and long tract signs should be investigated for an underlying cancer. The CSF is usually acellular in contrast with sensory neuropathy but the protein is usually raised. The unusual osteosclerotic form of myeloma can cause the combination of endocrine, dermatological and neurological features encapsulated within the acronym POEMS (polyneuropathy, organomegaly, endocrinopathy, M protein, skin changes). This neuropathy is typically demyelinating (Chapter 11).

Acute inflammatory demyelinating polyradiculoneuropathy Motor neuropathies are much less common than sensory neuropathies in paraneoplastic neurological disease. However, patients with Hodgkin's disease can present with acute inflammatory demyelinating polyradiculoneuropathy, a syndrome clinically and electrophysiologically indistinguishable from Guillain–Barré syndrome. Similarly, neuralgic amyotrophy (brachial plexitis) occasionally occurs in association with lymphoma, but a true paraneoplastic association is uncertain. Focal monomelic motor neuropathy has also been described.

Motor neuropathy A subacute lower motor neuropathy is occasionally seen with non-Hodgkin's lymphoma presenting as a slowly progressive lower motor neurone syndrome affecting the lower limbs.

Vasculitic neuropathy Vasculitis is occasionally associated with haematological malignancies and usually presents with rashes. Paraneoplastic vasculitic neuropathy has been described in patients with high grade B-cell lymphoma.

Autonomic neuropathy Paraneoplastic autonomic neuropathies are rare and patients present subacutely with gastrointestinal pseudo-obstruction, bladder dysfunction, orthostatic hypotension, labile blood pressure, pupillary abnormalities and pseudomotor dysfunction, impotence and xerophthalmia. Autonomic neuropathy can be the sole manifestation of an anti-Hu syndrome or part of a more widespread encephalomyelitis. In recent series of patients with anti-Hu antibodies, autonomic dysfunction was present in some 25% of cases and was the predominant symptom in approximately 5%.

Neuromyotonia

Neuromyotonia is a rare PND described with thymomas or SCLC. Muscle cramps, stiffness, twitching, sweating and abnormal relaxation after voluntary contraction occur. This is caused by hyperexcitability of peripheral nerve fibres. Electromyography shows abnormal doublet and triplet discharges with high intra-burst frequency as well as myokymic and neuromyotonic discharges. Fasciculations and fibrillation potentials are common.

Acquired neuromyotonia typically is not paraneoplastic but an immune-mediated disorder (Isaac's syndrome) with elevated antibody levels against presynaptic, voltage gated potassium channels. These antibodies may also be detected in the even rarer Morvan's syndrome, also non-paraneoplastic, characterised by neuromyotonia, hyperhidrosis, agitation, confusion and insomnia.

Lambert–Eaton myasthenic syndrome

LEMS (Chapter 10) is caused by SCLC in 60% of cases and is characterised by proximal weakness, predominantly affecting lower limbs in association with autonomic disturbance such as impotence, constipation and dry mouth. The paraneoplastic syndrome is usually more severe than the autoimmune form but is electrophysiologically indistinguishable. The characteristic finding, consistent with presynaptic neuromuscular dysfunction and impaired quantal release of neurotransmitter, is of small compound muscle action potentials that decrement at low-frequency stimulation but increment at high-frequency stimulation. The diagnosis of LEMS is confirmed by finding antibodies against P/Q type voltage gated calcium channels (VGCC). Some patients with LEMS also have a cerebellar syndrome – and some patients with cerebellar syndromes but without LEMS have anti-VGCC antibodies. A recent study of over 200 patients with LEMS identified seven clinical predictors of SCLC: age, smoking, weight loss, Karnofsky Performance Status, bulbar dysfunction, male impotence and Anti-SOX1 antibodies – a score higher than 3 indicated a probability of SCLC of greater than 80%. In new cases of LEMS, the current recommendation is screening for lung cancer for up to 2 years after diagnosis.

Myasthenia gravis

Myasthenis gravis is the prototypical autoimmune disease with antibodies to post-synaptic acetylcholine receptors at the neuromuscular junction. In some 10% of cases of myasthenis gravis there is an underlying thymoma. Myasthenis gravis can thus be considered a paraneoplastic condition. No other tumour is associated with myasthenis gravis.

Polymyositis and dermatomyositis

Polymyositis or dermatomyositis can be paraneoplastic conditions. In general, patients with paraneoplastic myositis are older and have a more severe course than their autoimmune counterparts. Dermatomyositis in the elderly is much more likely to be paraneoplastic than polymyositis in the same age group.

Acute necrotising myopathy

Acute necrotising myopathy is rare. It is proximal, rapidly progressive, associated with rhabdomyolysis and usually fatal.

Diagnosis of PND

Frequently, a PND will be suspected from the clinical features and confirmed by finding usually well-characterised paraneoplastic autoantibodies. A pattern of symptoms and signs can be diagnosed as possibly or definitely paraneoplastic using a descending hierarchy:

1 Presence or absence of known cancer
2 Presence or absence of a classic syndrome
3 Presence or absence of well-characterised antineuronal antibodies, and
4 Exclusion of other causes of a similar neurological syndrome, particularly malignant meningitis.

Paraneoplastic antineuronal autoantibodies

The detection of serum paraneoplastic antineuronal autoantibodies (PNA) is highly specific and forms the cornerstone of diagnosis of PND. Sensitivity varies between different syndromes. At best it is only 80–90% and therefore a diagnosis of PND cannot be excluded if PNA testing is negative. Tables 21.12 and 21.13 show the more common antineuronal antibodies, their clinical associations, immunohistochemical staining patterns and putative antigens. There is a bewildering array of PNA which can be divided into those against intracellular antigens (Table 21.12) and cell surface antigens (Table 21.13). It is therefore reassuring that a detailed knowledge of specific antibodies is rarely required as most laboratories test

Table 21.12 Well-characterised paraneoplastic autoantibodies against intracellular antigens and their clinical and immunological associations.

Antibody	Neurological syndrome	Immunohistochemistry	Western Blot	Antigen	Associated tumour
Hu (ANNA 1)	PEM/PSN, LE, PCD, LEMS, intestinal neuropathy	Neuronal nuclei in CNS and PNS	36–40 kD	Hu family triplet bands	SCLC, neuroblastoma, non-SCLC, prostate
Ri (ANNA 2)	POM, PEM, PCD	Neuronal nuclei in CNS	55 and 80 kD	Nova 1 and 2	Breast, SCLC, gynaecological
Yo (PCA 1)	PCD	Purkinje cell cytoplasm	34 and 62 kD	Cdr 1 and 2	Breast, ovary, uterus
Tr	PCD	Purkinje cell cytoplasm (molecular layer)	No reactive protein	DNER (delta/notch-like epidermal growth factor-related receptor)	Hodgkin's disease
Amphiphysin	Stiff person syndrome, rapidly progressive myelopathy	Synaptosomes	128 kD	Amphiphysin	Breast, SCLC
CV2/CRMP5	PEM, chorea, uveitis, optic neuropathy, intestinal neuropathy, chorea	Diffuse neuropil, cytoplasm of oligodendrocytes	66 kD	CRMP-5	SCLC, breast, thymoma
Ma	PEM, PCD, BE	Nuclei and cytoplasm	37 kD		Miscellaneous
Ma2 (Ta)	BE, LE, hypothalamic syndrome	Nucleolus, perikaryon	40 kD	Ma 2	Testicular cancer

BE, brainstem encephalitis; LE, limbic encephalitis; LEMS, Lambert–Eaton myasthenic syndrome; PCD, paraneoplastic cerebellar degeneration; PEM, paraneoplastic encephalomyelitis; POM, paraneoplastic opsoclonus/myoclonus; PSN, paraneoplastic sensory neuronopathy.

Table 21.13 Autoantibodies against cell surface or synaptic antigens associated with paraneoplastic neurological syndromes.

Antibody	Neurological syndrome	Immunohistochemistry	Antigen	Associated tumour
NMDA receptor	Diffuse encephalitis with prominent neuropsychiatric features, autonomic dysfunction, movement disorder	Hippocampal neurophil Membrane glutamate receptors Glial nuclei in cerebellum	NR1/NR2 heteromers	Ovarian teratoma
mGluR5	Limbic encephalitis	Membrane glutamate receptors	mGluR1	Hodgkin's disease (two cases reported)
mGluR1	Cerebellar ataxia	Membrane glutamate receptors	mGluR5	Hodgkin's disease (two cases reported)
$GABA_BR$	Limbic encephalitis	GABA receptors	GABA receptors	SCLC
CASPR2 (contactin associated protein 2)	Morvan's syndrome (neuromyotonia, muscle fasciculations, hyperhidrosis, insomnia, agitation and confusion)			Thymoma
AMPAR	Limbic encephalitis with prominent psychiatric symptoms and aggression	AMPA receptors	AMPA receptors	SCLC, breast, thymus

Table 21.14 Chemotherapy-related neurotoxicity.

Acute encephalopathy	Methotrexate, cisplatin, vincristine, asparaginase, ifosfamide
Chronic encephalopathy	Methotrexate, 5-fluorouracil/levamisole
Cerebellar syndrome	5-fluorouracil, cytosine arabinoside, ciclosporin, vincristine
Visual loss	Tamoxifen (retinopathy), cisplatin (cortical blindness)
Deafness	Cisplatin
Myelopathy/aseptic meningitis	Intrathecal methotrexate, cytosine arabinoside
Neuropathy	Vinca alkaloids, cisplatin, oxaliplatin, taxol

patients sera against crude homogenates of CNS tissue (usually rat or mouse) both by immunohistochemisty and Western immunoblotting. Further characterisation of the specific antigen can then be carried out using recombinant proteins.

Imaging

There is no single imaging modality that can identify a PND with a high degree of sensitivity and specificity. The role of MRI is predominantly to rule out structural disease. Body CT imaging of the thorax, abdomen and pelvis is used for detection of an underlying tumour. Whole body FDG-PET scanning is useful when conventional imaging is unremarkable or equivocal as it detects small (6–8 mm) tumours if metabolically active.

Treatment for PND

The treatment of PND is distinctly unsatisfactory. Early detection and treatment of the tumour seems to offer the greatest chance of stabilisation of PND. By contrast, immune-modulating therapies aimed at reducing levels of circulating antineuronal antibodies (e.g. plasma exchange, intravenous immunoglobulin, steroids and immunosuppressants) usually have no or modest effects on CNS syndromes, although they be helpful in LEMS (Chapter 10). Palliative symptom-directed therapy is usually the most appropriate management.

Neurological complications of chemotherapy

Many chemotherapeutic drugs are neurotoxic, causing particularly neuropathy and encephalopathy (Table 21.14). In many instances, diagnosis of treatment-induced disease is based on clinical experience and exclusion of other causes. Frequently, combination therapy causes previously unrecognised syndromes as some drugs act synergistically with others and with radiotherapy. Neurotoxicity from cancer chemotherapy tends to be frequent and severe in patients with pre-existing neurological disease.

Polyneuropathy

A pure sensory neuropathy, often painful, is most commonly associated with vinca alkaloids, taxol and cisplatin. Oxaliplatin, commonly used in metastatic colorectal cancer, causes a reversible syndrome characterised by tingling, painful dysaesthesiae on contact with cold, laryngospasm, thought to be caused by a reversible sodium channelopathy. It also causes a chronic sensory neuropathy or neuronopathy which may start some weeks after the end of chemotherapy. Motor neuropathies are rare but are occasionally seen with suramin and vincristine. They are usually reversible on cessation of the drug.

Encephalopathy

Almost any cancer chemotherapy can cause an acute encephalopathy characterised by seizures and confusion. The most notable example is the combination of methotrexate and cranial irradiation causing an irreversible leukoencephalopathy. Methotrexate can also cause an acute encephalopathy, mainly in children and teenagers, characterised initially by emotional lability and alternating hemiplegia such that the initial diagnosis is often thought to be psychogenic, particularly as standard MRI sequences are usually normal. However, high signal on diffusion-weighted imaging may occur confirming the diagnosis (Figure 21.20). Ifosfamide is the other drug, used mainly in the treatment of sarcomas, that can produce an encephalopathy.

Further reading

Epidemiology

Grant R. Overview: Brain tumour diagnosis and management/Royal College of Physicians Guidelines. *J Neurol Neurosurg Psychiatry* 2004; **75** (Suppl 2): 37–42.

Hardell L, Carlberg M, Sonderqvist F, Hansson Mild K. Case-control study of the association between malignant brain tumours diagnosed between 2007 and 2009 and mobile and cordless phone use. *Int J Oncol* 2013; **43:** 1833–1845.

Pobereskin LH, Chadduck JB. Incidence of brain tumours in two English counties: a population based study. *J Neurol Neurosurg Psychiatry* 2000; **69**: 464–471.

Clinical features

Bradley D, Rees J. Brain tumours: mimics and chameleons. *Pract Neurol* 2013; **13:** 359–371.

Pathology

Bailey P, Cushing H. *A Classification of Tumors of the Glioma Group on a Histogenetic Basis with a Correlation Study of Prognosis.* Philadelphia: Lippincott, 1926.

Cancer Genome Atlas Research Network. Comprehensive, integrative genomic analysis of diffuse lower-grade gliomas. *N Engl J Med* 2015; **372:** 2481–2498.

Louis DN, Chgaki H, Wiestler OD, *et al.* The 2007 WHO Classification of Tumours of the Central Nervous System. *Acta Neuropathol* 2007; **114**: 97–109.

Louis DN, Perry A, Burger P, *et al.* International Society of Neuropathology–Haarlem Consensus Guidelines for Nervous System Tumor Classification and Grading. *Brain Pathology* 2014; **24:** 429–435

Reya T, Morrison SJ, Clarke MF, Weissman IL. Stem cells, cancer, and cancer stem cells. *Nature* 2001; **414**: 105–111.

Imaging

Behin A, Hoang-Xuan K, Carpetier AF, Delattre JY. Primary brain tumours in adults. *Lancet* 2003; **361**: 323–331.

Cha S. Update on brain tumor imaging: from anatomy to physiology. *Am J Neuroradiol* 2006; **27**: 475–487.

Danchaivijitr N, Waldman AD, Tozer DJ, Benton CE, Brasil Caseiras G, Tofts PS, *et al.* Low-grade gliomas: do changes in rCBV measurements at longitudinal perfusion-weighted MR imaging predict malignant transformation? *Radiology* 2008; **2471:** 170–178.

Hygino da Cruz LC Jr, Rodriguez I, Domingues RC, Gasparetto EL, Sorensen AG. Pseudoprogression and pseudoresponse: imaging challenges in the assessment of posttreatment glioma. *AJNR Am J Neuroradiol.* 2011; **32:** 1978–1985. Review.

Jenkinson MD, Smith TS, Joyce KA, *et al.* Cerebral blood volume, notype and chemosensitivity in oligodendroglial tumours. *Neuroradiology* 2006; **48:** 703–713.

Khalid L, Carone M, Dumrongpisutikul N, Intrapiromkul J, Bonekamp D, Barker PB, Yousem DM. Imaging characteristics of oligodendrogliomas that predict grade. *Am J Neuroradiol* 2012; **33:** 852–857.

Kong DS, Kim ST, Kim EH, Lim DH, Kim WS, Suh YL, *et al.* Diagnostic dilemma of pseudoprogression in the treatment of newly diagnosed glioblastomas: the role of assessing relative cerebral blood flow volume and oxygen-6-methylguanine-DNA methyltransferase promoter methylation status. *Am J Neuroradiol* 2011; **32:** 382–387.

Law M, Yang S, Babb JS, *et al.* Comparison of cerebral blood volume and vascular permeability from dynamic susceptibility contrast-enhanced perfusion MR imaging with glioma grade. *Am J Neuroradiol* 2004; **25**: 746–755.

Law M, Yang S, Wang H, *et al.* Glioma grading: sensitivity, specificity, and predictive values of perfusion MR imaging and proton MR spectroscopic imaging compared with conventional MR imaging. *Am J Neuroradiol* 2003; **24**: 1989–1998.

Macdonald DR, Cascino TL, Schold SC Jr, Cairncross JG. Response criteria for phase II studies of supratentorial malignant glioma. *J Clin Oncol* 1990; **8:** 1277–1280.

Mong S, Ellingson BM, Nghiemphu PL, Kim HJ, Mirsadraei L, Lai A, *et al.* Persistent diffusion-restricted lesions in bevacizumab-treated malignant gliomas are associated with improved survival compared with matched controls. *Am J Neuroradiol* 2012; **33:** 1763–1770.

Sugahara T, Korogi Y, Kochi M, *et al.* Usefullness of diffusion-weighted MRI with echo-planar technique in the evaluation of cellularity in gliomas. *J Magn Reson Imaging* 1999; **9**: 53–60.

Tozer DJ, Jager HR, Danchaivijitr N, *et al.* Apparent diffusion coefficient histograms may predict low-grade glioma subtype. *NMR Biomed* 2006.

Vlieger EJ, Majoie CB, Leenstra S, Den Heeten GJ. Functional magnetic resonance imaging for neurosurgical planning in neurooncology. *Eur Radiol* 2004; **14:** 1143–1153.

Wen PY, Macdonald DR, Reardon DA, Cloughesy TF, *et al.* Updated response assessment criteria for high-grade gliomas: Response Assessment in Neuro-Oncology Working Group (RANO). *J Clin Oncol* 2010; **28:** 1963–1972.

Young RJ, Knopp EA. Brain MRI: tumor evaluation. *J Magn Reson Imaging* 2006; **24:** 709–724.

Surgery, radiotherapy and chemotherapy

Buckner JC, Shaw EG, Pugh SL, *et al.* Radiation plus Procarbazine, CCNU and Vincristine in Low-Grade Glioma. *N Engl J Med* 2016; **374**: 1344–1355.

Duffau H, Lopes M, Arthuis F, *et al.* Contribution of intraoperative electrical stimulations in surgery of low grade gliomas: a comparative study between two series without (1985–96) and with (1996–2003) functional mapping in the same institution. *J Neurol Neurosurg Psychiatry* 2005; **76**: 845–851.

Kocher M, Soffietti R, Abacioglu U. Adjuvant whole-brain radiotherapy versus observation after radiosurgery or surgical resection of one to three cerebral metastases: results of the EORTC 22952-26001 study. *J Clin Onc* 2011; **29:** 134–141.

Patchell RA, Tibbs PA, Regine WF, *et al.* Direct decompressive surgical resection in the treatment of spinal cord compression caused by metastatic cancer: a randomised trial. *Lancet* 2005; **366**: 643–648.

Patchell R, Tibbs PA, Walsh JW, *et al.* A randomized trial of surgery in the treatment of single metastases to the brain. *N Engl J Med* 1990; **322**: 494–500.

Stupp R, Hegi ME, Mason WP, *et al.* Effects of radiotherapy with concomitant and adjuvant temozolomide versus radiotherapy alone on survival in glioblastoma in a randomised phase III study: 5-year analysis of the EORTC-NCIC trial. *Lancet Oncol* 2009; **10:** 459–466.

Van den Bent MJ, Afra D, de Witte O, *et al.* Long-term efficacy of early versus delayed radiotherapy for low-grade astrocytoma and oligodendroglioma in adults: the EORTC 22845 randomised trial. *Lancet* 2005; **366:** 985–990.

Walker MD, Alexander E Jr, Hunt WE, *et al.* Evaluation of BCNU and/or radiotherapy in the treatment of anaplastic gliomas: a cooperative clinical trial. *J Neurosurg* 1978; **49**: 333–343.

Quality of life

Davies E, Clarke C, Hopkins A. Malignant cerebral glioma II: Perspectives of patients and relatives on the value of radiotherapy. *Br Med J* 1996; **313:** 1512–1516.

Fox S, Lantz C. The brain tumour experience and quality of life: a qualitative study. *J Neurosci Nurs* 1998; **30**: 245–252.

National Institute for Health and Clinical Excellence (NICE). Improving outcomes in brain and other central nervous system tumours. *The Manual.* London: The Stationery Office, 2006.

Taphoorn MJB, Klein M. Cognitive deficits in adult patients with brain tumours. *Lancet* 2004; **3**: 159–168.

Paraneoplastic neurological syndromes

Candler PM, Hart PE, Barnett M, Weil R, Rees JH. A follow-up study of patients with paraneoplastic neurological disease in the United Kingdom. *J Neurol Neurosurg Psychiatry* 2004; **75:** 1411–1415.

Graus F, Dalmau J. Paraneoplastic neurological syndromes. *Curr Opin Neurol* 2012; **25:** 795–801.

Graus F, Delattre JY, Antoine JC, *et al.* Recommended diagnostic criteria for paraneoplastic neurological syndromes. *J Neurol Neurosurg Psychiatry* 2004; **75**: 1135–1140.

Rees JH, Hain SF, Johnson MR, *et al.* The role of [^{18}F]fluoro-2-deoxyglucose-PET scanning in the diagnosis of paraneoplastic neurological disorders. *Brain* 2001; **124**: 2223–2231.

Shams'ili S, Grefkens J, de Leeuw B, *et al.* Paraneoplastic cerebellar degeneration associated with anti-neuronal antibodies: analysis of 50 patients. *Brain* 2003; **126**: 1409–1418.

Malignant meningitis

Kak M, Nanda R, Ramsdale EE, Lukas RV. Treatment of leptomeningeal carcinomatosis: current challenges and future opportunities. *J Clin Neurosci* 2015; **22:** 632–637.

Brain tumour charities and support services

Brain and Spine Foundation. T: 0808 808 1000. www.bbsf.org.uk

Brain Tumour Research. T: 01296 733011. www.braintumourresearch.org

Cancer Research UK. T: 0800 226 237. www.cancerresearchuk.org

International Brain Tumour Alliance. T: 01737 813872. www.theibta.org

Macmillan Cancer Relief. T: 0808 808202. www.macmillan.org.uk

National Brain Appeal T: 020 3448 4724. www.nationalbrainappeal.org

The Brain Tumour Charity. T: 0808 800 0004. www.thebraintumourcharity.org

CHAPTER 22

Neuropsychiatry

Eileen Joyce
UCL Institute of Neurology

Requests for neuropsychiatric consultations are usually for one of three reasons. The first is when patients present with neurological symptoms but no organic cause can be found and the features do not fit with a known neurological illness. Symptoms include convulsions, disordered movement such as apparent dystonia, paralysis or tremor, sensory disturbance, amnesia, blindness and dysphonia. In this context, these symptoms are described as 'functional' as opposed to 'organic' and they may be psychologically determined. This presentation is common – up to 30% of general neurology clinic attendees have functional neurological symptoms (FNS) – and they are a significant cause of disability.

The second type of request is for assessment of psychiatric symptoms in the context of a known neurological disorder. For example, depression is a common feature of many neurological disorders and leads to high rates of morbidity as it can worsen a patient's subjective experience of symptoms and interfere with response to treatment and the ability to participate in rehabilitation. Low mood may either be a premorbid feature, a consequence of the illness itself, or a reaction to the diagnosis or to the disability. It is therefore important to determine the nature of the depression in order to optimise its treatment and that of the underlying neurological condition. Another problem that falls into this category concerns the adverse effects of drug treatment for neurological disorders. Examples include steroids, which can induced mania, depression and psychosis; drugs for Parkinson's disease, which can induce psychosis or impulsive behaviour; certain antiepileptics, which can induce depression, suicidal ideation and psychosis; and sedative drugs such as opiates and benzodiazepines, which can cause delirium.

The third type of request is when patients develop prominent psychiatric symptoms but there is concern that these are the product of an underlying neurological process. Examples include an autoimmune encephalopathy presenting primarily as psychosis, as in NMDA receptor encephalitis, or a mood disorder, as in systemic lupus erythematosus (Chapter 20); a temporal lobe tumour presenting as severe anxiety; and multiple sclerosis presenting as depression (see Neuropsychiatric aspects of white matter disorders).

The key to understanding the interplay of neurological and psychiatric symptoms is to assess the patient within a biological, psychological and social context. This means taking a detailed history which addresses family history, personal development, life events and social circumstances, and performing a mental state examination. Often this process, the bread and butter of psychiatry, is enough to clarify and formulate the diagnosis and, if relevant, suggest a treatment plan.

The mental state examination

The mental state examination is a strictly laid-out process for systematically assessing psychiatric symptoms. It is analogous to the process of eliciting neurological signs. It is the cornerstone of determining whether abnormal behaviour is a feature, a consequence or an imitator of neurological disease. The essential elements are listed here.

Appearance and behaviour

This can give important clues to particular diagnoses and is valuable for ascertaining a patient's level of functioning:

- *Clothing and personal care:* self-neglect may point to depression, psychosis or dementia.
- *Behaviour:* agitation and distractability may indicate psychosis, delirium or dementia. Abnormal movements such as tremor, chorea or tics may indicate a neurological disorder.
- *Activity level:* retardation may point to depression and excitability to mania.
- *Appropriateness:* disinhibition may reflect a frontal syndrome and inappropriate crying or laughing may suggest pseudobulbar palsy.

Speech

How a patient speaks can provide a clue to diagnosis. Dysarthria and dysphasia (Chapter 4) are commonly seen with neurological conditions and affect the quality and clarity of a patient's voice. In a psychiatric assessment the qualities of speech that should be noted are as follows:

- *Quantity:* can be reduced in depression and dementia
- *Rate:* often rapid in mania and slow in depression
- *Tone:* can be monotonous in depression and Parkinson's disease
- *Rhythm:* normal intonation and rhythm can be lost in psychotic illnesses
- *Volume:* can be loud in mania and quiet in depression and Parkinson's disease.

Neurology: A Queen Square Textbook, Second Edition. Edited by Charles Clarke, Robin Howard, Martin Rossor and Simon Shorvon.

Mood and affect

Mood is documented both subjectively and objectively. Subjective feelings of depression may be described as 'down', 'low' or 'sad'. In mania this might be 'high'. Objectively, a patient may appear depressed, hypomanic/manic or euthymic (i.e. normal). Affect is how mood varies. This can be reactive in euthymia, flat and unchanging in depression, and labile or exaggerated in mania. Associated symptoms to ask about include:

- *Anhedonia:* the inability to enjoy usually pleasurable activities.
- *Sleep:* commonly disrupted in mood disorders; manic patients often report a decreased need for sleep and depressed patients can be troubled by initial insomnia, broken sleep or early morning waking.
- *Appetite:* poor appetite and weight loss are common in depression.
- *Energy levels and libido:* can be reduced in depression and elevated in mania.
- *Suicidal ideation:* it is important to ask about this and document findings clearly (see Identifying and managing risk secondary to abnormal mental states).

Thoughts

These are described in terms of form (i.e. the natural progression from one idea to the next) and content.

Formal thought disorder

- *Speed of thinking:* can be increased in mania with flight of ideas (rapid shifting between topics but with a logical flow), and slowed in depression and cognitive impairment.
- *Ordering of thoughts:* can be disrupted in organic brain syndromes and psychosis, for example perseveration (repetition of the same thought) in frontal lobe damage and thought block (abrupt cessation of speech) in psychosis.
- *Psychotic formal thought disorder:* can be difficult to follow what a patient is saying because of abnormal transitions in thought processes. This can be described as derailment (speech shifts gradually off the point); tangential speech (speech is related to the topic but off the point); or 'knight's move thinking' (abrupt illogical shifts between statements).

Thought content

Delusions are firmly held false beliefs. They can be persecutory, grandiose, nihilistic, hypochondriacal or bizarre (completely implausible). They can be elicited in the primary psychiatric disorders of schizophrenia, depression with psychosis and mania and as secondary phenomena in certain neurological disorders such as temporal lobe epilepsy, the neurodegenerative dementias and Parkinson's disease. Abnormalities of possession of thought (thought insertion, withdrawal and broadcasting) or beliefs that the body and emotions are under the control of an outside force can be experienced in psychosis.

Obsessional thoughts or images are recurrent and persistent ideas which the patient sees as senseless and coming from within (cf. hallucinations and delusions) but is unable to prevent intruding into the mind. They may then be compelled to carry out ritualistic acts to relieve the associated anxiety that the obsessive thought or image elicits (e.g. having to wash repeatedly because of intrusive thoughts about contamination).

Perceptions

These abnormalities can be in any sensory modality. Illusions are false perceptions in the presence of an external stimulus (i.e. misinterpretations). Misinterpretation of the surroundings, such as seeing faces in hospital curtains, are common in delirium and advanced Parkinson's disease. Hallucinations are perceptions in the absence of an external stimulus. Visual hallucinations are indicative of an organic cause such as delirium, epilepsy, Lewy body dementia, advanced Parkinson's disease and the Charles Bonnet syndrome (Chapter 14). Auditory hallucinations are typical of primary psychotic illnesses such as schizophrenia and the affective psychoses. When a patient experiences 'voices' it is important to ask about what exactly is being heard, as they may act on the content and put themselves at risk. For example, some patients with schizophrenia experience 'command hallucinations' where voices tell them to harm others and this may be difficult to resist. In psychotic depression voices may tell the patient that they are worthless or guilty of a crime and in mania the voice of 'God' might be experienced. Whereas illusions and hallucinations are perceived in external space, pseudo-hallucinations are experienced internally (i.e. 'inside the head'). They are indicative of severe distress and can be seen in anxiety or personality disorders.

Depersonalisation is a distorted sense of self in which patients describe feeling outside their body. Derealisation is a distorted sense of reality and is described as a feeling of looking on the world from the outside rather than being in it. These often occur together and can be indicative of a temporal lobe seizure. In temporal lobe epilepsy, depersonalisation and derealisation are normally transient experiences, lasting seconds to minutes; if they last longer (i.e. hours to weeks) they are suggestive of a dissociative or anxiety disorder. In some people depersonalisation and derealisation are persistent in the absence of other symptoms, a condition known as depersonalisation/derealisation disorder (see Depersonalisation/derealisation disorder). Similarly déjà vu, an abnormal feeling of familiarity, can be experienced in these conditions.

Cognition

A brief cognitive assessment is required to interpret any elicited mental phenomena. For example, anxiety in the context of mild memory impairment may point to incipient dementia (Chapter 8).

Insight

This refers to the patient's understanding of their symptoms and whether they believe them to be a sign of illness. Insight can be impaired in many conditions and make adherence with treatment problematic. Many organic illnesses can impair insight. For example, patients with parietal lesions may show anosognosia and fail to identify deficits caused by their illness such as hemiparesis and inattention. Lack of insight is common in dementia and psychosis.

Formulation

Having carried out a mental state examination, it is helpful to provide a formulation, which is a summary of the history and mental state with a diagnostic interpretation.

Identifying and managing risk secondary to abnormal mental states

Agitation and aggression

Agitation and aggression commonly occur together, have numerous causes and should be managed quickly to prevent harm to the patient or others. Often patients are frightened and confused because of hallucinations or paranoid delusions. De-escalation techniques should always be employed first; for example by assessing the patient in a quiet and calm environment, standing away from the patient to give them space, speaking clearly and slowly, and listening to the patient to try to understand what has triggered the situation. Medication should only be used if this fails and if the patient is risking the safety of themselves or others. Small doses of lorazepam orally or intramuscularly is a useful first choice. An antipsychotic can also be used if a longer action is needed, such as olanzapine orally and haloperidol or aripiprazole intramuscularly.

Lack of insight

Lack of insight and awareness of risk is especially common in dementia. Risks include wandering, leaving keys in the door or the house unlocked, leaving the gas and taps running, continuing to drive when it is not safe and not taking medication. If there is lack of insight, collateral information should be sought from a relative or carer. Risk can be reduced by home adaptations, care packages, 'dosette' boxes for medication or institutional care, if required.

Suicidal ideation/suicidal behaviour

Thoughts of suicide are common in neuropsychiatric conditions and should be actively identified. It is important to understand that asking about suicidal thoughts does not increase the risk of suicidal behaviour and patients often find it a relief to be able to speak about them. Risk of suicide is increased if there have been previous attempts and with chronic illness, older age, unemployment, social isolation, a past psychiatric history and drug and alcohol dependence. It is important to distinguish between a passive wish to die and active thoughts and plans to end life. The latter, being more serious, should trigger immediate intervention from the local psychiatry team.

Legal issues: use of mental health and capacity acts

There are legal frameworks in place to cover the treatment of patients who may lack capacity to make decisions or refuse treatment because of mental disorder. All doctors should be competent in assessing capacity, which is decision or issue specific (i.e. someone may have the capacity to agree to a blood test but not to decide on major surgery).

For a person to have capacity they must:

- Be able to understand relevant information
- Be able to weigh up the pros and cons of the decision
- Retain information long enough to come to a decision
- Be able to communicate their decision.

People are assumed to have capacity unless they have a disorder of mind that affects their decision-making ability. It is the responsibility of the treating team to assess capacity. The assessment and reasoning behind the decision must be clearly documented by the responsible medical doctor.

Psychiatric symptoms commonly seen in neurological disorders

Personality change

The DSM-5 classification of psychiatric conditions describes personality disorders as being 'associated with ways of thinking and feeling about oneself and others that significantly and adversely affect how an individual functions in many aspects of life.' Ten types of personality disorder are recognised and these are clustered according to common attributes. Patients often have attributes of more than one personality disorder, especially those within a cluster.

- *Cluster A* (odd or eccentric): paranoid, schizoid and schizotypal personality disorders.
- *Cluster B* (dramatic, emotional or erratic): antisocial, borderline, histrionic and narcissistic personality disorders.
- *Cluster C* (anxious or fearful): avoidant, dependent and obsessive–compulsive personality disorders (OCPD).

Each personality disorder represents a specific set of personality traits that are pervasive, maladaptive and present from young adulthood. Personality disorders are often preceded by childhood disorders of conduct or emotion. In neurology, it is important to differentiate these from newly acquired changes in behaviour or emotion as this may be indicative of an organic process. For example, the antisocial personality disorder is characterised by callousness, hostility and disinhibition. If such personality changes develop *de novo* later in life, it may be indicative of a frontal lobe tumour or of frontal neurodegenerative changes as seen in Huntington's disease or progressive supranuclear palsy. Typical personality changes seen in other neurological conditions include emotional lability in multiple sclerosis, apathy in Parkinson's disease and persistent dysphoria in epilepsy. Closed head injury can lead to a range of personality changes from apathy to disinhibition.

Functional, that is non-organic, neurological symptoms often develop in the context of a personality disorder, especially borderline and obsessive–compulsive types. Borderline personality disorder, also known as emotionally unstable personality disorder, is characterised by difficulty maintaining personal relationships, unstable mood and impulsivity which often leads to self-harm such as cutting or displays of intense anger. OCPD, also known as anankastic personality disorder, is characterised by maladaptive and rigid perfectionism, preoccupation with detail and persistence with fruitless behaviours. It is often associated with difficulty in expressing emotion (alexithymia). The recognition of these personality disorders in individuals with functional neurological symptoms is important as this will inform the approach to psychological treatment.

Obsessions and compulsions

OCPD is different from obsessive–compulsive disorder (OCD). Both disorders are associated with compulsive behaviours. In people with OCPD, these are performed to impose order on their environment, compatible with their way of thinking about how the world should be ordered. People with OCD, on the other hand, are highly anxious and preoccupied about perceived threats from the world and compulsive behaviours are performed to reduce this anxiety, for example repetitive hand washing to prevent contamination. Other sources of anxiety in OCD are obsessions which are unwanted, repetitive, intrusive thoughts or images and in many people with OCD, obsessions and compulsions coexist. Another distinguishing feature is that people with OCD realise that their thoughts and behaviours are irrational but cannot resist them whereas people with OCPD think that their way of thinking and behaving is correct.

OCD is normally a mental illness without antecedent but it can also be the sequel of basal ganglia disease with features that are indistinguishable. Compulsive behaviours, in the absence of the rigid perfectionism of OCPD and the anxiety of OCD, can also be witnessed as separate phenomena in neurological disorders. For example, compulsive behaviours are very common in Tourette's syndrome and it can be difficult to distinguish complex motor tics from compulsions as both are preceded by an urge and result in a coordinated stereotyped set of movements. One difference is that compulsions, unlike complex motor tics, are usually goal directed, for example touching, tapping and evening-up. Compulsions can also be seen in patients with Parkinson's disease secondary to levodopa or dopamine agonist therapy; this is witnessed in the so-called impulse control disorders (see Impulse control disorder).

Anxiety

Anxiety is characterised by the subjective emotion of fear accompanied by physical symptoms reflecting over-activation of the autonomic nervous system: palpitation, dyspnoea, throat constriction (globus) and abdominal sensations. Neurological symptoms may be prominent such as tremor, dizziness and paraesthesiae (e.g. secondary to hyperventilation). When disabling symptoms of anxiety are triggered by certain events or circumstances they are classified as specific disorders, for example post-traumatic stress disorder after a life-threatening experience and social anxiety disorder when meeting new people or performing in public.

People with neurological disorders are commonly anxious. If this anxiety is a source of disability, the diagnosis of a separate anxiety disorder may be appropriate. The anxiety disorders most commonly seen are panic disorder and generalised anxiety disorder where the symptoms are 'free floating' in that the triggers are no longer obvious. In the former, anxiety symptoms are paroxysmal whereas in the latter they are pervasive. On occasion, patients with these disorders and no pre-existing neurological disorder may be referred to a neurologist because the symptoms of anxiety may also be accompanied by prominent fatigue, poor concentration and memory and urinary retention. Particular constellations of symptoms in general anxiety disorder and panic disorder may be misinterpreted as complex partial seizures, neuro-otological dysfunction, multiple sclerosis, movement disorder or neurodegenerative disorders and require expert assessment to prevent over-investigation.

Mood

Disturbance of mood is a very common accompaniment of neurological disorders. This can be a reaction to receiving a diagnosis with a poor prognosis or to the disability or pain that ensues. In some conditions, mood disturbance appears to be a reflection of how the disease process interacts with the forebrain systems that mediate emotion and cognition, as in epilepsy, Parkinson's disease and multiple sclerosis.

Depression is both a specific and colloquial term. Often, people refer to being depressed when they have a transient and mild lowering of mood (dysphoria) in response to specific circumstances or events. It is only when depression is of sufficient frequency and severity and substantially affects quality of life that it becomes a specific disorder. Disorders of mood are classified as depressive disorders or bipolar disorders. Major depression refers to a specific syndrome characterised by persistent low mood, anhedonia (lack of enjoyment) and disturbances of the so-called vegetative functions of sleep and appetite. Cognitive function may be impaired, sometimes to the extent that it may resemble dementia, especially in the elderly (see Pseudodementia). Major depression is episodic but may be recurrent. When symptoms of major depression are persistent it is classified as 'persistent depressive disorder (dysthymia)'.

Mania is a state reflecting an excessive heightening of mood; hypomania is a less severe clinical presentation of mania. In both mania and hypomania there is an increased sense of well-being accompanied by euphoria, racing thoughts, pressure of speech and diminished need for sleep. In mania, there is also thought disorder with speech characterised by rhyming, punning and wordplay; patients may develop grandiose delusions and auditory hallucinations. In mania, dysphoric mood often follows a period of elation, associated with irritability or frank aggression. Bipolar disorder refers to a condition whereby major depression alternates with episodes of hypomania or mania. Cyclothymic disorder refers to a mild form of bipolar disorder which may appear as a constitutional state rather than a mental illness unless formally assessed.

Mood disorders are distinguished from disorders where there is a transient lability of mood. For example, unstable mood is a feature of borderline personality disorder (see Personality change). In pseudobulbar palsy or frontal lobe syndrome frequent changes in mood may be witnessed, such as excessive laughing and crying.

Pseudodementia

The term pseudodementia is most commonly used to describe cognitive impairment in elderly patients with depression. Depressive pseudodementia can resemble true dementia. It is important to distinguish the two as in depression, the cognitive impairment generally improves with treatment of the underlying condition (Table 22.1).

Psychosis

Psychosis refers to a set of symptoms that indicate that the patient has lost contact with reality and that their thought processes have become disconnected. Hallucinations and delusions are the most frequently encountered psychotic symptoms. Thought disorder can be seen in association with hallucinations and delusions or, less commonly, on its own (see The mental state examination for definitions). Psychosis can arise in the context of brain neurodegeneration as in Alzheimer's disease and Parkinson's disease, or brain neurotoxicity as in delirium, alcohol withdrawal and certain forms of substance abuse. People with epilepsy can also develop psychotic conditions either in relation to seizure activity (peri-ictal or ictal psychosis) or as an inter-ictal state presumed to reflect progressive and permanent brain changes. Psychosis can also arise in types of mental illness where there is no neurological antecedent, most commonly schizophrenia and the affective disorders.

The form of hallucinations and the content of delusions point to the nature of the underlying disorder. In the 'organic psychoses' (neurodegeneration, neurotoxcity, ictal or peri-ictal psychosis) hallucinations are usually visual, that is patients see objects that are not there. These can take the form of animals, people or even whole scenes which are often vivid and frightening. Hallucinations in other modalities are less common but notable types include tactile hallucinations, experienced as insects crawling under the skin

Table 22.1 Clinical features that help to distinguish dementia from depressive pseudodementia.

	Dementia	Depressive pseudodementia
Behaviour	Relatively unconcerned	Distressed and frightened
Memory	Greater impairment for recent than remote memories	Complaints of generalised memory impairment but performs better than described
Cognitive testing	Cooperative	Gives up easily, 'don't know' answers

(formication), seen in alcohol withdrawal or cocaine intoxication, and olfactory or gustatory hallucinations in complex partial seizures. Auditory hallucinations are less common in organic conditions and usually point to schizophrenia or an affective disorder. The exception to this is epilepsy, when psychosis can develop as an inter-ictal condition that typically resembles schizophrenia.

Psychosis can arise in the context of severe depression. Hallucinations are characteristically of a voice speaking directly to the patient (i.e. in the second person). The voice is usually highly critical (e.g. telling the patient that they are worthless). Delusions are 'mood congruent' and include beliefs about being guilty of some terrible act and deserving to be punished. Nihilistic delusions are also typical and take the form of believing the body is dysfunctional, rotting or even disappearing (Cotard's syndrome). In mania, hallucinations are less common than in both depression and schizophrenia, but if present resemble those of schizophrenia. Delusions are grandiose in nature and include beliefs about being a famous person or having special powers.

Psychosis is central to the concept of schizophrenia. A diagnosis of an affective disorder can be made without the presence of psychosis whereas in schizophrenia at least one psychotic symptom is mandatory – one of hallucinations, delusions and thought disorder. The psychotic symptoms of schizophrenia tend to be much more bizarre and 'ununderstandable' than in other disorders, so much so that Schneider listed symptoms of the 'first rank' which are highly indicative of schizophrenia (Table 22.2). First rank symptoms can also be present in the inter-ictal psychosis of epilepsy

There are some notable types of delusion that can be seen in schizophrenia and sometimes in dementia or following brain injury. These are the misidentification syndromes. For example, the Capgras delusion occurs when a patient believes that somebody familiar to the patient has been replaced by an imposter. In contrast, the Fregoli delusion, or delusion of doubles, occurs when a patient believes that different people are the same person in disguise. More commonly associated with brain injury than schizophrenia is reduplicative paramnesia, which occurs when the patient believes that he or she is in a familiar place (e.g. their house), at the same time admitting it is also located elsewhere.

Table 22.2 The first rank symptoms of Schneider.

If present in the setting of clear consciousness are highly supportive of a diagnosis of schizophrenia

Delusional perception: abnormal significance attached to a real perception with no logical explanation

Delusions of possession of thought: the belief that an outside force is inserting or withdrawing thoughts or that one's own thoughts are being broadcast to the world

Delusions of control
- **Somatic passivity**: belief that bodily sensations are imposed from outside
- **Made acts, thought or emotions**: belief that affects, impulses and motor actions are under outside control

Auditory hallucinations
- Hearing own thoughts spoken aloud (thought echo)
- Hearing voices arguing about or discussing the patients
- Hearing voices commenting on the patient's actions

Mental phenomena experienced during the transition from wakefulness to sleep (hypnogogia) or vice versa (hypnopompia) are common in narcolepsy but also occur in those who have neither psychiatric nor neurological disease. They can occur in any modality. Auditory hallucinations include simple noises (bumps in the night), one's name being called out loud or fragments of speech. They are experienced 'outside the head' and, although they can be vivid and frightening, insight is rapidly gained. Visual hallucinations are typically of geometric shapes but sometime hallucinations of people are reported as are olfactory and tactile phenomena.

Catatonia

Catatonia is a rare mental and behavioural state that can be seen in a range of psychiatric and neurological conditions including schizophrenia, severe depression and the encephalitides. Typically, the patient is mute and displays a range of bizarre motor abnormalities. An example is catatonic posturing whereby an unusual position is held for long periods of time but a body part can be passively moved to another position which is then maintained (waxy flexibility). This form of immobility can be interspersed by periods of purposeless hyperactivity (catatonic excitement). In its most severe form, patients can become rigid and immobile for prolonged periods (catatonic stupor) accompanied by an involuntary resistance to passive movement (geigenhalten). This can progress to a life-threatening state of 'lethal catatonia' where autonomic instability and hyperpyrexia develop and rigidity can give rise to dangerously elevated creatine kinase levels. This syndrome resembles the neuroleptic malignant syndrome and should be considered a medical emergency.

Non-organic disorders in neurology

Functional neurological symptoms

Functional neurological symptoms (FNS) manifest as neurological problems, for example tremor, paralysis, seizure or sensory disturbance, but the clinical examination points away from an organic cause and investigations fail to find one. They are clinically significant because of associated disability.

The term 'functional' therefore refers to the fact that the nervous system is not functioning normally despite there being no explanation in terms of known neurological disease. FNS are very common. Approximately 30% of patients referred to general neurology clinics from primary care have FNS. In the population at large, 4–12/100 000 are estimated as having clinically important FNS at any one time. Despite the health burden that these symptoms cause, the importance of FNS remains largely unrecognised with regards to treatment: all neurologists know that such symptoms are most difficult to help.

Terminology

For over a century FNS were considered to be associated with distressing psychological events or conflict occurring at some point in the individual's history. The term 'conversion' was coined by Freud to denote his theory that the mind defends against conscious psychic pain by unconsciously converting emotional symptoms into physical ones. The term 'conversion disorder' was subsequently incorporated into both the International Classification of Diseases (ICD) and the Diagnostic and Statistical Manual of Mental Disorders (DSM) classification systems of psychiatric illness as a collective descriptor of FNS; for example DSM-IV required the fulfillment of the diagnostic criterion: 'Psychological factors are

Table 22.3 Alternative terms used for functional neurological symptoms.

Hysteria An ancient term attributed to Hippocrates to describe the physical consequences of a 'wandering womb', a view that is hard to understand today. It was revived by Charcot in nineteenth century to describe functional symptoms which he saw as developing mainly in women. Hysteria remains in colloquial use, to describe florid emotional responsiveness in both sexes

Conversion disorder Conversion is an historical term coined by Freud to denote the hypothetical process by which the experience of psychological distress caused by conflict or trauma is avoided by the unconscious conversion of anxiety into physical symptoms. The term 'conversion disorder' is retained in DSM editions to denote physical functional neurological symptoms (e.g. paralysis, tremor); in DSM-5 the term 'functional neurological symptom disorder' is given as an alternative

Non-organic neurological symptoms This is essentially shorthand communication between doctors but says nothing about the nature of the problem for the patient

Psychogenic neurological symptoms This directly implies a psychological cause and can cause offence

Somatisation This is used to denote the attribution of anxiety to a physical problem. Somatisation can concern any organ or system of the body, not only the nervous system

Pseudoseizure Like 'non-organic', this term is used to communicate between clinicians that a seizure is false because it is not epileptic. Not useful for patients and can cause offence

Non-epileptic seizure, non-epileptic attack disorder, non-epileptic event These are common descriptors of functional convulsions. They are neutral in tone but like 'non-organic' say nothing about the nature of the problem

judged, in the clinician's belief, to be associated with the symptom or deficit because conflicts or other stressors precede the initiation or exacerbation of the symptom or deficit. A diagnosis where the stressor precedes the onset of symptoms by up to 15 years is not unusual'. However, while there may be a causative stressor, there is no research evidence to support such a psychodynamic formulation and clinicians often fail to elicit any history of psychological trauma or conflict. Patients themselves usually misinterpret the explanation of the term 'conversion disorder' as the clinician inferring that their symptoms are 'all in the mind' or even fabricated. This situation has not been helped by the use of other value-laden labels for FNS (Table 22.3). DSM-5 has retained 'conversion disorder' as the main label but the term 'functional neurological symptom disorder', which has no emotive connotations, is also given in parentheses as an alternative.

Diagnosis

Many patients with FNS are often told what they do *not* have, for example a brain tumour, multiple sclerosis or Parkinson's disease, but not what they *do* have. Although the exclusion of serious neurological disease is reassuring, it can leave the patient discontented because they still do not understand what is causing their symptoms. They may believe that the doctor has missed the proper diagnosis and then embark on a round of consultations with different specialists. As different specialists usually give different explanations of their symptoms, some contradictory, this can cause more confusion and the feeling that 'nobody is taking them seriously' and serve to maintain or worsen the symptom complex.

Table 22.4 Physical signs that help in the differentiation of organic and functional motor symptoms.

Functional tremor

Entrainment test: copying a 3-Hz tapping movement from the examiner with one hand either results in a significant shift in tremor frequency in the other hand or bizarre difficulty in performing the tapping task

Functional weakness

Give-way or collapsing weakness: the examined limb collapses from a normal position with a light touch. Normal power can often be achieved with encouragement. NB Organic weakness can also be collapsing in 30%.

Inconsistency (i.e. normal strength can be demonstrated)

- *Hoover's sign*: with the patient supine on a couch, the examiner places their hand under the subjectively weak leg and asks the patient to flex the contralateral hip (the strong leg) against resistance. If the examiner feels pressure from the apparently weak leg, the weakness is likely non-organic. This is a positive Hoover's sign (If no pressure is felt from the extensor muscles, this suggests that the weakness is organic.)
- *Chair test*: Patients with a disordered functional gait when walking may show that they can propel themselves with their legs when sitting in a chair with wheels, and/or imitate walking movements when sitting in a chair.

Fahn and Williams criteria (1988)

- Abrupt onset, inconsistency/incongruency, distractibility, false weakness, false sensory changes, pain, exhaustion, excessive startle, bizarre movements, concomitant somatisations
- 96% specificity, 97% sensitivity

Neurologists use particular physical signs to show and confirm that symptoms are not organic (Table 22.4). They often then refer to a psychiatrist to 'confirm the diagnosis' on the assumption that he or she can elicit a presumed underlying psychiatric disorder or relevant psychological factors. There are two problems with this approach. First, the diagnosis is essentially a neurological one based on the incongruity of symptoms and signs with known neurological disorders. Secondly, patients frequently do not have a major psychiatric illness such as major depression or generalised anxiety disorder. Any psychological component may be subtle and, if present, the link between it and the development of physical symptoms may not be evident to anyone. Thus, psychiatrists find themselves uncomfortable at labelling physical symptoms unfamiliar to them as psychologically determined. Patients can then fall between neurological and psychiatric stools, with neither side feeling confident to offer help.

The recent advance in providing the label 'functional neurological symptom (FNS) disorder' as an alternative to 'conversion disorder' has helped to resolve this impasse. In addition, DSM-5 has introduced a new diagnostic criterion requiring positive evidence that the clinical features are not compatible with a known neurological disorder, and has removed the need for a demonstrable psychological prerequisite (Table 22.5). This should enable neurologists and psychiatrists to work collaboratively, with neurologists making a positive diagnosis of FNS disorder, explaining to patients why this

Table 22.5 DSM-5 criteria for conversion disorder (functional neurological symptom disorder).

Criteria A, B, C and D must all be fulfilled to make the diagnosis
A One or more neurological symptoms such as altered voluntary motor, sensory function, cognition or seizure-like episodes
B The symptom, after appropriate medical assessment, is found not to be caused by a general medical condition, the direct effects of a substance or a culturally sanctioned behaviour
C The physical signs or diagnostic findings are internally inconsistent or incongruent with recognised neurological disorder
D The symptom causes clinically significant distress or impairment in social, occupational or other important areas of functioning or warrants medical evaluation

is so on the basis of symptoms and signs, and with psychiatrists treating any mental illness and coordinating therapy.

FNS can be present in isolation or as part of a more general disorder involving unexplained symptoms affecting other bodily systems (e.g. the gastrointestinal tract or the genitourinary system). Here, the older diagnostic terms include Briquet's syndrome and somatisation disorder. DSM-5 has abolished 'somatisation disorder' as a diagnosis, because the criteria were overly complex and ultimately not useful, and introduced 'somatic symptom disorder' instead. Another major change is that DSM-5 now acknowledges that organic and non-organic symptoms can coexist, something long recognised by neurologists. For example, patients with epilepsy can also have non-epileptic seizures.

In somatic symptom disorder, patients must have 'one or more chronic somatic symptoms about which they are excessively concerned, preoccupied or fearful. These fears and behaviours cause significant distress and dysfunction, and although patients may make frequent use of health care services, they are rarely reassured and often feel their medical care has been inadequate.' This is distinguished from illness anxiety disorder or hypochondriasis in which patients 'may or may not have a medical condition but have heightened bodily sensations, are intensely anxious about the possibility of an undiagnosed illness, or devote excessive time and energy to health concerns, often obsessively researching them. Like people with somatic symptom disorder, they are not easily reassured. Illness anxiety disorder can cause considerable distress and life disruption, even at moderate levels.'

Specific types of functional neurological symptoms

Functional seizures

Functional seizures are one of the most common functional neurological presentations. In the general population the best estimate of the prevalence is of 4.6/100 000. About 20% of patients referred to seizure clinics have functional seizures and it is not uncommon for patients admitted to intensive care units with apparent status epilepticus to eventually receive this diagnosis (23% in one study). Functional seizures occur more often in women than men by 4 : 1. They are associated with high rates of personality disorder, anxiety and dissociation. Functional seizures, contrary to other forms of FNS, are often associated with childhood physical or sexual abuse, estimated as 25%. It used to be thought that functional seizures commonly developed in people with epilepsy but recent estimates are that 5–10% of functional seizure cases have a double diagnosis.

As with other FNS, there are a number of different labels used for functional seizures (Table 22.3), the most common being 'non-epileptic seizures'.

Non-epileptic seizures are characterised by episodes of loss of motor control. The majority (60%) resemble grand mal seizures (i.e. convulsive attacks), and the rest are blank spells where the patient is motionless and uncontactable. There are a number of features that can usefully discriminate grand-mal epileptic seizures from the convulsive type of non-epileptic seizures. Seizures are most likely to be non-epileptic if the prodrome or seizure itself lasts longer than 5 minutes; the eyes are closed and resist passive opening; and there are side to side head movements. Importantly, non-epileptic seizures can be associated with features considered more typical of epilepsy, such as tongue biting; urinary incontinence; an aura; post-ictal confusion or drowsiness; attacks appearing to emerge from sleep; and apparent status epilepticus. These are not therefore discriminators. Injuries are also frequently seen in patients with non-epileptic attacks including cuts, bruises and even fractures. During an attack, the patients are conscious, though may appear not to be so. On questioning, they often describe their subjective experience during a non-epileptic attack, of being aware of their surroundings but feeling detached, as in depersonalisation/derealisation, and unable to speak.

It is important not to dismiss an apparent non-epileptic attack. In practice, non-epileptic attacks are often unrecognised panic attacks. This is especially so if the patient does not describe subjective fear but displays paroxysmal autonomic symptoms such as tremor and depersonalisation/derealisation. Other apparent non-epileptic attacks may be syncopal episodes especially if associated with brief myoclonic jerks.

A useful diagnostic finding is of a normal electroencephalogram (EEG) during a typical attack. However, in this circumstance it is important to consider the possibility of frontal seizures, in which seizures may manifest as bizarre uncoordinated movements with a normal EEG. The interictal EEG is not helpful, as 20% of patients with non-epileptic seizures have non-specific EEG abnormalities. Another distinguishing factor is that serum prolactin levels are often raised 10–20 minutes after a generalised epileptic seizure. However, this is an unreliable finding and other clues to the diagnosis should be sought. About 70% of patients with epilepsy respond well to standard antiepileptic therapy. Failure to respond, with continuing frequent attacks, should raise doubts about the diagnosis.

Fixed dystonia

Dystonia is characterised by sustained, often painful, contractions of groups of muscle. It causes repetitive involuntary movements or abnormal postures and can affect any body part. Dystonia-like movements can be functional and, as with other functional symptoms, differentiated by their incongruity. Fixed dystonia is an extreme form of functional dystonia in which an abnormal posture becomes permanent or fixed. Fixed dystonia has several characteristic features. There is often a history of a mild physical injury (e.g. being hit by a ball), followed by the rapid development and spread of abnormal movements. For example, in the upper limb, dystonia begins with contraction and flexion of the fingers, then affects the wrist and eventually moves up the arm. In the legs, classically, the foot becomes inverted. Eventually the patient begins to walk entirely on the lateral border of the foot and even on the dorsum, or is confined to a wheelchair as the contraction moves up the leg or across to the other leg.

On examination, the patient is unable to move the affected part voluntarily and an attempt at passive movement is met with resistance. Examination in the fixed posture at rest often shows that the muscles are not actively contracting and the patient is usually unable to contract opposing muscle groups. Patients with fixed dystonia can become dissociated from their affected limb in the sense that they feel that it is not part of them and they sometimes request amputation. Over time, the involved joints in fixed dystonia can become ankylosed, meaning there is no prospect of regaining movement. If this is suspected, examination under anaesthetic is indicated to determine the range of movements before embarking on physiotherapy.

Treatment of functional neurological symptoms

Many patients when confronted with the notion that there is no organic condition underlying their complaints are initially reluctant to accept the diagnosis because their symptoms are so physical; they feel offended at the concept of a non-organic cause. However, a clear presentation of the diagnosis, with the demonstration of positive signs, is often sufficient to significantly reduce symptoms, especially in the case of non-epileptic seizures. Psychotherapy is the cornerstone of treatment. There are few clinical trials comparing particular types but the evidence that does exist favours cognitive–behavioural therapy (CBT).

Inpatient treatments are available in a small number of centres in the United Kingdom. These provide multi-disciplinary therapy combining CBT with occupational and physiotherapy. The approach is similar to rehabilitation services for organic disorders but with a greater emphasis on CBT.

There is no evidence that drug treatment is effective. Antidepressant drugs can be helpful in patients with prominent symptoms of depression.

Dissociative disorders

Dissociation is a term derived from psychoanalytic theory to denote the separation of memory, sense of identity or sense of reality from consciousness. The most common precipitant is a psychological trauma. The dissociative disorders are categories that describe the behavioural expression of these phenomena. Although both conversion disorder and dissociative disorders refer to non-organic neurological symptoms, DSM-5 classifies them separately because conversion is a somatic complaint and dissociation is a mental complaint. In neurology, the most common dissociative disorders present as amnesia, fugue or depersonalisation/derealisation.

Dissociative amnesia

Dissociative amnesia is sometimes referred to as psychogenic amnesia and denotes the inability to recall important personal information, usually related to psychologically traumatic or stressful events, but is sometimes more global. There is preservation of the ability to comprehend environmental information and to perform complex learned skills.

Dissociative fugue

The word fugue refers to an episode of wandering in which the patient appears to be behaving normally in a goal-directed manner but has no recollection of the event and is confused about their personal identity. Rarely, a new identity may be adopted if autobiographical memory is not fully recovered. Episodes of dissociative fugue can last hours to days. Similar events may be seen in the context of other neurological disorders. In epileptic automatism, the episode is usually shorter in duration, the patient is in a more obvious state of altered consciousness and the behaviour is more stereotyped and purposeless. In transient global amnesia, the patient is aware, during the episode, that they cannot remember preceding events and they do not lose their sense of personal identity.

Depersonalisation/derealisation disorder

These two mental states are grouped together as a single disorder because they usually occur together. Patients describe depersonalisation as a feeling of disconnection from their body or not being fully inside their body; they may describe out-of-body experiences. These symptoms are very unpleasant and can be pervasive and associated with substantial risk of suicide. Depersonalisation and derealisation (a feeling of being cut-off from the world) can also be experienced in complex partial seizures and epilepsy should be considered as a possible diagnosis.

Dissociative disorders can be difficult treat. As they are sometimes considered a manifestation of anxiety, a common strategy is to recommend an anxiolytic antidepressant (i.e. an SSRI), and CBT, either separately or in combination.

Psychiatric disorders of epilepsy

Psychiatric symptoms are common in people with epilepsy, up to 50% in some studies. They can manifest either as transient phenomena directly related in time to the seizure (peri-ictal or ictal) or as more persistent inter-ictal conditions.

Peri-ictal and ictal psychiatric symptoms

Recognised prodromal symptoms are pre-ictal depression, labile mood and irritability. These can last for hours to days and are usually alleviated by the seizure.

Psychiatric symptoms during the ictus itself are most commonly witnessed in complex partial seizures. If they precede a secondary generalised tonic–clonic seizure, they are often referred to as an aura but in fact represent ictal phenomena arising from a temporal lobe focus. Patients may describe intense fear, depersonalisation/derealisation or déjà vu and they may hallucinate an unpleasant taste or smell. These symptoms are often accompanied by motor symptoms such as staring, stereotyped lip smacking or purposeless plucking movements. These ictal phenomena are usually short lived lasting a few minutes only.

The most common post-ictal psychiatric syndromes are delirium and psychosis. Post-ictal delirium usually presents with confusion and behavioural withdrawal. Agitation with hyperactivity can occur but is less common. Post-ictal delirium is usually self-limiting; patients with prolonged and frequent seizures tend to have longer episodes and these can last from hours to days. During the delirium the patient needs to be kept safe but no specific treatment is usually necessary. If delirium lasts longer than normal for that particular patient, non-convulsive status and other causes of delirium should be suspected.

The most significant risk factor for developing post ictal psychosis is temporal lobe epilepsy. The classic presentation is of a cluster of seizures followed by a 'lucid interval' lasting several hours to days. During this period the patients may exhibit unusual behaviour such as lethargy, irritability or restlessness. Psychotic symptoms then emerge, typically as visual and/or auditory hallucinations with delusional beliefs of a religious or paranoid nature. Patients can be floridly paranoid and aggressive and be a risk to themselves or others. Suicide is a particular risk and tends to be impulsive and violent, for example jumping in front of a train or jumping off buildings. The mean duration is 10 days but some people can remain psychotic for several months. Early and active treatment is required using a benzodiazepine (e.g. lorazepam) in combination with an antipsychotic (e.g. risperidone or haloperidol). If post-ictal psychosis is a regular occurrence following a cluster of seizures, immediate treatment before the onset of psychotic symptoms is often recommended. People with a history of post-ictal psychosis are at risk of developing an inter-ictal psychosis.

Inter-ictal psychiatric disorders

The most common inter-ictal psychiatric disorder is depression (estimated prevalence 22–40%). This has been particularly linked to temporal lobe epilepsy. Further, the risk of depression in the 3 months following neurosurgery for epilepsy, either *de novo* or as a recurrence is relatively high at 25%; this may become persistent in 10%. Depressive symptoms, such as pervasive low mood and biological disturbances of sleep and appetite, conforming to a DSM diagnosis of major depression, are well recognised. In addition, the presence of a group of more atypical symptoms has been recognised and labelled as 'inter-ictal dysphoric disorder'. This refers to a persistent state of irritability, anergia, depressed mood, insomnia, atypical pain and anxiety, sometimes with intermittent euphoria. It was initially thought that this syndrome was a specific disorder of temporal lobe epilepsy and linked to the underlying pathology. More recently this has been challenged with evidence that this symptom cluster is essentially a stable mood disorder variant and not specific to temporal lobe epilepsy. Depression in epilepsy can be effectively treated with psychotherapy, including CBT, antidepressants and electroconvulsive therapy (ECT). The newer antidepressants, such as selective serotonin re-uptake inhibitors (SSRIs), have a much lower liability to lower the seizure threshold (<0.5%) than the older tricyclic antidepressants and therefore should not be a barrier to their use.

Inter-ictal psychosis is well recognised, mainly in temporal lobe epilepsy, with a maximum estimated prevalence of 10%. This typically develops a long time after the onset of seizures, often more than 15 years. It has a schizophrenia-like presentation, often including Schneider's first rank symptoms (Table 22.2) and is therefore referred to as 'schizophrenia-like psychosis of epilepsy'. The reported difference between this and schizophrenia proper is a better preservation of personality and fewer negative symptoms. The risk factors for developing an inter-ictal psychosis are: early age of onset of seizures; left-sided epileptic focus and treatment resistance. Treatment is with long-term antipsychotic medication. Atypical antipsychotics, with the exception of clozapine, are less likely to lower the seizure threshold than older antipsychotics.

Forced normalisation

Forced normalisation refers to the observation by Landolt that psychosis, or more rarely depression, anxiety or agitation, can emerge when the EEG becomes normal. This EEG definition has since been extended to include the clinical observation that psychosis can emerge when seizures come under control with anticonvulsant medication. This can occur especially if there is an abrupt improvement in seizure control with the addition of a new drug in a patient with long-standing epilepsy. If seizures return, there is usually an improvement in psychosis and hence the term 'alternative psychosis' is often used to describe this clinical phenomenon.

Personality changes in epilepsy

The prevalence of a DSM-defined personality disorder is higher in people with epilepsy than in the general population (14%) with various studies estimating this as between 18% and 61%. In addition, there are behavioural traits that are characteristically seen in people with epilepsy, especially temporal lobe epilepsy. These do not conform to DSM diagnoses, suggesting that the pathological process that gives rise to seizures can also affect personality development. Certain traits have been grouped together as the Gastaut–Geschwind interictal behaviour syndrome and include viscosity or 'stickiness' of thought, when patients adopt circumstantial speech; hypergraphia or the tendency to compulsive and excessive writing often about minutiae; hyper-religiosity or the tendency to form deep and intense mystical or religious beliefs; and altered sexuality which is most often hyposexuality and decreased libido. Although personality changes are commonly seen in people with epilepsy, the concept of an inter-ictal syndrome is controversial and the elements of the syndrome rarely co-occur.

Psychotropic effects of anticonvulsants

When considering how to treat inter-ictal psychiatric disorders, it is important to recognise that the prescribed antiepileptic drug may have had psychotropic effects. For example, some studies have attributed 30% of cases of depression to antiepileptics and this has been reported with tiagabine, topiramate, vigabatrin and felbamate. Anticonvulsants that promote GABA neurotransmission, as a rule of thumb, tend to be sedative, anxiolytic and mood stabilising (e.g. pregabalin, gabapentin and sodium valproate) whereas those that inhibit glutamate neurotransmission tend to be activating and have antidepressant properties (e.g. lamotrigine). Other antiepileptics may increase the risk of developing psychosis (e.g. vigabatrin and topiramate).

Neuropsychiatric aspects of movement disorders

Parkinson's disease

Parkinson's disease is traditionally considered a movement disorder caused by degeneration of dopamine neurones in the midbrain substantia nigra. These neurones give rise to the dopaminergic nigrostriatal pathway which innervates the dorsal striatum. Here it modulates information flow through the opposing direct and indirect fronto-striato-thalamic motor output pathways and the net balance of output determines whether movement is initiated or inhibited. Reduced dopamine neurotransmission favours inhibition and, in Parkinson's disease, tonically diminished dopamine release results in the cardinal motor symptoms of bradykinesia, tremor and rigidity.

The neuropathology that is associated with cellular degeneration in Parkinson's disease – the Lewy body and Lewy neurite – is not restricted to the substantia nigra or even to dopaminergic neurones. Lewy pathology can be found in neurones throughout the central nervous system and even in peripheral nerves, for example the enteric, sympathetic and cardiac nervous systems and even in glandular tissue. As Lewy pathology can be widespread, non-motor symptoms associated with neuronal damage outside motor pathways are frequently present in people with Parkinson's disease and these include abnormalities of the mental state.

Anxiety, depression, apathy, psychosis and cognitive impairment, including dementia, are well-recognised neuropsychiatric syndromes of Parkinson's disease. Not all patients develop these complications and, if present, they develop at different time points.

For example, anxiety and depression tends to present early whereas dementia is a relatively late feature of the illness.

One way of conceptualising the development of psychiatric symptoms in Parkinson's disease is with respect to what we know about the spread of Lewy pathology. This has been found to occur in predictable stages, beginning in the medulla and olfactory bulb. From the medulla this spreads forward in the brain to successively involve the pons, midbrain, limbic cortex and neocortex. Because the appearance of motor symptoms has been shown to correlate with Lewy body pathology affecting the midbrain substantia nigra, it is likely that psychiatric non-motor symptoms of Parkinson's disease develop at a time when Lewy pathology affects the neural systems thought to be important for regulating cognition, mood and other emotions and behaviours.

Depression

The best estimate for the prevalence of all forms of depression in Parkinson's disease is 30–35%, when measured either by fulfilling diagnostic criteria or reaching specified levels of symptom severity on clinical scales. DSM-defined major depressive disorder accounts for 10–17%. Depression is a common disorder and the prevalence is also known to increase in people with chronic debilitating medical conditions. It is therefore likely that some people with Parkinson's disease would have become depressed anyway, as a result of a combination of genetic susceptibility and pre-morbid life events. Others may develop depression as a reaction to the impact of their illness on their quality of life. However, because depression is far more frequent in those with Parkinson's disease than in either the population at large or in populations with other disabling long-term conditions, it is likely to be intrinsic to the disorder in some people. Features of depression that seem to characterise a Parkinson's disease-specific mood disorder are lack of family history, onset within the 5 years preceding the development of motor symptoms and lack of symptoms of guilt or self-blame.

The observation from epidemiological studies that show that depression frequently precedes the onset of the motor symptoms of Parkinson's disease tallies with what is known about the spread of Lewy pathology. The brainstem nuclei of the serotonergic raphe and noradrenergic locus coeruleus can be involved before the midbrain dopamine nuclei. As antidepressants exert their action by increasing the neurotransmission of serotonin, noradrenaline, or both, the corollary is that early damage in these nuclei may precipitate a mood disorder. Neurochemical imaging studies have provided some evidence in support of this. Other evidence suggests that reduced neurotransmission of dopamine itself may cause depressed mood. The midbrain ventral tegmental nucleus, which is immediately adjacent to the substantia nigra, also contains dopaminergic cell bodies that can be affected by Lewy pathology. These cells bodies give rise to the mesolimbic and mesocortical pathways that innervate the ventral striatum (also known as the nucleus accumbens), limbic and frontal association cortex. In contrast to the dorsal striatum being involved in motor control, the ventral striatum is involved in reward processing. Thus, reduced dopamine neurotransmission at this site can arguably give rise to depressed affect. In support of this as a phenomenon, some patients on dopamine replacement therapy report a significant lowering of mood as the current dose of levodopa wears off with concomitant improvement following the next dose.

A difficulty with the diagnosis of depression in Parkinson's disease is that there is an overlap in clinical features such as reduced facial expression and psychomotor slowing. In practice, however, it has been shown that current DSM diagnostic criteria can be used unchanged to accurately distinguish patients with Parkinson's disease and depression from those with Parkinson's disease alone. Thus, careful assessment to include the whole range of DSM clinical criteria can reliably determine the presence of depression.

Given the varied aetiology of depression in Parkinson's disease, it is important to understand the context of depressive symptoms. Thus, it is crucial to take a full personal, family and social history to formulate the likely precipitants as this will guide the optimum type of intervention required. For example, when depression is secondary to social factors such as isolation or difficulty with dressing and bathing, changes to the immediate environment may significantly improve quality of life and therefore mood. The prescription of non-psychotropic medications may also help causes of low mood related to pain, urinary incontinence and sleep disturbance. Psychological interventions may also help; for example CBT has been shown to be very effective in helping a proportion of depressed patients with Parkinson's disease and it is worth considering this for those who have pessimistic thoughts and hopelessness about their future.

Between one-fifth and one-quarter of patients with Parkinson's disease take antidepressants, thus emphasising the significance of the problem in this disorder. When antidepressant medication is indicated, the choice is between drugs that specifically enhance serotonin neurotransmission (SSRIs); those that specifically improve both serotonin and noradrenaline neurotransmission (serotonin and noradrenaline reuptake inhibitors [SNRIs] or mirtazapine – a receptor antagonist) and those that have more diverse actions, including the older tricyclic drugs. There have been relatively few randomised controlled trials to guide pharmacotherapy. Further, the evidence from these is often contradictory, probably because of the small numbers of participants and the heterogeneous nature of depression in Parkinson's disease. As a rule of thumb, optimisation of dopamine replacement therapy should be the first tactic, especially for those patients whose mood fluctuates or dips as the current dose is wearing off. Smoothing of dopamine replacement therapy, by increasing the frequency of dosage and/or modifying the dose using motor function as a guide, can often stabilise and improve mood. Furthermore, some trials have shown that adding dopamine agonists to levodopa, such as pramipexole or rotigotine patches, can improve mood in depressed Parkinson's disease patients. There are also case studies showing the benefit of bupropion, an indirect dopamine agonist.

If this strategy does not help, either because of ineffectiveness or disruption of motor control, traditional antidepressants are then indicated. The evidence does not favour any particular class or particular antidepressant. Head to head studies have shown equivalent efficacy for SSRIs and SNRIs and for SSRIs and tricyclics, but again there are negative examples. The choice is therefore a pragmatic one and it is advisable to prescribe medications with the least potential for adverse effects first, such as SSRIs, then moving to SNRIs or mirtazapine and finally tricyclics. In severe depression, ECT can be effective and has the benefit of transiently improving motor control. A study has found repetitive transcranial magnetic stimulation beneficial but the evidence is insufficient to recommend this for clinical practice. Monoamine oxidase inhibitors (MAOIs) are rarely used these days to treat depression and are absolutely contraindicated in Parkinson's disease because of a potentially lethal interaction with levodopa.

Anxiety

Anxiety frequently accompanies low mood in affective disorders but general anxiety disorder, panic disorder and social phobia frequently present as separate disorders in Parkinson's disease.

The estimated point prevalence of all DSM anxiety disorders in Parkinson's is around 34%. Less is known about the specific pathophysiology and treatment of anxiety disorders in Parkinson's disease than depression. However, clinical experience suggests that as a levodopa wearing-off phenomenon, anxiety is more prominent than depression. Anxiety can be intense, especially at night. Like depression, a link between anxiety and reduced dopaminergic neurotransmission should be considered in patients whose anxiety fluctuates throughout the day, for example when marked anxiety is inter-dispersed with periods of calmness and normality of the mental state. Given this link and the fact that antidepressant medication is also anxiolytic, the same principles of treatment for depression also apply to anxiety, in other words, optimisation of treatment with levodopa or dopamine agonists, followed by the use of antidepressants if the response is unsatisfactory.

Apathy

Apathy has many features in common with depression but distinguishing factors include impaired motivation in the absence of low mood or sadness. In Parkinson's disease, there is some neuroimaging evidence that apathy and depressed mood are mediated by distinct neural systems, with depression reflecting abnormalities of the subgenual cingulate cortex, an area associated with major depression, and apathy being related to motor and frontal cortex dysfunction. In practice, pure apathy is rare and it is most often co-morbid with depression and/or cognitive impairment. Some studies suggest that apathy is a predictor of dementia in Parkinson's disease. There is no specific treatment for apathy; for example there is currently insufficient evidence for the use of stimulants such as modafinil.

Psychosis

Minor abnormal experiential phenomena commonly occur early in Parkinson's disease. They are regarded as benign because insight is retained and they are not frightening or distressing. These include visual illusions – the abnormal perception or misinterpretation of objects – whereby nearby objects are seen to 'morph' into living things. Another is a form of hallucination – a sensory perception without an object – in the form of people or animals moving past the periphery of the visual field. Yet another common phenomenon is the intense feeling of a benign human presence located outside of the visual field. This is sometimes referred to as an extracampine hallucination but this is not strictly correct as there is no abnormal sensory perception – the patient 'feels' the presence of the object but does not 'see' it.

Frank psychotic phenomena commonly develop later in the illness. These can be present in clear consciousness (i.e. in the absence of delirium), as in primary psychotic disorders. However, the conjunction of Parkinson's disease and an independent psychotic disorder, such as schizophrenia, is rare and the type of psychotic symptoms in Parkinson's disease is different from these and the range is more restricted. For example, the most prominent type of hallucination in Parkinson's disease is visual, as opposed to auditory. Cross-sectional estimates vary between 16% and 37% for visual hallucinations and 2% and 22% for auditory hallucinations. Delusions (i.e. fixed abnormal beliefs) can also occur in Parkinson's disease but again they are much less frequent than in the primary psychoses (1–14% in Parkinson's) and tend to be less bizarre, persecutory or grandiose. Other first rank psychotic symptoms, commonly witnessed in schizophrenia, such as passivity phenomena and abnormalities of thought control, are not seen in Parkinson's disease.

Visual hallucinations are usually stereotyped and commonly take the form of children or animals; they disappear if approached and, if multiple, they interact with each other but ignore the patient. They occur mostly in situations of diminished ambient light such as in the evening or in the context of visual impairment, in the periphery of vision. Again, if insight is retained these are non-threatening and usually ignored. However, as the disease progresses they usually worsen in intensity and frequency and become real to the patient, causing significant distress. This feature of late Parkinson's, estimated to develop in over 50% of cases, is the strongest factor causing admission to nursing homes because families are unable to cope.

It is often assumed that because hallucinations in Parkinson's disease occur mainly in treated patients, these are caused by medication-induced increased dopamine neurotransmission in limbic areas. However, the majority of studies have not found differences between non-psychotic and psychotic Parkinson's disease patients in the total dose of levodopa being received or in the types of drug being prescribed, including dopamine agonists. In addition, psychosis in Parkinson's disease was seen in the era before levodopa therapy. The factors associated with hallucinations are older age and longer illness duration; impaired visual input because of ophthalmic disease; abnormal cortical visual processing; sleep disturbance indicative of impaired brainstem dysfunction such as vivid dreams; and cognitive impairment.

The treatment of psychosis in Parkinson's disease is difficult. The use of first generation antipsychotics, such as haloperidol, runs the considerable risk of worsening motor symptoms and these are contraindicated. The second generation antipsychotic drugs were thought to be more promising because they are much less likely to produce extrapyramidal symptoms in non-Parkinson's disorders, especially olanzapine and quetiapine. However, this has not been borne out in practice. In placebo controlled trials, olanzapine was not effective for the treatment of psychosis and worsened motor symptoms. Similarly, there is no strong evidence for quetiapine ameliorating psychosis although it tends not to worsen motor symptoms and if given at night can improve sleep. The only medication with proven efficacy is clozapine, an atypical drug commonly used for patients with treatment-resistant schizophrenia. Clozapine has the potentially lethal adverse effect of neutropenia and therefore requires regular blood monitoring by a specialist service. Fortunately, the doses required in Parkinson's disease psychosis (50 mg maximum) are much lower than for schizophrenia, making leukopenia less likely, but the need to admit to hospital to initiate the drug and regular blood monitoring has made the uptake of this option uncommon. The use of the cholinesterase inhibitor rivastigmine has been shown to be effective in small studies, especially in patients showing signs of dementia where reduced acetylcholine neurotransmission is likely. As a rule of thumb, it is worth trying rivastigmine before moving on to clozapine in patients with troublesome hallucinations.

Cognitive impairment

It has been estimated that approximately 50% people with Parkinson's disease will ultimately develop dementia. The exact pathological basis may vary but it is highly likely that formation of Lewy bodies in the cortex is the main contributing factor. Another possible mechanism is degeneration of the acetylcholinergic neurones in the basal forebrain. As in Alzheimer's disease, reduced cortical acetylcholine is likely to contribute to impaired attention in addition to cortical pathology itself. This is supported by studies that have shown that drugs that enhance cholinergic neurotransmission, especially rivastigmine, improve cognitive function in Parkinson's disease.

The main predictors of dementia are age, severity of motor impairment and mild cognitive impairment especially visuospatial problems and reduced semantic fluency.

The presence of executive dysfunction alone, reflecting frontal cortical impairment, does not predict dementia. Executive impairment is frequently found in patients with Parkinson's disease on neuropsychological testing and reflects reduced dopaminergic input into non-motor cortex such as the dorsolateral prefrontal cortex and can improve with levodopa treatment.

Iatrogenic neuropsychiatric problems

Impulse control disorder The use of dopamine receptor agonists such as ropinirole as first-line treatment in Parkinson's disease, to spare the use of levodopa and thus delay development of dyskinesias, has highlighted a significant adverse effect of these drugs. This is the development of reduced impulsive control, known as impulse control disorder (ICD) with the emergence of features such as gambling, overspending, inappropriate sexual behaviour in men (e.g. seeking out pornography or prostitutes) and overeating. These behaviours can become compulsive and seriously affect the life of the individual and their family. Another type of compulsive behaviour is punding. This word describes a behaviour that was originally goal-directed, such as packing a bag or sorting out clothes, but becomes senseless, repetitive and time-consuming. Such ICDs are more common in men with young onset Parkinson's disease treated with dopamine agonists, with a family or premorbid personal history of sensation seeking. The main way of managing ICDs is to reduce and stop the dopamine agonist. Treatment with medications used for OCD, such as SSRIs, do not seem to help. In those patients where ICDs persist following reduction or cessation of dopamine antagonist, CBT shows modest benefit.

Deep brain stimulation Deep brain stimulation (DBS) has become a relatively common treatment for managing motor symptoms including drug-induced dyskinesias. The electrode placements are mainly in the motor section of the subthalamic nucleus (STN) but the globus pallidus interna is also used. As these sites are close by the non-motor circuitry mediating cognitive and emotional processes (Figure 22.1), the effect of DBS on cognition and mood

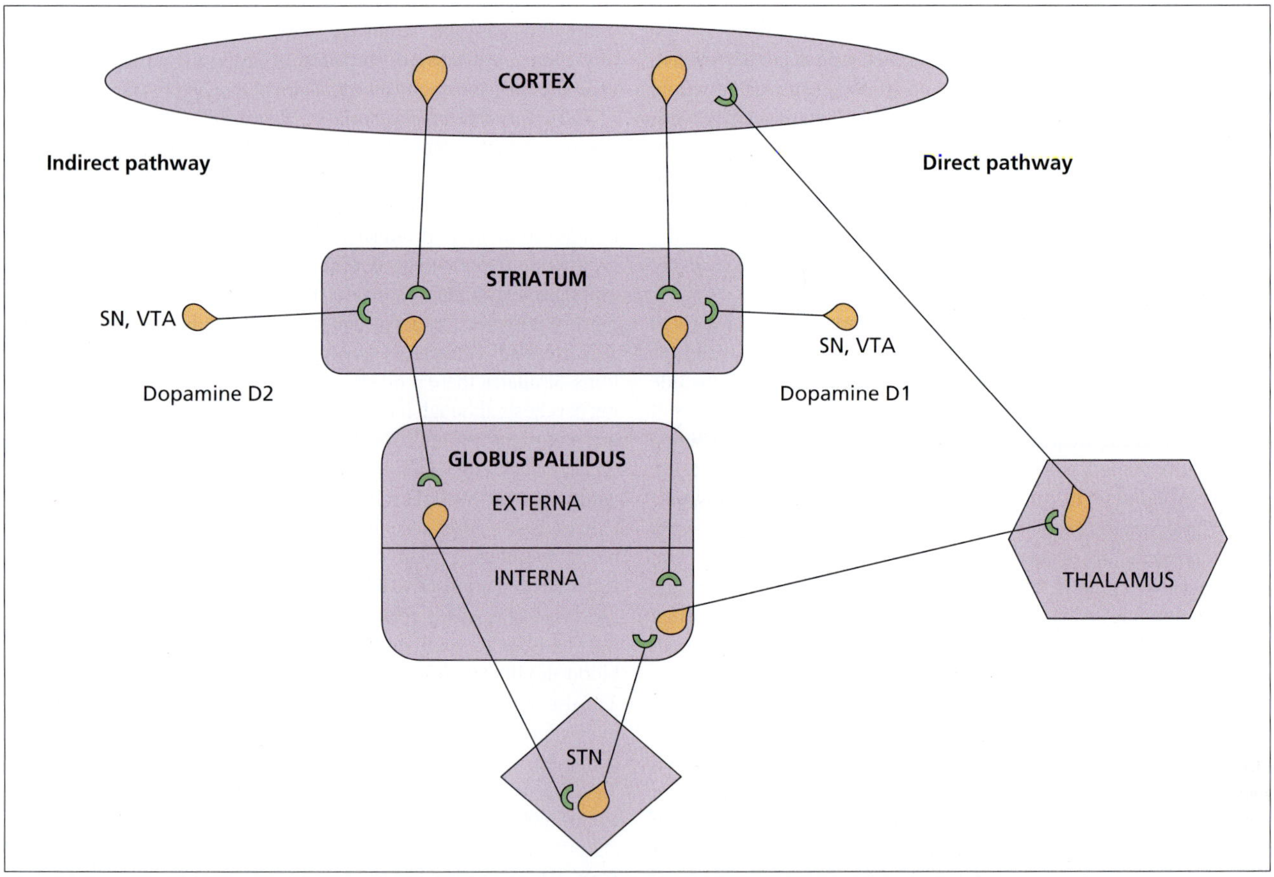

Figure 22.1 Generic schema of cortical-striato-thalamo-cortical feedback circuits. Information from cortex concerning movement, cognition and emotion is processed in direct and indirect pathways. Activation of the direct pathway facilitates the initiation and control of action and thought. Activation of the indirect pathway, via the subthalamic nucleus (STN), inhibits information in the direct pathway being relayed to the thalamus and inhibits action and thought. Dopamine innervation from substantia nigra (SN) or ventral tegmental area (VTA) to striatum modulates information processing in these pathways via D2 receptors (indirect) and D1 receptors (direct) neurotransmission. Increased dopamine release in striatum has the net result of increasing activity in the direct pathway. Reduced dopamine release, as in Parkinson's disease, facilitates the indirect pathway thereby causing bradykinesia and bradyphrenia. There are five circuits that follow the same general scheme; they project from different areas of frontal cortex and follow distinct but topographically parallel routes through the same structures. The cortical areas of origin are dorsolateral prefrontal and orbitofrontal cortex (cognitive circuits); anterior cingulate (emotional circuit); supplementary motor area (motor circuit); and frontal eye fields (oculomotor circuit). Neuropathology that involves any of these grey matter structures will cause a movement disorder and cognitive and emotional dysfunction.

has been a subject of interest. Cognitive decline has been reported but if DBS parameters are such as to restrict current spread to non-motor areas as much as possible, this can be prevented. The most common finding is impaired verbal fluency but this is usually mild and can be transient. The effect on mood is more controversial. Postoperative depression and apathy is a risk of DBS but this seems more a reflection of excessive reduction in levodopa therapy than the effect of stimulation per se. This is particularly predictable in patients with premorbid non-motor fluctuations in mood and can be averted by less drastic reduction in levodopa. There is a distinct increased risk of suicide following DBS thought to be 12–15 times higher than the general population. Risk factors are being single, a previous history of ICD and a current diagnosis of depression. STN DBS is associated with euphoria or even hypomania but this usually develops soon after the onset of stimulation and can be averted by reducing the stimulation parameters.

Other movement disorders

Understanding how the neuropsychiatric symptoms of Parkinson's disease are related to the dysfunction of neural networks mediating emotion and cognition is a model for understanding the symptom complex of other movement disorders (Figure 22.1). In addition to a movement disorder, most are additionally characterised by emotional and cognitive dysfunction and the expression over time mirrors the distribution and evolution of the particular pathology.

Like Parkinson's disease, Lewy body dementia (LBD) and multi-system atrophy (MSA) are alpha synucleinopathies associated with parkinsonian movement disorder. In LBD, pathology is prominent in the cerebral cortex giving rise to an early presentation of dementia and visual hallucinosis. In MSA, pathology is more posterior with early involvement of brainstem autonomic nuclei and the cerebellum causing ataxia, bladder problems and blood pressure instability. Frontal executive deficits can be demonstrated in MSA but frank dementia is rare and mood disturbance is best characterised by emotional lability.

Progressive supranuclear palsy is a tauopathy involving the amine and cholinergic neurotransmitter nuclei (substantia nigra, nucleus basalis, locus coeruleus and raphe nuclei), basal ganglia and oculomotor complex. This explains the development of a complex range of symptoms including motor symptoms of parkinsonism and ophthalmoplegia, frontal executive dysfunction, and psychiatic symptoms of apathy, mood lability, disinhibition and compulsive behaviour.

Wilson's disease is caused by copper deposition in the basal ganglia, thalamus and cerebellum. Rigidity dystonia and choreoathetosis is accompanied by cognitive impairment, personality change depression and even psychosis.

Huntington's disease is caused by the abnormal protein huntingtin being deposited in GABA neurones of the caudate nucleus and frontal cortex. The prominent abnormal movement is chorea and there is progressive cognitive impairment. Psychiatric problems develop early, even before chorea, and characteristically are of personality changes including irritability, aggression and disinhibition. Depression occurs in 40–50% of patients, often with psychotic features. Suicide is a major complication of depression and can occur in the absence of knowledge of the diagnosis. Psychosis occurs in 5–15% of patients with Huntington's disease and is typically paranoid rather than schizophrenia-like.

Other forms of chorea that are particularly relevant for neuropsychiatry include Sydenham's chorea and the paediatric autoimmune neuropsychiatric disorders associated with streptococcal infection (PANDAS). Sydenham's chorea is associated with the development of OCD, while PANDAS is characterised by tics and OCD. Affective disturbances and behaviour abnormalities are reported and patients sometimes appear hypomanic.

Tourette's syndrome is thought to be a neurodevelopmental abnormality of GABA and/or dopamine synaptic function in the striatum and is characterised by the onset of motor and vocal tics usually in or before teenage years. Tics are characterised by a build-up of the urge to perform them which can be resisted to varying degrees. Suppression of tics is invariably effortful and usually results in a period of rebound worsening. The symptoms characteristically wax and wane over the years. Tics can be simple and brief (e.g. blinking) or more complex coordinated movements. The latter can lead to secondary neurological damage. For example, repetitive head and neck tics can cause cervical spine damage, root lesions and myelopathy. Vocal tics are characteristic and necessary for the diagnosis and these can be so disturbing that the patient becomes socially reclusive. Coprolalia is often thought to be the hallmark of Tourette's but in fact occurs in about 10% of patients. Secondary forms of this disorder, tourettism, can be seen following stroke, the prescription of various stimulant drugs or after withdrawal from neuroleptics.

There are two co-morbidities associated with Tourette's syndrome. In childhood, attention deficit hyperactivity disorder (ADHD) is common, occurring in about 50% of patients. Obsessive–compulsive behaviours occur in 30–40% of patients. These can emerge during childhood but are more common in the teenage and adult years. The symptoms are not typical of OCD. For example, hand-washing rituals and phobias of contamination are not common. Instead, arithmomania (a strong need to count actions or objects) and the compulsive need for symmetry and order are more often found. Self-injurious tics may be seen whereby tics are performed to inflict pain, for example body punching or eye-poking. Compulsive touching is also often seen and can be directed at strangers thus causing social difficulty. Tic suppression can be helped with dopamine receptor antagonist drugs, in particular aripiprazole and risperidone, and clonidine which is more helpful in children than adults. Obsessive–compulsive behaviour, like OCD, is often helped with SSRIs, and ADHD, like the pure form, with methylphenidate.

Neuropsychiatric aspects of white matter disorders

While many neuropsychiatric disorders reflect grey matter dysfunction, psychopathology can also be seen in disorders affecting predominately white matter. The classic disorder is multiple sclerosis (MS) but other acquired disorders of white matter such as the leukoencephalopathies can also present clinically with psychiatric symptoms.

In MS, the main neuropsychiatric problem is disturbed cognition which occurs early in the course of the illness and can be detected in 40–65% of patients when tested formally. Demyelination most commonly affects speed of information processing, working memory and attention.

Psychiatric symptoms are also very common in MS and take the form of depression (50%), agitation (40%), anxiety (40%) and irritability (35%). Symptoms are often associated with the slow development of rigid and inflexible thinking. The prevalence of these symptoms is higher than that for patients with other chronic CNS conditions suggesting that they are not only a reaction to the effect of disability, but also are related to forebrain demyelination and cortical shrinkage. Mania is also more common in MS than the rest of the population. Of relevance to the aetiology of mood change in MS is the observation that, in general psychiatry practice, patchy deep white matter lesions seen on MRI scans are associated with bipolar disorder and treatment-resistant depression, especially after the age of 50 years. It is also important to recognise that severe depression is a side effect of β-interferon treatment where suicide is a distinct risk.

A mental state consisting of euphoria and eutonia (a sense of bodily well-being) has been described as being specific for MS and seen in about 10% of cases. This can be considered as a form of 'pseudobulbar affect', whereby mood and affect are disconnected leading to a denial of the severity of the illness. It is thought to reflect a physical disconnection between the frontal lobes and subcortical structures including the cerebellum.

Whereas MS is an acquired condition, the leukodystrophies are genetic demyelination disorders. In metachromatic leukodystrophy, patients with juvenile or adult onset forms characteristically present with personality changes and a schizophrenia-like illness which, if treated successfully, uncovers a progressive dementia. In adrenoleukodystrophy, dementia, learning difficulties and behaviour changes are the most frequent presenting psychiatric problems but again schizophrenia-like states have been reported.

Minor head injury and post-concussion syndrome

The neuropsychiatric features following severe traumatic brain injury and the value of multi-disciplinary rehabilitation are discussed in Chapter 18.

Post-concussion syndrome is often used as a term to infer that the physical symptoms that follow a minor closed head injury are psychological in origin. However, it is important to recognise that similar symptoms may be the result of shearing forces giving rise to subtle white matter damage. Typical complaints are of persistent headache, dizziness, blurred vision, fatigue, noise sensitivity and poor concentration. Recovery over several weeks is the norm but some remain symptomatic for months or years.

Acknowledgement

Professor Joyce gratefully acknowledges Professor Michael Trimble who wrote the first edition chapter and upon which this chapter is substantially based.

Further reading

General

American Psychiatric Association. *Diagnostic and Statistical Manual of Mental Disorders (DSM-5)*, 5th edn. Washington, DC: American Psychiatric Association, 2013.

Functional neurological symptoms

Carson AJ, Brown R, David AS, Duncan R, Edwards MJ, Goldstein LH, *et al*; UK-FNS. Functional (conversion) neurological symptoms: research since the millennium. *J Neurol Neurosurg Psychiatry* 2012; **83:** 842–850.

Edwards MJ, Bhatia KP. Functional (psychogenic) movement disorders: merging mind and brain. *Lancet Neurol* 2012; **11:** 250–260.

Fahn S, Williams DT. Psychogenic dystonia. In Fahn S, Mardsen CD, Calne DB, eds. *Dystonia: Advances in Neurology*, vol. **50**. New York: Raven Press, 1988: 431–455.

LaFrance WC Jr, Reuber M, Goldstein LH. Management of psychogenic nonepileptic seizures. *Epilepsia* 2013; **54** (Suppl 1): 53–67.

Neurosymptoms.org website. www.neurosymptoms.org (accessed 27 January 2016).

Non-Epileptic Attacks website. www.nonepilepticattacks.info/(accessed 27 January 2016).

Schrag A, Trimble M, Quinn N, Bhatia K. The syndrome of fixed dystonia: an evaluation of 103 patients. *Brain* 2004; **127:** 2360–2372.

Stone J, Carson A, Duncan R, Coleman R, Roberts R, Warlow C, *et al.* Symptoms 'unexplained by organic disease' in 1144 new neurology out-patients: how often does the diagnosis change at follow-up? *Brain* 2009; **132:** 2878–2888.

Epilepsy

Elliott B, Joyce E, Shorvon S. Delusions, illusions and hallucinations in epilepsy: 1. Elementary phenomena. *Epilepsy Res* 2009; **85:** 162–171.

Elliott B, Joyce E, Shorvon S. Delusions, illusions and hallucinations in epilepsy: 2. Complex phenomena and psychosis. *Epilepsy Res* 2009; **85:** 172–186.

Kanner AM. The treatment of depressive disorders in epilepsy: what all neurologists should know. *Epilepsia* 2013; **54** (Suppl 1): 3–12.

Krishnamoorthy ES, Trimble MR, Blumer D. The classification of neuropsychiatric disorders in epilepsy: a proposal by the ILAE Commission on Psychobiology of Epilepsy. *Epilepsy Behav* 2007; **10:** 349–353.

Trimble M, Kanner A, Schmitz B. Postictal psychosis. *Epilepsy Behav* 2010; **19:** 159–161.

Movement disorders

Gallagher DA, Anette Schrag A. Psychosis, apathy, depression and anxiety in Parkinson's disease. *Neurobiol Dis* 2012; **46:** 581–589.

Goedert M, Spillantini MG, Del Tredici K, Braak H. 100 years of Lewy pathology. *Nat Rev Neurol* 2012; **9:** 13–24.

Starkstein SE, Brockman S, Hayhow BD. Psychiatric syndromes in Parkinson's disease. *Curr Opin Psychiatry* 2012; **25:** 468–472.

Voon V, Krack P, Lang AE, Lozano AM, Dujardin K, Schüpbach M, *et al.* A multicentre study on suicide outcomes following subthalamic stimulation for Parkinson's disease. *Brain* 2008; **131:** 2720–2728.

Williams-Gray CH, Mason SL, Evans JR, Foltynie T, Brayne C, Robbins TW, *et al.* The CamPaIGN study of Parkinson's disease: 10-year outlook in an incident population-based cohort. *J Neurol Neurosurg Psychiatry* 2013; **84:** 1258–1264.

CHAPTER 23

Pain

Paul Nandi
National Hospital for Neurology & Neurosurgery

In neurology, as in all specialties within medicine, accurate diagnosis of the cause of symptoms is seen as an essential prerequisite for rational management. This is undoubtedly true, but in the assessment and management of pain, elucidating the primary neurological diagnosis is very much the beginning, not the end, of the evaluation of the problem. This is because the phenotypic characteristics of pain in the context of neurological disease are – with a few exceptions – not disease-specific, but occur in disorders of widely diverse aetiology. For example, neuropathic pain of burning quality can occur in the limb of a patient with peripheral neuropathy, syringomyelia or a cerebral infarct. Conversely, a patient with multiple sclerosis (MS) may have constricting neuropathic pain of the trunk, shooting neuropathic pain in the face and painful spasticity of the lower limbs. Knowing the diagnosis does not automatically inform the clinician of the nature of the pain; knowing the nature of the pain does not provide an automatic diagnosis. Confronted in the neurology clinic with a patient with pain, the clinician should aim to elucidate the likely mechanistic nature of the generation of the pain – or pains – before embarking on a management plan.

Definitions

For a phenomenon that is such a universal part of the human experience, it is perhaps surprising that pain is difficult to define. The International Association for the Study of Pain (IASP) defines it as 'an unpleasant sensory and emotional experience associated with actual or potential tissue damage, or described in terms of such damage'. This definition highlights the important points that pain can occur in the absence of damage and that there is an emotional component to it, but it has shortcomings.

The definition excludes those with severe cognitive impairment, infants and young children, patients with aphasia and animals. Some elements of the unpleasant sensory experience of those with neuropathic pain are not perceived as associated with tissue damage and are better covered by the term 'dysaesthesia'. In addition, the affective associations of pain are highly situational and, it can be argued, are not invariably unpleasant (consider eating chilli peppers). However, clinical pains generally are unpleasant, and may be especially so because of the patient's lack of control over the pain, and its association with disease and disability.

All pain may be classified into one of two categories: nociceptive (or nocigenic) and neuropathic (or neurogenic). Nociceptive pain is more common and more familiar, and is of the type experienced when tissue damage occurs (or is threatened), activating specific nociceptive neurones that transmit their signals within a functionally intact nervous system. Neuropathic pain is defined as 'pain arising as a direct consequence of a lesion or disease affecting the somatosensory system'; it is often qualitatively different from nociceptive pain, responds differently to various therapeutic interventions and is generally more difficult to treat.

Neuropathic pain can be further subdivided into peripheral or central, on the basis of the location of the lesion or disease. However, this may tend to engender an over-simplistic view in terms of pain mechanisms, because even when the lesion is initially entirely restricted to the periphery (e.g. trauma to a peripheral nerve), central mechanisms typically develop and may dominate the clinical picture.

Allodynia is pain produced in response to a stimulus that is normally innocuous. It may be mechanical (evoked by light touch or brushing) or thermal (evoked by application of gentle warmth or cooling). Hyperalgesia is an increase in pain response, with lowering of the pain threshold, to a stimulus that is normally painful (such as pinprick). Both allodynia and hyperalgesia may be subdivided into three types, depending on the pattern of applied stimulus that evokes the response: static (e.g. light sustained pressure); punctate (e.g. a single or repetitive pinprick at a single location); or dynamic (such as light brushing), where the stimulus is applied over a larger area.

Hyperpathia is a specific form of painful sensory disorder, pathognomonic of neuropathic pain and indicative of somatosensory neuronal loss. There is an increased threshold of sensory perception, so that a stimulus such as light touch or warmth may not be felt on initial application. However, with sustained or repetitive application of the stimulus, after a delay there is an explosive pain response reflecting central sensitisation.

Dysaesthesia is defined by IASP as any unpleasant abnormal sensation, whether spontaneous or evoked. The term is sometimes used as if to exclude pain in all its manifestations, but within the terms of this definition this is incorrect. Abnormal forms of pain (e.g. tactile allodynia associated with neuropathy) fall within the definition of dysaesthesia. However, many forms of dysaesthetic

Neurology: A Queen Square Textbook, Second Edition. Edited by Charles Clarke, Robin Howard, Martin Rossor and Simon Shorvon.

sensation that occur in a disordered somatosensory system fall outside the definition of pain. Examples include feelings of liquid running over an affected limb, or insects crawling on the skin. Patients frequently have difficulty describing dysaesthetic sensations, which is not surprising as these sensations are beyond normal experience.

Mechanisms of neuropathic pain

By no means all clinical pains encountered in the neurology clinic are neuropathic. However, pain is often of neuropathic type in patients with diseases affecting the somatosensory system, and aside from the obvious observation that such pains will commonly present to neurologists, the distinction between nociceptive and neuropathic pain is of practical importance because the treatment of each is different.

The following section focuses on some of the pathophysiological processes that may contribute to neuropathic pain (see also Chapter 2). However, it should be emphasised at the outset that most of the scientific literature on neuropathic pain mechanisms relates to data from animal (largely rodent) models measuring behavioural responses to sensory stimulation. Such studies therefore use models of stimulus-evoked pain and this is only one element of clinical neuropathic pain. Moreover, the models of nerve injury are usually to peripheral nerves (e.g. the various types of experimental rodent sciatic nerve injury). Caution should be exercised in extrapolating the findings of these studies uncritically to human disease and, in the account that follows, reference will be made to instances where evidence from human disease and pharmacotherapy give some support to the validity of such extrapolation. A recent exciting line of research is the development of a technique for transfecting human channel mutations into cell cultures.

A core concept in considering mechanisms of neuropathic pain is neuropathic hypersensitivity. At its most basic this means that in neuropathic pain states, neurones involved in nociception and pain exhibit increased excitability, manifest by spontaneous impulse discharge or discharge evoked by minimal (and normally sub-threshold) stimulation, producing the clinical phenomena of allodynia and hyperalgesia. A number of mechanisms can contribute to this.

Peripheral neuropathy

Abnormal ion channel expression

Voltage-gated sodium channels are subdivided into two groups based on their sensitivity or relative resistance to block by a potent neurotoxin found in puffer fish, tetrodotoxin (TTx). There are currently nine known subtypes, designated $Na_v1.1$–1.9, of which $Na_v1.7$ and $Na_v1.8$ (which are TTx resistant) probably have the greatest influence on nociception. In peripheral nerve injury a variety of changes occur, with combinations of up-regulation, down-regulation and translocation of individual subtypes at different locations on the neurone and characteristic changes involving the dorsal root ganglion. Recent work has also demonstrated gain of function mutations in painful diabetic neuropathy.

Drugs that produce use-dependent block at sodium channels, such as the local anaesthetics, show clear evidence of efficacy in treating clinical neuropathic pain. Mutations of the *SCN9A* gene, which encodes the $Na_v1.7$ sodium channel, occur in three disorders of pain in humans: a loss-of-function mutation gives rise to congenital insensitivity to pain, while gain-of-function mutation causes two painful conditions – primary erythromelalgia, a clinical syndrome of severe burning pain and erythema of the extremities, and the very rare paroxysmal extreme pain disorder.

Calcium channel activation is essential in the release of neurotransmitters, and antagonists of N-type calcium channels can reduce hypersensitivity to mechanical and thermal stimuli in models of neuropathic pain. There is also some evidence that L-type calcium channels may have an important role in pain and hypersensitivity phenomena. Cannabinoid receptor agonists, which are analgesic in nerve injury models, may exert their analgesic effect through an inhibitory action at these receptors. Of particular interest in terms of clinical relevance is the $\alpha_2\delta$-1 subunit, which exhibits up-regulation in dorsal root ganglion (DRG) nerve cells and within the dorsal horn of the spinal cord in rodent models of nerve injury, and which is the probable site of action of gabapentin and pregabalin.

Transient receptor potential (TRP) ion channels are normally present in nociceptive primary afferent neurones where they are involved in chemically and thermally evoked pain. The subtypes TRPV1 and TRPA1 are activated by noxious heat/capsaicin and noxious cold/mustard oil, respectively, in either case giving rise to a sensation of burning. Following nerve injury, these ion channels may be increased in small diameter fibres, giving rise to cold hyperalgesia, and in addition may be expressed in non-nociceptive sensory neurones, for example in Aβ fibres, providing a possible peripheral mechanism for mechanical allodynia.

Spinal cord

Central sensitisation and 'wind-up'

Hypersensitivity phenomena in neuropathic pain may be largely the result of changes in the central nervous system (CNS), even if the initiating event is entirely peripheral. Mechanisms may conveniently be divided into excitatory and inhibitory. The term 'central sensitisation' is frequently used to describe a state of hyperexcitability of second-order nociceptive neurones in the dorsal horn of the spinal cord, clinically manifest by allodynia and hyperalgesia. The term 'wind-up' is sometimes used as though synonymous with central sensitisation, but this is strictly incorrect; wind-up is the increasing response of dorsal horn neurones to repetitive C-fibre volleys (i.e. it is a neurophysiological event observed in the laboratory) and its relevance to persisting central sensitisation is uncertain. Evidence to date indicates that an ongoing afferent input is necessary to maintain wind-up; it is unclear whether this occurs via C fibres or sensitised large diameter afferents, or both.

Excitatory mechanisms

Glutamate is the principal excitatory neurotransmitter released in the dorsal horn in response to noxious stimulation. It acts on a number of different receptors including the *N*-methyl-D-aspartic acid (NMDA) receptor, activation of which appears to be a key element in producing central sensitisation. NMDA receptor activation is a complex process involving phosphorylation and removal of a magnesium ion channel block but, once activated, a positive feedback loop, induced through increased concentrations of glutamate, tends to maintain sensitisation. The NMDA antagonists MK-801 in animal studies, and ketamine in humans, are effective in reducing sensitisation.

There is also evidence that anatomical reorganisation occurs in the site of termination of Aβ afferents following nerve injury, with these afferents sprouting to terminate in lamina II of the dorsal horn, rather than their usual deeper location. This provides an additional explanation for the phenomenon of tactile allodynia.

Inhibitory mechanisms

GABA (γ aminobutyric acid) and glycine are the major neurotransmitters inhibitory to nociceptive activity present in the spinal cord. Decreased concentrations of GABA and loss of GABA receptors in the dorsal horn have both been demonstrated in peripheral nerve injury models. There is also evidence of loss of GABA interneurones, with reintroduction of GABA interneurones into the dorsal horn in experimental models of neuropathic pain reversing some of the behavioural manifestations of hypersensitivity.

The endogenous opioid system is also affected by nerve injury, with loss of μ receptors in the DRG and dorsal horn, accompanied by increased synthesis of cholecystokinin (CCK) which is an opioid antagonist. This provides an explanation of the relative ineffectiveness of opioids in the treatment of neuropathic pain. In contrast, the endogenous cannabinoid system appears unaffected by nerve damage in the periphery, providing a rational basis for the use of cannabinoids for neuropathic pain.

Role of inflammation and the immune system

There is now abundant evidence that there are major influences of non-neuronal cells in the development of neuropathic pain in traumatic nerve injury, largely the cells of the immune system and their associated chemical mediators, and these effects occur both in peripheral nerve and in the spinal cord. In peripheral nerve injury, a number of chemical mediators are released from macrophages, mast cells and Schwann cells, including the cytokines tumour necrosis factor-α (TNFα) and interleukins 1β and 6 (IL-β and IL-6), chemokines, prostaglandin and nerve growth factor (NGF).

The combined effects of these substances are complex and incompletely understood, but include local influences on ion channels and retrograde transport to the DRG where they may give rise to alteration of neuronal gene expression. In the dorsal horn of the cord, activation of microglia results in similar cascades of release of largely pro-inflammatory mediators with a net effect of increasing neuronal hypersensitivity. There is evidence for a role of the parasympathetic system in modulating and reducing inflammation and sensory neural hypersensitivity. It is interesting to speculate on the importance of these mechanisms in the clinical condition of complex regional pain syndrome.

Supraspinal influences

Descending pathways from the peri-aqueductal grey (PAG) and rostral ventromedial medulla (RVM) can modulate the transmission of pain at spinal level, in the form of either facilitation or inhibition. In conditions of neuropathic pain, there may be a shift in the normal balance of this system in favour of facilitation, resulting in an increase in central sensitisation.

Assessment of pain in the patient with neurological disease

The overall clinical assessment of the patient with neurological disease is set out in Chapter 4; this section highlights issues of particular relevance in the assessment of pain.

The pain history

The following information concerning the presenting pain – or pains – should be sought, with the main aim of establishing diagnosis.

- *Location:* in some cases, the patient's account of where their pain is located may be vague; in other cases, it may be quite precise in which case it should be recorded in detail. In a few conditions, the diagnosis can be made with near-certainty on the basis of this information alone (e.g. meralgia paraesthetica). In other situations, precise identification and documentation of the pain location may challenge preconceptions regarding diagnosis. For example, a patient with unilateral lower limb pain following a stroke may be presumed to have central post-stroke pain, but if the pain is restricted to a single dermatome it may be likelier to indicate a lumbar root lesion. It may be helpful for the patient to indicate the site of their pain on a line drawing of the body.
- *Onset:* was this sudden, rapid or insidious? A sudden onset should raise suspicion of an acute neurovascular event; a rapid early course of symptom development may suggest an inflammatory origin, while metabolic conditions typically are characterised by an insidious onset and slow deterioration. Sometimes there will be an obvious precipitating event (e.g. in cases of trauma).
- *Intensity:* likely to be at least moderate if pain is the presenting symptom, but variation in intensity is important.
- *Temporal pattern:* frequently yields useful information. Is the pain continuous or intermittent? Is it of constant intensity or fluctuating? Pain that is constantly present is frequently neuropathic. In addition, central pain is characteristically worse when the patient is trying to rest and relax, and better when active and concentrating on a task.
- *Quality:* burning, shooting or electric shock sensations are characteristic of neuropathic pain; nociceptive pain is more likely to be described as dull, aching or cramp-like. Difficulty in describing the pain is quite common with neuropathic pain.
- *Exacerbating/alleviating factors:* when asked about this, patients often focus on treatments, but in this context questioning is intended to identify pain modifiers that the patient has noticed – the effects of activity (both general and specific to the painful part), mechanical and thermal stimulation and the presence of allodynia, hyperalgesia or hyperpathia.
- *Current trend:* is the pain state static or evolving? If evolving, it may be improving or deteriorating over time, but may also be changing in other respects, for example becoming more widespread or changing in quality.

In addition, patients may identify more than one pain phenotype, in which case each pain should be analysed along the same lines.

The following questions should additionally be asked in patients presenting with pain to the neurology clinic:

- Is the pain in an area of sensory deficit?
- Is there accompanying paraesthesia/dysaesthesia?
- Are there, or have there been, associated abnormalities of skin colour, temperature or sweating, oedema or deformity?
- Is there evidence of an associated motor system disorder?

Treatment history

It is self-evident that a current drug history should be obtained as part of the assessment of every patient, but in the case of the patient with chronic pain more than this is required. It is important to obtain details of previous as well as present treatments, and non-pharmacological as well as drug therapy. The effectiveness of each treatment should be inquired into, as well as unwanted effects; drug dosages should be established if possible. This should enable the clinician to answer the question 'Why was this treatment stopped?' Possible answers are that it was ineffective, that it gave rise to adverse effects or that it was discontinued by default.

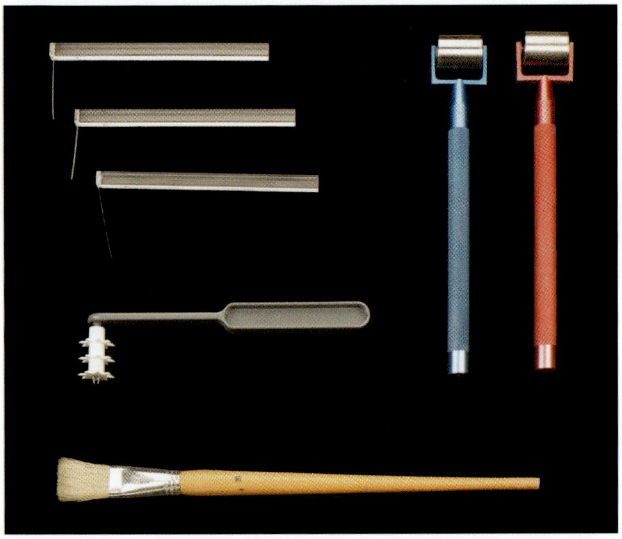

Figure 23.1 Quantitative sensory testing equipment.

Physical examination

In the general neurology clinic, sensory examination can often quite reasonably be kept to a minimal level, or even omitted if the patient denies any abnormality of sensation. However, in patients with neuropathic pain, far more emphasis on assessment of abnormalities of the somatosensory system is required. Full laboratory quantitative sensory testing is, in the author's view, not necessary as part of routine assessment, but some simple tools that can readily be used at the bedside can provide useful information, on hypersensitivity phenomena as well as deficits (Figure 23.1).

Von Frey hairs can be used to detect (and map) subtle degrees of tactile sensory deficit as well as static or punctate tactile allodynia; dynamic tactile allodynia can be assessed by stroking with a cotton wool ball or soft-haired brush. Mechanical hyperalgesia can be assessed with a pricking roller device. Appreciation of non-noxious cold and heat, and the presence of thermal allodynia, can be assessed with constant temperature thermorollers.

The next section gives an account of the manifestations of pain in some specific disorders, with emphasis on those conditions liable to be encountered in the neurology clinic. Neurological disorders have been subdivided into two groups, in line with the convention of disease classification on the basis of an origin in either the peripheral or CNS, but there is increasing recognition that such subdivision can be artificial and is not always helpful. Prior to considering individual central and peripheral diseases, some general issues of anatomy and pathology are discussed.

Central spinal pain: some anatomical and pathological considerations

How spinal, and indeed cerebral, lesions affecting somatosensory pathways cause central pain is unclear. Most theories invoke either excitation of damaged sensory pathways, or diminution of inhibitory processes, or perhaps both. There are tracts in the dorsal and ventral segments of the spinal cord that mediate transmission of excitatory and inhibitory influences to and from the brain.

Pain transmission reaches the brain mainly via two types of ascending spinal pathways:

1. *Spino-parabrachial pathway:* this originates in lamina I within the superficial dorsal horn and projects to the parabrachial region of the brainstem, peri-aqueductal grey matter and more rostral structures including hypothalamus and amygdala. The pathway appears mainly concerned with the affective component of pain.
2. *Classic spinothalamic pathway:* this ascends in the anterolateral quadrant of the spinal cord, terminates in the more posterolateral thalamus and projects to the sensory cortex. It is implicated in discrimination and localisation of pain.

Increasingly recognised as distinct entities, these ascending pathways mediate distinct sensory and affective components inherent in pain. There is also an ascending pathway running close to the central canal of the cord, thought to be the main transmission path for visceral and urogenital pain.

There are major descending pathways from the sensory cortex, thalamus, hypothalamus and brainstem to the spinal cord. Some of these pathways inhibit spinal nociceptive processes. Evidence in humans for central inhibition:

- Drugs with enhancing effects on noradrenaline and serotonin, neurotransmitters thought to inhibit pain and present in descending inhibitory pathways, may alleviate pain. Conversely, drugs and toxins such as reserpine, p-chlorophenylalanine and strychnine that block serotonin and GABA can produce pain.
- Stimulation of cerebral and spinal targets thought to be implicated in inhibitory processes can alleviate pain. This phenomenon is discussed further in the section on management of neuropathic pain.

Recently, the importance of descending excitatory pathways has been recognised, the key relay station being the rostroventromedial medulla, the output from which contributes to hyperalgesia. The evidence that excitation of the CNS can cause pain in humans:

- Pain can occur in an epileptic attack, including post-stroke epilepsy.
- Therapeutic stimulation of parts of the somatosensory CNS can inadvertently cause pain.
- Abnormal neural activity coinciding with pain has been recorded – for example, in the thalamus, midbrain and spinal cord in some patients with on-going central pain.
- Anticonvulsants and local anaesthetics can alleviate central pain.

Apart from excitation and inhibition, numerous other factors, including effects resulting from cortical and thalamic plasticity and changes in affective processing of pain, are of major importance.

Pain in individual disorders of the central nervous system

Multiple sclerosis

Pain in MS (Chapter 11) was until relatively recently considered rare and received little attention in standard neurology textbooks. It is now clear that pain in this condition is common and frequently severe; it probably occurs in 50% or more of cases and may be reported as the dominant symptom. Neuropathic pain can be extremely severe even in cases where other manifestations of the condition are mild.

MS provides a striking example of the diversity of pain presentation and mechanisms that may exist within a single disease diagnosis, summarised in Table 23.1; pain may be neuropathic or

Table 23.1 Acute and chronic pain in multiple sclerosis.

Acute	Chronic
<1 month	>1 month
Trigeminal neuralgia	Dysaesthetic lower extremity pain
Lhermitte's phenomenon	Back, joint and musculoskeletal leg pains
Paroxysmal neuralgic burning extremity pain	Painful leg spasms
Optic neuritis Painful tonic spasms	Visceral pain
Treatment: often responds to carbamazepine or phenytoin	Treatment: those used for neuropathic pain (including, rarely, intrathecal drugs, e.g. baclofen); standard treatments for back pain when present; antispastic agents for leg spasms
Mechanisms: in paroxysmal symptoms, ?ephaptic transmission at site of demyelination	Mechanisms of central pain: uncertain – spinothalamic tract fibre loss ± posterior column involvement probably implicated

nociceptive, and within each of these categories much variety is seen. However, there are a number of recognisable common presentations.

Neuropathic paroxysmal pain

MS is the most common cause of secondary trigeminal neuralgia (Chapter 13) and occurs in 1–5% of cases. The presentation may be indistinguishable from that of classic trigeminal neuralgia but may be atypical. Trigeminal neuralgia can occasionally be the presenting symptom in MS; suspicion of this is aroused by the development of trigeminal neuralgia in an unusually young patient or, if symptoms are bilateral, spread beyond the territory of the fifth cranial nerve or are accompanied by an obvious somatosensory deficit (which is usually very subtle or clinically absent in the classical condition). Lhermitte's phenomenon consists of spreading electrical sensations down the back and into the lower limbs provoked by neck flexion and attributable to a demyelinating plaque in the cervical cord; it may be described as painful, although not invariably so. In addition to these two well-recognised presentations, paroxysmal pain may occur at almost any site, reflecting the location of the CNS lesions, and may be spontaneous or evoked by tactile or other stimuli.

Neuropathic non-paroxysmal pain

This is perhaps the most common type of pain in MS and the presentation is usually consistent with a myelopathic origin, although lesions rostral to the cord can also produce pain, sometimes mimicking the picture of central post-stroke pain. It most commonly involves the lower limbs and trunk, but upper limb involvement also occurs. The pain may be of typical neuropathic character; an additional common complaint is of feelings of pressure or constriction, like wearing an over-tightened corset or an undersized boot. Feelings of unpleasant intense cold, particularly of the distal lower limbs, are also commonly reported.

Table 23.2 Pain in Parkinson's disease.

Musculoskeletal factors: shoulder stiffness, spinal deformity including scoliosis and camptocormia (bent spine), arthritis, contractures
Limb rigidity and stiffness
Dystonia, dyskinesia, akathisia
Restless legs and sleep-related pains
Visceral pains: abdominal pain. This is sometimes (but not necessarily) related to constipation. Also: non-cardiac chest pain
Central neuropathic pain

Nociceptive pain

This also takes a number of forms. Painful spasticity is a characteristic feature especially in the advanced stages of more severe disease. Management of spasticity is covered elsewhere (Chapter 18). Musculoskeletal pain in general may be more troublesome and more difficult to manage – although not necessarily more common – than in the general population, because the motor problems of weakness, spasticity and consequent poor posture can limit the effectiveness of physical therapies normally employed to manage pain of this type.

Parkinson's disease

Parkinson's disease (Chapter 6) provides a further example of a condition in which pain has traditionally received little attention, but in which it is very common (probably in excess of 50% of established cases). A range of non-motor symptoms, including pain, are increasingly recognised as common and distressing in patients with this disease. As in the case of MS, various characteristic types of pain are seen, reflecting different mechanisms, although central pain of Parkinson's disease remains poorly understood (Table 23.2).

Neuropathic (central) pain

The presumed central pain of Parkinson's disease comprises a variety of types, including burning and stabbing, and may be accompanied by other sensory phenomena including tingling, itching, tense feelings and restlessness. These symptoms can precede the onset of the motor symptoms, sometimes by several years. Pain is often bilateral but can sometimes be more marked on one side, either ipsilateral or contralateral to the predominant motor features. Of interest because of its midline distribution, pain can involve the mouth, throat or genital regions, suggesting in some instances a link with the burning mouth syndrome and vulvodynia (see Burning mouth syndrome and Vulvodynia).

The diurnal relationship between pain and any relief with levodopa or dopaminergic medication often seems unclear. Although levodopa has occasionally been used as an analgesic drug in other conditions, it is rare that pain experienced by a patient with Parkinson's disease can be switched off simply by antiparkinsonian drugs. While pain resulting from stiffness often improves when the stiffness improves, any temporal relationship between dystonia, dopaminergic deficiency and drug administration needs to be evaluated on an individual basis, but is unpredictable. Pain from focal dystonia, as might affect the hallux or produce a clenched fist, sometimes responds to botulinum toxin injections.

The mechanisms of central pain in Parkinson's disease are poorly understood. Compared with controls, these patients have lower pain thresholds to heat, especially in their affected limbs, and regardless of whether the patients are 'on' or 'off'. This is the opposite of the raised thresholds sometimes seen in central post-stroke pain (CPSP), suggesting there could be different mechanisms involved. Dopamine has analgesic properties and is present in descending spinal as well as ascending pathways. Furthermore, there are inhibitory pathways that project from the basal ganglia and brainstem to the spinal cord in which enkephalins, substance P, noradrenaline, serotonin and other neurotransmitters implicated in endogenous pain modulation are present.

It is therefore not surprising that degeneration of these extrapyramidal pathways in the brain and spinal cord could give rise to central pain, and conversely that pallidal deep brain stimulation might reduce pain. Mechanisms underlying the pain of such co-morbidities such as osteoarthritis, spinal deformity and muscle stiffness are of course entirely different; nocigenic musculoskeletal pain is common in patients with Parkinson's disease, who are also susceptible to osteoporosis with the attendant risk of crush fractures.

Dystonia/dyskinesia pain

Following diagnosis, Parkinson's disease is no longer seen in its unmodified state beyond the early stages as it is virtually always treated with levodopa or other dopaminergic therapy. This ultimately leads to alternating states of dyskinesia and bradykinesia ('on–off' fluctuations). Involuntary movements may be very pronounced during the 'on' phase in advanced cases, giving rise to mechanically induced nociceptive musculoskeletal pain.

Pain is also associated with other extrapyramidal and related degenerative disorders. In pure autonomic failure and multiple system atrophy (Chapter 24), intense discomfort known as 'coat-hanger' pain can occur. This pain around the shoulders and upper arms could be caused by ischaemia in suboccipital and paracervical muscles. The ischaemia is associated with increasing degrees of postural hypotension, and thus the pain occurs when the patient is upright, particularly in the mornings and after meals, and is relieved by lying flat.

Amongst various often ill-defined sensory symptoms, pain is an important feature of various dystonias and tics, in particular Tourette's syndrome and spasmodic torticollis – in which there is evidence of central pain in addition to pain related to musculoskeletal components. Other combinations of pain and involuntary movements are encountered in the syndrome of painful legs and moving toes, complex regional pain syndromes (CRPS), and stump and phantom phenomena.

Central post-stroke pain

Neuropathic pain following a stroke is common and appears to occur with equal frequency, and similar characteristics, whether the stroke is infarctive or haemorrhagic. The term 'thalamic pain' is often used for central pain following a stroke, doubtless because of the coining of the term 'thalamic syndrome' (Table 23.3) in the definitive 1906 paper by Déjerine and Roussy. However, central pain following vascular brain damage can result from injury from many structures other than the thalamus, and the term 'central post-stroke pain' (CPSP) is more appropriate.

Table 23.3 Classic features of central post-stroke pain (the thalamic syndrome).

A mild, rapidly improving hemiplegia without contractures
Persistent superficial hemi-anaesthesia or hyperaesthesia, with impaired deep sensation
Mild hemi-ataxia and astereognosis
Choreo-athetotic movements on the paralysed side
Sharp, enduring, paroxysmal, often intolerable pain on the hemiplegic side that does not respond to any analgesic treatment

Table 23.4 Clinical features of central pain.

Often very difficult for the patient to describe
Can be on-going, triggered, or a combination; superficial, deep, or a combination
Most often has a burning quality
May not disturb sleep
Patients may not appear to be in pain
May be in an odd distribution (e.g. a quadrant of the body; corner of mouth; ipsilateral mouth and hand – the cheiro-oral syndrome)
Onset may be delayed by weeks, months or years
Usually persistent, but influenced by factors such as movement, emotion, temperature change

Table 23.5 Clinical findings in central pain.

Pain is experienced within the area of the sensory deficit or a smaller area
The sensory deficit, if selective, is most typically thermal or for pain, and sometimes only detectable by quantitative sensory testing
There may be various spontaneous or evoked sensory phenomena (e.g. allodynia), typically seen with neuropathic pain
Rarely, central pain occurs in the absence of detectable sensory impairment; conversely, pain can occur in an anaesthetic area (anaesthesia dolorosa)
There may be variable accompanying motor and autonomic features

Not all pain following a stroke is central and the pain should fulfil certain criteria in order to make the diagnosis of CPSP:

- The pain should be located within an area of the body corresponding to the somatosensory lesion of the CNS.
- The history should be suggestive of a stroke and the onset of the pain should occur at, or after, the stroke.
- There should be confirmation of a CNS lesion by imaging and/or negative or positive somatosensory signs.
- Other causes of pain, such as nociceptive or peripheral neuropathic pain, should be excluded if possible; however, it is of course the case that other forms of pain may coexist with pain of central origin.

Central pain in general exhibits some characteristic clinical features and findings (Tables 23.4 and 23.5).

Approximately 10% of patients suffering a stroke will develop CPSP, making this the most common cause of central pain of supraspinal origin. The stroke may be of any degree of severity in terms of motor deficit (and in Déjerine and Roussy's original series of cases, weakness was minor in all); injury to the somatosensory pathways appears essential to the development of CPSP, but this can also be quite subtle. The pain is restricted generally to the area of sensory loss, but by no means has to be co-extensive with it; it can involve half of the body, or be restricted to a single digit. The likelihood of pain developing post-stroke appears to depend on location; it is particularly common (25%) following infarction in the posterior inferior cerebellar artery territory, producing lateral medullary (Wallenberg's) syndrome with ipsilateral facial sensory deficit and contralateral loss in the limbs and trunk.

There is usually some delay in the onset of CPSP following the stroke, and this can range from days to years, although in the latter case it is always possible that a more recent and silent cerebrovascular event may be responsible for the emergence of pain. In most cases, the pain develops in the few weeks after the stroke. Burning is the most frequently reported pain quality, and tactile/cold allodynia is common. Kinaesthetic allodynia, in which pain is mediated via the nerves of joint position sense, is rare but virtually pathognomonic of central pain.

Spinal cord injury

Over two-thirds of patients with spinal cord injury have chronic pain and in one-third this is severe. Severing the cord has no therapeutic benefit; central pain can occur in the presence of a functionally complete cord lesion and abnormal spontaneous firing in dorsal horn neurones has been recorded immediately above a lesion at L1 in a paraplegic patient. However, incomplete cord lesions and gun-shot injuries cause pain more frequently than other cord injuries.

Pain following spinal cord injury can arise from a variety of mechanisms (Table 23.6) and it is important to attempt to identify those mechanisms in the individual case in order to manage the pain appropriately. It is usually easier to deal with nociceptive (musculoskeletal) than neuropathic pain; for example, attention to abnormal spinal posture or management of a frozen shoulder is more likely to be rewarding than treating central neuropathic pain.

The central pain associated with spinal cord trauma has similar characteristics to the pain associated with other lesions of the spinal cord, not only including MS, but also expanding or compressive lesions such as tumours and syringomyelia, and vascular damage. Management of pain from spinal cord lesions is similar to that for other central pains. Surgery rarely has a part to play; the main exception is pain from post-traumatic syringomyelia (see Syringomyelia), which occasionally responds to decompression. Pain at the level of injury has been reported to respond to dorsal root entry zone (DREZ) lesioning, in which afferent impulses are interrupted as they enter the dorsal horn, but this procedure is now seldom performed as results are generally poor and unwanted neurological sequelae are common. Spinal cord stimulation can be helpful in patients with partial lesions but is of no value if the lesion is complete.

Table 23.6 Pain following spinal cord injury.

Musculoskeletal pains, including spinal pain from instability and deformity, shoulder disorders, muscle spasm, secondary overuse, and pressure syndromes
Segmental pain, sometimes with a band of hyperaesthesia, at the level of injury: central (from the spinal cord) ± peripheral (from nerve roots, including cauda equina damage)
Spinal cord pain below the level of injury: central pain, sometimes with persistent dysaesthesia. Like central post-stroke pain, onset may be delayed months or years. Spinothalamic dysfunction is probably a necessary but not a sufficient factor. Particular conditions include the central cord syndrome and post-traumatic syringomyelia
Deep visceral pain, which may be a form of central pain. There may be associated autonomic dysreflexia
Phantom pain below the level of injury
?Complex regional pain syndrome

Syringomyelia

In syringomyelia, a cystic cavity (syrinx) develops in the spinal cord, usually fairly centrally situated, but separate from the central canal. The general features and causes of syringomyelia are described in Chapter 16. Dissociated sensory loss typically occurs as the result of relatively selective damage to spino-thalamic tract fibres with sparing of the dorsal columns. Recurrent painless injury of the affected body parts, often the upper limb extremities, frequently occurs. However, although normal pain transmission is impaired, pathological central pain is very common, occurring in the majority of cases sometimes as the presenting symptom. The anatomical distribution of the pain typically reflects that of the somatosensory loss, commonly involving the upper limbs and trunk, but may be more extensive, affecting the lower limbs and perineum.

Phantom pain

It has long been recognised that whenever a body part is removed, a sensation of the missing part can persist (the phantom sensation) and sometimes there will be pain in that missing part (phantom pain). The phenomenon of phantom limb pain was recognised by Ambroise Paré in the sixteenth century, but the term was probably first used by Silas Weir Mitchell in the nineteenth century. Phantom pain most commonly develops in a missing limb, or part of a limb, but phantom teeth, breasts, eyes, genitalia and various viscera have been described.

Phantom pain can occur in a body part that has been denervated but not amputated; for instance, the body below a completely or partially transected spinal cord, or an arm following a brachial plexus avulsion injury. Phantom pains, and other phantom sensations, are liable to seem especially bizarre to the lay-person, and because patients may therefore suspect they will be disbelieved or thought insane, phantom sensations including pain are almost certainly under-reported.

Phantom pain in a limb needs to be distinguished from stump pain. In the latter, pain is in the region of the stump, where neuromas (although not necessarily painful) are commonly present, with other tissue abnormalities including scarring and musculoskeletal changes. In any individual case of post-amputation pain, there can therefore be a combination of neuropathic and nociceptive pains. Local measures are appropriate in some cases to address problems of poorly fashioned skin flaps or local infections; sometimes surgery is needed, but it is very rarely indicated for pain control itself. Surgery for a neuroma is seldom required unless there are particular circumstances, such as the neuroma being situated where pain is induced by pressure from wearing a prosthesis. This is because removing the neuroma frequently results in the formation of another neuroma more proximally.

Phantom pain has characteristic features:

- It occurs unpredictably in those with missing body parts, particularly when the missing part is distal.
- It is felt in, or within, the area of the missing part.
- The pain varies from the mild to the intolerable. Suicide has occasionally been reported.

The pain may have various qualities (e.g. burning, aching, crushing and gnawing); it can be continuous or intermittent, sometimes with brief paroxysms; and can be influenced by stimulation of other parts of the body, visceral influences such as micturition, and psychological factors. It may be associated with cramps, spasms, painful postures and distortions within the phantom. It is worse if the patient perceives they have no ability to move the phantom, although paradoxically pain may prevent this feeling of being able to move. Pain prior to amputation is sometimes a risk factor for the development of phantom pain, and in such cases the phantom pain may resemble the pre-amputation pain.

With time, the area of the phantom sometimes shrinks, particularly its proximal part, and this feature can also affect phantom pain. This 'telescoping' can give rise to curious phantom phenomena; for instance, a phantom hand may be felt tucked up near the shoulder with nothing intervening. Other forms of distortion of the phantom are common, such as the fingers or thumb being enlarged and twisted into an abnormal and painful posture.

Phantom pain may develop instantaneously, or soon after removal of the part, or may develop months or years later. It is often very long-lasting, but sudden resolution rarely occurs spontaneously, and even more rarely after a stroke affecting the phantom area represented in the brain. Phantom sensations and pain occur regardless of the cause of loss of the body part (i.e. whether from trauma, surgical removal or disease). Usually, loss of a body part will have been instantaneous or rapid, but the same phantom phenomena have been described in the slow loss that occurs with leprosy.

Phantom phenomena, including pain, are relatively rarely experienced in congenital absence of a limb, or after amputation of a body part in childhood, although childhood phantom pain may be more common than previously thought.

Some very curious temporal painful phantom phenomena have been reported. Phantom lower limbs felt after thoracic spinal cord transaction disappeared when cord compression from a cervical disc developed, only to return when the disc was removed. Conversely and paradoxically, phantom pain in a paraplegic became manifest following spinal anaesthesia. The author has recently encountered a case in which a phantom lower limb, which had spontaneously remitted, re-emerged following the implantation of a spinal cord stimulator.

Unfortunately, treatment of phantom pain remains extremely disappointing. Over 60 types of treatment have been reported, ranging from drugs to neurosurgical and other invasive treatments. Although the use of opioids is being explored further, currently treatment is usually ineffective. For those patients in whom amputation is therapeutic and elective, pre-emptive analgesia has not convincingly been shown to prevent the development of phantom pain, although this perhaps reflects inadequacy of the techniques employed to block the afferent barrage completely. It is hoped that recent studies on neural plasticity will lead to new approaches.

When a body part loses its sensory innervation, changes in somatosensory cortical and thalamic representation take place. Changes can be very rapid; for example, even a local anaesthetic ring block of a finger results in cortical changes within a few minutes. The area of brain from which input has been deprived is physiologically 'invaded' by innervation from adjacent areas. Such phenomena have been studied extensively in humans, and shifts in cortical representation may be more extensive in the presence of pain, normalise with treatment of the pain and account for peculiar referred patterns of sensation, for instance a touch on the face being felt in the phantom limb of amputees. The specific role of pain in these phenomena remains to be clarified.

In order to try to modify these neuroplastic changes, graded motor imagery techniques have been tried, as has the mirror box, particularly for patients with a phantom upper limb. In this ingenious technique, a mirror is placed in front of the patient, at right angles to the chest, such that the patient sees the reflection of the intact limb producing a simulation of the missing limb. The patient is asked to mimic the position of the phantom limb with the intact limb, and then to look into the mirror on the side of the intact limb. By attempting symmetrical movements of the two limbs, the patient can feel the phantom limb move. Intriguingly, the ability to exert apparent control over the phantom limb can result in pain relief. Beneficial results have been reported with these techniques, but pain relief is unpredictable and often transient. Further studies are needed.

Painful legs and moving toes syndrome

On the borderland between a central and peripheral neurological disorder and with movement-related and sensory components, the clinical features are summarised in the title: there is pain in the distal lower limbs accompanied by spontaneous movements of the toes, foot or lower leg. The pain varies from being a mild discomfort to a very severe intractable pain; rarely, instances of suicide have occurred.

The pain is often difficult to describe and can be burning, crushing, cramping or twisting. The movements are usually slow and irregular with sinuous fanning and clawing of the toes. The number of toes affected is very variable. Sometimes, the movements can briefly be stopped with effort, but break through again when concentration is relaxed. In some patients, pain precedes the onset of the movements; in others, vice versa. The condition can start unilaterally, although it tends to become bilateral, if sometimes asymmetrical. A similar phenomenon, 'painful arm and moving fingers', has also been described.

The cause is unknown, but the disorder has been described in association with lumbar root lesions in degenerative spine disease, peripheral neuropathy and peripheral limb trauma. Rarely, other involuntary movements are seen, which, as with the upper limb syndrome, suggests there is a central rather than peripheral cause in some patients – a distinction that might possibly be clarified in future from neurophysiological studies. The increasing recognition of movement abnormalities in CRPS suggests that painful legs and moving toes share common pathophysiological mechanisms with that condition, but without the objective signs of vasomotor or sudomotor instability.

Treatment is usually ineffective, for both the movements and the pain. For the pain, drugs including anticonvulsants such as gabapentin, antispasticity agents, benzodiazepines, phenothiazines, dopaminergic drugs and beta-blockers have not proven effective in the long term. There have been reports of sodium channel blocking agents such as carbamazepine being effective, possibly through blocking of ephaptic transmission across damaged axons. Epidural opiates and local anaesthetics have been tried, and while initially

Table 23.7 Painful legs and moving toes and restless legs syndromes.

Painful legs and moving toes	Restless legs syndrome
Spontaneous movements of toes and feet	Irresistible desire to move legs around
Present throughout day	Worse in evening and night, sometimes associated with periodic limb movements during sleep
No known family history	Often positive family history
Involuntary irregular, fanning, sinuous, dystonic movements affecting toes in particular	No spontaneous involuntary movements
Pain deep, diffuse, of various sorts	Pains of various sorts, also dysaesthesia, discomfort
Underlying causes sometimes seen, including peripheral neuropathy and radiculopathy, infections, and trauma; rarely, central causes	Underlying causes occasionally seen, including peripheral neuropathy and radiculopathy, iron deficiency anaemia, pregnancy, renal failure
Rarely responds to dopaminergic drugs	May respond to levodopa and dopaminergic drugs, benzodiazepines, opioids, anticonvulsants

lumbar sympathetic blockade was thought promising, this has not proved beneficial in most patients. The main disorder with which painful legs and moving toes is confused is the restless legs syndrome, although the distinction can usually be made with ease (Table 23.7).

Epilepsy

Pain can be a feature of an epileptic attack, as first noted by Gowers in 1901. Although rare, some studies have reported that about 2% of patients with epilepsy have painful seizures, but this figure is probably an overestimate resulting from selection bias. The pains have been divided into three categories:

1 *Unilateral pain in the face, arm, leg or trunk:* seizures tend to originate from the hemisphere contralateral to the pain, usually in the rolandic area. Parietal, or occasionally centro-parietal or other lesions can be responsible, but sometimes no obvious structural lesion is detectable. Pain can be caused by direct excitatory involvement of the primary sensory area or spread there from elsewhere. Ictal depression of inhibitory processes could provide an alternative explanation.
2 *Headache:* distinct from the common post-ictal headache, headache and other head pains, sometimes with a migrainous element, may be part of the seizure. Temporal lobe involvement may be more common in these patients although localising value is often poor. Increased cerebral blood flow occurs during a seizure, and it is thought that vascular factors could contribute to these pains.
3 *Abdominal pain,* rather than nausea, is a very rare feature of an epileptic attack and may be associated with temporal or frontal lobe seizures.

The treatment is that of the seizure disorder.

Fibromyalgia

Fibromyalgia syndrome (FMS) was originally described in the 1800s and has been known by a number of titles including muscular rheumatism and interstitial fibrositis. These labels imply that the condition is primarily a rheumatological disorder, an impression strengthened by the presence of myofascial tender points at characteristic locations. However, there are no diagnostic abnormalities of muscle in the condition, although there is possible evidence of non-specific changes related to microcirculation alteration giving rise to reduced oxygen delivery, and the widespread hyperalgesia of FMS appears likely to indicate a state of diffuse central sensitisation.

There is no evidence of either an inflammatory process or autoimmune disorder, but in addition to widespread pain there are a number of associated features, in particular poor sleep and daytime fatigue, and often coexistence of other painful conditions such as headache, irritable bowel syndrome and temporo-mandibular pain.

Many treatments have been tried, including drugs such as amitriptyline and newer antidepressants such as duloxetine, pregabalin and intravenous lidocaine, acupuncture, exercise and other physical measures, and behavioural techniques. Their efficacy is variable and unpredictable and a multi-disciplinary approach is probably best.

Peripheral pain: anatomical and pathological considerations (Chapter 2)

Pain from the periphery is conveyed to the CNS by primary afferent nociceptors – sensory neurones that are activated by noxious mechanical, thermal and chemical stimuli. These neurones contain thinly myelinated, faster conducting Aδ fibres and unmyelinated, slower conducting C fibres; the former mediate brief, acute, sharp 'first' pain, and the latter the delayed, more diffuse, dull 'second' pain. The majority of Aδ and C fibres are polymodal (i.e. they react to a variety of noxious stimuli), and these fibres use numerous signal transduction mechanisms in order to convert noxious environmental stimuli into electrochemical signals. C fibres have been further tentatively subdivided into:

- Fibres that, amongst other properties, express P2X3 purine receptors (one type of ATP-responsive channel) and receptors for glial cell line-derived neurotrophic factor (GDNF). These fibres are sensitive to GDNF, terminate deep in the substantia gelatinosa of the spinal cord, and may be important in mediating neuropathic pain.
- Fibres that contain peptides including substance P and calcitonin gene-related peptide (CGRP), and express the high affinity NGF receptor TrkA. These fibres are sensitive to NGF, terminate more superficially in the dorsal horn of the spinal cord and mediate plasma extravasation and vasodilatation – also called neurogenic inflammation. This inflammation, whether resulting from tissue damage or from release of peptides and neurotransmitters from the sensory nerve endings themselves, sensitises nociceptor endings. This results in peripheral sensitisation. These fibres are an important component of visceral afferents and have a more diffuse pattern of innervation than those fibres innervating skin. They also appear to regulate the behavioural sensitivity to pain through projections to deep central brain structures in the brainstem, hypothalamus and amygdala.

Both groups of C fibres respond to noxious stimulation and express the vanilloid (capsaicin) TRPV1 receptor which transduces noxious chemical and heat (>43 °C) stimuli. Noxious cold (<15 °C) is mediated by the menthol and a variety of other cold receptors. Chemicals such as bradykinin, serotonin, lipids and low pH stimulate other specific receptors. Mechanical stimuli are transduced by yet other receptors, less well characterised.

Some noxious stimuli affect ion channels and alter neuronal excitability directly; others involve metabotropic receptors and act through second-messenger processes. Several voltage-gated sodium, potassium and calcium ion channels are also expressed in sensory nerves, some specifically in C fibres, and a number of these are likely to be involved in transmission of nociceptive information. However, the selective properties of nociceptors change after damage or disease. For example, there are silent or 'sleeping' nociceptors that acquire mechanical sensitivity only during inflammation.

There are many ways in which these peripheral phenomena and their central sequelae can generate pain:

- *Ectopic discharges.* Discharges from damaged but also adjacent non-damaged neurones, the latter perhaps implicating Schwann cells, generate various pain-producing substances. These ectopic discharges not only generate spontaneous sensations, but also lead to changes in excitability of neurones in the CNS. The mechanisms responsible are likely to relate to changes in specific ion channels. Substances that block neuronal activity (e.g. local anaesthetics, mexiletine, some tricyclic antidepressants) which are sometimes effective for neuropathic pain work through effects on specific ion channels.
- *Changes in neuronal properties.* Genes expressed in primary sensory nerves are eventually responsible for transduction, conduction and synaptic transmission. Disorders affecting the sensory nerve result in changes in up- and down-regulation of these genes and their transcripts, and changes in the function and selectivity of the nerves. For example, the $\alpha 2\delta$ calcium channel subunit is up-regulated after nerve injury, which may explain the efficacy of gabapentin in neuropathic pain.
- *Loss of sensory neurones.* After peripheral damage, atrophy occurs that affects the whole of the sensory neurone. This loss particularly affects C fibres, and the resulting imbalance can contribute to abnormal sensations, as in some patients with post-herpetic neuralgia in whom areas of severe sensory loss occur. The central ends of C fibres atrophy in the dorsal horn; whether adjacent Aβ fibre terminals sprout into that area remains controversial, but innocuous mechanical stimuli become perceived as pain (mechanical allodynia). This is an example of central sensitisation.
- *Central sensitisation* after lesions of peripheral sensory nerves occur in the spinal cord and also at higher levels. Central sensitisation is associated with various features: enlargement of the area in the periphery where stimuli activate neurones; sub-threshold stimuli now reach threshold; increased response to supra-threshold stimuli; and pain from activity in non-nociceptive fibres. Some of these phenomena account for pain that spreads beyond the affected nerve territory, exaggeration and prolonged pain after peripheral stimulation, and other features including allodynia, hyperpathia and related sensory disturbances.
- *Disinhibition* can also be important, contrasting with these excitatory processes. Normally, GABA and glycine mediate inhibition of pain-subserving processes. Blocking these substances can cause pain. Nerve injury can result in impaired GABA inhibition in the spinal cord.
- *Microglia and other glial cells* are intimately involved in the neuro-immune responses that follow neurological lesions of the CNS and which can generate pain. There are also peripheral immune responses that are associated with peripheral nerve damage and a number of painful peripheral nerve disorders.

Pain in individual disorders of the peripheral nervous system

Painful peripheral neuropathies

It is puzzling why some patients with a specific neuropathy develop pain, while others do not. Furthermore, pain in some neuropathies can result from several different aetiologies. For example, in diabetic neuropathy there are vascular, inflammatory and metabolic factors. In HIV neuropathy, there are direct effects of the virus, nutritional factors, vasculitis, toxicity from antiretroviral agents, and co-infection. Painful neuropathies, a few examples of which are singled out later, can be roughly classified into causative groups:

- Inflammatory and vascular disorders – diabetes, collagen vascular disease and vasculitis, polyarteritis nodosa, Guillain–Barré syndrome and chronic inflammatory demyelinating polyradiculoneuropathy (CIDP). Many of these disorders cause mononeuritis multiplex, and to what extent vasa nervorum and nervi vasorum and sympathetic nerve fibres are implicated is uncertain. Changes in the neurochemical milieu surrounding damaged nerve endings, some of which follow leakage from damaged blood vessels, can be important.
- Infective – Lyme disease, HIV, leprosy and varicella zoster.
- Infiltration of nerves – sarcoid and tumours, particularly lymphoma.
- Metabolic factors – diabetes, alcohol, nutritional and vitamin deficiency states (especially thiamine and vitamin B_{12} deficiency), peripheral ischaemia and paraneoplastic states.
- Toxic and drug-induced causes – chemotherapeutic drugs (e.g. vincristine, cisplatin, taxols – especially docetaxol), thalidomide, antiretrovirals, nitrofurantoin, gold, isoniazid, disulfiram; toxic agents – arsenic, thallium.
- Trauma, including iatrogenic lesions after surgery.
- Hereditary peripheral neuropathies (see Absence of pain).

Many disorders span more than one category; for example, diabetes features in both the vascular and metabolic categories, and the pain of HIV-associated neuropathy appears in both the infective and chemotherapeutic categories.

Burning feet, and the small-diameter fibre neuropathies

Although autonomic and later large fibre involvement sometimes occur, burning pain, typically distal and affecting the feet, is often caused by a small fibre sensory neuropathy. While routine testing of nerve conduction is typically normal, there may be abnormalities of thermal thresholds. However, the latter is a psychophysical test requiring patient cooperation, and abnormalities do not prove that the neuropathy and hence the pain arises peripherally. Sometimes a small fibre neuropathy is only detectable on skin biopsy. It is striking how many of the painful neuropathies are accompanied by autonomic involvement, presumably because small-diameter fibres are those subserving both efferent autonomic and afferent sensory modalities. Causes of these small-fibre neuropathies include the following:

- Diabetes mellitus, which deserves particular mention because this may only be revealed by a glucose tolerance test. Thus, in an otherwise obscure case of peripheral neuropathy with burning pain, diabetes needs to be carefully excluded.
- Connective tissue diseases such as Sjögren's disease and monoclonal gammopathy.
- Acquired amyloidosis.
- Genetic causes, which perhaps account for an otherwise cryptogenic burning feet syndrome more frequently than usually suspected.

As with so many other painful conditions, non-neurological causes need to borne in mind, and with pain in the feet, even when burning, disorders such as plantar fasciitis need to be considered.

Erythromelalgia

First recognised and named in 1872 by Weir Mitchell, a physician during the American Civil War and author of *Injuries of Nerves and Their Consequences*, this term comprises a group of symptoms that appear to have variable combinations of vascular and neuropathic features. The characteristic features are episodes of heat, redness and pain in the extremities, predominantly the legs, worse and prolonged in the heat, and with improvement in the cold such that, for relief, patients sometimes immerse their feet in cold water to an extent that skin maceration and its complications develop. The episodic features and heat triggering differentiate erythromelalgia from small fibre neuropathies, CRPS and vascular insufficiency.

Erythromelalgia can be divided into:

1 Primary:
   - Sporadic
   - Hereditary (childhood onset, autosomal dominant).

2 Secondary, to thrombocythaemia and less commonly polycythaemia, collagen vascular disease, diabetes, peripheral neuropathy, drugs (e.g. calcium-channel blockers, pergolide, bromocriptine), following freezing and non-freezing cold injury, and rare toxic causes.

Whether the clinical features are caused by vascular factors, a small fibre neuropathy or a combination, the various components have a final common pathway in which there are abnormalities of microvascular perfusion of the skin, with a combination of skin hyper-perfusion together with hypoxia.

Neurological investigations have variously shown evidence of abnormalities in both afferent C fibres and efferent post-ganglionic sympathetic fibres in a number of patients, but the precise relationship between such abnormalities and the vasomotor changes remains unclear. There is evidence suggesting that, by different mechanisms depending on the cause, there is sensitisation of polymodal C nociceptors, with abnormally low thresholds and prolonged after-discharges, and involvement of mechano-insensitive fibres. The axon reflex results in vascular leakage and vasodilatation. The hereditary form results from a gain-of-function mutation in the *SCN9A* gene encoding the Na_v1.7 voltage-gated sodium channel. Recently, the very rare paroxysmal extreme pain disorder (familial rectal pain syndrome) has been shown to be a channelopathy resulting from a disorder affecting the same gene. How any of these mechanisms give rise to the episodic nature of the clinical features remains obscure.

Treatment

- Remove the offending drug: the condition often resolves.
- Low-dose aspirin when due to thrombocythaemia: often effective.
- Epidural analgesics and other symptomatic measures: rarely effective.
- High dose topical capsaicin to damage C fibres: experimental and unlicensed.
- In the hereditary condition, consider drugs with inhibitory action at voltage-gated sodium channels (intravenous local anaesthetics, class I anti-arrhythmics and antiepileptics such as carbamazepine).
- Avoid damage from cold immersion.

Neuropathy in diabetes mellitus (Chapter 10)

Pain occurs in over 10% of patients with type I and one-third of patients with type II diabetic peripheral neuropathy, but what characterises those patients with pain is unknown, even when their nerves are studied by microneurography. However, in a small study the glucose metabolite methygloxal has been shown to be a predictor of pain and appears associated with a gain-of-function in Na_v 1.8 channels. The classification shown in Table 23.8 is both arbitrary and a simplification, but illustrates the variety of types of painful neuropathies encountered. Individual patients often have more than one type of nerve involvement. In painful neuropathies of acute onset, vascular and inflammatory factors are particularly important and pain is more likely to be reversible; by comparison, metabolic factors probably predominate in those neuropathies of gradual onset, in which pain is often persistent.

Some of these diabetic neuropathies merit particular mention. Acute painful neuropathy, associated with rapid weight loss, has a good prognosis over months. 'Insulin neuropathy', a neuropathy that develops as insulin is introduced, again has a good prognosis. Both conditions are uncommon. About 50% of diabetic third cranial nerve palsies are painful. Pain presumably arises from involvement of associated trigeminal afferents and resolves over days or a few weeks. Truncal involvement can mimic acute cardiac or abdominal disorders, and shingles without a rash. Pain resolves over months. Lumbosacral radiculoplexopathy (diabetic amyotrophy; femoral neuropathy) is typically seen in late-onset diabetes in men over 60 years. There is severe aching thigh pain, worse at night. Gradual resolution occurs over months. The differential diagnosis includes lumbar root compression, pelvic malignancy, CIDP and vasculitis. A similarly painful plexopathy affecting the upper limb has been described.

Table 23.8 Varieties of painful diabetic neuropathy.

	Acute onset	Chronic onset
Symmetrical	Acute distal sensory neuropathy 'Insulin neuropathy'	Peripheral polyneuropathy, particularly with small-fibre involvement Associated with CIDP
Focal and multifocal	Cranial neuropathy – IIIrd nerve palsy Truncal neuropathy Lumbosacral radiculoplexopathy Isolated (compression) peripheral neuropathy	Lumbosacral radiculoplexopathy Isolated (compression) peripheral neuropathy Associated with asymmetric CIDP

CIDP, chronic inflammatory demyelinating polyradiculoneuropathy.

The most common and most intractable painful neuropathy is a distal polyneuropathy, often worse at night or with stress. Most information on treatment is derived from studies on this group of patients, in whom pain has a severe and long-lasting impact.

The painful diabetic foot can be caused by neuropathic or neuro-ischaemic factors. Infection, including osteomyelitis, needs to be excluded, and meticulous foot care is essential.

Treatment, usually with drugs, is as for any other painful peripheral neuropathy. Optimal control of blood sugar should always be attempted, but glycaemic control in late-onset diabetes does not appear to be a predictor of painful neuropathy.

Shingles and post-herpetic neuralgia: shingles

Shingles results from reactivation of the varicella-zoster virus (VZV) that has remained latent in a trigeminal or dorsal root ganglion following primary infection in the form of chickenpox, usually decades earlier. VZV, which is both epithelial and neurotrophic, causes a painful segmental neuropathy with skin changes that typically include small blisters from which the virus can be isolated. Although the clinical diagnosis of shingles is nearly always straightforward from its appearance, blisters with local pain and sensory disturbances are sometimes caused by herpes simplex rather than zoster infections. Definitive distinction can be made from viral identification in the blister fluid. Rarely, shingles can occur in the absence of a rash (*zoster sine herpete*). However, without viral confirmation during the initial stages, shingles remains a clinical diagnosis – suspected when there is segmental pain associated with concomitant sensory changes.

Reactivation is more likely when there is reduced cellular immunity as occurs with increasing age, immunosuppressive disorders and treatments, and in those with certain human leukoctye antigen (HLA) tissue types; it seems to occur less frequently in black people. In immunocompetent patients it is very rare that shingles signals an underlying malignancy or other predisposing factor. Investigation for an underlying cause is rarely necessary in isolated shingles. Both herpes simplex, and less commonly herpes zoster (in about 6% of cases), can recur. VZV is found in both small and large fibre sensory cell bodies in the dorsal root and trigeminal ganglia (i.e. it is not confined to nociceptive fibres), and it may cause pain through involvement of spinal NMDA receptors and possibly other mechanisms.

The pain of acute shingles can range from the trivial to the excruciating. Treatment during the acute stage is symptomatic with analgesics; sometimes strong opioids are required. Three practical questions then arise in respect of the pain.

First, what predicts the development of post-herpetic neuralgia? The incidence of post-herpetic neuralgia increases with increasing patient age. As a rule of thumb, the percentage affected is that of the age so 50% of patients aged 50 will develop this complication and 90% at age 90. This prediction is now considered a pessimistic over-estimate, but nevertheless old age is undoubtedly the most important factor. In addition, female sex, the presence of virus in peripheral blood, severity of rash, severity of the acute shingles pain, prodromal pain and possibly a specific HLA haplotype are also thought to be risk factors. Reducing the viral load with antiviral agents is the rationale for their use during the acute phase to diminish the likelihood of post-herpetic neuralgia.

Secondly, are antiviral drugs always indicated? These should be given if there is ocular involvement – when urgent referral for ophthalmic assessment is essential – and in the immuno-compromised. While there is little firm evidence, meta-analyses suggest that there may be less prolonged pain and possibly a reduction in the incidence of post-herpetic neuralgia following early use of antiviral drugs, including valaciclovir and famciclovir. These two drugs have better bioavailability than aciclovir with oral administration and also have the advantage of being taken three rather than five times daily. The largest study of aciclovir failed to demonstrate a reduction in the incidence of post-herpetic neuralgia. There are ongoing studies with brivudin, which can be given once daily, but it is not currently licensed in the United Kingdom. Brivudine can give rise to a serious and sometimes fatal interaction with 5-fluorouracil, so co-administration is contraindicated.

Thirdly, are there other measures that will prevent the development of post-herpetic neuralgia? Corticosteroids are ineffective. There is only one small study suggesting that early treatment with amitriptyline reduces the occurrence of post-herpetic neuralgia; large, appropriately controlled trials are needed. Furthermore, it is inevitably difficult to decide whether to recommend prophylactic drugs to prevent an uncertain but sometimes severe complication that might never occur, particularly in an elderly patient in whom drug-induced side effects are common. Neither sympathetic blockade nor a single injection of steroids with local anaesthetic is beneficial, and although prolonged somatic nerve blocks using an epidural catheter have been reported as being helpful, these are rarely a realistic prophylactic approach. Recent, impressive evidence suggests that a live attenuated vaccine reduces the incidence and morbidity of herpes zoster and also the incidence of post-herpetic neuralgia. The role of this vaccine as a preventative public health measure to protect a population as a whole remains to be clarified.

Post-herpetic neuralgia

Defining the time when pain from acute shingles becomes the chronic pain of post-herpetic neuralgia is arbitrary. The most generally applied point is 3 months after the rash. Pain and other sensory disturbances range from the trivial to the most severe. Severe post-herpetic neuralgia is a common reason for referral for pain management.

Post-herpetic neuralgia can comprise any form or multiple forms of pain, on-going or evoked, with or without itch, but two characteristic phenotypes are recognised although it should be emphasised that they represent opposite ends of a continuous spectrum. In one type, there is marked somatosensory deficit of the affected dermatome, and while paroxysmal pain can occur in addition to background pain, this is not usually stimulus-evoked. In the other type, sensory loss is much less pronounced, but allodynia and hyperalgesia can be severe. This heterogeneity relates to the different ways in which the virus damages nerves, the underlying pain-related processes being subserved by combinations of sensitisation and de-afferentation that give rise to various forms of sensory disturbance including sensory loss.

Skin biopsies suggest that patients with neuralgia have fewer cutaneous nerve endings than pain-free patients, but, in addition, a variety of neurochemical changes occur in the affected skin. The spinal cord is also affected. Focal atrophy of the dorsal horn sometimes occurs, together with surprisingly long-lasting chronic inflammatory changes which have been detected even 2 years after the shingles.

Acknowledging the numerous mechanisms that mediate the different forms of pain, treatment nevertheless remains as empirical as it is for most other similar pains. Systematic studies provide evidence of benefit for tricyclic antidepressants, gabapentin and pregabalin, and opioids including morphine, oxycodone and tramadol. Topical treatments are most likely to be of benefit in those cases in which cutaneous hypersensitivity phenomena dominate the clinical picture and include lidocaine patches, now licensed in the United Kingdom; aspirin in ether, benzydamine and capsaicin have also been used. While capsaicin is licensed, it produces a burning sensation and is often poorly tolerated; great care is needed to avoid contact with the eyes. A high-concentration (8%) topical capsaicin patch has become available recently. Prior application of local anaesthetic is required to reduce the otherwise frequently intolerable burning pain caused by applying capsaicin at this concentration.

Just as in the management of epilepsy, there is no reason why combinations of drugs should not be tried (e.g. nortriptyline and gabapentin), especially as their modes of action are different and lower doses of each can be used.

Despite reports of numerous other treatments, ranging from transcutaneous electrical nerve stimulation to invasive procedures, the long-term benefit of these other techniques has not yet been established. One of the more recent claims has been for pain relief from intrathecal methylprednisolone, which in one study was reported to provide excellent pain relief over follow-up of 2 years, without reported complications, but subsequent studies have failed to confirm the benefits of this treatment.

Guillain–Barré syndrome

Pain commonly affects patients with this condition and can sometimes be the first symptom, and a particularly prominent one. Pain affects mainly the low back, buttocks and backs of the thighs and although it often seems muscular in character – reminiscent of the pain seen in acute poliomyelitis, as well as in some of the inflammatory myopathies – there is evidence that gabapentin is an effective treatment, implying neurogenic mechanisms, and pain can be severe even in cases that are mild with respect to motor dysfunction. It has been postulated that the pain could be a consequence of radicular inflammation.

The pain is often under-recognised and can be difficult to manage in those severe cases in which the patient, although cognitively intact, is paralysed and ventilator-dependent. Opioids, particularly in the early stages, are sometimes required. Although complete, or near-complete, recovery has widely been considered the rule in this condition, recent data suggest that many patients experience pain years after the onset of symptoms, and that this correlates with persisting sensory (but not motor) deficits. (For a fuller account of Guillain–Barré syndrome see Chapter 10.)

Neuralgic amyotrophy (brachial neuritis)

This condition (Chapter 10) is almost always extremely painful. Characteristically, the patient experiences acute pain around the shoulder girdle, followed days or a few weeks later by weakness, often producing winging of the scapula, and there may be patchy areas of sensory loss. There is histological evidence for sensory as well as motor nerve involvement. The characteristics of the pain are its severity, its diffuse and nagging quality, and sometimes the worsening with limb movement. The pain almost invariably seriously affects sleep. It will usually subside over some days or weeks and strong analgesics may be required in the initial stages, but there is no specific treatment available. Steroids are unhelpful.

Painful inherited neuropathies

The inherited neuropathies (Chapter 10) associated with pain are rare. However, they have a particular importance because in some the underlying mechanisms are beginning to be clarified. Examples of these neuropathies include the following.

- *Hereditary sensory and autonomic neuropathy (HSAN) type I.* In most families there are *SPTLC1* gene mutations, and patients present with sensory symptoms including lightning pains during their teens or young adult life.
- *Fabry disease.* The paroxysmal painful symptoms, which date back to childhood, bear some resemblance to erythromelalgia. How the abnormal sphingomyelin accumulation in the nerves, and any vascular component, generate the pains is unclear. Pain may be improved after prolonged treatment with agalsidase alfa – a form of enzyme replacement therapy.
- *Familial amyloid neuropathies.*
- *Tangier disease.*
- *Primary erythromelalgia* (see Erythromelalgia).

Latrogenic painful peripheral nerve lesions

In contrast to the expected pain that often follows accidental injury to a peripheral nerve, painful peripheral nerve lesions following surgery are often under-recognised. For example, post-surgical neuralgia persisting after 1 year has been reported in 41–61% of patients after thoracotomy, 27% of patients after mastectomy and 28% of patients after saphenous vein surgery. Intriguingly, pain after caesarean section almost never occurs although in almost all other circumstances cases of chronic pain following surgery, if sought, will be found. While management follows along conventional lines, in certain instances nerve repair may be followed by satisfactory resolution of pain. A striking example is repair of the spinal accessory nerve, occasionally damaged during lymph node exploration in the posterior triangle of the neck. This example is also of interest in that it indicates an afferent component in a nerve considered to be solely motor.

Complex regional pain syndrome

This topic is one of the most confused and controversial in the entire field of pain medicine. There is no universally accepted unifying theory on the cause of CRPS. The development of reliable accepted diagnostic criteria has been challenging. There is no definitive diagnostic investigation. Perhaps because of this, there is a tendency for the label of CRPS to be applied indiscriminately to any 'funny-sounding pain in a funny-looking limb' or quite simply to pain in one part of the body that is unexplained. Nevertheless, there is a highly characteristic clinical picture in the most florid cases, and so this section begins with an account of a typical severe case.

A previously healthy young woman sustains an ankle sprain while jogging, with the expected local pain and swelling. The ankle is bandaged and the joint immobilised. However, over time the pain does not settle as anticipated, but persists and gradually increases. Oedema also persists and is accompanied initially by erythema and later by mottled pallor and coldness; local excessive sweating develops as well as thickening of the toe nails and coarsening of the hair of the distal limb. In addition to background pain, tactile and cold allodynia emerge and become increasingly severe. The foot adopts a posture of fixed plantar flexion and inversion. Two years after the original injury, the patient has a cold, blue, immobile and functionally useless leg and foot which she cannot bear to have touched. She perceives the limb as alien and malign and requests amputation.

The term 'complex regional pain syndrome' was proposed in 1995 following an IASP consensus conference, to replace the terms 'reflex sympathetic dystrophy' (RSD) and 'causalgia'. The old term RSD was clearly unsatisfactory, as the condition is not the result of a reflex, is not demonstrably caused by an abnormality of the sympathetic nervous system and is not invariable associated with dystrophic changes. The term 'causalgia' was first used by Weir Mitchell, applied to the characteristic pain and physical signs in soldiers who sustained nerve injuries during the American Civil War.

It is of some interest to examine the historical background to the belief, widely held until relatively recently, that the sympathetic nervous system was crucially involved in the development of these conditions. In 1916, Leriche reported the case of a patient with upper limb causalgia whose symptoms improved following surgical sympathectomy, performed for brachial artery thrombosis. This led him to perform sympathectomy on subsequent patients with causalgia, again with reported symptomatic improvement. Later, local anaesthetic sympathetic blocks became commonly used and, later still, intravenous regional sympathetic block with guanethidine and other agents, but without critical analysis of their effectiveness. Only recently has sympathetic block come under closer scrutiny in the form of systematic review which suggests that intravenous regional sympathetic block probably has no specific therapeutic effect, and that the data on ganglionic blockade are too poor to permit any robust conclusions.

The current diagnostic criteria for CRPS are shown in Table 23.9. Recent guidelines for the diagnosis, treatment and referral of CRPS in adults have been published by the Royal College of Physicians. Although the condition continues often to be sub-classified into type I (without a demonstrable major nerve injury) and type II (with a major nerve injury), the distinction appears to have no practical utility in guiding therapy, nor does it contribute to the understanding of the condition. It is also unclear what constitutes a 'major' nerve injury, or how the pathogenesis might differ in a 'minor' nerve injury. CRPS can also occur following a number of non-traumatic precipitants, shown in Table 23.10.

The features of CRPS fall into four more or less distinct domains: sensory changes, vasomotor changes, sudomotor changes and oedema, and movement disorders and dystrophy.

Sensory changes include a number of abnormalities in addition to pain. The pain itself can be of various qualities with tearing, burning, stinging and squeezing most frequently reported; tactile and cold allodynia occur in about one-quarter of cases, and hyperalgesia and spontaneous pain in a substantial majority. Somatosensory deficit is also frequently found if sought, to pinprick and touch. In addition to these features, there are often abnormalities that indicate central mechanisms, such as neglect of the affected part (reminiscent of the neglect observed in patients with parietal lobe lesions) and feelings of the affected extremity being swollen or enlarged, even when the patient can see objectively that it is not.

Vasomotor changes characteristically evolve over time. Early vasomotor instability can produce cutaneous vasodilatation resulting in 'warm CRPS' as well as vasoconstriction ('cold CRPS'). These states can alternate. Late in the course of the condition the cold state is usual. In the advanced case, local tissue atrophy and disuse contribute to reduced regional blood flow, independent of any sympathetically mediated effect. Microneuronography studies, and catecholamine assays in venous blood of affected parts, indicate that local sympathetic outflow is reduced, not increased, in patients with CRPS. The apparent excessive sympathetic activity in these patients can be explained by the development of increased sensitivity to the local effects of catecholamines.

Sudomotor changes and oedema frequently occur but are seldom quantified in clinical practice. They usually resolve with improvement of other features of CRPS; there is no specific treatment.

Table 23.9 Diagnostic criteria for complex regional pain syndrome ('Budapest criteria').

A–D must apply:
- A The patient has continuing pain which is disproportionate to any inciting event
- B The patient has at least one sign in two or more of the categories
- C The patient reports at least one symptom in three or more of the categories
- D No other diagnosis can better explain the signs and symptoms

Category		Sign	Symptom
1 'Sensory'	*Allodynia* (to light touch and/or temperature sensation and/or deep somatic pressure and/or joint movement) and/or *hyperalgesia* (to pinprick)	☐	☐
2 'Vasomotor'	Temperature asymmetry and/or skin colour changes and/or skin colour asymmetry	☐	☐
3 'Sudomotor/ oedema'	Oedema and/or sweating changes and/or sweating asymmetry	☐	☐
4 'Motor/trophic'	Decreased range of motion and/or motor dysfunction (weakness, tremor, dystonia) and/or trophic changes (hair/nail/skin)	☐	☐

Source: Goebel *et al.* 2012. Reproduced with permission of Royal College of Physicians.

Table 23.10 Non-traumatic causes of complex regional pain syndrome (CRPS) type I.

Disorders of the peripheral nervous system (e.g. herpes zoster)
Disorders of the central nervous system (e.g. stroke, multiple sclerosis, spinal trauma, cerebral tumour, brain injury)
Immobilisation
Systemic illness (e.g. after myocardial infarct and cardiac surgery), lung disease
Pregnancy
Electric shock
Drugs (e.g. phenobarbital, isoniazid)
Idiopathic

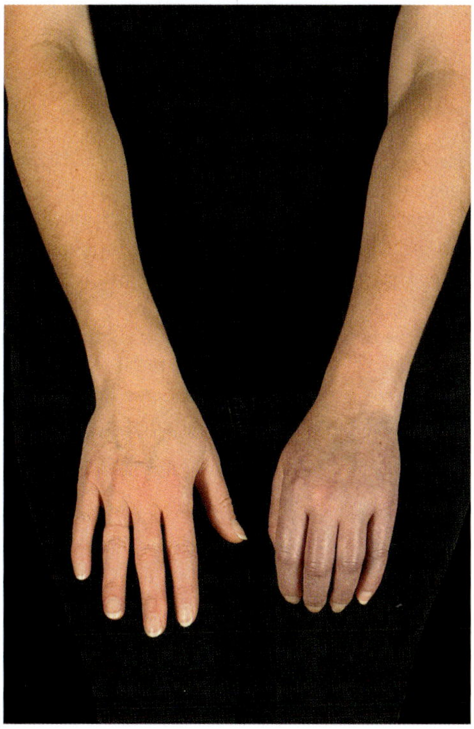

Figure 23.2 Complex regional pain syndrome (CRPS) showing dystrophic, vasomotor and oedematous changes in the left hand.

The dystrophic changes observed locally in CRPS have long been recognised, but a variety of disorders of movement also occur (Figure 23.2). Some of the dystrophic changes are explicable purely on the basis of disuse. The skin in the affected territory is typically thin and often shiny in appearance; the digits often taper towards their tips and the nails are thickened, brittle and ridged. Local hair growth exhibits loss or coarsening. Osteoporosis not surprisingly occurs, but in some cases appears disproportionately severe to be accounted for by disuse. Movement disorders are often present. Paucity of volitional movement of the affected part is almost universal, but in addition tremor and dystonia are sometimes seen.

The degree of prominence of the manifestations of the features of these four domains suggests that they are independent of one another. For example, in one case pain may be extremely severe but vasomotor changes trivial, whereas in another the reverse occurs. Some additional features associated with CRPS are listed in Table 23.11.

CRPS varies greatly in its severity; mild cases often resolve spontaneously, and fortunately few progress to resemble the case described at the beginning of this section. However, in order to prevent more severe cases developing, active management should be initiated early. In the absence of any specific treatment, the focus should be on combining effective pain relief with functional restoration. Although debate continues regarding whether CRPS can be defined as a neuropathic pain condition, it shares many features with conditions that are unequivocally neuropathic and therefore use of pharmacotherapy of demonstrated efficacy in neuropathic pain seems appropriate. Mediators of inflammation account for many of the features of CRPS, and corticosteroid therapy has been advocated. Sympathetic block can be effective in

Table 23.11 Various clinical features seen in complex regional pain syndromes (CRPS).

Skin erythematous, cyanosed, pale or blotchy	Excessive, reduced or absent sweating
Swelling or atrophy of skin	Inappropriate warmth or coldness
Excess or loss of hair	Loss of skin wrinkles or glossiness
Nails ridged, curved, thin, brittle or clubbed	Subcutaneous atrophy or thickening
Dupuytren's and other contractures	Joint stiffness, acute or chronic arthritis
Muscle wasting and weakness	Osteoporosis – spotty, localized or widespread
Involuntary movements – tremor, dystonia, spasms	Detrusor and urinary dysfunction
A syndrome comprising 'neglect' and other similar disturbances	Hemi-sensory impairment outside the painful area
Hyperacusis	Alterations in visuospatial perception

After Schott (1999) with permission from Oxford University Press.

some cases, but is not supported by case–control studies. Physical therapies and psychological interventions both have a major role in rehabilitation. In severe cases, spinal cord stimulation can be effective.

Pain associated with benign orthopaedic conditions

Glomus tumour and osteoid asteoma deserve mention here because patients may present to neurology clinics, and because they can be cured by appropriate treatment.

Glomus tumour

These uncommon benign tumours of bone, entirely unrelated to glomus jugulare tumours in the neck, are really hamartomas of the normal glomus body. The glomus body is an innervated arteriovenous anastomotic structure which has a temperature regulating function. The afferent arterioles are tortuous, associated with glomus (endothelial) cells, and innervated by myelinated and unmyelinated fibres. Some 50% of glomus tumours affect the hand, often subungually, where they may appear as a little blue nodule. Such an appearance is not diagnostic of a glomus tumour; the differential diagnosis includes melanomas, neuromas and neurofibromas. Glomus tumours occur anywhere over the body, including within bone, but they are usually subcutaneous. The key clinical triad comprises:

1 Severe and continuous pain
2 Extreme cold sensitivity (for instance, worsening pain by immersing the hand in cold water)
3 Extreme tenderness (for instance, even the slightest contact of the nodule with the end of an orange stick induces quite exquisite pain).

Diagnosis is often straightforward when tumours are visible, but otherwise can be difficult. Plain radiographs can reveal bony erosion; otherwise detection requires ultrasound, MRI or angiography. Surgical removal is usually immediately curative.

Osteoid osteoma

This bony disorder occasionally presents to the neurologist as a cause of unexplained pain, usually in a limb. The cardinal features are the often severe and sometimes localised pain, usually worse at night, and characteristically extremely good response to anti-inflammatory drugs. The good response only lasts for the duration of action of these drugs. The reason for this responsiveness is that the fine nerve terminals in this benign tumour of bone are exposed to prostaglandins present in the tumour. The abnormal bony tissue sometimes shows as a focal radiolucent or radio-opaque nidus, often with surrounding cortical thickening. On isotope bone scanning it produces a dramatic focal hot spot. CT scanning can also be useful. Gratifyingly, excision of the tumour is curative and immediate pain relief occurs.

Motor neurone disease

Although not typically classified within neuropathies, pain has been reported in 64% of 42 patients with motor neurone disease (MND) and in 57% of 124 patients admitted to a hospice. Pain is variously described as aching, cramping, burning, shock-like, or is indescribable. In some patients with MND pain can be a dominant symptom, especially when weakness is not advanced.

The cause of this pain is ill-understood, although musculoskeletal factors and skin pressure (only rarely with pressure sores) are likely to operate. Central mechanisms may also be important. Just as with Parkinson's disease, pain may be one of the subjective sensory symptoms that can occur even long before serious disability develops, and in occasional patients with MND there is objective evidence of sensory involvement both clinically and on investigation. In many patients with MND it is likely that the pain is caused by a combination of musculoskeletal and neuropathic factors, which may be partially or completely alleviated by medication, in particular opiates, especially in the later stages of the disease.

Painful peripheral viscero-somatic disorders

Some disorders referred to a neurologist appear to involve the interface between cutaneous and visceral innervations. These neuropathic disorders include the burning mouth syndrome and vulvodynia.

Burning mouth syndrome

Contrasting with the severe, usually unilateral, paroxysmal stabbing pains of glossopharyngeal neuralgia, sometimes accompanied by syncope, the burning mouth syndrome embraces various types of persistent and unpleasant sensations within the mouth and includes terms such as glossodynia. Women are affected more than men, and the mean age is 50–60 years. The clinical features comprise a burning sensation that is usually diffuse and bilateral, and any area within the mouth can be affected including the tongue.

The pain is usually constant but can fluctuate in severity during the day. Influencing factors in some patients include eating (making symptoms either better or worse), stress and previous dental procedures. There may be associated dryness of the mouth and loss or altered taste appreciation. The condition is usually long-lasting, although spontaneous improvement or recovery has been reported. Treatment remains empirical and includes drugs used for neuropathic pain, and cognitive behavioural and other psychological therapies that also help the depression and other psychological disturbances that often coexist.

Although routine oral and sensory examination is normal, quantitative sensory testing suggests abnormality of small fibre function. There is also a reduction of epithelial nerve fibres, suggesting a trigeminal small fibre neuropathy. In some patients, abnormalities of the blink reflex suggest more central involvement affecting the trigeminal system. Thus, at present the burning mouth syndrome appears to be a neuropathic disorder of unknown but probably various causes. These involve both peripheral and central components, and there is some suggestion of nigro-striatal system involvement in the latter. There is some limited evidence that zinc deficiency could be responsible for some cases and that correcting this can be therapeutic.

Vulvodynia

Different from many causes of perineal pain, vulvodynia comprises vulval pain associated with painful burning sensations, mechanical allodynia and hyperalgesia. Sometimes there is no spontaneous pain, allodynia only being provoked by touch and pressure. The disorder is likely to be multi-factorial and either primary or secondary to vulval or vaginal inflammatory or infective causes. While surgical excision of the affected tissue has sometimes been advocated, conservative treatment with topical local anaesthetic cream, or oral amitriptyline, gabapentin or pregabalin is generally more appropriate.

The syndrome is probably another example of a neuropathic pain disorder, in turn related to reduced sensory thresholds to a variety of sensory stimuli. These abnormalities are likely to result from factors including increased innervation secondary to nerve sprouting or neural hyperplasia, and sensitisation of thermoreceptors and nociceptors within the vaginal mucosa. The increased innervation in vulvodynia tissues is associated with increased expression of TRPV1 (vanilloid or capsaicin) receptors, a finding that might account for both the sensory disturbances and mild erythema sometimes seen. Some of the clinical and pathological features also occur in interstitial cystitis and related conditions.

Visceral pain

Visceral pain, mainly transmitted to the CNS through afferents running within sympathetic nerves, has characteristic features (Table 23.12). These features, clearly different from those encountered in typical somatic pain, can be explained by various factors:

- Different molecular mechanisms that selectively transduce the various different peripheral chemical and mechanical stimuli, including ischaemia or distension, all which affect viscera.
- The contribution of processes that sensitise visceral afferents.
- The important contribution of silent afferents, which only become active in the presence of inflammation.

Table 23.12 Characteristics of visceral pain.

Only evoked from some viscera (e.g. not from the liver)
Not always linked to injury
Diffuse and poorly localised
Referred to other sites
Accompanied by motor and autonomic responses

- Viscero-somatic convergence in the spinal cord, thalamus and cortex.
- Central spinal processes that result in amplification and persistence of afferent impulses from the damaged viscera.
- Ascending transmission of pain, via dorsal column and other non-spinothalamic pathways in the spinal cord, to specific brainstem nuclei, amygdala and hypothalamus – regions implicated more in affective than discriminative aspects of pain.

Patients with visceral pain caused by acute painful cardiac, gastrointestinal or urogenital disorders rarely present to the neurologist. However, other aspects of visceral pain have important practical significance. Examples include odd distributions of pain (e.g. ear pain from carcinoma of the lung), involvement of the viscera in shingles and perhaps post-herpetic neuralgia, and possibly various chronic painful conditions such as the irritable bowel syndrome, non-ischaemic cardiac pain, fibromyalgia, chronic pelvic pain and headache. Some patients have a number of these disorders at the same or different times. In these individuals particularly, underlying mechanisms include abnormal sensitisation of peripheral or spinal neurones or aberrant central processing of visceral sensation, so that stimuli usually innocuous to other people are perceived as painful.

Plexopathies

The dorsal root ganglia and proximal roots of peripheral sensory nerves can be affected by conditions that result in pain, and, depending on their location, sometimes affect the spinal cord as well. Causes commonly presenting to the neurologist include infection (e.g. shingles and post-herpetic neuralgia), inflammation (e.g. arachnoiditis) and compression (e.g. tumours and discs). However, more peripherally, it is painful plexus lesions that sometimes prove particularly difficult to diagnose and manage. Amongst the various painful conditions, including the thoracic outlet syndrome affecting the upper limb, the three most serious disorders resulting in painful plexopathies are:

1. Trauma
2. Malignancy
3. Following irradiation.

Traumatic brachial plexus lesions

The most common cause of traumatic brachial plexus lesions is a traction injury, most typically following a motor cycle accident, in which there has been stretching or avulsion of the brachial plexus and sometimes the extradural and intradural nerve roots. Paradoxically, the introduction of crash helmets has made these injuries more frequently seen in clinical practice, because without head protection the patient was more likely to be killed. Traumatic plexus lesions are also frequently seen during warfare and usually result from missile injuries. Of interest from the developmental viewpoint is that lesions sustained in infancy are rarely painful.

Pain following trauma often develops immediately, but can develop or increase in severity in the months following the initial trauma. The pain affects the limb in the distribution of the affected roots or plexus but is sometimes more widespread. It is often burning and very severe, dominating the patient's life. Despite attempts at treatment, the prognosis for improvement in the pain is very poor. Pain can persist indefinitely. Spinal cord stimulation is sometimes effective in partial plexus lesions, but in cases of complete brachial plexus avulsion it is of no value; deep brain stimulation may have a role in such cases.

Recently, studies of nerve repair following brachial plexus injuries have shown there is a correlation and temporal association between a reduction in de-afferentation pain and return of motor function, with the former preceding the latter. Such surgery, itself requiring exceptional surgical skills, has led to much interest in processes underlying recovery and pain relief, including the contribution of NGF and other growth factors.

Malignant and radiation-induced plexopathies

Metastatic disease or a primary tumour can infiltrate the cervical, but more commonly the brachial or lumbosacral plexus, causing severe and unremitting pain. Particularly if at the outset there are few or no neurological signs pointing to neural involvement, discovering the cause of the pain can be very difficult. Nevertheless, pain is often the presenting symptom, for example occurring in 75% of patients with brachial plexopathy resulting from cancer. It is caused by malignant infiltration of the nerves themselves or of surrounding blood vessels and connective tissue. Involvement of adjacent structures such as bone also causes pain. On other occasions pain will develop in a patient known to have, or have had, malignant disease, in which case a malignant cause will be suspected early.

Usually, plexus involvement will become obvious when there are motor and sensory signs. When the lower trunk of the brachial plexus is involved, and Horner's syndrome accompanies the pain, a relatively proximal cause around T1 should be suspected, because it signifies involvement of the sympathetic trunk or ganglia (Pancoast's syndrome). Generally, pain is a major feature of malignant plexopathies; the absence of pain should lead to review of the diagnosis. Imaging will be the first step in evaluation.

Treatment of the pain will generally be managed by the oncologist or palliative care physician. This is because treatment is largely symptomatic and palliative, sometimes with radiotherapy, and a multi-disciplinary approach is required.

A particularly challenging problem is to decide whether, in a patient with known malignant disease and who has had radiotherapy, the pain is caused by the radiotherapy or to tumour recurrence. The distinction between malignant and radiation plexopathies is often very difficult. Some features that are helpful, although not diagnostic, are shown in Table 23.13.

Frequently, neither the clinical features nor the results of imaging studies allow a definite distinction to be made in an individual patient who has previously received radiotherapy. Treatment of pain from radiation-induced plexopathies is unfortunately extremely limited and the outlook for pain relief is poor.

Management

Management of chronic pain per se is often difficult but pain in neurological disease presents particular challenges. Much, although by no means all, pain in neurological disease is neuropathic, and this is generally more resistant to treatment than nociceptive pain. Improving pain-contingent disability is often a major objective of cognitive behavioural pain management, but many neurological conditions limit the capacity for improving physical functioning and in some cases cognition is also impaired.

An essential first step in effective management is the evaluation of the nature of the pain (or pains) in the patient. Primary diagnosis is important, but usually does not of itself inform the clinician of the cause of the pain. However, a knowledge of the types of pain characteristically encountered in individual disorders focuses attention on the likely differential diagnosis regarding pain. An example is

Table 23.13 Pain due to malignant plexopathy and radiation-induced plexopathy.

	Neoplastic	Radiation
Presentation	Pain	Paraesthesias, weakness
Pain	Early, severe	Later in course
Plexus involvement		
Brachial	Often lower plexus	Usually whole plexus
Lumbosacral	Lower, usually unilateral	Commonly bilateral
Horner's syndrome (brachial plexopathy)	Common	Unusual
Local tissue necrosis	Not present	Common
Rectal mass (lumbosacral plexopathy)	Common	Absent
Myokymia	Unusual	Present
Nerve enhancement (MRI)	Present	Usually absent
PET scan	Positive	Usually absent

MRI, magnetic resonance imaging; PET, positron emission tomography.
Source: Jaeckle 2004. Reproduced with permission of Thieme.

the patient with hemiplegia following a stroke who complains of pain in the shoulder territory of the affected side. This may represent CPSP – but it may also have a local nociceptive origin. Nociceptive shoulder pain is well recognised in cases of stroke and is usually far more amenable to effective treatment than CPSP. It is also possible for both mechanisms of pain to coexist in the same patient. Another example is the patient with MS with back pain and pain in a lower limb. The lower limb pain might be the result of demyelinating myelopathy – but it could also be coincidentally caused by lumbar spinal nerve root compression, which might respond to quite different treatment. In the assessment of the patient with pain, the question 'What is the diagnosis?' should be swiftly followed by the question, 'What is causing this pain/these pains in this patient?'

Management of neuropathic pain

Systemic drug treatments

It is an interesting (if frustrating) observation that in neuropathic pain, none of the drug treatments available are effective in all cases, or even in a clear majority of cases. This is in marked contrast to most nociceptive pain. Even severe nociceptive pain, such as that encountered acutely following major surgery, will respond to treatment with a potent opioid analgesic provided that a sufficient dose is given, in almost every case. However, in neuropathic pain, not only can opioids be completely ineffective, but other types of drugs with clear evidence of efficacy derived from clinical trials (such as tricyclic antidepressants) can be highly effective in one patient and completely ineffective in another patient with the same neurological diagnosis and near-identical clinical presentation. Many drugs used to treat neuropathic pain give rise to troublesome side effects and are poorly tolerated, limiting their practical utility, but this is a separate issue from their simply not working.

The reasons for this marked variability in response to drugs are poorly understood, and there are usually no reliable indicators in any individual patient's presentation (or diagnosis, with a few exceptions) to suggest whether their pain will respond to a member of a particular drug group well, partially or not at all. Part of the explanation probably lies in genetically determined differences in drug metabolism between subjects, and genetic polymorphism in respect of the metabolism of some drugs has been clearly demonstrated. However, this cannot explain the wide variations in response to gabapentin and pregabalin, which are not metabolised. It seems likelier that most of the variability between patients' responses to drugs is attributable to differences in the activation and/or expression of nociception-inducing receptors and the neurotransmitters and neuromodulators acting on them. Whatever the prime reason, the clinical reality is that pharmacological treatment of neuropathic pain involves a considerable element of 'trial and error'. Pharmacological treatments with evidence of efficacy in neuropathic pain, together with ratings of evidence levels, are shown in Table 23.14. A recent meta-analysis of pharmacotherapy for neuropathic pain indicated that even those drugs with good quality evidence of efficacy were effective only in a minority of patients (number needed to treat for over 50% pain relief approximately four for tricyclic antidepressants, six for serotonin and noradrenaline re-uptake inhibitors and seven for gabapentin and pregabalin).

Opioids and other analgesics

While clearly and reliably effective in acute nociceptive pain, drugs in this group have tended traditionally to be dismissed as ineffective in neuropathic pain. However, there is evidence that opioids can be effective in treating neuropathic pain, at least in the short to medium term, in some cases, as well as tramadol, combined tramadol/paracetamol and the novel analgesic tapentadol. Conditions studied have largely been painful diabetic neuropathy and post-herpetic neuralgia.

In the past two decades, the use of potent opioids in the treatment of chronic non-malignant pain has increased dramatically in many countries including the United States and the United Kingdom. However, the practice of prescribing these drugs long-term for patients with non-cancer pain is currently under scrutiny as evidence of lack of long-term effectiveness is emerging, as well as increasing problem opioid use (especially prescription opioids), accompanied by a rising rate of fatalities attributable to opioids, particularly in the United States. Recent guidelines on appropriate opioid prescribing have been published.

Antidepressants

The tricyclic antidepressant (TCA) group of drugs have long been established as effective treatments in neuropathic pain, for both peripheral and central disorders. These drugs have complex actions which include central serotonin and noradrenaline reuptake inhibition and inhibition of voltage-gated sodium channels (all of which may contribute to their analgesic effects), and antimuscarinic activity which probably does not contribute to analgesia but is responsible for many of the unwanted effects. The noradrenergic action of TCAs may be more important than the serotonergic action so far as analgesic effect is concerned, as the serotonin-specific re-uptake inhibitors (SSRIs) seem relatively ineffective.

Table 23.14 Pharmacological treatments with evidence of efficacy in neuropathic pain, together with ratings of evidence levels.

Classification of evidence for drug treatments in commonly studied neuropathic pain conditions and recommendations for use. Treatments are presented in alphabetical order. Only drugs used at repeated dosages are shown here(with the exception of treatments with long lasting effects such as capsaicin patches). Drugs marked with an asterisk were found effective in single class II or III studies and are generally not recommended. Drugs marked with two asterisks are not yet available for use.

Aetiology	Level A rating for efficacy	Level B rating for efficacy	Level C rating for efficacy	Level A/B rating for inefficacy or discrepant results	Recommendations for first line	Recommendations for second or third line
Diabetic NP	Duloxetine Gabapentin-morphine TCA Gabapentin Nicotine agonist** Nitrate derivatives ** Oxycodone Pregabalin TCA Tramadol alone or with paracetamol Venlafaxine ER	Botulinum toxin* Dextromethorphan Gabapentin/ venlafaxine* Levodopa*	Carbamazepine Phenytoin	Capsaicin cream Lacosamide Lamotrigine Memantine Mexiletine Mianserin NK1 antagonist** Oxcarbazepine SSRI Topical clonidine Topiramate Valproate Zonisamide	Duloxetine Gabapentin Pregabalin TCA Venlafaxine ER	Opioids Tramadol
PHN	Capsaicin 8% patch Gabapentin Gabapentin ER** Lidocaine plasters Opioids (morphine, oxycodone, methadone) Pregabalin TCA	Capsaicin cream Valproate*		Benzydamine (topical) Dextromethorphan Fluphenazine Memantine COX-2 inhibitor Tramadol	Gabapentin Pregabalin TCA Lidocaine plasters	Capsaicin Opioids
Classical trigeminal neuralgia	Carbamazepine	Oxcarbazepine	Baclofen* Lamotrigine* Pimozide* Tizanidine*		Carbamazepine Oxcarbazepine	Surgery
Central pain	Cannabinoids (oro-mucosal, oral) (MS) Pregabalin (SCI)	Lamotrigine (CPSP) TCA (SCI, CPSP) Tramadol (SCI)* Opioids		Carbamazepine Gabapentin Lamotrigine (SCI) Levetiracetam Mexiletine S-ketamine iontophoresis Valproate	Gabapentin Pregabalin TCA	Cannabinoids (MS) Lamotrigine Opioids Tramadol (SCI)

CPSP, central post-stroke pain; ER, extended release; MS, multiple sclerosis; PHN, post-herpetic neuralgia; SCI, spinal cord injury; TCA, tricyclic antidepressants; SSRI, selective serotonin reuptake inhibitor.
Source: Adapted from Attal 2010 with permission from John Wiley & Sons.

Although undoubtedly effective in treating neuropathic pain, the TCAs possess several drawbacks. The antimuscarinic actions produce the familiar side-effects of dry mouth, blurred vision, constipation and a tendency to urinary retention. They are variably sedating, with amitriptyline, dosulepin and trimipramine being more sedating and imipramine and nortriptyline less so. In some circumstances the sedative action is useful if the patient suffers from disturbed sleep, but these drugs are long-acting and even if given as a single evening dose (as is usually the case), unwanted sedation is frequently present in the morning and can persist throughout the day. TCAs are highly protein-bound, resulting in potential for drug interactions with other protein-bound compounds, and they are cardiotoxic in overdose.

The newer selective serotonin and noradrenaline re-uptake inhibitors (SNRIs), duloxetine and venlafaxine, both show evidence of efficacy for treating neuropathic pain and appear comparable to TCAs in terms of efficacy but better tolerated, without the sedative and antimuscarinic actions and safer in overdosage.

Antiepileptics

This group of compounds is more diverse in the mode of action of individual drugs than the antidepressants, which all exert their effects through central actions of monoamines. An account of the individual characteristics of these drugs is given in Chapter 7, and the following section highlights issues relevant to their use in the treatment of pain.

The properties responsible for the analgesic effects of the antiepileptics are not fully understood but are probably mainly attributable to two broad categories of action:

1. Use-dependent block of sodium channels (phenytoin, carbamazepine and oxcarbazepine, lamotrigine, lacosamide)
2. Inhibitory action at the $\alpha2\delta$-1 subunit of pre-synaptic calcium channels (gabapentin, pregabalin).

It is often suggested that the antiepileptic drugs show a degree of selectivity of action on paroxysmal neuropathic pain, whereas burning continuous pain is more likely to respond to the antidepressants. Recent evidence suggests that there is some correlation between neuropathic pain phenotype (and hence putative pain-generator mechanisms) and response to oxcarbazepine.

Carbamazepine and oxcarbazepine remain the first line drugs for the treatment of trigeminal neuralgia (Chapter 13). Current evidence suggests that there is little to choose between them in terms of efficacy, with approximately 50% of patients becoming pain-free on titrating the dose to optimal level. Both drugs rarely cause serious adverse reactions including Stevens–Johnson syndrome, but less severe side effects of a dose-dependent nature are common, including nausea, dizziness, somnolence and fatigue, impaired concentration and memory, and headache. Oxcarbazepine appears on the whole to be better tolerated although it has a greater tendency to cause hyponatraemia. Evidence of benefit from these drugs in the management of other causes of neuropathic pain (e.g. painful diabetic neuropathy) is weak.

Gabapentin and pregabalin (sometimes referred to collectively as 'gabanoids') have both been demonstrated in systematic reviews to be effective in a range of neuropathic pain conditions. They both exert their action at the $\alpha2\delta$ type 1 subunit of pre-synaptic, voltage-dependent calcium channels. Their adverse effects are similar, including those listed for carbamazepine and oxcarbazepine, and in addition oedema, weight gain and dry mouth. However, serious adverse effects are uncommon, and the absence of either metabolism (both drugs are excreted unchanged by the kidneys) or plasma protein binding limits their capacity for adverse drug interactions, which is reassuring if they are being considered in the context of combination therapy.

Pregabalin exhibits linear pharmacokinetics whereas the kinetics of gabapentin are more complex; in practice this means that there is less inter-subject dose variability with pregabalin than with gabapentin, and titration to optimum dosage can generally be achieved more rapidly. Pregabalin also has the longer half-life, and is typically administered twice daily in contrast to the three or four times daily dose regime required for gabapentin.

Lamotrigine was reported in early studies as showing evidence of benefit in a range of neuropathic pain conditions, central as well as peripheral, but more recent evidence has tended to quell some of the earlier optimism. The usual dose-dependent side effects occur (although cognitive impairment seems relatively uncommon) but it can give rise to Stevens–Johnson syndrome, and slow and cautious up-titration is therefore recommended to minimise the risk of this, which creates the practical disadvantage that it can take months to attain a dose at the higher end of the therapeutic range. Its use should probably be reserved for cases of severe neuropathic pain resistant to antidepressants and the gabanoids.

Lacosamide, one of the newer antiepileptics, has randomised controlled trial evidence of benefit in painful diabetic polyneuropathy. It is generally well tolerated but may give rise to abnormalities of cardiac conduction and is contraindicated in patients with second or third degree heart block.

Other antiepileptics have been tried although the evidence to support their use is generally weak, and they should probably be used as third line drugs in cases where the first and second line options have proved ineffective. As with the TCAs, adverse effects often limit the practical usefulness of antiepileptic drugs in the treatment of pain.

Local anaesthetics and related compounds

There is good evidence that drugs with inhibitory actions at voltage-gated sodium channels are effective treatments for neuropathic pain. Inhibition of ectopic neuronal activity by systemically administered local anaesthetics and antiarrhythmics such as mexiletine has been demonstrated at multiple sites in the peripheral and central nervous systems, including peripheral neuromas, the dorsal root ganglia, dorsal horn, rostroventromedial medulla and peri-aqueductal grey matter. Rather more surprisingly, it appears that a single administration of a dose of intravenous local anaesthetic can produce analgesic effects lasting much longer than predicted on the basis of the drug's kinetics, for example several weeks. This observation accords with the author's experience and in his unit intravenous lidocaine infusion is a frequently employed intervention used to treat neuropathic pain, with some success.

While cardiac antiarrhythmic drugs such as mexiletine are usually less dramatically effective in the treatment of neuropathic pain than the local anaesthetics, they have the advantage of being effective when administered by the orogastric route (the local anaesthetics when taken by mouth are almost completely excluded from the systemic circulation by hepatic first-pass metabolism).

NMDA receptor antagonists

NMDA receptor antagonists, particularly ketamine, have been clearly demonstrated to be effective in treating neuropathic pain, with evidence to support their use in the treatment of both central and peripheral pain. Ketamine can cause several undesirable effects in addition to sedation, notably dysphoria, hallucinations and other transient psychotic effects; it is also in recent years increasingly being abused as a recreational drug. However, it may, in common with IV lidocaine, induce remissions of pain that long outlast its anticipated effect, and current evidence suggests that if used in relatively low dosage and with dose intervals of a week or more, it is safe. It is the author's practice to assess the response to ketamine initially with an intravenous infusion of 150 μg/kg over 30 minutes;

if effective and well tolerated, it can be administered subsequently via a number of routes, including sublingual.

Cannabinoids

Cannabinoids can relieve both neuropathic pain and painful spasticity. There are currently two preparations available in the United Kingdom; nabilone (synthetic tetrahydrocannabinol; THC) which is presented as a capsule, and an oromucosal spray (Sativex) consisting of a mixture of THC and cannibadiol. Neuropathic pain appears more responsive to cannabinoids than nociceptive pain, and both central and peripheral pain respond to treatment. The licenced indication for the oromucosal spray is at present limited to treatment of severe spasticity in MS. Major side-effects are uncommon, although anxiety concerning risk of abuse and addiction is undoubtedly a factor in restricting its use.

Topical agents

There is evidence supporting the use of 5% lidocaine patches, licensed in the United Kingdom for the treatment of post-herpetic neuralgia. Capsaicin cream, licensed for treatment of post-herpetic and diabetic neuropathic pains, may be useful, but side effects including burning and stinging at the site of application often occur, and great care has to be taken to avoid contact with the eyes. Recently, a high concentration (8%) capsaicin preparation, in the form of a self-adhesive patch, has become available for the treatment of post-herpetic neuralgia. It is liable to produce burning pain on initial application unless topical local anaesthetic is applied first; it should be administered by a clinician familiar with its use.

Botulinum toxin

Botulinum toxin has pain-relieving properties in addition to those resulting from treatment of muscle spasm and abnormal posture. Pain relief can occur well before, and outlast, improvement in these musculoskeletal abnormalities. There have been anecdotal reports, and some small placebo-controlled studies, of pain relief in various other disorders including post-herpetic neuralgia and trigeminal neuralgia, diabetic neuropathy, migraine and chronic facial pain. Botulinum toxin does not seem to improve acute pain, and the role of this toxin in relief of pain is uncertain. There is experimental evidence that, apart from effects on acetylcholine, the toxin blocks release of substance P, release of glutamate and other neurotransmitters involved in nociceptive sensory processing.

Intrathecal drugs

Several drugs have been used intrathecally for pain management. These include baclofen especially for central pain, clonidine, opioids and, most recently, ziconotide. Phenol has also been used, but as a neurolytic agent. The evidence base is poor, benefit unpredictable, and this form of treatment should only be carried out in specialised pain management units.

Neuro-ablative and neuro-stimulation procedures

Neuro-ablative procedures

Over the past century, except in the treatment of trigeminal neuralgia, there has been a steady decline in neurosurgical and other procedures designed to interrupt pain pathways, particularly in those whose pain has a non-malignant cause. Apart from the risks of the procedure itself and in particular of causing damage affecting other neurological functions, even successful procedures can result in painful sensory loss (termed 'anaesthesia dolorosa' after somatic nerve lesioning, and 'sympathalgia' after sympathectomy). Furthermore, paradoxically pain will often return, sometimes after a long interval, although obviously this is less important in management of those painful malignant conditions in which life expectancy is short. These sequelae are caused by a variety of often poorly understood adaptive central phenomena.

Certain destructive procedures are still occasionally performed, for instance dorsal root entry zone (DREZ) lesions for treatment of pain from spinal cord injury or brachial plexus lesions. Here too the evidence base for their efficacy is poor, and there is a substantial risk of ipsilateral lower limb weakness. The same reservations apply to destructive chemical procedures. The use of phenol and other neurolytic chemicals applied around nerve roots or intrathecally is rarely undertaken, apart from treating spasticity and its accompanying pain. Phenol applied peripherally can induce further pain (phenol neuritis).

Neuro-stimulation procedures

Every part of the somatosensory nervous system has been stimulated to try to relieve pain, but apart from transcutaneous electric nerve stimulation (TENS), these techniques are complex and only carried out in specialised centres. Much of the rationale for stimulation procedures is based on the seminal paper by Melzack and Wall (1965) which led to the gate control theory of pain. This paper, which reported physiological experiments on dorsal root potentials in rats, gave rise to the novel concept that stimulation of large diameter afferent fibres might inhibit (gate) the activity of small diameter, pain subserving fibres in the dorsal horn of the spinal cord, and possibly elsewhere. Although the subject of heated controversy, the paper led to the development of various techniques that provide innocuous neural stimulation, with the aim of alleviating pain.

Transcutaneous electrical nerve stimulation TENS involves applying electrodes to the skin with an interposed gel or other appropriate contacting substance. The electrodes are usually placed either side of the painful area, and are attached via wires to a small battery-operated stimulation unit. Impulses can be of variable frequency and intensity, the parameters usually being selected by the patient so as to cause non-painful tingling sensations. Stimulation can be continuous, intermittent or in bursts, and applied for minutes, hours or days. Side effects are infrequent and minor, usually comprising skin irritation beneath the electrodes. Contraindications include open or infected skin, pregnancy (other than in labour), and the presence of a pacemaker. TENS has no effect and can cause burns if applied to anaesthetic skin. Benefit is unpredictable, and may only develop some time after stimulation. Some pains are transiently worsened, particularly if there is tactile allodynia. Controlled trials are obviously difficult, but the technique is simple, safe and cheap, and patients can obtain devices over the counter.

The mechanism of action includes segmental inhibition at the dorsal horn, distinct from painful counter-irritation (pain inhibiting another pain) in which there is diffuse noxious inhibitory control through ascending and descending pathways. As a historical footnote, TENS was originally used as a screening tool for spinal cord stimulation (see Spinal cord stimulation), and only after some years was it introduced as a treatment in its own right.

Peripheral nerve stimulation Open implanting of stimulating electrodes around a peripheral nerve to obtain pain relief is rarely undertaken now. However, there is a growing trend in some specialist centres of using dorsal root ganglion stimulation for patients with appropriately anatomically restricted pain. There has also been increasing use of (and increasing literature on) the technique of pulsed radiofrequency stimulation since it was first described in 1998. Essentially, this entails a modification of the much older technique of radiofrequency lesioning. Radiofrequency thermocoagulation denervation remains an established treatment for trigeminal neuralgia (Chapter 13) but is seldom used for other indications, for the reasons stated earlier. However, if a radiofrequency current is applied to a nerve target in short bursts with a long recovery period (typically 20 ms stimulation time per 500 ms), the local tissues do not heat above 42 °C. No neurolysis occurs and the treatment should be considered a form of stimulation analgesia, although the physiological basis for the pain relief is unclear.

Occipital nerve stimulation has also rapidly become established in specialist centres in the treatment of some forms of intractable headache (Chapter 12).

Spinal cord stimulation Spinal cord stimulation (SCS; formerly known as dorsal column stimulation) was originally devised and trialed on the basis of Melzack and Wall's gate control theory of pain. An array of electrodes is implanted in the posterior epidural space, percutaneously or at open operation, so as to stimulate the spinal cord by means of electrical stimuli provided by a pulse generator. The aim is to stimulate the dorsal columns and the electrode array is placed so as to overlie them, but this stimulation is probably not its only mode of action. However, technically successful stimulation is generally deemed to require the production of paraesthesia in the painful territory (but with the proviso below).

Over the four and a half decades since its introduction, it has become clear that some types of pain respond better than others to this technique. Well-established indications include CRPS, neuropathic pain secondary to peripheral nerve damage or radicular lumbar or cervical spinal pain (often in the context of a poor outcome from decompressive surgery), and post irradiation and partial traumatic brachial plexus lesions. In general, neuropathic pains in which the lesion is in the periphery respond better than myelopathic pains, and – as would be expected – severe dorsal column damage in the territory of the attempted stimulation renders the technique ineffective. Pain arising rostral to the cord is generally completely unresponsive. There is growing use of SCS for a range of visceral pains, and a substantial body of literature supports its use in treatment-resistant angina pectoris.

Curiously, the results of conventional frequency SCS are very poor in all pains of nociceptive type. However, recently a modification of this treatment has been introduced that utilises much higher frequencies and early results indicate that this may be effective for nociceptive as well as neuropathic pain. This ultra-high frequency SCS does not induce paraesthesia, which may increase patient acceptability. More clinical data are required before this new form of SCS is established in terms of the indications for its use.

Up-to-date recommendations for best clinical practice, details of conditions that respond, contraindications, technical details and a literature review are well set out in a consensus document from the British Pain Society and the Society of British Neurological Surgeons.

Deep brain stimulation This highly specialised technique originated from two startling discoveries: in humans, stimulation of the fornix and septal regions during psychosurgery produced analgesia, and, in rats, stimulation of the central midbrain grey matter allowed them to be operated on without an anaesthetic. The three areas most frequently targeted include the peri-aqueductal grey matter, peri-ventricular grey matter and the somatosensory nuclei of the thalamus. While experimental pain relief has been attributed predominantly to stimulation of endogenous opioid systems at the first two sites, and stimulation of inhibitory pathways at the third, the underlying mechanisms in humans remain unclear. Debate continues on many aspects, including the indications for deep brain stimulation (probably patients with constant, burning or aching neuropathic pain unresponsive to other measures), appropriate targets and stimulation parameters.

Motor cortex stimulation This counter-intuitive procedure involves the extradural placement of electrodes over the motor cortex. Pain relief is thought to be subserved by effects on descending inhibition, in turn mediated by sensory nerves present in the motor cortex. Recently, repetitive transcranial magnetic stimulation over the motor cortex has been reported to provide analgesia in patients with central pain and trigeminal neuralgia, an effect that might usefully predict benefit from long-term motor cortex stimulation.

Other physical methods of treatment

Many treatment modalities are used, including different forms of physiotherapy for nociceptive pains, and treatment is usually carried out by physiotherapists, occupational therapists and other allied therapists such as osteopaths and chiropractors. TENS is one such procedure and has been discussed earlier. Another technique often used for musculoskeletal and other pains, and a form of peripheral stimulation, is acupuncture.

Acupuncture

Acupuncture, the insertion of needles into the body for pain relief, has been used for 5000 years. Various techniques are employed:

- Needle stimulation of local points in painful areas, such as for treatment of tennis elbow.
- Needle stimulation of distant points, sometimes multiple and sometimes situated along classic Chinese acupuncture lines. However, the importance of classic acupuncture points is doubtful.
- Needle(s) are simply inserted, repetitively rotated or stimulated electrically, and inserted to different depths.
- Treatment is often given for about 30 minutes, but the optimum duration is unclear.

Acupuncture has been used in treatment of acute and numerous chronic painful and other disorders. It is most commonly and perhaps most effectively used for musculoskeletal rather than neuropathic pain. Contraindications include local skin lesions, anticoagulation and pregnancy. Side effects are infrequent, but infection, bleeding, syncope, paraesthesia and, depending on the site and depth of needle insertion, pneumothorax and other internal complications very rarely occur. Attempts have been made to undertake controlled trials of efficacy using specially adapted needles, but in practice acupuncture is usually given on a trial and error basis.

Despite its potential for placebo effects, acupuncture provides a form of powerful peripheral stimulation. The physiological basis underpinning acupuncture is complex, and includes effects mediated by release of endogenous opioids, as demonstrated by the fact that acupuncture analgesia can be reversed by naloxone. Acupuncture also induces both segmental and supraspinal descending inhibitory effects.

Acupuncture carried out for prolonged periods and at a stimulus intensity sufficient to cause pain raises the pain threshold and can induce analgesia. This acupuncture-induced analgesia, different from treatment of pain, has been used in selected cases as a method for allowing surgery to take place without general anaesthesia.

Psychological approaches to management of chronic pain

The psychological components of pain are extraordinarily complex, but the tendency to assume that pain intensity correlates with perceived pain severity can easily be disproved. Rather than being closely linked to sensory dysfunction, from the psychological perspective it is the affective, cognitive, behavioural and social aspects for the patient as well as the family that are crucial. As consistently shown by functional imaging, magneto-encephalography and other investigative tools, non-sensory brain changes occur alongside the sensory phenomena that characterise acute and chronic pains. Structures, particularly including the anterior cingulate, prefrontal cortex and insula, are implicated in encoding pain affect. It is thus increasingly recognised that any firm division between psychological and somatosensory aspects of pain is probably meaningless.

Currently, normal psychological aspects of pain are thought to comprise four concepts: attention, catastrophising, avoidance and depression. The neurophysiological bases underlying these are starting to be investigated. Building on these concepts and coinciding with the decrease in invasive procedures, there has been a rapid increase in the use of psychological strategies for management of pain.

Patient management falls to pain psychologists, the majority of whom work as members of a multi-disciplinary pain management team. It is important for the patient to accept that pain psychologists are concerned with management and not cure of the pain. Individual psychologists tend to have expertise in one or more specific therapeutic approaches, and while it is difficult to compare different forms of psychological intervention, cognitive behavioural therapy is one of the most widely used techniques that meta-analyses have shown to be effective.

Psychiatric treatment is sometimes also required. It is usually unwise to attribute chronic pain to a psychological cause, and patients with significant depression will need appropriate treatment and when necessary referral to a psychiatrist. Malingering presenting as chronic pain is well recognised but rare.

The placebo phenomenon

The placebo phenomenon in treating pain encapsulates the concept that individuals receiving a pharmacologically inert substance, or other inherently inactive 'sham' therapy, but believing that they are receiving an effective analgesic treatment experience reduced pain. Although it is often stated that one-third of the population are 'placebo responders', this figure can generally be traced to a single paper by Beecher who cited a number of studies in which the average rate of placebo response was indeed around 30% but with huge departures from the average across the studies quoted. Subsequent studies have indicated rates of placebo response ranging from 0 to 100% and it is clear that there is no 'fixed fraction' of placebo responders. Moreover, there is experimental evidence that individuals can be converted from non-responders to responders through conditioning. Cultural, experiential, experimental and numerous other factors are relevant. It is often thought that pain relief following a sham treatment can only induce psychological change, but there is compelling evidence that placebo effects can have measurable, and sometimes substantial, physiological effects. This evidence, from acute pain studies, includes findings that:

- Placebo ultrasound can reduce swelling and trismus as well as pain, and reduce C reactive protein levels, after wisdom tooth extraction.
- Naloxone can in some cases reverse placebo analgesia, suggesting endogenous opioid mechanisms are important, although naloxone can also produce hyperalgesia that can offset the placebo effect.
- Placebo analgesia is associated with changed patterns of cerebral blood flow similar to those seen with opioids.
- Functional MRI evidence suggests that placebo decreases activity in pain-subserving brain regions; conversely, during anticipation of pain, brain activity increases in the prefrontal cortex.
- Placebo analgesic effects, including physiological phenomena, are seen following technically abortive surgery when the patient is under general anaesthesia and therefore unaware.
- Placebo is a phenomenon also seen in treatment of other, non-painful and chronic, disorders including Parkinson's disease, Alzheimer's disease and depression.

The placebo phenomenon is proving to be an intriguing and important phenomenon in pain and other conditions, and the mechanisms are likely to include those subserving expectancy and conditioning. It should be noted that nocebo responses, in which an inert treatment induces an adverse response (e.g. nausea following a saline injection believed to be an opioid), are also well recognised.

Although pain relief by means of placebo would appear to be an ideal outcome, there are major ethical considerations when using placebo in clinical practice and in clinical trials. The issue is controversial, but the prevailing consensus is that patients should not receive placebo without consent, even if that consent includes placebo being one of a number of treatment options offered.

Insensitivity to pain

In these conditions, stimuli that would normally be painful are not transmitted to the brain. This lack of pain input may be congenital and occurs in some rare hereditary small fibre neuropathies, notably, but not exclusively, HSAN type IV(Chapter 10). Patients with this autosomal recessive neuropathy develop serious painless injuries amongst other defects, and have absence of unmyelinated peripheral axons, small sensory neurones in the dorsal root ganglia, and Lissauer's tracts. The mechanisms for the lack of pain perception may relate to mutations in the *TrkA* gene that encodes the high affinity receptor for NGF, which in turn is crucial for development of nociceptive and sympathetic neurones.

Acquired causes include occasional cases of diabetes, syphilitic tabes dorsalis, and lesions interrupting second-order central crossing spino-thalamic fibres as seen in syringomyelia. As a result of the lack of protective innervation, patients can develop painless scars, burns and ulcers, inadvertently bite their tongue and otherwise self-mutilate, and have disorganised (Charcot) joints and osteomyelitis. Such injuries need to be contrasted with the self-mutilation that can occur in association with anaesthesia dolorosa, in which the positive sensory disturbances (possibly including itch) give rise to constant scratching and damage, the human equivalent of autotomy in animals.

Congenital insensitivity to pain

In congenital indifference to pain (also known as asymbolia for pain, congenital pure analgesia and congenital indifference to pain), patients appear to have absent pain recognition which dates from birth. They do not react to painful stimuli anywhere over the body, but other sensory modalities and reflexes seem to be normal. They sustain painless injuries including skin lesions and fractures dating from childhood. Autosomal dominant and recessive families have been reported. In some patients insular damage perhaps leading to sensori-limbic disconnection has been reported, but in most patients no consistent pathological abnormalities have been found in either the peripheral or central nervous system. The cause of these very rare disorders remains unknown, although the clinical features recall those patients with other conditions in which medial pain-subserving circuits may well be implicated – for example, patients with frontotemporal dementia, and patients who in previous decades had a frontal lobotomy for treatment of intractable pain. However, it is now evident that, in some patients, their supposed indifference to pain is caused by impaired function of the voltage-gated sodium channel gene *SCN9A*, encoding the Na_v 1.7 sodium channel, and is in reality a channelopathy-associated insensitivity to pain.

Transient indifference to pain

It has long been observed that in certain acute situations of severe tissue injury in which pain would be expected, quite paradoxically pain may not be experienced at all. Classic studies came from Beecher who described this in battle-injured soldiers in the Second World War, but the same phenomenon has been documented in other wartime situations and in occasional patients with very severe injuries admitted to a hospital A&E department.

Early in the history of the recognition of this condition in warfare, it was assumed by some that the absence of pain was in some way induced by relief at having escaped alive from a potentially lethal combat situation, but there is no evidence to bear this out; recipients of these injuries are generally distressed rather than elated. Moreover, the analgesia is localised to the site of injury; the soldier who reports no pain from his shattered leg may complain of pain from clumsy venous cannulation in the arm.

The mechanisms of this form of analgesia are thought to include cortical and spinal inhibitory processes. It is always short lived (hours). Presumably the response has evolved because it confers selective advantage, and it can be seen to have potential survival value, enabling an animal to run from a predator on a broken leg. Perhaps having a similar basis is the impaired pain perception in those patients with parasomnias who sustain injuries during sleep-related violence. Pain appreciation is also impaired as a result of the transient effects of drugs such as opiates.

Conclusions

Pain in disorders of the nervous system is common, and diverse in its pathophysiological mechanisms and clinical manifestations. It is widely underestimated in its prevalence and severity. It can be very difficult to treat effectively, but in practice is often inadequately treated even when effective therapies are available. Effective management depends on accurate diagnosis, not only of the primary neurological condition, but of the putative mechanisms of generation of the pain – or pains – in the individual patient. The optimal management of the more challenging cases frequently requires the input of a multi-specialist team comprising (amongst others) psychologists and physical therapists as well as physicians.

In recent years, understanding of the mechanisms that give rise to pathological pain have advanced greatly. However, it remains the case that the advances in our knowledge have not been matched by advances in effective treatment.

Acknowledgement

The author wishes to acknowledge his indebtedness to his retired friend and colleague Dr G.D. Schott, much of whose contribution to the first edition of this textbook has been retained in this chapter, and also his grateful thanks to Dr M.S. Chong for the generosity of his time spent reading the manuscript and his helpful comments and advice.

References

Melzack R, Wall PD. Pain mechanisms: a new theory. *Science* 1965; **150**: 971–979.
Déjerine J, Roussy G. Le syndrome thalamique. *Rev Neurol (Paris)* 1906; **14:** 521.

Further reading

General

Cervero F, Laird JMA. Visceral pain. *Lancet* 1999; **353**: 2145–2148.
Faber CG, Hoeijmakers JG, Ahn HS, *et al.* Gain of function Nav1.7 mutations in idiopathic small fiber neuropathy. *Ann Neurol* 2012; **71:** 26–39.
Graven-Nielsen T, Mense S. The peripheral apparatus of muscle pain: evidence from animal and human studies. *Clin J Pain* 2001; **17**: 2–10.
Hunt SP, Mantyh PW. The molecular dynamics of pain control. *Nat Rev Neurosci* 2001; **2**: 83–91.
Rainville P, Duncan GH, Price DD, Carrier B, Bushnell MC. Pain affect encoded in human anterior cingulate but not somatosensory cortex. *Science* 1997; **277**: 968–971.
Ramachandran VS. Plasticity and functional recovery in neurology. *Clin Med* 2005; **5**: 368–373.
Scherder E, Oosterman J, Swaab D, Herr K, Ooms M, Ribbe M, *et al.* Recent developments in pain in dementia. *Br Med J* 2005; **330**: 461–464.
Schott GD. Pain and the sympathetic nervous system. In: Mathias CJ, Bannister R, eds. *Autonomic Failure*, 4th edn. Oxford: Oxford University Press, 1999: 520.
Schweinhardt P, Lee M, Tracey I. Imaging pain in patients: is it meaningful? *Curr Opin Neurol* 2006; **19**: 392–400.
von Hehn CA, Baron R, Woolf CJ. Deconstructing the neuropathic pain phenotype to reveal neural mechanism. *Neuron* 2012; **73**: 638–652.
Yosipovitch G, Greaves MW, Schmelz M. Itch. *Lancet* 2003; **361**: 690–694.

Classic papers on pain

Beecher HK. The powerful placebo. *J Am Med Assoc* 1955; **159:** 1602–1606.
Mitchell SW, Moorehouse GR, Keen WW. *Gunshot Wounds and Other Injuries of Nerves*. Philadelphia: J.B. Lippincott, 1864.

Clinical assessment

Nandi PR, Newton-John T. History-taking and examination of the patient with chronic pain. In: Rice ASC (lead ed.) *Clinical Pain Management*, 2nd edn. *Practice and Procedures volume*. London: Hodder Arnold, 2008: 3–11.

Specific Conditions

Birklein F. Complex regional pain syndrome. *J Neurol* 2005; **252**: 131–138.
Boulton AJM. Management of diabetic peripheral neuropathy. *Clin Diabetes* 2005; **23**: 9–15.
Ford B. Pain in Parkinson's disease. *Mov. Disord* 2010; **25**(Suppl 1): S98–103.
Jaeckle KA. Neurological manifestations of neoplastic and radiation-induced plexopathies. *Semin Neurol* 2004; **24**: 385–393.
Johnson RW, Whitton TL. Management of herpes zoster (shingles) and postherpetic neuralgia. *Expert Opin Pharmacother* 2004; **5**: 551–559.
Kehlet H, Jensen TS, Woolf CJ. Persistent postsurgical pain: risk factors and prevention. *Lancet* 2006; **367**: 1618–1625.
Layzer RB. Hot feet: erythromelalgia and related disorders. *J Child Neurol* 2001; **16**: 199–202.
Musheb RM, Nash JM, Brondolo E, Kerns RD. Vulvodynia: an introduction and critical review of a chronic pain condition. *Pain* 2000; **86**: 3–10.
Nurmikko TJ, Gupta S, McIver K. Multiple sclerosis-related central pain disorders. *Curr Pain Headache Rep* 2010; **14**: 189–195.
O'Connor AB, Schwid SR, Herrmann DN, Markman JD, Dworkin RH. Pain associated with multiple sclerosis: systematic review and proposed classification. *Pain* 2008; **137**: 96–111.
Schott GD. From thalamic syndrome to central post-stroke pain. *J Neurol Neurosurg Psychiatry* 1996; **61**: 560–564.
Sommer C. Painful neuropathies. *Curr Opin Neurol* 2003; **16**: 623–628.

Spillane JD, Nathan PW, Kelly RE, Marsden CD. Painful legs and moving toes. *Brain* 1971; **94**: 541–556.

Waseem S, Gwinn-Hardy K. Pain in Parkinson's disease. *Postgrad Med* 2001; **110**: 33–40, 46.

Young GB, Blume WT. Painful epileptic seizures. *Brain* 1983; **106**: 537–554.

Zakrzewska JM. The burning mouth syndrome remains an enigma. *Pain* 1995; **62**: 253–257.

Treatment and the placebo response

Attal N, Cruccu G, Baron R, *et al.* EFNS guidelines on the pharmacological treatment of neuropathic pain: 2010 revision. *Eur J Neurol* 2010; **17**: e1113–1188.

Demant DT, Lund K, Vollert J, *et al.* The effect of oxcarbazepine in peripheral neuropathic pain depends on pain phenotype: a randomised, double-blind, placebo-controlled phenotype-stratified study. *Pain* 2014; **155**: 2263–2273.

Finnerup NB, Attal N, Haroutounian S, *et al.* Pharmacotherapy for neuropathic pain in adults: a systematic review and meta-analysis. *Lancet Neurol* 2015; **14**: 162–173.

Finnerup NB, Jensen TS. Spinal cord injury pain: mechanisms and treatment. *Eur J Neurol* 2004; **11**: 73–82.

Finniss DG, Benedetti F. Mechanisms of the placebo response and their impact on clinical trials and clinical practice. *Pain* 2005; **114**: 3–6.

Kalso E. Opioids for persistent non-cancer pain. *Br Med J* 2005; **330**: 156–157.

Morley S, Eccleston C, Williams A. Systematic review and meta-analysis of randomized controlled trials of cognitive behaviour therapy and behaviour therapy for chronic pain in adults, excluding headache. *Pain* 1999; **80**: 1–13.

Saarto T, Wiffen PJ. Antidepressants for neuropathic pain. *Cochrane Database Syst Rev* 2007; **4**: CD005454.

Simpson K, Stannard C, Raphael J. *Spinal cord stimulation for the management of pain: recommendations for best clinical practice*. London: British Pain Society, 2009.

Wolfe GI, Trivedi JR. Painful peripheral neuropathy and its nonsurgical treatment. *Muscle Nerve* 2004; **30**: 3–19.

Whitworth LA, Fernández J, Feler CA. Deep brain stimulation for chronic pain. *Semin Neurosurg* 2004; **15**: 183–193.

CHAPTER 24

Autonomic Aspects of Neurology

Christopher Mathias[1], Gordon Ingle[2] and Valeria Iodice[2]
[1] UCL Institute of Neurology
[2] National Hospital for Neurology & Neurosurgery

The last three decades have seen major advances in awareness and recognition of autonomic disorders, and in the investigation and treatment of a variety of diseases that cause or contribute to autonomic dysfunction; these have been a result of many factors. Many clinicians consulted by patients with symptoms that cannot be readily explained now consider autonomic disorders as a possible cause. Advances in non-invasive technology have resulted in more accurate and reproducible methods of investigation, thus aiding diagnosis, understanding pathophysiological mechanisms and enabling targeted therapy for autonomic dysfunction. Collaboration between specialties within neurology, such as with movement disorders groups and with other medical disciplines such as diabetology, cardiology and, more recently, rheumatology, has been helpful in understanding autonomic involvement in common neurological and medical diseases. Advances in basic science have enabled neurological repair (e.g. in the spinal cord) and have refocused attention on the many autonomic abnormalities that occur in patients with spinal cord injuries. Finally, new autonomic disorders have been described, examples being dopamine beta hydroxylase deficiency (DβH), immune disorders affecting autonomic ganglia and the postural tachycardia syndrome (PoTS), and in the latter its close association with the joint hypermobility (Ehlers–Danlos III) syndrome.

Autonomic investigation units began to be established in the United Kingdom during the 1970s. Their scope of activity varied, depending much upon research funding. Established units have seen exponential growth in clinical service and research activity, which have advanced greatly the recognition, investigation and management of autonomic disorders. Activities now encompass a wide range of disorders, from autonomic failure syndromes to common disorders such as parkinsonian syndromes, hyperhidrosis, autonomic mediated syncope (AMS) and, in the last few years, PoTS. This chapter summarises the usual diagnostic approach and the range of tests and treatments available.

Classification of autonomic dysfunction

The autonomic nervous system has cranio-sacral parasympathetic and thoraco-lumbar sympathetic pathways (Figure 24.1) and supplies every organ in the body. The system influences target organ function locally and also operates more centrally (i.e. it controls vital functions such as arterial blood pressure and body temperature). Specific neurotransmitters in each pathway influence ganglionic and post-ganglionic activity (Figure 24.2 and Figure 24.3). Thus, autonomic diseases may occur with lesions or dysfunction at different sites of the neural axis, in the brain, spinal cord or periphery.

Autonomic disorders may be classified in a variety of ways. One approach is to divide them into localised and generalised disorders. Localised disorders affect an organ or region of the body but they may be part of generalised disease, such as gustatory sweating in diabetes mellitus (Table 24.1). Generalised disorders often affect systems, such as those involved in blood pressure control and thermoregulation. They can be primary when the cause is unclear, or secondary when associated with a specific disease or its complications (Table 24.2a).

Damage to the autonomic nervous system often causes irreversible abnormalities. This contrasts with intermittent autonomic dysfunction, the common transient abnormalities that generate so much morbidity (Table 24.2b). These conditions include AMS, PoTS and essential hyperhidrosis. Drugs are a common cause of autonomic dysfunction, either because of their pharmacological effects or because of autonomic nerve damage (Table 24.3). Classification of disorders causing damage to the autonomic nervous system may also be considered under prognosis, based on natural history and/or possible interventional measures (Table 24.4).

Clinical features

Clinical features of autonomic disease cover a wide spectrum (Table 24.5) and result from underactivity or overactivity. The history is of particular importance in consideration and recognition of autonomic disease and in distinguishing dysfunction from other disorders. In brief:

- Sympathetic adrenergic failure causes orthostatic (postural) hypotension and ejaculatory failure in the male.
- Sympathetic cholinergic failure causes anhidrosis.
- Parasympathetic failure causes dilated pupils, fixed heart rate, sluggish urinary bladder, atonic large bowel and, in the male, erectile failure.

The extent of dysfunction is dependent on the degree of autonomic damage. With autonomic hyperactivity, the reverse occurs. In some disorders, particularly in AMS, there may be a combination of

Neurology: A Queen Square Textbook, Second Edition. Edited by Charles Clarke, Robin Howard, Martin Rossor and Simon Shorvon.

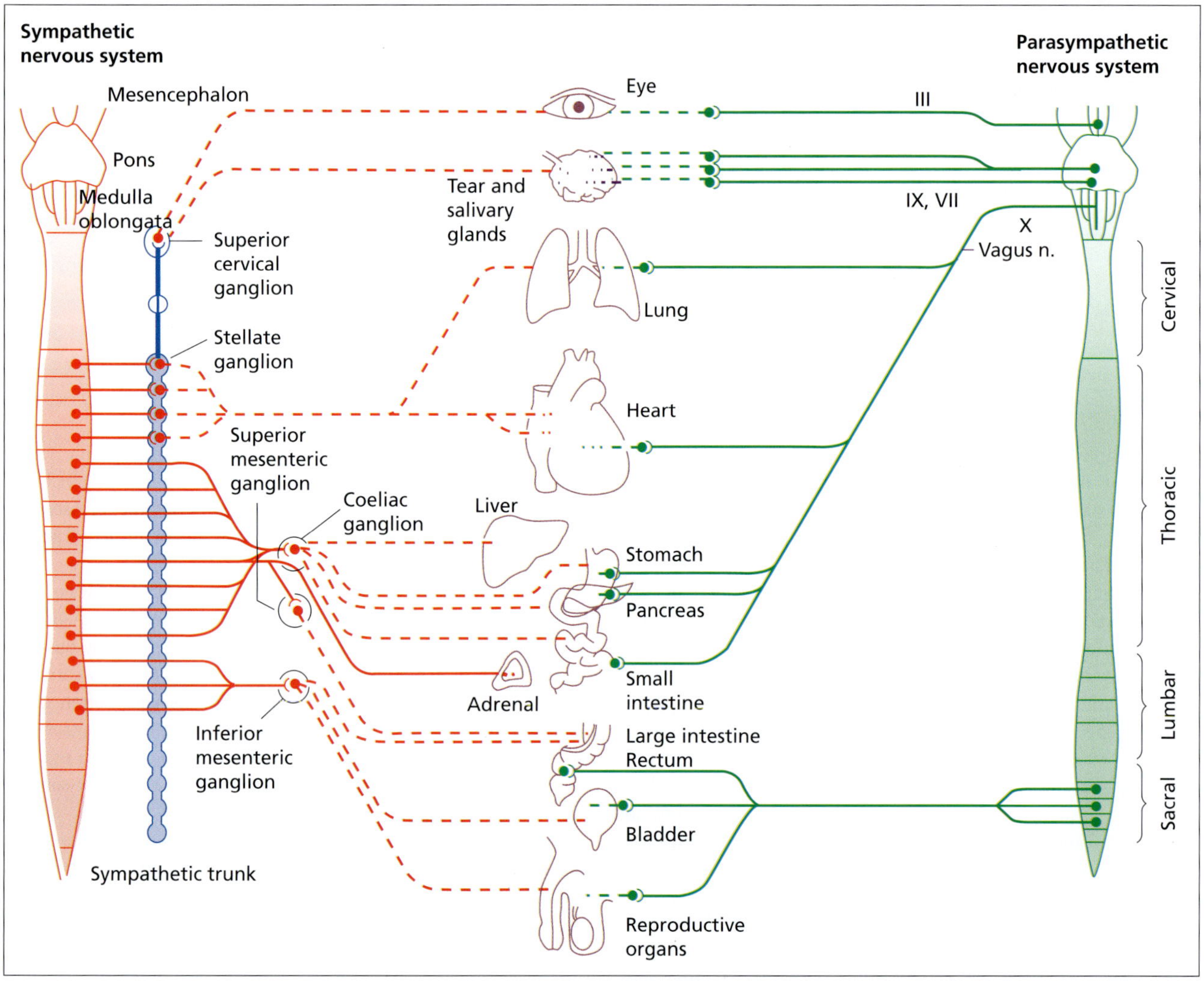

Figure 24.1 Cranio-sacral parasympathetic and thoraco-lumbar sympathetic outflow. Source: Janig 1987. Reproduced with permission of Springer Science + Business Media.

over-activity and under-activity, with bradycardia caused by increased parasympathetic activity and hypotension brought about by withdrawal of sympathetic activity.

Autonomic disease may occur in any age group. At birth it is seen in the rare condition familial dysautonomia (Riley–Day syndrome), in teenage years in the common disorder vasovagal syncope and between the ages of 30 to 50 in familial amyloid polyneuropathy (FAP). Neurodegenerative disorders affecting the autonomic nervous system often occur after the age of 50 years.

The majority of autonomic diseases are sporadic. However, genetically transmitted disorders include the Riley–Day syndrome and FAP. There often is a family history in vasovagal syncope, especially in those presenting below the age of 20 years. Drug-induced autonomic disease is caused by impaired metabolism or the production of toxic metabolites, as with perhexiline maleate neuropathy. A detailed history relating to drug usage, chemical and toxin exposure is always necessary (Table 24.3).

Autonomic involvement, even if it affects only a single organ or system (Table 24.5), may be an important feature of an underlying disease. For example, Horner's syndrome, with mainly cosmetic effects, can be the harbinger of underlying non-autonomic disease (such as apical tuberculosis or lung neoplasm in Pancoast's syndrome). The usually benign Holmes–Adie pupil sometimes occurs in isolation, or with absent tendon reflexes and other autonomic features, such as an afferent baroreceptor defect causing orthostatic hypotension and labile hypertension, sweating abnormalities and a dry cough (Holmes–Adie syndrome). In generalised disorders such as multiple system atrophy (MSA), a single system is sometimes involved initially. Thus, erectile failure in the male, and constipation or urinary bladder dysfunction in either gender, can pre-date other autonomic or neurological features. The clinical features are now considered under each major system.

Cardiovascular system

Orthostatic hypotension

Symptoms of orthostatic hypotension are often the reason for requesting medical advice and can provide initial clues to underlying autonomic disease. Orthostatic or postural hypotension is defined as a fall in blood pressure of 20 mmHg systolic or 10 mmHg diastolic on sitting, standing or during 60° head-up tilt (Figures 24.4 and 24.5). In neurogenic orthostatic hypotension, levels of plasma noradrenaline do not rise when upright, as occurs in

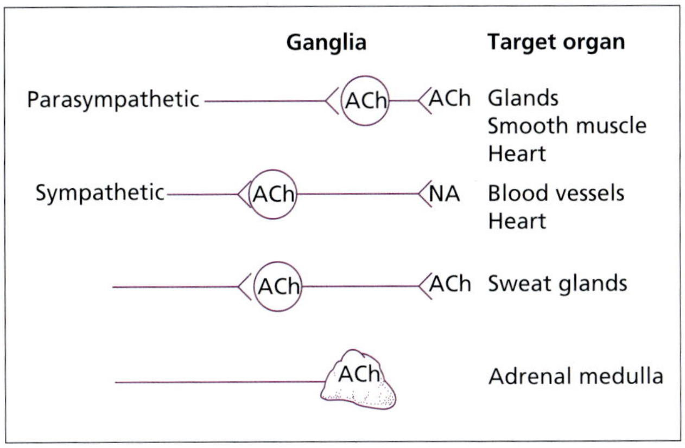

Figure 24.2 Outline of the major transmitters at autonomic ganglia and post-ganglionic sites on target organs supplied by the sympathetic and parasympathetic efferent pathways. The acetylcholine receptor at all ganglia is of the nicotinic subtype. Ganglionic blockers such as hexamethonium thus prevent both parasympathetic and sympathetic activation. However, atropine acts only on the muscarinic (ACh-m) receptor at post-ganglionic parasympathetic and sympathetic cholinergic sites. The co-transmitters along with the primary transmitters are also indicated (ACh, acetylcholine; NA, noradrenaline). Source: Adapted from Mathias 1998 with permission of Elsevier.

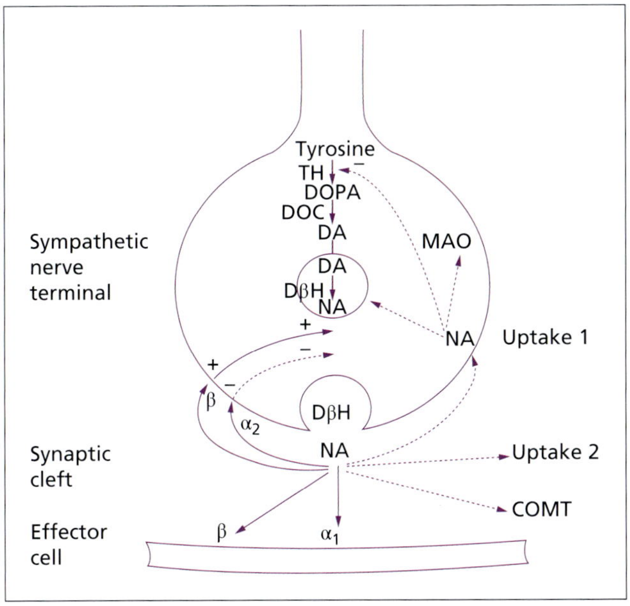

Figure 24.3 Formation of noradrenaline (NA) from tyrosine within a sympathetic nerve terminal (DA, dopamine; DβH, dopamine beta hydroxylase; DDC, dopadecarboxylase; DOPA, dihydroxyphenylalanine; TH, tyrosine hydroxylase). NA in granules is released by a process of exocytosis into the synaptic cleft, following which it acts on various alpha or beta adrenoreceptors, either pre- or post-synaptically. NA is subject to various processes which involve uptake 1 into the nerve terminal, following which it is either incorporated into granules, exerts negative feedback on TH or is metabolised by monoamine oxidase (MAO). Some is taken up into non-neuronal tissues (uptake 2), some metabolised by catechol-*O*-methyltransferase (COMT), while the rest spills over into the circulation. Source: Mathias 2004. Reproduced with permission of Elsevier.

Table 24.1 Examples of localised autonomic disorders.

Horner's syndrome
Holmes–Adie pupil
Crocodile tears (Bogorad's syndrome)
Gustatory sweating (Frey's syndrome)
Reflex sympathetic dystrophy
Idiopathic palmar or axillary hyperhidrosis
Chagas' disease (*Trypanosoma cruzi*)*
Surgical procedures†
Sympathectomy (regional)
Vagotomy and gastric drainage procedures in 'dumping' syndrome
Organ denervation following transplantation (heart, lungs)

*Listed here because the disease targets specifically intrinsic cholinergic plexuses in the heart and gut.

†Surgery also may cause other localised disorders, such as Frey's syndrome after parotid surgery.

Table 24.2 (a) Outline classification of autonomic disorders.

Primary
Acute/subacute dysautonomias
Pure pan-dysautonomia
Pan-dysautonomia with neurological features
Pure cholinergic dysautonomia
Chronic autonomic failure syndromes
Pure autonomic failure
Multiple system atrophy (Shy–Drager syndrome)
Autonomic failure with Parkinson's disease
Secondary
Congenital
Nerve growth factor deficiency
Hereditary
Autosomal dominant trait
Familial amyloid neuropathy
Autosomal recessive trait
Familial dysautonomia – Riley–Day syndrome
Dopamine β hydroxylase deficiency
Metabolic diseases
Diabetes mellitus
Chronic renal failure
Chronic liver disease
Alcohol-induced
Inflammatory
Guillain–Barré syndrome
Transverse myelitis

(continued)

Table 24.2 (continued)

Infections
Bacterial – tetanus
Viral – HIV infection
Neoplasia
Brain tumours – especially of 3rd and 4th ventricles or posterior fossa
Paraneoplastic, especially adenocarcinoma of lung and pancreas
Surgery
Vagotomy and drainage procedures – 'dumping syndrome'
Trauma
Cervical and high thoracic spinal cord transection
Drugs, chemical toxins (see also Table 24.3)
By direct effects
By causing a neuropathy

Source: Mathias and Bannister 2013. Reproduced with permission of Oxford University Press.

Table 24.2 (b) Examples of intermittent autonomic dysfunction.

Autonomic mediated syncope (AMS)
Vasovagal syncope
Carotid sinus hypersensitivity
Situational syncope
Postural tachycardia syndrome (PoTS)
Initial orthostatic hypotension
Autonomic dysfunction in spinal cord injury
Essential (idiopathic) hyperhidrosis

normal subjects (Figure 24.6), the lack of rise reflecting impaired sympathetic activity. Hypoperfusion of organs, especially above heart level such as the brain, cause the malaise, nausea, dizziness and visual disturbances that often precede loss of consciousness (Table 24.6).

The fall in blood pressure and associated symptoms during postural change often varies within the same individual. If blood pressure falls precipitously, syncope tends to occur instantly and is likely to cause injury. Occasionally, seizures occur as a result of cerebral hypoxia in syncope. With time and frequent exposure to orthostatic hypotension, some come to tolerate a low cerebral perfusion pressure with few or even no symptoms, presumably because of improved cerebrovascular autoregulation.

A variety of symptoms result from hypoperfusion elsewhere. Neck pain in a coat-hanger distribution (suboccipital and shoulder regions) differs from other types of neck pain by developing when upright. It is relieved by sitting or lying flat, when the blood pressure recovers. The pain probably is caused by reduced perfusion of neck muscles that need to be tonically active to maintain upright head posture. Using arm muscles especially when upright can increase cerebral symptoms of orthostatic hypotension by a subclavian steal-like mechanism further reducing brainstem blood flow. Central chest pain, suggestive of angina pectoris, sometimes occurs with normal coronary arteries and can be caused by chest wall ischaemia.

Oliguria, especially during the day when upright, is the result of reduced renal perfusion pressure. This can be difficult to separate from retention of urine resulting from urinary sphincter

Table 24.3 Drugs, chemicals, poisons, and toxins causing autonomic dysfunction.

Decreasing sympathetic activity
Centrally acting
Clonidine
Methyldopa
Moxonidine
Reserpine
Barbiturates
Anaesthetics
Peripherally acting
Sympathetic nerve endings (guanethidine, bethanidine)
α-Adrenoceptor blockade (phenoxybenzamine)
β-Adrenoceptor blockade (propranolol)
Increasing sympathetic activity
Amphetamines
Releasing noradrenaline (tyramine)
Uptake blockers (imipramine)
Monoamine oxidase inhibitors (tranylcypromine)
β-Adrenoceptor stimulants (isoprenaline)
Decreasing parasympathetic activity
Antidepressants (imipramine)
Tranquillisers (phenothiazines)
Antidysrhythmics (disopyramide)
Anticholinergics (atropine, probanthine, benztropine)
Toxins (botulinum)
Increasing parasympathetic activity
Cholinomimetics (carbachol, bethanechol, pilocarpine, mushroom poisoning)
Anticholinesterases
Reversible cholinesterase inhibitors (pyridostigmine, neostigmine)
Organophosphorous inhibitors (parathion, sarin)
Miscellaneous
Alcohol, thiamine (vitamin B_1) deficiency
Vincristine, perhexiline maleate
Thallium, arsenic, mercury
Mercury poisoning (pink disease)
Ciguatera toxicity
Jellyfish and marine animal venoms, scombroid poisoning
First dose of certain drugs (prazosin, captopril, propranolol)
Withdrawal of chronically used drugs (clonidine, opiates, alcohol)

Table 24.4 Classification based on natural history and intervention.

Fixed and irreversible	Pure autonomic failure Spinal cord injury
Progressive and irreversible	Multiple system atrophy
Progressive but stoppable	Familial amyloid polyneuropathy Diabetes mellitus
Reversible	Immune-mediated autonomic neuropathies

Table 24.5 Some clinical manifestations of autonomic dysfunction.

Cardiovascular
Postural hypotension
Supine hypertension
Lability of blood pressure
Paroxysmal hypertension
Tachycardia
Bradycardia
Sudomotor
Hypohidrosis or anhidrosis
Hyperhidrosis
Gustatory sweating
Hyperpyrexia
Heat intolerance
Alimentary
Xerostomia
Dysphagia
Gastric stasis
Dumping syndromes
Constipation
Diarrhoea
Urinary
Nocturia
Frequency
Urgency
Retention
Incontinence
Sexual
Erectile failure
Ejaculatory failure
Retrograde ejaculation
Eye
Pupillary abnormalities
Ptosis
Alachryma
Abnormal lachrymation with food ingestion
Respiratory system
Stridor, involuntary inspiratory gasps, apnoeic periods

abnormalities (e.g. in high spinal cord lesions). The reverse – polyuria – occurs when supine, especially at night when blood pressure is restored or even elevated. In the elderly, falls occur even without other symptoms of orthostatic hypotension. Other less specific symptoms include weakness, tiredness and fatigue.

A key component in the history is the relationship between symptoms and head-up postural change. Symptoms may be more prominent with rapid head-up change (e.g. getting out of bed in the morning) and on rising after a large meal, excessive alcohol or exercise (Figures 24.7 and 24.8). A variety of factors influence orthostatic hypotension and should be sought in the history (Table 24.7). Many patients recognise the association with head-up postural change and either sit down, lie flat, stoop or assume curious postures, such as squatting. These positions can prevent the fall in blood pressure or even elevate blood pressure. Orthostatic hypotension is often worsened by drugs that have vasodilator effects used to treat associated disease (levodopa or insulin), alleviate symptoms (nitrates) or reverse organ failure (sildenafil).

Syncope without orthostatic hypotension

Syncope has many causes (autonomic, cardiac, neurogenic and metabolic). In AMS orthostatic hypotension is not present but there is transient hypotension and bradycardia, often with a provoking factor. There are three major forms: vasovagal syncope, carotid sinus hypersensitivity and situational syncope. Blood pressure falls because of sympathetic withdrawal while heart rate falls because of increased vagal activity. This is more likely to occur when upright. There are usually no autonomic abnormalities detected between attacks. The history of the syncopal attack and its recovery often separates AMS from other neurological diseases, such as epilepsy. Recovery on lying flat usually is rapid, as this restores blood pressure and cerebral perfusion. Tongue biting normally does not occur. In some, convulsions result from hypoxia, especially if the subject is not laid flat and blood pressure recovery is delayed. Urinary incontinence can occasionally occur.

In vasovagal syncope (common faints or emotional syncope) provoking factors include fear, pain, the sight of blood and medical procedures, especially involving needles. Nausea and other gastrointestinal upsets, probably through activation of visceral afferents, may be causative. Palpitations and sweating occur in the pre-syncopal phase. In those with an adequate warning, sitting or lying flat prevents syncope. The reverse, prolonged standing or assumption of the upright position on a tilt table, may provoke a response; the latter is the basis for the laboratory investigation. Tilt table testing is usually for 10 minutes, with a provocative stimulus such as venepuncture; sometimes prolonged tilt testing for 45 minutes is needed. It is important to determine the underlying mechanism contributing to syncope as this influences the management of vasovagal syncope (Figures 24.9, 24.10 and 24.11).

In the elderly, carotid sinus hypersensitivity is increasingly recognised as a cause of falls (Figure 24.12). There may be a classic history of syncope induced while shaving, turning the head or buttoning the collar, when carotid afferents are stimulated. However, this history may not be obtained. Falls and syncope that remain unexplained should arouse suspicion of this disorder.

In situational syncope, various factors predispose the individual to syncope: induction of a Valsalva manoeuvre and hyperventilation. This occurs in weight-lifters, trumpet-blowers, in mess tricks

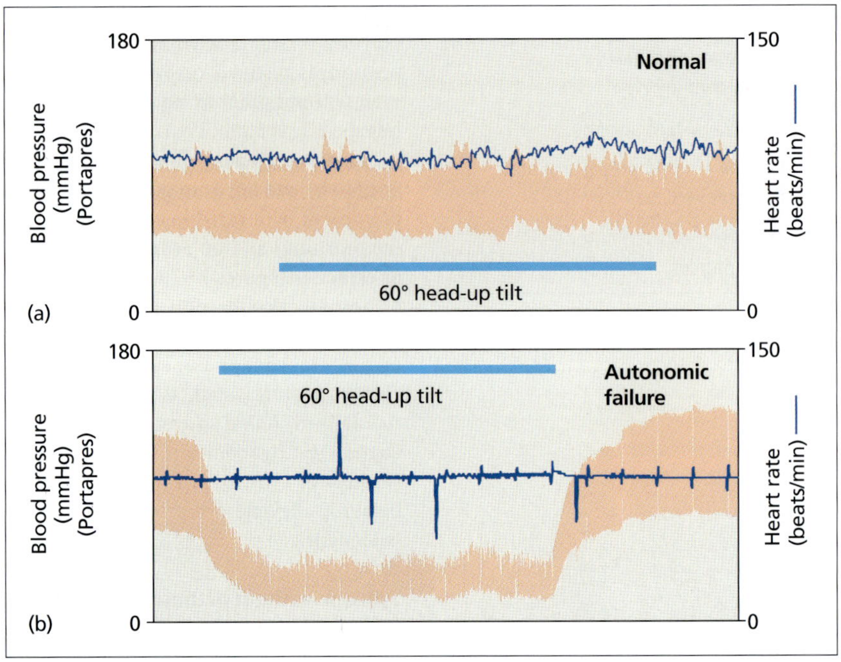

Figure 24.4 Blood pressure and heart rate before, during and after head-up tilt in (a) a normal subject, and (b) a patient with autonomic failure. In the normal subject there is no fall in blood pressure during head-up tilt, unlike a subject with autonomic failure in whom blood pressure falls promptly and remains low with a blood pressure overshoot on return to the horizontal. In this subject there is only a minimal change in heart rate despite the marked blood pressure fall. In both subjects continuous blood pressure and heart rate was recorded with the Finometer. Source: Mathias 2006. Reproduced with permission of Elsevier.

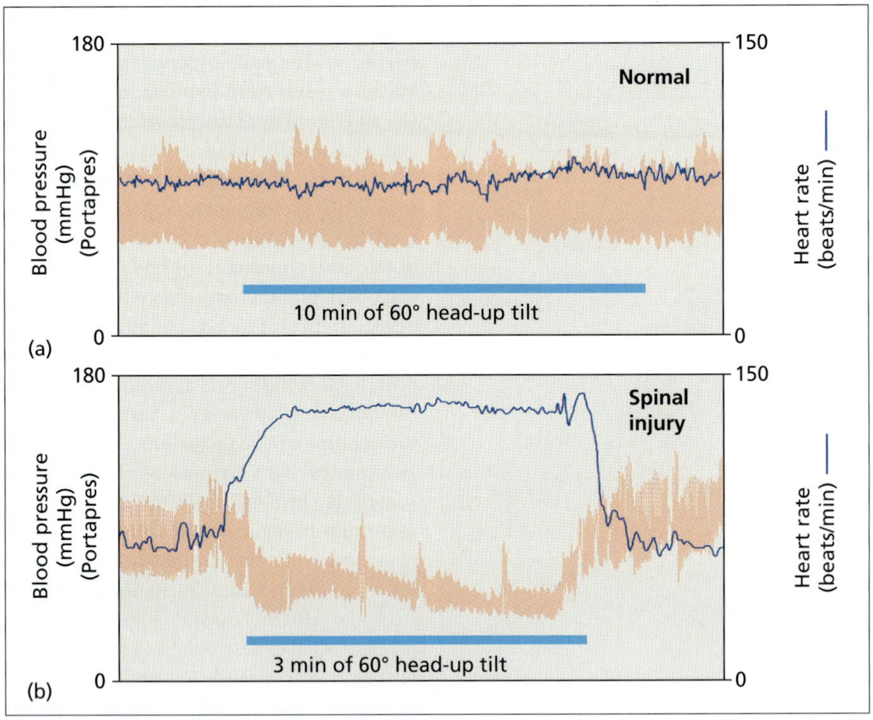

Figure 24.5 (a,b) Blood pressure and heart rate measured continuously with the Finometer in a patient with a high cervical spinal cord lesion. There is a fall in blood pressure because of impairment of the sympathetic outflow disrupted in the cervical spine. Heart rate rises because of withdrawal of vagal activity in response to the rise in pressure. Source: Mathias 2006. Reproduced with permission of Elsevier.

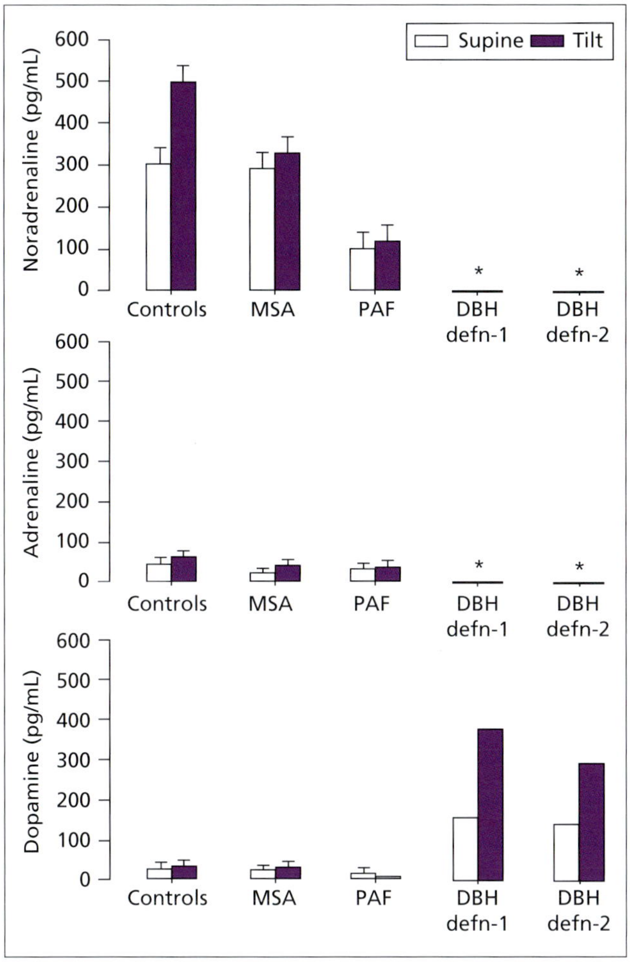

Figure 24.6 Plasma noradrenaline, adrenaline and dopamine levels (measured by high pressure liquid chromatography) in normal subjects (controls), patients with multiple system atrophy (MSA), pure autonomic failure (PAF) and two individual patients with dopamine β-hydroxylase (DBH) deficiency while supine and after head-up tilt to 45° for 10 minutes. The asterisk indicates levels below the detection limits for the assay, which are less than 5 pg/mL for noradrenaline and adrenaline and less than 20 pg/mL for dopamine. Bars indicate ± standard error of mean (SEM). Source: Mathias and Bannister 2013. Reproduced with permission of Oxford University Press.

(deliberate manoeuvres) and following paroxysms of coughing. In micturition syncope, hypotension results probably from a combination of vasodilatation caused by warmth and/or alcohol and straining during micturition (which raises intrathoracic pressure and induces a Valsalva manoeuvre), compounded by release of the pressor stimulus arising from a distended bladder while standing upright. Swallowing-induced syncope sometimes occurs with glossopharyngeal neuralgia.

Orthostatic intolerance with posturally induced tachycardia

When orthostatic intolerance occurs without orthostatic hypotension, but with a substantial rise in heart rate (of over 30 beats/minute), the term postural tachycardia syndrome (PoTS) is used

Table 24.6 Symptoms resulting from orthostatic hypotension and impaired perfusion.

Cerebral hypoperfusion
Dizziness
Visual disturbances
Blurred – tunnel
Scotoma
Greying out – blacking out
Colour vision defects
Syncope
Cognitive deficits
Muscle hypoperfusion
Paracervical and suboccipital ('coat-hanger') ache
Lower back/buttock ache
Subclavian steal-like syndrome
Renal hypoperfusion
Oliguria
Non-specific
Weakness, lethargy, fatigue
Falls

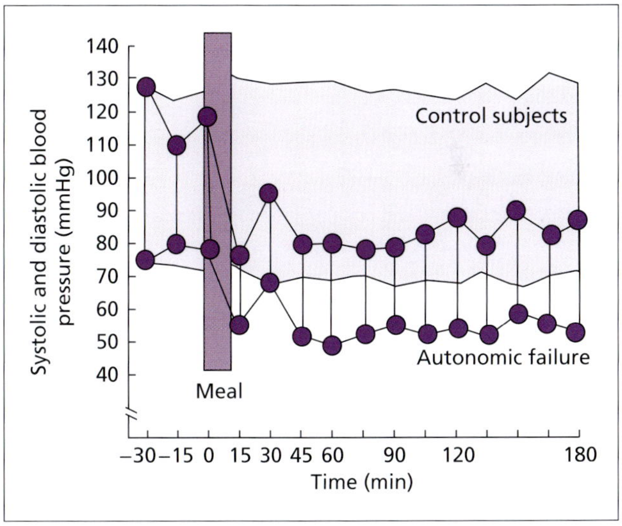

Figure 24.7 Changes in BP before and after a standard meal in a group of normal subjects (stippled area) and in a patient with autonomic failure (IR), while in the supine and horizontal position. Bars indicate ± standard error of mean (SEM). In the normal subjects there is no change in BP. In the patient with autonomic failure there is a marked fall in BP soon after food ingestion, with levels falling to around 80/50 mmHg and remaining low for 3 hours, even in the supine position. Source: Mathias and Bannister 2013. Reproduced with permission of Oxford University Press.

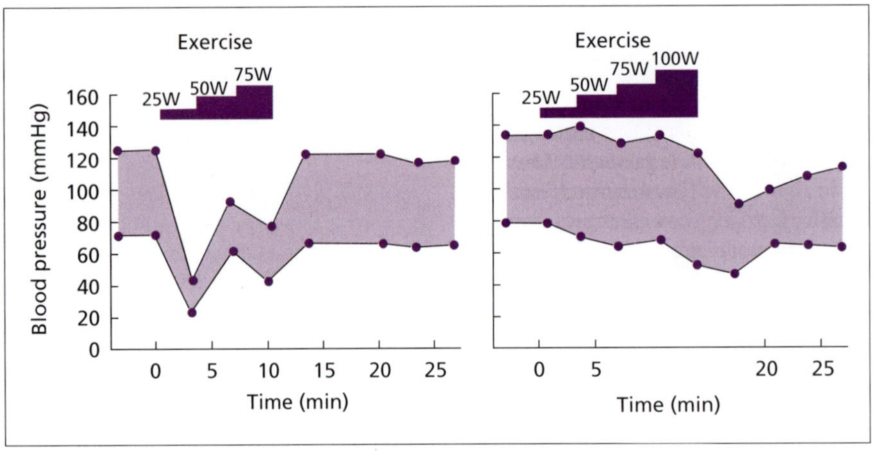

Figure 24.8 Systolic and diastolic blood pressure in two patients with autonomic failure before, during and after bicycle exercise performed with the patient in the supine position at different workloads, ranging from 25 to 100W. In the patient on the left there is a marked fall in blood pressure on initiating exercise; she had to crawl upstairs because of severe exercise-induced hypotension. In the patient on the right, there are minor changes in blood pressure during exercise, but a marked decrease soon after stopping exercise. This patient was usually asymptomatic while walking, but developed postural symptoms when he stopped walking and stood still. It is likely that the decrease in blood pressure post-exercise was a result of vasodilatation in exercising skeletal muscle, not opposed by the calf muscle pump. Source: Mathias 1994. Reproduced with permission of Elsevier.

Table 24.7 Factors influencing orthostatic hypotension.

Speed of positional change
Time of day (worse in the morning)
Prolonged recumbency
Warm environment (hot weather, central heating, hot bath)
Raising intrathoracic pressure – micturition, defaecation or coughing
Food and alcohol ingestion
Water ingestion*
Physical exertion
Physical manoeuvres and positions (bending forward, abdominal compression, leg crossing, squatting, activating calf muscle pump)†
Drugs with vasoactive properties (including dopaminergic agents)

*This raises blood pressure in autonomic failure.

†These manoeuvres usually reduce the postural fall in blood pressure, unlike the others.

(Figure 24.13). It predominantly affects women below the age of 50 years. Symptoms include marked dizziness on postural change or modest exertion; syncope may occur. There are usually no features of generalised autonomic failure. Associated disorders include the joint hypermobility syndrome (Ehlers–Danlos III; Figures 24.14 and 24.15), chronic fatigue syndrome, mitral valve prolapse and hyperventilation. A relationship to disorders described in wartime, such as da Costa's syndrome and soldier's heart, now often grouped with chronic fatigue syndrome, when dizziness and syncope on effort is accompanied by exhaustion, dyspnoea, headache, palpitations and pain over the heart, seems probable.

Hypertension

Unlike hypotension, hypertension typically causes few symptoms other than headaches – and these only occasionally. In high spinal cord lesions, severe paroxysmal hypertension can develop as part of autonomic dysreflexia, when an uninhibited increase in spinal sympathetic activity is caused by contraction of the urinary bladder, irritation of the large bowel, noxious cutaneous stimulation or skeletal muscle spasms. This can cause hypertension, a throbbing pounding headache, palpitations with bradycardia and sweating/flushing over the face and neck. The limbs tend to be cold as a result of peripheral vasoconstriction. In tetanus, hypertension in ventilated patients can be precipitated by muscle spasms or tracheal suction. Intermittent hypertension can occur in Guillain–Barré syndrome, porphyria, posterior fossa tumours and phaeochromocytoma (Figure 24.16), often without any evident precipitating cause.

Sustained hypertension resulting from increased sympathetic activity may occur in subarachnoid haemorrhage. Hypertension in the supine position can complicate orthostatic hypotension in pure autonomic failure (PAF). The mechanisms include impaired baroreflex activity, adrenoceptor supersensitivity, an increase in central blood volume because of a shift from the periphery and the effects of drugs used to prevent orthostatic hypotension.

Heart rate disturbances

Bradycardia, along with hypertension, sometimes occurs in cerebral tumours with or without raised intracranial pressure and during autonomic dysreflexia in high spinal cord injuries. In the latter, the afferent and vagal efferent components of the baroreflex arc are intact, and the heart slows in an attempt to control the rise in blood pressure. In phaeochromocytoma, bradycardia with escape rhythms and atrioventricular dissociation occurs in response to a rapid rise in blood pressure.

Severe bradycardia can occur in artificially ventilated high cervical cord injuries with diaphragmatic paralysis. The patients' intact vagal nerves are sensitive to hypoxia and stimuli such as

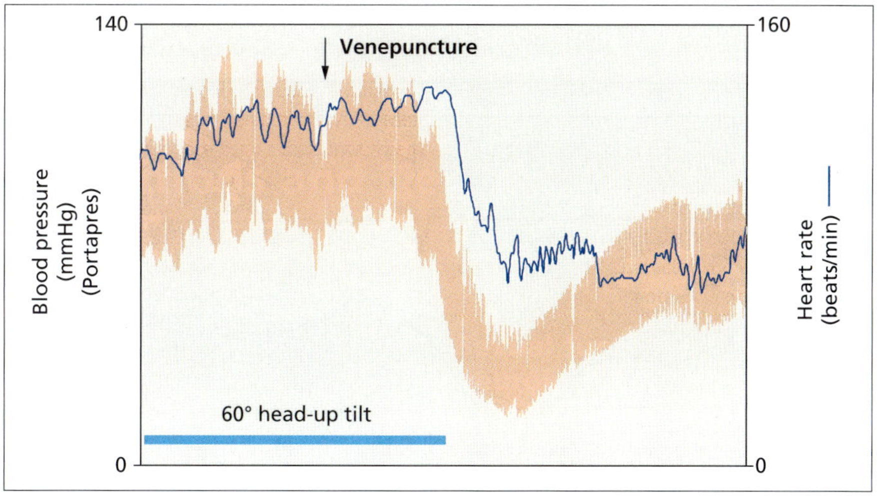

Figure 24.9 Blood pressure and heart rate with continuous recordings from the Finometer in a patient with the mixed (cardio-inhibitory and vasodepressor) form of vasovagal syncope. Source: Mathias and Galizia 2010. Reproduced with permission of Elsevier.

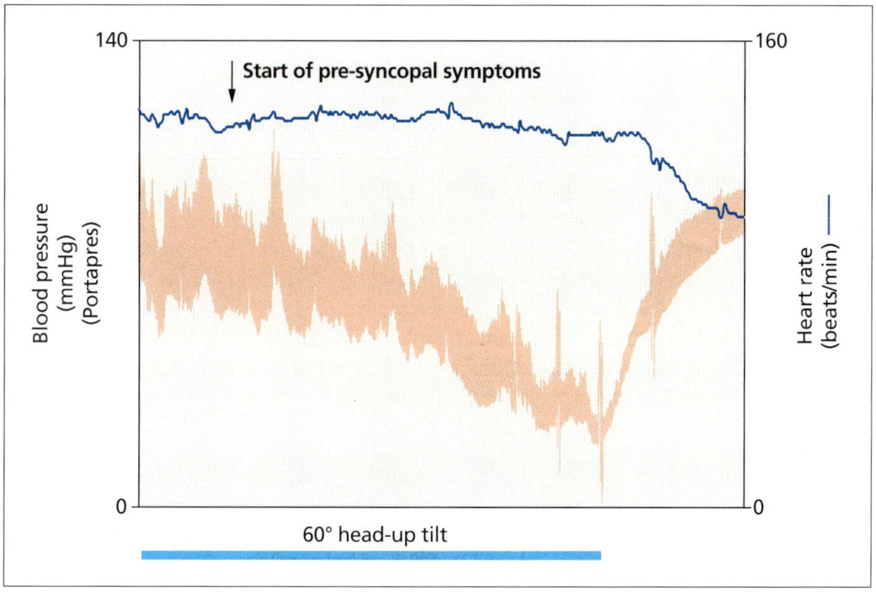

Figure 24.10 Blood pressure and heart rate with continuous recordings from the Finometer in a patient with the predominantly vasodepressor form of vasovagal syncope. Source: Mathias and Galizia 2010. Reproduced with permission of Elsevier.

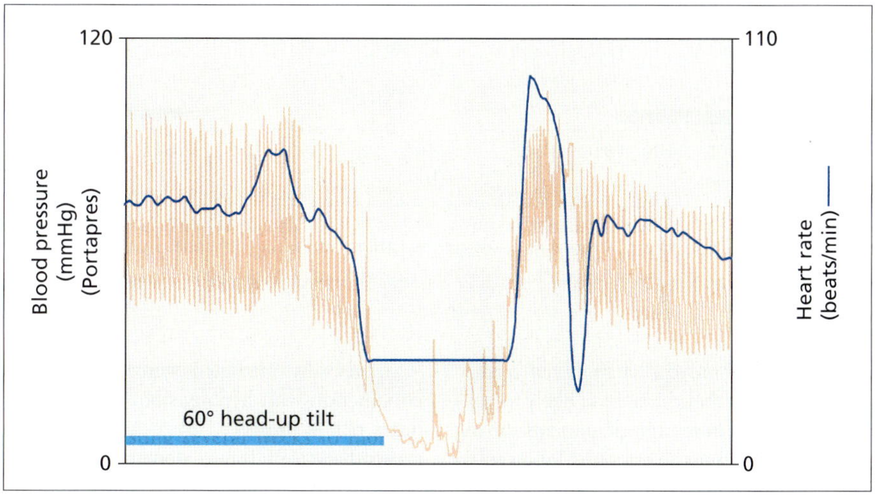

Figure 24.11 Blood pressure and heart rate with continuous recordings from the Finometer in a patient with the cardio-inhibitory form of vasovagal syncope. Source: Mathias and Galizia 2010. Reproduced with permission of Elsevier.

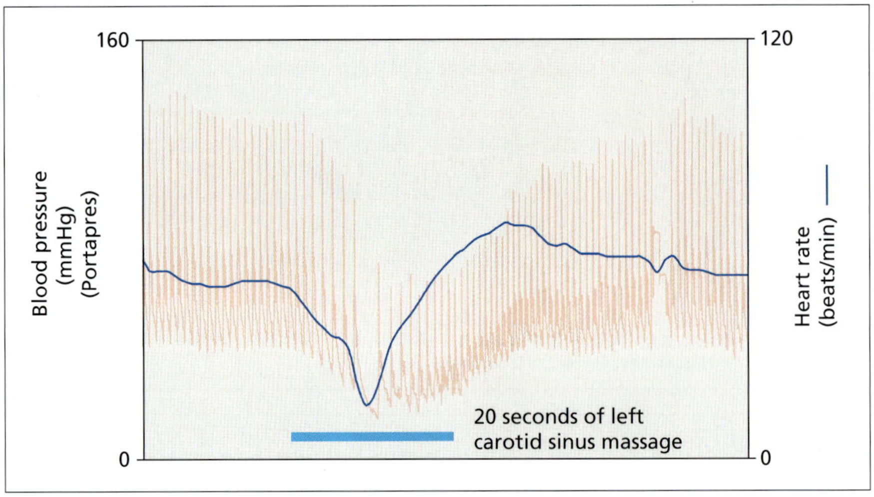

Figure 24.12 Continuous blood pressure and heart rate measured non-invasively (by Portapres) in a patient with falls of unknown aetiology. Left carotid sinus massage caused a fall in both heart rate and blood pressure. The findings indicate the mixed (cardio-inhibitory and vasodepressor) form of carotid sinus hypersensitivity. Source: Mathias 2013. Reproduced with permission of Oxford University Press.

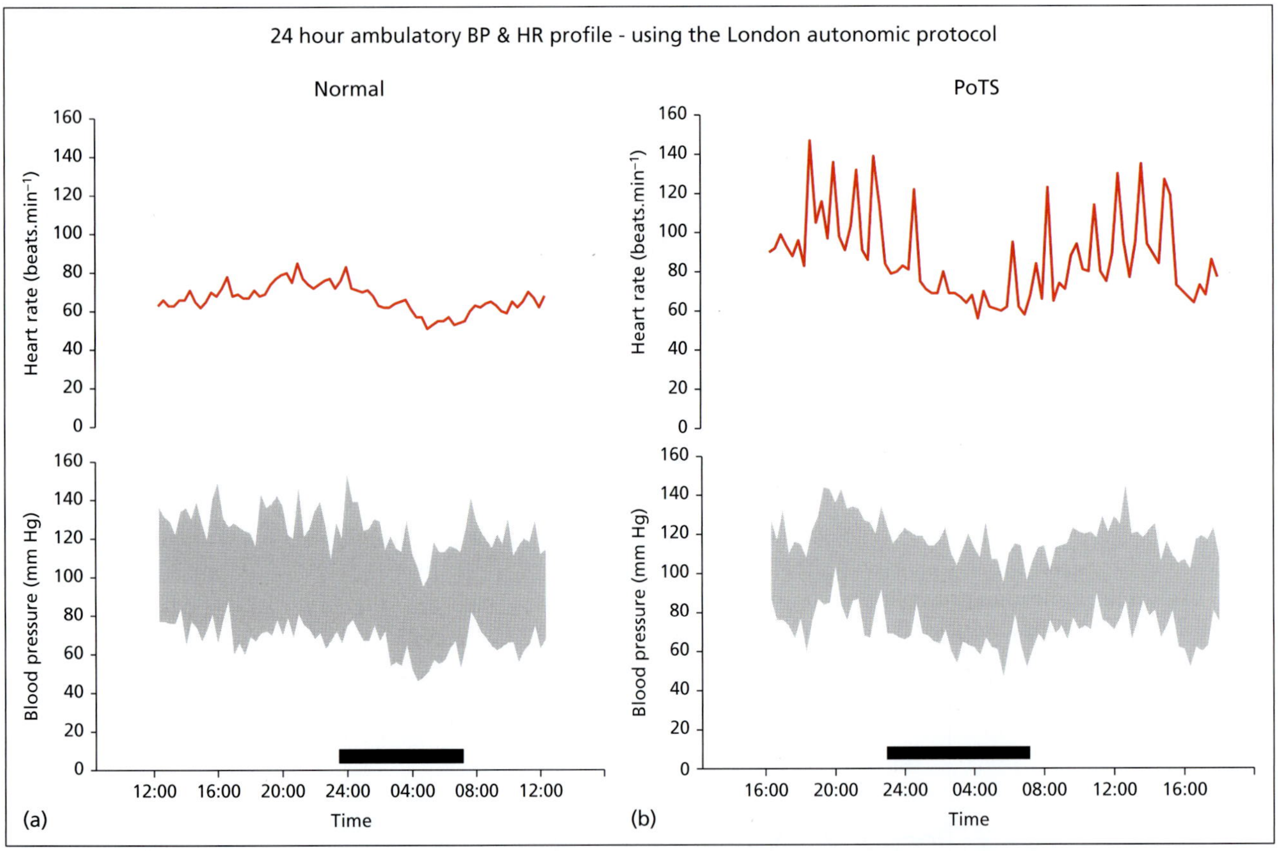

Figure 24.13 Blood pressure and heart rate measured continuously before, during and after 60° head-up tilt by the Finometer in (a) a normal subject, and (b) in subject with the postural tachycardia syndrome (PoTS). Source: Mathias *et al*. 2012. Reproduced with permission of Macmillan.

tracheal suction can readily induce bradycardia and even cardiac arrest. The inability to increase sympathetic activity is likely to contribute. Similar responses also occur in tetraplegic patients during general anaesthesia, especially when muscle paralysis followed by intubation is performed without atropine.

In neurally mediated syncope, severe bradycardia occurs in conjunction with hypotension. Syncope can even occur when the heart rate is preserved by a cardiac demand pacemaker, because sympathetic withdrawal alone can cause substantial vasodilatation resulting in hypotension.

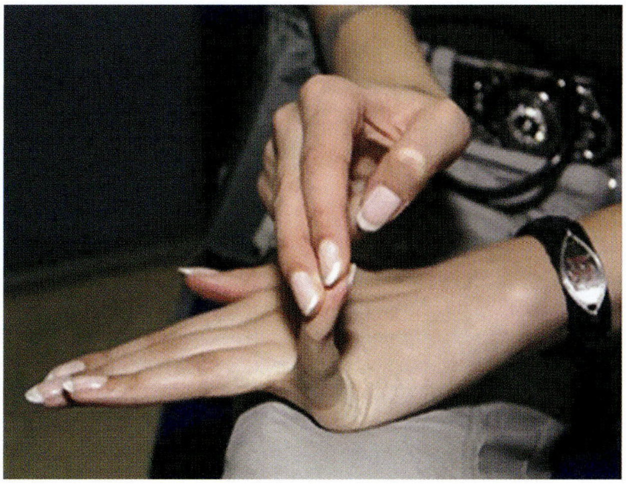

Figures 24.14 Clinical signs of joint hypermobility in a patient with PoTS and joint hypermobility syndrome/Ehlers–Danlos syndrome type III (also known as EDS hypermobility type). Source: Mathias *et al.* 2012. Reproduced with permission of Macmillan.

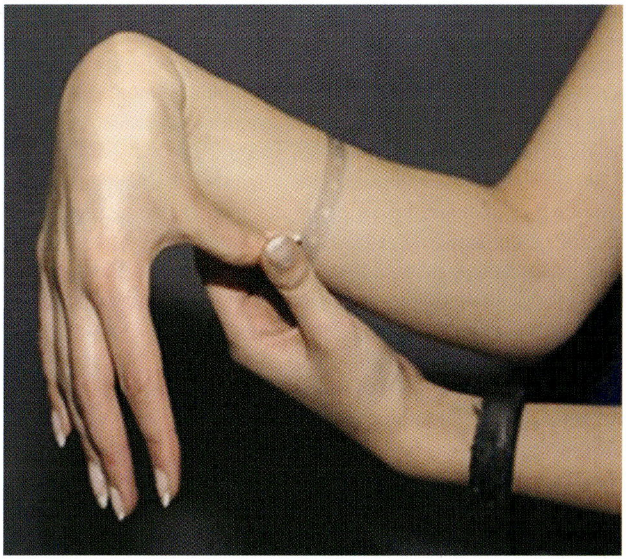

Figure 23.15 Clinical signs of joint hypermobility in a patient with PoTS and joint hypermobility syndrome/Ehlers–Danlos syndrome type III (also known as EDS hypermobility type). Source: Mathias *et al.* 2012. Reproduced with permission of Macmillan.

In diabetes mellitus, the presence of a cardiac vagal neuropathy can result in higher resting heart rate and impaired sinus arrhythmia and abnormalities on other tests of cardiac parasympathetic function (Figure 24.17). Disorders of cardiac conduction are common in Chagas' disease (South American trypanosomiasis) and sometimes in amyloidosis.

In PoTS, tachycardia is usually associated with head-up postural change and exertion. Tachycardia resulting from increased sympathetic discharge occurs along with hypertension in the Guillain–Barré syndrome and in tetanus. In phaeochromocytoma, tachycardia results from catecholamine release and β-adrenoceptor stimulation.

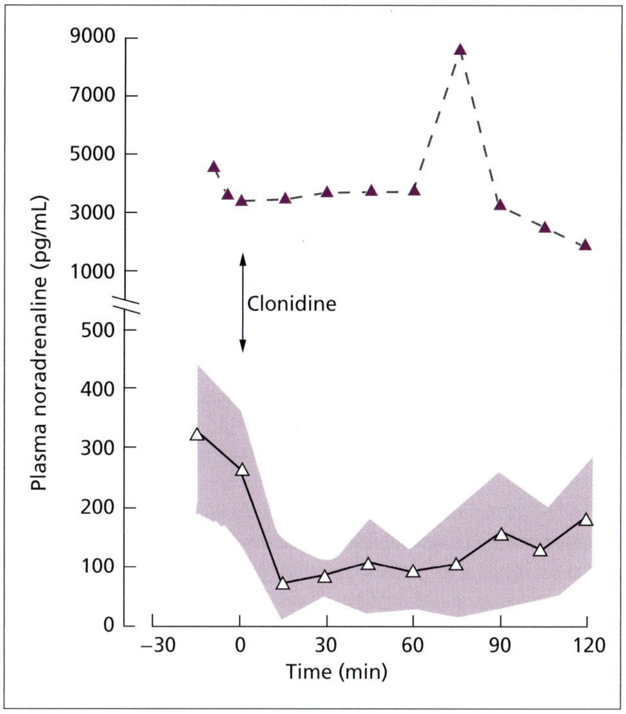

Figure 24.16 Plasma noradrenaline levels in a patient with a phaeochromocytoma (black triangles) and in a group of patients with essential hypertension (open triangles) before and after intravenous clonidine, indicated by an arrow (2 μg/kg over 10 minutes). Plasma noradrenaline levels fall rapidly in the essential hypertensives after clonidine and remain low over the period of observation. The stippled area indicates the ± standard error of mean (SEM). Plasma noradrenaline levels are considerably higher in the phaeochromocytoma patient and are not affected by clonidine. Source: Mathias and Bannister 2013. Reproduced with permission of Oxford University Press.

Facial and peripheral vascular changes

When blood pressure falls in postural hypotension or neurally mediated syncope, there is usually facial pallor with an ashen appearance. Restoration of colour follows promptly on assuming the supine position when blood pressure rises. Facial pallor can also occur during an attack in phaeochromocytoma but usually is accompanied by sweating, headache and hypertension. In long-standing tetraplegia, hypertension during autonomic dysreflexia is often accompanied by flushing and sweating over the face and neck. The precise mechanisms are unknown.

In Harlequin syndrome there is vasodilatation and anhidrosis on one side of the face caused by sympathetic impairment, with sparing of the pupil. The lesion spares the first thoracic segment (from which oculomotor fibres often leave) but affects sympathetic fibres of the second and third thoracic roots.

Raynaud's phenomenon can be seen in both PAF and MSA, for reasons that are unknown. In the latter, cold purplish blue hands and feet can be particularly troublesome. Livedo reticularis can accompany sympathetic over-activity, as in phaeochromocytoma. In erythromelalgia there is limb discomfort with vascular changes. The precise reasons for the cutaneous, vascular and sudomotor changes in reflex sympathetic dystrophy (chronic region pain disorder) remain debatable.

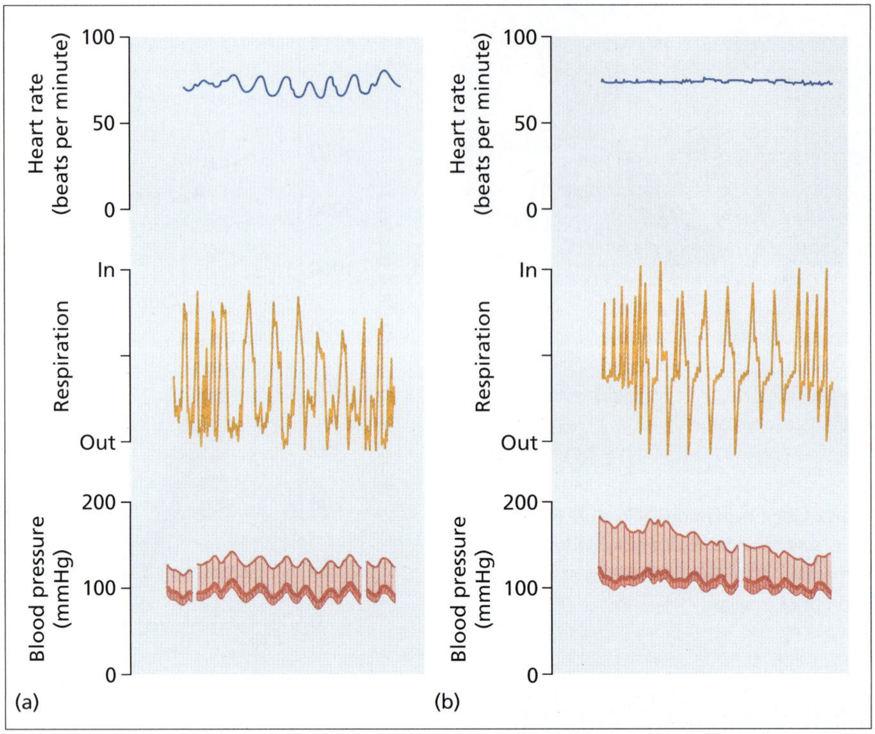

Figure 24.17 The effect of deep breathing on heart rate and blood pressure in (a) a normal subject, and (b) a patient with autonomic failure of the sort seen in diabetes. There is no sinus arrhythmia in the patient, despite a fall in blood pressure. Respiratory changes are indicated in the middle panel. Source: Mathias and Bannister 2013. Reproduced with permission of Oxford University Press.

Sudomotor system

The eccrine glands concerned with temperature regulation are innervated by sympathetic cholinergic fibres, unlike apocrine glands on palms and soles which are influenced by circulating substances, predominantly catecholamines. Anhidrosis or hypohidrosis is common in PAF and differences in sweating may first be noticed during exposure to warm temperatures. Occasionally, hyperhidrosis in segmental areas can be a disconcerting symptom, as a compensatory response to diminished sudomotor activity elsewhere. Anhidrosis may be congenital and occur without any other deficit. It can be an integral component of certain hereditary sensory and autonomic neuropathies, such as congenital insensitivity to pain with anhidrosis (HSAN type IV; Chapter 23).

Localised or generalised anhidrosis, sometimes with compensatory hyperhidrosis, can be associated with the Holmes–Adie pupil. This association is known as Ross's syndrome. In spinal cord injuries, there is often a band of hyperhidrosis above the lesion with anhidrosis below. During autonomic dysreflexia in high spinal lesions sweating occurs mainly over the face and neck. Facial and truncal hyperhidrosis can occur in Parkinson's disease. Hyperhidrosis is seen intermittently in phaeochromocytoma and accompany hypertension in tetanus.

Localised hyperhidrosis over the face and neck caused by food (gustatory sweating) can be socially distressing. It occurs in diabetes mellitus, following Bell's palsy and after parotid surgery, as a result of aberrant connections between nerve fibres supplying the salivary and sweat glands. Minimally invasive endoscopic techniques for sympathectomy often are successful in reducing axillary and palmar hyperhidrosis, but some develop troublesome compensatory hyperhidrosis over innervated areas of the trunk and lower limbs. The mechanisms are unclear.

Hypothermia can occur in hypothalamic disorders and in the elderly, in whom degenerative hypothalamic lesions are sometimes postulated. In high spinal injuries, especially in the early phases, the absence of 'shivering thermogenesis' and inability to vasoconstrict and thus prevent heat loss can readily result in hypothermia. Hypothermia can be missed if oral temperature only is recorded without a low-reading thermometer. Measurement of core tympanic or rectal temperature is essential.

Hyperpyrexia may be a problem with anhidrosis, with exposure to high ambient temperatures. Heat also increases vasodilatation and can enhance orthostatic hypotension leading to collapse.

Alimentary system

Reduced salivation and a dry mouth (xerostomia) occur in autonomic disease, especially in pure cholinergic dysautonomia. It can cause dysphagia, prominent when eating dry food. The lower two-thirds of the oesophagus contains smooth muscle that is autonomically innervated. Diseases affecting these pathways often cause dysphagia. Dysphagia is unusual in PAF, but often occurs in the later stages of MSA, where the problem is usually in the oropharyngeal region and can result in tracheal aspiration. The oesophagus is involved in Chagas' disease, with achalasia and mega-oesophagus causing vomiting. Gastric stasis in diabetes mellitus can cause abdominal distension and vomiting of undigested food.

Constipation is common in PAF but diarrhoea can also occur as result of overflow. Diarrhoea, especially at night, can be a distressing problem in diabetes mellitus. Reasons postulated include incomplete digestion, altered bowel flora and abnormal motility, but the cause remains poorly understood. Gastro-intestinal disturbances (reflux, abdominal bloating, low transit and constipation) previously classed as the irritable bowel syndrome are being increasingly recognised in association with PoTS and Ehlers–Danlos III.

Kidneys and urinary tract

Nocturnal polyuria is a frequent symptom in PAF. The causes include restitution of blood pressure sometimes to elevated levels while supine, redistribution of blood from the peripheral into the central compartment, and alteration in release of hormones that influence salt and water handling (such as renin, aldosterone and atrial natriuretic peptide). In MSA, where there is additional autonomic impairment of bladder and sphincter control, nocturia can be particularly troublesome. By day, the low level of blood pressure when upright is likely to cause oliguria.

Autonomic disease can cause urinary frequency, urgency, incontinence or retention. Loss of sacral parasympathetic function, as in the early phase of spinal cord injury, causes an atonic bladder with urinary retention, whereas recovery of isolated spinal cord function results in a neurogenic bladder. Dyssynergia, with detrusor contraction but without sphincter relaxation, causes autonomic dysreflexia. Ureteric reflux predisposes to renal damage, especially in the presence of infection. In PAF, urinary symptoms initially may be attributed in older men to prostatic hypertrophy and in women to pelvic muscle weakness, especially in those who are multiparous. In MSA, surgery in suspected prostate enlargement usually is of no benefit. The use of drugs with anticholinergic effects sometimes unmasks urinary bladder dysfunction in autonomic failure.

Infection is common when bladder dysfunction causes urinary stasis. Some patients, such as those with spinal injuries, are prone to urinary calculi, especially when immobility increases calcium excretion. In PoTS and joint hypermobility syndrome (Ehlers–Danlos III), female patients have a greater tendency to recurrent urinary tract infections, sometime difficult to eradicate when there is interstitial cystitis. Whether laxity of the bladder wall contributes is unclear.

Sexual function

In the male, failure of erection, dependent partly on the parasympathetic system, can cause impotence. Ejaculation is controlled by the sympathetic system. Retrograde ejaculation can occur, especially if there are urinary sphincter abnormalities. Dissociating the effects of increasing age, systemic illness and depression from definable organic causes of impotence can be difficult and the effect of concomitant drug therapy needs consideration (Chapter 25). The 5-HT uptake inhibitor, fluoxetine, prolongs ejaculation. Other drugs normally not considered to have autonomic side effects, such as thiazides used in hypertension, can diminish sexual potency.

Priapism resulting from abnormal spinal reflexes sometimes occurs in patients with spinal cord lesions. In women, autonomic impairment does not appear directly to affect sexual function, although this has been inadequately studied.

Eyes and lacrimal glands

The non-striated component of the levator palpebrae superioris (Müller's muscle) is innervated by sympathetic fibres and a mild ptosis is part of Horner's syndrome. If sympathetic lesions are bilateral, as in high spinal cord transection, Horner's syndrome is difficult to detect. A variety of pupillary abnormalities occur with autonomic involvement; both the miosis of Horner's syndrome and dilated myotonic pupils in Holmes–Adie syndrome. Symptoms directly relating to ocular function can be minimal in such disorders. Night vision is impaired in sympathetic denervation. There is reduced tolerance to sunlight when pupils are dilated following parasympathetic failure. The ciliary muscle is innervated by parasympathetic nerves; blurred vision caused by cycloplegia may follow disease or anticholinergic drugs. The latter can also raise intra-ocular pressure and cause glaucoma.

Impaired tear production can occur in PAF, sometimes as part of a presumed sicca or Sjögren's syndrome, along with diminished salivary secretion. Excessive and inappropriate lacrimation occurs in crocodile tears syndrome (gusto-lacrimal reflex).

Respiratory system

Involuntary inspiratory sighs, stridor and snoring of recent onset are more frequent in MSA than in Parkinson's disease. Stridor results from weakness of the crico-arytenoid muscles, the main laryngeal abductors. Nocturnal apnoea, which occurs in the later stages of the disorder, is caused by involvement of brainstem respiratory centres.

Abnormal responses following activation of reflexes from the respiratory tract, such as during tracheal suction, can cause profound cardiovascular disturbances. Thus, for example, severe hypertension and tachycardia can occur in tetanus, and bradycardia and cardiac arrest with high cervical cord transection.

Additional features of neurological conditions: MSA and Parkinson's disease

In the parkinsonian form of MSA, bradykinesia and rigidity with minimal tremor are more likely than in idiopathic Parkinson's disease (Figure 24.18). This causes difficulties in mobility, especially turning in bed and changing direction. Facial expression is affected to a lesser degree in MSA than in idiopathic Parkinson's disease. In MSA there often is a response to antiparkinsonian agents in the early stages but drug side effects, such as orthostatic hypotension, are likely to occur as the disease progresses. In Parkinson's disease with autonomic failure, extrapyramidal features have often been present for a long period and usually remain responsive to levodopa therapy.

In the non-parkinsonian forms of MSA, cerebellar features predominate with an ataxic gait, intention tremor, scanning speech and

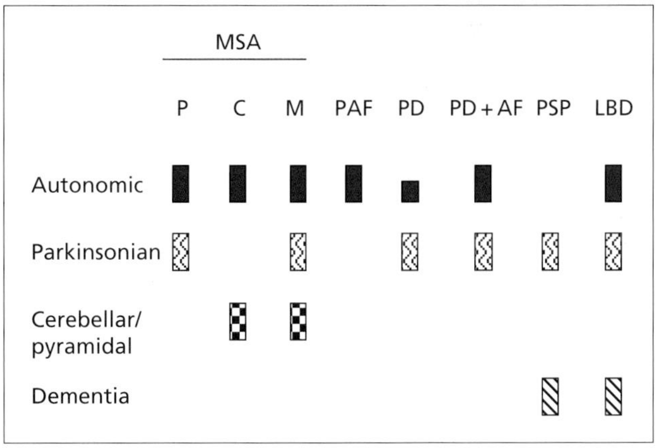

Figure 24.18 The major clinical features in parkinsonian syndromes and allied disorders with autonomic failure. These include the three major neurological forms of multiple system atrophy (MSA); the parkinsonian form (MSA-P, also called striatonigral degeneration), the cerebellar form (MSA-C, also called olivopontocerebellar atrophy) and the multiple or mixed form (MSA-M, which has features of both other forms), pure autonomic failure (PAF), idiopathic Parkinson's disease (IPD), Parkinson's disease with autonomic failure (PD + AF), progressive supranuclear palsy (PSP) and diffuse Lewy body disease (LBD). After Mathias (1997, 2005).

nystagmus. Ataxia can be difficult to separate from or perhaps be compounded by unsteadiness caused by orthostatic hypotension. There also may be pyramidal involvement with increased tone, exaggerated tendon reflexes and extensor plantar responses. In the mixed form of MSA, a varying combination of extrapyramidal, cerebellar and pyramidal features is seen. Sensory deficits are uncommon in MSA. Patients with secondary autonomic failure have neurological features that are a part of, or a complication of, a primary disease. In diabetes mellitus, a sensorimotor neuropathy often coexists with, or precedes the autonomic neuropathy.

Psychological and psychiatric disturbances

Dementia is unusual in PAF. Most patients with MSA are not clinically depressed, despite their disabilities and the probable deficit in central catecholamine levels. Overall, they tend to have a normal affective state, especially when comparisons are made with Parkinson's disease. In PAF there is no psychological disorder, but the absent autonomic responses can result in subtle emotional deficits. They appear less emotional than normal subjects and, when compared with similarly disabled patients with Parkinson's disease without autonomic failure, are less anxious. Cognitive function may transiently be affected when blood pressure falls below critical cerebral perfusion pressure limits. Whether this affects certain tasks (e.g. involving attention) rather than others, is unclear.

Anxiety and tremulousness may occur in phaeochromocytoma. Psychological factors contribute to vasovagal syncope (hence the term 'emotional syncope') and also to essential hyperhidrosis. Whether this is the cause, or result, of the autonomic condition can be difficult to determine. Anxiety is frequently observed in PoTS and joint hypermobility syndrome (Ehlers–Danlos III), especially in those with multiple morbidities who have been undiagnosed for many years with symptoms attributed to psychological factors. Psychiatric disturbances can also complicate conditions associated with autonomic dysfunction such as porphyria.

Clinical examination

A detailed physical examination is essential and, with the symptoms elicited, provides important clinical pointers towards autonomic disease. Features on general examination include dryness of skin, hyperhidrosis or cold hands in Raynaud's disease, and pupillary changes. Measurement of blood pressure, both lying and standing (or sitting), is needed to determine if orthostatic hypotension is present, as is recording the pulse rate changes in patients with PoTS. The extent and distribution of the neurological abnormalities provide important clues to underlying central or peripheral autonomic disorders. Examination of other systems, as in hepatic disease, diabetes and joint hypermobility syndrome (Ehlers–Danlos III), is necessary along with urine testing for glucose and protein.

The combination of a detailed history and physical examination is crucial in determining if autonomic disease is present, in ascertaining the probable underlying diagnosis and also for interpreting the results of autonomic tests in the context of the associated disorder.

Investigations

The aims of investigations in autonomic dysfunction are twofold. The first relates to diagnosis. The second is to understand the pathophysiological basis of disturbed autonomic function, as this often forms the basis of treatment strategies and their evaluation. An outline of investigations is provided in Table 24.8.

Management

The management of autonomic dysfunction encompasses a number of aspects. Of immediate and practical importance is alleviation of symptoms. The ideal is to rectify the autonomic deficit and cure the underlying disorder but this rarely is achieved. Autonomic

Table 24.8 Outline of investigations in autonomic disease.

Cardiovascular
Physiological
Head-up tilt (60°);* standing;* Valsalva maneouvre*
Pressor stimuli* (isometric exercise, cold pressor, mental arithmetic)
Heart rate responses – deep breathing,* hyperventilation,* standing,* head-up tilt,* 30 : 15 R–R interval ratio
Liquid meal challenge
Exercise testing
Carotid sinus massage
Biochemical
Plasma noradrenaline: supine and head-up tilt or standing; urinary catecholamines; plasma renin activity and aldosterone
Pharmacological
Noradrenaline: alpha-adrenoceptors, vascular
Isoprenaline: beta-adrenoceptors, vascular and cardiac
Tyramine: pressor and noradrenaline response
Edrophonium: noradrenaline response
Atropine: parasympathetic cardiac blockade
Imaging
Cardiac sympathetic innervation with MIBG or fluoro-dopamine
Endocrine
Clonidine – alpha-2 adrenoceptor agonist: noradrenaline suppression; growth hormone stimulation
Sudomotor
Central regulation thermoregulatory sweat test
Sweat gland response to intradermal acetylcholine, quantitative sudomotor axon reflex test, localised sweat test
Sympathetic skin response
Gastrointestinal
Video-cine fluoroscopy, barium studies, endoscopy, gastric emptying studies, lower gut studies
Renal function and urinary tract
Day and night urine volumes and sodium/potassium excretion
Urodynamic studies, intravenous urography, ultrasound examination, sphincter electromyography
Sexual function
Penile plethysmography
Intracavernosal papaverine
Respiratory
Laryngoscopy
Sleep studies to assess apnoea and oxygen desaturation
Eye and lacrimal function
Pupil function, pharmacological and physiological
Schirmer's test

*Screening tests widely used.

disease often involves various systems. Basic principles in relation to management of the major clinical features are provided here. Specific aspects vary in different diseases and always should be directed to the needs of the individual patient.

Cardiovascular system

Orthostatic hypotension

Orthostatic hypotension causes few symptoms in some but can cause considerable distress in others. It can contribute to disability and even death because of the potential risk of substantial injury. Treatment may be needed even in those who are asymptomatic, as they are at risk in situations such as fluid depletion or treatment with vasodilator drugs when there may be marked falls in blood pressure.

No single drug or treatment can effectively replace the actions of the sympathetic nervous system in different situations. A multi-pronged approach, combining non-pharmacological and pharmacological measures, is usually needed (Table 24.9).

The doctor and patient should be aware of the limitations of treatment and associated deficits (such as cerebellar features in MSA) can limit mobility in some patients, despite effective treatment of orthostatic hypotension.

Increasing patient awareness of factors that lower blood pressure is important. Rapid postural change, especially in the morning when getting out of bed, must be avoided because the supine blood pressure often is lowest at this time. Prolonged bed rest and recumbency through factors that include decompensation can contribute to orthostatic intolerance even in healthy individuals and can considerably worsen orthostatic hypotension in autonomic failure. Head-up tilt at night is beneficial and reduces salt and water loss by stimulating the renin–angiotensin–aldosterone system. Straining during micturition and defaecation lowers blood pressure further by inducing a Valsalva manoeuvre. In toilets in small enclosed areas (e.g. in aircraft), the severe hypotension induced can be dangerous because of the inability to fall to the floor and thereby recover blood pressure and consciousness. In hot weather, because of impairment of thermoregulatory mechanisms, the rise in body temperature will increase cutaneous vasodilatation and worsen orthostatic hypotension. Ingestion of alcohol or large meals, especially those with a high carbohydrate content, causes splanchnic vasodilatation and postprandial hypotension which can aggravate orthostatic hypotension. Various physical manoeuvres, such as leg crossing, squatting, sitting in the knee–chest position and abdominal compression, reduce orthostatic hypotension (Figure 24.19). Drugs needed for associated symptoms (such as dopaminergic drugs) or to improve quality of life (sildenafil for erectile failure) lower blood pressure further.

Table 24.9 Approaches to management of orthostatic hypotension (e.g. in chronic autonomic failure).

Non-pharmacological measures
To be avoided
Sudden head-up postural change (especially on waking)
Prolonged recumbency
Straining during micturition and defaecation
High environmental temperature (including hot baths)
Severe exertion
Large meals (especially with refined carbohydrate)
Alcohol
Drugs with vasodepressor properties
To be introduced
Head-up tilt during sleep
Small frequent meals
High salt intake
Judicious exercise (including swimming)
Body positions and manoeuvres
To be considered
Elastic stockings
Abdominal binders
Water ingestion
Pharmacological measures
Starter drug (fludrocortisone)
Sympathomimetics (ephedrine, midodrine, L-DOPS)
Specific targeting (octreotide, desmopressin, erythropoietin)

L-DOPS, L-dehydroxyphenylserine.

Lower limb elastic compression stockings, abdominal binders and positive-gravity suits reduce venous pooling during standing. Each has its limitations and increases susceptibility to orthostatic hypotension when not in use. Water ingestion (250–500 mL) raises blood pressure substantially in PAF by mechanisms that remain unclear (Figures 24.20 and 24.21). The ensuing diuresis can be troublesome, especially in MSA with associated urinary bladder disturbances.

Drugs that act in a variety of ways to raise blood pressure are often needed in association with non-pharmacological measures in moderate to severe orthostatic hypotension (Table 24.10). A valuable first line drug is fludrocortisone in a dosage of 50–100 μg at night or twice daily. It acts by retaining salt and water and increasing the sensitivity of blood vessels to pressor substances. In some patients ankle oedema, and with higher doses hypokalaemia, are unwanted effects.

The second line drugs include those that mimic actions of noradrenaline. Ephedrine (15 mg three times daily to a maximum of 45 mg three times daily), which acts both directly and indirectly, raises blood pressure in central and incomplete autonomic lesions, including MSA. In peripheral sympathetic lesions, such as PAF, it can have minimal effects. Tachycardia, tremor and insomnia limit use of higher doses. In peripheral lesions, where ephedrine may not be effective, midodrine (2.5 μg to a maximum of 10 μg three times daily) is used. It is converted to the active metabolite, desglymidodrine, which acts on α-adrenoceptors. Side effects include a tingling scalp, goose pimples and, in the male, urinary retention. The ergot alkaloid, dihydro-ergotamine, acts predominantly on venous capacitance vessels, but its effects are limited by its poor absorption necessitating high oral doses (5–10 mg three times daily).

In dopamine beta-hydroxylase (DβH) deficiency, a rare genetic disorder, there is an absence of plasma noradrenaline and adrenaline with increased plasma dopamine levels, resulting in severe orthostatic hypotension (Figure 24.22). Symptoms noted during infancy include hypotension, hypotonia and hypothermia. Children with DβH deficiency cannot exercise fully because their blood pressure falls, causing syncope. Symptoms usually worsen during the first two decades and severe orthostatic hypotension becomes prominent in adulthood. DβH deficiency is caused by changes in *DBH* gene expression and is inherited as an autosomal recessive disorder. Restoration of plasma noradrenaline is achieved by treatment with the precursor of noradrenaline, L-threo-3-4-dihydroxyphenylserine

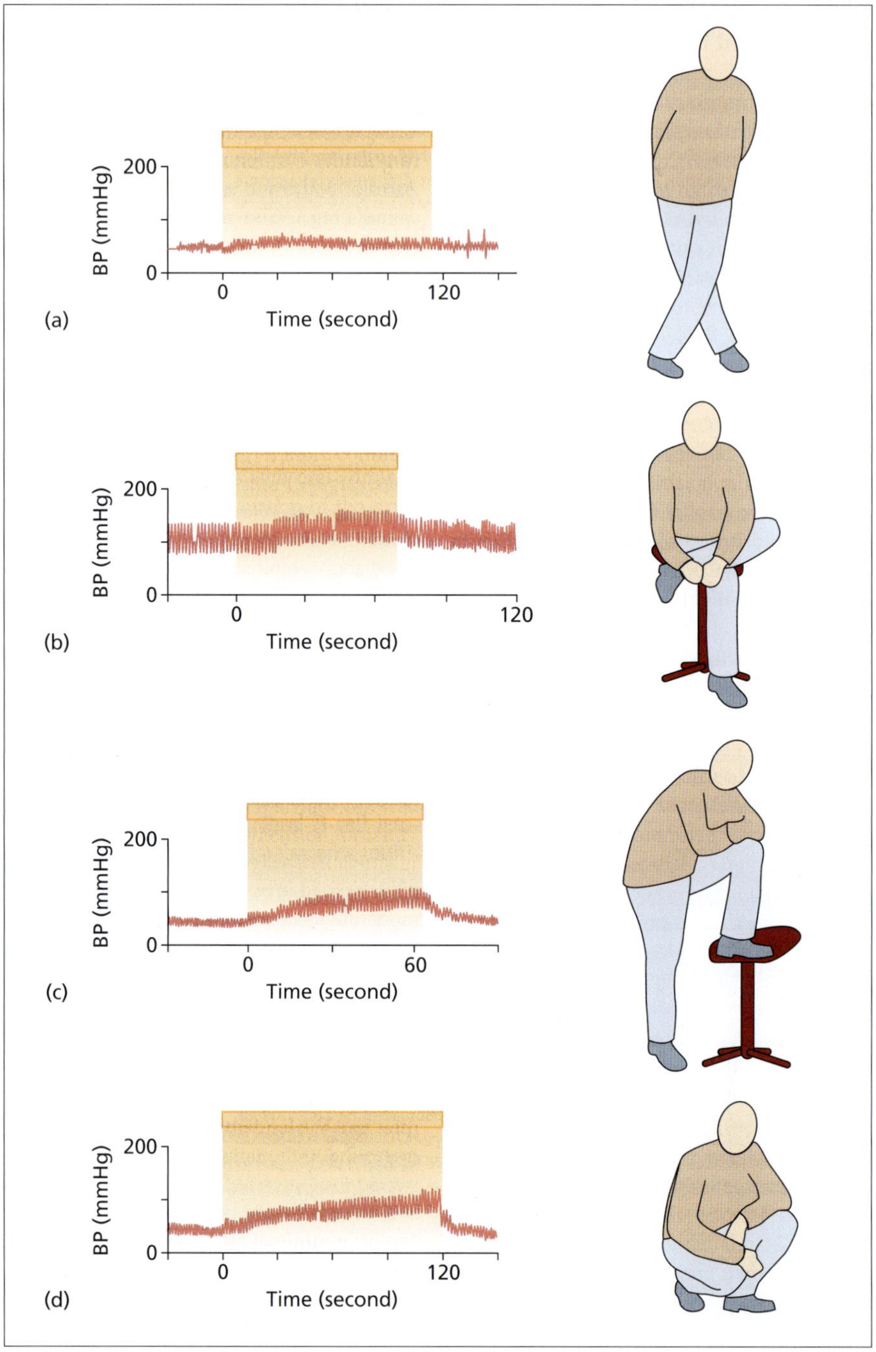

Figure 24.19 (a–d) Physical counter-manoeuvres using isometric contractions of the lower limbs and abdominal compression. The effects of leg crossing in standing and sitting positions, placing a foot on a chair and squatting, on blood pressure in a 54-year-old male patient with PAF and incapacitating OH. The patient was standing (sitting) quietly prior to the manoeuvres. Bars indicate the duration of the manoeuvres. Source: Smit *et al.* 1997. Reproduced with permisison from John Wiley & Sons.

(DOPS), which has a structure similar to noradrenaline but with a carboxyl group. It can be given by mouth and is converted from the inert form to noradrenaline by the enzyme dopa decarboxylase, thus bypassing the DβH deficiency. It thus replaces the deficient neurotransmitter and has been remarkably effective in this condition (Figure 24.23). DOPS can benefit other patient groups with PAF.

Specific targeting of pathophysiological mechanisms should be introduced when the combination of fludrocortisone and sympathomimetics is not effective. Nocturnal polyuria often worsens morning orthostatic hypotension. The vasopressin-2 receptor agonist, desmopressin, orally at night (e.g. 5–40 μg intranasally) is a potent antidiuretic with minimal direct pressor activity. In MSA with nocturia also caused by bladder disturbances, desmopresssin can be of considerable benefit in allowing less disturbed rest. Smaller doses are needed in PAF patients who appear more sensitive than those with MSA. Plasma sodium should be measured at intervals to exclude hyponatraemia. Water intoxication can be reversed by stopping the drug, and withholding water.

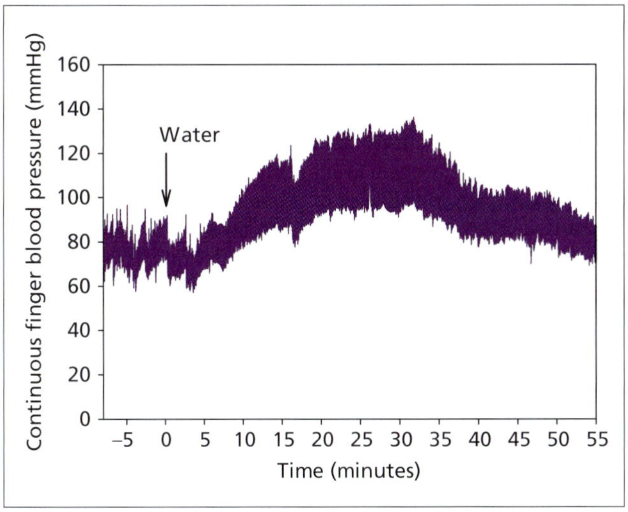

Figure 24.20 Changes in blood pressure before and after 500 mL distilled water ingested at time '0' in a patient with pure autonomic failure. Blood pressure is measured continuously using the Portapres II. Source: Cariga and Mathias 2001. Reproduced with permission of Portland Press and the Biochemical Society.

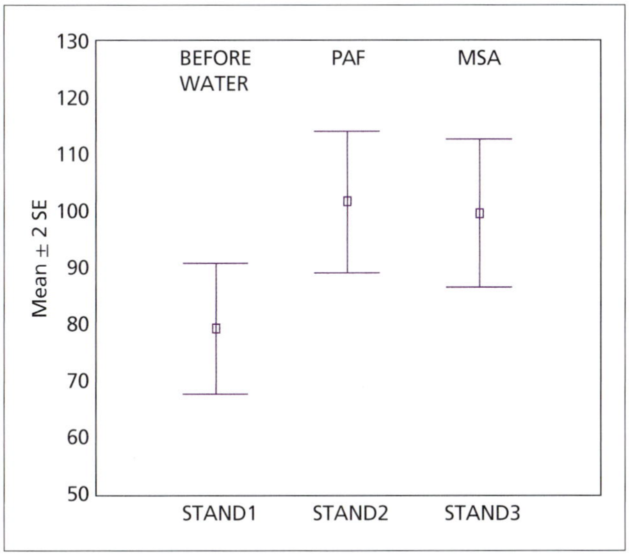

Figure 24.21 Standing blood pressure in seven pure autonomic failure (PAF) and seven multiple system atrophy (MSA) patients before and 15 and 30 minutes after ingestion of 500 mL water. Source: Young and Mathias 2004. Reproduced with permission of BMJ.

In postprandial hypotension, large meals should be avoided; instead small meals with low carbohydrate content should be eaten at frequent intervals. Drinking coffee after meals can help as caffeine blocks vasodilatatory adenosine receptors. A dose of 250 mg (present in two cups of typical espresso) can be used although tolerance sometimes develops. The somatostatin analogue, octreotide (25 or 50 μg, ideally 30 minutes before food) prevents postprandial hypotension by inhibiting release of a variety of vasodilatatory gastrointestinal peptides. It also reduces postural and exercise-induced hypotension. Side effects include abdominal colic and loose stools which respond to spasmolytics (Buscopan) and opiates (codeine phosphate and loperamide). Octreotide does not appear to enhance supine nocturnal hypertension.

Table 24.10 Outline of mechanisms by which drugs reduce postural hypotension.

Reducing salt loss/plasma volume expansion
Mineralocorticoids (fludrocortisone)
Reducing nocturnal polyuria
V_2-receptor agonists (desmopressin)
Vasoconstriction
Sympathetic
On resistance vessels (ephedrine, midodrine, phenylephrine, noradrenaline, clonidine, tyramine with monoamine oxidase inhibitors, yohimbine, L-dihydroxyphenylserine)
On capacitance vessels (dihydroergotamine)
Non-sympathomimetic
V_1-receptor agents (terlipressin)
Increasing acetylcholine
Acetylcholine esterase inhibitors (pyridostigmine)
Preventing vasodilatation
Prostaglandin synthetase inhibitors (indometacin, flurbiprofen)
Dopamine receptor blockade (metoclopramide, domperidone)
$Beta_2$-adrenoceptor blockade (propranolol)
Preventing postprandial hypotension
Adenosine receptor blockade (caffeine)
Peptide release inhibitors (somatostatin analogue: octreotide)
Increasing cardiac output
Beta-blockers with intrinsic sympathomimetic activity (pindolol, xamoterol)
Dopamine agonists (ibopamine)
Increasing red cell mass
Erythropoietin

Anaemia worsens symptoms of orthostatic hypotension and can occur in PAF and with renal impairment, in diabetes mellitus and in systemic amyloidosis. Erythropoietin (given subcutaneously) stimulates red cell production, raises red cell mass and haemoglobin levels. This reduces orthostatic hypotension and its symptoms in such situations.

Difficulties in the management of orthostatic hypotension have resulted in an array of drugs that have been reported to provide benefit in individual cases or in certain disorders (Tables 24.11 and 24.12). As with all drugs they should be used cautiously. Some have serious side effects such as cardiac failure with pindolol, and gastric ulceration and haemorrhage with indometacin. The use of a noradrenaline pump in extreme cases has been used with benefit.

Drugs should be used to reduce the side effects of therapy that is essential for associated disease. When levodopa is used to treat parkinsonism, higher doses of dopa-decarboxylase inhibitors should be used. The dopamine antagonists metoclopramide and domperidone also reduce the peripheral effects of dopamine.

Supine hypertension

Supine hypertension occurs frequently in PAF and can be worsened by drug treatment. It is unclear if certain drugs, such as higher doses of fludrocortisone, are more likely to cause it. Supine

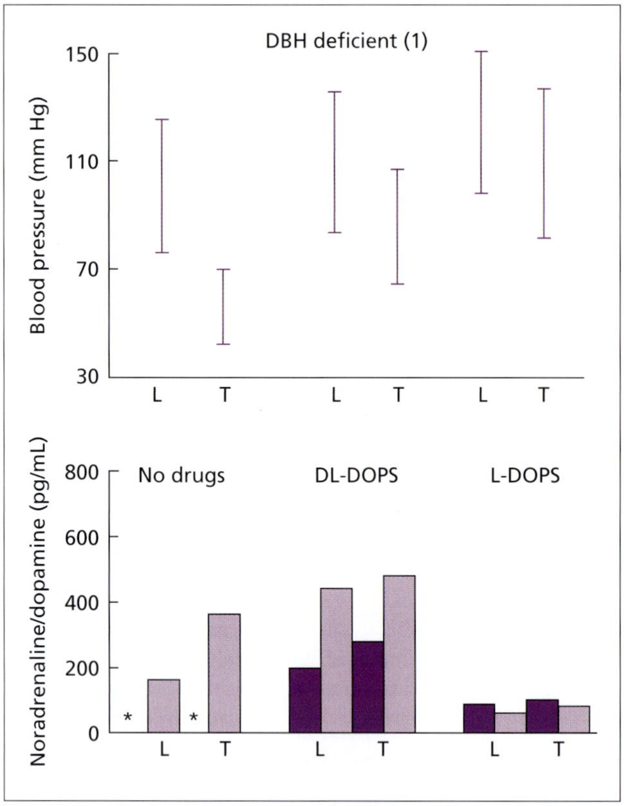

Figure 24.22 Blood pressure (systolic and diastolic) while lying (L) and during head-up tilt (T) in one of two siblings with dopamine beta hydroxylase (DβH) deficiency (1) before, during and after treatment with DL-DOPS (racemic mixture; DOPS, dihydroxyphenylserine) and L-DOPS (laevo form). The laevo form causes a greater rise in blood pressure and a greater reduction in postural hypotension than the racemic mixture. (From Mathias *et al.* 1990, with permission.)

hypertension increases symptoms of cerebral ischaemia during postural change through an unfavourable resetting of cerebral autoregulatory mechanisms. Head-up tilt especially at night is probably the most practical method to prevent nocturnal supine hypertension. Omission of the evening dose of vasopressor agents, a pre-bedtime snack or alcohol to induce postprandial hypotension, and sometimes even use of short-acting antihypertensive drugs should be considered.

The long-term possible effects of supine hypertension include cardiac hypertrophy and damage to subcortical cerebral vessels. This can occur in PAF; these patients have a good prognosis and drugs can be used over many years. The benefits of treating orthostatic hypotension effectively, thus reducing the likelihood of trauma and improving their quality of life, should be weighed against the long-term risks.

Autonomic mediated syncope

Management is dependent on the cause, provoking factors, disability caused and whether the episodes are of the cardio-inhibitory, vasodepressor or mixed type. Vasovagal syncope usually carries an excellent prognosis. Once the diagnosis is confirmed, an important component is positive reassurance. Advice on non-pharmacological measures includes ensuring salt repletion, an adequate fluid intake and techniques to enhance sympathetic activity and prevent pooling. These include the use of isometric hand exercise and activation of the calf muscle pump. If necessary, subjects should lie flat with their legs upright or with their head between the knees. Each subject should decide on which methods to use effectively in different situations. This is of particular value when there is a window of warning before the loss of consciousness. In vasodepressor syncope, low-dose fludrocortisone and sympathomimetics can be used if needed. Ephedrine is contraindicated if tachycardia is a problem; midodrine is the alternative. In those with a predominant cardio-inhibitory component, a demand pacemaker needs consideration especially when there is minimal warning before fainting. Cognitive behavioural psychotherapy is helpful if there is coexisting phobia, panic attack or anxiety disorder. 5-HT and noradrenaline uptake inhibitors such as fluoxetine, sertraline and venlafaxine have also been used.

In carotid sinus hypersensitivity, a cardiac demand pacemaker often is needed in the cardio-inhibitory and mixed forms. When the vasodepressor component is present and persists following pacemaker insertion, vasopressor agents including midodrine should be considered. Caution should be exercised as these patients often are elderly and sometimes have vascular disease and prostatic hypertrophy which increase the tendency to side-effects. In unilateral hypersensitivity, carotid sinus denervation is sometimes carried out.

In situational syncope, management should be directed towards the underlying cause and pathophysiological basis. In micturition syncope, occuring mainly in males, advice is needed to avoid contributing factors (e.g. alcohol). The bladder should be emptied while sitting rather than standing, especially if the patient has to pass urine during the night.

Postural tachycardia syndrome

Patients with postural tachycardia syndrome often need a combination of measures. Tachycardia is often associated with a low supine level of blood pressure, and a substantial number also have vasovagal syncope. Treatment is similar to the vasodepressor form of vasovagal syncope, with non-pharmacological measures and if needed drugs such as fludrocortisone and sympathomimetics. Ephedrine is contraindicated. Midodrine does not cause tachycardia and is the sympathomimetic of choice. Beta-adrenoceptor blockers, especially cardioselective ones such as bisoprolol, have a role. In those with blood pressure lability or more sustained elevations there is a role for the central sympatholytic drug, clonidine. A selective sinus node blocker, ivabradine, has also been used to reduce tachycardia.

Hypertension

Hypertension resulting from increased sympathetic nervous activity in the Guillain–Barré syndrome and following subarachnoid haemorrhage often responds to propranolol and sympatholytic agents. In high spinal cord injuries, determining and rectifying the provoking cause of autonomic dysreflexia is crucial, as the key is prevention. A range of drugs, based on knowledge of the pathophysiological mechanisms, can be used to prevent or reduce hypertension in such patients (Table 24.11).

Sudomotor disorders

Anhidrosis

The ensuing problems include dry skin, hyperthermia and vasomotor collapse in hot weather. Dry skin is helped by suitable emollients. Prevention of hyperthermia is important by avoiding exposure to heat and ensuring a suitable micro-environment, ideally by air conditioning. Mechanisms to aid heat loss include tepid sponging to aid evaporation, fans to enhance convection loss and

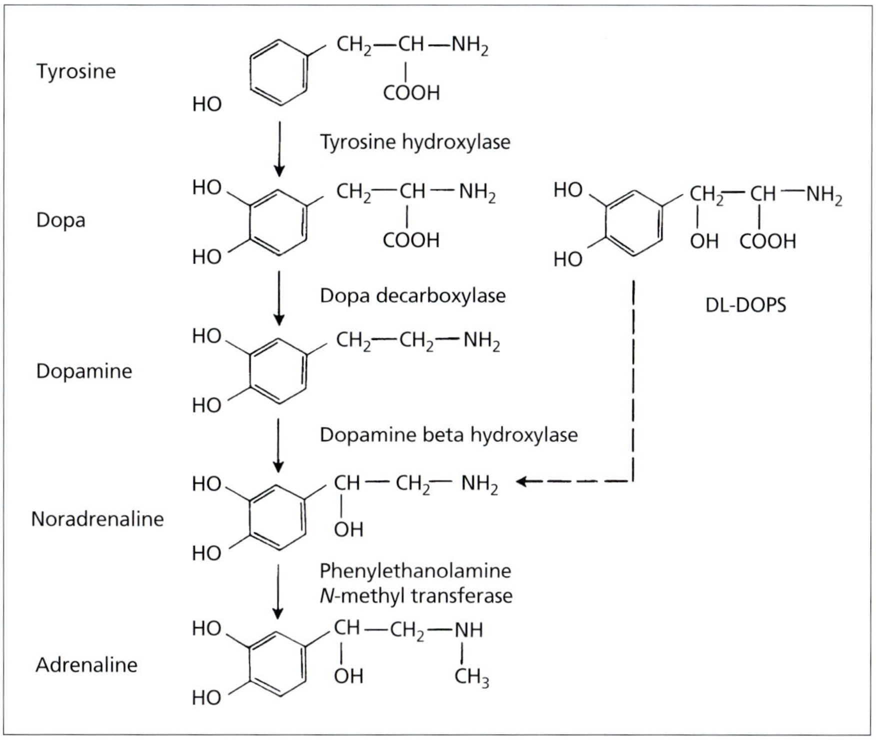

Figure 24.23 Biosynthetic pathway in the formation of adrenaline and noradrenaline. The structure of DL-DOPS is indicated on the right. It is converted directly to noradrenaline by dopa decarboxylase, thus bypassing dopamine β-hydroxylase.

Table 24.11 Drugs used for reducing hypertension in autonomic dysreflexia.

Afferent		**Topical lidocaine**
Spinal cord		Clonidine*
		Reserpine*
		Spinal anaesthetics
Efferent	Sympathetic ganglia	Hexamethonium
	Sympathetic nerve terminals	Guanethidine
	Alpha-adrenoceptors	Phenoxybenzamine
Target organs	Blood vessels	Glyceryl trinitrate
		Nifedipine

*Clonidine and reserpine have multiple effects, some of which are peripheral.

Table 24.12 Management strategy in autonomic failure.

Specific
For orthostatic hypotension and bladder, bowel, sexual dysfunction: non-pharmacological and pharmacological therapy
For respiratory abnormalities: consider tracheotomy
For oropharyngeal dysphagia: consider percutaneous endoscopic gastrostomy (PEG)
For depression: drug treatment
General education
Of patients and partners, relatives, carers, medical practitioners, supportive therapists, to include physiotherapists, occupational therapists, speech therapists and dietitians
Patient support groups and information sites
Dysautonomia Information Network (www.dinet.org) Dysautonomia International (www.dysautonomiainternational.org) Dysautonomia SOS (www.dysautonomiasos.com) Ehlers Danlos Support UK (www.ehlers-danlos.org) Familial Dysautonomia – UK (www.fd-uk.org) Hypermobility Syndromes Association (www.hypermobility.org) MSA Trust (UK) (www.msatrust.org.uk) PoTS UK (www.potsuk.org) STARS – for Syncope Trust and Reflex Anoxic Seizures (www.stars.org.uk) The MSA Coalition (US) (www.multiplesystematrophy.org) UK Potsies (www.ukpotsies.org.uk)
Autonomic nurse specialist or autonomic liaison nurse
To link, coordinate and streamline specialist care with the patient, carers and community

the ingestion of cool drinks. In severe hyperpyrexia, immersion in a cold bath may be needed.

Hyperhidrosis

Management depends upon the underlying cause, the sites involved and the functional and emotional disability. In hyperhidrosis over the palms and soles, local application of astringents containing glutaraldehyde and antiperspirants containing aluminium salts reduces sweating as does iontophoresis (a local treatment that works by introducing an ionised substance through intact skin by the application of direct current). Low-dose oral pharmacotherapy includes anticholinergics (propantheline bromide 15 mg three times daily) and centrally acting sympatholytics (clonidine 25–50 μg three times daily). Side effects include a dry mouth. Glaucoma should be excluded prior to use of anticholinergics. Clonidine can reduce facial flushing. Topical anticholinergic cream (hyoscine hydrobromide or glycopyrrolate) may be helpful over small areas. Botulinum toxin is successful in hyperhidrosis affecting the axillae, palms and face. Injections may need to be repeated.

When these measures fail, surgical intervention using percutaneous endoscopic transthoracic sympathectomy, with ablation of prevertebral sympathetic ganglia from T2 to T4 should be considered. Ablation of T1/T2 is also used in facial flushing. In some, compensatory hyperhidrosis below the anhidrotic region can be extremely troublesome.

Alimentary system

Xerostomia is helped by artificial saliva. Excessive salivation responds to botulinum injection. Achalasia of the oesophagus may require dilatation, botulinum injection or surgery. In MSA with oropharyngeal dysphagia, advice should be provided on the type and consistency of food; severe dysfunction increases the risk of tracheal aspiration and a feeding percutaneous gastrostomy is sometimes needed.

The dopamine antagonists metoclopramide and domperidone increase gastric emptying in gastroparesis, as does the macrolide erythromycin which stimulates motilin receptors. Peptic ulceration occurs in the early stages after high spinal cord injury and prophylaxis includes H_2 antagonists (cimetidine and ranitidine) and proton-pump inhibitors (omeprazole).

In diarrhoea caused by bacterial overgrowth, as in the blind loop syndrome, broad-spectrum antibiotics (neomycin or tetracycline) may be the initial step before using codeine phosphate or other opiate-based antidiarrhoeal agents. Octreotide, the somatostatin analogue, can reduce diarrhoea in amyloidosis and diabetic autonomic neuropathy. Aperients and laxatives, together with a high-fibre diet, are needed in constipation.

Urinary tract

In outflow tract obstruction, procedures which include prostatectomy, transurethral resection or sphincterotomy are sometimes needed. Surgical procedures often induce or worsen incontinence in MSA. Bladder dysfunction is helped by drugs that influence detrusor muscle activity (anticholinergics) or sphincter malfunction (alpha-adrenergic blockers). Intermittent or in-dwelling catheterisation may be necessary. Nocturia in PAF is often helped by intranasal or oral desmopressin given in the evening.

Sexual function and the reproductive system

Erectile failure in men can be treated by suction devices, an implanted prosthesis or drugs. The latter can be given locally (intracavernosal or urethral) or orally (sildenafil). Sildenafil and allied drugs have the potential through vasodilatation to lower blood pressure substantially, especially in patients with orthostatic hypotension. In DβH deficiency, difficulty in ejaculation is improved by treatment with DOPS. Pregnant women with high spinal injuries can develop severe hypertension with cardiac dysrhythmias and eclampsia during uterine contractions and delivery. Spinal anaesthesia, which reduces spinal sympathetic discharge, often permits a normal delivery.

Respiratory system

A tracheostomy is sometimes necessary in severe inspiratory stridor resulting from laryngeal abductor paresis, especially when oxygen desaturation occurs at night. With periodic apnoea, timed or triggered bi-level positive airway pressure ventilation may be useful. In high spinal cord lesions on artificial ventilation particular care should be taken during tracheal suction and toilet to avoid bradycardia and even cardiac arrest. In ventilated tetanus patients, the reverse – tachycardia and hypertension – may occur.

Eye and lacrimal glands

In alachryma, tear substitutes such as hypromellose eye drops are needed. Cycloplegia can be reduced by local cholinomimetics such as pilocarpine. Patients should be made aware of night blindness in sympathetic denervation and of a low threshold to sunlight in parasympathetic denervation.

Treatment in MSA and Parkinson's disease

In the parkinsonian forms of MSA, levodopa is sometimes of benefit in the early stages. However, it can cause or enhance orthostatic hypotension and should be used with higher doses of dopa decarboxylase inhibitors. The monoamine oxidase-B inhibitor, selegiline, has been used in combination with levodopa but may also worsen orthostatic hypotension. It can cause hypotension also in Parkinson's disease by mechanisms that include the central effects of its metabolites, methyl-amphetamine. Amantidine can provide motor benefit without lowering blood pressure. Dopaminergic agonists may be effective but it is unclear if they worsen orthostatic hypotension. With time there is often refractoriness to anti-parkinsonian drugs in MSA. There is no effective pharmacotherapy for cerebellar deficits in MSA. Supportive therapy using disability aids should be provided.

The management of autonomic dysfunction needs to consider local organ dysfunction, the underlying or associated disease and integrative components often needing specialist care (Table 24.12).

Of particular importance, especially in generalised disorders, is the need for a holistic approach which includes the management of the autonomic deficits and the underlying disorder. Management should involve not only the patient, but the family, carers and community.

References

Cariga P, Mathias CJ. Haemodynamics of the pressor effect of oral water in human sympathetic denervation due to autonomic failure. *Clin Sci* 2001; **101**: 313–319.

Janig W. 1987. Autonomic nervous system. In: Schmidt RF, Thews G, eds. *Human Psychology*, 2nd edn. Berlin: Springer, 1989: 333–370. Fig. 16.1.

Mathias CJ. Autonomic disorders. In: Bogousslavsky J, Fisher M, eds. *Textbook of Neurology*. Boston, MA: Butterworth-Heinemann, 1998: 519–545.

Mathias CJ. Disorders of the autonomic nervous system. In: Bradley WG, Daroff RB, Fenichel GM, Jancovich J, eds. *Neurology in Clinical Practice*, 4th edn. Boston, MA: Butterworth-Heinemann, 2004: 2403–2240.

Mathias CJ. Orthostatic hypotension and orthostatic intolerance. In: *Endocrinology*, 5th edn. DeGroot LJ, Jameson JL, de Kretser D, Grossman AB, Marshall JC, Melmed S, Potts JT, Weir GC, eds. Elsevier Saunders, Philadelphia PA, USA 2006, 2613–2632.

Mathias CJ, Bannister R, eds. *Autonomic Failure: A Textbook of Clinical Disorders of the Autonomic Nervous System*, 5th edn. Oxford: Oxford University Press, 2013.

Mathias CJ, Galizia G. Orthostatic hypotension and orthostatic intolerance. In: De Groot LJ, Jameson JL, de Kretser D, Grossman AB, Marshall JC, Melmed S, *et al*., eds. *Endocrinology*, 6th edn. Philadelphia, PA: Elsevier, 2010: 2063–2082.

Mathias CJ, Low DA, Iodice V, Owens A, Kirbiš M, Grahame R. The Postural Tachycardia Syndrome (PoTS): current experiences and concepts. *Nat Rev Neurol* 2012; **8**: 22–34.

Smit AAJ, Hardjowijona MA, Wieling W. Are portable folding chairs useful to combat orthostatic hypotension? *Ann Neurol* 1997; **42**: 975–978.

Young TM, Mathias CJ. The effects of water ingestion on orthostatic hypotension in two groups with chronic autonomic failure: multiple system atrophy and pure autonomic failure. *J Neurol Neurosurg Psychiatry* 2004, **75**: 1737–1741.

Further reading

Johnson RH, Lambie DG, Spalding JMK. *Neurocardiology: The Interrelationship Between Dysfunction in the Nervous and Cardiovascular Systems*. London: W.B. Saunders, 1984.

Low PA, Benarroch EE, eds. *Clinical Autonomic Disorders*, 3rd edn. Philadelphia: Lippincott Raven, 2008.

Mathias CJ, Bannister R, Cortelli P, Heslop K, Polak J, Raimbach SJ, *et al*. Clinical autonomic and therapeutic observations in two siblings with postural hypotension and sympathetic failure due to an inability to synthesize noradrenaline from dopamine because of a deficiency of dopamine beta-hydroxylase. *Q J Med* 1990; **75**: 617–633.

Mathias CJ, Jones K. Postprandial hypotension in autonomic disorders. In: Mathias CJ, Bannister R, eds. *Autonomic Failure: A Textbook of Clinical Disorders of the Autonomic Nervous System*, 5th edn. Oxford: Oxford University Press, 2013: 254–370.

Mathias CJ, Low DA, Iodice V, Bannister R. Investigation of autonomic disorders. In: Mathias CJ, Bannister R, eds. *Autonomic Failure: A Textbook of Clinical Disorders of the Autonomic Nervous System*, 5th edn. Oxford: Oxford University Press, 2013: 259–289.

Mathias CJ, Williams AC. The Shy Drager syndrome (and multiple system atrophy). In: Donald B, Calne DB, ed. *Neurodegenerative Diseases*. Philadelphia, PA: W.B. Saunders, 1994: 743–768.

CHAPTER 25

Uroneurology

Jalesh Panicker
National Hospital for Neurology & Neurosurgery

Urogenital dysfunction is common in neurological disease and has a significant impact on patients' health and quality of life. The investigations and management of disorders of urogenital function were formerly regarded as the preserve of urologists. However, as specialists in neurology increasingly enquire about urogenital symptoms, and become aware of the range of effective non-surgical treatments, they are taking a more active interest in uroneurology – a specialty that focuses on bladder and sexual dysfunction viewed from the neurological perspective.

This chapter covers the neural control of lower urinary tract and sexual functions, followed by a description of the effects of neurological disease at different levels of the nervous system, and the essentials a neurologist should be aware of when managing these conditions.

The lower urinary tract and its neurological control

The lower urinary tract (bladder and urethra) has essentially two functions: storage and periodic elimination of urine. This requires the synergistic activity of smooth and striated muscles of the bladder, bladder neck and urethra. This coordination is mediated by complex neural circuits located in the brain, spinal cord and peripheral ganglia.

The lower urinary tract differs from other visceral organs in many ways. Micturition is under voluntary control and depends upon learned behaviours. This reflects the critical role that the central nervous system (CNS) has in controlling lower urinary tract functions but renders the lower urinary tract susceptible to dysfunction whenever there is neurological disease. However, many of the other visceral organs are regulated involuntarily and can maintain a level of functioning even after damage to the extrinisic innervation. The pattern of activation of the lower urinary tract is unusual in that it has only two modes of operation, and therefore the neural circuits involved in regulating micturition have a phasic or switch-like activity. This is in contrast to the tonic pattern of activity that regulates the cardiovascular system.

The bladder is in the *storage phase* for 98% of the time. The frequency of micturition in a person with a bladder capacity of 400–600 mL is once every 3–4 hours and switching to a *voiding phase* is initiated by a conscious decision which is determined by the perceived state of bladder fullness and an assessment of the social appropriateness of voiding. To effect storage and voiding, connections between the pons and the sacral spinal cord must be intact, as must the peripheral innervation that originates from the most caudal segments of the cord. During the storage phase, the pressure within the bladder outlet is raised to maintain continence, and this is mediated through sympathetic and pudendal nerve activation of the internal and external urethral sphincters, respectively. Inhibition of the parasympathetic outflow prevents detrusor contractions. Throughout the storage phase, our perception of bladder fullness enables us to make the necessary planned strategies to achieve the next appropriately located void before reaching an uncomfortable degree of bladder distension or the sensation of 'severe urge to void'.

Whereas the voluntary control of micturition originates from the cerebral cortex, the switch is operated from the brainstem via neurones that run to the sacral cord segments S2–S3, where they synapse on neurones innervating the lower urinary tract. In recent years, functional brain imaging has contributed greatly to our understanding of the central input into lower urinary tract control and a consistent finding of all these studies is activation of the peri-aqueductal grey matter during bladder filling. This is in keeping with experimental studies in the cat, and it is thought that the peri-aqueductal grey matter serves as a central relay centre for afferent activity from the pelvic organs and is an interface between the afferent and efferent limbs of bladder control circuits, 'informing' the pontine micturition centre, in the dorsal tegmentum of the pons, about the degree of bladder fullness. The peri-aqueductal grey matter has multiple connections with higher centres such as the thalamus, insula, cingulate and prefrontal cortices. Activation of the insula is consistent with what is known about regions of activation involved in interoceptive awareness of visceral sensations.

The prefrontal cortex, the seat of planning complex cognitive behaviours and of appropriate social behaviours, is activated on bladder filling and it is likely that this region of the brain is involved in the conscious and social control of bladder function. It has been proposed that the task of the prefrontal cortex is to make a decision as to whether or not micturition should take place at a particular place or time.

With the decision to void, activation is seen in the prefrontal cortex, insula, hypothalamus and peri-aqueductal grey matter and the pontine micturition centre. The pontine micturition centre is

Neurology: A Queen Square Textbook, Second Edition. Edited by Charles Clarke, Robin Howard, Martin Rossor and Simon Shorvon.

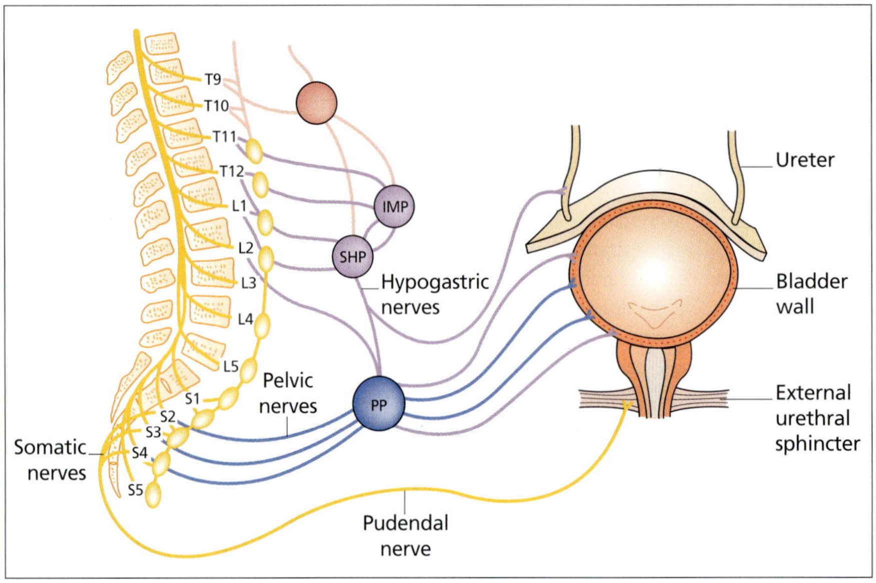

Figure 25.1 Innervation of the lower urinary tract. IMP, inferior mesenteric plexus; PP, pelvic plexus; SHP, superior hypogastric plexus. Source: http://www.deckerpublishing.com/SlideMenuLinks/permissionsIntroPage.aspx

no longer tonically inhibited and the pattern of reciprocal activation–inhibition of the sphincter–detrusor reverses. Voiding is achieved by relaxation of the urethral sphincter and pelvic floor muscles, and parasympathetic mediated contraction of the detrusor muscle, resulting in effective bladder emptying. Intact neural circuitry between the pontine micturition centre and bladder ensures coordinated activity between the detrusor and sphincter muscles. Figure 25.1 depicts the peripheral innervation of the bladder.

Lower urinary tract dysfunction following neurological disease

Both central and peripheral lesions of the nervous system can result in characteristic patterns of bladder dysfunction which depend upon the level of the lesion in the nervous system. The patterns of lower urinary tract dysfunction and findings during commonly performed tests are outlined in Table 25.1.

Cortical disease

When the lesion is above the level of the pons, inhibitory control of the pontine micturition centre is lost and this results in involuntary spontaneous or induced contractions of the detrusor muscle (detrusor overactivity), which can be identified during the filling phase of cystometry. The importance of the anterior regions of the frontal lobes in bladder control was established by Andrew and Nathan. A series of patients was reported with disturbed bladder control from various frontal lobe pathologies including tumours, damage following rupture of an intracranial aneurysm, penetrating brain wounds or leukotomy. The typical clinical picture was of a patient with severe urgency and frequency of micturition and urge incontinence, who is both socially aware and embarrassed by their incontinence. Only if frontal lobe pathology is more extensive, causing loss of social inhibition, do patients become unconcerned about their loss of bladder control.

Urinary retention has occasionally been described in patients with brain lesions. In the series by Andrew and Nathan (1964) two of the patients were in urinary retention at some stage and there have been a small number of case histories of patients with right frontal lobe pathology with urinary retention.

Cerebrovascular disease

Incontinence following stroke is not a straightforward problem. Cystometric studies in patients following stroke generally conclude that detrusor overactivity is the most common urodynamic abnormality, although patients with haemorrhagic stroke more often develop urinary retention asa result of detrusor underactivity. There does not appear to be any definite lateralisation of lesions causing detrusor overactivity, although possibly the pathology is more often right-sided, nor are there any specific locations; however, anteriorly situated damage is more likely to result in incontinence. At admission, approximately 50% of patients with stroke will have incontinence, but the prevalence declines over the following 6 months to approximately 5%. Long-term incontinence is commonly caused by detrusor overactivity and is seen in patients with severe neurological deficits (aphasia particularly) and a high level of persistent disability.

Increasingly, cerebral small vessel disease is being recognised as a cause of incontinence. Sakakibara *et al.* first observed a correlation between the extent of white matter changes and incidence of detrusor overactivity. Kuchel *et al.* analysed the location of white matter changes and urinary dysfunction in community-dwelling elderly individuals and demonstrated the presence of white matter change in the right frontal and right inferior frontal regions to predict incontinence severity. In a functional imaging study involving a paradigm of repeated bladder filling and emptying, regional activations and deactivations became more prominent with increasing global white matter change and the main effect activations and deactivations were superimposed with the anterior thalamic radiation. The results of a study by Tadic *et al.* indicated that the white matter changes, particularly the anterior portion that includes the anterior thalamic radiation, were related to an overactive bladder in cognitively intact, elderly women.

Another approach to looking at stroke and urinary incontinence has been epidemiological. Following a stroke, the presence of

Table 25.1 The pattern of lower urinary tract dysfunction differs according to the site of neurological lesion.

	Suprapontine lesion (e.g. stroke, Parkinson's disease)	Infrapontine suprasacral lesion (e.g. myelopathy)	Infrasacral lesion (e.g. conus medullaris, cauda equina, peripheral nerve)
History/ bladder diary	Urgency, frequency, urgency incontinence	Urgency, frequency, urgency incontinence, hesitancy, retention	Hesitancy, retention
Post-void residual urine	No PVR	± Elevated PVR	PVR >100 mL
Uroflowmetry	Normal flow	Interrupted flow	Poor/absent flow
Urodynamics	Detrusor overactivity	Detrusor overactivity Detrusor sphincter dyssynergia	Detrusor underactivity Sphincter insufficiency

PVR: postvoid residual, measured using a bladder scan or by in–out cathetersiation.
Source: Fowler *et al.* 2009. Reproduced with permission of BMJ Publishing Group Ltd.

Table 25.2 Incontinence in the patient with dementia may be multi-factorial.

Neurogenic detrusor overactivity
Specific cognitive deficits – memory impairment, visuo-spatial disorientation, dysphasia, compulsive behaviour, apraxia, amotivation, social disinhibition
Urological causes – bladder outlet obstruction (e.g. prostate enlargement, stress incontinence)
Functional incontinence – impaired mobility
Medications – antidepressants, cholinesterase inhibitors
The ageing bladder – 'detrusor hyperactivity with impaired contractile function'

urinary incontinence within 7 days appears to be the most powerful prognostic indicator for poor survival and eventual functional dependence, more so than a depressed level of consciousness in this period. The explanation for this is not known but it has been suggested that either incontinence is the result of a severe general rather than specific loss of function reflecting the severity of brain damage, or that those who remain incontinent are less motivated, both to recover continence and more general functions.

Dementia

Urinary incontinence in dementia is a major socio-economic problem of ever-increasing proportions and incontinence is also common in the frail elderly and has many causes. In a large group of elderly patients who were institutionalised because of their general frailty, the same underlying pathophysiologies were found in those with cognitive impairment as those without. Although detrusor overactivity was the most common cause of incontinence in 40% there were other causes and in nearly one-third incontinence was related to disorders of the urethral outlet (i.e. potentially surgically correctable conditions). There are several causes for incontinence in the individual with dementia which should be considered during the evaluation; these are listed in Table 25.2.

There is also evidence of a specific disorder of the detrusor muscle characterised by ultra-structural changes of smooth muscle and axonal degeneration that has an increasing incidence in the elderly. This is thought to result in detrusor overactivity and incomplete emptying: detrusor hyperactivity with impaired contractile function (DHIC). It seems highly likely that with loss of general 'coping abilities' because of cognitive impairment, DHIC becomes a prominent cause of incontinence.

The relationship of symptoms to cerebral pathology is unclear. Frontal lobe pathology would be expected to cause detrusor overactivity and there is some evidence that this is a contributing factor. One of the differences between symptoms in those with and those without dementia is that urgency preceding episodes of incontinence is more frequently reported by those without.

In a study of patients with cognitive decline, incontinence was associated with severe Alzheimer's disease but preceded cognitive impairment in diffuse Lewy body disease. A cross-sectional study by Ransmayr *et al.* suggests that urgency and urge incontinence, indicative of detrusor overactivity, is more common in dementia with Lewy bodies than in Alzheimer's disease.

Since the advent of cholinesterase inhibitors to treat symptoms in mild to moderate Alzheimer's disease, it is not uncommon to find a patient on such a treatment who has also been prescribed an antimuscarinic to treat their urinary urgency. No systematic study has yet been published that looks at interactions of these medications, but on theoretical grounds it would seem sensible to use an antimuscarinic to treat the bladder that does not cross the blood–brain barrier, such as tolterodine or trospium chloride, or possibly an antimuscarinic that is relatively more selective for the M3 rather than the M1 receptor such as darifenacin (Table 25.6).

Low-pressure hydrocephalus, a much less common cause of dementia, has incontinence as a cardinal feature. Improvement in cystometric function has been demonstrated within hours of lumbar puncture in patients with this disorder.

Parkinson's disease

Non-motor symptoms in Parkinson's disease (PD) are thought to be the consequence of widespread dopaminergic and non-dopaminergic neurodegeneration. The resulting 'vegetative symptoms' have a very negative impact on the patient and their carer as the condition advances.

Nocturia is the most common non-motor symptom. How common bladder symptoms are in patients with clearly defined idiopathic PD is uncertain. Studies report prevalence figures between 38 and 71% but some early studies of prevalence were based on patients presenting in urology clinics, in elderly patient populations or were published before the diagnosis of multiple system atrophy (MSA) was recognised as often as it is today. In the most recent study of patients with PD diagnosed according to modern criteria, and using validated questionnaires, the prevalence of urinary symptoms was found to be 27–39%, considerably higher than in healthy controls. A clear correlation with the neurological disability and stage of disease suggests a relationship between dopaminergic degeneration and symptoms of urinary dysfunction.

Typically, PD patients with bladder dysfunction have advanced disease and describe how the bladder symptoms came on many years after treatment for PD started. Cystometry commonly shows a reduced capacity and detrusor overactivity, usually with complete emptying, although sometimes an apparently obstructed voiding picture may be seen. It has been suggested that there may be an impaired relaxation of the urethral sphincter ('pseudo-dyssynergia') which could be reduced by subcutaneous apomorphine. The most common complaint is of nocturia and urinary urgency, and urgency incontinence can occur if poor mobility compounds the bladder disorder. A particular difficulty arises because symptoms of outflow obstruction can also occur in males with PD, making the distinction between neurogenic and bladder outflow obstruction resulting from benign prostatic enlargement difficult. The reputation for a poor outcome following prostatic surgery in men with PD is probably because of the inclusion of some patients with MSA in studies of 'Parkinson's disease and the bladder'. If there is convincing evidence of prostatic occlusion and obstructed voiding on cystometry, a prostatectomy should be considered.

The commonly accepted hypothesis to explain bladder symptoms in PD is that degeneration of dopaminergic neurones leads to loss of the substantia nigra tonically D1-mediated inhibition of the pontine micturition centre. Detrusor overactivity has been demonstrated in experimentally induced parkinsonism in marmosets, and selective dopamine D1 receptor agonists alleviated the abnormality. In rats, dopaminergic neurones originating in the ventral tegmental area (VTA) control the micturition reflex biphasically, with a facilitatory effect from low-dose stimulation of dopamine D2 receptors, while high-dose stimulation of the dopamine D1 receptors has an inhibitory effect on micturition. Patients with PD and bladder symptoms have less uptake of dopamine transporter tracer (DAT scan) in the striatum than patients with PD but without bladder dysfunction, indicating a correlation between urinary dysfunction and degeneration of the nigrostriatal dopaminergic cells. Furthermore, recent studies have shown that the presence of bladder symptoms is related to the decrease in the total number of dopaminergic neurones in the striatum and that relative degeneration of the caudate correlates with severity of symptoms.

The effect of antiparkinsonian medication on bladder function is complex and studies of the effect of levodopa or apomorphine on bladder behaviour have produced conflicting results. In one study of patients with more advanced disease showing 'on–off' phenomena, detrusor overactivity lessened with levodopa in some patients and worsened in others. A recent study suggests that in advanced PD, levodopa exacerbates detrusor overactivity in the filling phase, but also improves bladder emptying through increased detrusor contractility, so that the post-micturition residual volumes diminish. The effects of medication on bladder control are complex and it has been suggested that the effect of dopamine occurs through cortical mechanisms, by improvement in the ability to separate and integrate sensory input.

Multiple system atrophy

MSA selectively involves neural components specifically involved in the innervation of the urogenital tract; bladder control may therefore be affected early in the course of the disease, often before symptoms and signs of postural hypotension. Corticotrophin-releasing factor staining cells in the pontine region have been shown to undergo selective atrophy and it has been postulated that these cells are in the region of the pontine micturition centre. Axons of the intermediolateral cell column conveying autonomic innervation to the sacral segments are known to atrophy, as do the cells in Onuf's nucleus which innervate the sphincters. Single-photon emission computed tomography (SPECT) studies have shown reduced cerebellar vermis activation during urinary storage and micturition in MSA.

The functional effects of these deficits include detrusor overactivity, incomplete emptying, an open bladder neck in men and sphincter weakness, all compounding to produce early and severe incontinence. Incomplete emptying commonly occurs (unlike the situation in PD), although the symptoms are predominantly those of incontinence. Very occasionally, a complete failure to void (i.e. retention) can be a presenting feature in both men and women. Bladder dysfunction may change during the course of MSA, with a progressive reduction in the degree of detrusor overactivity and increasingly high post-micturition residual volume. This is a situation that is highly amenable to treatment and many patients with MSA can regain bladder control for several years before their general neurological disability becomes overwhelming.

There are characteristic differences in the pattern of urogenital dysfunction between PD and MSA (Table 25.3). The diagnostic role of sphincter electromyography (EMG) to identify re-innervation, secondary to the loss of anterior horn cells in Onuf's nucleus in MSA (Figure 25.2), has been contentious. In a retrospective post-mortem study, a very high proportion of patients who were subsequently shown to have died of MSA had an abnormal sphincter EMG – often early in the course of their disease – but sufficient EMG data were lacking on patients who had alternative diagnoses, including PD, for the specificity of the test to be calculated. Some groups have shown sphincter EMG abnormalities in patients with long-standing PD. The author is a proponent of the value of sphincter EMG if found to be highly abnormal in a patient with early parkinsonism or in patients with a cerebellar syndrome of late onset. The test is method-sensitive and centres that carry out individual motor unit analysis by manual methods seem to find it more valuable than those that use an automated analysis technique.

Bladder symptoms in other parkinsonian syndromes are generally less prominent and are rarely as severe, or occur at a stage of the disease when a neurological diagnosis is clearly evident.

Brainstem lesions

The location of the micturition centre in the pons means that occasionally pathology affecting the dorsal tegmentum can result in disturbances of micturition, most commonly difficulties voiding. Voiding difficulty is a rare but recognised symptom of a posterior fossa tumour in children and has been reported in series of patients with brainstem pathologies including strokes. An analysis of urinary symptoms of 39 patients who had brainstem strokes showed that lesions that resulted in disturbance of micturition were usually dorsally situated. There have also been a number of sporadic case reports describing urinary retention resulting from brainstem lesions. The proximity in the dorsal pons of the medial longitudinal fasciculus to the pontine micturition centre means that an

Table 25.3 Differences in urogenital dysfunction between multiple system atrophy (MSA) and Parkinson's disease (PD).

	MSA	PD
Time of onset of urogenital dysfunction	Often precedes other neurological deficits	Usually follows other neurological deficits
Bladder dysfunction	Early and severe incontinence. Overactive bladder symptoms initially, progresses to urinary retention	Less severe incontinence Overactive bladder symptoms, nocturnal polyuria
Post void residual	Elevated	Usually normal
Urodynamics	Detrusor overactivity, acontractile detrusor In men, the finding of an open bladder neck may be relevant (video-urodynamics)	Detrusor overactivity
Sphincter EMG	Early signs of re-innervation (prolonged duration motor units mean >10 ms)	Usually normal, especially in the early stages
Sexual dysfunction	ED (often first manifestation)	ED, sometimes sexual compulsive behaviour as part of an impulse control disorder

ED, erectile dysfunction; EMG, electromyogram.

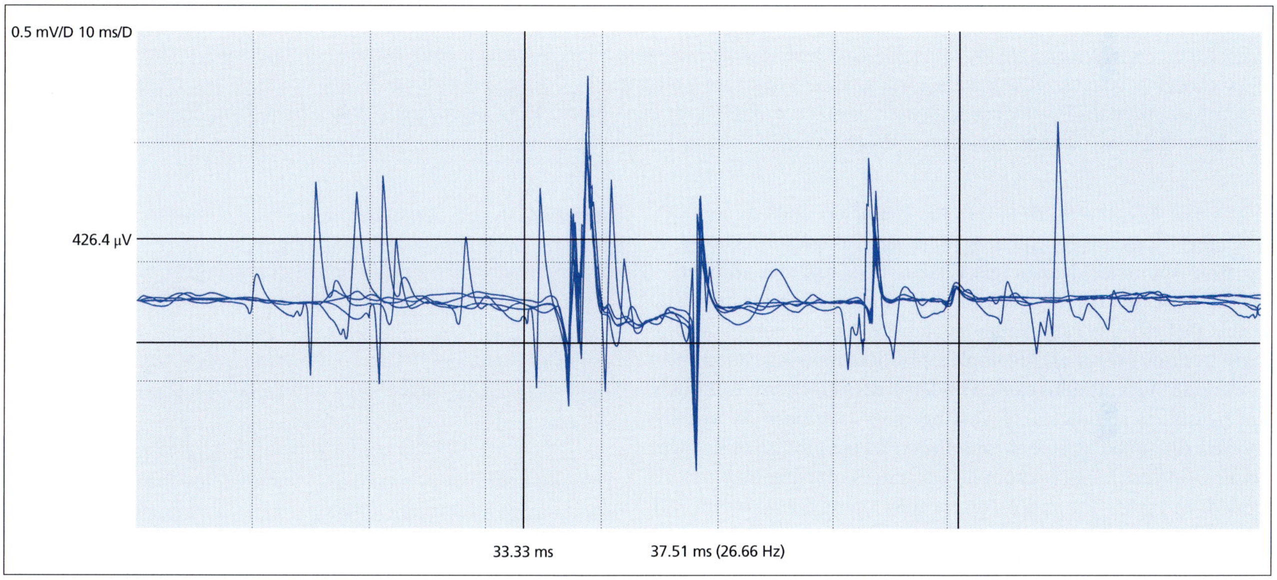

Figure 25.2 Concentric needle electromyogram (EMG) recording from the external anal sphincter (gain 0.5 mV, sweep speed 10 ms per division). The duration of the weighted motor unit potential (MUP) is 37.5 ms (normal <10 ms). Abnormally prolonged MUPs suggest re-innervation and may be seen in multiple system atrophy; however, this finding should be interpreted within the clinical context.

internuclear opthalmoplegia is highly likely in patients with pontine pathology causing a voiding disorder.

Spinal cord disease

Following acute spinal cord injury (SCI), the bladder may become acontractile during the stage of spinal shock. Over the course of weeks, reflex detrusor contractions gradually develop in response to low volumes of filling. Neurophysiological studies of recovery in the cat reveal that formerly quiescent C fibres emerge as the major afferent from the bladder and activation of this aberrant C fibre mediated spinal reflex drives detrusor overactivity (Figure 25.3). It is assumed that the same pathophysiology occurs in humans, and the improvement in detrusor overactivity following intravesical instillation of C fibre neurotoxins, capsaicin and resiniferatoxin, supports this view. The same spinal lesion that causes the emergence of the C fibre reflex often causes upper motor neurone symptoms and signs in the lower limbs, and urge incontinence is particularly likely to affect patients with spastic paraparesis and detrusor overactivity. This is the basis of a valuable clinical point: when considering whether or not a patient has a neurogenic bladder resulting from spinal cord involvement, an absence of neurological signs in the legs makes such a diagnosis unlikely.

Spinal pathways that connect the pontine micturition centre to the sacral cord are responsible for a coordinated reciprocal activity of the detrusor and sphincter muscles. Following disconnection from the pons, the synergistic activity between sphincter and the

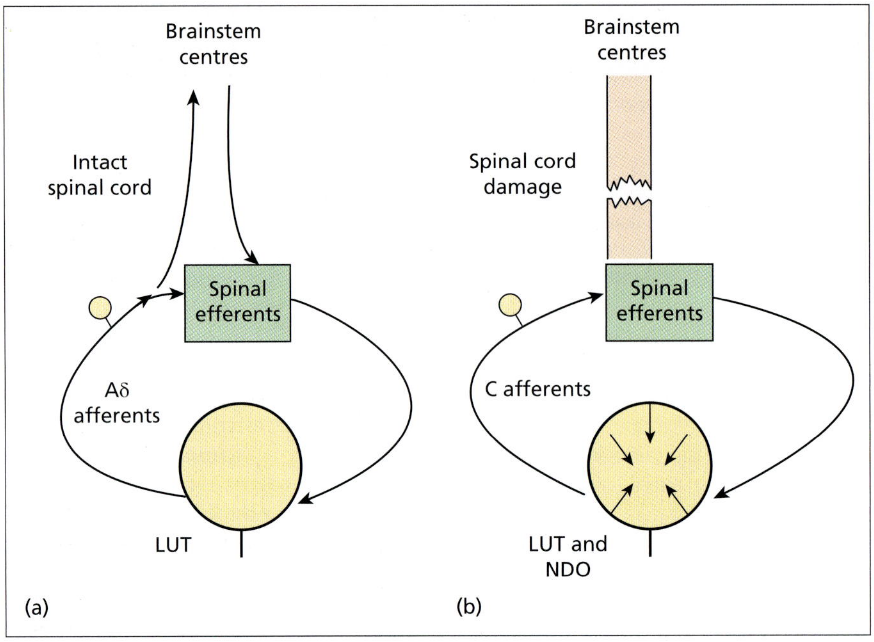

Figure 25.3 C fibres and the emergence of detrusor overactivity following spinal cord damage. (a) In health, thinly myelinated Aδ fibres have a lower threshold for activation and are responsible for conveying sensations of bladder filling. Whereas, unmyelinated C fibres have a greater threshold for activation and are thought to be quiescent. (b) Following spinal cord damage, C fibres become sensitised and are mechanosensitive at lower bladder volumes. A segmental spinal reflex emerges that is mediated by C fibres afferents nerves and results in involuntary detrusor contractions, the basis for neurogenic detrusor overactivity. LUT, lower urinary tract; NDO, neurogenic detrusor overactivity. Source: Panicker and Seth 2013. Reproduced with permission of Wiley.

detrusor is lost; the result is that the sphincter tends to contract when the detrusor is contracting, resulting in a condition known as detrusor–sphincter dyssynergia (DSD). This, together with poor neural drive on the detrusor muscle during attempts to void, means that there is likely to be incomplete bladder emptying and high detrusor pressures. Incomplete bladder emptying can in turn exacerbate the symptoms caused by detrusor overactivity. Although the neurological process of voiding may have been as equally severely disrupted by spinal cord disease as the process of storage, voiding difficulties and incomplete bladder emptying may not be evident and often it is only on direct questioning that a patient will admit to difficulty initiating micturition, an interrupted stream or a sensation of incomplete emptying. Table 25.4 summarises the pathophysiological consequences of a spinal cord lesion on the lower urinary tract.

Following SCI, detrusor overactivity, loss of compliance (the expansile property of the bladder) and DSD can be of such severity as to cause ureteric reflux, hydronephrosis and eventual upper renal tract damage. Before the introduction of modern treatments, renal failure was a common cause of death following SCI. The bladder problems of those with SCI must therefore be managed in such a way as to lessen the possibility of upper tract disease as well as provide the patient with adequate bladder control for a fully rehabilitated life. These patients need to remain under the care of a urologist who can regularly monitor the upper urinary tract and it may be better for the patients, who are often young and have no progressive disease, to undergo definitive surgery on their lower urinary tract with a view to protecting the upper tracts and restoring continence. It was in patients with complete spinal cord transection that the 'Brindley stimulator', which applied electrical stimulation directly to each of the sacral roots, S2, 3 or 4 was implanted, with considerable clinical improvement, but at the cost of sectioning of the dorsal roots.

Table 25.4 The possible pathophysiological consequences of spinal lesions on lower urinary tract functions.

Dysfunction	Symptoms
Detrusor overactivity: involuntary detrusor contractions at low filling volumes	Urgency Frequency Urge urinary incontinence
Detrusor–sphincter dyssynergia: concomitant contraction of the sphincter muscles when the detrusor is contracting during voiding	Interrupted stream Incomplete bladder emptying
Detrusor underactivity: impaired detrusor contractions during voiding	Poor stream Incomplete bladder emptying
Loss of central connections	Impaired initiation of voluntary voiding Inability to suppress urgency

Multiple sclerosis

The pathophysiological consequences of multiple sclerosis (MS) affecting the spinal cord are similar to those of SCI, but the medical context of increasing disability is such that the patient's management must be quite different. In patients with MS there is a strong association between bladder symptoms and the presence of clinical spinal cord involvement including paraparesis (i.e. any upper motor neurone signs in the lower limbs). Furthermore, bladder symptoms become increasingly resistant to treatment as lower limb mobility deteriorates.

The most common urinary symptom is urgency and all series of urodynamic studies of patients with MS have shown that this is caused by underlying detrusor overactivity. However, patients may also volunteer or admit on direct questioning to difficulty with voiding such as hesitancy of micturition and an interrupted urinary stream. Evidence of incomplete emptying is commonly based on the patient's observation that having passed urine once, they are able to do so again within 5–10 minutes, rather than a reported sensation of continued fullness.

Unlike the bladder dysfunction that follows SCI, MS and other progressive neurological diseases very rarely cause upper urinary tract involvement. The reason for this is not known, but it means that in such diseases the emphasis of management needs to be on symptomatic relief.

Other (non-traumatic) spinal cord diseases

A consistent feature of transverse myelitis is that although there may be an excellent clinical recovery from a tetraplegia of such severity that at its nadir artificial ventilation was necessary, bladder dysfunction is often the major residual neurological sequel. The explanation for this is not known but it may relate to the emergence of spinal segmental reflexes (Figure 25.3) during the period of 'spinal shock' which then persist as a dominant functional mechanism. This observation must inevitably cause a certain degree of pessimism about the prospect of restoration of bladder function if 'spinal repair' becomes a reality. Bladder dysfunction is common following acute disseminated encephalomyelitis (ADEM) and correlates with neurological deficits, especially in the lower limbs.

Detrusor overactivity occurs as an early feature and may even be a presenting symptom in patients with tropical spastic paraparesis caused by infection by human T-lymphotropic virus type 1 (HTLV-1).

Neurosyphilis, once a common cause of bladder dysfunction, is now rarely seen but tabes dorsalis classically resulted in an areflexic hyposensitive bladder because of involvement of the dorsal columns and roots, although a variety of abnormal urodynamic findings have been described.

Arteriovenous (AV) malformations of the spinal cord may be difficult to recognise clinically but commonly cause bladder disturbance as a prominent early feature. Although the majority of AV malformations occur in the thoraco-lumbar region, alterations to cord blood flow and subsequent conus ischaemia mean that the patient may present with what appears to be a conus or cauda equina lesion. Symptoms of voiding difficulty are common at an early stage followed by urinary retention.

A combination of upper and lower motor neurone signs in the legs together with urinary symptoms is characteristic of spinal dysraphism and a tethered cord. Typically, asymmetric wasting of the calves and intrinsic muscles of the feet occurs, but the prominent bladder symptoms and possibly extensor plantar responses suggest a diagnosis of a conus lesion rather than peripheral neuropathy or previous poliomyelitis. Although the majority of cases present in childhood, it is a condition that should be considered even in adults with the appropriate clinical features. Urodynamic studies show a mixed picture of detrusor overactivity and incomplete bladder emptying, and although an improvement in bladder function following a de-tethering procedure has been claimed, the operation is usually carried out to treat pain or prevent progression of neurological deficit.

Sacral and infrasacral lesions

Following damage to the conus medullaris, cauda equina or peripheral nerves voiding dysfunction predominates, caused by poorly sustained detrusor contractions and/or non-relaxing urethral sphincters.

Conus or cauda equina lesions

Damage to the cauda equina and S2–4 roots leaves the detrusor 'decentralised' but not 'denervated' because the post-ganglionic parasympathetic innervation is unaffected. This may explain why the bladder dysfunction following a cauda equina lesion is unpredictable and even detrusor overactivity has been described. Loss of voluntary control is usually a symptom and there are sometimes pronounced defects of anal sphincter control with incontinence for flatus or liquid stools in addition to an inability to evacuate the bowel without digital assistance. Loss of control over bladder, bowel and loss of sexual function is particularly difficult for patients to bear psychologically when they are otherwise ambulant and mobile.

Although there are a number of series reporting the urodynamic changes that can occur following a cauda equina lesion, there have been only limited analyses of the effect a cauda equina lesion can have on quality of life. However, the levels of compensation awarded in medico-legal cases reflect the fact that the loss of control of the pelvic organs resulting from a cauda equina injury is catastrophic.

Diabetic neuropathy

Bladder involvement was once considered an uncommon complication of diabetes but the greater use of techniques for studying bladder function have shown that the condition is often asymptomatic and discovered incidentally. Bladder dysfunction in isolation does not occur and other symptoms and signs of generalised neuropathy must be present in affected patients. The onset of the disorder is insidious, with progressive loss of bladder sensation and impairment of bladder emptying over years, eventually culminating in chronic low-pressure urinary retention. It seems likely that there is involvement of both the vesical sensory afferent fibres causing reduced awareness of bladder filling and also of parasympathetic efferent fibres to the detrusor decreasing the ability of the bladder to contract.

Other neuropathies

About one-quarter of patients with Guillian–Barré syndrome have bladder symptoms. These usually occur in patients with more severe neuropathy and appear after limb weakness is established. Both detrusor areflexia and bladder overactivity have been described.

Recessively inherited type II congenital sensory neuropathy and familial dysautonomias with involvement of small nerve fibres have bladder dysfunction amongst their associated disabilities.

Pelvic nerve injury

The peripheral innervation of the pelvic organs can be damaged by extirpative pelvic surgery such as resection of rectal carcinoma, radical prostatectomy or radical hysterectomy. The dissection necessary in the surgery of rectal cancer is likely to damage the parasympathetic innervation to the bladder and genitalia as the pelvic nerves take a medio-lateral course through the pelvis either side of the rectum and the apex of the prostate. The nerves are either removed together with the fascia that covers the lower rectum or can be damaged by a traction injury as the rectum is mobilised prior to excision.

Urinary incontinence following a radical prostatectomy or a radical hysterectomy that includes the upper part of the vagina is probably also caused by damage to the parasympathetic innervation of the detrusor. In the case of a radical prostatectomy, there can be additional direct damage to the innervation of the striated urethral sphincter.

Myotonic dystrophy

Although myotonic EMG activity has not been found in the sphincter or pelvic floor of patients with myotonic dystrophy, bladder symptoms can be quite prominent and difficult to treat, presumably because of involvement of bladder smooth muscle. With advancing disease resulting from involvement of the internal anal sphincter, faecal incontinence can become a problem.

Urinary retention

Although a failure of storage and detrusor overactivity leading to urinary incontinence is the most common bladder dysfunction seen with neurological disease, failure to empty and urinary retention also occur. When referred a patient in retention where the cause is not known, examination can reveal findings that betray a neurological lesion. Examining the sacral dermatomes for loss of sensation perianally and over the perineum ('saddle' area) can be helpful, although 10% of patients with a long-standing cauda equina syndrome have no peri-anal sensory loss. The examination should include assessing the tone and stength of voluntary contractions of the anal sphincter muscle, as well as assessing polysynaptic reflexes with centres in the sacral spinal segments (anal and bulbocavernosus reflexes). Innervation of the lower bowel and genitalia is shared through the second, third and fourth sacral spinal segments, and therefore patients in urinary retention because of a lesion of the cauda equina or conus lesion often report bowel and sexual dysfunction. However, if a urologist has referred a man or, more commonly, a young woman with urinary retention and there is no evidence of neurological disease on clinical examination, it is unlikely that imaging or other neurological investigations will be abnormal. Table 25.5 lists the differential diagnoses to consider in a patient presenting with urinary retention once a structural urological lesion has been excluded.

Table 25.5 Differential diagnosis of a patient in urinary retention referred from the urologist.

Lesions of the conus medullaris or cauda equina
Compressive lesions
Trauma
Intervertebral disc prolapse
Tumour
Granuloma
Abscess
Non-compressive lesions
Vascular: infarction, ischaemia (arteriovenous malformation)
Inflammation: myelitis, meningitis retention syndrome
Infection: herpes simplex, varicella zoster, cytomegalovirus, Elsberg's syndrome (viral aseptic meningitis)
Other neurological conditions
Spina bifida
Multiple system atrophy
Conditions associated with dysautonomia (e.g. pure autonomic failure, autonomic neuropathies)
Miscellaneous causes
Medications (e.g. opiates, anticholinergics, retigabine)
Fowler's syndrome: primary disorder of urethral sphincter relaxation in young women
Radical pelvic surgery
Chronic intestinal pseudo-obstruction, with additional involvement of the lower urinary tract
Primary detrusor myogenic failure
Cause unknown

Source: Panicker 2010. Reproduced with permission of BMJ Publishing Group Ltd.

Urinary retention in women

Women with unexplained non-neurogenic urinary retention were, until quite recently, often thought to have a psychogenic cause for their complaint and indeed this is still a common medical misconception. However, in 1985 an EMG abnormality of the striated urethral sphincter was described which, it was hypothesised, impairs urethral relaxation resulting in obstructed voiding and incomplete bladder emptying or complete retention. It was observed that many of the young women also had a history or clinical features of polycystic ovaries and over the years this condition has become known as Fowler's syndrome. Although an association with polycystic ovaries is often found this is not essential for the diagnosis, whereas exclusion of underlying urological or neurological pathology is. The syndrome is characterised by painless urinary retention, with a bladder capacity in excess of 1 L, and often difficulty in removing any catheter used for self-catheterisation. Anecdotally, many of these women have had a clinical incident that triggered the onset of their symptoms, such as a surgical procedure under general anaesthesia, a urinary tract infection or childbirth. The pathophysiology remains to be fully elucidated but it has been postulated that the disorder is brought about by a hormonally sensitive channelopathy of the striated urethral sphincter causing the muscle to be in a state of involuntary continuous contraction. The constant contraction of the sphincter has an inhibitory effect on the detrusor. Investigations demonstrate a raised resting urethral pressure and abnormal urethral sphincter EMG characterised by complex repetitive discharges and decelerating bursts, and sometimes an increased sphincter volume on ultrasound.

The cause for urinary retention often remains elusive even after extensive investigations. A prospective study of 61 women in urinary retention referred to the uroneurology department over 1 year revealed that only in 40% was a probable aetiology identified, the most common being Fowler's syndrome. Interestingly, nearly 40% of women in the study had been receiving treatment with opiates for various pain syndromes. Based on this, a more recent hypothesis is that Fowler's syndrome is the result of spinal cord intoxication by enkephalins. These have the effect of suppressing sensations from the bladder and inducing detrusor areflexia. In fact, the bladder of a woman with Fowler's syndrome shares many characteristics with that of someone who has developed urinary retention as a result of taking opiates.

There is also an uncommon condition in men where painless urinary retention is not associated with constipation, and sexual function is preserved, but in whom extensive investigation fails to reveal any underlying abnormality. It has been speculated that this disorder is caused by some abnormality of the intrinsic afferent innervation, possibly loss of the 'myofibroblast' or interstitial cell, thought to be an integral part of the bladder stretch sensing mechanism. This condition might make up a proportion of the women with unexplained urinary retention.

Management of lower urinary tract dysfunction

From the foregoing sections it will be evident that the most common bladder problem caused by neurological disease is a failure of storage and therefore incontinence. Because the bladder has such a limited repertoire of behaviour, incontinence can be the end product of several different pathophysiologies, but chief amongst these are either a failure of inhibition of the pontine micturition centre because of a suprapontine cortical lesion, or the emergence of an abnormal segmental spinal reflex as a result of disconnection between the sacral cord and the pons.

Non-pharmacological measures are generally helpful in the early stages when bladder symptoms are mild. A fluid intake of around 1–2 L a day is suggested, although this should be individualised. Caffeine reduction may reduce urgency and frequency, especially in patients who drink coffee or tea in excess. Bladder retraining, whereby patients void by the clock and voluntarily 'hold on' for increasingly longer periods, aims to restore the normal pattern of micturition.

Figure 25.4 shows a simple algorithm based on the two main interventions directed at the dual problems of detrusor overactivity and incomplete emptying that has proved to be a convenient low-cost effective management scheme. Urodynamic testing should be selectively employed to supplement clinical assessment in determining management of neurogenic lower urinary tract dysfunction. There is a hierarchy of treatment that may need to be employed as urinary incontinence worsens (e.g. with deteriorating spinal function in MS). The first line treatment is antimuscarinics, and if necessary then in combination with intermittent self-catheterisation. If these measures are insufficient, detrusor injection of botulinum toxin would then be considered. These various treatments and interventions are described next.

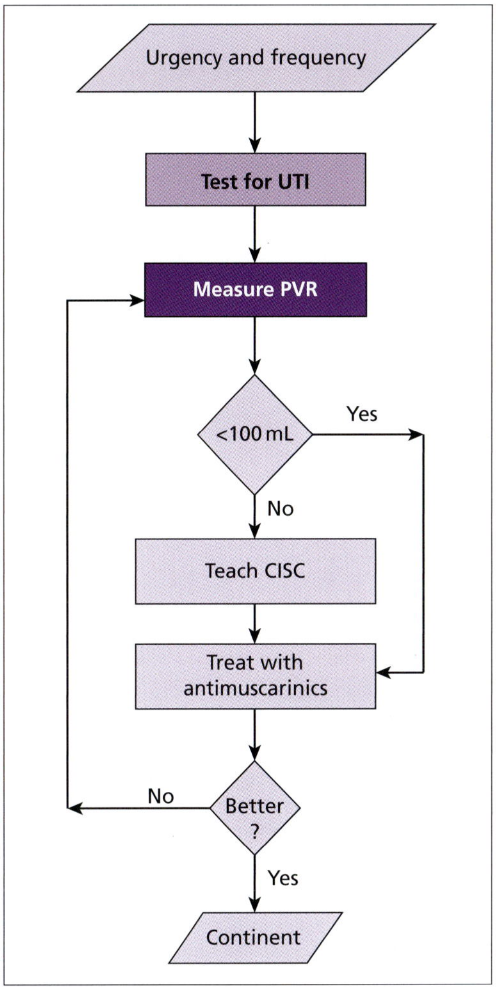

Figure 25.4 Algorithm for management of neurogenic incontinence. CISC, clean intermittent self-catheterisation; PVR, post void residual; UTI, urinary tract infection. Source: Fowler *et al.* 2009.

Management of storage dysfunction

Antimuscarinics (anticholinergics)

Antimuscarinic medications are the first line treatment for overactive bladder symptoms and their use is associated with better patient-reported cure and/or improvement and significant reduction of maximum detrusor pressures in patients with neurological disease. The premise for treatment of detrusor overactivity with an antimuscarinic agent was that this blocked the parasympathetic innervation effect on the M2/M3 receptors of the detrusor muscle. However, it is now being recognised that there may be a more complex mode of action during the storage phase, and mediated through a muscarinic afferent mechanism, thus explaining the observed effects of increased bladder capacity and reduction of urinary urgency with treatment. Not all the antimuscarinics currently available have been systematically investigated and their use is often by inference of efficacy. Dual therapy (combinations of oxybutynin, tolterodine and trospium) has been shown to be effective and well tolerated in a few patients. There are now a number of such agents available (Table 25.6), and the long-acting extended-life (XL) formulations of these medications have the significant advantage of only needing to be taken once a day to provide 24-hour cover.

Side effects associated with all of these agents are common, a dry mouth in particular reduces patient compliance. These drugs can also block central muscarinic M1 receptors and cause impairment in cognition and consciousness in susceptible individuals. In the cognitively impaired, antimuscarinics should be prescribed with a warning for carers to be vigilant about possible deterioration in cognitive function or the onset of confusion. In the absence of positive evidence it seems sensible at this time to recommend the use of antimuscarinics that do not cross the blood–brain barrier (i.e. trospium chloride, or darifenacin, a selective blocker of the M3 receptor which is not known to be involved in cognition).

Desmopressin

Desmopressin, a synthetic analogue of arginine vasopressin, temporarily reduces urine production and volume determined detrusor overactivity by promoting water reabsorption at the distal and collecting tubules of the kidney. It is useful for the treatment of urinary frequency or nocturia in patients with MS, providing symptom relief for up to 6 hours. It is also helpful in managing nocturnal polyuria, which is sometimes seen in patients with PD and various

Table 25.6 Antimuscarinic medications available in the United Kingdom.

Generic name	Trade name	Dose (mg)	Frequency
Darifenacin	Emselex	7.5–15	o.d.
Fesoterodine	Toviaz	4–8	o.d.
Oxybutynin	Ditropan, Cystrin	2.5–20	b.d. – q.d.s.
Oxybutynin modified release	Lyrinel XL	5–20	o.d.
Oxybutynin transdermal	Kentera	36 mg (releasing 3.9 mg/24 hours)	one patch twice weekly
Propiverine	Detrunorm	15–60	o.d. – q.d.s.
Solifenacin	Vesicare	5–10	o.d.
Tolterodine	Detrusitol	2–4	b.d.
Tolterodine modified release	Detrusitol XL	4	o.d.
Trospium	Regurin	20–40	b.d. (before food)
Trospium modified release	Regurin XL	60	o.d.

b.d., twice daily; o.d., once daily; q.d.s., four times daily; t.d.s., three times daily.

neurological conditions associated with dysautonomia. However, it should be prescribed with caution in patients over the age of 65 years or with dependent leg oedema, and should not be used more than once in 24 hours for fear of hyponatraemia or congestive heart failure.

Botulinum toxin

The most significant recent development in the treatment of neurogenic bladder dysfunction has been the use of botulinum toxin A (BTX-A), injected into multiple sites of the detrusor muscle. The treatment was introduced on the theoretical basis that botulinum toxin would temporarily block the presynaptic release of acetylcholine from the parasympathetic innervated muscles and produce a paralysis of the detrusor smooth muscle; however, it is now known that it has a more complex action that is likely to involve the intrinsic afferent innervation as well.

The toxin is cystoscopically injected into the bladder wall, resulting in significant improvement in cystometric capacity, detrusor pressures and bladder compliance. This is accompanied by an improvement in storage symptoms – reduced frequency, urgency, nocturia and incontinence episodes – and quality of life. Pivotal Phase III studies of onabotulinumtoxinA have shown clear benefit in managing neurogenic detrusor overactivity; however, no clinically relevant benefit in efficacy or duration was seen between dosages of 300 and 200 U, whereas the likelihood of developing urinary retention requiring self-catheterisation was dose dependent. Based upon these studies, onabotulinumtoxinA is now licensed for use in neurogenic detrusor overactivity in several countries. The beneficial effects last between 8 and 11 months, at which point the patient is eligible for further injections. Despite its success, patients must be counselled about a risk of performing clean intermittent self-catheterisation (CISC), because of the resultant voiding dysfunction and raised post void residual volume. Therefore patients being considered for this should be shown how to perform CISC so that they can demonstrate the ability and willingness to do this should it become necessary.

Neuromodulation

Tibial nerve stimulation is effective in treating patients with overactive bladder symptoms. The mechanism of action is unclear, but is thought to involve rebalancing the inhibitory and excitatory impulses travelling to the bladder. Tibial nerve stimulation therefore inhibits bladder activity by modulation of sacral and lumbar afferent nerves. Studies that examined the effect of percutaneous tibial nerve stimulation in a cohort of patients with MS showed improved urodynamic parameters as well as improvement in overactive bladder symptoms. Transcutaneous tibial nerve stimulation has also been shown to be successful in patients with MS. Additional studies are required to demonstrate long-term efficacy of tibial nerve stimulation in neurological patients.

Sacral neuromodulation can be used to treat detrusor overactivity and urgency incontinence, as well as non-obstructive chronic urinary retention. This is a surgical procedure, which takes place over two stages, to introduce a stimulating electrode in the sacral extradural space. The first stage is a test phase, where the stimulating lead is inserted through the S3 foramen and is connected to an external stimulator. Over the subsequent weeks, the patient is assessed to see if the stimulation has been beneficial by reducing symptoms documented by bladder diaries and measured residual volumes. If there has been significant benefit, the patient is eligible for a second stage which involves the implantation of a more permanent small subcutaneous stimulator connected to the stimulating lead. The continuous stimulations are maintained at a level that is subsensory for the patient, who remains unaware of its ongoing action.

Sacral neuromodulation has been tried in small numbers of patients with MS with limited success but, being a progressive neurological condition, it may lose its efficacy as the disease progresses. Moreover, currently available implants are not MRI compatible and therefore it is likely that the procedure would be an option only in patients whose MS has a benign indolent course and who report bladder symptoms that are not responsive to less invasive treatments. A systematic review of sacral neuromodulation for neurogenic lower urinary tract dysfunction concluded that the number of patients investigated so far is low, and there is a lack of randomised controlled trials, which would be needed before further guidance can be issued. Interestingly, it has been shown that in patients with SCI, early sacral neuromodulation prevented the development of neurogenic detrusor overactivity and high detrusor pressures compared with control patients who did not receive early intervention.

In patients with Fowler's syndrome the mainstay of treatment had been indefinite intermittent or in-dwelling catheterisation, but sacral neuromodulation has been shown to restore voiding in these women, probably by resetting brainstem functions. Sacral neuromodulation was first described as a treatment for urinary retention in the mid-1990s. At the time, it had been introduced for the management of bladder dysfunction, paradoxically for both intractable incontinence and retention. Of an initial cohort of 60 women with Fowler's syndrome who underwent a successful initial test procedure, percutaneous nerve evaluation (PNE) and subsequently underwent implant with a permanent sacral electrode, 70% were voiding spontaneously when followed up after a mean interval of 7 years.

Management of voiding dysfunction

Prior to prescribing an antimuscarinic for patients complaining predominantly of symptoms of detrusor overactivity, it is important to measure their post-void residual urine volume, particularly if the patient's symptoms suggest there is incomplete voiding. This can be performed with 'in–out' catheterisation or alternatively using a small hand-held ultrasound device (bladder scanner) which many specialist nurse continence advisers now have access to. The importance of recognising incomplete emptying is that any residual volume in the bladder can trigger volume-determined reflex detrusor contractions, exacerbating the clinical situation through worsening of the symptoms of frequency, urgency and urgency incontinence. If a symptomatic patient has a residual volume of over 100 mL, CISC is advocated.

A specialist nurse or continence adviser is the most suitable person to instruct the patient, or if necessary their carer, how to carry out intermittent catheterisation. Women find the procedure more difficult initially and often require a mirror to help locate the urethral orifice but, once learnt, even blind or partially sighted patients can become proficient. Many void a variable amount before passing the catheter, but after commencing antimuscarinic medication effective voiding may be so compromised that the patient relies mostly on intermittent self-catheterisation. Frequency of catheterisation will best be determined by the patient, but initially they should be advised to perform the procedure three or four times a day. Contact and support by the specialist nurse, particularly in the early stages of learning the technique, increases the patient's confidence and careful follow-up ensures compliance to a prescribed regimen. Asymptomatic bacteriuria is a common finding in those using intermittent self-catheterisation and is not an indication for antibiotic treatment.

Catheter technology has advanced significantly in recent years. Various innovative features have been incorporated into the design, although mostly of single-use catheters, with consequent increases in cost. The new catheters are manufactured from various materials, and of differing lengths and diameters. The continence adviser or specialist nurse can advise on the types of catheter available and put the patient in touch with suppliers.

Catheter choice depends on factors such as ease of use and storage, discomfort and minimisation of damage on insertion and the risk of urinary tract infection. Trauma and discomfort are reduced by using gel on the catheter, although many of those that are now available are hydrophilic coated so that on contact with water they develop a highly lubricated surface; some now come packed 'pre-wetted'. Convenience of use has improved as they are now disposable and can be secreted in a pocket or small bag. Those for use in women have been compacted into a tube similar in size to a lipstick container.

Unfortunately, there are few other effective methods for improving bladder emptying. There have been studies demonstrating that alpha blockers can reduce residual volumes in patients with MS, but the clinical impression is that alpha blockers are not effective in individual patients, possibly because incomplete bladder emptying is thought to be the result of a combination of poorly sustained and ill-coordinated detrusor contractions, or of an inappropriate contraction of the striated urethral sphincter.

The application of a suprapubic vibrating stimulus improves bladder emptying, and has benefited some patients. In patients with reflex detrusor overactivity, the vibrating stimulus might help to initiate micturition and possibly improve bladder emptying by triggering a detrusor contraction. Several devices are commercially available for suprapubic vibration, including small hand-held battery-operated vibrators.

Sexual functions and its neurological control

Physiology

Human sexual function depends on the integrity of the nervous system at many levels: higher centres determine the cognitive and emotional aspects of sexuality, hormonal levels drive libido and desire through the hypothalamus, and the ability to effect a sexual response depends on spinal autonomic reflexes. Malfunction of some aspect of this highly distributed system is therefore common in neurological disease.

Functional imaging techniques have been applied to examine brain responses on sexual arousal. Figure 25.5 shows a meta-analysis of four studies that used erotic visual stimulation compared with erotically neutral viewing in healthy subjects of both genders. Activation of the prefrontal cortex, the anterior cingulate, occipito-temporal cortex, thalamus, amygdala, hypothalamus, insula and claustrum is seen, those regions being part of the limbic and paralimbic system long known to be important in mediating sexual motivation. The hypothalamus has been linked to most aspects of sexual behaviour in both humans and animals. A study of brain activation during penile stimulation by the subjects' female partners showed strong activation predominantly on the right side of the insula and secondary somatosensory cortex and de-activation of the amygdala but no activation of the hypothalamus. The same group reported brain activation during male ejaculation and showed prominent activity in the dopamine-rich mesodiencephalic junction–ventral tegmentum, an area that was also seen to be activated with the 'rush' experienced by heroin and cocaine addicts who describe an orgasmic-like sensation with heroin use.

Animal and human studies following SCI have pointed to the existence of two independent pathways for the male erectile response: a psychogenic pathway mediated by the thoraco-lumbar sympathetic outflow (T12–L2) and a sacral spinal reflex pathway, whereby genital stimulation results in a short-lived erection. In neurological health these two responses appear to fuse to produce an erection adequate for intercourse. Comparable pathways mediate vaginal lubrication, the female sexual response being analogous to penile erection.

Erection results from increased blood flow into the corpus cavernosum, a response mediated by the efferent parasympathetic pathway originating in the intermediolateral aspect of the sacral cord (S2–S4) travelling in the pelvic nerve (nervi erigentes). The preganglionic neurotransmitter in these fibres is acetylcholine but the post-ganglionic nerve fibres, which terminate either on the vascular smooth muscle of the corporeal arterioles on the non-vascular smooth muscle of trabecular tissue surrounding the corporeal lacunae, release nitric oxide (NO).

In women, sexual arousal results in an increased vaginal blood flow, erection of the cavernous tissue of the clitoris and the outer part of the vagina. As in men, the erectile response of these tissues is NO dependent; neuronal NO synthetase has been detected in both the body and glans of the clitoris. Nerve fibres containing

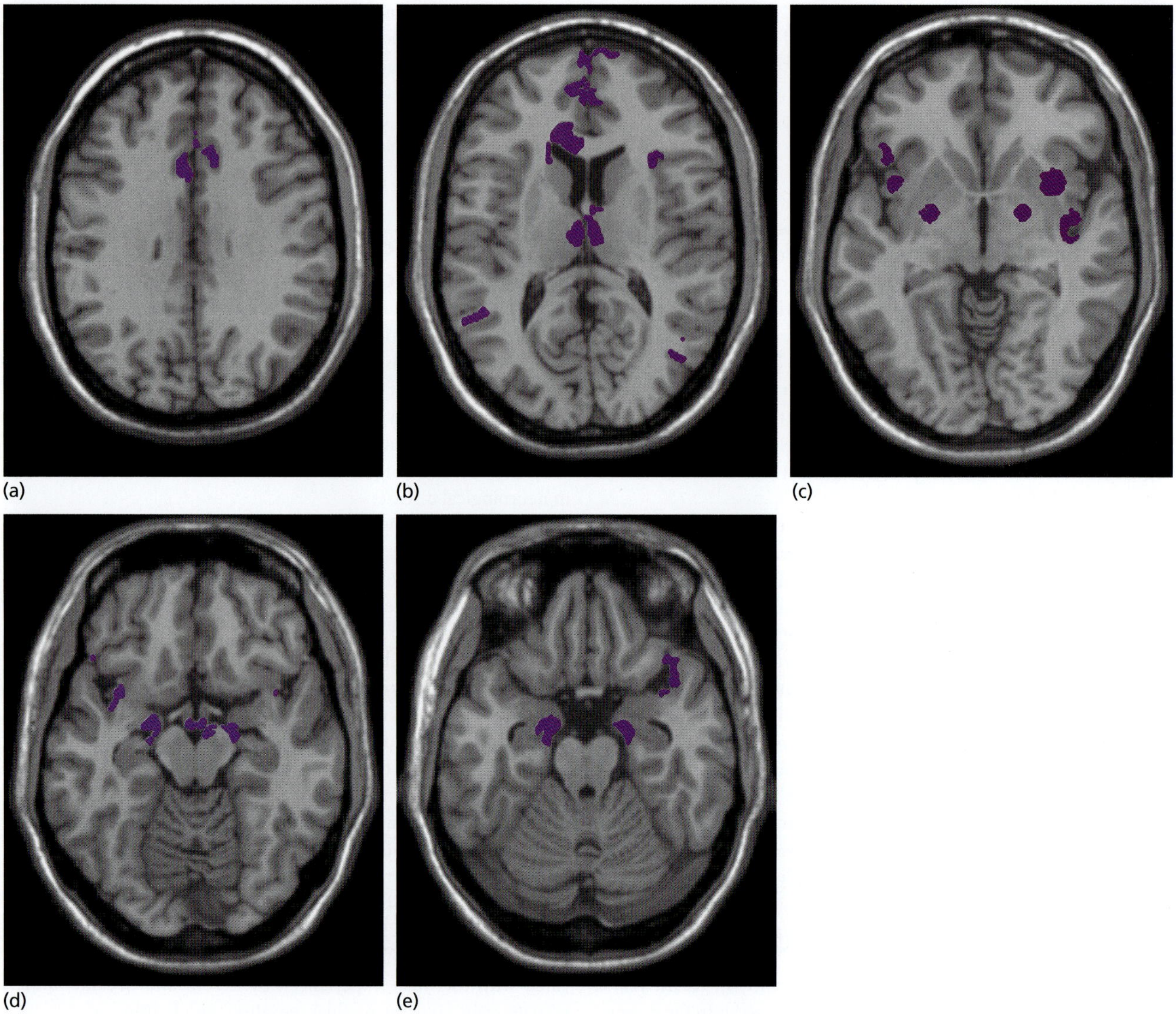

Figure 25.5 Meta-analysis of functional magnetic resonance studies that showed responses to erotic visual stimulation.

vasoactive intestinal polypeptide (VIP), calcitonin gene-related peptide (CGRP) and substance P (SP) have also been described in human clitoral tissue. Normal vaginal lubrication, which is dependent both on intact innervation and normal oestrogen levels, is also NO mediated.

Detumescence after orgasm is mediated by noradrenaline in the sympathetic system and in the absence of sexual arousal it maintains the penis in the flaccid state. In men, orgasm and ejaculation are not the same process. Ejaculation involves emission of semen from the vas deferens and seminal vesicles into the posterior urethra, and closure of the bladder neck, under sympathetic control, whereas orgasm involves contraction of the pelvic floor muscles under somatic nerve control from the perineal branch of the pudendal nerve. In neurological disease the two processes can be separately affected.

During female orgasm there can be a series of synchronous contractions of the sphincter and vaginal muscles, with associated sensory changes which are generally described as being intensely pleasurable pelvic events.

Sexual dysfunction following neurological disease

Sexual dysfunction is a significant, but often underestimated, symptom in patients with neurological disease.

Traumatic brain injury

Sexual dysfunction, usually reduced sexual desire, is common following traumatic brain injury particularly if there has been substantial cognitive damage. Both the extent and the location of damage determine the outcome. Damage to prefrontal areas can result either in erotic apathy or conversely disinhibition with inappropriate sexually demanding behaviour. Similar problems can be seen following encephalitis. Partner dissatisfaction plays an important part in influencing sexual activity following traumatic brain injury.

The importance of hypothalamic and pituitary damage following head injury and resulting hypopituitarism has recently been recognised, and full endocrine evaluation some months after a significant brain injury is often appropriate.

Stroke

Although pre-existing sexual dysfunction resulting from diseases such as hypertension, diabetes and myocardial infarction can mean that there is less impact of stroke on sexual behaviour, the frequency and spectrum of sexual problems can be comparable to those seen following traumatic brain injury.

Epilepsy

Temporal lobe disease causing epilepsy is particularly likely to have sexual manifestations. Sexual auras can occur as part of complex partial seizures and genital automatisms were observed in 11% of patients undergoing diagnostic video-telemetry. Although various sexual behaviours and occasionally hypersexuality have been described in patients with temporal lobe epilepsy (TLE), the picture most commonly seen is that of a profound failure of arousal.

There is sufficient evidence from studies that have compared sexual dysfunction in patients with generalised epilepsy and those with TLE to suggest that the deficit is a result of a specific temporolimbic involvement rather than a consequence of epilepsy, psychosocial factors or antiepileptic medication. The problem is usually that of a low or even absent libido – something that is a presenting complaint either because of its effect on sexual relationships formed prior to the onset of the disorder or because lack of sexual motivation prevents the formation of adult relationships. In a study that looked at changes in sexuality following epilepsy surgery, extratemporal resections usually resulted in no change whereas temporal lobe resection resulted more commonly in a change in sexuality.

Parkinson's disease

Whether or not specific genital dysfunction is a feature of PD is not entirely resolved. Using questionnaire surveys, several studies have shown that dissatisfaction with the quality of sexual experiences in men with PD is more likely than in control subjects. A survey of young patients with PD and their partners revealed a high level of dissatisfaction, with the most severely affected couples being those in which the patient was male and who complained of erectile dysfunction (ED) and premature ejaculation. Although ED, premature ejaculation in men and difficulty in arousal and reaching orgasm in women with PD may be significant problems, unless age and disability matched groups are compared it is difficult to know how specific these complaints are to PD. Early studies that found a high incidence of ED in men with PD may not have excluded MSA. A study that compared a group of married men with PD with a group with arthritis found a similar pattern of sexual functioning in the two groups, suggesting that although sexual dysfunction was common in PD, it was not more so than in men with a chronic illness that does not involve the nervous system. Age, severity of disease and depression, as well as testosterone levels, seem to be major determinants of sexual dysfunction, as they are in other neurological diseases.

Sexual compulsive behaviour may occur in patients with PD in the setting of an impulse control disorder (ICD). In a recent large multicentric cross-sectional study of patients with PD, the overall incidence of ICDs was found to be 13.6%. The most common syndromic presentations were compulsive buying (5.7%), pathological gambling (5.0%), binge-eating disorder (4.3%) and compulsive sexual behaviour (3.5%). Nearly one-quarter of patients have more than one impulse disorder and 3.9% had three or more.

There is experimental and clinical evidence that dopaminergic mechanisms are involved both in determining libido and inducing penile erection. In animal studies, the medial preoptic area of the hypothalamus has been shown to regulate sexual drive and selective stimulation of D2 dopaminergic receptors in this region increases sexual activity in rats. The pro-erectile effect of sublingual apomorphine was exploited as a licensed worldwide treatment for ED in 2001. Although some men with PD being treated with apomorphine had been taking advantage of this effect, no large-scale study of its effect in men with PD or MSA was carried out and since its licensing other therapies have been shown to be more effective.

Men with PD respond satisfactorily to treatment with sildenafil citrate and recently a small but positive response in sexual well-being was reported in men, but not women, after deep brain stimulation of the subthalamic nucleus.

Multiple system atrophy

ED may be a prodromal symptom of MSA. Initially, erectile response becomes intermittent and over the course of months or years erectile failure becomes complete. This can certainly pre-date the onset of recognised neurological features by several years. This was previously thought to be part of the symptom complex of autonomic failure, but the occurrence of this complaint is clearly separate from postural hypotension; it has been speculated that there is some more central, possibly dopamine-dependent, underlying process. Initially, libido remains intact and men treated with phosphodiesterase inhibitors who already have postural hypotension appear to be at particular risk of exacerbation. It is not clear whether ejaculation is equally affected and little information exists about whether or not sexual function in women is equally seriously disrupted.

Spinal cord injury

The earliest reports of human neurogenic sexual dysfunction were large series of war veterans who had sustained SCI. These early studies showed that the level and completeness of a lesion determined the extent of preserved erectile and ejaculatory capacity of a paraplegic man and it was from these observations that the concept of there being both spinal reflex and psychogenic pathways for erection originated. Following a complete cervical lesion, psychogenic erections were lost but spontaneous or reflex erections remained intact. In low lesions, particularly if the cauda equina was involved, there was poor or absent erectile capacity, because the thoracolumbar sympathetic outflow originates between T12 and L2 and it is through this pathway that psychogenic erectile responses are mediated. Occasionally, men with low lumbar cord lesions but intact sacral roots find that they are still able to obtain psychogenically driven erectile responses.

Ejaculation also depends on spinal cord integrity. Studies of men who have undergone bilateral anterolateral cordotomies for relief of pain and who have lost orgasmic sensation suggest that 'erotically coloured' sensation is conveyed in spinal pathways that travel in close proximity to the spinothalamic tracts. Anorgasmia has been described following an anterior cord syndrome where patients have been demonstrated to have loss of small myelinated nerve fibre function while large fibre dorsal column functions were spared. Preserved ejaculation function following a spinal cord lesion is unusual and it was found that only 4% of men following SCI were still able to ejaculate, a matter of the greatest concern to paraplegic young men who wish to father children.

Much less is known about sexual dysfunction in women with SCI but it seems that all aspects of genital neurology are affected; the women have little or no genital sensation, experience poor vaginal lubrication and have difficulty in reaching orgasm. As with erectile function in men, the analogous process of vaginal lubrication appears in health to be determined by psychogenic and reflex pathways and thus the level and completeness of an SCI determines what responses are preserved. A sensory level above T11–L2, the segmental origin of the thoraco-lumbar sympathetic outflow, was found to be associated with a failure to achieve psychogenic lubrication. By contrast, reflex genital vasocongestion in response to manual stimulation occurred despite a lack of subjective arousal, whereas women with cauda equina damage cannot usually achieve reflex lubrication. In women with preservation of sensory function in T11–L2, the psychogenic genital vasocongestion response is maintained. This suggests that the sympathetic outflow in the female is as important as it is in the male. Women with complete or incomplete suprasacral injury can achieve reflex genital response by manual stimulation but not when there is involvement of the sacral roots. Failure to reach orgasm is common in women with SCI and correlates poorly with the type of injury. Although their ability to reach orgasm is diminished, the written descriptions of the experience of orgasm in women with SCI were indistinguishable from those without, although they took much longer to achieve orgasm. It has been hypothesised that this preserved responsiveness is mediated through intact vagal innervation of the cervix.

Multiple sclerosis

The evidence points to spinal cord involvement as the major cause of ED in MS. Cord involvement in MS can initially result in a partial deficit so that ED is variable, with preserved nocturnal penile erections and erections on morning waking. It is only in the last 10–20 years that neurological teaching has recognised the error of the dictum that 'if a man can get an erection at any time, impotence is likely to be psychogenic'. The experience of men with SCI obviously belied that statement, but early studies put the incidence of 'organic impotence' in men with MS as low as 4%. Now it known to be a common problem, with estimates that it affects 50–75% of men with MS, depending on the severity of disability of the group studied.

A study that analysed the type of sexual dysfunction that affected men with MS who were still ambulant found that ED was the most common complaint (63%), followed by ejaculatory dysfunction and/or orgasmic dysfunction (50%) and reduced libido (40%). Other non-specific effects of MS also have adverse effects on sexual function, including fatigue, depression, spasticity and anxiety about incontinence. Prior to the advent of the oral erectogenic medications, men with MS were being successfully treated with intracavernosal injection therapy. Subsequently, a multicentre placebo controlled trial demonstrated an excellent response to sildenafil citrate by men with MS. Orgasmic capacity was also increased, a fact that was attributed to the men being able to sustain an erection for longer. Although many men are helped through that mechanism, a significant number continue to have difficulty with ejaculation for which there is no effective medication, although yohimbine can be tried. Probably the best recourse is to a vibrating sex aid.

Women with MS appear to report sexual dysfunction less frequently than men, but nevertheless it is a problem that is thought to affect more than 50%, the incidence increasing with increasing disability. A questionnaire survey of 133 women with mild disability found that although half reported voiding symptoms, 70% still enjoyed sexual intercourse, felt aroused and could experience orgasm. These figures are consistent with other questionnaire surveys that show that approximately one-third of women with MS experience loss of orgasm, reduced libido or decreased lubrication. Sensory dysfunction in the genital area was experienced by 62% of women with advanced MS. The nature of the sensory dysfunction is usually loss of sensation but, occasionally, particularly early in the course of the disease, dysaesthesia can make genital contact with their partner unbearable. Loss of orgasmic capacity is the complaint for which women seek treatment. Following the success of sildenafil citrate in the treatment of sexual function with men with MS, 19 women were recruited to a double-blind placebo controlled trial. A questionnaire was used to measure sexual response and although there was a significant improvement in the lubrication and some improvement in sensation, there was no overall change in orgasmic response to sildenafil compared with placebo. The responses to the 'global efficacy question' reflect limited overall subjective improvement following sildenafil. This was disappointing although perhaps not surprising. Despite the absence of specific treatment, the opportunity to discuss problems with a health care professional was found to be beneficial.

Lesions of the sympathetic thoraco-lumbar outflow

The fibres that travel from the thoraco-lumbar sympathetic pathway emerge from spinal levels T10–L2 and course through the retroperitoneal space to the bifurcation of the aorta, from where they enter the pelvic plexus. Loss of sympathetic innervation of the genitalia causes disorders of ejaculation with either failure of emission or retrograde ejaculation, although the ability to experience the sensation of orgasm can be retained. The sympathetic thoraco-lumbar fibres are particularly likely to be injured by the procedure of retro-peritoneal lymph node dissection and complaints of loss of ejaculation are common after such surgery.

Conus or cauda equina lesions

The cauda equina contains the sacral parasympathetic outflow together with the somatic efferent and afferent fibres. A lesion of the cauda equina therefore results in sensory loss as well as a parasympathetic defect and both men and women complain of perineal sensory loss and loss of erotic genital sensation – for which there is no effective treatment. In men ED is also a complaint.

A recent detailed study of 36 men with long-standing cauda equina damage of various aetiologies used a self-administered questionnaire to gauge sexual dysfunction and found severe dysfunction in 35%, moderate in 24% and slight sexual dysfunction in the remainder, with only one man highly confident of achieving and maintaining an erection. Orgasmic function was slightly more impaired than erectile function and sexual desire slightly less. The patients' age, but not findings on clinical neurological, even perineal sensation or EMG of the anal sphincter, correlated with sexual dysfunction. There had been very little recovery of function since onset and only five men had received medical attention for their problem.

Peripheral neuropathies

Diabetes is the most common cause of ED. Surveys of andrology clinics have found 20–31% of men attending to be diabetic. The prevalence of ED increases with age and duration of diabetes and the problem is known to be associated with severe retinopathy, a history of peripheral neuropathy, amputation, cardiovascular disease, raised glycosylated haemoglobin, use of antihypertensives and higher body mass index. A large population study of men with younger onset diabetes found 20% to have ED. Whether the pathogenesis of ED in diabetics is caused mainly by neuropathy or whether there is a significant microvascular contribution or the two processes are co-dependent is not yet resolved, but at a cellular level the evidence suggests there is a depletion of neurotransmitters. Age-matched studies of women with and without diabetes suggest that diabetic women are also affected by specific disorders of sexual function including decreased vaginal lubrication and capacity for orgasm.

Guillain–Barré syndrome (GBS) does not appear specifically to affect the innervation involved in sexual function over and above the extent to which it causes general disability. In about 25%, bladder symptoms appear after onset of weakness, but it is unknown if these are the patients who on recovery are likely to have sexual dysfunction. GBS patient support groups report anecdotally of sexual dysfunction in both genders as part of general disability.

Table 25.7 Factors that influence sexual functions in patients with neurological disease.

Primary
Neurological lesions interfering with the sexual response and/or sexual feelings
Secondary
Fatigue
Difficulties in attention and concentration
Bladder/bowel incontinence
Physical immobility: muscle weakness, leg spasms
Dysaesthesia/allodynia
Other factors: incoordination, tremor, pain
Tertiary
Depression, anxiety
Anger, guilt and fear
Altered self-image, low self-esteem
Relationship with the partner, change in family role
Others
Medications: antidepressants, baclofen, gabapentin
Use of urethral indwelling catheter

By contrast, neuropathies that involve selectively the small and unmyelinated nerve fibres, such as amyloid and some other rare inherited neuropathies, have urogenital symptoms as prominent features. Amyloid neuropathy, either familial or secondary, has a marked effect on urogenital function and symptoms are common. ED can be an early symptom of autonomic involvement.

Management of sexual dysfunction

There are several factors that influence sexual functions in patients with neurological disease (Table 25.7) and these should be individually addressed. Measures such as pelvic floor exercises or electrical stimulation feedback with cognitive therapy, which can improve symptoms in the neurologically intact, have not been found to be as effective in those with neurogenic sexual dysfunction. In men with neurogenic ED, corporeal injections of first papaverine and then alprostadil were the mainstay of treatment until the advent of sildenafil citrate, the type 5 phosphodiesterase inhibitor (PDE-5), in 1998.

Normal erectile function is dependent on the smooth-muscle relaxing effects of NO which is mediated by the cyclic nucleotide signalling pathway. Down-regulation of this pathway is central to the pathophysiology of many forms of ED. Hence, selective inhibition of PDE-5 which catalyses the degradation of cyclic guanosine monophosphate (cGMP) promotes erectile responses to sexual stimulation. The efficacy of sildenafil citrate transformed the treatment of ED, not only by providing an effective well-tolerated oral therapy, but also by introducing open discussion about the problem. The advent of vardenafil, which has the highest *in vitro* potency, may improve responsiveness, and tadalafil, which has a prolonged half-life of 18 hours, is enabling couples to have sexual activity with less planning (Table 25.8). ED will affect the female partner, and in an ideal world it is recommended that evaluation of the woman should be addressed within the context of the couple in a sexual medicine clinic.

Female sexual dysfunction is less satisfactorily treated. Growing realisation of the problem has resulted in the problem being better addressed and strategies considered (Table 25.8).

Table 25.8 Sexual dysfunction in men and women with neurological disease and potential treatment strategies.

Dysfunction	Symptoms	Potential management strategies
Sexual interest/desire	Diminished or absent feelings of sexual interest or motivation; rarely hypersexuality	Relationship counselling, psychotherapy ?Hormonal replacement
Sexual arousal	Poor/absent erections (males) (erectile dysfunction)	Treatment for erectile dysfunction – PDE5 inhibitors, Vacuum constriction devices, Intracavernous/ intraurethral prostaglandin therapy Vaginal lubricants
	Diminished/absent feelings of sexual excitement and sexual pleasure (sexual arousal dysfunction) and/or vulval swelling or vaginal lubrication (genital arousal dysfunction) (females)	?Sildenafil
Orgasm/ejaculation	Delayed or absent ejaculation (males)	?Yohimbine, midodrine
	Reduced or absent orgasms (males and females)	Therapy: sensate focus techniques, sex therapy, cognitive–behavioural therapy Sex aids
Pain	Dyspareunia (females)	Anaesthetic gels, pain modulation

PDE5, phosphodiesterase 5.

References

Andrew J, Nathan PW. Lesions of the anterior frontal lobes and disturbances of micturition and defaecation. *Brain* 1964; **87**: 233–262.

Fowler CJ, Panicker JN, Drake M, Harris C, Harrison SCW, Kirby M, *et al.* A UK census on the management of the bladder in multiple sclerosis. *J Neurol Neurosurg Psychiatry* 2009; **80:** 470–477.

Panicker JN, Seth JH. C-fibre sensory nerves – not so silent as we think? *BJU Int* 2013; **112:** 129–130.

Further reading

Abercrombie JF, Rogers J, Swash M. Faecal incontinence in myotonic dystrophy. *J Neurol Neurosurg Psychiatry* 1998; **64**: 128–130.

Andersson KE. Neurophysiology/pharmacology of erection. *Int J Impot Res* 2001; **13** (Suppl. 3): S8–S17.

Andersson KE. Pharmacology of penile erection. *Pharmacol Rev* 2001; **53**: 417–450.

Andersson KE. Antimuscarinics for treatment of overactive bladder. *Lancet Neurol* 2004; **3**: 47–53.

Araki I, Kuno S. Assessment of voiding dysfunction in Parkinson's disease by the international prostate symptom score. *J Neurol Neurosurg Psychiatry* 2000; **68**: 429–433.

Araki I, Kitahara M, Oida T, Kuna S. Voiding dysfunction and Parkinson's disease: urodynamic abnormalities and urinary symptoms. *J Urology* 2000; **164**: 1640–1643.

Aranda B, Cramer P. Effect of apomorphine and L-dopa on parkinsonian bladder. *Neurourol Urodyn* 1993; **12**: 203–209.

Arnow BA, Desmond JE, Banner LL, *et al.* Brain activation and sexual arousal in healthy, heterosexual males. *Brain* 2002; **125**: 1014–1023.

Athwal BS, Berkley KJ, Hussain I, *et al.* Brain responses to changes in bladder volume and urge to void in healthy men. *Brain* 2001; **124** (Part 2): 369–377.

Baird AD, Wilson SJ, Bladin PF, Saling MM, Reutens DC. Sexual outcome after epilepsy surgery. *Epilepsy Behav* 2003; **4**: 268–278.

Baird AD, Wilson SJ, Bladin PF, Saling MM, Reutens DC. The amygdala and sexual drive: insights from temporal lobe epilepsy surgery. *Ann Neurol* 2004; **55**: 87–96.

Bakke A, Myhr KM, Grønning M, Nyland H. Bladder, bowel and sexual dysfunction in patients with multiple sclerosis: a cohort study. *Scand J Urol Nephrol* 1996; **179** (Suppl): 61–66.

Beck RO, Betts CD, Fowler CJ. Genito-urinary dysfunction in multiple system atrophy: clinical features and treatment in 62 cases. *J Urol* 1994; **151**: 1336–1341.

Benarroch EE. Brainstem in multiple system atrophy: clinicopathological correlations. *Cell Mol Neurobiol* 2003; **23**: 519–526.

Berger Y, Blaivas JG, DeLaRocha ER, Salinas JM. Urodynamic findings in Parkinson's disease. *J Urol* 1987; **138**: 836–838.

Beric A, Light J. Anorgasmia in anterior spinal cord syndrome. *J Neurol Neurosurg Psychiatry* 1993; **56**: 548–551.

Betts CD, D'Mellow MT, Fowler CJ. Urinary symptoms and the neurological features of bladder dysfunction in multiple sclerosis. *J Neurol Neurosurg Psychiatry* 1993; **56**: 245–250.

Betts CD, Jones SJ, Fowler CG, Fowler CJ. Erectile dysfunction in multiple sclerosis: associated neurological and neurophysiological deficits, and treatment of the condition. *Brain* 1994; **117**: 1303–1310.

Blok B, Sturms L, Holstege G. Brain activation during micturition in women. *Brain* 1998; **121**: 2033–2042.

Blok B, Weer H, Holstege G. Ultrastructural evidence for a paucity of projections from the lumbosacral cord to the pontine micturition centre of M-Region in the cat: a new concept for the organization of the micturition reflex with the periaqueductal gray as central relay. *J Comp Neurol* 1995; **359**: 300–309.

Blok B, Willemsen T, Holstege G. A PET study of brain control of micturition in humans. *Brain* 1997; **120**: 111–121.

Blumer D. Hypersexual episodes in temporal lobe epilepsy. *Am J Psychiatry* 1970; **126**: 1099.

Bors E, Comarr A. Neurological disturbances of sexual function with special references to 529 patients with spinal cord injury. *Urol Surv* 1960; **10**: 191–222.

Bronner G, Royter V, Korczyn AD, Giladi N. Sexual dysfunction in Parkinson's disease. *J Sex Marital Ther* 2004; **30**: 95–105.

Chandiramani VA, Palace J, Fowler CJ. How to recognize patients with parkinsonism who should not have urological surgery. *Br J Urol* 1997; **80**: 100–104.

Chandler BJ, Brown S. Sex and relationship dysfunction in neurological disability. *J Neurol Neurosurg Psychiatry* 1998; **65**: 877–880.

Critchley HD, Wiens S, Rotshtein P, Ohman A, Dolan RJ. Neural systems supporting interoceptive awareness. *Nat Neurosci* 2004; **7**: 189–195.

Dasgupta R, Critchley HD, Dolan RJ, Fowler CJ. Changes in brain activity following sacral neuromodulation for urinary retention. *J Urol* 2005; **174**: 2268–2272.

Dasgupta R, Wiseman OJ, Kanabar G, Fowler CJ, Mikol DD. Efficacy of sildenafil in the treatment of female sexual dysfunction due to multiple sclerosis. *J Urol* 2004; **171**: 1189–1193; discussion 1193.

Dasgupta R, Wiseman OJ, Kitchen N, Fowler CJ. Long-term results of sacral neuromodulation for women with urinary retention. *BJU Int* 2004; **94**: 335–337.

Fowler CJ, Beck RO, Gerrard S, Betts CD, Fowler CG. Intravesical capsaicin for treatment of detrusor hyperreflexia. *J Neurol Neurosurg Psychiatry* 1994; **57**: 169–173.

Fowler CJ, Christmas TJ, Chapple CR, *et al.* Abnormal electromyographic activity of the urethral sphincter, voiding dysfunction, and polycystic ovaries: a new syndrome? *Br Med J* 1988; **297**: 1436–1438.

Fowler CJ, Dasgupta R. Electromyography in urinary retention and obstructed voiding in women. *Scand J Urol Nephrol* 2003; **210**: 55–58.

Fowler CJ, Griffiths D, de Groat WC. The neural control of micturition. *Nat Rev Neurosci* 2008; **9**: 453–466.

Fowler CJ, Griffiths DJ. A decade of functional brain imaging applied to bladder control. *Neurourol Urodyn* 2010; **29**: 49–55.

Fowler CJ, Kirby R, Harrison M. Decelerating bursts and complex repetitive discharges in the striated muscle of the urethral sphincter associated with urinary retention in women. *J Neurol Neurosurg Psychiatry* 1985; **48**: 1004–1009.

Fowler CJ, Miller JR, Sharief MK, *et al.* A double blind, randomised study of sildenafil citrate for erectile dysfunction in men with multiple sclerosis. *J Neurol Neurosurg Psychiatry* 2005; **76**: 700–705.

Georgiadis JR, Holstege G. Human brain activation during sexual stimulation of the penis. *J Comp Neurol* 2005; **493**: 33–38.

Ginsberg D, Gousse A, Keppenne V, et al. Phase 3 efficacy and tolerability study of onabotulinumtoxinA for urinary incontinence from neurogenic detrusor overactivity. *J Urol* 2012; **187:** 2131–2139.

Griffiths DJ. The pontine micturition centres. *Scand J Urol Nephrol Suppl* 2002; **210:** 21–26.

Grosse J, Kramer G, Stohrer M. Success of repeat detrusor injections of botulinum-A toxin in patients with severe neurogenic detrusor overactivity and incontinence. *Eur Urol* 2005; **47**: 653–659.

Hahn K, Ebersbach G. Sonographic assessment of urinary retention in multiple system atrophy and idiopathic Parkinson's disease. *Mov Disord* 2005; **20**: 1499–1502.

Hamann S, Herman RA, Nolan CL, Wallen K. Men and women differ in amygdala response to visual sexual stimuli. *Nat Neurosci* 2004; **7**: 411–416.

Han KS, Heo SH, Lee SJ, Jeon SH, Yoo KH. Comparison of urodynamics between ischemic and hemorrhagic stroke patients; can we suggest the category of urinary dysfunction in patients with cerebrovascular accident according to type of stroke? *Neurourol Urodyn* 2010; **29:** 387–390.

Hussain I, Brady CM, Swinn MJ, Mathias CJ, Fowler CJ. Treatment of erectile dysfunction with sildenafil citrate (Viagra) in parkinsonism due to Parkinson's disease or multiple system atrophy with observations on orthostatic hypotension. *J Neurol Neurosurg Psychiatry* 2001; **71**: 371–374.

Jonas U, Fowler CJ, Chancellor MB, *et al.* Efficacy of sacral nerve stimulation for urinary retention: results 18 months after implantation. *J Urol* 2001; **165**: 15–19.

Kavia R, Dasgupta R, Fowler CJ. Functional imaging and central control of the bladder. *J Comp Neurol* 2005: **493**: 27–32.

Kavia RB, Datta SN, Dasgupta R, Elneil S, Fowler CJ. Urinary retention in women: its causes and management. *BJU Int* 2006; **97**: 281–287.

Kessler TM, La Framboise D, Trelle S, *et al.* Sacral neuromodulation for neurogenic lower urinary tract dysfunction: systematic review and meta-analysis. *Eur Urol* 2010; **58:** 865–874.

Kirchhof K, Apostolidis AN, Mathias CJ, Fowler CJ. Erectile and urinary dysfunction may be the presenting features in patients with multiple system atrophy: a retrospective study. *Int J Impot Res* 2003; **15**: 293–298.

Komisaruk BR, Whipple B, Crawford A, *et al.* Brain activation during vaginocervical self-stimulation and orgasm in women with complete spinal cord injury: fMRI evidence of mediation by the vagus nerves. *Brain Res* 2004; **1024**: 77–88.

Kuchel GA, Moscufo N, Guttmann CR, *et al.* Localization of brain white matter hyperintensities and urinary incontinence in community-dwelling older adults. *J Gerontol A Biol Sci Med Sci* 2009; **64:** 902–909.

Matsumoto S, Levendusky MC, Longhurst PA, Levin RM, Millington WR. Activation of mu opioid receptors in the ventrolateral periaqueductal gray inhibits reflex micturition in anesthetized rats. *Neurosci Lett* 2004; **363**: 116–119.

Matsuura S, Kakizaki H, Mitsui T, *et al.* Human brain region response to distension or cold stimulation of the bladder: a positron emission tomography study. *J Urol* 2002; **168**: 2035–2039.

Melis MR, Argiolas A. Nitric oxide synthase inhibitors prevent apomorphine- and oxytocin-induced penile erection and yawning in male rats. *Brain Res Bull* 1993; **32**: 71–74.

Minderhoud JM, Leemhuis JG, Kremer J, Laban E, Smits PM. Sexual disturbances arising from multiple sclerosis. *Acta Neurol Scand* 1984; **70**: 299–306.

Mochizuki H, Saito H. Mesial frontal lobe syndromes: correlations between neurological deficits and radiological localizations. *J Exp Med* 1990; **161**: 231–239.

Morrison J, *et al.* Neural control. In: Abrams P, Andersson K, Brubaker LT, *et al.*, eds. *Incontinence*. Plymouth: Health Publication, 2005: 373–374.

Mouras H, Stoléru S, Bittoun J, *et al.* Brain processing of visual sexual stimuli in healthy men: a functional magnetic resonance imaging study. *Neuroimage* 2003; **20**: 855–869.

Nakayama H, Jørgensen HS, Pedersen PM, Raaschou HO, Olsen TS. Prevalence and risk factors of incontinence after stroke. The Copenhagen Stroke Study. *Stroke* 1997; **28**: 58–62.

Nour S, Svarer C, Kristensen JK, Paulson OB, Law I. Cerebral activation during micturition in normal men. *Brain* 2000; **123**: 781–789.

Panicker JN, Fowler CJ. The bare essentials: uro-neurology. *Pract Neurol* 2010; **10:** 178–185.

Panicker JN, Game X, Khan S, *et al.* The possible role of opiates in women with chronic urinary retention: observations from a prospective clinical study. *J Urol* 2012; **188:** 480–484.

Panicker JN, Nagaraja D, Kovoor JM, Nair KP, Subbakrishna DK. Lower urinary tract dysfunction in acute disseminated encephalomyelitis. *Mult Scler* 2009; **15:** 1118–1122.

Podnar S, Fowler CJ. Sphincter electromyography in diagnosis of multiple system atrophy: technical issues. *Muscle Nerve* 2004; **29**: 151–156.

Podnar S, Oblak C, Vodusek DB. Sexual function in men with cauda equina lesions: a clinical and electromyographic study. *J Neurol Neurosurg Psychiatry* 2002; **73**: 715–720.

Podnar S, Trsinar B, Vodusek DB. Bladder dysfunction in patients with cauda equina lesions. *Neurourol Urodyn* 2006; **25**: 23–31.

Popat R, Apostolidis A, Kalsi V, *et al.* A comparison between the response of patients with idiopathic detrusor overactivity and neurogenic detrusor overactivity to the first intradetrusor injection of botulinum-A toxin. *J Urol* 2005; **174**: 984–989.

Ransmayr GN, Holliger S, Schletterer K, *et al.* Lower urinary tract symptoms in dementia with Lewy bodies, Parkinson disease, and Alzheimer disease. *Neurology* 2008; **70:** 299–303.

Rapp DE, Lucioni A, Katz EE, *et al.* Use of botulinum-A toxin for the treatment of refractory overactive bladder symptoms: an initial experience. *Urology* 2004; **63**: 1071–1075.

Remillard GM, Andermann F, Testa GF, *et al.* Sexual ictal manifestations predominate in women with temporal lobe epilepsy: a finding suggesting sexual dimorphism in the human brain. *Neurology* 1983; **33**: 323–330.

Resnick N, Yalla S. Detrusor hyperactivity with impaired contractile function: an unrecognized but common cause of incontinence in elderly patients. *JAMA* 1987; **257**: 3076–3081.

Resnick N, Yalla S, Laurino E. The pathophysiology of urinary incontinence among institutionalized elderly persons. *N Engl J Med* 1989; **1989**: 1–7.

Saenz de Tejada I, Goldstein I, Azadzoi K, Krane RJ, Cohen RA. Impaired neurogenic and endothelium-mediated relaxation of penile smooth muscle from diabetic men with impotence. *N Engl J Med* 1989; **320**: 1025–1030.

Sakakibara R, Hattori T, Kuwabara S, Yamanishi T, Yasuda K. Micturitional disturbance in patients with Guillain-Barre syndrome. *J Neurol Neurosurg Psychiatry* 1997; **63**: 649–653.

Sakakibara R, Hattori T, Tojo M, *et al.* Micturitional disturbance in myotonic dystrophy. *J Auton Nerv Syst* 1995; **52**: 17–21.

Sakakibara R, Hattori T, Uchiyama T, Yamanishi T. Urinary function in elderly people with and without leukoaraiosis: relation to cognitive and gait function. *J Neurol Neurosurg Psychiatry* 1999; **67:** 658–660.

Sakakibara R, Hattori T, Yasuda K, Yamanishi T. Micturitional disturbance after acute hemispheric stroke: analysis of the lesion site by CT and MRI. *J Neurol Sci* 1996; **137**: 47–56.

Sakakibara R, Shinotoh H, Uchiyama M, *et al.* SPECT imaging of the dopamine transporter with [(123)I]-beta-CIT reveals marked decline of nigrostriatal dopaminergic function in Parkinson's disease with urinary dysfunction. *J Neurol Sci* 2001; **187**: 55–59.

Sakakibara R, Uchiyama T, Lui Z, *et al.* Meningitis-retention syndrome: an unrecognized clinical condition. *J Neurol* 2005; **252**: 1495–1499.

Sakakibara R, Uchida Y, Uchiyama T, Yamanishi T, Hattori T. Reduced cerebellar vermis activation during urinary storage and micturition in multiple system atrophy: 99mTc-labelled ECD SPECT study. *Eur J Neurol* 2004; **11**: 705–708.

Sandel M, Williams KS, Dellapietra L, Derogatis LR. Sexual functioning following traumatic brain injury. *Brain Injury* 1996; **10**: 719–728.

Sipski ML. Sexual function in women with neurologic disorders. *Phys Med Rehabil Clin North Am* 2001; **12**: 79–90.

Sipski ML, Alexander CJ, Rosen RC. Sexual response in women with spinal cord injuries: implications for our understanding of the able bodied. *J Sex Marital Ther* 1999; **25**: 11–22.

Sipski ML, Alexander CJ, Rosen R. Sexual arousal and orgasm in women: effects of spinal cord injury. *Ann Neurol* 2001; **49**: 35–44.

Sipski ML, Behnegar A. Neurogenic female sexual dysfunction: a review. *Clin Auton Res* 2001; **11**: 279–283.

Smith MD, Seth JH, Fowler CJ, Miller RF, Panicker JN. Urinary retention for the neurologist. *Pract Neurol* 2013; **13**: 288–291.

Spark RF, Wills CA, Royal H. Hypogonadism, hyperprolacinaemia, and temporal lobe epilepsy in hyposexual men. *Lancet* 1984; **1**: 413–417.

Swinn MJ, Kitchen ND, Goodwin RJ, Fowler CJ. Sacral neuromodulation for women with Fowler's syndrome. *Eur Urol* 2000; **38**: 439–443.

Tadic SD, Griffiths D, Murrin A, Schaefer W, Aizenstein HJ, Resnick NM. Brain activity during bladder filling is related to white matter structural changes in older women with urinary incontinence. *Neuroimage* 2010; **51**: 1294–1302.

Uchiyama T, Sakakibara R, Hattori T, Yamanishi T. Short-term effect of a single levodopa dose on micturition disturbance in Parkinson's disease patients with the wearing-off phenomenon. *Mov Disord* 2003; **18**: 573–578.

Wade D, Langton Hewer R. Outlook after an acute stroke: urinary incontinence and loss of consciousness compared in 532 patients. *Q J Med* 1985; **56**: 601–608.

Weintraub D, Koester J, Potenza MN, *et al.* Impulse control disorders in Parkinson disease: a cross-sectional study of 3090 patients. *Arch Neurol* 2010; **67**: 589–595.

Winge K, Werdelin LM, Nielse, KK, Stimpel H. Effects of dopaminergic treatment on bladder function in Parkinson's disease. *Neurourol Urodyn* 2004; **23**: 689–696.

Yamamoto T, Sakakibara R, Uchiyama T, Liu Z, Ito T, Awa Y, *et al.* Neurological diseases that cause detrusor hyperactivity with impaired contractile function. *Neurourol Urodyn* 2006; **25**: 356–360.

Zorzon M, Zivadinov R, Bosco A, *et al.* Sexual dysfunction in multiple sclerosis: a case-control study. I. Frequency and comparison of groups. *Mult Scler* 1999; **5**: 418–427.

CHAPTER 26

Systemic Conditions and Neurology

David Werring[1], Robin Howard[2] and Simon Shorvon[1]
[1] UCL Institute of Neurology
[2] National Hospital for Neurology & Neurosurgery

Neurology has developed somewhat separately from the body of general medicine. However, the subjects remain inextricably linked, because diseases of all body systems can profoundly influence the nervous system. About one in five acute medical admissions to district general hospitals in the United Kingdom are caused by neurological illness. General physicians often lack first-hand experience in managing patients with neurological symptoms; neurologists can make important contributions to optimising management, often assisting with accurate diagnosis, appropriate investigation and treatment. Effective communication between neurologists and general physicians is thus critical.

In this context, a working knowledge of the neurological aspects of general medical conditions is invaluable and this chapter aims to summarise neurological manifestations of disorders of other body systems, outlining some basic elements of pathophysiology, diagnosis and management. It is intended neither to be exhaustive, nor a comprehensive and detailed guide to treatment. Rather, we aim to give a broad overview of the range of neurological disease encountered in general medicine.

Aortic and cardiac disorders

The neurological consequences of aortic or cardiac disorders can be devastating. Ischaemic stroke and transient ischaemic attack (TIA) – the main clinical result of embolism from the heart or great vessels – are briefly considered here but also dealt with in detail in Chapter 5. An understanding of the effects of vascular disease of the great vessels and spinal cord requires an understanding of basic vascular anatomy, outlined here.

Aortic pathology

Anatomy

The whole body, including the nervous system, is supplied by the aorta. Disease processes affecting the aorta and surgical instrumentation can therefore cause damage to the brain, spinal cord and peripheral nervous system. The neurological syndrome caused depends more on the part of the aorta affected, rather than the nature of the pathology.

Blood supply

Cerebral The aorta leaves the heart to become the aortic arch; the great vessels supply the brain, brainstem and cervical spinal cord (Figure 26.1). From the heart, the order in which these vessels arise is as follows: innominate (brachiocephalic) artery – continuing as the right subclavian artery and giving rise to the right common carotid; then the left common carotid, and finally the left subclavian artery. Each vertebral artery arises from the subclavian of that side.

Spinal The anterior spinal artery is formed from paired branches arising from the vertebral arteries which descend at the level of the medulla. The anterior spinal artery is joined by radiculo-medullary arteries at various segmental levels. The upper and mid-thoracic anterior spinal artery is generally supplied by a small feeding vessel. The anterior spinal artery at the level of the lumbar enlargement is supplied by a single large vessel, the great anterior medullary artery of Adamkiewicz (Albert Adamkiewicz, 1850–1921, professor of general and experimental pathology, Cracow). This artery usually runs alongside a nerve root on the left side, usually between T9 and L2. The posterior spinal arteries are also formed from the intracranial vertebral arteries rostrally but after their origin become mixed with a posterior pial arterial plexus joined at various levels by posterior radiculo-medullary vessels (Figure 26.2).

Cerebral ischaemia resulting from aortic disease

Aortic disease, such as atherosclerosis, aortitis or aneurysm, can cause cerebral ischaemia (i.e. stroke, TIA and hypoperfusion syndromes). Aortic atheroma is an increasingly recognised source of embolic material to the brain and, although difficult to detect by non-invasive imaging, it can be well visualised by trans-oesophageal echocardiography. Neurological syndromes caused by aortic disease are often indistinguishable from those produced by emboli from other sources.

Steal syndromes can result from occlusive disease of the innominate or subclavian vessels proximal to the origin of a vertebral artery. The left side is three times more likely to be affected than the right, probably because the different vertebral–subclavian angle, predisposes to atheroma. The word steal describes reverse flow, usually in a vertebral artery, typically exacerbated by exercising the ipsilateral arm, thus increasing blood flow to the arm and metabolic

Neurology: A Queen Square Textbook, Second Edition. Edited by Charles Clarke, Robin Howard, Martin Rossor and Simon Shorvon.

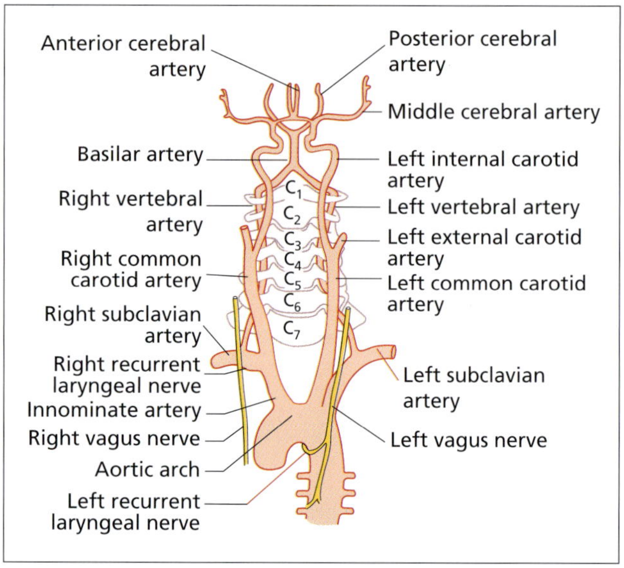

Figure 26.1 Vessels arising from the aorta. Source: Aminoff 1992. Reproduced with permission of Elsevier.

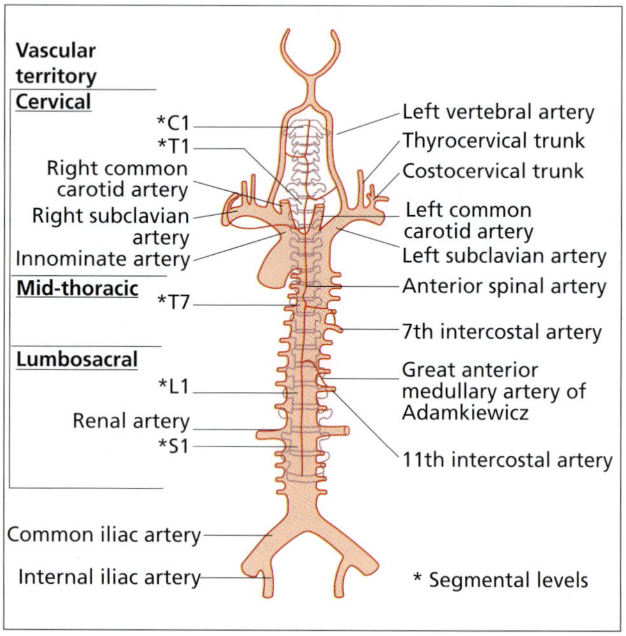

Figure 26.2 Blood supply of the spinal cord. Source: Aminoff 1992. Reproduced with permission of Elsevier.

demand or, less commonly, neck movement. Non-invasive imaging of these phenomena suggests that in the vast majority of cases such a steal is asymptomatic, but surgical or endovascular intervention may be considered if symptoms are troublesome. The term subclavian steal syndrome should only be used if symptoms are present; these are usually of posterior circulation ischaemia including vertigo, visual disturbances and ataxia.

Spinal cord ischaemia resulting from aortic disease

The most common spinal cord ischaemic lesion is an anterior spinal artery syndrome, characterised by loss of spinothalamic sensation (pain and temperature), paralysis (usually bilateral) below the level

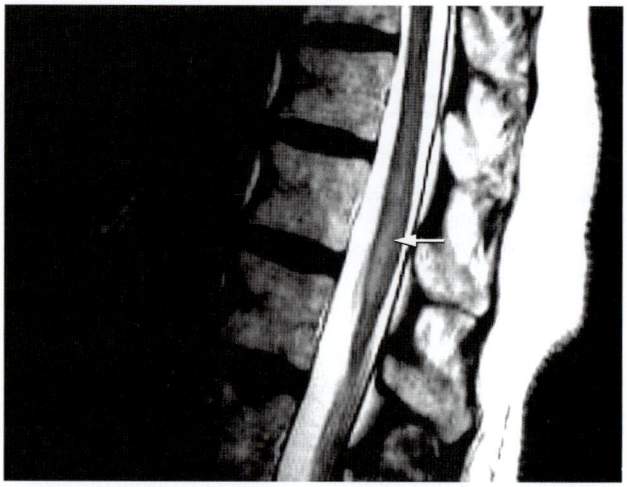

Figure 26.3 Spinal cord infarction. A 60-year-old woman presented with sudden radicular low back pain radiating around the umbilicus with sudden leg weakness and numbness. This progressed over a several hours with loss of sphincter function. T2 coronal MRI shows abnormal high signal in the central portion of the lower dorsal cord (arrow).

of the lesion with preserved dorsal column function (vibration and joint position) and loss of sphincter control. This develops abruptly or evolve over several hours. Clinically, at the onset radicular thoracic pain occurs and is often severe. The cervical spinal cord has a more robust vascular supply than the thoracic and lumbar regions, from collateral feeders, so that cervical cord infarction is uncommon. Very rarely, dissection of the extracranial vertebral arteries can cause cervical cord ischaemia with brachial diplegia and neck pain. The mid to lower thoracic region is selectively vulnerable to ischaemia, and this is the authors' experience, although not confirmed in all studies. Atherosclerosis and thrombo-embolism in the anterior spinal artery is rare; infarction in this territory is often a result of aortic disease or surgery. However, no cause is identified in more than 50% of cases. The diagnosis of spinal infarction is clinical, but magnetic resonance imaging (MRI) shows signal abnormalities in the cord in the majority (Figure 26.3). Diseases of the aorta including atherosclerotic occlusive disease, aortitis, dissection, aneurysms or coarctation can cause spinal cord ischaemia. In order to produce cord ischaemia, the pathological process generally must involve the suprarenal aorta, because the most important radiculomedullary arteries that feed the cord usually originate above this level.

Although the spinal cord syndrome caused will generally be similar regardless of the underlying pathology, patients with dissection of the thoracic aorta present classically with searing interscapular pain, shock and asymmetric arm pulses. The dissection commonly causes ischaemia of the mid-thoracic spinal cord, producing a thoracic sensory level. Cardiac or aortic surgery requiring clamping of the aorta for over half an hour, and aortic angiography, can also cause an anterior spinal artery syndrome. The likelihood of spinal infarction is up to 1 in 10 following a surgical procedure involving the suprarenal aorta, but is rare following infra-renal procedures. In some post-instrumentation cases the mechanism is a cholesterol embolus arising from an atheromatous aorta. Spinal cord ischaemia can result from endovascular stent graft repairs of thoracic and thoraco-abdominal aortic aneurysm. Peri-operative cerebrospinal fluid (CSF) drainage, with augmentation of systemic blood pressure, sometimes has a beneficial role in reducing the risk of paraplegia in patients undergoing surgical or endovascular procedures involving the aorta.

Inflammation of the aorta can cause neurological symptoms directly or indirectly via the development of aneurysms, aortic stenosis or atherosclerosis. Syphilitic aortitis was common prior to the introduction of penicillin but is now rare. It typically affects the thoracic aorta, causing aneurysmal dilatation and cerebral embolism. Atherosclerosis, by contrast, causes aneurysmal dilatation of the abdominal aorta. Takayasu's disease is a large vessel vasculitis that can cause aortitis, typically in female patients under 30 years of age. This rare condition has a pre-pulseless phase with systemic symptoms of fever, weight loss, arthralgia, myalgia, night sweats and chest pain. This develops into the pulseless phase, in which there is occlusion of the major vessels of the aortic arch with aortic regurgitation, aneurysm formation and hypertension. Cerebral ischaemia is uncommon.

Neurological complications of cardiac surgery

Cardiac surgery, particularly coronary artery bypass grafting (CABG) is one of the most common thoracic operations performed in developed countries. Early neurological sequelae include acute stroke (1–5% of patients), delirium and confusion. Later on, an encephalopathy can become apparent. The mechanisms underlying these complications include particulate microemboli and hypoperfusion during surgery and postoperative atrial fibrillation. Embolism is the most common mechanism of postoperative stroke, accounting for some 60% of cases. Pre-existing symptomatic cerebrovascular disease is a strong risk factor for postoperative stroke. Carotid stenosis (asymptomatic or symptomatic) may be identified, leading to the question of intervention. Although carotid stenosis is associated with an increased risk of postoperative stroke, studies show that in most cases it is not directly causal; it is likely that the stenosis is simply one marker of generalised vascular disease. For this reason the management of asymptomatic carotid stenosis pre-operatively is controversial; randomised trials are needed to guide such management decisions. The available data do not support routine intervention in patients with asymptomatic carotid stenosis, but if the stenosis is high grade (>90% or occlusion) or bilateral, intervention may be considered. Generally, in symptomatic patients with carotid stenosis greater than 70% intervention prior to cardiac surgery is recommended. It is not known whether intervention on the carotid is best performed before or simultaneously with the cardiac surgery; some advocate a joint procedure to avoid two potential peri-operative stroke risks. Other complications of cardiac surgery include short- and long-term cognitive impairment, acute delirium and seizures. Cognitive abnormalities of executive function, memory, attention and processing speed occur in between 5–80% of patients in the first few post-operative weeks. The mechanisms underlying such deficits are unknown but it is speculated that changes in perfusion, oxygenation or microparticle embolisation during pump bypass are relevant. The natural history of early cognitive impairment is for resolution over months, but about 25% of patients have detectable long-term deficits on formal psychological testing.

Neurological complications of acquired cardiac disease

Cardiac embolism

Ischaemic stroke is caused by large vessel atherosclerosis and thromboembolism, small vessel occlusion, cardiac embolism and a miscellany of many rarer causes including arterial dissection, haematological abnormalities and metabolic conditions. Cardiac embolism accounts for up to one-quarter of all ischaemic strokes. Clinical and radiological findings suggestive of cardio-embolism include abrupt and maximal deficit at onset (rather than stepwise) and haemorrhagic transformation (because of rapid reperfusion) or multiple vascular territory infarcts on imaging, with an identified potential cardiac source on echocardiography. About 80% of cardiac emboli enter the anterior cerebral vessels; an anterior circulation branch occlusion and striatocapsular infarction is highly suggestive of a cardio-embolic source. Although cardio-embolism to the posterior circulation is less common, certain stroke syndromes are characteristic, including the 'top of the basilar syndrome' (reduced conscious level, visual field loss, limb sensory or motor symptoms) and unilateral posterior cerebral artery occlusion causing hemianopia. Of course, none of these features are specific, and it must be remembered that a definitive diagnosis of cardiac embolism can be difficult in the presence of coexisting large vessel athero-thrombotic or cerebral small vessel disease. Common sources of cardiac embolism are shown in Table 26.1.

Rhythm disturbances

Atrial fibrillation Atrial fibrillation (AF; Chapter 5) is associated with a sixfold increase in stroke risk. There is a cumulative risk of stroke in patients with AF, which can be stratified according to the number of additional factors. Important factors increasing the stroke risk in patients with AF include age, history of previous stroke, hypertension and left ventricular dysfunction. The presence of one or more of these risk factors should lead to strong consideration of anticoagulant treatment, which reduces the risk of stroke by about 70%. Warfarin has recently been shown to be superior to aspirin in older patients as well as those under 75 years of age. In addition to warfarin, non-vitamin K oral anticoagulants (NOACs) are now available, including direct thrombin and factor Xa inhibitors. Large-scale randomised trials indicate that NOACs are as effective as warfarin but with an approximately 50% lower risk of intracranial haemorrhage. Long-term observational data on NOAC use in clinical practice will help more clearly establish their efficacy and safety.

Sick sinus syndrome Sick sinus syndrome is defined by sinus node dysfunction, often idiopathic and common in the older population. Patients are often asymptomatic, although syncope, palpitations or dizziness occur. Rhythm disturbances include sinus bradycardia,

Table 26.1 Common sources of cardiac embolism.

Rhythm disturbances
Atrial fibrillation
Sick sinus syndrome
Cardiomyopathy
Congenital
Acquired – alcohol, recreational drugs (cocaine), amyloid, ischaemic heart disease
Valve disease
Endocarditis
Rheumatic heart disease
Mitral valve prolapse
Prosthetic valves
Structural cardiac lesions
Atrial myxoma
Ventricular aneurysm
Patent foramen ovale
Ventricular akinesia (e.g. following myocardial infarction)

sinus arrest, sino-atrial block and bradycardia–tachycardia syndrome. Cardio-embolic stroke occurs in up to 20% of patients, and is more common in those with tachyarrhythmias. Pacemakers do not definitively reduce the risk of stroke. If atrial fibrillation occurs, anticoagulation should be considered to reduce the risk of stroke.

Cardiomyopathies

Primary cardiomyopathies (i.e. not caused by diseases such as ischaemic heart disease) are associated with arrhythmias and a tendency for stasis of blood within the heart, which can lead to left ventricular thrombus formation and embolism to the brain. Dilated or restrictive types are far more likely to be a cause of embolism than hypertrophic cardiomyopathies, in which cerebral embolism is rare. Primary cardiomyopathies have a genetic component, and family screening is usually indicated. Anticoagulation should be considered in those with a very low ejection fraction (e.g. <30%) because this may help prevent recurrent events.

Valve disease

Infective endocarditis (Chapter 9) is an important cause of embolism to the brain, which occurs in about one-fifth of patients. Usually, emboli occur during active infection, when the patient will usually be systemically unwell with fever, malaise and evidence of emboli to other organs such as the skin, eyes and kidneys. Patient groups at particular risk of endocarditis include those with immunosuppression, intravenous drug use, prosthetic heart valves or structural heart valve disease. Embolic material may cause infection or vasculitis of vessels where septic emboli impact, with or without the development of a mycotic aneurysm (often in the distal branches of the middle cerebral artery). Thus, in a high risk patient evidence of multiple cerebral emboli (or systemc emboli) should alert the physician to the possibility of infective endocarditis. The disease can also cause intracerebral haemorrhage (Figure 26.4). Anticoagulation is not recommended in native valve endocarditis because of the high risk of haemorrhagic complications. However, in the case of prosthetic valve endocarditis anticoagulants may need to be continued, although it is probably safe to discontinue them for 1–2 weeks temporarily. Early cerebral angiography is generally advised in symptomatic haemorrhage to exclude mycotic aneurysm, which can be treated by endovascular methods. Conversely, angiography is probably not necessary in cases of asymptomatic unruptured mycotic aneurysms. Because endocarditis often remains undetected by blood cultures and even echocardiography, a high index of suspicion is needed in any patient with unexplained haemorrhagic or ischaemic stroke and a cardiac murmur. Cerebral microbleeds, small rounded lesions best seen on blood-sensitive MRI (e.g. T2*gradient echo or susceptibility-weighted sequences), are common in infective endocarditis and may provide another diagnostic clue. Meningeal involvement is common in endocarditis, and CSF analysis, if safe following careful clinical and radiological assessment, will suggest the diagnosis if a markedly high polymorph count is found (>100 cells/mm^3). Rheumatic fever can also cause valvular damage leading to embolism to the brain, particularly if the mitral valve is affected or atrial fibrillation develops during the illness. Sydenham's chorea is discussed in Chapter 6.

Atrial myxoma

The diagnosis of atrial myxoma is challenging. A myriad of symptoms can occur, and this often leads to long delays in diagnosis and treatment. About 30% of atrial myxomas cause cerebral emboli – accounting for about 0.4% of all strokes and stroke is the most common neurological presentation (Figure 26.5). The majority of patients (up to 90%) present with constitutional symptoms of fatigue, fever, myalgia, arthralgia and weight loss. Cardiac symptoms are often present and include breathlessness in association with congestive failure and syncope. Investigations show elevated erythrocyte sedimentation rate (ESR) and C-reactive protein (CRP), anaemia and thrombocytosis or thrombocytopenia. Chest X-ray shows left

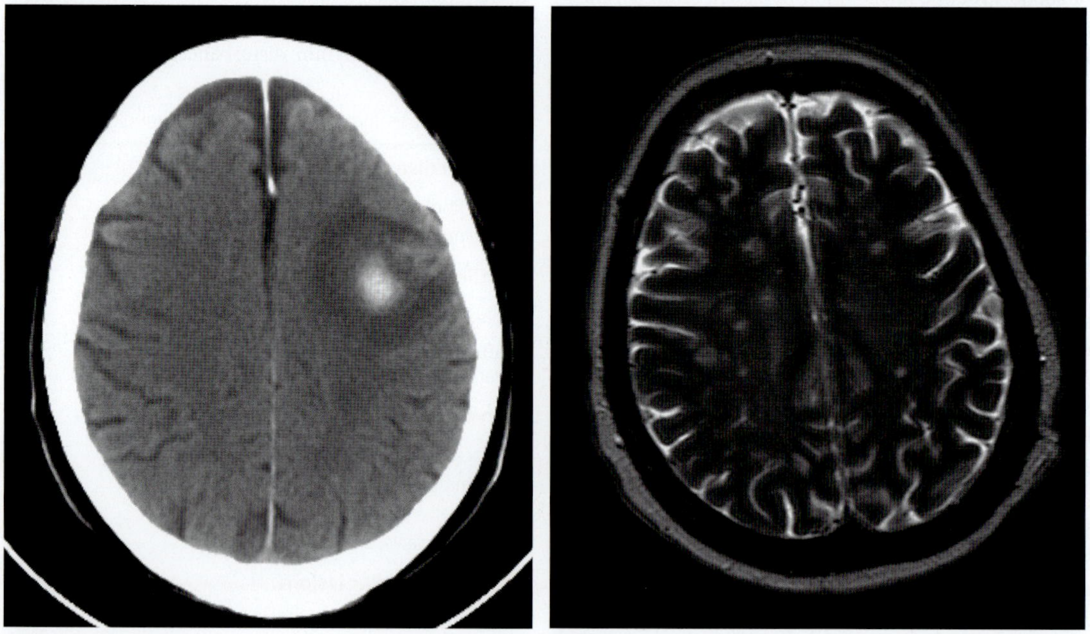

(a) (b)

Figure 26.4 Bacterial endocarditis. (a) Left frontal intracerebral haemorrhage in a patient with bacterial endocarditis and sudden non-fluent dysphasia. Haemorrhage may have come from a ruptured mycotic aneurysm, although no aneurysm was detected on formal angiography in this case. (b) Scattered foci of high signal caused by disseminated septic emboli caused by endocarditis (T1 axial images).

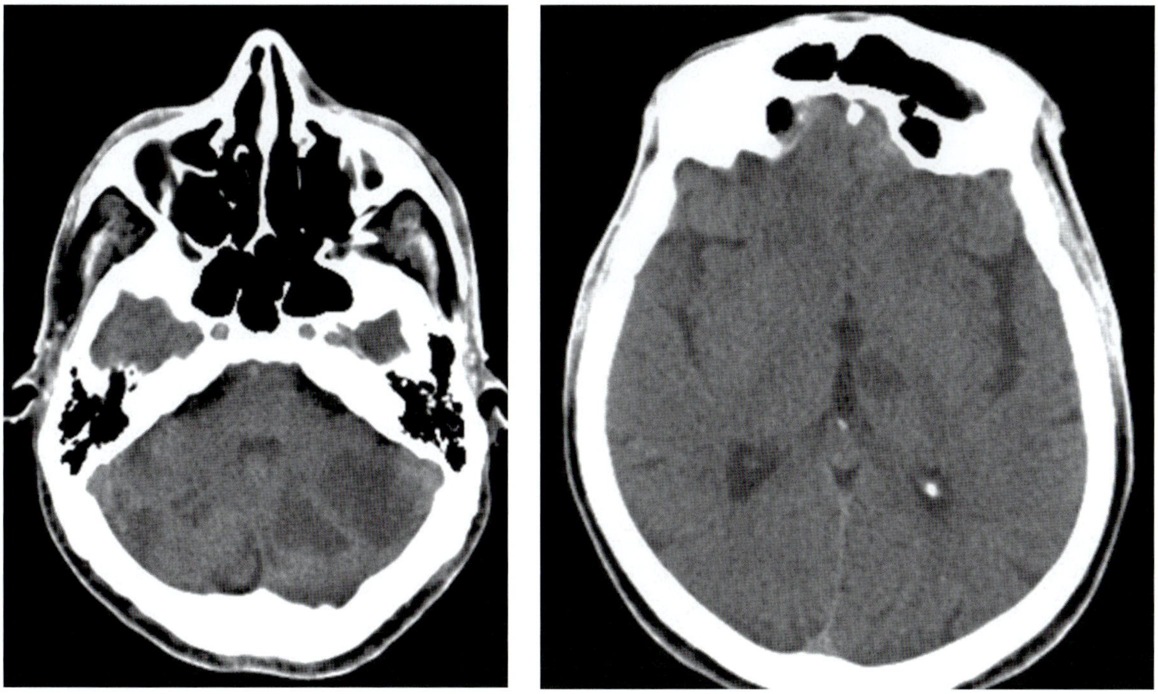

Figure 26.5 Axial CT brain scans from a patient with an atrial myxoma showing low attenuation in both cerebellar hemispheres and the left thalamus resulting from embolic material.

atrial or ventricular enlargement and occasionally intracardiac tumour calcification. Echocardiography is the investigation of choice, but transthoracic studies have a false negative rate of about 20%. For this reason, if clinical suspicion is high, transoesophageal echocardiography must be performed.

Stroke can result from embolic tumour fragments rather than fibrin thrombus, so anticoagulation may not be helpful and is probably best avoided, particularly as delayed cerebral aneurysm formation, often fusiform, in distal branches, can lead to cerebral haemorrhage. The treatment of atrial myxoma is optimisation of cardiac function and urgent surgical removal. Follow-up with transoesophageal echocardiography is recommended as recurrence can occur, especially within the first 2 years – but occasionally more than 10 years later.

Endocrine conditions

Thyroid disorders

Thyroid disorders can have a major impact on neurological function; they affect any part of the central nervous system (CNS), peripheral nerves or muscle, mainly via high or low levels of circulating T4 and T3 or immune-mediated damage. It is especially important to recognise neurological manifestations of thyroid disease, as the symptoms will usually respond to appropriate treatment.

Hyperthyroidism

Hyperthyroidism is most often brought about by immune mechanisms (Graves' disease), but other causes include thyroiditis, multinodular goitre or, rarely, pituitary tumours. A myopathy is present to some extent in almost all patients with hyperthyroidism, although this may be asymptomatic. The onset is usually subacute, with proximal limb muscles typically affected, leading to difficulties ascending stairs, rising from a chair and raising the arms. Bulbar involvement is less common, although this may be a prominent feature in the rare acute form of thyrotoxic myopathy. Pain is common. Clinical findings are of proximal wasting especially involving shoulder and pelvic girdle muscles including quadriceps with hyper-reflexia but usually normal tone. The investigation findings usually include a normal creatine kinase (CK), in contrast to the raised CK of hypothyroid myopathy; electromyographic (EMG) abnormalities are seen, such as polyphasic motor potentials and sometimes a decrement in compound muscle action potential (CMAP) on repetitive stimulation. Rarely, hyperthyroidism is associated with a form of hypokalaemic periodic paralysis, a condition seen particularly in South-East Asia (Chapter 10).

Thyroid disease is strongly associated with myasthenia gravis, probably because susceptible individuals are genetically predisposed to autoimmune disorders. About 10% of patients with myasthenia have a thyroid disorder, more commonly hyperthyroidism than hypothyroidism.

Hyperthyroidism can occasionally cause a dramatic upper motor neurone syndrome, particularly affecting the legs, with spasticity, weakness, clonus and extensor plantars. This can cause diagnostic confusion by mimicking spinal cord compression. A mixed upper and lower motor neurone picture can also be present causing an amyotrophic lateral sclerosis-like presentation.

Tremor is a near-invariable feature of hyperthyroidism, often most apparent in the outstretched arms. Myoclonus, chorea and even parkinsonism have also been described.

Peripheral neuropathy is an uncommon but described feature of hyperthyroidism. A flaccid paraparesis with areflexia rarely occurs (Basedow's paraplegia).

Thyroid eye disease is a common feature of Graves' disease, occurring in up to 70% of patients depending on criteria used. The features of Graves' ophthalmopathy are lid retraction, inflammation of orbital soft tissues, causing redness and swelling of the lids and conjunctivae, proptosis, extraocular muscle involvement causing ophthalmoplegia, corneal damage and, rarely, optic nerve compression.

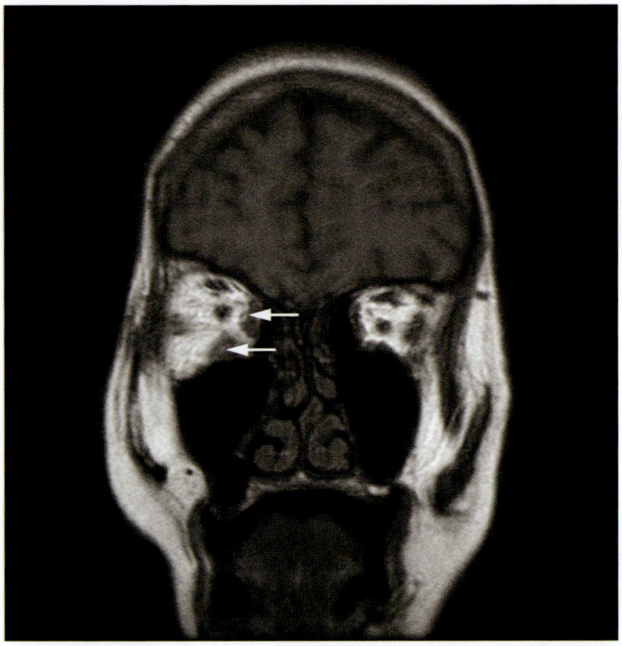

Figure 26.6 Graves' disease. Graves' disease with progressive diplopia and restriction of right eye movements. MRI shows enlarged inferior and medial recti on the right (arrows).

MRI or CT scanning are helpful in showing enlarged extraocular muscles, particularly the medial and inferior recti (Figure 26.6). Although usually both eyes are affected, some patients have markedly asymmetric involvement. Treatment includes steroids, botulinum toxin, radiotherapy or surgery.

Hyperthyroid encephalopathy is now rare, but can occur in untreated patients, after radio-iodine treatment, during intercurrent illness or following surgical procedures. Florid signs of thyrotoxicosis, confusion, agitation, fever, seizures and upper motor neurone signs may all be present. Mortality from this disorder remains high.

Hypothyroidism

Hypothyroidism, resulting from immune-mediated mechanisms or following surgical or radiotherapy thyroid ablation, is an important treatable cause of neurological dysfunction affecting many parts of the nervous system.

An encephalopathy characterised by slowness, lethargy and impaired attention is commonly seen in hypothyroidism. In its most severe form, myxoedema coma, there is a substantial mortality if not recognised early and treated. Clinical features of myxoedema coma include hypothermia, depressed conscious level and usually a precipitating event such as sepsis or trauma. Early recognition and treatment with thyroid replacement (T4 and T3), antibiotics and steroids are often life-saving.

Hypothyroidism should be carefully excluded in all patients presenting with any dementing illness, because it is so readily amenable to treatment. Neuropsychiatric features can also occur, for example psychosis with paranoia and hallucinations (myxoedema madness).

Cerebellar ataxia is well described and does occur, if rarely, in hypothyroidism, involving gait and the limbs, but with normal eye movements. Muscular weakness is common in hypothyroidism and sometimes an early clinical feature; it occurs in some 80% of cases if carefully sought. Weakness (usually fairly mild) is accompanied by depressed or slow-relaxing reflexes (pseudomyotonia), and typically involves the pelvic and shoulder girdles. Percussion of the muscle may cause a slow rippling effect termed myoedema. Pain during or following muscle activity is typical of hypothyroid myopathy, and all patients presenting with unexplained muscle pains, especially related to exertion, should be screened for hypothyroidism; early treatment prevents development of more severe symptoms. The CK level is usually raised, sometimes markedly so (<10 times normal). Treatment with thyroxine improves the weakness, usually promptly but in advanced cases it is sometimes over a year before the situation recovers fully.

Hypothyroidism also causes peripheral nerve problems. An entrapment neuropathy, most frequently carpal tunnel syndrome, is seen in some 10% of hypothyroid patients. A useful working rule is to check the thyroid function in all patients with suspected carpal tunnel syndrome. Treatment is restoration of the euthyroid state rather than surgical decompression. A polyneuropathy develops in up to two-thirds of hypothyroid patients, usually mild and mainly sensory.

Neurological aspects of Hashimoto's thyroiditis

The possible relationship between thyroid antibodies and encephalopathy has been debated since the 1960s. The term Hashimoto's encephalopathy describes a subacute, sometimes relapsing encephalopathy, responding well to corticosteroids and associated with a high titre of antithyroid antibodies. The encephalopathy in such cases is not explained by thyroid status, which may be normal. The term Hashimoto's encephalopathy has been criticised as it implies that the antibodies are pathogenic in the development of encephalopathy, a link for which there is little convincing evidence. It has been suggested that the thyroid antibodies may be epiphenomena, and indeed they may be seen in encephalopathies known to have an alternative cause. It is therefore important to try to establish a definitive diagnosis for an encephalopathy associated with antithyroid antibodies. For example, the syndromes of encephalopathy with antibodies to voltage-gated potassium channels or *N*-methyl-D-aspartate (NMDA) receptors, or amyloid-beta related angiitis, may also need to be considered. Sometimes, invasive tests including cerebral biopsy are needed to exclude treatable causes of encephalopathy.

Diabetes mellitus

Diabetes mellitus can cause multiple effects on the nervous system. Rare congenital causes of diabetes that may be encountered by neurologists include mitochondrial cytopathies, particularly patients with sensorineural deafness but also those with MELAS or Kearns–Sayre syndrome (Chapter 10), Friedreich's ataxia and Wolfram's syndrome (type 1 diabetes, diabetes insipidus, optic atrophy and deafness [DIDMOAD]). The other main neurological conditions associated with diabetes are acute metabolic disturbances (related to hyperglycaemia or hypoglycaemia) and the diabetic neuropathies.

Acute metabolic disturbances

Diabetic ketoacidosis occurs because of insufficient insulin levels in patients with type 1 diabetes, usually because of undertreatment with insulin or its omission, with or without an intercurrent illness such as sepsis. Drowsiness occurs but not usually coma. Very rarely, cerebral oedema can develop during treatment because of over-rapid correction of hyperosmolality, especially in children. This can cause death from raised intracranial pressure (ICP). Hyper-osmolar non-ketotic coma (HONK) occurs mainly in patients with type 2 diabetes and can lead to very high blood glucose with high sodium levels and therefore high osmolality. Reduced conscious level or seizures also occur. Conversely, low blood glucose can result from excessive doses of oral hypoglycaemics or insulin. With a low blood sugar, there is often a warning prodrome, allowing the patient to react and correct the problem, but in some patients with type 1 diabetes the warning is absent, placing them at much greater risk of prolonged hypoglycaemia. Early warning symptoms include sweating, trembling, tingling hands and palpitations. Neurological features include confusion, dysarthria, altered behaviour and agitation, seizures and, albeit rarely, focal neurological features (e.g. hemiparesis or hemiplegia) that can mimic a TIA or stroke. If profound hypoglycaemia is unrecognised coma and permanent hypoglycaemic brain injury can occur.

Diabetic neuropathies

The neuropathies caused by diabetes are covered in detail in Chapter 10. The most common is a distal sensorimotor neuropathy, affecting over 50% of patients with long-standing disease. Rarer variants include diabetic autonomic neuropathy, acute painful neuropathy, cranial neuropathy (especially oculomotor), thoraco-abdominal neuropathy and painful proximal neuropathy (diabetic amyotrophy).

Pituitary disorders

Pituitary tumours are discussed in Chapter 21. Pituitary neoplasms either produce an excess of hormone secretion (in about two-thirds) or are non-functioning – sometimes causing deficiency by mass effects (in about one-third). Tumours secreting prolactin (prolactinomas) cause secondary amenorrhoea, galactorrhoea, infertility and impotence. Other clinical syndromes include acromegaly (resulting from growth hormone secretion) and Cushing's disease (resulting from adenocorticotrophic hormone [ACTH] secretion). Patients with pituitary tumours can present with visual disturbances, including visual failure, headaches, and endocrine features, or simply with an unexplained high serum prolactin level. Non-secreting tumours cause hypopituitarism, with secondary amenorrhoea, infertility or impotence, loss of secondary sexual characteristics or hypothyroidism.

Diabetes insipidus results from dysfunction of the posterior pituitary. Reduced secretion of arginine vasopressin and antidiuretic hormone cause symptoms of thirst, polyuria and polydipsia. The common causes are trauma, tumours, sarcoidosis and other granulomatous conditions, and infections.

Pituitary apoplexy (Sheehan's syndrome) is a dramatic clinical syndrome of severe headache, nausea, vomiting and often hypotensive collapse with sudden bilateral visual loss. The usual cause is haemorrhage into a pituitary macroadenoma.

Inappropriate antidiuretic hormone secretion and cerebral salt wasting

Inappropriate antidiuretic hormone secretion (SIADH) and cerebral salt wasting are discussed in Chapter 20.

Parathyroid disorderss

In cases of hypoparathyroidism (or pseudohypoparathyroidism, a rare familial form with skeletal and developmental anomalies), the reduction in serum ionic calcium causes sensory disturbances, tetany, chorea or seizures (Table 26.2); basal ganglia or cerebellar calcification may also occur. Hyperparathyroidism resulting from parathyroid adenoma or hyperplasia causes muscle weakness, fatiguability and amyotrophy with preserved reflexes, and has been reported on occasion to resemble motor neurone disease.

Adrenal disorders

Cushing's disease Cushing's disease results from pituitary hypersecretion of ACTH and thus high plasma cortisol, most often from a pituitary microadenoma. Cushing's syndrome is the result of treatment with exogenous steroids or primary hyperadrenalism and ACTH levels are low. Clinically, the disease and the syndrome are indistinguishable, both being characterised by centripetal obesity, hypertension, hirsutism, abdominal striae, acne, menstrual irregularity, immunosuppression, myopathy and psychosis. Cushing's disease is usually caused by a microadenoma that typically does not cause visual symptoms.

Addison's disease

Addison's is caused by adrenal insufficiency. In the past, tuberculosis was a common cause, but now an autoimmune mechanism is the cause in most cases. A rare cause is adrenoleukodystrophy, in which brain and spinal cord involvement results in other neurological features of varying severity (Chapter 19). The important features of Addison's disease are a tendency to faint, episodes of unexplained coma or episodes of stupor, weight loss, apathy and vomiting with pigmentation of the skin and mucous membranes. Addison's disease can be mistaken for 'ME'. The condition can be life-threatening, especially during intercurrent illnesses. The laboratory findings are of low serum sodium, high potassium and low serum cortisol and high ACTH. Primary adrenal failure (Addison's disease) needs to be differentiated from secondary causes of ACTH deficiency, both iatrogenic and resulting from pituitary failure.

Phaeochromocytoma Phaeochromocytoma is a neuroendocrine catecholamine secreting tumour of the adrenal medulla and is an important cause of hypertension, especially in younger people. Tumours are often multiple and sometimes extramedullary (paragangliomas). Other clinical features include panic, anxiety, palpitations, headaches and weight loss. Neurological features are rare, but can include those of accelerated hypertension, including intracranial haemorrhage and hypertensive encephalopathy.

Electrolyte disturbances

Electrolyte abnormalities are extremely common in acute and outpatient practice; their effects range from being asymptomatic to causing profound disturbance of function in the central and peripheral nervous systems. As a general principle, the clinical severity of any electrolyte disturbance is greatest when the abnormality has developed rapidly. Treatment is aimed at not only correcting the electrolyte disturbance itself, but also identifying and treating the cause. The CNS effects of electrolyte imbalance, often including altered consciousness and seizures, are related to fluid shifts and brain volume changes. Serum hyperosmolality causes brain shrinkage, while hypo-osmolality causes brain swelling. Other mechanisms include disordered transmembrane potentials and neurotransmission. The clinical features of abnormalities in serum sodium, potassium, calcium and magnesium are summarised in Table 26.2 and are briefly discussed here.

Sodium

Neurological effects of sodium disturbances are covered in detail in Chapter 20. SIADH is a consequence of a number of intracerebral pathologies including meningo-encephalitis or subarachnoid haemorrhage. Because the diagnosis can be made only when the serum is dilute and the urine inappropriately concentrated, osmolality

Table 26.2 Causes and features of common electrolyte disturbances.

Electrolyte disturbance	Some causes	Neurological features
Hyponatraemia	SIADH Cerebral salt wasting Diuretic use Diarrhoea, vomiting Addison's disease Drug induced (e.g. carbamazepine, antidepressants, tobutamide) Liver disease Cardiac failure Psychogenic polydipsia	Coma Confusion Convulsions (<115 mmol/L)
Hypernatraemia	Diabetes insipidus HONK Diarrhoea Dehydration Sweating, inadequate water intake Cushing's syndrome, Conn's syndrome	Reduced conscious level Seizures Tremor Movement disorders
Hypokalaemia	Diarrhoea Vomiting Renal tubular disease Drug/toxin induced (e.g. alcohol, diuretics, antibiotics, theophylline, steroids, laxatives) Diabetic ketoacidosis	Generalised muscle weakness
Hyperkalaemia	Renal disease Addison's disease Drug induced Excessive intake Burns Metaboic acidoisis	Generalised muscle weakness ECG changes Cardiac arrest
Hypocalcaemia	Hypoparathyroidism Vitamin D deficiency Chronic renal failure Pseudohypoparathyroidism Eating disorders Acute pancreatitis, septic shock Magnesium deficiency	Paraesthesias Tetany Seizures, chorea Encephalopathy Papilloedema and ICP Coma
Hypercalcaemia	Hyperparathyroidism Other endocrine diseases Osteolytic bone malignancy Immobility Sarcoidosis Drug induced Vitamin D intoxication Renal disease	Anorexia, abdominal pain Nausea Fatigue Reduced conscious level Constipation Myoclonus, rigidity Elevated CSF protein
Hypomagnesaemia	Rarely isolated – usually part of complex electrolyte derangement Calcium deficiency states	
Hypermagnesaemia	Renal disease Iatrogenic (e.g. treatment of eclamptic seizures)	

CSF, cerebrospinal fluid; ECG, electrocardiography; HONK, hyper-osmolar non-ketotic coma; ICP, intracerebral pressure; SIADH, syndrome of inappropriate antidiuretic hormone.

measurements are critical in the evaluation of hyponatraemia. The over-rapid correction of chronic hyponataemia can cause the distinct syndrome of central pontine myelinolysis (Chapter 20); the fully developed syndrome of a quadriparesis with brainstem signs carries a high mortality. This syndrome is more common in high risk groups such as alcoholics.

Hyponatraemia can be a clue to the development of limbic encephalitis associated with antibodies against voltage-gated potassium channels. This syndrome is associated with SIADH and consequent hyponatraemia.

Potassium

Patients with hyperkalaemia or hypokalaemia do not usually present to neurologists. However, both conditions are features of periodic paralysis (Chapters 3 and 10), and whatever the cause, the main neurological effect of low (or sometimes high) serum potassium is muscle weakness. Serum potassium must always be checked in anyone with weakness.

Calcium and magnesium

Disturbances of calcium metabolism sometimes present to a neurologist and should be sought in patients with tetany, seizures or occasionally chorea. Tetany is the classic clinical manifestation of acute hypocalcaemia, reflecting neuromuscular irritability. Symptoms of tetany include tingling or numbness (peri-oral or in the hands and feet), muscle cramps and, when severe, carpopedal spasm, laryngospasm, seizures or generalised tonic muscle contractions. Less specific symptoms include fatigue, hyperirritability, anxiety and depression, and some patients, even with severe hypocalcaemia, have no neuromuscular symptoms. Key causes of hypocalcaemia are hypoparathyroidism, pseudohypoparathyroidism and vitamin D deficiency. Chronic hypocalcaemia can lead to calcification in the basal ganglia, usually found coincidentally on imaging. Treatment of severe symptomatic acute tetany (e.g. carpopedal spasm seizures) is with intravenous calcium. For milder symptoms of neuromuscular irritability (paresthesias), oral calcium supplementation may be sufficient. Vitamin D deficiency must be corrected.

Isolated hypomagnaesaemia is uncommon. Clinical manifestations of hypomagnesaemia overlap with those of hypocalcaemia and include features of neuromuscular hyperexcitability (e.g. tetany, convulsions), weakness, apathy, delirium and coma. Encephalographic (ECG) changes include QRS complex widening, peaking of T waves and, with more severe hypomagnesaemia, PR prolongation and arrhythmias. Abnormalities of calcium metabolism, including hypocalcaemia and hypoparathyroidism, may be associated. Hypomagnesaemia may be a feature of eclamptic seizures and should be treated in this context.

Haematological disorders

This section considers anaemias, haematological proliferative disorders, bleeding diatheses and coagulation disorders. Haematological disorders and stroke are discussed in Chapter 5 and are briefly mentioned here.

Anaemias

Anaemias generally cause rather non-specific symptoms including fatigue, dizziness, impaired concentration, faintness and syncope, irritability and headache; a full blood count should always be performed to exclude anaemia as a cause of these symptoms, and those of chronic daily headache. Occasionally, severe anaemia (less than 8 g/dL) can cause focal neurological deficits, and TIAs (usually in the presence of a significant atherosclerotic stenosis in an extracranial or intracranial vessel). Iron deficiency anaemia has been reported to be associated with idiopathic intracranial hypertension, with response to treatment of the anaemia. Iron deficiency is also associated with the restless leg syndrome (Chapters 6 and 20), sometimes with normal haemoglobin but a reduced serum ferritin level. Retinal haemorrhages are sometimes seen with very severe anaemias, especially with B_{12} deficiency.

Vitamin B_{12} deficiency, one cause of megaloblastic anaemia, is an important and potentially treatable cause of neurological symptoms and signs and discussed in detail elsewhere (Chapters 16 and 19). Vitamin B_{12} deficiency can cause many different neurological syndromes: peripheral neuropathy with or without myelopathy (together known as subacute combined degeneration of the cord), encephalopathy, dementia, optic neuropathy and ophthalmoplegia. Folic acid can mask the anaemia without preventing the neurological sequelae. Before the discovery of vitamin B_{12}, subacute combined degeneration of the cord was fatal. Treatment is with long-term hydrocobalamin injections. Measurement of serum homocysteine should be carried out if the serum vitamin B_{12} level is non-diagnostic and there is clinical suspicion of deficiency. Nitrous oxide exposure and low serum copper are also rare causes of a syndrome resembling subacute combined degeneration of the cord.

Sickle cell disease causes neurological symptoms from intravascular sickling of erythrocytes via a number of mechanisms including large vessel arteriopathy, small perforating vessel occlusion, haemolysis, abnormal vasomotor tone and promotion of a hypercoagulable state. The incidence of stroke in sickle cell disease is much higher than in the general population. Sickling is exacerbated by low oxygen saturation and/or intercurrent illness. Small vessels can be occluded to cause subcortical infarction (usually not acutely symptomatic) while large vessels (especially the supraclinoid intracranial internal carotid and proximal middle cerebral arteries) can develop intimal proliferation causing stenosis and thrombo-embolism (often symptomatic). In patients with overt large artery stroke there is commonly distal collateral formation (secondary Moyamoya changes). Subacute or chronic symptoms include headaches, which may be migrainous, and cognitive impairment caused by the accumulation of ischaemic damage. Haemorrhagic complications of sickle cell disease can occur in adults, especially subarachnoid haemorrhage. Neurological symptoms have been found to occur in some 25% of patients with sickle cell disease, while up to one-third have imaging evidence of cerebrovascular disease. Migrainous headaches are common. Treatments available to prevent the neurological consequences of sickle cell disease include partial-exchange transfusion, hydroxyurea and bone marrow transplantation.

Thalassaemia is a rare cause of neurological symptoms. Haematopoeisis outside the marrow occurs in lymphoid tissue, spleen, liver and bone. Myelopathy has been described and attributed to haematopoietic tissue in the epidural space. Corticosteroids, radiotherapy, blood transfusions and surgical decompression have been used in this situation.

Proliferative conditions

Leukaemias

Leukaemia can cause neurological symptoms by direct infiltration of nervous tissue or indirectly by haemorrhage related to low platelets, from infection resulting from impaired immunity, electrolyte disturbances or hyperviscosity.

Leukaemic cells enter the nervous system by haematogenous seeding, lymphatic spread or direct invasion by spread along the meninges. Meningeal leukaemia is most commonly associated with acute lymphocytic leukaemia (ALL) and presents as a subacute meningitic syndrome with headache, drowsiness, neck stiffness, irritability and cranial neuropathy, especially affecting the optic, oculomotor, abducens, facial and vestibulocochlear nerves. Papilloedema is commonly seen. Raised CSF protein may impair CSF resorption leading to hydrocephalus. The CSF contains leukaemic cells and usually a high protein, although repeated lumbar puncture may be needed to establish a diagnosis.

Solid leukaemic deposits may occur in any part of the CNS, although the brain is more commonly affected than the spine. Peripheral nerve involvement is unusual.

Plasma cell dyscrasias

Plasma cell dyscrasias are conditions resulting from the proliferation of a single clone of immunoglobulin-secreting plasma cells (activated B cells). The antibodies secreted by the proliferating clone are classified into IgM, IgG and IgA types according to their heavy-chain class, from which are derived various terms including monoclonal gammopathy, M-protein and other paraproteins. All patients with neuropathy should be tested for a paraprotein.

The plasma cell dyscrasias include myeloma (multiple myeloma and osteosclerotic myeloma), Waldenstrom's macroglobulinaemia, monoclonal gammopathy of undetermined significance (MGUS), plasmacytoma and plasma cell leukaemia.

Multiple myeloma affects bones causing pain, fractures and sometimes compression of neural tissue. Myeloma involving the vertebrae is a common cause of spinal cord compression; the development of the paraparesis is usually preceded by back pain for several months. The cauda equina and nerve roots are sometimes compromised by direct infiltration. Meningeal involvement can also cause cranial neuropathies; occasionally such meningeal infiltration may be the only manifestation of myeloma. A peripheral neuropathy can result from a paraneoplastic mechanism, amyloid deposition compromising nerve blood supply or direct infiltration of nerves.

Waldenstrom's macroglobulinaemia is a a syndrome secondary to lymphoplasmacytoid lymphoma, causing hyperviscosity associated with an IgM gammopathy; it involves the nervous system in about 25% of cases. A progressive sensori-motor neuropathy results from IgM antibody binding and/or lymphocytic infiltration. The hyperviscosity can cause focal neurological deficits including strokes and an encephalopathy with headache. Patients also have a bleeding tendency and may develop bruising, purpura and subarachnoid haemorrhage. The Bing–Neel syndrome describes CNS infiltration by neoplastic lymphoplasmacytoid and plasma cells with or without CSF hyperglobulinaemia. The increased blood viscosity caused by cellular infiltration impairs circulation through small vessels in the brain and the eye causing central venous thrombosis. The abnormal cells may involve the brain parenchyma, leptomeninges, dura and/or CSF. Patients present with a variety of neurological symptoms and signs including seizures, hearing loss, cognitive impairment, gait instability and lower limb weakness. It is important to distinguish the condition from CNS involvement resulting from hyperviscosity, vasculitis or malignant transformation. Treatment of the underlying lymphoma includes systemic or intrathecal chemotherapy and cranial irradiation.

MGUS is a benign condition, but some patients ultimately develop a malignant plasma cell dyscrasia; the paraprotein level should be monitored 6–12 monthly. A chronic inflammatory demyelinating peripheral neuropathy (CIDP) may be associated.

Lymphomas

Lymphoma, both of Hodgkin's and non-Hodgkin's type, can affect the nervous system. Usually, patients will have evidence of lymphoma elsewhere and the disease spreads directly to CNS tissue (Figure 26.7). Spinal cord disease (solid tumours) and meningeal infiltration are common manifestations of lymphoma. Extradural deposits compromise the blood supply of the cord to cause an ischaemic myelopathy or exert a direct compressive effect. The cauda equina and lumbosacral roots can be infiltrated causing

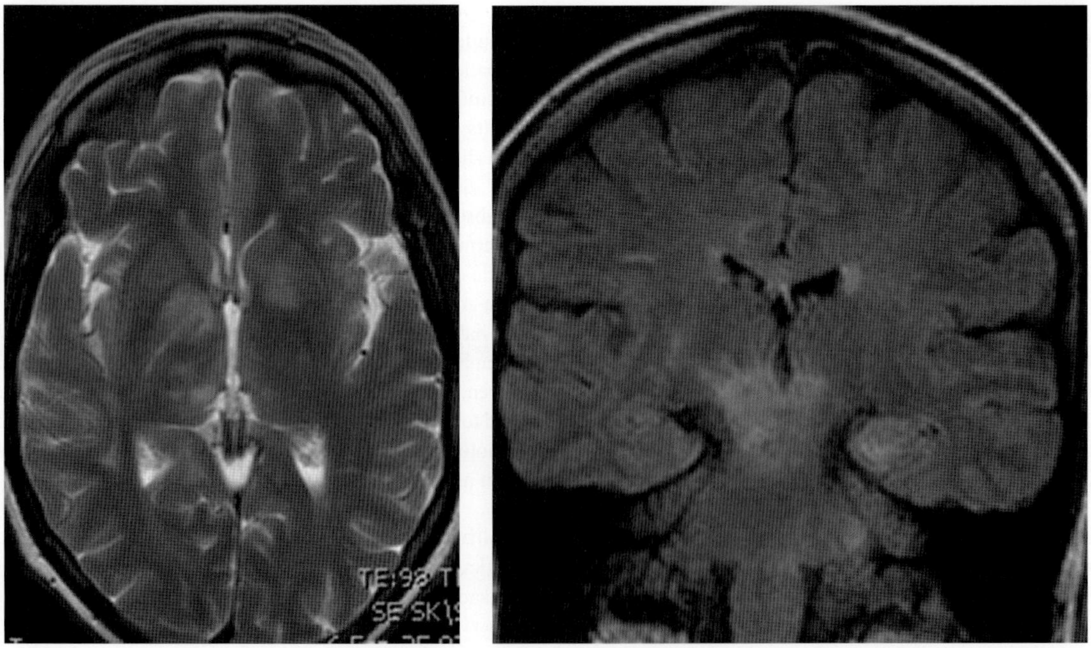

Figure 26.7 Metastatic intracerebral lymphoma. Axial T2 and coronal T1 MRI scans showing multiple hypointense intracranial lesions affecting both grey and white matter structures including the temporal lobes, brainstem and cerebellum.

painful radicular syndromes. Meningeal lymphoma can have a chronic clinical course, sometimes with spontaneous temporary remission. The hemispheres, cerebellum or brainstem may be infiltrated to cause focal signs and elevated ICP. A number of lymphoma-associated paraneoplastic syndromes have been described, including peripheral neuropathy, necrotising myelopathy, leukoencephalopathy and polymyositis.

Primary CNS lymphomas are rare, constituting only 1% of primary brain neoplasms (Figure 26.8). They are typically of B-cell origin and affect principally individuals with impaired immunity, including transplant recipients, patients with HIV and inherited immunodeficiency disorders. The tumours are usually ill-defined lesions in the cerebral hemispheres, ventricles, corpus callosum, basal ganglia and cerebellum. Lymphoma can respond dramatically but temporarily to corticosteroids in the early stages, which can cause diagnostic confusion. Lymphoma also presents with focal symptoms or encephalopathy and/or seizures and nodular enhancing lesions in the ventricular wall. Intravascular lymphoma is a rare subtype of large B-cell lymphoma that is characterised by the proliferation of lymphoma cells within the lumina of small blood vessels, particularly capillaries and post-capillary venules, without an obvious extravascular tumor mass or detectable circulating lymphoma cells in the peripheral blood (Figure 26.9).

The differential diagnosis of cerebral lymphoma is wide and includes metastatic carcinoma, glioma, tuberculosis, toxoplasmosis, neuro-cysticercosis and sarcoidosis. A tissue diagnosis is usually essential. For a more detailed discussion of primary CNS lymphoma see Chapter 21.

Langerhans cell histiocytosis

Langerhans cell histiocytosis (LCH) is a histiocytic cell disorder that occurs in all age groups. Histiocytes are derived from macrophages or dendritic cells in the skin and mucosa. LCH is characterised by single or multiple osteolytic bone lesions which may be associated with extraskeletal lesions affecting multiple organs and the CNS.

The most frequent site of lytic bone lesions are the skull, particularly involving the calvaria, maxillofacial bones and the sella affecting the hypothalamus–pituitary axis. Patients with LCH present with localised bony pain, skull or facial swelling, hearing loss, seizures or

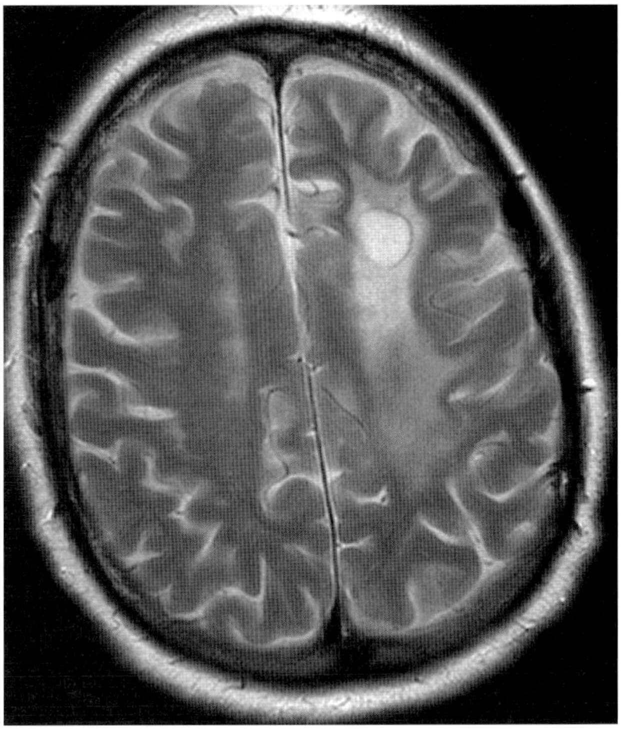

Figure 26.9 Intravascular cerebral B-cell lymphoma. Axial T2 MRI showing extensive white matter high signal and haemorrhage.

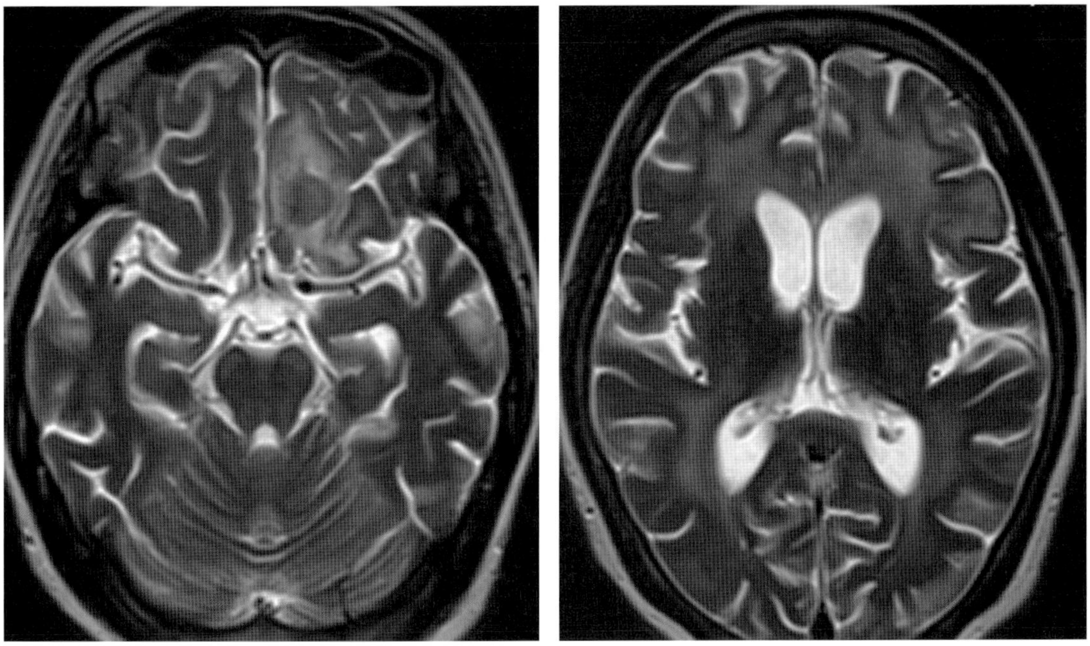

Figure 26.8 Intracerebral B-cell lymphoma. Left inferior frontal lesion with extensive, diffuse signal change in cerebral white matter and diffuse volume loss (MRI T2-weighted images).

cranial nerve palsies. Involvement of the CNS is particularly associated with the presence of bone lesions affecting the anterior or middle cranial fossa. There may be ataxia, cognitive dysfunction, hypopituitarism or diabetes insipidus. Mass lesions or granulomas develop in the parenchyma or choroid plexus leading to obstruction of CSF flow and hydrocephalus. Imaging shows lytic bone lesions or bilateral T2 high signal changes in the basal ganglia and cerebellum. Treatment is with varying chemotherapy regimens.

Related conditions include Erdheim–Chester disease which is a multisystem, infiltrative, histiocytc disorder in which granulomatous lesions affect the long bones, skull, pituitary and CNS in addition to multiple systemic organs. Rosai–Dorfman disease (sinus hitiocytosis with massive lymphadenopathy) is a predominantly macrophage-related disorder associated with extensive lymphadenopathy involving mediastinum, axillary and inguinal sites as well as the head and neck.

Polycythaemia

Polycythaemia is an increased red cell mass causing a raised haematocrit. It may be primary (polycythaemia vera) or secondary to another condition (e.g. chronic hypoxia). The symptoms of polycythaemia can be generalised and rather ill-defined (including poor concentration, feelings of cephalic fullness, tinnitus, paraesthesias) or acute focal vascular syndromes, either permanent or transient. These may be caused by arterial or venous events. Chorea is associated with polycythaemia vera (related to a mutation in the erythropoietin receptor gene, *JAK2*) and may respond to treatment of the polycythaemia. Polycythaemia vera can transform into other haematological malignancies (e.g. leukaemias, myelofibrosis). The mainstay of treatment of polycythaemia is repeated venesection.

Thrombocythaemia

Thrombocythaemia (platelet count >800 000/mm^3) is associated with an increased risk of thrombosis and haemorrhage within the CNS. It may be associated with leukaemia or myelodysplasia. Thrombosis can occur in arteries, veins or venous sinuses and is related to hyperviscosity. Haemorrhage can also occur (subdural, extradural, intracerebral, subarachnoid); the mechanism presumably involves abnormal platelet function. Treatment with hydroxyurea is usually recommended to prevent neurological symptoms.

Bleeding disorders

Thrombotic thrombocytopenic purpura

Thrombotic thrombocytopenic purpura (TTP) is a rare disorder of early adulthood characterised by recurrent and widespread occlusion of small vessels. The pathophysiology involves micro-angiopathic haemolysis and formation of platelet micro-thrombi throughout the body including the CNS. TTP may be familial or acquired but in both cases endothelial cells secrete abnormally large von Willebrand factor multimers that are not degraded because of the lack of the cleavage enzyme ADAMTS-13. This allows the formation of platelet thrombi in small vessels. The clinical hallmarks are fevers, hepatic and renal disease and a low platelet count. Fragmented red cells on the blood film, elevated lactate dehydrogenase, bilirubin and reticulocyte count also point towards the diagnosis. Fluctuating neurological symptoms of altered conscious level, seizures, headache or encephalopathy can be the presenting features in half of the patients and may be preceded by a provoking factor such as an intercurrent illness. The majority of patients will at some stage of the illness develop neurological symptoms. Low platelets lead to haemorrhage including intracerebral haemorrhage. Ischaemic stroke from large or small vessel occlusion also occurs. The mainstay of treatment is plasma exchange. Antiplatelet agents or anticoagulants can be used although evidence for efficacy is lacking. Other immunomodulatory treatments have been used including ciclosporin. Rituximab is the subject of ongoing investigation.

Haemophilia, disseminated intravascular coagulation and von Willebrand's disease are also rare causes of intracerebral haemorrhage.

Coagulation disorders

The antiphospholipid antibody syndrome (Chapter 5), although usually characterised by venous thromboses, is also an important rare cause of arterial cerebrovascular events, sometimes in association with skin rashes, migraine and recurrent miscarriage. Thrombophilias including protein C and S deficiency, antithrombin III deficiency, factor V Leiden and the *MTHFR* mutation are associated with cerebral venous thrombosis, but not strongly with arterial events. These disorders are also discussed in more detail in Chapters 5 and 19.

Primary immunodeficiency

Primary immunodeficiency describes conditions caused by inherited defects of the immune system and can be divided into disorders affecting humoral immunity, cell-mediated immunity, phagocytic or complement function. Combined immunodeficiency is caused by mutations of the genes coding for the development and function of both T and B cells and the most severe form causes early death from overwhelming infection. Incomplete forms are milder and present in late childhood with recurrent or chronic respiratory tract infections (including bronchiectasis), chronic viral disease, opportunistic infection, chronic lymphoma, a family history of immunodeficiency or the new onset of autoimmune disease. T-cell disorders include ataxia-telangiectasia (see Neurocutaneous syndromes), Wiskott–Aldrich syndrome and X-linked lymphoproliferative disease.

Common variable immunodeficiency (CVID) is characterised by impaired B-cell differentiation with defective immunoglobulin production. The clinical manifestations are heterogeneous and include recurrent infections (including meningitis), chronic lung disease, autoimmune disorders, gastrointestinal disease and a heightened susceptibility to lymphoma. CVID is a collection of hypogammaglobulinaemia syndrome and is associated with multiple genetic defects. The condition is defined by reduced serum concentration of IgG, IgA and/or IgM with a poor response to immunisation in the absence of other immune deficiency states. Patients with CVID can develop diffuse infiltration with non-caseating granuloma affecting lymphoid or solid organs including the brain and the eyes. There is an increased risk of malignancy, and, in particular, non-Hodgkin's lymphoma which is usually extranodal, well differentiated and of B-cell origin and can lead to meningeal or parenchymatous involvement.

Gastrointestinal disorders

Hepatic encephalopathy

In severe hepatic failure, toxins are not removed from portal blood and thus enter the systemic circulation. The toxins responsible for hepatic encephalopathy include ammonia, aromatic amino acids, mercaptans, short-chain fatty acids and endogenous benzodiazepines. The speed of onset of encephalopathy parallels that of the underlying hepatic failure; this may vary from hours to very slow progression over months. Delirium typically fluctuates during the day and may be accompanied by euphoria and neurological signs including a flapping postural tremor of the hands (asterixis) and constructional apraxia. Hepatic foetor is the sickly sweet odour on the breath found in many cases. Untreated, delirium progresses to stupor and coma. Treatment is mainly aimed at reducing the nitrogen burden in the bowel – a low protein diet, regular large doses of lactulose and sometimes neomycin. Hepatic transplantation is sometimes required.

Vitamin deficiencies causing neurological disorders (Chapter 19)

Vitamin B_1 deficiency

Vitamin B_1 (thiamine) deficiency causes Wernicke's encephalopathy, Korsakoff's syndrome and beri-beri (Chapter 19). Wernicke's encephalopathy is a subacute illness causing delirium, nystagmus – with or without ophthalmoplegia – and ataxia, typically of gait more than limbs. The syndrome is underdiagnosed and potentially treatable. Korsakoff's syndrome can follow Wernicke's encephalopathy and is characterised by a more restricted syndrome of anterograde and retrograde amnesia without delirium. Although classically a result of chronic alcoholism, Wernicke's encephalopathy and Korsakoff's syndrome are well known to result from other causes, such as intractable vomiting (e.g. anorexia nervosa, hyperemesis gravidarum). One of the three patients originally reported by Wernicke suffered from severe vomiting from pyloric stenosis induced by sulfuric acid poisoning.

The extent of recovery is influenced by the time to diagnosis and treatment with thiamine. Some of the eye signs and ataxia often resolve but a residual amnestic syndrome is common. In any patient with cognitive disturbance or delirium in the context of heavy alcohol use, prompt treatment with high dose intravenous B vitamins is recommended – it rarely causes harm.

Vitamine B_3 (niacin) deficiency (Pellagra)

Endemic niacin deficiency is rarely seen in developed countries, but is characterised by dementia, dermatitis and diarrhoea (the three D's). The most common cause of pellagra now is chronic alcoholism, which usually presents with acute and isolated delirium. There can also be generalised rigidity (sometimes cogwheeling), dysarthria and myoclonus.

Vitamin D deficiency

Proximal muscle weakness can develop as a result of vitamin D malabsorption. The symptoms usually start in the legs, affecting hip movements but with preservation of distal power, reflexes and sensation. EMG shows myopathic features with short duration polyphasic potentials. The degree of muscle weakness is not correlated with plasma calcium concentration and the underlying mechanism is unclear. Vitamin D treatment is generally helpful. Causes include lack of sunlight, chronic malabsorption syndromes, coeliac and Crohn's disease, renal and hepatic disease, cystic fibrosis. Genetic factors are important and people with dark skin are particularly susceptible, and some drug therapies – including the enzyme-inducing antiepileptic drugs – are associated with a decrease in vitamin D levels.

Vitamin E deficiency

Vitamin E deficiency results from cholestatic liver disease, fat malabsorption, abetalipoproteinaemia or as a familial absorption disorder. The clinical features include neuropathy, ataxia, ophthalmoplegia and muscle weakness. A familial condition with poor conservation of plasma α-tocopherol in very low density lipoproteins is characterised by ataxia, cerebellar signs, dysarthria, leg areflexia, impaired proprioception, bilateral extensor plantar responses, pes cavus and scoliosis. These signs are strikingly similar to those seen in Friedreich's ataxia (Chapter 17). All patients presenting with an unexplained spinocerebellar syndrome or tremor should have vitamin E concentrations measured, as the symptoms can respond to treatment.

Malabsorption

Malabsorption is the result of gluten sensitivity or many other processes affecting the small bowel, including surgical resection.

Coeliac disease

Many neurological syndromes affecting the central and peripheral nervous systems have been reported in association with coeliac disease, including epilepsy, myoclonus, cerebellar atrophy and ataxia, multifocal leukoencephalopathy, dementia and peripheral neuropathies, both axonal and demyelinating. It is speculated that immunological mechanisms or trace vitamin deficiency underlie these associations. Substantial neurological features can occur in the absence of overt coeliac disease. Coeliac disease should certainly be considered in cryptogenic ataxias and neuropathies (Chapter 17).

Inflammatory bowel disease

Both ulcerative colitis and Crohn's disease are associated with thrombo-embolic complications including cerebral venous thrombosis and spinal cord ischaemia caused by arterial and venous thrombosis. Scattered white matter lesions are seen on T2-weighted MRI more frequently than in control subjects and patients receiving anti-tumour necrosis factor (anti-TNF) biological agents are at risk of developing progressive multifocal leukoencephalopathy and possibly lymphoma. Inflammatory bowel disease is associated with a sensory axonal and demyelinating polyneuropathy and also dermatomyositis.

Renal disease

Renal diseases are relevant to neurologists in two main ways. First, certain diseases affect both the kidneys and the nervous system – these include the vasculitides and connective tissue diseases as well as serious conditions including genetic disorders (Fabry's disease, Wilson's disease, von Hippel–Lindau disease), infections and plasma cell dyscrasias. Secondly, renal failure, dialysis and renal transplantation can affect neurological function in a variety of ways.

Conditions affecting both renal and neurological function

These conditions are mainly covered in other sections; the key features of some selected conditions are briefly summarised in Table 26.3. A neurologist should remember that renal disease in its early stages causes few or no symptoms and that renal function must therefore be screened when there is even a small degree of clinical suspicion. Vigilance is important; the consequences of progressive renal disease are severe and potentially avoidable. Routine biochemistry (urea and creatinine) are crude measures of renal impairment. If renal disease is questioned (e.g. a patient with a mononeuritis multiplex), urine microscopy for casts and detailed urinalysis, close monitoring of blood pressure and renal ultrasound should all be performed without delay.

Table 26.3 Conditions affecting renal and neurological function.

Condition	Renal effects	Neurological effects
Vasculitis		
PAN	Proteinuria, granular casts, hypertension	Peripheral neuropathy, encephalopathy, stroke (infarction and SAH)
Eosinophilic granulomatosis with polyangiitis (EGPA)(previously Churg–Strauss syndrome)	Rarely involved	Mononeuritis multiplex encephalopathy, SAH
Granulomatosis with polyangiitis (GPA) (previously Wegener's granulomatosis)	Proteinuria, haematuria, red cell casts, renal failure	Cranial neuropathies, mononeuropathies, polyneuropathy, ischaemic stroke
Connective tissue disorders		
Rheumatoid disease	Glomerulonephritis (rare)	Polyneuropathy, mononeuropathies, cervical cord damage due to bony disease
SLE	Haematuria, proteinuria, nephritic syndrome, renal failure	Neuropsychiatric symptoms, encephalopathy, seizures, ischaemic stroke, chorea
Sjögren's syndrome	Tubular disorders	Dorsal roots ganglionopathy, neuropathy, cranial neuropathy (especially V), encephalopathy, MS-like symptoms
Myeloproliferative disorders		
Multiple myeloma	Proteinuria, Bence-Jones protein, nephrotic syndrome	Nerve root/cord compromise
MGUS	Rarely abnormal	Demyelinating sensory > motor peripheral neuropathy
Waldenstrom's macroglobulinaemia	Proteinuria, nephrotic syndrome	Sensorimotor neuropathy, encephalopathy, SAH, stroke, myelopathy
POEMS	Rarely, M protein in urine	Demyelinating neuropathy (sensory > motor) resembling CIDP (50%)

CIDP, chronic inflammatory demyelinating polyradiculoneuropathy; MGUS, monoclonal gammopathy of undetermined significance; MS, multiple sclerosis; PAN, polyarteritis nodosa; POEMS, (syndrome of) polyneuropathy, organomegaly, endocrinopathy, M protein, skin changes.

Neurological consequences of renal disease and its treatment

Uraemic encephalopathy (Chapter 20)

Neurological manifestations are usually associated with the rapid development of uraemia in acute renal failure. The onset is with subtle clouding of consciousness that may progress rapidly to apathy, irritability, confusion and disorientation. A coarse irregular tremor with asterixis can develop. Severe metabolic encephalopathy associated with uraemia is also associated with a progressive stimulus-sensitive multi-focal myoclonus and eventually the development of generalised tonic–clonic or focal motor seizures. Frank psychosis and agitation with hallucinations sometimes supervene before the development of uraemic coma, Cheyne–Stokes respiration and respiratory arrest. Uraemic encephalopathy is generally reversible with recovery from acute uraemia.

Dialysis encephalopathy

Dialysis encephalopathy (dialysis dementia) is the rare but potentially fatal condition that previously complicated chronic dialysis and is still occasionally seen. Patients develop subacute progression of fluctuating symptoms in the early stages which either become fixed or progress. The condition is characterised by dysarthria, dysphasia and progressive metabolic encephalopathy with myoclonus and asterixis, culminating in generalised seizures and intellectual decline. The syndrome is caused by the aluminium content in gels and dialysate solution. Treatment with purified dialysate has led to the disappearance (almost) of this condition. Chronic haemodialysis can also lead to Wernicke's encephalopathy, sensorimotor axonal polyneuropathy and occasionally subdural haematoma.

Dialysis disequilibrium syndrome

This is related to changing osmotic gradients between plasma and brain during rapid dialysis. Patients present with non-specific symptoms of nausea, visual blurring and headache prior to development of worsening mental confusion, clouding of consciousness, seizures and tremor. The symptoms are usually mild and can be alleviated with slow flow rates during dialysis and the addition of osmotically active solutes to the dialysate.

Neuropathy associated with renal disease

Uraemic neuropathy is a distal axonal degeneration with secondary myelin loss. This occurs in the majority of patients with chronic renal failure; the severity is related to the extent and duration of renal failure. Onset is often with periodic limb movements or restless legs and established neuropathy is characterised by a distal paraesthetic sensory disturbance. The neuropathy is reversible with treatment of the renal failure.

Neurological aspects of organ transplantation

Organ transplantation is now widely undertaken. Kidney, liver, heart, lung, pancreas and bone marrow are successfully transplanted with relatively low morbidity and mortality. The neurological complications of these procedures are related to the effects of the underlying organ failure, immunosuppression leading to secondary infection, allograft rejection, effects of drug treatment or consequences of the surgical procedure. The neurological complications vary with time following surgery.

CNS infections

CNS infections develop in less than 10% of transplant recipients and in immunosuppressed patients; these can be severe and carry a high mortality. Infections in the immunosuppressed patient are discussed in Chapter 9 but a number of issues relate specifically to post-transplant patients. The risk of infection depends on the degree of immunosuppression, the intensity of exposure to potential pathogens and the time since transplantation. It is rare for opportunistic infection to develop within 1 month of surgery and commencing immunosuppression. During this period, infection is unrelated to the degree of immunosuppression, and is usually caused by the regular nosocomial organisms such as Gram-negative bacteria, staphylococci and *Candida*. Patients are predisposed to these infections, as is anyone critically ill, by contamination of vascular access or drainage catheters, prolonged intubation, stents or other foreign bodies and fluid collections. Rarely, active toxoplasmosis and viral infections can be passed with the graft.

More than 1 month after transplantation, as effective immunosuppression develops, the patient is at increased risk of infection with viruses: cytomegalovirus (CMV); Epstein–Barr virus (EBV); herpes simplex virus (HSV); varicella-zoster virus (VZV); human herpesvirus (HHV), and fungi (*Aspergillus* and *Candida*). Most patients with successful transplants are maintained on low-dose immunosuppression and are not at particularly high risk of late opportunistic infection.

More than 6 months after transplantation, infection can occur if the degree of immunosuppression has been increased because of recurrent or chronic allograft rejection. These patients are at particular risk of opportunistic infections listed above but also with other viruses (e.g. JC virus), fungi (*Aspergillus, Cryptococcus, Nocardia, Histoplasmosis, Mucor*), protozoa (toxoplasmosis) or bacteria (*Listeria monocytogenes, Pneumocystis carinii,* mycobacteria).

Viral infection

The pattern of opportunistic viral infection following transplantation is highly variable. The most frequent pathogens are EBV, VZV, adenoviruses and herpes viruses HSV1 and HSV2; HHV6 is less common. CMV and EMV can cause severe encephalitis which can be difficult to diagnose. Reactivation of VZV can lead to cutaneous dissemination (chickenpox) and/or a generalised meningo-encephalitis, transverse myelitis and cranial neuropathy. Progressive multi-focal leukoencephalopathy (Chapter 9) is associated with JC virus infection and must be distinguished in the post-transplant encephalopathic patient from central pontine myelinolysis and posterior reversible leukoencephalopathy related to treatment.

Bacterial infection

Bacterial infection in the transplant patient is less common than viral but can be caused by *Listeria monocytogenes* which causes meningo-encephalitis, often with a brainstem emphasis, multiple abscess formation or myelitis. Mycobacteria can cause pulmonary tuberculosis, TB meningitis or atypical TB CNS infection. Haemophilus or staphylococcal pneumonia and/or meningitis also occur in post-transplant patients. *Nocardia* infection is associated with cerebral abscess formation and often with pleural disease.

Fungal infection

Fungal meningitis (Chapter 9) is most commonly caused by *Aspergillus* in the first 6 months, while typically *Cryptococcus* develops later than 6 months. *Aspergillus* species occur commonly in the environment. Primary infection is usually airborne and established in the lungs. Spread to the CNS occurs in some 50% of cases. This carries an extremely poor prognosis because of the development of severe meningitis, focal aspergilloma brain abscesses and invasion of the cerebral vessels leading to intracerebral haematomas. The spinal cord can also be occasionally affected. Disseminated cryptococcosis involves the CSF and can cause severe chronic relapsing meningitis with raised ICP. There is a high mortality in transplant recipients. *Candida* meningitis is a rare post-transplant infection with chronic relapsing meningitis and/or brain abscess formation; this usually responds well to aggressive antifungal treatment. *Mucor* is an occasional CNS infection.

Parasitic infection

Toxoplasma gondii is the most frequent protozoa to infect transplant recipients. The pattern of single or multiple enhancing cerebral abscesses is similar to that described in other immunosuppressive situations in Chapter 9. There may also be an acute encephalitis, occasionally with myocardial involvement. The CSF shows marked mononuclear pleocytosis with elevated protein, sometimes with depressed glucose. MRI shows characteristic ring enhancing abscesses, often in the basal ganglia.

Neurological sequelae of transplantation

Seizures

Seizures are relatively common in transplant recipients and have a number of causes. They commonly occur as a manifestation of drug toxicity (especially with ciclosporin and OKT3). Seizures can also be associated with drug withdrawal, metabolic derangements, hypoxic–ischaemic injury, cerebrovascular disease and sepsis. The initial management is correction of the underlying disturbance but in patients with ongoing impairment of consciousness it is essential to exclude non-convulsive status epilepticus. Status epilepticus should be treated conventionally, with benzodiazepines and a barbiturate or levetiracetam. However, titration of these drugs can be difficult because of renal and hepatic impairment, and hypoalbuminaemia. Isolated seizures following organ transplantation rarely lead to long-term epilepsy and therefore anticonvulsant medications are seldom required when the acute episode has resolved.

Encephalopathy

Encephalopathy develops commonly following transplantation and varies from a mild confusional state to psychosis with obtundation and coma. In the acute postoperative situation it is often brought about by a surgical complication (e.g. hypoxic–ischaemic insult), the development of a metabolic encephalopathy, acute allograft rejection, isolated or multiple organ failure, sepsis, seizures or drug toxicity (particularly ciclosporin).

Stroke

Stroke following transplantation is an important cause of morbidity and mortality. It is often related to the underlying disease process and in particular accelerated cerebrovascular atherosclerosis in diabetes mellitus. Stroke can also be a consequence of cardiogenic emboli and CNS infections that cause vasculopathy or vasculitis. Cardiac transplantation carries the complications of bypass – cardio-embolic stroke, air embolism and bacterial endocarditis.

Fungal CNS infections (particularly aspergillosis and mucormycosis) are associated with invasion and occlusion of the cerebral vessels resulting in haemorrhagic infarction.

Medication including ciclosporin and sirolimus and, to a lesser extent, tacrolimus can also lead to hypercholesterolaemia, potentially increasing the risk of vaso-occlusive events.

Intracerebral haemorrhage is usually seen in the setting of haemorrhagic transformation of an ischaemic stroke, resulting from coagulopathy or following CNS infection. Subdural haematoma can occur with thrombocytopenia, particularly following bone marrow transplantation. Subarachnoid haemorrhage is particularly associated with the increased incidence of berry aneurysms which may rupture following renal transplantation for polycystic disease. Cerebral venous thrombosis can occur as a consequence of a hypercoagulable state, dehydration or CNS infection.

Medication

Complications of immunosuppressive drugs are also discussed in Chapters 19 and 21. The drugs most frequently causing neurotoxicity are ciclosporin, tacrolimus, steroids and OKT3.

Ciclosporin neurotoxicity occurs in some 25% of patients and includes tremor, headache and, less commonly, posterior reversible encephalopathy. The complications are lessened with oral administration and are usually reversible with discontinuation of the drug. Profound impairment in cognitive function has also been reported to be associated with tacrolimus and ciclosporin. OKT3 is a murine E monoclonal antibody used in the treatment of rejection and has been associated with aseptic meningitis, encephalopathy and seizures.

The combination of steroids with neuromuscular junction blocking agents can cause prolonged neuromuscular blockade or a critical illness myopathy.

CNS malignancy

There is an increased incidence of CNS malignancy in allograft recipients who are immunosuppressed. Intracerebral B-cell lymphoma affecting the brain and spinal cord and glioblastoma multiforme are the most common CNS cancers. They may be associated with previous EBV infection.

Neuro-ophthalmological problems

Cortical blindness, complex visual disturbances and hallucinations, not uncommon in all critically ill patients, can be caused by dose-related toxicity from tacrolimus or ciclosporin. This is often reversible.

Movement disorders

Both ciclosporin and tacrolimus are associated with a high incidence of tremor. Occasionally, parkinsonism has been described in bone marrow transplant recipients. Rarely, chorea has occurred as a manifestation of rejection following cardiac transplantation. It is usually steroid responsive.

Neuromuscular problems

Mononeuropathies follow surgery and anaesthesia and can occur as a consequence of positioning, traction or the mechanical complications of surgery. Phrenic nerve damage can follow cold plegia of the heart (induced hypothermia) during cardiac transplantation. Rarely, systemic infection may lead to a form of polymyositis.

Acute myopathy sometimes follows liver transplantation, particularly in those receiving intravenous steroids and neuromuscular blocking agents. In general, the prognosis for neuromuscular complications following most transplantation is good providing there is no major structural damage, but this is not true for graft versus host disease (GvHD, see Bone marrow transplantation).

Complications related to specific allograft transplantation

Renal transplantation

Renal transplantation is now undertaken routinely but neurological complications remain relatively frequent. Uraemic encephalopathy can develop suddenly following acute tubular necrosis, acute accelerated rejection or renal vein thrombosis. Spinal cord ischaemia occurs when the iliac artery is diverted for graft re-vascularisation; this is a particular risk when there is an anomalous vascular supply to the spinal cord from the internal iliac artery rather than the intercostals. There is an increased frequency of cerebrovascular disease related to the underlying vasculopathy and hypertension, particularly in the presence of diabetes or systemic lupus erythematosus (SLE). However, there is evidence that combined kidney and pancreas transplantation decreases the subsequent incidence of stroke in diabetic patients. Compressive neuropathies involving the femoral nerve are often related to haematoma formation. Rejection encephalopathy is extremely rare.

Liver transplantation

Liver transplantation carries a relatively high incidence of complications. These are related to the underlying hepatic disease including viral hepatitis, alcoholic liver disease, primary biliary cirrhosis, acute liver failure or toxic hepatic damage. Patients with hepatic encephalopathy have usually been critically ill and carry all the consequences of their underlying disorders following surgery. Delayed rejection or failing graft function may lead to recurrent encephalopathy or central pontine myelinolysis, impairment of coagulation and failure of synthetic and metabolic hepatic functions. Encephalopathy is also a common complication – associated with drug toxicity, metabolic derangement, hypoxic–ischaemic injury and sepsis. Coagulopathies can also lead to intracerebral or subarachnoid haemorrhage. The postoperative period is frequently complicated by the development of severe sepsis and critical care myopathy.

Cardiac transplantation

Cardiac transplantation complications are usually related to bypass. Cannulation of the diseased ascending aorta can dislodge atheromatous material leading to cerebral emboli and there is a risk of introducing air emboli when bypass is discontinued. There remains a significant instance of ischaemic and haemorrhagic stroke, ischaemic hypoxic brain injury, encephalopathy and peripheral nerve injury often affecting the lower brachial plexus because of stretching during chest wall retraction. The recurrent laryngeal nerve can also be damaged leading to vocal cord paralysis; phrenic nerve paralysis, from direct trauma or cold plegia, can cause diaphragmatic weakness.

Lung transplantation

Lung transplantation is often undertaken in combination with heart transplantation. Encephalopathy is usually a result of metabolic causes, drug toxicity or seizures. The cerebrovascular and neuromuscular complications are similar to those described earlier.

Bone marrow transplantation

Bone marrow transplantation is now widely undertaken both for the treatment of haematological malignancies but also as an adjunct in the treatment of other malignancies or autoimmune disorders. Neurological complications usually occur after allogenic bone marrow transplant requiring immunosuppression. Following bone marrow infusion, pancytopenia can be present for 2–5 weeks before a significant response is mounted. During this critical period, overwhelming Gram-negative sepsis, severe bleeding from thrombocytopenia and disseminated intravascular coagulation are the most serious complications. Transplantation is combined with radiotherapy or intrathecal chemotherapy. There may be an associated posterior reversible leukoencephalopathy. However, the most serious complication is the development of GvHD.

Acute GvHD occurs in the first 100 days following transplantation and primarily affects the skin, liver and intestines. Chronic GvHD is a different entity and develops at any time later than 80 days following transplantation. The condition strongly resembles a vasculitic syndrome with scleroderma-like skin involvement, bronchiolitis, Sjögren's syndrome, polymyositis, myasthenia gravis and neuropathy.

Polymyositis develops up to 4–5 years after allogenic bone marrow transplantation in association with GvHD. Seropositive myasthenia occurs sometimes with severe bulbar and respiratory muscle weakness. The use of neuromuscular blocking agents can lead to prolonged blockade and the development of critical illness myopathy. Acute demyelinating neuropathy has also been described in chronic GvHD. Reduction of immunosuppression usually results in improvement of the symptoms but there remains a high morbidity and mortality associated with the condition.

Neurological involvement in systemic vasculitides and related disorders

Neurological involvement in systemic vasculitic disorders is common although, with the exception of giant cell arteritis (GCA) and isolated cerebral angiitis (ICA), it is rare for patients with this group of disorders to present solely with neurological symptoms. As such, many neurological episodes occur in patients who already have an established rheumatological or systemic vasculitis diagnosis and who may consequently be receiving some form of immunomodulatory therapy. Neurological symptoms presenting in such patients can be split into three broad aetiological groups, each requiring different therapeutic approaches. First, neurological symptoms or signs can develop with increased underlying systemic disease activity, needing prompt escalation of the immunomodulatory therapy. Secondly, the symptoms may be iatrogenic and related to side effects of disease modifying or other agents (e.g. a proximal myopathy associated with steroid therapy or reversible posterior leukoencephalopathy associated with immunomodulatory treatments). Thirdly, the symptoms can be caused by a separate and possibly associated disease process which requires attention on its own merits (e.g. ischaemic stroke in a patient with rheumatoid arthritis and diabetes).

Any part of the nervous system can be affected by the diseases described here, but the propensities vary across these conditions as do the causative mechanisms. For each disease mentioned, the different sites of neurological involvement are ranked depending on how commonly they occur. Many of the disease mechanisms, and thus related therapeutic considerations are shared across these conditions and are discussed first. Vasculitic disorders can be classified according to the predominant size and type of the vessel affected and/or whether there is associated granuloma. A further division is between vasculitides associated with the presence or absence of antineutrophil cytoplasmic antibodies (ANCA). The three ANCA associated forms of vasculitis are granulomatosis with polyangiitis (GPA; previously known as Wegener's granulomatosis); microscopic polyangiitis (MPA) and eosinophilic granulomatosis with polyangiitis (EGPA; previously known as Churg–Strauss; Table 26.4).

Table 26.4 Classification of vasculitis.

Large vessel vasculitis
Giant cell arteritis (GCA)
Takayasu's arteritis (TAK)
Medium-sized vessel vasculitis
Polyarteritis nodosa
Kawasaki's disease
Small vessel vasculitis (SVV)
ANCA-associated vasculitis (AAV)
Granulomatosis with polyangiitis (Wegener's) (GPA)
Eosinophil granulomatosis with polyangiitis (Churg–Strauss) (EGPA)
Microscopic polyangiitis (MPA)
Immune complex vasculitides
Antiglomerular basement membrane disease
IgA vasculitis (Henoch–Schönlein purpura)
Vasculitis secondary to immune complex disease (SLE, dysproteinaemias, cryoglobulinaemia, chronic infection)
Variable vessel vasculitis
Behçet's disease
Cogan's syndrome
Single organ vasculitis
Central nervous system, peripheral nerve, cutaneous, testicular
Vasculitis associated with systemic disease

SLE, systemic lupus erythematosus.

Pathological mechanisms

Regardless of the lesion site within the neuraxis, the final common pathway of vasculitis is ischaemic damage to neural tissue, usually with permanent damage. Histological examination of tissue from both the central and peripheral nervous systems often reveals a necrotising arteritis affecting blood vessels with a transmural infiltrate initially consisting of a variety of reactive leukocytes, typically a mixture of polymorphs, lymphocytes and eosinophils. The proportions, subtypes and behaviour of these cells vary both within and across the different types of systemic vasculitides, with granulomas (a nodular aggregation of mononuclear inflammatory cells or modified macrophages usually surrounded by a rim of lymphocytes) more common in GPA and GCA. The cell populations at the lesion site also vary with the age of the lesion: neutrophils in the acute phase and intimal proliferation and fibrosis in the chronic phase. All these cellular responses conspire to reduce blood flow through the affected vessel. When individual nerves are involved the arteritis usually affects the pre-capillary arteries. In the CNS the calibre of blood vessel affected is associated with disease type, but overlap is common. A nosology based primarily on vessel size is desirable but problematic, especially as immunotherapy is not yet at the stage where different populations of inflammatory cells can be targeted.

With inflammatory and reactive stromal cells narrowing the arterial lumen, secondary thrombotic events can occur causing distal embolism to terminal portions of the arterial tree. However, in some systemic disorders the vasculopathy is primarily or even solely caused by thrombotic occlusion of arteries, capillaries or veins, in which case anticoagulation may be appropriate (see Systemic lupus erythematosus). Other causes of secondary vasculitis affecting the nervous system include:

- *Infections:* fungi, TB, other bacteria, spirochaetes, viruses including VZV, HIV.
- *Drugs:* amphetamine, cocaine.
- *Malignancy:* either via direct involvement such as in lymphoma or as part of a paraneoplastic vasculitis.

Isolated cerebral angiitis (ICA) is a rare but well-recognised disorder. The existence of its peripheral equivalent, an isolated peripheral nervous system vasculitis, is less certain because many vasculitic neuropathies are secondary to an underlying disease (e.g. Sjögren's syndrome).

Compressive spinal cord or root pathology can occur in any of the systemic disorders, especially as steroid-related osteopenia has a predilection for the vertebral bodies. However, this is most commonly seen in patients with rheumatoid arthritis (RA). Entrapment neuropathies can be caused by nodule formation in RA (typically ulnar or median nerve) or granulomas (typically cranial nerves).

Ophthalmoplegia occurs in approximately 5% of patients with GPA. The causes of this are varied and multifactorial:

- Contiguous extension of a granulomatous mass from a nasal or paranasal site into the orbit causing pseudotumour.
- Vasculitis of the extraocular muscles.
- Oculomotor palsy secondary to vasculitis.
- Granulomatous compression at some point along a cranial nerve.

Dedicated MRI scanning protocols with contrast can help to demonstrate the cause.

Diagnosis and treatment of vasculitides involving the nervous system

Immunosuppressive therapies for vasculitis are relatively toxic, and the decision to administer them should be supported by a tissue diagnosis, if at all possible. When neurological symptoms and signs occur alongside multi-system disease activity, a diagnostic biopsy may well be from affected skin, kidney or lung. However, if the neurological syndrome occurs while disease remains quiescent in other organs then brain, nerve or muscle biopsy may be the only reasonable option.

Immunosuppressive treatment of neurological involvement in systemic disorders is unlikely to be based directly on prospective randomised trials; however, indirect evidence is available from controlled trails of patients with systemic vasculitis. Given that the underlying pathology is similar in non-neurological organs, extrapolation is reasonable. In general, the majority of vasculitic disorders can be reversed or controlled in some 90% of patients with a combination of high-dose oral corticosteroids and oral cyclophosphamide. Cyclophosphamide is usually given for 3 months with less toxic drugs such as azathioprine to sustain remission while steroid therapy is gradually reduced. Newer agents or non-pharmacological treatments such as plasma exchange are sometimes needed in resistant or persistently relapsing conditions. Many of the current immunosuppressive drugs and their associated side effect monitoring parameters are included in Table 26.5 and the newer biological agents are shown in Table 26.6.

Polyarteritis nodosa and related conditions

Polyarteritis nodosa (PAN) is the prototype necrotising vasculitis. Medium-sized vessels are those usually affected and can be associated with aneurysm formation, seen on angiography. Middle-aged men are most commonly affected. Systemic symptoms include abdominal pain (from hepatic or other visceral infarcts), hypertension (from renal involvement, although glomerulonephritis is not a feature), fever and weight loss. Diagnosis is based on the clinical features and either positive angiography or biopsy of affected tissue (skin, kidney or nerve). The only serological marker clearly associated with PAN is hepatitis B infection (20–40% HbsAg-positive). PAN is considered to be an ANCA-negative syndrome.

Table 26.5 Drug treatments for vasculitis.

Drug	Class/action	Side-effects	Monitor (prophylaxis)
Acute, induction or rescue therapy			
Methylprednisolone	Corticosteroid	Diabetes, neuropsychiatric, hypotension	Glucose, BP
Cyclophosphamide	Alkylating agent	Haemorrhagic cystitis, bone marrow suppression, neutropenia, sepsis	FBC (mesna for cystitis)
IVIG	Pooled antibodies from ~1000 human donors	As for any blood product, renal failure rarely	Check IgA levels before therapy, (absent IgA = absolute contraindication), U&E
Long-term therapy			
Prednisolone	Corticosteroid	Diabetes, osteopenia, adrenal suppression	DEXA scan (bisphosphanates for osteoprophylaxis)
Mycophenolate mofetil	Inhibitor of inosine monophosphate dehydrogenase	Bone marrow suppression, gastrointestinal intolerance, chronic viral infections	FBC; (ideally) monitor mycophenolic acid levels
Methotrexate	Folate antagonist/adenosine agonist	Pulmonary fibrosis, liver failure, bone marrow suppression	FBC, U&E, LFT (folate prophylaxis)
Azathioprine	Blocks purine synthesis	Bone marrow suppression, squamous-cell carcinoma, chronic viral infections, hypersensitivity	FBC + (ideally) check TMPT pre-Rx. (absent TMPT = absolute contraindication; reduced level = reduce dose)
Tacrolimus	Calcineurin inhibitor	Diabetes, hypertension	FBC, U&E, glucose, tacrolimus levels

FBC, full blood count; Ig, immunoglobulin; IVIG, intravenous immunoglobulin; LFT, liver function test; TMPT, thiopurine methyltranferase; TNF, tumour necrosis factor; U&E, urea and electrolytes.

Table 26.6 Biological agents currently being used or studied.

	Drug	Adverse reaction
Anti TNF therapies		
TNF receptor fusion protein	Etanercept	Cytopenia, infection, liver dysfunction, injection site reactions
Monoclonal antibodies	Adalimumab SC Golimumab SC Certolizumab SC Infliximab IV	All as above
B-cell depletion (monoclonal anti-CD20)	Rituximab IV	Cytopenia, infection, liver dysfunction, infusion reactions
IL-6 inhibitor	Tocilizumab IV	Cytopenia, infection, liver dysfunction, infusion reactions, hypercholesterolaemia
T-cell co-stimulatory molecule inhibitor	Abatacept IV/SC	Cytopenia, infection, liver dysfunction, infusion reactions

IL, interleukin; IV, intravenous; SC, subcutaneous.

The most common neurological problem is a progressive mononeuritis multiplex which occurs in up to 50% of patients with PAN. In common with other causes of vasculitic mononeuritis this tends to present with a painful sensory or sensorimotor picture. More central involvement occurs in 25% of cases, in a variety of patterns – encephalopathy, seizures, stroke, aseptic meningitis, rarely an ischaemic myelopathy and sometimes cranial nerves palsies.

MPA is related to PAN and is also more commonly seen in males. Unlike PAN, the kidneys are most commonly affected and when the lungs are simultaneously involved it is one of the causes of 'pulmonary–renal syndrome', along with GPA, SLE, EGPA and Goodpasture's syndromes. Other less specific features include arthralgia, purpuric rashes, myalgia and conjunctival haemorrhage. Like PAN, diagnosis rests primarily on the clinical syndrome with histological support from affected tissue (usually kidney, skin or lung). Angiography has less of a role in MPA because, as its name suggests, it tends to affect arterioles, capillaries or venules below the resolution of direct angiography. MPA, like GPA, is associated with circulating ANCA. There are two main ANCA staining patterns: peri-nuclear (pANCA) associated with the myeloperoxidase antigen, and cytoplasmic (cANCA), associated with the neutrophil enzyme proteinase 3. Both these forms are seen in microscopic polyangiitis (60–70% pANCA and 30–40% cANCA); combined they have a sensitivity of 90% with a specificity of 70%. ANCA can also be positive in patients with RA and SLE. The pattern of neurological involvement seen in MPA is similar to that of PAN.

Like MPA, EGPA affects the lungs and kidneys and also has an association with ANCA, albeit a weaker one. Unlike other systemic vasculitides, EGPA produces symptoms of asthma and is almost always associated with a peripheral eosinophilia ($>1.5 \times 10^9 L^{-1}$). Cardiac, gastrointestinal and skin involvement is also common. Histology of affected tissue usually shows three cardinal features: necrotising vasculitis, granulomas and infiltration by eosinophils. Typically, a vasculitic neuropathy is seen in EGPA and sometimes with GPA and MPA.

Granulomatosis with polyangiitis (Wegener's granulomatosis)

GPA is characterised by the triad of upper respiratory tract granuloma (typically affecting the nasal mucosa and/or inner ear), lower respiratory tract granuloma (typically pulmonary nodules) and a necrotising glomerulonephritis. Non-specific generalised skin and joint symptoms akin to those described for MPA also occur. cANCA is usually found in this condition and has a specificity of 95% and a sensitivity of 80%. Some physicians use circulating levels as an indirect disease marker against which immunomodulatory therapy can be titrated.

The best data for neurological complications associated with GPA come from a large series from the Mayo Clinic, of over 300 cases. Patients rarely died of neurological complications, but one-third had neurological involvement at one or more sites in the nervous system at some point in their illness:

- Peripheral polyneuropathy 50%
- Cranial neuropathy, including hearing loss 20%
- Ophthalmoplegia 15%
- Stroke 12%
- Seizures 10%, and
- Cerebritis 5%.

Peripheral nerve involvement is heavily skewed towards mononeuritis multiplex (80% of neuropathy patients) with 10% having an insidious distal symmetrical polyneuropathy; a further 10% were unclassified. The most common nerve affected by mononeuritis multiplex is the common peroneal nerve, followed by the tibial, ulnar, median, radial and femoral nerves. Fifty per cent of those with cranial nerve involvement have optic nerve pathology, usually an arteritic anterior ischaemic optic neuropathy. Cranial nerves VI and VII were the next most commonly affected. Ophthalmoplegia can be the presenting symptom in GPA, and can be caused by several mechanisms. All call for an increase in immunomodulatory therapy. Acute or subacute hearing loss is associated with GPA; this is often because of a combination of conduction hearing loss (otitis media or otitis interna) and sensorineural loss (granuloma or vasculitic processes affecting the auditory nerve).

Giant cell arteritis

GCA, widely known as temporal arteritis, is the most common primary vasculitis affecting those over 50 years. Typically, the extracranial branches of the aorta and the aorta itself are involved, with intracranial involvement much more rarely, probably because intracranial vessels lack the internal elastic lamina that appears to be the focus of the inflammatory response. Headache is the most common symptom, but can be absent. Other symptoms caused by involvement of extracranial arteries include jaw claudication and scalp tenderness. Constitutional symptoms are present in at least one-third of cases as this condition overlaps with polymyalgia rheumatica (weight loss, fever and myalgia). Blindness is the most common serious neurological sequel and can present with either monocular (or bilateral) or homonymous visual loss (Chapter 14). The former is caused by arteritic involvement of the posterior ciliary arteries, leading to optic nerve head infarction which may be partial causing sector or altitudinal field defects. The latter is caused by thrombo-embolism of the posterior cerebral arteries, which are preferentially affected. Sequential ischaemic optic neuropathies or bilateral occipital infarction can lead to permanent blindness. Strokes affecting the MCA territory also occur, although they are rarer. Sometimes the arteritis is clinically apparent to palpation. Affected arteries feel thickened, pulseless and cord-like, such as the superficial temporal artery or other extracranial branches of the external carotid artery, the facial artery as it runs under the mandible, or the occipital arteries as they run over the inion. The ESR is almost always raised as is the CRP; anaemia is present in two-thirds of cases with a leukocytosis and raised transaminases in one-third. Temporal artery biopsy is the most specific finding but often a diagnosis will have to be made without this confirmation as skip lesions occur. The diagnostic yield drops with the interval following initiation of steroid therapy, although this fact should not delay initiating steroids; perusing a biopsy after the oft-quoted 2-week window of opportunity post-steroids is occasionally fruitful. Patients started on steroids are not completely protected from ischaemic events; there is good evidence for starting patients also on low-dose aspirin when GCA is suspected.

Isolated cerebral angiitis

ICA or primary cerebral vasculitis is especially difficult to diagnose. Unlike most of the diseases mentioned earlier, there are neither extra diagnostic clues from involvement of non-neurological organ systems, nor specific serological nor CSF tests. ICA can present in a wide variety of ways with an acute or subacute, relapsing or even chronic time course. Three main patterns of presentation are proposed: an encephalopathic picture with accompanying headache, confusion and coma; isolated or multiple intracranial mass lesions with a mixture of focal and general CNS signs and raised ICP; an atypical MS-like syndrome with a relapsing–remitting course, optic nerve involvement, sometimes with stroke-like episodes and seizures (Figure 26.10).

Although brain MRI is usually abnormal in patients with ICA, there are no pathognomic findings; intra-arterial cerebral angiograms have a disappointing specificity and sensitivity, of the order of 30%. This leaves brain biopsy as the diagnostic test of choice. Brain biopsy (including meninges) leads to a diagnosis in over 75% of cases, even when targeted at radiologically normal-looking brain tissue. However, about half of positive biopsies for presumed ICA show an alternative, unsuspected cause of the problem. Infection, lymphoma and multiple sclerosis (MS) are high on this list.

Treatment of ICA is not and may never be based on prospective placebo-controlled trials. However, as with treatment for the systemic vasculitides, more potent immunosuppression than can be provided by steroids alone is almost certainly warranted. A current reasonable therapy regimen would be: intravenous methylprednisolone 1 g/day for 3 days followed by 60 mg/day prednisolone tapering over months and eventually being superseded by a steroid-sparing agent such as azathioprine, with oral cyclophosphamide 2 mg/kg/day for 9–12 weeks, or pulsed intravenous cyclophosphamide 0.5 g/m^2 every 2 weeks for 3–6 months, starting after the 3 days of intravenous steroid.

Rheumatoid arthritis

RA, also known as rheumatoid disease, is a multi-system disorder usually presenting with a symmetrical distal polyarthropathy. Stiffness of the joints is usually prominent, especially in the morning and the diagnosis is usually supported by the presence of rheumatoid nodules, positive rheumatoid factor in serum and characteristic juxta-articular changes on X-rays of affected joints. Inflammatory or vasculitic neurological complications also occur but are rare. More common are entrapment neuropathies and, most worrying, spinal cord or lower brainstem syndromes secondary to erosive skeletal involvement of the atlanto-axial, odontoid or other vertebral components. The cervical spine is most often affected by erosive disease but extradural pannus can cause compression at any spinal location, including the cauda equina (Chapter 16).

A group of rheumatological disorders overlap with RA, the mixed connective tissue diseases (MCTD) consisting of RA, scleroderma, Sjögren's syndrome, SLE and myositis. Patients with this disorder are often positive for the U1-RNP antibody which is associated with the main threat to life: pulmonary hypertension. Neurological manifestations are similar to those seen in RA or SLE; an inflammatory myopathy is present in up to 50% of cases. MCTD-associated myopathy is particularly responsive to steroids.

Systemic lupus erythematosus

SLE is a multi-system disorder like RA, which commonly affects the joints and almost any other organ system, although the arthritis is less erosive than that seen in RA and mucocutaneous involvement more common. Antinuclear antibodies (ANA) are often present in SLE, but the test has a high false positive rate and detection of more specific antibodies to intracellular antigens is often required (e.g. double and single stranded DNA). Neurological complications of SLE usually occur within the CNS. In the largest unselected cohort to date, up to 50% had so-called neuropsychiatric lupus (NPSLE).

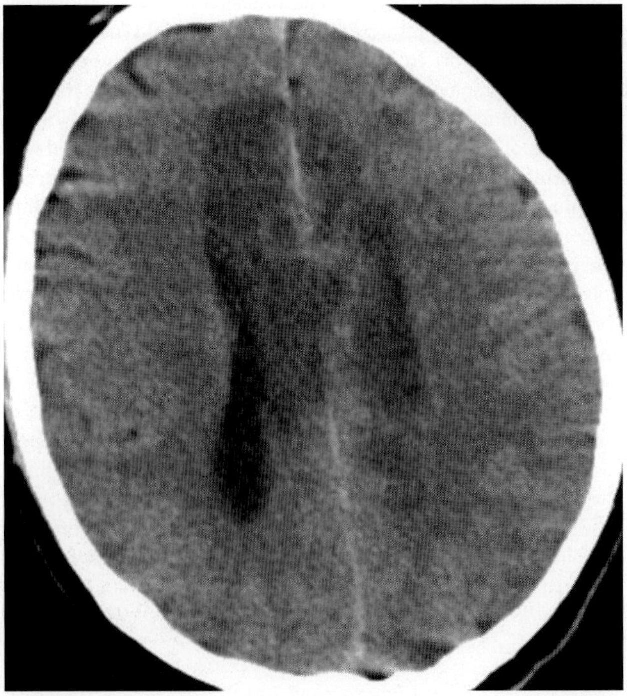

Figure 26.10 Primary CNS vasculitis. Axial CT scan showing multiple confluent cerebral infarcts.

This proportion is closer to 30% if all those with headache alone are excluded, as they probably should be because headache is no more common in SLE patients than controls. Mood disorders, strokes and cognitive disorders occur in 10–15% of patients; seizures, frank psychosis and acute confusional states are less common, as are disorders of the nerve or muscle.

The exact mechanism(s) involved in NPSLE are still unclear. A key feature seems to be a primary vasculopathy not fulfilling criteria for a true 'vasculitis', with mild to moderate peri-vascular mononuclear cell infiltration (but not destructive fibrinoid necrosis) sometimes causing occlusion and small infarcts. Clinically, stroke has been reported to affect 19% of patients with SLE, making this potentially an important cause of stroke in younger individuals. Cohort studies confirm that those with SLE are at higher risk of stroke than an age-matched population. Other factors than the vasculopathy (e.g. accelerated atherosclerois or hypertension), can be caused by long-term corticosteroid use.

Antibodies contribute to various components of NPSLE; for example, antiphospholipid antibodies are associated with stroke. Furthermore, anticardiolipin antibodies have been detected in 55% of patients with NPSLE compared to 20% with SLE alone. The therapeutic implication is that NPSLE should be treated with antithrombotic rather than immunosuppressive therapy. The indications for anticoagulation (e.g. with warfarin rather than aspirin) for secondary stroke prevention remains controversial. If stroke occurs and there are high levels of antiphospholipid antibodies, long-term anticoagulation with warfarin is generally recommended.

Antiphospholipid syndrome

Antiphospholipid syndrome (APS) is characterised by thrombosis (venous and/or arterial or microvascular) and/or pregnancy loss in association with a heterogeneous group of antibodies known as antiphospholipid antibodies (aPL). Positive aPL consists of the presence of one or more of the following antibodies:

- Lupus anticoagulant (LA) which causes prolongation of *in vitro* phospholipid-dependent clotting assays
- Anticardiolipin antibodies (aCL)
- Anti-β2 glycoprotein-1 (β2-GPI) antibodies.

aPL are present in autoimmune disorders (including SLE, RA, systemic sclerosis, Behçet's syndrome and Sjögren's syndrome); and in association with lymphoproliferative disorders, drugs and infections. The presence of aPL in patients with SLE is approximately 30% and <40% of patients with SLE and aPL will develop APS. aPL is directly prothrombotic and accounts for <10% of cases of acute venous thrombo-embolism (VTE), usually affecting the deep veins of the lower limbs.

The most frequent site of arterial occlusion is the cerebral vasculature which may be thrombotic or embolic. Ischaemic stroke resulting from arterial thrombosis is the most common neurological manifestation in APS, and aPL have also been noted in the presence of Sneddon's syndrome. A wide range of neurological manifestations have been described in association with aPL: an MS-like syndrome, migraine, cognitive impairment, epilepsy, psychiatric disorders and visual disturbances. However, a causal relationship remains unproven. The conventional initial management of VTE in patients with APS involves standard therapy with low molecular weight heparin followed by indefinite oral anticoagulation using standard intensity (target INR 2.5). However, high-intensity anticoagulation (target INR 3.5) is recommended for patients with APS-related stroke.

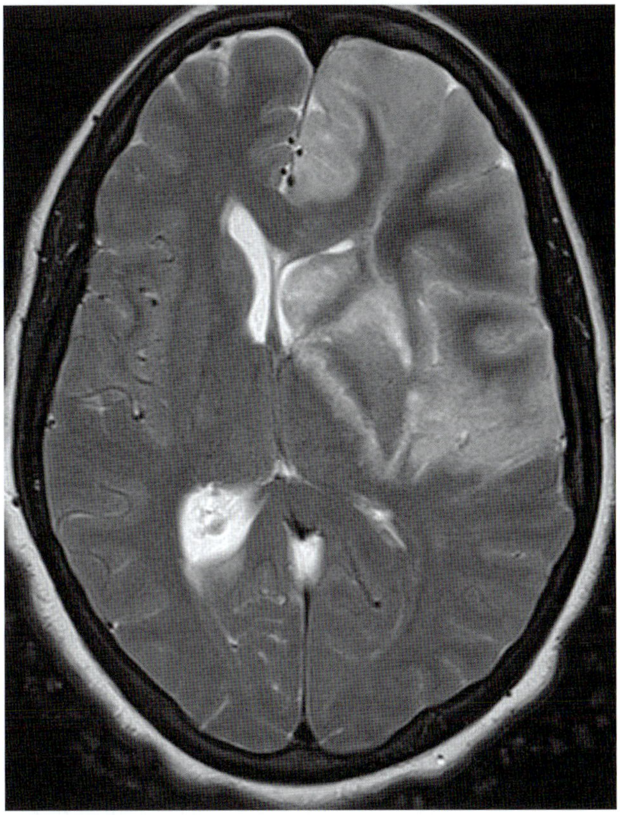

Figure 26.11 Catastrophic antiphospholipid syndrome. Axial MRI (T2-weighted) showing left anterior and middle cerebral artery infarction.

Catastrophic APS (CAPS) is a rare but potentially life-threatening condition characterised by sudden extensive microvascular thrombosis leading to multi-organ failure (Figure 26.11). CAPS carries a high mortality. Treatments have included anticoagulation, intravenous immunoglobulin and immunosuppressive therapy including high-dose corticosteroids, cyclophosphamide and rituximab.

Sjögren's syndrome

Sjögren's syndrome is characterised by lymphocytic infiltrates and destruction of epithelial exocrine glands. The main symptoms are dry eyes (keratoconjunctivitis sicca) and dry mouth (xerostomia). Sjögren's syndrome is classified as primary (where dry eyes and dry mouth with systemic complications are more common), or secondary to other connective tissue disorders such as RA, SLE or overlap syndromes (mixed connective tissue diseases [MCTD]). Systemic involvement is characterised by chronic fatigue, arthralgia, oesophageal hypomotility, haematological disorders and, rarely, a cutaneous vasculitis, alopecia and vitiligo.

The primary syndrome usually affects females (9 : 1 female : male ratio), develops slowly and is associated with B-cell lymphoma in 5% of cases. Lymphocytic infiltration leads to cutaneous purpura, lymphocytic alveolitis/interstitial pneumonitis and malabsorption. There may also be renal tubular necrosis, nephritis and Raynaud's syndrome. Antinuclear antibodies, rheumatoid factor and various anti-extractable nuclear antigen antibodies (ENAs, specifically anti-Ro and anti-La antibodies) are associated with Sjögren's syndrome. Schirmer's test for objective evidence of dry eyes and minor salivary gland biopsy showing focal lymphocytic sialadenitis (usually of the lip) also has a role in the most recent diagnostic criteria.

In Sjögren's syndrome, several different types of neuropathy have been described. The most common pattern (approximately 50%) is of an asymmetric, segmental or multi-focal sensory neuropathy starting with distal paraesthesia but often progressing to involve the trunk or face. A large proportion of these patients have an associated sensory ataxia, severe in some cases; they are likely to have high signal intensity in the posterior columns of the spinal cord on T2 MRI. In some subjects, ataxia is less prominent but neuropathic pain more so; the general progression of symptoms tends to be over months to years. A less common pattern of peripheral nerve involvement is one of a sensory and motor syndrome indistinguishable from mononeuritis multiplex seen in other connective tissue disorders; the progression tends to be acute or subacute rather than slowly progressive. Neuropathological studies suggest that the sensory–ataxic pattern is caused by a ganglioneuronitis with lymphocytic infiltration of the dorsal root ganglia similar to that seen in the glandular tissues of the mouth. While a vasculitic pathology is more likely to underlie the mononeuritis multiplex type, overlap forms clearly occur.

Cranial neuropathies are also associated with Sjögren's syndrome and again tend to follow one of two patterns mirroring involvement of the peripheral nerves: either a sensory neuropathy affecting one or both trigeminal nerves with no motor features, or a cranial polyneuropathy that can affect any nerve with little discrimination between motor and sensory nerve populations. Hearing loss is sensorineural because of a lesion of the VIIIth nerve and this may develop suddenly or progressively. Autonomic features are often associated with Sjögren's syndrome neuropathies (60%): abnormalities of pupillary function (Holmes–Adie pupils), sweating and orthostatic hypotension are the most common manifestations; a pure autonomic neuropathy also occurs, but is much rarer. Many older patients who are diagnosed with Sjögren's syndrome turn out to have had a chronic, apparently idiopathic, neuropathy for many years, so it is worth screening for Sjögren's syndrome in this group, especially if the symptoms are patchy or associated with autonomic features.

CNS involvement is increasingly recognised and may be severe. MS-like features are often associated with a cutaneous vasculitis and optic neuropathy. Other manifestations include meningo-encephalitis with stroke-like episodes, intracerebral or subarachnoid haemorrhage resulting from vasculitis and focal abnormalities including sensorineural deafness, internuclear ophthalmoplegia, nystagmus, dystonia, athetosis, parkinsonism, focal and generalised seizures. Rarely, affective symptoms develop as a consequence of an encephalopathic-like presentation with depression, anxiety and cognitive impairment. Spinal cord involvement can develop with an acute transverse myelitis of sudden onset, usually associated with a vasculitis; more progressive forms of spinal cord involvement also occur. A neuromyelitis optica-like syndrome has been reported in several cases. The MRI changes are of focal high signal abnormalities on T2 images in the brain white matter and cortex and in the spinal cord. These can be indistinguishable from those seen in MS.

If there is involvement of the peripheral or central nervous system, aggressive treatment for underlying vasculitis is indicated. The first line is with intravenous corticosteroid therapy but if progression continues an alternative immunosuppressant may be indicated. The sensory axonal ganglioneuropathy responds poorly to immunosuppression. Other agents that may augment steroids include azathioprine and hydroxychloroquine. TNF inhibitors (e.g. infliximab) have not been shown to have benefit in Sjögren's syndrome.

Miscellaneous cerebral arteriopathies

CADASIL

CADASIL (cerebral autosomal dominant arteriopathy with subcortical infarcts and leukoencephalopathy) is an autosomal dominant disease of small cerebral vessels caused by mutations in the *notch 3* gene on chromosome 19q13. *Notch 3* is a large gene coding for a transmembrane protein involved in intracellular signalling. The condition is characterised by episodic migraine-like headaches and recurrent subcortical ischaemic strokes usually beginning in mid-adulthood. A multi-focal motor and sensory deficit develops often with cognitive impairment, incoordination and progression to pseudobulbar palsy and subcortical dementia (Chapter 8).

CT or MRI shows confluent white matter disease and multiple small deep infarcts with myelin loss usually sparing the U fibres (Figure 26.12). White matter change characteristically involves the anterior temporal horn and external capsule, areas that are less frequently affected in sporadic cerebral small vessel disease. Genetic testing for *Notch 3* mutations allows non-invasive confirmation of the diagnosis in many cases. Skin biopsy reveals pathological changes of a non-amyloid angiopathy with deposition of eosinophilic electron dense granular material within the media of the small arteries and arterioles. This leads to concentric arterial wall thickening, narrowing of the vessel lumen and impaired reactivity of the vessel culminating in chronic arterial insufficiency, ischaemia and infarction.

The prognosis for CADASIL is poor, with progressive stepwise deterioration leading to severe impairment of sensory and motor function and progressive dementia. However, recent data suggest that treatment of modifiable vascular risk factors including hypertension, lipid abnormalities and hyperhomocysteinaemia is appropriate and may limit the severity of expression of the disease.

CARASIL

CARASIL (cerebral autosomal recessive arteriopathy with subcortical infarcts and leukoencephalopathy) is a rare single-gene small vessel disorder, mainly affecting individuals of Japanese ancestry (although Chinese and Caucasian pedigrees have been reported). CARASIL is caused by mutations in the *HTRA1* gene encoding HtrA serine peptidase/protease 1. Progressive cognitive impairment and focal neurological symptoms from recurrent ischaemic subcortical strokes are typical, though migraine is not. Hypertension is not a feature. Distinctive extracerebral manifestations include premature alopecia and severe low back pain, sometimes with herniation of vertebral discs or spondylosis deformans. T2-weighted MRI shows extensive areas of hyperintensity in the hemispheric white matter, thalami and brainstem (Figure 26.13). Pathologically, there is severe widespread loss of arterial medial smooth muscle cells. Treatment is with standard best medical preventive therapy including antihypertensive agents, antiplatelet agents and lipid-lowering agents.

Fabry's disease

Fabry's disease is an X-linked lysosomal storage disease resulting from deficient alpha-galactosidase A enzyme levels and accumulation of globotriaosylceramide in various cells, including the vascular endothelium and smooth muscle cells, resulting in an arteriopathy affecting both small and large vessels. The characteristic skin rash (angiokeratoma corporis diffusum) is caused by ecstatic vessels and usually involves the bathing trunk region although it may be more widely distributed (Figure 26.14). Vascular involvement can cause ischaemic stroke from mechanisms

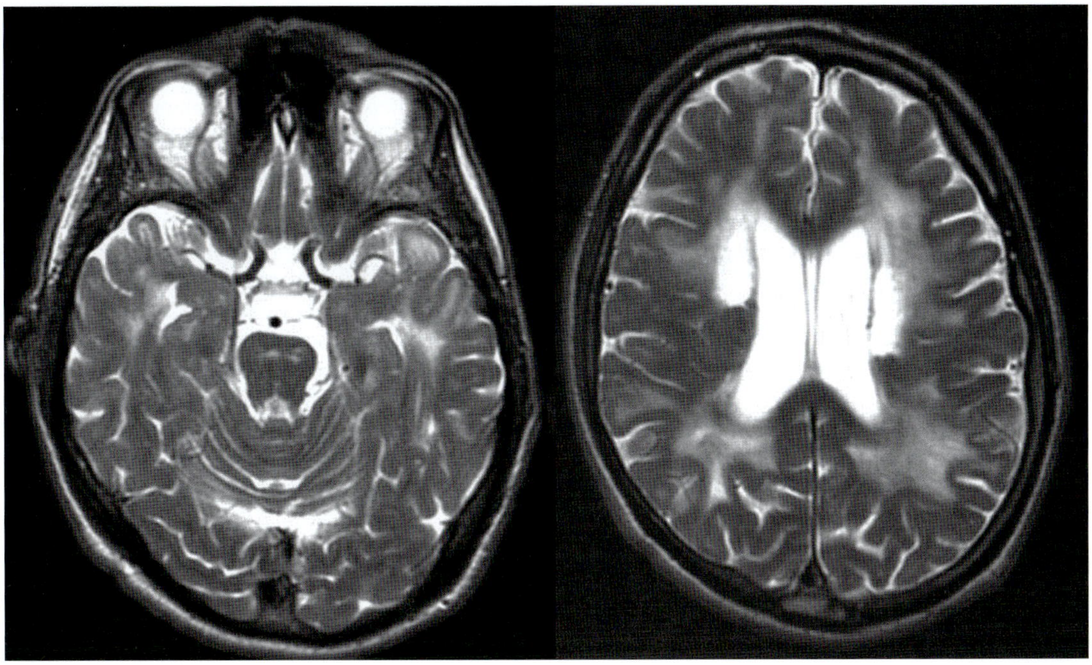

Figure 26.12 CADASIL. T2 axial MRI from a 54-year-old man with recurrent migraine, transient ischaemic attacks (TIAs), subcortical stroke syndromes and progressive cognitive impairment. Note the low attenuation in both anterior temporal lobes, extensive and confluent low attenuation in the deep cerebral white matter, and bilateral subcortical infarcts. Genetic testing confirmed the diagnosis of CADASIL.

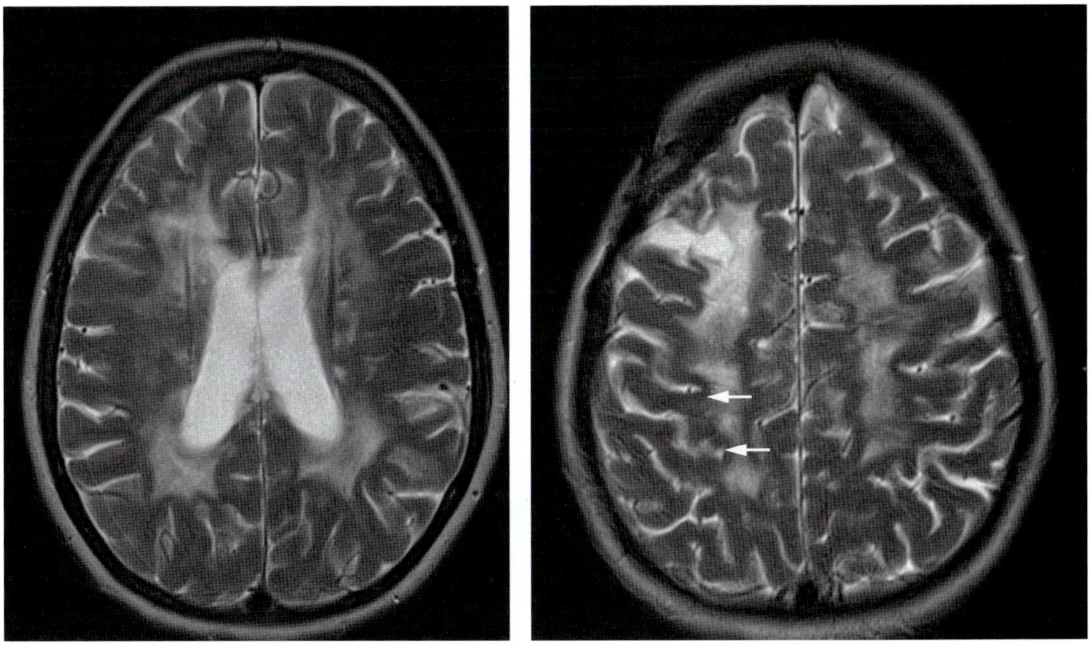

Figure 26.13 CARASIL. Multiple T2 hyperintensities in the peri-ventricular, deep white matter sparing subcortical U fibres (arrows).

including small vessel occlusion or cardio-embolism. The Fabry vasculopathy has been reported to show a predilection for the vertebrobasilar circulation, causing posterior circulation infarction. The multi-system manifestations of Fabry's disease include cardiomyopathy and renal failure. Although isolated neurological involvement at presentation is unusual, it is now realised that stroke can be the first symptom. Indeed, a study suggested that Fabry's disease could be responsible for up to 5% of cryptogenic strokes in young men. Subsequent large studies suggest that definite or probable Fabry's disease accounts for only about 1% of strokes in younger individuals (<55 years). Early recognition is vital to permit early therapeutic intervention and family screening, and could prevent clinical progression and recurrent stroke. The MRI findings of Fabry's disease include white matter hyperintensities, lacunar infarcts, basilar dilochoectasia and pulvinar hyperientensity on T1-weighted images (specific but not sensitive;

Figure 26.15). The white matter MRI changes, in combination with recurrent focal neurological symptoms (especially brainstem disturbances) in younger individuals, can frequently lead to confusion with MS. Fabry's disease is discussed further in Chapters 5 and 19.

Susac's syndrome

Susac's syndrome is a micro-angiopathy of unknown aetiology affecting the brain, cochlea and retina. It manifests as a triad of encephalopathy, sensorineural hearing loss and branch retinal artery occlusion. The condition predominantly affects women. At presentation not all of the clinical triad may be present. The onset of encephalopathy is typically associated with prodromal headache that may last for several months before the development of cognitive and psychiatric symptoms, sometimes with seizures and myoclonus. The hearing loss is often acute, bilateral and symmetrical suggesting infarction because of occlusion of the cochlear end arteries. Sometimes, hearing loss is asymmetric or even asymptomatic, being detectable only on audiometry. Visual loss is characteristically segmental, and fundoscopy reveals multiple branch retinal artery occlusions and a macular cherry red spot. The electroencephalogram (EEG) shows diffuse encephalopathic changes and MRI confirms multiple small high signal white matter lesions on T2 imaging typically involving the corpus callosum, and sometimes the posterior fossa and brain parenchyma (Figure 26.16). CSF shows elevated protein with normal cells or a minimal pleocytosis; oligoclonal bands are absent. Histological changes on brain biopsy confirm micro-infarcts resulting from arteriolar occlusion but the mechanism is unclear as there is neither vasculitis nor fibrinoid necrosis. There is no clear guidance to treatment particularly given the tendency for spontaneous remission. The rarity of the condition precludes clinical trials. Antiplatelet agents and steroids are widely used and second line immunosuppression with cyclophosphamide and azathioprine has been recommended. Rarely, plasma exchange and intravenous immunoglobulin have been used.

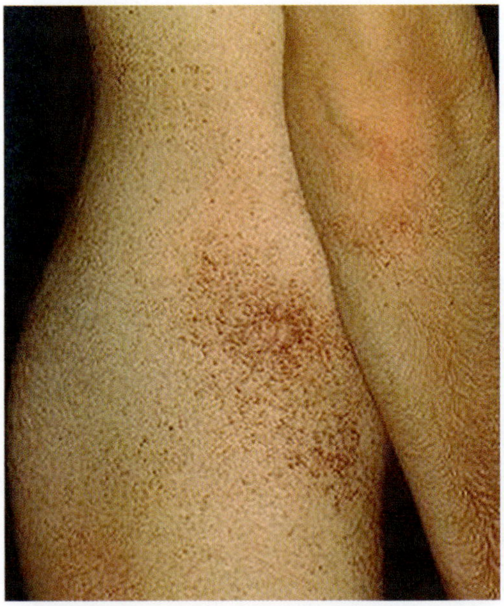

Figure 26.14 Angiokeratomas in a 'bathing trunks' distribution in a patient with Fabry's disease. Source: Ginsberg *et al.* 2005. Reproduced with permission of BMJ.

Sneddon's syndrome

Sneddon's syndrome is a rare disorder characterised by recurrent strokes (typically in the middle cerebral artery territory) in young patients, often with a history of migraine. Cognitive impairment sometimes develops. There is livedo reticularis (a fixed violaceous and net-like rash on the limbs and trunk); antiphospholipid antibodies are sometimes elevated. The pathology is of an arteriopathy affecting small and medium-sized vessels. Some MRI studies have shown extensive cortical high signal lesions and atrophy. The condition is associated with antiendothelial cell and antiprothrombin antibodies. Treatment is of standard vascular risk factors including hypertension. Anticoagulation may be considered, particularly in the presence of antiphospholipid antibodies.

Degos' disease

Degos' disease is a multi-system small vessel occlusive arteriopathy leading to ischaemia, initially involving the skin causing erythematous pink or red papules which heal to leave scars with characteristic white atrophic centres. Gastrointestinal and CNS complications can develop as the disease progresses. Ischaemic and haemorrhagic stroke can occur in the absence of vasculitis. Neurological involvement is characterised by the development of paraesthesiae, visual symptoms, weakness and myelopathy. MRI demonstrates multifocal ischaemic abnormalities or dural enhancement; skin biopsy shows vasculopathy but no active vasculitis.

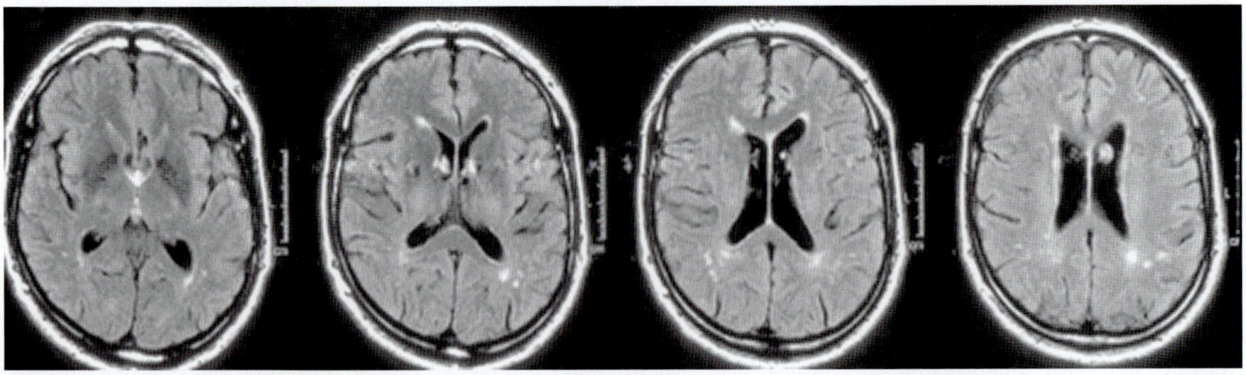

Figure 26.15 Four contiguous axial MRI sections with FLAIR weighting, demonstrating numerous white matter lesions in the cerebral hemispheres in Fabry's disease. Lesion load generally increases with patient age and the lesions may ultimately become confluent. Source: Ginsberg *et al.* 2005. Reproduced with permission of BMJ.

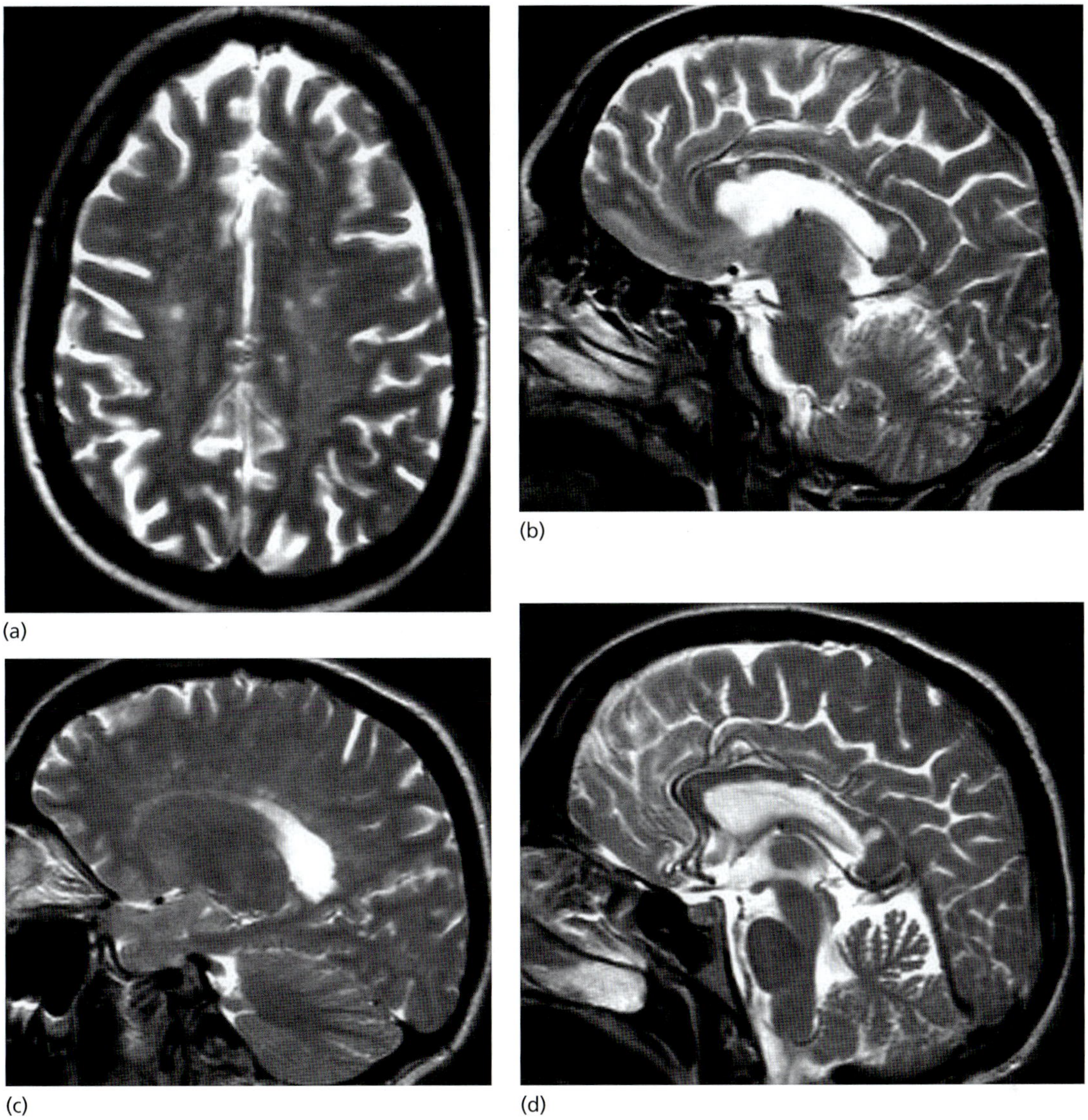

Figure 26.16 Susac's syndrome. A 24-year-old woman who presented with encephalopathy. Fundoscopy showed branch retinal arterial occlusions. Her family gave the history of hearing problems. These T2-weighted MRIs (a, axial; b, c, parasagittal; and d, sagittal) show small round foci of high T2 signal in the deep white matter and centre of the corpus callosum, consistent with microinfarctions. Gadolinium-enhanced T1-weighted parasagittal. Source: Renowden 2014. Reproduced with permission of BMJ.

HANAC

HANAC (hereditary angiography with neuropathy, aneurysms and cramps) is caused by a mutation in the *COL4A1* gene which encodes type IV collagen alpha 1 chain, which is a crucial component of basement membranes including vasculature, renal glomerulus and ocular structures. Neurological involvement is manifest as a diffuse leukoencephalopathy associated with intracranial aneurysms, muscle cramps, peripheral neuropathy, retinal tortuosities and haemorrhage and optic nerve abnormalities.

Reversible cerebral vasoconstriction syndrome

Reversible cerebral vasoconstriction syndrome (RCVS) describes a collection of clinical and radiological features: sudden, severe ('thunderclap') headache; transient, multi-focal, segmental vasoconstriction of cerebral arteries lasting several weeks to months; and focal neurological symptoms, sometimes with stroke (which may be caused by infarction or haemorrhage). The same syndrome has been variously described as thunderclap headache with vasospasm; migrainous vasospasm or angiitis; drug-induced angiitis; postpartum angiopathy; and benign angiopathy of the CNS. It seems likely that there are many causes (or triggers) for RCVS, and probably more than one underlying pathophysiological mechanism causing abnormal vascular tone. Multiple aetiologies for RCVS are suggested by the many and varied associations, including sympathomimetic, serotonergic or other drugs, pregnancy and the puerperium, though no obvious cause can be found in about 50% of cases. Ischaemic stroke can complicate RCVS, but it is also increasingly recognised that intracranial haemorrhage, especially cortical subarachnoid bleeding, can accompany RCVS. The clinical hallmark is *recurrent* thunderclap headache over days to weeks (a presentation that is extremely suggestive of, and possibly pathognomonic of, this disorder). Women are more often affected than men. The syndrome is important to recognise because the outcome is generally good, although less favourable when stroke occurs. A clinical challenge is that the syndrome cannot be confidently disgnosed until follow-up demonstration of resolution of vasoconstriction, and exclusion of other potential causes (e.g. CNS vasculitis). Treatment includes careful observation for complications, expert supportive care (e.g. in a stroke or neurosciences unit) and avoiding triggers (e.g. sympathomimetic drugs). Calcium channel blockers (e.g. nimodipine) are often given for 4–8 weeks, with some evidence of benefit on the headache. Steroids have not been shown to be effective.

Sarcoidosis

Sarcoidosis is a multi-system granulomatous disorder of unknown aetiology that affects the nervous system in some 5% of patients. Its hallmarks are non-caseating epitheloid cell granulomas with associated inflammation and the development of secondary fibrotic change which causes irreversible tissue damage.

Clinical features and investigation

The clinical presentation depends upon the pattern of organ involvement. Systemic sarcoid affects the lungs in 90% of patients; involvement varies from asymptomatic bilateral hilar lymphadenopathy to severe interstitial lung disease causing respiratory failure. Other organs often involved are the liver, lymph nodes, skin, endocrine and musculoskeletal system. The diagnosis in the presence of hilar lymphadenopathy can be confirmed by bronchoscopy, broncho-alveolar lavage or tissue biopsy. The presence of elevated serum angiotensin-converting enzyme and characteristic imaging appearances can help but have limited specificity. CSF ACE may be elevated. Gallium scans can show characteristic increased uptake in parotid salivary glands. However, in the absence of tissue evidence of non-caseating granulomas the diagnosis is sometimes extremely difficult and is often one of exclusion. Acute presentation is associated with a good prognosis but poorer prognostic features include a later age of onset, Afro-Caribbean extraction, the presence of lupus pernio, chronic uveitis, chronic hypercalcaemia, progressive pulmonary pathology, nasal mucosal disease or cardiac involvement. Neurological involvement is uncommon but carries a worse prognosis than pulmonary disease and may be associated with ocular and cardiac involvement. In approximately 15% of patients with neurosarcoidosis the presenting features are neurological but in others neurological involvement develops within 2 years of presentation. Chronic neurosarcoidosis can cause multiple cranial nerve palsies, parenchymatous cerebral involvement, hydrocephalus and encephalopathy or peripheral nervous system manifestations.

Cranial neuropathy

The most common neurological manifestations are isolated cranial neuropathy or aseptic meningitis. Up to 50% of neurosarcoid patients present with an isolated or bilateral facial palsy. This can be associated with dysgeusia, indicating a proximal lesion affecting the chorda tympani. Deafness from VIIIth nerve involvement occurs in 10–20% of cases; bilateral involvement strongly suggests neurosarcoidosis. Optic neuropathy occurs in up to 40% of patients and is often subacute, presenting with a progressive visual field defect, impaired acuity and pupillary dysfunction. Examination shows anterior uveitis, papillitis, papilloedema or optic atrophy secondary to granulomatous infiltration or compression of the optic nerve. Oculomotor abnormalities or bulbar weakness occur as a result of a diffuse meningeal infiltration. Infiltration is common at the base of the brain and can lead to hydrocephalus in 6–30% of neurosarcoidosis patients, which may be either obstructive or communicating. CSF diversion procedures are sometimes necessary but tend to fail.

Meningeal and parenchymatous sarcoid

Meningeal involvement commonly presents as an aseptic meningitis or occasionally as a meningeal mass lesion. The CSF shows a mononuclear pleocytosis with an elevated protein and a reduced glucose level. Parenchymal lesions are unusual. Clinical manifestations depend on their location and size. They can mimic tumours or demyelination, cause raised ICP with headache and papilloedema, seizures or focal involvement of the brainstem, basal ganglia or cerebellum (Figure 26.17). Isolated spinal lesions (often cervical) present as a progressive myelopathy with paraparesis and sphincter dysfunction (Figure 26.18). Pituitary and hypothalamic involvement occurs and can result in neuroendocrine disorders including diabetes insipidus, pan-hypopituitarism and hyperprolactinaemia.

Sarcoid encephalopathy

A diffuse or relapsing sarcoid encephalopathy can present with cognitive impairment or a confusional state often associated with memory disturbance. T2-weighted MRI shows diffuse contrast enhancement of the meninges with increased signal. Encephalopathy can coexist with a diffuse vasculopathy characterised by arteritis, external compression of arteries by an inflammatory mass lesion or multiple cardiac emboli. Rarely, dural venous thrombosis may occur. Neuropsychiatric features are also well described, presenting with psychosis or bipolar affective disorder. There is occasionally an isolated progressive amnesia or dementia without evidence of other neurological or systemic involvement. These patients appear to respond well to steroids.

Peripheral neuromuscular sarcoid

Peripheral neuromuscular involvement occurs in some 20% of patients with neurosarcoidosis. Peripheral nerve involvement is an isolated mononeuritis or a mononeuritis multiplex caused by granulomatous vasculitis or compression from granulomas. A symmetrical chronic axonal neuropathy occurs in some 25% of neurosarcoid patients. This is usually mild and of a mixed sensorimotor pattern but a more acute form indistinguishable from Guillain–Barré syndrome with demyelinating features can also develop. Muscle involvement is common but usually asymptomatic with non-caseating granulomas found on biopsy in more than 25% of patients. Symptomatic involvement varies from acute to chronic myopathy with an inflammatory component and occasionally palpable intramuscular nodules.

Diagnosis

Diagnosis can be challenging; histological confirmation should be sought if possible. MRI shows parenchymatous mass lesions – hyperintense lesions on T2 sequences – with linear enhancement of thickened meninges and focal nodular enhancement. CSF findings are non-specific but can be helpful if there is meningeal involvement. There may be a pleocytosis of up to 100 cells/mm^2 and elevated protein <2 g/dL (occasionally higher). Glucose is also occasionally reduced in active aseptic meningitis, CSF pressure is increased and oligoclonal bands present variably. Muscle biopsy can be diagnostic. Biopsy of cerebral lesions and the meninges is sometimes helpful, and the non-caseating granulomatous changes are diagnostic.

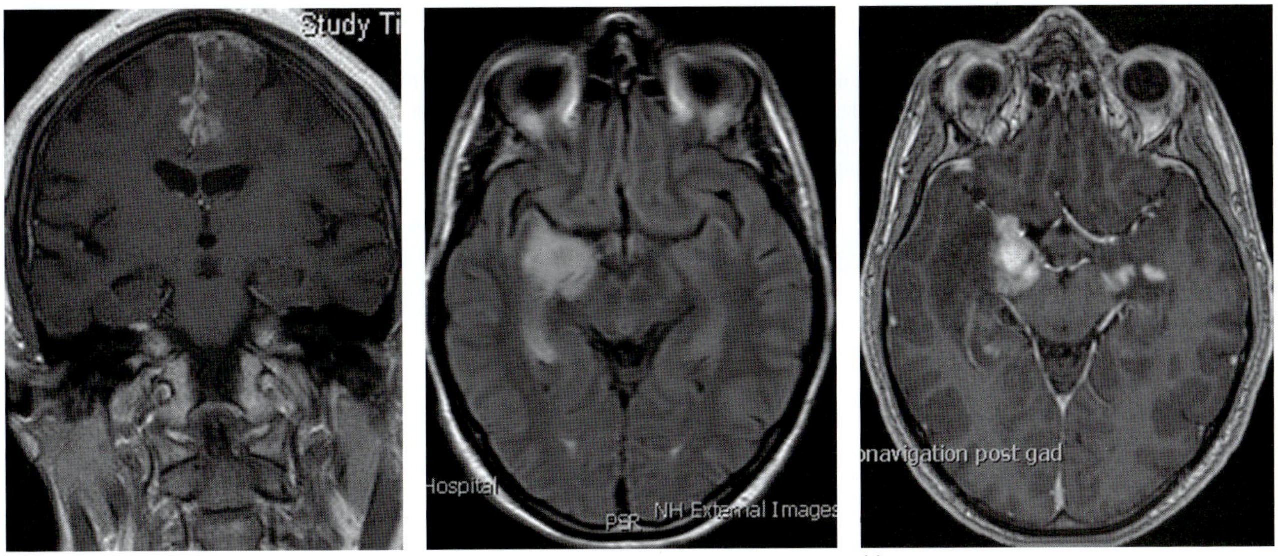

(a) (b) (c)

Figure 26.17 Neurosarcoid. MRI from patients showing lesions of neurosarcoidosis. (a) T1 coronal image showing extensive meningeal thickening with parenchymal involvement. (b) T1 axial imaging showing extensive focal intraparenchymal temporal lobe sarcoid lesion. (c) T1 axial lesion showing enhancement of temporal lesion and thickened meninges.

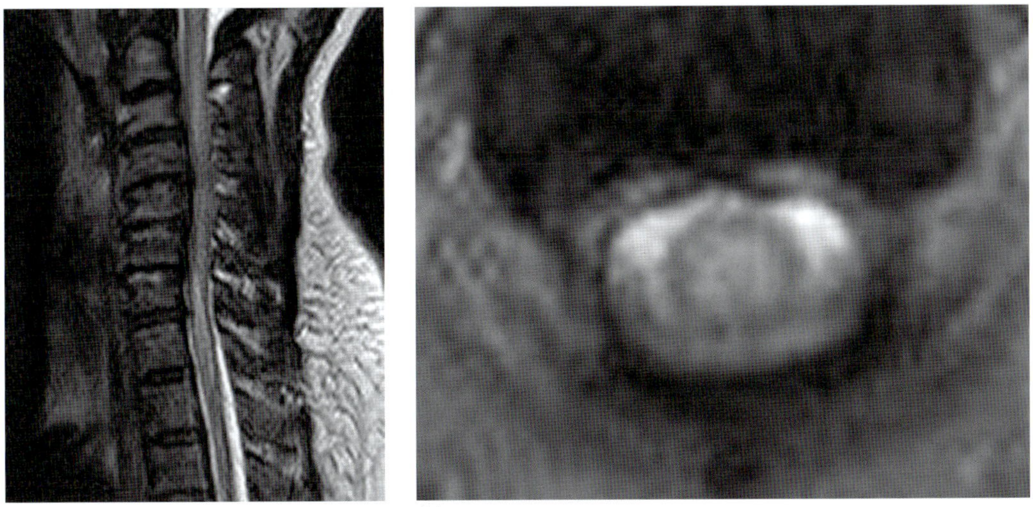

(a) (b)

Figure 26.18 Extensive intrinsic sarcoid of the cervical spinal cord: (a) T2 sagittal; and (b) axial image.

Prognosis

The prognosis is variable but generally neurosarcoidosis is a serious disease. Involvement of the peripheral nervous system tends to carry a better prognosis than central involvement. One-third of neurosarcoid cases have progressive disease despite immunosuppression with steroids and other agents.

Steroids are the principal treatment for neurosarcoidosis; the dose and duration are determined by the disease location, severity and time course. Treatment aims to reduce the inflammatory component and prevent progression to fibrosis and ischaemia. Steroids should be built up rapidly to high doses and the dosage tapered only after clinical response has been established. Occasionally, it is possible to withdraw steroids completely but many patients require long-term steroids and some require additional immunosuppressive agents such as azathioprine, methotrexate, ciclosporin, mycophenolate, cyclophosphamide, chlorambucil or cladribine, all of which have been reported to have efficacy in neurosarcoidosis. Infliximab is an antibody that specifically blocks TNF-alpha, and may have a role in neurosarcoidosis that is refractory to corticosteroids. Small case series have reported clinical and MRI improvement or stabilisation of neurosrcoidosis with this agent and also with rituximab (a B-cell directed monoclonal antibody).

Behçet's syndrome

Behçet's syndrome is a multi-system disease consisting of recurrent oral ulceration (at least three times in a year) and two of the following: recurrent genital ulcers, skin lesions, ocular lesions and a positive pathergy test. Neurological involvement occurs in approximately 5% of cases and falls into two distinct patterns, which rarely overlap:

- Parenchymal CNS lesions, most commonly affecting the brainstem, although any part of the CNS can be involved, known as neuro-Behçet's syndrome (NBS); and
- Cerebral venous sinus thrombosis (CVST).

The former is associated with relapsing-remitting and progressive disease patterns often culminating in moderate or severe disability; the latter tends to occur as a single episode. Features of the multiple systems affected by Behçet's syndrome are shown in Table 26.7.

Epidemiology and pathology

Behçet's syndrome usually occurs in the third decade and is seen most commonly in regions along the ancient Silk Route, thus extending from the Eastern Mediterranean to Japan; the prevalence in Turkey and Japan is 20 times that in the United Kingdom. Men are more commonly affected than women (1.4 : 1), a ratio that rises to 3 : 1 when considering cases of NBS. HLA B51 is associated in 50% of patients with Behçet's syndrome, especially those with uveitis.

There is still a debate whether the neuropathology of Behçet's syndrome is primarily one of vasculitis. While active CNS lesions often contain peri-vascular inflammatory infiltrates, the arteriolar vessel wall itself is rarely involved; associated fibrinoid necrosis is not reported in CNS pathological specimens. Blood vessels with characteristic changes suggesting vasculitis have been encountered in non-CNS organs, but usually on the venous side of the circulation.

Patterns of nervous system involvement

Of patients with Behçet's syndrome and neurological symptoms or signs other than isolated headache, roughly 80% present with NBS while the remaining 20% have CVST. Headache is the most common neurological symptom in Behçet's syndrome, even given its high prevalence in the general population. Both migraine and tension-type patterns are seen. New or severe headache in patients with known Behçet's syndrome should prompt imaging as CVST or parenchymal lesions will sometimes be found.

CNS involvement: parenchymal

The most common pattern of NBS is of a subacute brainstem syndrome that may be associated with lesions elsewhere in the CNS or, more rarely, cranial neuropathies (V, VII or VIII). Spinal cord and hemispheric presentations are also common but peripheral neuropathy is unusual. Symptoms not easily localisable are also seen (impaired consciousness, epilepsy, neuropsychiatric Behçet's syndrome). Ophthalmological involvement is discussed in Chapter 14, isolated optic neuropathy is rare (>1%) but raised intracranial pressure can occur following CVST or due to isolated idiopathic

Table 26.7 Multi-system manifestations of Behçet's syndrome.

Ocular (present in 70–95%) (loss of vision occurring approximately 3 years after onset of ocular symptoms)	Acute pan-uveitis usually associated with hypopyon Scleral and corneal involvement Conjunctival aphthous lesions Glaucoma Posterior segment changes Alteration in macular pigment epithelium Peri-venous sheathing Retinal and vitreous haemorrhages and exudates Occlusion of retinal arteries and veins Retinal detachment Optic and retrobulbar neuritis (becomes bilateral in 50% within 1 year and 80% within 2 years)
Mucocutaneous	Oral ulceration: small round oval painful crops on gums, lips, tongue, palette, posterior pharynx Genital ulcers: deep, painful and scarring Skin lesions: pustules, vesicles, folliculitis, acneiform lesions and erythema nodosum
Arthritis	Non-erosive, non-migrating, oligoarticular involvement of large joints especially knees, ankles and wrists
Gastrointestinal	Constipation, diarrhoea, abdominal pain and vomiting Ulcers may occur in any part of the gastrointestinal tract especially distal ileum and caecum
Vascular involvement	Arterial and venous malformations Venous – superficial thrombo-phlebitis, DVT, superior venocaval obstruction, Budd–Chiari syndrome and cerebral venous sinus thrombosis Arterial inflammatory change presenting as occlusion or aneurysm formation of the pulmonary, renal, subclavian, femoral and carotid arteries
Pulmonary	Recurrent haemoptysis, cough, chest pain and dyspnoea
Cardiac	Peri-myocarditis or endocarditis or coronary arteritis
Gastrointestinal	Dysphagia, epigastric pain, colicky abdominal pain and bloody diarrhoea

DVT, deep venous thrombosis.

intracranial hypertension. Most authors do not accept the existence of isolated NBS without pre-existing Behçet's syndrome, arguing that those patients who present with neurological symptoms have a history of recurrent oral ulcers at least.

NBS can mimic a variety of disease states, with MS being high on the differential list in Western practice. Although NBS can have a relapsing remitting or progressive course like MS, it is usually differentiated on the following grounds:

- MRI in NBS often reveals symptomatic lesion(s) below the tentorium, as opposed to the multiple, clinical silent, peri-ventricular lesions commonly seen in MS.
- CSF protein and lymphocyte counts are similar in both disorders, but oligoclonal bands are either absent or matched with serum in NBS and, if present, disappear on remission, compared to the persistently present unpaired intrathecal oligoclonal bands found typically in MS.
- Optic neuritis is rare in NBS and, when associated VEPs are abnormal, the pattern is of reduced amplitude and preserved latency rather than normal amplitude and prolonged latency encountered in demyelination.
- Systemic symptoms and headache are seldom present in an acute attack of MS.

Although NBS rarely complicates Behçet's syndrome, parenchymal disease is sometimes a cause of major disability. Of patients with NBS, 45% have a single neurological episode, while half each of the remainder have either a relapsing-remitting or a progressive course. NBS is a serious disease. Half of all NBS patients have an Expanded Disability Status Scale (EDSS) of <6 at 10 years from diagnosis.

Cerebral venous sinus thrombosis

Symptomatic CVST should be treated with anticoagulation (either low molecular weight heparin or warfarin) in the short to medium term but, given that it rarely recurs, long-term anticoagulation is not warranted. The main caveat to this statement is that Behçet's syndrome in general and Behçet's syndrome complicated by CVST in particular, are associated with coexisting pulmonary artery aneurysms (PAA). These aneurysms, which can occur at other sites in the vascular tree, are probably caused by inflammatory changes in the vasa vasorum of the larger pulmonary vessels, which can result in necrosis of the vessel wall causing true aneurysms or dissection causing false ones. It is therefore prudent to screen patients with Behçet's syndrome and CVST for PAA (usually with a CT pulmonary angiogram), before starting anticoagulation. PAA in Behçet's syndrome can be treated with immunosuppression, endovascular intervention or surgery.

Investigation

Peripheral blood is often but not always normal, with an absence of acute phase reactants. CSF examination shows pleocytosis (neutrophils and lymphocytes with an elevated protein but normal glucose). The opening pressure is increased if there is venous sinus thrombosis but oligoclonal bands are only present in a minority. The pathergy test is somewhat variable in its sensitivity. MRI in the acute stage can show lesions that appear iso- or hypo-intense on T1 images and hyper-intense on T2 and FLAIR, because of venous thrombosis with reversible oedema; lesions may be single or multiple. They are seen most commonly in the mesodiencephalic junction (Figure 26.19), cerebellar peduncle, basal ganglia and brainstem but can also occur in the optic nerve and hemispheres. In chronic disease brainstem atrophy with gliosis can develop.

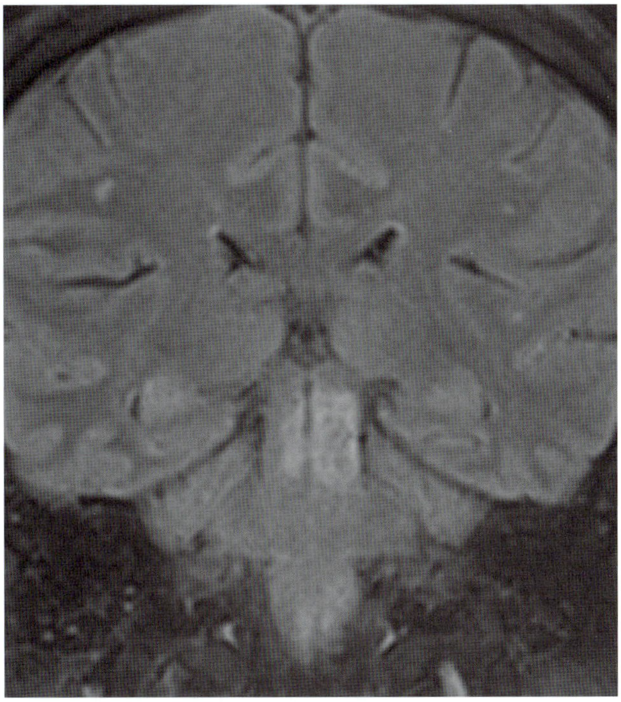

Figure 26.19 Coronal FLAIR MRI in a patient with Behçet's syndrome showing extensive brainstem and also some diffuse parenchymal signal change.

Pathergy test in Behçet's disease

The forearm is pricked with a fine sterile needle. With a positive pathergy test, a small red bump at the site of needle insertion develops 1–2 days later. Histologically, there is a largely lymphocytic reaction. Not all patients with Behçet's disease have positive pathergy tests. Behçet's patients from the Mediterranean littoral tend to have positive tests, around 50% from the Middle East and Japan but fewer from western Europe and the United States. A positive test is not diagnostic for Behçet's disease.

Treatment

Unfortunately, drug treatment for NBS has a limited evidence base. Common practice at centres experienced with treating NBS is to treat acute episodes with high dose, usually intravenous, steroids for 3–7 days, with many experts preferring to continue with a tapering dose of oral prednisolone over the next 3 months. Patients with relapsing or progressive NBS are usually treated with azathioprine, methotrexate or pulsed cyclophosphamide, with or without added prednisolone. Some of the newer immunomodulatory therapies such as tacrolimus and infliximab have been tried with NBS because there is some evidence of their efficacy in controlling systemic Behçet's syndrome symptoms. Thalidomide and colchicine are widely used for the mucocutaneous manifestations. Neurovascular disease is managed conventionally with antiplatelet agents; the role of anticoagulation remains uncertain.

IgG4-related disease

IgG4-related disease is an increasingly recognised fibroinflammatory condition characterised by tumour-like dense lymphoplasmacytic infiltrates rich in IgG4 -positive plasma cells with variable fibrosis. Elevated serum concentrations of IgG4 is found in 60–70% of patients.

IgG4 lesions can be found in most organ systems of the body. The condition is particularly associated with autoimmune pancreatitis and salivary gland disease. Patients present with subacute development of a mass in an affected organ or diffuse enlargement of the organ (e.g. pancreas, salivary gland, biliary tree, kidney, lungs, breast, lymph nodes, thyroid and skin). Neurological involvement generally involves the development of lesions in the pituitary gland, a meningeal mass or a pachymeningitis.

The diagnosis is based upon biopsy findings showing a lymphoplasmacytic infiltration of mainly IgG4 positive plasma cells and lymphocytes accompanied by fibrosis. Serum IgG4 levels are generally elevated. The condition generally response to steroids and second line immunosuppression over several weeks or months but surgical removal of the mass is often necessary (Figure 26.20).

CLIPPERS

Chronic lymphocytic inflammation with pontine peri-vascular enhancement (CLIPPERS) is an inflammatory condition associated with the characteristic appearance on MRI of nodular or punctate enhancement in the brachium pontis, pons and cerebellum (Figure 26.21), with biopsy showing a marked perivascular and

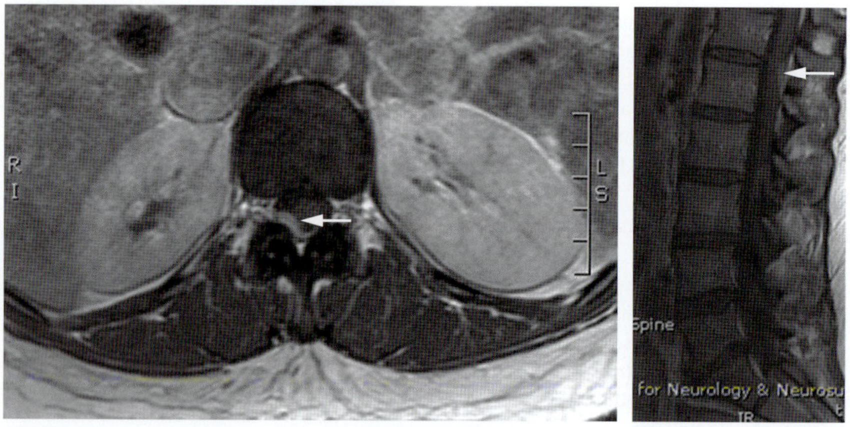

(a) (b)

Figure 26.20 IgG4 disease. Sessile enhancing intradural lesion (indicated by arrows) based on the right posterolateral dura at T12–L1 level: (a) axial T2; (b) sagittal T1 image.

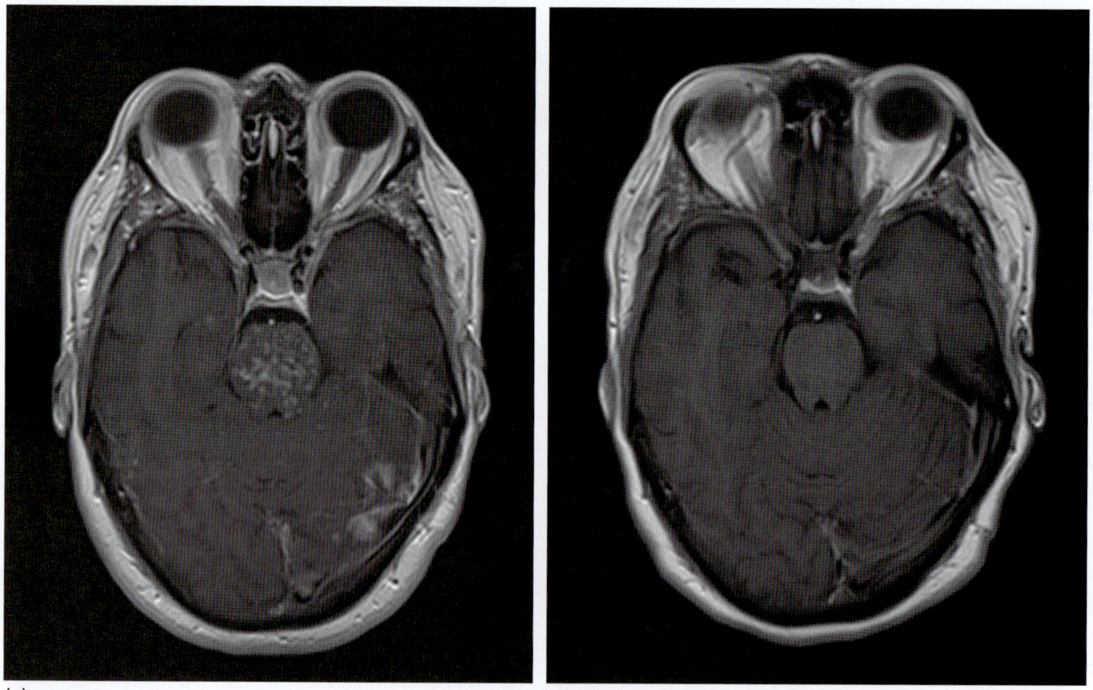

(a) (b)

Figure 26.21 Axial gadolinium-enhanced T1-weighted images at the time of subsequent presentation with a new brainstem syndrome demonstrating extensive punctate/linear areas of enhancement within the pons, characteristic of CLIPPERS: (a) occipital lesion with scattered areas of enhancement surrounding it and (b) 7 days after treatment with intravenous steroids, demonstrating dramatic improvement to the previous changes.

Table 26.8 Differential diagnosis of CLIPPERS.

Neurosarcoidosis
Lymphoma
Multiple sclerosis and ADEM
Sjögren's syndrome
Histiocytosis
Vasculitis (isolated angiitis of the CNS)
Lyme disease
Bickerstaff brainstem encephalitis
Whipple's disease
Behçet's disease

ADEM, acute disseminated encephalomyelitis; CLIPPERS, chronic lymphocytic inflammation with pontine peri-vascular enhancement.

parenchymal CD3+ T-cell infiltrate. Lesions also occur in the spinal cord, basal ganglia and cerebral white matter. Patients with CLIPPERS can present with local brainstem features including cranial nerve lesions and long tract signs. However, gait ataxia and dysarthria also occur and occasionally a more insidious cognitive impairment develops. Lesions characteristically respond to corticosteroids. There is no evidence of systemic involvement. The important differential diagnosis is summarised in Table 26.8.

Neurocutaneous syndromes

Neurocutaneous syndromes (also sometimes termed phakomatoses) are multi-system disorders that have characteristic CNS and skin manifestations. The features of these diseases are important to recognise for neurologists, because the skin manifestations are an important clue to potential neurological complications.

Neurofibromatosis type 1 (von Recklinghausen's disease)

Neurofibromatosis type 1 (NFI) is an autosomal dominant disorder caused by a mutation in the NF1 gene (17q11.2), encoding the protein neurofibromin which acts as a tumour suppressor. The clinical diagnosis is based on the presence of at least two diagnostic features: six or more café-au-lait patches, axillary or groin freckling, two or more neurofibromas or one plexiform neurofibroma, Lisch nodules in the iris, optic pathway glioma, bony dysplasia of the sphenoid wing, pseudoarthrosis of the long bones or a first degree relative with NF1. The birth frequency is 1 in 2500, with a prevalence of 1/4000–5000. The condition is also discussed in Chapters 14 and 16.

Neurological complications affect both the peripheral and central nervous systems. Neurofibromas are benign peripheral nerve sheath tumours that contain a mixture of Schwann cells, fibroblasts, mast cells and axons embedded in an extracellular matrix. Neurofibromas can be:

- *Cutaneous:* these develop in 99% of patients usually in early adulthood and consist of soft fleshy pedunculated skin tags. They increase in size and number during pregnancy. These are associated with considerable psychological distress but do not undergo malignant change (Figure 26.22).
- *Subcutaneous:* these are firm peripheral nerve tumours that frequently cause pain and neurological deficit. They also develop in adolescence (Figure 26.23).
- *Plexiform*: about 60% of patients with NF1 have plexiform neurofibromas (PN). These develop during adolescence and adulthood and cause both neurological deficit and disfigurement. They develop in deep tissues and are therefore difficult to remove. PN can transform into malignant peripheral nerve sheath tumours (Figure 26.24).

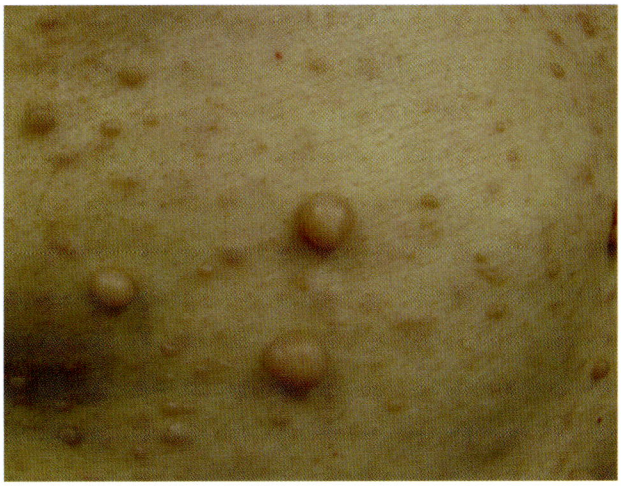

Figure 26.22 Cutaneous neurofibromas in an adult male with neurofibromatosis type 1. Subcutaneous: these are firm peripheral nerve tumours that frequently cause pain and neurological deficit. They also develop in adolescence (Figure 26.23). Source: Ferner 2010. Reproduced with permission of BMJ.

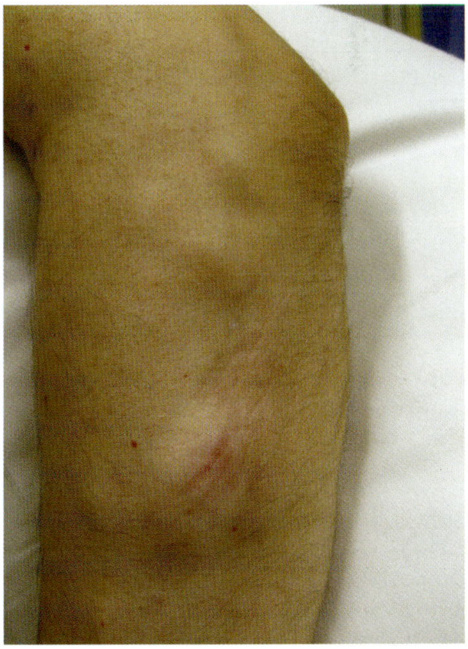

Figure 26.23 Subcutaneous neurofibromas in an adult male with neurofibromatosis type 1. Source: Ferner 2010. Reproduced with permission of BMJ.

Malignant peripheral nerve sheath (MPNSTs) usually arise from pre-existing focal subcutaneous neurofibromas or PNs but can arise *de novo*. Patients with MPNSTs present with persistent or nocturnal pain, a rapid increase in the size of a neurofibroma, new neurological deficit and a change in the texture of the pre-existing neurofibroma. The goal of treatment is complete removal of the tumour with clear margins. Radiotherapy is administered for high grade or

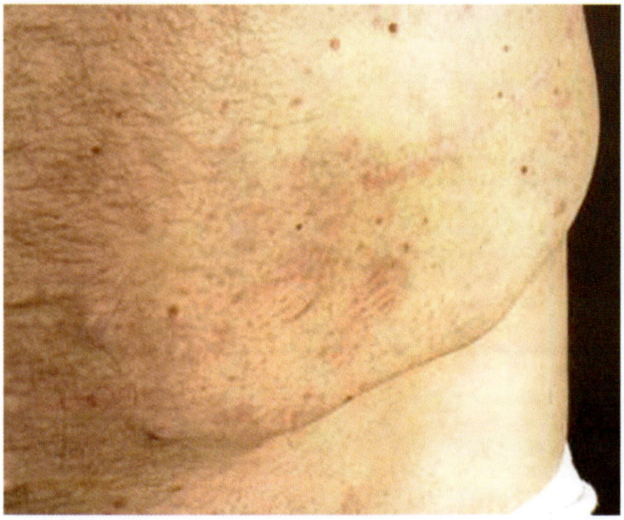

Figure 26.24 Plexiform neurofibroma of the abdominal wall in an adult male with neurofibromatosis. Source: Ferner 2010. Reproduced with permission of BMJ.

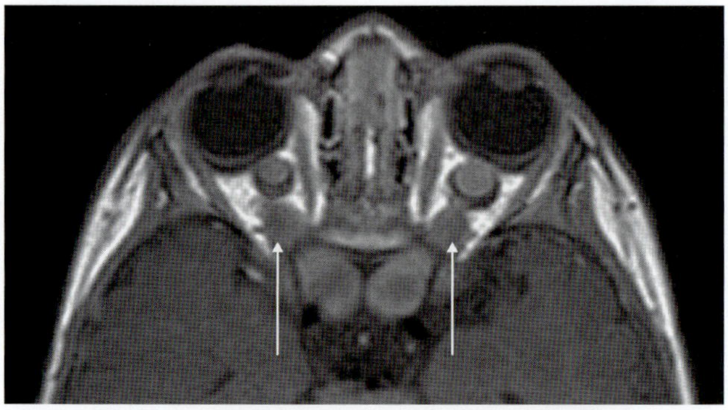

Figure 26.25 Optic pathway gliomas in a child with neurofibromatosis type 1 involving both optic nerves which are grossly enlarged (arrows): axial MR scan. Source: Ferner 2010. Reproduced with permission of BMJ.

incompletely excised lesions and chemotherapy with ifosfamide and doxarubicin can provide palliative support.

Other neurological manifestations of NF1 include:

- Cognitive impairment, characterised by an IQ in the low average range, specific learning difficulties and behavioural problems including attention deficit–hyperactivity disorder.
- Epilepsy, which occurs in 4–13% of cases and may be caused by cerebral dysgenesis, mesial temporal sclerosis or tumours including glioma or dysembryoplastic neuroepithelial tumours or have no obvious cause.
- Cerebral malformations, which include macrocephaly, Chiari 1 malformation and aqueduct stenosis caused by subependymal glial cell proliferation.
- Spinal nerve root neurofibromas may be asymptomatic but can cause pressure on the adjacent nerve root of spinal cord.
- Peripheral neuropathy is relatively uncommon. It presents with mild distal motor and sensory impairment associated with nerves thickened by infiltration with neurofibroma tissue.
- Brain and optic pathway tumours: gliomas generally occur in the optic pathways (Figure 26.25), cerebellum and brainstem. Most slow-growing tumours are pilocytic astrocytomas but higher grade gliomas are common.
- Other tumours can occur – rhabdomyosarcoma is encountered more frequently in NF1, often at an earlier age and frequently arising in the genitourinary tract.
- Bone abnormalities are common and include short stature, scoliosis and osteoporosis.
- Primary progressive and relapsing multiple sclerosis occurs with increased frequency in NF1.
- Systemic manifestations are common and include cardiovascular disease (hypertension and congenital heart disease), renal artery stenosis and cerebrovascular disease. Respiratory compromise can be caused by a restrictive deficit as a result of scoliosis or direct compression by PN. Mesenchymal gastrointestinal stromal tumours occur mainly in the small bowel. Pheochromocytoma is also rarely associated with NF1.

Genetic counselling is recommended for everyone with NF1 and both prenatal mutation testing and pre-implantation genetic diagnoses are available. Surveillance should involve lifelong annual follow-up with developmental assessment, transitional planning and prompt access to specialist advice from nationally commissioned specialist centres.

Neurofibromatosis type 2

Neurofibromatosis type 2 (NF2) is characterised by the development of multiple tumours of the nervous system. The most common manifestation is bilateral vestibular schwannoma but other tumours including cranial or orbital meningioma, spinal and cutaneous schwannoma also occur. NF2 is an autosomal dominant condition caused by a mutation in the *NF2* gene (22q11.2) which produces merlin, a tumour suppressor. However, <30% of patients with NF2 without a family history are mosaic.

Schwannomas are benign tumours arising from peripheral nerve sheaths and are comprised entirely of Schwann cells. Unlike neurofibromas, they rarely undergo malignant change. Vestibular schwannomas occur in 95% of patients with NF2 (Figure 26.26), generally presenting with unilateral or bilateral sensorineural deafness, tinnitus and impaired balance. Raised ICP and brainstem compression can develop. Surgical removal is generally indicated but this usually causes sensorineural hearing loss. Most patients with NF2 develop spinal tumours. Bevacizumab, a monoclonal antibody against vascular endothelial growth factor (VEGF), is reported to induce both tumour regression and hearing improvement in patients with NF2-associated vestibular schwannomas. Extramedullary schwannomas and meningiomas are common but only cause symptoms in approximately 30% of patients. Schwannomas arise from the dorsal root and have a characteristic dumb bell shape. Intramedullary tumours, particularly ependymomas, are seen in <30% of patients. Ependymomas and pilocytic astrocytomas occur predominantly in the upper cervical cord and brainstem, and are commonly associated with a syrinx. Schwannomas of other cranial nerves are slower growing and do not usually require surgical intervention. Cranial meningiomas develop in 45% of patients and are frequently multiple.

NF2 is also associated with the development of an axonal peripheral neuropathy which can be severe and progressive. Focal amyotrophy can occur in the affected limb and vision can be impaired by cataract or the effects of orbital meningiomas, retinal hamartomas or epiretinal membranes. *NF2* gene mutation testing is routinely undertaken and prenatal and pre-implantation diagnosis are available. Routine annual clinical and radiological surveillance is essential for at risk individuals.

Xeroderma pigmentosa

Xeroderma pigmentosa is an uncommon autosomal recessive disorder caused by mutations in the nucleotide repair genes. There is severe solar sensitivity leading to the development of basal and squamous cell carcinoma and melanomas beginning in early childhood. Ocular abnormalities include keratitis, opacification of the cornea, iritis and melanoma of the choroid. Up to 20% of patients with xeroderma pigmentosa have neurological abnormalities of varying severity caused by primary neuronal degeneration.

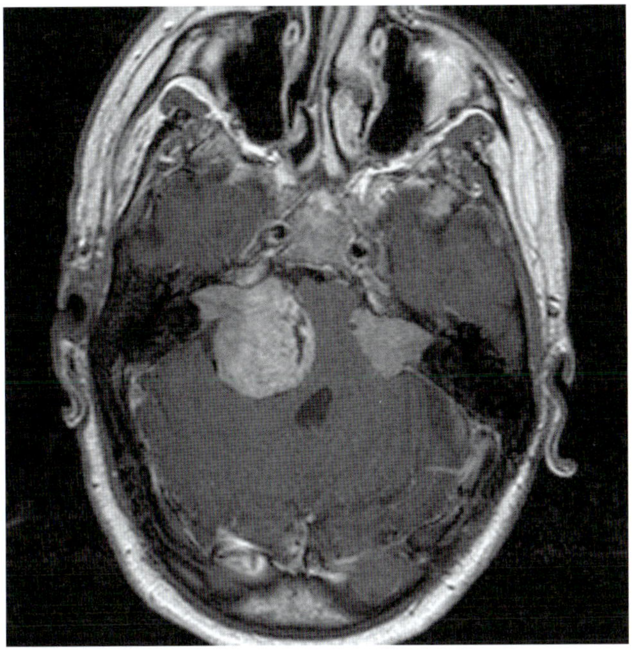

Figure 26.26 Bilateral vestibular schwannomas distorting the brainstem in a young man with neurofibromatosis type 2: enhanced axial MR scan. Source: Ferner 2010. Reproduced with permission of BMJ.

Tuberous sclerosis

Tuberous sclerosis (Chapter 16) is characterised by multiple hamartomatous lesions which affect virtually any organ but particularly involve the brain, skin, eye, kidney, heart and lung. It is autosomal dominant and caused by mutations in either the *TSC1* or *TSC2* genes. Penetrance is complete but expression of tuberous sclerosisis highly variable. Characteristic skin lesions include hypopigmented macules (ash leaf spots), adenoma sebaceum (angiofibromas typically involving the malar region of the face), shagreen patches (which usually involve the lower trunk), peri-ungual fibromas and fibrous plaques (often seen on the forehead). Neurological involvement is characterised by the presence of subependymal nodules, subependymal giant cell tumours (Figure 26.27), white matter heterotopia and glioneuronal hamartomas (cortical tubers). The severity of neurological dysfunction (i.e. seizures and cognitive function) is related to the extent of glioneuronal hamartomas. Subependymal giant cell tumours are slow-growing tumours of mixed glioneuronal origin that arise in peri-ventricular areas. There is a risk of malignant transformation, particularly affecting subependymal giant cell tumours in the brain, kidneys and soft tissues.

Epilepsy occurs in <90% of patients, often developing in the first year as infantile spasms or partial epilepsy but patients remain at risk. Cognitive impairment and behavioural difficulties including autistic spectrum disorders are common. Ophthalmic abnormalities include retinal hamartomas, which may be calcified (mulberry appearance), chorioretinal depigmentation and angiofibromatosis of the eyelids. Systemic involvement is characterised by cardiac rhabdomyoma, aortic coarctation and aneurysm formation, renal angiomyolipomas and diffuse interstitial pulmonary fibrosis.

Von Hippel–Lindau disease

Von Hippel–Lindau disease (VHL) is an autosomal dominant condition caused by a germline mutation in the *VHL* gene. Two forms of the condition are recognised depending on the risk of developing pheochromocytoma. Neurological involvement is characterised by the development of haemangioblastoma (HBO), particularly affecting the cerebellum, brainstem or spinal cord, often at a young age.

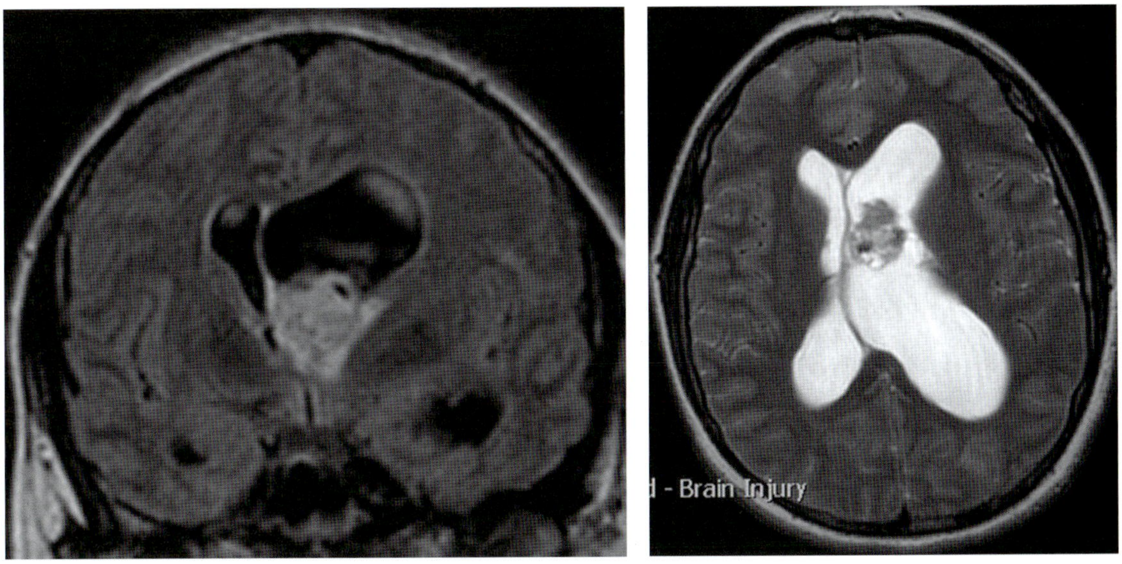

(a) (b)

Figure 26.27 Left subependymal giant cell astrocytoma in a patient with tuberosclerosis: (a) T1-weighted coronal; (b) T2 axial MRI.

HBO are well-circumscribed capillary-rich benign neoplasms which cause symptoms by direct compression of adjacent structures. They are often infratentorial and multiple in VHL. Surgical intervention is generally reserved until lesions become symptomatic or they develop accelerated growth. Retinal capillary haemangioblastomas (RCH) are typically found in the peripheral retina and/or juxtapapillary region. They are often multifocal and bilateral and occur in <70% of VHL by the age of 60. Visual loss is a result of exudation from the tumour causing retinal oedema or by traction effects, in which glial proliferation causes retinal striae and distortion. However, haemorrhage can occur leading to retinal detachment, glaucoma and loss of vision. Any patient presenting with seemingly sporadic HBO or RCH (particularly aged less than 40) should be screened for VHL.

VHL is associated with a number of important systemic features including the development of pheochromocytoma, multiple renal cysts (often considered premalignant) and renal clear celll carcinoma (RCC), endolymphatic sac tumours of the middle ear, serous cystadenomas and neuroendocrine tumours of the pancreas and papillary cystadenomas of the epididymis. Routine annual screening should include imaging of the kidneys, estimation of plasma metanephrins and biannual imaging of the brain and spinal cord. Meticulous genetic counselling must be undertaken in women with VHL and they should be closely monitored during pregnancy because of the risk of accelerated tumour growth.

Ataxia telangiectasia

Ataxia telangiectasia is a rare autosomal recessive condition associated with defective DNA repair mechanisms caused by a gene mutation at 11q 22.3. Patients develop progressive cerebellar ataxia, abnormal eye movements (oculomotor apraxia), oculocutaneous telangiectasia, immunodeficiency affecting both cellular and humoral immunity with particular impairment of IgA and IgG and other neurological abnormalities including progressive impairment of motor development often leading to wheelchair dependency by the age of 10, particularly in homozygotes. Dysphagia, aspiration and respiratory muscle weakness also occur. Other systemic features include pulmonary disease (recurrent infections, bronchiectasis and pulmonary fibrosis), an increased incidence of malignancy (generally lymphoma or acute leukaemia) and diabetes mellitus resulting from insulin resistance.

Sturge–Weber syndrome

Sturge–Weber syndrome is characterised by a facial capillary malformation (port wine stain) and an associated capillary–venous malformation affecting the brain and the eye. Sturge–Weber syndrome can lead to progressive neurological deficits including seizures, which may be associated with cortical malformations including polymicrogyria and cortical dysplasia; intellectual impairment; behavioural problems; and focal neurological signs often caused by stroke-like episodes. Hydrocephalus is common, probably associated with thrombosis in the deep cerebral veins or extensive arteriovenous anastomoses. Visual field deficits are caused by occipital cortex lesions. Vascular abnormalities also occur in the conjunctive, episclera, choroid and retina. The predominant ocular manifestation is glaucoma which presents in newborns with enlargement of the globe (buphthalmos). MRI with gadolinium contrast demonstrates the presence of leptomeningeal capillary venous malformations and the extent of brain involvement. Cranial CT imaging identifies the extent of calcification.

Other neurocutaneous syndromes are described in Table 26.9.

Table 26.9 Other neurocutaneous disorders.

Parry–Romberg	Hemifacial atrophy of the skin, soft tissues, muscles and bones of the face below the forehead EEG and MRI abnormalities often ipsilateral to the affected side of the face
Basal cell naevus syndrome	Autosomal dominant Developmental anomalies and post nasal tumours especially multiple basal cell carcinomas Medulloblastoma in 3–5% (occasionally meningioma)
Gardner's syndrome	Autosomal dominant Familial adenomatous polyposis Multiple skin epidermoid cysts, lipomas, osteomas, gastric polyps CNS tumour including medulloblastoma
Incontinentia pigmenti	X-linked dominant (lethal in males) Symptoms develop in the neonatal period Linear papules, vesicles, hyperpigmented whorls which lose pigmentation and become atrophic CNS involvement in one-third (seizures, intellectual impairment, spastic weakness)

Neurological aspects of pregnancy

Pregnancy is associated with a range of physiological changes including dynamic alterations in hormone levels. These changes can either change the presentation or severity of pre-existing neurological diseases, including migraine, epilepsy, multiple sclerosis and myasthenia gravis; or they may be associated with a conditions arising *de novo* during pregnancy, in particular cerebrovascular disorders. The management of epilepsy in women of childbearing age is of particular importance and is dealt with in some detail here.

Epilepsy and women of childbearing age

Fertility

Fertility rates are lower in women with treated epilepsy than in an age-matched control population. In a study of a general population of over 2 million persons in England and Wales, an overall fertility rate was found of 47.1 (95% CI 42.3–52.2) live births/1000 women with epilepsy per year compared with a national rate of 62.6. The difference in rates was found in all age categories between the ages of 25 and 39 years (Figure 26.28). There are probably several reasons for this. Women with epilepsy have low rates of marriage, marry later, suffer social isolation and stigmatisation. Some avoid having children because of the risk of epilepsy in the offspring, and some because of the teratogenic potential of antiepileptic drugs. Biological factors that may be relevant include genetic influences on fecundity and adverse antiepileptic drug effects. One-third of menstrual cycles in women with temporal lobe epilepsy can be anovulatory, compared with 8% in control populations. It has been suggested that valproate results in polycystic ovarian syndrome, possibly by causing obesity, peripheral insulin resistance, hyperandrogenism and hyperinsulinaemia, although this finding has not been widely replicated.

Pregnancy

Effects of epilepsy on pregnancy and delivery There are 3–4 live births per 1000 women of childbearing age with epilepsy in Western populations, and epilepsy is one of the most common medical

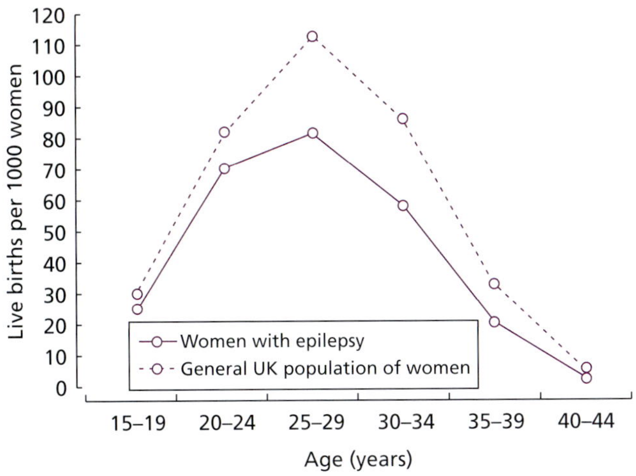

Figure 26.28 Fertility rates amongst women with epilepsy compared with that in the general population in a unselected UK population of 2 052 922 persons. Source: Wallace *et al.* 1998. Reproduced with permission of Elsevier.

Table 26.10 Complications of pregnancy reported with increased frequency in women with epilepsy.

Bleeding *in utero*
Premature separation of the placenta
Toxaemia of pregnancy and pre-eclampsia
Miscarriage and stillbirth
Intrauterine growth retardation, low birth weight
Perinatal mortality
Premature labour
Breech and other abnormal presentations
Forceps delivery, induced labour, caesarean section
Precipitant labour
Psychiatric disorders
Seizures and status epilepticus

conditions encountered in obstetric units. Epilepsy increases by up to threefold the risks of various common complications (Table 26.10). The perinatal mortality rate has been found to be twice that of the general population. It is said that 1–2% of all women with active epilepsy will have tonic–clonic seizures during delivery and this can clearly complicate labour. The fetal heart rate can be dramatically slowed by a seizure, and fetal monitoring is recommended during vaginal delivery. Home birth should not generally be contemplated and obstetricians are more likely to recommend caesarean section. Epilepsy from pre-existing neurological disorders can be worsened during pregnancy, including seizures caused by multiple sclerosis, ateriovenous malformations and meninigiomas.

Effect of pregnancy on the rate of seizures and on antiepileptic drug levels Pregnancy has a little effect on seizure frequency in most patients, although there are patients whose seizures stop only during pregnancy and others, usually with severe epilepsy, whose seizures worsen. There are a number of potential causes for changes in seizure frequency: hormonal effects, non-compliance with medication, inappropriate dose reductions, changing drug disposition and serum levels, fluid retention, vomiting, stress, anxiety and sleep deprivation. The levels of many antiepileptic drugs fall in later pregnancy. This effect occurs most notably with lamotrigine, where levels on an unchanged dosage can fall to less than half the pre-pregnancy levels. Regular blood level checks and incrementation of dosage is often required, and lamotrigine particularly is a difficult drug to use in late pregnancy for this reason.

New-onset epilepsy during pregnancy The annual incidence of epilepsy at childbearing age is about 20–30 cases per 100 000 persons, and so the chance development of epilepsy during pregnancy is not uncommon. Occasionally, presumably because of hormonal or metabolic influences, some women experience epileptic seizures exclusively during pregnancy (gestational epilepsy) but this is a rare pattern.

Symptomatic epilepsy presents in pregnancy from various underlying causes. Pregnancy can stimulate an increase in size of meningiomas because of oestrogenic stimulation, resulting in newly presenting epilepsy. Arteriovenous malformations can also present more commonly in pregnancy. The risk of ischaemic stroke increases in pregnancy. The underlying causes include arteriosclerоisis, cerebral angiitis and Moyamoya disease, Takayasu's arteritis, embolic disease from a cardiac or infective source, sickle cell disease, antiphospholipid antibody syndrome, thrombotic thrombocytopenic purpura, deficiencies in antithrombin, protease C and S factor V Leiden and posterior reversible leukoencephalopathy syndrome (PRES). There is also a higher incidence of subarachnoid haemorrhage and of cerebral venous thrombosis. Pregnancy can also predispose to cerebral infections from bacteria (including *Listeria*), fungi (coccidioides), protozoa (*Toxoplasma*), viruses and HIV infection.

The extent of investigation of newly developing epilepsy in pregnancy will depend on the clinical setting. X-rays, and thus CT, should be avoided whenever possible. There are no known risks to the developing fetus from MRI and this is the brain imaging modality of choice. In the non-urgent situation, investigation is often deferred until pregnancy is completed.

Eclampsia and pre-eclampsia Most new-onset seizures in the late stages of pregnancy (after 20 weeks) are caused by eclampsia. Pre-eclampsia is characterised by hypertension, proteinuria, oedema, abnormalities of hepatic function, platelets and clotting parameters. About 5% of cases, if left untreated, progress to eclampsia. The eclamptic encephalopathy results in confusion, stupor, focal neurological signs and cerebral haemorrhage as well as seizures. The epilepsy can be severe and progress rapidly to status epilepticus. The incidence of eclampsia in Western Europe is about 1/2000 pregnancies, but it is more common in some developing countries with rates as high as 1/100. It carries a maternal mortality rate of 2–5% and also significant infant morbidity and mortality.

Traditionally, obstetricians have used magnesium sulfate in the treatment of seizures in eclampsia, and the superiority of magnesium over phenytoin and/or diazepam has been clearly demonstrated in recent randomised controlled studies. Not only does magnesium confer better seizure control, but there are fewer complications of pregnancy and infant survival is improved. Magnesium seems also to lessen the chance of cerebral palsy in low birth weight babies and has also been shown to decrease secondary neuronal damage after experimental traumatic brain injury. The mechanism by which magnesium sulfate acts in eclampsia is unclear; it may do so via its influence on NMDA receptors or on free radicals, prostacyclines, other neurochemical pathways or, more likely, by reversing the intense eclamptic cerebral vasospasm. It is possible that patients would benefit from both magnesium and a conventional antiepileptic, but this has not been investigated. Magnesium should be administered as an intravenous infusion of 4 g, followed by 10 g intramuscularly, and then 5 g intramuscularly every 4 hours as required.

Management of labour Regular antiepileptic drugs should be continued during labour. If oral therapy is not possible, intravenous replacement therapy can be given for at least some drugs. Tonic–clonic seizures occur in about 1–2% of susceptible mothers. In patients at risk, oral clobazam (10–20 mg) is useful given at the onset of labour as additional seizure prophylaxis. Fetal monitoring is advisable. Most women have a normal vaginal delivery, but sleep deprivation, over-breathing, pain and emotional stress can greatly increase the risk of seizures. Elective caesarean section should be considered in patients at particular risk. A history of status or life-threatening tonic–clonic seizures are an indication for caesarean section, and if severe seizures or status occur during delivery, an emergency caesarean section should be performed. Intravenous lorazepam or phenytoin should be given during labour if severe epilepsy develops and the patient prepared for caesarean section.

There is a maternal as well as infant mortality associated with severe seizures during delivery. The hypoxia consequent on a seizure is sometimes more profound in gravid than in non-gravid women because of the increased oxygen requirements of the fetus, and resuscitation facilities should be immediately at hand in the delivery suite.

Vitamin K Maternally ingested enzyme-inducing antiepileptic drugs can induce a relative deficiency of infantile vitamin-K dependent clotting factors (factors II, VII, IX and X) and protein C and S, predisposing to infantile haemorrhage, including cerebral haemorrhage. The neonate should therefore receive 1 mg vitamin K intramuscularly at birth and at 28 days of life. It is also sometimes recommended that the mother take oral vitamin K (20 mg/day) in the last trimester, although the evidence that this improves neonatal clotting is rather contradictory. If any two of the clotting factors fall below 50% of their normal values, intramuscular vitamin K will be insufficient to protect against haemorrhage and fresh frozen plasma should be given intravenously. Similarly, if there is evidence of neonatal bleeding, or if concentrations of factors II, VII, IX or X fall below 25% of normal, an emergency infusion of fresh frozen plasma is required.

Epilepsy and the fetus

Effect of seizures on the fetus The exact risks are not established. Clearly, in the latter stages of pregnancy, a convulsion carries the risk of trauma to the placenta and/or fetus, especially if the women falls. However, most debate has revolved around the suggestion that seizures damage the fetus through lactic acidosis or hypoxia. The hypoxia is usually very short-lived and the placenta is a well-buffered system; intuitively these risks seem likely to be small. More than five tonic–clonic seizures during pregnancy has, in a retrospective study, been found to be associated with lower IQ in the offspring. Another study has found that first trimester seizures are accompanied by a higher risk of fetal malformation than seizures at other times, although the reliability of these conclusions is in doubt. Stillbirth has been recorded after a single seizure or series of seizures, although this must be very rare. However, status epilepticus during pregnancy or delivery is extremely hazardous, and a study of status epilepticus during delivery reported a 50% infant mortality and 30% maternal mortality. Partial seizures have no known effects upon a fetus.

Teratogenicity of antiepileptic drugs

There is no doubt that some maternally ingested antiepileptic drugs carry the risk of teratogenicity. This has been shown clearly both in animals and in clinical practice. However, assessment is complicated by the fact that seizures themselves can cause malformations, although this effect is probably small. Also, social, dietary and socio-economic factors increase the risk both of epilepsy and of malformations. Evidence is therefore difficult to assess, and accurate clinical advice difficult to give. Nevertheless, it is generally considered that of the commonly prescribed antiepileptic drugs, the use of carbamazepine, lamotrigine and possibly levetiracetam during pregnancy carries a lower teratogenic risk than valproate, barbiturates, phenytoin or topiramate.

Major malformations associated with antiepileptic drugs The most common major malformations associated with traditional antiepileptic drug therapy (phenytoin, phenobarbital, primidone, benzodiazepines, valproate, carbamazepine, topiramate) are cleft palate and cleft lip, cardiac malformations, neural tube defects, hypospadias, renal anomalies and skeletal abnormalities. Different drugs have a different range of associated abnormality and the highest rates are found with valproate. Cerebral malformations can also occur. Polytherapy carries higher risks than monotherapy, and the individual risks of some drugs have not been fully established. Phenytoin as monotherapy has a relatively low incidence of major defects although earlier studies with the drug in polytherapy showed much higher levels. One particular association is the increased risk of neuroblastoma although the absolute risk is very small. One study purported to demonstrate smaller head circumference in babies of mothers on carbamazepine, but the statistical basis of this observation was not well founded. It is unclear whether or not the benzodiazepines carry any teratogenic potential, although there are case reports of facial clefts, cardiac and skeletal abnormalities. The risk of spina bifida has been particularly well studied. The background population risk of spina bifida is approximately 0.2–0.5% with geographical variation. Valproate is associated with a 1–2% risk of spina bifida aperta, a risk that is strongly dose-related. Carbamazepine carries a risk of spina bifida aperta of about 0.5–1%. It is instructive to note that the induction of neural tube defects by valproate, and to a lesser extent carbamazepine, were not noticed initially during animal toxicology testing.

Other developmental abnormalities and neurodevelopmental delay In addition to the major malformations, less severe dysmorphic changes occur ('fetal syndromes'), although there is little agreement about their frequency or indeed in some cases their existence. The fetal phenytoin syndrome was the first to be described, and is said to consist of a characteristic pattern of facial and limb disturbances (Table 26.11). However, most of these features are minor and overlap with the normal variation seen in children born to healthy mothers. Recent prospective and blinded studies have shown that only hypertelorism and distal digital hypoplasia occurred at any greater frequency, and even these associations are weak. Furthermore, the nail hypoplasia tends to disappear during childhood. Cases of a 'carbamazepine syndrome' are reported with cranio-facial abnormalities, growth retardation, neural tube defects and fingernail hypoplasia. Reports of primidone

Table 26.11 Fetal anticonvulsant syndromes. This is a list of reported abnormalities, although many are uncontrolled observations and the frequency of the anomalies is unclear. Genetic, environmental and socio-economic factors also have a role in their development.

Growth
Cranio-facial
Short nose, low cranial bridge
Hypertelorism
Epicanthic fold
Strabismus and other ocular abnormalities
Low-set ears and other aural abnormalities
Wide mouth and prominent lips
Wide fontenelles
Cleft palate and cleft lip
Limbs
Hypoplasia of nails
Transverse palmar crease
Short fingers
Extra digits
Cerebral
Learning disability
Developmental delay
General
Short neck, low hairline
Rib, sternal and spinal anomalies
Widely spaced hypoplastic nipples
Hernias
Undescended testes
Neuroblastoma and neural ridge tumours
Cardiac and renal abnormalities
Hypospadias
Neural tube defects

and phenobarbital 'syndromes' have been published, consisting of facial changes and developmental delay. The problem of determining risk is further complicated by the confounding influences of socio-economic and genetic factors. Recent interest has focused on a 'valproate syndrome' said to occur in up to 40% of infants born to mothers on valproate although no robust controlled and blinded studies have been carried out to demonstrate the true frequency. The valproate syndrome comprises cranio-facial and skeletal abnormalities, characteristic dysmorphic features and craniostenosis. Neurodevelopmental delay, cognitive problems and learning disability can be part of the valproate syndrome, although again the frequency is unclear. It has also been suggested that children exposed to valproate monotherapy, even if they have no other features of a valproate syndrome, can have significantly lower verbal IQ scores and cognitive problems which become apparent only later in childhood when compared with children exposed to carbamazepine or phenytoin monotherapy.

The teratogenic effects of most of the newer antiepileptic drugs have not been established. This does not imply safety, however, and three points from experience with traditional therapies are worth making. First, even today, the full range of the teratogenicity has not been not established. Secondly, the risk of even major malformations were not noticed until the drugs had been in extensive use for decades. Thirdly, negative results from animal models are not a reliable indicator of safety.

Puerperium

Maternal seizures and antiepileptic drug doses There is an increased risk of seizures in the puerperium. Clobazam 10 mg taken during delivery and for a few days after delivery can be useful to prevent seizures in this vulnerable period. If antiepileptic drug dosage has been increased because of falling levels during pregnancy, the dosage should be reduced in the first week after delivery to its previous levels. Drugs circulating in the mother's serum cross the placenta. If maternal antiepileptic drug levels are high, the infant may experience drowsiness or withdrawal symptoms and neonatal serum levels should be measured in patients at risk.

Breastfeeding The concentration of most antiepileptic drugs in breast milk is less than 30% that of plasma; although exceptions are lamotrigine, levetiracetam and phenobarbital. Furthermore, even if a drug is present in significant concentrations in breast milk, the amount ingested by the infant is usually much less than would normally be considered needed for clinical effects. Only lamotrigine, levetiracetam and phenobarbital require special precautions. Maternal phenobarbital ingestion is a particular problem, as in neonates the half-life of phenobarbital is long (up to 300 hours) and the free fraction is higher than in adults; neonatal levels can therefore sometimes exceed maternal levels.

Maternal epilepsy A mother at risk from seizures with altered consciousness should not be left alone with a small child. There is a danger of dropping the child or leaving the child unattended, and maternal epilepsy probably poses a greater risk to infants and toddlers than to the fetus. Sensible precautions should be taken. These include avoiding carrying the child unaccompanied, changing and feeding the infant at ground level and bathing the infant only when someone else is present.

Reducing risks of pregnancy to mother and child

Preconception review of drug therapy The patient's antiepileptic drug regimen should be reviewed if possible before conception is contemplated, as many major malformations are established within the first 8 weeks of pregnancy.

It is important to establish whether antiepileptic therapy is needed at all. This will be an individual decision, based on the risks of teratogenicity against the risks of worsening epilepsy. If tonic–clonic seizures are occurring, it is usual to continue drug therapy, as such seizures carry significant risk both to the mother and child. However, some women with partial or non-convulsive seizures will elect to withdraw therapy even if seizures are active or likely to become more frequent. Conversely, other women who are seizure-free will wish to continue therapy because of the social and physical risks of seizure recurrence.

All women should be counselled fully about the risks of seizures and of antiepileptic drugs during pregnancy. A specialist review should be offered to all women with epilepsy who are contemplating pregnancy.

Drug therapy during pregnancy Because of the teratogenic risks of antiepileptic drugs, in some patients, it is reasonable to withdraw therapy for the whole pregnancy or for the first half of pregnancy. The latter approach is based upon the fact that the teratogenic risk is greatest in the first trimester and the physical risk of seizures greatest in the later stages of pregnancy. The relative risks need to carefully assessed, however, and a specialist review is needed before embarking upon this unusual course.

If the woman elects to continue therapy, it is best to strive for monotherapy and to aim for the minimum effective dose. A few women with severe epilepsy will need combination therapy, but this should be avoided wherever possible. It is useful to measure the serum drug concentrations that give optimal control of the epilepsy before conception. These values form a useful starting point on which to base subsequent drug dosage adjustments. The choice of drug to use can be difficult. It is important to recognise that all therapy is a balance between risk and benefit. In most cases, monotherapy with either carbamazepine, lamotrigine or levetiracetam should be aimed for. Difficulties arise particularly in the treatment of idiopathic generalised epilepsy, a syndrome in which seizures are often best controlled by valproate. In this situation, replacing valproate by levetiracetam or even carbamazepine (which will control tonic–clonic seizures even if exacerbating absence or myoclonic seizures) is often recommended. However, there are a few patients in whom valproate has to be continued, and if so the drug should be given in the slow-release form and its dosage regimens changed to two or three times daily to minimise blood level peaks.

Dosage increases of lamotrigine (and to a lesser extent carbamazepine, phenytoin and phenobarbital) may be necessary as serum antiepileptic drug levels can fall in the second half of pregnancy. The mechanisms of the changing dose reqirement include reduced drug absorption, reduced serum albumin, protein binding changes, increased clearance and fluid retention. In the case of lamotrigine, levels can fall precipitously, and monthly or even fortnightly blood level estimations are needed in some cases.

Screening for fetal malformations Some malformations can be detected by prenatal ultrasound screening. If therapeutic termination of pregnancy is acceptable, screening procedures should include, where appropriate, a high quality ultrasound scan at 10, 18–20 and 24 weeks, measurement of α-fetoprotein levels and amniocentesis. About 95% of significant neural tube defects can be detected prenatally, as well as cleft palate and other midline defects, and major cardiac and renal defects. However, the mother should be informed that not all malformations are detectable even with the most sophisticated screening methods.

Folic acid supplementation The fetus of an epileptic women is at a greater than expected risk of a neural tube defect, particularly if the mother is taking valproate. A recent Medical Research Council trial of folic acid supplementation during pregnancy showed a 72% protective effect against neural tube defects in women who had conceived a fetus previously with neural tube defects. Although there has been no specific study in epilepsy, it would seem reasonable for all epileptic women to be given folic acid supplementation during pregnancy. A dose of at least 4 mg/day is recommended on an empirical basis, as lower doses may not fully restore folate levels. Folic acid supplementation is generally recommended for all women who may become pregnant.

Cerebrovascular disorders in pregnancy

Pregnancy is associated with an increased risk of ischaemic and haemorrhagic stroke. Ischaemic stroke in pregnancy is caused by arterial occlusion in about two-thirds of cases (most often in the middle cerebral artery territory), and venous occlusion of cortical veins or venous sinuses in the remaining third. Thus, venous events are over-represented in pregnancy and a high index of suspicion is required. Arterial stroke is most often in the third trimester or in the first week postpartum. Venous sinus thrombosis is most common in the first 2 weeks postpartum but can occur in the third trimester; presentation differs from arterial stroke in that headache, seizures and behavioural changes may be prominent, in addition to focal neurological symptoms.

Cerebral haemorrhage in pregnancy can be caused by pre-existing aneurysm or arteriovenous malformation, or in association with venous infarction or uncontrolled hypertension (e.g. in the context of eclampsia). Rupture of arteriovenous malformations is most common in the second trimester, while there is no particular peak timing for aneurysmal haemorrhage. There is no evidence that vaginal delivery increases the risk of rupture from arteriovenous malformation or aneurysm; decisions on the method of delivery should be based on obstetric factors.

Pre-eclampsia and eclampsia are discussed earlier. They are defined by pregnancy-associated proteinuria and hypertension with multi-system involvement (renal, hepatic, neurological). The neurological manifestations include seizures (usually generalised without focal features), visual disturbance and reduced conscious level. These symptoms require urgent investigation to exclude intracranial haemorrhage or other vascular causes. Treatment of hypertension and of seizures with intravenous magnesium is appropriate, sometimes with conventional anticonvulsant drugs. Eclampsia is characterised by persistent frontal and occipital headache, blurred vision, photophobia, epigastric pain and altered mental state followed by tonic–clonic seizures. Hypertension (>140/90 mmHg) is common but may be absent at presentation in less than one-third of patients. More than 90% of cases of eclampsia develop after 28 weeks' gestation and >30% occur at term or in the peripartum or immediate postpartum period (48 hours). MRI is essential to exclude PRES, RCVS, venous thrombosis, acute infarction or dissection. Aggressive treatment with magnesium and antihypertensive therapy is essential for eclampsia.

The pathophysiology of eclampsia overlaps with several neurovascular syndromes associated with pregnancy, including PRES and RCVS. PRES characteristically occurs in the first postpartum week, and is characterised by seizures, uncontrolled hypertension and visual symptoms. The pathophysiology is thought to be disruption of the blood–brain barrier, perhaps because perfusion exceeds the autoregulation threshold. The predilection for the posterior circulation is suggested to result from a reduced sympathetic innervation compared to the anterior circulation. The symptoms of PRES mimic those of cerebral venous sinus thrombosis and eclampsia; neuro-imaging is essential to make an accurate diagnosis. In PRES, the findings on MRI are characteristic, showing altered signal in the occipito-parietal regions, usually without a major component of restricted diffusion on diffusion-weighted MRI in contrast to acute ischaemia (Figure 26.29). Urgent treatment is required for the hypertension and seizures; good recovery is the rule if treatment is started promptly. The imaging abnormalities usually resolve, and if this is the case and ongoing seizures have not occurred then anticonvulsants can be stopped. It has been suggested that the term PRES be abandoned because the condition is not only posterior in location, not always reversible and not always associated with encephalopathy (Chapter 20).

RCVS is commonly observed in the postpartum period and clinically causes a thunderclap headache followed by focal neurological deficit. Definitive diagnosis requires the demonstration of vasospasm on angiographic imaging. Areas of ischaemic change may be seen on MRI as infarction can result from vasospasm. There is clearly potential overlap because of a lack of firm diagnostic criteria

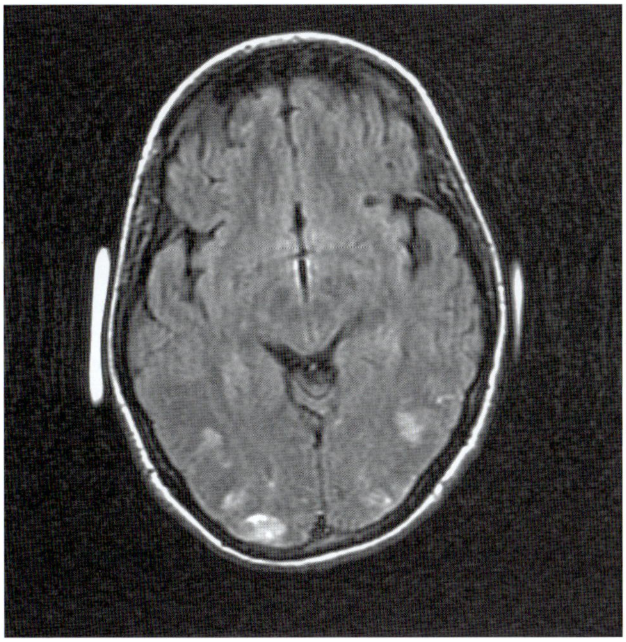

Figure 26.29 Posterior reversible leukoencephalopathy syndrome (PRES): axial FLAIR MRI of a 17-year-old woman who presented with seizures and complete visual loss in the context of uncontrolled hypertension 1 week after delivery. Note patchy high signal abnormalities bilaterally in the parieto-occipital regions. One month later these imaging abnormalities had fully resolved.

for both PRES and RCVS, and there is a need for further clarification of these diagnostic terms.

Pregnancy and other neurological diseases

Pituitary disorders

Pregnancy causes the pituitary gland to enlarge. Sheehan's syndrome is a rare condition of pituitary infarction, usually caused by postpartum haemorrhage and systemic hypotension, or by the vascular demands of an enlarging pituitary gland exceeding the available vascular supply. Infarction may transform into haemorrhage. In some cases, primary haemorrhage arises in an enlarged pituitary for reasons that are unclear. Infarction or haemorrhage can result in acute pituitary insufficiency and shock, hence the term pituitary apoplexy.

Lymphocytic hypophysitis may develop in pregnancy. It is thought to be of autoimmune origin and usually self-limited. If the pituitary enlargement is causing symptoms (e.g. visual loss), corticosteroids may be indicated.

Headache

Migraine is reported to improve in up to 80% of cases during pregnancy, presumably because of altered oestrogen levels. However, because migraine is so common, there are large numbers of women with significant migraine requiring treatment during pregnancy. Headache arising for the first time in pregnancy is of greater concern and requires further investigation. If migraines are frequent and disabling then propranolol can be used in pregnancy. Paracetamol is the safest acute treatment. Ergotamine is contraindicated and there is insufficient information on the safety of triptans to recommend them in pregnancy. The most common type of headache in pregnancy is tension-type headache.

Neuromuscular disorders

Restless leg syndrome affects up to 30% of women during the third trimester. Oral folate reduces the frequency of symptoms. Pregnancy has an unpredictable effect on myasthenia gravis, with no particular trend for worsening or improvement in symptoms. Bell's palsy is several times more common in pregnancy and the puerperium than at other times. Carpal tunnel syndrome affects about one-fifth of patients in the third trimester and is likely to resolve after delivery. Meralgia paraesthetica can occur late in pregnancy because of stretching or compression of the lateral cutaneous nerve of the thigh and can be expected to improve following delivery. Gestational polyneuropathy is related to nutritional deficiency because of general malnourishment or hyperemesis gravidarum. The latter can also cause Wernicke's encephalopathy. Damage to the nerves of the lumbosacral plexus is a rare complication of delivery, particularly if there are complicating factors including cephalopelvic disproportion, shoulder dystocia or instrumentation with forceps (see complications of obsteric anaesthesia).

Multiple sclerosis

Unless there are complicating factors (e.g. severe motor disability and contractures), MS has no known effects on fertility, pregnancy, recommended mode of delivery, congenital malformations or perinatal death rates. Overall, pregnancy does not affect the frequency of MS relapses or rate of disease progression. There are no studies of the efficacy or safety of disease-modifying agents including the interferons and glatiramer acetate in pregnancy. Corticosteroids can be safely used to treat relapses of MS in pregnancy.

Chorea gravidarum

Chorea gravidarum (CG) simply refers to any type of chorea occurring in pregnancy. It is extremely uncommon and is characterised by regular brief unpredictable jerk movements of the limbs and trunk. It typically begins in the first trimester but can present postpartum. The term does not imply a specific cause; this condition is a clinical syndrome not a distinct disease. About one-third of patients have a history of rheumatic fever or Syndenham's chorea. It is therefore speculated that CG results from the reactivation of previous subclinical basal ganglia damage; the mechanism involves ischaemia or increased dopamine sensitivity mediated by elevated hormone levels during pregnancy. CG can occur secondary to other known causes of chorea including Syndenham's chorea, lupus or Huntington's disease. Symptoms generally resolve spontaneously and CG seldom requires drug treatment. If CG is mild the patient may even be unaware of the involuntary movements. Drug treatment is only used if its severity puts the mother or fetus in danger (e.g. because of poor nutrition, disturbed sleep or injury). If treatment is necessary dopamine blockers including haloperidol are used. Wernicke's encephalopathy can complicate hyperemesis gravidosum. Abnormal eye movements (e.g. ophthalmoplegia and nystagmus causing diplopia) are commonly present but confusion and gait abnormalities are less frequent and a metabolic acidosis sometimes occurs. There is an immediate response to thiamine.

Tumours

Overall, brain and spine tumours are no more common in pregnant than non-pregnant women of similar age. Meningiomas present more often than expected by chance during the second half of pregnancy as they may enlarge because of the effects of changes in circulating oestrogen levels on tumour oestrogen receptors. Gliomas and arteriovenous malformations can also grow more aggressively during pregnancy. The symptoms of meningiomas often improve spontaneously postpartum, so that treatment can be delayed until after delivery. However, surgery for large or aggressive brain tumours during pregnancy is needed urgently if there are signs of raised ICP or papilloedema. Most women with brain tumours presenting in pregnancy are managed by caesarean section to avoid possible cerebral herniation during labour. Choriocarcinoma is a malignancy seen in pregnancy and often metastasises to the brain. Pituitary adenomas are slightly more common in pregnancy and large tumours can be associated with the onset of visual failure; careful visual field assessment is therefore mandatory in every pregnant woman presenting with new headache symptoms.

Idiopathic intracranial hypertension

Idiopathic intracranial hypertension (Chapter 14) is more common during pregnancy than at other times, and patients often present in the second trimester. If already present it usually deteriorates in pregnancy. Treatment is guided by close monitoring of visual function including visual fields. Weight control is recommended. A short course of corticosteroids may be considered, along with serial lumbar puncture or more invasive procedures such as lumboperitoneal shunting or optic nerve fenestration if vision is threatened. The teratogenic potential of acetazomlamide is unknown, but it should be avoided in the first trimester.

Complications of obstetric anaesthesia

Regional anaesthesia, particularly when used peripartum, can lead to complications; systemic toxicity can cause hypotension, pruritus, nausea and vomiting. A failed block causes inadequate analgesia or anaesthesia following epidural or spinal injection and may be a result of inadequate dose, poor catheter placement, subsequent displacement or anatomical variation. High spinal anaesthesic is caused by cephalad progression of the level of anaesthesia with neuraxial block. It is usually caused by accidental injection of local anaesthesia into the intrathecal rather than the epidural space. If a high concentration of anaesthetic is used a serious reaction can develop, characterised by profound hypotension with a lack of compensatory tachycardia, and is caused by massive sympathetic discharge with block of cardiac accelerator fibres. Hypoperfusion of the brainstem causes respiratory depression, dyspnoea from block of the intercostal muscles and diaphragm, and there may be aspiration caused by bulbar weakness, impaired consciousness and impaired airway reflexes. The fetus can also be affected if maternal hypotension leads to reduced placental perfusion. Management includes ventilation and inotropic support until the anaesthetic has dissipated.

Pneumocephalus occurs if air is introduced into the intrathecal space and the CSF during placement of the neuraxial block if the dura is inadvertently punctured. It causes acute onset of severe headache.

Spinal epidural haematoma is uncommon but occurs if a vascular structure is punctured and is a particular risk in those receiving anticoagulants or with disorders of coagulation. Haematoma compresses the nerve roots or the spinal cord leading to radicular pain and loss of sensory, motor and sphincter function. Urgent surgical intervention is essential to prevent permanent impairment of neurological function. Rarely, if the needle entry level is too high, epidural or spinal anaesthesia can cause direct needle trauma to the nerve root or to the spinal cord itself, occasionally leading to syrinx formation.

Post delivery sequelae following neuraxial analgesia include postspinal headache due to dural puncture causing CSF leakage, traction on the cranial structures and cerebral vasodilation. Epidural blood patch is the treatment of choice for severe and debilitating post-spinal headache. Infective complications are extremely uncommon but epidural abscess can develop after epidural puncture and meningitis if the dura is breached either intentionally in spinal anaesthesia or unintentionally after an epidural procedure.

Postpartum compression neuropathies

Postpartum neuropathy is usually caused by compression of the lumbosacral plexus by the descending fetal head, by extrinsic neural compression (e.g. stirrup supports) or from ischaemia because of prolonged stretch of the nerves during the second stage of labour. Rarely, it can result from trauma to the nerve root cause by spinal epidural needle or catheter. The femoral and lateral femoral cutaneous nerves are vulnerable and most commonly affected. Predisposing factors include enlarged fetal skull size, malpresentation, sensory impairment, the use of forceps, prolonged lithotomy or second stage or improper use of legs stirrups and retractors. Patients with femoral neuropathy develop weakness of the quadriceps with sparing of adduction. There may be sensory loss over the anterior thigh and medial calf, foot and big toe. Involvement of the lateral femoral cutaneous nerve is restricted to sensory change and characterised by pain, paraesthesiae and sensory loss over the upper outer thigh. Peroneal nerve compression results in foot drop resulting from weakness of ankle and toe dorsiflexion and ankle eversion. Obturator neuropathy causes medial knee pain and adductor weakness.

The sciatic nerve is vulnerable in the lithotomy position because it may become stretched as the hip is flexed. Compression of the sciatic nerve can also be caused by the fetal head in the pelvis near the sciatic notch. Sciatic neuropathy presents with weakness, numbness and paraesthesiae. Foot drop is the most prominent sign although more generalised weakness occurs if the lesion is severe. This is because the peroneal division is fixed in the sciatic notch and lies superior to the tibial division in the hip and proximal thigh, it is therefore more vulnerable to injury leading to signs of distal weakness. The ankle reflexes are usually lost and sensory loss reflects sciatic nerve distribution. Most peripheral nerve injuries incurred during delivery progressively improve and usually recover completely.

Other conditions causing acute neurological symptoms during pregnancy

Amniotic fluid embolism presents with agitation, confusion, seizures and encephalopathy in the context of cardiovascular and respiratory collapse during or immediately after labour. Choriocarcinoma metastasises to the brain in 20% of patients. It is a rare cancer of trophoblastic tissue which may be haemorrhagic or invade cerebral vessels. Air embolism occurs if air enters the myometrium during delivery and then enters the venous circulation and right ventricle. This leads to reduced cardiac output and pulmonary embolism. A right-to-left intracardiac shunt from a patent foramen ovale will result in systemic embolism leading to stroke, seizures and abnormal cognition during or just after delivery.

Thrombotic thrombocytopenic purpura commonly presents in the second or third trimester and is characterised by the acute onset of thrombocytopenia, microangiopathic haemolytic anaemia, fever, neurological and renal dysfunction. Neurological features include headache, seizures and focal deficits. PRES may also be present. Pituitary apoplexy is caused either by infarction or haemorrhage into the gland in the setting of a known adenoma. Patients present with headache, visual loss, ophthalmoplegia and an impaired level of consciousness. More chronic presentation of panhypopituitarism may be a result of Sheehan's syndrome following postpartum haemorrhage or lymphocytic hypophysitis.

Palliative and end of life care in neurology

Palliative care is also discussed in Chapter 21. It is an important aspect of the treatment of many neurological disorders, and involves the management of symptoms and psycho-social and spiritual issues which may arise from the time of diagnosis and influence the course of the disease. The aim is to provide holistic support in the context of the patient's personal situation. Palliative care involves the relief of pain and distressing symptoms but intends neither to hasten nor postpone death in terminal disease. It affirms life and regards death as a normal process but provides support to allow patients to be as active as possible until death. It integrates their psychological and spiritual care and supports the family in coping with illness and bereavement. The introduction of palliative care is entirely compatible with active medical treatment of the underlying condition and its complications such as secondary infection.

Specialist palliative care services provide care and support in the home, in a hospice as day care or resident, or in hospital. Multidisciplinary palliative care teams are involved throughout the course of the disease to provide respite care or in the final weeks or days of life. Palliative care requires the involvement of multiple expertise including medical practitioner, specialist nurse, social worker, occupational therapist, physiotherapist, speech and language therapist, dietitian, religious representative, clinical psychologist, pharmacist and complementary therapist. The range of neurological conditions requiring palliative care is considerable but many of the symptomatic and end of life issues are shared. These conditions include stroke, demyelinating disease, tumours, Parkinson's disease, dementia, motor neurone disease, infectious disorders, muscular dystrophy, epilepsy and inherited metabolic disorders.

The techniques of symptom management and the ethical difficulties of care apply particularly to patients in states of reduced consciousness and awareness or profound disability: persistent vegetative state, minimally aware states, locked in syndrome or immobility resulting from quadriplegia or paraplegia. Management of the major symptomatic issues has been considered in the relevant chapters. These are briefly summarised in Table 26.12.

Considerable ethical issues have been raised in neurological practice concerning the maintenance of autonomy and decision-making, the provision of artificial hydration and nutrition for the dying and the profoundly disabled patient and the role of advanced directives, refusal of treatment, physician assisted suicide and euthanasia. Each of these remains actively debated in different societies and particularly in the neurological community. It is unlikely that a complete resolution will ever be reached as society's values and expectations constantly evolve. There remains a spectrum of opinion; practice should always continues to be tailored to the individual, respecting their different hopes, expectations and aspirations.

Table 26.12 Summary of major symptoms and their management in palliative care neurology.

Symptom	Modality of treatment	Detail of treatment
Spasticity	Primary	Treat underlying factors including infection, ulcers
	Medication	Anti-spasticity agents – baclofen, tizanidine, dantrolene, memantine, benzodiazepines
	Procedures	Baclofen pump Local injections of botulinum toxin microsurgery to the dorsal root entry zone tendon surgery
Dysphagia		Swallowing techniques Dietary modification Adaptions Augmented feeding (PEG, RIG)
Communication impairment		SALT techniques Augmentive and alternative communication aids (Light writer, ipad, Tobi systems)
Pain	Primary	Treat underlying factors including decubitus ulcers. Joint contractures and osteoporosis
	Psychological support	
	Medication	Non-opioid Adjuvent (e.g. antidepressant, anticonvulsants) Opioid analgesics
	Procedures	Neural blockade Myofascial injection Neurostimulation Neuraxial drug infusion
Nausea and vomiting	Primary	Treat underlying factors (e.g. hypercalcaemia, hyperglycaemia, hypocortisolism, hyponatraemia, uraemia, constipation, raised intracranial pressure)
	Medication	Antiemetics (metoclopramide, phenothiazines, butyrophenones, anticholinergics, ondansetron, cisapride, antihistamine). Others: steroids, octreotide

(continued)

Table 26.12 (continued)

Symptom	Modality of treatment	Detail of treatment
Fatigue	Primary	Treat underlying factors including anaemia, depression, thyroid, malnutrition, dehydration
	Non-pharmacological	Exercise programme Modification of activity Stress Cognitive–behavioural therapy
	Medication	Modafanil Amantidine Corticosteroids
Acute confusional state	Primary	Treat underlying factors including (e.g. toxic/drug factors, sepsis, electrolytes, organ failure, endocrine and metabolic factors)
	Medication	Haloperidol Benzodiazepines (lorazepam, midazalam) Chlorpromazine Risperidone/olanzapine
Respiratory	Primary	Treat underlying factors (e.g. bronchospasm, heart failure, abdominal distension, pulmonary oedema)
	Non-pharmacological	Ventilatory support: CPAP, NIV, tracheostomy
	Medication	Oxygen (if no CO_2 retention) Benzodiazepines Opioids
Mucus secretions	Non-pharmacological	Insufflator – exsufflator Physiotherapy Botulinum toxin injected into salivary glends Radiotherapy to salivary glands
	Medication	Nebuliser or saline Bronchodilator Mucolytic agent – carbocysteine Amitriptyline Anticholinergics – atropine, hyoscine, glycopyrrolate
Constipation	Prophylaxis	Fibre Hydration
	Medication	Stimulants – senna Softeners – lactulose, docusate Bulking agents – methyl cellulose Rectal suppositories
Diarrhoea	Primary	Treat underlying factors (e.g. leakage past faecal impaction)
	Medication	Codeine Loperamide Bulking agents (methyl cellulose)

CPAP, continuous positive airway pressure; NIV, non-invasive ventilation; PEG, percutaneous endoscopic gastrostomy; RIG, radiologically inserted gastrostomy; SALT, speech and language therapy.

The dying patient

The key symptom areas include managing fear, respiratory problems, pain, restlessness and agitation. Dyspnoea and cough can easily be managed by the use of opioids and benzodiazepines in carefully titrated doses. A sensation of choking is commonly experienced but choking is rarely a cause of death. Anxiety often accompanies and exacerbates breathlessness, benzodiazepines (lorazepam or midazalam given subcutaneously or occasionally intravenously) act as muscle relaxants and anxiolytics. Anticholinergics are valuable in the relief of noisy breathing. Although life may rarely be shortened by the appropriate use of opioids to control severe breathlessness there is no ethical objection as long as the physician does not intend to cause death by this treatment, although the process must be explained to those closest to the patient.

Restlessness, agitation and myoclonus are common with increasing metabolic disturbance and reduced level of consciousness. The patient sometimes appears to relatives to be in distress. Primary causes such as hypoxic, constipation or urinary retention should be excluded and hydration should be maintained. Sedation is occasionally necessary if the patient does not settle with a soothing and supportive environment. The aim is to relieve distress rather than induce sleep and careful dose titration is essential to ensure it is not associated with life shortening. It is essential that the aims and methods of treating distress are understood by all involved with the patient. The principal sedating drugs include haloperidol and midazalam. Rarely, phenobarbital or propofol can be used to establish sleepiness in a patient who is calm yet conscious, but titration of the dose is extremely difficult. The provision of appropriate support for families and carers is an essential part of management.

Palliative care seeks to provide a comprehensive approach to the management of disease when the opportunity for cure has passed. The appropriate management of the later stages of many neurological disorders increasingly requires the expertise of the multi-disciplinary palliative care team at home and in the hospital and hospice.

References

Aminoff MJ, ed. Thyroid disease and the nervous system. In: *Neurology and General Medicine*. New York: Churchill Livingstone, 1992.

Ferner RE. The neurofibromatoses. *Pract Neurol* 2010; **10:** 82–93.

Ginsberg L, Valentine A, Mehta A. Fabry diease. *Pract Neurol* 2005; **5:** 110–113.

Renowden S. Imaging in stroke and vascular disease – part 2: intracranial haemorrhage and related pathologies. *Pract Neurol* 2014; **14:** 159–175.

Wallace H, Shorvon SD, Tallis R. Age-specific incidence and prevalence rates of treated epilepsy in an unselected population of 2,052,922 and age specific fertility rates of women with epilepsy. *Lancet* 1998; **352:** 1970–1974.

Further reading

Cardiovascular disorders

Goodin DS. Neurological complications of aortic disease and surgery. In: Aminoff MJ, ed. *Neurology and General Medicine*. New York: Churchill Livingstone, 1992: 27–52.

Kanter MC, Hart RG. Neurologic complications of infective endocarditis. *Neurology* 1991; **41:** 1015–1020.

Selim M. Peri-operative stroke. *N Engl J Med* 2007; **356:** 706–713.

Endocrine disorders

Watkins PJ, Thomas PK. Diabetes mellitus and the nervous system. *J Neurol Neurosurg Psychiatry* 1998; **65:** 620–632.

Haematological disorders

Austin S, Cohen H, Losseff N. Haematology and neurology and the blood. *J Neurol Neurosurg Psychiatry* 2007; **78:** 334–341.

Gastro-intestinal disorders

Perkin GD, Murray-Lyon I. Neurology and the gastrointestinal system. In: Hughes RAC, Perkin GD, eds. *Neurology and Medicine*. BMJ Books, 1999: 185–209.

Renal disease

Zandi MS, Coles AJ. Notes on the kidney for the neurologist. *J Neurol Neurosurg Psychiatry* 2007; **78:** 444–449.

Vasculitis

Arachillage DJ, Cohen H. Antiphospholipid syndrome. *Medicine* 2014; **42:** 156–161.

Fox RI. Sjögren's syndrome. *Lancet* 2005; **366:** 321–331.

Giannakopoulos B, Krilis SA. The pathogenesis of the antiphospholipid syndrome. *N Engl J Med* 2013; **368:** 1033–1044.

Holle JU, Gross WL. Neurological involvement in Wegener's granulomatosis. *Curr Opin Rheumatol* 2011; **23:** 7–11.

Jennette JC, Falk RJ, Bacon PA, et al. Revised International Chapel Hill Consensus Conference Nomenclature of vasculitides. *Arthritis Rheum* 2013; **65:** 1–11.

Jones RB, Savage COS. Systemic vasculitides: an overview. *Medicine* 2014; **42:** 134–137.

Keeling D, Mackie I, Moore GW, Greer IA, Greaves M. Guidelines on the investigation and management of antiphospholipid syndrome. *Br J Haematol* 2012; **157:** 47–58.

Nesher G, Berkun Y, Mates M, Baras M, Nesher R, Rubinow A, *et al.* Risk factors for cranial ischemic complications in giant cell arteritis. *Medicine (Baltimore)* 2004; **83:** 14–22.

Nishino H, Rubino FA, DeRemee RA, Swanson JW, Parisi JE. Neurological involvement in Wegener's granulomatosis: an analysis of 324 consecutive patients at the Mayo Clinic. *Ann Neurol* 1993; **33:** 4–9.

Pons-Estel GJ, Alarcón GS, Scofield L, Reinlib L, Cooper GS. Undrerstanding the epidemiology and progression of systemic lupus erythematosis. *Semin Arthritis Rheum* 2010; **39:** 257–268.

Scolding NJ, Joseph FG. The neuropathology and pathogenesis of systemic lupus erythematosis. *Neuropathol Appl Neurobiol* 2002; **28:** 173–189.

Tsokos GC. Systemic lupus erythematosis. *N Engl J Med* 2011; **365:** 2110–2121.

Younger DS. Vasculitis of the nervous system. *Curr Opin Neurol* 2004; **17:** 317–336.

Neurosarcoidosis, Sjögren

Berkowitz AL, Samuels MA. The neurology of Sjögren's synderome and the rheumatology of peripheral neuropathy and myelitis. *Pract Neurol* 2013; **14:** 14–22.

Mori K, Iijima M, Koike H, *et al.* The wide spectrum of clinical manifestations in Sjögren's syndrome-associated neuropathy. *Brain* 2005; **128:** 2518–2534.

Pawate S, Moses H, Sriram S. Presentations and outcomes of neurosarcoidosis: a study of 54 cases. *Q J Med* 2009; **102:** 449–460.

Segal BM. Neurosarcoidosis: diagnostic approaches and therapeutic strategies. *Curr Opin Neurol* 2013; **26:** 307–313.

Stone JH, Zen Y, Deshpande V. IgG4-related disease. *N Engl J Med* 2012; **366:** 539–551.

Behçet's syndrome

Kidd D, Steuer A, Denman AM, Rudge P. Neurological complications in Behçet's syndrome. *Brain* 1999; **122:** 2183–2194.

Siva A, Altintas A, Saip S. Behçet's syndrome and the nervous system. *Curr Opin Neurol* 2004; **17:** 347–357.

Neurocutaneous disorders

Warburton KL, Wakerley B. Dermatological clues to neurological diagnoses. *Pract Neurol* 2011; **11:** 289–295.

Pregnancy

Lim SY, Evangelou N, Jürgens S. Postpartum headache: diagnostic considerations. *Pract Neurol* 2014; **14:** 92–99.

Shah AK, Rajamani K, Whitty JE. Eclampsia: a neurological perspective. *J Neurol Sci* 2008; **271:** 240–245.

Palliative care

Oliver D, Borasio GD, Walsh D, eds. *Palliative Care in Amyotrophic Lateral Sclerosis: From Diagnosis to Bereavement*, 2nd edn. Oxford: Oxford University Press, 2006.

Voltz R, Bernat JL, Borasio GD, Maddocks I, Oliver D, Portenoy RK, eds. *Palliative Care in Neurology*. Oxford: Oxford University Press, 2004.

Index

Page numbers in *italics* refer to figures; those in **bold** to tables.

Neurology: A Queen Square Textbook, Second Edition. Edited by Charles Clarke, Robin Howard, Martin Rossor and Simon Shorvon.

Discovery Library
Tel: 01752 439111